CW01499076

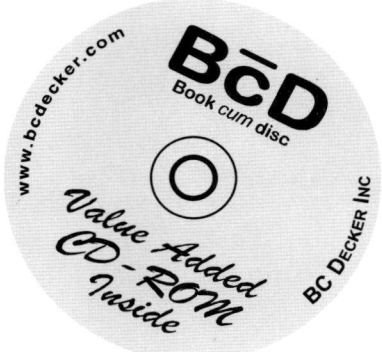

Every Decker book is accompanied by a CD-ROM.

The disc appears in the front of each copy, in its own sealed jacket. Affixed to the front of the book will be a distinctive Bc̄D sticker **"Book *cum* disc."**

The disc contains the complete text and illustrations of the book, in fully searchable PDF files. The book and disc are sold *only* as a package; neither is available independently, and no prices are available for the items individually.

BC Decker Inc is committed to providing high-quality electronic publications that complement traditional information and learning methods.

We trust you will find the book/CD package invaluable and invite your comments and suggestions.

Brian C. Decker
CEO and Publisher

Fourth Edition

Interstitial Lung Disease

MARVIN I. SCHWARZ, MD
Department of Medicine
University of Colorado Health Sciences Center
Denver, Colorado

TALMADGE E. KING JR, MD
Department of Medicine
University of California
San Francisco, California

2003
BC Decker Inc
Hamilton • London

BC Decker Inc
P.O. Box 620, LCD 1
Hamilton, Ontario L8N 3K7
Tel: 905-522-7017; 1-800-568-7281
Fax: 905-522-7839; 1-888-311-4987
E-mail: info@bcdecker.com
www.bcdecker.com

02 03 04 05 / GSA / 9 8 7 6 5 4 3 2 1

ISBN 1–55009–179–4
Printed in Spain

Sales and Distribution

United States
BC Decker Inc
P.O. Box 785
Lewiston, NY 14092-0785
Tel: 905-522-7017; 800-568-7281
Fax: 905-522-7839; 888-311-4987
E-mail: info@bcdecker.com
www.bcdecker.com

Canada
BC Decker Inc
20 Hughson Street South
P.O. Box 620, LCD 1
Hamilton, Ontario L8N 3K7
Tel: 905-522-7017; 800-568-7281
Fax: 905-522-7839; 888-311-4987
E-mail: info@bcdecker.com
www.bcdecker.com

Foreign Rights
John Scott & Company
International Publishers' Agency
P.O. Box 878
Kimberton, PA 19442
Tel: 610-827-1640
Fax: 610-827-1671
E-mail: jsco@voicenet.com

Argentina
CLM (Cuspide Libros Medicos)
Av. Córdoba 2067 – (1120)
Buenos Aires, Argentina
Tel: (5411) 4961-0042/(5411) 4964-0848
Fax: (5411) 4963-7988
E-mail: clm@cuspide.com

Japan
Igaku-Shoin Ltd.
Foreign Publications Department
3-24-17 Hongo
Bunkyo-ku, Tokyo, Japan 113-8719
Tel: 3 3817 5680
Fax: 3 3815 6776
E-mail: fd@igaku-shoin.co.jp

U.K., Europe, Scandinavia,
Middle East
Elsevier Science
Customer Service Department
Foots Cray High Street
Sidcup, Kent
DA14 5HP, UK
Tel: 44 (0) 208 308 5760
Fax: 44 (0) 181 308 5702
E-mail: cservice@harcourt.com

Singapore, Malaysia, Thailand,
Philippines, Indonesia, Vietnam,
Pacific Rim, Korea
Elsevier Science Asia
583 Orchard Road
#09/01, Forum
Singapore 238884
Tel: 65-737-3593
Fax: 65-753-2145

Australia, New Zealand
Elsevier Science Australia
Customer Service Department
STM Division
Locked Bag 16
St. Peters, New South Wales, 2044
Australia
Tel: 61 02 9517-8999
Fax: 61 02 9517-2249
E-mail: stmp@harcourt.com.au
Web site: www.harcourt.com.au

Mexico and Central America
ETM SA de CV
Calle de Tula 59
Colonia Condesa
06140 Mexico DF, Mexico
Tel: 52-5-5553-6657
Fax: 52-5-5211-8468
E-mail: editoresdetextosmex@prodigy.net.mx

Brazil
Tecmedd
Av. Maurílio Biagi, 2850
City Ribeirão Preto – SP – CEP: 14021-000
Tel: 0800 992236
Fax: (16) 3993-9000
E-mail: tecmedd@tecmedd.com.br

DEDICATION

This book is dedicated to:

My mother Claire Schwarz
and
my wife Kathleen Post

MIS

— ❖ —

My wife Mozelle Davis King
and
my children Consuelo and Malaika

TEK

CONTENTS

Preface vii

Acknowledgment viii

PART 1: CLINICAL APPROACHES

1   Approach to the Evaluation and Diagnosis of Interstitial Lung Disease 1
     Marvin I. Schwarz, Talmadge E. King Jr, Ganesh Raghu

2   Anatomic Distribution and Histopathologic Patterns of Interstitial Lung Disease 31
     Kevin O. Leslie, Thomas V. Colby, Stephen J. Swensen

3   Physiology of Interstitial Lung Disease 54
     Denis E. O'Donnell, Michael F. Fitzpatrick

4   Imaging of Diffuse Parenchymal Lung Diseases 75
     David Lynch

5   Bronchoalveolar Lavage 114
     Ulrich Costabel, Josune Guzman

6   Pediatric Interstitial Lung Disease 134
     Leland L. Fan

7   Genetic Basis of Interstitial Lung Disease 152
     Francis X. McCormack

PART 2: BASIC MECHANISMS

8   Inflammation in the Pathogenesis of Interstitial Lung Diseases 187
     David W. H. Riches, G. Scott Worthen, Andrei Augustin, Razvan Lapadat,, Edward D. Chan

9   Role of the Alveolar Epithelium in the Pathogenesis of Pulmonary Fibrosis 221
     Francis X. McCormack, John M. Shannon

10 Cytokine Biology and the Pathogenesis of Interstitial Lung Disease 245
     Michael P. Keane, John A. Belperio, Robert M. Strieter

11 Extracellular Matrix in the Pathogenesis of Lung Injury and Repair 276
     Jesse Roman

12 Immunologic Events in the Development of Interstitial Lung Disease: The Paradigm of Sarcoidosis . . . 300
     Gianpietro Semenzato, Carlo Agostini

13 The Future of Medical Therapy for Lung Fibrosis 323
     Marvin I. Schwarz, Kevin K. Brown

PART 3: CLINICAL ENTITIES

14 Sarcoidosis 332
     Glen P. Westall, R. G. Stirling, Paul Cullinan, Roland M. du Bois

15 Silicosis 387
     David N. Weissman, Daniel E. Banks

16 Coal Workers' Pneumoconiosis 402
     Daniel E. Banks

17 Asbestosis and Asbestos-Induced Pleural Fibrosis 418
    Mark P. Steele, Michael W. Peterson, David A. Schwartz

18 Beryllium Disease 435
    Lee S. Newman, Lisa A. Maier

19 Hypersensitivity Pneumonitis 452
    Moisés Selman

20 Drug-Induced Infiltrative Lung Diseases 485
    Philippe Camus

21 Connective Tissue Diseases 535
    Michelle M. Freemer, Talmadge E. King Jr

22 Pulmonary Vasculitis 599
    Ulrich Specks

23 Diffuse Alveolar Hemorrhage 632
    Andrew P. Fontenot, Marvin I. Schwarz

24 Eosinophilic Pneumonias 657
    Jean-François Cordier

25 Idiopathic Interstitial Pneumonias 701
    Talmadge E. King Jr

26 Bronchiolitis 787
    Talmadge E. King Jr

27 Lymphoplasmocytic Infiltrations of the Lung 825
    Gregory P. Cosgrove, Michael B. Fessler, Marvin I. Schwarz

28 Pulmonary Langerhans Cell Histiocytosis 838
    Robert Vassallo, Andrew H. Limper

29 Lymphangioleiomyomatosis 851
    Arnold S. Kristof, Joel Moss

30 Pulmonary Alveolar Proteinosis 865
    Jason S. Vourlekis, Kelly E. Greene

31 Miscellaneous Interstitial Lung Diseases 877
    Marvin I. Schwarz

Index 917

PREFACE

This is the fourth edition of this book that has become a standard reference work in our field. Since the appearance of third edition, substantial progress has been made in our understanding of the pathogenesis of lung fibrosis. In addition, several international consensus panels have issued statements defining the diagnosis, evaluation, and management of patients with interstitial lung diseases. However, the diagnosis and management of patients with interstitial lung disease continues to pose significant challenges to clinicians. As a result, it has been increasingly emphasized that the final diagnosis should be rendered only after the pulmonologist, radiologist, and pathologist have reviewed all of the clinical, radiologic, and pathologic data obtained from evaluation of the patient. Consequently, one of the major changes in this edition is the expanded attention to a multidisciplinary approach to diagnosis.

The editors have recruited international experts from these disciplines to contribute to this edition. A number of new chapters have been included and all previous chapters have been extensively revised. Each chapter includes helpful tables and figures, and as in the previous edition, each chapter is extensively referenced.

The book is divided into three sections. Part 1, *Clinical Approaches*, provides an overview of the clinical, pathologic, physiologic, and radiologic manifestations of the interstitial lung diseases. The approach in these chapters is to provide the basis for recognizing the key features that allow a specific diagnosis to be achieved.

The seven chapters in Part 2, *Basic Mechanisms*, emphasize the many advances in genetics and cellular and molecular biology that have greatly expanded our understanding of the biologic processes involved in the pathogenesis of the interstitial lung diseases. The roles of the various components of the pathogenetic process of lung fibrosis are discussed including those of the fibroblast, epithelium, cytokine biology, and matrix accumulation and breakdown, as well as the key immunologic events. Finally, a chapter describes how this improved understanding of the fibrogenic mechanisms in the lung is likely to yield more effective therapies.

Part 3, *Clinical Entities*, provides a detailed review of each of the interstitial lung diseases. Each chapter describes the clinical manifestations, radiologic patterns, histopathologic features, and management of the specific process.

This fourth edition of *Interstitial Lung Disease* is geared primarily toward clinicians; however, we are certain that it will be a valuable tool for radiologists, pathologists, and scientists interested in this field.

The Editors
December 2003

ACKNOWLEDGMENTS

The editors wish to express their appreciation to the authors for their outstanding contributions to this book. We would also like to acknowledge the helpfulness and patience of the staff at BC Decker Inc. We thank the faculties and fellows of the Divisions of Pulmonary and Critical Care Medicine at the University of Colorado Health Sciences Center and the University of California, San Francisco for their helpful discussions. We would like to express our appreciation to Reuben Cherniack, MD for his years of encouragement and support. We express our gratitude to our wives and families for their unwavering support. Finally, we remain forever grateful to our patients for allowing us to participate in their care.

CONTRIBUTORS

CARLO AGOSTINI, MD
Department of Clinical and Experimental Medicine
University of Padua
Padova, Italy

ANDREI AUGUSTIN, MD
Department of Immunology
National Jewish Medical and Research Center
Denver, Colorado

DANIEL E. BANKS, MD
Department of Internal Medicine
Louisiana State University Health Science Center
Shreveport, Louisiana

JOHN A. BELPERIO, MD
Department of Internal Medicine
David Geffen School of Medicine at UCLA
Los Angeles, California

KEVIN K. BROWN, MD
Department of Medicine
University of Colorado Health Sciences Center
Denver, Colorado

PHILIPPE CAMUS, MD
Department of Pulmonary Pharmacology/Toxicology
Université de Bourgogne
Dijon, France

EDWARD D. CHAN, MD
Department of Medicine
National Jewish Medical and Research Center
Denver, Colorado

THOMAS V. COLBY, MD
Department of Laboratory Medicine and Pathology
Mayo Clinic, Scottsdale
Scottsdale, Arizona

JEAN-FRANÇOIS CORDIER, MD
Department of Respiratory Medicine
Claude Bernard University
Lyon, France

GREGORY P. COSGROVE, MD
Department of Medicine
University of Colorado Health Sciences Center
Denver, Colorado

ULRICH COSTABEL, MD, FCCP
Faculty of Medicine
University of Essen
Essen, Germany

PAUL CULLINAN, MD, FRCP
Department of Occupational Medicine
Imperial College School of Medicine
London, United Kingdom

ROLAND M. DU BOIS, MA, MD
National Heart and Lung Institute
Imperial College School of Medicine
London, United Kingdom

LELAND L. FAN, MD
Department of Pediatrics
Baylor College of Medicine
Houston, Texas

MICHAEL B. FESSLER, MD
Department of Medicine
University of Colorado Health Sciences Center
Denver, Colorado

MICHAEL F. FITZPATRICK, MD
Department of Medicine
Queen's University
Kingston, Ontario, Canada

ANDREW P. FONTENOT, MD
Department of Medicine and Immunology
University of Colorado Health Sciences Center
Denver, Colorado

MICHELLE M. FREEMER, MD
Department of Medicine
University of California
San Francisco, California

KELLY E. GREENE, MD
Department of Medicine
University of Colorado Health Sciences Center
Denver, Colorado

JOSUNE GUZMAN, MD
Department of General and Experimental Pathology
Ruhr-University Bochum
Bochum, Germany

MICHAEL P. KEANE, MD
Department of Medicine
David Geffen School of Medicine at UCLA
Los Angeles, California

TALMADGE E. KING JR, MD
Department of Medicine
University of California
San Francisco, California

ARNOLD S. KRISTOF, MD
Pulmonary-Critical Care Medicine Branch
National Institute of Health
Bethesda, Maryland

RAZVAN LAPADAT, MD
Department of Pharmacology
University of Colorado Health Sciences Center
Denver, Colorado

KEVIN O. LESLIE, MD
Department of Laboratory Medince and Pathology
Mayo Clinic, Scottsdale
Scottsdale, Arizona

ANDREW H. LIMPER, MD
Department of Internal Medicine
Mayo Medical School
Rochester, Minnesota

DAVID LYNCH, MD
Department of Radiology
University of Colorado Health Sciences Center
Denver, Colorado

LISA A. MAIÉR, MD, MSPH
Department of Medicine and Preventative Medicine/Biometrics
University of Colorado Health Sciences Center
Denver, Colorado

FRANCIS X. MCCORMACK, MD
Department of Internal Medicine
University of Cincinnati
Cincinnati, Ohio

JOEL MOSS, MD
Pulmonary-Critical Care Medicine Branch
National Institutes of Health
Bethesda, Maryland

LEE S. NEWMAN, MD, MA
Department of Medicine and Preventative Medicine/Biometrics
University of Colorado Health Sciences Center
Denver, Colorado

DENIS E. O'DONNELL, MD
Department of Medicine
Queen's University
Kingston, Ontario, Canada

MICHAEL W. PETERSON, MD
Department of Medicine
University of California, San Francisco–Fresno
Fresno, California

GANESH RAGHU, MD
Department of Medicine
University of Washington School of Medicine
Seattle, Washington

DAVID W. H. RICHES, PhD
Department of Pediatrics
National Jewish Medical and Research Center
Denver, Colorado

JESSE ROMAN, MD
Department of Medicine
Emory University School of Medicine
Atlanta, Georgia

DAVID A. SCHWARTZ, MD
Department of Medicine
Duke University Medical Center
Durham, North Carolina

MARVIN I. SCHWARZ, MD
Department of Medicine
University of Colorado Health Sciences Center
Denver, Colorado

MOISÉS SELMAN, MD
Faculty of Medicine
National Autonomous University of Mexico
Mexico, Distrito Federal

GIANPIETRO SEMENZATO, MD
Department of Clinical and Experimental Medicine
University of Padua
Padova, Italy

JOHN M. SHANNON, PhD
Department of Pediatrics
Cincinnati Children's Hospital Medical Center
Cincinnati, Ohio

ULRICH SPECKS, MD
Division of Pulmonary and Critical Care Medicine
Mayo Medical School
Rochester, Minnesota

MARK P. STEELE, MD
Department of Medicine
Duke University Medical Center
Durham, North Carolina

R. G. STIRLING, MD
Department of Respiratory Medicine
Monash Medical School, The Alfred Hospital
Melbourne, Victoria, Australia

ROBERT M. STRIETER, MD
Department of Medicine and Pathology
David Geffen School of Medicine at UCLA
Los Angeles, California

STEPHEN J. SWENSEN, MD
Department of Radiology
Mayo Clinic
Rochester, Minnesota

ROBERT VASSALLO, MD
Department of Internal Medicine
Mayo Medical School
Rochester, Minnesota

JASON S. VOURLEKIS, MD
Division of Pulmonary Sciences and Critical Care Medicine
University of Colorado Health Sciences Center
Denver, Colorado

DAVID N. WEISSMAN, MD
Health Effects Laboratory Division
National Institute for Occupational Safety and Health
Morgantown, West Virginia

GLEN P. WESTALL, MD
Department of Medicine
Monash Medical School, The Alfred Hospital
Melbourne, Victoria, Australia

G. SCOTT WORTHEN, MD
Department of Medicine
National Jewish Medical and Research Center
Denver, Colorado

1

APPROACH TO THE EVALUATION AND DIAGNOSIS OF INTERSTITIAL LUNG DISEASE

MARVIN I. SCHWARZ
TALMADGE E. KING JR
GANESH RAGHU

The interstitial lung diseases (ILDs), also referred to as diffuse parenchymal lung diseases, are a diverse group of pulmonary disorders that are classified together because of similar clinical, roentgenographic, physiologic, or pathologic manifestations (Tables 1–1 to 1–9[1–208]). Diffuse lung diseases such as emphysema or chronic obstructive lung disease (COPD) and pulmonary hypertension are excluded from this classification. One of the difficulties with understanding this group of diseases is the confusing terminology. In fact, the term interstitial is somewhat misleading in that most of these disorders have extensive alteration of airways, lung parenchyma, blood vessels, or pleura as well. Also, other terms can be confusing: *idiopathic* indicates an unknown cause and *interstitial pneumonia* refers to involvement of the lung parenchyma by varying combinations of fibrosis and inflammation, in contrast to air space disease typically seen in bacterial pneumonia.[209] For the purposes of this book, the following terms are viewed as synonymous: *idiopathic* and *cryptogenic* as well as *pneumonia* and *pneumonitis*.[209]

In general, the major abnormality in interstitial lung disorders is disruption of the distal lung parenchyma. The lung has two interstitial connective tissue compartments: the parenchymal interstitium (alveolar wall or the alveolar septae) and the loose-binding connective tissue (peribronchovascular sheaths, interlobular septa, and visceral pleura). The parenchymal interstitium represents an anatomic space that is lined by alveolar epithelial cells and capillary endothelial cells. The epithelium and endothelium share a common basement membrane. The interstitium contains the lung's connective tissue elements (collagen, elastin, and reticulin fibrils), extracellular matrix—ground substance or matrix of glycosaminoglycans including a complex mixture of polysaccharide molecules (eg, proteoglycans, glycoproteins), and noncollagenous proteins (fibronectin and laminin).[210,211] Small numbers of interstitial cells reside in the connective tissue spaces of the lung—macrophages, mast cells, plasma cells, fibroblasts, and myofibroblasts.

When the lung is injured, epithelial cell basement membranes lose their integrity, heralding the appearance, depending on the injury, of a variety of inflammatory cells, regenerating type II epithelial cells, and increasing the expression of fibroblasts resulting in the accumulation of extracellular matrix components. (See Chapter 8, "Inflammation in the Pathogenesis of Interstitial Lung Diseases.") Continuation of this process can be fueled by persistent injury (blood borne or inhaled) or by profibrotic cytokines released from the regenerating alveolar epithelium, inflammatory cells, and the proliferating fibroblasts themselves. (See Chapter 10, "Cytokine Biology and the Pathogenesis of Interstitial

---

TABLE 1–1   Clinical Classification of Interstitial Lung Disease: Collagen Vascular Disease Associated

Scleroderma[1–3]
Polymyositis/dermatomyositis[4,5]
Systemic lupus erythematosus[6–8]
Rheumatoid arthritis[9–11]
Ankylosing spondylitis[12]
Mixed connective tissue disease[13,14]
Primary Sjögren's syndrome[15,16]
Behçet's syndrome[17,18]

TABLE 1–2   Clinical Classification of Interstitial Lung Disease: Drug and Treatment Induced Partial Listing

Antibiotics
  Nitrofurantoin[19]
  Sulfasalazine[20,21]
  Cephalosporin[22]
  Minocycline[23–25]
  Ethambutol[26]
Antiarrhythmic
  Amiodarone[27,28]
  Angiotensin converting enzyme-inhibitors[29]
  Tocainide[30]
  Beta-blocking agents[31–33]
Anti-inflammatory
  Gold[34–36]
  Penicillamine[37]
  Nonsteroidal anti-inflammatory agents[38–40]
Neurotropic and psychotropic
  Dilantin[41]
  Fluoxetine[42]
  Carbamazepine[43]
  Antidepressants[44,45]
Chemotherapeutic agents[46]
  Antibiotics
    Mitomycin C[47,48]
    Bleomycin[49,50]
  Alkalating agents
    Busulfan[51]
    Cyclophosphamide[52]
    Chlorambucil [53]
    Melphalan[54]
    Antimetabolites
    Methotrexate[55,56]
    Azathioprine[57]
    Cytosine arabinoside[58,59]
  Nitrosoureas[60]
    Carmustine (BCNU)[61]
    Lomustine (CCNU)[62]
  Others
    Procarbazine[63]
    Nilutemide[64]
    Alpha interferon[65,66]
    Paclitaxel[67]
    Interleukin-2[68]
  L-Tryptophan[69]
  Dopaminergic drugs
    Bromocryptine[70]
  Radiation[71,72]
  Oxygen[73,74]
  Paraquat[75,76]
  Bacille Calmette-Guérin[77]
  Cocaine[78]

mative interstitial pneumonia, alter the lung interstitium but are more accurately classified as an alveolar filling process with prominent accumulation of macrophages. In other instances, the alveolar lumens are defaced by the following: proliferating fibroblasts (organizing pneumonia), red blood cells (diffuse alveolar hemorrhage), proteinaceous material (alveolar proteinosis); obliterated by coalescing granulomas (sarcoidosis), calcium microliths (alveolar microlithiasis), or a hamartomatous proliferation of smooth muscle cells in the alveolar septa, around vessels and lymphatics, and in the pleura, without clearly evident alveolitis (lymphangioleiomyomatosis).

CLASSIFICATION

Interstitial lung diseases can be classified into clinical groups (see Tables 1–1 to 1–5) or by their underlying pattern of lung injury/repair based on lung histology (see Tables 1–6 to 1–8). A single clinical entity, such as drug-induced ILD or collagen vascular disease–associated ILD can be associated with several distinct histologic patterns. In general, the histologic appearance dictates therapeutic responsiveness. Processes with more a cellular histology (inflammation) tend to be more responsive to treat-

TABLE 1–3   Clinical Classification of Interstitial Lung Disease: Primary or Unclassified Disease Related

Sarcoidosis[79]
Eosinophilic granuloma[80]
Amyloidosis[81]
Lymphangioleiomyomatosis[82]
Tuberous sclerosis[83]
Neurofibromatosis[84]
Lymphangitic carcinomatosis[85]
Gaucher's disease[86]
Niemann-Pick disease[87]
Hermansky-Pudlak syndrome[88]
Adult respiratory distress syndrome[89,90]
Bone marrow transplantation[91,92]
Acquired immunodeficiency syndrome (AIDS)[93]
Postinfection[94–97]
Pulmonary vasculitis[98,99]
Respiratory bronchiolitis[100]
Interstitial cardiogenic pulmonary edema
Pulmonary veno-occlusive disease[101]
Agnogenic myeloid metaplasia[102]
Familial hemophagocytic lymphohistiocytosis[103]
Diabetes mellitus[104]
Lysinuric protein deficiency[105,106]
Alveolar filling diseases
  Alveolar proteinosis[107]
  Diffuse alveolar hemorrhage syndromes[108]
  Lipoid pneumonia[109]
  Bronchioloalveolar carcinoma[110]
  Pulmonary lymphoma[111]
  Chronic aspiration[112]
  Eosinophilic pneumonia[113–115]
  Alveolar microlithiasis[116]
  Alveolar sarcoidosis[79]
  Bronchiolitis obliterans organizing pneumonia[117–119]
Metastatic pulmonary calcification or ossification[120,121]

Lung Disease".) This is reflected pathologically as either inflammation and/or fibrosis. (See Chapter 9, "Role of the Alveolar Epithelium in the Pathogenesis of Pulmonary Fibrosis.") In some ILDs, malignant cells, amyloid fibrils, or granulomas infiltrate the interstitial space and interfere with lung function.

Several of the ILDs are bronchiolocentric (hypersensitivity pneumonitis, eosinophilic granuloma of the lung) implying inflammation or fibrosis of respiratory and terminal bronchioles and the adjacent alveolar structures. In addition, several of the ILDs, such as desqua-

TABLE 1–4   Clinical Classification of ILD: Occupational and Environmental Exposure Related

Inorganic
    Silicosis[122–124]
    Asbestosis[125,126]
    Talc pneumoconiosis[127,128]
    Kaolin pneumoconiosis[129]
    Diatomaceous earth pneumoconiosis[130]
    Aluminum oxide fibrosis[131]
    Berylliosis[132,133]
Hard metal fibrosis[134]
Coal workers' pneumoconiosis[135]
Baritosis (barium)[136]
Antimony pneumoconiosis[137]
Siderosilicosis (iron oxide)[138]
Polyvinylchloride pneumoconiosis[139]
Shale pneumoconiosis[140]
Siderosis (arc welder's lung)[141]
Stannosis (tin)[142]
Silicone pneumonitis[143]
Wood burning interstitial fibrosis[144]
Textile worker's pneumonitis[145]
    Flock Lung (nylon)[146]
Organic (hypersensitivity pneumonitis)[147–174]
    Bagassosis (sugar cane)
    Bird breeder's lung (pigeons, parakeets, etc.)
    Chicken handler's lung
    Duck fever
    Dove handler's disease
    Farmer's lung
    Coffee worker's lung
    Tobacco grower's lung
    Coptic disease (mummy wrappings)
    Cheese worker's lung
    Fishmeal worker's lung
    Furrier's lung
    Meat worker's lung
    Mushroom worker's lung
    Paprika splitter's lung
    Miller's lung (wheat flour)
    Wood worker's disease
    Sequoiosis
    Maple bark stripper's lung
    Malt worker's lung
    Tea grower's lung
    Suberosis (cork)
    Lycoperdonosis (*Lycoperdon* puffballs)
    Compost lung
    Humidifier lung
    Sauna taker's lung
    Woodman's disease (oak and maple)
    Pauli's hypersensitivity pneumonitis (reagent)
    Pituitary snuff disease
    Detergent worker's lung (isocyanates)
    Japanese summer-type hypersensitivity
    Thatched roof lung
    Familial hypersensitivity pneumonitis (wood dust)
    Vineyard sprayer's lung
    Laboratory worker's lung (rat urine)
    Mollusk shell hypersensitivity pneumonitis
    Goose down hypersensitivity pneumonitis
    Ceramic tile worker's pneumoconiosis
    Toluene diisocyanate hypersensitivity pneumonitis
    Machine operator's lung

TABLE 1–5   Clinical Classification of ILD: Idiopathic Interstitial Pneumonias and Autoimmune Diseases

Acute interstitial pneumonia[175] (Hamman-Rich syndrome)
Idiopathic pulmonary fibrosis[176]
Familial pulmonary fibrosis[177]
Lymphocytic interstitial pneumonitis[178]
Cryptogenic organizing pneumonia[117–119]
Nonspecific interstitial pneumonitis[179]
Desquamative interstitial pneumonitis[180]
Autoimmune hemolytic anemia[181]
Idiopathic thrombocytopenic purpura[182]
Cryoglobulinemia[183]
Inflammatory bowel disease[184]
Celiac disease[185]
Whipple's disease[186]
Primary biliary cirrhosis[187]
Chronic active hepatitis[188]
Cryptogenic cirrhosis[188]

TABLE 1–6   Histologic Classification and Response to Therapy: Treatment Responsive

Chronic eosinophilic pneumonia[113]
Acute eosinophilic pneumonia
    Idiopathic[114,115]
    Drug induced[20–25,38–40,78,189]
Nonspecific interstitial pneumonia
    Collagen vascular disease[1–11]
    Idiopathic[176]
    Drug induced[19,22,26–36,42,43,45]
    Hypersensitivity pneumonitis[148]
Bronchiolitis obliterans organizing pneumonia
    Idiopathic (cryptogenic organizing pneumonia)[117,118]
    Collagen vascular disease[4–9]
    Drug induced[34–36,65,66,78,190,191]
    Radiation[192,193]
    Graft-versus-host disease[194,195]
    Infection[196,197]
Desquamative interstitial pneumonia
Lymphocytic interstitial pneumonitis
    Idiopathic[178]
    Primary Sjögren's syndrome[15,16]
    Collagen vascular disease[1–8]
    Other autoimmune disease[178]
    Hypogammaglobulinemia[178]
    Acquired immunodeficiency syndrome[178]
Pulmonary capillaritis
    Wegener's granulomatosis[198,199]
    Microscopic polyangiitis[200]
    Other small vessel vasculitis[201,202]
    Collagen vascular disease
    Goodpasture's syndrome[203]
    Isolated pulmonary capillaritis[204]
Granulomatous interstitial pneumonitis
    Sarcoidosis[79]
    Hypersensitivity pneumonitis[148]
    Drug induced[43,55,56]
    Mycobacterial and fungal infections
    Berylliosis
Alveolar proteinosis
    Idiopathic variety[107]
Vasculitis
    Wegener's granulomatosis
    Churg-Strauss syndrome

TABLE 1–7   Histologic Classification and Response to Therapy: Sometimes Treatment Responsive

Diffuse alveolar damage
    Acute respiratory distress syndrome (ARDS) (all causes)[89,90]
    Cytotoxic drugs[47–67]
    Idiopathic pneumonia syndrome (bone marrow transplantation)[205]
    Collagen vascular disease[4–8]
    Acute interstitial pneumonitis (Hamman-Rich syndrome)[175,206]
    Toxic gas inhalation[89,90]
Diffuse alveolar hemorrhage (bland)
    Goodpasture's syndrome[203]
    Idiopathic pulmonary hemosiderosis[207]
    Systemic lupus erythematosus[208]
    Pulmonary veno-occlusive disease[101]
Granulomatous interstitial lung disease
    Eosinophilic granuloma[80]
    Berylliosis[132,133]

ment, whereas those with a more fibrotic histology tend not to respond to current therapies.

EPIDEMIOLOGY

Although the incidence of ILD in the United States is difficult to determine, it has been estimated that ILD accounts for 100,000 hospital admissions yearly and represents 15% of patients seen by pulmonologists nationwide.[212,213] Current statistics support the contention that ILD is far more prevalent than previously thought. Prior underestimation of the incidence and prevalence of ILD (5/100,000) in the United States was most likely due to inaccurate data obtained from death certificates.[214] An epidemiologic study from a county in New Mexico found that the overall prevalence of ILD was 80.9 per 100,000 in males and 67.2 per 100,000 in females and the incidence of ILD was 31.5 per 100,000 in men and 26.1 per 100,000 in women. Idiopathic pulmonary fibrosis represented 45% of the patient base.[215]

TABLE 1–8   Histologic Classification and Response to Therapy: Unresponsive to Therapy

Usual interstitial pneumonitis
    Idiopathic pulmonary fibrosis[176]
    Collagen vascular disease[1–16]
    Asbestosis
    Chronic hypersensitivity pneumonitis[148]
    Chronic eosinophilic pneumonia
Fibrotic nonspecific interstitial pneumonia
    Idiopathic[209]
    Collagen vascular disease[1–16]
    Hypersensitivity pneumonitis[148]
    Drug induced
    Progressive diffuse alveolar damage[89,90]
    Progressive organizing pneumonia
    Progressive lymphocytic pneumonitis[178]
    Progressive desquamative insterstitial pneumonia
Smooth muscle deposition
    Lymphangioleiomyomatosis[82]

TABLE 1–9   Acute Noninfectious Interstitial Lung Disease and their Underlying Histology

Acute idiopathic interstitial pneumonia (Hamman-Rich syndrome)
    Organizing diffuse alveolar damage (acute)
    Fibrotic nonspecific interstitial pneumonia (progressive)
Acute eosinophilic pneumonia
    Eosinophilic pneumonia
    Diffuse alveolar damage
    Organizing pneumonia
Hypersensitivity pneumonitis
    Granulomatous interstitial pneumonitis
    Nonspecific interstitial pneumonitis (cellular)
    Organizing pneumonia
    Usual interstitial pneumonitis (chronic)
    Nonspecific interstitial pneumonitis (fibrotic)
Drug-induced ILD
    Diffuse alveolar damage (cytotoxic drugs)
    Organizing pneumonia (amiodarone, gold)
    Eosinophilic pneumonia (NSAIDs, minocycline)
    Nonspecific interstitial pneumonia (nitrofurantoin, amiodarone)
    Usual interstitial pneumonitis (progressive)
Bronchiolitis obliterans organizing pneumonia (idiopathic)
    Organizing pneumonia
    Nonspecific interstitial pneumonia (cellular)
    Nonspecific interstitial pneumonia (fibrotic)
Acute immunologic pneumonia (collagen vascular disease)
    Pulmonary capillaritis (SLE, PM-DM, MCTD, Scl, RA)
    Organizing pneumonia (PM-DM, RA)
    Cellular/fibrotic nonspecific interstitial pneumonia (PM-DM, RA, SLE, Scl)
    Diffuse alveolar damage (SLE, PM-DM, MCTD, Scl)
    Usual interstitial pneumonitis (SLE, PM-DM, RA, Scl)
Diffuse alveolar hemorrhage syndromes
    Pulmonary capillaritis (CVD, Vas, Drugs, GPS)
    Bland pulmonary hemorrhage (IPH, GPS, Coag, MS)
    Diffuse alveolar damage (Drugs, ARDS, Hamman-Rich syndrome)

NSAIDs = nonsteroidal anti-inflammatory drugs; SLE = systemic lupus erythematosus; PM-DM = polymyositis/dermatomyositis; MCTD = mixed connective tissue disease; Scl = scleroderma; RA=rheumatoid arthritis; CVD = collagen vascular disease; Coag = coagulopathy; MS = mitral stenosis; ARDS = acute respiratory distress syndrome; ILD = interstitial lung disease; Vas = vasculitis; GPS = Goodpasture's syndrome; IPH = idiopathic pulmonary hemosiderosis.

In the United Kingdom, it was estimated that 1 in every 3,000 to 4,000 of the population had ILD and that each year 3,000 people die, half of these from idiopathic pulmonary fibrosis.[216,217]

The ILDs are rare in children. (See Chapter 6, "Pediatric Interstitial Lung Disease.") The incidence appears to increase with age, especially for idiopathic pulmonary fibrosis, which approaches 160 per 100,000 in those over the age of 75 years. Also, the prevalence of ILD varies among certain specific disease entities. For example, the incidence of ILD among patients with scleroderma has been reported to be as high as 100%.[3] Approximately 33% of patients with rheumatoid arthritis have radiographic or physiologic evidence of ILD.[218] In sarcoidosis, a disease that affects 70 of every 100,000 African Americans, there is residual pulmonary fibrosis in 33% of patients.[79] It is also estimated that 30 to 40%

of ILD falls into the category of the idiopathic interstitial pneumonias.[176]

If one considers the continued development of cytotoxic drugs with the potential for lung injury (eg, for the treatment of malignant disease and preconditioning therapy for bone marrow transplantation), the increased recognition of nonspecific interstitial pneumonitis in acquired immunodeficiency syndrome (AIDS), and the detection of occupation-related ILD, the incidence of ILD will increase. Furthermore, using methods that detect subclinical ILD in patients at risk, such as bronchoalveolar lavage, high-resolution computed tomography, or extensive physiologic testing, more patients will be identified—hopefully at an earlier stage of disease.

PATHOGENESIS

The pathogenesis of most ILDs, especially the idiopathic interstitial pneumonias, remains unknown. Current understanding of the basic mechanisms of injury and repair are discussed in Part 2 of this book.

It is generally agreed that for many of the ILDs some form of injury to the alveolar epithelial cells initiates the pathogenetic sequence. This could result in an inflammatory response and coupled with the lung's attempts at repair result in scarring and the eventual structural changes that are responsible for clinical symptoms and physiologic abnormalities. The initiating injury can be introduced through the airways by inhalation of mineral fibers or dusts as occurs in occupational lung diseases. The injury can also occur as a result of sensitization to inhaled antigens, from both environmental and occupational sources, which is the case in hypersensitivity pneumonitis. Alternately, the route of injury can be via the circulation as most likely occurs in collagen vascular diseases, drug-induced ILD, and other immunologic diseases. If the injury is limited, it is possible to reverse the trend toward collagen deposition and fibrosis, restore the integrity of the epithelial basement membrane, and reverse the physiologic abnormalities. With continuing injury, however, the repair process continues driven by proinflammatory and profibrotic cytokines released by inflammatory cells, proliferating epithelial cells, and matrix components, resulting in continued proliferation of fibroblasts, collagen deposition, and obliteration of the interstitial capillaries. This is likened to the healing of a wound, but in this case the repair process, heralded by uncontrolled fibroproliferation is not turned off. In a skin wound, re-establishment of the overlying epithelium turns off the repair process.

The clinical and physiologic consequences appear early in the acute injury during the inflammatory stage as well as in the more chronic stages. During the chronic stage, interstitial and intra-alveolar fibrosis occur, and alveolar collapse ensues.[210,211,219] Although this pathologic sequence is applicable for many entities (see Tables 1–1 to 1–5), there are notable exceptions. For example,

in lymphangioleiomyomatosis,[82] amyloidosis,[81] and lymphangitic carcinomatosis,[85] the interstitium is infiltrated with smooth muscle, amyloid fibrils, and malignant cells, respectively. In several of the alveolar-filling disorders, prior to the appearance of interstitial and intra-alveolar fibrosis, red blood cells (diffuse alveolar hemorrhage syndrome), eosinophils (eosinophilic pneumonia), lipoproteinaceous exudate (alveolar proteinosis), or malignant cells (bronchoalveolar cell carcinoma) fill the alveolar spaces. Note that the collagen deposition, which typically involves the alveolar wall, may also be intraluminal in location.[117,118,220–222] Intracellular collagen deposition often occurs in idiopathic pulmonary fibrosis, bronchiolitis obliterans organizing pneumonia, hypersensitivity pneumonitis, eosinophilic pneumonia, and during the organizing phase of the acute respiratory distress syndrome, to mention a few.

CLINICAL EVALUATION

The clinical assessment of a patient with ILD requires a combination of history and physical examination, laboratory investigation, lung function testing, chest imaging studies, bronchoalveolar lavage, and histologic examination.

History

Length Of Illness And Clinical Course

Although the rate of symptomatic progression and physiologic deterioration for the individual patient with ILD is variable, it generally runs a chronic course that ranges from 6 months from the time of diagnosis to up to 10 or more years, depending on the specific etiology.

In contrast to this clinical course, Table 1–9 lists a number of clinical entities with underlying histology in which the onset of respiratory symptoms is acute (1 to 14 days). These are the so-called acute (noninfectious) interstitial pneumonias.[223–225] Diffuse radiographic alveolar opacities are found in this group of diseases (Figure 1–1). In addition to cough and dyspnea, fever, an elevated sedimentation rate, and mild-to-moderate leukocytosis can be detected. Recurrences are common, particularly in patients with the Hamman-Rich syndrome,[175,206] hypersensitivity pneumonitis, and acute immunologic pneumonias associated with collagen vascular diseases and diffuse alveolar hemorrhage syndromes. The acute noninfectious interstitial pneumonias must be distinguished from community-acquired pneumonias caused by viruses, *Mycoplasma* species, and *Legionella* species in the immunocompetent host, and from diffuse viral and fungal infections in the immunosuppressed patient. Also predisposing conditions for the acute respiratory distress syndrome must be excluded, since its presentation is similar.

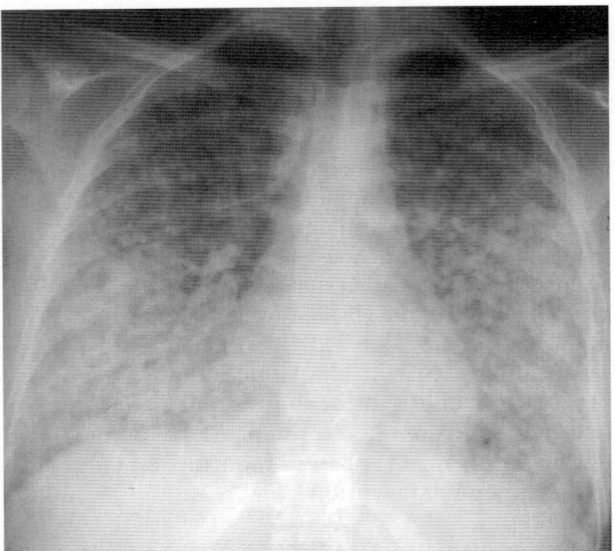

Figure 1–1   Chest radiograph of acute noninfectious interstitial pneumonitis. Diffuse alveolar filling in an acute presentation of idiopathic bronchiolitis obliterans organizing pneumonia.

Although most cases of collagen vascular disease–associated ILD are detected in previously established cases, the pulmonary disease, on occasion, may precede the more typical manifestations by months or even years.[2,4] The acute presentation of either an immunologic pneumonia or diffuse alveolar hemorrhage may be the initiating event in this group of diseases.

Occupational and Environmental History

A detailed lifelong occupational history must be obtained because the latency period between occupational exposure and onset of symptoms and radiographic abnormalities may be prolonged. There is an extensive and growing list of antigens both in the workplace and in the home environment that can cause hypersensitivity pneumonitis (see Table 1–4). The symptoms of hypersensitivity pneumonitis may be acute, disappear when contact with the offending antigen is interrupted, and reappear with re-exposure to the responsible environmental antigen. On the other hand, an insidious progressive form of hypersensitivity pneumonitis is clinically indistinguishable from idiopathic pulmonary fibrosis or other progressive fibrotic lung diseases.

Drug History

A careful drug history must also be obtained (see Table 1–2). Patients often neglect to mention past medications taken for prolonged periods. In most cases, the onset of a drug-induced ILD is temporally related to the administration of that drug. There are reports, however, that describe a variable latency period ranging from weeks, and in the case of carmustine (BCNU), to many years.[226,227] An adjuvant effect from either radiation treatment or the inhalation of high concentrations of inspired oxygen associated with diffuse alveolar damage is associated with bleomycin and other lung cytotoxic drugs.[46]

A history of gastroesophageal reflux that is associated with nocturnal cough and wheezing is important because a variety of gastroesophageal disorders may result in gastric acid aspiration and insidious development of lower-zone pulmonary fibrosis.[112,228] Patients should also be questioned about the nasal instillation of mineral oil drops or petroleum products, which can cause lipoid pneumonia and, with chronic use, fibrosis.[109] In a recent study, occult acid gastroesophageal reflex (GERD) was detected in 90% of patients with idiopathic pulmonary fibrosis (ILP).[330]

Age and Gender

Age and gender are sometimes useful in the general evaluation of ILD. Between the ages of 20 and 40 years, sarcoidosis, eosinophilic granuloma, collagen vascular disease–associated ILD, lymphangioleiomyomatosis, the inherited interstitial lung diseases such as Gaucher's disease and alveolar microlithiasis, and familial forms of idiopathic pulmonary fibrosis are more likely to occur. Above the age of 50 years, idiopathic pulmonary fibrosis must be considered. For most other etiologies of ILD there are no age or gender considerations above this age. There are a few exceptions, women are somewhat more likely to have collagen vascular disease–associated ILD; lymphangioleiomyomatosis and tuberous sclerosis–associated ILDs are exclusively seen in women. Men are more likely to have pneumoconiosis, although asbestosis and berylliosis have been reported to cause bystander pneumoconiosis in wives and children of workers who are exposed to contaminated clothing.[229,230]

Smoking History

There is a relationship with the development of ILD and tobacco consumption. In eosinophilic granuloma > 90% of patients are active smokers at the time of diagnosis.[231,232] In fact, the diagnosis of eosinophilic granuloma is unlikely in the absence of a smoking history. Respiratory bronchiolitis is another ILD in which almost all affected individuals are smokers.[100] In Goodpasture's syndrome, which is one cause of diffuse alveolar hemorrhage, 100% of smokers experience pulmonary hemorrhage compared with only 20% of affected nonsmokers.[233] It is more likely that individuals exposed to asbestos who smoke will develop asbestosis.[234] In patients with idiopathic pulmonary fibrosis,

66% are former or current smokers.[235] On the other hand, hypersensitivity pneumonitis is less likely to develop in active smokers.[236] In sarcoidosis, another granulomatous lung disease, the incidence is lower in a smoking cohort.[237]

Family History

A family history is important since genetic factors play a role in the development of some ILDs.[238] A familial form of idiopathic pulmonary fibrosis affecting family members and usually for several generations, is transmitted via an autosomal dominant pattern of inheritance with variable penetrance. This has suggested the possible presence of a fibrotic gene.[239,240] Mutations of the surfactant protein C gene in family members with familial pulmonary fibrosis have been described.[241,242] Interestingly, in clinically unaffected relatives of patients with familial idiopathic pulmonary fibrosis, the bronchoalveolar lavage cellular constituents can be abnormal, indicating subclinical disease.[243] Other ILDs with autosomal-dominant inheritance include tuberous sclerosis,[83] neurofibromatosis,[84] and Hermansky-Pudlak syndrome (ILD with oculocutaneous albinism).[88]

Lymphangioleiomyomatosis, a disease characterized by smooth muscle proliferation in the lung, occurs primarily in premenopausal women,[82] but there is no familial predisposition. More than 450 cases of familial sarcoidosis have been reported, often among sibling pairs with similar pulmonary and extrapulmonary manifestations.[238] It remains unclear whether this is genetically based or due to common environmental exposure.

Respiratory Symptoms and Signs

Dyspnea

The most recognizable presentation of ILD is a symptomatic patient with an abnormal chest radiograph. Progressive dyspnea, initially with exercise and then at rest, is by far the most common complaint, but cough and fatigue may also be prominent. As many as 10% of patients with ILD may also present with dyspnea but have a normal chest radiograph.[244] After more common lung conditions such as pulmonary embolus and obstructive lung diseases are excluded, ILD should be considered. In this situation, high-resolution computed tomography and extensive lung physiologic testing, to include gas exchange with exercise, often point to an ILD and lead to a lung biopsy. Alternately, patients with ILD may be asymptomatic and have an abnormal chest radiograph. In this situation standard lung physiologic testing may or may not indicate abnormalities. Dyspnea is only relevant to the amount of physical activity performed by the individual. An abnormal chest radiograph indicating ILD in an asymptomatic patient should not

be ignored because almost all forms of ILDs progress and eventually cause symptomatic and functional impairment. It is also likely that early identification of an ILD makes it more amenable to therapeutic intervention. Even with normal spirometry and lung volumes, measurement of rest and exercise gas exchange reveals physiologic abnormalities in asymptomatic patients with abnormal chest radiographs.

Cough

A particularly irritating cough occurs in lymphangitic carcinomatosis, which, in addition to invading the lymphatics of the lung parenchyma, can also involve the bronchial submucosal lymphatics; in sarcoidosis, granulomas often infiltrate the bronchial submucosa. In the bronchiolocentric diseases, such as hypersensitivity pneumonitis, bronchiolitis obliterans organizing pneumonia, eosinophilic granuloma, and bronchiolitis, cough is a frequent complaint.

Chest Pain

Substernal or pleuritic chest pain is an uncommon symptom for most ILDs but is reported by patients with sarcoidosis.[79] In the collagen vascular diseases, particularly rheumatoid arthritis and systemic lupus erythematosus, as well as in several of the drug-related ILDs (eg, nitrofurantoin), pleurisy can occur. Acute pleuritic chest pain can also result from a spontaneous pneumothorax. Pneumothorax is often the first manifestation of eosinophilic granuloma, lymphangioleiomyomatosis, tuberous sclerosis, or neurofibromatosis.

Wheezing

Wheezing, an unusual complaint in ILD, is sometimes reported by patients with either hypersensitivity pneumonitis or chronic eosinophilic pneumonia in which 50% of patients have asthma or respiratory bronchiolitis.

Hemoptysis

Hemoptysis, most often the presenting complaint of patients with one of the diffuse alveolar hemorrhage syndromes or lymphangioleiomyomatosis, is an infrequent symptom in other ILDs. If it appears in the presence of a known ILD, consideration should be given for the development of a malignancy, a pulmonary embolus, or an infection.[245] Hemoptysis, although expected in the diffuse alveolar hemorrhage syndromes, may initially be absent in as many as 33% of these patients, even in the face of a falling hematocrit, radiographic diffuse pulmonary infiltrates, and a bloody bronchoalveolar lavage.[246]

Physical Examination

The characteristic physical sign in ILD is bibasilar inspiratory crackles. This is not, however, a consistent finding. For example, in granulomatous ILD (eg, sarcoidosis, hypersensitivity pneumonitis, silicosis, eosinophilic granuloma), crackles are less frequently present compared with idiopathic pulmonary fibrosis, asbestosis, or collagen vascular disease–associated ILD.[247] Resting tachypnea and tachycardia may be present.

Digital clubbing, a marker of advanced fibrotic disease, is most often found in patients with idiopathic pulmonary fibrosis. Rarely, the syndrome of hypertrophic pulmonary osteodystrophy appears, causing severe pain in the distal extremities.[248] Digital clubbing is asymptomatic, although its appearance in a patient with a known ILD could indicate a complicating bronchogenic carcinoma.

An increased pulmonic component of the second heart sound, tricuspid insufficiency, peripheral edema, and cyanosis are manifestations of secondary pulmonary hypertension and cor pulmonale. Other nonpulmonary physical findings are listed in Table 1–10. Platypnea-orthodeoxia, dyspnea, and hypoxemia accentuated by the upright position have been reported in patients with severe pulmonary fibrosis, particularly with extensive lower lobe fibrosis.[251]

Physical examination may indicate a collagen vascular disease or a systemic vasculitis (eg, musculoskeletal pain, weakness, fatigue, fever, joint pains or swelling, photosensitivity, Raynaud's phenomenon, pleuritis, dry eyes, dry mouth, or skin rash).

Laboratory Investigation

Laboratory evaluation can help confirm or suggest the possibility of a diagnosis in the ILDs (Table 1–11). A negative result, however, does not necessarily exclude a specific diagnosis. The potential problems of laboratory test results are best demonstrated in hypersensitivity pneumonitis in which the diagnosis is often confirmed by finding precipitating antibodies to the causative agent in the patient's serum. Results of serum precipitin testing can be affected by certain situations: (1) the antigen may not be included in the panel of serum precipitins tested for; (2) a new antigen may be responsible for the patient's lung disease; (3) the presence of a serum precipitin does not necessarily indicate disease activity (since most agents responsible for hypersensitivity pneumonitis are ubiquitous, and exposed populations can have positive antibody titers without evidence of lung disease); and (4) there is a causative relationship between the ILD and the serum test.

Anemia is more likely to occur with the diffuse alveolar hemorrhage syndromes, but leukocytosis is nonspecific. Peripheral eosinophilia supports the diagnosis of acute eosinophilic pneumonia; however, more often it is

absent at presentation. For all cases of suspected acute noninfectious interstitial pneumonitis, a microscopic examination of the urinary sediment and measurement of the serum antinuclear factor, rheumatoid factor, and antibody to double-stranded DNA are indicated. If diffuse alveolar hemorrhage is suspected, serum antineutrophil cytoplasmic antibodies (ANCA) and antibasement membrane antibodies (ABMA) are indicated.[198–202]

Physiologic Testing

Although there are differences in the severity and rate of progression of physiologic disturbances in ILD, the

TABLE 1–10   Associated Systemic Signs Accompanying Interstitial Lung Disease

Systemic hypertension	CVD, NF, GPS, WG, MPA
Erythema nodosum	Sarc, BS, CVD
Maculopapular rash	CVD, DI, Lip, Amyl
Heliotrope rash	DM
Café au lait spots	NF
Albinism	HPS
Discoid lupus	IPF, SLE
Neurofibromas	NF
Telangiectasia	Scl
Calcinosis	Scl, PM-DM
Raynaud's phenomena	CVD, IPF
Cutaneous vasculitis	WG, RA, MPA, SLE
Subcutaneous nodules	RA, NF, Vas
Scleritis	SLE, Scl, Sarc, WG, MPA
Keratoconjunctivitis sicca	SS, CVD
Uveitis	Sarc, BS, AS
Lacrimal gland enlargement	Sarc
Salivary gland enlargement	Sarc, SS
Lymphadenopathy	Sarc, LC, LIP, Lym
Pericarditis	CVD, Rad, GPS, Vas
Hepatosplenomegaly	Sarc, EG, CVD, Amyl, LIP, Lym
Myositis	CVD, Sarc
Bone involvement	EG, Sarc, LC, LIP
Arthritis	Sarc, CVD, WG, MPA
Diabetes insipidus	EG, Sarc
Glomerulonephritis	CVD, WG, GPS, Sarc, MPA
Nephrotic syndrome	Amyl, DI, SLE, Sarc
Renal mass	LAM, TS
Neurologic abnormalities	Sarc, LC, NF, TS, CVD, WG, MPA

Adapted from James DGJ and Graham E;[249] Sharma OP and Nam H.[250] CVD = collagen vascular disease; NF = neurofibromatosis; GPS = Goodpasture's syndrome; WG = Wegener's granulomatosis; MPA = microscopic polyangiitis; Sarc = sarcoidosis; BS = Behçet's syndrome; DI = drug induced; Lip = lipoidosis; Amyl = amyloidosis; DM = dermatomyositis; HPS = Hermansky-Pudlak syndrome; IPF = idiopathic pulmonary fibrosis; SLE = systemic lupus erythematosus; Scl = scleroderma; PM-DM = polymyositis/dermatomyositis; RA = rheumatoid arthritis; Vas = vasculitis; SS = Sjögren's syndrome; AS = ankylosing spondylitis; LC = lymphangitic carcinomatosis; Lym = lymphomas; Rad = radiation pneumonitis; EG = eosinophilic granuloma; TS = tuberous sclerosis; LAM = lymphangioleiomyomatosis; LIP = lymphocytic interstitial pneumonia.

characteristic pattern is one of gradual loss of lung volume (restrictive ventilatory impairment); preservation of flow rates; reduction in the diffusing capacity for carbon monoxide; stiff nondistensible lungs with increased elastic recoil; and gas exchange abnormalities both at rest and accentuated by exercise. (See Chapter 3, "Physiology of Interstitial Lung Disease.") The dyspnea these patients experience is a consequence of the increased effort required to breathe due to decreased lung compliance (stiff lungs); this compromises ventilatory ability and is characterized by resting tachypnea, small tidal volumes, and respiratory alkalosis. There is also compromise of the pulmonary circulation due to alveolar scarring with resultant capillary destruction. These changes contribute significantly to the exercise intolerance these patients experience.[252]

Abnormalities in pulmonary function testing do not point to a specific diagnosis nor do specific physiologic abnormalities pinpoint the underlying histologic change (eg, differentiating between inflammation and fibrosis).[253,254] The severity of physiologic disarrangements do, however, correlate with the overall extent of pathologic abnormalities.[255] Abnormalities of pulmonary function also verify the presence of disease, particularly in those patients with normal chest roentgenograms; they are also useful in monitoring disease progression and response to therapy.

In the dyspneic patient with or without radiographic evidence of ILD, it would not be unusual for lung volumes, flow rates, diffusing capacity, and resting arterial blood gases to be within the normal range. The evaluation of such a patient is not complete until rest and exercise gas exchange studies are performed. Frequently, physiologic abnormalities are revealed only after the additional oxygen requirements necessary for exercise indicate a fall in the partial pressure of oxygen, a widening of the alveolar-arterial oxygen gradient, and an increase in deadspace ventilation. These are consequences of physiologic shunting and deadspace ventilation.[255–257] The pathologic alterations in some ILDs involve not only the alveolar structures but also the terminal airways (terminal bronchioles, respiratory bronchioles, and alveolar ducts). It is likely that disease involving these structures contributes significantly to the ventilation-perfusion mismatching and resultant hypoxemia.[258] The inability of the lung to correct the ventilation-perfusion mismatching and the increase in the effort of breathing during exercise account for the characteristic symptoms in this group of diseases; this also prompts early use of oxygen therapy, particularly with exertion. Interestingly, abnormal sleep quality in patients with ILD with hypoxemia indicates the need for nocturnal oxygen as well.[259,260] A few patients with ILD do not respond as expected. Rather than improving, the arterial desaturation in the upright position worsens, a condition known as orthodeoxia.[251,261] This may occur with extensive lower lobe fibrosis.

Airflow is preserved in most ILDs, unless the patient has an accompanying obstructive lung disease. ILD may, of course, be superimposed on pre-existing obstructive lung disease. There are, however, several ILDs that, because of their bronchiolocentric propensity, can eventually cause reduction in flow rates and increase rather than decrease the functional residual capacity and thoracic gas volume. These include sarcoidosis, hypersensitivity pneumonitis, eosinophilic granuloma, lymphangioleiomyomatosis, tuberous sclerosis, and neurofibromatosis.

Radiographic Features

Chest Radiograph

The chest radiograph remains the most practical first step for the detection, verification, and classification of ILDs, although a high-resolution computed tomography

TABLE 1–11   Laboratory Results in Intersititial Lung Disease

Hemolytic anemia	SLE, MCTD, DI, Lym, IPF, Sarc
Normocytic normochromic anemia	CVD, LC
Iron deficiency anemia	DAH
Leukopenia	CVD, DI, Sarc, Lym
Leukocytosis	HSP, Lym, Vas
Eosinophilia	Sarc, DI, EP, Vas
Thrombocytopenia	CVD, IPF, DI, Sarc
Abnormal urinary sediment	SLE, GPS, WG, MPA, Vas
Hypergammaglobulinemia	CVD, IPF, Sarc, LIP, Sil, SS, WG, MPA
Hypogammaglobulinemia	LIP
Autoantibodies (rheumatoid factor, antinuclear factors, cryoglobulins)	CVD, Sil, Asb, IPF, Sarc, LIP, WG, MPA, Vas
Serum angiotensin converting enzyme	Sarc, HSP, Sil, LIP, ARDS
Serum immune complexes	IPF, HSP, RA, SLE, EG, WG
Hypercalcemia	Sarc, LC
Antibasement membrane antibody	GPS
Antineutrophilic cytoplasmic antibody	WG, MPA
Increased serum lactic dehydrogenase	IPF, PAP, AIP

SLE = systemic lupus erythematosus; MCTD = mixed connective tissue disease; DI = drug induced; Lym = lymphoma; IPF = idiopathic pulmonary fibrosis; Sarc = sarcoidosis; CVD = collagen vascular disease; LC = lymphangitic carcinomatosis; DAH = diffuse alveolar hemorrhage; HSP = Henoch Shoenlein purpura; Vas = vasculitis; EP = eosinophilic pneumonia; GPS = Goodpasture's syndrome; WG = Wegener's granulomatosis; MPA = microscopic polyangiitis; LIP = lymphocytic interstitial pneumonia; Sil = silicosis; SS = Sjögren's syndrome; Asb = abestosis; ARDS = acute respiratory distress syndrome; RA = rheumatoid arthritis; EG = eosinophilic granuloma; PAP = pulmonary alveolar proteinosis; AIP = acute interstitial pneumonitis.

(HRCT) scan clearly has improved utility for detection and classification. (See Chapter 4, "Imaging of Diffuse Parenchymal Lung Diseases.") Traditionally, the ILDs are either alveolar filling or interstitial opacities. Although this classification has its limitations, it provides a logical starting point for the work-up of a patient with ILD.[262] Ziskind and colleagues deserve much of the credit for this classification.[263,264] The major criticism of this classification, however, is that many ILDs appear both interstitial and alveolar and thus produce a mixed radiographic pattern. As mentioned previously, 10% of symptomatic patients who are subsequently diagnosed as having ILD have normal chest radiographs.[244] In this case, other causes for symptoms and abnormal physiology must first be excluded; these include pulmonary vascular disease and chronic obstructive lung disease. Also, the HRCT scan plays an important role in the detection of ILD in a symptomatic patient with a normal chest radiograph.[265,266] Desquamative interstitial pneumonia, type I sarcoidosis, and hypersensitivity pneumonitis are conditions that most often present with symptoms and physiologic alterations in the face of a normal chest radiograph.[244,267–269] Any ILD, however, may present in this fashion.

Alveolar Opacities.   Alveolar filling disorders produce either homogeneous consolidations with air bronchograms (Figure 1–2) or variably sized nodular densities with ill-defined borders associated with acinar rosettes (air alveolograms) (Figures 1–3 and 1–4). Air bronchograms appear when cells or fluid producing an air-fluid contrast fills alveoli adjacent to an unobstructed air-filled bronchus. Similarly, acinar rosettes evolve when sublobular consolidation of terminal alveolar units are adjacent to an open-terminal bronchiole.[264] Another important radiographic feature of an

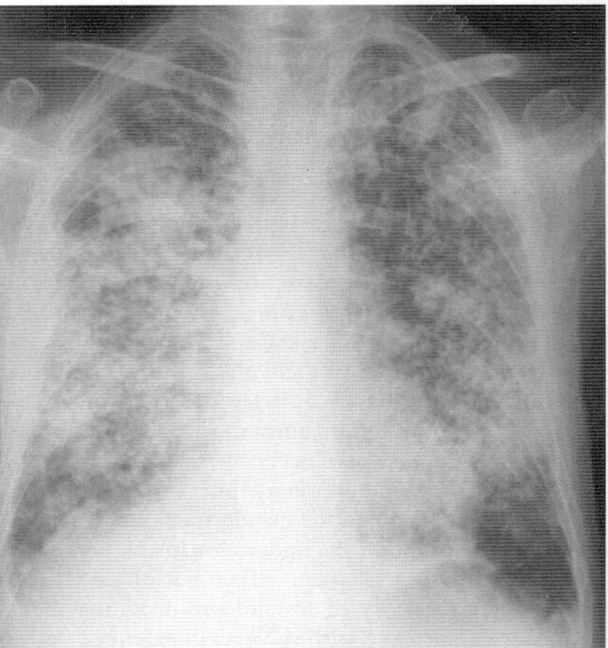

Figure 1–3   Chest radiograph of diffuse alveolar filling. A patient with bronchioloalveolar cell carcinoma. Note the poorly defined alveolar nodules, areas of coalescence of alveolar nodules, and obliteration of portions of the heart border and diaphragm, and pulmonary vessels.

alveolar filling process is the obliteration or silhouetting of structures that are usually visible; these include the diaphragm, the pulmonary blood vessels, and the cardiac borders. Roentgenographic features of alveolar filling disorders are listed below:

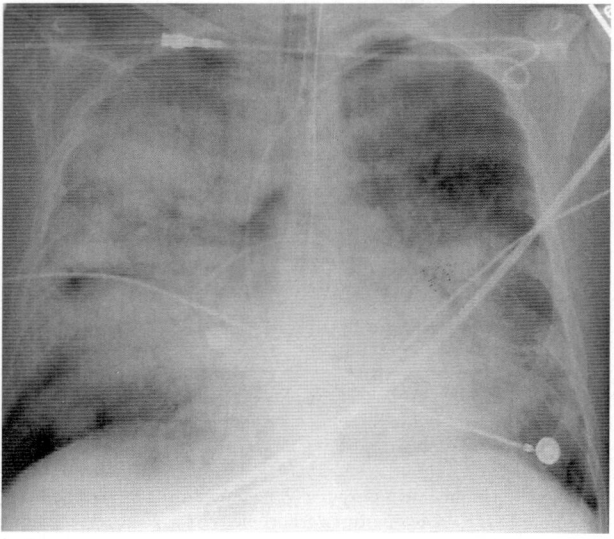

Figure 1–2   Chest radiograph of diffuse alveolar filling. A patient with respiratory failure in which lung biopsy revealed alveolar proteinosis. Note the air bronchograms and the silhouetting of portions of the heart border, diaphragm, and intraparenchymal blood vessels.

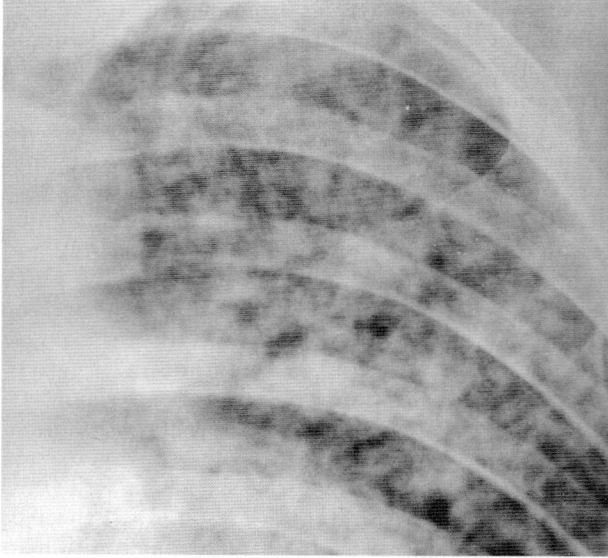

Figure 1–4   Chest radiograph of diffuse alveolar filling. Bronchioloalveolar cell carcinoma with alveolar nodules and distal air bronchograms.

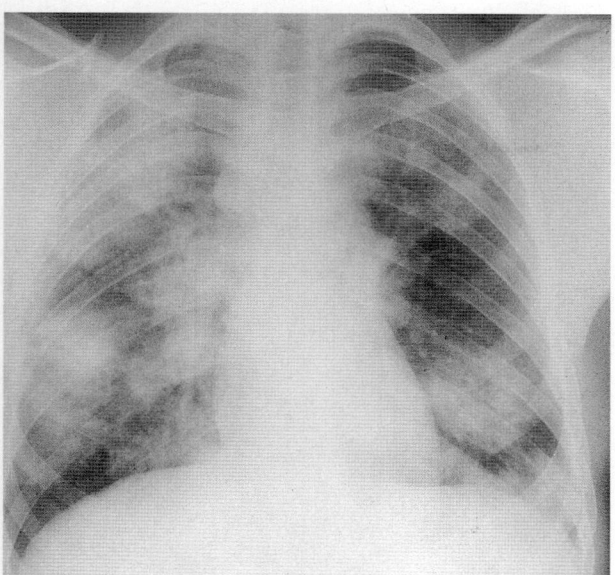

Figure 1–5   Chest radiograph of diffuse patchy alveolar filling and lymphadenopathy. A patient with type II sarcoidosis with bilateral hilar and mediastinal adenopathy as well as poorly defined areas of consolidation in the lung parenchyma.

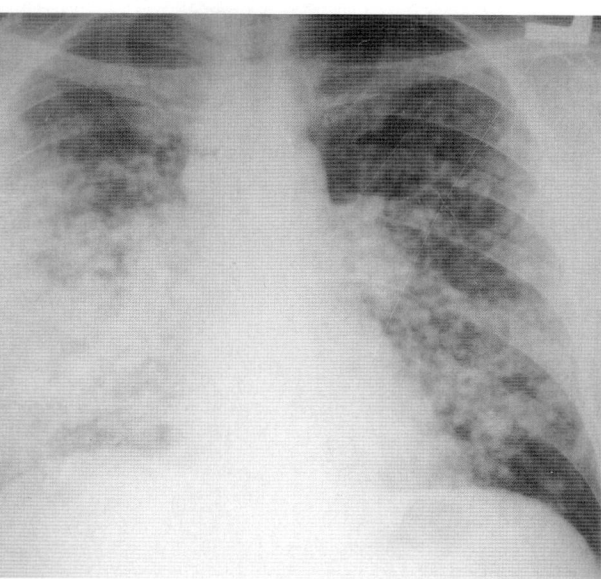

Figure 1–7   Chest radiograph of diffuse alveolar filling with lymphadenopathy. Patient with Hodgkin's disease demonstrating areas of dense consolidation as well as smaller alveolar nodules. Also note the proximal and distal air bronchograms.

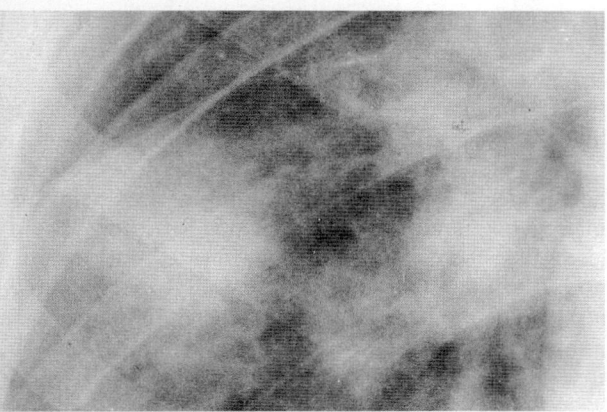

Figure 1–6   Chest radiograph of diffuse alveolar filling. Close-up view of patient described in Figure 1–5.

- Air bronchograms
- Acinar rosettes
- Diffuse consolidation
- Nodule-like configuration with poorly defined borders
- Obliteration (silhouetting) of normal structures (eg, diaphragm, heart borders, pulmonary vasculature)

Interstitial lung diseases can produce radiographic diffuse alveolar filling. Four of these disorders can be associated with hilar and mediastinal adenopathy: sarcoidosis (Figures 1–5 and 1–6), lymphoma (Figure 1–7), lymphocytic interstitial pneumonia, and less commonly with idiopathic pulmonary hemosiderosis.[270] The chest

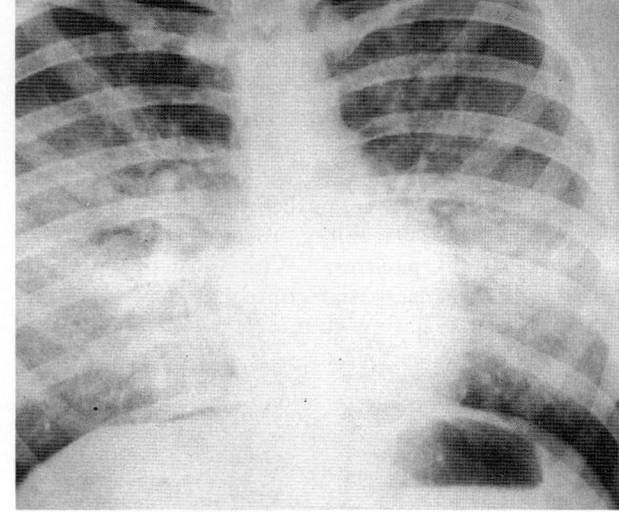

Figure 1–8   Chest radiograph of diffuse alveolar filling with sparing of the lung parenchyma adjacent to the diaphragm in a patient with alveolar proteinosis.

roentgenogram of alveolar proteinosis, another alveolar filling disorder, typically shows sparing of the lung parenchyma immediately adjacent to the diaphragm (Figure 1–8). In desquamative interstitial pneumonia, the typical appearance is that of a triangular alveolar filling process with its apex at the pulmonary hilum and its base extending to the level of the diaphragm (Figure 1–9).[271,272] It can also appear as a diffuse, hazy density

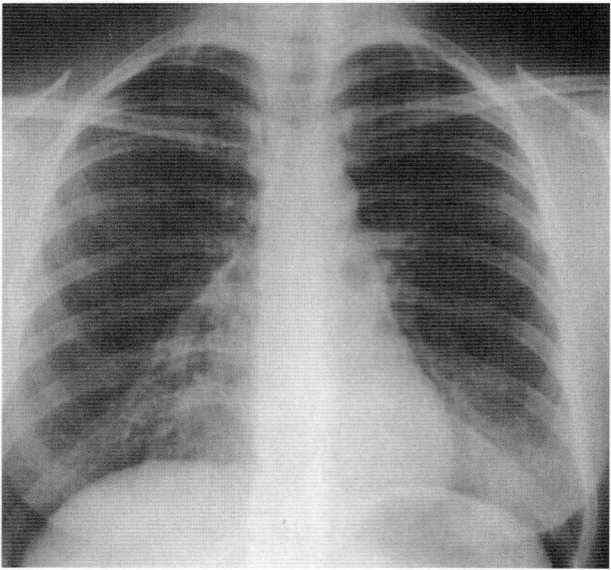

Figure 1–9   Chest radiograph of alveolar filling. A patient with primary desquamative interstitial pneumonia demonstrating a triangular alveolar filling process with apices at the pulmonary hilum and extending down to the level of the diaphragm.

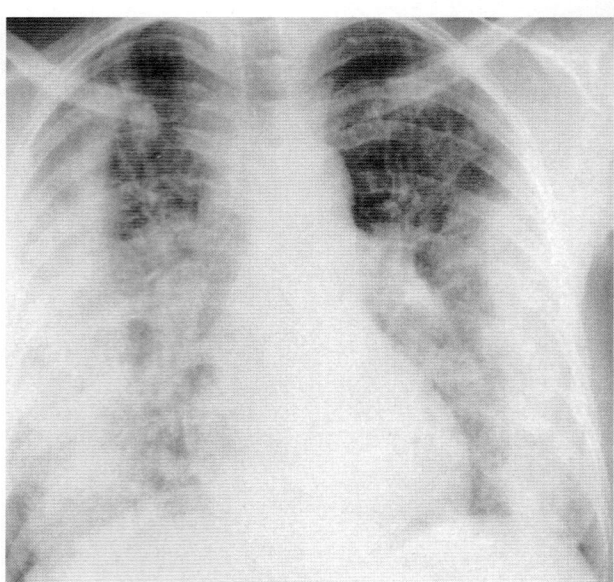

Figure 1–11   Chest radiograph of alveolar filling. A patient with chronic eosinophilic pneumonia whose radiograph shows predominantly peripheral infiltrates.

(Figure 1–10). The pattern described in chronic eosinophilic pneumonia has been referred to as the radiographic "negative" of pulmonary edema because the alveolar infiltrate is more prominent in the peripheral portions of the lung fields (Figures 1–11 and 1–12).[187,273] Some cases of idiopathic bronchiolitis obliterans organizing pneumonia (cryptogenic organizing pneumonia) can produce a similar radiographic distribution. Acute eosinophilic pneumonia, on the other hand, appears as a more diffuse alveolar filling process (Figure 1–13).

Interstitial Opacities.   With broadening and distortion of the interstitial compartment by edema, inflammatory cells, smooth muscle proliferation, gran-

ulomas, or collagen, a radiographic change that is recognized as an interstitial infiltrate appears. The interstitial infiltrate is nodular, varying in size from 2 to 3 mm (miliary) to 10 mm, or linear (reticular). In most ILDs, linear and nodular infiltrates coexist. Miliary nodules (Table 1–12) result from a blood-borne process, such as hematogenous infectious granulomas and metastatic malignancy (Figures 1–14 and 1–15). The nodules coalesce as the miliary process progresses, resulting in a nonuniform nodule size (Figure 1–16). Interstitial nodules, which are not miliary in character and larger than 3 mm, are most often the result of sarcoidosis, silicosis, eosinophilic granuloma, and berylliosis (Figure 1–17). It

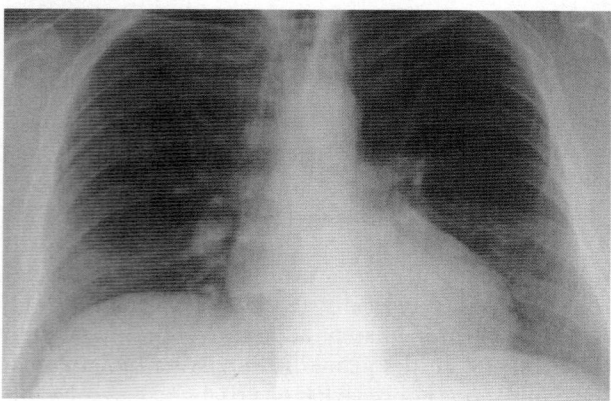

Figure 1–10   Chest radiograph of alveolar filling. Another patient with desquamative interstitial pneumonia whose radiograph demonstrates a poorly defined haziness over both lung bases.

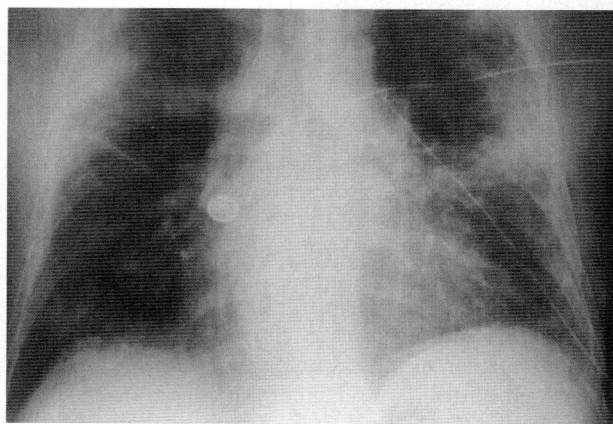

Figure 1–12   Chest radiograph of alveolar filling. Peripheral infiltrates in a patient with bronchiolitis obliterans organizing pneumonia.

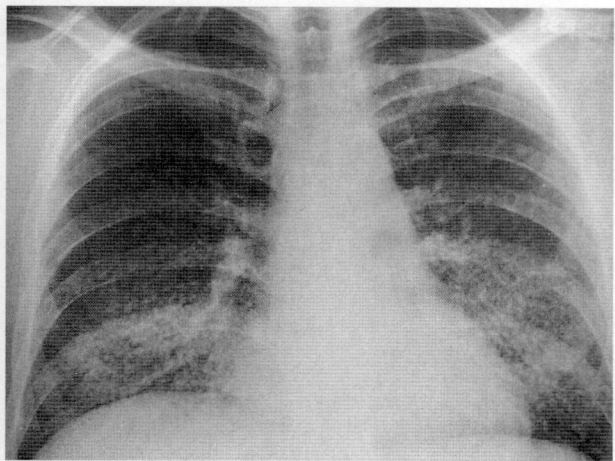

Figure 1–13   Chest radiograph of acute alveolar filling. Patient with acute eosinophilic pneumonia.

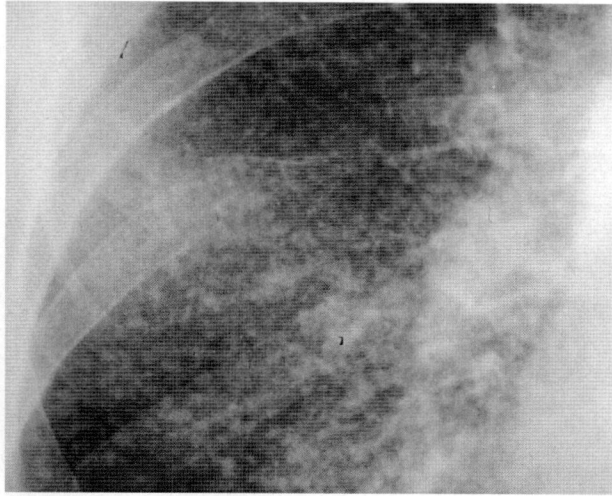

Figure 1–15   Chest radiograph of diffuse interstitial nodules. Miliary and larger-size nodules in a patient with disseminated coccidioidomycosis.

is unusual for nodular interstitial infiltrates to appear without reticular infiltrates except in the miliary diseases. The major roentgenographic distinction between the alveolar and the interstitial nodule is that in the former the margins are indistinct.

Linear (reticular) interstitial infiltrates occur with many ILDs, and, as is the case of nodular infiltrates, it is unusual to find linear interstitial infiltration alone (Figures 1–18 and 1–19). There are, however, patterns of linear infiltration, which narrow the differential diagnosis. Kerley's B lines, which represent thickened intralobular septa due to edema, most frequently result from left ventricular failure and also appear in diseases that cause intralobular lymphatic obstruction (eg, lymphangitic carcinomatosis, lymphoma, and lymphangioleiomyomatosis) (Figure 1–20). Kerley's B lines are best seen as horizontal lines extending to the pleural surface producing a "stepladder" appearance.[274,275] Honeycomb change is another recognizable reticular interstitial pattern (Figure 1–21). Any ILD associated with an under-

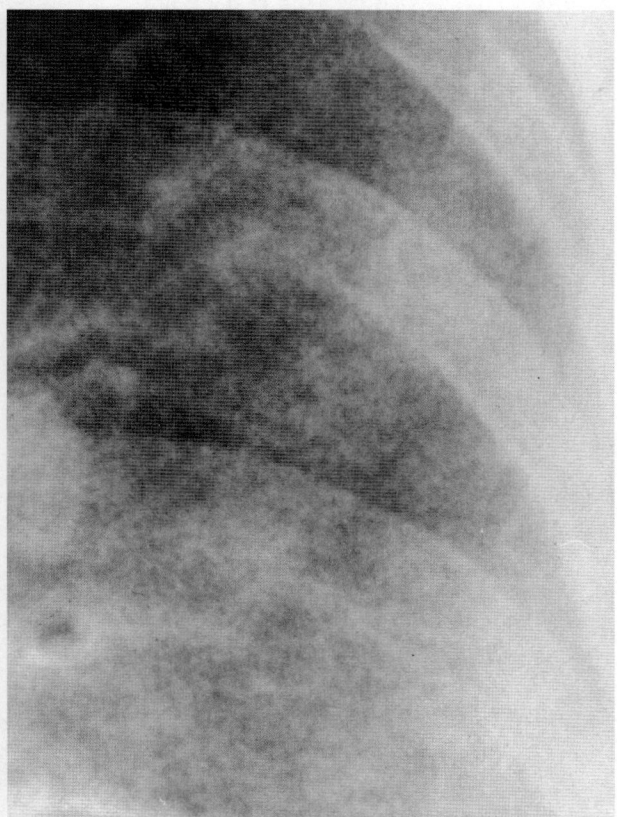

Figure 1–14   Chest radiograph of miliary nodules. Fine miliary nodulation in a Native American man with disseminated tuberculosis.

TABLE 1–12   Interstitial Lung Diseases Producing a Miliary Pattern on Chest Radiograph

Infectious granulomatous disease
   Mycobacterial diseases
   Fungal diseases
Noninfectious granulomatous disease
   Sarcoidosis (types II and III)
   Silicosis
   Eosinophilic granuloma
   Hypersensitivity pneumonitis (acute)
   BCGosis
Metastatic malignant disease
   Hypernephroma
   Breast cancer
   Malignant melanoma
   Thyroid cancer
Lipoid pneumonia (eg, complication of lymphangiogram)
Bronchiolitis
Amyloidosis
Gaucher's disease

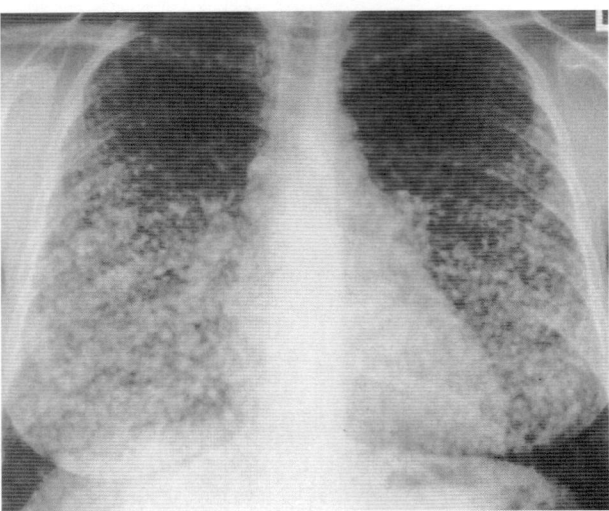

Figure 1–16   Chest radiograph of diffuse interstitial nodules. Coalescence of nodules in a woman with metastatic thyroid cancer.

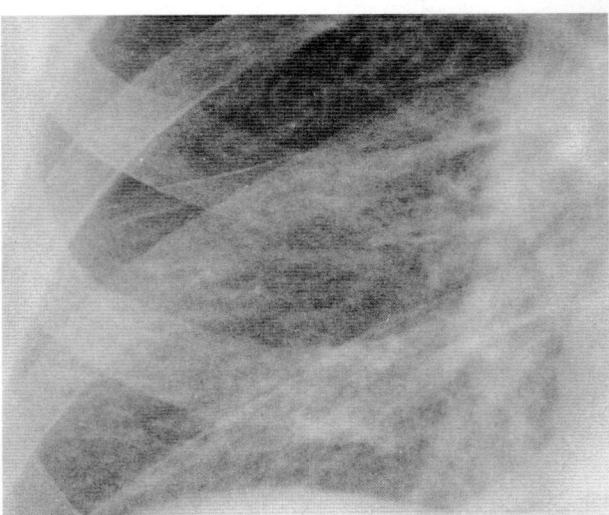

Figure 1–18   Chest radiograph of reticular (linear) interstitial infiltrates in a patient with a cellular interstitial pneumonitis.

lying histologic pattern of usual interstitial pneumonitis, most often due to idiopathic pulmonary fibrosis, can cause marked disruption of the distal lung architecture appearing as broad bands of collagen producing a network of small cysts. These cysts are referred to as honeycomb changes and can also occur in the collagen vascular diseases, asbestosis, and hypersensitivity pneumonitis. Lower-zone honeycomb changes associated with lower lung zone volume loss typify the entities associated with usual interstitial pneumonia (Figures 1–22

to 1–24). Moreover, the finding of honeycomb change on the chest radiograph or computed tomography (CT) scan has a high correlation with histologic honeycombing[276] and indicates advanced irreversible disease.[176]

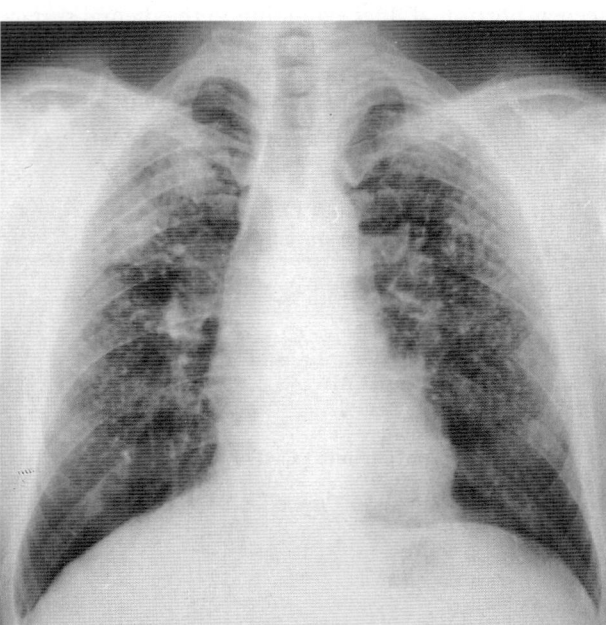

Figure 1–17   Chest radiograph of multiple interstitial nodules. Multiple nodules with coalescence in the upper lobes in this patient with sarcoidosis.

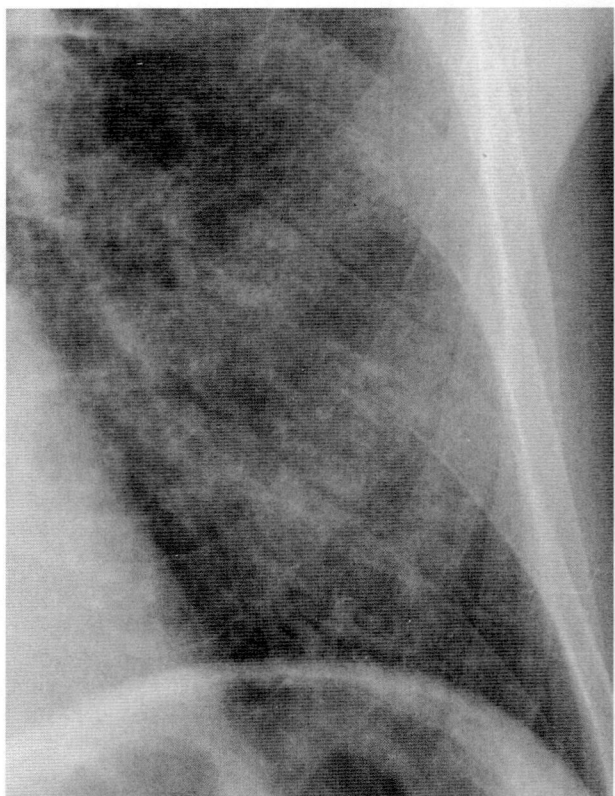

Figure 1–19   Chest radiograph of reticulonodular interstitial infiltrates. A patient with idiopathic pulmonary fibrosis whose chest radiograph demonstrates both nodules and lines.

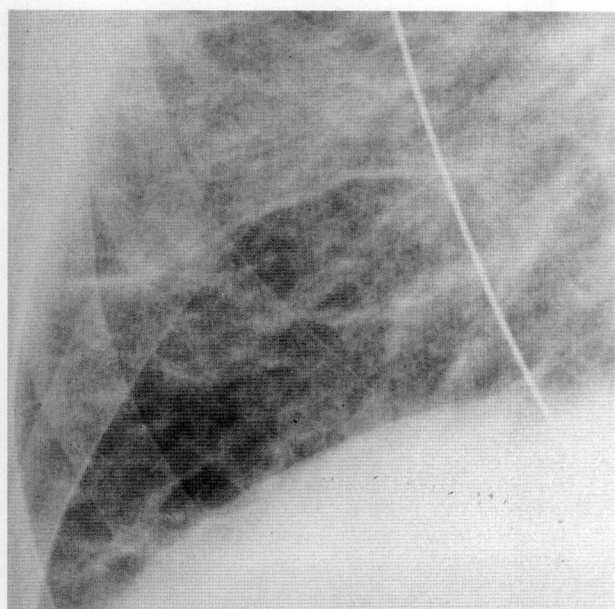

Figure 1–20 Chest radiograph of a patient with lymphangitic carcinomatosis whose radiograph demonstrates peripheral linear densities that extend to the pleural surface producing a "stepladder" appearance (Kerley's B lines).

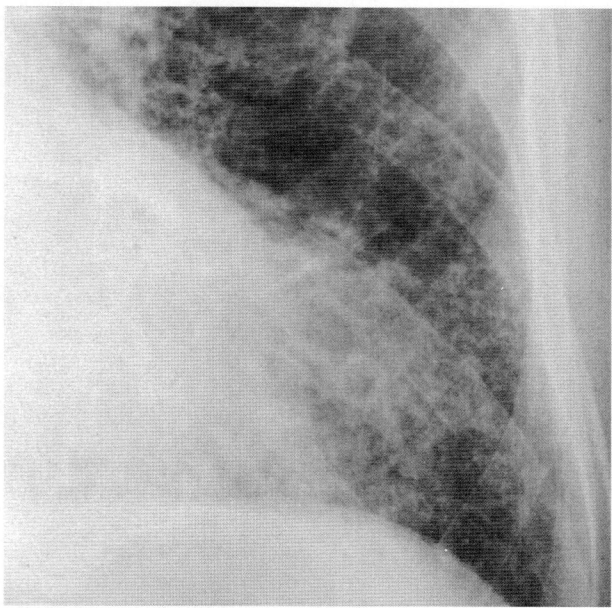

Figure 1–21 Chest radiograph of honeycomb lung. A patient with far-advanced idiopathic pulmonary fibrosis whose chest radiograph reveals a linear pattern with multiple small cysts resembling a honeycomb.

Occasionally, other features of the chest radiograph in ILD point to a diagnosis or exclude other diagnostic possibilities (Table 1–13). Pleural disease often appears with asbestosis or collagen vascular disease–associated ILD. Pleural involvement in an asbestos-exposed individual may appear with or without evidence of ILD (asbestosis). Pleural involvement in asbestos-related disease can represent a chronic lymphocytic effusion, a malignant mesothelioma, or, most often, fibrotic pleural plaques.[277–279] The pleural plaques appear on the radiograph as linear calcifications, which characteristically involve the diaphragmatic and mediastinal pleural surfaces (Figure 1–25). Asbestos exposure may also cause pericardial calcification. Pleurisy and pleural effusion are common manifestations of all the collagen vascular diseases; the exception is polymyositis/dermatomyositis. Spontaneous pneumothorax can result from any ILD that causes lung cysts, but it is most common in and often the presenting manifestation of eosinophilic granuloma,[280] lymphangioleiomyomatosis,[82] and tuberous sclerosis.[83] A pneumothorax occurring with underlying fibrotic lung is often a significant problem because the lung is noncompliant preventing re-expansion and subsequent sealing of the bronchopleural fistula. This leads to the formation of a chronic bronchopleural fistula, persistent pneumothorax, partially collapsed lung, and worsening of symptoms.

Although most interstitial processes result in a progressive reduction of lung volume, the discovery of an increased lung volume as well as airflow obstruction and increased functional residual capacity and thoracic gas volume in the face of interstitial radiographic changes,

should alert the physician to the possibility of several conditions. Lymphangioleiomyomatosis and tuberous sclerosis, two conditions that are associated with smooth muscle obliteration of bronchioles and smooth muscle infiltration of the alveolar walls, produce a radiographic pattern of hyperinflation and interstitial infiltrates (Figure 1–26). Advanced sarcoidosis, chronic hypersensitivity pneumonitis, and the late stages of eosinophilic granuloma probably due to the bronchiolocentric location of

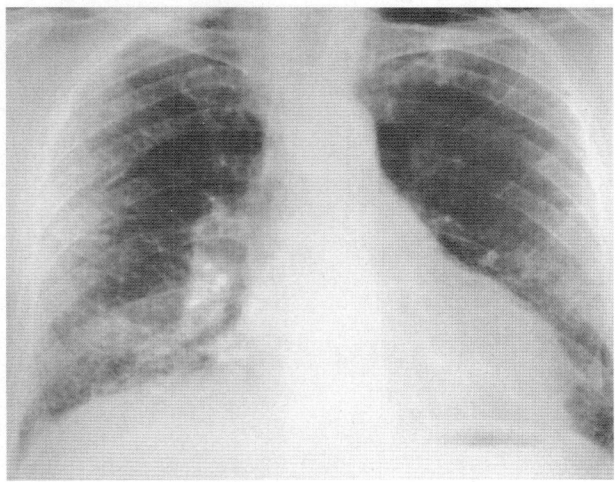

Figure 1–22 Chest radiograph of advanced interstitial infiltrates. A patient with scleroderma whose chest radiograph shows diffuse reticulonodular infiltrates with a lower-zone and peripheral distribution. There is also right lower lobe volume loss (note the position of the right pulmonary artery) and lower-zone honeycomb changes.

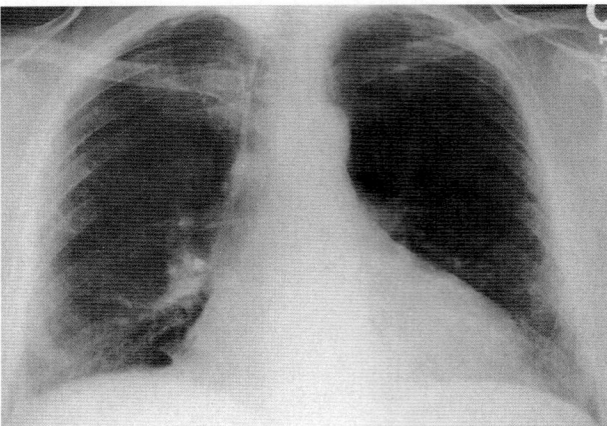

Figure 1–23   Chest radiograph of a patient with rheumatoid arthritis and usual interstitial pneumonitis. There are lower-zone and peripheral reticulonodular interstitial infiltrates.

the granulomatous processes, result in fibrous obliteration of the distal bronchioles with progressive hyperinflation on chest radiograph and spirometric airflow limitation. An ILD may also be superimposed on pre-existing emphysema (Figure 1–27). The combination of smoking-related obstructive lung disease and idiopathic pulmonary fibrosis results in interstitial infiltrates superimposed on the hyperinflated lung.[281] Subcutaneous calcium deposits in the chest wall can be seen as part of the general calcinosis in both scleroderma and dermatomyositis (Figure 1–28).

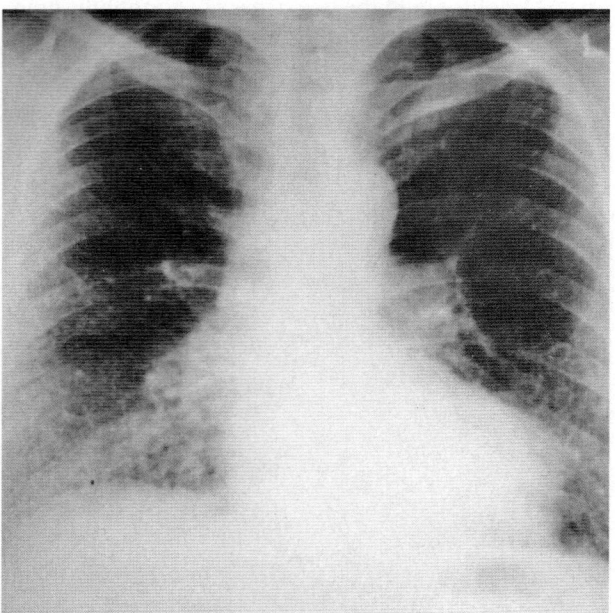

Figure 1–24   Chest radiograph of idiopathic pulmonary fibrosis with underlying usual interstitial pneumonitis. There is lower-zone honeycombing and peripheral reticular opacities. Lung volume is preserved due to coexistant chronic obstructive lung disease.

TABLE 1–13   Other Chest Radiographic Features of Interstitial Lung Disease

Pleural effusion and/or pleural thickening
   Lymphangitic carcinomatosis
   Lymphangioleiomyomatosis (chylous)
   Drug induced (nitrofurantoin)
   Sarcoidosis
   Chronic radiation pneumonitis
   Asbestosis
      Effusion
      Pleural thickening
      Calcified pleural plaques
      Mesothelioma
   Collagen vascular disease (excluding polymyositis)
Hilar or mediastinal lymphadenopathy
   Common
      Sarcoidosis
      Lymphoma
      Lymphangitic carcinomatosis
   Uncommon
      Lymphocytic interstitial pneumonia
      Amyloidosis
      Gaucher's disease
      Berylliosis
Hilar nodal eggshell calcification
   Silicosis
   Sarcoidosis
Kerley's B lines
   Chronic left ventricular failure
   Lymphangitic carcinomatosis
   Lymphoma
   Lymphangioleiomyomatosis
   Pulmonary veno-occlusive disease
Pneumothorax
   Eosinophilic granuloma
   Lymphangioleiomyomatosis
   Tuberous sclerosis
   Neurofibromatosis
Increased lung volumes
   Lymphangioleiomyomatosis
   Tuberous sclerosis
   Sarcoidosis (type III)
   Eosinophilic granuloma (chronic)
   Neurofibromatosis
   Chronic hypersensitivity pneumonitis
   Interstitial lung disease superimposed on chronic obstructive
      pulmonary disease
Subcutaneous calcinosis
   Scleroderma
   Polymyositis/dermatomyositis

In general, the radiographic changes of ILDs are most prominent in the lower lung zones. In fact, volume loss that defines the restrictive process of ILD primarily affects the lower lobes. This is true of idiopathic pulmonary fibrosis, the collagen vascular diseases, some drug-induced lung diseases, and asbestosis. All lung zones eventually become involved as the disease progresses. As previously mentioned, in some ILDs, particularly idiopathic pulmonary fibrosis, the subpleural or distal lung parenchyma is prominently involved. Moreover, radiographic signs of pulmonary hypertension appear with prolonged hypoxemia. There are a group of ILDs, however, that have a radiographic predilection for

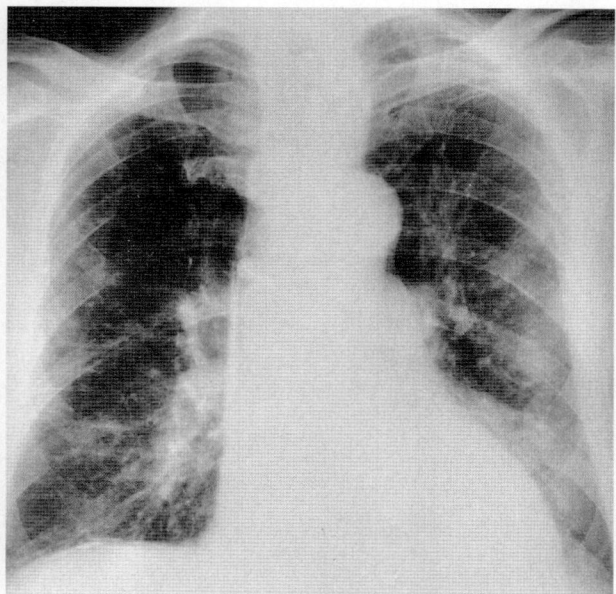

Figure 1–25 Chest radiograph of interstitial lung disease with pleural involvement. A man with a long history of asbestos exposure reveals reticular and nodular opacities with predilection for the lung bases. There is also linear calcification of the right diaphragmatic pleural surface and calcification of the right mediastinal pleural surface. This individual also has obstructive lung disease with left lower lobe pneumonia and a history of untreated systemic hypertension that accounts for the cardiomegaly.

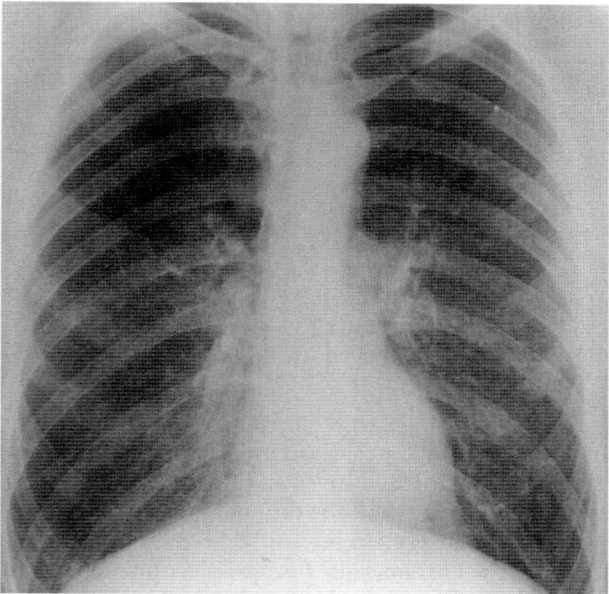

Figure 1–27 Chest radiograph of interstitial lung disease and hyperinflation. A man with both idiopathic pulmonary fibrosis and tobacco-related obstructive lung disease. Pulmonary function tests indicated preservation of lung volumes but marked reduction of diffusing capacity for carbon monoxide.

the upper lung zones and result in upper lobe volume loss (Table 1–14) (Figures 1–29 and 1–30). As Table 1–14 indicates, many of these disorders are granulomatous in nature. Mediastinal mantle field irradiation for malignancy protects the majority of exposed lung parenchyma. The radiation fibrosis that develops in the upper lung zones is paramediastinal in location and has a vertical orientation (Figure 1–31).

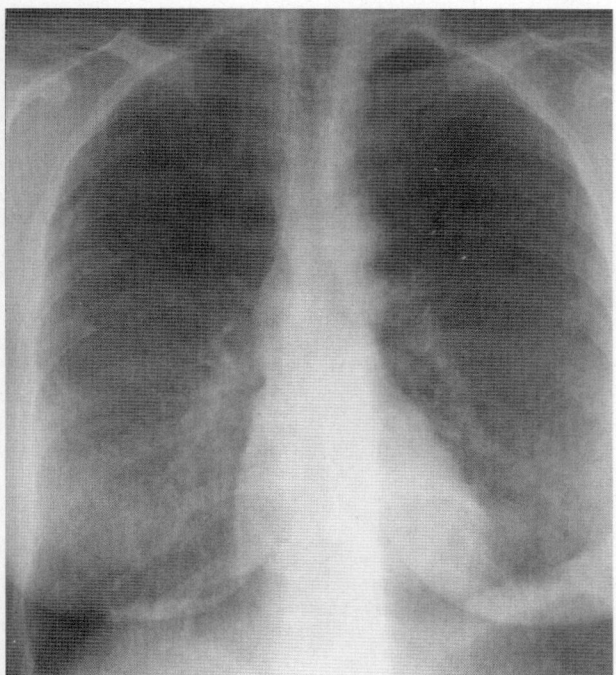

Figure 1–26 Chest radiograph of interstitial lung disease and hyperinflation. Chest radiograph of a woman with lymphangioleiomyomatosis. Note the loculated pneumothorax at the right base. The left pleural reaction is secondary to a talc slurry instilled into the left pleural space for control of recurrent pneumothorax.

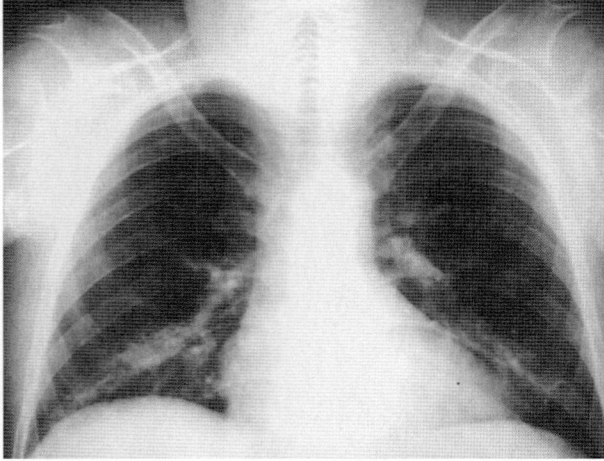

Figure 1–28 Chest radiograph of interstitial lung disease and subcutaneous calcifications. A woman with polymyositis/dermatomyositis–related interstitial lung disease with subcutaneous calcifications in both axilla.

TABLE 1–14   Interstitial Lung Diseases with Radiographic Predilection for Upper Lung Zones

Sarcoidosis (type III, IV)
Chronic hypersensitivity pneumonitis
Eosinophilic granuloma
Silicosis
Nodular rheumatoid arthritis (necrobiotic nodules, Caplan's syndrome)
Chronic infectious granulomatous disease
Berylliosis
Ankylosing spondylitis
Radiation fibrosis
Drug induced (amiodarone, gold, carmustine)
Chronic eosinophilic pneumonia

Recognizing a mixed pattern (alveolar and interstitial) is more difficult. Alveolar filling diseases such as alveolar proteinosis and the diffuse alveolar hemorrhage syndromes may result in interstitial fibrosis because these may be recurrent and cause fibrosis.[282] Diffuse interstitial processes are often associated with alveolar filling. For example, intra-alveolar macrophages and intraluminal fibrosis can be superimposed on interstitial inflammation and collagen deposition in idiopathic pulmonary fibrosis, the collagen vascular diseases, and drug-induced lung diseases. Sarcoidosis, a disease characterized by interstitial granulomas, often demonstrates radiographic alveolar filling either owing to coalescence of the interstitial granulomas with compression of the air spaces or to an

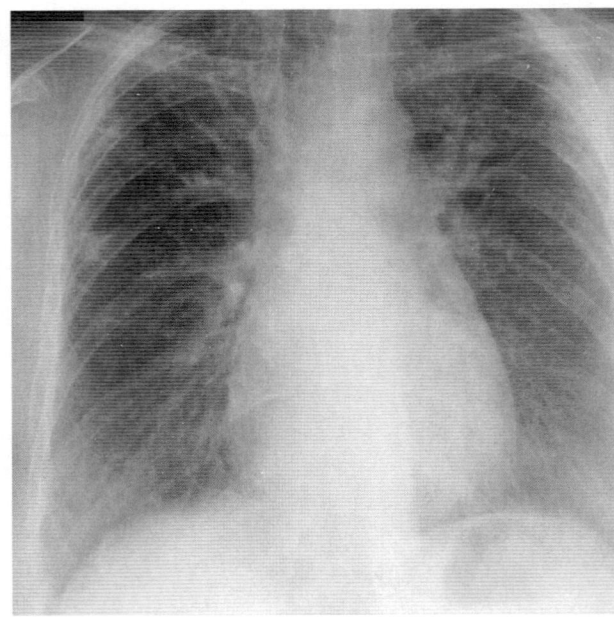

Figure 1–30   Chest radiograph of a patient with biopsy-proven hypersensitivity pneumonitis who had symptoms for many years showing interstitial lung disease with upper lung zone predominance.

outpouring of lymphocytes and macrophages into the alveolar lumens.[283] Dense fibrosis from any ILD can collapse the adjacent lung and obliterate alveolar spaces,

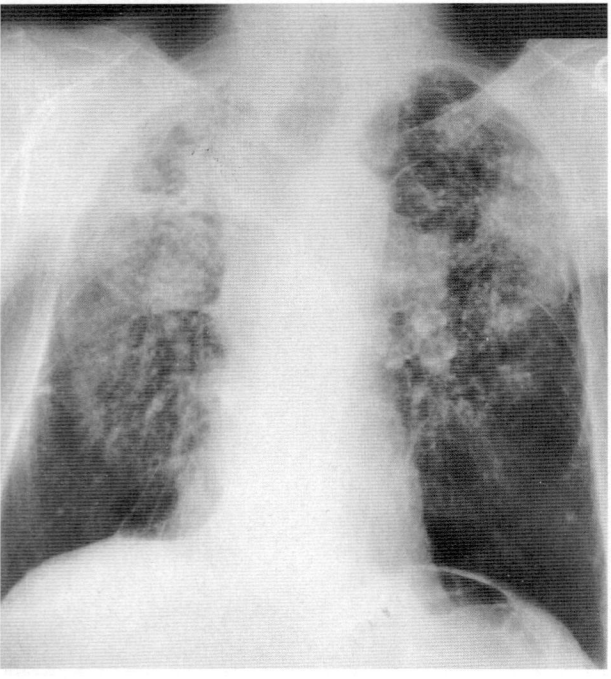

Figure 1–29   Chest radiograph of a patient with silicosis whose chest radiograph shows primarily nodular interstitial lung disease with coalescence. Note retraction of the hilar structures, egg-shell calcifications and a right upper lobe cavity that harbored tuberculosis.

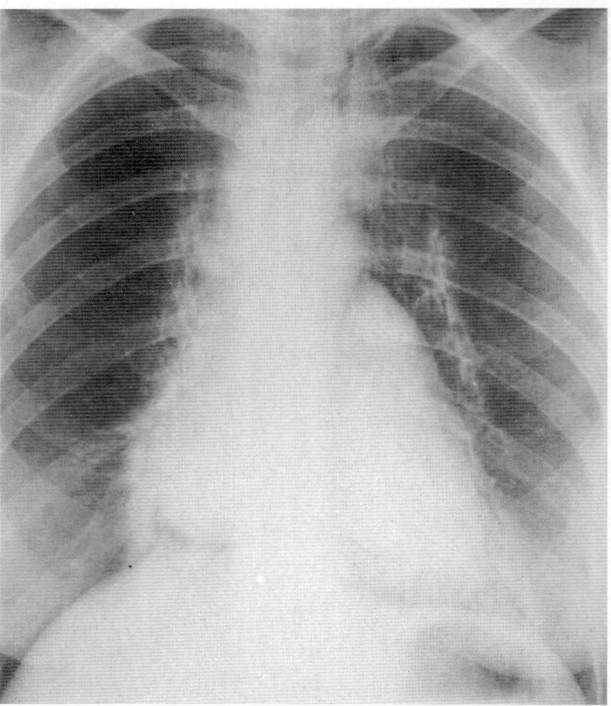

Figure 1–31   Chest radiograph of a woman with Hodgkin's disease who had received mantle field irradiation 3 years earlier showing vertical orientation of paramediastinal reticular infiltrates.

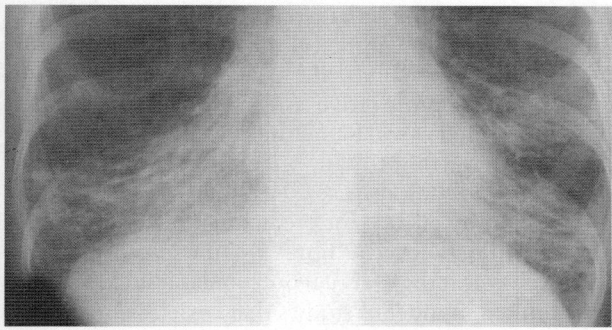

Figure 1–32 Chest radiograph of an individual with rheumatoid arthritis with dense fibrosis involving the lower lobes simulating an alveolar filling (air space) process.

thereby producing what appears to be an alveolar filling pattern on the chest radiograph (Figure 1–32). The gradual appearance of a diffuse alveolar filling pattern on the chest radiograph of a patient with prior ILD should raise concern that diffuse bronchioloalveolar cell carcinoma may develop in the finely scarred lung (Figures 1–33 and 1–34).[252] More acute alveolar disease superimposed on a chronic disease may be secondary to an infectious process or may represent an acute exacerbation of the chronic disease, which is often the case in idiopathic alveolar damage superimposed on usual interstitial pneumonia.

High-Resolution Computed Tomography

High-resolution computed tomography is valuable in detecting ILD and should precede lung biopsy in the investigation of ILD. HRCT has several significant advantages over standard chest radiography. Greater resolution permits better definition of the extent, location, and pattern of disease. For example, honeycomb change is more obvious and widespread on HRCT compared with conventional chest radiographs.[284] CT may also be useful in selecting the site(s) for lung biopsy. HRCT may offer greater accuracy in ILD diagnosis, compared with standard radiography.[285,286] Accuracy increases significantly for the end stages of different ILDs.[287] In the proper clinical setting, HRCT may be sufficiently diagnostic as to preclude the need for lung biopsy. See Chapter 4, "Imaging of Diffuse Parenchymal Lung Disease" for a full discussion on HRCT patterns in ILD.

Two important uses of HRCT are staging and detection of disease, both in symptomatic patients with negative chest radiographs and in cohorts of patients who are predisposed to ILD. Evidence in idiopathic pulmonary fibrosis suggests the finding of hazy areas of air space disease as opposed to reticular changes, and honeycomb cysts point to an earlier disease stage as opposed to a fibrotic process.[271,285,288,289] Both in scleroderma[290] and in asbestos-exposed workers,[291] HRCT has identified patients with ILD who had normal chest radiography. It does, however, appear that physiologic testing, specifically gas exchange with exercise, is more sensitive than HRCT in detecting ILD, eventually proven by open lung biopsy.[292]

Bronchoalveolar Lavage

Bronchoalveolar lavage (BAL) performed through the fiberoptic bronchoscope allows determination of the cellular contents, cellular products, and proteins of the

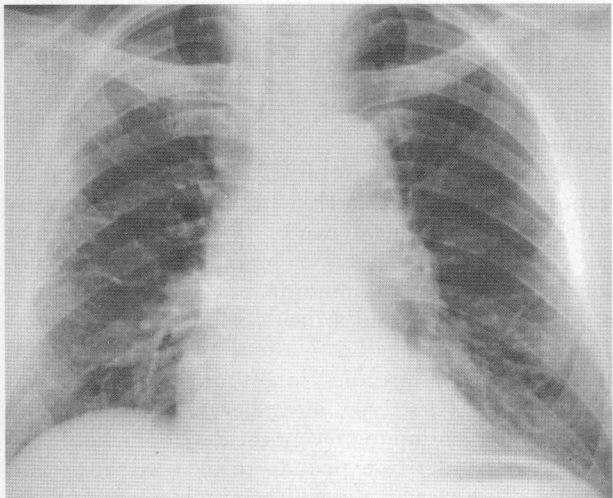

Figure 1–33 Chest radiograph of an individual with idiopathic pulmonary fibrosis demonstrating reticular opacities with lower zone and peripheral lung field predilection.

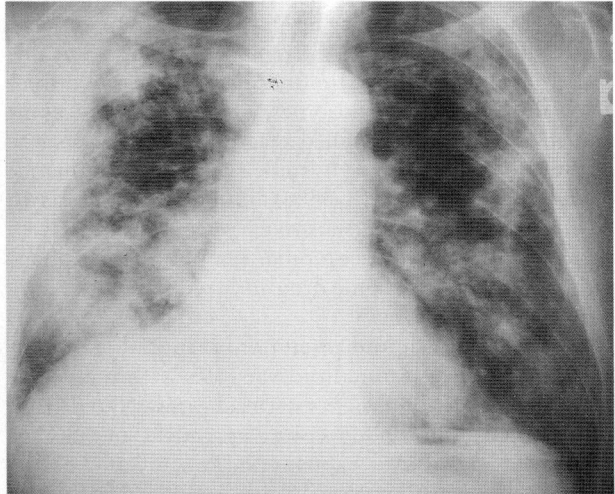

Figure 1–34 Chest radiograph of same patient as in Figure 1–33, now with superimposed bronchoalveolar cell carcinoma. Chest radiograph shows alveolor opacities superimposed on reticular opacities.

distal air spaces of the lung. (See Chapter 5, "Bronchoalveolar Lavage.") Initially, BAL studies in ILDs were performed only for investigational purposes, but there now is some clinical application. It has been difficult to validate this procedure due to the lack of standardized techniques for performance and analysis of the subsequent data. Previous studies often did not consider smoking or the treatment status of the patient.[293] Correlative studies between lavage and open lung biopsies were frequently not available. A large cohort, four-center cooperative study in which lavage techniques and analysis of results of normal subjects and patients with ILD were similar, has established guidelines for clinical use of BAL in ILD.[294] Other major stumbling blocks for the use of BAL in clinical studies have been the differing amounts of instilled lavagate, inconsistent methods of cellular analysis, and considerable differences in lavage results when comparing cigarette smokers to nonsmoking normal subjects and patients with ILD. The well-designed study mentioned above demonstrated marked expansion of the macrophage populations as well as smaller increases in the number of eosinophils in subjects who smoke, with and without ILD.[294] Similarly, smoking affects protein distribution and T-cell subsets in BAL. The relative safety of BAL has been documented; transient low-grade fever, pulmonary infiltration due to retained fluid, and mild hypoxemia do, however, occasionally occur.[295]

Bronchoalveolar lavage is a useful diagnostic tool for evaluating acute diffuse pneumonic processes by excluding infection, particularly in unsuspected cases of AIDS. Bronchoalveolar lavage has some clinical utility for the diagnosis and management of ILD. For example, the finding of malignant cells may indicate bronchioloalveolar carcinoma, lymphoma, or lymphangitic carcinomatosis[296–299] and lavage eosinophilia (> 35%) secures the diagnosis of acute eosinophilic pneumonia.[113–115] It was previously thought that the finding of periodic acid–Schiff (PAS)-staining lipoproteinaceous material in BAL fluid was indicative of alveolar proteinosis, but this could also be a nonspecific finding.[300–302] In the diffuse alveolar hemorrhage syndromes, a bloody lavage accompanied by hemosiderin-filled macrophages suggests one of the etiologies of this syndrome.[108] The predominance of BAL lymphocytes (> 35%) limits the diagnosis to either sarcoidosis, hypersensitivity pneumonitis,[156] lymphocytic interstitial pneumonia, lymphoma, lymphangitic carcinomatosis, some drug-induced interstitial lung diseases, or berylliosis.[302–308]

In suspected lipoid pneumonia, special stains for fat disclose cytoplasmic lipid vacuoles within alveolar macrophages.[309] In patients with asbestos-related ILD, when the asbestos body count exceeds 1 per mL of BAL fluid, significant exposure has occurred.[310] This, however, does not necessarily confirm asbestos-related disease.[311] The diagnosis of berylliosis can be established after a positive BAL lymphocyte transformation test in exposed patients.[133] In eosinophilic gran-

uloma of the lung, ultrastructural studies of BAL mononuclear cells will reveal the typical Birbeck granule of the Langerhans' cell.[80] The expense of electron microscopy is prohibitive and should be performed only in selected cases. Langerhans' cells also stain positively with S-100 protein, but they can be present in other fibrotic lung diseases.[312]

The utility of BAL for predicting underlying histology (inflammation versus fibrosis)—the so-called staging of disease—and the eventual outcome is less clear. There are a limited number of studies that correlate BAL cellular constituents with underlying pathology. Idiopathic pulmonary fibrosis is typified by increased proportions of BAL neutrophils and eosinophils. It is now understood that these acute inflammatory cells were washed from endstage honeycombed lung in which there is mucostasis. In approximately 20% of idiopathic pulmonary fibrosis cases, there were BAL lymphocytes. This was correlated with cellular infiltration of the alveolar wall rather than fibrosis.[313] Recent data show that these cellular cases of pulmonary fibrosis represent the underlying lesion of nonspecific interstitial pneumonia rather than usual interstitial pneumonia. In another common ILD, sarcoidosis, it has been suggested that clinical deterioration over a 6-month period could be expected when initial BAL lymphocytes exceeded 28%.[314] Several studies have refuted this finding and indicate that the initial level of BAL lymphocytes has no bearing on the clinical outcome in sarcoidosis.[315–317]

Response to treatment in the idiopathic interstitial pneumonias is variable when BAL neutrophilia is present but is more predictable if the initial BAL demonstrates lymphocytosis representing nonspecific interstitial pneumonia.[311,318] The presence of lymphocytes in BAL fluid predicts therapeutic responsiveness and an improved survival compared with usual interstitial pneumonia. The combination of neutrophilia and, in particular, eosinophilia typical of usual interstitial pneumonia points to a poorer prognosis and lack of response to corticosteroid treatment.[313,319] In general, a similar relationship between lavage cellular contents and outcome holds up for the collagen vascular disease–associated ILD.[320]

Another potential use of BAL is for prospective evaluation of populations at risk. In scleroderma, a disease with a very high incidence of ILD, bronchoalveolar lavage cellular abnormalities precede clinical, physiologic, and radiographic abnormalities.[321,322] There is also a group of rheumatoid arthritis patients who demonstrate BAL lymphocytosis without evidence of clinical disease.[323] In these studies, longitudinal follow-up was not available. These types of studies raise the possibility of early intervention to prevent the development of ILD in these disorders. In primary biliary cirrhosis and Crohn's disease, entities in which granulomatous inflammation is prominent and in which pulmonary involvement is unusual, BAL fluid demonstrates lymphocytosis in asymptomatic patients.[324,325]

TABLE 1–15   Characteristics Determining Need For Surgical Lung Biopsy In Patients With Diffuse Parenchymal Lung Disease

Characteristic	Lung Biopsy Advisable	Lung Biopsy Not Essential
Age	< 50 years	> 50 years
Duration of illness	Less than 3 months	Longstanding and stable (> 2 years)
Systemic symptoms	Fever, weight loss, sweats	No systemic symptoms
Clinical or exposure history	No cause defined	Known collagen vascular disease, drug, occupational or environmental cause present
Unusual pulmonary or extrapulmonary manifestations	Hemoptysis Unexplained pulmonary hypertension Peripheral vasculitis	No extrapulmonary manifestation except clubbing
Pneumothorax	Recurrent	Absent
Family history of fibrosing alveolitis	Absent	Documented familial cryptogenic fibrosing alveolitis in at least two first-degree relatives
Chest Radiograph	Normal Kerley's B lines (in absence of identifiable cause) Rapid progression over several months	Stable or very slow progression of bibasilar interstitial opacities over several years; No hilar or mediastinal lymphadenopathy
High Resolution Computed Tomography of Chest (HRCT)	Nodular or patchy opacities; Ground glass opacities Hilar/mediastinal lymphadenopathy Pleural effusion/scar	No pleural abnormalities; Endstage disease (eg., severe honeycombing) Characteristic HRCT findings (See text)
Physiological changes	Rapid deterioration in lung function	No change in gas exchange (DL_{CO} and PaO_2) over several years.
Transbronchial lung biopsy or bronchoalveolar lavage	Normal or nonspecific (showing no features to support a specific diagnosis)	Features found consistent with a known cause of ILD (eg., infection; cancer; lipoid pneumonia; hemorrhage; eosinophilic pneumonia; asbestos-bodies; positive lymphocyte transformation test, etc.) (See Table 1–16)

Adapted after: Chan-Yeung M, Müller N. Cryptogenic fibrosing alveolitis. Lancet 1997; 350:651–6.

Lung Biopsy

The final step in the diagnostic evaluation of a patient with ILD is to decide whether it is necessary to obtain lung tissue (Table 1–15). A transbronchial lung biopsy and BAL can be performed at the same time. It is our practice to perform thoracoscopic lung biopsy under the following situations: if the diagnosis remains questionable after review of the clinical, radiographic, and BAL data; if a transbronchial biopsy does not yield a specific histologic diagnosis; and if the patient is not a high-risk candidate for this procedure due to advanced age or medical comorbidities. Table 1–16 lists the ILDs in which transbronchial biopsy tissue is useful for establishing a diagnosis. If, however, the histology is considered nonspecific or shows primarily fibrosis or chronic inflammation but without a specific diagnosis, an open or thoracoscopic lung biopsy should be considered.[326,327] The mortality rate for both video-assisted thoracoscopic and open lung biopsy is < 1%, the morbidity rate is < 3%, and a specific diagnosis is established in > 92%.[327,328] For many of the diagnoses listed in Tables 1–1 to 1–5, including drug-induced, collagen vascular disease–related, and occupational- and environmental exposure–related ILD, the diagnosis is often obvious. To establish a diagnosis in the idiopathic interstitial pneumonias, tissue is often required. Since 30 to 40% of all ILDs are due to idiopathic pulmonary fibrosis,[176] thoracoscopic or open lung biopsy is recommended unless the

clinicoradiographic picture is typical—an older individual without an occupational, drug, or collagen vascular disease history with insidious dyspnea and a chest radiograph and HRCT indicating lower-zone and peripheral reticular opacities often with honeycombing—or the patient is considered to be at a high risk for this procedure.

TABLE 1–16   Usefulness of Transbronchial Lung Biopsy for Diagnosis of Interstitial Lung Disease

Very useful
  Sarcoidosis
  Lymphangitic carcinomatosis
  Alveolar proteinosis
  Bronchioloalveolar carcinoma
  Eosinophilic pneumonia
  Berylliosis
Occasionally useful
  Eosinophilic granuloma
  Amyloidosis
  Wegener's granulomatosis
  Pulmonary lymphoma
  Hypersensitivity pneumonitis
  Pulmonary capillaritis
  Lymphocytic interstitial pneumonia
  Bronchiolitis obliterans organizing pneumonia
Not useful
  Idiopathic pulmonary fibrosis
  Other disease categories with underlying idiopathic interstitial pneumonitis
  Non-specific interstitial pneumonias

TREATMENT AND FOLLOW-UP

The diagnosis and subsequent treatment dictate the interval required for follow-up evaluation. We have revised the clinical-radiographic-physiologic scoring system that has been used for assessing initial disease severity, therapeutic response, and rate of disease progression.[329,330] The new scoring system for the prediction of survival includes age at presentation, smoking history, profusion of radiographic infiltrates, radiographic presence of pulmonary hypertension, reduced total lung capacity, and PaO$_2$ at the end of maximal exercise.[331]

Treatment-responsive ILDs are listed in Tables 1–6 to 1–7. Corticosteroids with and without other immunosuppressives remain the mainstay of therapy. For the responsive ILD, corticosteroids are a highly appropriate form of treatment. Many patients with ILD, however, first receive these drugs during the poorly responsive fibrotic stage of their disease; therein lies the frustration in the management of ILDs. New therapies are being developed (See Chapter 13, "The Future of Medical Therapy for Lung Fibrosis."), and these offer hope for the future.[331–334]

The following key points concerning ILD need to be emphasized:

- The extent and perceived severity of the radiographic changes often do not correlate with symptoms or physiologic abnormalities. The discovery of an abnormal chest radiograph that shows interstitial infiltrates should not be ignored simply because the patient is asymptomatic and the screening pulmonary function studies do not demonstrate an abnormality.
- Although the rate of disease progression is variable, the great majority of ILDs are relentlessly progressive. It is not unusual to discover a series of previ-

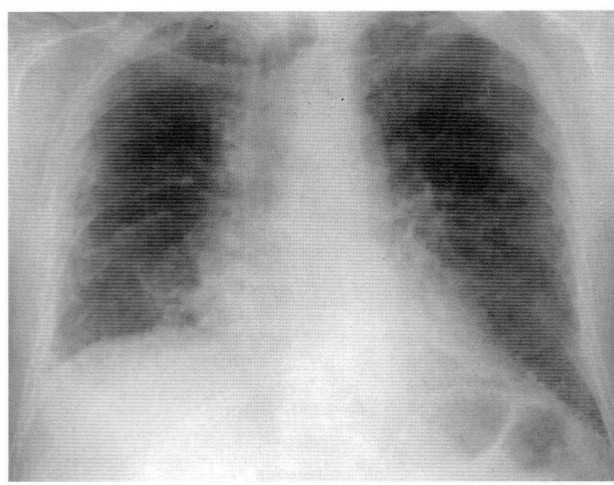

Figure 1–36   Chest radiograph of same patient as in Figure 1–35, who is now asymptomatic with significant physiologic impairment. Note the progressive reticular opacities and right lower lobe volume loss. Thoracoscopic lung biopsy revealed usual interstitial pneumonitis. The clinical picture was compatible with idiopathic pulmonary fibrosis.

ously abnormal chest radiographs in patients presenting for the first time with symptomatic ILD (Figures 1–35 and 1–36). Therefore, it is important not to ignore or dismiss incidental interstitial

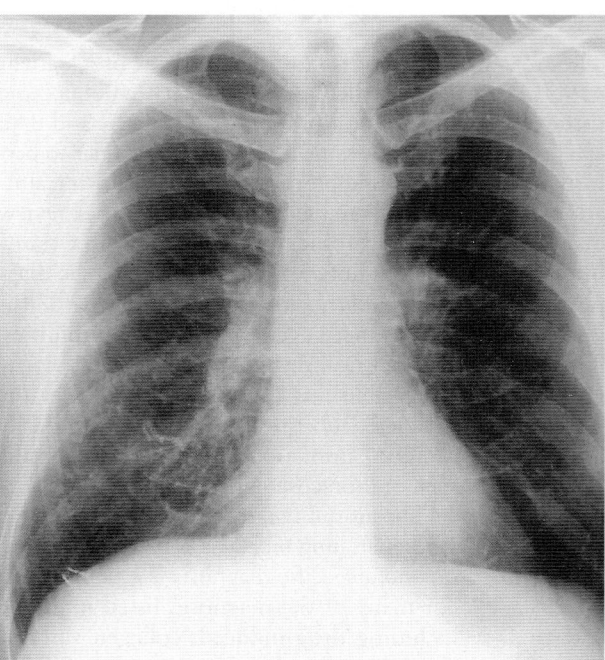

Figure 1–37   Chest radiograph shows interstitial infiltrates with hyperinflated lungs in a patient with obstructive lung disease and interstitial lung disease. Patient was asymptomatic with gas exchange abnormalities. An open lung biopsy revealed emphysema and usual interstitial pneumonitis compatible with idiopathic pulmonary fibrosis. He refused any form of treatment.

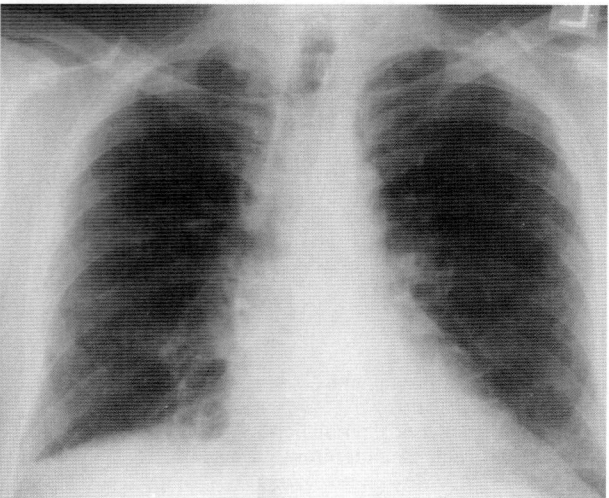

Figure 1–35   Chest radiograph shows minimal interstitial opacities in an asymptomatic patient with normal spirometry and diffusing capacity.

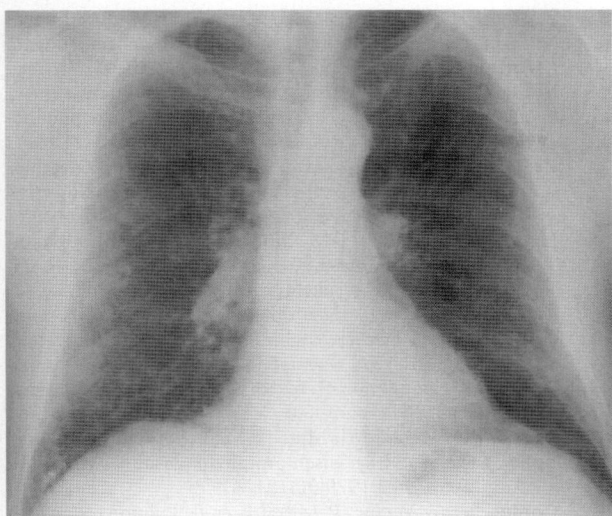

Figure 1–38   Chest radiograph shows stable interstitial infiltrates in the same patient as in Figure 1–37 ten years later. Symptoms and physiologic testing revealed little or no change.

changes on screening chest radiographs or HRCT scans. In the unusual case there may be long periods of stability with or without treatment, but there are no predictive tests that determine those patients who will follow this course (Figures 1–37 and 1–38).

- A normal chest roentgenogram in a symptomatic patient must be addressed. At present, three methods (physiologic testing, bronchoalveolar lavage, and particularly HRCT) are useful for detection, staging, and follow-up as well as assessing the response to therapy of an ILD.
- Clinical and physiologic deterioration in a patient with interstitial lung disease most often represents disease progression. Other considerations, however, including pulmonary embolic disease, the development of complicating diffuse bronchioloalveolar carcinoma, and infectious pneumonia in the patient treated with immunosuppressive medications, must be considered.[245]
- These conditions are uncommon and few physicians have substantial experience with their diagnosis and management. Therefore, patients with ILD or suspected ILD should be under the direct or joint care of a pulmonologist. The clinician, radiologist, and pathologist should meet regularly to evaluate chest imaging studies in patients with ILD.

REFERENCES

1. Owens GR, Follansbee WP. Cardiopulmonary manifestations of systemic sclerosis. Chest 1987;91:118–27.
2. Lomeo RM, Cornella RJ, Schabel S, et al. Progressive systemic scleroses sine scleroderma presenting as pulmonary interstitial fibrosis. Am J Med 1989;87:525–7.
3. Greenwald GI, Tashkin DP, Gong H, et al. Longitudinal changes in lung function and respiratory symptoms in progressive systemic sclerosis. Am J Med 1987;83:83–92.
4. Schwarz MI, Matthay RA, Sahn SA, et al. Interstitial lung disease in polymyositis and dermatomyositis: analysis of six cases and review of the literature. Medicine 1976;55:89–104.
5. Tazelaar HD, Viggiano RW, Pickersgill J, et al. Interstitial lung disease in polymyositis and dermatomyositis. Am Rev Respir Dis 1990;141:727–33.
6. Eisenberg H, Dubois EL, Sherwin RP, et al. Diffuse interstitial lung disease in systemic lupus erythematosus. Ann Intern Med 1973;79:37–45.
7. Haupt HM, Moore GW, Hutchins GM. The lung in systemic lupus erythematosus: analysis of the pathological changes in 120 patients. Am J Med 1981;71:791–8.
8. Boulware DW, Hedgpeth MT. Lupus pneumonitis and anti-SSA (Ro) antibodies. J Rheumatol 1989;16:479–81.
9. Walker WC, Wright V. Pulmonary lesions and rheumatoid arthritis. Medicine 1968;47:501–20.
10. Yousem SA, Colby TV, Carrington CB. Lung biopsy in rheumatoid arthritis. Am Rev Respir Dis 1985;131:770–7.
11. Garcia JG, James HL, Zinkgraf S, et al. Lower respiratory tract abnormalities in rheumatoid interstitial lung disease. Am Rev Respir Dis 1987;136:811–7.
12. Cohen AA, Natelson EA, Fechnar RE. Fibrosing interstitial pneumonitis in ankylosing spondylitis. Chest 1971;59:369–71.
13. Sullivan WD, Hurst DJ, Harmon CE, et al. A prospective evaluation emphasizing pulmonary involvement in patients with mixed connective tissue disease. Medicine 1984;63:92–107.
14. Prakash VB, Luthra HS, Divertie MB. Intrathoracic manifestations in mixed connective tissue disease. Mayo Clin Proc 1985;60:813–21.
15. Constantopoulos SH, Papadimitriou CS, Moutsopoulos HM. Respiratory manifestations in primary Sjögren's syndrome. Chest 1985;88:226–9.
16. Vitali C, Tavoni A, Viegi G, et al. Lung involvement in Sjögren's syndrome: a comparison between patients with primary and with secondary syndrome. Ann Rheum Dis 1985;44:455–61.
17. Efthimiou J, Johnston C, Spiro SG, et al. Pulmonary disease in Behçet's syndrome. QJM 1986;227:259–80.
18. Fairley C, Wilson JW, Barraclough D. Pulmonary involvement in Behçet's syndrome. Chest 1989;96:1428–9.
19. Rosenow EC, DeRemee RA, Dines DE. Chronic nitrofurantoin pulmonary reaction. N Engl J Med 1968;279:1258–62.
20. Wang KK, Bowyer BA, Fleming CR, et al. Pulmonary infiltrates and eosinophilia associated with sulfasalazine lung. Mayo Clin Proc 1984;59:343–6.
21. Salerno SM, Ormseth EJ, Roth BJ, et al. Sulfasalazine pulmonary toxicity in ulcerative colitis mimicking clinical features of Wegener's granulomatosis. Chest 1996;110:556–9.
22. Dries DF, Winterbauer RH, Van Norman GA. Cephalosporin-induced interstitial pneumonitis. Chest 1984;86:130–40.
23. Sitbon O, Bidel N, Dussop TC, et al. Minocycline pneumonitis and eosinophilia: a report on eight patients. Arch Intern Med 1994;154:1633–40.
24. Piperno D, Donn EC, Loire R, Cordier JF. Bronchiolitis obliterans organizing pneumonia associated with minocycline therapy: a possible cause. Eur Respir J 1995;8:1018–20.
25. Dyhuizen RS, Legge JS. Minocycline induced pulmonary eosinophilia. Respir Med 1995;89:61–2.
26. Wong PC, Yew WW, Wong CF, Choi HY. Ethambutol induced pulmonary infiltrates with eosinophilia and skin involvement. Eur Respir J 1995;8:866–8.
27. Oren S, Turkot S, Golzman B, et al. Amiodarone induced bronchiolitis obliterans organizing pneumonia (BOOP). Respir Med 1996;90:167–9.
28. Martin WJ, Rosenow EC. Amiodarone pulmonary toxicity: recognition and pathogenesis. Part 1. Part 2. Chest 1988;93:1067–74, 1242–8.

29. Bernard A, Melloni B, Gosselin B, et al. Perpindopril associated pneumonitis. Eur Respir J 1996;9:1314–6.

30. Feinberg L, Travis WD, Ferrans V, et al. Pulmonary fibrosis associated with tocainide: report of a case with literature review. Am Rev Respir Dis 1990;141:505–8.

31. Akoun GM, Milleron BD, Mayaud CM, et al. Provocation test coupled with bronchoalveolar lavage in diagnosis of propranolol induced hypersensitivity pneumonitis. Am Rev Respir Dis 1989;139:247–9.

32. Gauthier-Rahman S, Akoun GM, Milleron BJ, et al. Leucocyte migration inhibition in propranolol induced pneumonitis. Chest 1990;97:238–41.

33. Lombard JN, Bonnotte B, Maynadie M, et al. A lipoid pneumonitis. Eur Respir J 1993;6:588–91.

34. Winterbauer RH, Wilske KR, Wheelis RF. Diffuse pulmonary injury associated with gold treatment. N Engl J Med 1976;294:919–21.

35. Partanen J, van Assendelft AHW, Koskimies S, et al. Patients with rheumatoid arthritis and gold induced pneumonitis express two high risk histocompatibility complex patterns. Chest 1987;92:277–81.

36. Agarwal R, Sharma SK, Malaviya AN. Gold induced hypersensitivity pneumonitis in a patient with rheumatoid arthritis. Clin Exp Immunol 1989;7:89–90.

37. Camus P, Degat OR, Justrabo E, et al. D-penicillamine-induced severe pneumonitis. Chest 1982;81:376–8.

38. Khalil H, Molinari E, Stoller JK. Diclofenac (Voltarin)-induced eosinophilic pneumonitis. Arch Intern Med 1993;153:1649–52.

39. Goodwin SD, Glenny RW. Nonsteriodal anti-inflammatory drug-associated pulmonary infiltrates with eosinophilia. Arch Intern Med 1992;152:1521–4.

40. Pfitzenmeyer P, Meier M, Zuck P, et al. Piroxicam induced pulmonary infiltrates and eosinophilia. J Rheumatol 1994;21:1573–7.

41. Michael JR, Rudin ML. Acute pulmonary disease caused by phenytoin. Ann Intern Med 1981;95:452–4.

42. Gonzalez-Rothi RJ, Zander DS, Ros PR. Fluoxetine hydrochloride (Prozac) induced pulmonary disease. Chest 1995;107:1763–5.

43. King GG, Barnes DJ, Hayes MJ. Carbamazepine-induced pneumonitis. Med J Aust 1994;160:126–7.

44. Salerno SM, Strong JS, Roth BJ, Sakata V. Eosinophilic pneumonia and respiratory failure associated with a trazodone overdose. Am J Respir Crit Care Med 1995;152:2170–2.

45. de Kerviler E, Tredaniel J, Revlon G, et al. Fluoxetine-induced pulmonary granulomatosis. Eur Respir J 1996;9:615–7.

46. Cooper JAD, White DA, Matthay RA. Drug induced pulmonary disease. Part 1. Cytotoxic drugs. Am Rev Respir Dis 1986;133:321–40.

47. Andrews AT, Bowman HS, Patel S, et al. Mitomycin and interstitial pneumonitis. Ann Intern Med 1971;90:127.

48. Castro M, Veeder MT, Mailliard JA, et al. A prospective study of pulmonary function in patients receiving mitomycin. Chest 1996;109:939–44.

49. Luna MA, Bedrossian CWM, Lichtiger B, et al. Interstitial pneumonitis associated with bleomycin therapy. Am J Clin Pathol 1972;58:501–10.

50. White DA, Kris MG, Stover DE. Bronchoalveolar lavage cell populations in bleomycin lung toxicity. Thorax 1987;42:551–2.

51. Kirschner RH, Esterly JR. Pulmonary lesions associated with busulfan therapy of chronic myelogenous leukemia. Cancer 1971;27:1074–80.

52. Siemann DW, Macler L, Penney DP. Cyclophosphamide-induced pulmonary toxicity. Br J Cancer 1986;53:343–6.

53. Cole SR, Myers TJ, Ktalsky AV. Pulmonary disease with chlorambucil therapy. Cancer 1978;4:455–9.

54. Goucher G, Rowland V, Hawkins J. Melphelan-induced pulmonary interstitial fibrosis. Chest 1980;77:805–6.

55. Elsasser S, Dalquen P, Soler M. Methotrexate-induced pneumonitis: appearance four weeks after discontinuation of therapy. Am Rev Respir Dis 1989;140:1089–92.

56. White DA, Rankin JA, Stover DE, et al. Methotrexate pneumonitis: bronchoalveolar lavage findings suggest an immunological disorder. Am Rev Respir Dis 1989;139:18–21.

57. Bedrossian CWM, Sussman J, Conklin RH, et al. Azathioprine-associated interstitial pneumonitis. Am J Clin Pathol 1984;82:148–54.

58. Haupt HM, Hutchins GM, Moore GW. ARA-C lung: noncardiogenic pulmonary edema complicating cytosine arabinoside therapy of leukemia. Am J Med 1981;70:256–61.

59. Tham RT, Peters WG, de Bruine FT, et al. Pulmonary complications of cytosine arabinoside therapy: radiographic findings. AJR Am J Roentgenol 1987;149:23–7.

60. Smith AC. The pulmonary toxicity of nitrosoureas. Pharmacol Ther 1989;41:443–60.

61. Durant JR, Norgard MJ, Murad TM, et al. Pulmonary toxicity associated with bischloroethylnitrosourea (BCNU). Ann Intern Med 1979;90:191–4.

62. Cordonnier C, Verant JP, Mitral P, et al. Pulmonary fibrosis subsequent to high doses of CCNU for chronic leukemia. Cancer 1983;51:1814–8.

63. Lewis LD. Procarbazine associated alveolitis. Thorax 1984;39:206–7.

64. Akown GM, Liote HA, Liote F, et al. Provocation test coupled with bronchoalveolar lavage in the diagnosis of drug (nilutamide) induced hypersensitivity pneumonitis. Chest 1990;97:495–8.

65. Chin K, Tabata C, Satake N, et al. Pneumonitis associated with natural and recombinant interferon alpha therapy for chronic hepatitis C. Chest 1994;105:939–41.

66. Ogata K, Koga T, Yagawa K. Interferon related bronchiolitis obliterans organizing pneumonia. Chest 1994;106:612–3.

67. Ramanathan RK, Reddy V, Holbert JM. Pulmonary infiltrates following administration of paclitaxel. Chest 1996;110:289–92.

68. Berthiaume Y, Boiteau P, Fick G, et al. Pulmonary edema during IL-2 therapy: combined effect of increased permeability and hydrostatic pressure. Am J Respir Crit Care Med 1995;152:329–35.

69. Tazelaar HD, Myers JL, Drage CW, et al. Pulmonary disease associated with L-tryptophane-induced eosinophilic myalgia syndrome. Chest 1990;97:1032–6.

70. Kinnunen E, Viljanen A. Pleuropulmonary involvement during bromocriptine treatment. Chest 1988;94:1034–6.

71. Gross NJ. Pulmonary effects of radiation. Ann Intern Med 1977;86:81–92.

72. Gibson PG, Bryant DH, Morgan GW, et al. Radiation induced lung injury: a hypersensitivity pneumonitis? Ann Intern Med 1988;109:288–91.

73. Davis WB, Rennard SI, Bitterman PB, et al. Pulmonary oxygen toxicity: early reversible changes in human alveolar structures induced by hyperoxia. N Engl J Med 1983;309:873–8.

74. Crapo JD. Morphologic changes in pulmonary oxygen toxicity. Ann Rev Physiol 1986;48:721–31.

75. Copland GM, Kolin A, Shulman HS, et al. Pulmonary intraalveolar fibrosis after paraquat ingestion. N Engl J Med 1974;291:290–2.

76. Parkinson C. The changing pattern of paraquat poisoning in man. Histopathology 1980;4:171–83.

77. LeMense GP, Strange C. Granulomatous pneumonitis following intravesical BCG: what therapy is needed? Chest 1994;106:1624–6.

78. Haim DY, Lippmann ML, Goldberg SK, Walkenstein MD. The pulmonary complications of crack cocaine: a comprehensive review. Chest 1995;107:233–40.

79. James DG. Sarcoidosis of the respiratory system. Semin Respir Med 1986;8:1–111.

80. Hance AJ, Cadranel J, Soler P, et al. Pulmonary and extra pulmonary Langerhans' cell granulomatosis (histiocytosis X). Semin Respir Med 1988;9:349–68.

81. Gertz MA, Greipp RR. Clinical aspects of pulmonary amyloidosis. Chest 1986;90:790–1.

82. Taylor JR, Ryu J, Colby TV, et al. Lymphangiomyomatosis: clinical course in 32 patients. N Engl J Med 1990;323:1254–60.

83. Dwyer JH, Hickie JB, Garvan J. Pulmonary tuberous sclerosis. Report of three patients and a review of the literature. QJM 1971;40:115–25.

84. Patchefsky AS, Atkinson WG, Hoch WS. Interstitial pulmonary fibrosis and von Recklinghausen's disease: an ultrastructural and immunofluorescent study. Chest 1973;64:459–64.

85. Yang SP, Lin CC. Lymphangitic carcinomatosis of the lung: the clinical significance of its roentgenographic classification. Chest 1972;62:179–87.

86. Schneider EL, Epstein CJ, Kaback MJ, et al. Severe pulmonary involvement in Gaucher's disease: report of three cases and review of the literature. Am J Med 1977;63:475–80.

87. Lachman R, Crocker A, Schulman J, et al. Radiologic findings in Niemann-Pick disease. Radiology 1973;108:656–64.

88. White DA, Walker-Smith GT, Cooper JAD, et al. Hermansky-Pudlak syndrome and interstitial lung disease: report of a case with lavage findings. Am Rev Respir Dis 1984;130:138–41.

89. Peters JI, Bell RC, Prihoda TJ, et al. Clinical determinants of abnormalities in pulmonary function in survivors of the adult respiratory distress syndrome. Am Rev Respir Dis 1989;139:1163–8.

90. Burkhardt A. Alveolitis and collapse in the pathogenesis of pulmonary fibrosis. Am Rev Respir Dis 1989;140:513–24.

91. Wingard JR, Mellits DE, Sostrin MB, et al. Interstitial pneumonitis after allogeneic bone marrow transplantation. Medicine 1988;67:175–86.

92. Wingard JR, Sostrin MB, Vtiesendorp HM, et al. Interstitial pneumonitis following autologous bone marrow transplantation. Transplantation 1986;42:515–8.

93. Ognibene FP, Masur H, Rogers P, et al. Non-specific interstitial pneumonitis without evidence of *pneumocystis carinii* in asymptomatic patients infected with human immunodeficiency virus. Ann Intern Med 1988;109:874–9.

94. Jekat GJ, Astry CL, Warr GA. Alveolitis induced by influenza virus. Am Rev Respir Dis 1983;128:730–9.

95. Vastro JA, Littner MR, Taskkin DP, et al. Diffuse pulmonary interstitial infiltrate and mycoplasmal pneumonia. Am Rev Respir Dis 1974;110:659–62.

96. Hurter T, Rumpelt HJ, Ferlinz R. Following alveolitis responsive to corticosteroids following Legionnaires disease pneumonia. Chest 1992;101:281–3.

97. Lin AL, Kessimian N, Benditt JO. Restrictive lung disease due to interlobar septal fibrosis associated with disseminated infection by *Strongyloides stercoralis*. Am J Respir Crit Care Med 1995;151:205–9.

98. Shasby DM, Schwarz MI, Forstot JZ, et al. Pulmonary immune complex deposition in Wegener's granulomatosis. Chest 1982;81:338–40.

99. Doyle L, McWilliam L, Hasleton PS. Giant cell arteritis with pulmonary involvement. Br J Dis Chest 1988;82:88–92.

100. Myers JL, Veal CF, Myung SS, et al. Respiratory bronchiolitis causing interstitial lung disease: a clinicopathologic study of six cases. Am Rev Respir Dis 1987;135:880–4.

101. Palevsky HI, Pietra GG, Fishman AP. Pulmonary veno-occlusive disease and its response to vasodilator agents. Am Rev Respir Dis 1990;142:426–9.

102. Asa Kura S, Colby TV. Agnogenic myeloid metaplasia with extramedullary hematopoiesis and fibrosis in the lung. Chest 1994;105:1866–8.

103. Popper HH, Zenz W, Mache C, Ohlinger W. Familial haemophagocytic lymphohistiocytosis. A report of three cases with unusual lung involvement. Histopathology 1994;25:433–9.

104. Farina J, Furio V, Fernandez-Aenero MJ, Muzas MA. Nodular fibrosis of the lung in diabetes mellitus. Virchows Arch 1995;427:61–3.

105. Parto K, Svedstrom E, Majurin ML, et al. Pulmonary manifestations in lysinuric protein intolerance. Chest 1993;104:1176–82.

106. Parto K, Kallajoki M, Aho H, Simell O. Pulmonary alveolar proteinosis and glomerulonephritis in lysinuric protein intolerance: case reports and autopsy findings of four pediatric patients. Hum Pathol 1994;25:400–7.

107. Clague HW, Wallace AC, Morgan WKC. Pulmonary interstitial fibrosis with alveolar proteinosis. Thorax 1983;38:865–6.

108. Leatherman JW. Immune alveolar hemorrhage. Chest 1987;91:891–7.

109. Kennedy JD, Costello P, Balikian JP, et al. Exogenous lipoid pneumonia. AJR Am J Roentgenol 1981;136:1145–9.

110. Harpole DH, Bigelow C, Young WG. Alveolar cell carcinoma of the lung: a retrospective analysis of 205 patients. Ann Thorac Surg 1988;46:502–7.

111. Colby TV, Carrington CB. Lymphoreticular tumors and infiltrates of the lung. Pathol Annu 1983;18:27–70.

112. Sladen A, Zanc AP, Hadnott WH. Aspiration pneumonitis: the sequela. Chest 1971;59:448–50.

113. Jederlinic PJ, Sicilian L, Gaensler EA. Chronic eosinophilic pneumonia: a report of 19 cases and review of the literature. Medicine 1988;67:154–62.

114. Badesch DB, King TE Jr, Schwarz MI. Acute eosinophilic pneumonia: a hypersensitivity phenomenon? Am Rev Respir Dis 1989;139:249–52.

115. Allen JN, Pacht ER, Gadek JE, et al. Acute eosinophilic pneumonia as a reversible cause of non-infectious respiratory failure. N Engl J Med 1989;321:569–74.

116. Prakash VBS, Barham SS, Rosenow EC, et al. Pulmonary alveolar microlithiasis: a review including ultrastructural and pulmonary functional studies. Mayo Clin Proc 1983;58:290–300.

117. Epler GR, Colby TV, McCloud TL, et al. Bronchiolitis obliterans organizing pneumonia. N Engl J Med 1985;312:152–8.

118. Davison AG, Heard BC, McAllister WAC, et al. Cryptogenic organizing pneumonitis. QJM 1983;52:382–94.

119. Costabel U, Guzman J, Teschler H. Bronchiolitis obliterans with organizing pneumonia. Thorax 1995;50:559–64.

120. Gevenois PA, Abehsera M, Knopp C, et al. Disseminated pulmonary ossification in endstage pulmonary fibrosis: CT demonstration. AJR Am J Roentgenol 1994;162:1303–4.

121. Brodeur FJ, Kazerooni EA. Metastatic pulmonary calcification mimicking air-space disease: technetium-99m-MDP SPECT imaging. Chest 1994;106:620–2.

122. Davis GS. Pathogenesis of silicosis. Current concepts and hypothesis. Lung 1986;164:139–54.

123. McDonald JC. Silica, silicosis and lung cancer. Br J Ind Med 1989;46:289–91.

124. Begin R, Ostiguy G, Cantin A, et al. Lung function in silica exposed workers: a relationship to disease severity assessed by CT scan. Chest 1988;54:539–45.

125. Mossman BT, Gee JBL. Asbestos-related diseases. N Engl J Med 1989;320:1721–30.

126. Staples CA, Gamsu G, Carolyn SR, et al. High resolution computed tomography and lung function in asbestos-exposed workers with normal chest radiographs. Am Rev Respir Dis 1989;139:1502–8.

127. Vallyathan NV, Craighead JE. Pulmonary pathology in workers exposed to non-asbestos form of talc. Hum Pathol 1981;12:28–35.

128. Hopkins GB, Taylor DG. Pulmonary talc granulomatosis. Am Rev Respir Dis 1970;101:101–4.

129. Seaton A. Silicates and disease. In: Morgan WKC, Seaton A, editors. Occupational lung diseases. Philidelphia: WB Saunders; 1984. p. 250.

130. Davies D, Cotton R. Mica pneumoconiosis. Br J Ind Med 1983;40:22–7.

131. Jederlinic PJ, Abraham JL, Churg A, et al. Pulmonary fibrosis in aluminum oxide workers. Am Rev Respir Dis 1990;142: 1179–84.

132. Kriebel D, Brain JD, Sprince NL. The pulmonary toxicity of beryllium. Am Rev Respir Dis 1988;137:464–73.

133. Newman LS, Kreiss K, King TE Jr, et al. Pathologic and immunologic alterations in early stages of beryllium disease. Am Rev Respir Dis 1989;139:1479–86.

134. Davison AG, Haslam PL, Corrin B, et al. Interstitial lung disease and asthma in hard-metal workers: bronchoalveolar lavage, ultrastructural and analytic findings and results of bronchial provocation tests. Thorax 1983;38:119–28.

135. Parkes WR. Pneumoconiosis due to coal and carbon. In: Parkes WR, editor. Occupational lung disorders. Boston: Butterworths; 1982. p. 175.

136. Pendergrass E, Greening R. Baritosis: report of a case. Arch Ind Hyg 1953;7:44–7.

137. Cooper DA, Pendergrass EP, Volwald AK, et al. Pneumoconiosis in workers in an antimony industry. AJR Am J Roentgenol 1968;103:495–500.

138. Stewart MJ, Faulds JS. The pulmonary fibrosis of hematite miners. J Pathol Bacteriol 1934;39:233–5.

139. Soutar CA, Copeland LH, Thornby PE, et al. Epidemiological study of respiratory disease in workers exposed to polyvinyl chloride dust. Thorax 1980;35:644–51.

140. Seaton A, Lamb D, Rhind Brown W. Pneumoconiosis of shale miners. Thorax 1981;36:412–4.

141. Morgan WKC. Other pneumoconiosis. In: Morgan WKC, Seaton A, editors. Occupational lung disease. 2nd ed. Philadelphia: WB Saunders; 1984. p. 449–97.

142. Robertson AJ, Rivers D, Nagelschmidt G, et al. Stannosis. Lancet 1961;i:1089–91.

143. Chastre J, Brun P, Soler P, et al. Acute and latent pneumonitis after subcutaneous injections of silicone in transsexual men. Am Rev Respir Dis 1987;135:236–40.

144. Ramage JE, Roggli VL, Bell DY, Piantadosi CA. Interstitial lung disease and domestic wood burning. Am Rev Respir Dis 1988;137:1229–32.

145. Lougheed MD, Roos JO, Waddell WR, Munt PW. Desquamative interstitial pneumonitis and diffuse alveolar damage in textile workers: potential role of mycotoxins. Chest 1995;108:1196–200.

146. Kern DG, Crausman RS, Durand KTH, et al. Flock workers lung: chronic interstitial lung disease in the nylon flocking industry. Ann Intern Med 1998;129:261–72.

147. Richerson HB, Bernstein LI, Fink JN, et al. Guidelines for the clinical diagnosis of hypersensitivity pneumonitis. J Allergy Clin Immunol 1989;84:839–44.

148. Coleman A, Colby TV. Histologic diagnosis of extrinsic allergic alveolitis. Am J Surg Pathol 1988;12:514–8.

149. Weill H, Buechner HA, Gonzalez E, et al. Bagassosis: a study of pulmonary function in 20 cases. Ann Intern Med 1966;64:737–58.

150. Fink JN, Sosman AJ, Barboriak JJ, et al. Pigeon breeders disease: a clinical study of hypersensitivity pneumonitis. Ann Intern Med 1968;68:1205–19.

151. Bourke SJ, Banham SW, Carter R, et al. Longitudinal course of extrinsic allergic alveolitis in pigeon breeders. Thorax 1988;44:415–8.

152. Warren CPW, Tsek S. Extrinsic allergic alveolitis owing to hypersensitivity to chickens—significance of sputum precipitins. Am Rev Respir Dis 1974;109:672–7.

153. Burdon JGW, Stone C. Bird fancier's lung after an unusual exposure to avian protein. Am Rev Respir Dis 1986;134: 1319–20.

154. Emanuel DA, Wenzel FJ, Bowerman LI, et al. Farmer's lung: clinical pathologic and immunologic study of seventy four patients. Am J Med 1964;37:392–401.

155. Salvaggio JE. Recent advances in pathogenesis of allergic alveolitis. Clin Exp Immunol 1990;20:137–44.

156. Reynolds HY. Hypersensitivity pneumonitis. Clin Chest Med 1982;3:503–19.

157. Campbell JA, Kryda MJ, Treuhaft MW, et al. Cheese workers hypersensitivity pneumonitis. Am Rev Respir Dis 1983; 127:495–6.

158. Avila R. Extrinsic allergic alveolitis in workers exposed to fish meal and poultry. Clin Allergy 1971;1:343–6.

159. Stewart CT. Mushroom workers lung—two outbreaks. Thorax 1974;29:252–7.

160. Villar TG. Vineyard sprayers lung: clinical aspects. Am Rev Respir Dis 1974;110:545–55.

161. Pimentel JC, Avila R. Respiratory disease in cork workers (suberosis). Thorax 1973;28:409–23.

162. Harper LO, Burrell RG, Lapp NL, et al. Allergic alveolitis due to pituitary snuff. Ann Intern Med 1970;73:581–4.

163. Bauer X, Behr J, Dewair M, et al. Humidifier lung and humidifier fever. Lung 1988;166:113–24.

164. Sosman AJ, Schlueter DP, Fink JN, et al. Hypersensitivity to wood dust. N Engl J Med 1969;281:977–80.

165. Yoshizawa Y, Ohtsuka M, Noguchi K, et al. Hypersensitivity pneumonitis induced by toluene diisocyanate—sequelae of continuous exposure. Ann Intern Med 1989;110:31–4.

166. Fink JN, Banaszak EF, Baroriak JJ, et al. Interstitial lung disease due to contamination of forced air systems. Ann Intern Med 1976;84:406–13.

167. Jacobs RL, Thorner RE, Holcomb JR, et al. Hypersensitivity pneumonitis caused by *Cladosporium* in an enclosed hot tub area. Ann Intern Med 1986;105:204–6.

168. Orriols R, Manresa JM, Aliaga JL, et al. Mollusk shell hypersensitivity pneumonitis. Ann Intern Med 1990;113:80–1.

169. Hogan MB, Patterson R, Pore RS, et al. Basement showers hypersensitivity pneumonitis secondary to *Epicoccium nigrum*. Chest 1996;110:855–6.

170. Suda T, Sato A, Ida M, et al. Hypersensitivity pneumonitis associated with home ultrasonic humidifiers. Chest 1995;107:711–7.

171. Haitjema TJ, van Velzen-Blad H, van den Bosch JM. Extrinsic allergic alveolitis caused by goose feathers in a duvet. Thorax 1992;47:990–1.

172. Lippo KK, Sisko AL, Talkina-Aho O, et al. Hypersensitivity pneumonitis and exposure to zirconium silicate in a young ceramic tile worker. Am Rev Respir Dis 1993;148:1089–92.

173. Vandenplas O, Malo JL, Dugas M, et al. Hypersensitivity pneumonitis-like reaction among workers exposed to piphenylmethane diisocyanate (MDI). Am Rev Respir Dis 1993;147:338–46.

174. Bernstein DI, Lummus ZL, Santilli G, et al. Machine operators lung: a hypersensitivity pneumonitis disorder associated with exposure to metalworking fluid aerosols. Chest 1995;108:636–41.

175. Katzenstein AL, Myers JL, Mazur MT. Acute interstitial pneumonia: a clinicopathologic, ultrastructural, and cell kinetic study. Am J Surg Pathol 1986;10:256–67.

176. Schwarz MI. Idiopathic pulmonary fibrosis. West J Med 1988;149:199–203.

177. Musk AW, Zilko PJ, Manners P, et al. Genetic studies in familial fibrosing alveolitis: possible linkage with immunoglobulin allotypes (gm). Chest 1985;89:206–10.

178. Koss MN, Hochholzen L, Langloss JM, et al. Lymphoid interstitial pneumonia: clinicopathologic and immunopathologic findings in 18 cases. Pathology 1987;19:178–85.

179. Katzenstein ALA, Fiorelli RF. Non-specific interstitial pneumonia/fibrosis. Am J Surg Pathol 1994;18:136–47.

180. Liebow AA. Desquamative interstitial pneumonia. Am J Pathol 1962;41:127–41.

181. Scadding JW. Fibrosing alveolitis with autoimmune hemolytic anemia: two case reports. Thorax 1977;32:134–9.

182. Meduri GV, Reynaso G. Idiopathic interstitial pneumonitis occurring with idiopathic thrombocytopenic purpura. Chest 1989;96:253S.

183. Bombardieri S, Pasletti P, Ferri C, et al. Lung involvement in essential mixed cryoglobulinemia. Am J Med 1979;66: 748–56.

184. Heatly RV, Thomas P, Prokipchuk EJ, et al. Pulmonary function abnormalities in patients with inflammatory bowel disease. QJM 1982;203:241–50.

185. Tarlo SM, Broder I, Prokipchuk EJ, et al. Association between coeliac disease and lung disease. Chest 1981;80:715–8.

186. Pollack JJ. Pleuropulmonary Whipple's disease. South Med J 1985;78:216–7.

187. Leff JA, Ready JB, Repetto C, et al. Co-existence of primary biliary cirrhosis and sarcoidosis. West J Med 1990;153:439–41.

188. Turner-Warwick M. Fibrosing alveolitis and chronic liver disease. QJM 1968;37:133–39.

189. Salerno SM, Strong JS, Roth BJ, Sakata V. Eosinophilic pneumonia and respiratory failure associated with a trazodone overdose. Am J Respir Crit Care Med 1995;152:2170–2.

190. Valle JM, Alverez D, Antunez J, Valdes L. Bronchiolitis obliterans organizing pneumonia secondary to amiodarone: a rare etiology. Eur Respir J 1995;8:470–1.

191. Oren S, Turkot S, Golzman B, et al. Amiodarone induced bronchiolitis obliterans organizing pneumonia (BOOP). Respir Med 1996;90:167–9.

192. King TE Jr. BOOP: an important cause of migratory pulmonary infiltrates? Eur Respir J 1995;8:193–5.

193. Crestani B, Kambouchner M, Soler P, et al. Migratory bronchiolitis obliterans organizing pneumonia after unilateral radiation therapy for breast carcinoma. Eur Respir J 1995; 8:318–21.

194. Alasaly K, Miller N, Ostrow DN, et al. Cryptogenic organizing pneumonia: a report of 25 cases and a review of the literature. Medicine 1995;74:201–11.

195. Siddiqui MT, Garrity ER, Husain AN. Bronchiolitis obliterans pneumonia-like reactions: non-specific response or an atypical form of rejection or infection in lung allograft recipients. Hum Pathol 1996;27:714–9.

196. Sanito AJ, Morley TF, Condoluci DV. Bronchiolitis obliterans organizing pneumonia in an AIDS patient. Eur Respir J 1995;8:1021–4.

197. Diehl JL, Gisselbrecht M, Meyer G, et al. Bronchiolitis obliterans organizing pneumonia associated with chlamydial infection. Eur Respir J 1996;9:1320–2.

198. Mark EJ, Ramierez JF. Pulmonary capillaritis and hemorrhage in patients with systemic vasculitis. Arch Pathol Lab Med 1985;109:413–8.

199. Travis WD, Carpentier HA, Lie ST. Diffuse pulmonary hemorrhage: an uncommon manifestation of Wegener's granulomatosis. Am J Surg Pathol 1987;11:702–8.

200. Savage COS, Winearls CG, Evans DV, et al. Microscopic polyarteritis. Presentation, pathology, and prognosis. QJM 1985;56:467–83.

201. Myers JL, Katzenstein ALA. Microangiitis in lupus-induced pulmonary hemorrhage. Am J Clin Pathol 1986;85:552–6.

202. Schwarz MI, Suturik JM, Nick JA, et al. Pulmonary capillaritis and diffuse alveolar hemorrhage: a primary manifestation of polymyositis. Am Rev Respir Crit Care Med 1995;151:2037–40.

203. Lombard CM, Colby TV, Elliot CG. Surgical pathology of the lung in anti-basement antibody disease associated with Goodpasture's syndrome. Hum Pathol 1989;20:445–51.

204. Jennings CA, King TE, Tuder R, et al. Diffuse alveolar hemorrhage with underlying isolated paucci-immune pulmonary capillaritis. Am Rev Respir Crit Care Med 1997;155:1101–9.

205. Clark JG, Hansen JA, Hertz MI, et al. Idiopathic pneumonia syndrome after bone marrow transplantation: NHLBI workshop summary. Am Rev Respir Dis 1993;147:1601–6.

206. Vourlekis JS, Brown KK, Cool CD, et al. Acute interstitial pneumonia: case series and review of the literature. Medicine 2000;79:369–78.

207. Katzenstein ALA. Idiopathic pulmonary hemosiderosis. In: Katzenstein ALA, Askin FB, editors. Surgical pathology of non-neoplastic lung disease. Philadelphia: WB Saunders; 1982. p. 133.

208. Zamora MR, Warner ML, Tuder R, Schwarz MI. Diffuse alveolar hemorrhage in systemic lupus erythematosus: clinical presentation, histology, survival, and outcome. Medicine 1997;76:192–202.

209. American Thoracic Society/European Respiratory Society International Multidisciplinary consensus classification of the idiopathic interstitial pneumonias. Am J Respir Crit Care Med 2002;165:277–304.

210. Clark JG, Kuhn C, McDonald JA, et al. Lung connective tissue. Int Rev Conn Tissue Res 1983;10:231–49.

211. Campbell EJ, Senior RM, Welgus HG. Extracellular matrix injury during lung inflammation. Chest 1987;92:161–7.

212. Stulberg MS. Interstitial (diffuse parenchymal) lung disease: etiologic, clinical and roentgenological considerations. In: Baum GL, Wolinsky E, editors. Textbook of pulmonary diseases. 4th ed. Boston, Toronto: Little, Brown; 1989. p. 967–78.

213. National Heart and Lung Institute. Task force on research in respiratory diseases. Report on problems, research approaches, and needs. Washington: The Lung Program, Natl Heart and Lung Inst; 1972 October. Washington: 1973 DHEW No: 73–432.

214. Coultas DB, Hughes MP. Accuracy of mortality data for interstitial lung disease in New Mexico USA. Thorax 1996; 51:717–20.

215. Coultas DB, Zumualt RE, Black W, Sobonya RE. The epidemiology of interstitial lung diseases. Am J Respir Crit Care Med 1994;150:967–72.

216. du Bois RM. Diffuse lung disease: an approach to management. BMJ 1994;309:175–9.

217. Johnston I, Britton J, Kinnear W, Logan R. Rising mortality of cryptogenic fibrosing alveolitis. BMJ 1990;301:1017–21.

218. Popper MS, Bogdonoff ML, Hughes RL. Interstitial rheumatoid lung disease: a reassessment and review of the literature. Chest 1977;62:243–9.

219. Kumar R, Lykke AWJ. Messages and handshakes: cellular interactions in pulmonary fibrosis. Pathology 1995;27:18–26.

220. Snyder LS, Hertz MI, Peterson MS, et al. Acute lung injury: the pathogenesis of intraalveolar fibrosis. J Clin Invest 1991;88:663–73.

221. Fukuda Y, Ishizaki M, Masuda Y, et al. The role of intraalveolar fibrosis in the process of pulmonary structural remodeling in patients with diffuse alveolar damage. Am J Pathol 1987;126:171–82.

222. Basset F, Ferrans VJ, Soler P, et al. Intraluminal fibrosis in interstitial lung disorders. Am J Pathol 1986;122:443–61.

223. Hamman L, Rich AR. Fulminating diffuse interstitial fibrosis of the lungs. Bull Johns Hopkins Hosp 1944;74:154–63.

224. Schwarz MI. The acute (non-infectious) interstitial lung diseases. Compr Ther 1996;22:622–30.

225. Pratt DS, Schwarz MI, May JJ, et al. Rapidly fatal pulmonary fibrosis: the accelerated variant of interstitial pneumonitis. Thorax 1979;34:587–93.

226. O'Driscoll BR, Haselton PS, Taylor PM, et al. Active lung fibrosis up to 17 years after chemotherapy with carmustine (BCNU) in childhood. N Engl J Med 1990;323:378–82.

227. Elsasser S, Dalquen P, Soler M, et al. Methotrexate induced pneumonitis: appearance four weeks after discontinuation of therapy. Am Rev Respir Dis 1989;140:1089–92.

228. Tobin RW, Pope CE, Pellegrini CA, et al. Increased prevalence of gastroesophageal reflux in patients with idiopathic pulmonary fibrosis. Am J Respir Crit Care Med 1998;158: 1804–8.

229. Kriebel D, Brain JD, Sprince NL, Kazemi H. The pulmonary toxicity of beryllium. Am Rev Respir Dis 1988;137:464–73.

230. Mossman BT, Gee JBL. Asbestos-related diseases. N Engl J Med 1989;320:1721–30.

231. Soler P, Moreau A, Basset F, et al. Cigarette smoking-induced changes in the number and differentiated state of pulmonary dendritic cells/Langerhans' cells. Am Rev Respir Dis 1989;139:1112–7.

232. Hance AJ, Basset F, Saumon G, et al. Smoking and interstitial lung disease. The effect of cigarette smoke in the incidence of pulmonary histiocytosis X and sarcoidosis. Ann N Y Acad Sci 1986;465:643–56.

233. Donaghy M, Rees AJ. Cigarette smoking and lung hemorrhage in glomerulonephritis caused by autoantibodies to glomerular basement membrane. Lancet 1983;2:1390–3.

234. Weiss W. Cigarette smoke, asbestos, and small irregular opacities. Am Rev Respir Dis 1984;130:293–301.

235. de Cremoux H, Bernaudin JF, Laurent P, et al. Interactions between cigarette smoking and the natural history of idiopathic pulmonary fibrosis. Chest 1990;98:71–6.

236. Kusaka H, Homma Y, Ogasawara H, et al. Five year follow up of *Micropolyspora faeni* antibody in smoking and non-smoking farmers. Am Rev Respir Dis 1989;140:695–9.

237. Valeyre D, Soler P, Clericci C, et al. Smoking and pulmonary sarcoidosis: effect of cigarette smoking on prevalence, clinical manifestations, alveolitis, and evolution of disease. Thorax 1988;43:516–24.

238. Raghu G. Genetic susceptibility to pulmonary fibrosis. Pulm Perspect 1995;12:5–8.

239. Libby DM, Gibofsky A, Fotino M, et al. Immunogenetic and clinical findings in idiopathic pulmonary fibrosis: association with the B-cell alloantigen HLA-DR2. Am Rev Respir Dis 1983;127:618–22.

240. Musk AW, Zilko PJ, Manners P, et al. Genetic studies in familial fibrosing alveolitis. Chest 1986;89:206–10.

241. Nogee LM, Dunbar AE, Wert SE, et al. A mutation in the surfactant protein C gene associated with familial interstitial lung disease. N Engl J Med 2001;344:573–9.

242. Thomas AO, Lane K, Phillips J, et al. Heterozygosity for a surfactant protein C gene mutation associated with usual interstitial pneumonitis and non-specific interstitial pneumonitis in one kindred. Am J Respir Crit Care Med 2002;165:1322–8.

243. Bitterman PB, Rennard SI, Keogh BA, et al. Familial idiopathic pulmonary fibrosis: evidence of lung inflammation in unaffected family members. N Engl J Med 1986;314:1343–7.

244. Epler GR, McCloud TC, Gaensler EA, et al. Normal chest roentgenograms in chronic diffuse interstitial lung disease. N Engl J Med 1978;298:934–9.

245. Panos RJ, Mortenson RL, Niccoli SA, King TE Jr. Clinical deterioration in patients with idiopathic pulmonary fibrosis: causes and assessment. Am J Med 1990;88:396–404.

246. Schwarz MI, Cherniack RM, King TE Jr. Diffuse alveolar hemorrhage and other rare infiltrative disorders. In: Murray JF, Nadel JA, editors. Respiratory medicine. 2nd ed. Philadelphia: WB Saunders; 1994. p. 1889–912.

247. Epler GR, Carrington CB, Gaensler EA. Crackles in the interstitial pulmonary diseases. Chest 1978;73:333–7.

248. Galko B, Grossman RF, Day A, et al. Hypertrophic pulmonary osteodystrophy in four patients with interstitial pulmonary disease. Chest 1985;88:94–7.

249. James DGJ, Graham E. Occulopulmonary syndromes. Semin Respir Med 1988;9:380–4.

250. Sharma OP, Nam H. Cutaneous manifestations of pulmonary disease. Semin Respir Med 1988;9:385–94.

251. Bourke SJ, Munro NC, White JES, et al. Platypnea-orthodeoxia in cryptogenic fibrosing alveolitis. Respir Med 1995;89:387–9.

252. Hansen JE, Wasserman K. Pathophysiology of activity limitation in patients with interstitial lung disease. Chest 1996;109:1566–76.

253. Haddad R, Massaro D. Idiopathic diffuse interstitial fibrosis: atypical epithelial proliferation and lung cancer. Am J Med 1968;45:211–9.

254. Fulmer JD, Roberts WC, Von Gal R, et al. Morphologic-physiologic correlates of severity of fibrosis and degree of celllular infiltration in idiopathic pulmonary fibrosis. J Clin Invest 1979;63:665–76.

255. Chinet T, Sanbert F, Dusser D, et al. Effects of inflammation and fibrosis on pulmonary function in diffuse lung fibrosis. Thorax 1990;45:675–8.

256. Jernudd-Wilhelmsson Y, Hoinblad Y, Hederstierna G. Ventilation-perfusion relationships in interstitial lung disease. Eur J Respir Dis 1986;68:39–49.

257. Miller A, Brown LK, Sloane MF, et al. Cardiorespiratory responses to incremental exercise in sarcoidosis patients with normal spirometry. Chest 1995;107:323–9.

258. Fulmer JD, Roberts WC, Von Gal ER, et al. Small airways in idiopathic pulmonary fibrosis: comparison of morphologic and physiologic observations. J Clin Invest 1977;60:595–610.

259. Bye PTP, Issa F, Berthon-Jones M, et al. Studies of oxygenation during sleep in patients with interstitial lung disease. Am Rev Respir Dis 1984;129:27–32.

260. Perez-Padilla R, West P, Lertzman M, et al. Breathing during sleep in patients with interstitial lung disease. Am Rev Respir Dis 1985;132:224–9.

261. Tenholder MF, Russell MD, Knight E, et al. Orthodeoxia: a new finding in interstitial fibrosis. Am Rev Respir Dis 1987;136:170–3.

262. McCloud TC, Gaensler EA, Carrington CB. Chronic diffuse infiltrative lung disease. Clin Chest Med 1984;5:329–44.

263. Ziskind MM, Weill H, Buechner HA, Brown M. Recognition of distinctive radiologic patterns in diffuse pulmonary disease. Arch Intern Med 1964;114:108–12.

264. Ziskind MM, Weill H, George RB. Diffuse pulmonary disease. Medicine 1967;254:95–117.

265. Webb RW. High resolution CT of the lung parenchyma. Radiol Clin North Am 1989;27:1085–97.

266. Schurawitzke H, Stiglbauer R, Graninger W. Interstitial lung disease in progressive systemic sclerosis: high resolution CT versus radiography. Radiology 1990;1776:755–9.

267. Young RC Jr, Caron C, Krumholz RA, et al. Pulmonary sarcoidosis (1) pathophysiologic correlations. Am Rev Respir Dis 1968;97:997–1008.

268. Sahn SA, Schwarz MI. Desquamative interstitial pneumonia with a normal chest radiograph. Br J Dis Chest 1974;68:228–34.

269. Unger GF, Scarlon GT, Fink JN, et al. A radiologic approach to hypersensitivity pneumonia. Radiol Clin North Am 1973;11:339–56.

270. Bronson SM. Idiopathic pulmonary hemosiderosis in adults: report of a case review of the literature. AJR Am J Roentgenol 1960;83:260–71.

271. Vedal S, Welsh EV, Miller RR, et al. Desquamative interstitial pneumonia: computed tomographic findings before and after treatment with corticosteroids. Chest 1988;93:215–7.

272. Liebow AA, Steer A, Billingsley JG. Desquamative interstitial pneumonia. Am J Med 1965;39:369–404.

273. Carrington CB, Addington WW, Goffam, et al. Chronic eosinophilic pneumonia. N Engl J Med 1969;280:787–98.

274. Trapnell DH. Radiologic appearances of lymphangitis carcinomatosa of the lung. Thorax 1964;19:251–60.

275. Corrin B, Liebow AA, Friedman RI. Pulmonary lymphangiomyomatosis: a review. Am J Pathol 1975;79:348–82.

276. Fulmer JD. An introduction to the interstitial lung diseases. Clin Chest Med 1982;3:457–73.

277. Chahinian AP, Pajak TF, Holland JF, et al. Diffuse malignant mesothelioma. Ann Intern Med 1982;96:746–55.

278. Gaensler EA, Kaplan AI. Asbestos pleural effusion. Ann Intern Med 1971;74:178–91.

279. Becklake MR. Asbestos-related diseases of the lung and other organs; their epidemiology and implications for clinical practice. Am Rev Respir Dis 1976;114:187–227.

280. Laronique J, Roth C, Battestic JP, et al. Chest radiologic features of pulmonary histocytosis X: a report based upon 50 adult cases. Thorax 1982;37:104–9.

281. Schwartz DA, Merchant RK, Helmers RA, et al. The influence of cigarette smoking in lung function in patients with idiopathic pulmonary fibrosis. Am Rev Respir Dis 1991; 144:504–6.

282. Claque HW, Wallace AC, Morgan WKC. Pulmonary interstitial fibrosis associated with alveolar proteinosis. Thorax 1983;38:865–6.

283. Sahn SA, Schwarz MI, Lakshminarayan S. Sarcoidosis: the significance of an acinar pattern on chest roentgenogram. Chest 1974;65:684–7.

284. Muller NL, Miller RR. Computed tomography of chronic diffuse lung disease. Part 1; 2. Am Rev Respir Dis 1990;142: 1206–15, 1440–8.

285. Muller NL, Staples CA, Miller RR, et al. Disease activity in idiopathic pulmonary fibrosis: computed tomographic-pathologic-correlation. Radiology 1987;165:731–4.

286. Mathieson JR, Mayo JR, Staples CA, et al. Chronic diffuse infiltrative lung disease: comparison of diagnostic activity of CT and chest radiography. Radiology 1989;171:111–6.

287. Primack SL, Hartman TE, Hansell DM, Muller NL. Endstage lung disease: CT findings in 61 patients. Radiology 1993;189:681–6.

288. Lee JS, Im JG, Ahn JM, et al. Fibrosing alveolitis prognostic implication of ground glass attenuation on high resolution CT. Radiology 1992;184:451–4.

289. Wells AU, Hansell DM, Rubens MB, et al. The predictive value of appearance on thin-section computed tomography of fibrosing alveolitis. Am Rev Respir Dis 1993;148:1076–82.

290. Schurawitzki H, Stiglbauer R, Graninger W, et al. Interstitial lung disease in progressive systemic sclerosis: high resolution CT versus radiography. Radiology 1990;176:755–9.

291. Aberle DR, Gamsu G, Ray CS. High resolution computed CT of benign asbestos related disease: clinical and radiographic correlation. AJR Am J Radiol 1988;151:883–91.

292. Orens JB, Kazerooni EA, Martinez JF, et al. The sensitivity of high resolution CT in detecting idiopathic pulmonary fibrosis proved by open lung biopsy: a prospective study. Chest 1995;108:109–15.

293. Watters LC, King TE, Cherniack RM, et al. Bronchoalveolar lavage fluid neutrophils increase after corticosteroid therapy in smokers with idiopathic pulmonary fibrosis. Am Rev Respir Dis 1988;133:104–9.

294. The BAL Cooperative Steering Committee. Bronchoalveolar lavage constituents in healthy individuals, idiopathic pulmonary fibrosis, and selected comparison groups. Am Rev Respir Dis 1990;141:S199–S202.

295. Stumpf IV, Feld MK, Cornelius M, et al. Safety of fiberoptic bronchoalveolar lavage in elevation of interstitial lung disease. Chest 1981;80:268–71.

296. Sestini P, Rottoli L, Gotti G, et al. Bronchoalveolar lavage diagnosis of bronchioloalveolar carcinoma. Eur J Respir Dis 1985;66:55–88.

297. Myers JL, Fulmer JD. Bronchoalveolar lavage in the diagnosis of pulmonary lymphomas. Chest 1987;91:642–3.

298. Miller KS, Sahn SA. Mycosis fungoides presenting as ARDS and diagnosed by bronchoalveolar lavage: radiologic and pathologic pulmonary manifestations. Chest 1986;89:312–4.

299. Morales FM, Matthews JI. Diagnosis of parenchymal Hodgkin's disease using bronchoalveolar lavage. Chest 1987;91:785–90.

300. Martin RJ, Coalson JJ, Rogers RM, et al. Pulmonary alveolar proteinosis: the diagnosis by segmental lavage. Am Rev Respir Dis 1980;121:819–25.

301. Haslam PL, Hughes DA, Dewar A, et al. Lipoprotein macroaggregates in bronchoalveolar lavage fluid from patients with diffuse interstitial lung disease: comparison with idiopathic alveolar lipoproteinosis. Thorax 1988;43:140–6.

302. Hunninghake GW, Gadek JE, Kawanami O, et al. Inflammatory and immune processes in the human lung in health and disease: evaluation by bronchoalveolar lavage. Am J Pathol 1979;97:149–206.

303. Turner-Warwick ME, Haslam PL. Clinical applications of bronchoalveolar lavage: an interim view. Br J Dis Chest 1986;80:105–21.

304. Fedullo AJ, Ettensohn DB. Bronchoalveolar lavage in lymphangitic spread of adenocarcinoma of the lung. Chest 1985;87:129–32.

305. Helmers RA, Hunninghake GW. Bronchoalveolar lavage in the nonimmunocompromised patient. Chest 1989;96:1184–90.

306. Ettensohn DB, Roberts NJ, Condemi JJ. Bronchoalveolar lavage in gold lung. Chest 1984;85:569–70.

307. Brutinel WM, Martin WJ. Chronic nitrofurantoin reaction associated with T-lymphocyte alveolitis. Chest 1986;89:150–2.

308. Akoun GM, Gauthier-Rahman S, Milleron BG. Amiodarone induced hypersensitivity pneumonitis: evidence of an immunological cell-mediated mechanism. Chest 1984;85: 133–5.

309. Lauque D, Dongay G, Levade T, et al. Bronchoalveolar lavage in liquid paraffin pneumonitis. Chest 1990;98:1149–55.

310. Sebastien P, Armstrong B, Monchaux G, et al. Asbestos bodies in bronchoalveolar lavage fluid and in lung parenchyma. Am Rev Respir Dis 1988;137:75–8.

311. De Vuyst P, Dumortier P, Moulin E, et al. Diagnostic value of asbestos bodies in bronchoalveolar lavage fluid. Am Rev Respir Dis 1987;136:1219–24.

312. Kawanami O, Basset F, Ferrans VJ, et al. Pulmonary Langerhans' cells in patients with fibrotic lung disorders. Lab Invest 1981;44:227–33.

313. Watters LC, Schwarz MI, Cherniack RM, et al. Idiopathic pulmonary fibrosis: pretreatment bronchoalveolar lavage cellular constituents and their relationships with lung pathology and clinical response to therapy. Am Rev Respir Dis 1987;135:696–704.

314. Keogh BA, Hunninghake GW, Line BR, et al. The alveolitis of pulmonary sarcoidosis—evaluation of natural history and alveolitis dependent changes in lung function. Am Rev Respir Dis 1983;128:236–65.

315. Israel-Biet D, Venet A, Chretien J. Persistant high alveolar lymphocytosis as a predictive criterion of chronic pulmonary sarcoidosis. Ann N Y Acad Sci 1986;465:395–406.

316. Costabel V, Bross KJ, Guzman J, et al. Predictive value of bronchoalveolar T cell subsets for the course of pulmonary sarcoidosis. Ann N Y Acad Sci 1986;465:418–26.

317. Verstraeten A, Demedts M, Verwilghen J, et al. Predictive value of bronchoalveolar lavage in pulmonary sarcoidosis. Chest 1990;98:560–7.

318. Turner-Warwick M, Haslam PL. The value of serial bronchoalveolar lavage in assessing the clinical progress of patients with cryptogenic fibrosing alveolitis. Am Rev Respir Dis 1987;135:26–34.

319. Peterson MW, Monick M, Hunninghake GW. Prognostic role of eosinophils in pulmonary fibrosis. Chest 1987;92:51–6.

320. Rudd RM, Haslam PL, Turner-Warwick M. Cryptogenic fibrosing alveolitis: relationships of pulmonary physiology and bronchoalveolar lavage to response to treatment and prognosis. Am Rev Respir Dis 1981;124:1–8.

321. Greene NB, Solinger AM, Baughman RD. Patients with collagen vascular disease and dyspnea: the value of gallium scanning and bronchoalveolar lavage in predicting response to steroid therapy and clinical outcome. Chest 1987; 91:698–703.

322. Silver RM, Miller KS, Kinsella MB, et al. Evaluation and management of scleroderma lung disease using bronchoalveolar lavage. Am J Med 1990;88:470–6.

323. Garcia JGN, Parhamic N, Killam D, et al. Bronchoalveolar lavage fluid evaluation in rheumatoid arthritis. Am Rev Respir Dis 1986;133:450–4.

324. Smiejan JM, Cosnes J, Chollet-Martin S, et al. Sarcoid-like lymphocytosis of the lower respiratory tract in patients with active Crohn's disease. Ann Intern Med 1986; 104:17–21.

325. Waller TB, Bonniere P, Prin L, et al. Primary biliary cirrhosis: subclinical inflammatory alveolitis in patients with normal chest roentgenograms. Chest 1986;90:842–8.

326. Wall CP, Gaensler EA, Carrington CB, et al. Comparison of transbronchial and open biopsies in chronic infiltrative lung diseases. Am Rev Respir Dis 1981;123:280–5.

327. Krassna MJ, White CS, Aisner SC, et al. The role of thoracoscopy in the diagnosis of interstitial lung disease. Ann Thorac Surg 1995;59:348–51.

328. Gaensler EA, Carrington CB. Open lung biopsy for chronic diffuse infiltrative lung disease: clinical, roentgenographic, and physiologic correlations in 502 patients. Ann Thorac Surg 1980;30:411–26.

329. Watters LC, King TE Jr, Schwarz MI, et al. A clinical radiographic and physiologic scoring system for the longitudinal assessment of patients with idiopathic pulmonary fibrosis. Am Rev Respir Dis 1986;133:97–103.

330. King TE Jr, Tooze JA, Schwarz MI, et al. Predicting survival in idiopathic pulmonary fibrosis: scoring system and survival model. Am J Respir Crit Care Med 2001;164:1171–84.

331. Fox DA. Biological therapies: a novel approach to the treatment of autoimmune disease. Am J Med 1995;99:82–8.

332. Hunninghake GW, Kalica AR. Approaches to the treatment of pulmonary fibrosis. Am J Respir Crit Care Med 1995; 151:915–8.

333. Goldstein RH, Fine A. Potential therapeutic initiatives for fibrogenic lung diseases. Chest 1995;108:848–55.

334. Mapel DW, Samet J, Coultas DB. Corticosteroids and the treatment of idiopathic pulmonary fibrosis: past, present, and future. Chest 1996;110:1058–67.

2 ANATOMIC DISTRIBUTION AND HISTOPATHOLOGIC PATTERNS OF INTERSTITIAL LUNG DISEASE

KEVIN O. LESLIE
THOMAS V. COLBY
STEPHEN J. SWENSEN

Interstitial lung disease (ILD) encompasses a large and diverse group of pathologic conditions that share many clinical, radiologic, and physiologic features.[1] The method of diagnosis in cases of ILD varies with the specific entities. Surgical biopsy specimens of the lung are required for diagnosis in most cases. For some ILDs, biopsy findings alone may establish a specific etiologic diagnosis, whereas in others, the histopathology requires correlation with clinical and radiologic findings. Unfortunately, a small number of patients with diffuse lung disease (mainly inflammatory ILD) elude a specific diagnosis since the histopathologic features are often nonspecific. By their nature, the histologic changes in inflammatory diseases tend to overlap. Problems of overlap in reaction patterns are compounded by the range of histologic changes in terms of both severity and age.

Despite these limitations, histologic findings provide information about etiology, activity, age, reversibility, and prognosis. For example, some histologic patterns may be reversible and reflect both a favorable response to treatment and a good prognosis (eg, eosinophilic pneumonia), whereas others may portend an unfavorable response and ultimate outcome to medical intervention (diffuse fibrosis and structural lung remodeling). In many TLDs, tissue examination is the only way to obtain some of this relevant information.

Experienced pathologists generally rely on the low power magnification pattern of disease using "gestalt" in arriving at a histologic diagnosis or ILD. For less experienced observers and in cases where experience and gestalt do not provide an answer, it is helpful to have a conceptual framework in the approach to a lung biopsy specimen. This chapter explores the concept of anatomic distribution of histopathologic changes and associated reaction patterns of tissue injury for the development of a differential diagnosis. Then, the applied clinical and radiologic findings can further narrow the possibilities.[2,3] This approach is viable because, in their pure and unadulterated forms, ILDs tend to affect certain anatomic compartments preferentially, a feature best appreciated at scanning magnification under the microscope. In other cases, the anatomic distribution may be unclear, sometimes as a result of another disease which obscures the underlying pattern. When this occurs, a descriptive diagnosis encompassing the findings will be reported. Finally, in some ILDs, specific histologic clues (eg, organisms, malignant cells) can be identified that allow a definitive diagnosis.

ASSESSMENT OF DIFFUSE PULMONARY DISEASE ACCORDING TO ANATOMIC DISTRIBUTION OF LESIONS

The two-dimensional presentation of lung anatomy, as seen in tissue sections under the microscope, is complex and nearly overwhelming to the inexperienced eye. To define an anatomic distribution for a pathologic condition, one must first have a working knowledge of the normal anatomic landmarks in lung tissue. These are easily recognized in a stylized schematic (Figure 2–1), but may be more difficult to identify in poorly processed or inadequate biopsy specimens. Again, experience plays a large role in the accuracy of diagnosis. The recognition of an anatomic distribution generally requires examination of the slide at scanning magnification (2 × or 4 × objective lens) or even with the naked eye. With some practice, even atelectatic biopsy specimens can be analyzed for anatomic distribution of disease. Identifying an anatomic distribution is useful in correlating the histopathology of ILDs with radiologic changes, particularly those seen in high-resolution computed tomog-

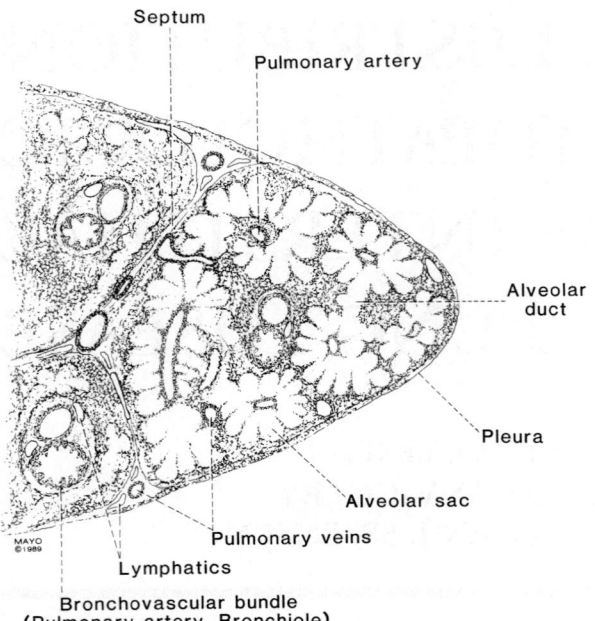

Septum

Pulmonary artery

Alveolar duct

Pleura

Alveolar sac

Pulmonary veins

Lymphatics

Bronchovascular bundle
(Pulmonary artery, Bronchiole)

MAYO ©1989

Figure 2–1   This schematic representation of a lung biopsy shows normal anatomic structures that can be recognized histologically. From Colby TV et al.[4]

raphy (HRCT) scans. Recognizable patterns according to anatomic landmarks (and their HRCT correlates) are shown in Table 2–1.

Bronchocentric/Bronchiolocentric Distribution

A bronchocentric/bronchiolocentric pattern of distribution (Figure 2–2) implies preferential involvement of the airways, including the bronchi, bronchioles, and alveolar ducts. In some cases, the modifiers "centrilobular" or "centriacinar" are appropriate. Among ILDs, this pattern may be found with infections (especially those caused by viruses or mycoplasma), other forms of bronchiolitis (eg, diffuse panbronchiolitis and obliterative bronchiolitis), extrinsic allergic alveolitis (eg, hypersensitivity pneumonitis), pulmonary Langerhans cell histiocytosis (pulmonary eosinophilic granuloma, especially in early stages), respiratory bronchiolitis-associated interstitial lung disease (RBILD), the collagen vascular diseases (especially Sjögren's syndrome and rheumatoid arthritis), pneumoconioses (eg, dust macules, cobalt/hard metal disease), and others.[2,3]

Bronchiolocentric lesions primarily affect the small airways but may manifest themselves clinically and radiologically as diffuse interstitial/infiltrative lung disease. Furthermore, the pathologic recognition of small airway pathology may not correlate with physiologic evidence of "airway disease." In fact, from the radiologic and histologic points of view, the time-honored separation of interstitial disease from airway disease is too simplistic.

Angiocentric Distribution

An angiocentric distribution refers to pathologic changes centered on blood vessels (arteries and veins), and, as a pure process, it is an uncommon manifestation of ILD. Examples include primary and secondary vasculitis, angioinvasive infections, pulmonary arterial thrombi and thromboemboli, pulmonary hypertension, lung transplant rejection, intravenous drug abuse, and some primary and secondary tumors that preferentially involve the vessels of the lung (especially lymphomas, metastatic angiosarcoma, pulmonary artery sarcoma, and some intra-arterial metastatic carcinomas).[4]

Pleural Distribution

Lung disease preferentially involving the pleura and subpleural lung tissue is an uncommon manifestation of ILD. In some cases of sarcoidosis, amyloidosis, and asbestosis, pleural involvement dominates the pathologic findings. Moreover, some tumors may show preferential pleural involvement, particularly lymphomas. In this category, the distinction of a pleural disease from an interstitial parenchymal disease may be somewhat arbitrary.

Lymphatic Distribution

The pulmonary lymphatics are found beside veins and bronchovascular bundles in the pleura and in the interlobular septa. Therefore, a lymphatic distribution (Figures 2–3 and 2–4) will show pathologic changes in these distributions. A lymphatic distribution is a relatively common pattern among ILDs, although the lymphatic vessels themselves may or may not be appreciated because of

TABLE 2–1   Anatomic Distribution in Diffuse Lung Disease*

Histologic	Radiologic (HRCT)
Broncho/bronchiolocentric	Centrilobular
	Bronchovascular
Angiocentric	Bronchovascular (arterial)
	Interlobular septal (venous)
Pleural/subpleural	Pleural/subpleural
Lymphatic	Bronchovascular
	Interlobular septal
	Pleural/subpleural
Peripheral acinar	Subpleural peripheral distribution (paraseptal)
Septal	Septal (interlobular septal)
Random nodular	Random nodular
Parenchymal consolidation	Consolidation
Diffuse interstitial	Diffuse interstitial, ground-glass attenuation
Mixed and unclassified	Mixed/unclassifiable

*Adapted from Colby TV and Swensen SJ.[3]
HRCT = high-resolution computed tomography.

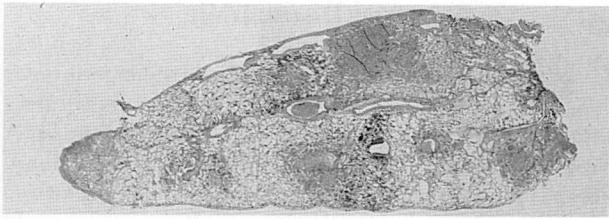

A

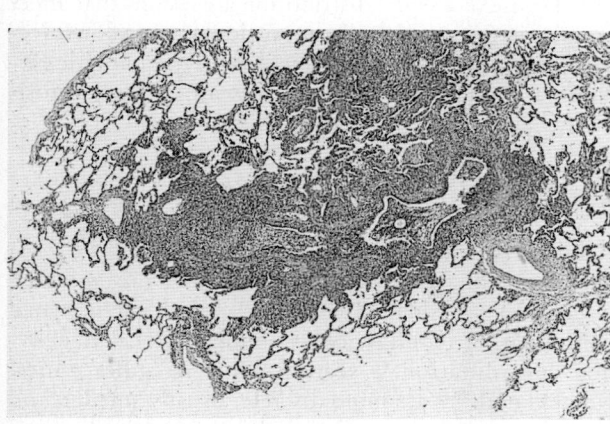

B

Figure 2–2 *A, B,* Bronchocentric distribution as illustrated by these two cases of *Mycoplasma pneumoniae* pneumonia. Note the patchy nature of the process reflecting bronchiolar involvement and the sparing of the peripheral alveoli.

overshadowing by the pathologic process. A lymphatic distribution often occurs with sarcoidosis, lymphangitic carcinoma (and occasionally some sarcomas), lymphoreticular infiltrates (both primary and secondary lymphomas, leukemias, and lymphoid hyperplasias), pneumoconioses, Erdheim-Chester disease, and diffuse pulmonary lymphangiomatosis.[2–7] It is not surprising that lymphoreticular processes would involve the lymphatic routes of the lung; similarly, the pathways by which dust is cleared from the lungs by lymphatic routes explains the lymphatic distribution in many pneumoconioses. Difficulty in recognizing a lymphatic distribution in a given patient can occur when there is disproportionate involvement of one component of the lymphatic system. For example, marked pathologic changes distributed along bronchovascular bundles (appearing angiocentric or bronchiolocentric) with relatively little involvement of interlobular septa or pleura, may obscure the underlying lymphatic distribution; this is common in sarcoidosis, for example. Nevertheless, in the majority of cases, perusal of reasonably sized lung biopsy specimens permits appreciation of the lymphatic distribution.

Peripheral Acinar Distribution

The periphery of the acinus is a difficult anatomic compartment to visualize given the three-dimensional relationship that exists between acini and the likeli-

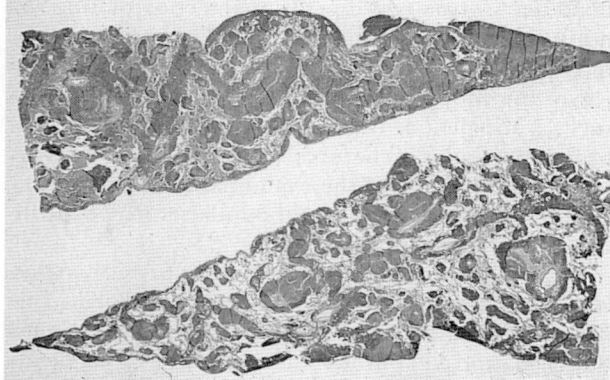

A

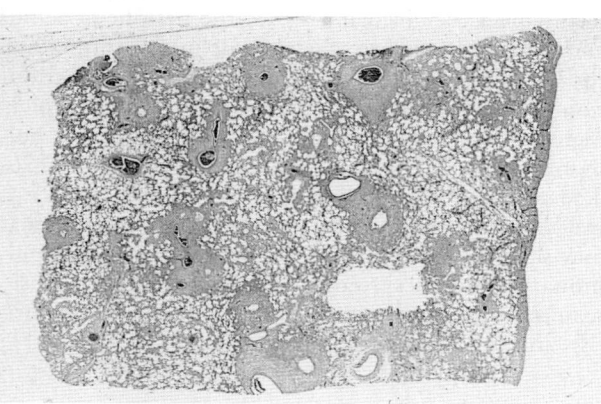

B

Figure 2–3 Lymphatic distribution illustrated in a case of *A,* diffuse small lymphocytic lymphoma and *B,* acute myelosclerosis. *A,* The neoplastic lymphoid cells outline the lymphatic routes in the pleura, septa, and along bronchovascular bundles. *B,* The case of acute myelosclerosis shows a similar distribution with a cuff of myelosclerotic tissue that follows lymphatic routes.

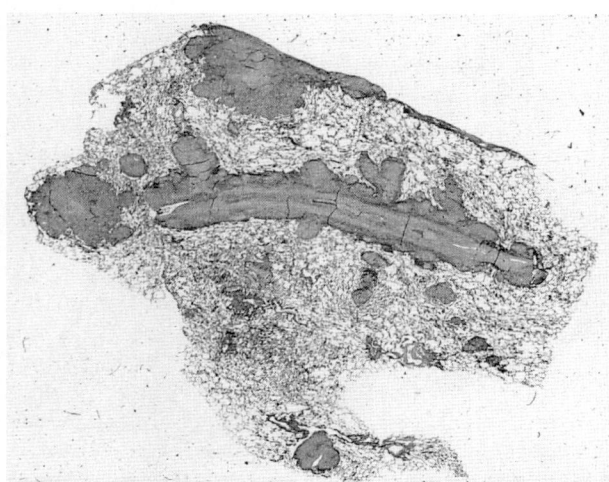

Figure 2–4 A lymphatic distribution is illustrated in sarcoidosis where a bronchovascular bundle cut longitudinally has a beaded appearance due to the granulomas along it; there is also a pleural granulomatous nodule.

hood that a given two-dimensional section of lung will not uniformly bisect these spherical structures in one plane. The periphery of the acinus can be best seen where the lung parenchyma abuts specific structures such as the pleura, the interlobular septa, and larger bronchovascular structures (larger than respiratory bronchioles). Between these landmarks, acini abut one another and their peripheral boundaries may be difficult to distinguish.

The peripheral acinar distribution pattern is illustrated in Figure 2–5. A predominantly peripheral acinar distribution can mimic a lymphatic distribution because of the relationship of the acinar periphery to the pleura and bronchovascular bundles. Lymphatic and peripheral acinar patterns can be distinguished since the latter involves the alveolar walls of the peripheral acinus and not the lymphatic channels or interstitium along the lymphatic routes.[4,5] The peripheral acinar distribution has not been systematically studied, but its involvement is prominent in many cases of idiopathic pulmonary fibrosis (IPF) and other interstitial pneumonias. The propensity for subpleural involvement in IPF is well known. Other fibrosing interstitial pneumonias may show a similar distribution including familial pulmonary fibrosis, systemic collagen vascular diseases manifesting in the lung (particularly rheumatoid arthritis), and certain fibrotic drug reactions.

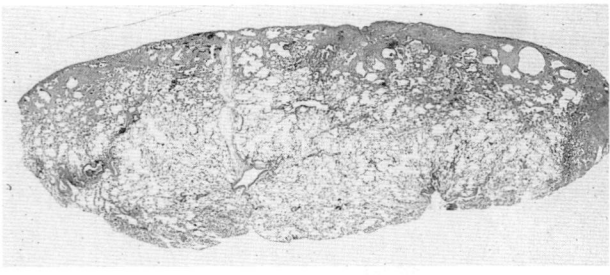

A

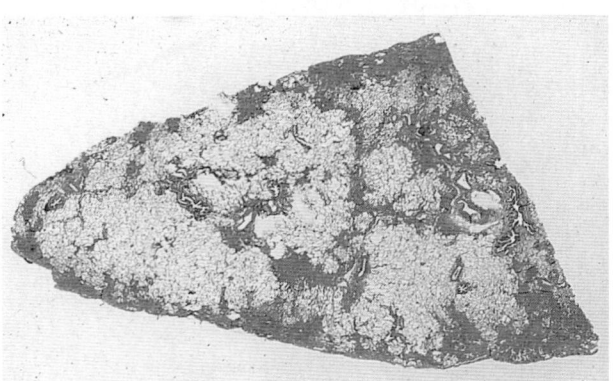

B

Figure 2–5   A peripheral acinar distribution is shown in these two cases of usual interstitial pneumonia (idiopathic pulmonary fibrosis) in which the fibrosis is *A*, predominantly subpleural or *B*, subpleural and adjacent to the septa and bronchovascular bundles.

Septal Distribution

Disease processes that primarily affect the interlobular septa are unusual,[3,4] and a septal distribution is not necessarily useful in establishing a differential diagnosis. A septal distribution is seen in some cases of pulmonary edema, pulmonary veno-occlusive disease, and chronic passive congestion of the lung. The most frequently noted cause of a septal distribution are lesions that affect lymphatic routes with disproportionate septal involvement, such as that seen in sarcoidosis, lymphangitic carcinoma, and Erdheim-Chester disease (a histiocytosis with characteristic bone lesions).

Nodular Lesions

Random distribution of nodular lesions (Figure 2–6) occurs in miliary tuberculosis and other disseminated infections.[3,4] As such, there is overlap with parenchymal consolidation (confluence of nodular foci). Parenchymal consolidation is seen as large irregular zones, whereas nodules are more discrete, usually smaller, and sometimes necrotic or fibrotic. The nodular lesions of pulmonary Langerhans cell histiocytosis (PLCH) and silicosis can be randomly distributed late in their course, although early on, these lesions develop in a bronchiolocentric and lymphatic distribution, respectively. The nodular lesions of PLCH tend to be stellate and have a mixed composition, including fibroblasts, collagen, Langerhans cells, eosinophils, and pigmented alveolar macrophages. In contrast, the nodules of silicosis are round with a whorled, lamellar, and hyaline character to the fibrosis, with variable admixed polarizable silicates. Many nodular processes, such as sarcoidosis and certain neoplasms, are not randomly distributed, but show a lymphatic pattern on scanning magnification.

Parenchymal Consolidation

Parenchymal consolidation (filling of air spaces) can be either diffuse or patchy (Figure 2–7). This pattern of lung disease occurs with many ILDs such as acute and organizing infections, pulmonary hemorrhage, pulmonary alveolar proteinosis, chronic eosinophilic pneumonia, desquamative interstitial pneumonia, RBILD, and many others.[3,5] Parenchymal consolidation alone is not helpful in establishing a diagnosis unless the constituent pathologic elements are nearly diagnostic, such as pulmonary alveolar proteinosis and chronic eosinophilic pneumonia. For most diseases with this distribution, the observer must try to recognize the pattern and then establish a differential diagnosis. In satellite lesions distant to large foci of consolidation, and in less affected regions of the lung, one may discern a recognizable distribution other than the consolidation. This is particularly true of lymphoreticular infiltrates and certain infectious pneumonias (eg, bronchopneumonia in a bronchiolocentric pattern).

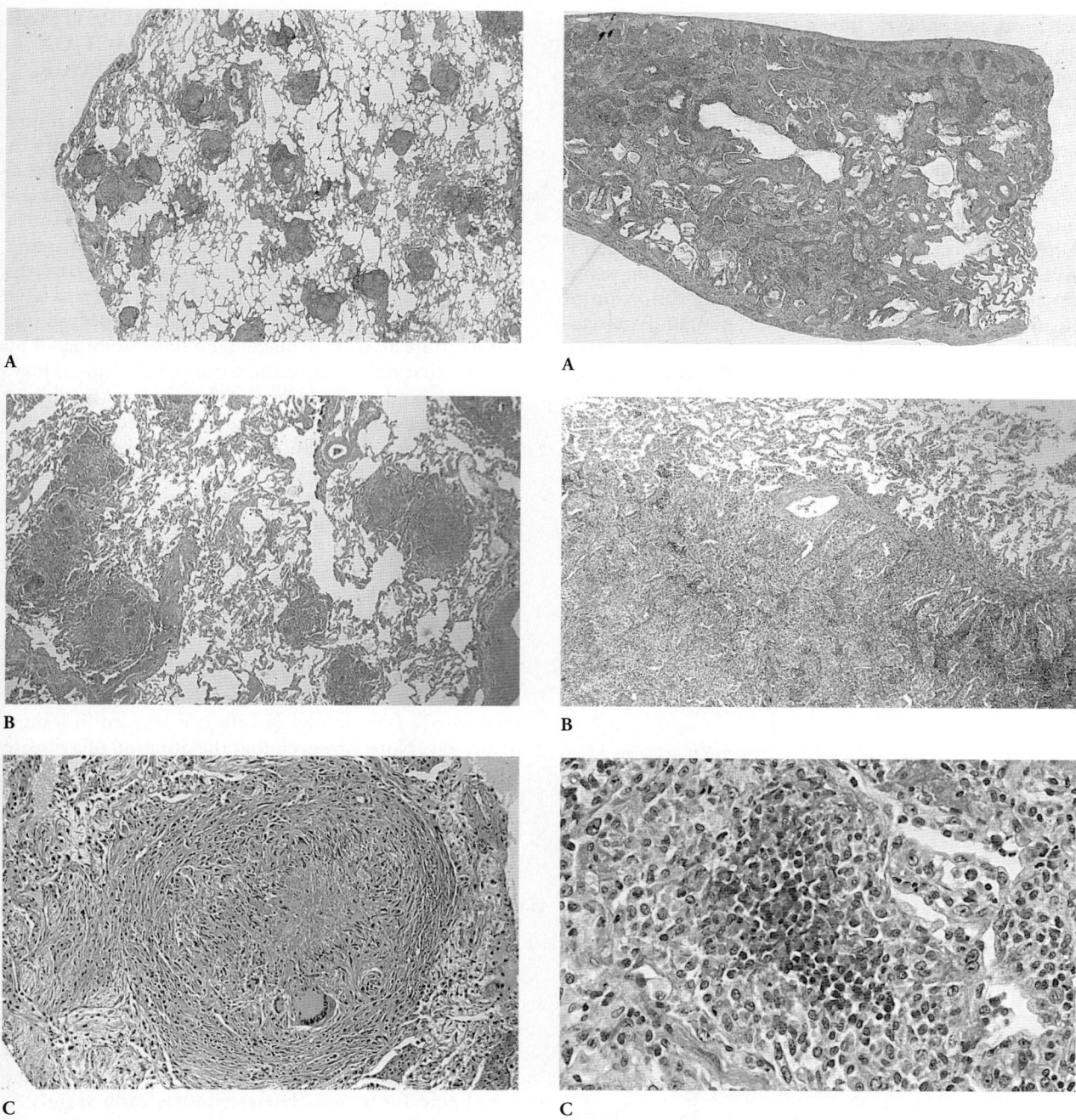

A

B

C

C

Figure 2–6   Randomly distributed nodules are typical of miliary granulomatous infections shown here in a case of *Mycobacterium avium-intracellulare* infection in a previously healthy young woman in *A,* and in miliary tuberculosis, *B* and *C,* with necrosis of the granulomas in an immunosuppressed host. Compare the randomly scattered granulomas in *A* and *B* with those of sarcoidosis in Figures 2–4 and 2–18.

Figure 2–7   *A* and *B,* Parenchymal consolidation is typical of eosinophilic pneumonia, which sometimes shows a *B,* sharp cut off at an interlobular septum. *C,* Distinctive features at higher power are the large numbers of eosinophils and associated histiocytes.

Diffuse Interstitial Infiltrates

Diffuse infiltration of the lung parenchyma by inflammatory cells (mononuclear cells, including lymphocytes and plasma cells) is a common pattern in ILD (Figure 2–8) and often not particularly helpful in arriving at a specific diagnosis. Nevertheless, diseases that produce mononuclear interstitial infiltrates often have similar responses to therapy and similar prognosis. Diseases in this category include hypersensitivity pneumonitis, drug reactions, lymphocytic interstitial pneumonia, systemic collagen vascular diseases manifesting in the lung, and some lymphoreticular infiltrates.[3–5] When the pathologic changes indicate an acute process, accompanied by reactive type II cells and air space fibrin with hyaline membranes, the diffuse interstitial infiltrative pattern can reflect diffuse alveolar damage.

For both parenchymal consolidation and diffuse interstitial infiltrates, the distribution of disease by scanning magnification may narrow the differential diagnosis but may not always result in a specific diagnosis. A variety of potential problems, including distortion of tissue, small biopsy size, sample location, and atelectasis, may lead to difficulty in recognition of landmarks. Comorbid processes occurring in the same patient, either or incidentally superimposed, further complicate the interpretation. *Because of this, it is often necessary to go beyond anatomic distribution and identify a reaction pattern in order to narrow the differential diagnosis.* The common reaction patterns in lung disease are shown in Table 2–2.

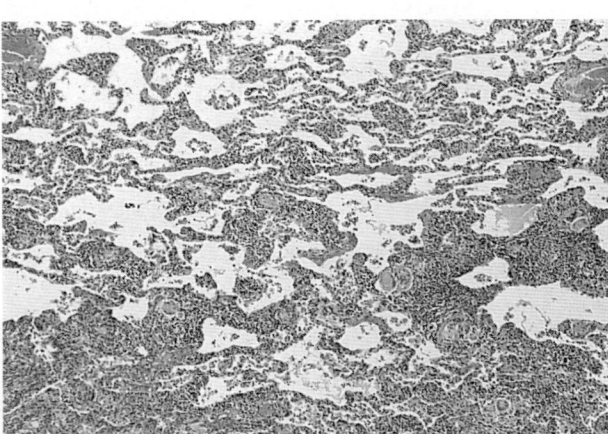

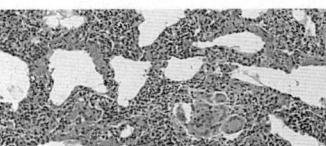

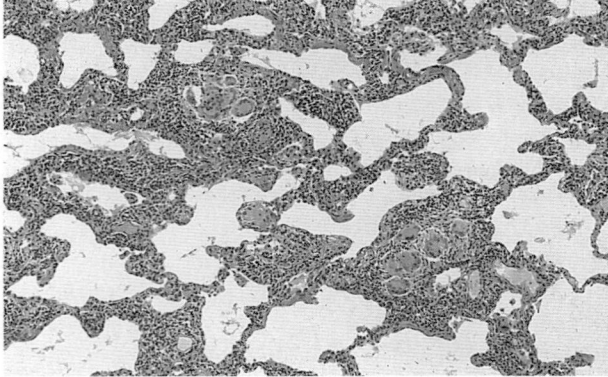

Figure 2–8 *A*, Diffuse interstitial infiltrates with little fibrosis are characteristic of extrinsic allergic alveolitis. *B*, Scattered small granulomas, seen in this case as clusters of giant cells, are associated with diffuse interstitial inflammation.

HISTOLOGIC EVALUATION OF INTERSTITIAL DISEASES BY IDENTIFYING A REACTION PATTERN OF LUNG INJURY AND REPAIR

The lung has a limited repertoire in response to injury and a histological pattern may have different causes. A specific diagnosis usually requires clinicopathologic correlation. The anatomic distribution of the most common reaction patterns shows a mixture of both parenchymal consolidation and interstitial infiltrates. Considerable overlap occurs frequently among patterns as illustrated in Table 2–2. Some of these patterns have temporal variablity or "life cycles." Acute processes (eg, acute diffuse alveolar damage) tend to be dominated by features that reflect the acute nature of the lung injury: fibrinous exudates, hyaline membranes, and combined interstitial and intra-alveolar edema. Subacute organizing processes (eg, organizing pneumonia pattern) are reflected histologically by the organization of exudates, reactive type II cell repopulation of alveolar walls, and interstitial/air space fibroblastic proliferation with minimal mature collagen deposition. This occurs in organizing diffuse alveolar damage and bronchiolitis obliterans with organizing pneumonia. Microscopic honeycombing, dense interstitial fibrosis, and smooth muscle proliferation suggest chronicity; these features can be seen in the pattern of interstitial fibrosis with honeycombing. Granulomas and interstitial infiltrates comprised of mononuclear cells can be seen in lesions of any age. Note, however, that the duration of a disease based on clinical history is one of the best indicators of the age of the process and is useful for correlation with the histopathologic pattern identified.

Diffuse Alveolar Damage Pattern

Diffuse alveolar damage (DAD) (Figure 2–9) is a very common histologic injury pattern in acute ILD, particularly in patients with adult respiratory distress syndrome (ARDS) and those who are immunosuppressed.[8–12] Edema, epithelial necrosis and epithelial sloughing, fibrinous exudate in air spaces, and hyaline membrane formation characterize the early stages. As the process organizes and undergoes repair (organizing diffuse alveolar damage), there is proliferation of type II

TABLE 2–2   Common Reaction Patterns of Interstitial Lung Diseases

Diffuse alveolar damage (acute or organizing)

Alveolar hemorrhage (clinically—alveolar hemorrhage syndrome)

Bronchiolitis obliterans with organizing pneumonia (OP pattern)

Interstitial fibrosis (usually with honeycombing)

Desquamative interstitial pneumonia-like (DIP pattern)

Cellular interstitial infiltrates

Granulomatous interstitial pneumonias (with or without necrosis)

cells along the alveolar walls, absorption of hyaline membranes and air space exudates, and fibroblastic proliferation both in the interstitium and in the air spaces. Hyaline membranes may no longer be seen.

DAD is usually a relatively uniform process in degree of severity, being similar in all fields examined. In some early cases of ARDS, radiographic infiltrates may start in one portion of the lung and progress to diffuse involvement. Diffuse alveolar damage is associated with the following:

1. Infections (viral, fungal, bacterial, parasitic)
2. Toxic inhalation
3. Drugs
4. Shock
5. Collagen vascular diseases
6. Radiation reactions (acute)
7. Acute allergic reactions (eg, hypersensitivity pneumonitis)
8. Alveolar hemorrhage syndromes
9. Other miscellaneous conditions
10. Idiopathic disease (acute interstitial pneumonia/The Hamman-Rich Syndrome)

Immunosuppressed patients with acute interstitial lung disease often show diffuse alveolar damage in biopsy specimens. In this case, infections and drug reactions are most frequent. The diffuse alveolar damage pattern can also be seen superimposed on endstage idiopathic pulmonary fibrosis (the so-called acute exacerbation of IPF).[13]

Alveolar Hemorrhage Pattern

The alveolar hemorrhage syndromes (Figure 2–10) can overlap with diffuse alveolar damage, although clinically, pulmonary hemorrhage is recognized often as the problem. Recent and remote evidence of hemorrhage are the most prominent histologic features that help distinguish hemorrhage syndromes from other forms of acute lung injury.[3,14] Histologically, hemorrhagic parenchymal consolidation is the most prominent change at low magnification. Large numbers of hemosiderin-filled macrophages can be present within the air spaces in chronic hemorrhage, and these may mimic desquamative interstitial pneumonia (DIP) (see "Desquamative Interstitial Pneu-

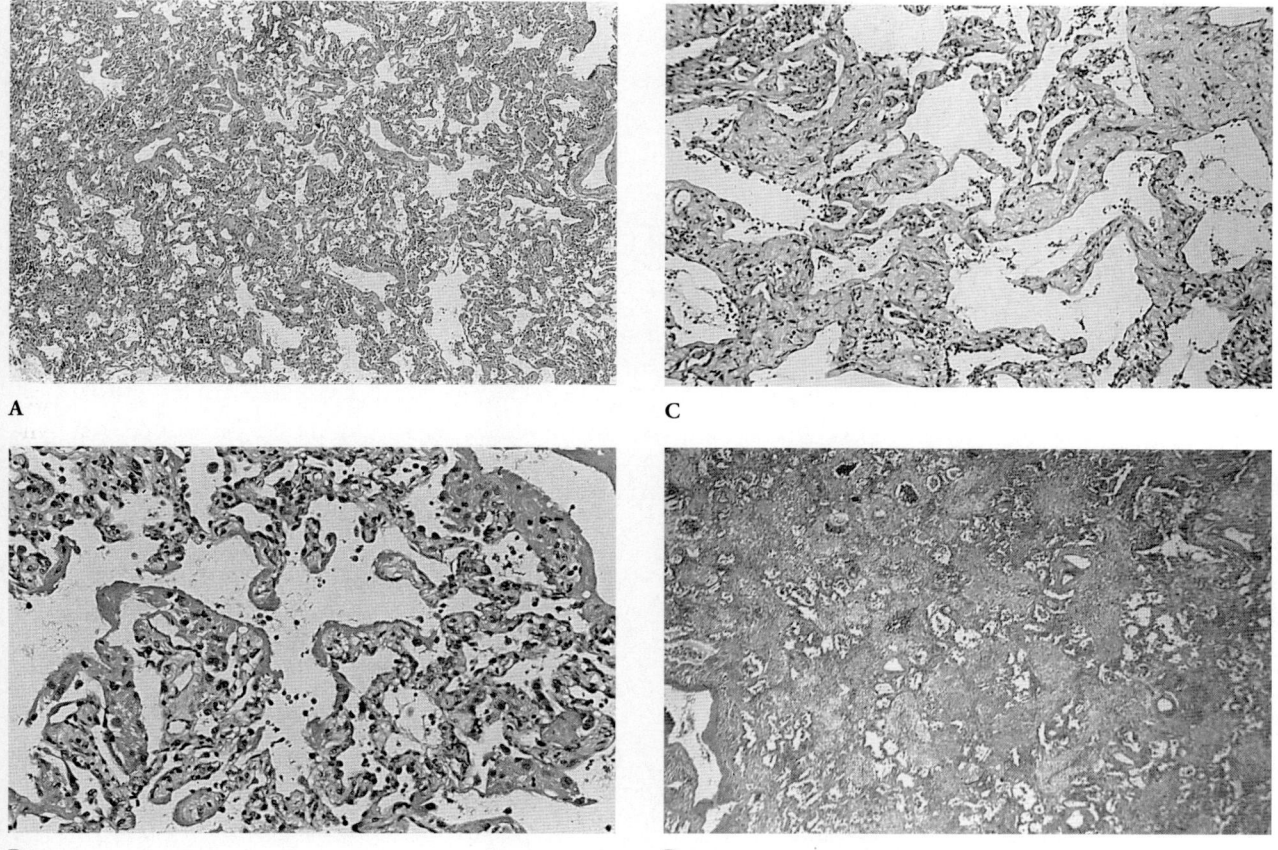

Figure 2–9   Diffuse alveolar damage *A*, and *B*, may be acute with hyaline membranes or may show *C*, evidence of organization after resorption of hyaline membranes with interstitial fibroblastic tissue, or *D*, extensive air space organization. In all figures the underlying lung architecture is intact. Despite the marked air space organization shown in *D*, this patient with bleomycin-induced diffuse alveolar damage recovered completely without sequelae.

monia Pattern"). Capillaritis is a distinctive histologic feature seen in some alveolar hemorrhage syndromes. Capillaritis is characterized by infiltrates of neutrophils within and around the capillaries of the alveolar walls and small pulmonary veins (see Figure 2–10). Capillaritis can be seen with many causes of diffuse alveolar hemorrhage. There may be small tufts of organizing connective tissue within air spaces if organization of the hemorrhage has begun. Varying degrees of interstitial fibrosis may also accompany this process in its chronic form. Many of the causes of alveolar hemorrhage syndromes also manifest in the kidney, causing glomerulonephritis. The most common pulmonary hemorrhage syndromes and disease processes associated with diffuse pulmonary hemorrhage include[4,14]:

1. Goodpasture's syndrome (anti–glomerular basement membrane antibody disease)
2. Vasculitides (especially Wegener's granulomatosis)
3. Mitral stenosis
4. IgA nephropathy
5. Behçet's syndrome
6. Certain collagen vascular diseases (especially systemic lupus erythematosus)
7. Human immunodeficiency virus (HIV) infection
8. Antiphospholipid syndrome
9. Pulmonary veno-occlusive disease
10. Idiopathic pulmonary hemosiderosis
11. Drug reactions, including toxic reactions and anticoagulants
12. Acute lung allograft rejection
13. Unclassified forms

In evaluating the presence of blood within the alveolar spaces, the pathologist should first separate artifactual or traumatic hemorrhage (resulting from the biopsy procedure itself) from true alveolar hemorrhage. Traumatic hemorrhage is not associated with hemosiderin deposition in macrophages, fibrin aggregates within the air spaces, or capillaritis. It is important to note that neutrophilic margination, related to the surgical procedure, may simulate capillaritis, and capillaritis with neutrophilic shedding into the air spaces can, on occasion, simulate acute pneumonia. Clinical correlation is usually

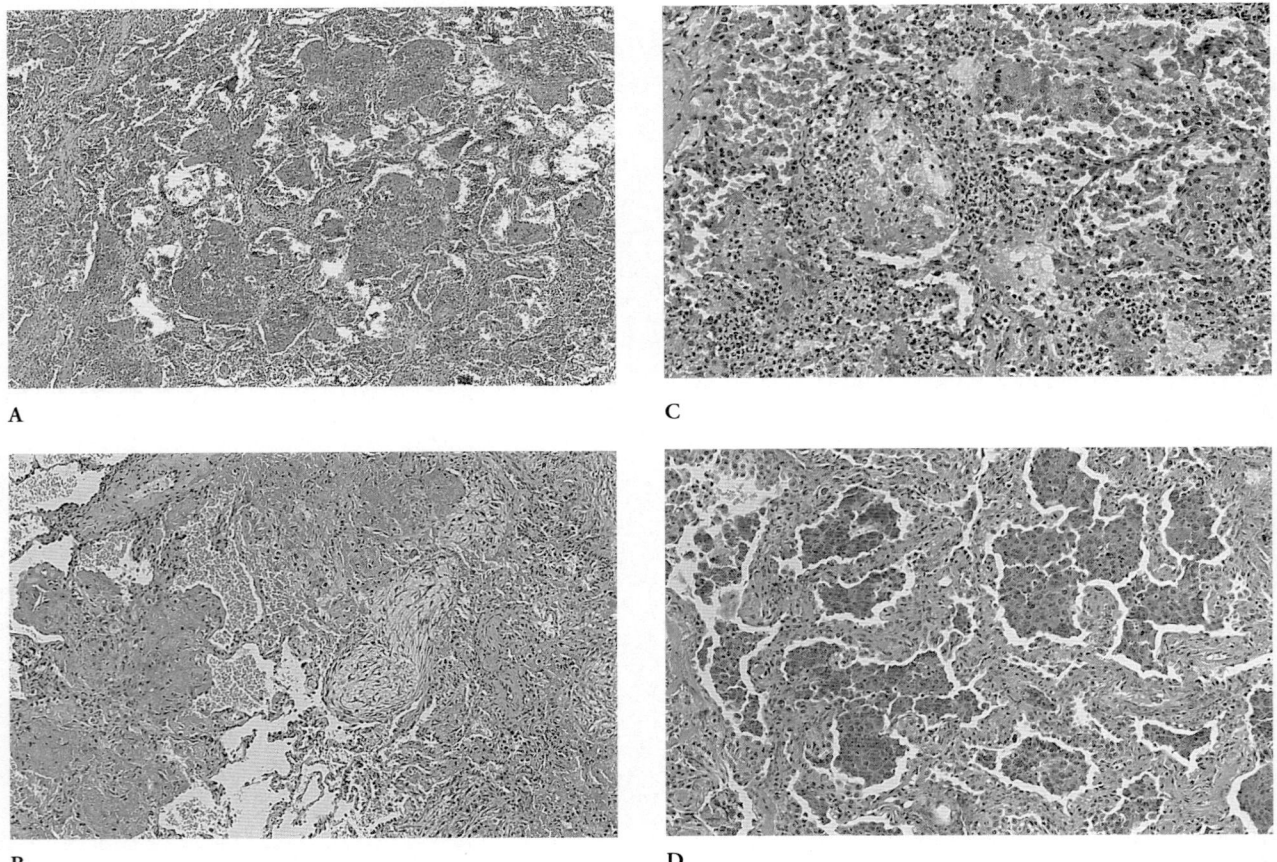

A   **B**   **C**   **D**

Figure 2–10   Alveolar hemorrhage is characterized acutely by *A*, air space fibrin and red blood cells, *B*, sometimes with foci of organization, right center. *C*, center, Regardless of the cause, alveolar hemorrhage may be associated with capillaritis, in which neutrophils permeate and ultimately destroy the alveolar septum. *D*, Chronic alveolar hemorrhage, is associated with hemosiderin-filled air spaces and modest associated interstitial thickening.

helpful in confirming the presence of true alveolar hemorrhage (hemoptysis, anemia, renal findings, etc). When in doubt, serologic studies may help substantiate an immunologic mechanism and provide information on any specific hemorrhage syndrome that may be involved. Finally, smoker's alveolar macrophages can have considerable amounts of finely granular pigment that can be Prussian blue positive, thereby simulating the siderophages of pulmonary hemorrhage. In most instances, these can be distinguished from true hemosiderin-laden macrophages by their lack of coarsely crystalline, golden brown cytoplasmic pigment.

Bronchiolitis Obliterans Organizing Pneumonia Pattern (Organizing Pneumonia)

Bronchiolitis obliterans with patchy organizing pneumonia (BOOP pattern) is a common reaction pattern in the lung (Figure 2–11). A BOOP pattern is prominent in organizing acute lung injury from any cause.[2–9,15] It is seen in a number of settings, most notably in idiopathic bronchiolitis obliterans organizing pneumonia (so-called "idiopathic BOOP" or "cryptogenic organizing pneumonia"), a form of idiopathic ILD. The most prominent finding is patchy involvement of the air spaces by small polypoid tufts of organizing connective tissue distributed within terminal bronchioles, alveolar ducts, and alveoli. Organization is most prominent within the alveolar ducts. The term bronchiolitis obliterans has been applied to the bronchiolar lesion, but it is a histologically descriptive term and does not imply clinical airflow obstruction. The presence of intraluminal tufts of organizing connective tissue within alveolar ducts and more distal air spaces has been traditionally referred to as "bronchiolitis obliterans organizing pneumonia" or simply "BOOP" by pathologists, hence we used the term "BOOP pattern" as a more generic descriptor of the lesion. Recently, an American Thoracic Society/European Respiratory Society (ATS/ERS) working group has suggested replacing the term BOOP with organizing pneumonia (OP). Other findings that may accompany an OP pattern include mononuclear interstitial infiltrates, fibrinous exudates, foam cells in air spaces, and

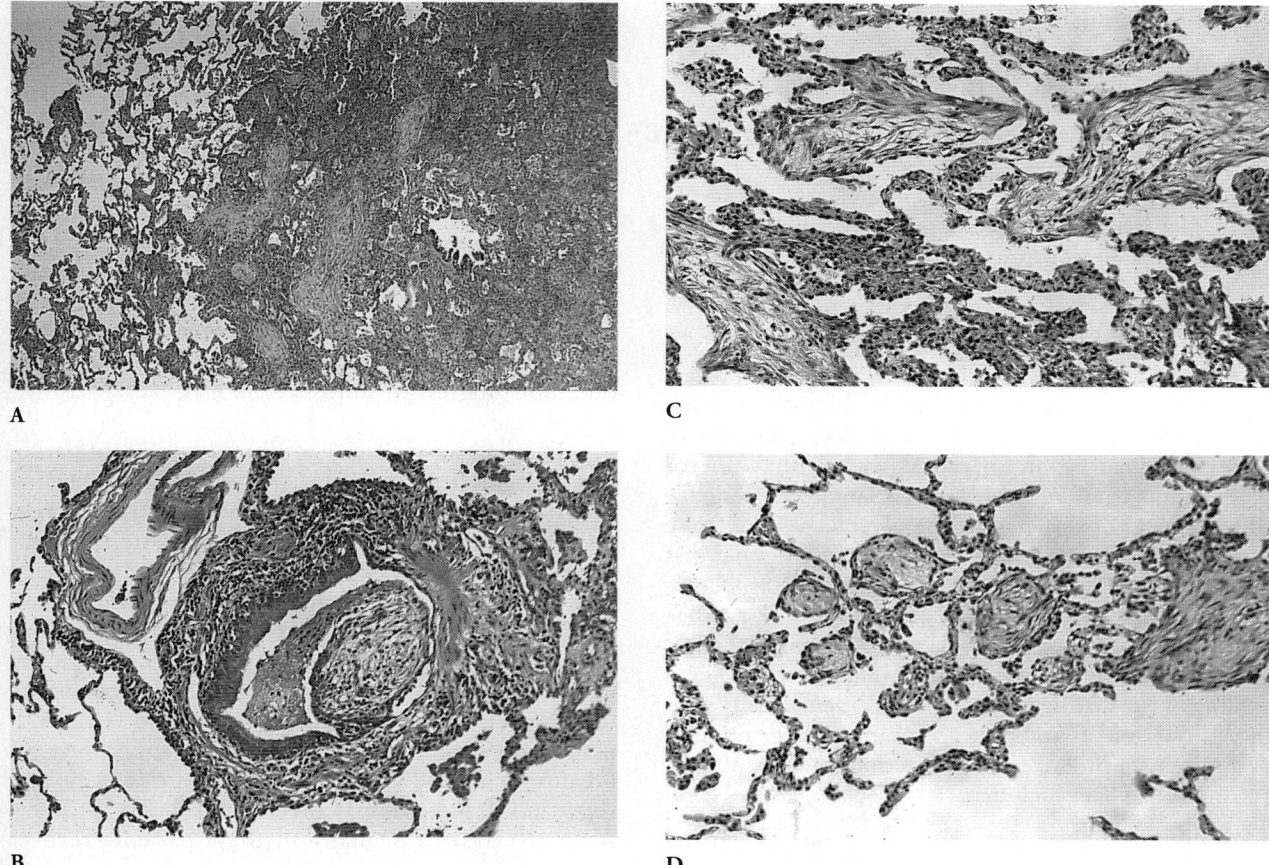

Figure 2–11   Organizing pneumonia (OP) shows *A*, patchy involvement of lung parenchyma by air space organization associated with *B*, bronchiolitis obliterans with intraluminal polyps. *C*, The more distal lung parenchyma shows slight interstitial thickening and type 2 cell metaplasia with tufts of organizing tissue within the alveolar ducts and, *D*, sometimes even within the alveoli.

prominent type II pneumocytes. Common causes of an OP pattern include:

1. Organizing infections (viral, bacterial, fungal, other)
2. Organizing diffuse alveolar damage (regardless of the cause)
3. Drug and toxic reactions
4. Collagen vascular diseases
5. Extrinsic allergic alveolitis (hypersensitivity pneumonitis)
6. Chronic eosinophilic pneumonia
7. Organizing infectious pneumonias complicating chronic bronchitis and emphysema, bronchiectasis, cystic fibrosis, aspiration pneumonia, and chronic bronchiolitis
8. Airway obstruction
9. The peripheral reaction around abscesses, infarcts, Wegener's granulomatosis, and others
10. An idiopathic form (cryptogenic organizing pneumonia)

Interstitial Fibrosis Pattern

Interstitial fibrosis is frequently accompanied by permanent and irreversible alteration of lung architecture. One of the hallmarks of irreversability is "honeycombing," in reference to the large interconnected cystic spaces that can be seen on computed tomography (CT) scans and in whole lung sections. Such gross or macroscopic honeycombing is often recapitulated at the microscopic level, where it is referred to as "microscopic honeycombing."

Usual interstitial pneumonia (UIP), illustrated in Figure 2–12, is the prototypical chronic interstitial pneumonia showing interstitial fibrosis and honeycombing (both microscopic and macroscopic).[4,5,16,17] Patients with idiopathic pulmonary fibrosis have UIP on surgical lung biopsy.[19] UIP is characterized by a variegated histologic appearance in the biopsy specimen that includes zones of normal lung tissue adjacent to zones of advanced architectural remodeling (microscopic honeycombing), with intervening zones of active fibrosis in association with the alveolar walls. These three elements are related, as a transition from old disease (fibrosis) to normal lung, with active "fibroblastic foci" forming a leading edge between them. A peripheral acinar pattern can often be recognized in UIP,[3,4] accompanied by relative centriacinar sparing. These findings help distinguish UIP from other lesions with interstitial fibrosis and honeycombing. A large number of diseases can produce some degree of fibrosis and honeycombing. These include:

1. Idiopathic pulmonary fibrosis (usual interstitial pneumonia)
2. Desquamative interstitial pneumonia
3. Lymphocytic interstitial pneumonia
4. Systemic collagen vascular disease
5. Drug reaction
6. Pneumoconioses (asbestosis, berylliosis, silicosis, hard metal pneumoconiosis, and others)
7. Sarcoidosis
8. Pulmonary Langerhans cell histiocytosis (histiocytosis X)
9. Chronic granulomatous infections
10. Chronic aspiration
11. Chronic hypersensitivity pneumonitis
12. Organized chronic eosinophilic pneumonia
13. Organized and organizing diffuse alveolar damage
14. Chronic interstitial pulmonary edema/passive congestion
15. Radiation (chronic)
16. Healed infectious pneumonias and other inflammatory processes
17. Nonspecific interstitial pneumonia/fibrosis (NSIP/F)

The entities listed above have considerable variation in the patterns of scarring. For example, sarcoidosis can produce scarring along lymphatic routes, hypersensitivity pneumonia and aspiration can produce centriacinar scarring, and pulmonary Langerhans cell histiocytosis tends to form patchy stellate scars associated with cystic change. In addition, many of the conditions have historic features that point to a specific diagnosis, although the fibrosis is nonspecific.

UIP is now the required pattern for a diagnosis of clinical "idiopathic pulmonary fibrosis." DIP represents a distinct pathologic entity that has clinical, radiologic, and prognostic differences from UIP. The hypothesis that DIP represents an early (cellular) phase of UIP is untenable based on incidence alone. A more appealing notion is that some forms of NSIP represent early manifestations of UIP, or alternately are examples of poorly sampled UIP. Furthermore, a number of cases previously classified as DIP have been reclassified as RBILD, an interstitial lung disease of smokers that does not progress to fibrosis. The DIP pattern is discussed below.

The relative maturity of fibroblastic proliferation and collagen deposition can help distinguish forms of interstitial fibrosis. Immature fibroblastic tissue is present in organizing DAD and in the OP pattern; conditions that are reversible to some extent. Interstitial pneumonias with any degree of fibrous proliferation have often been lumped together as "pulmonary fibrosis." Such cases invariably represent a histologically diverse group and can be better classified into one of the three patterns presented earlier: organizing DAD, OP pattern, and interstitial fibrosis.[4] Biopsy specimens of organizing diffuse alveolar damage, and diseases that show an OP pattern, may include fibroblastic proliferation. Nevertheless, many of these patients recover without apparent deficit and do not develop progressive lung disease. On the other hand, the "mature" interstitial fibrosis and honeycomb lung remodeling that characterize IPF represent endpoints of a progressive disease

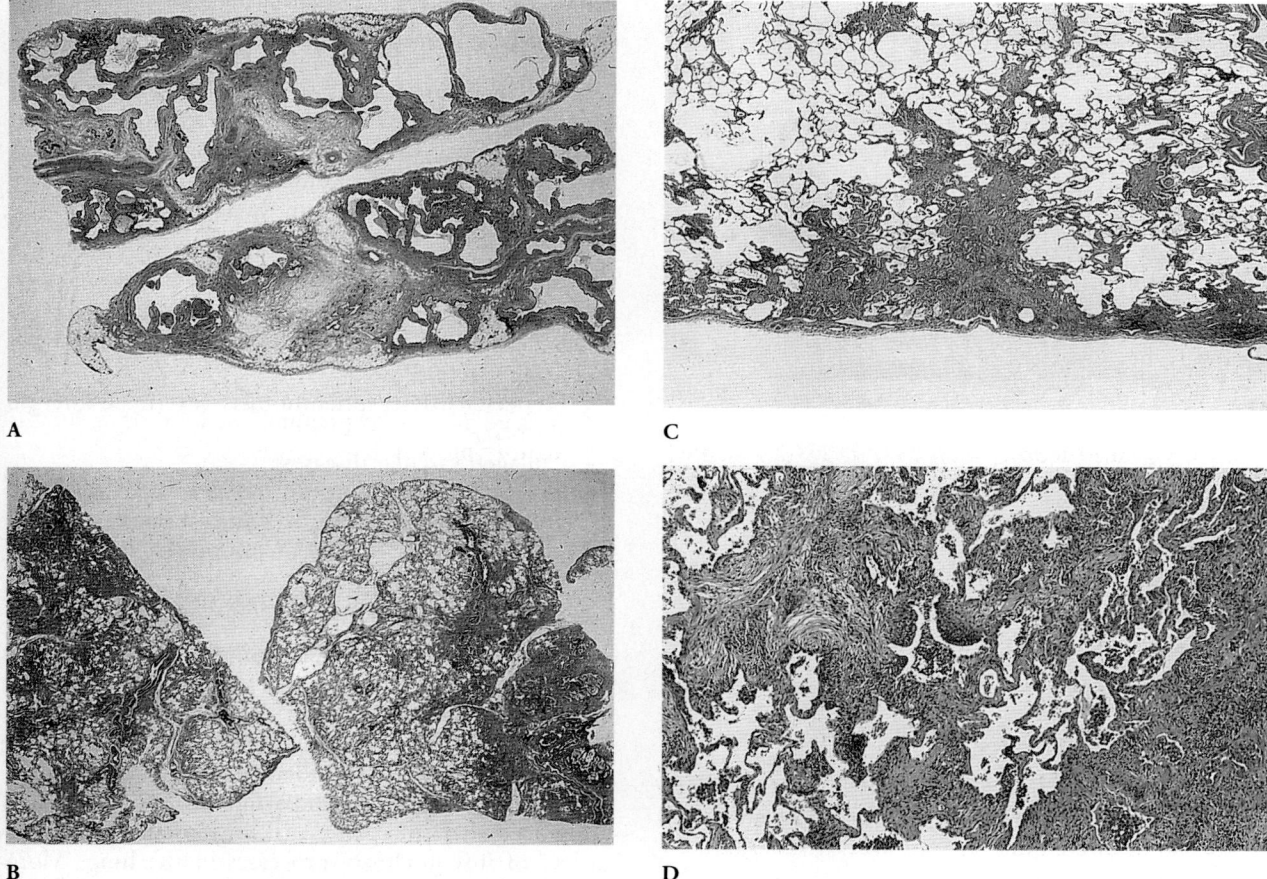

Figure 2–12   Interstitial fibrosis and honeycombing in usual interstitial pneumonia. *A*, Some biopsy specimens show complete honeycomb change, and, as such reflect sampling from the most severely affected regions of the lung. *B*, Typically, biopsy specimens should show patchy interstitial fibrosis in which zones of scarring alternate with relatively unaffected lung tissue. The fibrosis in usual interstitial pneumonia typically starts in the peripheral acinar regions (*C*, particularly in the subpleural regions) and shows *D*, older scarring, lower right, associated with more active and recent fibroblastic proliferation, upper left, reflecting recent activity of the process.

process which accumulates over time. Thus, the character of the fibrotic or fibroblastic proliferation is prognostically important, and all cases of pulmonary fibrosis are not identical.[12] In light of these inherent differences, a general morphologic approach to ILDs should include an assessment of the character of the fibrotic or fibroblastic reaction, the degree and extent of mature interstitial scarring, and the presence or absence of honeycomb remodeling.[4,5]

Desquamative Interstitial Pneumonia Pattern

A desquamative interstitial pneumonia (DIP) pattern (Figure 2–13) is characterized by increased numbers of alveolar macrophages, with mild inflammation in alveolar walls.[3-5] Entities demonstrating this pattern (in some cases focally) include:

1. Idiopathic DIP
2. Respiratory bronchiolitis-associated interstitial lung disease

3. Pulmonary Langerhans cell histiocytosis (pulmonary histiocytosis X)
4. Drug reactions (especially that associated with amiodarone)
5. Chronic alveolar hemorrhage
6. Eosinophilic pneumonia (especially after corticosteroid therapy)
7. Pneumoconioses (talcosis, hard metal disease, and asbestosis)
8. Obstructive pneumonias (with foamy alveolar macrophages)
9. Exogenous lipoid pneumonia and lipid storage diseases
10. Infection in the immunosuppressed patient (histiocytic pneumonia)
11. A focal microscopic finding in many unrelated conditions

The cytologic features of the macrophages in these conditions vary. In RBILD, the macrophages contain fine, light-brown cytoplasmic pigmentation with deli-

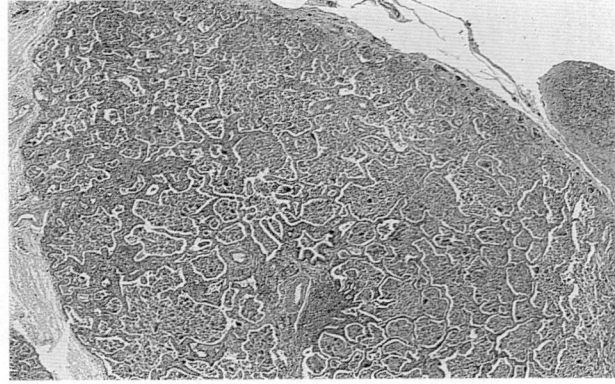

A

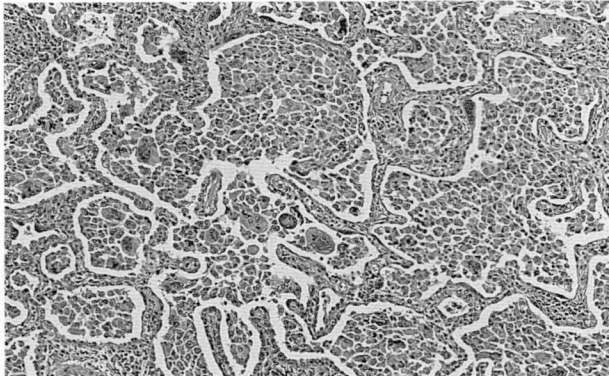

B

Figure 2–13   *A,* Desquamative interstitial pneumonia differs from UIP by the diffuse involvement of the lung parenchyma with air space filling by macrophages and mild associated interstitial changes. *B,* Sometimes, relatively numerous giant cells are present that reflect the presence of large numbers of histiocytes.

cate black punctation, characteristic of smoker's macrophages. In amiodarone reactions, obstructive pneumonias, lipoid pneumonia, and lipid storage diseases, foamy or vacuolated histiocytes predominate. In hard metal pneumoconiosis (cobalt), distinctive multinucleated intra-alveolar histiocytes are the dominant finding.

Respiratory bronchiolitis associated with interstitial lung disease is characterized by a distinctive bronchiolocentricity; pulmonary Langherhans cell histiocytosis (histocytosis X) is characterized by discrete nodular lesions that contain variable numbers of Langerhans histiocytes with a DIP pattern at the edge of nodular lesions. Chronic alveolar hemorrhage is associated with extensive hemosiderin-laden macrophage accumulation. The distinctive features of eosinophilic pneumonia are the presence of interstitial and air space eosinophils, markedly reactive type II cells, and dense alveolar macrophages. Birefringent material can be identified within the DIP-like reaction in many of the pneumoconioses. Large clear spaces with associated fibrosis characterize exogenous lipoid pneumonia.

Cellular Interstitial Infiltrates (Including Nonspecific Interstitial Pneumonia)

Cellular interstitial infiltrates consisting of lymphocytes and plasma cells (usually with little fibrosis and preservation of underlying lung alveolar architecture) are non-specific.[3,4] For example, a mild cellular interstitial infiltrate is common in the late phase of diffuse alveolar damage. Other entities that demonstrate this reaction include:

1. Certain infections (particularly *Pneumocystis carinii* pneumonia and healing viral pneumonias)
2. Drug reactions
3. Hypersensitivity pneumonitis (extrinsic allergic alveolar)
4. Collagen vascular diseases
5. Late or nearly resolved diffuse alveolar damage
6. Evolving chronic interstitial pneumonia, in particular, early phase idiopathic pulmonary fibrosis
7. Many other ILDs
8. Nonspecific interstitial pneumonia (idiopathic)

Katzenstein and Fiorelli reported 64 patients with cellular interstitial inflammatory changes that did not fit in the spectrum of diseases originally described in Liebow's classification of the idiopathic interstitial pneumonias.[18] In their report, they coined the term "nonspecific interstitial pneumonia/fibrosis (NSIP/F)" and recognized that this pattern likely represented a wide variety of inflammatory processes in the lung. More recently, the simplified term "NSIP" has been adopted.

NSIP occurred mainly in middle-aged adults. The average age at onset was 46 years (range 9 to 78 years) and in distinction to UIP, there was a slight female predominance. The average duration of symptoms prior to biopsy was 8.1 months (range 0.25 to 60 months), and the presenting symptoms included dyspnea (51%), cough (21%), and fever (14%). Radiologically, bilateral interstitial opacities (alveolar and alveolar-interstitial) were seen, often with a bibasilar distribution (21 patients), although 4 of the 64 patients in their series had normal chest radiographs.

Biopsy findings included variable amounts of interstitial chronic inflammation (lymphoplasmocytic) and fibrosis. Importantly, extensive OP-like air space organization or significant honeycomb fibrosis, were not present. The main emphasis was on the temporally uniform appearance of the disease process; that is, the pathology reflected a single injury in time (ie, lacking a spectrum ranging from new disease to old). Because the term nonspecific interstitial pneumonia/fibrosis implies an "unclassifiable" process, a number of patterns were evident in their series.

Katzenstein and Fiorelli subdivided their cases into three groups: group I had diffuse interstitial inflammation alone (Figure 2–14), group II had interstitial inflammation and early interstitial fibrosis in a similar distribution (Figure 2–15), and group III had denser, diffuse interstitial fibrosis without significant inflammation (Figure 2–16). These uniform injury patterns were distinguished from the temporally heterogeneous injury seen in UIP (Figure 2–17).

Group I disease is perhaps the least controversial pattern and the easiest to identify pathologically, because it corresponds to what others for many years have called "cellular interstitial pneumonia." With the addition of fibrosis to groups II and III, potential confusion arises for many pathologists, especially in consistently separating NSIP/F from IPF on biopsy. In Katzenstein and Fiorelli's study, emphasis was placed on the uniform distribution of fibrosis, which was interstitial in location and there was preservation of lung architecture. If fibrous obliteration of parenchyma with scarring occurred, it was only a minor component and not in a distribution suggestive of UIP (compare Figures 2 –16 and 2–17).

Some patients in the Katzenstein and Fiorelli series had idiopathic interstitial lung disease, most had either systemic autoimmune disease or hypersensitivity pneumonitis. For example, connective tissue disease was identified in 16% of patients, including rheumatoid arthritis, systemic lupus erythematosus, polymyositis/dermatomyositis, scleroderma, and Sjögren's syndrome. Interestingly, pulmonary disease preceded the development of systemic collagen vascular disease in some of their cases; a phenomenon well documented for some collagen vascular diseases, such as polymyositis/dermatomyositis.[19,20] Other autoimmune diseases occurred in this series included Hashimoto's thyroiditis, glomerulonephritis, and primary biliary cirrhosis. Hypersensitivity reactions were evident in a subset of patients found to have a history of chemical, organic antigen, or drug exposures. Two patients were post ARDS and two had pneumonia several months prior.

Perhaps the most important finding in this study was that the morbidity and mortality rate was significantly different from that of UIP. Only 5 of 48 patients with clinical follow-up died of progressive lung disease (11%), while 39 patients either recovered or were alive and stable. During follow-up, no deaths were reported in group I patients, whereas 3 patients from group II and 2 patients from group III, died. Unfortunately a significant number of patients were lost and mean follow-up periods were variable. Nevertheless, the mortality data contrast sharply with UIP, in which mortality figures are 90%, with a median survival of 2.5 years.[21]

Other series of NSIP have been reported with variable survival rates (Table 2–3).[21–28] NSIP deaths occurred in those with fibrosis (groups II and III), analogous to Katzenstein and Fiorelli's results. One new and important criterion, initiated by Nagai and colleagues in a 1998 study, was to restrict the scope of NSIP to those patients with idiopathic disease, primarily by excluding patients with known collagen vascular diseases and environmental exposures.[24] Two of 31 patients in their study (6.5%) died of progressive lung disease, both of whom had group

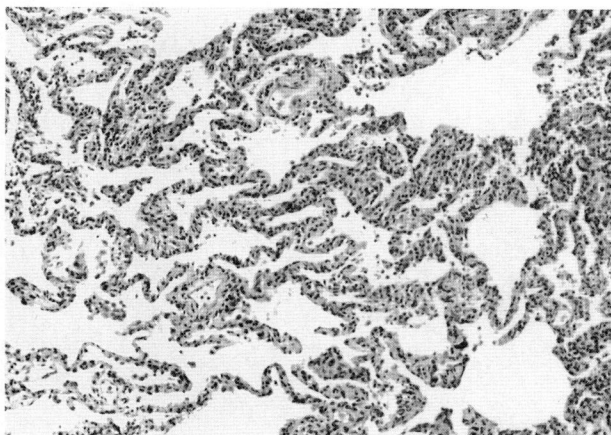

Figure 2–14   NSIP/cellular interstitial pneumonia (Katzensteins and Fiorelli's group I). Lymphocytes and plasma cells expand alveolar septae without fibrosis.

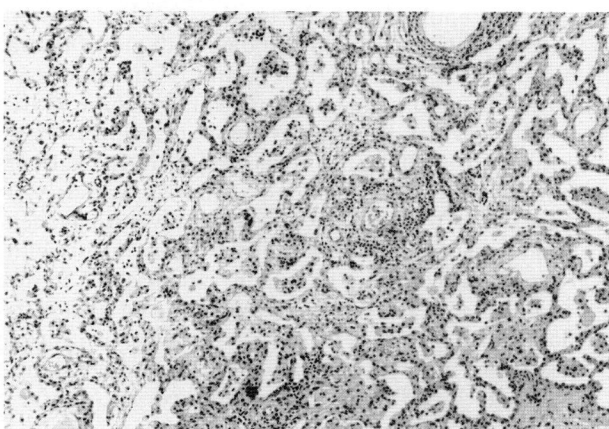

Figure 2–15   NSIP (Katzenstein and Fiorelli's group II). There is mixed cellular interstitial pneumonia with mild interstitial fibrosis.

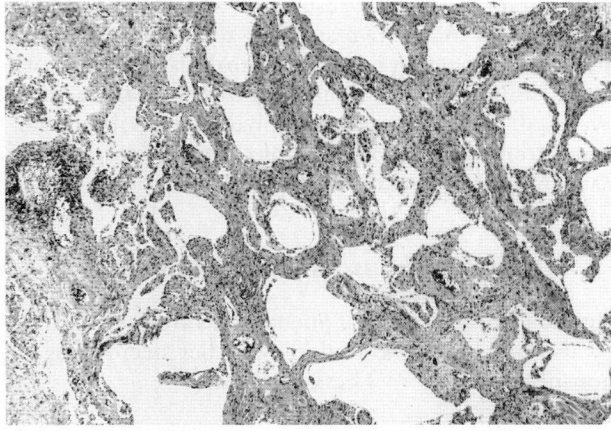

Figure 2–16   NSIP (Katzenstein and Fiorelli's group III). Note the uniform interstitial fibrosis without evidence of ongoing injury (lack of fibroblastic foci). The absence of transition from peripheral fibrosis to normal lung is helpful in distinguishing this pattern from that of UIP.

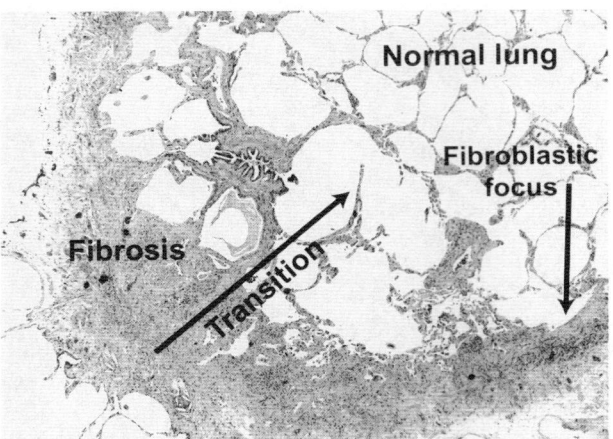

Figure 2–17   Classic UIP with typical heterogeneity.

III disease. The highest mortality rate was reported in the most recently published series by Travis and colleagues, in which 9 of 22 patients (41%) died with group II and III disease.[28] Importantly, these deaths occurred 5 years following diagnosis, again distinguishing fibrotic NSIP from UIP. Travis and colleagues reported 5- and 10-year survival rates of 90% and 35%, respectively, in their patients with NSIP, compared to 5- and 10-year survival rates for UIP of 43% and 15%, respectively.[28] It has been speculated that the higher mortality rate for patients with NSIP in the Travis series represents case bias due to the selection of more aggressive disease occurring in a referral population. Of note is that a significant percent of their patients' biopsy specimens showed honeycombing.

With each additional patient studied, the nonspecific interstitial pneumonia/fibrosis may evolve into a more specific idiopathic entity. NSIP is now included by Katzenstein and Myers as a new category of idiopathic interstitial pneumonia.[29]

Since NSIP is a diagnosis of exclusion, it is difficult to accurately compare results of different groups of investigators. A positive step has been taken by some authors in excluding nonidiopathic disease,[24] but a serious dilemma will arise if the diagnosis of NSIP becomes overused, especially without applying the discipline garnered from the past 30 years of studying morphologic patterns of inflammatory lung disease.

Granulomatous Inflammation Pattern

Several diffuse interstitial pneumonias are characterized by the presence of granulomas, either necrotizing or non-necrotizing.[3,4,11] These include:

1. Sarcoidosis
2. Hypersensitivity pneumonitis
3. Drug reactions
4. Granulomatous infections
5. Intravenous talcosis

6. Pneumoconioses (eg, inhalation talcosis, berylliosis)
7. Sjögren's syndrome
8. Aspiration pneumonia
9. Tumors, especially lymphomas

Clues to the etiology of granulomatous interstitial pneumonias depend on the anatomic distribution and the qualitative features of the granulomas themselves. In intravenous talcosis, perivascular giant cell clusters with birefringent particulate material are characteristic. In sarcoidosis (Figure 2–18) and berylliosis, conglomerates of non-necrotizing granulomas are present in a distribution which follow the lymphatic routes. These granulomas tend to be surrounded by dense, eosinophilic lamellar collagen, and adjacent granulomas have a tendency to coalesce within this matrix.[4,30] Drug reactions and hypersensitivity pneumonitis (Figure 2–19) tend to have small, scattered (nonconfluent) granulomas without necrosis. The granulomas of hypersensitivity pneumonitis are poorly defined and may be overlooked by the untrained eye. Infectious granulomas may be solitary or confluent and may or may not be associated with necrosis.[3–5] Necrosis appearing as microabscess suggests infection. Although necrosis rarely occurs in sarcoidosis and berylliosis, when it does it has a more fibrinoid or hyaline appearance and is likely a degenerative phenomenon.[4,5,30] When miliary microscopic granulomas with necrosis are identified in the immunocompetent patient, consideration should be given to the possibility of *Mycobacterium avium-intracellulare*-associated infection that may occur with bioaerosol exposure (so-called "hot tub lung").[46]

Regardless of etiology, all granulomas can be associated with distinctive inclusions, such as the hematoxyphilic Schaumann body, lucent oxalate crystals, and eosinophilic asteroid bodies in the cytoplasm of multinucleate giant cells.[4,5,31] Oxalate crystals are brightly birefringent in polarized light and should not be confused with foreign material or a pneumoconiosis. Inhalational talcosis is characterized by the massive accumulation of plate-like birefringent material within alveolar macrophages and granulomas within the air spaces. There may be marked ferruginous body formation around the talc particles.

TABLE 2–3   Deaths or Progression Related to NSIP/F

Lead Author (yr) Reference	No. of Patients	Age/ Gender	Progression (%)	Deaths (NSIP) (%)
Katzenstein (1994)[18]	64	26/M 38/F	13	11
Bjoraker (1998)[19]	14	8/M 6/F	Not given	25 (5 yr)
Park (1996)[22]	7	1/M 6/F	29	29
Midthun (1998)[23]	39	16/M 23/F	19	29
Nagai (1998)[24]	31	15/M 16/F	16	6
Kim (1998)[25]	23	1/M 22/F	Not given	Not given
Cottin (1998)[26]	12	6/M 6/F	33	0
Daniil (1999)[27]	15	7/M 8/F	33	13
Travis (2000)[28]	29	20/M 9/F	41 (at least)	41

NSIP/F = nonspecific interstitial pneumonia/fibrosis.

Hsu and colleagues[32] studied 92 cases of granulomas identified on transbronchial biopsy with special stains negative for organisms. Subsequent microbiologic cultures from tissue samples obtained at the initial bronchoscopy (all 93 cases were cultured), showed positive results in 10 (9 mycobacterial and 1 fungal), and these were ultimately diagnosed as granulomatous infection. The remainder of the cases were classified as sarcoidosis. Necrosis in the granulomas was observed in 20% of the cases of sarcoidosis and in only 40% of the infectious cases. Also, the granulomas in sarcoidosis tended to be present in greater number than those seen in the infectious cases. Schaumann's bodies were also more likely to be present in association with sarcoidosis.

MORE SPECIFIC HISTOLOGIC FEATURES OF INTERSTITIAL LUNG DISEASE

Careful analysis of the anatomic distribution and pathologic reaction pattern will result in an accurate diagnosis in the majority of lung biopsies for ILD. Further subclassification, and sometimes a definitive diagnosis, can be achieved by identifying specific morphologic clues. Examples of some specific (or nearly so) histologic findings in ILDs are shown in Table 2–4.

The features listed in Table 2–4 vary in their specificity. For example, pulmonary alveolar microlithiasis and lymphangioleiomyomatosis are histologically unique in their morphologic appearance.[4,5] Foreign materials including asbestos bodies, talc, silica, and silicates must be evaluated in their clinicopathologic context to insure an accurate final diagnosis. For example, the presence of foreign material alone, does not establish a diagnosis of pneumoconiosis.[33] All urban dwellers have small amounts of silica and silicates among the anthracotic pigment deposited in their lungs; other features (nodules and/or infiltrates of dust-filled histiocytes along lymphatic routes) must be identified and correlated with clinical and radiologic findings before a diagnosis of silicosis can be rendered.[4,31] The finding of isolated dense aggregates of eosinophils in the lung parenchyma occurs in a relatively small number of ILDs, which considerably narrows down the differential diagnosis. Chronic eosinophilic pneumonia is the most common situation in which this occurs.

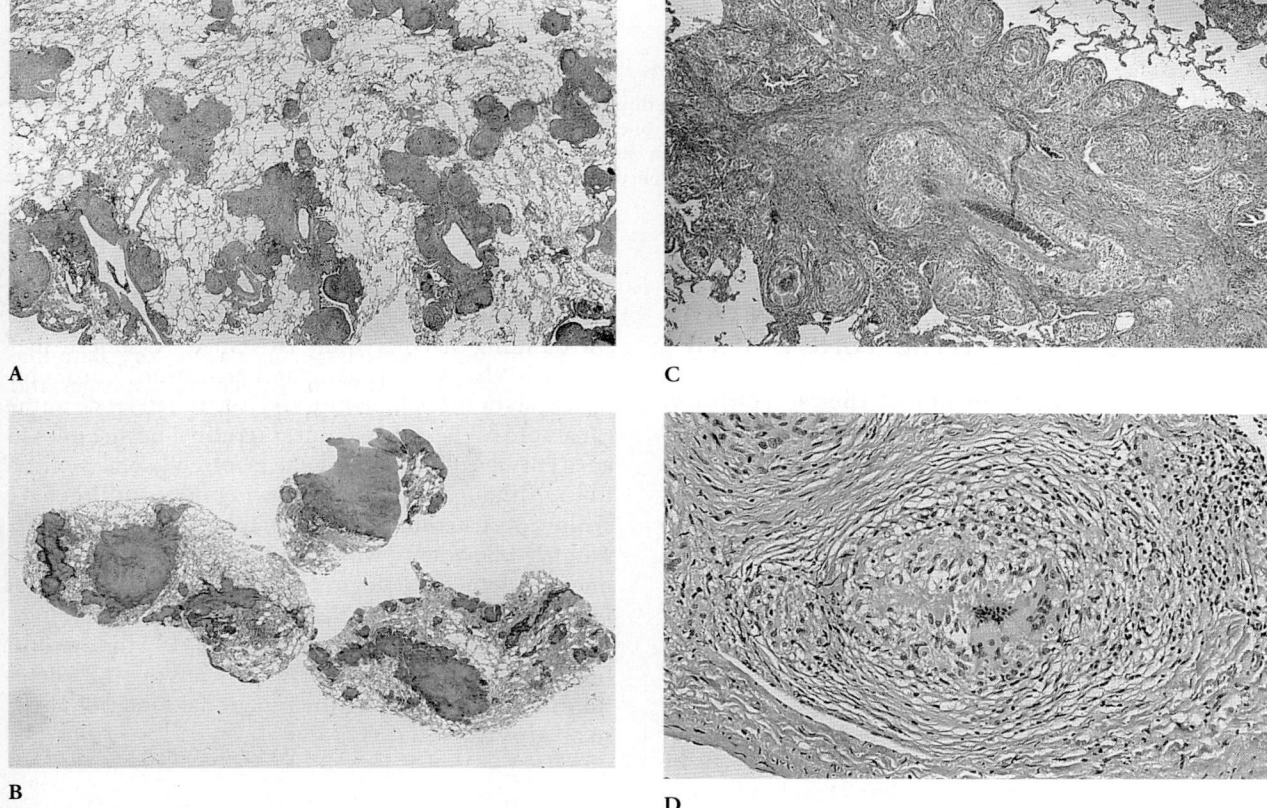

A

B

C

D

Figure 2–18   A, and B, Sarcoidosis is characterized by "naked" granulomas in which the granulomas have relatively little surrounding inflammatory change, and the lung tissue appears relatively normal. A, The distribution is typically along the lymphatic routes, with involvement of the pleura, septa, and bronchovascular bundles. B, Coalescence of granulomas leads to large nodules for which the distribution is difficult to discern; although, the distribution may be identified when looking away from the largest lesions. Granulomas of sarcoidosis may C, extensively involve vessels, and are D, commonly associated by lamellar eosinophilic collagen. D, Small foci of fibroid necrosis may also be seen, center.

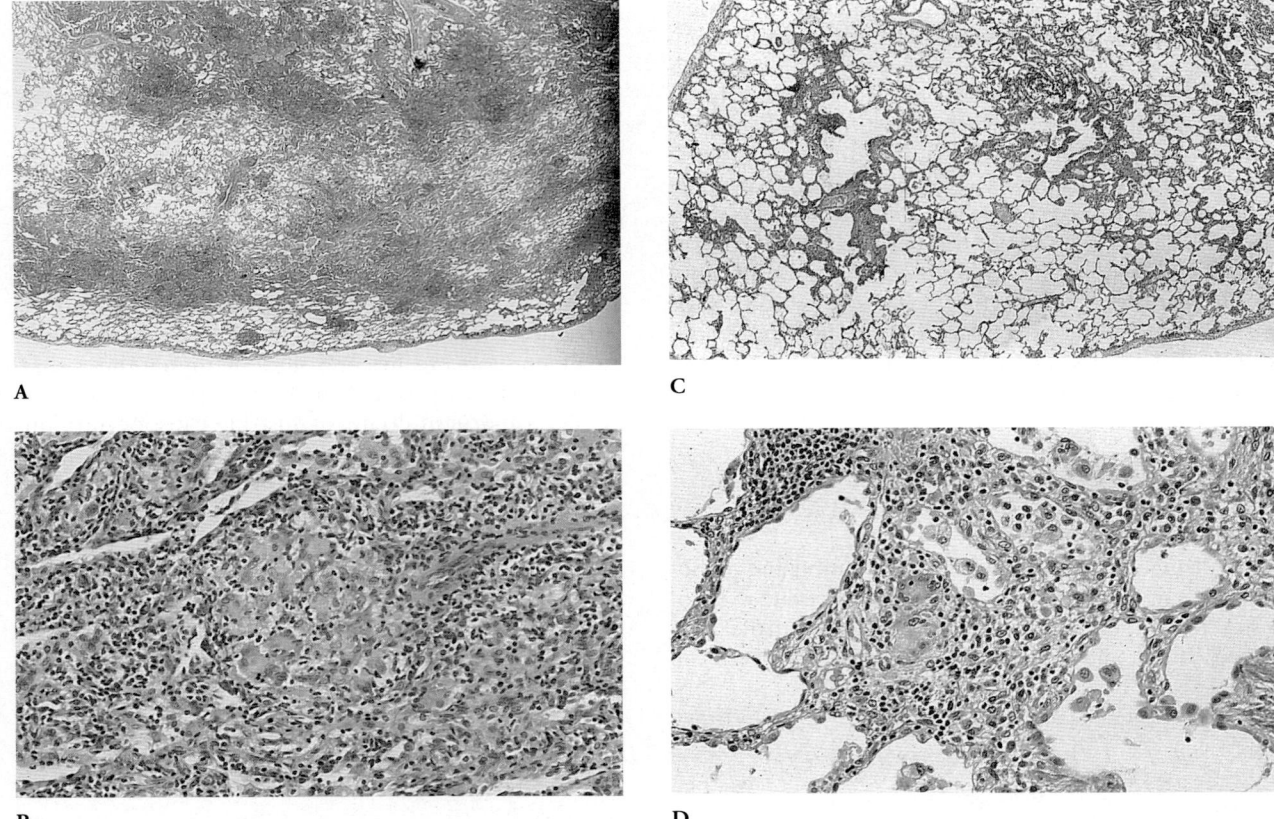

Figure 2–19   *A*, Hypersensitivity pneumonitis sometimes shows a distinct nodularity with inflammatory tissue that involves and obscures small airways. *B*, The granulomas are typically solitary and "loose," in comparison with sarcoidosis, and surrounded by relatively abundant inflammation. *C*, In some cases, the bronchiolocentric distribution is very easily appreciated; inflammation is more marked in the regions of the respiratory bronchioles. *D*, The granulomas in hypersensitivity pneumonitis may be subtle and sometimes comprise only a small cluster of epithelioid histiocytes, left lower center.

AN APPARENTLY NORMAL BIOPSY IN THE SETTING OF INTERSTITIAL LUNG DISEASE

The lung biopsy from a patient with clinical evidence of ILD may appear normal.[3,4,31] Table 2–5 lists the possibilities to explain this occurrence. A "normal" biopsy in a patient with clinical evidence of ILD should lead to a review of the clinical findings, and of the histology, with particular reference to the lesions in Table 2–5. Chronic passive congestion and pulmonary veno-occlusive disease may manifest as ILD. Early pulmonary edema or early diffuse alveolar damage may feature endothelial vacuolization, lymphatic dilatation, and interstitial thickening. Embolic diseases (eg, fat and fibrin) should be considered in the appropriate clinical setting.

Pathologic changes in the small airways may be quite subtle, despite significant clinical and radiologic evidence of ILD.[3,4] Changes include a decrease in airway lumen size or frank obliteration of terminal airways to a variable degree, muscular hypertrophy, submucosal fibrous thickening, mild chronic inflammation, ectasia with mucostasis, peribronchiolar scarring, and meta-

plastic bronchiolar epithelium that extends along the surrounding alveolar walls (so-called "Lambertosis," which is also known as "Lambertization," bronchiolization, or bronchiolar metaplasia, in reference to the canals of Lambert that connect terminal bronchioles to adjacent alveoli as a mechanism of collateral ventilation). Although some cases showing these features have airflow obstruction and radiographic hyperinflation, a number of patients with small airways disease alone, presents with physiologic and radiographic features of interstitial lung disease that is clinically and radiologically indistinguishable from other ILDs.[4] High-resolution inspiratory and expiratory CT scans may be a helpful first step in assessing the functional integrity of the small airways.[35]

CLINICOPATHOLOGIC CORRELATION IN INTERSTITIAL LUNG DISEASE

Clinicopathologic correlation is necessary for the pathologic assessment and diagnosis of the patient with

TABLE 2–4   Examples of Specific Morphologic Clues for Interstitial Lung Diseases

Microorganisms (bacteria, fungal, other); viral inclusions

Langerhans histiocytes of pulmonary Langerhans cell histiocytosis (Figure 2–20)

Malignant cells (specific morphologic features for subclassification are often identified)

"Cannibalistic" multinucleated giant cells and multinucleated alveolar lining cells of hard metal (cobalt) pneumoconiosis[33,34] (Figure 2–21)

Exogenous material (asbestos bodies, talc, silica, silicates)[33] (Figure 2–22)

Microliths of pulmonary alveolar microlithiasis[5]

Granular eosinophilic material within alveoli in pulmonary alveolar proteinosis[5] (Figure 2–23)

Eosinophils in pools[5] in eosinophilic pneumonia (see Figure 2–7)

"Holes" and smooth muscle fascicles in lymphangioleiomyomatosis[5]

TABLE 2–5   Causes of a "Normal" Biopsy in Interstitial Lung Disease*

Sampling error (eg, Langerhans cell histiocytosis)

A very subtle interstitial infiltrate or early diffuse alveolar damage

Airway disease (especially bronchiolar)

Pulmonary edema

Pulmonary emboli (including fat emboli)

Lymphangioleiomyomatosis with inconspicuous lesions

Pulmonary vascular disease

*Adapted from Colby TV and Yousem SA.[31]

ILD.[2–5,11,15,36] The clinical history of interstitial lung disease or diffuse interstitial infiltrates is insufficient for the accurate (and informed) interpretation of biopsy material. Combined clinical and radiologic information greatly enhance the pathologic interpretation, just as they enhance clinical evaluation, diagnosis, and management of patients with ILD. Readily available information, such as age, sex, duration of symptoms, radiologic findings (including character and distribution of disease), any therapies administered, and pulmonary function data are often critical in the evaluation of the lung biopsy specimen.

CORRELATION OF PATHOLOGY AND RADIOLOGY IN THE STUDY OF INTERSTITIAL LUNG DISEASE

The advent of high-resolution computed tomography (HRCT) scanning has made it possible to better define radiologic findings in the context of specific ILDs,[37] especially with regard to anatomic distribution of disease. Characteristics recognized on HRCT usually combine anatomic distribution with other distinctive features such as the presence of honeycombing in idiopathic pulmonary fibrosis, ground glass opacities in hypersensitivity pneumonitis, plaques in asbestosis, and cystic change in lymphangioleiomyomatosis or pulmonary Langerhans cell histiocytosis. In sarcoidosis and lymphangitic carcinoma, HRCT shows nodular thickening along the septa, pleura, and bronchovascular bundles, just as one would expect from the histologic involvement of lymphatic routes in biopsies. High-resolution computed tomography of IPF shows a predilection for pathologic changes at the periphery of the lung, which correlates with a peripheral acinar distribution recognized histologically. Radiologic study of ILD and HRCT are discussed further in chapter 6.

EXAMPLES OF SPECIFIC INTERSTITIAL LUNG DISEASES

1. Idiopathic pulmonary fibrosis (usual interstitial pneumonia) (see Figures 2–5, 2–12, and 2–17).[4]
   a) Anatomic distribution—peripherally accentuated fibrosis, especially in subpleural regions with evidence of centrilobular sparing
   b) Pathologic pattern—interstitial fibrosis with microscopic honeycombing showing crescent-like air space fibroplasia abutting older zones of fibrosis. Transitions to normal lung are present in the biopsy specimen.
   c) Specific morphologic clues—transitions from honeycomb remodeled lung through active air space fibroplasia to normal uninvolved lung parenchyma
   d) HRCT—pulmonary infiltrates characterized by a peripheral, bibasilar, subpleural distribution, often with honeycomb change; intralobular reticulation as well as interlobular septal thickening; patchy foci of ground-glass change, which, on follow-up studies, may progress to honeycombing

2. Nonspecific interstitial pneumonia/fibrosis (see Figures 2–14 through 2–16).[18–28]
   a) Anatomic distribution—interstitial infiltrates in lower lung zones most consistently but diffuse infiltrates and randomly distributed disease also described
   b) Pathologic pattern—cellular interstitial infiltrates with histiocytes, lymphocytes, and plasma cells. Fibrotic forms have variable interstitial fibrosis
   c) Specific morphologic clues—none; absence of characteristics of other ILDs; when fibrosis is present it uniformly thickens the alveolar walls.
   d) HRCT findings—patchy ground-glass attenuation and/or consolidation with variable reticular changes; relatively little, if any, honeycombing; variable distribution characteristic

3. Respiratory bronchiolitis-associated interstitial lung disease (see Figure 2–24).[4,5,38,39]
   a) Anatomic distribution—bronchiolocentric with bronchiolocentric parenchymal consolidation

b) Pathologic pattern—DIP reaction (in region of respiratory bronchioles)

c) Specific morphologic clues—smoker's macrophages (but they reflect only cigarette smoking, not the disease per se)

d) HRCT—multifocal regions of ground-glass attenuation; mild reticular and linear interstitial abnormalities; vague centrilobular nodular ground glass change

4. Cryptogenic organizing pneumonia (formerly known as idiopathic bronchiolitis obliterans organizing pneumonia [see Figure 2–12]).[4,5,11,15,40]

   a) Anatomic distribution—patchy mixed interstitial infiltrates and parenchymal consolidation; some bronchiolocentricity may be apparent

   b) Pathologic pattern—OP pattern

   c) Specific morphologic clues—none

   d) HRCT findings—bilateral (usual) multifocal regions of consolidation or small nodular opacities; ground-glass change may be seen; bronchial wall thickening, and bronchiolocentric nodular opacities may be seen; consolidated foci tend to be in the periphery of the lung

5. Methotrexate reaction in rheumatoid arthritis[4,5,11]

   a) Anatomic distribution—patchy mixed interstitial infiltrate and parenchymal consolidation

   b) Pathologic pattern—OP pattern and/or cellular interstitial infiltrate

   c) Specific morphologic clues—often none; small granulomas present in some cases

   d) HRCT findings—patchy ground-glass attenuation and/or consolidation with reticular changes

6. Chronic eosinophilic pneumonia (see Figure 2–7).[4,5,11,42]

   a) Anatomic distribution—parenchymal consolidation with sharp demarcation at septa

   b) Pathologic pattern—DIP pattern, OP pattern, or mixtures thereof

   c) Specific morphologic clues—eosinophils in dense aggregates

   d) HRCT findings—peripheral bilateral regions and consolidation, often with sharp demarcation at septa; upper lobe distribution is common; ground-glass change may be present; may be indistinguishable from OP

7. Hypersensitivity pneumonitis (extrinsic allergic alveolitis) (see Figures 2–8 and 2–19).[4,5,11,43]

   a) Antatomic distribution—bronchiolocentricity in some cases, mixed bronchiolocentric/diffuse interstitial in others

   b) Pathologic pattern—granulomatous interstitial pneumonia, OP pattern, cellular interstitial infiltrates, or mixtures

   c) Specific morphologic clues—histologic triad of cellular bronchiolitis, interstitial mononuclear cell infiltrate (often many plasma cells), and small, poorly formed interstitial granulomas. The presence of well-formed, discrete granulomas argues against hypersensitivity pneumonitis

   d) HRCT findings—patchy or diffuse bilateral ground-glass attenuation; diffuse bilateral tiny poorly circumscribed nodular opacities that may be bronchiolocentric; the bronchiolitis may result in lobular sparing and air trapping (mosaic pattern)

8. Pulmonary Langerhans cell histiocytosis (histiocytosis X) (see Figure 2–20).[4,5,44]

   a) Anatomic distribution—bronchiolocentric (early); randomly scattered fibrotic nodules (late)

   b) Pathologic pattern—cellular and/or fibrotic nodules; DIP pattern adjacent to the nodules

   c) Specific morphologic clues—stellate fibrous lesions rimmed by Langerhans histiocytes and pigmented macrophages, with variable numbers of eosinophils

   d) HRCT findings—upper lobe nodular and cystic change; cysts may become confluent and have bizarre shapes; some cases manifest only small nodules; unlike lymphangioleiomyomatosis, the bases are relatively spared

9. Sarcoidosis (see Figures 2–4 and 2–18).[4,5,45]

   a) Anatomic distribution—lymphatic

   b) Pathologic pattern—granulomatous interstitial pneumonia

   c) Specific morphologic clues—confluent, nonnecrotizing granulomas, often with surrounding lamellar fibrosis; although characteristic, these findings are not specific

   d) HRCT findings—nodularity showing a central, perihilar and peribronchovascular distribution; pleural/subpleural and interlobular septal nodularity also seen; scarring present in later stages with architectural distortion possible; traction bronchiectasis, honeycombing, and conglomerate mass lesions may be seen late; foci of ground-glass opacity occasionally seen in early stages

10. Silicosis (see Figure 15–2)[3,4,34]

   a) Anatomic distribution—accumulations of dust-filled histiocytes along lymphatic routes in which fibrotic nodules arise (early); randomly scattered hyalinized fibrotic nodules (late)

   b) Pathologic pattern—cellular interstitial infiltrate of histiocytes (early); fibrotic nodules (late)

   c) Specific morphologic clues—weakly birefringent silicate particles seen in histiocytes and/or periphery of nodules. Interstitial silicate particles may also be present diffusely

   d) HRCT findings—Dorsal and upper lung zones predominantly involved with diffuse small nodular opacities; nodules are well-defined and generally randomly distributed but may be centrilobular or subpleural; conglomerate masses may be seen in later stages

11. Hard metal (cobalt) pneumoconiosis/giant cell interstitial pneumonia (see Figures 2–21 and 2–25).[4,5,34,47]
    a) Anatomic distribution—bronchiolocentric fibrotic zones and diffuse interstitial infiltrates
    b) Pathologic pattern—ill-defined bronchiolocentric cellular and fibrotic nodules, interstitial cellular infiltrates

    c) Specific morphologic clues—intra-alveolar multinucleated giant cells, termed "cannibalistic" because they contain phagocytosed histiocytes within their cytoplasm
    d) HRCT findings—interstitial infiltrates with small ill-defined nodular opacities; middle to lower zone predominance in changes

12. Wegener's granulomatosis (see Figure 22–12)[4,48,49]
    a) Anatomic distribution—mixed angiocentric and parenchymal consolidation

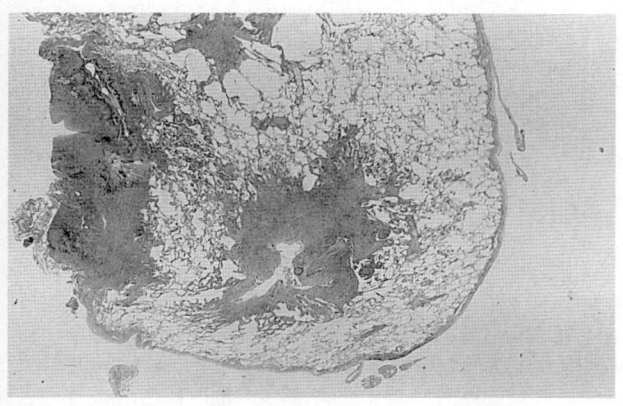

A

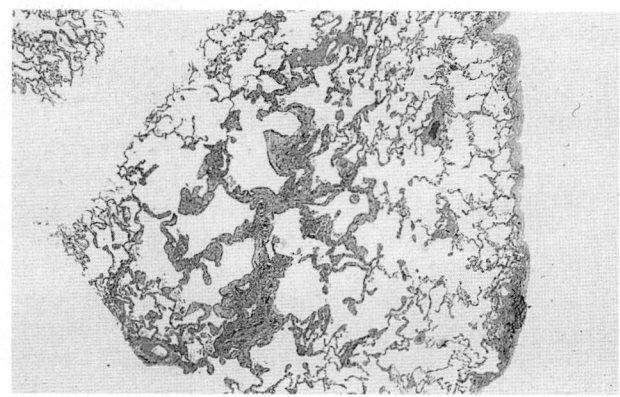

D

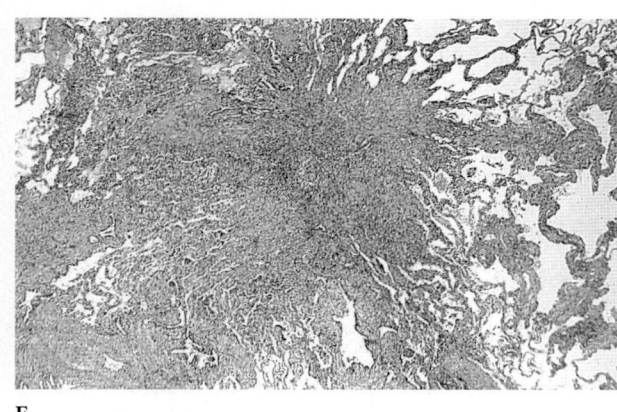

E

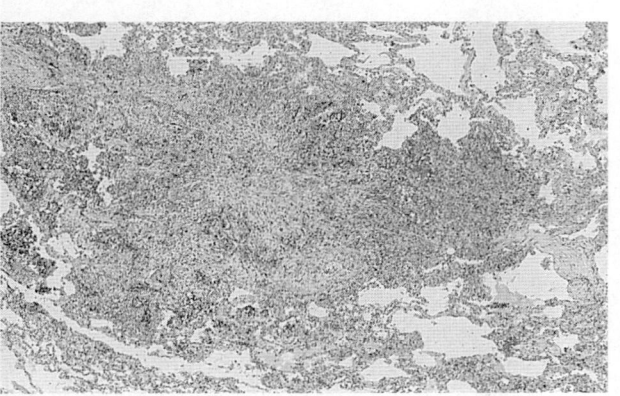

B

C

Figure 2–20 *A*, Langerhans cell histiocytosis typically manifests as scattered nodules with intervening relatively normal (or emphysematous) lung parenchyma. Nodules may show central cavitation or holes, lower center, and pericicatricial emphysema around the nodules may be present, upper center. The lesion is due to a proliferation of Langerhans histiocytes, which are identified as pale histiocytic cells with interspersed eosinophils. *B*, Langerhans cells show delicate folded nuclear membranes and inconspicuous cell borders. *C*, They are antibody S-100 positive, and sometimes large numbers of them comprise the nodules seen at low power as illustrated by positive (red) staining in an S-100 stain. *D*, The earliest lesions of pulmonary histiocytosis X are central in distribution; even late lesions may show residual centrilobular scarring. *E*, The classic lesion of pulmonary histiocytosis X is a stellate nodule in which the distribution may not be apparent at all.

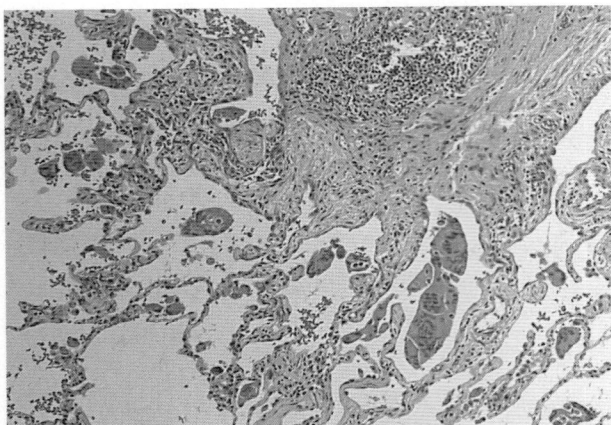

Figure 2–21   *A,* Huge multinucleated giant cells are the characteristic feature of giant cell interstitial pneumonia/hard metal pneumoconiosis.

  b) Pathologic pattern—alveolar hemorrhage with hemosiderosis, OP pattern, zonal necrosis with associated histiocytic reaction, or mixtures of these findings. Well-defined granulomas without necrosis are uncommon
  c) Specific morphologic clues—geographic basophilic necrosis is characteristic but not specific. The earliest lesion involves neutrophilic necrosis of collagen
  d) HRCT findings—multifocal masses and/or regions of consolidation, often cavitary

13. Malignant lymphoma presenting as ILD[4,50]
  a) Anatomic distribution—lymphatic routes along larger bronchovascular bundles and peripherally in pleura and interlobular septae
  b) Pathologic pattern—generally not applicable, but for many lymphomas, nodular lesions can be seen
  c) Specific morphologic clue—histologic and cytologic features of specific lymphoma subtypes
  d) HRCT findings—multifocal nodules and/or regions of consolidation; peribronchovascular and intralobular septal involvement may be smooth or nodular

14. Lymphangitic carcinoma[4]
  a) Anatomic distribution—lymphatic routes along larger bronchovascular bundles and peripherally in pleura and interlobular septae
  b) Pathologic pattern—not applicable
  c) Specific morphologic clues—some carcinomas can be specifically recognized on morphologic grounds, especially after comparison with previous biopsy material
  d) HRCT findings—smooth and/or nodular thickening of pleura, septa, and bronchovascular structures

15. Lymphangioleiomyomatosis (see Figure 28–2)[3–5]
  a) Anatomic distribution—usually not readily discernible
  b) Pathologic pattern—not applicable
  c) Specific morphologic clues—distinctive cystic spaces in the lung tissue; in the walls of cysts

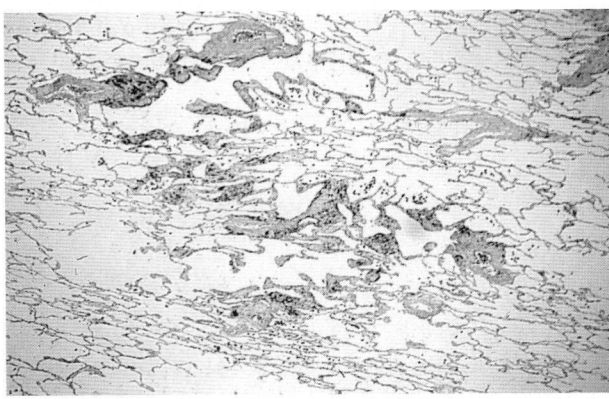

A

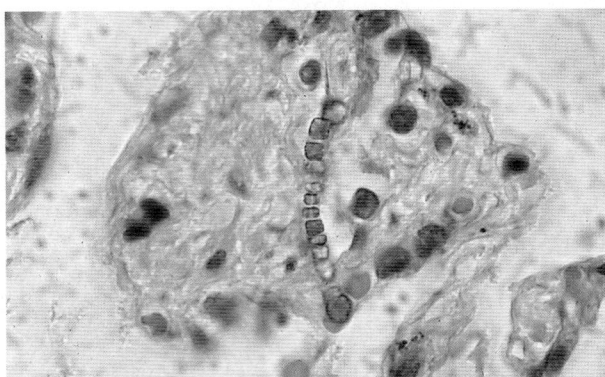

B

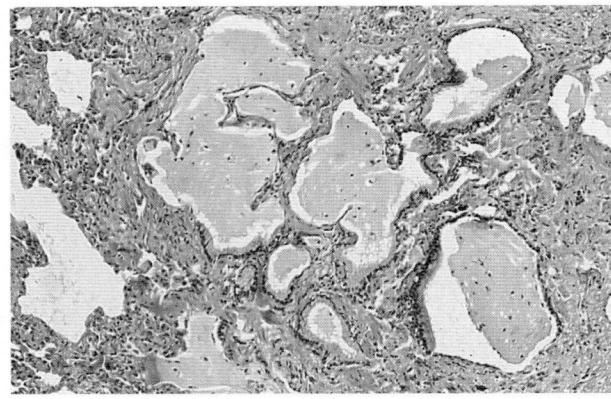

C

Figure 2–22   *A,* Asbestosis in its early/mild stages shows thickening of the interstitial tissue around respiratory bronchioles and alveolar ducts, often with associated anthracotic pigment. *B,* The diagnosis is confirmed by the finding of asbestos bodies. *C,* Severe cases of asbestosis show nonspecific honeycombing, and, in such cases, many asbestos bodies are usually found.

there are fascicles of immature-appearing (antimelanoma antibody, HMB-45, positive) smooth muscle

d) HRCT findings—uniformly distributed thin-walled cysts involving the lung parenchyma; intervening lung tissue appears normal

SUMMARY

An organized approach to the diagnosis of ILD relies on the anatomic distribution and specific histologic patterns. The anatomic distribution may not correlate with the clinical features. For example, bronchiolocentricity is an important and prominent feature in hypersensitivity pneumonitis and respiratory bronchiolitis-associated ILD, but neither is considered an airway disease. There is overlap between anatomic distribution and specific patterns, but the approach presented allows the development of a conceptual framework from which to approach ILDs.

For obvious reasons, an approach to interstitial lung disease that relies on anatomic distribution and pathologic pattern recognition is facilitated by the examination of larger tissue specimens, including surgical (usually thoracoscopic) wedge biopsy specimens, resected lung specimens, and autopsy lung tissue. Nevertheless, even generous transbronchial biopsy specimens commonly yield sufficient tissue to enable the pathologist to identify distinctive patterns when they are present and apply the principles outlined above.

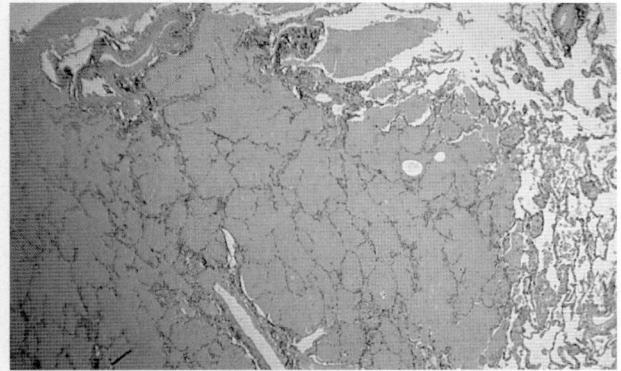

A

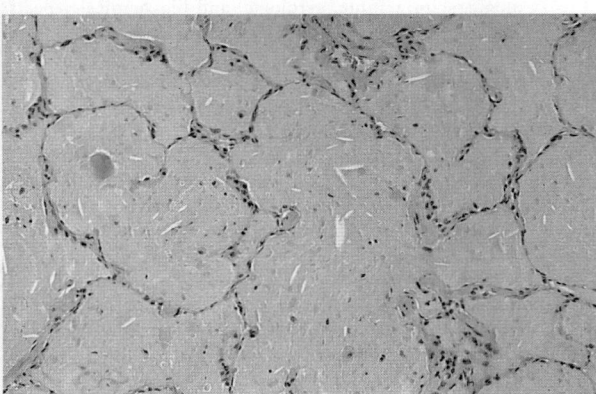

B

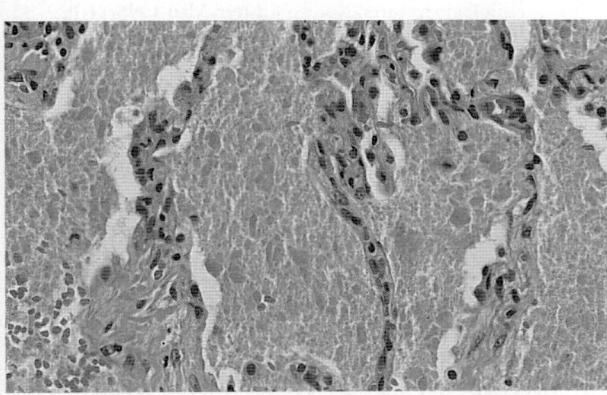

C

Figure 2–23 *A*, and *B*, Pulmonary alveolar proteinosis is an air space filling disease, with dense granular eosinophilic material filling the alveoli. *B*, Cholesterol clefts and hyaline globules may be prominent. *C*, The most distinctive feature of pulmonary alveolar proteinosis is granularity, which usually allows the differentiation of pulmonary alveolar proteinosis from other lesions (such as pulmonary edema and *Pneumocystis carinii* infection) on routine sections.

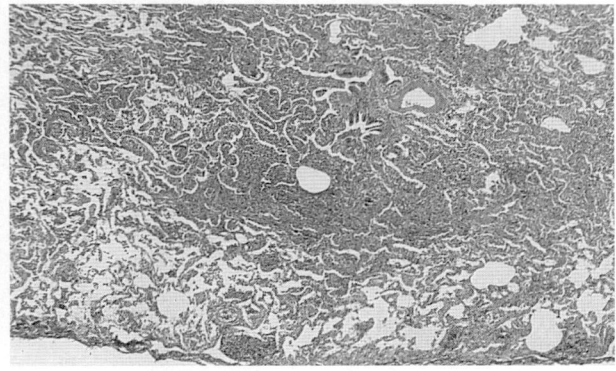

A

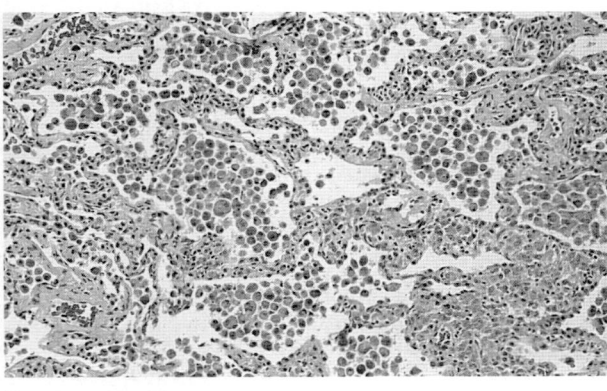

B

Figure 2–24 Respiratory bronchiolitis-associated interstitial lung disease is an exaggerated inflammatory reaction around respiratory bronchioles caused by smoking. *A*, At low power, a bronchiolocentric consolidated process is apparent, which, *B*, at higher magnification, shows a DIP pattern. *B*, The tan pigmentation, is apparent in the macrophages, which is characteristic of cigarette smoking.

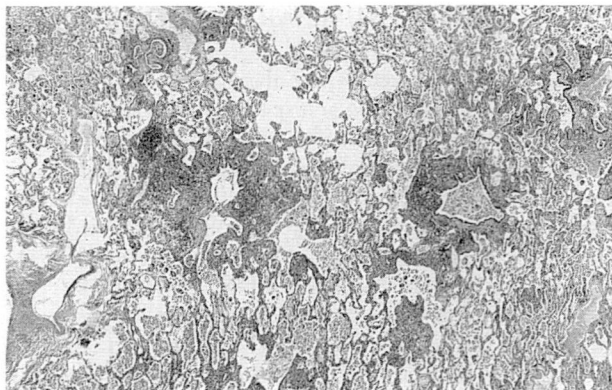

A

B

Figure 2–25   *A,* Giant cell interstitial pneumonia/hard metal pneumoconiosis typically shows centrilobular inflammation and scarring as shown by thickening of the walls of the bronchioles at low power. *B,* The distinctive high magnification finding is numerous multinucleated giant cells that may show apparent "cannibalism," as though other histiocytes have been engulfed.

REFERENCES

1. Crystal RG, Bitterman PB, Rennard SI, et al. Interstitial lung diseases of unknown cause. Part I. N Engl J Med 1984;310:154–66.
2. Colby TV, Churg AC. Patterns of pulmonary fibrosis. (Part 2). Pathol Annu 1986;21:277–310.
3. Colby TV, Swensen SJ. Anatomic distribution and histolopathologic patterns in diffuse lung disease: correlation with HRCT. J Thorac Imaging 1996;11:1–26.
4. Colby TV, Lombard CM, Yousem SA, Kitaichi M. Atlas of pulmonary surgical pathology. Philadelphia: W.B. Saunders; 1991. p. 1–11, 357–72.
5. Colby TV, Carrington CB. Infiltrative lung disease. In: Thurlbeck WM, editor. Pathology of the lung. New York: Thieme Medical Publishers; 1988. p. 425–518.
6. Tazelaar HD, Kerr D, Yousem SA, et al. Diffuse pulmonary lymphangiomatosis. Hum Pathol 1993;24:1313–22.
7. Colby TV. Miscellaneous conditions and lung diseases of unknown origin. In: Hassleton PS, editor. Spencer's pathology of the lung. 5th ed. New York: McGraw-Hill; 1996. p. 767–803.
8. Katzenstein A, Bloor C, Liebow A. Diffuse alveolar damage. The role of oxygen, shock, and related factors. Am J Pathol 1976;85:210–28.
9. Pratt PC. Pathology of adult respiratory distress syndrome. In: Thurlbeck WM, Abell MR, editors. The lung. Baltimore: Williams & Wilkins; 1978. p. 43–57.
10. Blennerhassett JB. Shock lung and diffuse alveolar damage. Pathological and pathogenetic considerations. Pathology 1985;17:239–47.
11. Katzenstein ALA, Askin FB. Surgical pathology of nonneoplastic lung disease. Philadelphia: W.B. Saunders; 1990. p. 9–57.
12. Olson J, Colby TV, Elliott CG. Hamman-Rich syndrome revisited. Mayo Clin Proc 1990;65:1538–48.
13. Kondoh Y, Taniguchi H, Kawabata Y, et al. Acute exacerbation in idiopathic pulmonary fibrosis. Chest 1993;103:1808–12.
14. Travis WD, Colby TV, Lombard C, Carpenter HA. A clinicopathologic study of 34 cases of diffuse pulmonary hemorrhage with lung biopsy confirmation. Am J Surg Pathol 1990;14:1112–25.
15. Colby TV, Myers JL. Clinical and histologic spectrum of bronchiolitis obliterans including bronchiolitis obliterans organizing pneumonia (BOOP). Semin Respir Med 1992;13:119–33.
16. Carrington CB, Gaensler EA, Coutu RE, et al. Natural history and treated course of usual and desquamative interstitial pneumonia. N Engl J Med 1978;298:801–10.
17. Crystal RG, Fulmer JD, Roberts WC, et al. Idiopathic pulmonary fibrosis – clinical, histologic, radiographic, physiologic, scintigraphic, cytologic, and biochemical aspects. Ann Intern Med 1976;85:769–88.
18. Katzenstein AL, Fiorelli RF. Nonspecific interstitial pneumonia/fibrosis: histologic features and clinical significance. Am J Surg Pathol 1994;18:136–47.
19. Bjoraker JA, Ryu JH, Edwin MK, et al. Prognostic significance of histopathologic subsets in idiopathic pulmonary fibrosis. Am J Respir Crit Care Med 1998;157:199–203.
20. Travis WD, Koss MN, Ferrans BJ. The lung in connective tissue disorders. In: Hasleton PS, editor. Spencer's pathology of the lung. 5th ed. New York: McGraw-Hill; 1997. p. 803–34.
21. Tazelaar HD, Viggiano RW, Pickersgill J, Colby TV. Interstitial lung disease in polymyositis and dermatomyositis: clinical features and prognosis as correlated with histologic findings. Am Rev Respir Dis 1990;141:727–33.
22. Park CS, Jeon JW, Park SW, et al. Nonspecific interstitial pneumonia/fibrosis: clinical manifestations, histologic and radiologic features. Korean J Intern Med 1996;11:122–32.
23. Midthun DE, Ryu JH, Myers, JL, et al. Nonspecific interstitial pneumonia: clinical, radiographic, and pathologic features. Am J Respir Crit Care Med 1998;157:A277.
24. Nagai S, Kitaichi M, Itoh H, et al. Idiopathic nonspecific interstitial pneumonia/fibrosis: comparison with idiopathic pulmonary fibrosis and bronchiolitis obliterans organizing pneumonia. Eur Respir J 1998;12:1010–9.
25. Kim TS, Lee KS, Chung MP, et al. Nonspecific interstitial pneumonia with fibrosis: high-resolution CT and pathologic findings. AJR Am J Roentgenol 1998;171:1645–50.
26. Cottin V, Donsbeck A-V, Revel D, et al. Nonspecific interstitial pneumonia. Individualization of a clinicopathologic entity in a series of 12 patients. Am J Respir Crit Care Med 1998;158:1286–93.
27. Daniil ZD, Gilchrist FC, Nicholson AG, et al. A histologic pattern of nonspecific interstitial pneumonia (NSIP) is associated with a better prognosis than usual interstitial pneumonia (UIP) in patients with cryptogenic fibrosing alveolitis (CFA). Am J Respir Crit Care Med 1999;160:899–905.
28. Travis WD, Matsui K, Moss J, Ferrans VJ. Idiopathic nonspecific interstitial pneumonia (NSIP): prognostic significance of cellular and fibrosing patterns. Survival comparison with usual interstitial pneumonia and desquamative interstitial pneumonia. Am J Surg Pathol 2000;24:19–33.

29. Katzenstein AL, Myers JL. Idiopathic pulmonary fibrosis: clinical relevance of pathologic classification. Am J Respir Crit Care Med 1998;157:1301–15.

30. Colby TV. Berylliosis. In: Churg A, Green FHY, editors. Pathology of occupational lung disease. New York: Igaku-Shoin; 1988. p. 73–88.

31. Colby TV, Yousem SA. The lungs. In: Sternberg SS, editor. Histology for pathologists. New York: Raven Press; 1992.

32. Hsu RM, Connors AF, Tomashefski JF. Histologic microbiologic and clinical correlates of the diagnosis of sarcoidosis by transbronchial biopsy. Arch Pathol Lab Med 1996; 120:364–8.

33. Churg A, Green FHY, editors. Pathology of occupational lung disease. New York: Igaku-Shoin; 1988. p. 56–61.

34. Abraham JL. Lung pathology in 21 cases of giant cell interstitial pneumonia (GIP) suggests GIP is pathognomonic of cobalt (hard metal) disease [abstract]. Chest 1987;91:312.

35. Hansell DM, Rubens MB, Padley SPG, Wells AU. Obliterative bronchiolitis: individual CT signs of small airways disease and functional correlation. Radiology 1997;203:721–6.

36. Carrington CB, Gaensler EA. Clinical-pathologic approach to diffuse infiltrative lung disease. In: Thurlbeck WM, Abell MR, editors. The lung: structure, function, and disease. Baltimore: Williams & Wilkins; 1978. p. 58–87.

37. Muller NL, Miller RR. Computed tomography of chronic diffuse infiltrative lung disease. Parts I and II. Am Rev Respir Dis 1990;142:1206–15, 1440–8.

38. Myers JL, Veal CF Jr, Shin MS, Katzenstein ALA. Respiratory bronchiolitis causing interstitial lung disease. A clinicopathologic study of six cases. Am Rev Respir Dis 1987; 135:880–6.

39. Yousem SA, Colby TV, Gaensler EA. Respiratory bronchiolitis-associated interstitial lung disease and its relationship to DIP. Mayo Clin Proc 1989;64:1373–80.

40. Epler G, Colby TV, McCloud TC, et al. Bronchiolitis obliterans organizing pneumonia. N Engl J Med 1985;312:152–8.

41. Hartman TE, Swensen SJ, Hansell DM, et al. Nonspecific interstitial pneumonia: variable appearance at high-resolution chest CT. Radiology 2000;217:701–5.

42. Jederlinic PJ, Sicilian L, Gaensler EA. Chronic eosinophilic pneumonia: a report of 19 cases and review of the literature. Medicine 1988;67:154–62.

43. Colby TV, Coleman A. Histological differential diagnosis of extrinsic allergic alveolitis. Prog Surg Pathol 1989;10:11–26.

44. Colby TV, Lombard C. Pulmonary eosinophilic granuloma: a review for the pathologist. Hum Pathol 1983;14:847–56.

45. Carrington CB, Gaensler EA, Mikus JP, et al. Structure and function in sarcoidosis. Ann N Y Acad Sci 1976;278:265–83.

46. Khoor A, Leslie KO, Tazelaar HD, et al. Diffuse pulmonary disease caused by nontuberculous mycobacteria in immunocompetent people (Hot tub lung). Am J Clin Pathol 2001;115:755–62.

47. Austenfeld JL, Colby TV. Hard metal asthma and interstitial lung disease. J Respir Dis 1989;10:65–75.

48. Colby TV. Diffuse pulmonary hemorrhage in Wegener's granulomatosis. Semin Respir Med 1989;10:136–9.

49. Travis WD, Hoffman GS, Leavitt RY, et al. Surgical pathology of the lung in Wegener's granulomatosis: review of 87 open lung biopsies in 67 patients. Am J Surg Pathol 1991;15: 315–33.

50. Colby TV, Carrington CB. Pulmonary lymphoreticular infiltrates. Pathol Annu 1983;1:27–70.

3

PHYSIOLOGY OF INTERSTITIAL LUNG DISEASE

DENIS E. O'DONNELL
MICHAEL F. FITZPATRICK

Although interstitial lung disease (ILD) is characterized by diverse clinical and histopathologic manifestations, they share a common basic pattern of physiologic dysfunction. In this chapter, we will examine the mechanical derangements peculiar to this group of diseases and explain the basis for pulmonary function test abnormalities that typically occur. We will review exercise pathophysiology, discuss the nature and mechanisms of gas exchange impairment, and probe the mechanisms of exertional breathlessness, the most common symptom in ILD. Finally, we will review the clinical use of physiologic measurements, both at rest and during exercise, in the management of ILD.

PULMONARY MECHANICS

Static Lung Compliance

Interstitial lung disease is characterized by restrictive ventilatory deficit: the static expiratory pressure-volume (P-V) curve of the lung is shifted downward and to the right compared with normal subjects (Figure 3–1).[1–4] Lung recoil is increased over the entire range of the reduced inspiratory capacity. Thus, the P-V relation of the lung is contracted along its volume axis, and both total lung capacity (TLC) and vital capacity are diminished.[1–4] In a number of studies, the chord compliance, expressed as percent vital capacity per centimeter of water pressure, has been shown to be lower (< 50%) than normal over the operating tidal breathing range (functional residual capacity + 0.5 L).[5,6] The coefficient of retraction (pleural pressure at TLC divided by lung volume at TLC) is consistently elevated in ILD compared with normal.[2,7–9] Similarly, the transpulmonary pressure near TLC is increased (see Figure 3–1), which reflects the greater mechanical advantage of the inspiratory muscles, particularly the diaphragm, whose force-generating capacity is enhanced at the lower absolute volume in ILD.[10,11]

The mechanisms of reduced lung compliance in ILD are multifactorial and include: (1) loss of lung volume, (2) reduced alveolar distensibility, (3) changes in the elastic properties of the lung, and (4) increased alveolar surface tension. The relative contribution of reduced alveolar distensibility (lung shrinkage) and loss of functioning alveoli to reduce static lung compliance, probably varies among

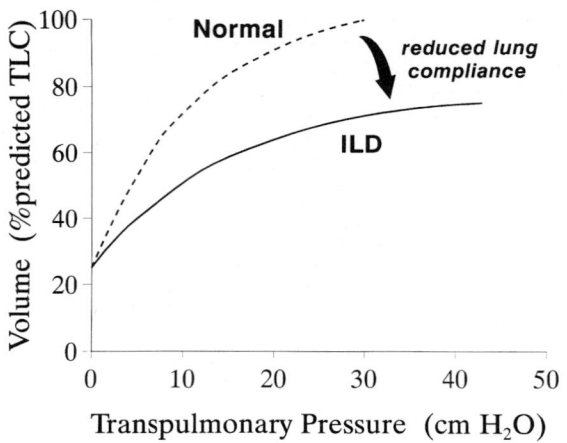

Figure 3–1 Static compliance of the lungs (represented by the slope of the pressure-volume curve) is reduced in interstitial lung disease (ILD), compared to normal.

patients with different types of ILD and within individual patients over the course of the disease. A decrease in lung volume is probably the most important explanation for reduced static compliance in ILD.[7,10–13] Gibson and Pride[10] have argued that in patients with more advanced ILD and fibrosis, reduced static lung compliance can be explained primarily by the loss of functioning alveoli that occurs heterogeneously throughout the lungs. These authors expressed static expiratory P-V curves when lung volume was expressed as either a percentage of the predicted TLC (which corrects for differences in body size) or as a percentage of the actual TLC (which corrects for differences in lung size). They found that in many patients, P-V curves were normalized when expressed as percentages of the actual TLC. This implies that a reduced number of functioning alveolar units is an important determinant of reduced static lung compliance.[10] Additional factors that potentially contribute to decreased lung compliance in ILD include alterations in tissue elastic elements,[4,14–17] reduced alveolar size,[18,19] and increased surface tension due to abnormal quantities or composition of pulmonary surfactant.[20,21] Although the relative importance of these latter mechanisms in contributing to reduced compliance is not precisely known, they are believed to be less important than the effects of reduced lung volume.

Static Lung Volumes

From the preceding considerations of lung mechanics, it is evident that static lung volumes are typically reduced in ILD (Figure 3–2). Vital capacity (VC) is variably diminished, with a wide standard deviation in the measurement among patients. Reduced VC is, of course, not specific for ILD and may occur (1) in obstructive lung diseases, (2) in the presence of inspiratory muscle weakness, (3) with chest wall restriction, (4) with lung resection, or (5) merely as a reflection of poor volitional effort by the patient during the measurement. Vital capacity may be within the normal range early in the course of the disease.[22,23] Reduced VC primary reflects fewer functioning alveolar units due to obliteration by the disease process and filling of the alveoli with exudate, edema, or inflammatory material.[24–26] Altered tissue elasticity as a result of ILD is believed to contribute little to the reduced volume expansion.[17]

Functional residual capacity (FRC) is, on average, also reduced in ILD but relatively less so than are VC and TLC. Combining data from several large series in ILD in which plethysmographic lung volumes were measured,[5,18,23,27,28] Gottlieb and Snider[29] reported that the mean reduction of FRC was to 79% predicted normal compared with mean VC and TLC reductions to 63% and 72% predicted normal, respectively. The FRC is determined by the balance between the outward chest wall recoil and the inward elastic recoil of the lung. Functional residual capacity is relatively preserved in ILD because the reduction in thoracic gas volume is usually accompanied by an increase in lung tissue volume. To the extent that a reduced FRC (gas volume) is associated with an increased outward chest wall recoil, then intrapleural pressure (P_{pl}) would be expected to be diminished (more negative) at that volume. Several studies have, however, shown P_{pl} to be normal or actually increased at FRC in ILD,[7,10,12] confirming that total thoracic gas volume is normal in association with a normal chest wall recoil pressure. Preservation of chest wall configuration in ILD may be related to adaptive changes in diaphragmatic length in response to chronically diminished lung volumes.[30] The FRC/TLC ratio has been shown to be increased in ILD with a consequent reduction in the inspiratory capacity (IC) (see Figure 3–2).[27–29,31]

The decrease in total lung capacity is relatively less than in vital capacity.[5,8,23,27–29,31] The TLC is determined by the balance between inspiratory muscle strength and the combined recoil of the lung and chest wall. The TLC is relatively well preserved despite reduced lung compliance due to the inspiratory muscles' mechanical advantage and the normal chest wall recoil pressure.[10,29] In some patients with ILD, plethysmographic TLC may be augmented toward normal values if there is concomitant small airways disease with air trapping, particularly when the history includes cigarette smoking.[32–34]

Residual volume (RV) is relatively well preserved (> 80% predicted normal) in ILD, and the RV/TLC ratio is often elevated.[5,8,23,27–29,31] The preservation of RV appears to be due to (1) the presence of poorly ventilated cystic air space (ie, honeycombing) that contribute to lung volumes measured by body plethysmography[35] and (2) the coexistence of small airways disease as part of the disease process or as a result of damage from smoking.[32,34–36] Plethysmographic TLC and FRC measurements are partially derived from RV measurements, therefore, all these volume measurements tend to increase together in patients with an obstructive component or extensive cystic changes.[32,34–36]

Airway Function

Airway function is generally well preserved in ILD. Spirometric measurements, including the forced expiratory volume in 1 second/forced vital capacity (FEV_1/FVC) ratio and the mean expiratory flow rate between 25% and 75% of the FVC (forced expiratory flow [FEF]$_{25–75}$), are typically normal or abnormal normal.[5,9,23,27–29,31] Examination of the maximal expiratory flow-volume loop shows that although peak expiratory flows may be reduced in absolute terms, flow rates are consistently increased at a given volume compared with normals (see Figure 3–2). This behavior is explained by the increased driving pressure for expiratory flow as a result of increased lung recoil pressures at volumes above FRC and by attendant preservation of static airway dimensions.

Histologic abnormalities of the bronchial walls of segmental and larger bronchi have frequently been documented in ILD of various etiologies.[37,38] Peribronchial inflammation and fibrosis with narrowing of small (< 2 mm) airways, also commonly accompany ILD.[37,38] Clinical suspicion of small airway dysfunction arises if, for example, $FEF_{25–75}$ is reduced or if the maximal expiratory flow curve is oriented concave to the horizontal volume

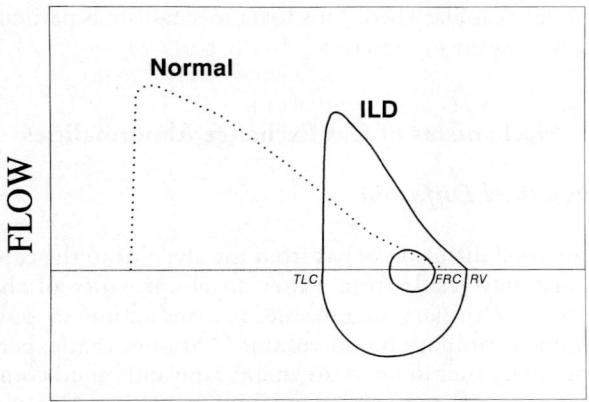

Figure 3–2 Maximal and tidal flow-volume curves are shown at rest in interstitial lung disease (ILD) (*solid lines*) compared with the normal predicted maximal expiratory flow-volume curve (*dotted line*).

axis. Several studies have shown that plethysmographic measurements of total airway conductance are usually in the normal range,[6,7,9,10,39–41] even in the presence of documented pathologic involvement of the small airways. This suggested that tests of total airway resistance are not sufficiently sensitive to detect increased resistance in small airways, where conditions of laminar flow prevail.[42]

More sophisticated tests to evaluate small airway dysfunction in ILD include: (1) isovolume pressure-flow measurements,[43] (2) the ratio of dynamic to static compliance measurements,[44] and (3) closing volume measurements.[45] Since these tests are technically difficult to perform and have not been adequately standardized, it is not surprising that several studies have yielded conflicting results. The calculation of resistance in smaller airways upstream from the equal pressure point (R_{us}) (which is obtained by dividing the maximal expiratory flow rate by the transpulmonary pressure at lung volumes where expiratory flow limitation prevails, ie, flow is effort independent), has determined increased values compared with normals in some studies[9,39,40] but not consistently in others.[7,10] It has been shown that increased R_{us} values are more likely to occur if a coexistent significant smoking history is present in patients with ILD.[7,46]

Fulmer and colleagues[37] have shown a strong correlation between reduced dynamic lung compliance and the extent of small airways disease in lung biopsy specimens in patients with ILD. In diseases of small airways or in any condition where there are significant time constant inequalities, dynamic compliance decreases below static compliance values when breathing frequency is increased.[17,44,47] Increased time constants for airflow are present because of the inhomogeneity in compliance of different alveolar units and because of a heterogeneous distribution of increased resistance in small airways throughout the lung.[17,44,47] Some studies in ILD have shown a frequency-dependent fall in dynamic compliance confirming time-constant inequalities and, thus, small airways dysfunction.[44,47,48] Similarly, closing volume measurements have been used in the research setting by a number of investigators in an attempt to detect small airways involvement in ILD.[32,33,45,49,50] These have met with similarly wide variations due, in part, to technical difficulties that arise when this technique is used in the population with ILD.[37,45] For these reasons, it has been a challenge to draw definitive conclusions about the extent of involvement of small airways in ILD and their functional significance. Clearly, however, small airways disease may occur in ILD as part of the disease process or as a result of a concurrent cigarette-smoking history. It is also well known that small airway dysfunction may contribute to decreased dynamic compliance and, thus, to the elastic load on the ventilatory muscles. Moreover, time-constant inhomogeneity can adversely affect the distribution of ventilation and result in gas exchange abnormalities (see below). Despite extensive involvement of the small airways, volume matched maximal expiratory flow rates (FEV_1/FVC) are, nevertheless, typically normal or above normal in ILD.

GAS EXCHANGE ABNORMALITIES

The characteristic arterial blood gas abnormalities in ILD are resting hypoxemia and an increased alveolar-arterial oxygen tension gradient ($P_{(A-a)}O_2$). Arterial CO_2 tension ($PaCO_2$) is usually normal but may be reduced at rest in a proportion of patients because of alveolar hyperventilation. Arterial pH is typically normal. Elevation of $PaCO_2$ is distinctly unusual except in the terminal phase of the disease, as airway function is relatively preserved and eucapnia is ensured by increased minute ventilation, even in the presence of substantial gas exchange derangements at the alveolar-capillary interface.

Resting PaO_2 measurements correlate poorly with disease severity and in many instances, particularly early in the disease, PaO_2 may be in the normal range[23,28,51] whereas $P_{(A-a)}O_2$ is elevated. Diffusion capacity (DL_{CO}) or transfer factor is characteristically diminished in ILD and to a greater extent than the lung volume (TLC) at which it is measured.[5,9,23,27–29,31] Single-breath DL_{CO} measurements have been shown to predict arterial oxygen desaturation in several studies[52–55]; however, significant oxygen desaturation can occur in the presence of a normal resting DL_{CO} and PaO_2.[56–58] Thus, DL_{CO} measurements do not take the place of formal exercise testing with arterial blood gas measurements to evaluate the nature and severity of gas exchange impairment in individuals with ILD.[58]

Factors that contribute to reductions in both DL_{CO} and PaO_2 include loss of available alveolar capillary bed, abnormal thickness of the alveolar capillary membrane, and reduced pulmonary capillary blood volume. Other factors, independent of reduce DL_{CO}, that potentially contribute to resting and exercise hypoxemia include ventilation-perfusion inequalities, right-to-left shunting, and rapid red blood cell transit through the pulmonary capillary bed. This latter mechanism is particularly relevant to exercise.

Mechanisms of Gas Exchange Abnormalities

Impaired Diffusion

Impaired diffusion of gas from the alveolus to the capillary may result from either an abnormality of the alveolar-capillary membrane or a reduction in pulmonary capillary blood volume.[59] Studies that experimentally fractionated the membrane and blood components of reduced diffusion in ILD[60–63] have established that their relative contribution can vary but that membrane conductance abnormalities often predominate in ILD.[62,63] Reduction in the membrane component has been shown, from morphometric studies of lung biopsy specimens, to be due more to reduced mean alveolar surface area than to increased membrane thickness per se.[35,64,65]

Ventilation-Perfusion Inequalities

The pathological process in ILD generally has a patchy distribution throughout the lungs as shown by high-resolution computed tomography (CT) imaging. This patchy involvement results in substantial regional variation in lung compliance and in time constants for airflow. These, in turn, lead to a nonuniform distribution of ventilation.[66] Radionucleotide lung scanning techniques[67,68] and, more recently, multiple inert gas elimination techniques,[69,70] have confirmed marked interregional heterogeneity of the ventilation-perfusion ($\dot{V}/\dot{Q}$) distribution in ILD. Abnormal $\dot{V}/\dot{Q}$ ratios have been shown in some studies to explain much of the resting hypoxemia.[67] Wagner and colleagues[70] using multiple inert gas elimination techniques, showed that the distribution of $\dot{V}/\dot{Q}$ relationships in ILD was bimodal; the majority of alveolar units have normally preserved $\dot{V}/\dot{Q}$ ratios (ie, $\dot{V}/\dot{Q}$ ratio = 1.0), and the remaining units (9% of total) show markedly reduced ventilation ($\dot{V}/\dot{Q}$ ratio < 0.1).[70] These studies have shown that virtually all arterial hypoxemia at rest in patients with ILD could be explained on the basis of the above-mentioned $\dot{V}/\dot{Q}$ derangements.[70,71] Other studies using radionucleotide scanning have shown that a small proportion of the elevated resting $P_{(A-a)}O_2$ in ILD was explained by impaired diffusion.[54,72]

Right-to-Left Shunting

It is believed that intrapulmonary right-to-left shunting contributes minimally to resting arterial hypoxemia in ILD. Shunt fractions from 2 to 5% have been reported in three studies in this population.[54,70,71] In some patients, however, large clinically significant shunts may develop at some stage during the course of illness.[35,73,74] These shunts may be related to one or more of the following: (1) the development of an anastomosis between the bronchial and pulmonary circulation, (2) raised pulmonary artery pressure, and (3) the development of right-to-left intracardiac shunts accompanied by severe pulmonary hypertension with right ventricular hypertrophy.

EXERCISE PATHOPHYSIOLOGY

The previously outlined pathophysiologic derangements of ILD become even more pronounced when the cardiorespiratory system is stressed during exercise. As disease severity increases, exercise performance becomes increasingly curtailed. Therefore, exercise testing can precisely identify the nature and severity of the physio-

logic impairment in any given individual. In the following section, we will discuss the abnormalities in the cardiorespiratory response to exercise in ILD (Table 3–1). Cardiorespiratory responses to exercise in normal patients and in patients with ILD are graphically illustrated in Figure 3–3.

Ventilatory Responses to Exercise

Peak ventilation is usually diminished in ILD as a result of abnormal ventilatory mechanics. Compared with normal subjects, minute ventilation ($\dot{V}E$) in ILD is greater at rest[12,75,76] and at any given external power output O_2 consumption ($\dot{V}O_2$) during exercise[12,75,76] (see Figure 3–3). Respiratory drive, as measured by mouth occlusion pressure ($P_{0.1}$) or mean inspiratory flow rate (V_T/T_I), has been shown to be elevated both at rest or at any given ventilation during exercise.[77,78] Factors contributing to the increased ventilation during exercise include: (1) high physiologic dead space, (2) exercise-induced hypoxemia, (3) excessive metabolic acidosis, and (4) possible neurogenic mechanisms.

High Physiologic Deadspace

In the majority of patients with ILD, physiologic deadspace (deadspace volume/tidal volume [V_D/V_T]) has been shown to be elevated at rest.[79,80] Moreover, these patients' V_D/V_T fails to decline during exercise as it does in normal subjects (see Figure 3–3); elevated V_D/V_T measurements of 36 to 50% have been recorded in larger series of patients with ILD.[79,80] The principal explanation for the elevated V_D/V_T is low perfusion of normally ventilated alveolar units caused by capillary disruption that occurs as part of the interstitial disease process. Lack of a normal decline in V_D/V_T during exercise occurs partly as a consequence of failure to recruit increased tidal volumes as the exercise progresses compared with

---

TABLE 3–1 Typical Exercise Responses in ILD

1. Reduced peak oxygen consumption and work rate
2. Increased dyspnea ratings at submaximal work rates
3. Diminished ventilatory reserve: high peak ventilation to maximal ventilatory capacity ratio
4. High submaximal ventilation level:
   - High resting and exercise physiologic deadspace
   - Arterial oxygen desaturation
5. Breathing pattern: high frequency, low tidal volume
6. Increased mechanical restriction: high submaximal tidal volume to inspiratory capacity ratio (reduced submaximal inspiratory reserve volume)
7. Adequate cardiac reserve: low peak heart rates ± high submaximal heart rates
8. Normal efficiency: normal oxygen consumption to work rate relation

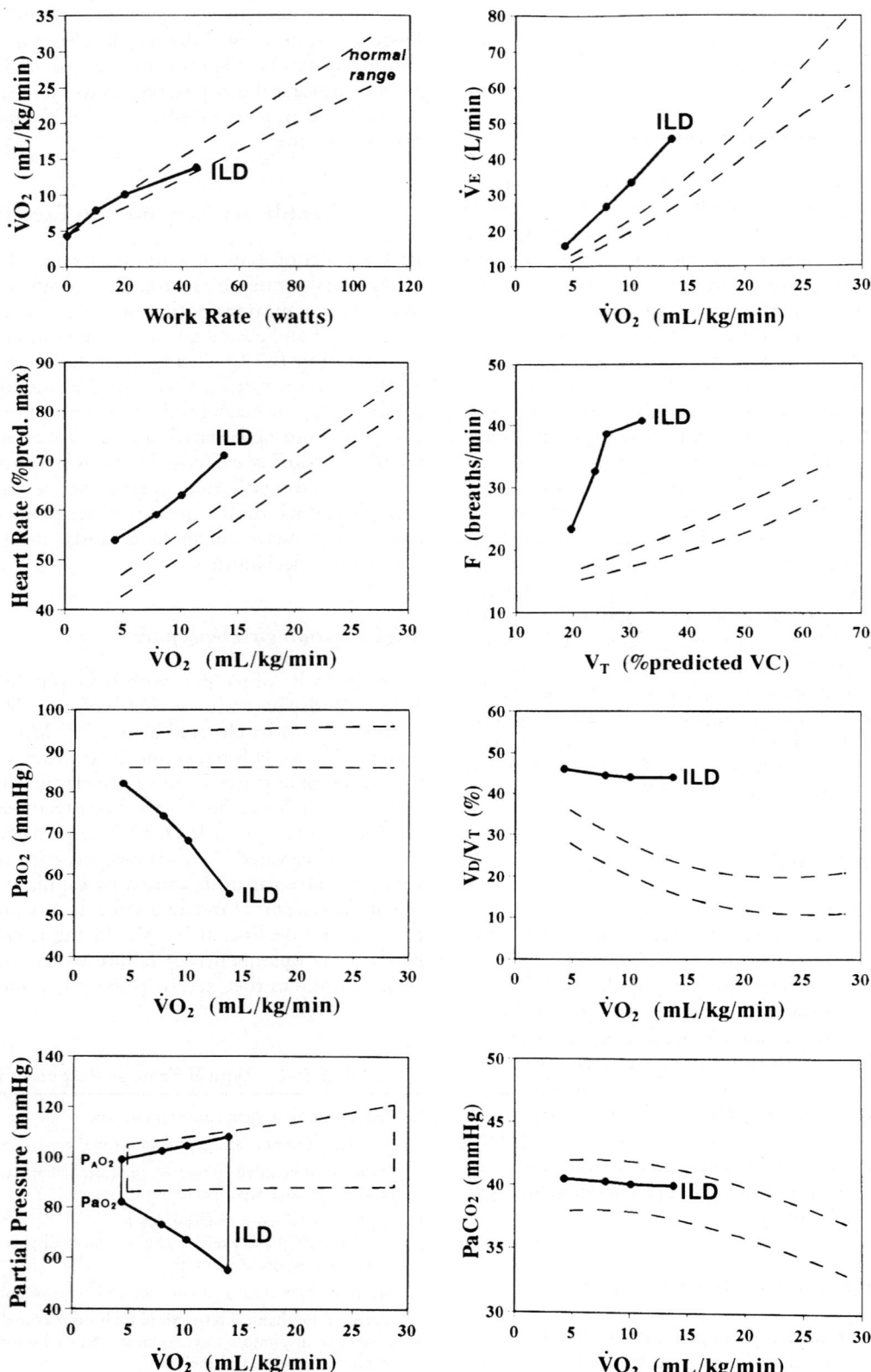

Figure 3–3   Exercise responses in interstitial lung disease (ILD) compared with normal (*dotted lines* indicate ± 1 SEM from an age-matched normal mean value established in our laboratory). The bottom four graphs represent responses obtained from stage III exercise testing. See text for explanation. Abbreviations: $\dot{V}O_2$ = oxygen consumption; $\dot{V}_E$ = ventilation; F = breathing frequency; V_T = tidal volume; PaO_2 = arterial oxygen tension; $PaCO_2$ = arterial carbon dioxide; $P_{A}O_2$ = alveolar oxygen tension; V_D/V_T = physiologic deadspace.

normal. The breathing pattern of these patients is characteristically rapid and shallow,[81,82] reflecting the response to the increased elastic load and the mechanical constraints on tidal volume expansion during exercise. Minute ventilation must increase to maintain eucapnia in ILD in the setting of high V_D/V_T.

Exercise-Induced Hypoxemia

The mechanisms of resting hypoxemia in ILD have been outlined above. Worsening hypoxemia typically occurs during exercise in ILD[54,56,57,83] and can occur in patients who have early disease and normal resting arterial blood gases. Arterial oxygen desaturation during exercise, if sufficiently severe, may contribute to the heightened ventilatory response in these patients. Exercise further stresses the already compromised gas exchange capabilities of the cardiorespiratory system. Exercise-induced hypoxemia results from a combination of (1) poor recruitment of alveolar capillaries during exercise and consequent increased red blood cell transit times across the gas exchange surface of the lung and (2) reduced mixed venous oxygen (P_vO_2) concentrations in the setting of low $\dot{V}/\dot{Q}$ ratios and shunt.

Diffusion capacity normally increases during exercise as a result of increasing distention and recruitment of unperfused alveolar capillaries, with a consequent increase in capillary blood volume.[84] This results in a large surface area available for gas exchange during exercise. Several studies in ILD have demonstrated the failure of DL_{CO} to increase normally during exercise. This is probably due to inadequate recruitment of pulmonary capillaries and relatively reduced capillary blood volume.[76,83,85] Decreased capillary blood volume, in turn, results in excessive reduction of the contact time between the alveolar gas and the capillary red blood cells. Normally, the contact time between blood and alveolar gas is in the range of 0.75 to 1.0 seconds.[86] Reductions in contact time to 0.1 to 0.6 seconds has been shown to occur in ILD[61] because the reduced ratio of blood volume in the capillary to blood flow is more pronounced during exercise. Reduction in the contact time below a critical level (< 0.2 s) compromises the equilibration of the partial pressure of O_2 between the alveolar gas and capillary blood and undoubtedly leads to increases in $P_{(A-a)}O_2$ in some patients during exercise. It is estimated that during maximal exercise, 20 to 30% of the widening of the $P_{(A-a)}O_2$ above resting values may be explained by impairment of oxygen diffusion.[70]

The P_vO_2 may be normal in ILD at rest but generally falls during exercise, reflecting reduced oxygen delivery to the exercising muscles.[51,72] In some patients, P_vO_2 may be further diminished by coexistent cardiac dysfunction either as a manifestation of the underlying disease process or as a separate entity. Reduced P_vO_2 contributes further to the elevated $P_{(A-a)}O_2$ during exercise

that is characteristic of ILD and is caused by $\dot{V}/\dot{Q}$ mismatching and diffusion limitation.

In contrast to healthy subjects, in whom $\dot{V}/\dot{Q}$ inequalities become more pronounced during exercise,[87] $\dot{V}/\dot{Q}$ inequalities in patients with ILD have been shown to contribute less to hypoxemia during exercise than during rest.[54,71,72] The $\dot{V}/\dot{Q}$ relationships and the $P_{(A-a)}O_2$ may actually improve,[54,71,72] particularly in patients with coexistent obstructive lung disease.[88] Hypoxemia during exercise is very rarely due to alveolar hypoventilation,[89] except in very advanced disease or were an additional obstructive ventilatory deficit or inspiratory muscle weakness is present. The $PaCO_2$ levels at the peak of incremental exercise are either at resting levels or below in the majority of patients with ILD, despite the heightened V_D/V_T and a characteristically rapid shallow breathing pattern.

Studies that have shown that the prevention of arterial O_2 desaturation with supplemental oxygen reduced ventilation at a given $\dot{V}O_2$, with consequent delay in ventilatory limitation and improved exercise endurance,[90,91] support the importance of arterial hypoxemia in contributing to the accelerated ventilatory response to exercise in ILD. Oxygen therapy improves oxygen delivery and possibly use at the peripheral muscle level. Thus, supplemental O_2 delays the rate of lactate accumulation and reduced ventilatory stimulation.[91] In patients with an increased hypoxic drive, supplemental O_2 reduces ventilation and worsens hypercapnia by altering chemoreceptor activation.

Excessive Metabolic Acidosis

In some patients with ILD, early onset of metabolic acidosis may contribute to the hyperventilatory response, particularly if cardiac performance[92] is impaired or the patient is severely deconditioned. The corollary to this is that therapeutic interventions such as cardiac drugs or supervised exercise training can result in diminished metabolic acidosis and ventilatory demand as well as improvement in exercise performance.

Neurogenic Mechanisms

Neurogenic factors may contribute to the increased ventilatory response to exercise in ILD. In the past, vagally mediated J-receptor stimulation was believed to contribute to exercise-induced tachypnea in ILD.[93–95] Our knowledge of the nature of these reflex responses is, however, imprecise,[93] and the role of such receptors in the nonmetabolic stimulation of ventilation remains conjectural.

Ventilatory Mechanics During Exercise

In ILD, the P-V relationship of the respiratory system is contracted along its volume axis but it retains its sigmoid shape (Figure 3–4).[96] The IC represents the operational limits of expansion for V_T and is often markedly diminished. Thus, V_T expansion is seriously constrained under conditions of high ventilatory demand such as exercise (Figure 3–5).[97] As a result, V_T increases during exercise, so the dynamic end-inspiratory lung volume (EILV) encroaches on the upper nonlinear extreme of the contracted P-V relation where there is substantial elastic loading of the inspiratory muscles. The inspiratory work of breathing is increased at rest in patients with ILD due to increased minute ventilation.[12,13] With exercise, the work of breathing increases further as a result of increased elastic loading due to reduced lung compliance: the work per liter of ventilation has been calculated as four to six times higher than normal at any given external power output.[12,13] The flow-resistive work of breathing is normal in ILD, so the elastic work constitutes the major component and is due to both reduced static compliance[12,13] and to a further frequency-dependent reduction in dynamic compliance as exercise progresses.[5,37,47] Thus, at any given work rate, esophageal pressure excursions required for a given change in V_T are higher in ILD than in age-matched normal subjects,[5,12,13] and represent a significantly greater fraction of their dynamic maximal force generating capacity (PI_{max}).[97] Dynamic PI_{max} is reduced below static levels because the increased mean inspiratory flow rates reflect the greater velocity of shortening of the inspiratory muscles in tachypneic patients with ILD during exercise.[98] Thus, greater dynamic functional weakness of the inspiratory muscles results from the greater velocity of shortening in ILD (compared with normal subjects).

Patients have few options to keep pace with the increased ventilatory demands of exercise due to the mechanical constraints on V_T expansion. Possible strategies to combat this include increasing breathing frequency and encroachment of the V_T on the expiratory reserve volume (ERV) by expiratory muscle recruitment. Several studies demonstrate clearly that ILD patients use the former strategy and rely, to a greater extent than do normal subjects, on increasing frequency of breathing to increase ventilation (see Figure 3–3).[81,82] Maximal respiratory rates in the order of 50 to 60 breaths per minute are not unusual at relatively low metabolic loads in ILD.[81,82,97] Increased breathing frequency occurs as a result of reduction in both inspiratory timing (TI) and expiratory timing (TE).[81,82] In ILD, the ratio of inspiratory duty cycle (TI/TTOT) has been reported to be lower than in normal subjects at peak exercise.[81] Although V_T in absolute terms is reduced, the V_T/VC ratio at peak exercise reaches 50 to 60% of the (reduced) VC, as is the case in normal subjects.[81,82] In patients with more advanced disease, however, V_T/VC and particularly V_T/IC ratios approach unity at rest or very early in exercise.[97] In the absence of expiratory flow limitation, increasing breathing frequency remains an effective strategy to increase ventilation and reduces intrathoracic pressure perturbations and the work of breathing.[98] Thus, the rapid, shallow breathing pattern characteristically adopted in ILD is an appropriate compensatory strategy for elastic loading; it probably reduces the associated unpleasant respiratory sensations (see section on Mechanisms of Dyspnea).

The second possible strategy to increase ventilation in ILD is to increase V_T by encroaching on the expiratory reserve volume by expiratory muscle recruitment. Younger normal subjects employ this strategy during exercise; this ensures that V_T and EILV are positioned on the linear compliant portion of the respiratory systems P-V relation,

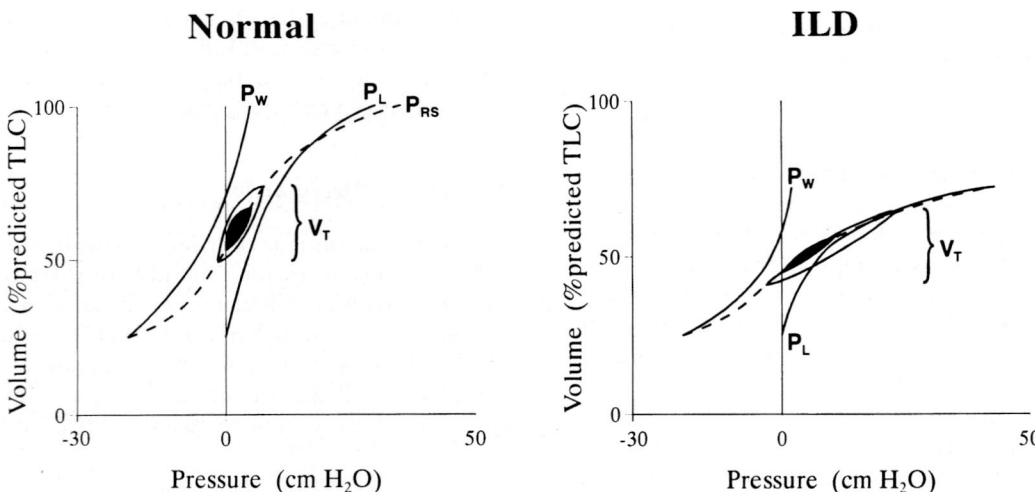

Figure 3–4   Schematic diagram of static pressure-volume relationships for the chest wall (P_W), lung (P_L), and total respiratory system (P_{RS}) (*dashed lines*) are shown for a normal subject and a patient with interstitial lung disease (ILD). Tidal loops at rest and at a given tidal volume during exercise are shown (*shaded areas*). Patients with ILD must expend a significantly greater effort to achieve an equivalent tidal volume compared with normal subjects because of high-end P-V alinearities (see text for further explanation).

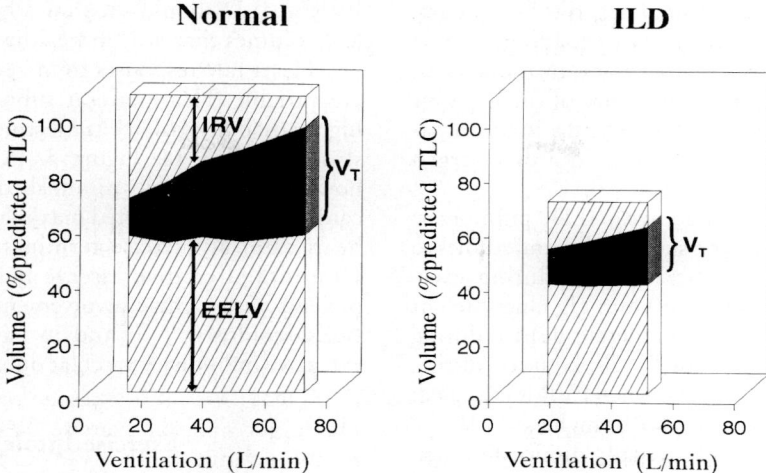

Figure 3–5 Operational lung volumes expressed over ventilation from rest to peak for interstitial lung disease (ILD) patients and age-matched normal subjects. Note minimal tidal volume expansion during exercise in ILD. Abbreviations: EELV = end-expiratory lung volume; IRV = inspiratory reserve volume; V_T = tidal volume. Adapted from reference 97.

(see Figure 3–4), thus reducing elastic loading by avoiding its upper nonlinear extreme.[99–101] Expiratory muscle recruitment during exercise takes the burden off the inspiratory muscles in normal subjects.[98] Currently available information suggests that dynamic end-expiratory lung volume ($EELV_{dyn}$) does not appreciably diminish from rest to peak exercise in ILD.[97,102] We have recently found that the behavior of $EELV_{dyn}$ is no different in ILD patients from that of age-matched normal subjects (see Figure 3–5).[97] The lack of change in the $EELV_{dyn}$ may reflect concomitant expiratory flow limitation (age related, as part of the disease, or related to smoking). Alternately, expiratory muscle weakness may in some patients result in an unchanged $EELV_{dyn}$ from rest to peak exercise. Failure to reduce $EELV_{dyn}$ in ILD during exercise is probably helpful because it may obviate the accentuation of expiratory flow limitation at the further reduced lung volume.

Ventilatory Muscle Function

Reduced lung volumes and improved length-tension relationships should increase the force-generating capacity of the diaphragm and other inspiratory muscles in ILD. De Troyer and Yernault[11] have demonstrated that maximal inspiratory P_{pl} is normal relative to lung volume over much of the inspiratory capacity in ILD. In contrast, other investigators have demonstrated significant reductions in both maximal inspiratory P_{pl}, transdiaphragmatic pressures, and maximal inspiratory and expiratory mouth pressures in patients with ILD.[78,103] For lack of definitive studies, the true prevalence of static inspiratory muscle weakness remains to be determined. It is well known, however, that ventilatory muscle weakness may occur in

ILD in relation to coexisting factors such as chronic hypoxemia, steroid myopathy, collagen vascular disorders that involve skeletal muscle (ie, scleroderma, polymyositis), electrolytic disturbances, and nutritional problems, particularly in patients with more advanced disease.

During exercise, the ventilatory muscles may become functionally compromised and predisposed to fatigue as a result of (1) increased elastic loading (increased lung recoil and dynamic compliance), (2) altered force-velocity relations (ie, increased V_T/T_I), (3) the inability to effectively recruit expiratory muscles, and (4) worsening arterial oxygen desaturation.[90] The extent to which inspiratory muscle fatigue develops during exercise in ILD is unknown. The authors of one study concluded, on the basis of a breathing pattern analysis that failed to show a fatiguing pattern in the recovery phase, that fatigue did not occur after incremental exercise to tolerance in ILD.[104]

Cardiovascular Responses to Exercise

The characteristic cardiac abnormality in ILD is increased pulmonary vascular resistance (PVR) with consequent right ventricular hypertrophy that ultimately leads to the development of cor pulmonale during the terminal phase of the illness.[105,106] Left ventricular ejection fraction and pressures are usually preserved, as are pulmonary artery occlusion pressures.[107,108] Cardiac output is usually normal at rest and during low levels of exercise in ILD, but the rate of rise of cardiac output is diminished at higher levels of exercise,[107,108] due in part to increased PVR. Left ventricular afterload also may be increased significantly during exercise, an effect of the substantial negative intrapleural pressure swings that result from elastic loading in these patients.[109,110] Thus, the left ventricular transmural pressure gradient is elevated in the presence of the negative intrathoracic (juxtacardiac) pressures; this is accompanied by an increased heart rate and myocardial oxygen consumption.[110]

In the majority of patients with ILD, pulmonary artery pressures (P_{pa}) have been shown in several studies to be high at rest and to further increase during exercise.[51,105,111] Values for P_{pa} in the 40 mm Hg range are not unusual in patients with even moderate disease during minimal activity. High levels of P_{pa} are required during exercise to maintain cardiac output when PVR is increased; P_{pa} is often double the normal value or higher.[35,105,106]

In the normal lung, PVR actually diminishes during exercise due to recruitment of previously unperfused capillaries, and P_{pa} does not increase despite a two- to three-fold increase in pulmonary blood flow.[112] In ILD, PVR is increased at rest due to near-maximum recruitment of the pulmonary capillary bed.[113] Thus, flow resistance does not fall during exercise as it does in normal subjects, and P_{pa} must increase substantially to increase cardiac output to keep pace with the increased metabolic demands of exercise.[35,105–108] Factors contributing to the increased PVR are (1) vascular obliteration of the pulmonary capillary bed, (2) hypoxic vasoconstriction, and (3) reduced lung volume. Obliteration of the vascular bed by progressive parenchymal fibrosis is the main explanation for the reduced vascular bed and the increased PVR in ILD.[113,114] Longstanding pulmonary hypertension may itself result in further irreversible changes in the small pulmonary arteries (ie, medial hypertrophy, intimal fibrosis, and proliferation), which lead to further augmentation of PVR.[113]

The role of hypoxemia in contributing to increased PVR during exercise has been studied extensively.[54,106,115] Alveolar oxygen tension correlates poorly with PVR, and administration of supplemental oxygen has minimal effects in reducing PVR and P_{pa} during exercise in ILD.[54,106,113,115] Although oxygen therapy does not reduce PVR, one study demonstrated improved perfusion to low $\dot{V}/\dot{Q}$ areas within the lung in patients with ILD receiving O_2, suggesting some inhibition of hypoxic vasoconstriction.[54] It has been demonstrated that vasoconstriction resulting from low mixed venous oxygen tensions occurs independently of the alveolar oxygen tension in ILD.[116] This mechanism of vasoconstriction may be important in contributing to the increased PVR in patients with serious cardiac impairment where oxygen delivery is critically diminished.[72,107,116]

The role of reduced lung volumes in contributing to raised PVR in ILD remains uncertain. It is believed that reduced lung volume in normal patients causes increased resistance in extra-alveolar vessels due to reduced elastic tractions.[117] In ILD, however, blood vessel dimensions probably stabilize at the low lung volumes due to disease-associated increased elastic traction forces. It follows that PVR in ILD should theoretically be less influenced by low volumes than it is in healthy subjects.[117]

Heart rate responses to incremental exercise in ILD are variable. Heart rate at submaximal loads is often higher than normal,[92,118] reflecting the relatively reduced stroke volume (see Figure 3–3). Maximal heart rates, however, are generally diminished, and there is adequate cardiac reserve (predicted maximal heart rate minus peak heart rate) at exercise termination (see Figure 3–3). Diminished cardiac reserve may become evident in patients with cardiac involvement in the disease process (ie, sarcoidosis)[118–120] and in patients with additional extensive pulmonary vascular disease (ie, scleroderma).[121]

Exercise Intolerance

Exercise limitation in ILD is multifactorial. Limiting factors, both physiologic and psychological, vary greatly among patients and even within patients through the course of disease. As is the case in other chronic pulmonary conditions (eg, chronic obstructive pulmonary disease [COPD]), it is evident from clinical experience that exercise is often limited by exertional symptoms such as dyspnea or leg discomfort before the physiologic boundaries dictated by the ventilatory and cardiovascular systems are reached.[122] To understand the basis of exercise intolerance in many patients with ILD, clinicians should have a greater understanding of the source and mechanisms of exertional symptoms. Factors that may contribute to exercise intolerance in ILD include (1) reduced ventilatory capacity and/or increased ventilatory demand; (2) mechanical factors; (3) ventilatory muscle weakness; (4) general musculoskeletal deconditioning and weakness; (5) cardiovascular impairment; and (6) coexistent problems such as peripheral vascular insufficiency, musculoskeletal problems, or lack of motivation.

Reduced Ventilatory Capacity

Ventilatory limitation has traditionally been regarded as an important, if not preeminent, contributor to exercise limitation in ILD. Peak $\dot{V}E$ during incremental exercise is almost invariably reduced (compared with normal) as a result of the significant mechanical derangements associated with these diseases.[12,75,76,97] Additionally, $\dot{V}E$ is higher at any given external power output in ILD compared with normal,[12,75,76,97] causing some patients to reach their reduced ventilatory "ceiling" prematurely. Several studies have shown that patients with ILD have minimal ventilatory reserve (calculated as maximal ventilatory capacity minus peak $\dot{V}E$) at the end of incremental exercise, which suggests that ventilatory limitation is the proximate limiting factor in ILD.[81,123] A study that compared selective loading of the ventilatory muscles by adding deadspace in normal subjects and in patients with ILD adds evidence of a true ventilatory limitation.[123] In normal subjects, the addition of deadspace resulted in increased ventilation at a given work rate and higher peak ventilation during incremental testing with no change in the peak oxygen consumption ($\dot{V}O_2$).[123] This suggests that in normal subjects, ventilatory limitation is not instrumental in limiting the maximum $\dot{V}O_2$ during control conditions, because selective muscle loading stimulated ventilation further and did not impair exercise performance. In contrast, patients with ILD challenged with deadspace loading did not increase peak $\dot{V}E$, and their exercise performance was further impaired as demonstrated by a reduced peak $\dot{V}O_2$ below control levels.[123] These results suggested that such patients had minimal ventilatory reserve at exercise cessation during unloaded control.

Despite the evidence outlined above, there is considerable debate on whether ventilatory limitation is the most proximate contributor to exercise intolerance in the majority of patients with ILD. Ventilatory capacity is determined by ventilatory muscle performance and characteristics that include their strength, force velocity, and length-tension relationships, as well as the impedances (elastic loading) against which they must act. Other factors that determine maximal ventilatory capacity include the status of the neuroregulatory control system and the prevailing mechanical conditions (eg, extent of expiratory flow limitation). The $FEV_{1.0}$, however, is a poor indicator of ventilatory muscle performance, neural control, and intrinsic mechanical loading, which explains why estimates of the maximal voluntary ventilation (MVV) derived from spirometric measurements (ie, $FEV_{1.0} \times 35$) are often inaccurate in ILD. Even direct measurements of MVV often do not correspond with the maximal ventilatory capacity achieved at peak exercise due to significant differences in breathing patterns and, in some cases, in operational lung volumes under the two conditions (ie, exercise and resting hyperventilation).

More rigorous analysis of ventilatory limitation, in which tidal flow–volume loops at the peak of symptom-limited exercise are compared with the maximal postexercise flow-volume curve, show that tidal inspiratory flows at a matched volume rarely reach the maximal inspiratory flow envelope, indicating adequate ventilatory reserve (Figure 3–6).[97,102] Studies have shown variable encroachment of the tidal expiratory flow curve on the maximal expiratory flow envelope at a given volume, suggesting expiratory flow limitation in some patients with ILD (see Figure 3–6).[97,102]

The relative contribution of the mechanical load to exercise limitation in ILD has not been precisely defined. Such an evaluation is difficult, particularly since patients develop effective compensatory strategies (ie, rapid, shallow breathing pattern) to diminish the negative effects of elastic loading on the ventilatory muscles. Studies that employ elastic/mechanical unloading during exercise may provide new insights into the role of mechanical factors in exercise limitation in ILD. Similarly, the specific contribution of cardiac impairment,[124] exercise deconditioning, and ventilatory muscle weakness to exercise intolerance in ILD has not been determined; it is probably highly variable.

It is evident that any quest for a single limiting factor to explain exercise intolerance in ILD is misdirected. Clearly, a combination of factors ultimately culminates in impairing exercise performance in a given individual. Evidence for the complex and multifactorial nature of exercise limitation in ILD is derived from studies of the effects of therapeutic interventions that successfully improve exercise performance in such patients. The administration of supplemental oxygen therapy to hypoxemic patients is one such example.[91] Oxygen therapy improves oxygen delivery to exercising muscles, reduces reliance on anerobic metabolism, and reduces metabolic acid accumulation.[91] This, in turn, reduces ventilation at a given work rate,[91] relieves exertional dyspnea, and improves exercise tolerance. Oxygen may also improve cardiac performance and, by altering the metabolic milieu at the peripheral muscle level,[91] may reduce leg discomfort that contributes to exercise limitation in many patients with ILD.[122] Although the effects of oxygen on each of these individual components is relatively

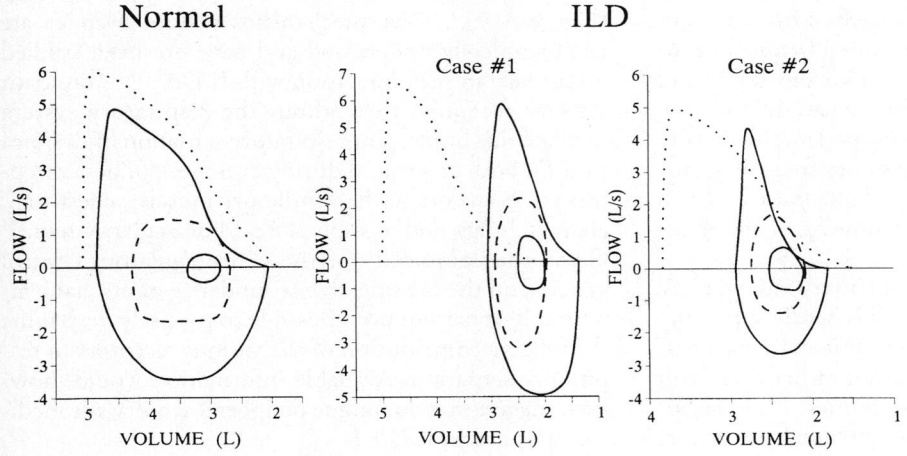

Figure 3–6 Typical flow-volume curves are shown in a normal subject and in two patients with interstitial lung disease (ILD). Case 1 has no expiratory flow limitation and adequate reserves of inspiratory and expiratory flow at the end exercise. In Case 2, tidal loops at peak exercise exceed the maximal expiratory envelope. Note the markedly reduced inspiratory reserve volume (IRV=TLC–EILV) in ILD compared with normal. Maximal and tidal loops at rest (*solid lines*), tidal loops at peak exercise (*dotted lines*), predicted normal maximal expiratory loops (*dotted lines*). Adapted from reference 97.

modest, cumulative favorable effects result in clinically meaningful improvements in exercise performance.

Supervised exercise training is another intervention that has been shown to improve exercise performance in ILD.[125] Based on our knowledge of the effects of exercise training in other chronic pulmonary disease (eg, COPD),[126,127] improved exercise performance in ILD probably results from improved aerobic capacity and reduced lactate accumulation, improved mechanical efficiency, improved breathing pattern, reduced ventilatory demand with reduced exertional dyspnea, as well as improved cardiac performance, increased strength, and endurance of peripheral muscles with reduced leg discomfort. Finally, exercise training leads to positive psychological benefits such as increased tolerance to exertional symptoms or improved motivation.[126,127]

SLEEP AND INTERSTITIAL LUNG DISEASE

There is an important interaction between interstitial lung disease and sleep. Changes in respiratory function occur during sleep in patients with interstitial lung disease, and, reciprocally, interstitial lung disease is associated with disruption of the normal sleep pattern. When breathing patterns during wakefulness and sleep were compared between 11 patients with ILD and 11 age- and sex-matched controls, the patients with ILD were noted to sustain much of their higher waking respiratory frequency during sleep.[128] Patients with ILD in the latter study had a higher breathing frequency (21/min vs 16/min) with consequent shorter TI, TE, and TTOT than normal subjects during wakefulness and sleep (but similar TI/TTOT values), but there was no systematic change in the respiratory pattern of the group with ILD during sleep. Hypoxic ventilatory stimulation in the group with ILD may have obscured changes in the breathing pattern during sleep in the latter study. Shea and colleagues[129] administered supplemental oxygen to patients with ILD to alleviate nocturnal hypoxemia. In comparison with wakefulness, patients with ILD demonstrated a fall in minute ventilation, a decrease in breathing frequency, and prolongation of TE during deep (slow wave, delta) sleep.[129] Interestingly, although patients with ILD continued to demonstrate a higher breathing frequency during wakefulness in the latter study, with shorter TI and TE than normal subjects, these differences did not persist during sleep. Thus, hypoxemic patients with ILD maintain their higher waking respiratory frequency during sleep, but the addition of supplemental oxygen in these patients is associated with a slowing of the respiratory rate during (deep) sleep. Since V/Q inequalities are the primary mechanism responsible for hypoxemia in ILD, it is hardly surprising that the degree of nocturnal hypoxemia correlates best with resting awake oxygen saturation, rather than with derangements in awake lung mechanics.[130–132] Sleep-related hypoxemia in ILD is generally much less severe than that observed during exercise,[133] and although brief episodes of hypoxemia are common, prolonged periods of clinically significant hypoxemia during sleep are unusual in patients with ILD.[133,134] Several possible mechanisms are likely to contribute to nocturnal hypoxemia in patients with ILD, although it must be emphasized that, to date, these mechanisms remain largely unexplored in this patient group. There is a fall in the functional residual capacity of approximately 20% on changing from the erect to the supine position in normal subjects,[135] and a further fall in the FRC of approximately 10% during sleep.[136] The existing ventilation-perfusion inhomogeneity in the recumbent sleeping patient with ILD would reasonably be expected to worsen as the FRC approaches or descends below the closing volume. In addition, minute ventilation and tidal volume are highly variable during rapid eye movement (REM) sleep in patients with ILD,[131] just as in normal subjects. The nadir of the overnight oxygen saturation in patients with ILD coincides with transient decrements in the tidal volume during REM sleep.[131] Thus, it seems likely that the physiologic mechanism for the transient episodes of hypoxemia observed during REM sleep in patients with ILD, is episodic alveolar hypoventilation superimposed on existing V̇/Q̇ inequalities.

Sleep quality is worse in patients with ILD, with more arousals and time spent in stage 1 (very light) sleep and less time spent in REM sleep compared with normal subjects.[128] Patients with more severe hypoxemia had worse sleep quality in the latter study. More recently, in a survey of 48 patients with ILD, the presence of nocturnal hypoxemia was strongly associated with an increase in subjective complaints of decreased energy levels and impaired daytime social and physical functioning, and this effect was independent of the measured vital capacity.[132]

MECHANISMS OF DYSPNEA

Exertional dyspnea is the principal presenting symptom in ILD.[137] Dyspnea, leg discomfort, or a combination of both, contribute heavily to exercise intolerance in ILD (Figure 3–7).[122] The mechanisms behind dyspnea are not completely understood and have not been studied extensively in the population with ILD.[138,139] Abundant sensory receptors throughout the respiratory system mediate this unpleasant respiratory sensation of dyspnea in ILD, both at rest and during exercise.[140] These receptors are in the brain, the ventilatory muscles, chest wall, airways, lungs, and possibly the cardiovascular system.[131] Given the complexity of the neuroregulatory control system and the considerable redundancy of mechanisms within it, it has not been possible to precisely determine the relative contribution of the various receptors to respiratory sensation. Available information would, however, suggest that no unique peripheral sensory site mediates dyspnea in ILD.[138]

Current unitary concepts of the origins of dyspnea emphasize the importance of (1) central mechanisms such as increased respiratory motor command output[98,141–143] and (2) a mismatch in the relationship between motor command (or efferent) output and multiple afferent inputs from activated peripheral mechanoreceptors throughout the respiratory system.[97,138] The latter disparity of motor command output to the mechanical response has been termed "neuromechanical dissociation" (Figure 3–8).[138] Several recent studies suggest a potential basis for the conscious appreciation of central motor command output (via corollary discharge) and of afferent information from mechanoreceptors in the muscles, chest wall, airways, and lung.[144–148]

In ILD, strong statistical correlations have been demonstrated between ratings of dyspnea intensity during exercise and physiologic indices of motor output, such as esophageal pressure expressed as a fraction of maximal inspiratory pressure (Pes/PI_{max}).[148] Such correlations suggest that exertional dyspnea in ILD is a function of the heightened inspiratory muscle contractile effort (relative to maximal possible effort) that occurs as a consequence of increased elastic load.[98,148] The sense of inspiratory effort is believed to share the same neurophysiologic basis as the sense of muscular effort in general; it is readily distinguishable from the sense of muscle tension and displacement.[146,147] Some propose that inspiratory effort at a certain critical level is perceived as discomfort by patients with ILD. Whereas there is little doubt that dyspnea in ILD is a function of the absolute level of respiratory effort or amplitude of medullary respiratory drive, we have recently argued that some of the most important qualitative dimensions of dyspnea in ILD result from the disparity between the increased expended effort and the resultant blunted mechanical response (ie, instantaneous changes in respiratory flow or volume) (see Figure 3–8).[97]

The relationship between effort (Pes/PI_{max}) and the mechanical response (ie, extent of inspiratory muscle shortening as expressed by V_T as a fraction of VC or IC) is an index of "neuromechanical coupling" (see Figure 3–8). In normal subjects, from rest to symptom-limited peak exercise, this relationship is constant since V_T throughout exercise is positioned on the linear portion of the respiratory systems P-V relation (see Figure 3–4). Although normal subjects report an increased sense of effort at higher levels of exercise, they very rarely report the distressing sensation of unsatisfied inspiratory effort and inspiratory difficulty that are the predominant qualitative sensation in ILD.[97] In patients with ILD, the relationship between Pes/PI_{max} and V_T/VC or V_T/IC becomes increasingly disparate as exercise progresses because IC is markedly reduced; the V_T/IC ratio approaches unity, and $EILV_{dyn}$ increasingly encroaches on the upper nonlinear extreme of the contracted respiratory systems P-V curve. It appears that neuromechanical dissociation contributes to the distressing sensations of unsatisfied inspiratory effort and inspiratory difficulties commonly experienced in ILD. Unsatisfied inspiratory effort may have its psychophysical basis in the conscious awareness of a disparity between corollary discharge and afferent feedback from multiple mechanoreceptors. These mechanoreceptors provide precise proprioceptive information about muscle and chest wall displacement (muscle spindles and joint receptors), inspiratory muscle tension development (Golgi tendon organs), and changes in respiratory flow or volume (vagal airway and pulmonary receptors).[140]

Clinical studies on the causes of dyspnea in ILD have determined that the intensity of dyspnea during exercise rises as a function of the $\dot{V}E/MVV$ ratio.[97,102] This correlation can be predicted, since high $\dot{V}E/MVV$ ratios crudely reflect increased respiratory drive. The DL_{CO} is a coarse indicator of the degree of $\dot{V}/\dot{Q}$ inhomogeneity and a predictor of arterial oxygen desaturation during exercise.[52,53,58] It has been shown to correlate significantly with chronic activity-related dyspnea ratings, such as the Baseline Dyspnea Index.[149] Thus, the DL_{CO} is one of the best resting physiologic correlates of dyspnea.[149]

The role of chemoreceptor activation in dyspnea in ILD is not fully understood. There is evidence that chemoreceptor activation in response to hypoxia or hyper-

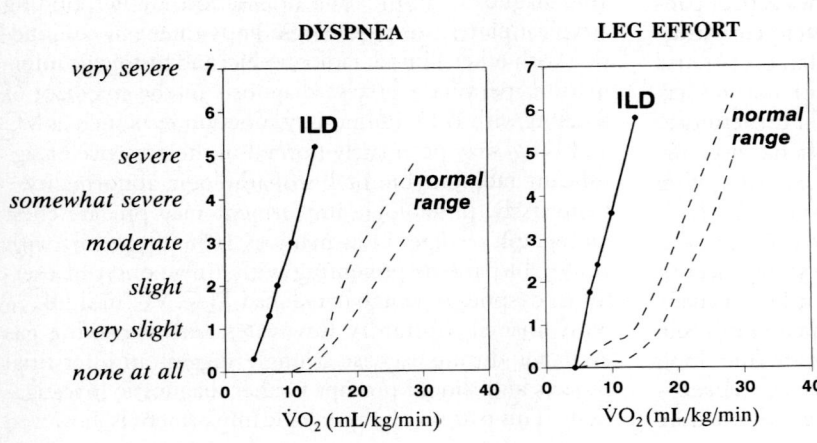

Figure 3–7 The intensity of exertional symptoms of dyspnea and perceived leg effort are shown for patients with interstitial lung disease (ILD) and age-matched normal subjects (range shown is ±1 SEM). Ratings were measured using the modified Borg scale. Adapted from reference 97.

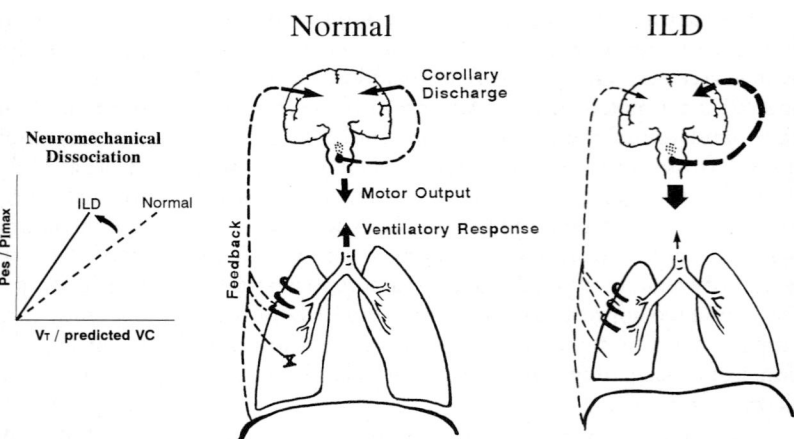

Figure 3–8 Neuromechanical coupling occurs normally when respiratory effort (Pes/PI_{max}) is proportional to the mechanical response (change in respired flow and/or volume). Neuromechanical dissociation occurs in ILD when the respiratory effort is dysproportionally high for the mechanical response achieved; this may form the basis for the distressing sensations of inspiratory difficulty and unsatisfied inspiratory effort in ILD.

capnia causes dyspnea only in proportion to the increase in ventilation.[150,151] Supplemental oxygen has been shown to relieve dyspnea both at rest[152] and during exercise[90] in ILD perhaps due to improved oxygen delivery, delayed anerobic threshold, and reduced ventilation.[91]

The contribution of mechanical factors to exertional dyspnea in ILD has only recently received attention. Exertional dyspnea ratings in ILD correlate well with the V_T/IC ratio, which is a measure of the mechanical constraints on volume expansion.[97] Marciniuk and colleagues[102] have shown that patients with ILD and concomitant expiratory flow limitation during exercise (as assessed by exercise flow-volume curve analysis) have greater levels of exertional breathlessness than those with a comparable baseline restrictive ventilatory deficit but who do not have flow limitation.[102] There is little information to implicate peripheral mechanoreceptors in the airways (or lungs), whose afferent information is carried in the vagus nerve, in the causation of dyspnea in ILD.[93,94,140] Juxtacapillary (J) receptors, are supplied by unmyelinated C fibers and are thought to be activated in response to interstitial fluid accumulation or mechanical distortion.[93,94,140] Juxtacapillary receptor stimulation has been shown to have a tachypneic influence on ventilation in animals.[140] The importance of vagal pathways, in general and in mediating ventilatory responses to exercise, has, however, recently been questioned, particularly in view of the findings of an intact ventilatory response to exercise in vagally denervated (ie, post-transplantation) subjects.[153] In addition, vagal blockade has highly variable effects on dyspnea at rest.[95] Furthermore, inhalation of aerosolized topical anesthesia has no consistent effect on perceived dyspnea in patients with restrictive lung disease[154] or in normal subjects.[155]

The conditions under which dyspnea occurs in the clinical setting are well established. Dyspnea occurs when ventilatory demand is increased relative to capacity, when the ventilatory muscles are impeded in their action, and when the ventilatory muscles are functionally weakened. All these conditions apply in the exercising patient with ILD. Thus, any intervention that would reduce ventilatory demand, improve ventilatory capacity, reduce the mechanical load, or increase the functional strength of weakened ventilatory muscles, should alleviate dyspnea. Therapeutic interventions that have the potential to relieve exertional dyspnea by reducing ventilatory demand include oxygen therapy,[90] exercise training,[125–127] and opiate medication[156] (Figure 3–9). Interventions that reduce the mechanical load include steroids, which reduce the elastic load, and bronchodilators, which decrease the resistive load in patients with coexistent reversible airways obstruction. Finally, specific inspiratory muscle training may strengthen the ventilatory muscles in patients with ILD who have overt inspiratory muscle weakness.[157] Strengthening ventilatory muscles should translate in the sensory domain to reduced dyspnea because less motor output means less effort is required by the muscles to generate a given force.[158,159]

CLINICAL UTILITY OF PHYSIOLOGIC MEASUREMENT

Clinicians use physiologic measurements extensively to (1) aid diagnosis, (2) assess disease severity, (3) evaluate the response to therapy, and (4) follow the course of the illness. Pulmonary function tests do not provide specific diagnostic information in isolation. Rather, finding a typical pattern of physiologic impairment in conjunction with other clinical, radiographic, and histologic information, permits a precise diagnosis in the majority of patients with ILD. Pulmonary function tests such as VC and DI_{CO} may be entirely normal in the presence of significant radiographic or histopathologic abnormality.[23] Conversely, physiologic impairment may predate chest radiograph changes in as many as 10% of patients with ILD.[22] In patients presenting with a new onset of exertional dyspnea or cough, a reduced TLC, VC, and DL_{CO}, with normal expiratory flow rates and worsening gas exchange during exercise strongly suggest an interstitial process and should prompt further diagnostic investigations. This pattern of physiologic impairment is, however, nonspecific for ILD and may occur in a number of other disorders characterized by a restrictive ventilatory deficit. Vital capacity is reduced in chest wall restriction, lung resection, neuromuscular disease, and in nonfibrotic interstitial processes within the lung. In addition, DL_{CO} may be reduced in pulmonary vascular disease, anemia, and emphysema. Similarly, although arterial oxygen desaturation with increased $P_{(A-a)}O_2$ during exercise in the presence of normal resting arterial blood gases is characteristic of ILD,[52-54] it is not specific and can occur in other disorders such as emphysema and pulmonary vascular disease.

More extensive mechanical studies such as static expiratory pressure-volume curves have been employed as a means of differentiating among the restrictive diseases category (ie, ILD versus neuromuscular disease).[96] Peak transpulmonary pressures are much lower at TLC in patients with restriction that results from inspiratory muscle weakness, whereas these pressures are greatly elevated if the restriction is the result of ILD (increased recoil).[96] In patients with chest wall disorder, the slope of the static P-V relation is normal compared with the reduced slope in ILD. Such tests currently have little practical utility, particularly since more direct tests of static inspiratory muscle strength are available and because advances in radiographic imaging technology (ie, high-resolution CT scans) delineate incipient interstitial disease. Similarly, the utility of invasive physiologic measurements of upstream resistance[39] or closing volume[45] that assess small airway function or tests of ventilation perfusion inhomogeneity[70] is questionable. Although these tests provide valuable, quantitative information about a given individual's level of physiologic impairment, they have no diagnostic specificity.

Thus, simple pulmonary function tests such as the static lung volumes and DI_{CO} provide reliable information about disease severity at the time of measurement; reference values have been provided by the American Thoracic Society.[160] Trend graphs that plot changes in the various relevant physiologic parameters over time are, of course, more useful in profiling an individual's disease behavior than are "spot" tests.

Differential Diagnosis

Many attempts have been made to identify distinguishable patterns of physiologic impairment among the different interstitial diseases. Although intriguing differences among various diseases in the ILD designation have been uncovered in some studies, the considerable overlap in the findings preclude any diagnostic specificity or sensitivity. Examples of physiologic differences in ILD include elevation of the RV (in absolute terms) as a result of small airway involvement in diseases such as asbestos,[15,161,162] silicosis,[40] and hypersensitivity pneumonitis,[48] compared with the RV in idiopathic pulmonary fibrosis, which is relatively decreased in some studies.[18] Patients with pulmonary sarcoidosis are more likely to have a reduced FEV_1/FVC ratio compared with other ILDs, because the granulomatous process is more likely to involve the bronchial tree.[9,163,164] Some studies show that patients with idiopathic pulmonary fibrosis (IPF) have greater gas exchange abnormalities than those with sarcoidosis or histiocytosis X for a similar degree of reduction in VC and DL_{CO}.[79,83,165] Reduction in DL_{CO} was shown to be greater in IPF than sarcoidosis or asbestosis for a similar reduc-

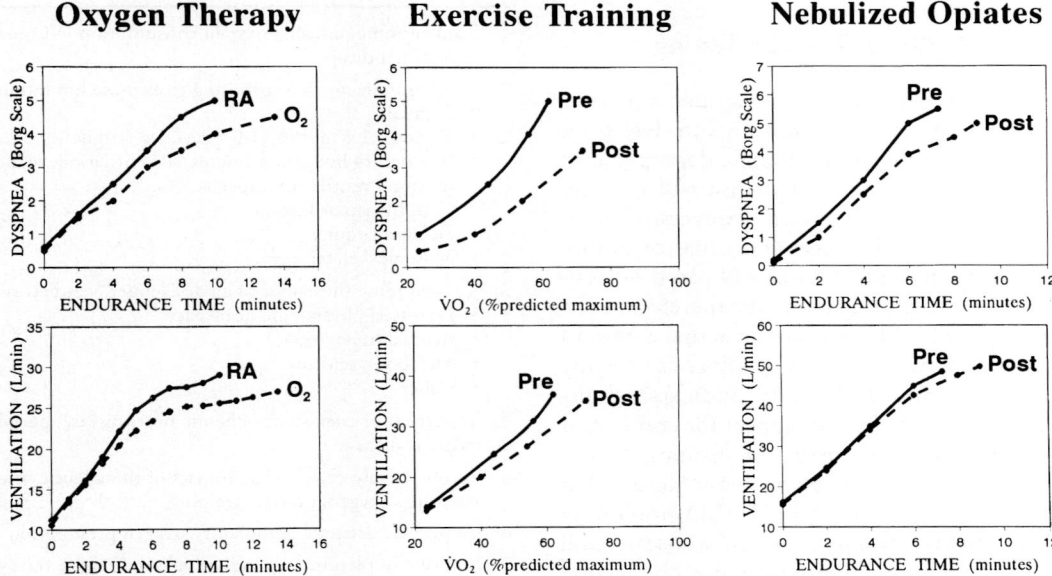

Figure 3–9 Typical responses to therapeutic interventions (oxygen, exercise training, nebulized morphine) are shown in patients with interstitial lung disease. Dyspnea was reduced in all cases despite the presence or absence of significant changes in ventilation. Abbreviations: RA=room air; O_2=60% oxygen.

tion in VC.[55] Hanley and colleagues[36] have shown differences in the shape and position of the static P-V curve of the lung in sarcoidosis compared with IPF. These differences are believed to be due to the different effects of cigarette smoking in the two conditions: in IPF, smoking causes an upward shift to the left, whereas in sarcoidosis, it causes a downward shift to the right in the P-V relation.[36] The apparent mechanical advantage in patients with IPF who smoke (ie, reduced elastic loading) is very probably negated by the combined detrimental effects of smoking and the native lung disease process on gas exchange. It is generally accepted that such mechanical studies do not provide sufficient diagnostic specificity to justify their routine use in clinical practice.

Other patterns of physiologic impairment that are typical but not diagnostic include the propensity for a mixed obstructive-restrictive ventilatory deficit in conditions such as bronchiolitis obliterans (where hyperinflation and an upward left shift of the P-V curve may occur),[166] eosinophilic granuloma,[167,168] and lymphangioleiomyomatosis.[169] Mixed obstructive-restrictive patterns can, however, occur in other interstitial diseases and in people with a coexistent smoking history. It has been shown that additional inspiratory muscle weakness can contribute to pulmonary restriction in ILD as a result of connective tissue disorders such as systemic lupus erythematosus (SLE)[170,171] and polymyositis/dermatomyositis. Again, concomitant reduction in static muscle strength is nondiagnostic because inspiratory muscle weakness can occur for a variety of reasons (ie, steroids, malnutrition, etc) in other disorders within ILD. The pattern of abnormalities in the cardiorespiratory responses to exercise is also not significantly different among the various interstitial disorders and is not useful in differential diagnosis.

Clinical Utility of Exercise Testing

Exercise testing has repeatedly demonstrated superiority over resting pulmonary function tests in determining the nature and extent of physiologic derangements in ILD (Table 3–2).[53,79,83,165,168] Exercise will uncover problems of gas exchange not evident from resting arterial blood gases.[55,79,83,165] Exercise performance cannot be predicted in any individual with ILD based on resting pulmonary function measurements, therefore, exercise tests are required to determine the actual extent of exercise curtailment (ie, peak $\dot{V}O_2$). Exercise testing also objectively measures the level of handicap and disability in patients with ILD who appeal for compensation from employers, government, or insurance companies. It reveals unsuspected physiologic factors that contribute to exercise intolerance in ILD, including coexistent heart disease, peripheral vascular disease, and musculoskeletal problems. In addition, exercise testing is necessary to accurately prescribe ambulatory oxygen. It is also helpful in the evaluation of subjective or objective physiologic response to therapeutic intervention

(to follow). Although the role of exercise testing in evaluating the therapeutic response to steroid medication has not been determined conclusively, many clinicians believe that because gas exchange abnormalities during exercise correlate well with histopathologic severity,[37] serial exercise tests can be useful in evaluating the response to therapy over the course of the illness.

Response to Therapy: The Value of Physiologic Measurement

A preponderance of inflammatory features (ie, increased cellularity) versus fibrosis on lung biopsy specimens is the best predictor of the response to steroid therapy in ILD.[27,29] No physiologic parameter has been shown to reliably predict the extent of cellularity or the likelihood of a positive therapeutic response within a given individual with ILD. Although the VC correlates with the extent of fibrosis and pathophysiologic severity on lung biopsy in some studies,[7,27,172] baseline VC is a poor predictor of therapeutic response in both IPF[27,173,174] and sarcoidosis.[175] Similarly, the DL_{CO} is not useful in predicting the response to treatment in these diseases.[174,175] In IPF, mechanical measurements (ie, lung compliance, coefficient of retraction, maximal transpulmonary pressures) have been shown to correlate well with the degree of fibrosis.[7] These measurements cannot, however, exclude coexisting active inflammation and have not been shown to predict therapeutic response.[176] The

TABLE 3–2   Clinical Utility of Exercise Testing in Interstitial Lung Disease

1. To determine maximal oxygen consumption ($\dot{V}O_2max$) and level of handicap

2. To identify factors contributing to exercise limitation in a given individual:
   - Exertional symptoms (dyspnea, leg fatigue)
   - Ventilatory limitation (increased ventilation, reduced maximal ventilatory capacity)
   - Cardiovascular factors
   - Deconditioning
   - Musculoskeletal factors

3. To determine the causes of an accelerated ventilatory response:
   - Increased physiologic deadspace
   - Arterial hypoxemia
   - Metabolic acidosis
   - Other

4. To screen for coexistent ischemic heart disease, peripheral vascular disease

5. To objectively evaluate the impact of therapeutic interventions (steroids, oxygen, exercise training)

6. To provide accurate ambulatory oxygen prescription

7. To assist in planning an individualized exercise training schedule

8. To assess for lung transplantation

9. To provide objective disability assessment

change in $P_{(A-a)}O_2$ during exercise shows a significantly better correlation with the indices of pathologic severity on biopsy specimens than chest radiography, VC, DL_{CO}, and resting PO_2.[7,27] The exercise $P_{(A-a)}O_2$ has not, however, been shown to reliably predict the response to therapy.[27,177,178] Documented improvement in exercise gas exchange measurements following steroid therapy may persuade clinicians (and patients) to persevere with steroid therapy for a longer duration, particularly in those patients with more marginal improvements of mechanics and resting gas exchange. These theoretical advantages of exercise testing over resting measurements notwithstanding, sufficient data to recommend the routine use of exercise testing in clinical management does not exist.

In practice, clinicians rely on simple serial measurements of static lung volume and DL_{CO} to determine a therapeutic response in the context of a broader clinical evaluation, including radiography. Improvements in the VC and DL_{CO} in the range of 10 to 20% are generally considered clinically meaningful. It has been suggested that VC is superior to DL_{CO} in monitoring the response to steroid therapy in patients with sarcoidosis[179,180] and asbestosis,[181] since improvement in VC is often more common and of greater magnitude than improvement in DL_{CO} in these conditions.[179–181] In many patients, however, these parameters improve together following therapy.[179–181] Ideally, evaluation of therapy should depend on a composite index, which includes a semiquantitative analysis of dyspnea relief, improvement in mechanics and gas exchange, and improved pathophysiology.

A recent International Consensus Statement[182] has suggested criteria for determining a favorable treatment response in patients with IPF. The criteria include two or more of the following, documented on two consecutive visits over a 3- to 6-month period:

- A decrease in symptoms, specifically an increase in the level of exertion required before the patient must stop because of breathlessness or a decline in the frequency or severity of cough
- Reduction of parenchymal abnormalities on chest radiograph or high-resolution CT scan
- Physiologic improvement defined by two or more of the following:
  - $\geq$ 10% increase in TLC or VC (or at least 200 mL change)
  - $\geq$ 15% increase in DL_{CO} (or at least 3 mL/min/mm Hg)
  - An improvement or normalization of the oxygen saturation ($\geq$ 4% increase in measured oxygen saturation) or PaO_2 ($\geq$ 4 mm Hg increase from the previous measurement) achieved during a formal cardiopulmonary exercise test

In patients with more advanced, irreversible ILD, alleviation of dyspnea and improvement in exercise tolerance should be the primary goals of management.

Exercise testing with concomitant dyspnea evaluation (Borg scale) can be useful in objectively assessing therapeutic responses to such interventions as oxygen, opiates, exercise training, and other measures in this group (see Figure 3–9). Using n = 1 case studies employing constant-load submaximal exercise test (ie, treadmill, cycle, six-minute walking distance), with the patient blinded to the intervention (ie, nebulized opiates versus saline; supplemental oxygen versus room air), clinicians can readily identify true subjective and objective responses to treatment. Slopes of dyspnea (Borg scale values) over time during exercise are highly reproducible and responsive to interventions (see Figure 3–7), and cardiorespiratory responses to incremental exercise in ILD have also been shown to be highly reproducible.[183]

Physiologic Measurements and Prognosis

The highly variable course of ILD and the factors that determine length of survival are complexly inter-related. Several studies have examined physiologic measurements and other factors in predicting morbidity and mortality.[23,28,177,178,183,184] The importance of the various physiologic and nonphysiologic factors in prognosis await the results of longitudinal studies in large well-defined populations of ILD. Such analyses should help to clarify the relationship between severity of pulmonary pathology, level of physiologic impairment, symptomatology, and survival. Important prognostic factors in ILD include (1) disease-specific factors (eg, propensity to develop lung malignancy), (2) gender issues,[28,184] (3) intensity of dyspnea,[184] (4) extent of radiographic interstitial change,[184] (5) age of onset,[28,184] and (6) baseline pulmonary function tests.[178] Favorable prognostic factors include female gender, younger age of onset, early diagnosis, response to corticosteroids, and minor radiographic abnormalities.[28,184] Differences in prognostic factors between various studies may, in part, reflect differences in the mean age of study populations, which tend to vary greatly between studies.[28,178,184] Thus, some differences in the prognostic factors between studies may disappear if pulmonary function parameters, including resting PaO_2, are expressed as a percent of predicted (or are age corrected) rather than as absolute measurements.

Generally speaking, reduced VC and DL_{CO} in IPF predict reduced survival.[23,174,177,178] Furthermore, studies have shown that patient groups who fail to improve the VC in response to steroid therapy within the first year of treatment have reduced survival.[174,177,185] Hanson and colleagues[177] have recently shown a survival advantage if the VC increased by more than 10% or if the DL_{CO} increased by more than 20% after one year of therapy.[177] In a number of studies, decreased resting PaO_2 has predicted decreased survival.[28,111,183] The PaO_2 also correlates with the level of pulmonary hypertension. Panos and colleagues[186] have shown that a VC less than 50% predicted and a DL$_{CO}$ less than 45% predicted appear to be associated with significant pulmonary hypertension. A P$_{pa}$ greater than 30 mm Hg has been shown to be associated with a poor 2-year survival in both IPF[23] and silicosis.[187] Erbes and colleagues[178] have recently demonstrated that in IPF, TLC and VC held greater prognostic value than the DL$_{CO}$ alone, when the latter is expressed in absolute terms or has been corrected for lung volume. The PaO$_2$ at rest and during exercise and the exercise P$_{(A-a)}$O$_2$ were not of useful prognosis value in that study.[178] Similarly, Hanson and colleagues[177] did not find correlation between changes in P$_{(A-a)}$O$_2$ after one year of therapy and survival in 58 patients with IPF. Collectively, these studies suggest that simple VC and DL$_{CO}$ measurement may yield more useful information than more invasive measurements in the follow-up of patients with ILD.[188] These measurements provide important prognostic information and help evaluate therapeutic responsiveness.

SUMMARY

Interstitial lung diseases, despite their diversity, show a common pattern of physiologic impairment. The hallmark of the disease is increased lung recoil, which is principally the result of a reduction in functional alveolar units as a result of the disease process. Reduced lung compliance accounts for the typically reduced static lung volume measurements in ILD; VC is relatively more decreased than TLC, FRC, and RV. Airway function is generally well preserved in ILD, as reflected by the normal or increased expiratory flow rates at a given volume. Small airway involvement in various interstitial diseases is not uncommon and contributes to the exaggerated frequency-dependence of dynamic compliance found in ILD. This, in turn, leads to regional inhomogeneity in ventilation. Resting hypoxemia, with or without alveolar hyperventilation, in association with a reduced volume-corrected DL$_{CO}$, is typically found in ILD. Worsening hypoxemia during exercise is characteristic and occurs as a result of diffusion limitation and high mixed venous P$_v$O$_2$ in the setting of low $\dot{V}/\dot{Q}$ abnormalities. Hypercapnia is distinctly unusual, except in end-stage ILD. Exercise intolerance is invariable in advanced disease and is multifactorial. Potentially reversible factors can be identified on exercise testing. Ventilatory limitation is more likely to contribute to exercise intolerance than is cardiac limitation. Patients with ILD have an accelerated ventilatory response due to high V$_D$/V$_T$, hypoxemia, and, in some cases, early metabolic acidosis. Peak ventilation is diminished due to mechanical derangement. The elastic work of breathing is increased and patients adopt a rapid, shallow breathing pattern that reflects the serious mechanical constraints on volume expansion as a result of high-end P-V alinearities. The true prevalence of inspiratory muscle weakness in ILD is unknown, but many patients have preserved their inspiratory muscle strength. Exertional dyspnea, the most common symptom in ILD, has its basis in the increased amplitude of central motor command output in the setting of a restricted mechanical response of the ventilatory system. The main cardiovascular abnormality is increased pulmonary vascular resistance with increased pulmonary artery pressure, eventual right ventricular hypertrophy, and cor pulmonale. Left ventricular function is preserved except in situations in which there is cardiac involvement in the disease process.

The prognosis in ILD is highly variable and multifactorial. Physiologic measurements that predict mortality include reduced static lung volumes, resting arterial hypoxemia, and pulmonary hypertension. Vital capacity and DL$_{CO}$ are useful in following the course of ILD and appear to be more useful than other, more invasive measurements. A response to therapy cannot reliably be predicted from baseline physiologic measurements. Although the extent of gas exchange impairment during exercise correlates well with histopathologic severity in lung biopsy specimens, such tests have not been shown to predict morbidity, mortality, or therapeutic response. Physiologic measurements do not provide diagnostic specificity or sensitivity, but in conjunction with the broader clinical, radiographic, and histopathologic evaluations, they allow physicians to optimally manage patients with ILD.

REFERENCES

1. Macklem PT, Becklake MR. The relationship between mechanical and diffusing properties of the lung in health and disease. Am Rev Respir Dis 1963;87:47–56.
2. Schlueter DP, Immekus J, Stead WW. Relationship between maximal inspiratory pressure and total lung capacity (coefficient of retraction) in normal subjects and in patients with emphysema, asthma, and diffuse pulmonary infiltration. Am Rev Respir Dis 1967;96:656–65.
3. Glaister DH, Schroter RC, Sudlow MF, Milic-Emili J. Bulk elastic properties of excised lungs and the effect of a transpulmonary pressure gradient. Respir Physiol 1973;17:347–64.
4. Gibson GN, Pride NB, Davis J, Schroter RC. Exponential description of the static pressure-volume curve of normal and diseased lung. Am Rev Respir Dis 1979;120:799–811.
5. Yernault JC, deJonghe M, de Coster A, Englert M. Pulmonary mechanics in diffuse fibrosing alveolitis. Bull Eur Physiopathol Respir 1975;11:231–44.
6. Dutton RE, Renzi PM, Lopez-Majano V, Renzi GD. Total and regional lung function in sarcoidosis. Ann N Y Acad Sci 1986;465:502–14.
7. Fulmer JD, Roberts WC, von Gal ER, Crystal RG. Morphologic-physiologic correlates of the severity of fibrosis and degree of cellularity in idiopathic pulmonary fibrosis. J Clin Invest Med 1979;63:665–76.
8. Bjerke RD, Tashkin DP, Clements PJ, et al. Small airways in progressive systemic sclerosis (PSS). Am J Med 1979;66:201–9.
9. Levinson S, Metzger LF, Stanley NN, et al. Airway function in sarcoidosis. Am J Med 1977;62:51–9.
10. Gibson GJ, Pride NB. Pulmonary mechanics in fibrosing alveolitis: the effects of lung shrinkage. Am Rev Respir Dis 1977;116:637–47.

11. De Troyer A, Yernault J-C. Inspiratory muscle force in normal subjects and patients with interstitial lung disease. Thorax 1980;35:92–100.

12. West JR, Alexander JK. Studies on respiratory mechanics and the work of breathing in pulmonary fibrosis. Am J Med 1959;27:529–44.

13. Snider GL, Doctor LR. The mechanics of ventilation in sarcoidosis. Am Rev Respir Dis 1964;89:897–908.

14. Salazar E, Knowles JH. An analysis of pressure-volume characteristics of the lungs. J Appl Physiol 1964;19:97–104.

15. Colebatch HJH, Ng CKY, Nikov N. Use of an exponential function for elastic recoil. J Appl Physiol 1979;46:387–93.

16. Knudson RJ, Kaltenborn WT. Evaluation of lung elastic recoil by exponential curve analysis. Respir Physiol 1981;46:29–42.

17. Mead J. Mechanical properties of the lung. Physiol Rev 1961;41:281–330.

18. Thompson MJ, Colebatch HJH. Decreased pulmonary distensibility in fibrosing alveolitis and its relation to decreased lung volume. Thorax 1989;44:725–31.

19. Haber PS, Colebatch HJH, Ng CKY, Greaves IA. Alveolar size as a determinant of pulmonary distensibility in mammalian lungs. J Appl Physiol 1983;54:837–45.

20. McCormack FX, King TE Jr, Voelker DR, et al. Idiopathic pulmonary fibrosis: abnormalities in the bronchoalveolar lavage content of surfactant protein A. Am Rev Respir Dis 1991;144:160–6.

21. Robinson PC, Watters LC, King TE, Mason RJ. Idiopathic pulmonary fibrosis: abnormalities in bronchoalveolar lavage fluid phospholipids. Am Rev Respir Dis 1988;137:585–91.

22. Epler GR, McLoud TC, Gaensler EA, et al. Normal chest roentgenograms in chronic diffuse infiltrative lung disease. N Engl J Med 1978;298:934–9.

23. Jezek V, Fucik J, Michaljanic A, Jezkova L. The prognostic significance of functional tests in kryptogenic fibrosing alveolitis. Bull Eur Physiolpathol Respir 1980;16:711–20.

24. Spencer H. Pathogenesis of interstitial fibrosis of the lung. Prog Respir Res 1975;8:34–44.

25. Liebow AA. Definition and classification of interstitial pneumonias in human pathology. Prog Respir Res 1975;8:1–33.

26. Flint A. Pathologic features of interstitial lung disease. In: Schwarz MI, King TE Jr, editors. Interstitial lung disease. Toronto: BC Decker; 1988. p. 45–62.

27. Carrington CB, Gaensler EA, Coutu RE, et al. Natural history and treated course of usual and desquamative interstitial pneumonia. N Engl J Med 1978;298:801–9.

28. Tukiainen P, Taskinen E, Holsti P, et al. Prognosis of cryptogenic fibrosing alveolitis. Thorax 1983;38:349–55.

29. Gottlieb DJ, Snider GL. Lung function in pulmonary fibrosis. In: Phan SH, Thrall RS, editors. Pulmonary fibrosis. Lung biology in health and disease. New York: Marcel Dekker; 1985. p. 80, 85–135.

30. Brennan NJ, Morris AJR, Green M. Thoracoabdominal mechanics during tidal breathing in normal subjects and in emphysema and fibrosing alevolitis. Thorax 1983;38:62–6.

31. Turner-Warwick M, Burrows B, Johnson A. Cryptogenic fibrosing alveolitis: clinical features and their influence on survival. Thorax 1980;35:171–80.

32. Seal RME. Pathology of extrinsic allergic bronchiolo-alveolitis. Prog Respir Res 1975;8:66–73.

33. Gaensler EA, Mikus JP, Schachter AW, et al. Structure and function in sarcoidosis. Ann N Y Acad Sci 1976;278:265–83.

34. Davis GS, Calhoun WJ. Occupational and environmental causes of interstitial lung disease. In: Schwarz MI, King TE Jr, editors. Interstitial lung disease. Philadelphia: BC Decker; 1988. p. 68–109.

35. Bignon J, Hem B, Molinier B. Morphometic and angiographic studies in diffuse interstitial pulmonary fibrosis. Prog Respir Res 1975;8:141–60.

36. Hanley ME, King TE Jr, Schwarz MI, et al. The impact of smoking on mechanical properties of the lungs in idiopathic pulmonary fibrosis and sarcoidosis. Am Rev Respir Dis 1991;144:1102–6.

37. Fulmer JD, Roberts WC, von Gal ER, Crystal RG. Small airways in idiopathic pulmonary fibrosis: comparison of morphologic and physiologic observations. J Clin Invest 1977;60:595–610.

38. Edward CW, Carlisle A. The larger bronchi in cryptogenic fibrosing alveolitis: a morphometric study. Thorax 1982;37:828–33.

39. Ostrow D, Cherniack RM. Resistance to airflow in patients with diffuse interstitial lung disease. Am Rev Respir Dis 1973;108:205–10.

40. Bohadana AB, Peslin R, Poncelet B, Hannhart B. Lung mechanical properties in silicosis and silicoanthracosis. Bull Eur Physiopathol Respir 1980;16:521–32.

41. Jodoin G, Gibbs GW, Macklem PT, et al. Early effects of asbestos exposure on lung function. Am Rev Respir Dis 1971;104:525–35.

42. Mead J. The lung's "quiet zone." N Engl J Med 1970;282:1318–9.

43. Mead J, Turner JM, Macklem PT, Little JB. Significance of the relationship between lung recoil and maximum expiratory flow. J Appl Physiol 1967;22:95–108.

44. Woolcock AJ, Vincent NJ, Macklem PT. Frequency dependence as a test for obstruction in the small airways. J Clin Invest 1969;48:1097–106.

45. McCarthy DS, Spencer R, Greene R, Milic-Emili J. Measurement of "closing volume" as a simple and sensitive test for early detection of small airway disease. Am J Med 1972;52:747–53.

46. Finucane KE, Prichard MG. Mechanical properties of the lung in diffuse interstitial lung disease. Aust N Z J Med 1984;14:755–61.

47. Seaton A, Lapp NL, Morgan WKC. Lung mechanics and frequency dependence of compliance in coal miners. J Clin Invest 1972;51:1203–11.

48. William JV. Pulmonary function in patients with farmer's lung. Thorax 1963;18:255–363.

49. Todisco T, Matthys H, Cegla UH. Clinical determination of airway closure, comparison of three methods in patients with lung fibrosis. Respiration 1977;34:197–204.

50. Reyes CN, Wenzel FJ, Lawton BR, Emanuel DA. The pulmonary pathology of farmer's lung disease. Chest 1982;81:142–6.

51. Hawrylkiewicz I, Izdebska-Makosa Z, Grebska E, Zielinski J. Pulmonary hemodynamics at rest and on exercise in patients with idiopathic pulmonary fibrosis. Bull Eur Physiopathol Respir 1982;18:403–10.

52. Kelley MA, Panettieri RA Jr, Krupinski AV. Resting single-breath diffusing capacity as a screening test for exercise-induced hypoxemia. Am J Med 1986;80:807–12.

53. Athos L, Mohler JG, Sharma OP. Exercise testing in the physiologic assessment of sarcoidosis. Ann N Y Acad Sci 1986;465:491–501.

54. Agusti AGN, Roca J, Gea J, et al. Mechanisms of gas-exchange impairment in idiopathic pulmonary fibrosis. Am Rev Respir Dis 1991;143:219–25.

55. Dunn TL, Watters LC, Hendrix C, et al. Gas exchange at a given degree of volume restriction is different in sarcoidosis and idiopathic pulmonary fibrosis. Am J Med 1988;85:221–4.

56. Brown LK, Sloane MF, Bauprani A, et al. Cardiorespiratory responses to incremental exercise in sarcoidosis patients with normal spirometry. Chest 1995;107:323–9.

57. Karevzky M, McDonough M. Exercise and resting pulmonary function in sarcoidosis. Sarc Vasc Diffuse Lung Dis 1996;13:43–9.

58. Sue DY, Oren A, Hansen JE, Wasserman K. Diffusion capacity for carbon monoxide as a predictor or gas exchange during exercise. N Engl J Med 1987;316:1301–6.

59. Roughton FJW, Forster RE. Relative importance of diffusion

and chemical reaction rates in determining rate of exchange of gases in the human lung, with special reference to true diffusing capacity of pulmonary membrane and volume of blood in the lung capillaries. J Appl Physiol 1957;11: 291–302.

60. McNeill RS, Rankin J, Forster RE. The diffusing capacity of the pulmonary membrane and the pulmonary capillary blood volume in cardiopulmonary disease. Clin Sci 1958;17:465–82.

61. Hamer J. Cause of low arterial oxygen saturation in pulmonary fibrosis. Thorax 1964;19:507–14.

62. Georges R, Saumon G, Lafosse JE, Turiaf J. Membrane-diffusing capacity and pulmonary capillary blood volume. Prog Respir Res 1975;8:198–212.

63. Lafosse JE, Saumon G, Georges R. Gas exchange model of the lung. Prog Respir Res 1975;8:186–97.

64. Weibel ER. Morphological basis of alveolar-capillary gas exchange. Physiol Rev 1973;53:419–95.

65. Cassan SM, Divertie MB, Brown AL Jr. Fine structural morphometry on biopsy specimens of human lung. Chest 1974;65:275–8.

66. Read J, Williams RS. Pulmonary ventilation. Blood flow relationships in interstitial diseases of the lungs. Am J Med 1959;27:545–50.

67. McCarthy D, Cherniack RM. Regional ventilation-perfusion and hypoxia in cryptogenic fibrosing alveolitis. Am Rev Respir Dis 1973;107:200–8.

68. Ewan PW, Ronchetti R, Hughes JMB. Regional ventilation and ventilation-perfusion ratios in pulmonary fibrosis. Prog Respir Res 1975;8:161–5.

69. Evans JW, Wagner PD. Limits on VA/Q distributions from analysis of experimental inert gas elimination. J Appl Physiol 1977;42:889–98.

70. Wagner PD, Dantzker DR, Dueck R, et al. Distribution of ventilation-perfusion ratios in patients with interstitial lung disease. Chest 1976;69:256–7.

71. Jernudd-Wilhelmsson Y, Hornblad Y, Hedenstierna G. Ventilation-perfusion relationships in interstitial lung disease. Eur J Respir Dis 1986;68:39–49.

72. Eklund A, Broman L, Broman M, Holmgren A. V/Q and alveolar gas exchange in pulmonary sarcoidosis. Eur Respir J 1989;2:135–144.

73. Turner-Warwick M. Precapillary systemic pulmonary anastomoses. Thorax 1963;18:225–37.

74. Livingstone JL, Lewis JG, Reid L, Jefferson KE. Diffuse interstitial pulmonary fibrosis. Q J Med 1964;129:71–103.

75. Kaltreider NL, McCann WS. Respiratory response during exercise in pulmonary fibrosis and emphysema. J Clin Invest 1937;16:23–40.

76. Austrian R, McClement JH, Renzetti AD, et al. Clinical and physiologic features of some types of pulmonary diseases with impairment of alveolar-capillary diffusion. Am J Med 1951;2:267–85.

77. VanMeerhaeghe A, Scane G, Sergysels R, et al. Respiratory drive and ventilatory pattern during exercise in interstitial lung disease. Bull Eur Physiopathol Respir 1981;17:15–26.

78. DiMarco AF, Kelsen SG, Cherniack NS, Goethe B. Occlusion pressure and breathing pattern in patients with interstitial lung disease. Am Rev Respir Dis 1983;127:425–30.

79. Keogh BA, Lakatos E, Price D, Crystal RG. Importance of the lower respiratory tract in oxygen transfer. Exercise testing in patients with interstitial and destructive lung disease. Am Rev Respir Dis 1984;129:S76–80.

80. Spiro GS, Dowdeswell IRG, Clark TJH. An analysis of submaximal exercise responses in patients with sarcoidosis and fibrosing alveolitis. Br J Dis Chest 1981;75:169–80.

81. Burdon JGW, Killian KJ, Jones NL. Pattern of breathing during exercise in patients with interstitial lung disease. Thorax 1983;38:778–84.

82. Jones NL, Rebuck AS. Tidal volume during exercise in patients

with diffuse fibrosing alveolitis. Bull Eur Physiopathol Respir 1979;15:321–7.

83. Risk C, Epler GR, Gaensler EA. Exercise alveolar-arterial oxygen pressure difference in interstitial lung disease. Chest 1984;85:69–74.

84. Johnson RL Jr, Spice WS, Bishop JM, Forster RE. Pulmonary capillary blood volume, flow and diffusing capacity during exercise. J Appl Physiol 1960;15:893–902.

85. Hughes JMB, Lockwood DNA, Jones HA, Clark RJ. DL_{CO}/Q and diffusion limitation at rest and on exercise in patients with interstitial fibrosis. Respir Physiol 1991;83:155–66.

86. Staub NC. Alveolar-arterial oxygen tension gradient due to diffusion. J Appl Physiol 1963;18:673–80.

87. Gale GE, Torre-Bueno JR, Moon RE, et al. Ventilation-perfusion inequality in normal humans during exercise at sea level and simulated altitude. J Appl Physiol 1985;58:978–88.

88. Agusti AGN, Barbera JAR, Wagner PD, et al. Hypoxic pulmonary vasoconstriction and gas exchange during exercise in chronic obstructive pulmonary disease. Chest 1990; 97:268–75.

89. Marciniuk DD, Gallagher CG. Clinical exercise testing in interstitial lung disease. Clin Chest Med 1994;15:287–303.

90. Bye PTB, Anderson SD, Woolcock AJ, et al. Bicycle endurance performances of patients with interstitial lung disease breathing air and oxygen. Am Rev Respir Dis 1982;126: 1005–12.

91. Harris-Eze AO, Sridhar G, Clemens RE, Gallagher CG. Oxygen improves maximal exercise performance in interstitial lung disease. Am J Respir Crit Care Med 1994;150:1616–22.

92. Widimsky J, Riedel M, Stonek V. Central hemodynamics during exercise in patients with restrictive pulmonary disease. Bull Eur Physiopath Respir 1977;13:369–79.

93. Widdicombe JG. Nervous receptors in the respiratory tract and lung. In: Hornbein TD, editor. Regulation of breathing. Vol I. 17th ed. Lung biology in health and disease. New York: Marcel Dekker; 1981. p. 429–72.

94. Paintal AS. Vagal sensory receptors and their reflex effects. Physiol Rev 1973;53:159–227.

95. Guz A, Novel MIM, Eisele JH, Trechard D. Experimental results in vagal block in cardio-pulmonary disease. In: Porter R, editor. Breathing. Hering-Breuer Centenary Symposium. London: Churchill; 1970. p. 15–28.

96. Pride NB, Macklem PT. Lung mechanics in disease. In: Fishman AP, editor. Handbook of physiology. Section 3, Vol III, Part 2. The respiratory system. Bethesda MD: American Physiological Society; 1986. p. 659–92.

97. O'Donnell DE, Chau LKL, Webb KA. Qualitative aspects of exertional dyspnea in patients with interstitial lung disease. J Appl Physiol 1998;84:2000–9.

98. Younes M. Determinants of thoracic excursions during exercise. In: Whipp BJ, Wasserman K, editors. Lung biology in health and disease. Vol 52. Exercise, pulmonary physiology and pathophysiology. New York: Marcel Dekker; 1991. p. 1–65.

99. Younes M, Kininen G. Respiratory mechanics and breathing pattern during and following maximal exercise. J Appl Physiol 1984;57:1773–82.

100. Henke KG, Sharratt M, Pegelow DF, Dempsey JA. Regulation of end-expiratory lung volume during exercise. J Appl Physiol 1988;64:135–46.

101. Lind F, Hesser CM. Breathing pattern and lung volumes during exercise. Acta Physiol Scand 1984;120:123–9.

102. Marciniuk DD, Sridhar G, Clemens RE, et al. Lung volumes and expiratory flow limitation during exercise in interstitial lung disease. J Appl Physiol 1994;77:963–73.

103. Laporta D, Grassino A. Assessment of transdiaphragmatic pressure in humans. J Appl Physiol 1985;58:1469–76.

104. Gallagher CG, Younes M. Breathing pattern during and after maximal exercise in patients with chronic obstructive lung disease, interstitial lung disease and cardiac disease in normal subjects. Am Rev Respir Dis 1986;133:581–6.

105. Weitzenblum E, Ehrhart M, Rasaholinjanahary I, Hirth C. Pulmonary hemodynamics in idiopathic pulmonary fibrosis and other interstitial pulmonary diseases. Respiration 1983;44:118–27.

106. Sturani C, Papiris S, Galavotti V, Gunella G. Pulmonary vascular responsiveness at rest and during exercise in idiopathic pulmonary fibrosis: effects of oxygen and nifedipine. Respiration 1986;50:117–29.

107. Lupi-Herrera E, Seoane M, Verdejo J, et al. Hemodynamic effects of hydralazine in interstitial lung disease patients with cor pulmonale. Chest 1985;87:564–73.

108. Bush A, Busst CM. Cardiovascular function at rest and on exercise in patients with cryptogenic fibrosing alveolitis. Thorax 1988;43:276–83.

109. Pinsky MR. Effects of change in intrathoracic pressure. In: Lenfant C, Scharf SM, Cassidy SS, editors. Lung biology in health and disease: heart-lung interactions in health and disease. New York: Marcel Dekker; 1989. p. 839–76.

110. Rodarte JR. Lung and chest wall mechanics. In: Lenfant C, Scharf SM, Cassidy SS, editors. Lung biology in health and disease: heart-lung interactions in health and disease. New York: Marcel Dekker; 1989. p. 221–42.

111. Jezek V, Michalnanik A, Fucik J, Ramaisl R. Long-term development of pulmonary arterial pressure in diffuse interstitial lung fibrosis. Prog Respir Res 1985;20:170–5.

112. Gurtner HP, Walser P, Fassler B. Normal values for pulmonary hemodynamics at rest and during exercise in man. Prog Respir Res 1975;9:295–315.

113. Enson Y, Thomas HM, Bosken CH, et al. Pulmonary hypertension in interstitial lung disease: relation of vascular resistance to abnormal lung structure. Trans Assoc Am Phys 1975;88:248–55.

114. McLees B, Fulmer J, Adair N, et al. Correlative studies of pulmonary hypertension in idiopathic pulmonary fibrosis. Am Rev Respir Dis 1977;115:354A.

115. Todisco T, Cegla UH, Matthys H. Oxygen breathing during exercise in patients with diffuse interstitial lung fibrosis. Bull Eur Physiopathol Respir 1977;13:387–97.

116. Hyman AL, Higashida RT, Spannhake EW, Kadowitz PJ. Pulmonary vasoconstrictor responses to graded decreases in precapillary blood PO_2 in intact-chest cat. J Appl Physiol 1981;51:1009–16.

117. McDonald IG, Butler J. Distribution of vascular resistance in the isolated perfused dog lung. J Appl Physiol 1967;23:463–74.

118. Baughman PR, Gerson M, Bosken CH. Right and left ventricular function at rest and with exercise in patients with sarcoidosis. Chest 1984;85:301–6.

119. Siverman KJ, Hutchins GM, Bulkey BH. Cardiac sarcoid: a clinicopathologic study of 84 unselected patients with systemic sarcoid. Circulation 1978;58:1204–11.

120. Gibbons WJ, Levy RD, Nava S, et al. Subclinical cardiac dysfunction in sarcoidosis. Chest 1991;100:44–50.

121. Guttadauria M, Ellman H, Kaplan D. Progressive systemic sclerosis: pulmonary involvement. Clin Rheum Dis 1979;5:151–66.

122. Rampulla C, Baiocchi S, Dacosto E, Ambrosino N. Dyspnea on exercise: pathophysiologic mechanisms. Chest 1992;101:248S–52S.

123. Marciniuk DD, Watts RE, Gallagher CG. Dead space loading and exercise limitation in patients with interstitial lung disease. Chest 1994;105:183–9.

124. Morrison DA, Stovall JR. Increased exercise capacity in hypoxemic patients after long-term oxygen therapy. Chest 1992;102:542–50.

125. Foster S, Thomas HM. Pulmonary rehabilitation in lung disease other than chronic obstructive pulmonary disease. Am Rev Respir Dis 1990;141:601–4.

126. Casabrur R, Patessio A, Ioli F, et al. Reductions in exercise lactic acidosis and ventilation as a result of exercise training in patients with obstructive lung disease. Am Rev Respir Dis 1991;143:9–18.

127. O'Donnell DE, McGuire M, Samis L, Webb KA. Impact of exercise reconditioning on breathlessness in severe chronic airflow limitation. Am J Respir Crit Care Med 1995;142:2005–13.

128. Perez-Padilla R, West P, Lertzman M, Kryger MH. Breathing during sleep in patients with interstitial lung disease. Am Rev Respir Dis 1985;132:224–9.

129. Shea SA, Winning AJ, McKenzie E, Guz A. Does the abnormal pattern of breathing in patients with interstitial lung disease persist in deep, non-rapid eye movement sleep. Am Rev Respir Dis 1989;139:653–8.

130. Midgren B, Hansson L. Changes in transcutaneous PCO_2 with sleep in normal subjects and in patients with chronic respiratory diseases. Eur J Respir Dis 1987;71:388–94.

131. Tatsumi K, Kimura H, Kunitomo F, et al. Arterial oxygen desaturation during sleep in interstitial pulmonary disease. Correlation with chemical control of breathing during wakefulness. Chest 1989;95:962–7.

132. Clark M, Cooper B, Singh S, et al. A survey of nocturnal hypoxaemia and health related quality of life in patients with cryptogenic fibrosing alveolitis. Thorax 2001;56:482–6.

133. Midgren B, Hansson L, Eriksson L, et al. Oxygen desaturation during sleep and exercise in patients with interstitial lung disease. Thorax 1987;42:353–6.

134. McNicholas WT, Coffey M, Fitzgerald MX. Ventilation and gas exchange during sleep in patients with interstitial lung disease. Thorax 1986;41:777–82.

135. Agostoni E, Hyatt RE. Static behaviour of the respiratory system. In: Macklem PT, Mead J, editors. Handbook of physiology. Section 3. The respiratory system. Bethesda: Williams & Wilkins; 1986. p. 120.

136. Hudgel DW, Devadatta P. Decrease in functional residual capacity during sleep in normal humans. J Appl Physiol 1984;57:1319–22.

137. Turner-Warwick M, Burrows B, Johnson A. Crytogenic fibrosing alveolitis: clinical features and their influence on survival. Thorax 1980;35:171–80.

138. O'Donnell DE. Mechanism of exertional dyspnea in chronic lung diseases. In: Mahler DA, editor. Dyspnea. Lung biology in health and disease. New York: Marcel Dekker 1998;11:97–147.

139. Ogosvoni P, Smith DD, Schoene RB, et al. Evaluation of breathlessness in asbestos workers. Results of exercise testing. Am Rev Respir Dis 1987;135:812–6.

140. Zechman FW Jr, Wiley RL. Afferent inputs to breathing: respiratory sensation. In: Fishman AP, editor. Handbook of physiology. Section 3, Vol II, Part 2. The respiratory systems. Bethesda (MD): American Physiological Society; 1986. p. 149–74.

141. Altose M, Cherniack N, Fishman AP. Respiratory sensations and dyspnea: perspectives. J Appl Physiol 1985;58:1051–4.

142. Gandevia SC. Neural mechanisms underlying the sensation of breathlessness: kinesthetic parallels between respiratory and limb muscles. Aus N Z J Med 1988;18:83–91.

143. Chen Z, Eldridge FL, Wagner PG. Respiratory-associated rhythmic firing of mid-brain neurons in cats: relation to level of respiratory drive. J Physiol (Lond) 1991;437:305–25.

144. Chen Z, Eldridge FL, Wagner PG. Respiratory-associated thalamic activity is related to level of respiratory drive. Respir Physiol 1992;90:99–113.

145. Davenport PW, Friedman WA, Thompson FJ, Franzen O. Respiratory-related cortical potentials evoked by inspiratory occlusion in humans. J Appl Physiol 1986;60:1843–8.

146. Matthews PBC. Where does Sherrington's "muscular sense" originate: muscles, joints corollary discharges? Ann Rev Neurosci 1982;5:189–218.

147. Roland PE, Ladegaard-Pederson HA. A quantitative analysis of sensation of tension and kinaesthesia in man. Evidence

for peripherally originating muscular sense and for a sense of effort. Brain 1977;100:671–92.

148. Leblanc P, Bowie DM, Summers E, et al. Breathlessness and exercise in patient with cardio-respiratory disease. Am Rev Respir Dis 1986;133:21–5.

149. Mahler DA, Harver A, Rosiello R, Daubenspeck JA. Measurements of respiratory sensation in interstitial lung disease: evaluation of clinical dyspnea ratings and magnitude scaling. Chest 1989;96:767–71.

150. Adams L, Lane R, Shea SA, et al. Breathlessness during different forms of ventilatory stimulation: a study of mechanisms in normal subjects and respiratory patients. Clin Sci 1985;69:663–72.

151. Lane R, Adams L, Guz A. The effects of hypoxia and hypercapnia on perceived breathlessness during exercise in humans. J Physiol (Lond) 1990;429:579–93.

152. Swinburn CR, Mould H, Stone TN, et al. Symptomatic benefit of supplemental oxygen in hypoxemic patients with chronic lung disease. Am Rev Respir Dis 1991;143:913–5.

153. Kimoff RJ, Cheong TH, Cosio MG, et al. Pulmonary denervation: effects on dyspnea and ventilatory pattern during exercise. Am Rev Respir Dis 1990;142:1034–40.

154. Winning AM, Hamilton RD, Guz A. Ventilation and breathlessness on maximal exercise in patients with interstitial lung disease after local anesthetic aerosol. Clin Sci 1988;74:275–81.

155. Winning AJ, Hamilton RD, Shea SA, et al. The effect of airway anesthesia on the control of breathing and the sensation of breathlessness in man. Clin Sci 1985;68:215–25.

156. Light RW, Muro JR, Sako RI, et al. Effects of oral morphine on breathlessness and exercise intolerance in patients with chronic obstructive pulmonary disease. Am Res Respir Dis 1989;129:126–33.

157. Celli BR, Gill HS. Respiratory muscle training. In: Fishman AP, editor. Pulmonary rehabilitation. Vol 91. Lung biology in health and disease. New York: Marcel Dekker; 1996. p. 524–43.

158. Killian KJ, Campbell EJM. Dyspnea. In: Roussos C, Macklem PT, editors. Lung biology in health and disease. Vol 29, Part B. The thorax. New York: Marcel Dekker; 1985. p. 787–828.

159. Harver A, Mahler DA, Daubewspect JA. Targeted inspiratory muscle training improves respiratory muscle function and reduces dyspnea in patients with chronic obstructive pulmonary disease. Ann Intern Med 1989;111:117–24.

160. Official statement of the American Thoracic Society. Lung function testing. Selection of reference volumes and interpretative strategies. Am J Respir Crit Care Med 1991;144:1202–18.

161. Becklake MR, Fournier-Massey G, Rossiter CE, McDonald JE. Lung function in chrysotile asbestos mine and mill workers of Quebec. Arch Environ Health 1972;24:401–9.

162. Williams R, Hugh-Jones P. The significance of lung function changes in asbestosis. Thorax 1960;15:109–19.

163. Miller A, Tierstein AS, Jackler I, et al. Airway function in chronic pulmonary sarcoidosis with fibrosis. Am Rev Respir Dis 1974;109:179–89.

164. Dutton RE, Renzi PM, Lopez-Majano V, Renzi GD. Airway function in sarcoidosis: smokers versus nonsmokers. Respiration 1982;43:164–73.

165. Agusti AGN, Roca J, Rodriguez-Roisin R, et al. Different patterns of gas exchange response to exercise in asbestosis and idiopathic pulmonary fibrosis. Eur Respir J 1988;1:510–6.

166. Begis R, Masse S, Contin A, et al. Airway disease in a subset of nonsmoking rheumatoid patients. Characterizations after disease and evidence for auto-immune pathogenesis. Am J Med 1982;72:743–50.

167. Hoffman L, Cohn JE, Gaensler EA. Respiratory abnormalities in eosinophilic granuloma of the lung: long term study of five cases. N Engl J Med 1962;267:577–89.

168. Cransman RS, Jennings CA, Tuder RM, et al. Pulmonary histiocytosis X: pulmonary function and exercise pathophysiology. Am J Respir Crit Care Med 1996;153:426–35.

169. Taylor JR, Rhes J, Colby TV, Raffin TA. Lymphangioleiomyomotosis: clinical course in 32 patients. N Engl J Med 1990;323:1254–60.

170. Thompson PJ, Dhillon DP, Ledingham J, Turner-Warwick M. Shrinking lungs, diaphragmatic dysfunction and systemic lupus erythematosus. Am Rev Respir Dis 1985;132:926–8.

171. Martens J, Demedts M, Vanmeenen MT, Dequeker J. Respiratory muscle dysfunction in systemic lupus erythematosus. Chest 1984;84:170–5.

172. Gaensler EA, Carrington CB. Open biopsy for chronic diffuse infiltrative lung disease: clinical, roentgenographic, and physiological correlations in 502 patients. Ann Thorac Surg 1980;30:411–26.

173. Winterbauer RH, Hammar SP, Hallman KO, et al. Diffuse interstitial pneumonitis: clinicopathologic correlations in 20 patients treated with prednisone/azathioprine. Am J Med 1978;65:661–72.

174. Rudd RM, Haslam PL, Turner-Warwick M. Cryptogenic fibrosing alveolitis: relationships of pulmonary physiology and bronchoalveolar lavage to response to treatment and prognosis. Am Rev Respir Dis 1981;124:1–8.

175. Colp C, Park SS, Williams MH Jr. Pulmonary function follow-up of 120 patients with sarcoidosis. Ann N Y Acad Sci 1976;278:301–7.

176. Kanensinger LC, Rapaport DM, Epstein H, Goldring RM. Volume adjustment of mechanics and diffusion in interstitial lung disease: lack of clinical relevance. Chest 1989;96:1036–42.

177. Hanson D, Winterbauer RH, Kirkland SH, Wu R. Changes in pulmonary function test results after one year as a predictor of survival in patients with idiopathic pulmonary fibrosis. Chest 1995;108:305–10.

178. Erbes R, Schabers T, Lodden-Kemper R. Lung function tests in patients with idiopathic pulmonary fibrosis: are they helpful for predicting outcome? Chest 1997;111:51–7.

179. Johns CJ. The management of pulmonary sarcoidosis. Pulm Perspect 1992;9:4–7.

180. Johns CJ, MacGregor MI, Zachary JB, Ball WC. Extended experience in the long-term corticosteroid treatment of pulmonary sarcoidosis. Ann N Y Acad Sci 1976;278:722–31.

181. Becklake MR. Asbestos-related disease of the lung and other organs: their epidemiology and implications for clinical practice. Am Rev Respir Dis 1976;114:187–227.

182. International Consensus Statement. Idiopathic pulmonary fibrosis: diagnosis and treatment. Am J Respir Crit Care Med 2000;161:646–64.

183. Marciniuk DD, Watts RE, Gallagher CG. Reproducibility of incremental maximal cycle ergometer testing in patients with restrictive lung disease. Thorax 1993;48:894–8.

184. Schwartz DA, Helmers RA, Galvin JR, et al. Determinants of survival in idiopathic pulmonary fibrosis. Am J Respir Crit Care Med 1994;149:450–4.

185. Wells AU, Hansell DM, Rubens MB, et al. The predictile value of appearances on thin section computer tomography in fibrosin alveolitis. Am Rev Respir Dis 1993;148:1076–82.

186. Panos RJ, Mortenson RL, Niccoli SA, King TE. Clinical deterioration in patients with idiopathic pulmonary fibrosis. Am J Med 1990;88:396–404.

187. Jandova R, Widimsky J, Nikodymova L. Long-term prognosis of pulmonary hypertension in chronic lung disease. Prog Respir Res 1985;20:157–69.

188. Kirland SH, Winterbauer RH. Pulmonary function tests and idiopathic pulmonary fibrosis. Simple may be better. Chest 1997;111:7–8.

4   IMAGING OF DIFFUSE PARENCHYMAL LUNG DISEASES

DAVID LYNCH

Radiologic imaging has a central role in the detection, diagnosis, and follow-up of parenchymal lung diseases. In particular, high-resolution chest computed tomography (CT) is becoming an indispensable clinical tool. The past 15 years have led to a great increase in our understanding of the utility of CT in the evaluation of parenchymal disease. The purpose of this chapter is to outline the uses and limitations of imaging techniques in patients with diffuse parenchymal lung disease.

TECHNIQUES

Chest Radiograph

Evaluation of diffuse lung disease on the chest radiograph is critically dependent on the use of a reproducible high-quality technique. Standard technique includes the use of a wide-latitude screen-film combination with a grid to reduce scatter. The usual kVp (peak kilovoltage) is 120 to 140. Tube current and exposure time are usually determined by a phototimer, which allows correction for the size of the patient.

Because of its ready availability and relatively low cost, the chest radiograph still has a role in the detection, characterization, and follow-up of diffuse parenchymal lung disease. About 90% of subjects with biopsy-proven interstitial lung disease have an abnormal chest radiograph.[1] Indeed, an abnormal chest radiograph is often the first indication of an abnormality in subjects with interstitial lung disease, before the development of symptoms or of spirometric impairment. Evidence of lung fibrosis on a chest radiograph should not be ignored, even if the patient is asymptomatic or has normal spirometry. High-resolution CT (HRCT) scanning can be useful in demonstrating the presence of fibrosis in patients who have abnormal radiographs but few or no symptoms.

Limitations of the chest radiograph include the fact that it is relatively insensitive for early interstitial lung disease. A normal chest radiograph is seen in at least 10% of subjects with biopsy-proven interstitial disease.[1] Though the frequency of normal chest radiographs is greatest in subjects with sarcoidosis, desquamative interstitial pneumonitis, and hypersensitivity pneumonitis, a normal chest radiograph may be seen with any interstitial lung disease, including idiopathic pulmonary fibrosis.[2] Population-based studies have shown that a normal chest radiograph may be seen in over 90% of subjects with hypersensitivity pneumonitis.[3] Therefore, the presence of a normal chest radiograph cannot be used as evidence against the presence of interstitial lung disease (Figure 4–1). Conversely, extensive chest radiographic abnormality does not imply physiologically significant disease. This is particularly true for nodular lung diseases such as sarcoidosis or coal workers' pneumoconiosis, where extensive lung nodularity may be associated with minimal or no symptoms or physiologic impairment.

The chest radiograph gives little useful information regarding the severity of inflammation in interstitial lung disease. Ground-glass opacity, which sometimes indicates acute or reversible lung disease, is difficult to appreciate on the chest radiograph, particularly in obese patients.

Evaluation of serial chest radiographs may give useful information regarding progression or regression of disease. Since the radiographic lung volume is related to the total lung capacity, the observation of decreasing lung volumes on serial radiographs usually indicates progressive, restrictive lung disease (Figure 4–2). Appreciation of other changes on chest radiographs is subjective, and is influenced by the technical factors used in obtaining the study.

Digital imaging of the thorax (computed radiography) is being increasingly used in place of analog imaging, because it improves access to the patients' images. Detection of subtle diffuse lung disease depends on the availability of high-resolution digital images. The resolution of conventional chest radiographs corresponds to approximately 4,000 by 4,000 pixels. Most available digital modalities have resolutions of about 2,000 by 2,000 pixels, leading to concern about the visibility of subtle interstitial lung disease on the resultant images. Digitization of radiographs for purposes of transmission to a central reading site (teleradiology) does not seem to lead to a loss of diagnostic sensitivity for subtle interstitial lung disease.[4] Images should be digitized using a high-resolution digitizer and viewed at a resolution of at least 2,000 by 2,000 pixels.[5] Similarly, com-

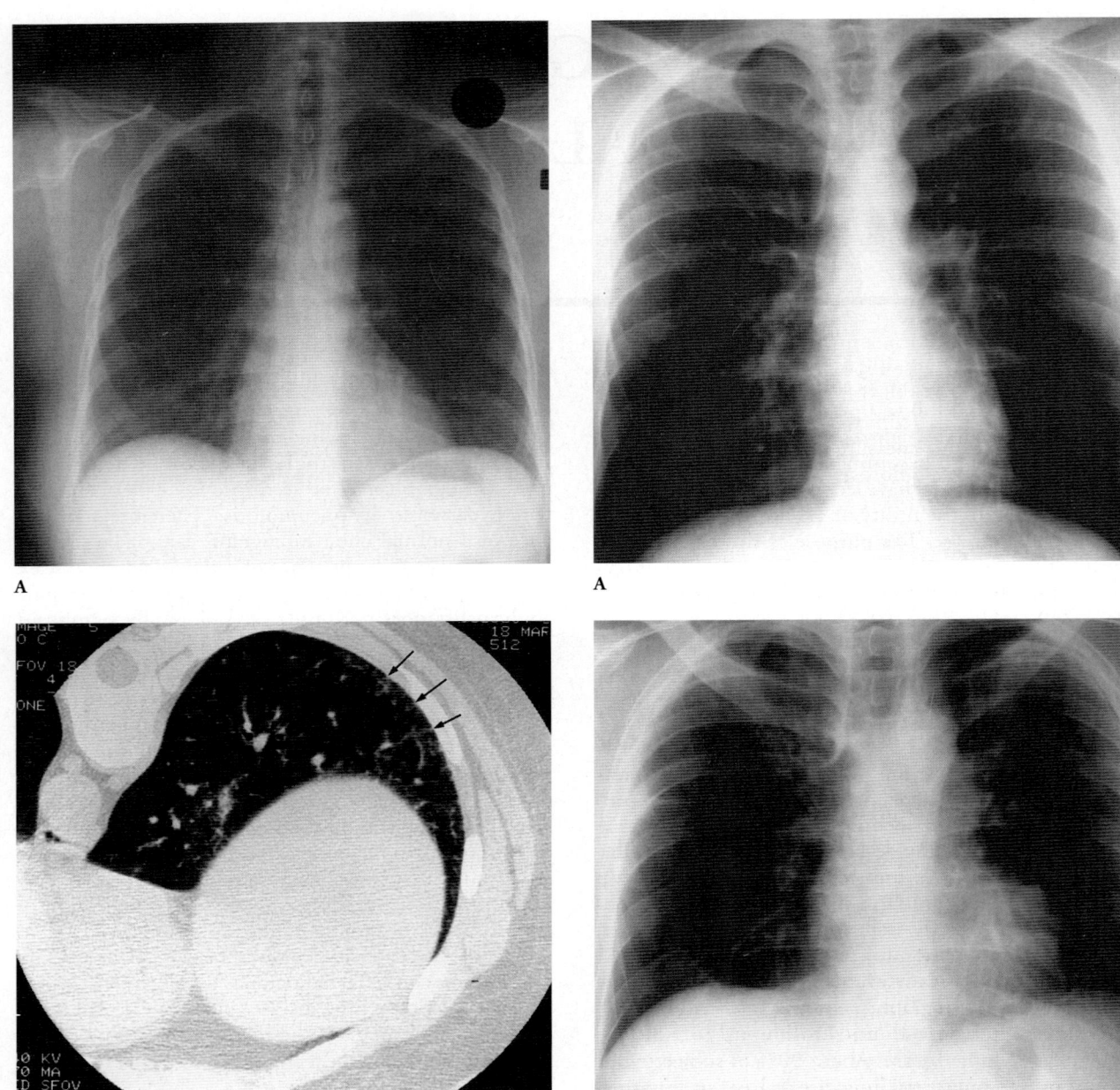

Figure 4–1   Early pulmonary fibrosis in scleroderma. *A*, Chest radiograph is normal. *B*, Prone HRCT scan shows widespread thickening of interlobular septa (*arrows*), centrilobular thickening, and some reticular lines typical for early pulmonary fibrosis associated with scleroderma.

Figure 4–2   Delayed lung fibrosis following BCNU treatment for brain tumor. *A*, Chest radiograph at time of treatment is normal. *B*, Chest radiograph at time of symptoms 15 years later shows no appreciable parenchymal abnormality but marked decrease in lung volumes due to restrictive lung disease.

puted radiographic acquisition, with a resolution of 2,000 by 2,000 pixels, does not appear to impair detection of diffuse lung disease.[6,7] The effect of image digitization on the characterization of lung disease has not been evaluated. Newer technologies such as selenium-based imaging and advanced multiple-beam equilization radiography (AMBER) may enhance the conspicuity of interstitial abnormalities.[8,9] Digital imaging

may also facilitate textural analysis of chest radiographs to assist in the characterization of lung disease.[10]

Nuclear Imaging Techniques

The role of nuclear imaging in the evaluation of a patient with interstitial lung disease is very limited. Gallium scanning was widely used in the past but has little value in the detection or characterization of lung disease. In rare cases, whole-body scanning with gallium may assist in the diagnosis of sarcoidosis when the patient presents with extrapulmonary symptoms and a normal or equivocal chest radiograph.[11] Scanning of the lungs following the administration of technetium-labeled pentetic acid (DTPA) is used in some centers but is limited by the fact that the clearance of DTPA is markedly increased in cigarette smokers. Clearance of the labeled DTPA appears to be more rapid in patients with diffuse lung disease due to fibrosing alveolitis or scleroderma.[12–14] Positron emission tomography (PET) with fluorodeoxyglucose F 18 may show some increase in metabolic activity in the lungs of patients with interstitial disease, but the clinical utility of this is unclear. PET has been used to measure neutrophil activation in animal models of lung fibrosis.[15]

Computed Tomography Imaging

Thick-section CT scanning of the lung, performed using 5 to 10 mm thick, contiguous slices is insensitive for the subtle changes of interstitial lung disease, particularly ground-glass attenuation and fine bronchial and parenchymal abnormalities.[16] This is because structures of many different densities may be contained within the slice thickness of conventional CT scans (partial volume averaging). Therefore conventional CT assessment of interstitial lung disease must be supplemented with or replaced by thin-section imaging. Thick-section imaging of the lung is important for nodule detection, because nodules may be missed between noncontiguous HRCT slices.

Spiral (helical) CT scanning is increasingly used to acquire CT data from the entire thorax. With spiral CT scanning, the scan time is significantly reduced, and the scans form a contiguous dataset, which allows construction of a three-dimensional model of the lung. An exciting aspect of this evolving technology is the ability to measure lung volumes.[17] Inspiratory lung volumes calculated from spiral CT correlate well (r = .88) with total lung capacity (TLC), although the TLC is underestimated by about 10%. Expiratory lung volumes correlate well with residual volume, although with some overestimation. The newer technique of multitrack or multidetector spiral CT can provide the ideal situation of acquiring high-quality thin sections from the entire lung. The limiting factors are radiation dose and the requirement for a prolonged breath-hold (between 10 and 30 seconds, depending on the acquisition parameters).

High-Resolution Computed Tomography

Two technical factors are essential for HRCT of the lung parenchyma.[18,19] The first is the use of narrow slice thickness (usually about 1 mm, compared with 5 to 7 mm for conventional CT). The decreased slice thickness means that small, fine abnormalities such as interstitial lines are less likely to be "averaged" out within a slice. Secondly, the image must be reconstructed using a high-spatial-frequency (high-resolution) algorithm, distinct from the smoothing algorithm used for most conventional CT imaging. The high-spatial-frequency algorithm allows better visualization of fine parenchymal detail, such as small bronchi or branching vessels and interlobular septae (Figure 4–3). Inevitably, the use of the high-resolution algorithm and the decreased slice thickness causes a moderate increase in image noise, which does not usually interfere significantly with image interpretation.[18] Occasionally, in obese patients, the artifact due to image noise is significant and may require an increase in radiation dose to create an image of diagnostic quality. It is possible to further increase the resolution of the scan by targeting to one lung or even a portion of one lung or, on newer scanners, by narrowing the slice collimation to 0.75 mm or 0.5 mm, but the clinical benefit of doing this has not been evaluated.

In a study performed by Mayo and colleagues,[20] the mean radiation dose delivered to the skin at the level of the breasts by a limited HRCT was 4.4 mGy for scans performed every 10 mm and 2.1 mGy for scans performed every 20 mm. A more recent study showed radiation exposures of less than 10 mGy for a full spiral CT acquisition and 2.2 mGy for HRCT scans obtained at 10 mm intervals.[21] This compares with a dose of 0.5 mGy for frontal chest radiographs and 0.8 mGy for lateral chest radiographs. The breasts are the most radiation-sensitive organs in the imaging field, but the precise risk of radiation in such low doses is unclear. Clearly there is a trade-off between acquiring adequate diagnostic information and minimizing the radiation dose to the patient, particularly in younger patients.

The increasing sensitivity of currently available CT detectors is likely to lead to a further decrease in the radiation dose from HRCT scanning. HRCT images obtained using low radiation doses (10 to 40 milliampere-second [mAs]) have been shown to be adequate for characterizing interstitial lung disease.[22,23] HRCT images obtained using a dose of 80 mAs have been shown to provide a diagnostic accuracy similar to that of conventional-dose (340 mAs) images.[24] However these images show an increase in linear streak artifact and may fail to demonstrate subtle emphysema or ground-glass density. In clinical practice, a dose of 140 to 160 mAs demonstrates parenchymal detail well in most patients.[25,26] This dose must be substantially increased in larger patients. Lower dose CT scanning may be of value in the follow-up evaluation of infiltrative lung disease and in the diagnosis of bronchiectasis.[21]

HRCT scans of the lung are usually performed at full inspiration, allowing maximal contrast between inflated normal lung and areas of lung disease. For purposes of reproducibility it would be useful to document

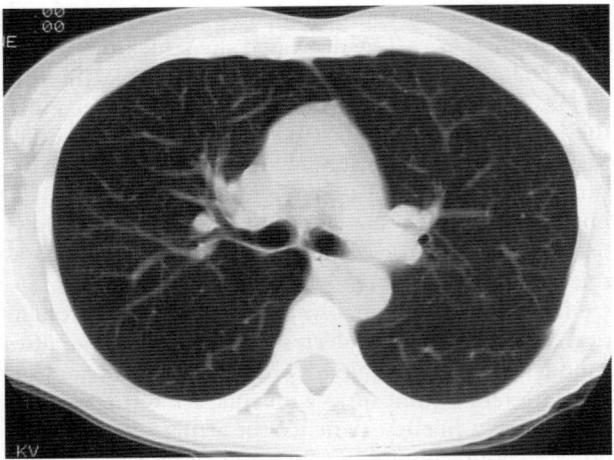

A

B

Figure 4–3   Normal conventional and high resolution CT scans. *A,* Conventional CT (10 mm thickness) shows most of the pulmonary vessels and bronchi as long branching structures. The interlobar fissure is seen as a hypodense avascular area. *B,* Normal high resolution CT (1.5 mm thickness) shows the vessels as short lines or dots. The fissure is seen as a thin white line (*arrow*). Scattered short branching structures 5 to 10 mm deep to the pleural surface represent normal centrilobular structures (*arrowheads*). No interlobular septa are seen.

the level of inspiration for each scan. Although it is possible to use spirometry to monitor the level of inspiration for each scan,[27–29] the technology has not been supported by American manufacturers of CT scanners and is not widely used. As discussed above, the increasing availability of spiral CT scanners and associated image analysis software should allow routine calculation of lung volumes at the time of the examination along with other measurements such as the amount of soft tissue and air per unit volume of lung.[30,31]

Respiratory motion artifact is a common problem when imaging patients with diffuse lung disease. Almost all patients, with adequate coaching, can suspend respiration for 1 to 2 seconds (all that is required for a single HRCT image). However, patients with severe lung disease may require an interval of up to 30 seconds to recover between slices. The CT technologist must interact closely with the patient to ensure that an adequate interval is allowed between slices. The automated scanning feature (autovoice) available on many CT scanners usually does not allow an adequate interslice delay and results in substantial motion artifact. This feature should not be used when performing HRCT of the lungs.[32] Clinicians should work with the radiologist and the technologist to ensure that adequate motion-free images are obtained.

HRCT examination of young children is difficult because motion artifact obliterates subtle changes of airways disease or interstitial lung disease. Ultrafast CT scanning can eliminate motion artifact by producing diagnostic images at scan times of 100 msec.[33] However, the ultrafast CT scanner is relatively expensive, and the resolution of its images does not yet equal that of conventional CT scanners. It is available in relatively few centers. In pediatric centers that do not have access to ultrafast CT, motion artifact may be minimized by the use of subsecond scanning and careful coaching of the older child.[34,35] In the newly described "stop ventilation" technique, a sedated child is given several deep breaths, resulting in a respiratory pause of up to 15 seconds.[36]

Although the technical factors used for high-resolution CT lung imaging have been well-documented, the number of scans performed varies widely. Some institutions employ full conventional CT scanning with contiguous 10 mm scans followed by high-resolution sections at selected levels.[37] Further HRCT sections are performed through areas where an abnormality is suspected on conventional CT scanning. At other sites, HRCT imaging is used alone and is performed at 4 cm intervals in supine and prone positions.[38] This screening technique is clearly faster, results in a lower radiation dose to the patient, and can be done at significantly lower cost to the patient. Although this technique is probably adequate for screening for diffuse lung diseases, it must be realized that significant focal disease may be missed in the gap between slices. It is often important to perform prone as well as supine HRCT scans, because dependent lung density may mask significant interstitial abnormalities, and also because interlobular septal thickening may be mimicked by engorgement of pulmonary veins in the dependent lung.[39] The only significant abnormalities on HRCT are those that persist in the nondependent lung.[40] Indeed, some sites perform HRCT only in the prone position. Most centers routinely obtain a limited number of expiratory thin-section CT scans in addition to the inspiratory evaluation, because the detection of air-trapping can be very useful in the differential diagnosis of diffuse lung diseases and may help explain the patient's physiology.[41–44]

Careful written or verbal communication from the clinician is important to ensure that the examination performed is appropriate to the clinical question being asked. The HRCT examination can be tailored to the specific disease being sought. For instance, in asbestos-exposed subjects, scans may focus on the lung bases.[45] In patients with suspected obstructive lung disease (emphysema or bronchiolitis obliterans), expiratory CT scanning may be very important to identify areas of air-trapping not evident on inspiratory images (Figure 4–4).[46] Other technical modifications include the use of spiral CT scans to create thin 3-dimensional "slabs" of data. The use of minimal intensity projections derived from these spiral slabs may enhance the demonstration of fine nodules and allow discrimination between vessels and nodules.[47,48]

HRCT images should usually be viewed or photographed at a relatively narrow (contrasty) window width (usually 1,000 to 1,500 Hounsfield Units). This narrow setting is optimal for identifying subtle areas of emphysema, ground-glass opacity, or air-trapping. The window level is set around the normal attenuation of the lung (between –700 and –800 Hounsfield Units). Variability in settings of laser cameras may cause substantial differences in the brightness and contrast of the printed images, even if the same window and level settings are used.

Magnetic Resonance Imaging

There are several theoretical reasons to advocate the use of magnetic resonance imaging (MRI) in the lung. MRI uses nonionizing radiation, can quantify the amount of lung water,[49,50] and can distinguish fibrosis from active inflammation.[51–53] However, MRI of the lung has been gravely hampered by the problems of respiratory motion and induced inhomogeneity of the magnetic field within individual voxels. The magnetic inhomogeneity problem arises because the lung is composed of innumerable air-soft tissue interfaces. Magnetic field inhomogeneity is created at each of these interfaces, causing a dramatic loss of signal with standard MRI techniques. Despite the development of ingenious and innovative techniques,[54–57] there is still no clinical role for MRI of the lungs.[58] The use of inhaled hyperpolarized helium[59,60] or oxygen[61,62] as contrast agents to image pulmonary ventilation is the latest technical advance in MRI, which is currently under evaluation in patients with obstructive lung diseases.

COMPUTED TOMOGRAPHY SCANNING IN NORMAL PATIENTS

Computed tomography densities are recorded on a standard scale of Hounsfield Units (HU). Air has a density of –1,000 HU, whereas water has a density of 0 HU. Soft-tissue structures have a density between 40 and 80 HU. The mean CT density of normal lung is around –820 to –860 HU on both conventional CT and

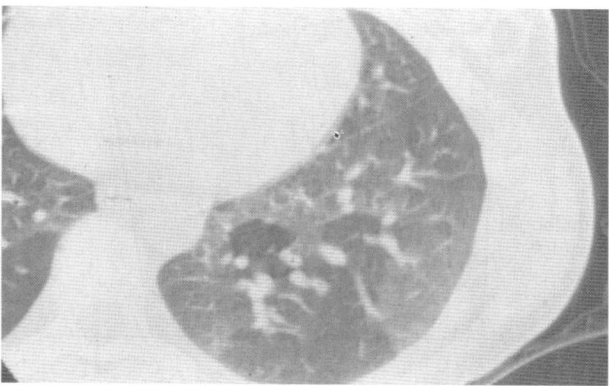

Figure 4–4 A 60-year-old female with asthma. Inspiratory CT scan was normal, apart from bronchial wall thickening. Expiratory CT scan shows bronchial wall thickening with multifocal lobular air-trapping in left lower lobe. Reproduced with permission from Lynch DA, Newell JD, Lee JS, editors. Imaging of diffuse lung disease. Hamilton: B.C. Decker; 2000.

HRCT,[63,64] but this value is critically dependent on the volume of inspired air.[27] Scans performed at twenty percent of vital capacity give a mean lung CT density of –760 HU, whereas at eighty percent of vital capacity the CT density decreases to –860 H. In children, mean lung density appears to decrease with increasing age,[65] though this decrease may be partly due to improving ability to comply with breathing instructions. An anteroposterior gradient of increasing lung density is seen in normal lungs, because the dependent posterior lung has relatively less air and more blood flow than the nondependent lung.

On HRCT scans, vessels are usually identified as dots or short lines, a feature that readily distinguishes thin sections from conventional 8 to 10 mm sections, where vessels are usually seen as longer branching lines because more vessel is included within the 10 mm voxel thickness (see Figure 4–3). Vessels that accompany the bronchi usually represent pulmonary arteries. Any vessel that reaches the pleural surface is usually a pulmonary vein running in an interlobular septum.

An appreciation of normal and abnormal HRCT findings in the lung requires an understanding of the anatomy of the secondary pulmonary lobule, which is the basic anatomic and physiologic unit of the mammalian lung (Figure 4–5).[66] In humans, the irregular polyhedral secondary pulmonary lobule is composed of several acini, each supplied by a terminal bronchiole. The secondary lobules are separated from each other by interlobular septa, which contain branches of the pulmonary veins and lymphatics. The septa are best developed in the peripheral anterior lung and less well developed posteriorly and in the central lung. Interlobular septa become visible as septal (Kerley's) lines on the chest radiograph when they are thickened by interstitial fluid, cellular infiltration, or fibrosis. On HRCT,[66] the interlobular septa may be visible in the normal anterior

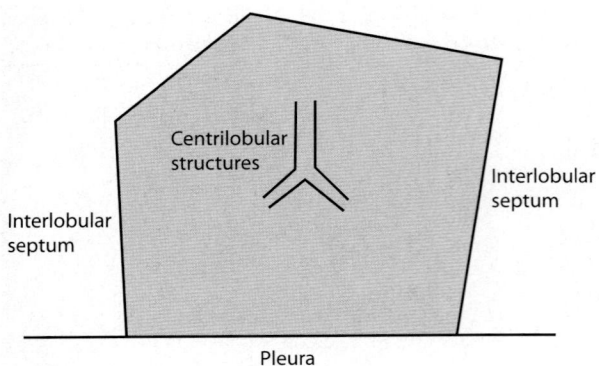

Figure 4–5 Schematic diagram of the secondary pulmonary lobule, an irregularly shaped polyhedral structure outlined by interlobular septa that are roughly perpendicular to the pleura. At the center of the lobule, about 5 mm deep to the pleural surface, are the centrilobular structures.

lung as scattered, thin nontapering lines, 1 to 2 cm long, perpendicular to the pleura and often contacting the pleural surface.

In the center of the secondary pulmonary lobule are the distal bronchus and its terminal bronchioles with the associated distal pulmonary artery branches. These structures are often called centrilobular or core structures and may be visible on HRCT as a dot or branching structure 5 to 10 mm deep to the pleural surface. This visualized centrilobular structure represents the distal pulmonary artery branch; its accompanying bronchus is not normally seen.

The interlobar fissures, usually not seen as distinct structures on conventional CT, are well demonstrated on HRCT as fine white lines (see Figure 4–3). The anatomy of the pleura and extrapleural structures by HRCT scanning was well described by Im and colleagues.[67] HRCT allows identification of extrapleural fat, intercostal muscles, intercostal vessels, and subtle pleural plaques.

PATTERN RECOGNITION IN DIFFUSE LUNG DISEASES

Chest Radiograph

In approaching the radiograph of a patient with diffuse lung disease, it is possible to recognize distinct patterns, which may be of value in characterization of the disease (Table 4–1). Lung disease may be categorized into interstitial disease, air space disease, airways disease, and emphysema. All of these disease groups may be recognized by their radiographic signs.

Interstitial disease is characterized on the chest radiograph by nodules, lines, honeycombing, and ground-glass opacification. The first three of these signs are easy to recognize on the chest radiograph, but detection of ground-glass opacity can be difficult, particularly in

patients with dense overlying soft tissues or in those with underpenetrated radiographs. These useful signs of interstitial lung disease must be clearly distinguished from "increased interstitial markings," a loosely used term that usually refers to prominent bronchovascular structures radiating from the hila, usually due to airway

Table 4–1   Differential Diagnosis of Infiltrative Lung Disease Based on Chest Radiographic Pattern

Pattern	Radiographic Findings	Differential Diagnosis

Air space (alveolar) disease	Poorly defined opacities Coalescence Air bronchograms	Acute
		  Pneumonia
		  Edema
		  Aspiration
		  Hemorrhage
		
		Chronic
		  Chronic infection (TB, fungal)
		  BOOP
		  Sarcoidosis (pseudoalveolar)
		  Pulmonary alveolar proteinosis
		  Cellular infiltrations
		  Bronchioloalveolar cell carcinoma
		  Lymphoma
		  Eosinophilic pneumonia
		  Vasculitis
		  Chronic aspiration (esp. lipid)

Nodular disease	Well-defined nodules	Malignancy pneumoconiosis
		  Silicosis
		  Coalworkers' pneumoconiosis
		
		Granulomas
		  Infectious (miliary)
		  Sarcoidosis
		  Berylliosis
		  Langerhans cell histiocytosis

	Poorly defined nodules	Malignancy
		  Bronchioloalveolar
		  Lymphoma
		  Hemorrhagic metastases
		
		Granulomas
		  Infection (TB/fungal)
		  Sarcoidosis
		  Langerhans cell histiocytosis
		
		Infection
		  Viral (varicella, CMV)

Fibrotic disease	Reticular lines Honeycombing	Idiopathic pulmonary fibrosis Asbestosis Collagen vascular disease Sarcoidosis Chronic hypersensitivity pneumonitis
Septal thickening	Kerley's lines A, B, C	Lung edema Lymphangitic spread Infection (PCP, mycoplasma) Drug reaction

TB = tubercolosis; BOOP = bronchiolitis obliterans with organizing pneumonia; CMV = cytomegalovirus; PCP = *Pneumocystis carinii* pneumonia.

wall thickening. Airways disease may be specifically recognized on the chest radiograph by ring shadows representing end-on airways, or "train-tracking," which refers to thin parallel lines that represent the thickened walls of airways coursing from the hila. Air space disease is characterized by poorly defined opacities, which tend to be confluent and may contain air bronchograms. The lung destruction of emphysema may be recognized by hyperlucency (increased lung blackness) and by abnormality of the pulmonary vessels, which are usually sparse and thin, with a decreased number of branches.

The pattern recognition approach on the chest radiograph has substantial limitations.[68] First, any radiographic opacity represents a summation of all structures traversed by the x-ray beam on its course through the patient. A beam that traverses a series of perfectly superimposed linear densities will therefore cause the appearance of a nodule on the radiograph. Likewise, a linear density may be produced on the chest radiograph by a series of almost superimposed nodules. Therefore, it may be very difficult to accurately identify and characterize individual parenchymal structures on the radiograph. Secondly, the patterns recognized on the chest radiograph for individual patients may not fall neatly into one category. Thirdly, of course, the pathologic distribution of lung disease may not be confined neatly to one anatomic compartment: many "interstitial" diseases have a substantial alveolar component, whereas others such as sarcoidosis may be distributed along the airways. Despite these limitations, a correct diagnosis may be made by recognition of the chest radiographic pattern of disease in 40 to 80% percent of cases.[69–73]

High-Resolution Computed Tomography Scanning

There are two complementary approaches to the differential diagnosis of interstitial disease on HRCT scanning. One approach emphasizes the anatomic distribution of disease within the lung, and the other relies on recognition of the radiographic pattern of abnormality.

Anatomic Distribution of Disease

A valuable approach to the differential diagnosis of interstitial lung disease involves assessment of the distribution of disease in relation to bronchovascular structures, the pleura, and the secondary pulmonary lobule (Table 4–2).[74,75] In patients with inflammation or plugging of small airways, the normally invisible centrilobular structures become visible as short branching structures. When these branching structures terminate in a nodule, the "tree-in-bud" sign is present (Figure 4–6). The tree-in-bud sign is usually due either to small airway inflammation or to disease that spreads by the airways, such as tuberculosis.[76] Nodules that are centrilobular without a tree-in-bud appearance are usually

TABLE 4–2 Differential Diagnosis of Infiltrative Lung Diseases on HRCT by Evaluation of Lobules

Bronchovascular thickening	Sarcoidosis Lymphangitic carcinoma
Centrilobular nodules	Pneumoconiosis Sarcoidosis Hypersensitivity pneumonitis
Centrilobular thickening with tree-in-bud pattern	Bronchiolitis
Dominant septal thickening	Lymphangitis carcinomatosa Left heart failure
Mixed septal and centrilobular thickening	Sarcoidosis Lymphangitic carcinoma
Panlobular increased density	Hypersensitivity pneumonitis Drug toxicity Desquamative interstitial pneumonitis
Panlobular decreased density	Pulmonary embolism Constrictive bronchiolitis Panlobular emphysema

due to some form of inhalational disease. Thickening of interlobular septa (Figure 4–7) is usually due to edema or infiltration of the lymphatic structures and is often associated with thickening of the other lymphatic pathways (subpleural and peribronchovascular). Panlobular ground-glass attenuation (Figure 4–8), often associated with sparing of one or more lobules, commonly represents an active inflammatory process. A limitation of analysis of the secondary pulmonary lobule is that many common interstitial lung diseases such as idiopathic pulmonary fibrosis, sarcoidosis, and lymphangiomyomatosis are associated with distortion of lobular

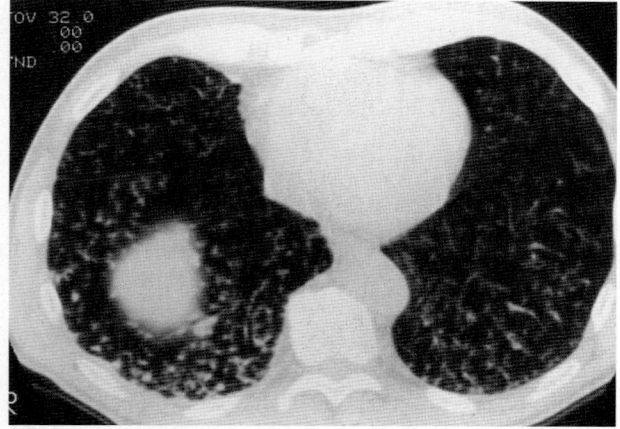

Figure 4–6 Centrilobular nodules. Conventional CT scan in a non-Asian patient with panbronchiolitis shows extensive centrilobular nodules. These are recognized as being centrilobular by their short distance from the pleural surface and their connection to more central branching structures.

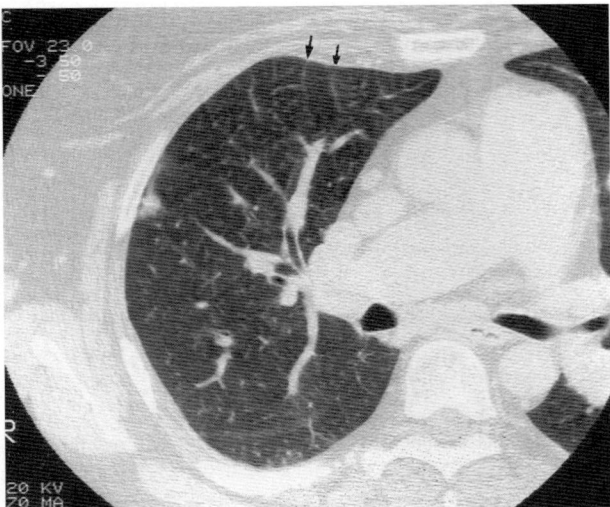

Figure 4–7 Septal thickening. Chronic interstitial pulmonary edema associated with mitral valve disease. Mild smooth thickening of intralobular septa is noted in the anterior lung (*arrows*), readily distinguished from the nodular septal thickening seen in lymphangitic spread of carcinoma and sarcoidosis.

anatomy,[77] so that assessment of the lobular anatomy is not very useful in these individuals.

In addition to the distribution of disease within the secondary lobule, it is important to observe the distribution of disease within the lung. Many interstitial lung diseases have a peripheral predominance (Table 4–3). In particular, the characteristic peripheral distribution of idiopathic pulmonary fibrosis[78] (Figure 4–9) and eosinophilic pneumonia[79] (Figure 4–10) is much better demonstrated on CT than on conventional radiographs. The upper lobe predominance of the cysts and nodules of pulmonary Langerhans cell histiocytosis[80,81] helps to

distinguish this entity from the diffuse cysts seen in lymphangiomyomatosis.[82]

A very useful standard terminology for describing the CT findings in parenchymal lung diseases has been published by the Fleischner Society.[83] Some of the more important features are to follow and are listed in Table 4–4.

Nodules. Nodules are defined as round, discrete, parenchymal densities. It is sometimes difficult to differentiate nodules from vessels on HRCT scans, because both are seen as round dots. This distinction may be easier on conventional CT,[84] where vessels are usually more linear than nodules. On HRCT, one may distinguish nodules from vessels by examining the anatomy of the secondary pulmonary lobule or by detecting the presence of "too many dots" (Figure 4–11). Contiguous thin-section spiral CT acquisitions may facilitate discrimination of vessels from nodules by allowing vessels to be followed through a slab of acquired images.[47,48]

Nodules seen on HRCT can be classified according to their size (micronodules or larger nodules), density (ground-glass, soft-tissue, or calcific densities), definition (well defined or poorly defined), and distribution. Micronodules measure less than 3 mm in diameter.[85] Gruden and colleagues[86] classified nodules on the basis of their location (random, perilymphatic, centrilobular, or airways-associated). Perilymphatic micronodules are seen in subpleural and septal locations and are most profuse in subjects with lymphangitic carcinomatosis and sarcoidosis but may also be seen in pneumoconiosis. Scattered subpleural micronodules may be seen in normal subjects. Centrilobular nodules differ from small-airways–associated nodules in that the small-airways nodules are frequently patchy, tend to be related to small branching structures (tree-in-bud phenomenon), and are often associated with patches of air space opacification.

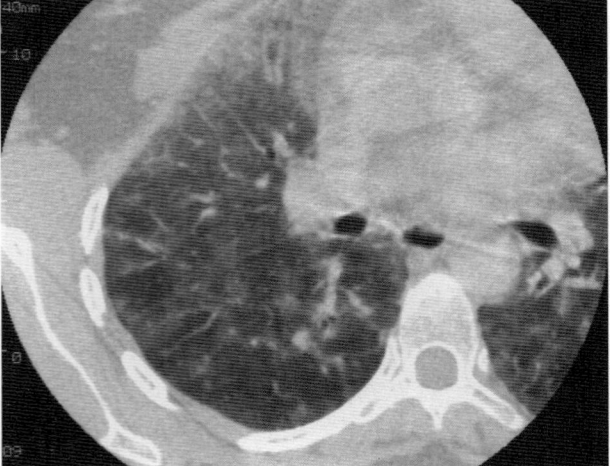

Figure 4–8 Panlobular ground-glass opacity. Prone HRCT scan in patient with hypersensitivity pneumonitis shows widespread panlobular, ground-glass opacity. The distribution of the ground-glass opacity is patchy, with sparing of some secondary pulmonary lobules.

TABLE 4–3   Differential Diagnosis of Infiltrative Lung Diseases by Distribution Within the Lung on HRCT

Peripheral disease	UIP, OP
	Asbestosis
	Collagen vascular disease
	Eosinophilic pneumonia
Central/peribronchovascular disease	Sarcoidosis
	Lymphangitis carcinomatosa
	Lymphoproliferative disorders
	Organizing pneumonia
Upper lobe predominance	Sarcoidosis
	Coal workers' pneumoconiosis
	Silicosis
	Eosinophilic pneumonia
	Langerhans cell histiocytosis
	Hypersensitivity pneumonitis
Lower lobe predominance	UIP, NSIP, OP
	Asbestosis
	Collagen vascular disease

UIP = usual interstitial pneumonia; OP = organizing pneumonia; NSIP = nonspecific interstitial pneumonia.

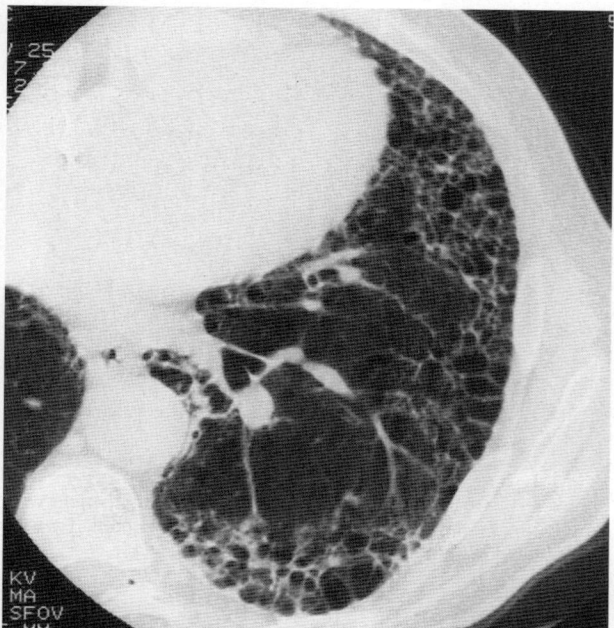

Figure 4–9   Peripheral honeycombing in IPF. HRCT scan in a patient with idiopathic pulmonary fibrosis shows a peripheral rim of honeycombing with clustered cysts measuring 3 to 10 mm. All of the honeycomb cysts have a well-defined wall. More centrally, there are scattered, poorly defined lucencies consistent with emphysema. The peripheral distribution of the honeycombing is characteristic of IPF.

Nodules may also be distinguished according to their pattern of attenuation. Nodules of ground-glass density are typically seen in hypersensitivity pneumonitis (Figure 4–12) but may also be seen in respiratory bronchiolitis (Figure 4–13). Soft-tissue density nodules are seen in patients with granulomatous lung diseases, malignancy, or pneumoconiosis. Calcific nodules are seen in prior granulomatous infection or in pulmonary alveolar microlithiasis.

Lines.   A variety of linear densities may be seen on HRCT. Thickened interlobular septa are identified because they are perpendicular to the pleura (see Figure 4–7),[39] or by the fact that they form polygonal structures (Figure 4–14).[87] Reticular lines are probably the commonest type of linear abnormality (Figure 4–15). These lines are less than 5 mm long, forming a fine lace-like network that usually does not conform to lobular anatomy. They are seen in all types of fibrotic lung conditions, particularly idiopathic pulmonary fibrosis,[88] collagen vascular disease, and asbestosis. Reticular lines are also a prominent CT feature in patients with the crazy paving pattern (see "Crazy Paving Pattern").

The curvilinear subpleural line was emphasized in the literature as an early sign of asbestosis.[89] It is a curved line, 2 to 10 mm deep to the pleural surface and parallel to the pleural surface (Figure 4–16). In subjects with asbestosis, this line appears to correspond to linear interstitial fibrosis, extending from one secondary lobule to

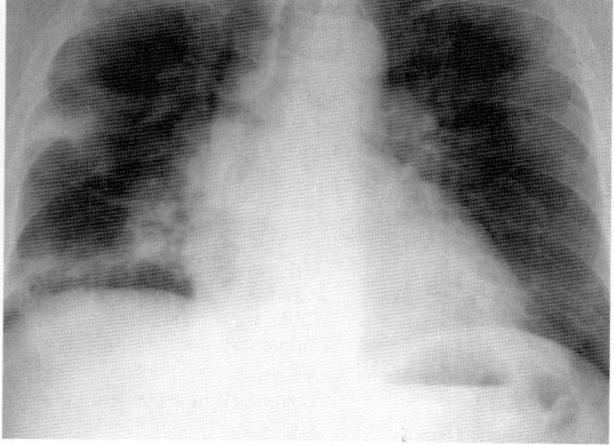

A

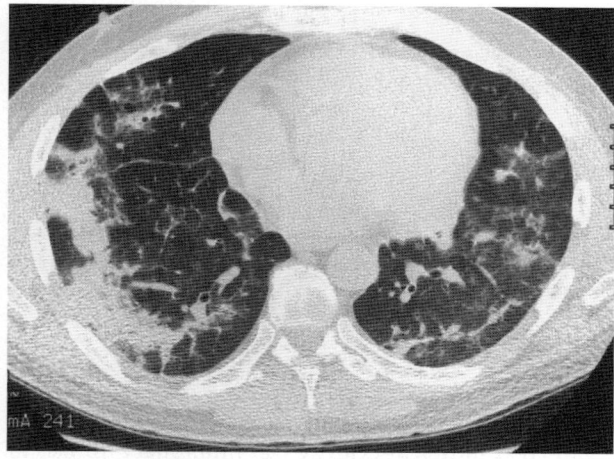

B

C

Figure 4–10   Chronic eosinophilic pneumonia. *A*, Chest radiograph shows typical distribution of air space consolidation, the classic "negative pulmonary edema" pattern. *B*, Chest radiograph 7 days later shows progression to more diffuse air space abnormality. *C*, HRCT confirms predominantly peripheral consolidation and also shows a curvilinear density about 1 cm deep to the pleural surface in the left posterior lung. This line is often seen as eosinophilic pneumonia resolves.

TABLE 4–4   CT Features of Common Lung Diseases

Nodules	Sarcoidosis
	Langerhans cell histiocytosis
	Hypersensitivity pneumonitis
	Silicosis
	Metastatic cancer
Centrilobular nodules	See Table 4–2
Lines	
Thickened Septa	See Table 4–2
Intralobular or reticular lines	UIP, NSIP
	Asbestosis
	Collagen vascular disease
	Pulmonary alveolar proteinosis
Curvilinear subpleural line	Asbestosis
	Congestion in dependent lung
Parenchymal band	Asbestosis
	Scarring from pleural disease
Lung cysts	Distinguish from emphysema
	Langerhans cell histiocytosis
	Lymphangiomyomatosis
	Lymphoid interstitial pneumonitis
Honeycombing	Asbestosis
	UIP
	Collagen vascular disease
	Sarcoidosis
	Hypersensitivity pneumonitis
Parenchymal opacification Ground-glass attenuation	Organizing pneumonia
	Hypersensitivity pneumonitis
	Drug toxicity
	Desquamative interstitial pneumonitis
	Pulmonary alveolar proteinosis
	Sarcoidosis
Consolidation	Organizing pneumonia
	Eosinophilic pneumonia
	Alveolar cell carcinoma
	Lipoid pneumonia
	Pulmonary alveolar proteinosis
Decreased lung attenuation	Pulmonary embolism
	Constrictive bronchiolitis
	Panlobular emphysema
Mosaic pattern	Constrictive bronchiolitis
	Pulmonary thromboembolism
	Diseases causing ground-glass attenuation

UIP = usual interstitial pneumonia; NSIP = nonspecific interstitial pneumonia.

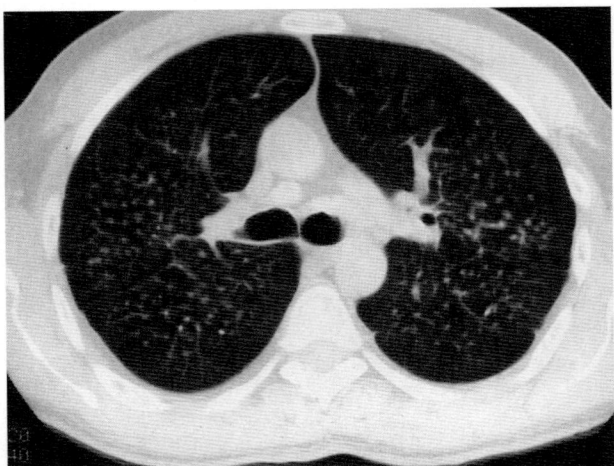

Figure 4–11   Simple silicosis. Conventional CT of a patient with simple silicosis shows moderate diffuse pulmonary nodularity with upper lobe predominance.

ease and should not be regarded as being due to diffuse lung fibrosis without other supportive evidence.

Cysts.   The cysts of interstitial lung disease are air-containing lucencies with a well-defined, complete wall (Figure 4–18). They are usually round, but may sometimes be irregular in shape, particularly in Langerhans cell histiocytosis. They must be distinguished from the "moth-eaten" lucencies of centrilobular emphysema, which are usually irregular in outline and do not have a definable wall (Figure 4–19). Cysts may be distinguished from bronchiectatic bronchi by the fact that

the next.[89,90] However, the subpleural curvilinear line is a nonspecific finding and probably should not be regarded as sufficient evidence for pulmonary fibrosis in the absence of other CT signs of lung disease.

Parenchymal bands of fibrosis or lung scars have been reported predominantly in asbestosis[39,45] but are also seen in idiopathic pulmonary fibrosis or collagen vascular disease. These bands are coarse strands of soft-tissue density, usually extending to a pleural surface and commonly irregular in outline (Figure 4–17). Parenchymal bands sometimes represent areas of scarring related to pleural dis-

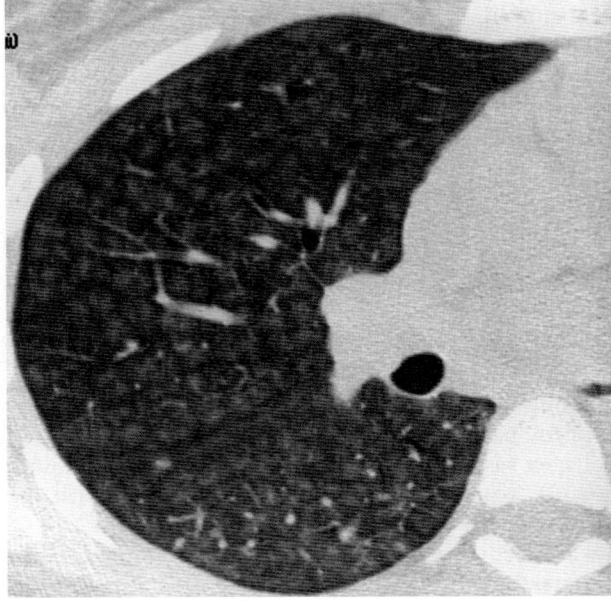

Figure 4–12   Acute hypersensitivity pneumonitis. A 23-year-old female with unexplained breathlessness, thought to be due to asthma. HRCT shows profuse, poorly defined ground-glass nodules typical for acute hypersensitivity pneumonitis.

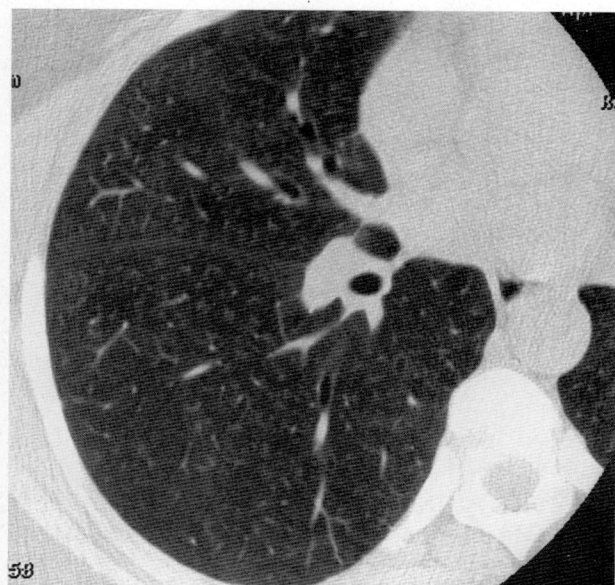

Figure 4–13   Respiratory bronchiolitis (RB)-ILD. CT of a cigarette smoker with symptoms of cough and dyspnea shows widespread fine centrilobular nodularity similar to that found in hypersensitivity pneumonitis. Biopsy showed respiratory bronchiolitis-interstitial lung disease.

bronchi are usually accompanied by a smaller pulmonary artery and can usually be traced back to the hilum on serial CT sections.

Honeycombing is defined as a cluster or row of cysts (see Figure 4–9). Honeycomb cysts are usually very small (less than 5 mm in diameter). This CT finding correlates with histologic honeycombing and is found in end-stage lung disease of any cause.[91] Larger honeycomb cysts may sometimes be found in patients with sarcoidosis.

Traction Bronchiectasis/Bronchiolectasis.   Traction bronchiectasis and bronchiolectasis refers to dilatation and distortion of the bronchi and bronchioles in areas of fibrosis, presumed to be due to the forces of increased elastic recoil acting on these structures (Figure 4–20).[92] It is usually associated with a reticular pattern or

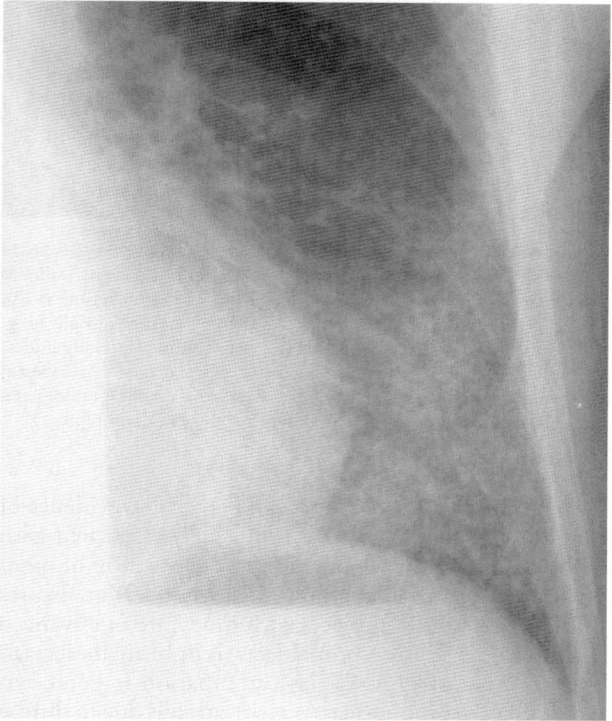

A

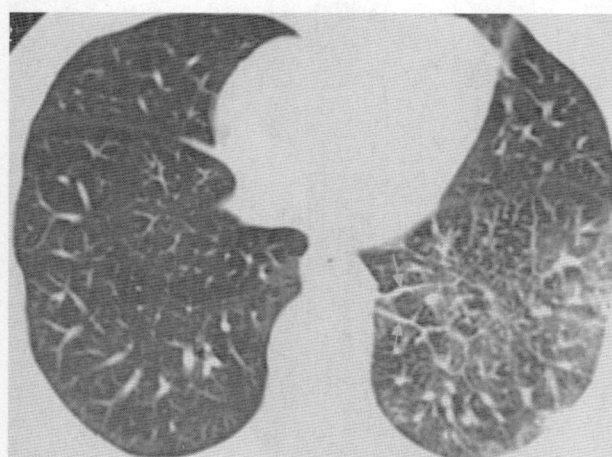

Figure 4–14   A 70-year-old male with lymphangitic carcinomatosis. High-resolution chest CT through the left lower lobe shows irregular septal thickening, forming polygonal structures that correspond to secondary pulmonary lobules, with beading of intralobular septa (*arrows*). The asymmetry of this process and the irregular nodularity of the septa are characteristic for lymphangitic carcinomatosis.

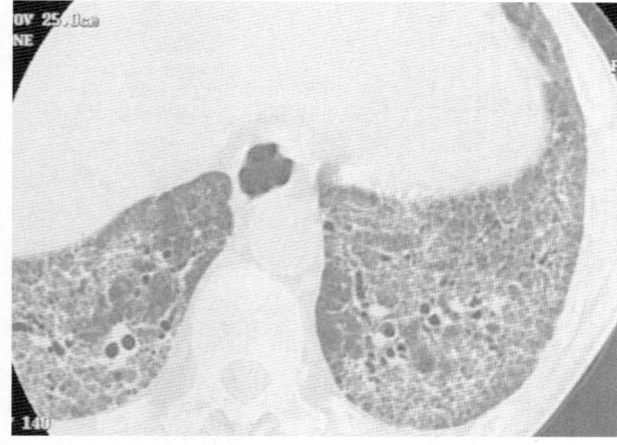

B

Figure 4–15   A 72-year-old male with chronic hypersensitivity pneumonitis. *A*, Chest radiograph shows a basal reticular pattern. *B*, HRCT through the left lower lung shows a diffuse reticular pattern with bronchial dilation due to traction bronchiectasis. Reproduced with permission from Lynch DA, Newell JD, Lee JS, editors. Imaging of diffuse lung disease. Hamilton: B.C. Decker; 2000.

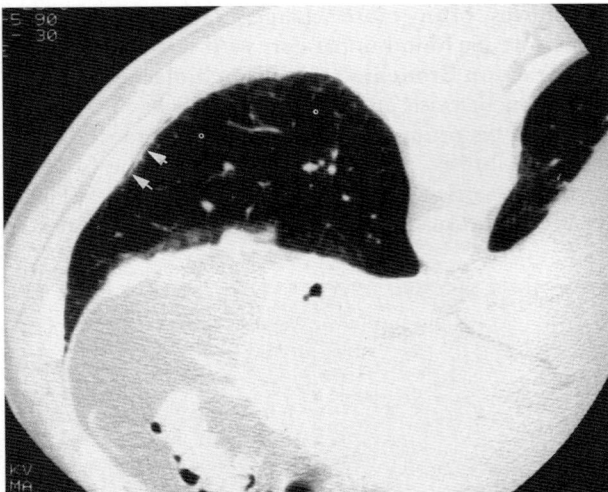

Figure 4–16 Early asbestosis. Prone HRCT of an asbestos-exposed worker shows a subtle curvilinear subpleural line (*arrows*) parallel to the chest wall in the posterior left lung. Mild septal thickening is also present, and there is reticular opacity in the posteromedial right lung. Although the findings are subtle, they were found bilaterally and at multiple levels; they are therefore adequate for the diagnosis of asbestosis, even though the parenchyma appeared normal on chest radiograph. A focal pleural plaque is present along the left hemidiaphragm.

with ground-glass attenuation and is reliable evidence of lung fibrosis. This finding is not usually associated with clinical symptoms of bronchiectasis. Distortion of other anatomic features of the lung such as vessels or fissures may also be seen in subjects with moderate or advanced lung fibrosis. Traction bronchiectasis or bronchiolectasis seen in areas of ground-glass attenuation is good evidence that the ground-glass opacification is due to diffuse lung fibrosis rather than to active lung inflammation (alveolitis).[93]

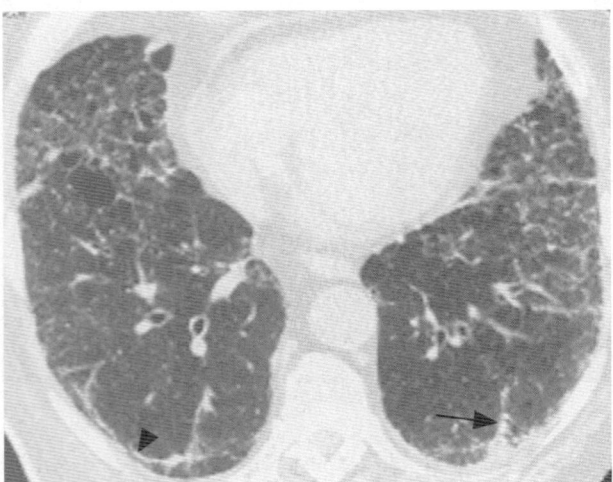

Figure 4–17 A 62-year-old male with asbestosis. HRCT shows a parenchymal fibrotic band (*arrow*) and a subpleural curvilinear line (*arrow head*) as well as a bilateral reticular abnormality compatible with asbestosis.

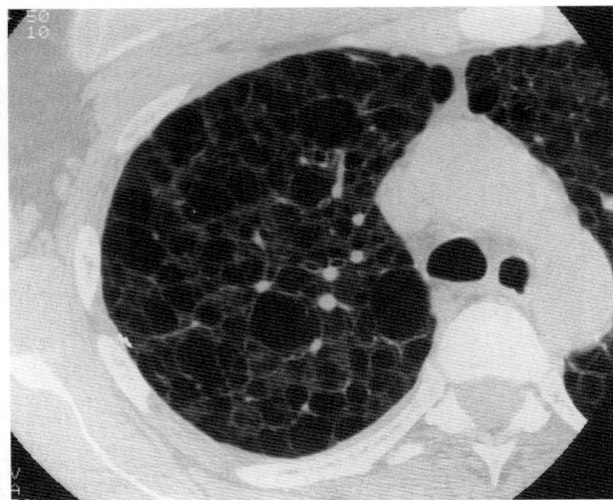

Figure 4–18 Lymphangiomyomatosis. HRCT scan shows profuse round lucencies. In contrast to centrilobular emphysema, the cysts all have well-defined walls with vessels along these walls rather than centrally.

Pleural Abnormalities. Other CT signs of interstitial lung disease[94] include irregular pleural interfaces and pleural or subpleural thickening, usually representing subpleural fibrosis. These findings are seen along the chest wall or interlobar fissures in patients with moderate or advanced pulmonary fibrosis and are not usually of value in the differential diagnosis. The irregular pleural thickening of lung fibrosis must be distinguished from the smoother pleural parietal thickening caused by pleural plaques.

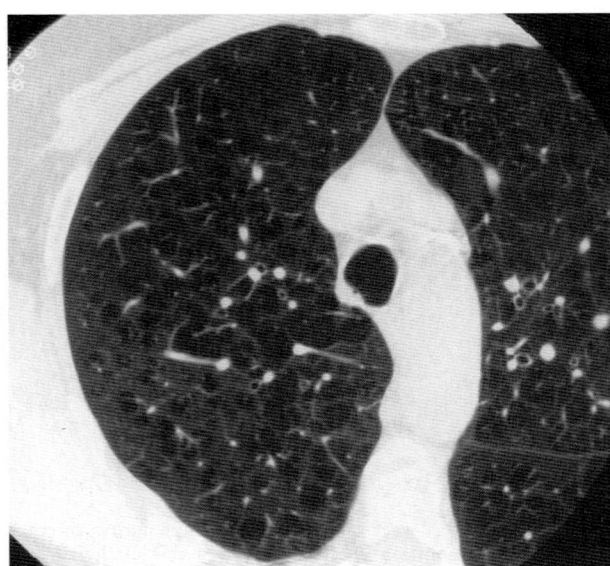

Figure 4–19 Centrilobular emphysema. HRCT scan through the upper lung shows round lucencies, none of which have a well-defined wall. Most of the lucencies have vessels coursing through them, a finding typical for centrilobular emphysema.

Parenchymal Opacification.   The term parenchymal opacification[83,95] is applied to any homogeneous increase in lung density on chest radiographs or chest CT. When this parenchymal opacification is dense enough to obscure the vessels and other parenchymal structures, it is called consolidation (see Figure 4–10). Ground-glass attenuation (sometimes called hazy increase in lung density) is defined as an increase in lung density not sufficient to obscure vessels (see Figure 4–8). The term parenchymal opacification is preferable to the previously used term "air space opacification," as it may sometimes be due to pure interstitial thickening. Ground-glass attenuation is commonly, though not always, associated with reversible or potentially reversible lung disease.

Decreased Lung Attenuation/Mosaic Pattern. The attenuation (density) of a given area of lung depends on the amount of parenchymal tissue, air, and blood in that area. Therefore, decreased attenuation of the lung may be due to lung destruction (in panlobular emphysema), decreased blood flow (in vascular disease such as pulmonary thromboembolism), or decreased ventilation with air-trapping and reflex pulmonary oligemia (in small airways diseases with constrictive bronchiolitis) (Figure 4–21). Panlobular emphysema differs from vascular lung disease and small airway disease in that it usually causes a diffuse decrease in lung attenuation (increased blackness), whereas thromboembolic disease and obliterative bronchiolitis are commonly (though not always) more patchy in distribution. Vascular disease can often be distinguished from airways disease by comparing inspiratory and expiratory scans. In airways disease, one will expect to see air-trapping on the expiratory scans, resulting in an increase in the number of areas of decreased attenuation. In patients with occlusive vascular disease, the areas of decreased attenuation should not increase on expiration.[96]

Because patients with thromboembolic disease and obliterative bronchiolitis commonly have a patchy decrease in lung attenuation, they may present with a mosaic pattern, with lobules of normal attenuation adjacent to lobules or subsegments of decreased attenuation. A similar mosaic pattern may be caused by parenchymal disease, which causes lobular areas of ground-glass attenuation. With the mosaic pattern, it can be difficult to decide whether the abnormal areas are those of decreased attenuation or those of increased attenuation. This distinction can be made by observing the pulmonary vessels, which will be reduced in size in areas affected by vascular occlusive disease or obliterative bronchiolitis but will be normal in size in patients with parenchymal infiltrative lung diseases.[96] One can then use expiratory images to distinguish between airway obstruction and thromboembolic disease.[41] Physiologic evaluation will also help to distinguish between vascular disease, airways obstruction, and parenchymal infiltration.

Crazy Paving Pattern.   In the crazy paving pattern, thickened intralobular and interlobular lines form a fine geographic network superimposed on a background of ground-glass attenuation.[97] In the correct clinical context, this pattern is virtually pathognomonic of pulmonary alveolar proteinosis. The pattern can also be seen in patients with other lung diseases including resolving pneumonia, acute respiratory distress syndrome (ARDS), lipoid pneumonia, and mucinous bronchioloalveolar carcinoma, but in those conditions it is usually associated with other types of CT abnormalities.[98–100]

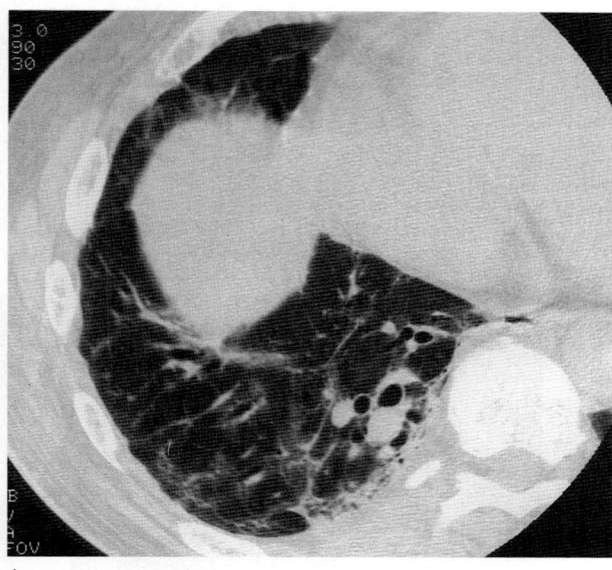

A

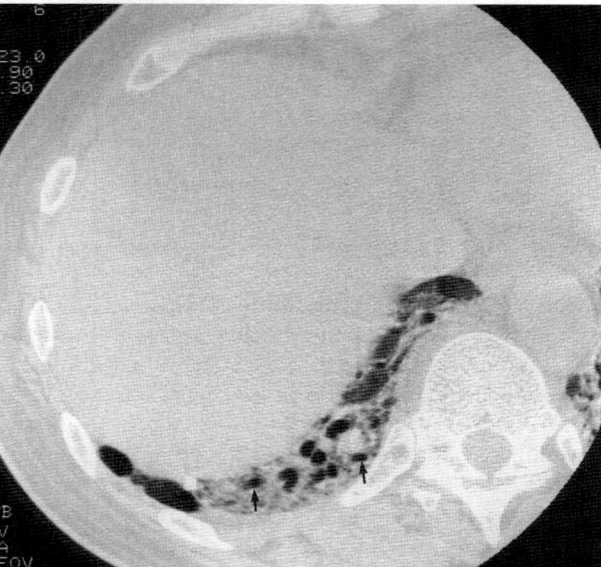

B

Figure 4–20 A, B   Traction bronchiectasis in idiopathic pulmonary fibrosis. Two HRCT scans obtained through the right lung base demonstrate linear bands of fibrosis. A posteromedial area of dense fibrosis contains multiple dilated bronchi (*arrows*). The areas of ground-glass attenuation in the posterolateral lung are associated with reticular opacity, and therefore are more likely to represent areas of lung fibrosis rather than alveolitis.

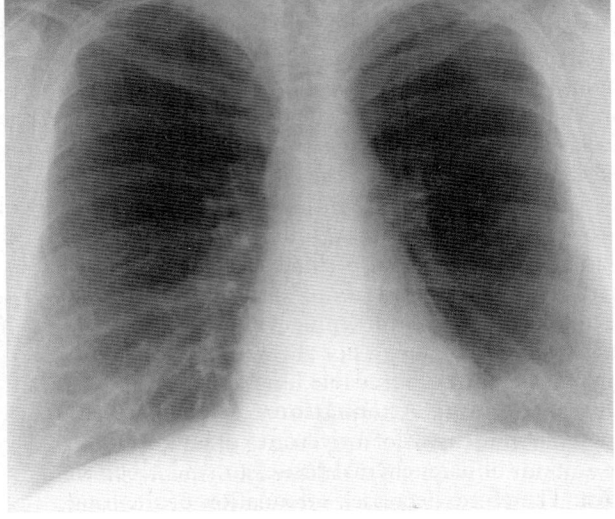

Figure 4–21 Unilateral, postinfectious constrictive bronchiolitis (Swyer-James syndrome). *A*, Chest radiograph shows hyperlucency of the left lung. *B*, *C*, HRCT scans show near-complete absence of vessels in the left lung, and sharply defined, lobular areas of decreased density in the right lung. The sharply defined areas of decreased density seen in the right lung are typical for constrictive bronchiolitis. Note the decreased size of vessels in the hyperlucent areas.

A

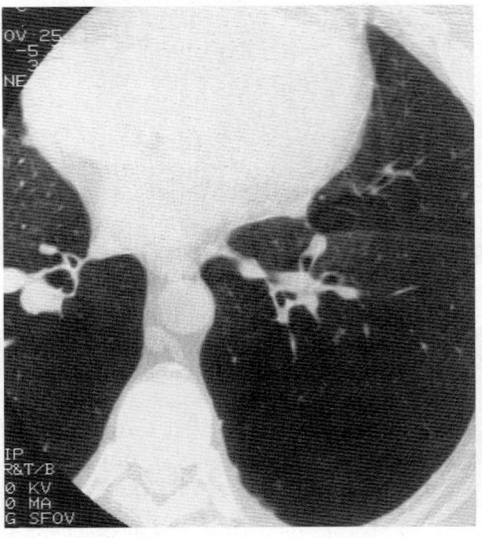

B

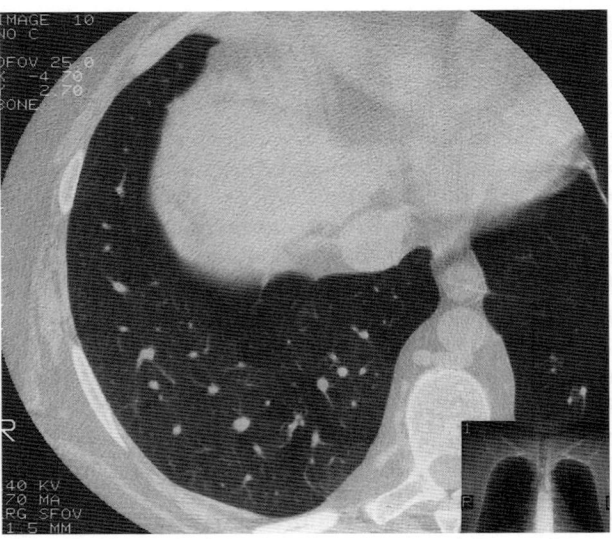

C

Mediastinal Lymphadenopathy.   Mediastinal lymph node enlargement is a common CT finding in usual interstitial pneumonitis (UIP) and may also occur in asbestosis. Lymph node enlargement was seen in 13 of 14 subjects with UIP studied by Bergin and Castellino.[101] Nodes as large as 2 × 3 centimeters were identified in three of their subjects. In a large series of 175 patients with diffuse lung diseases, mediastinal lymphadenopathy was found in 84% of patients with sarcoidosis, 67% of patients with idiopathic pulmonary fibrosis (IPF), 70% of patients with collagen vascular disease, 53% of patients with hypersensitivity pneumonitis, and 36% of patients with organizing pneumonia (OP). In a study of subjects with systemic sclerosis,[102] mediastinal adenopathy was uncommon in patients without parenchymal abnormality, and the extent of adenopathy increased with the extent of lung disease,

suggesting that the lymph nodes are reactive. A more recent study similarly suggested that the extent of adenopathy was reflective of the extent of lung disease.[103]

The reactive adenopathy seen in diffuse lung disease is never visible on the chest radiograph. Sarcoidosis, silicosis, or lymphangitic carcinoma should be the primary considerations if a patient with an interstitial parenchymal abnormality has hilar or mediastinal lymphadenopathy visible on the chest radiograph.

CT AND HRCT FEATURES OF SPECIFIC INTERSTITIAL LUNG DISEASES

Idiopathic Interstitial Pneumonias

The diverse histologic features of the idiopathic interstitial pneumonias are reflected in their CT appearances, which are often suggestive of the correct diagnosis. In this section, the CT features of each of the idiopathic interstitial pneumonias will be discussed, beginning with the most common, usual interstitial pneumonia.

Usual Interstitial Pneumonia

Idiopathic pulmonary fibrosis is characterized on the chest radiograph by a predominantly peripheral, basal reticular opacity. Lower lobe volume loss, evident from fissural and hilar displacement, is often marked and is sometimes the only radiographic sign of disease (Figure 4–22). Though this disease is often asymmetric, it is rarely unilateral. Chest radiographic abnormality is frequently the earliest sign of lung disease in patients with IPF. Evaluation of sequential radiographs usually shows progression of disease, often over several years, associated with progressive loss of lung volumes.

The diagnostic features of IPF on CT are peripheral reticular opacities and honeycombing, predominating in the lower lobes (see Figures 4–9 and 4–20).[71,88] Asymmetric or patchy fibrosis is common. Although thickening of interlobular septa may be seen in early IPF, it is much more common to see intralobular or nonlobular reticular opacities without recognizable lobular anatomy. Advanced IPF is characterized by honeycombing that is usually subpleural and is frequently associated with traction bronchiectasis (see Figure 4–20) and bronchiolectasis. A prospective, multicenter study of the accuracy of the diagnosis of UIP found that a confident CT diagnosis of UIP, based on typical features, was correct in 96% of cases,[104] consistent with the results of several other studies indicating that the correctness of a confident first choice diagnosis of UIP, made by an experienced radiologist, is greater than 90%.[70,105,106] Univariate and multivariate analysis showed that radiologic features were the primary discriminants between UIP and other causes of diffuse lung disease.[107] Among clinical features, an elevated forced expiratory volume in 1 second/forced vital capacity (FEV_1/FVC) ratio was found to be associated with UIP on univariate analysis but not on multivariate analysis. None of the other classic clinical features of IPF were useful in diagnosis. However, it should be noted that in this study, a confident CT diagnosis of UIP was made in only about 50% of cases. In other cases of histologically confirmed UIP, the CT features were not typical enough to make a confident diagnosis.

A much-discussed feature of HRCT in IPF has been its reported ability to assess disease activity. Several studies performed between 1987 and 1995 suggested that the presence of ground-glass attenuation in patients with fibrosing alveolitis or idiopathic pulmonary fibrosis was associated with a substantial probability of reversibility on treatment with steroids, whereas patients with a more fibrotic pattern usually progressed despite treatment.[108–111] It now seems likely that most of the patients in these studies who had a predominant ground-glass

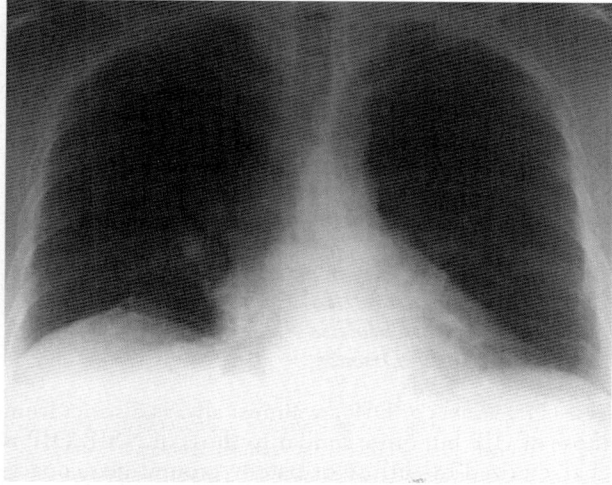

Figure 4–22   Lower lobe volume loss in IPF. Chest radiograph of a patient with IPF shows marked bilateral lower lobe volume loss with depression of the hila.

attenuation pattern on CT had nonspecific interstitial pneumonia rather than UIP. In true UIP, ground-glass attenuation is usually associated with early fibrosis, which progresses over time to a fibrotic pattern with traction bronchiectasis and reticular abnormality. Pathologists no longer describe active alveolar inflammation in UIP, but emphasize that fibroblastic foci are early lesions.[112]

The histologic pattern of UIP is not always idiopathic. It may be seen in patients with collagen vascular disease, asbestosis, and chronic hypersensitivity pneumonitis.[113] Not surprisingly, the CT features of these conditions are often identical to those of UIP.[71,106,114] Differentiation between idiopathic pulmonary fibrosis and fibrosis related to inhalational exposure or collagen vascular disease is an important task for the clinician.

Nonspecific Interstitial Pneumonia

We are still learning about nonspecific interstitial pneumonia. Reports of its CT appearances have varied, but all studies have agreed that it tends to have a peripheral and lower lobe predominance.[115–120] Ground-glass attenuation is the most common CT feature, often associated with a reticular pattern and traction bronchiectasis (Figure 4–23). The prevalence of consolidation, honeycombing, and nodules has varied substantially among different series. The reasons for this variation in CT descriptions are unclear but may relate to the variation in pathologic criteria for establishing this diagnosis and also, perhaps, to the inclusion in some series of nonspecific interstitial pneumonia (NSIP) related to collagen vascular disease.

In our practice, we have found that NSIP is almost always associated with a predominant basal reticular and ground-glass pattern, without honeycombing. In a recent study comparing the CT features of UIP with those of NSIP, MacDonald and colleagues found that a confident diagnosis of NSIP based on these appearances was correct in 69% of cases.[118] The CT appearances of NSIP overlap with those of desquamative interstitial pneumonitis (DIP) and with some cases of UIP. The CT abnormality of NSIP is usually at least partly reversible on steroid treatment.[119,121]

Desquamative Interstitial Pneumonitis/ Respiratory Bronchiolitis-Associated Interstitial Lung Disease

The CT features of DIP are almost always distinct from those of UIP but quite similar to those of NSIP. DIP is characterized by diffuse or patchy ground-glass opacification, often with a peripheral predominance (Figure 4–24).[122] In contrast to UIP, the ground-glass opacification of DIP is frequently reversible.[123] An uncommon feature of DIP is the presence of multiple small

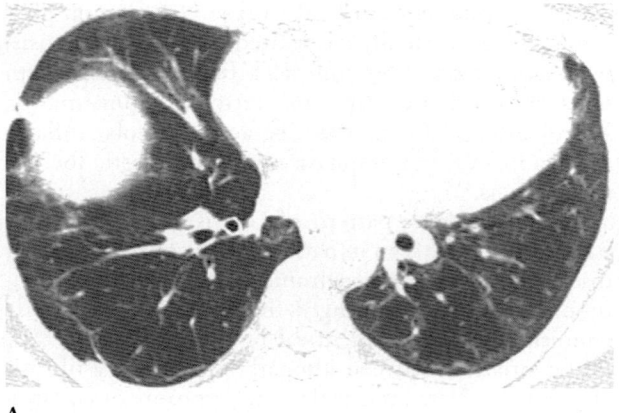

A

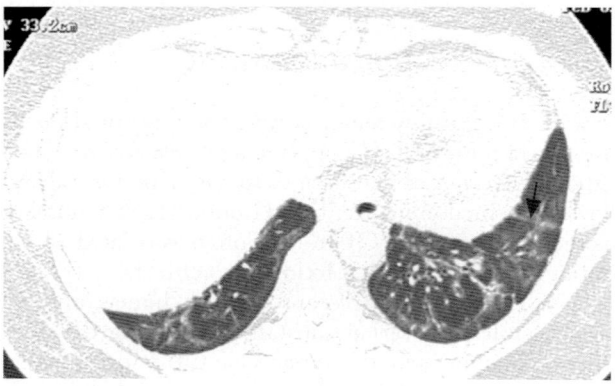

B

Figure 4–23 A 37-year-old female with nonspecific interstitial pneumonia related to progressive systemic sclerosis. High-resolution chest CT through the lower lungs shows peripheral predominant ground-glass attenuation. The posterior displacement of the left major fissure (*arrow*) and the mild bronchial dilation suggest that there is probably some associated lung fibrosis.

cysts within the areas of ground-glass attenuation.[124] The presence of cysts within areas of ground-glass attenuation should suggest either DIP or lymphoid interstitial pneumonia (LIP).

The entity of respiratory bronchiolitis-associated interstitial lung disease (RBILD) is closely related to DIP, and many observers believe that a spectrum of smoking-related lung diseases extends from respiratory bronchiolitis (which is usually asymptomatic) to respiratory bronchiolitis-associated interstitial lung disease to DIP.[125] Respiratory bronchiolitis is characterized on CT primarily by centrilobular nodularity (see Figure 4–13). The CT appearances of RBILD exhibit a combination of patchy ground-glass attenuation and poorly defined centrilobular nodularity. In heavy cigarette smokers, these findings are strongly suggestive of RBILD. A study by Park and colleagues,[126] correlating imaging and pathology in patients with RBILD, showed that the extent of centrilobular nodules correlated with the extent of macrophages in respiratory bronchioles and with the severity of respiratory bronchiolitis, whereas the extent of ground-glass opacity correlated with the extent of macrophage accumulation in the alveoli and alveolar ducts.

Organizing Pneumonia

The most prominent CT finding in cryptogenic organizing pneumonia (COP) is patchy consolidation, which was present in 79% of 43 patients studied by Lee and colleagues (Figure 4–25).[127] The consolidation is often peripheral or peribronchovascular in distribution, and may predominate in the lower lobes. Ground-glass attenuation is also common. Other less frequent findings included poorly defined or well-defined nodules. The nodular pattern of COP appears to correlate with localized organizing pneumonia, centered on obliterated bronchioles, whereas the consolidated pattern appears to correlate with more diffuse organizing pneumonia. Although OP is commonly reversible, it may progress to lung fibrosis in a minority of cases. Progression appears to be more likely if a reticular pattern is present on the initial chest radiograph or CT scan.[128] As with the other interstitial pneumonias, the OP pattern may be seen with a variety of causes of lung injury, including collagen vascular disease, infection, resolving ARDS, resolving pulmonary hemorrhage, and drug toxicity.

Acute Interstitial Pneumonia

The CT appearances of acute interstitial pneumonia (AIP) are similar to those of idiopathic ARDS. In the acute phase, AIP is characterized by patchy, geographic ground-glass attenuation with consolidation in the more dependent portions of the lung. In the organizing phase of ARDS, architectural distortion and traction bronchiectasis are frequent. The CT pattern can be used to distinguish between the acute and organizing phases of this disease.[129-131]

Lymphoid Interstitial Pneumonia

Lymphoid interstitial pneumonia is the least common form of idiopathic pneumonia. Its CT appearances are quite varied, but ground-glass attenuation is the most frequent feature. A more specific finding is the presence of multiple perivascular and subpleural cysts,[132] which, in the correct clinical context (eg, Sjögren's syndrome), should suggest the diagnosis.

Sarcoidosis

The chest radiographic findings in sarcoidosis are often sufficiently characteristic to be diagnostic. Adenopathy is usually most prominent in the pulmonary hila, right paratracheal region, and aortopulmonary window. The adenopathy is usually symmetric but may be apparently unilateral in 5% of cases. Parenchymal abnormalities seen on the chest radiograph include discrete nodules. Linear abnormalities are usually less prominent. A later stage of sarcoidosis is characterized by marked conglomerate lung fibrosis with perihilar masses and marked upward displacement of the hila. The chest radiographic appearances of sarcoidosis (Siltzbach staging) can have substantial prognostic significance. The most widely used radiographic staging system, based on that of Siltzbach, is as follows:

- stage 0: normal chest radiograph
- stage 1: mediastinal and hilar lymphadenopathy
- stage 2: lymphadenopathy with lung parenchymal abnormality
- stage 3: lung parenchymal abnormality in the absence of lymphadenopathy
- stage 4: significant lung fibrosis with architectural distortion or bullae

This classification scheme has substantial prognostic significance. Untreated patients with stage 1 disease experience resolution of symptoms and radiographic abnormalities in 50 to 90% of cases, compared with 30 to 70% for stage 2, 10 to 20% with stage 3, and 0% with stage 4.[133]

Typical CT and HRCT findings in pulmonary sarcoidosis include nodules, hazy increase in lung density, irregular linear densities, and hilar and mediastinal adenopathy.[134-137] The nodules are characteristically deposited along the bronchovascular bundles, interlobular septa, and along the pleura (including the fissures) (Figure 4–26). These nodules presumably correspond to coalescent granulomas, which are commonly seen histologically in these areas.[138,139] Both the nodules and hazy density may be partially reversible on steroid therapy. In subjects with fibrosis due to sarcoidosis one sees irregular linear densities, distortion of lobular anatomy, and

cysts or honeycombing. Conglomeration of segmental or subsegmental vessels and bronchi is a characteristic feature of advanced disease (Figure 4–27). Masslike fibrosis, similar to that seen in silicosis, may also occur.

Use of CT can help to clarify the appearance of "pseudoalveolar sarcoidosis," in which clusters of granulomata cause a radiographic appearance of poorly defined masses, often associated with air bronchograms. On CT scanning, these masses are shown to lie along the bronchovascular axis, have an irregular nodular outline, and be surrounded by numerous satellite nodules.[140] Associated findings of parenchymal sarcoidosis are commonly found.

The potential benefits of HRCT scanning in pulmonary sarcoidosis include the early detection of disease, improved characterization of the type of pulmonary disease, identification of CT features that indicate progression of disease (eg, hazy increase in lung density), and accurate quantification of the extent of pulmonary disease, which aid in the determination of progression or response to therapy.[141]

The morphologic appearance of sarcoidosis helps to predict the extent and type of physiologic impairment. In general, patients with nodules, focal consolidation, or spherical opacities have less physiologic impairment than those with linear opacities[142,143] or conglomerate masses, suggesting that focal sarcoid granulomas probably cause minimal pulmonary dysfunction. Abehsera and colleagues classified fibrotic sarcoidosis into three distinct patterns based on HRCT appearances.[144] Central bronchial distortion (often associated with conglomerate perihilar masses) was the most common pattern, occurring in 47% of 80 patients in their series, and was asso-

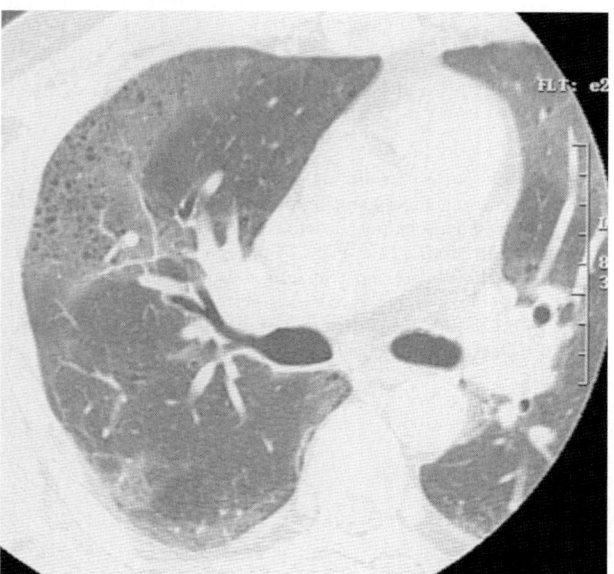

Figure 4–24 A 45-year-old male with desquamative interstitial pneumonitis. High-resolution CT shows patchy ground-glass opacity. The areas of ground-glass attenuation contain multiple cysts. Reproduced with permission from Lynch DA, Newell JD, Lee JS, editors. Imaging of diffuse lung disease. Hamilton: B.C. Decker; 2000.

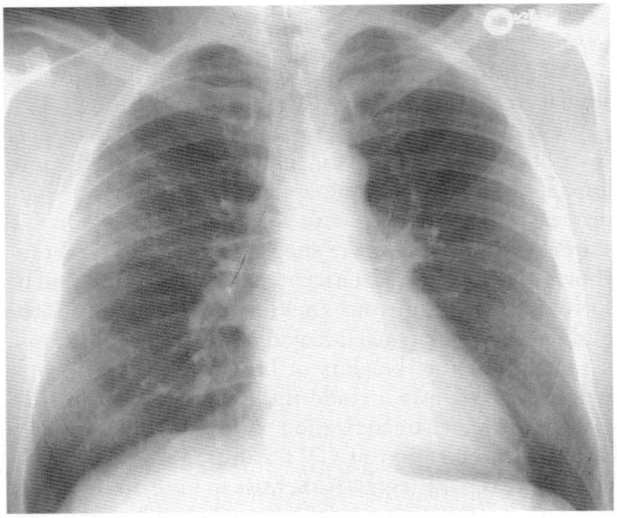

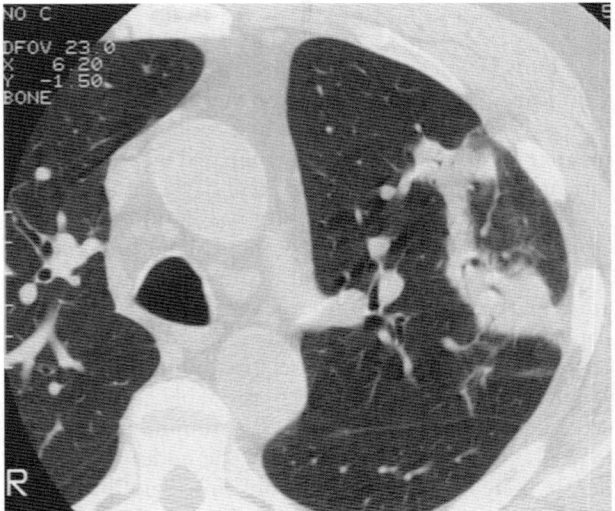

Figure 4–25   A 62-year-old male with recurrent migratory opacities due to cryptogenic organizing pneumonia. *A, B, C,* Chest radiographs show migratory, poorly defined lung opacities of cryptogenic organizing pneumonia. *D, E,* HRCT images obtained during another exacerbation show bilateral patchy lung consolidation typical of organizing pneumonia. Reproduced with permission from Lynch DA, Newell JD, Lee JS, editors. Imaging of diffuse lung disease. Hamilton: B.C. Decker; 2000.

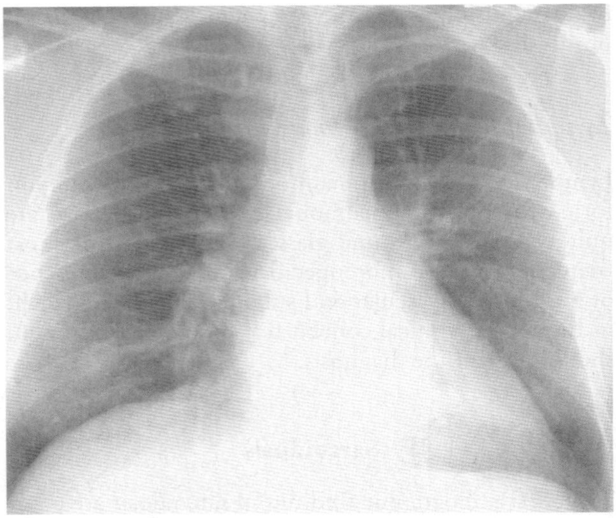

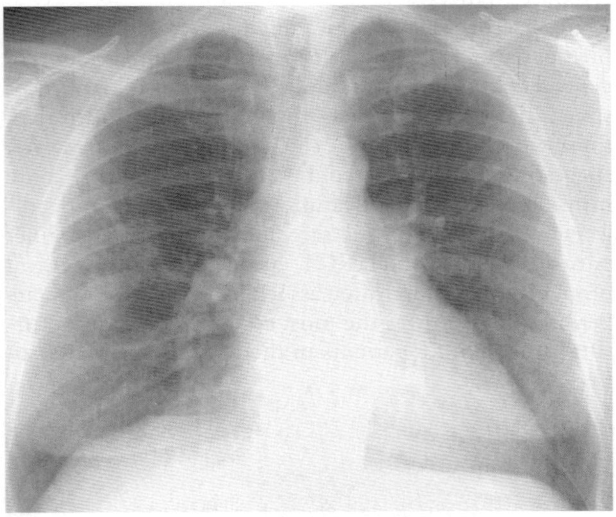

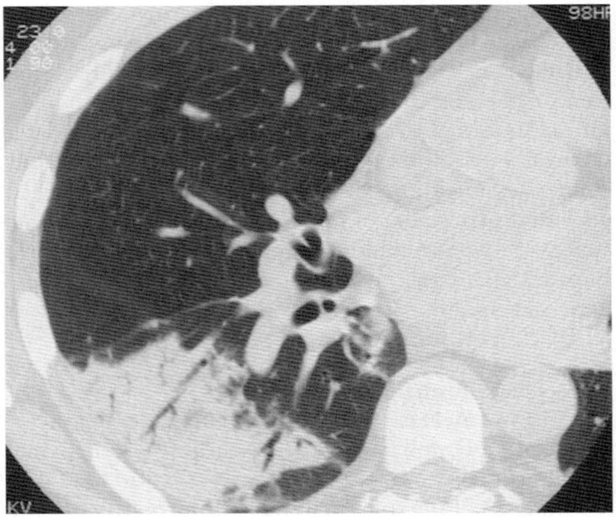

ciated with physiologic evidence of airflow obstruction. A peripheral honeycomb pattern, found in 29%, was associated with pulmonary restriction, whereas a diffuse linear pattern, seen in 24%, was associated with less marked physiologic impairment. Physiologic airways obstruction in sarcoidosis may be due either to central bronchial distortion,[144] endobronchial airway granulomas, or air-trapping at the lobular or subsegmental level, as detected on expiratory CT images.[42,145]

The role of CT scanning in patients with known or suspected pulmonary sarcoidosis remains unclear. Recog-

nition of the characteristic CT patterns may help to suggest the diagnosis and may provide a "road-map" in identifying high-yield areas for biopsy sampling by the bronchoscopist. In patients with unilateral adenopathy, in whom there is concern for the presence of lymphoma or other abnormality, CT may help by identifying bilateral nodal and parenchymal abnormalities more suggestive of sarcoidosis. The CT features in some cases of sarcoidosis (see Figure 4–26) can be sufficiently specific to obviate the need for bronchoscopy. However, CT adds little to the diagnostic evaluation of patients with typical clinical and chest radi-

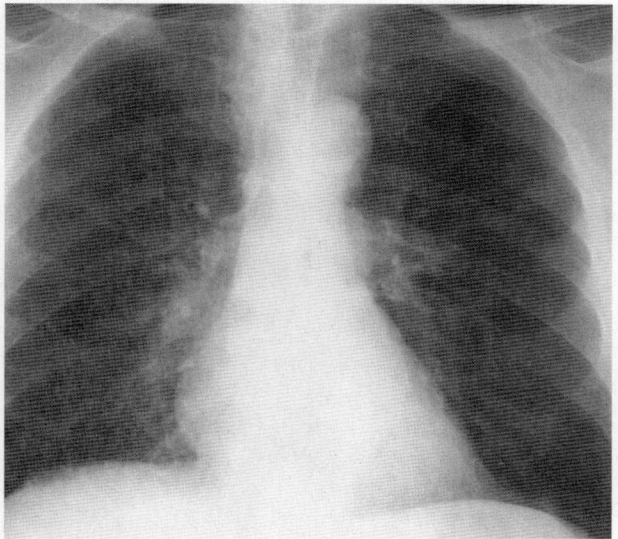

A

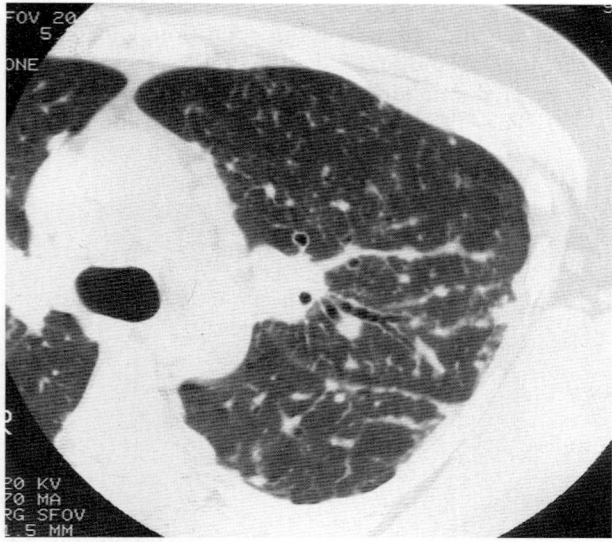

C

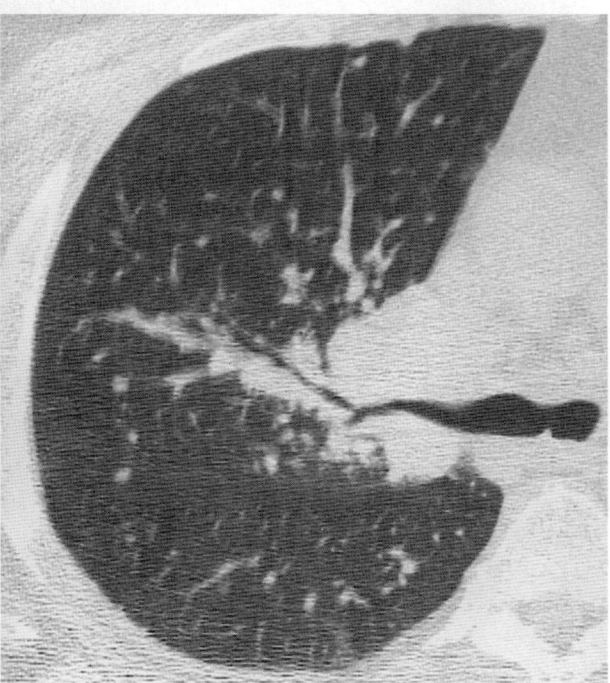

B

Figure 4–26 Sarcoidosis. *A*, Chest radiograph shows widespread fine pulmonary nodules, most marked in middle and lower zones, associated with bilateral hilar and mediastinal adenopathy. *B*, HRCT scan shows a nonrandom distribution of nodules in contrast to the more diffuse pattern of silicosis. The nodules are clustered along the bronchovascular bundle. *C*, HRCT scan in another patient shows nodules studded along the bronchovascular bundles, and along the major fissure, interlobular septa, and subpleural regions. Coalescence of nodules along the pleural surfaces simulates pleural thickening (pseudoplaques). This distribution is typical for sarcoidosis.

ographic findings of sarcoidosis. A study by Mana and colleagues suggests that CT does little to change the management of patients in whom it is performed.[146] However, in individual cases, CT may be helpful in determining the extent of abnormality, identifying large and small airways obstruction, and in following response to treatment in patients in whom the physiologic evaluation is equivocal.

Lymphangitic Carcinomatosis

Several studies have reported on the CT appearances of pulmonary lymphangitic spread of tumor.[87,91,147] Irregular thickening of bronchovascular bundles and interlobular septa is the hallmark of this condition. Unlike most other interstitial diseases, lymphangitic carcinomatosis may be predominantly or entirely unilateral (see Figure 4–14). The "beaded chain" appearance of interlobular septa is characteristic and usually correlates with tumor infiltration, rather than edema or fibrosis (desmoplastic reaction).[147] Coarse thickening of interlobular septa without architectural distortion allows the polygonal secondary pulmonary lobules to be seen to a degree rarely found in other conditions. Prominence of centrilobular tissues is also common. These features are quite different from the fine, smooth interlobular thickening and hazy increase in lung density seen in interstitial pulmonary edema (see Figure 4–7). The changes of lymphangitic carcinomatosis may persist or progress slowly over years in long-term survivors.[148] The CT differential diagnosis of lymphangitic carcinoma includes sarcoidosis, which may similarly involve the axial and interlobular interstitium of the lung. However lymphangitic carcinoma tends to be more asymmetric than sarcoidosis, and shows greater involvement of the interlobular septa and subpleural interstitium.[149]

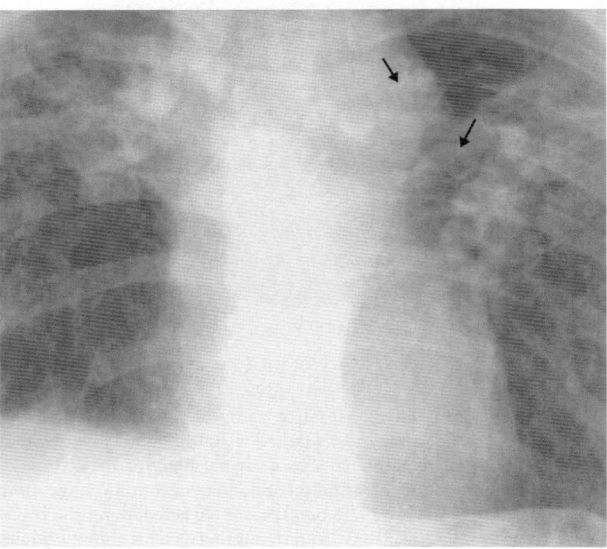

A

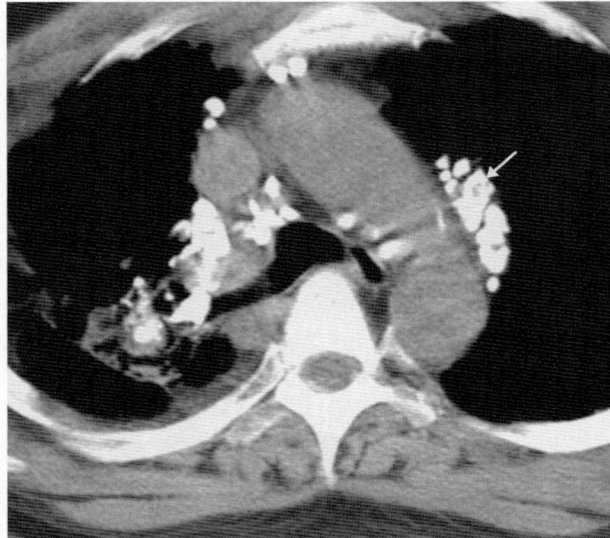

B

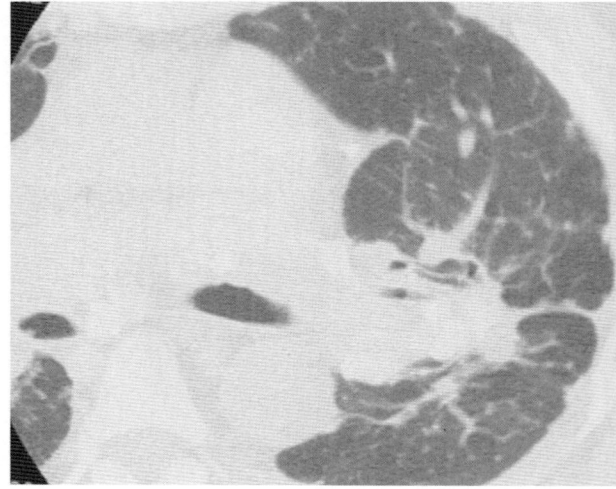

C

Figure 4–27   A 52-year-old female with long-standing sarcoidosis and eggshell nodal calcification. *A*, Chest radiograph shows marked volume loss in the upper lobes. Multiple calcified mediastinal nodes are shown with eggshell calcification (*arrows*). *B*, CT scan photographed at soft-tissue windows shows extensive nodal calcification with eggshell calcification. *C*, HRCT shows left upper lobe mass-like opacity with associated bronchial distortion. Reproduced with permission from Lynch DA, Newell JD, Lee JS, editors. Imaging of diffuse lung disease. Hamilton: B.C. Decker; 2000.

Pneumoconiosis

The radiographic and CT features of coal workers' pneumoconiosis[150] and silicosis[151,152] are similar (see Figure 4–11). On the chest radiograph, both conditions present with predominantly upper lobe nodules, which may later coalesce to form mass-like opacities (progressive massive fibrosis). However, the CT findings in these diseases vary with the size of the opacities seen on the chest radiograph. Opacities classified as type p by the International Labor Office (ILO) criteria are characterized on HRCT by tiny branching structures or a cluster of small dots. Centrilobular emphysema is a frequent association. By contrast, opacities of the q and r type are characterized by sharply demarcated round nodules or irregular contracted nodules. The nodules may be centrilobular or subpleural in location and tend to predominate in the posterior upper lobes. Subpleural micronodules may become confluent to form a "pseudoplaque."[85] A small proportion (perhaps 10%) of patients with coal workers' pneumoconiosis develops basal reticular opacity similar to that of idiopathic pulmonary fibrosis.[153–155] These patients with diffuse interstitial fibrosis seem to be at higher risk for the development of lung cancers.[155]

In silicosis, pulmonary function correlates poorly with the profusion of nodules on CT, but the CT-determined extent of emphysema correlates well with FEV_1 and diffusing capacity.[151] In a study by Begin and colleagues of workers with silicosis,[152] CT demonstrated unsuspected early conglomeration in one-third of patients who were classified as having simple silicosis on the basis of the chest radiograph. These subjects had corresponding abnormalities of lung function. A further study by Begin and colleagues showed that combined use of conventional CT and HRCT was the most sensitive technique for detection of pulmonary opacities in subjects with silicosis.[156] The interobserver agreement for CT scan readings was markedly higher than for radiographic interpretations.

Several papers have shown that emphysema develops in a substantial proportion of life-long nonsmokers exposed to silica. In a CT study of 207 miners with normal or near-normal chest radiographs, emphysema was seen in 8 of 11 nonsmokers with pneumoconiosis but in only 1 of 20 nonsmokers without pneumoconiosis.[157] The presence of pneumoconiosis on CT was a predictor of emphysema extent, and exposure to silica was a significant predictive factor for emphysema even in patients without CT evidence for pneumoconiosis. A study of 70 gold miners by Cowie and colleagues reached similar conclusions.[158]

In coal workers' pneumoconiosis,[150] CT is more sensitive than chest radiography for the detection of pulmonary nodules, and HRCT is more sensitive for the detection of nodules less than 3 mm in diameter than is conventional CT. Importantly, in subjects in whom small round opacities were identified on the chest radiograph, HRCT was normal in 20% and was minimally abnormal in a further 42%. Similarly, Gevenois and colleagues[159] demonstrated that opacities thought to represent pneumoconiosis on the chest radiograph can often be ascribed by CT to bronchiectasis or emphysema. Thus, the chest radiograph may both underestimate and overestimate the extent of pneumoconiosis. With progression of disease, the nodules increase both in size and in profusion.

Progressive massive fibrosis (PMF) may occur in coal workers' pneumoconiosis or in silicosis. Synonyms for this entity include complicated pneumoconiosis and conglomerate pneumoconiosis. It is much more common in silicosis than in coal workers' pneumoconiosis. On the chest radiograph, PMF presents with mass-like or sausage-shaped opacities, typically seen in the posterior upper lobes, with associated hilar retraction (Figure 4–28). Sequential evaluation of these masses often shows apparent migration toward the hila, leaving a peripheral rim of cicatricial emphysema. Although usually symmetric, masses may be unilateral. Unilateral PMF may be distinguished from lung cancer by the presence of lobar volume loss and peripheral emphysema. On CT, PMF typically appears as an upper lobe mass (often bilateral) with irregular borders, frequent calcification, and surrounding paracicatricial emphysema (see Figure 4–28). Thickening of the adjacent extrapleural fat is common. A central area of low density is often seen in masses that are greater than 4 cm in diameter and likely represents necrosis. Cavitation is a less frequent finding. The presence of cavitation should always raise the suspicion of tuberculous or atypical mycobacterial superinfection.

The ILO classification system for radiographs of patients with pneumoconioses was developed over 50 years ago, with several subsequent revisions, the most recent being in 1980.[160] It requires systematic comparison of radiographs with standard films to evaluate the presence, type, and extent of radiographic opacity. Initially intended as an epidemiologic tool, it has become enshrined in law as a method for determining the extent of disease and even the level of compensation for individual workers. The system is limited by the inherent lack of sensitivity and specificity of the chest radiograph and also by a moderate amount of interobserver variation, but it remains the only systematic radiographic classification.[161] There is an ongoing international effort to standardize the acquisition and scoring of CT scans for occupational lung disease,[162] using standard images similar to those used for chest radiographs. Such a system, if validated, should provide a more sensitive and specific method for the evaluation of occupational lung disease.

Asbestosis

The role of radiology in the assessment of asbestos exposure is to document the presence or absence of pleural disease, to index asbestos exposure, and to ascertain the presence and extent of complications including asbestos-related lung fibrosis (asbestosis), lung cancer, and mesothelioma.[163]

The chest radiograph has substantial limitations in the diagnosis of asbestos-related pleural and lung fibrosis. Noncalcified plaques are difficult to identify on the chest radiograph, except when the x-ray beam is tangential to the plaque. Also it may sometimes be difficult to differentiate between noncalcified plaques and extrapleural fat.[164] The chest radiograph is abnormal in a minority of cases of pathologically demonstrated asbestosis.[165] A further limitation of chest radiographic assessment of asbestosis is the questionable physiologic and pathologic significance of the small irregular opacities that are the chest radiographic hallmark of early asbestosis.[166–169] In at least some cases, these small irregular opacities appear to be related to cigarette smoking.

CT scanning is more sensitive than the chest radiograph for the detection of pleural plaques,[67,170] particu-

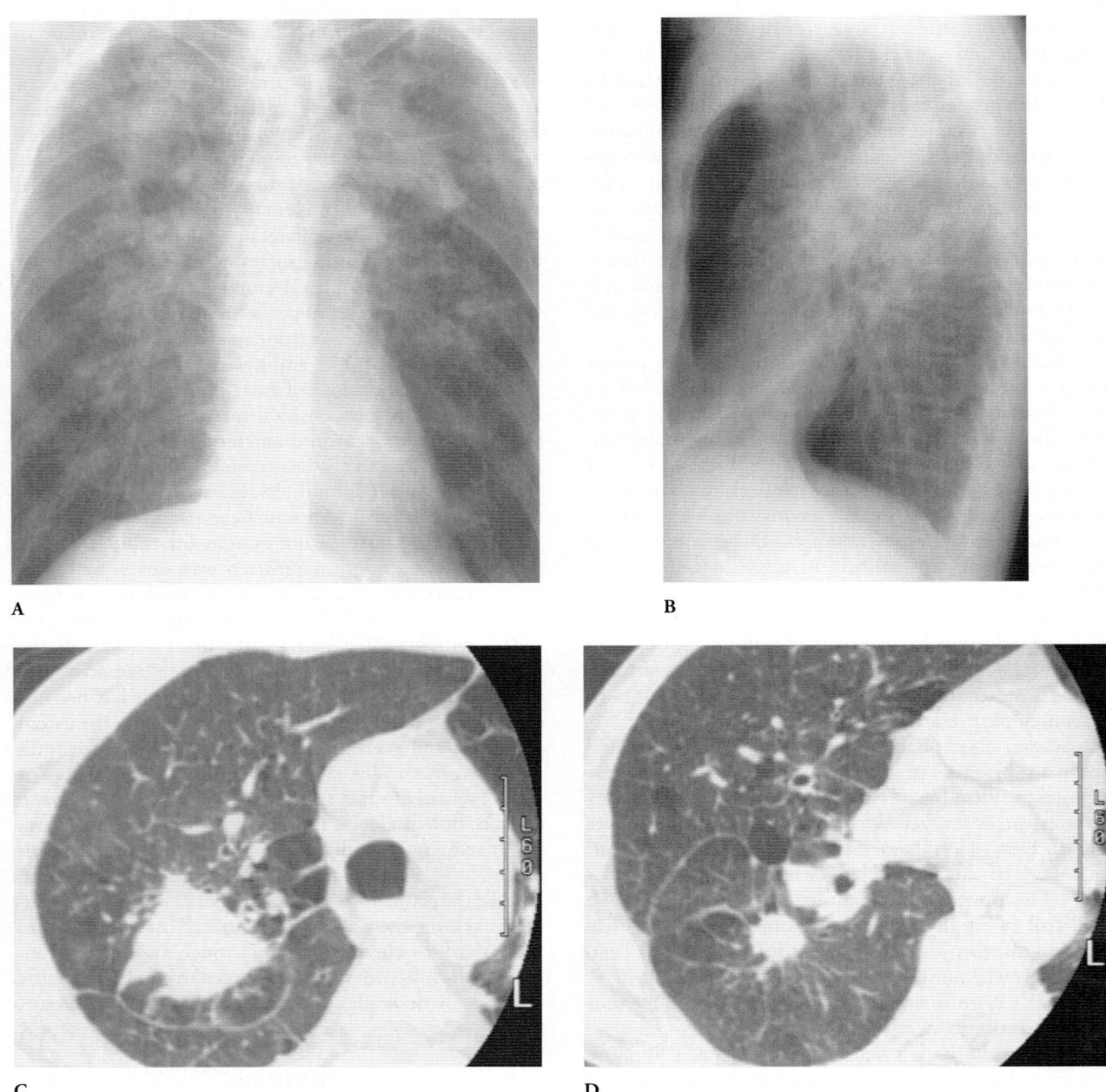

A   B

C   D

Figure 4–28   A 69-year-old coal miner with progressive massive fibrosis. *A, B,* Frontal and lateral chest radiographs show bilateral posterior upper lobe masslike opacities with peripheral bullae. Small nodules are present in the remainder of the lungs. Both hila are displaced superiorly. *C,* HRCT shows a fibrotic mass of the posterior right upper lobe with peripheral emphysema. *D,* HRCT shows a smaller fibrotic mass in the superior segment of the right lower lobe. Reproduced with permission from Lynch DA, Newell JD, Lee JS, editors. Imaging of diffuse lung disease. Hamilton: B.C. Decker; 2000.

larly noncalcified pleural plaques. HRCT can also eliminate false-positive radiographic diagnoses of pleural plaques caused by extrapleural fat and false positive diagnoses of asbestosis caused by extensive overlying plaques or by emphysema.[171] Plaques are identified on CT by the presence of smooth soft tissue thickening along the chest wall (see Figure 4–16). Plaques can be distinguished from intercostal muscles and intercostal vessels by HRCT. The sensitivity of CT for detection of pleural plaques depends on the sampling interval. A paper by Gamsu and colleagues affirms that asbestosis may be present even when plaques are not seen on HRCT (performed at 4 cm intervals). To optimize the detection of plaques on CT, one must image the thorax contiguously by conventional CT, in addition to selective high-resolution imaging.[172,173]

It is clear that the presence of diffuse pleural thickening on chest radiograph or chest CT is associated with significant decreases in FVC and the diffusion capacity of carbon monoxide (DL_{CO}).[174] However, the relationship between pleural plaques, lung function, and the amount of asbestos exposure remains controversial. A quantitative study by Schwartz and colleagues suggested that the extent of pleural plaque is independently associated with a decrease in total lung capacity.[175] However, a more similar recent study by Van Cleemput and colleagues[176] found that the volume of plaque determined at CT was unrelated to the degree of asbestos exposure and to lung function.

HRCT is more sensitive than the chest radiograph for diagnosis of the early changes of asbestosis (Figure 4–16).[39,170,177] HRCT is also useful in diagnosing other diseases such as emphysema, which may significantly impair lung function in asbestos-exposed subjects.[177] Early asbestosis is manifested on HRCT by peripheral reticular opacities, intralobular lines, prominent centrilobular core structures, and interlobular septal thickening. Because of the posterior and basal predominance of the lesions of early asbestosis, examination of the lung bases in the prone position is critical for confirming the fixed nature of septal thickening and curvilinear subpleural lines. More advanced asbestosis is characterized by parenchymal bands of fibrosis (see Figure 4–17), honeycombing, and traction bronchiectasis. Clearly, none of these features is specific for asbestosis, and similar changes may be seen in other lung diseases such as IPF.[178] When the CT scans of patients with asbestosis are compared with those of patients with IPF, patients with asbestosis have a higher prevalence of parenchymal bands and a lower prevalence of ground-glass opacities.[179]

A study by Aberle and colleagues evaluated HRCT in 100 asbestos-exposed subjects.[170] They assigned scores for the probability of asbestosis based on the signs mentioned above. This HRCT probability score correlated with forced vital capacity and weakly with lung diffusing capacity. Forty-five of the subjects satisfied clinical criteria for asbestosis: 43 of these had an intermediate or high probability HRCT score, including 8 of 10 subjects with a normal chest radiograph. Interestingly 30 of the 55 subjects who did not meet the clinical criteria for asbestosis had an intermediate or high probability HRCT score. This suggests that the disease detected by HRCT may sometimes be too localized to cause a radiographic abnormality or to affect resting pulmonary function, but it does raise the concern that CT-detected abnormalities may not reflect real disease. However, several studies of asbestos workers with normal lung parenchyma by chest radiograph have shown that an abnormal HRCT is associated with physiologic impairment (decreased total lung capacity, vital capacity, and diffusing capacity).[177,180,181] Akira and colleagues,[182] in a serial study of 23 asbestos-exposed patients with minimal or no abnormalities on chest radiographs demonstrated that the changes of early asbestosis progressed in 2 of 7 patients who were reexamined between 10 and 19 months after the first CT scan, and in 6 of 8 patients who were examined between 20 and 39 months after the first CT examination. This evidence of progression on CT was accompanied by a decrease in lung diffusing capacity in 3 of 4 patients in whom serial pulmonary function tests were available. Progression of disease by HRCT criteria appeared to be more prominent in cigarette smokers. Using postmortem HRCT scans these authors also demonstrated that the centrilobular nodules and branching structures corresponded histologically to fibrosis around the bronchioles, which subsequently involved the alveolar ducts. Pleural-based nodular irregularities corresponded histologically to subpleural fibrosis. Hazy patches of increased attenuation tended to correspond to fibrotic thickening of the alveolar walls and interlobular septa.

A study by Gamsu and colleagues showed that the CT findings of early asbestosis are neither sensitive nor specific.[172] In a series of 30 patients who had pathologic evaluation for asbestosis, 5 of 9 subjects who had no evidence of asbestosis on CT had histologic asbestosis. Of 5 further subjects who had minor parenchymal opacities, deemed insufficient in extent and severity for the diagnosis of asbestosis, 4 had asbestosis. Because most patients in this study had the diagnosis made at autopsy or at lobectomy for malignancy, the population is not representative of the general population with asbestosis. Nevertheless, it reminds us that the borderline between normal and disease is blurred. The paper affirms that asbestosis can be diagnosed with confidence when parenchymal changes are bilateral or present at multiple levels. Also, scoring of the profusion of abnormality on CT correlated significantly (r = .78) with the severity of lung fibrosis on histologic evaluation.

CT and HRCT scanning may be helpful in the evaluation of focal pulmonary masses associated with asbestosis. Although asbestos exposure is associated with a markedly increased incidence of lung cancer, the incidence of benign lung masses is also high.[183] These benign masses include rounded atelectasis,[184–186] intrapulmonary fibrotic bands, and fissural pleural plaques.[187] The typical CT features of rounded atelectasis include the relationship to an area of pleural thickening, lobar volume loss, and a swirl of bronchi and vessels curving toward the medial or lateral aspects of the pleural-based mass. However, as with all other lung masses, the best index of benignity is a lack of change over a 2-year interval. Therefore careful sequential follow-up of all asbestos-related lung masses (by chest radiographs or by CT) is recommended, with a low threshold for biopsy in atypical or changing masses.

The major unresolved issue in the evaluation of asbestos-exposed workers is the role of CT screening for pleural disease, asbestosis, and lung cancer. Tiitola and colleagues[188] screened 602 asbestos workers with spiral CT and found that 111 (18%) had nodules measuring more than 5 mm in diameter. Five patients (1%) were found to have lung cancer, with three patients being stage I or II. These workers were also evaluated for asbestosis using a standardized HRCT scoring system. It is difficult to develop selection criteria for CT screening, because neither the chest radiograph, level of exposure, nor physiology can predict the presence of abnormality on CT.[189] However, it is increasingly clear that we need to move beyond the chest radiograph in the evaluation of workers at risk.

Hypersensitivity Pneumonitis

On the chest radiograph, the features of hypersensitivity pneumonitis (HP) are relatively nonspecific. Indeed, the chest radiograph is frequently normal even in patients with physiologically significant disease. One may sometimes detect ground-glass opacity or fine nodularity. In patients with chronic HP, volume loss in the upper lobes or less commonly in the lower lobes may be associated with reticular or linear opacities due to fibrosis.

The most typical CT finding in patients with HP is the presence of profuse poorly defined micronodules (see Figure 4–12).[190–195] These micronodules may be found in those with acute, subacute, or chronic disease and, in the correct clinical context, are strongly suggestive of HP. The nodules usually appear to be at the center of the secondary pulmonary lobule, where the larger bronchioles are located, and they are therefore termed centrilobular. They differ from nodules seen in most other diseases in that they are not of soft-tissue density but instead are of ground-glass density. Since the poorly formed granulomas seen on histology in HP are too small to be seen individually on CT, these centrilobular nodules are most likely to be due to the inflammatory cellular infiltrate that centers on the terminal bronchiole. In other subjects with HP, ground-glass attenuation is the predominant or only finding. This is usually diffuse but sometimes spares the periphery of the secondary lobule.

Focal areas of hyperlucency, similar to those seen in obliterative bronchiolitis, may be a prominent feature in some patients with HP, presumably because the bronchiolocentric inflammation causes areas of air-trapping. Hansell and colleagues[43] have shown that such areas are associated with decreased residual volume, whereas areas of ground-glass opacity and reticular opacity are independently associated with restrictive physiology.

In chronic HP there are signs of lung fibrosis: lobar volume loss, linear/reticular opacities, or honeycombing (Figure 4–29).[192,194,196] These findings may be more prominent in the upper lobes or in the lower lobes. If poorly defined nodules are also present, then HP can be suggested. Some nonsmoking patients with chronic HP have been reported to show emphysema,[192,196] perhaps related to bronchiolar inflammation and obstruction. In a long-term study of 88 patients in whom farmer's lung had been diagnosed a mean of 14 years previously, emphysema was found in 18% of nonsmokers and in 44% of smokers and was significantly more prevalent than in a control group without a history of farmer's lung.[197] In this study, and in another by Cormier and colleagues,[198] emphysema was the most frequent finding in patients with chronic farmer's lung. The imaging characteristics of emphysema related to chronic HP remain unclear.

Because patients with mild or focal HP may not have sufficient lung abnormalities to cause a visible increase in lung density, the high-resolution CT scan may be normal in subjects with HP. In one population-based study,[191] only 5 of 13 patients with biopsy-proven HP had an abnormal CT scan. Thus, a normal high-resolution CT scan cannot be used to exclude HP. However, CT may still be useful in screening studies because an abnormal CT scan can provide strong support for the diagnosis of HP, perhaps obviating the need for a biopsy.

Some cases of chronic HP have basal-predominant lung fibrosis similar to that of UIP. Radiologic features that can be helpful in differentiating between UIP and chronic HP include: the predominance of fibrosis in mid or upper lung zones (see Figure 4–29),[192,199] the presence of micronodules, and the absence of honeycombing.[106] Because the management of hypersensitivity pneumonitis is substantially different from that of IPF, a thorough clinical history is critical, and in some cases a biopsy may be necessary to distinguish between these two disorders. The contribution of HRCT to the evaluation of patients with HP is to demonstrate the features that suggest the diagnosis and to follow patients for evidence of improvement.

Cystic Lung Diseases

Langerhans Cell Histiocytosis

High-resolution computed tomography contributes greatly to the accuracy of the diagnosis of Langerhans cell histiocytosis. Grenier and colleagues[69] showed that a first choice diagnosis of Langerhans cell histiocytosis had a 60% likelihood of being correct when made from the chest radiograph but had a 90% likelihood of correctness on CT scanning. The combination of pulmonary nodules and cysts is virtually diagnostic of pulmonary Langerhans cell histiocytosis (Figure 4–30).[80,81,200] The nodules may be poorly defined or well defined and are typically most prominent in the upper lobes. They are usually less than 5 mm in diameter and may appear cavitary.[201] The cysts in this disorder are invariably well defined and again are usually most profuse in the upper lobes. The cysts may be round or irregular in outline and may be thin walled or thickwalled. Some patients with "burnt-out" Langerhans cell histiocytosis show no lung nodules, only cysts. These patients may be distinguished from lymphangiomatosis by the fact that the cysts spare the lung bases. Many patients with burnt-out Langerhans cell histiocytosis will have pulmonary arterial enlargement due to pulmonary hypertension,[202] related to the pulmonary vasculopathy found in this condition.

The CT-determined extent of lung abnormality in Langerhans cell histiocytosis correlates well with diffusing capacity. The HRCT is also useful in following the progression or regression of pulmonary histiocytosis X. Regression of the nodules of pulmonary Langerhans cell histiocytosis is a well-known phenomenon.[203] Follow-up by HRCT has shown that regression of these nodules leaves multiple thin-walled cysts, not apparent on the chest radiograph.[200] Similarly, a study of patients with childhood histiocytosis showed pulmonary cysts in about 20%, mainly in those who were cigarette smokers.[204]

Lymphangiomyomatosis

The CT appearance of lymphangiomyomatosis (LAM) is diagnostic in the correct clinical context.[82,205–207] Virtually all subjects demonstrate thin-walled, round, or geographic cysts, distributed evenly through all lung zones, with apical sparing (see Figure 4–18). Vessels are typically seen at the margins of the cysts, rather than at their centers, as is characteristically seen with emphysema. Nodularity is uncommon. LAM may be distinguished from Langerhans cell histiocytosis by the diffuse lung involvement, the regular shape of the cysts, and the absence of nodules. Scoring of the extent of LAM by CT correlates with lung diffusing capacity, and in the study by Aberle and colleagues[82] disease extent also correlated with the FEV_1/FVC ratio. Quantitative assessment of the extent of LAM is possible using the CT density mask technique,[208] and shows strong correlations with measures of airflow, air-trapping, and gas exchange. The density mask technique, or similar methods may be useful in following patients with LAM for the progression of disease or response to treatment. HRCT is significantly more sensitive than the chest radiograph for demonstration of the cysts in LAM. Other abnormalities demonstrated by CT in LAM may include pneumothoraces, chylous pleural effusions, and mediastinal or abdominal lymph node enlargement, due to the proliferation of smooth muscle. CT demonstrates renal angiomyolipomas in 50 to 55% of cases of LAM.[209,210] Other abdominal findings include adenopathy, lymphangiomyomas, ascites, and a dilated thoracic duct.

LAM occurs in 25 to 35% of adult females with tuberous sclerosis.[211,212] In subjects with the lung disease CT findings of tuberous sclerosis are identical to those seen in lymphangiomyomatosis.[206]

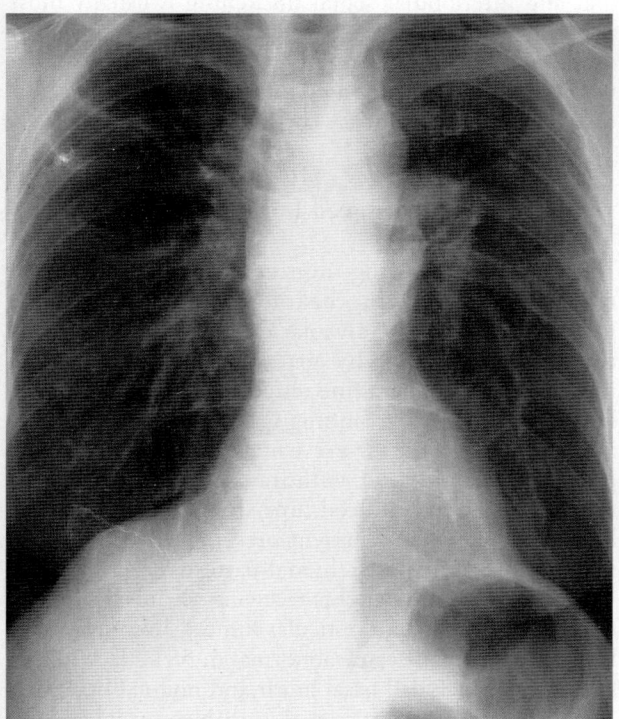

A

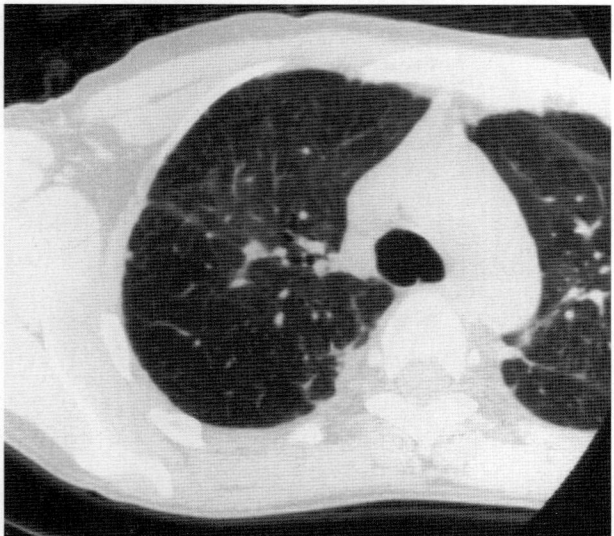

B

Figure 4–29   Chronic hypersensitivity pneumonitis. *A*, Chest radiographs shows bilateral pulmonary fibrosis predominantly in the upper lobes associated with marked hilar retraction. *B*, HRCT scan shows a combination of interlobular septal thickening, patchy hazy increase in lung density, and scattered fine peripheral nodules. This combination of findings suggests chronic hypersensitivity pneumonitis.

Chronic Air Space Diseases

The chronic air space lung diseases all have a rather similar appearance on high-resolution CT scanning. They are characterized by poorly marginated or well-defined opacities that are dense enough to obscure the underlying vessels and may be associated with air bronchograms.[213] Possible causes for this appearance include eosinophilic pneumonia,[79] COP,[214] chronic infection, lipoid pneumonia, pulmonary vasculitis, and alveolar cell carcinoma or lymphoma.

CT can assist in the differential diagnosis of air space diseases in several ways. "Alveolar" sarcoidosis may present with poorly defined masses, which on CT will usually have a nodular, irregular outline.[140] Statistically, the most common cause of air space opacification in patients with infiltrative lung disease will be COP, which may be recognized by its predominant subpleural and peribronchovascular distribution (see Figure 4–24). The CT pattern of chronic eosinophilic pneumonia[79] is similar to the classic chest radiographic pattern, with patchy air space consolidation, usually most marked in the mid and upper zones (see Figure 4–10). The characteristic peripheral distribution of the consolidation is much easier to recognize on CT than on chest radiographs. It differs from COP by the fact that it predominates in the upper lungs. The CT pattern of acute eosinophilic pneumonia may be diagnostic in the correct clinical context.[215] It differs from the other causes of acute diffuse lung disease in that it is associated with septal thickening and effusions (Figure 4–31).

Pulmonary alveolar proteinosis differs from all of the other alveolar lung diseases in that it is almost always associated with the crazy paving pattern (Figure 4–32). Although the crazy paving pattern can be found in other conditions such as ARDS or resolving pneumonia, it is rarely the sole finding in those entities, and the intralobular and interlobular septal thickening is usually most pronounced in patients with alveolar proteinosis. If dense consolidation, nodules, or masses are present, the possibility of a superimposed infection with *Nocardia* or other organisms should be considered.[97]

Drug-Induced Lung Disease

The CT pattern of drug-induced lung disease typically reflects the underlying histology, which may range from NSIP to diffuse alveolar damage. Common patterns include a patchy ground-glass abnormality indicative of OP and a fine reticular pattern suggesting lung fibrosis. Honeycombing is relatively uncommon, and the abnormalities are usually partially or completely reversible after withdrawal of the drug. The diagnosis of drug-induced lung disease should always be considered when a patient presents with these relatively nonspecific parenchymal patterns.

A study of 100 patients receiving bleomycin for the treatment of malignant testicular tumors showed that the lung parenchyma became abnormal in 38%.[216] Minimal CT changes included basal linear and nodular opacities. Peripheral nodular densities due to bleomycin toxicity may sometimes be difficult to distinguish from metas-

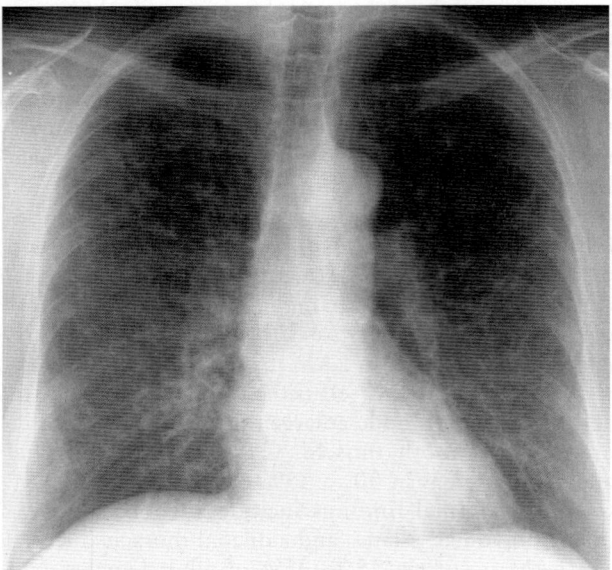

A

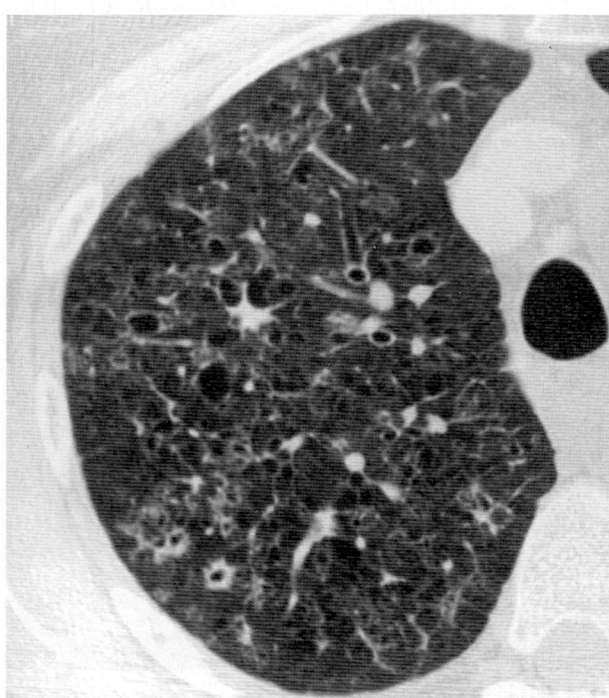

B

Figure 4–30   Pulmonary histiocytosis X. *A*, Chest radiograph shows profuse nodules with sparing of the costophrenic sulci and preservation of lung volumes. *B*, HRCT shows irregular shaped but well-defined cysts and scattered nodules. The combination of nodules and cysts strongly suggests pulmonary histiocytosis X.

tases.[217] Moderate changes of bleomycin injury were characterized by coarse reticular and nodular shadowing (Figure 4–33), whereas severe bleomycin-related lung damage was characterized by confluent irregular opacities extending through the lung, though the lung apices were relatively spared. Follow-up CT examinations showed that many or all of the pulmonary changes reversed over several months after withdrawal of therapy. However those with severe lung damage tended to remain unchanged.

Pulmonary toxicity due to amiodarone is sometimes associated with high-density pleuroparenchymal lesions on CT.[218] This rather specific CT appearance, seen in 8 of 11 cases in one study, is thought to be due to the high concentration of iodine-containing amiodarone present in alveolar macrophages and type 2 pneumocytes in these lesions. The increased density of the liver or spleen seen in these subjects is likely due to a similar mechanism. Recognition of these characteristic opacities may be helpful in distinguishing between amiodarone pulmonary toxicity and congestive heart failure (Figure 4–34).[219]

Exogenous lipoid pneumonia due to aspiration of lipid material is uniquely recognizable on CT by the presence of areas of consolidation or mass-like opacities containing areas of fat attenuation (Figure 4–35). The fat attenuation is helpful if present, but lipoid pneumonia is not excluded by the absence of fat attenuation.

A paper by Padley and colleagues[220] divided the CT findings of patients with drug-induced disease into four categories (see Figure 4–35). Reticular opacity with architectural distortion was the most frequent finding and was most frequently due to bleomycin or nitrofurantoin (see Figure 4–33). The second most frequent pattern was ground-glass opacification, frequently due to chemotherapeutic drugs (methotrexate,

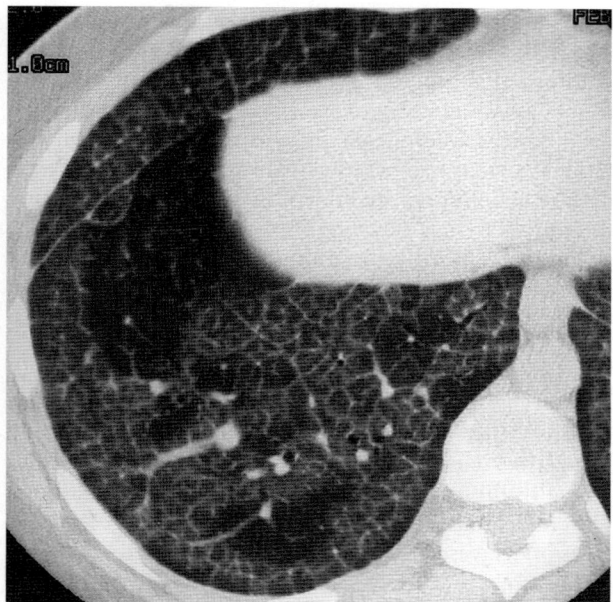

Figure 4–32 Pulmonary alveolar proteinosis. HRCT scan shows a classic pattern of ground-glass opacity with superimposed marked septal thickening and reticulation, the "crazy-paving" pattern. The septal thickening is thought to be due to accumulation of proteinaceous material in the interlobular septa.

carmustine, cyclophosphamide, or bleomycin) (Figure 4–36). This was felt to be due to a hypersensitivity phenomenon. An ARDS pattern of widespread consolidation was seen in two cases, related to chemotherapy. A bronchiolitis pattern (patchy hyperlucency) was seen in two cases, both related to penicillamine treatment for rheumatoid arthritis.

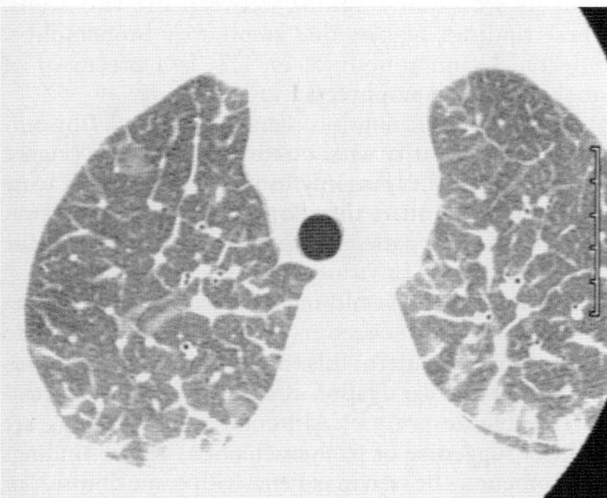

Figure 4–31 A 42-year-old female with acute eosinophilic pneumonia. HRCT shows marked intralobular septal thickening. A small pleural effusion was also evident. Reproduced with permission from Lynch DA, Newell JD, Lee JS, editors. Imaging of diffuse lung disease. Hamilton: B.C. Decker; 2000.

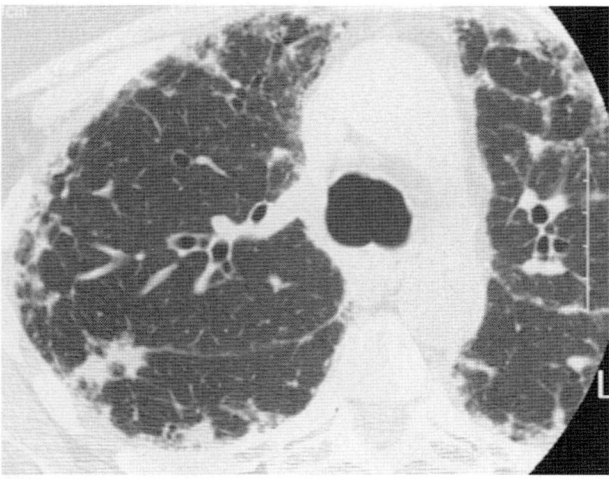

Figure 4–33 Bleomycin lung in a 63-year-old woman who developed shortness of breath shortly after receiving treatment for Hodgkin's lymphoma. HRCT shows irregular nodular abnormalities with peripheral reticular abnormality and honeycombing. Reproduced with permission from Lynch DA, Newell JD, Lee JS, editors. Imaging of diffuse lung disease. Hamilton: B.C. Decker, 2000.

Bronchiolar Disease

Computed tomography has contributed substantially to our understanding of small airways diseases and has resulted in numerous changes in the classification system. A current CT-based classification of small airways disease is presented in Table 4–5. Although organizing pneumonia (proliferative bronchiolitis, bronchiolitis obliterans organizing pneumonia) has long been included as a small airway disease, there is agreement that this should now be considered as an interstitial pneumonia.

In patients with constrictive bronchiolitis (Figure 4–37), the primary CT finding is a dramatic decrease in lung density in the affected lobules or subsegments, associated with narrowing of the pulmonary vessels. These findings are presumed to be due to air-trapping with reflex pulmonary vasoconstriction. The geographic areas of decreased density may be interspersed with areas of relatively increased density, due perhaps to overperfusion of normal lung lobules (Figure 4–38). These changes have been described in children with postviral obliterative bronchiolitis,[33,221] in patients with bronchiolitis due to cystic fibrosis, in Swyer-James syndrome[222] (see Figure 4–21), in adults with cryptogenic bronchiolitis obliterans,[223] and in patients who develop bronchiolitis obliterans after lung transplantation.[224] In most of these subjects, bronchiolitis obliterans is associated with peripheral or central bronchiectasis of varying severity, demonstrating that diseases that affect small airways also frequently affect larger airways (see Figure 4–37). Padley and colleagues showed that in patients with obliterative bronchiolitis, the extent of hyperlucency is a predictor of the degree of obstruction found on physiologic evaluation.[225]

The main CT signs of bronchiolitis obliterans following lung transplantation or bone marrow transplantation are bronchial dilation, vascular narrowing, and

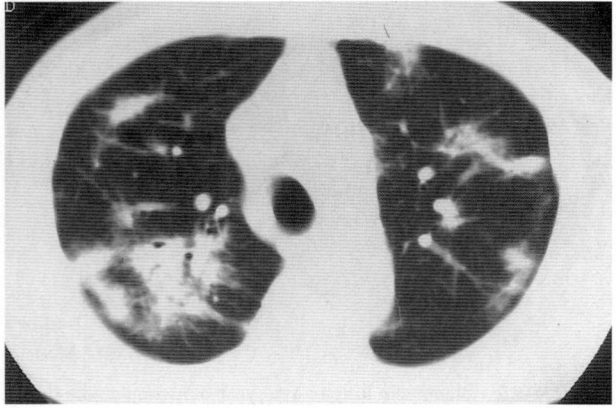

Figure 4–34 Amiodarone lung. HRCT viewed at lung windows shows air space consolidation. The CT attenuation of the areas of consolidation was greater than that of soft tissues, suggesting amiodarone accumulation in the lung parenchyma.

expiratory air-trapping.[224,226–230] For unclear reasons, the sensitivity of CT for the detection of bronchiolitis obliterans based on these signs is quite low (at most 75%). It is possible that quantitative techniques might result in improved sensitivity for detection of the bronchiolitis obliterans syndrome.

Cryptogenic bronchiolitis obliterans is characterized by geographic or diffuse hyperlucency sometimes associated with bronchial dilation, on inspiratory scans, and by air-trapping on expiratory imaging. One clinical problem that may arise is the differentiation between constrictive bronchiolitis and refractory asthma. In a study by Jensen and colleagues of 30 patients with severe refractory asthma and 14 with constrictive bronchiolitis obliterans, the presence of a mosaic pattern on inspiratory scans was a useful discriminant between these two entities, as it was found in 50% of those with bronchiolitis obliterans and 3% of cases with asthma.[231]

Smoking-related respiratory bronchiolitis (see Figure 4–13) is undoubtedly the commonest form of bronchiolitis as it was found in all cigarette smokers at autopsy. As discussed above, a small number of smokers develop respiratory bronchiolitis-associated interstitial lung disease or DIP. A study by Remy-Jardin and colleagues in 111 healthy volunteers found abnormal CT scans in 36 (54%) of 67 smokers, mainly comprising micronodules, ground-glass attenuation, and emphysema.[232] Such abnormalities were found in 2 (15%) of 13 smokers and in none of 31 nonsmokers. On follow-up CT 4.5 to 7.5 years later, the 57 subjects who continued to smoke had an increasing prevalence of ground-glass attenuation and emphysema, with micronodules being replaced by areas of emphysema in 5 patients.[233] Ground-glass attenuation and micronodules tended to decrease in extent or resolve in the 10 smokers who quit smoking between the two scans. These findings suggest that respiratory bronchiolitis, reflected by micronodules on CT, is a precursor of smoking-related emphysema.

Cellular bronchiolitis is characterized on CT by centrilobular nodularity with a tree-in-bud pattern (Figure 4–39). It is most commonly seen in patients with acute or chronic pulmonary infection. In the acute context, it is usually seen in patients with atypical pneumonia due to mycoplasma[234] or viruses.

Panbronchiolitis, although typically seen in Asian patients, may also be seen in Caucasians. In addition to the tree-in-bud pattern, this entity is uniquely characterized by bronchiolar dilation associated with bronchiectasis (see Figure 4–6).[235] Although these findings are strongly suggestive of panbronchiolitis, similar findings may sometimes be seen in patients with cystic fibrosis[33] or other causes of chronic bronchial infection such as immunodeficiency. The centrilobular abnormalities, airway wall thickening, and mucoid impaction may all regress with appropriate treatment, but the airway dilation is usually irreversible.[236,237]

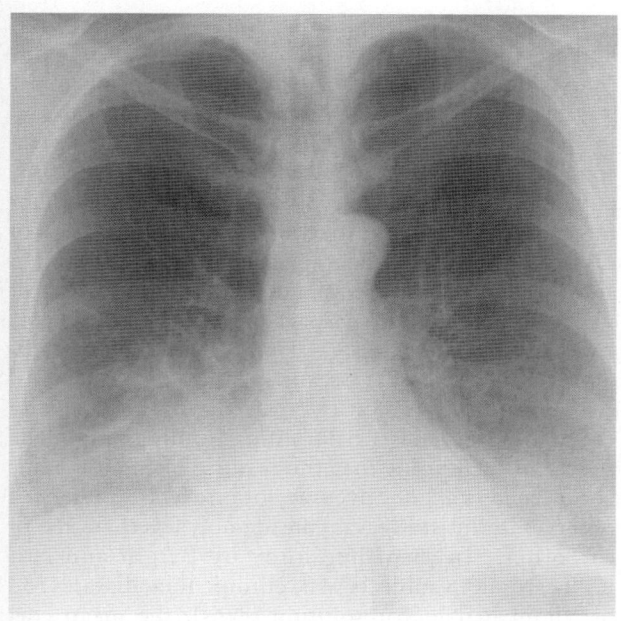

A

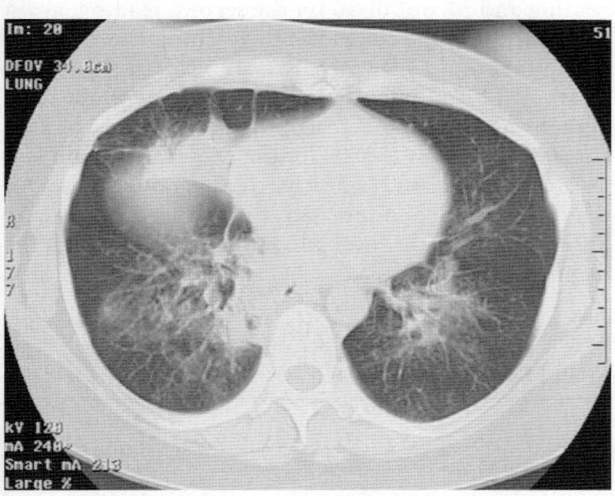

B

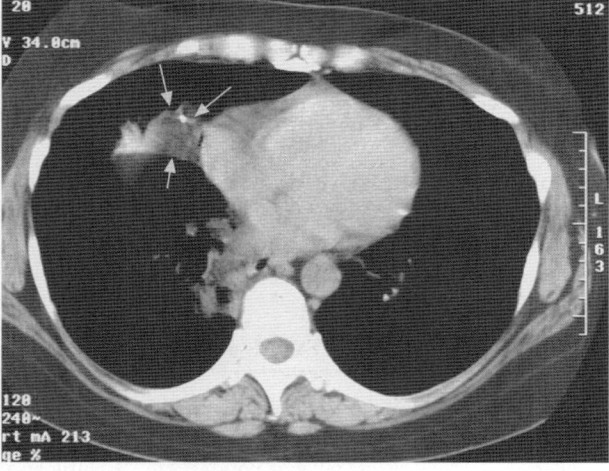

C

Figure 4–35   A 50-year-old female with lipoid pneumonia. *A,* Chest radiograph shows bilateral poorly defined masslike opacities in the lower lungs. *B,* CT scan shows that the masses are irregular in outline with surrounding ground-glass attenuation. *C,* Soft-tissue windows show that the CT attenuation of the right middle lobe mass is similar to that of fat (*arrows*). Reproduced with permission from Lynch DA, Newell JD, Lee JS, editors. Imaging of diffuse lung disease. Hamilton: B.C. Decker, 2000.

CLINICAL APPLICATIONS OF HRCT IN EVALUATION OF INTERSTITIAL LUNG DISEASE

Some current indications for HRCT are listed in Table 4–6.

Detection of Early Interstitial Lung Disease

The ability of HRCT scanning to detect interstitial disease in subjects with normal chest radiographs has been demonstrated in many diseases including asbestosis (see Figure 4–16), silicosis,[156] sarcoidosis,[143] scleroderma (see Figure 4–1),[238,239] and HP (see Figure 4–8).[190,195] In asbestosis, HRCT may detect an abnormality before resting pulmonary function tests become abnormal.[170,177] It

is also clear that the HRCT scan may be normal despite the presence of biopsy-proven interstitial disease. In a population-based study of subjects with HP who had normal resting pulmonary function, the sensitivity of HRCT was 38%.[191] Similarly, in the paper by Gamsu and colleagues, CT scanning was normal or near normal in 5 of 25 patients with histologic asbestosis.[172] These studies emphasize the fact that there is a phase in the evolution of any lung disease when the degree of parenchymal infiltration is too slight or too focal to cause a recognizable increase in lung attenuation on CT. Therefore, although CT is substantially more sensitive than the chest radiograph for ILD, normal findings on HRCT cannot be used to exclude ILD. In the future, it is possible that computer-based characterization systems might help to detect lung disease in patients with visually normal CT scans.

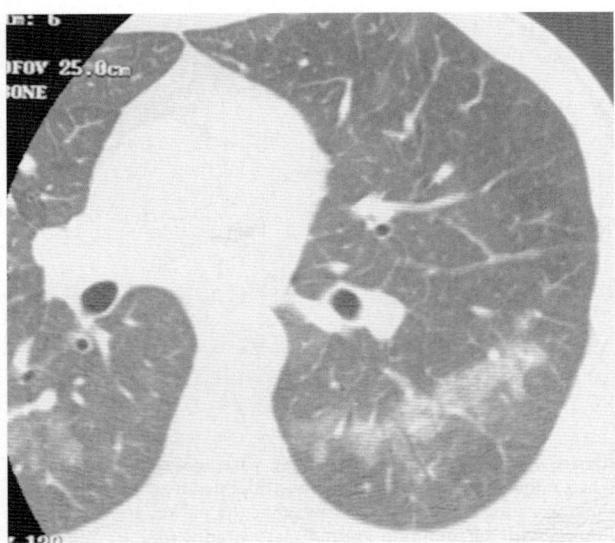

Figure 4–36 Drug toxicity due to BCNU following high-dose chemotherapy with bone marrow transplantation for breast cancer. CT scan shows a focal area of ground-glass abnormality in the superior segment of left lower lobe. More patchy ground-glass abnormality is present elsewhere. Reproduced with permission from Lynch DA, Newell JD, Lee JS, editors. Imaging of diffuse lung disease. Hamilton: B.C. Decker; 2000.

Characterization of Interstitial Lung Disease

Several large retrospective studies have compared the diagnostic accuracy of chest CT and chest radiography for the diagnosis of specific lung diseases. The first, by

Mathieson and colleagues,[71] examined the chest radiographs and CT scans of 118 patients with diffuse infiltrative lung diseases. For UIP, the first choice diagnosis was correct in 75% of the cases on chest radiograph and in 89% of the cases on CT. For silicosis, the corresponding figures were 63% and 93%, and sarcoidosis, 61% and 77%, respectively. For lymphangitic carcinomatosis, the first choice diagnosis was correct in 56% of cases on the chest radiograph and in 85% on CT. In addition, interobserver variation appeared to be less for CT scanning than for chest radiographs. Overall, a correct first choice diagnosis was made with 57% of radiographs and 76% of CT scans.

A similar study of 140 patients by Grenier and colleagues[69] gave essentially similar findings and made the additional point that the reading of HRCT scans is a learned skill. The accuracy of one less-experienced observer in this study was considerably less than that of the others. In a smaller study by Bergin and colleagues[240] of 48 subjects with chronic lung diseases (30 of whom had high-resolution scans), the mean correctness of two observers was 50 out of 56 on the first reading and 52 out of 56 on the second reading, again demonstrating the evidence of a learning curve. When Nishimura and colleagues used 20 readers (10 radiologists and 10 pulmonologists) to evaluate chest radiographs and chest CT scans, the accuracy of the first choice diagnosis was 38% for the chest radiograph and 46% for CT scans.[73] Clearly, the overall accuracy of diagnosis is dependent on the experience of the observer and on the level of confidence with which the diagnosis is made.

TABLE 4–5   Radiologic Classification of Small Airways Diseases

Radiologic Pattern	Pathologic Features	Characteristic Radiologic Features	Prototype Disease	Other Causes
Cellular bronchiolitis	Acute inflammatory infiltration of bronchiolar wall	Centrilobular nodularity Tree-in-bud pattern	Acute infection (viral, mycoplasma)	Chronic infection (mycobacterial) Hypersensitivity pneumonitis
Constrictive bronchiolitis	Circumferential thickening of bronchiolar wall with narrowing or obliteration of lumen	Diffuse or geographic air-trapping/mosaic pattern	Cryptogenic bronchiolitis obliterans	Rheumatoid disease Chronic rejection Prior viral mycoplasma infection Prior toxic fume exposure
Panbronchiolitis	Severe transmural inflammation of bronchiolar wall	Tree-in-bud pattern Bronchiolectasis Bronchiectasis	Diffuse panbronchiolitis	Cystic fibrosis Immune deficiency Atypical mycobacterial infection
Respiratory bronchiolitis	Macrophage accumulation in bronchiolar lumen and adjacent alveoli	Poorly defined centrilobular nodules Patchy ground-glass attenuation	Smoker's lung	None
Follicular bronchiolitis	Lymphoid follicles adjacent to bronchioles	Centrilobular nodules Peribronchial nodules Ground-glass opacity	Rheumatoid disease	Other collagen vascular diseases Immunodeficiency

One of the defects of these earlier studies was that they may have included patients with well-established disease. In a more recent study of 85 patients who were scanned prior to surgical lung biopsy, the accuracy of a confident first choice diagnosis of disease was 90%, but such a confident diagnosis was made in only about 25% of cases.[105] This relatively low level of diagnostic confidence was most likely due to selection bias (patients in whom confident CT diagnoses could be made would likely not undergo biopsy). However, it is also possible that confident diagnoses are more difficult to make in those with earlier disease.

It must be clearly understood that even a confident CT diagnosis should be integrated with the available clinical information. Patients with discrepant findings on clinical evaluation and CT should usually undergo biopsy. Biopsy is also indicated in patients with nonspecific CT findings. HRCT can be valuable for predicting whether a transbronchial biopsy would be helpful (in suspected sarcoidosis or lymphangitic carcinoma) and for identifying a suitable site for biopsy by the bronchoscopist or surgeon. When a biopsy is performed, it is important to review the biopsy in conjunction with the CT findings. Discrepancies between the CT pattern and the biopsy findings may be due to sampling of a nonrepresentative part of the lung.

Quantification of Interstitial Lung Disease

There are numerous schemes for visual quantification of diffuse lung disease. Interobserver variation improves sub-

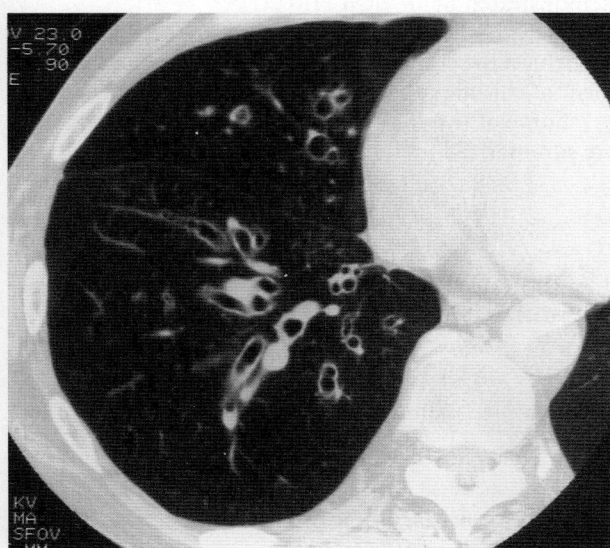

A

Figure 4–37 Bronchiolitis obliterans with bronchiectasis in a patient with rheumatoid arthritis. *A,* Chest radiograph shows widespread bronchial wall thickening that is more marked in the lung bases. *B,* High resolution CT shows extensive bronchiectasis, predominately cylindric in pattern, with diffuse decrease in lung density and attenuation of the peripheral pulmonary vasculature that is probably due to air-trapping with pulmonary oligemia.

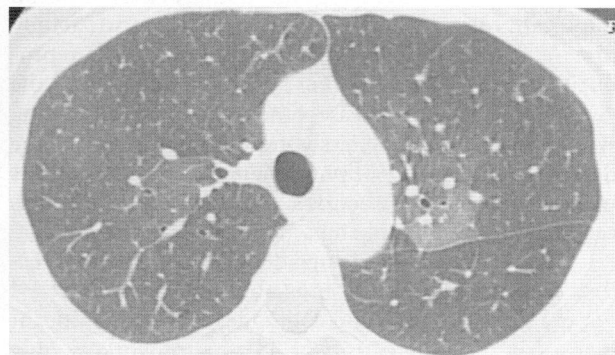

A

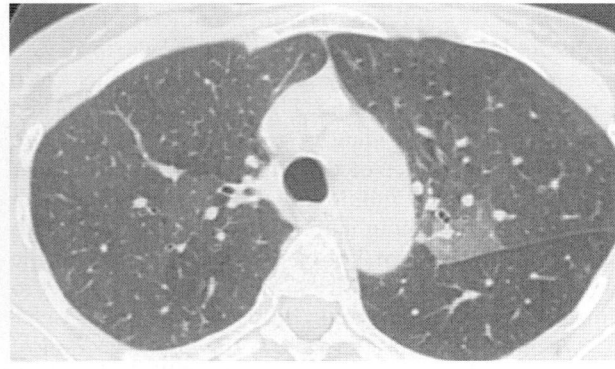

B

Figure 4–38 A 48-year-old male with cryptogenic bronchiolitis obliterans. *A,* Inspiratory CT scan through the upper lungs shows diffusely decreased attenuation with a focal area of normal or increased attenuation in the medial left upper lobe. *B,* Expiratory imaging shows little change in the attenuation of the hypoattenuating areas, confirming the presence of air-trapping.

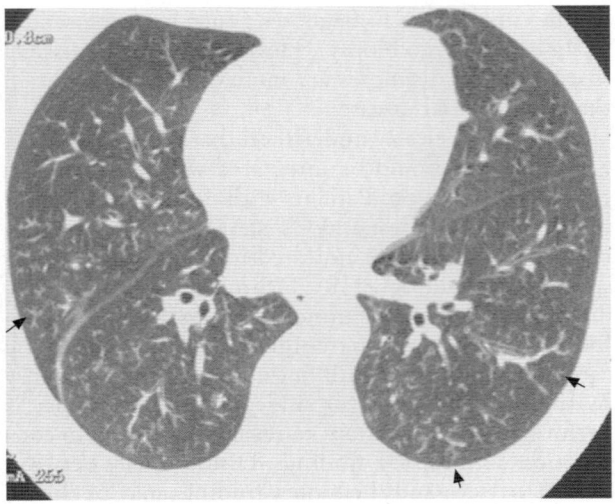

Figure 4–39   Cellular bronchiolitis due to mycoplasma infection in a 64-year-old male. High-resolution CT through the lower lungs shows centrilobular thickening with a tree-in-bud pattern (*arrows*).

stantially when the extent of interstitial lung disease is assessed by CT rather than conventional radiographs.[69,156,241] This suggests that CT may have an important role in following patients with interstitial lung disease. However, there is no widely accepted, reproducible, standardized scoring system for describing the visual extent of lung disease. Studies using visual scoring systems have been moderately successful in predicting the degree of abnormality of pulmonary function in subjects with sarcoidosis,[69,156] asbestosis,[170] pulmonary Langerhans cell histiocytosis, lymphangiomyomatosis,[82] and IPF.[82]

Measurements of CT lung density offer a more objective, quantitative index of lung abnormality.[63,64,216,242–244] For example, Wollmer and colleagues found a significant increase in CT lung density in 33 asbestos workers, only 3 of whom had evidence of asbestosis on chest radiographs.[245] They found that lung density correlated inversely with static lung volumes. Subjects with idiopathic pulmonary fibrosis have been shown to have a moderate but variable increase in lung density when compared with normal subjects. They also have a decreased anteroposterior lung density gradient, perhaps due to decreased compliance of the anterior lung.[246] Although visual assessment of pulmonary damage in subjects with bleomycin-related lung damage does not correlate with the degree of abnormality of pulmonary function, the increase in CT lung density in these subjects appears to correlate with the decrease in diffusing capacity.[216]

A more detailed approach to the quantification of lung disease by CT is based on the CT density histogram. In normal subjects, the first order histogram of CT density is sharply peaked (kurtotic) and skewed to the left, by comparison with the normal Gaussian distribution. In IPF, because of increased amounts of fibrotic or inflammatory tissue in the lung, the mean lung attenuation is increased, and the histogram

becomes less skewed and less kurtotic. Measurements of mean CT lung density, skewness, and kurtosis in patients with IPF correlate with the degree of impairment as measured by pulmonary function testing.[247]

More sophisticated techniques for image analysis allow for the estimation of lung volumes and simultaneous calculation of the relative amounts of soft tissue and air present in the lung.[30] Lung surface area may also be calculated.[248] Textural analysis of images may use multiple image features to differentiate between features of lung fibrosis and ground-glass attenuation,[249] or to distinguish different types of lung disease such as emphysema, sarcoidosis, and IPF.[250]

Other Uses

A combination of obstructive and restrictive lung disease frequently occurs in cigarette smokers who have interstitial lung disease. It is often difficult to determine whether the patient's disability is attributable primarily to interstitial fibrosis or to emphysema. HRCT is an elegant method for delineating the extent of emphysema and fibrosis (Figure 4–40).[251] This application is particularly useful in subjects with asbestosis or idiopathic pulmonary fibrosis.

In children with diffuse lung disease, HRCT can be invaluable for separating diffuse airways disease from infiltrative lung disease and for characterizing the pattern of infiltration present.[35,36]

The correlation between HRCT abnormalities and pathologic findings is close and may be exquisitely demonstrated by in vitro HRCT.[66,90,252,253]

HRCT is 90 to 95% accurate in the diagnosis of bronchiectasis[254] and therefore may be useful in the assessment of chronic cough or hemoptysis of unknown cause.

Some of the current clinical indications for HRCT are summarized in Table 4–6.

SUMMARY

The limitations of chest radiographic assessment of interstitial lung disease are well known. However,

---

TABLE 4–6   Clinical Indications for HRCT Scanning

Suspected interstitial disease with a normal chest radiograph

Nonspecific increased markings on the chest radiograph

Characterization of known interstitial lung disease

Unexplained dyspnea, chronic productive cough, or hemoptysis

Unexplained low diffusing capacity or other pulmonary function abnormality

Guidance for selection of mode of biopsy sampling (transbronchial or open) and of biopsy site

Suspected mixed interstitial lung disease and emphysema

Suspected small airways disease

Follow-up of interstitial lung changes for resolution or progression because of its ready availability and low cost, the chest radiograph remains valuable as a primary screening tool for initial diagnosis and follow-up of subjects with interstitial lung disease.

HRCT scanning has a clearly defined role in the early diagnosis of interstitial lung disease and in the differential diagnosis of established interstitial disease. In idiopathic pulmonary fibrosis, HRCT may be used to suggest the diagnosis, to determine the extent of lung disease and associated emphysema, and, perhaps, to determine the intensity of lung inflammation. In sarcoidosis, HRCT seems to be useful in predicting pulmonary dysfunction based on the CT pattern and extent of disease. In the cystic lung diseases, it readily distinguishes between emphysema, eosinophilic granuloma, and LAM. In asbestosis, it helps to identify pleural plaques, parenchymal fibrosis, and associated emphysema. HRCT improves the accuracy of diagnosis of pneumoconioses and may be of considerable value in the diagnosis and differentiation of small airways diseases. In chronic air space diseases, CT will rarely provide a specific diagnosis but may suggest a diagnostic pathway.

For HRCT imaging to continue to contribute to the management of interstitial lung disease, accurate and reproducible scoring techniques should be developed and applied. In addition, studies are needed to determine the prognostic significance of abnormalities identified on HRCT scanning.

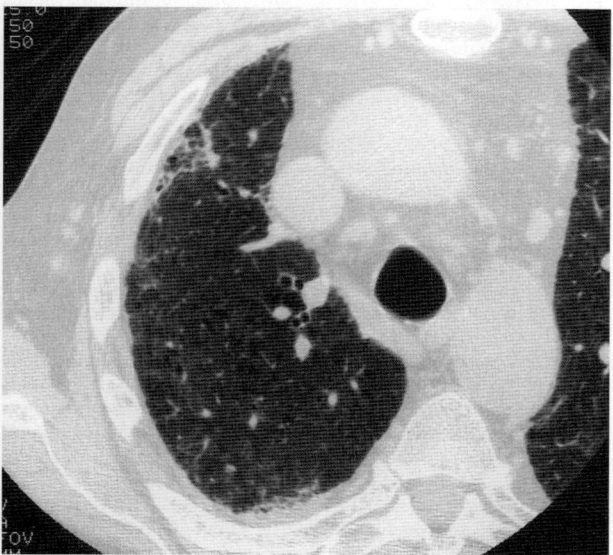

A

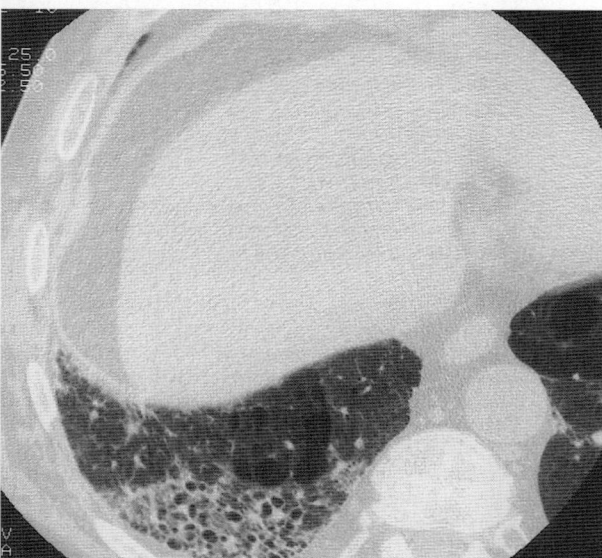

B

Figure 4–40   Mixed emphysema and idiopathic pulmonary fibrosis. *A,* HRCT scan through the upper right lung shows widespread small lucencies with poorly defined walls typical for centrilobular emphysema. Some peripheral areas of linear fibrosis are seen. *B,* A scan through the lung base shows several small bullae, and patchy fibrosis, honeycombing, and traction bronchiectasis. The patient's dominant disease is lung fibrosis.

REFERENCES

1. Epler G, McLoud T, Gaensler E, et al. Normal chest roentgenograms in chronic diffuse infiltrative lung disease. N Engl J Med 1978;298:934–9.
2. Orens JB, Kazerooni EA, Martinez FJ, et al. The sensitivity of high-resolution CT in detecting idiopathic pulmonary fibrosis proved by open lung biopsy. A prospective study. Chest 1995;108:109–15.
3. Hodgson M, Parkinson D, Karpf M. Chest x-rays in hypersensitivity pneumonitis: meta-analysis of a secular trend. Am J Ind Med 1989;16:45–53.
4. Kido S, Ikezoe J, Kondoh H, et al. Detection of subtle interstitial abnormalities of the lungs on digitized chest radiographs: acceptable compression ratios. AJR Am J Roentgenol 1996;167:111–5.
5. Larson A, Lynch DA, Zeligman B, et al. Accuracy of diagnosis of subtle chest disease and subtle fractures with a teleradiology system. AJR Am J Roentgenol 1998;170:19–22.
6. Ishikagi T, Endo T, Ikeda M, et al. Subtle pulmonary disease: detection with computed radiography versus conventional chest radiography. Radiology 1996;201:51–60.
7. Miro SP, Leung AN, Rubin GD, et al. Digital storage phosphor chest radiography: an ROC study of the effect of 2K versus 4K matrix size on observer performance. Radiology 2001;218:527–32.
8. van Heesewijk HP, van der Graaf Y, de Valois JC, et al. Chest imaging with a selenium detector versus conventional film radiography: a CT-controlled study. Radiology 1996; 200:687–90.
9. Bernhardt TM, Otto D, Reichel G, et al. Detection of simulated interstitial lung disease and catheters with selenium, storage phosphor, and film-based radiography. Radiology 1999;213:445–54.
10. Katsuragawa S, Doi K, MacMahon H, et al. Classification of normal and abnormal lungs with interstitial diseases by rule-based method and artificial neural networks. J Digit Imaging 1997;10:108–14.
11. Israel H, Albertine K, Park C, Patrick H. Whole-body gallium scans: role in diagnosis of sarcoidosis. Am Rev Respir Dis 1991;144:1182–6.
12. Labrune S, Chinet T, Collignon MA, et al. Mechanisms of increased epithelial lung clearance of DTPA in diffuse fibrosing alveolitis. Eur Respir J 1994;7:651–6.

13. Yeh SH, Liu RS, Wu LC, et al. 99Tcm-HMPAO and 99Tcm-DTPA radioaerosol clearance measurements in idiopathic pulmonary fibrosis. Nucl Med Commun 1995;16:140–4.

14. Pantin CF, Valind SO, Sweatman M, et al. Measures of the inflammatory response in cryptogenic fibrosing alveolitis. Am Rev Respir Dis 1988;138:1234–41.

15. Jones HA, Schofield JB, Krausz T, et al. Pulmonary fibrosis correlates with duration of tissue neutrophil activation. Am J Respir Crit Care Med 1998;158:620–8.

16. Remy-Jardin M, Remy J, Deffontaines C, Duhamel A. Assessment of diffuse infiltrative lung disease: comparison of conventional CT and high-resolution CT. Radiology 1991;181:157–62.

17. Kauczor HU, Heussel CP, Fischer B, et al. Assessment of lung volumes using helical CT at inspiration and expiration: comparison with pulmonary function tests. AJR Am J Roentgenol 1998;171:1091–5.

18. Mayo J, Webb W, Gould R, et al. High-resolution CT of the lungs: an optimal approach. Radiology 1987;163:507–10.

19. Strickland B, Brennan J, Denison DM. Computed tomography in diffuse lung disease: improving the image. Clin Radiol 1986;37:335–8.

20. Mayo J, Jackson S, Müller N. High resolution CT of the chest: radiation dose. AJR Am J Roentgenol 1993;160:479–81.

21. Jung KJ, Lee KS, Kim SY, et al. Low-dose, volumetric helical CT: image quality, radiation dose, and usefulness for evaluation of bronchiectasis. Invest Radiol 2000;35:557–63.

22. Naidich DP, Marshall CH, Gribbin C, et al. Low-dose CT of the lungs: preliminary observations. Radiology 1990;175:729–31.

23. Zwirewich CV, May JR, Müller NL. Low-dose high-resolution CT of lung parenchyma. Radiology 1991;180:413–7.

24. Lee KS, Primack SL, Staples CA, et al. Chronic infiltrative lung disease: comparison of diagnostic accuracies of radiography and low- and conventional-dose thin-section CT. Radiology 1994;191:669–73.

25. Majurin ML, Varpula M, Kurki T, Pakkala L. High-resolution CT of the lung in asbestos-exposed subjects. Comparison of low-dose and high-dose HRCT. Acta Radiol 1994;35:473–7.

26. Mayo JR, Hartman TE, Lee KS, et al. CT of the chest: minimal tube current required for good image quality with the least radiation dose. AJR Am J Roentgenol 1995;164:603–7.

27. Kalender W, Rienmüller R, Seissler W, et al. Measurement of pulmonary parenchymal attenuation: use of spirometric gating with quantitative CT. Radiology 1990;175:265–8.

28. Kohz P, Stabler A, Beinert T, et al. Reproducibility of quantitative, spirometrically controlled CT. Radiology 1995;197:539–42.

29. Rienmuller RK, Behr J, Kalender WA, et al. Standardized quantitative high resolution CT in lung diseases. J Comput Assist Tomogr 1991;15:742–9.

30. Coxson HO, Hogg JC, Mayo JR, et al. Quantification of idiopathic pulmonary fibrosis using computed tomography and histology. Am J Respir Crit Care Med 1997;155:1649–56.

31. Uppaluri R, Mitsa T, Sonka M, et al. Quantification of pulmonary emphysema from lung computed tomography images. Am J Respir Crit Care Med 1997;156:248–54.

32. Bankier AA, Fleischmann D, Dantendorfer K, et al. Automatic patient-instruction devices in thin-section CT of the thorax: impact on image quality. Radiology 1995;196:841–4.

33. Lynch D, Brasch R, Hardy K, Webb W. Pediatric pulmonary disease: assessment with high-resolution ultrafast CT. Radiology 1990;176:243–8.

34. Copley SJ, Coren M, Nicholson AG, et al. Diagnostic accuracy of thin-section CT and chest radiography of pediatric interstitial lung disease. AJR Am J Roentgenol 2000;174:549–54.

35. Lynch DA, Hay T, Newell JD Jr, et al. Pediatric diffuse lung disease: diagnosis and classification by high-resolution CT. AJR Am J Roentgenol 1999;173:713–8.

36. Kuhn J, Brody A. High resolution CT of pediatric lung disease. Radiol Clin North Am 2002;40:89–110.

37. Müller N, Miller R. Computed tomography of chronic diffuse infiltrative lung disease. Part 2. Am Rev Respir Dis 1990;142:1440–8.

38. Klein J, Gamsu G. High resolution computed tomography of diffuse lung disease. Invest Radiol 1989;24:805–12.

39. Aberle DR, Gamsu G, Ray CS, Feuerstein IM. Asbestos-related pleural and parenchymal fibrosis: detection with high-resolution CT. Radiology 1988;166:729–34.

40. Aberle DR. Current imaging of asbestosis. Curr Opin Radiol 1989;1:9–15.

41. Arakawa H, Webb WR, McCowin M, et al. Inhomogeneous lung attenuation at thin-section CT: diagnostic value of expiratory scans. Radiology 1998;206:89–94.

42. Bartz RR, Stern EJ. Airways obstruction in patients with sarcoidosis: expiratory CT scan findings. J Thorac Imaging 2000;15:285–9.

43. Hansell DM, Wells AU, Padley SP, Müller NL. Hypersensitivity pneumonitis: correlation of individual CT patterns with functional abnormalities. Radiology 1996;199:123–8.

44. Lucidarme O, Coche E, Cluzel P, et al. Expiratory CT scans for chronic airway disease: correlation with pulmonary function test results. AJR Am J Roentgenol 1998;170:301–7.

45. Lynch D, Gamsu G, Aberle D. Conventional and high resolution CT in the diagnosis of asbestos-related diseases. Radiographics 1989;9:523–51.

46. Stern EJ, Frank MS. Small-airway diseases of the lungs: findings at expiratory CT. Am J Roentgenol 1994;163:37–41.

47. Remy-Jardin M, Remy J, Artaud D, et al. Diffuse infiltrative lung disease: clinical value of sliding-thin-slab maximum intensity projection CT scans in the detection of mild micronodular patterns. Radiology 1996;200:333–9.

48. Bhalla M, Naidich DP, McGuinness G, et al. Diffuse lung disease: assessment with helical CT—preliminary observations of the role of maximum and minimum intensity projection images. Radiology 1996;200:341–7.

49. Cutillo AG, Morris AH, Ailion DC, et al. Quantitative assessment of pulmonary edema by nuclear magnetic resonance methods. J Thorac Imaging 1988;3:51–8.

50. Cutillo AG, Morris AH, Ailion DC, Durney CH. Clinical implications of nuclear magnetic resonance lung research. Chest 1989;96:643–52.

51. Glazer HS, Lee JK, Levitt RG, et al. Radiation fibrosis: differentiation from recurrent tumor by MR imaging. Radiology 1985;156:721–6.

52. Glazer HS, Levitt RG, Lee JK, et al. Differentiation of radiation fibrosis from recurrent pulmonary neoplasm by magnetic resonance imaging. AJR Am J Roentgenol 1984;143:729–30.

53. Vinitski S, Pearson MG, Karlik SJ, et al. Differentiation of parenchymal lung disorders with in vitro proton nuclear magnetic resonance. Magn Reson Med 1986;3:120–5.

54. Gefter WB, Hatabu H, Dinsmore BJ, et al. Pulmonary vascular cine MR imaging: a noninvasive approach to dynamic imaging of the pulmonary circulation. Radiology 1990;176:761–70.

55. O'Callaghan C, Small P, Chapman B, et al. Determination of individual and total lung volumes using nuclear magnetic resonance echo-planar imaging. Ann Radiol (Paris) 1987;30:470–2.

56. Bergin CJ, Pauly JM, Macovski A. Lung parenchyma: projection reconstruction MR imaging. Radiology 1991;179:777–81.

57. King MA, Bergin CJ, Ghadishah E, et al. Detecting pulmonary abnormalities on magnetic resonance images in patients with usual interstitial pneumonitis: effect of varying window settings and gadopentetate dimeglumine. Acad Radiol 1996;3:300–7.

58. Primack SL, Mayo JR, Hartman TE, et al. MRI of infiltrative lung disease: comparison with pathologic findings. J Comput Assist Tomogr 1994;18:233–8.

59. Kauczor HU, Hofmann D, Kreitner KF, et al. Normal and abnormal pulmonary ventilation: visualization at hyperpolarized He-3 MR imaging. Radiology 1996;201:564–8.

60. de Lange EE, Mugler JP 3rd, Brookeman JR, et al. Lung air spaces: MR imaging evaluation with hyperpolarized 3He gas. Radiology 1999;210:851–7.

61. Edelman RR, Hatabu H, Tadamura E, et al. Noninvasive assessment of regional ventilation in the human lung using oxygen-enhanced magnetic resonance imaging. Nat Med 1996;2:1236–9.

62. Kauczor HU, Kreitner KF. Contrast-enhanced MRI of the lung. Eur J Radiol 2000;34:196–207.

63. Wegener O, Koeppe P, Oeser H. Measurement of lung density by computed tomography. J Comput Assist Tomogr 1978;2:263–73.

64. Hedlund L, Vock P, Effmann E. Evaluating lung density by computed tomography. Semin Respir Med 1983;5:76–87.

65. Vock P, Malanowski D, Tschaeppeler H, et al. Computed tomographic lung density in children. Invest Radiol 1987; 22:627–31.

66. Webb W, Stein M, Finkbeiner W, et al. Normal and diseased isolated lungs: high resolution CT. Radiology 1988; 166:81–87.

67. Im J-G, Webb W, Rosen A, Gamsu G. Costal pleura: appearances at high-resolution CT. Radiol 1989;171:125–31.

68. Felson B. A new look at pattern recognition of diffuse pulmonary disease. AMJ Am J Roentgenol 1979;133:183–9.

69. Grenier P, Valeyre D, Cluzel P, et al. Chronic diffuse interstitial lung disease: diagnostic value of chest radiography and high-resolution CT. Radiology 1991;179:123–32.

70. Tung KT, Wells AU, Rubens MB, et al. Accuracy of the typical computed tomographic appearances of fibrosing alveolitis. Thorax 1993;48:334–8.

71. Mathieson JR, Mayo JR, Staples CA, Müller NL. Chronic diffuse infiltrative lung disease: comparison of diagnostic accuracy of CT and chest radiography. Radiology 1989; 171:111–6.

72. Padley S, Hansell D, Flower C, Jennings P. Comparative accuracy of high resolution computed tomography and chest radiography in diagnosis of chronic diffuse infiltrative lung disease. Clin Radiol 1991;44:222–6.

73. Nishimura K, Izumi T, Kitaichi M, et al. The diagnostic accuracy of high-resolution computed tomography in diffuse infiltrative lung diseases. Chest 1993;104:1149–55.

74. Murata K, Khan A, Herman PG. Pulmonary parenchymal disease: evaluation with high-resolution CT. Radiology 1989;170:629–35.

75. Noma S, Khan A, Herman PG, Rojas KA. High-resolution computed tomography of the pulmonary parenchyma. Semin Ultrasound CT MR 1990;11:365–79.

76. Murata K, Itoh H, Todo G, et al. Centrilobular lesions of the lungs: demonstration by high-resolution CT and pathologic correlation. Radiology 1986;161:641–5.

77. Bergin C, Roggli V, Coblentz C, Chiles C. The secondary pulmonary lobule: normal and abnormal CT appearances. AJR Am J Roentgenol 1988;151:21–5.

78. Staples C, Müller N, Vedal S, et al. Usual interstitial pneumonia: correlation of CT with clinical, functional, and radiographic findings. Radiology 1987;162:377–81.

79. Mayo JR, Müller NL, Road J, et al. Chronic eosinophilic pneumonia: CT findings in six cases. AJR Am J Roentgenol 1989;153:727–30.

80. Brauner MW, Grenier P, Mouelhi MM, et al. Pulmonary histiocytosis X: evaluation with high-resolution CT. Radiology 1989;172:255–8.

81. Moore A, Godwin J, Müller N, et al. Pulmonary histiocytosis X: comparison of radiographic and CT findings. Radiology 1989;172:249–54.

82. Aberle DR, Hansell DM, Brown K, Tashkin DP. Lymphangiomyomatosis: CT, chest radiographic, and functional correlations. Radiology 1990;176:381–7.

83. Austin J, Müller N, Friedman P, et al. Glossary of terms for CT of the lungs: recommendations of the nomenclature committee of the Fleischner Society. Radiology 1996;200:327–31.

84. Müller NL, Kullnig P, Miller RR. The CT findings of pulmonary sarcoidosis: analysis of 25 patients. AMJ Am J Roentgenol 1989;152:1179–82.

85. Remy-Jardin M, Beuscart R, Sault MC, et al. Subpleural micronodules in diffuse infiltrative lung diseases: evaluation with thin-section CT scans. Radiology 1990;177:133–9.

86. Gruden JF, Webb WR, Naidich DP, McGuinness G. Multinodular disease: anatomic localization at thin-section CT—multireader evaluation of a simple algorithm. Radiology 1999;210:711–20.

87. Stein M, Mayo J, Müller N, et al. Pulmonary lymphangitic spread of carcinoma: appearance on CT scans. Radiology 1987;162:371–5.

88. Müller NL, Miller RR, Webb WR, et al. Fibrosing alveolitis: CT-pathologic correlation. Radiology 1986;160:585–8.

89. Yoshimura H, Hatakeyama M, Otsuji H, et al. Pulmonary asbestosis: CT study of subpleural curvilinear shadow. Radiology 1986;158:653–8.

90. Akira M, Yamamoto S, Yokoyama K, et al. Asbestosis: high-resolution CT-pathologic correlation. Radiology 1990;176:389–94.

91. Meziane M, Hruban R, Zerhouni E, et al. High resolution CT of the lung parenchyma with pathologic correlation. Radiographics 1988;8:27–54.

92. Westcott JL, Cole SR. Traction bronchiectasis in end-stage pulmonary fibrosis. Radiology 1986;161:665–9.

93. Remy-Jardin M, Giraud F, Remy J, et al. Importance of ground-glass attenuation in chronic diffuse infiltrative lung disease: pathologic-CT correlation. Radiology 1993;189:693–8.

94. Zerhouni E, Naidich D, Stitik F, et al. Computed tomography of the pulmonary parenchyma. Part 2: Interstitial disease. J Thorac Imaging 1985;1:54–64.

95. Leung A, Miller R, Müller N. Parenchymal opacification in chronic infiltrative lung disease: CT-pathologic correlation. Radiology 1993;188:209–14.

96. Stern E, Swensen S, Hartman T, Frank M. CT mosaic pattern of lung attenuation: distinguishing different causes. AJR Am J Roentgenol 1995;165:813–6.

97. Godwin J, Müller N, Takasugi J. Pulmonary alveolar proteinosis: CT findings. Radiology 1988;169:609–13.

98. Tan RT, Kuzo RS. High-resolution CT findings of mucinous bronchioloalveolar carcinoma: a case of pseudopulmonary alveolar proteinosis. AJR Am J Roentgenol 1997;168:99–100.

99. Laurent F, Philippe JC, Vergier B, et al. Exogenous lipoid pneumonia: HRCT, MR, and pathologic findings. Eur Radiol 1999;9:1190–6.

100. Murayama S, Murakami J, Yabuuchi H, et al. "Crazy paving appearance" on high resolution CT in various diseases. J Comput Assist Tomogr 1999;23:749–52.

101. Bergin C, Castellino RA. Mediastinal lymph node enlargement on CT scans in patients with usual interstitial pneumonitis. AMJ Am J Roentgenol 1990;154:251–4.

102. Garber SJ, Wells AU, duBois RM, Hansell DM. Enlarged mediastinal lymph nodes in the fibrosing alveolitis of systemic sclerosis. Br J Radiol 1992;65:983–6.

103. Jung JI, Kim HH, Jung YJ, et al. Mediastinal lymphadenopathy in pulmonary fibrosis: correlation with disease severity. J Comput Assist Tomogr 2000;24:706–10.

104. Hunninghake GW, Zimmerman MB, Schwartz DA, et al. Utility of a lung biopsy for the diagnosis of idiopathic pulmonary fibrosis. Am J Respir Crit Care Med 2001;164:193–6.

105. Swensen S, Aughenbaugh G, Myers J. Diffuse lung disease: diagnostic accuracy of CT in patients undergoing surgical biopsy of the lung. Radiology 1997;205:229–34.

106. Lynch D, Newell J, Logan P, et al. Can CT distinguish idio-

pathic pulmonary fibrosis from hypersensitivity pneumonitis? AMJ Am J Roentgenol 1995;165:807–11.

107. Hunninghake G, Lynch D, Galvin J, et al. Radiological findings are most strongly associated with a pathological diagnosis of IPF. 2002 [Submitted]

108. Müller NL, Staples CA, Miller RR, et al. Disease activity in idiopathic pulmonary fibrosis: CT and pathologic correlation. Radiology 1987;165:731–4.

109. Lee J, Im J-G, Ahn J, et al. Fibrosing alveolitis: prognostic implication of ground-glass attenuation at high-resolution CT. Radiology 1992;184:451–4.

110. Wells AU, Hansell DM, Corrin B, et al. High resolution computed tomography as a predictor of lung histology in systemic sclerosis. Thorax 1992;47:508–12.

111. Wells AU, Rubens MB, du Bois RM, Hansell DM. Serial CT in fibrosing alveolitis: prognostic significance of the initial pattern. AJR Am J Roentgenol 1993;161:1159–65.

112. Katzenstein AL, Myers JL. Idiopathic pulmonary fibrosis: clinical relevance of pathologic classification. Am J Respir Crit Care Med 1998;157(4 Pt 1):1301–15.

113. Perez-Padilla R, Salas J, Chapela R, et al. Mortality in Mexican patients with chronic pigeon breeder's lung compared with those with usual interstitial pneumonia. Am Rev Respir Dis 1993;148:49–53.

114. Johkoh T, Ikezoe J, Kohno N, et al. High-resolution CT and pulmonary function tests in collagen vascular disease: comparison with idiopathic pulmonary fibrosis. Eur J Radiol 1994;18:113–21.

115. Hartman TE, Swensen SJ, Hansell DM, et al. Nonspecific interstitial pneumonia: variable appearance at high-resolution chest CT. Radiology 2000;217:701–5.

116. Kim T, Lee K, Chung M, et al. Nonspecific interstitial pneumonia with fibrosis: high resolution CT and pathologic findings. AMJ Am J Roentgenol 1998;171:1645–50.

117. Nagai S, Kitaichi M, Itoh H, et al. Idiopathic nonspecific interstitial pneumonia/fibrosis: comparison with idiopathic pulmonary fibrosis and BOOP. Eur Respir J 1998;12:1010–9.

118. MacDonald S, Rubens M, Hansell D, et al. Nonspecific interstitial pneumonia and usual interstitial pneumonia: comparative appearances and diagnostic accuracy of high-resolution computed tomography. Radiology 2001;221:600–5.

119. Nishiyama O, Kondoh Y, Taniguchi H, et al. Serial high resolution CT findings in nonspecific interstitial pneumonia/fibrosis. J Comput Assist Tomogr 2000;24:41–6.

120. Park JS, Lee KS, Kim JS, et al. Nonspecific interstitial pneumonia with fibrosis: radiographic and CT findings in seven patients. Radiology 1995;195:645–8.

121. Kim EY, Lee KS, Chung MP, et al. Nonspecific interstitial pneumonia with fibrosis: serial high-resolution CT findings with functional correlation. AJR Am J Roentgenol 1999;173:949–53.

122. Hartman TE, Primack SL, Swensen SJ, et al. Desquamative interstitial pneumonia: thin-section CT findings in 22 patients. Radiology 1993;187:787–90.

123. Hartman TE, Primack SL, Kang EY, et al. Disease progression in usual interstitial pneumonia compared with desquamative interstitial pneumonia. Assessment with serial CT. Chest 1996;110:378–82.

124. Akira M, Yamamoto S, Hara H, et al. Serial computed tomographic evaluation in desquamative interstitial pneumonia. Thorax 1997;52:333–7.

125. Heyneman LE, Ward S, Lynch DA, et al. Respiratory bronchiolitis, respiratory bronchiolitis-associated interstitial lung disease, and desquamative interstitial pneumonia: different entities or part of the spectrum of the same disease process? AJR Am J Roentgenol 1999;173:1617–22.

126. Park J, Brown K, Tuder R, et al. Respiratory bronchiolitis-associated interstitial lung disease: radiologic features with clinical and pathologic correlation. J Comput Assist Tomogr 2002;26:13–20.

127. Lee KS, Kullnig P, Hartman TE, Müller NL. Cryptogenic organizing pneumonia: CT findings in 43 patients. AJR Am J Roentgenol 1994;162:543–6.

128. Cordier JF, Loire R, Brune J. Idiopathic bronchiolitis obliterans organizing pneumonia. Definition of characteristic clinical profiles in a series of 16 patients. Chest 1989;96:999–1004.

129. Ichikado K, Johkoh T, Ikezoe J, et al. Acute interstitial pneumonia: high-resolution CT findings correlated with pathology. AJR Am J Roentgenol 1997;168:333–8.

130. Johkoh T, Müller N, Taniguchi H, et al. Acute interstitial pneumonia: thin section CT findings in 36 patients. Radiology 1999;211:859–63.

131. Primack SL, Hartman TE, Ikezoe J, et al. Acute interstitial pneumonia: radiographic and CT findings in nine patients. Radiology 1993;188:817–20.

132. Ichikawa Y, Kinoshita M, Koga T, et al. Lung cyst formation in lymphocytic interstitial pneumonitis: CT features. J Comput Assist Tomogr 1994;18:745–8.

133. Lynch JP 3rd, Kazerooni EA, Gay SE. Pulmonary sarcoidosis. Clin Chest Med 1997;18:755–85.

134. Dawson WB, Müller NL. High-resolution computed tomography in pulmonary sarcoidosis. Semin Ultrasound CT MR 1990;11:423–9.

135. Kuhlman JE, Fishman EK, Hamper UM, et al. The computed tomographic spectrum of thoracic sarcoidosis. Radiographics 1989;9:449–66.

136. Hamper UM, Fishman EK, Khouri NF, et al. Typical and atypical CT manifestations of pulmonary sarcoidosis. J Comput Assist Tomogr 1986;10:928–36.

137. Henry DA, Kiser PE, Scheer CE, et al. Multiple imaging evaluation of sarcoidosis. Radiographics 1986;6:75–95.

138. Lynch D, Webb W, Gamsu G, et al. Computed tomography in sarcoidosis. J Comput Assist Tomogr 1989;13:405–10.

139. Nishimura K, Itoh H, Kitaichi M, Nagai S, Izumi T. Pulmonary sarcoidosis: correlation of CT and histopathologic findings. Radiology 1993;189:105–9.

140. Johkoh T, Ikezoe J, Takeuchi N, et al. CT findings in "pseudoalveolar" sarcoidosis. J Comput Assist Tomogr 1992;16:904–7.

141. Austin JH. Pulmonary sarcoidosis: what are we learning from CT? Radiology 1989;171:603–4.

142. Müller N, Mawson J, Mathieson J, et al. Sarcoidosis: correlation of extent of disease at CT with clinical, functional, and radiographic findings. Radiology 1989;171:613–8.

143. Bergin C, Bell D, Coblentz C, et al. Sarcoidosis: correlation of pulmonary parenchymal pattern at CT with results of pulmonary function tests. Radiology 1989;171:619–24.

144. Abehsera M, Valeyre D, Grenier P, et al. Sarcoidosis with pulmonary fibrosis: CT patterns and correlation with pulmonary function. AJR Am J Roentgenol 2000;174:1751–7.

145. Gleeson F, Traill Z, Hansell D. Evidence on expiratory CT scans of small-airway obstruction in sarcoidosis. AJR Am J Roentgenol 1996;166:1052–4.

146. Mana J, Teirstein AS, Mendelson DS, et al. Excessive thoracic computed tomographic scanning in sarcoidosis. Thorax 1995;50:1264–6.

147. Munk P, Müller N, Miller R, Ostrow D. Pulmonary lymphangitic carcinomatosis: CT and pathologic findings. Radiology 1988;166:705–9.

148. Ikezoe J, Godwin J, Hunt K, Marglin S. Pulmonary lymphangitic carcinomatosis: chronicity of radiographic findings in long-term survivors. AJR Am J Roentgenol 1995;165:49–52.

149. Honda O, Johkoh T, Ichikado K, et al. Comparison of high resolution CT findings of sarcoidosis, lymphoma, and lymphangitic carcinoma: is there any difference of involved interstitium? J Comput Assist Tomogr 1999;23:374–9.

150. Akira M, Higashihara T, Yokoyama K, et al. Radiographic type P pneumoconiosis: high-resolution CT. Radiology 1989;171:117–23.

151. Bergin CJ, Müller NL, Vedal S, Chan-Yeung M. CT in silicosis: correlation with plain films and pulmonary function tests. AJR Am J Roentgenol 1986;146:477–83.

152. Begin R, Bergeron D, Samson L, et al. CT assessment of silicosis in exposed workers. AJR Am J Roentgenol 1987; 148:509–14.

153. Brichet A, Wallaert B, Gosselin B, et al. Idiopathic-like pulmonary fibrosis in coal workers. Am J Resp Crit Med 1997;155:A331.

154. Remy-Jardin M, Degreef JM, Beuscart R, et al. Coal worker's pneumoconiosis: CT assessment in exposed workers and correlation with radiographic findings. Radiology 1990; 177:363–71.

155. Katabami M, Dosaka-Akita H, Honma K, et al. Pneumoconiosis-related lung cancers: preferential occurrence from diffuse interstitial fibrosis-type pneumoconiosis. Am J Respir Crit Care Med 2000;162:295–300.

156. Begin R, Ostiguy G, Fillion R, Colman N. Computed tomography in the early detection of silicosis. Am Rev Respir Dis 1991;144:697–705.

157. Begin R, Filion R, Ostiguy G. Emphysema in silica- and asbestos-exposed workers seeking compensation. A CT scan study. Chest 1995;108:647–55.

158. Cowie RL, Hay M, Thomas RG. Association of silicosis, lung dysfunction, and emphysema in gold miners. Thorax 1993; 48:746–9.

159. Gevenois PA, Pichot E, Dargent F, et al. Low grade coal worker's pneumoconiosis. Comparison of CT and chest radiography. Acta Radiol 1994;35:351–6.

160. Guidelines for the use of ILO international classification of radiographs of pneumoconioses. Revised Edition 1980. Occupational Safety and Health Series. No.22 (Rev.). Geneva: International Labour Office, 1980.

161. Henry D. The ILO classification system in the age of imaging: relevant or redundant? J Thorac Imaging 2002. [In press]

162. Tossavainen A. International expert meeting on new advances in the radiology and screening of asbestos-related diseases. Scand J Work Environ Health 2000;26:449–54.

163. Gamsu G. High resolution CT in the diagnosis of asbestos-related pleuroparenchymal disease [editorial]. Am J Ind Med 1989;16:115–7.

164. Sargent E, Boswell W, Ralls P, Markovitz A. Subpleural fat pads in patients exposed to asbestos: distinction from non-calcified pleural plaques. Radiology 1984;152:273–7.

165. Kipen HM, Lilis R, Suzuki Y, et al. Pulmonary fibrosis in asbestos insulation workers with lung cancer: a radiological and histopathological evaluation. Br J Ind Med 1987;44:96–100.

166. Weiss W. Cigarette smoke, asbestos, and small irregular opacities. Am Rev Respir Dis 1984;130:293–301.

167. Weiss W. Presentation of data on pulmonary fibrosis and cigarette smoking [letter]. Am J Ind Med 1984;5:417–9.

168. Blanc PD, Gamsu G. The effect of cigarette smoking on the detection of small radiographic opacities in inorganic dust diseases. J Thorac Imaging 1988;3:51–6.

169. Blanc P, Golden J, Gamsu G. Asbestos exposure-cigarette smoking interactions among shipyard workers. JAMA 1988;259:370–3.

170. Aberle DR, Gamsu G, Ray CS. High-resolution CT of benign asbestos-related diseases: clinical and radiographic correlation. AJR Am J Roentgenol 1988;151:883–91.

171. Friedman AC, Fiel SB, Fisher MS, et al. Asbestos-related pleural disease and asbestosis: a comparison of CT and chest radiography. AJR Am J Roentgenol 1988;150:269–75.

172. Gamsu G, Salmon CJ, Warnock ML, Blanc PD. CT quantification of interstitial fibrosis in patients with asbestosis: a comparison of two methods. AJR Am J Roentgenol 1995;164:63–8.

173. Gevenois PA, De Vuyst P, Dedeire S, et al. Conventional and high-resolution CT in asymptomatic asbestos-exposed workers. Acta Radiol 1994;35:226–9.

174. Gamsu G, Kee ST, Blanc P. Causes of pulmonary impairment in asbestos-exposed individuals with diffuse pleural thickening. Am J Respir Crit Care Med 1996;154:789–93.

175. Schwartz DA, Galvin JR, Yagla SJ, et al. Restrictive lung function and asbestos-induced pleural fibrosis. A quantitative approach. J Clin Invest 1993;91:2685–92.

176. Van Cleemput J, De Raeve H, Verschakelen JA, et al. Surface of localized pleural plaques quantitated by computed tomography scanning: no relation with cumulative asbestos exposure and no effect on lung function. Am J Respir Crit Care Med 2001;163(3 Pt 1):705–10.

177. Staples CA, Gamsu G, Ray CS, Webb WR. High resolution computed tomography and lung function in asbestos-exposed workers with normal chest radiographs. Am Rev Respir Dis 1989;139:1502–8.

178. Bergin CJ, Castellino RA, Blank N, Moses L. Specificity of high-resolution CT findings in pulmonary asbestosis: do patients scanned for other indications have similar findings? AJR Am J Roentgenol 1994;163:551–5.

179. al Jarad N, Strickland B, Pearson MC, et al. High resolution computed tomographic assessment of asbestosis and cryptogenic fibrosing alveolitis: a comparative study. Thorax 1992;47:645–50.

180. Oksa P, Suoranta H, Koskinen H, et al. High-resolution computed tomography in the early detection of asbestosis. Int Arch Occup Environ Health 1994;65:299–304.

181. Neri S, Boraschi P, Antonelli A, et al. Pulmonary function, smoking habits, and high resolution computed tomography (HRCT) early abnormalities of lung and pleural fibrosis in shipyard workers exposed to asbestos. Am J Ind Med 1996;30:588–95.

182. Akira M, Yokoyama K, Yamamoto S, et al. Early asbestosis: evaluation with high-resolution CT. Radiology 1991; 178:409–16.

183. Lynch D, Gamsu G, Ray C, Aberle D. Asbestos-related focal lung masses: manifestations on conventional and high-resolution CT scans. Radiology 1988;169:603–7.

184. Doyle TC, Lawler GA. CT features of rounded atelectasis of the lung. AJR Am J Roentgenol 1984;143:225–8.

185. Franzblau A. Asbestos-associated rounded atelectasis: a case report and review of the literature. Mt Sinai J Med 1989; 56:321–5.

186. Hillerdal G. Rounded atelectasis. Clinical experience with 74 patients. Chest 1989;95:836–41.

187. Rockoff SD. CT demonstration of interlobar fissure calcification due to asbestos exposure. J Comput Assist Tomogr 1987;11:1066–8.

188. Tiitola M, Kivisaari L, Huuskonen MS, et al. Computed tomography screening for lung cancer in asbestos-exposed workers. Lung Cancer 2002;35:17–22.

189. Michel JL, Catilina P, Laubignat JF, Gabrillargues D. Is there criteria to allow the selection of patients exposed to asbestos which is relevant to thoracic computed tomography screening? J Radiol 1999;80:141–5.

190. Hansell D, Moskovic E. High-resolution computed tomography in extrinsic allergic alveolitis. Clin Radiol 1991;43:8–12.

191. Lynch DA, Rose CS, Way D, King TJ. Hypersensitivity pneumonitis: sensitivity of high-resolution CT in a population-based study. AMJ Am J Roentgenol 1992;159:469–72.

192. Adler BD, Padley SP, Müller NL, et al. Chronic hypersensitivity pneumonitis: high-resolution CT and radiographic features in 16 patients. Radiology 1992;185:91–5.

193. Akira M, Kita N, Higashihara T, et al. Summer-type hypersensitivity pneumonitis: comparison of high-resolution CT and plain radiographic findings. Am J Roentgenol 1992; 158:1223–8.

194. Buschman DL, Gamsu G, Waldron JJ, et al. Chronic hypersensitivity pneumonitis: use of CT in diagnosis. AJR Am J Roentgenol 1992;159:957–60.

195. Silver S, Müller N, Miller R, Lefcoe M. Hypersensitivity pneumonitis: evaluation with CT. Radiology 1989;173:441–5.

196. Remy-Jardin M, Remy J, Wallaert B, Müller NL. Subacute and chronic bird breeder hypersensitivity pneumonitis: sequential evaluation with CT and correlation with lung function tests and bronchoalveolar lavage. Radiology 1993;189:111–8.

197. Erkinjuntti-Pekkanen R, Rytkonen H, Kokkarinen JI, et al. Long-term risk of emphysema in patients with farmer's lung and matched control farmers. Am J Respir Crit Care Med 1998;158:662–5.

198. Cormier Y, Brown M, Worthy S, et al. High-resolution computed tomographic characteristics in acute farmer's lung and in its follow-up. Eur Respir J 2000;16:56–60.

199. Primack SL, Hartman TE, Hansell DM, Müller NL. End-stage lung disease: CT findings in 61 patients. Radiology 1993;189:681–6.

200. Kulwiec E, Lynch D, Aguayo S, et al. Imaging of pulmonary histiocytosis X. Radiographics 1992;12:515–26.

201. Taylor DB, Joske D, Anderson J, Barry WC. Cavitating pulmonary nodules in histiocytosis-X high resolution CT demonstration. Australas Radiol 1990;34:253–5.

202. Fartoukh M, Humbert M, Capron F, et al. Severe pulmonary hypertension in histiocytosis X. Am J Respir Crit Care Med 2000;161:216–23.

203. Marcy T, Reynolds H. Pulmonary histiocytosis X. Lung 1985;163:129–150.

204. Bernstrand C, Cederlund K, Sandstedt B, et al. Pulmonary abnormalities at long-term follow-up of patients with Langerhans cell histiocytosis. Med Pediatr Oncol 2001; 36:459–68.

205. Horwitz T, Friedman L. Findings on computed tomography of the chest in lymphangiomyomatosis [letter]. S Afr Med J 1991;79:53–4.

206. Lenoir S, Grenier P, Brauner MW, et al. Pulmonary lymphangiomyomatosis and tuberous sclerosis: comparison of radiographic and thin-section CT findings. Radiology 1990; 175:329–34.

207. Müller NL, Chiles C, Kullnig P. Pulmonary lymphangiomyomatosis: correlation of CT with radiographic and functional findings. Radiology 1990;175:335–9.

208. Crausman R, Lynch D, Mortenson R, et al. Quantitative CT predicts the severity of physiologic dysfunction in patients with lymphangioleiomyomatosis. Chest 1996;109:131–7.

209. Bernstein SM, Newell JD Jr, Adamczyk D, et al. How common are renal angiomyolipomas in patients with pulmonary lymphangioleiomyomatosis? Am J Respir Crit Care Med 1995;152:2138–43.

210. Avila NA, Kelly JA, Chu SC, et al. Lymphangioleiomyomatosis: abdominopelvic CT and US findings. Radiology 2000; 216:147–53.

211. Costello LC, Hartman TE, Ryu JH. High frequency of pulmonary lymphangioleiomyomatosis in women with tuberous sclerosis complex. Mayo Clin Proc 2000;75:591–4.

212. Moss J, Avila NA, Barnes PM, et al. Prevalence and clinical characteristics of lymphangioleiomyomatosis (LAM) in patients with tuberous sclerosis complex. Am J Respir Crit Care Med 2001;164:669–71.

213. Naidich D, Zerhouni E, Hutchins G, et al. Computed tomography of the pulmonary parenchyma. Part 1. Distal airspace disease. J Thorac Imaging 1985;1:39–53.

214. Müller NL, Staples CA, Miller RR. Bronchiolitis obliterans organizing pneumonia: CT features in 14 patients. AJR Am J Radiol 1990;154:983–7.

215. King MA, Pope-Harman AL, Allen JN, et al. Acute eosinophilic pneumonia: radiologic and clinical features. Radiology 1997;203:715–9.

216. Bellamy E, Nocholas D, Husband J. Quantitative assessment of lung damage due to bleomycin using computed tomography. Br J Radiol 1987;60:1205–9.

217. Santrach PJ, Askin FB, Wells RJ, et al. Nodular form of bleomycin-related pulmonary injury in patients with osteogenic sarcoma. Cancer 1989;64:806–11.

218. Kuhlman J, Teigen C, Ren H, et al. Amiodarone pulmonary toxicity: CT findings in symptomatic patients. Radiology 1990;177:121–5.

219. Nicholson A, Hayward C. The value of computed tomography in the diagnosis of amiodarone-induced lung toxicity. Clin Radiol 1989;40:564–7.

220. Padley SP, Adler B, Hansell DM, Müller NL. High-resolution computed tomography of drug-induced lung disease. Clin Radiol 1992;46:232–6.

221. Chang AB, Masel JP, Masters B. Post-infectious bronchiolitis obliterans: clinical, radiological and pulmonary function sequelae. Pediatr Radiol 1998;28:23–9.

222. Marti-Bonmati L, Ruiz Perales F, Catala F, et al. CT findings in Swyer-James syndrome. Radiology 1989;172:477–80.

223. Sweatman MC, Millar AB, Strickland B, Turner-Warwick M. Computed tomography in adult obliterative bronchiolitis. Clin Radiol 1990;41:116–9.

224. Morrish WF, Herman SJ, Weisbrod GL, Chamberlain DW. Bronchiolitis obliterans after lung transplantation: findings at chest radiography and high-resolution CT. Radiology 1991;179:487–90.

225. Padley SP, Adler BD, Hansell DM, Müller NL. Bronchiolitis obliterans: high resolution CT findings and correlation with pulmonary function tests. Clin Radiol 1993;47:236–40.

226. Ikonen T, Kivisaari L, Taskinen E, et al. High-resolution CT in long-term follow-up after lung transplantation. Chest 1997;111:370–6.

227. Lau DM, Siegel MJ, Hildebolt CF, Cohen AH. Bronchiolitis obliterans syndrome: thin-section CT diagnosis of obstructive changes in infants and young children after lung transplantation. Radiology 1998;208:783–8.

228. Ooi GC, Peh WC, Ip M. High-resolution computed tomography of bronchiolitis obliterans syndrome after bone marrow transplantation. Respiration 1998;65:187–91.

229. Lee ES, Gotway MB, Reddy GP, et al. Early bronchiolitis obliterans following lung transplantation: accuracy of expiratory thin-section CT for diagnosis. Radiology 2000;216:472–7.

230. Miller WT Jr, Kotloff RM, Blumenthal NP, et al. Utility of high resolution computed tomography in predicting bronchiolitis obliterans syndrome following lung transplantation: preliminary findings. J Thorac Imaging 2001;16:76–80.

231. Jensen S, Lynch D, Brown K, et al. High resolution CT features of severe asthma and bronchiolitis obliterans. Radiology 2000;217:595.

232. Remy-Jardin M, Remy J, Gosselin B, et al. Lung parenchymal changes secondary to cigarette smoking: pathologic-CT correlations. Radiology 1993;186(3):643–51.

233. Remy-Jardin M, Edme JL, Boulenguez C, et al. Longitudinal follow-up study of smoker's lung with thin-section CT in correlation with pulmonary function tests. Radiology 2002;222(1):261–70.

234. Reittner P, Müller NL, Heyneman L, et al. *Mycoplasma pneumoniae* pneumonia: radiographic and high-resolution CT features in 28 patients. AJR Am J Roentgenol 2000; 174:37–41.

235. Akira M, Kitatani J, Yong-Sik L, et al. Diffuse panbronchiolitis: evaluation with high-resolution CT. Radiology 1988; 168:433–8.

236. Akira M, Higashihara T, Sakatani M, Hara H. Diffuse panbronchiolitis: follow-up CT examination. Radiology 1993;189:559–62.

237. Ichikawa Y, Hotta M, Sumita S, et al. Reversible airway lesions in diffuse panbronchiolitis. Detection by high-resolution computed tomography. Chest 1995;107:120–5.

238. Harrison NK, Glanville AR, Strickland B, et al. Pulmonary involvement in systemic sclerosis: the detection of early changes by thin section CT scan, bronchoalveolar lavage and 99mTc- DTPA clearance. Respir Med 1989;83:403–14.

239. Schurawitzki H, Stiglbauer R, Graninger W, et al. Interstitial lung disease in progressive systemic sclerosis: high-

resolution CT versus radiography. Radiology 1990;176:755–9.

240. Bergin CJ, Coblentz CL, Chiles C, et al. Chronic lung diseases: specific diagnosis by using CT. AJR Am J Roentgenol 1989;152:1183–8.

241. Collins CD, Wells AU, Hansell DM, et al. Observer variation in pattern type and extent of disease in fibrosing alveolitis on thin section computed tomography and chest radiography. Clin Radiol 1994;49:236–40.

242. Gilman M, Laurens R, Somogyi J, Honig E. CT attenuation values of lung density in sarcoidosis. J Comput Assist Tomogr 1983;7:407–10.

243. Robinson P, Kreel L. Pulmonary tissue attentuation with computed tomography: comparison of inspiration and expiration scans. J Comput Assist Tomogr 1979;3:740–8.

244. Van Dyk J, Hill R. Postirradiation lung density changes as measured by computerised tomography. Int J Radiat Oncol Biol Phys 1983;9:847–52.

245. Wollmer P, Jakobsson K, Albin M, et al. Measurement of lung density by x-ray computed tomography: relation to lung mechanics in workers exposed to asbestos cement. Chest 1987;91:865–9.

246. Millar AB, Denison DM. Vertical gradients of lung density in supine subjects with fibrosing alveolitis or pulmonary emphysema. Thorax 1990;45:602–5.

247. Hartley PG, Galvin JR, Hunninghake GW, et al. High-resolution CT-derived measures of lung density are valid indexes of interstitial lung disease. J Appl Physiol 1994;76:271–7.

248. Coxson HO, Rogers RM, Whittall KP, et al. A quantification of the lung surface area in emphysema using computed tomography. Am J Respir Crit Care Med 1999;159:851–6.

249. Goldin J. Quantitative CT of the lung. Radiol Clin North Am 2002;40:145–62.

250. Uppaluri R, Hoffman EA, Sonka M, et al. Interstitial lung disease: a quantitative study using the adaptive multiple feature method. Am J Respir Crit Care Med 1999;159:519–25.

251. Wiggins J, Strickland B, Turner WM. Combined cryptogenic fibrosing alveolitis and emphysema: the value of high resolution computed tomography in assessment. Respir Med 1990;84:365–9.

252. Hruban R, Meziane M, Zerhouni E, et al. High resolution computed tomography of inflation-fixed lungs: pathologic-radiographic correlation of centrilobular emphysema. Am Rev Respir Dis 1987;136:935–40.

253. Naidich DP, Weinreb JC, Schinella R. MR imaging of pulmonary parenchyma: comparison with CT in evaluating cadaveric lung specimens. J Comput Assist Tomogr 1990;14:595–9.

254. Grenier P, Maurice F, Musset D, et al. Bronchiectasis: assessment by thin-section CT. Radiology 1986;161:95–9.

5

BRONCHOALVEOLAR LAVAGE

ULRICH COSTABEL
JOSUNE GUZMAN

Bronchoalveolar lavage (BAL) is a technique used to collect cells, inhaled particles, infectious organisms, and solutes from the lower respiratory tract and in particular from the alveolar spaces of the lung.[1] To achieve this, a sufficient volume of lavage fluid must be instilled to ensure a sufficient aspirate. In adults, a minimum of 100 mL of lavage fluid should be instilled.[2] The procedure is performed during fiberoptic bronchoscopy, is only minimally invasive, and usually well tolerated.

BAL differs from other lavage techniques in the following ways:

- Bronchial lavage (or bronchial washing) requires relatively little instilled fluid (10 to 30 mL) and samples material from large airways for bacteriologic study and/or tumor cytology.
- Therapeutic lavage, which uses small volumes as in bronchial lavage, is used to remove sticky bronchial secretions in patients with asthma and cystic fibrosis. With very large volumes (10 to 30 L) instilled through a double-lumen endotracheal tube during general anaesthesia it also is used as a whole-lung lavage to wash out an entire lung in patients with alveolar proteinosis.[3]

Since its introduction in the 1970s[4] as a valuable research tool to study local immune and inflammatory mechanisms,[5,6] BAL has gained widespread acceptance as a powerful investigative tool in the field of pulmonary medicine. It has become a standard diagnostic procedure in patients with interstitial lung disease (ILD).[3,7–9]

It is thought that alterations in lavage fluid and cells reflect pathologic changes in the corresponding parenchymal constituents. A number of studies have shown a good correlation between the type and number of inflammatory cells obtained by BAL and those observed in histologic lung biopsy sections or derived from mechanically dispensed lung tissue in several ILDs such as idiopathic pulmonary fibrosis, sarcoidosis, and hypersensitivity pneumonitis.[10–14]

Thus, this technique serves as a "window to the lung." The information gained from BAL is regarded as complementary to histopathology from biopsy specimens but, nevertheless, has several advantages over biopsy procedures. It is safe and associated with virtually no morbidity; therefore, it can be used repeatedly to investigate serial changes. In addition, BAL collects samples from a much larger area of the lungs than can be obtained by the small tissue fragments of transbronchial biopsy or even by surgical biopsy, thereby giving a more representative picture of inflammatory and immunologic changes.

Even less invasive than BAL is the technique of induced sputum. Its diagnostic role in ILD, particularly in comparison with BAL, has not yet been well defined; however, further studies are necessary.[15,16]

TECHNICAL PRINCIPLES

The details of different steps of the prodecure may vary between institutions and laboratories, but the principles are the same for each procedure. Attempts have been made to standardize the performance, laboratory processing, and analysis of the recovered constituents. Guidelines and recommendations for a standardized approach have been published.[2,3,17,18] These set a framework based on the principle of the so-called smallest common denominator, which allows for a number of technical variations in the different steps of the BAL procedure. Sometimes these differences give rise to problems when comparing data. When the guidelines are followed, however, the results of BAL are sufficiently valid for practical diagnostic purposes. For example, the correct information on cell differentials is important for clinical purposes. In this regard, the total volume of instilled fluid can range from 100 to 250 mL without affecting the results of cell differentials.[19–21]

Bronchoscopic Procedure

Bronchoalveolar lavage is usually performed during fiberoptic bronchoscopy with topical anesthesia following general inspection of the tracheobronchial tree. BAL can also be done under general anesthesia and in ventilated patients by passing the fiberoptic bronchoscope through either a rigid bronchoscope or an endotracheal tube. To avoid coughing, local anesthesia must be adequate, but superfluous lidocain, which might otherwise affect cell harvest, viability, and function, must be carefully suctioned off before the actual lavage.[22,23] To prevent iatrogenic bleeding and consecutive lavage contamination by blood, BAL should always be performed before any concomitant procedure (eg, biopsy or bronchial brushing). If the bronchoscopy shows signs of airway inflammation, especially putrid secretions, the results will be greatly influenced by the contribution of the bronchial spaces. BAL should not be performed until the patient has been treated with antibiotics if undertaken for the assessment of noninfectious ILD. This may be different if an infectious etiology is suspected.

Site

The fiberoptic bronchoscope is gently introduced until impacted or "wedged" in a segmental or subsegmental bronchus. Localized disease naturally requires lavage of the radiographically involved area. In diffuse lung disease, the middle or lingular lobe is recommended as a standard site for BAL. When the patient is supine, the anatomy favors maximal recovery from these sites, and $\geq 20\%$ more fluid and cells are recovered from these lobes compared with the the lower lobes.[24] If anatomic difficulties are encountered, the anterior segment of either the upper or lower lobe may be used. Lavage in one site seems adequate. Several studies have evaluated the interlobar variation of lavage cell differentials, lymphocyte subpopulations, and asbestos body counts by performing a bilateral lavage and analyzing both sides independently. In general, these studies have shown a good interlobar correlation in patients with nonfocal disease on the chest radiograph.[25–27] These observations indicate that in patients with diffuse lung disease, BAL at one site should yield representative information on the whole lung. Nevertheless, some centers routinely instill 100 mL of fluid into each of two or three different regions, which may be particularly useful in patients with marked radiographic heterogeneity.

Fluid Instillation

The most commonly used instillate is sterile, unbuffered isotonic saline (0.9% NaCl solution). Prior warming of the fluid to body temperature may decrease coughing and increase the cellular yield, but many groups continue to use room temperature saline.[24] The fluid is instilled with syringes through the biopsy channel of the bronchoscope using a standard number of input aliquots of 20 to 60 mL (4 to 5 aliquots are recommended as the most common) up to a total volume of 100 to 300 mL. Smaller instilled volumes (less than 100 mL) increase the likelihood of contamination by the

bronchial spaces, including inflammatory cells derived from the larger airways, which may skew the differential cell counts.[28]

Fluid Recovery

After each instillation, the aliquot is immediately recovered by gentle hand suction into a syringe or gentle wall suction into a fluid trap. Suction that is too strong can cause collapse of the distal airways or trauma to the airway mucosa, which reduces the recovery or changes the BAL fluid profile. The first aspirated volume is commonly smaller than the following ones. Usually, 40 to 70% of the instilled volume is recovered. In obstructive airway disease and emphysema, the recovery rate is significantly lower and may be less than 30%.[29] The yield is also reduced in healthy smokers and in the elderly.[17] In addition, fluid recovery may be low with a poor wedge position, leading to leakage of lavage fluid around the bronchoscope, which is associated with cough.

Differential evaluation of the "bronchial" (first aliquot) and "alveolar" (subsequent aliquots) samples may be useful in airway diseases. Siliconized and plastic containers should be used for collection and processing of BAL fluid to avoid loss of cells through adhesion to glass surfaces.

Technical Aspects in Children

In children, different sizes of bronchoscopes are used. The instillation volume has to be adapted to the different ages and sizes of children, and various protocols have been applied. Some investigators use two or four fractions of the same volume (10 to 20 mL) irrespective of body weight and age. Others adjust BAL volume to body weight using $3\ mL \times kg^{-1}$ of normal saline divided into three equal fractions in children weighing less than 20 kg and 20 mL portions in children weighing more than 20 kg.[30,31] The normal values for cellular components are slightly different in children; the major difference between children and adults is seen in the CD4/CD8 ratio, which has been found to be lower in children in two studies.[30,32] Detailed recommendations on BAL in children have recently been published by the European Respiratory Society (ERS) Task Force on BAL in children.[33] BAL is widely applied in pediatric patients with ILD. A recent multicentric survey on the diagnostic approach to ILD in children showed that BAL is the most frequently applied invasive technique, having been used in 63% of the 131 children studied.[34]

Side Effects

Bronchoalveolar lavage is generally well tolerated and its side effects are more or less comparable with those of routine fiberoptic bronchoscopy under local anesthesia. The procedure is associated with practically no mortality and carries a low complication rate between 0 to 2.3% compared with 7% with transbronchial biopsy and 13% with surgical lung biopsy.[35,36] There are no absolute contraindications for the performance of BAL beyond those noted for bronchoscopy.

Fever, some hours after BAL, is by far the most frequent adverse effect, occurring in 3 to 30% of patients, depending on the instilled volume. If a total volume below 150 mL is used, fever is seen in less than 3% of patients. Larger volumes will increase the frequency to 30% or more.[37,38] Other side effects include short-lasting alveolar infiltration, a transient decrease in lung function parameters, and, rarely, wheezing and bronchospasm in patients with hyperreactive airways (Table 5–1). These side effects do not last longer than 24 hours. Patients with severe heart failure can develop pulmonary edema from stress and hypoxia. The side effects can be reduced by limiting the instilled volume to 100 to 200 mL. Major or late complications are only seen in patients with severe lung or heart disease. Bleeding is reported just anecdotally even in patients with clotting disorders or thrombocytopenia. Severe complications are extremely rare.[2]

Risk factors for developing adverse effects are extensive pulmonary infiltrates, arterial oxygen pressure (PaO$_2$) < 8.0 kPa (< 60 mm Hg), oxygen saturation below 90%, forced expiratory volume in 1 second (FEV$_1$) below 1.0 L, prothrombin time < 50 sec, platelet count < 20,000 × mL^{-1}, significant comorbidity, and bronchial hyperreactivity. Patients with such conditions should be monitored carefully following the procedure.[2,39]

Laboratory Processing

It is important that the total fluid recovered is transported to the laboratory as quickly as possible (if kept at room temperature, in less than 1 hour) because the cells are not well preserved in the saline solution.[40] The fluid should be pooled into a single container and the total volume should be measured. The lavage fluid frequently contains large amounts of mucus; therefore, filtration through cotton gauze or nylon mesh is often performed. Filtration leads to a preferential loss of bronchial epithelial cells (in one study filtration reduced the proportion of epithelial cells from 10 to 6%) without a significant effect on the total cell count and cell differentials. After filtration, the fluid is centrifuged for 10 minutes at 500 g. The supernatant can be stored frozen at –20°C or –70°C for subsequent analysis of soluble components.

Cell Studies

The total number of cells are counted in a hemocytometer, either in a sample of the pooled native fluid or in a resuspension of the cells after the first centrifugation. Washing procedures result in a loss of total cells but lead to an increase in cell viability of the remaining cells. The Coulter counter has been used for the determination of the total cell count but is less accurate than the hemocytometer because BAL cells often form clumps. The total cell count is usually expressed as the total number of cells recovered per lavage and also as the concentration of cells per mL of recovered fluid. Cell viability is assessed by trypan blue exclusion and should range from 80 to 95%.

A number of different methods have been developed for the preparation of BAL cells for cytologic examination including cytocentrifugation, membrane filtration, and a cell smear technique. The differential cell counts, which are enumerated on these preparations, can be significantly affected by the applied method. For example, the two most frequently used methods, cytocentrifugation and membrane filtration, underestimate the percentage of lymphocytes (cytocentrifugation) or neutrophils (membrane filtration).[42,43] Advantages of cytocentrifugation, the more commonly used method, include a lower cost and superior morphology of cells compared with filtration methods. The disadvantage is the selective loss of lymphocytes that may not adhere to the glass slides, which

TABLE 5–1   Side Effects of Bronchoalveolar Lavage

Side Effect	Occurrence and Duration
Fever	In 3 to 30%, depending on instilled volume, occurring within 24 h
Alveolar infiltation on radiograph or CT	Segmental or subsegmental shadowing resolving within 48 h
Lung function decrement	Transient decrease in FEV$_1$, VC, PaO$_2$
Bronchospasm and wheezing	In < 1% of patients, more frequent in hyperreactive patients; may be prevented by prewarming the instillate
Crackles	Over involved area, within 24 h
Pulmonary edema	Rarely in patients with preexisting heart failure
Bleeding	Reported only anecdotally
Local inflammatory response	Increase in BAL neutrophils, resolved within 72 h

CT = computed tomography; FEV$_1$ = forced expiratory volume in 1 second; VC = vital capacity; PaO$_2$ = arterial oxygen pressure; BAL = bronchoalveolar lavage.

results in an artificially low lymphocyte count. In our laboratory, a cell smear technique is routinely performed. This is done, as in routine cytology and hematology, by streaking cells onto a microscope slide with the aid of a straight edge, typically a second microscope slide. As we have shown, this technique yields a well-preseved morphology of BAL fluid cells and produces significantly higher percentages of lymphocytes compared with cytocentrifugation.[44] The smear is better for tumor cell identification because more cells are present than on cytocentrifuged preparations. Also, when the BAL fluid is bloody, inflammatory cells in cytocentrifuged preparations can be obscured by a mass of red blood cells. Thus, we routinely apply this simple and accurate method for cell differentials and for detection of specific cytologic features that can occasionally aid in the diagnosis.

For the enumeration of cell differentials, at least 600 cells are counted after staining with May-Grünwald-Giemsa (MGG) stain. As we have shown, this number of cells is needed to achieve sufficient reproducibility and low variability in the differential cell counts.[29,44] The diff-quick stain should not be used because it does not stain mast cells. Ciliated or squamous epithelial cells should be noted but not included in the differential cell count. A high percentage of epithelial cells (> 5%) is indicative of contamination of the alveolar samples by bronchial cells. Such BAL probes may not be representative for the diagnosis of diffuse parenchymal lung disease. At least three unstained slides should be stored so that special stains (eg, iron, periodic acid–Schiff, silver, toluidine blue, fat, or Ziehl-Neelsen) can be performed if clinically indicated or is indicated from specific observations on the MGG slides.

If infection is suspected, a complete microbiologic assessment, including cultures, should be performed. To document asbestos exposure, quantitative determination of asbestos bodies can be made after vacuum filtration of the native BAL fluid through a 0.45 to 1.20 µm Millipore membrane.[9] Lymphocyte subpopulations are identified by immunocytochemical methods, immunofluorescence, or flow cytometry using monoclonal antibody techniques.[45]

In addition, for research purposes, functional studies of viable BAL cells can be performed. The cells can be cultivated in appropriate culture medium, and the release of mediators can be determined, along with the mechanisms that appear to regulate the mediator release. It is possible to study cell-cell interactions with cocultures of two different types of cells. Cells can also be probed with tools of molecular biology to investigate gene activation and intracellular signaling pathways.

Soluble Components

A large and increasing number of soluble components have been measured in lavage fluid. Their role for routine performance in clinical practice remains to be elucidated. Currently, none of them has proven useful in clinical settings. Solutes are too nonspecific to be of diagnostic value. The prognostic significance of solutes is also uncertain. In general, the quantitative expression of noncellular lavage constituents is hampered by the lack of satisfactory reference standards, to correct for the variable and unpredictable dilutional effects of the epithelial lining fluid. A reasonable pragmatic approach was recently taken by the ERS Task Force on measurement of acellular components. This Task Force concluded that the results of acellullar components should be expressed as amounts per mL of recovered BAL fluid, to facilitate comparison of data from different workers until a reliable external marker can be defined.[46] The report of the ERS Task Force provides detailed information on the measurement of soluble components including pulmonary surfactant components[57]; immunoglobulins[48]; proteases and antiproteases[49]; angiotensin converting enzyme[50]; antioxidants, oxidants, and oxidation products[51]; lipid mediators[52]; cytokines[53]; soluble adhesion molecules[54]; markers of fibrosis[55]; granulocyte-derived markers[56]; tumor markers[57]; markers of cell death[58]; and other acellular components.[59]

Interpretation of Cytology

Changes in the profile of cell differentials of BAL fluid have been described in various ILDs. Clearly, an abnormal BAL cell differential count does not allow a specific diagnosis, just as with conventional differential blood counts. But BAL studies should not be limited to counting cell differentials. At least as important as examining cell differentials is to note the morphologic appearances of cells and particles. Examples are the different morphology in hypersensitivity pneumonitis (foamy macrophages, heterogeneous macrophage size, presence of plasma cells) versus that of sarcoidosis (more monomorphous appearance of macrophages, less activated lymphocytes), the presence of malignant cells, the charateristic features of alveolar proteinosis, or the detection of dust particles such as asbestos bodies in occupational exposure conditions.[39]

Therefore, BAL cell differentials cannot not be used as an isolated finding for making a diagnosis but should always be interpreted in the context of disease history and clinical, laboratory, and radiologic findings. Combining BAL results with high-resolution computed tomography (HRCT) has surely increased the diagnostic power of both methods (see below).

BRONCHOALVEOLAR LAVAGE IN HEALTHY ADULTS

The BAL fluid obtained from healthy, nonsmoking adults without lung disease contains only small percentages of lymphocytes, neutrophils, and other inflammatory cells.[3,7,17] The alveolar macrophages are the predominant cell population (Figure 5–1A).

Cigarette smoking is a strong confounding factor with significant effects on BAL samples.[17,60,61] The alveolar macrophages from smokers show a characteristic appearance; many of them are much larger than those in nonsmokers and contain cytoplasmic inclusion bodies (smoker's inclusion bodies) consisting of tar products, lipids, lipofuscin, and other substances (Figure 5–1B). Thus, on gross examination, the recovered BAL fluid has a light to dark brown and turbid appearance caused by the color of the tar-laden macrophages. The total cell yield is three- to five-fold higher in smokers due to a three- to five-fold numeric increase in the number of macrophages. This leads to a relative decrease in the percentage of lymphocytes, which are unchanged in absolute numbers. Although the proportion of neutrophils is low, with average values of 2% in both nonsmokers and smokers, there is a tenfold increase in the absolute numbers of neutrophils in lavage from smokers. The eosinophil number is also increased but to a lesser extent. These changes must be known for the interpretation of cell differentials in patients with ILD.

BAL performed in healthy volunteers has permitted the determination of the normal composition of BAL fluid.[17] The normal values of BAL differential cytology that have been proposed in the literature are somewhat variable. One problem is that in most of the published studies there are only small numbers of normal persons (mostly volunteers) available for comparison. The other problem is that cigarette smoking changes the pattern of cell distribution by increasing the number of neutrophils. For practical reasons, the following percentages can be expected as normal in nonsmokers[2]:

- Macrophages > 80%
- Lymphocytes ≤ 15%
- Neutrophils ≤ 3%
- Eosinophils ≤ 0.5%
- Mast cells ≤ 0.5%

BRONCHOALVEOLAR LAVAGE IN THE DIFFERENTIAL DIAGNOSIS OF INTERSTITIAL LUNG DISEASE

Bronchoalveolar lavage has become a widely accepted diagnostic tool in pulmonary medicine. This holds true for both infectious and noninfectious infiltrative and immunologic lung diseases. In ILD, the application of BAL for diagnostic purposes has improved the diagnostic work-up, and some investigators use BAL even more frequently than transbronchial lung biopsy. In two recently published international statements on the major ILDs, BAL was considered helpful in strengthening the diagnosis in patients with sarcoidosis in the absence of a biopsy,[62] and BAL and/or transbronchial biopsy were considered requirements for the exclusion of other diseases in a patient with idiopathic pulmonary fibrosis (IPF) who did not undergo surgical biopsy (one of the four major criteria for making a clinical diagnosis of the disease).[63]

BAL is broadly indicated in every patient with unclear ILD or unclear pulmonary shadowing, no matter what cause is suspected. The underlying disorders may be of infectious, noninfectious immunologic, or malignant etiology.

BAL may also be indicated in patients with normal chest radiographs when clinical and lung function tests are abnormal and point toward a diffuse lung disease, or in patients with unexplained pulmonary symptoms in whom a normal BAL finding may exclude significant, active ILD.

Changes in the morphologic appearance of cells, in the cell yield, and in cell differentials have been described in a variety of diffuse lung diseases. BAL findings may be, on occasion, very specific, so that they can directly confirm a particular diagnosis and can then replace the lung biopsy. In other selected lung diseases, BAL findings are not diagnostic but may help narrow the differential diagnosis in the appropriate clinical setting. Some-

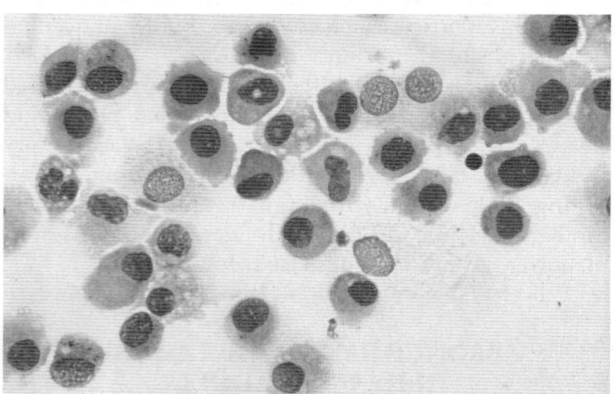

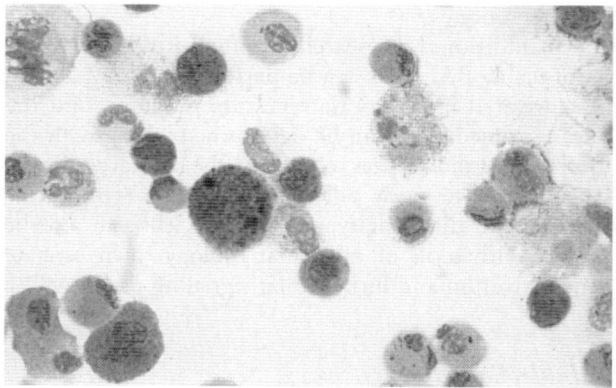

A   B

Figure 5–1   BAL cell differentials in healthy adults. May-Grünwald-Giemsa stain, ×400. *A,* Normal BAL cytology in a non-smoker. The predominant cells are alveolar macrophages, lymphocytes are seen only occasionally. *B,* Normal BAL cytology in a smoker. The alveolar macrophages are polymorphic, variable in size and display characteristic cytoplasmic smoker's inclusions.

times, a normal lavage may be useful to make certain disorders highly unlikely (eg, extrinsic allergic alveolitis, eosinophilic pneumonia, alveolar hemorrhage) and to focus attention in another direction.

Diagnostic Findings

There are a few lung diseases where BAL has a high diagnostic value. These diseases show a number of findings that are highly specific and present in almost every patient with such a disorder, such that if present, such findings obviate the need of a biopsy (Table 5–2). It is of interest to note that many of these disorders are included in the group of alveolar filling syndromes. Obviously, the abnormal material that accumulates in the alveolar spaces in these syndromes can easily be washed out by lavage and is so characteristic that a specific BAL diagnosis is possible.

Pulmonary Alveolar Proteinosis

In this disease, the gross appearance of the BAL fluid is milky and turbid (Figure 5–2A). This is so characteristic that the diagnosis can be suspected in the bronchoscopy room. Light microscopy reveals (1) characteristic acellular oval bodies composed of surfactant-derived lipoproteins that are basophilic on MGG staining and positive with PAS staining, (2) a few foamy macrophages, and (3) a dirty background due to large amounts of amorphous debris, which represents myelin-like multilamellated structures and lamellar bodies (Figure 5–2B).[39,64] Electron microscopy for confirmation is not necessary in the routine clinical setting. As a nonspecific reaction, an increase in lymphocytes with the tendency toward an elevated CD4/CD8 ratio can be seen in this disorder.[65]

Diffuse Alveolar Hemorrhage

Diagnosis by BAL is possible in all patients, even if the bleeding is occult, by the demonstration of numerous hemosiderin-laden macrophages and, in patients with fresh bleeding episodes, free red blood cells in the fluid and fragments of red blood cells in the cytoplasm of macrophages.[66–70] Because many syndromes are part of this group of disorders, other clinical and laboratory findings must establish the cause of the bleeding (see Chapter 23 "Diffuse Alveolar Hemorrhage").

On gross examination, the BAL fluid has a bloody or pink to orange-brown color, depending on the age and intensity of the bleeding, caused by red blood cells and hemosiderin-laden macrophages in the fluid. The recovered fluid stains more intensely from fraction to fraction (Figure 5–3). This is characteristic of alveolar hemorrhage and is not seen when the blood is aspirated from the central airways (then the first fraction is the most bloody one).

In severe hemorrhage, the iron stain shows that more than 90% of the macrophages are iron positive, (ie, hemosiderin-laden) (see Figure 5–3). The severity of the bleeding can be quantified using the Golde score (Table 5–3). The maximum score is 400 and a normal score is below 20. Scores between 20 and 100 indicate mild, between 100 and 300 moderate, and between 300 and 400 severe bleeding.[66] Hemosiderin-laden macrophages do not appear earlier than 48 hours after bleeding.[71] Thus, very early bleeding only shows numerous red blood cells. After a single episode of acute alveolar hemorrhage, the following chronologic changes can be observed:

1. Within the first hours, the only evidence is a high number of red blood cells; the macrophages still appear normal.
2. Within 48 hours, the macrophages show roundish, yellow-brown fragments of phagocytosed red blood cells.
3. Not earlier than 48 to 70 hours, hemosiderin becomes apparent in the macrophages which stain intensely blue with iron staining.

Endogenous bleeding has to be differentiated from exogenous iron load of the lungs, which may be caused

---

TABLE 5–2   Diagnostic Bronchoalveolar Lavage Findings

Finding	*Diagnosis*
Pneumocystis carinii, fungi, CMV-transformed cells	Opportunistic infections
Milky effluent, PAS-positive noncellular corpuscles, amorphous debris, foamy macrophages	Alveolar proteinosis
Hemosiderin-laden macrophages, intracytoplasmic fragments of red blood cells in macrophages, free red blood cells	Alveolar hemorrhage syndrome
Malignant cells of solid tumors, lymphoma, leukemia	Malignant infiltrates
Dust particles in macrophages, quantifiable asbestos bodies	Dust exposure
Eosinophils greater than 25%	Eosinophilic lung disease
Positive lymphocyte transformation test to beryllium	Chronic beryllium disease
CD1-positive Langerhans' cells increased	Langerhans cell histiocytosis
Atypical hyperplastic type II pneumocytes	Diffuse alveolar damage, drug toxicity

CMV = cytomegalovirus; PAS = periodic acid–Schiff.

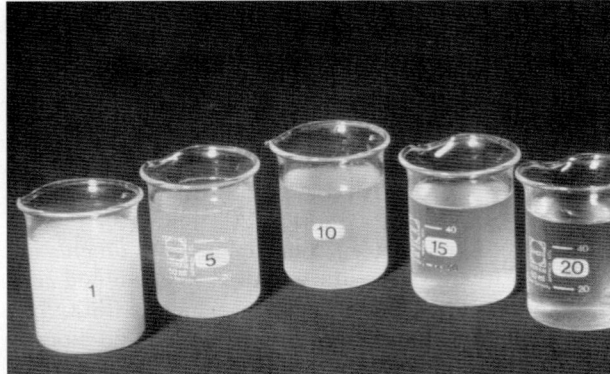

A

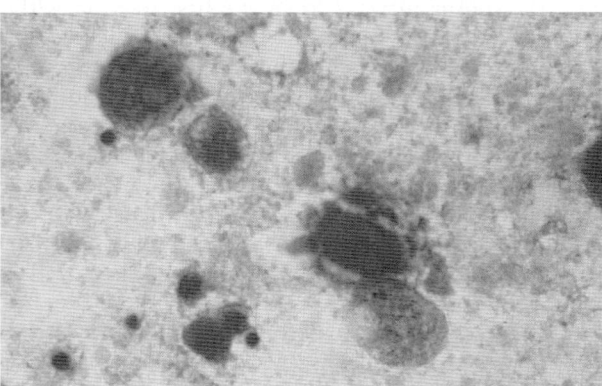

B

Figure 5–2 BAL in alveolar proteinosis (adapted from ref. 39). *A,* Gross appearance of recovered fluid before (*left*) and after (*right*) therapeutic whole lung lavage with 20 L. *B,* Light microscopic aspect on PAS stain (×400).

by inhalation of iron-rich dust particles in certain occupations, such as in metal grinders and welders. Exogenous siderosis does not show roundish fragments of erythrocytes but, instead, irregularly shaped dust particles engulfed by macrophages.[39]

Malignant Diseases

For the diagnosis of primary, solid bronchogenic carcinoma, BAL is not the method of choice as bronchoscopic biopsy techniques and brush cytology are superior to BAL. In primary lung cancer, the diagnostic yield of BAL ranges from 14 to 69% depending on the histologic type of cancer, the size and location of the lesion, and the experience of the investigators.[3]

Diffuse malignant infiltrates can be reliably diagnosed in 60 to 90% of cases.[72–77] The highest yield is seen in widespread malignancies, such as primary bronchoalveolar carcinoma or lymphangitic carcinomatosis due to adenocarcinoma (Figure 5–4). The presence of clusters of type II pneumocytes in the BAL fluid can be misinterpreted as tumor cells (Figure 5–5). In this

regard, even experienced investigators may have difficulties in distinguishing hyperplastic type II cells, appearing mainly in diffuse alveolar damage, from tumor cells.[78] Even tumor markers like carcinoembryonic antigen (CEA) are not helpful because they also react with type II pneumocytes.[78,79]

BAL can also provide diagnostic cytologic material in hematologic malignancies of the lung including

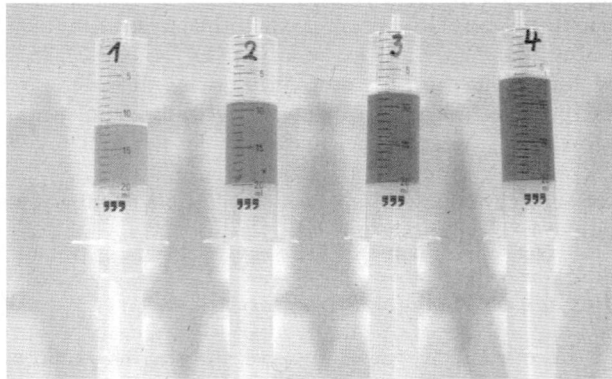

A

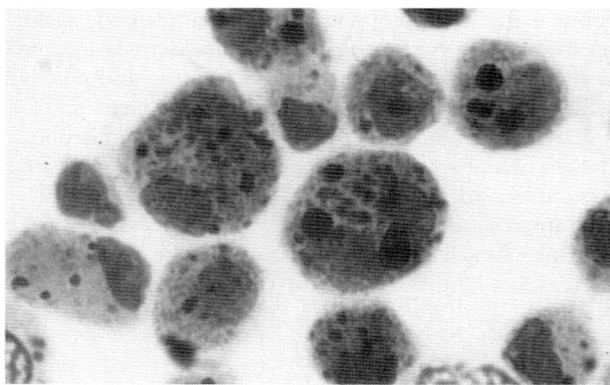

B

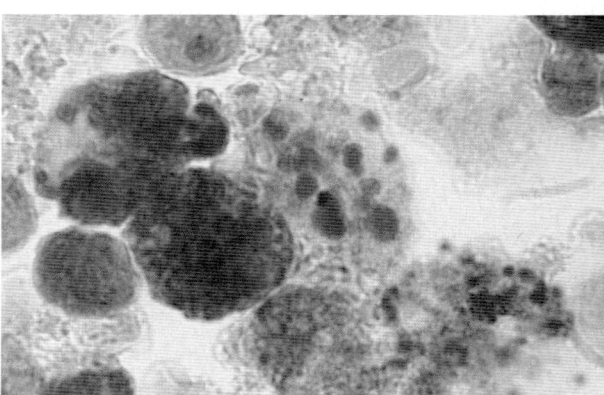

C

Figure 5–3 BAL in alveolar hemorrhage. *A,* Recovered fluid becomes more intensely orange-stained from fraction to fraction. *B,* Roundish fragments of red blood cells in the cytoplasm of macrophages. MGG ×1000. *C,* Iron staining shows most macrophages to be iron-positive, with blue staining of cytoplasm. Iron ×1000.

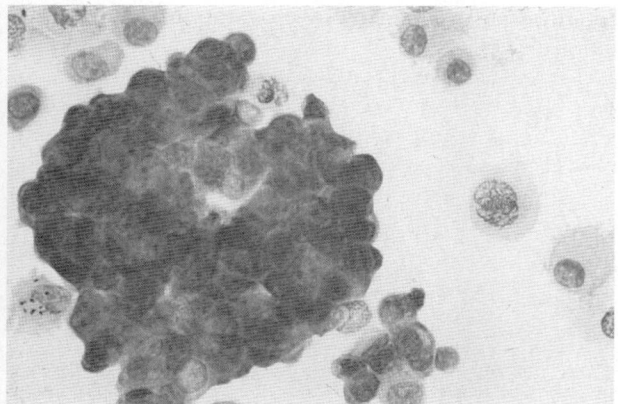

Figure 5–4 Tumor cells of adenocarcinoma in BAL. MGG ×400.

TABLE 5–3   Golde Score for the Quantification of Alveolar Hemorrhage

Hemosiderin Scale*	Blue Staining of Macrophage Cytoplasm
0	No blue color
1	Faint staining
2	Dense in minor portion or medium throughout cytoplasm
3	Deep blue in most parts of cytoplasm
4	Dark blue throughout cytoplasm

*200 to 300 macrophages are counted, and each cell is graded on the above scale. The mean score for 100 cells is calculated, with 400 being the maximum (if all cells are graded with 4).[66]

Hodgkin's disease, non-Hodgkin's lymphoma, leukemia, Waldenström's macroglobulinemia, myeloma, and mycosis fungoides.[76,77,80,81] In malignant B-cell lymphoma, the immunocytologic demonstration of a monoclonal B-cell population, expressing only one immunoglobulin type and either kappa or lambda light chains, can confirm the diagnosis of malignancy.[76]

Pneumoconioses

In diffuse lung disease due to exposure to mineral dust, BAL can confirm exposure by the detection of dust particles in alveolar macrophages. This is particularly useful in patients who may not be aware of being at increased risk of dust inhalation and in those with known exposure with new radiographic changes where other causes of ILD arise in the differential diagnosis. There is some relationship between the amount of mineral dust recovered (if quantified by specific techniques) and the severity of exposure, but considerable overlap occurs among exposed workers without disease and those with clinical disease. The diagnosis of pneumoconiosis cannot be made by BAL alone but requires compatible radiographic changes and/or functional impairment.

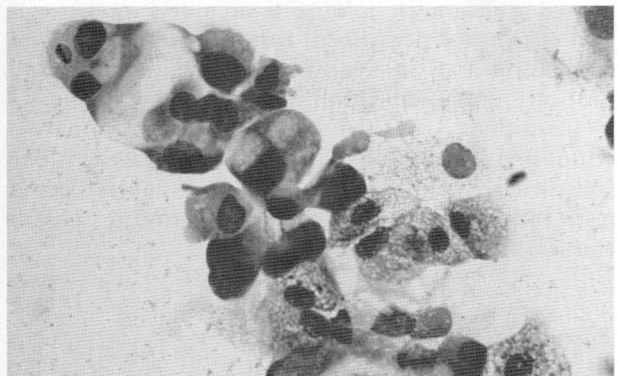

Figure 5–5 Hyperplastic activated type II pneumocytes and foamy macrophages in BAL. MGG ×400 (adapted from ref. 39).

Asbestos-Related Disease.   Asbestos bodies can be detected in smears or cytocentrifuged preparations of BAL fluid (Figure 5–6A). More sensitive, however, is the quantification of asbestos bodies by a specific Millipore filtration technique (Figure 5–6B).[9,27,82–87] The results are given as number of asbestos bodies per mL of BAL fluid which have a relatively good correlation with the asbestos body count in lung tissue analysis.[27,85–87] An asbestos body count of greater than 1.0 asbestos bodies per mL of BAL fluid corresponds to more than 100 asbestos bodies per cm³ of lung tissue, thus indicating an asbestos burden high enough to produce pulmonary asbestosis.[85,86] On the other hand, it is important to know that 10 to 15% of subjects with known occupational asbestos exposure may have no detectable asbestos bodies in their BAL fluid.[86,88] Thus, a negative BAL asbestos body count does not exclude asbestos-related disease.

It is important to differentiate between true and pseudoasbestos bodies, both in conventional BAL studies and in filtration preparations. Ferruginous bodies represent over 98% true asbestos bodies when they appear as a thin, regularly segmented rod with a fine central fiber almost invisible in the light microscope.[89] Pseudoasbestos bodies are formed around fibers that are thicker or irregularly shaped, including talc, glass fibers, and coal dust particles but not asbestos fibers (Figure 5–6C). In this regard, electron microscopic study with x-ray spectral analysis to identify true asbestos fibers is not necessary for routine purposes. Patients with asbestos-related diseases may show a moderate increase in BAL lymphocytes and/or neutrophils, occasionally with an elevated CD4/CD8 ratio. The clinical and prognostic value of this alveolitis is uncertain at present.[90–92]

Silicosis and Mixed Dust Pneumoconiosis.   In coal miners, characteristic large polygonal dark-brown carbon particles can easily be identified in alveolar macrophages (Figure 5–6D). The morphology of particles included in the cytoplasm of alveolar macrophages may vary according to the inhaled dust, such as crystalline silica, hard metals, aluminum, iron-rich particles, and alloys used in dentistry. Energy dispersive x-ray microanalysis allows the identification of the chemical

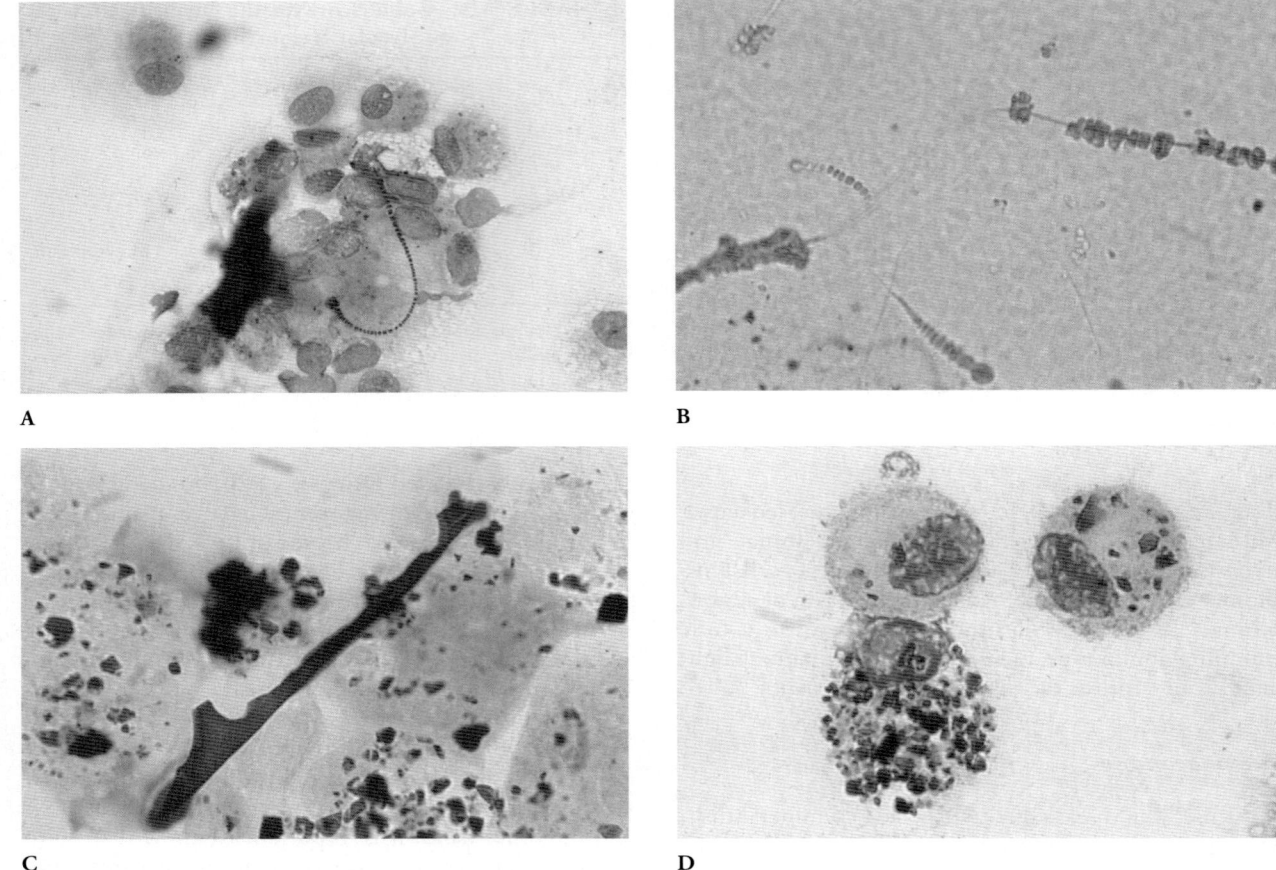

A

B

C

D

Figure 5–6   BAL in pneumoconiosis (adapted from ref. 39). *A*, Asbestos exposure. A curved asbestos body showing the characteristic segmentation around the invisible central fiber. *B*, Asbestos exposure. Several asbestos bodies on a millipore filter. ×1000. *C*, Pseudoasbestos body. Coal dust fiber with irregular edge. Iron ×1000. *D*, Coal dust exposure. Many coal dust particles in the cytoplasm of macrophages. MGG ×1000.

composition of mineral particles and may be useful to determine the type of exposure. Even a large amount of quartz in a BAL specimen does not necessarily indicate that a patient has silicosis—there is no difference in the amount of quartz between subjects with silicosis and those with exposure but no disease.[93] Patients with silicosis may show a mixed lymphocytic/granulocytic alveolitis in BAL differentials, but, in contrast to those exposed to asbestos, the CD4/CD8 ratio is generally reduced. Again, the diagnostic or prognostic value of this finding is uncertain.[91,94–97]

Hard Metal Lung Disease.   A characteristic but, unfortunately, nonspecific finding, is the presence of multinucleate giant cells in BAL; the proportion may range from 3 to 15% of total cells.[91,98] This feature is consistent with the histology of giant cell interstitial pneumonia, the characteristic histopathology of hard metal ILD. In this condition, radiochemical neutron activation analysis can confirm the diagnosis by demonstrating increased levels of the relevant trace metals in BAL fluid, such as cobalt, wolfram, titanium, tantalum, nickel, chromium, niobium, vanadium, and others.[99]

The associated alveolitis usually is mixed lymphocytic/granulocytic with a decreased CD4/CD8 ratio.

Chronic Beryllium Disease.   This condition is clinically, radiologically, and histologically indistinguishable from sarcoidosis. BAL findings are also similar, characterized by an increase in lymphocytes bearing the CD4+ phenotype. Because the antigen is known, a diagnostic in vitro lymphocyte transformation test can be performed. Lymphocytes from blood or BAL fluid are incubated with beryllium salts, and the beryllium-specific proliferation of the lymphocytes is quantified. A positive lymphocyte transformation test of BAL T cells to beryllium salts is highly sensitive and specific (definitely more sensitive than the blood test) and always recommended in doubtful cases to confirm the diagnosis.[100,101]

Eosinophilic Lung Disease

Eosinophilic infiltrates usually show more than 25% eosinophils in cell differentials if the lavage is performed

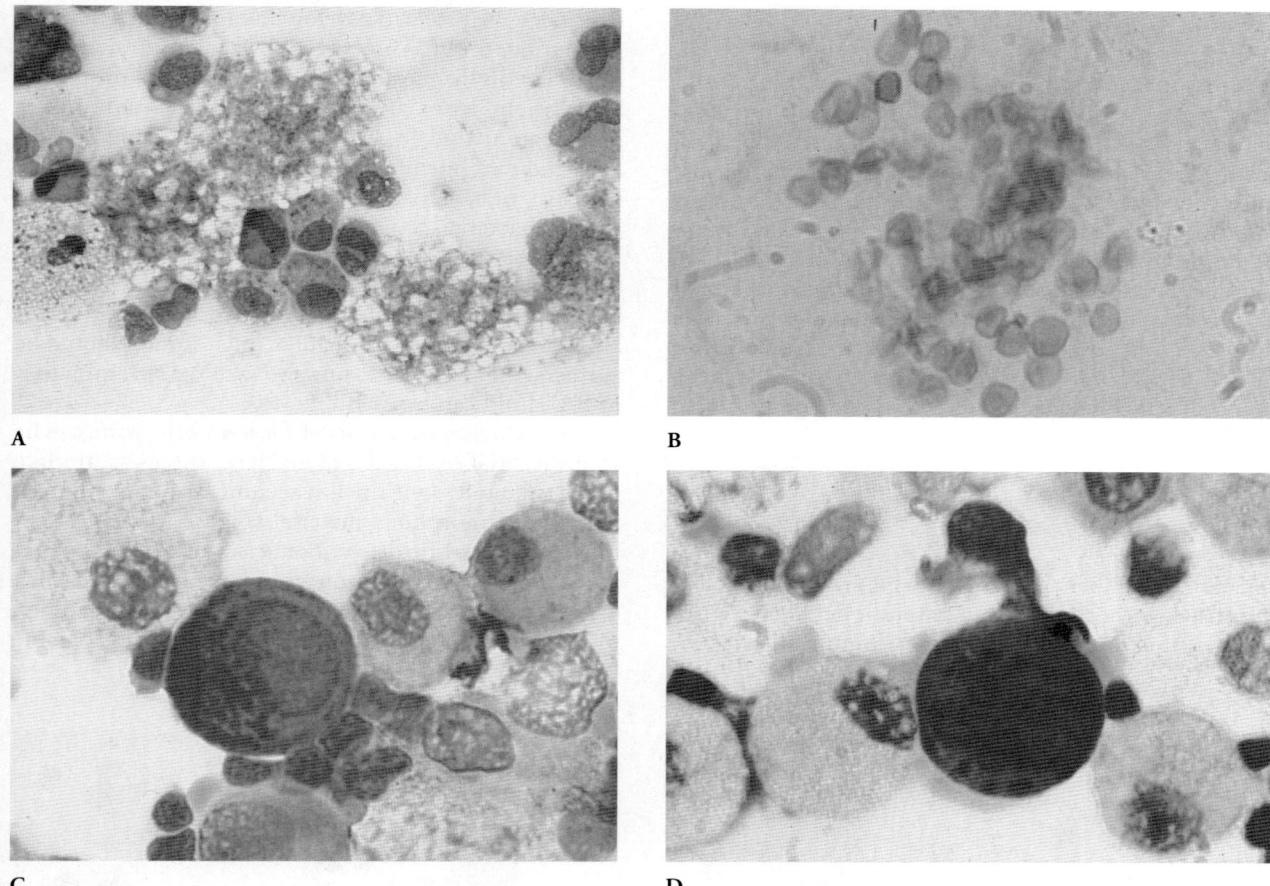

A

B

C

D

Figure 5–7   BAL in opportunistic infections (adapeted from ref. 39). *A, Pneumocystis carinii* pneumonia. Several groups of organisms appearing as foamy vacuoles within slightly basophilic material. MGG ×400. *B, Pneumocystis carinii* stained with modified toluidine blue. The typical spherical cysts are visible. Modified toluidine blue ×1000. *C,* CMV infection. Characteristic CMV transformed cell (owl eye cell) showing the perinuclear halo and cytoplasmic inclusions. MGG ×1000. *D,* CMV infection. Another CMV transformed cell with more prominent inclusions, stretching also over the area of the nucleus. MGG ×1000.

in the involved segment.[102] In eosinophilic pneumonia, either acute or chronic, the eosinophil count may range from 20 to 90% (in our laboratory mean ± SD is 46 ± 22%) and is always higher than the neutrophil count (in contrast with Wegener's granulomatosis).[103–105] In addition, a mild to moderate increase in lymphocytes with a low CD4/CD8 ratio, and a few plasma cells may be present.[3,103,105] The findings in Churg-Strauss syndrome are very similar. However; such high eosinophil counts are rarely seen in allergic bronchopulmonary aspergillosis, IPF, bronchiolitis obliterans organizing pneumonia (BOOP), histiocytosis X, Wegener's granulomatosis, and bronchial asthma. When correctly performed, a normal BAL finding generally excludes eosinopilic pneumonia and the Churg-Strauss syndrome. Eosinophilic lung disease is a group of disorders in which BAL, in the context of consistent clinical symptoms and signs (see Chapter 24 "Eosinophilic Pneumonias"), can give sufficient clues to the diagnosis to avoid surgical lung biopsy in many cases.

Langerhans Cell Histiocytosis

Because the disease is strongly associated with cigarette smoking, the BAL differential shows the typical smoker constellation, with increased total cell counts and macrophages with smokers' inclusions. Additionally, a mild increase in neutrophils and eosinophils may be seen. The specific finding is an increase in Langerhans' cells to more than 3% of the total BAL cell count.[105–107] Although this finding is very specific, the sensitivity is low (only about 50% in our institution) because in late cases of disease the number of Langerhans' cells decreases in the tissue, and only early cases show the characteristic elevations. The Langerhans' cells can be most easily identified in BAL by their staining with the monoclonal antibody CD1a.[105–107] The intracytoplasmic reaction with the polyclonal antibody S100 is not so specific. Electron microscopic demonstration of the specific inclusion bodies (x-bodies or Birbeck granules) is not needed for routine diagnosis, and the method is very time consuming.

Chronic Aspiration

Gastroesophageal reflux with aspiration is often considered in the differential diagnosis of recurrent pneumonia or atypical diffuse pulmonary infiltrates. The BAL cell differential shows a mixed pattern, with an increase in lymphocytes, neutrophils and eosinophils. The characteristic diagnostic finding is the presence of large numbers of lipid-laden macrophages.[108–110] On MGG stain, the macrophages show marked vacuolization of their cytoplasm. The proof that these vacuoles are lipid droplets is obtained by a positive fat stain (Sudan III or oil red O). Demonstration of these lipid-laden macrophages is highly suggestive of lipoid pneumonia caused by chronic aspiration.

Opportunistic Infections

Increasing numbers of patients who are immunocompromised, either by human immunodeficiency virus (HIV) infection or by receiving immunosuppressive treatment, are prone to develop pulmonary infections. In this setting, BAL has probably achieved the greatest practical value in diagnosing such infections and differentiating them from alveolar hemorrhage, pulmonary involvement due to the underlying malignancy, and drug-induced pneumonitis. The sensivity of BAL in the diagnosis of bacterial infections ranges from 60 to 90%; in mycobacterial, fungal, and most viral infections from 70 to 80%; and in *Pneumocystis carinii* pneumonia from 90 to 95% or higher.[3,111,112] A detailed description of the bacteriologic or virologic laboratory techniques is beyond the scope of this chapter. Such studies should be performed in every case, but also cytologic examination of BAL fluid can be useful.

The characteristic cysts of *Pneumocystis carinii* can be seen on MGG-stained slides. Here, the cysts are like foamy vacuoles within an accumulation of slightly basophilic amorphous material (Figure 5–7A). Sometimes, characteristic deoxyribonucleic acid (DNA) material of up to eight trophozoites can be recognized as small dark-blue dots within the cysts. Staining with modified toluidine blue (our preferred method) or silver methamine

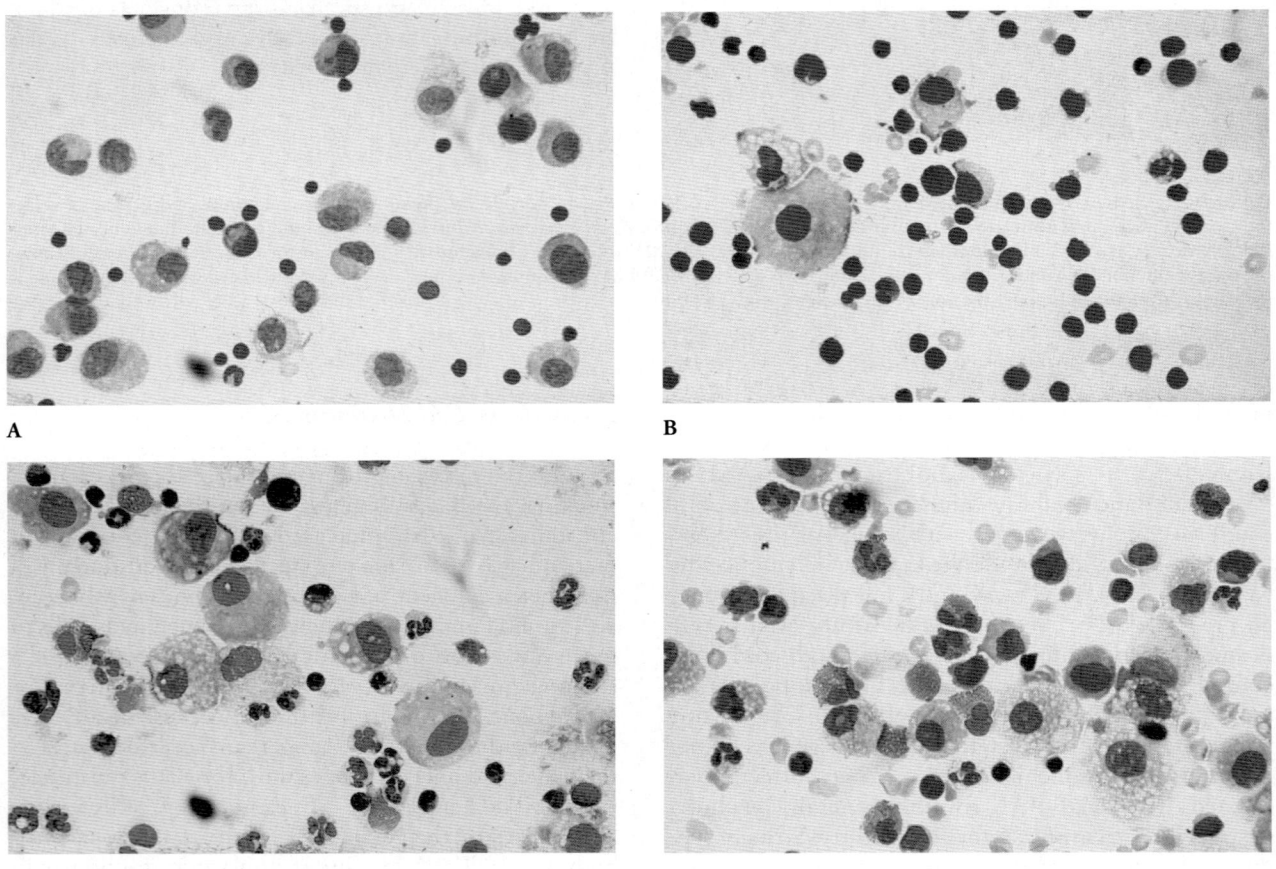

A

B

C

D

Figure 5–8   Representative BAL cellular patterns of interstitial lung disease. MGG ×400. *A,* Lymphocytic alveolitis of sarcoidosis. Monomorphous appearance of macrophages. *B,* Lymphocytic alveolitis of hypersensitive pneumonitis. Striking predominance of lymphocytes, many of them being activated. Foamy macrophages and heterogeneous size of macrophages. *C,* Neutrophilic alveolitis of IPF. *D,* Eosinophilic alveolitis of chronic eosinophilic pneumonia.

visualizes the cyst wall.[113] The typical spherical cysts are dark colored and a characteristic line crosses the surface. The cyst size is 4 to 6 µm, approximately the size of an erythrocyte (Figure 5–7B).

In cytomegalovirus pneumonia, the characteristic cytomegalic-transformed cell (the owl eye cell) with typical nuclear or cytoplasmic inclusions can be seen on light microscopy in 30 to 50% of cases. Thus, this finding is not very sensitive, but highly specific (Figure 5–7C, D).[114]

BRONCHOALVEOLAR LAVAGE AS AN ADJUNCT TO DIAGNOSIS

In a number of the more common ILDs, BAL findings are not specific but can be used as an adjunct to diagnosis together with a thorough clinical investigation. There are many diseases with a lymphocytic, neutrophilic, eosino-

TABLE 5–4 Bronchoalveolar Lavage Cellular Patterns as an Adjunct to Diagnosis

Lymphocytic
  Hypersensitivity pneumonitis
  Berylliosis
  Sarcoidosis
  Tuberculosis
  Connective tissue disorders
  Drug-induced pneumonitis
  Malignant infiltrates
  Silicosis
  Early asbestosis
  Crohn's disease
  Primary biliary cirrhosis
  Human immunodeficiency virus infection
  Viral pneumonia
Neutrophilic (+/– eosinophilic)
  Idiopathic pulmonary fibrosis
  Desquamative interstitial pneumonia (DIP)
  Acute interstitial pneumonia (AIP)
  Acute respiratory distress syndrome
  Bacterial pneumonia
  Connective tissue disorders
  Asbestosis
  Wegener's granulomatosis
  Diffuse panbronchiolitis
  Transplant bronchiolitis obliterans
  Idiopathic bronchiolitis obliterans
  Drug-induced reaction
Eosinophilic
  Eosinophilic pneumonia
  Churg-Strauss syndrome
  Hypereosinophilic syndrome
  Allergic bronchopulmonary aspergillosis
  Idiopathic pulmonary fibrosis
  Drug-induced reaction
Mixed cellularity
  Bronchiolitis obliterans organizing pneumonia
  Connective tissue disorders
  Nonspecific interstitial pneumonia (NSIP)
  Drug-induced reaction
  Inorganic dust disease

Adapted from Costabel U.[39]

philic, or mixed cellular pattern (Table 5–8, Figure 5–8). In these settings, BAL may be helpful to narrow the differential diagnosis. In general, the pattern of inflammatory cell populations in cell differentials will differentiate the fibrosing lung conditions (characterized by neutrophils and/or eosinophils) from the granulomatous or drug-induced lung diseases (characterized by an excess of lymphocytes with or without granulocytes).[115] The CD4/CD8 ratio in BAL may also be helpful. Low ratios are commonly observed in the more acute stages of hypersensitivity pneumonitis, certain drug-induced lung diseases, silicosis, HIV infection, and also BOOP. The CD4/CD8 ratio is usually not elevated in tuberculosis or Hodgkin's disease, which are important differential diagnoses of hilar or mediastinal lymphadenopathy.[116] A CD4/CD8 ratio of more than 3.5 supports the diagnosis of sarcoidosis in the right clinical setting (see "Sarcoidosis" below).

In these conditions, BAL analysis may be the key to diagnosis, together with a careful clinical/radiologic evaluation, making a lung biopsy unnecessary in many cases. However, if despite this thorough investigation the diagnosis remains unclear, a biopsy should be considered as the final diagnostic step. The definite place of the various tests (ie, a clinical assessment, HRCT, BAL, transbronchial biopsy, and surgical lung biopsy) as diagnostic procedures, also in regard to cost effectiveness, has not been studied prospectively.

Sarcoidosis

In sarcoidosis, BAL reveals a lymphocytic alveolitis in 90% of patients at the time of diagnosis (Figure 5–8A). This is a finding common to all stages of sarcoidosis.[3,6,117,118] Patients with clinically active disease tend to have higher lymphocyte counts than those with inactive disease (mean values 50% vs 30%), but the range is wide and the overlap is significant.[118] In late or advanced sarcoidosis, neutrophils also may be increased, as well as the number of mast cells.[119] In patients with primary extrathoracic sarcoidosis (eg, uveitis), BAL may demonstrate pulmonary involvement even when the imaging findings are normal.[120]

The value of the CD4/CD8 ratio has been debated recently because of the high variability of this ratio in sarcoidosis.[121] In fact, only about 55% show the characteristic elevated CD4/CD8 ratio and 15% of patients may even show a decrease in this ratio below 1.0 at the time of diagnosis. Nevertheless, three independent research groups found almost identical values for the sensitivity and specificity of an elevated ratio for diagnosing sarcoidosis.[122–124] Although the sensitivity was rather low, reaching only 55%, the specificity was high at 95%. The specificity of the CD4/CD8 ratio was even higher than the specificity of transbronchial biopsy in one of these studies.[123] An elevated CD4/CD8 ratio would obviate the need for a biopsy in the appropriate clinical setting, but this occurs in only approximately 50% of patients with sarcoidosis because of the low sensitivity. The CD4/CD8 ratio is particularly high in Löfgren's syndrome and in other patients with an acute stage of disease.[125] In inactive disease, the CD4/CD8 ratio is usually in the normal range.

A recent study indicated that increased numbers of neutrophils in BAL fluid can reliably distinguish patients with sarcoidosis who will experience remission from those who will deteriorate, but this needs to be confirmed by other groups.[126]

Hypersensitivity Pneumonitis

This disease shows, by far, the most striking BAL fluid lymphocytosis of all the interstitial diseases (Figure 5–8B, Table 5–5), usually with a relative predominance of CD8+ T cells resulting in a low CD4/CD8 ratio.[3,127] The CD4+ T cells are also significantly elevated in absolute numbers. In fact, the total cell yield is very high, usually above 20 million from a BAL of 100 mL total instillation. The lymphocyte count is usually greater than 50% of total cells, the reported mean values from the literature range between 50 and 70%.[128–136] In addition, neutrophils, eosinophils, and mast cells may be mildly elevated.[134,136,137] A more specific finding is the increase in plasma cells.[138,139] This cell type was found in a low percentage in 18 of 30 patients with bird keeper's disease; values ranged from 0.1 to 3.9% in this study.[139] Other morphologic features include signs of T-cell activation (folded nuclei, broad cytoplasm) and foamy macrophages.[103] The number of activated, human leukocyte antigen (HLA)-DR+ T lymphocytes is high.[130] A normal BAL cytology or an isolated increase in neutrophils or eosinophils is very much exclusive of extrinsic allergic alveolitis. On the other hand, BAL cannot differentiate between patients with overt disease and healthy subjects who have been exposed and sensitized.[3,127,137]

In regard to the CD4/CD8 ratio, the different series reported in the literature show no consistent behavior. Most studies show a significant decrease in the CD4/CD8 ratio, with mean values ranging between 0.5 and 1.0.[127,129,131,134,135,140] Two studies found that CD4/CD8 ratios were borderline (1.3 and 1.5, respectively).[141,142] In Japan, a normal ratio of 2.0 has been reported for ventilation hypersensitivy pneumonitis and even an increased mean ratio of 4.4 for farmer's lung.[140] The reasons for this discrepancy in reported CD4/CD8 ratios are unclear. Several explanations are possible and include different disease manifestations (acute vs chronic form), the timing of BAL investigations in relation to the last antigen exposure, and the type of antigen causing the disease. When analyzing major literature reports, CD4/CD8 ratios are higher in the acute[141,142] versus the chronic form,[103,127] are higher very shortly after the last antigen exposure (within 24 hours), and lowest between 7 and 30 days after the last exposure.[134,141] The type of antigen (farmer's antigens, birds, etc) does not seem to play a role. Although mean values of the CD4/CD8 ratio in most studies are low, in an individual patient the ratio may be within the normal range or even increased. Our data show that in 18 of 30 patients with hypersensitivity pneumonitis the ratio was decreased (below 1.0), in 11 of 30 in the normal range (1.0 to 3.5), and in 1 patient, elevated.[143] Similarly, Drent and colleagues showed that in 21 of 45 patients the ratio was below 1.0, in 25 of 45 patients in the above-mentioned normal range, and in 5 of 45 patients increased above 3.5.[141]

Acute episodes of extrinsic allergic alveolitis are associated with an influx of neutrophils into the lungs, lasting for up to 1 week.[144] After this period, the cellular profile of the BAL fluid returns to the significant increase in lymphocytes that was previously seen. In the follow-up, persistent BAL abnormalities indicate that complete avoidance has not been achieved.

TABLE 5–5   Cell Differentials in Bronchoalveolar Lavage

	Total Cells*	Macrophages (%)	Lymphocytes (%)	Neutrophils (%)	Eosinophils (%)	Mast cells (%)	Plasma cells (%)	Foamy macrophages (%)
Control nonsmokers	7 ± 3	92 ± 4	7 ± 3	1 ± 1	0.1 ± 0.3	0.1 ± 0.1	–	–
Control smokers	23 ± 12	96 ± 3	3 ± 2	1 ± 1	0.4 ± 0.6	0.1 ± 0.3	–	–
Sarcoidosis	16 ± 17	55 ± 21	41 ± 21	3 ± 5	1 ± 1	0.4 ± 0.5	–	–
Extrinsic allergic alveolitis	34 ± 22	18 ± 10	78 ± 10	2 ± 2	1 ± 1	0.9 ± 0.9	0.8 ± 0.9	22 ± 17
Idiopathic pulmonary fibrosis (IPF)	14 ± 11	66 ± 23	15 ± 15	14 ± 16	5 ± 5	0.3 ± 0.7	–	14 ± 13
Bronchiolitis obliterans organizing pneumonia (BOOP)	14 ± 9	39 ± 19	44 ± 19	10 ± 13	6 ± 8	1.0 ± 0.4	0.1 ± 0.1	25 ± 10
Chronic eosinophilic pneumonia	18 ± 22	27 ± 18	22 ± 18	6 ± 6	46 ± 22	1.0 ± 0.9	0.7 ± 0.4	6 ± 11

Adapted from Costabel U.[39]
Values are mean ± standard deviation.
*×10⁶/100 mL instillation volume.

Asymptomatic Exposed Individuals

In these individuals, although regularly exposed to antigens on the farm or as pigeon breeders, neither clinical features nor radiologic or functional abnormalities are present. Frequently, however, serum precipitins are positive, and BAL shows signs of a lymphocytic alveolitis.[103,131,135,142,145] This subclinical alveolitis is more frequent in farmers with positive serum precipitins than in precipitin-negative subjects.[145] The mean value of the BAL lymphocyte percentage is usually lower than in symptomatic disease.[103,131,135,142,145] The CD4/CD8 ratio tends to be somewhat higher than in patients with manifest disease.[131,135,142] Follow-up studies showed that the BAL lymphocytosis persisted in these individuals, and that no subject developed manifest farmer's lung disease.[146,147]

Drug-Induced Pneumonitis

Many drugs can induce an interstitial lung reaction, either toxic or immune mediated (see Chapter 20 "Drug Induced Infiltrative Lung Diseases"). In addition to toxic changes of the type II pneumocytes, any type of alveolitis may be present in BAL (lymphocytic, neutrophilic, eosinophilic, or mixed) and also diffuse alveolar hemorrhage (Table 5–6).[3,39,148–150] The most frequent finding is a lymphocytic alveolitis with a predominance of CD8+ cells, just as in extrinsic allergic alveolitis. In methotrexate-induced pneumonitis, the CD4+ cells may be pref-

TABLE 5–6 Bronchoalveolar Lavage Findings in Drug-Induced Interstitial Lung Disease

Lymphocytosis	Eosinophilia
Methotrexate	Bleomycin
Azathioprine	Nitrofurantoin
Cyclophosphamide	Cotrimazole
Bleomycin	Penicillin
Busulfan	Sulfasalazine
Vincristine	Ampicillin
Nitrofurantoin	Tetracycline
Minocycline	Maloprim
Gold	Minocycline
Sulfasalazine	L-Tryptophan
Amiodarone	
Acebutolol	Hemorrhage
Atenolol	D-Penicillamine
Celiprolol	Amphotericin B
Propranolol	Cytotoxic drugs
Flecainide	
Diphenylhydantoin	Cytotoxic reaction
Nilutamide	Bleomycin
	Methotrexate
Neutrophilia	Nitrosoureas
Bleomycin	Busulfan
Busulfan	Cyclophosphamide
Minocycline	
Amiodarone	

Adapted from Costabel U.[39]

erentially increased[151,152]; however, another study reported the opposite results.[153] Amiodarone causes characteristic changes in the alveolar macrophage population, which show foamy intracytoplasmic alterations corresponding to a form of phospolipidosis.[149] This feature is also seen in patients treated with amiodarone but who are free of clinical lung involvement. If foamy macrophages are not present in BAL, an amiodarone-induced pneumonitis can likely be excluded.

BAL findings are not, however, specific for any drug-induced lung disease, and the definitive diagnosis needs additional clinical investigations. BAL is useful, however, to exclude other pulmonary problems that are commonly associated with chemotherapeutic agents.

Idiopathic Pulmonary Fibrosis

In IPF, the characteristic BAL pattern is an increase in neutrophils, usually to a moderate degree (10 to 30% of total cells), with or without an additional increase in eosinophils (Figure 5–8C).[128,154–156] Usually, the neutrophils are twice as high as the eosinophils. Such an increase in neutrophils is noted in 70 to 90% of patients, an associated increase in eosinophils in 40 to 60% of patients, and an additional increase in lymphocytes in 10 to 20% of patients.[3] However, these findings are seen in a wide variety of fibrosing lung conditions other than IPF.[39] An isolated and marked increase in lymphocytes is uncommon in IPF (< 10% of patients), so when present, other disorders should be excluded (eg, granulomatous disease, sarcoidosis, extrinsic allergic alveolitis, BOOP, nonspecific interstitial pneumonia [NSIP]).

As our understanding of the idiopathic ILD changed with the new histologic classification of idiopathic interstitial pneumonia, we now recognize the important difference between the usual interstitial pneumonia (UIP) seen with IPF and the changes of NSIP, which is associated with a better prognosis.[157,158] The improved prognosis for a lymphocytic lavage in IPF may be an indication that cases with NSIP have been included in the older series.

The limited data available on BAL cell differentials in NSIP show that this entity is characterized by a predominant lymphocytosis in BAL in addition to a mild increase in neutrophils and eosinophils.[158–160] This is probably only true for the cellular type of NSIP but not for the fibrotic type that was studied in the series reported by Daniil and colleagues,[161] which demonstrated no difference in the lymphocyte counts between NSIP and UIP (Table 5–7). The BAL pattern in cellular NSIP seems similar to BOOP and contrasts with the predominant neutrophil and eosinophil increase in UIP or the excessive increase of neutrophils in acute interstitial pneumonia (AIP), thus allowing a certain discrimination between favorable prognostic entities (eg, BOOP and NSIP) and the more unfavorable diagnoses (eg, UIP or AIP).

TABLE 5–7   Bronchoalveolar Lavage Findings in NSIP versus UIP

	Lymphocytes (%)		Neutrophils (%)	
Author	NSIP	UIP	NSIP	UIP
Nagai et al[158]	37	7	8	6
Daniil et al[161]	9	8	8	10
Park et al[159]	46	8	23	13
Suga et al[160]	21	6	7	7
Own data	34	19	12	9

Adapted from Costabel U and Guzman J.[8]
Data are mean values given as % of total cells.
NSIP = nonspecific interstitial pneumonia; UIP = usual interstitial pneumonia.

Bronchiolitis Obliterans Organizing Pneumonia

In this disorder, the BAL profile is characterized by a mixed pattern, usually with a predominance of lymphocytes and a more moderate increase in neutrophils, eosinophils, and mast cells as well as the presence of foamy macrophages and, occasionally, plasma cells. Other BAL findings include a decrease in the CD4/CD8 ratio and an increase in activated HLA-DR+ T lymphocytes.[103,162]

BAL may be of value in distinguishing between BOOP and other ILDs.[103] In comparison with IPF, patients with BOOP have higher lymphocyte proportions. A lone increase in neutrophils and/or eosinophils, which is characteristic of IPF, was not seen in any of our patients with BOOP. In chronic eosinophilic pneumonia, BAL eosinophils usually exceed 25% and are below this threshold in BOOP. In a patient with typical signs and symptoms and patchy peripheral infiltrates, after infection and malignancy have been excluded by lavage, a BAL cell profile with more than 20% lymphocytes, between 2 and 25% eosinophils, and a CD4/CD8 ratio less than 1.0, is highly suggestive of idiopathic BOOP and may warrant a therapeutic trial of corticosteroid therapy.

Collagen Vascular Disease

In collagen vascular diseases (CVD), pulmonary involvement can be associated with various histopathologic patterns. The pathology may be similar to IPF, but many of the cases of CVD-associated pulmonary fibrosis show a pattern that is in the category of NSIP, based on CT scan or histology.[163,164] The BAL findings are also somewhat different from IPF. The general pattern is increased neutrophils, with or without eosinophils, but increased lymphocytes are more commonly seen than in IPF.[3,164,165] In general, BAL seems to have a limited value in the diagnosis of CVDs affecting the lungs because the BAL profile is very nonspecific. BAL may be useful, however, to detect other pulmonary problems that may arise in these disorders, including drug-induced toxicity, infection, pulmonary hemorrhage associated with vasculitis, and malignancy.[166]

An abnormal BAL may be the first evidence of pulmonary involvement in CVD. If radiographic signs are absent and pulmonary function tests are normal, this abnormal finding indicates a subclinical alveolitis. It is still not clear whether such a subclinical alveolitis needs treatment. It is also not clear whether the pattern of BAL cells (increase in neutrophils or lymphocytes) in a setting of subclinical alveolitis reflects the prognosis. In manifest ILD, however, increased lymphocytes are rather associated with a better prognosis, whereas increased neutrophils/eosinophils may be indicative of progressive disease.[165]

BRONCHOALVEOLAR LAVAGE IN THE DIFFERENTIAL DIAGNOSIS OF DIFFUSE PARENCHYMAL LUNG DISEASE

As outlined above, there are several rare disorders with specific BAL findings and sufficiently high sensitivity such that a biopsy is usually not necessary, including alveolar proteinosis, *Pneumocystis carinii* pneumonia, alveolar hemorrhage, and other conditions.

In many diffuse lung diseases, the cellular BAL profile is abnormal, with either a lymphocytic, neutrophilic, eosinophilic, or mixed cellularity. Some of these disorders almost always show an abnormal BAL (high sensitivity), although the specificity is low; however, in combination with clinical and HRCT features, the diagnosis may be possible without a biopsy (Table 5–8). In this

TABLE 5–8   Diagnostic Yield of Bronchoalveolar Lavage in Diffuse Parenchymal Lung Disease

BAL without biopsy usually sufficient (high sensitivity and high specificity)
  Alveolar proteinosis
  Pneumocystis carinii pneumonia
  Bronchoalveolar carcinoma
  Alveolar hemorrhage
  Eosinophilic pneumonia

BAL in combination with clinical and HRCT features frequently sufficient (high sensitivity, low specificity)
  IPF (neutrophils ± eosinophils)
  Extrinsic allergic alveolitis (lymphocytes, plasma cells, foamy macrophages)
  RB/ILD (smokers' macrophages)
  BOOP (mixed cellularity, CD4/CD8 ↓)
  Lymphangioleiomyomatosis (alveolar hemorrhage)

BAL typical in only 50% of patients, biopsy often needed (if CT atypical) (moderate sensitivity, high specificity)
  Sarcoidosis (CD4/CD8 ↑)
  Langerhans cell histiocytosis (CD1)

BAL mostly not diagnostic, biopsy required (low sensitivity ± low specificity)
  Hodgkin's disease
  Invasive aspergillosis

BAL = bronchoalveolar lavage; HRCT = high-resolution computed tomography; IPF = idiopathic pulmonary fibrosis; RB/ILD = respiratory bronchiolitis-associated interstitial lung disease; BOOP = bronchiolitis obliterans organizing pneumonia.

regard, if clinical criteria for IPF are met and the CT scan shows the characteristic pattern and distribution of UIP, a lone increase in neutrophils/eosinophils supports the diagnosis of IPF, as stated in the major and minor criteria of the recent ATS/ERS Statement.[63] Also, if the CT scan shows a patchy ground glass-pattern, BAL may be able to reveal that this patient suffers from hypersensitivity pneumonitis (high lymphocyte count), a smoking-related respiratory bronchiolitis/ILD (high smoker's macrophage count and normal cell differential), or possibly from alveolar hemorrhage (high count of hemosiderin-laden macrophages). In a patient with predominantly peripheral consolidation, plus some ground-glass infiltrates on CT scan, BAL may be suggestive of BOOP (mixed cellular pattern with a relatively low eosinophil count), chronic eosinophilic pneumonia (major increase in eosinophils), bronchoalveolar carcinoma (malignant cells of adenocarcinoma), or malignant lymphoma (monoclonal B-cell population).

Finally, if the CT scan reveals a cystic pattern, BAL may point toward either lymphangioleiomyomatosis (alveolar hemorrhage, CD1 count normal, female nonsmoker) or Langerhans cell histiocytosis (CD1 count elevated, smoker).

ASSESSING DISEASE ACTIVITY AND PROGNOSIS

It was initially hoped that BAL cell differentials would be able to provide a measure of disease activity over time. However, the debate is still ongoing as to whether BAL is useful for assessing the activity of disease processes with respect to obtaining prognostic information. It is also not proven if serial BAL has a role in monitoring the course of disease and guiding therapy better than other indices of change. Use of BAL to monitor therapy has not been widely used in pulmonary fibrosis. Some have proposed BAL as a method to help direct therapy with drugs other than corticosteroids. Treatment with cyclophosphamide has been shown to reduce the neutrophil percentage in IPF patients undergoing serial BAL studies.[167] In IPF, a marked increase in neutrophils and/or eosinophils was reported to adversely affect prognosis, whereas elevated lymphocyte counts were found to be more likely associated with a good response to corticosteroid treatment.[154,155,168,169] Today, such patients with increased lymphocyte counts most likely represent patients with an idiopathic NSIP variant of idiopathic interstitial pneumonia and not IPF (UIP) patients. In sarcoidosis, although differences were observed for several BAL parameters between clinically active and inactive patient groups, the range of overlap between groups is large, and none of the investigated findings was able to indicate prognosis reliably enough in a given individual patient.[119,170-172]

For scleroderma-associated pulmonary involvement, a recent study asked the question whether lung inflammation (alveolitis) as assessed by BAL may cause lung fibrosis and whether cyclophosphamide treatment is associated with a better prognosis in scleroderma patients with alveolitis.[173] This was a retrospective cohort study of 103 patients with scleroderma who had BAL or lung biopsy, and most of the patients with alveolitis had a moderate to severe restrictive lung disease and severe impairment in gas transfer. It is important to understand than these were not patients with a subclinical alveolitis. Those patients with alveolitis and cyclophosphamide therapy had a better outcome than those with alveolitis and no cyclophosphamide therapy. The group with no alveolitis did not receive cyclophosphomide treatment and remained stable in regard to pulmonary function tests. Similar data have previously been published by another group.[174]

BAL may be useful during the development of new drugs. Because new drugs such as interferon-γ for IPF or monoclonal antibodies to tumor necrosis factor for sarcoidosis are directed toward the inhibition of abnormal immune responses, BAL is suitable to study the cellular and biologic changes induced by the drugs. In this regard, BAL can be used for "proof-of-concept" studies in the clinical development of new drugs.

Whether repeated lavage measurements give better information to assess the evolution of disease activity and the natural history is not clear for the moment. Larger prospective studies are required to clarify this issue before BAL should be routinely applied for this purpose. At present, serial BAL cannot be routinely recommended.

REFERENCES

1. Reynolds HY. Use of bronchoalveolar lavage in humans—past necessity and future imperative. Lung 2000;178:271–93.
2. Klech H, Pohl W. Technical recommendations and guidelines for bronchoalveolar lavage (BAL). Report of the ERS Task Group. Eur Respir J 1989;2:561–85.
3. Klech H, Hutter C. Clinical guidelines and indications for bronchoalveolar lavage (BAL): report of the European Society of Pneumology Task Force on BAL. Eur Respir J 1990;3:937–74.
4. Reynolds HY, Newball HH. Analysis of proteins and respiratory cells obtained from human lungs by bronchial lavage. J Lab Clin Med 1974;84:559–73.
5. Yeager HC, Williams MC, Beckman JF, et al. Sarcoidosis: analysis of cells obtained by bronchial lavage. Am Rev Respir Dis 1976;113:96–100.
6. Crystal RG, Roberts WG, Hunninghake GW, et al. Pulmonary sarcoidosis: a disease characterized and perpetuated by activated lung T-lymphocytes. Ann Intern Med 1981;94:73–94.
7. American Thoracic Society. Clinical role of bronchoalveolar lavage in adults with pulmonary disease. Am Rev Respir Dis 1990;142:481–6.
8. Costabel U, Guzman J. Bronchoalveolar lavage in interstitial lung disease. Curr Opin Pulm Med 2001;7:255–61.
9. Guzman J, Costabel U. Bronchoalveolar lavage in diagnostic cytology. In: Wied GL, Keebler CM, Koss LG, et al. editors. Compendium on diagnostic cytology. Tutorials of cytology. Chicago (IL): 1992. p. 251–65.
10. Hunninghake GW, Kawanami O, Ferrans VJ, et al. Characterisation of the inflammatory and immune effector cells

in the lung parenchyma of patients with interstitial lung disease. Am Rev Respir Dis 1981;123:407–12.

11. Abe S, Munakata M, Nishimura M, et al. Gallium-67 scintigraphy, bronchoalveolar lavage, and pathologic changes in patients with pulmonary sarcoidosis. Chest 1984;85:650–5.

12. Semenzato G, Chilosi M, Ossi E, et al. Bronchoalveolar lavage and lung histology: comparative analysis of inflammatory and immunocompetent cells in patients with sarcoidosis and hypersensitivity pneumonitis. Am Rev Respir Dis 1985;132:400–4.

13. Campbell DA, Poulter LW, duBois RM. Immunocompetent cells in bronchoalveolar lavage reflect the cell populations in transbronchial biopsies in pulmonary sarcoidosis. Am Rev Respir Dis 1985;132:1300–6.

14. Paradis IL, Dauber JH, Rabin BS. Lymphocyte phenotypes in bronchoalveolar lavage and lung tissue in sarcoidosis and idiopathic pulmonary fibrosis. Am Rev Respir Dis 1986;133:855–60.

15. Olivieri D, D'Ippolito R, Chetta A. Induced sputum: diagnostic value in interstitial lung disease. Curr Opin Pulm Med 2000;6:411–4.

16. Fireman E, Lerman Y. Possible future of induced sputum in interstitial lung disease. Eur Respir J 2000;15:240–2.

17. BAL Cooperative Steering Group. Bronchoalveolar lavage constituents in healthy individuals, idiopathic pulmonary fibrosis, and selected comparison groups. Am Rev Respir Dis 1990;141:S169–202.

18. Haslam PL, Baughman RP. Report of European Respiratory Society (ERS) Task Force: guidelines for measurement of acellular components and recommmendations for standardization of bronchoalveolar lavage (BAL). Eur Respir Rev 1999;9:25–157.

19. Helmers RA, Dayton CS, Floerchinger C, Hunninghake GW. Bronchoalveolar lavage in interstitial lung disease: effect of volume of fluid infused. J Appl Physiol 1989;67:1443–6.

20. Dohn MN, Baughman RP. Effect of changing instilled volume for bronchoalveolar lavage in patients with interstitial lung disease. Am Rev Respir Dis 1985;132:390–2.

21. Davis GS, Giancola MS, Costanza MC, Low RB. Analysis of sequential bronchoalveolar lavage samples from healthy human volunteers. Am Rev Respir Dis 1982;126:611–6.

22. Baser Y, deShazo RD, Barman HW, et al. Lidocaine effects on immunocompetent cells. Implications for studies of cells obtained by bronchoalveolar lavage. Chest 1982;82:323–8.

23. Duddridge M, Kelly CA, Ward C, et al. The reversible effect of lignocaine on the stimulated metabolic activity of bronchoalveolar lavage cells. Eur Respir J 1990;3:1168–72.

24. Pingleton SK, Harrison GF, Stechschulte DJ, et al. Effect of location, pH and temperature of instillate in bronchoalveolar lavage in normal volunteers. Am Rev Respir Dis 1983;128:1035–7.

25. Garcia JGN, Wolven RG, Garcia PL, Keogh BA. Assessment of interlobar variation of bronchoalveolar lavage cellular differentials in interstitial lung diseases. Am Rev Respir Dis 1986;133:444–9.

26. Peterson MW, Nugent KM, Jolles H, et al. Uniformity of bronchoalveolar lavage in patients with sarcoidosis. Am Rev Respir Dis 1988;137:719–84.

27. Teschler H, Konietzko N, Schoenfeld B, et al. Distribution of asbestos bodies in the human lung as determined by bronchoalveolar lavage. Am Rev Respir Dis 1993;147:1211–5.

28. Lam S, Leriche JC, Kijek K, Phillips D. Effect of bronchial lavage volume on cellular and protein recovery. Chest 1985;88:856–9.

29. Costabel U. Technik und Methodik der bronchoalveolären Lavage bei interstitiellen Lungenkrankheiten. Schweiz Med Wochenschr 1986;116:1238–44.

30. Riedler J, Grigg J, Stone C, et al. Bronchoalveolar lavage cellularity in healthy children. Am J Respir Crit Care Med 1995;152:163–8.

31. Grigg J, van den Borre C, Malfroot A, et al. Bilateral fiberoptic bronchoalveolar lavage in acute unilateral lobar pneumonia. J Pediatr 1993;122:606–8.

32. Ratjen F, Bredendiek M, Zheng L, et al. Lymphocyte subsets in bronchoalveolar lavage fluid of children without bronchopulmonary disease. Am J Respir Crit Care Med 1995; 152:174–8.

33. ERS Task Force. Bronchoalveolar lavage in children. Eur Respir J 2000;15:217–31.

34. Barbato A, Panizzolo C, Cracco A, et al. Interstitial lung disease in children: a multicentre survey on diagnostic approach. Eur Respir J 2000;16:509–13.

35. Baughman RP. Bronchoalveolar lavage. 1st ed. St. Louis: Mosby Year Book; 1992.

36. Costabel U. CD4/CD8 ratios in bronchoalveolar lavage fluid: of value for diagnosing sarcoidosis? Eur Respir J 1997;10:2699–700.

37. Strumpf IJ, Feld MK, Cornelius MJ, et al. Safety of fiberoptic bronchoalveolar lavage in evaluation of interstitial lung disease. Chest 1981:80:268–71.

38. Dhillon DP, Haslam PL, Townsend PJ, et al. Bronchoalveolar lavage in patients with interstitial lung diseases: side effects and factors affecting fluid recovery. Eur J Respir Dis 1986; 68:342–50.

39. Costabel U. Atlas of bronchoalveolar lavage. London: Chapman and Hall; 1998.

40. Costabel U, Bross R, Baur R, et al. Differentialzytologie und Lymphozytensubpopulationen der bronchoalveolären Lavage unter verschiedenen Aufbewahrungsbedingungen. Prax Klin Pneumol 1988;42:103–5.

41. Lam S, Leroche JC, Kijek K. Effect of filtration and concentration on the composition of bronchoalveolar lavage fluid. Chest 1985;87:740–2.

42. Saltini C, Hance AJ, Ferrans VJ, et al. Accurate quantification of cells recovered by bronchoalveolar lavage. Am Rev Respir Dis 1984;130:650–8.

43. Thompson AB, Robbins RA, Ghafouri MA, et al. Bronchoalveolar lavage fluid processing. Effect of membrane filtation preparation on neutrophil recovery. Acta Cytol 1989;33:544–9.

44. Thompson AB, Teschler H, Wang YM, et al. Preparation of bronchoalveolar lavage fluid with microscope slide smears. Eur Respir J 1996;9:603–8.

45. Costabel U, Bross KJ, Matthys H. The immunoperoxidase slide assay: a new method for the demonstration of surface antigens on bronchoalveolar lavage cells. Bull Eur Physiopathol Respir 1985;21:381–7.

46. Haslam PL, Baughman RP. Report of ERS Task Force: guidelines for measurement of acellular components and standardization of BAL. Eur Respir J 1999;14:245–8.

47. Haslam PL, Postle TD, Raymondos K, Baker CS. Measurement of pulmonary surfactant components and function in bronchoalveolar lavage fluid. Report of ERS Task Force: guidelines for measurement of acellular components and recommendations for standardization of bronchoalveolar lavage (BAL). Eur Respir Rev 1999;66:43–69.

48. Merrill WW, Out TA. Measurement of immunoglobulins in bronchoalveolar lavage fluid. Report of ERS Task Force: guidelines for measurement of acellular components and recommendations for standardization of bronchoalveolar lavage (BAL). Eur Respir Rev 1999;69:70–5.

49. Braun J, O'Connor C. Measurement of proteases and antiproteases in bronchoalveolar lavage. Report of ERS Task Force: guidelines for measurement of acellular components and recommendations for standardization of bronchoalveolar lavage (BAL). Eur Respir Rev 1999;69:76–85.

50. Juillerat-Jeanneret L, Soubrier F, Aubert JD, Leuenberger P. Measurement of angiotensin converting enzyme in bronchoalveolar lavage fluid. Report of ERS Task Force: guidelines for measurement of acellular components and rec-

ommendations for standardization of bronchoalveolar lavage (BAL). Eur Respir Rev 1999;69:86–92.

51. Kelly FJ, Buhl R, Sandström T. Measurement of antioxidants, oxidants and oxidation products in bronchoalveolar fluid. Report of ERS Task Force: guidelines for measurement of acellular components and recommendations for standardization of bronchoalveolar lavage (BAL). Eur Respir Rev 1999;69:93–8.

52. Chavis C, Arnoux B, Bousquet J. Detection of lipid mediators in bronchoalveolar lavage fluid. Report of ERS Task Force: guidelines for measurement of acellular components and recommendations for standardization of bronchoalveolar lavage (BAL). Eur Respir Rev 1999;69:99–105.

53. Strieter RM, Miller EJ, Kurdowska AK, et al. Measurement of cytokines in bronchoalveolar lavage fluid. Report of ERS Task Force: guidelines for measurement of acellular components and recommendations for standardization of bronchoalveolar lavage (BAL). Eur Respir Rev 1999;69:106–12.

54. Dentener MA, Bouma MG, Drent M, et al. Measurement of soluble adhesion molecules (s-ICAM-I and sE-selectin) in bronchoalveolar lavage fluid. Report of ERS Task Force: guidelines for measurement of acellular components and recommendations for standardization of bronchoalveolar lavage (BAL). Eur Respir Rev 1999;69:113–7.

55. Pohl WR, Kummer F, Bjermer LH. Measurement of markers of fibrosis and extra-cellular matrix components in bronchoalveolar lavage fluid. Report of ERS Task Force: guidelines for measurement of acellular components and recommendations for standardization of bronchoalveolar lavage (BAL). Eur Respir Rev 1999;69:118–25.

56. Bjermer LH, Ahlstedt S, Braun J. Measurement of granulocyte derived markers in bronchoalveolar lavage fluid. Report of ERS Task Force: guidelines for measurement of acellular components and recommendations for standardization of bronchoalveolar lavage (BAL). Eur Respir Rev 1999;69:126–34.

57. Pirozynski M, Spatafora M, Rennard SI. Measurement of tumour markers in bronchoalveolar lavage fluid. Report of ERS Task Force: guidelines for measurement of acellular components and recommendations for standardization of bronchoalveolar lavage (BAL). Eur Respir Rev 1999;69:135–40.

58. Drent M, Cobben NAM, Henderson R, et al. Measurement of markers of cell damage or death in bronchoalveolar lavage fluid. Report of ERS Task Force: guidelines for measurement of acellular components and recommendations for standardization of bronchoalveolar lavage (BAL). Eur Respir Rev 1999;69:141–4.

59. Albera C, Cordeiro CR, Crosa F, Ghlo P. New fields in measurement of acellular components in bronchoalveolar lavage fluid. Report of ERS Task Force: guidelines for measurement of acellular components and recommendations for standardization of bronchoalveolar lavage (BAL). Eur Respir Rev 1999;69:145–57.

60. Maier KL, Leuschel L, Costabel U. Increased oxidized methionine residues in BAL fluid proteins in acute or chronic bronchitis. Eur Respir J 1992;5:651–8.

61. Costabel U, Guzman J. Effect of smoking on bronchoalveolar lavage constituents. Eur Respir J 1992;5:776–9.

62. Hunninghake GW, Costabel U, Ando M, et al. ATS/ERS/WASOG statement on sarcoidosis. Sarc Vasc Diffuse Lung Dis 1999;16:149–73.

63. ATS/ERS Statement. Idiopathic pulmonary fibrosis: diagnosis and treatment. Am J Respir Crit Care Med 2000;161:646–64.

64. Martin RJ, Coalson JJ, Rogers RM, et al. Pulmonary alveolar proteinosis: the diagnosis by segmental lavage. Am Rev Respir Dis 1980;121:819–25.

65. Milleron BJ, Costabel U, Teschler H, et al. Bronchoalveolar lavage cell data in alveolar proteinosis. Am Rev Respir Dis 1991;144:1330–2.

66. Golde D, Drew L, Klein H, et al. Occult pulmonary hemorrhage in leukemia. BMJ 1975;2:166–8.

67. Drew L, Finley T, Golde D. Diagnostic lavage and occult pulmonary hemorrhage in thrombocytopenic immunocompromised patients. Am Rev Respir Dis 1977;116:215–21.

68. Kahn F, Jones J, England D. Diagnosis of pulmonary hemorrhage in the immunocompromised host. Am Rev Respir Dis 1987;136:155–60.

69. Sherman J, Winnie G, Thomassen MJ, et al. Time course of hemosiderin production and clearance by human pulmonary macrophages. Chest 1984;86:409–11.

70. Vincent B, Flahault A, Antoine M, et al. AIDS-related alveolar hemorrhage. Chest 2001;120:1078–84.

71. Grebski E, Hess T, Hold G, et al. Diagnostic value of hemosiderin-containing macrophages in bronchoalveolar lavage. Chest 1992;102:1794–9.

72. Semenzato G, Poletti V. Bronchoalveolar lavage in lung cancer. Respiration 1992;59 Suppl 1:44–6.

73. Levy H, Horak DA, Lewis MI. The value of bronchial washing and bronchoalveolar lavage in the diagnosis of lymphangitic carcinomatosis. Chest 1988;94:1028–30.

74. Linder J, Radio SJ, Robbins RA, et al. Bronchoalveolar lavage in the cytologic diagnosis of carcinoma of the lung. Acta Cytol 1987;31:796–801.

75. De Gracia J, Bravo C, Miravitlles M, et al. Diagnostic value of bronchoalveolar lavage in peripheral lung cancer. Am Rev Respir Dis 1993;147:649–52.

76. Costabel U, Bross KJ, Matthys H. Diagnosis by bronchoalveolar lavage of cause of pulmonary infiltrates in haematological malignancies. BMJ 1985;290:1041.

77. Saito H, Anaissie EJ, Morice RC, Dekmezian R, Bodey GP. Bronchoalveolar lavage in the diagnosis of pulmonary infiltrates in patients with acute leukemia. Chest 1988;94:745–50.

78. Biyoudi-Vouenze R, Tazi A, Hance AJ, et al. Abnormal epithelial cells recovered by bronchoalveolar lavage: are they malignant? Am Rev Respir Dis 1990;142:686–90.

79. Guzman J, Izumi T, Nagai S, Costabel U. Immunocytochemical characterization of isolated human type II pneumocytes. Acta Cytol 1994;38:539–42.

80. Weynants P, Cordier JF, Chapuis Cellier C, et al. Primary immunocytoma of the lung: the diagnostic value of bronchoalveolar lavage. Thorax 1985;40:542–3.

81. Miller S, Sahn SA. Mycosis fungoides presenting as ARDS and diagnosed by bronchoalveolar lavage. Chest 1986;89:312–4.

82. Jaurand MC, Gaudichet A, Atassi K, et al. Relationship between the number of asbestos fibres and the cellular and enzymatic content of bronchoalveolar fluid in asbestos exposed subjects. Bull Eur Physiopathol Respir 1980;16:595–606.

83. De Vuyst P, Jedwab J, Dumortier P, et al. Asbestos bodies in bronchoalveolar lavage. Am Rev Respir Dis 1982;126:972–6.

84. Xaubet A, Rodriguez-Roisin R, Bombi JA, et al. Correlation of bronchoalveolar lavage and clinical and functional findings in asbestosis. Am Rev Respir Dis 1986;133:848–54.

85. Sebastien P, Armstrong B, Monchaux C, Bignon J. Asbestos bodies in bronchoalveolar lavage fluid and in lung parenchyma. Am Rev Respir Dis 1988;137:75–8.

86. De Vuyst P, Dumortier P, Moulin F, et al. Asbestos bodies in bronchoalveolar lavage reflect lung asbestos body concentration. Eur Respir J 1988;1:362–7.

87. Teschler H, Friedrichs KH, Hoheisel GB, et al. Asbestos fibers in bronchoalveolar lavage and lung tissue of former asbestos workers. Am J Respir Crit Care Med 1994;149:641–5.

88. De Vuyst P, Dumortier P, Moulin E, et al. Diagnostic value of asbestos bodies in bronchoalveolar lavage fluid. Am Rev Respir Dis 1987;136:1219–24.

89. Moulin E, Yourassowsky N, Dumortier P, et al. Electron microscopic analysis of asbestos body cores from the Belgian urban population. Eur Respir J 1988;1:818–22.

90. Churg A, Warnock ML, Green N. Analysis of the cores of ferruginous (asbestos) bodies from the general population. II. True asbestos bodies and pseudoasbestos bodies. Lab Invest 1989;40:31–8.

91. Costabel U, Donner CF, Haslam PL, et al. Clinical role of BAL in occupational lung diseases due to mineral dust exposure. Eur Respir Rev 1992;2:89–96.

92. Gellert AR, Langford JA, Winter RJD, et al. Asbestosis: assessment by bronchoalveolar lavage and measurement of pulmonary epithelial permeability. Thorax 1985;40:508–14.

93. Lusuardi M, Capelli A, Donner CF, et al. Semi-quantitative x-ray microanalysis of bronchoalveolar lavage samples from silica-exposed and nonexposed subject. Eur Respir J 1992;5:798–803.

94. Bégin R, Cantin AM, Boileau RD, Bisson CY. Spectrum of alveolitis in quartz-exposed human subjects. Chest 1987; 92:1061–7.

95. Rom WN, Bitterman PB, Rennard SI, et al. Characterization of the lower respiratory tract inflammation of nonsmoking individuals with interstitial lung disease associated with chronic inhalation of inorganic dusts. Am Rev Respir Dis 1987;136:1429–34.

96. Costabel U, Bross KJ, Huck E, et al. Lung and blood lymphocyte subsets in asbestosis and in mixed dust pneumoconiosis. Chest 1987;91:110–2.

97. Wallaert B, Lassalle P, Fortin F, et al. Superoxide anion generation by alveolar inflammatory cells in simple pneumoconiosis and in progressive massive fibrosis of nonsmoking coal workers. Am Rev Respir Dis 1990;141:129–33.

98. Antilla S, Sutinen S, Paananen M, et al. Hard metal lung disease: a clinical, histological, ultrastructural and x-ray microanalytical study. Eur J Respir Dis 1986;69:83–94.

99. Rizzato G, Lo Cicero S, Barberis M, et al. Trace of metal exposure in hard metal lung disease. Chest 1986;90:101–6.

100. Rossmann MD, Kern JA, Elias JA, et al. Proliferative response of BAL lymphocytes to beryllium. Ann Intern Med 1988;108:687–93.

101. Newman LS, Bobka C, Schumacher B, et al. Compartmentalized immune response reflects clinical severity of beryllium disease. Am J Respir Crit Care Med 1994;150:135–42.

102. Allen JN, Bruce Davis W, Pacht ER. Diagnostic significance of increased bronchoalveolar lavage fluid eosinophils. Am Rev Respir Dis 1990;142:642–7.

103. Costabel U, Teschler H, Guzman J. Bronchiolitis obliterans organizing pneumonia (BOOP): the cytological and immunocytological profile of bronchoalveolar lavage. Eur Respir J 1992;5:791–7.

104. Schnabel A, Reuter M, Gloeckner K, et al. Bronchoalveolar lavage cell profiles in Wegener's granulomatosis. Respir Med 1999;93:498–506.

105. Danel C, Israel-Biet D, Costabel U, et al. The clinical role of BAL in rare pulmonary diseases. Eur Respir Rev 1991;2:83.

106. Chollet S, Soler P, Dournovo P, et al. Diagnosis of pulmonary histocytosis X by immunodetection of Langerhans cells in bronchoalveolar lavage fluid. Am J Pathol 1984;115:225–32.

107. Auerswald U, Barth J, Magnussen H. Value of CD1 positive cells in bronchoalveolar lavage fluid for the diagnosis of pulmonary histiocytosis X. Lung 1990;169:305–9.

108. Corwin RW, Irwin RS. The lipid-laden alveolar macrophage as a marker of aspiration in parenchymal lung disease. Am Rev Respir Dis 1985;132:576.

109. Silverman JF, Turner RC, West R, Dillard TA. Bronchoalveolar lavage in the diagnosis of lipoid pneumonia. Diagn Cytopathol 1989;5:3.

110. Lauque D, Dongay G, Levade T, et al. Bronchoalveolar lavage in liquid paraffin pneumonitis. Chest 1990;98:1149–50.

111. Bjermer L, Rust M, Heurlin N, et al. The clincial use of bronchoalveolar lavage in patients with pulmonary infections. Eur Respir Rev 1992;2:106–13.

112. Huaringa J, Leyva FJ, Signes-Costa J, et al. Bronchoalveolar lavage in the diagnosis of pulmonary complications of bone marrow transplant patients. Bone Marrow Transplant 2000;25:975–9.

113. Gosey L, Howard RM, Witebsky FG, et al. Advantages of a modified toluidine blue O stain and bronchoalveolar lavage for the diagnosis of Pneumocystis carinii pneumonia. J Clin Microbiol 1985;22:803–7.

114. Woods GI, Thompson AB, Rennard SI, Linder J. Detection of cytomegalovirus in bronchoalveolar lavage specimens. Chest 1990;98:568–75.

115. Drent M, van Nierop MA, Gerritsen FA, et al. A computer program using BALF-analysis results as a diagnostic tool in interstitial lung diseases. Am J Respir Crit Care Med 1996;153:736–41.

116. Drent M, Wagenaar SS, Mulder PH, et al. Bronchoalveolar lavage fluid profiles in sarcoidosis, tuberculosis, and non-Hodgkin's and Hodgkin's disease. An evaluation of differences. Chest 1994;105:514–9.

117. Hunninghake GW, Crystal RG. Pulmonary sarcoidosis: a disorder mediated by excess helper T- lymphocyte activity at sites of disease activity. N Engl J Med 1981;305:429–32.

118. Costabel U, Bross KJ, Matthys H. Pulmonary sarcoidosis: assessment of disease activity by lung lymphocyte subpopulations. Klin Wochenschr 1983;61:349–56.

119. Bjermer L, Rosenhall L, Angström T, Hällgren R. Predictive value of bronchoalveolar lavage cell analysis in sarcoidosis. Thorax 1988;43:284–8.

120. Takahashi T, Azuma A, Abe S, et al. Significance of lymphocytosis in bronchoalveolar lavage in suspected ocular sarcoidosis. Eur Respir J 2001;18:515–21.

121. Kantrow SP, Meyer KC, Kidd P, et al. The CD4/CD8 ratio in BAL fluid is highly variable in sarcodosis. Eur Respir J 1997;10:2716–21.

122. Costabel U, Zaiss AW, Guzman J. Sensitivity and specificity of BAL findings in sarcoidosis. Sarcoidosis 1992;9 Suppl 1: 211–4.

123. Winterbauer RH, Lammert J, Selland M, et al. Bronchoalveolar lavage cell populations in the diagnosis of sarcoidosis. Chest 1993;104:252–61.

124. Thomeer M, Demedts M. Predictive value of CD4/CD8 ratio in bronchoalveolar lavage in the diagnosis of sarcoidosis [abstract]. Sarc Vasc Diffuse Lung Dis 1997;14 Suppl 1:36.

125. Ward K, O'Connor C, Odlum C, Fitzgerald MX. Prognostic value of bronchoalveolar lavage in sarcoidosis: the critical influence of disease presentation. Thorax 1989;44:6–12.

126. Drent M, Jacobs JA, de Vries J, et al. Does the cellular bronchoalveolar lavage fluid profile reflect the severity of sarcoidosis? Eur Respir J 1999;13:1338–44.

127. Costabel U. The alveolitis of hypersensitivity pneumonitis. Eur Respir J 1988;1:5–9.

128. Reynolds HY, Fulmer JD, Kazmierowski JA, et al. Analysis of cellular and protein content of broncho-alveolar lavage fluid from patients with idiopathic pulmonary fibrosis and chronic hypersensitivity pneumonitis. J Clin Invest 1977; 59:165–75.

129. Leatherman JW, Michael AF, Schwartz BA, Hoidal JR. Lung T cells in hypersensitivity pneumonitis. Ann Intern Med 1984;100:390–2.

130. Costabel U, Bross JK, Rühle KH, et al. Ia-like antigens on T-cells and their subpopulations in pulmonary sarcoidosis and in hypersensitivity pneumonitis. Analysis of bronchoalveolar and blood lymphocytes. Am Rev Respir Dis 1985;131:337–42.

131. Semenzato G, Agostini C, Zambello R, et al. Lung T cells in hypersensitivity pneumonitis: phenotypic and functional analyses. J Immunol 1986;137:1164–72.

132. Semenzato G, Bjermer L, Costabel U, et al. Clinical guidelines and indications for bronchoalveolar lavage (BAL): extrinsic allergic alveolitis. Eur Respir J 1990;3:945–9.

133. Guzman J, Costabel U. Bronchoalveolar lavage in diagnostic cytology. In: Wied GL, Keebler CM, Koss LG, et al., editors. Transparencies and explanatory text. Tutorials of Cytology. Chicago: International Acadamy of Cytology: 1992.

134. Soler P, Nioche S, Valeyre D, et al. Role of mast cells in the pathogenesis of hypersensitivity pneumonitis. Thorax 1987;42:565–72.

135. Johnson MA, Nemeth A, Condez A, et al. Cell mediated immunity in pigeon breeders' lung: the effect of removal from antigen exposure. Eur Respir J 1989;2:445–50.

136. Pesci A, Bertorelli G, Olivieri D. Mast cells in bronchoalveolar lavage fluid and in transbronchial biopsy specimens of patients with farmer's lung disease. Chest 1991;100: 1197–202.

137. Haslam PL, Dewar A, Butchers P, et al. Mast cells, atypical lymphocytes and neutrophils in bronchoalveolar lavage in extrinsic allergic alveolitis. Am Rev Respir Dis 1987;135:35–47.

138. Costabel U, Bross KJ, Guzman J, Matthys H. Plasmazellen und Lymphozyten-subpopulationen in der bronchoalveolären Lavage bei exogen-allergischer Alveolitis. Prax Klin Pneumol 1985;39:925–6.

139. Drent M, Wagenaar S, Ven Velzen-Blad H, et al. Relationship between plasma cell levels and profile of bronchoalveolar lavage fluid in patients with subacute extrinsic allergic alveolitis. Thorax 1993;48:835–9.

140. Ando M, Konishi K, Yoneda R, Tamura M. Difference in the phenotypes of bronchoalveolar lavage lymphocytes in patients with summer-type hypersensitivity pneumonitis, farmer's lung, ventilation pneumonitis, and bird fancier's lung: report of a nationwide epidemiologic study in Japan. J Allergy Clin Immunol 1991;87:1002–9.

141. Drent M, Ven Velzen-Blad H, Diamant M, et al. Bronchoalveolar lavage in extrinsic allergic alveolitis: effect of time elapsed since antigen exposure. Eur Respir J 1993;5:1276–81.

142. Keller RH, Swartz S, Schlueter DP, et al. Immunoregulation in hypersensitivity pneumonitis: phenotypic and functional studies of bronchoalveolar lavage lymphocytes. Am Rev Respir Dis 1984;130:766–71.

143. Costabel U, Teschler H, Bauer CP. Stellenwert der bronchoalveolären Lavage bei exogen-allergischer Alveolitis. Atemw Lungenkrhk 1989;15:598–604.

144. Fournier E, Tonnel AB, Gosset P, et al. Early neutrophil alveolitis after antigen inhalation in hypersensitivity pneumonitis. Chest 1985;88:563–5.

145. Solal-Celigny P, Laviolette M, Hebert J, Cormier Y. Immune reactions in the lungs of asymptomatic dairy farmers. Am Rev Respir Dis 1982;126:964–67.

146. Cormier Y, Belanger J, Laviolette M. Persistent bronchoalveolar lymphocytosis in asymptomatic farmers. Am Rev Respir Dis 1986;133:843–7.

147. Gariepy L, Cormier Y, Laviolette M, Tardif A. Predictive value of bronchoalveolar lavage cells and serum precipitins in asymptomatic dairy farmers. Am Rev Respir Dis 1989; 140:1386–9.

148. Huang MS, Colby T, Goellner JR, Martin WJ Jr. Utility of broncholveolar lavage in the diagnosis of drug-induced pulmonary toxicity. Acta Cytol 1989;33:533–8.

149. Israel-Biet D, Venet A, Caubarrere I, et al. Bronchoalveolar lavage in amiodarone pneumonitis. Cellular abnormalities and their relevance to pathogenesis. Chest 1987;91:214–21.

150. White DA, Kris MG, Stover DE. Bronchoalveolar lavage cell populations in bleomycin lung toxicity. Thorax 1987;42: 551–2.

151. Schnabel A, Richter C, Bauerfeind S, Gross WL. Bronchoalveolar lavage cell profile in methotrexate induced pneumonitis. Thorax 1997;52:377–9.

152. White DA, Rankin JA, Stover DE, et al. Methotrexate pneumonitis. Am Rev Respir Dis 1989;139:18–21.

153. Akoun G, Mayaud C, Touboul JL, et al. Use of bronchoalveolar lavage in the evaluation of methotrexate lung disease. Thorax 1987;42:652–5.

154. Haslam PL, Turton CWG, Lukoszek A, et al. Bronchoalveolar lavage fluid cell counts in cryptogenic fibrosing alveolitis and their relation to therapy. Thorax 1980;35:328–39.

155. Peterson WMW, Monick M, Hunninghake GW. Prognostic role of eosinophils in pulmonary fibrosis. Chest 1987;92: 51–6.

156. Lynch JP, Standiford TJ, Rolfe MW, et al. Neutrophilic alveolitis in idiopathic pulmonary fibrosis. The role of interleukin-8. Am Rev Respir Dis 1992;145:1433–9.

157. Bjoraker JA, Ryu JH, Edwin MK, et al. Prognostic significance of histopathology subsets in idiopathic pulmonary fibrosis. Am J Respir Crit Care Med 1998;157:199–203.

158. Nagai S, Kitaichi M, Itoh H, et al. Idiopathic nonspecific interstitial pneumonia/fibrosis: comparison with idiopathic pulmonary fibrosis and BOOP. Eur Respir J 1998;12:1010–9.

159. Park CS, Chung SW, Ki SY, et al. Increased levels of interleukin-6 are associated with lymphocytosis in bronchoalveolar lavage fluids of idiopathic nonspecific interstitial pneumonia. Am J Respir Crit Care Med 2000;162:1162–8.

160. Suga M, Iyonaga K, Okamoto T, et al. Characteristic elevation of matrix metalloproteinase activity in idiopathic interstitial pneumonias. Am J Respir Crit Care Med 2000;162: 1949–56.

161. Daniil ZD, Gilchrist FC, Nicholson AG, et al. A histologic pattern of nonspecific interstitial pneumonia is associated with a better prognosis than usual interstitial pneumonia in patients with cryptogenic fibrosing alveolitis. Am J Respir Crit Care Med 1999;160:899–905.

162. Cazzato S, Zompatori M, Baruzzi G, et al. Bronchiolitis obliterans-organizing pneumonia: an Italian experience. Respir Med 2000;94:702–8.

163. Chan TY, Hansell DM, Rubens MB, et al. Cryptogenic fibrosing alveolitis and the fibrosing alveolitis of systemic sclerosis: morphological differences on computed tomographic scans. Thorax 1997;52:265–70.

164. Nagao T, Nagai S, Kitaichi M, et al. Usual interstitial pneumonia: idiopathic pulmonary fibrosis versus collagen vascular diseases. Respiration 2001;68:151–9.

165. Greene NB, Solinger AM, Baughman RP. Patients with collagen vascular disease and dyspnea. The value of gallium scanning and bronchoalveolar lavage in predicting response to steroid therapy and clinical outcome. Chest 1987;91:698–703.

166. Schnabel A, Reuter M, Csermok E, et al. Subclinical alveolar bleeding in pulmonary vasculitides: correlation with indices of disease activity. Eur Respir J 1999;14:118–24.

167. O'Donnell K, Keogh B, Cantin A, Crystal RG. Pharmacologic suppression of the neutrophil component of the alveolitis in idiopathic pulmonary fibrosis. Am Rev Respir Dis 1987;136:288–92.

168. Rudd RM, Haslam PL, Turner-Warwick M. Cryptogenic fibrosing alveolitis: relationships of pulmonary physiology and bronchoalveolar lavage to treatment and prognosis. Am Rev Respir Dis 1981;124:1–8.

169. Turner-Warwick M, Haslam PL. The value of serial bronchoalveolar lavages in assessing the clinical progress of patients with cryptogenic fibrosing alveolitis. Am Rev Respir Dis 1987;135:26–34.

170. Costabel U, Bross KJ, Guzman J, et al. Predictive value of bronchoalveolar lavage T cell subsets for the course of pulmonary sarcoidosis. Ann N Y Acad Sci 1986;465:418–23.

171. Israel-Biet D, Venet A, Chretien J. Persistent high alveolar lymphocytosis as a predictive criterion of chronic pulmonary sarcoidosis. Ann N Y Acad Sci 1986;465:395–406.

172. Verstraeten A, Demedts M, Verwilghen J, et al. Predictive value of bronchoalveolar lavage in pulmonary sarcoidosis. Chest 1990;98:560–7.

173. White B, Moore WC, Wigley FM, et al. Cyclophosphamide is associated with pulmonary function and survival benefit in patients with scleroderma and alveolitis. Ann Intern Med 2000;132:947–54.

174. Behr J, Vogelmeier C, Beinert T, et al. Bronchoalveolar lavage for evaluation and management of scleroderma disease of the lung. Am J Respir Crit Care Med 1996;154:400–6.

6 PEDIATRIC INTERSTITIAL LUNG DISEASE

LELAND L. FAN

As in adults, interstitial lung disease (ILD) in children includes a large heterogeneous group of mostly rare conditions characterized by restrictive lung disease and disordered gas exchange.[1-5] Not only does ILD occur far less frequently in children than in adults, the spectrum and distribution of disease is also somewhat different in children.

Our current understanding of pediatric ILD is limited. Much of what is known has been derived from anecdotal case reports and small series of patients. Although attempts have been made to apply concepts derived from the adult ILD experience to children, it is far from clear that the disease mechanism, clinical presentation, natural history, and response to treatment of pediatric and adult ILD are similar. Specifically, there are unique forms of ILD in infants that are not found in adults. Although the models of lung injury and repair that have been developed for adult ILD[6-9] may be valid for pediatric ILD, the process is more complex in children because it occurs in the context of lung growth and differentiation.

This chapter summarizes the current understanding of ILD in children with regard to classification, clinical presentation, evaluation, treatment, and outcome.

CLASSIFICATION

Although no categorization of pediatric ILD is entirely satisfactory, a general classification of pediatric ILD is presented in Tables 6–1 through 6–3. A complete description of each disorder is beyond the scope of this chapter. Many, however, deserve emphasis, particularly those that are unique to infants and children.

Pediatric Interstitial Lung Diseases of Known Etiology

Aspiration

Inhalation of food, saliva, or foreign material into the airways from gastroesophageal reflux, tracheoesophageal fistula, and swallowing disorders, is a common cause of

TABLE 6–1 Pediatric Interstitial Lung Diseases of Known Etiology

Aspiration syndromes

Chronic infection (viral, bacterial, fungal, parasitic)
  Immunocompetent host
  Immunocompromised host

Bronchopulmonary dysplasia

Hypersensitivity pneumonitis (and other environmental exposures)

Lipid storage diseases

chronic lung disease in children.[10-13] In a recent study of children with recurrent pneumonia, aspiration was the etiology in 48% of 220 cases.[14] Children with neuromuscular disorders are particularly vulnerable to aspiration as are infants given oral mineral oil for constipation (Figure 6–1)[15] and older children who use lip gloss.[16]

It can be difficult to prove conclusively that a patient is aspirating without direct evidence of aspiration, such as tracheal penetration on barium swallow, radioactivity in the lung on scintigraphy, or a foreign body reaction on

TABLE 6–2 Pediatric Interstitial Lung Diseases of Unknown Etiology

Primary pulmonary disorders
  Usual interstitial pneumonitis (UIP)
  Desquamative interstitial pneumonitis (DIP)
  Lymphocytic interstitial pneumonitis (LIP) and related disorders
  Nonspecific interstitial pneumonitis
  Pulmonary hemosiderosis
  Pulmonary infiltrates with eosinophilia
  Bronchiolitis obliterans
  Bronchiolitis obliterans with organizing pneumonia (BOOP)
  Alveolar proteinosis
  Pulmonary vascular disorders (proliferative and congenital)
  Pulmonary lymphatic disorders
  Pulmonary microlithiasis

Systemic disorders with pulmonary involvement
  Connective tissue disease
  Malignancies
  Histiocytosis
  Sarcoidosis
  Neurocutaneous syndromes

**TABLE 6–3   Unique Forms of
Interstitial Lung Disease in Infancy**

Persistent tachypnea of infancy (PTI)/neuroendocrine cell
 hyperplasia of infancy (NEHI)

Follicular bronchitis/chronic bronchiolitis

Cellular interstitial pneumonitis of infancy

Acute idiopathic pulmonary hemorrhage of infancy (AIPHI)

Chronic pneumonitis of infancy

Idiopathic pulmonary fibrosis of infancy

Familial desquamative interstitial pneumonitis (DIP)

Surfactant protein abnormalities/congenital alveolar proteinosis

lung biopsy. The finding of increased numbers of lipid-laden macrophages in the bronchoaveolar lavage (BAL) fluid is a sensitive marker for aspiration,[17–22] but it may not be specific for aspiration.[23,24] The detection of specific

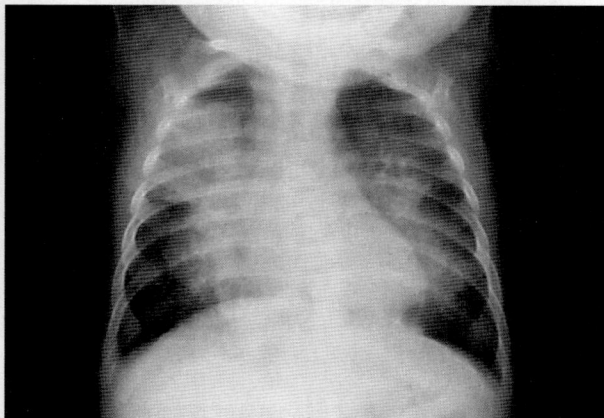

A

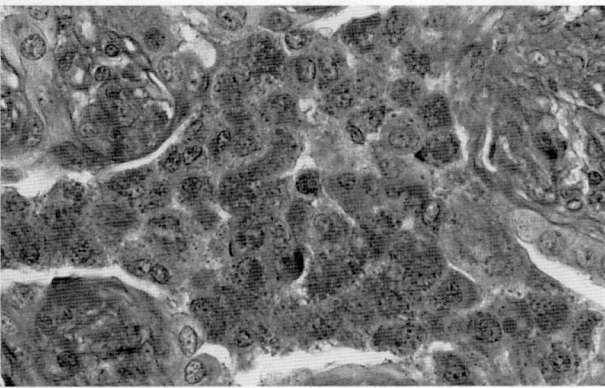

B

Figure 6–1   Lipoid pneumonia in an infant given mineral oil for constipation. *A,* Chest roentgenogram shows bilateral central air space consolidation. *B,* Lung biopsy shows dense consolidation of alveolar air spaces with lipid-laden macrophages (hematoxylin and eosin; ×100 original magnification). Reproduced with permission from Fan LL and Graham LM.[15]

milk proteins in alveolar macrophages recovered from BAL fluid using immunocytochemistry may prove to be a more specific marker for aspiration in children.[25] Although reflux is often demonstrated in children with ILD and other chronic respiratory disorders, it is often difficult to determine if reflux causes, exacerbates, or is caused by the lung disease itself.

Infection

The role of infectious agents, such as adenovirus,[26,27] influenza,[28] *Mycoplasma,*[29,30] and *Chlamydia,*[31] in the development of chronic lung disease in children has been well documented. Virtually any organism that infects the lower respiratory tract is capable of producing chronic diffuse lung disease, although most infected children have acute self–limited disease that resolves completely.

Probably the best example of postinfectious chronic lung disease is found in children who develop bronchiolitis obliterans (BO) after severe adenovirus infection.[26] BO is characterized by a fibrosis process of the small airways resulting in severe, nonreversible airways obstruction. Occasionally, severe involvement of one lung leads to the development of a unilateral, small, hyperlucent lung, known as Swyer-James syndrome.[26] Patients with severe adenovirus pneumonia have recently been shown to have immune complexes that contain adenovirus antigen in the lung as well as increased serum levels of interleukin (IL)-6, IL-8, and tumor necrosis factor alpha (TNF-α).[32,33] These studies suggest that in infants and young children, abnormal or excessive host immunologic and inflammatory responses may be important factors in the development of chronic lung disease from adenovirus. Other infectious agents known to cause BO include *Mycoplasma,* measles, parainfluenza, pertussis, and respiratory syncytial virus.[34,35] Although the majority of patients have persistent, nonprogressive symptoms, approximately 10% ultimately die from this disease.[36]

Other organisms have been associated with pediatric chronic lung disease. Perinatal infection or colonization with *Ureaplasma urealyticum* has been implicated in inducing pulmonary inflammation and subsequent development of bronchopulmonary dysplasia in premature neonates.[37] Finally parvovirus has been linked to autoimmune disease associated with ILD and other organ involvement.[38]

In a prospective study of immunocompetent children with chronic diffuse infiltrates, this author found an infectious agent as the underlying cause of chronic ILD in 20% (10/51) of pediatric ILD cases.[39] Identified agents included adenovirus alone in 4 patients, adenovirus and cytomegalovirus (CMV) in 2, varicella in 1, Epstein-Barr virus (EBV) in 1, *Chlamydia* in 1, and *Toxocara* in 1. Thus, infection, either chronic or acute with long-term sequelae, accounts for many cases of ILD of known etiology in children.

Hypersensitivity Pneumonitis

An immunologic response to the inhalation of organic dusts, hypersensitivity pneumonitis (HP) is an under-recognized cause of ILD in children; the youngest reported patient developed symptoms at 8 months of age.[40] HP in children is mainly caused by exposure to an array of domestic birds (83%) and fungi (17%), based on a review of 83 reported pediatric cases.[40–66] HP has also been reported in a child receiving methotrex-ate.[67] Familial cases have been identified, with a recent report describing a mother (who died from the disease) and all of her 5 children who developed HP from exposure to city pigeons.[66]

Most of these 83 children were quite ill at presentation, exhibiting symptoms of exercise intolerance, hypoxemia, and weight loss; reticulonodular infiltrates on chest films and high-resolution computed tomography (Figure 6–2); and moderate to severe restrictive lung disease by pulmonary function testing. Diagnosis was established by exposure history, positive precipitins, and, in some cases, lung biopsy. Treatment consisted of eliminating exposure to the offending antigen in all cases and administering corticosteroids in approximately half. In the reported cases, all but two children improved, and to date, there has been one recorded pediatric death from HP.[53]

Pediatric Interstitial Lung Diseases of Unknown Etiology

The classic forms of ILD, originally described in adults by Liebow[68] and still recognized as important today, are usual interstitial pneumonitis (UIP), desquamative interstitial pneumonitis (DIP), and lymphocytic interstitial pneumonitis (LIP). These forms of interstitial lung disease also occur in childhood, but their frequency differs from that found in adults. In a retrospective study of 48 immunocompetent children with ILD evaluated during a 12-year period (1980 to 1991) at the University of Colorado, only two patients had UIP, four had DIP, and five had LIP.[69] In a subsequent prospective study of 51 different children with ILD evaluated from 1992 to 1994 at the same institution, no cases of DIP or UIP were found, and one case of LIP associated with EBV infection was identified.[39] In another retrospective series of 38 cases of pediatric ILD from the Royal Brompton Hospital, Nicholson and colleagues[70] found 11 cases of reactive lymphoid hyperplasia (either LIP or follicular bronchiolitis) and four cases of DIP, but no cases of UIP. Thus, the classic forms of ILD in children are truly rare.

Usual Interstitial Pnuemonitis

The term UIP, initially described in adults, refers to a specific pathologic process characterized by ongoing and progressive lung disease that is patchy in distribution and variable in histology.[71] This patchy distribution and variable histology are due to the recruitment of initially normal lung units by an inflammatory and later fibrotic process. The most important histologic features of UIP are fibroblastic foci, which are thought to be the sites from which this process originates. As this recruitment progresses over time, all stages of reaction coexist from early acute lesions with hyaline membrane formation, through chronic inflammatory lesions with a mixed mononuclear infiltrate, to late fibrotic lesions. Thus, examination of lungs with UIP shows areas of normal

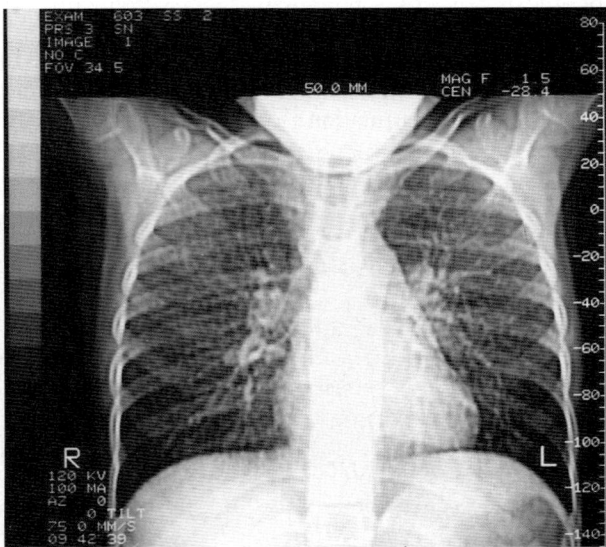

A

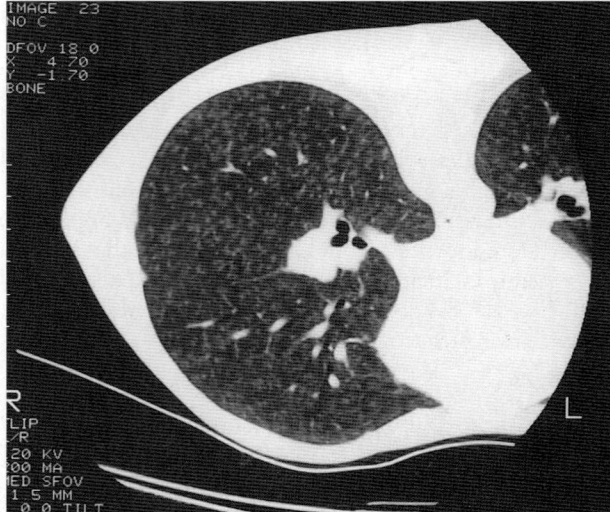

B

Figure 6–2   Hypersensitivity pneumonitis from cockatiel antigens in an adolescent. *A*, Chest roentgenogram shows bilateral reticulonodular infiltrates. *B*, HRCT scan shows diffuse multiple fine nodules. Courtesy of Robin Deterding, MD, University of Colorado, Denver.

lung intermixed with areas of acute change, areas of chronic inflammation, and areas of end-stage fibrosis or honeycombing. In children, true examples of this process are exceedingly rare, and some have questioned whether UIP occurs at all.[71] As mentioned previously, no cases of UIP were recorded in two recent series of children with ILD.[39,70]

Unfortunately, this term is sometimes used for less specific histologic processes and has been applied to a number of other less well-defined interstitial processes as well. The tendency to use this term for a wider variety of nonspecific processes in children may account for the better prognosis of children diagnosed with UIP as compared with adults with UIP, who generally have a poor prognosis. Although more than 100 children with UIP, cryptogenic fibrosing alveolitis, or idiopathic pulmonary fibrosis have been reported in the literature, many did not have biopsy confirmation of the diagnosis.[72–77] The inclusion of heterogeneous conditions in a single diagnostic category may significantly impair the evaluation of potential etiologies and therapeutic regimens.

Desquamative Interstitial Pneumonitis

As in adults, DIP in children is a uniform and monotonous histologic process, characterized by hyperplasia of alveolar epithelial cells and by an abundance of macrophages within air spaces. These cells within the air spaces, initially misidentified as desquamated epithelial cells, give this condition its name (see "Familial Desquamative Interstitial Pneumonitis"). Inflammatory cells, including histiocytes, lymphocytes, plasma cells, and eosinophils are present but usually only in small numbers. There may be minimal and generally uniform widening of alveolar septa by increased connective tissue, but fibrosis is not a notable feature. In some cases, DIP-like reactions occur in association with more specific lesions and may obscure the picture. Although it has been suggested that DIP and UIP represent different stages of the same disease process, this association has not been convincingly demonstrated in children. Desquamative interstitial pneumonitis in childhood appears to be a different process from DIP in adults, in that it is not decreasing in incidence, and it is not linked to smoking.[77–88] DIP has occasionally been associated with infection, particularly congenital rubella[83] and CMV.[88]

Lymphocytic Interstitial Pneumonitis

This is the most common of the classically described interstitial pneumonias in childhood. It is not truly an interstitial pneumonitis but rather a form of pulmonary lymphoproliferative disease. Lymphocytic interstitial pneumonia is characterized histologically by a diffuse infiltrate of mature lymphocytes, with smaller numbers of plasma cells and histiocytes in the pulmonary interstitium, including the alveolar wall.[89,90] The infiltrate may also be found along lymphatic pathways and is thus evident in the bronchovascular and interlobular septa; it usually spares the pleura. The lymphocytes, which are small noncleaved cells, may accumulate as small nodules, sometimes with germinal centers. They tend to be polyclonal, with B cells and a variety of T cells.[91,92] Fibrosis is generally not a feature, nor is air space disease significant.

Lymphocytic interstitial pneumonitis is distinguished histologically from the other benign lymphoid disorders of the lung, which include intraparenchymal lymph nodes, hyperplasia of the bronchial-associated lymphoid tissue, nodular lymphoid hyperplasia, and angioimmunoblastic lymphadenopathy.[89,90] Although many clinicians or pathologists assume that hyperplasia of the bronchial-associated lymphoid tissue and nodular lymphoid hyperplasia are stages in the evolution of LIP, this has not been conclusively established. Lymphocytic interstitial pneumonitis may exist as an isolated and sometimes familial disorder,[93–95] but it usually occurs in association with abnormalities of immune status that include autoimmune disorders[96,97] and immunodeficiency states.[98–101] This disease is a well-described complication of pediatric acquired immunodeficiency syndrome (AIDS), and occurs in up to 30% of children affected perinatally with human immunodeficiency virus-1 (HIV-1) (Figure 6–3).[91,92,102–108] Children with AIDS and LIP tend not to develop opportunistic infections such as *Pneumocystis carinii*. This group's better prognosis is probably related to less immune compromise. Although Epstein-Barr virus has been isolated from the lungs of some AIDS[109–112] and non-AIDS[113] patients with LIP, its role in the development of LIP is unclear.

Unique Forms of Interstitial Lung Disease in Infancy

Infants with chronic tachypnea, crackles, and hypoxemia present enormous diagnostic challenges. Although several distinct syndromes have been recently identified, the terminology is confusing and some of these conditions may overlap. The following entities are described in order of prognosis from favorable to poor.

Persistent Tachypnea of Infancy/Neuroendocrine Cell Hyperplasia of Infancy

This author and colleagues recently described a group of ten infants with chronic tachypnea, crackles, and hypoxemia.[114] Findings were present at birth in four. Chest films revealed minimal to no increase in interstitial markings, peribronchial thickening, and hyperinflation. Each patient's lung biopsy demonstrated hyperplasia of neuroendocrine cells in the distal airways.[115] Otherwise, there were very mild, nonspecific changes mainly of airway and vascular smooth muscle, with little or no interstitial involvement and no inflammation. No infectious disease agents were recovered from the patients. There was a striking discrepancy between the infants' clinical appearance (they seemed quite ill) and the lack of demonstrably significant abnormalities in the chest films, high-resolution computed tomography, and biopsy specimens. Response to corticosteroids was variable. Although the patients remained symptomatic and often required oxygen for months to years, the clinical condition of the patients remained static or gradually improved over time. Originally, the term *persistent tachypnea of infancy* (PTI) was used to described this condition, but since the identification of excessive neuroendocrine cells in the distal airways

was appreciated, the condition is now known as *neuroendocrine cell hyperplasia of infancy* (NEHI). Although these infants do not have true ILD, their clinical presentation is similar to those with it.

Follicular Bronchitis/Bronchiolitis

Although not true ILD, chronic airways obstruction in infants, not due to asthma or cystic fibrosis, often presents with respiratory signs and symptoms indistinguishable from ILD. Kinane and colleagues[116] reported five infants with follicular bronchitis/bronchiolitis presenting with tachypnea, fine crackles, and chronic cough by 6 weeks of age. Lung biopsy revealed follicular lymphocytic infiltration surrounding and locally infiltrating the bronchial walls; no organisms were recovered. All patients improved gradually over several years' time. Similar features were reported more recently by Hull and colleagues[117] in 8 infants, although 2 had normal biopsies.

It is tempting to speculate that chronic airways obstruction in infants is a continuum of disease from the more inflammatory follicular bronchiolitis to the more fibrotic or constrictive BO. Also, NEHI might be a milder form of this continuum, although infants with NEHI do not have inflammation of the airway walls on lung biopsy. The continuum concept would be consistent with models of inflammation and repair in both airways and interstitial lung disease in adults, but the relationship between follicular bronchiolitis and BO remains unproven in children.

Cellular Interstitial Pneumonitis

Schroeder and colleagues[118] described five infants with tachypnea since birth and diffuse infiltrates of unknown etiology. Lung biopsy changes included interstitial proliferation of bland, nondescript histiocytic-type cells and minimal or no inflammation. Although the patients remained tachypneic for prolonged periods of time (4 to 18 months after diagnosis), the overall clinical course was marked by general improvement in 4 of the 5 infants. The fifth infant died at 3 1/2 years of age. Another case of cellular interstitial pneumonitis was recently reported in a 4-month-old.[119]

Acute Idiopathic Pulmonary Hemorrrhage of Infancy

A group of 20 African American infants, most of them male from the inner-city areas of Cleveland[120] and Detroit,[121] with unexplained pulmonary hemorrhage and hemosiderosis was recently described, after an earlier report of 4 infants with acute alveolar hemorrhage.[122] All but 2 of the 20 infants in the combined studies required

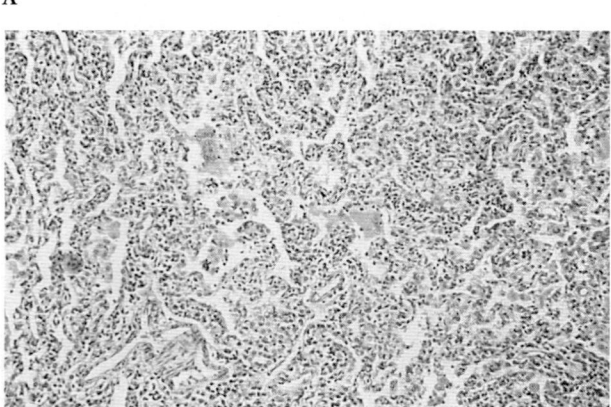

A

B

Figure 6–3 Lymphocytic interstitial pneumonitis in a young child with AIDS. *A*, Chest roentgenogram shows bilateral interstitial infiltrates. *B*, Lung biopsy shows diffuse mononuclear infiltration of the interstitium with predominantly lymphocytes (hematoxylin and eosin).

assisted ventilation, and 2 died of respiratory failure. Although no specific etiology was found, a case-controlled study of the Cleveland infants suggested that environmental risk factors, specifically water damage[120] and growth of toxogenic fungi, notably *Stachybotrys chartarum* (also known as *S. atra*),[123] in the homes may have contributed to the pulmonary hemorrhage. Since this series was published, a number of case reports have supported this association. In a report by Elidemir and colleagues, a case of *S. chartarum* was isolated from the bronchoalveolar lavage fluid of a child with pulmonary hemorrhage.[124] Due to the concern for this possible health risk, many public buildings have been closed, environmental cleanups imposed, and personal injury claims filed.[125]

As a result of this growing problem, a Centers for Disease Control and Prevention (CDC) task force was assembled to review the role of *S. chartarum* in acute idiopathic pulmonary hemorrhage of infancy (AIPHI). An internal group of senior CDC investigators and outside experts conducted separate reviews of the Cleveland research. Both groups found that due to limitations of the studies, the evidence was not sufficient to support an association between pulmonary hemorrhage and *S. chartarum*.[125] Subsequent to this report, Vesper and colleagues[126] reported that strains of *S. chartarum* from the homes of Cleveland infants with AIPHI as well as from the child from Houston reported by Elidemir and colleagues[124] had increased siderophore and hemolysin production compared with the control group. Thus, at this time, the association between AIPHI and environmental exposures, including *S. chartarum*, remains highly controversial.

Chronic Pneumonitis of Infancy

Katzenstein and colleagues[127] described nine infants with ILD characterized by marked alveolar septal thickening, striking pneumocyte hyperplasia, and an alveolar exudate containing numerous macrophages and foci of eosinophilic debris. As this pattern was markedly different from the previously described classic patterns of ILD (DIP, UIP, LIP) and from the cellular interstitial pneumonitis of infancy described by Schroeder and colleagues[118] they chose the term *chronic pneumonitis of infancy* to reflect the uniqueness of this entity. Of the 6 whose clinical course was known, 2 died and 1 required lung transplantation. Actually, Fisher and colleagues[128] had previously described a similar process in eight children, although the majority were much older. Although not studied, a defect in surfactant regulation might have played a role in some of these cases.

Idiopathic Pulmonary Fibrosis of Infancy

Osika and colleagues[129] recently described ten infants with severe, progressive chronic lung disease characterized by increased neutrophils in BAL and intense to moderate fibrosis on lung biopsy. All of the infants died, with the exception of one patient who appeared to respond to pulse methylprednisolone therapy. In a sequel study, the same group reported favorable outcomes in three other affected infants with pulse methylprednisolone therapy.[130] Apparently, not all patients have a poor outcome; Hacking and colleagues[131] reported on 11 infants, all of whom survived with conservative management, and some did not receive corticosteroids. The histologic descriptions of these cases are not very specific, therefore, it is difficult to know how this condition relates to the other diffuse lung diseases described in infants. Again, a defect in surfactant regulation might have played a role in some of these cases, although this possibility was not investigated in these studies.

Familial Desquamative Interstitial Pneumonitis

There are several reports of infant siblings with biopsy-proven DIP presenting early in life with progressive respiratory disease leading to respiratory failure and death in all but one of the reported cases.[69,132–134] In this author's experience, although the lung biopsy showed typical changes of DIP, immunohistochemical techniques demonstrated that the cells in the air spaces were macrophages, not desquamating epithelial lining cells (Figure 6–4), thus confirming that the term DIP is a misnomer. It has become increasingly clear that some forms of familial ILD, including DIP, are associated with surfactant protein abnormalities (see the following section).

Surfactant Protein Abnormalities/Congenital Alveolar Proteinosis

Since Nogee and colleagues[135] first reported 2 siblings with congenital alveolar proteinosis due to surfactant protein B (SP-B) deficiency, 30 infants with SP-B deficiency from 16 families have been identified and reported.[136] The most common mutation observed in this autosomal recessive disorder results from a substitution and a 2 base pair insertion in exon 4 of the SP-B gene (121ins2), which leads to a frameshift and premature signal for the termination of translation of the SP-B transcript.[137] Phenotypic heterogeneity suggests that variable degrees of SP-B deficiency may be more common than previously suspected.[138]

Although lung biopsies from the original patients contained frothy, periodic acid–Schiff (PAS) staining material in air spaces typical of alveolar proteinosis,[135] subsequent cases have been associated with alveolar epithelial hyperplasia, exudates of PAS-positive material intermixed with cellular debris, and a paucity of inflammatory cells.[136,139] In some cases, the histology is suggestive of DIP. Variations of surfactant abnormalities associated with DIP exist. In one fatal case, a deficiency of lamellar bodies in alveolar type II cells without mutations in the coding sequence of the SP-B gene was identified.[140]

Infants with these disorders lack functional pulmonary surfactant and usually develop early respiratory failure that is unresponsive to lung lavage, surfactant replacement therapy, corticosteroids, and extracorporeal life support; the disorder leads to death.[139] Recently, prolonged survival has been reported in 2 of 3 infants who had lung transplantation.[136] Following transplantation, all survivors exhibited normal SP-B expression and pulmonary surfactant function.

Two recent reports have linked familial ILD with surfactant protein C abnormalities (SP-C). In one report, a mutation in the SP-C gene was associated with interstitial lung disease in an infant and her mother.[141]

In another report of an 11-year-old girl, her sister, and her mother, SP-C was absent in BAL fluid and decreased immunostaining for SP-C in lung tissue was found.[142] No known mutations for SP-B or SP-C coding were identified. In summary, it has become increasingly clear that many cases of infant and familial ILD are linked to abnormalities of surfactant proteins.

Pulmonary Vascular Disorders

Alveolar capillary dysplasia is another form of congenital lung disease. It is uniformly fatal and defined histologically by the presence of anomalous pulmonary veins in the bronchovascular bundles, anomalous capillarization of alveolar septa, and increased muscularization of the arterioles.[143] Reported cases in siblings suggest a

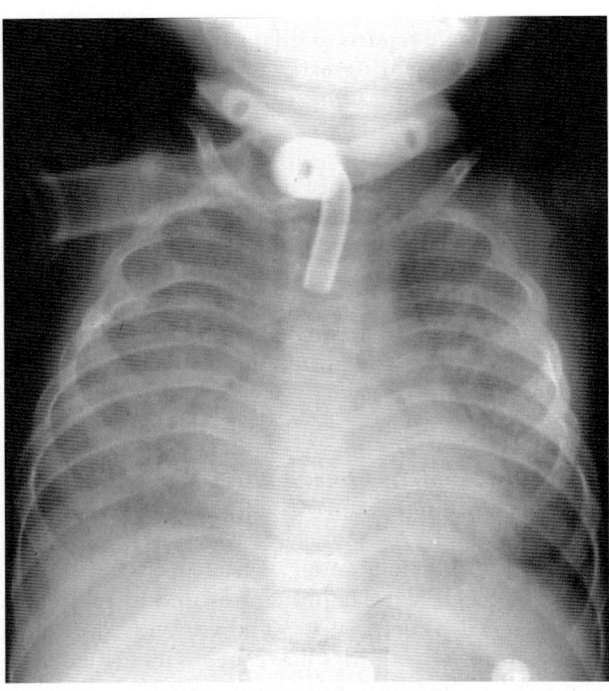

A

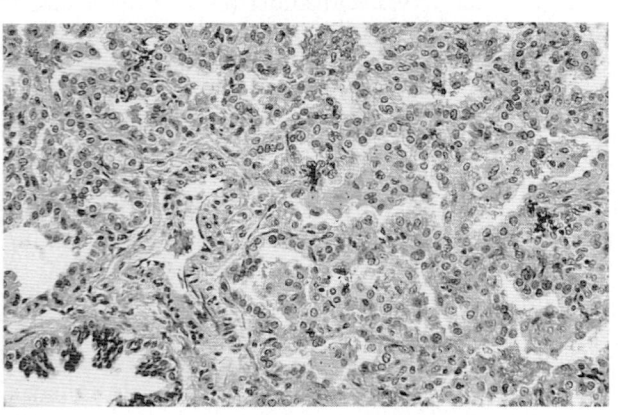

B

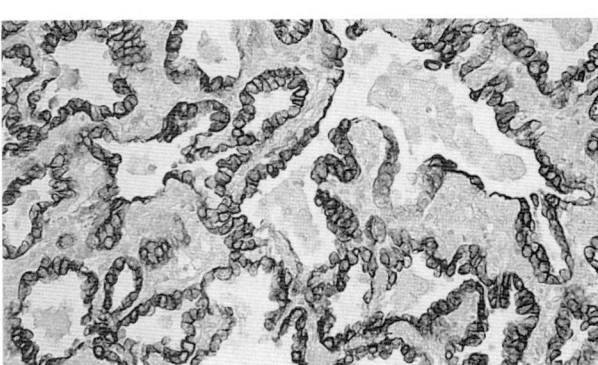

C

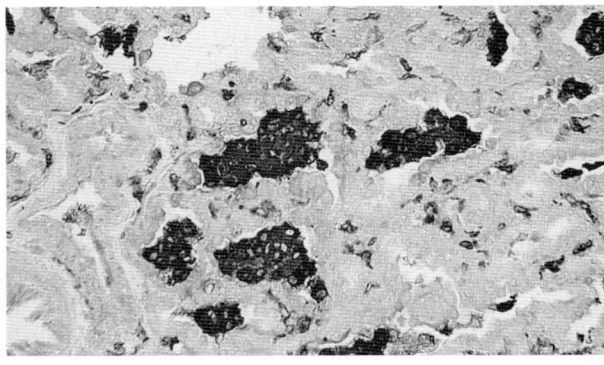

D

Figure 6–4 Familial desquamative interstitial pneumonitis in an infant. *A*, Chest roentgenogram shows bilateral diffuse ground-glass densities. *B*, Lung biopsy shows hyperplasia of alveolar lining cells and accumulation of mononuclear cells in air spaces (hematoxylin and eosin; ×20 original magnification). *C*, The cells in the lumen are negative and hence not epithelial cells (CAM 5.2, an antibody to cytokeratin to demonstrate alveolar epithelial cells; ×20 original magnification). *D*, The cells in the air spaces are positive for CD-68 and hence are macrophages not desquamated epithelial cells (CD-68, a lysosomal antigen to identify pulmonary macrophages; ×20 original magnification). Courtesy of Robert Mason, MD, National Jewish Medical and Research Center, Denver, Colorado. Reproduced with permission from Fan LL and Langston C.[1]

familial predisposition.[144] Inhaled nitric oxide enhances oxygenation but not survival in these infants.[145]

Other congenital vascular lesions associated with a poor prognosis include diffuse pulmonary arteriovenous malformations,[146] veno-occlusive disease,[147] and pulmonary vein atresia/stenosis.[39,69] Although not true ILD, these lesions usually present with diffuse infiltrates and are often misdiagnosed as ILD.[148]

CLINICAL PRESENTATION

Most children with ILD share a common presentation with signs and symptoms of restrictive lung disease. A careful history should be taken to assess the severity and to elicit information that may contribute to the diagnosis. The onset of symptoms is often insidious; many children may have had symptoms for years prior to the diagnosis of ILD.

Some children with ILD have been misdiagnosed as having asthma and treated with bronchodilators.[69] Although a history of wheezing can be elicited in 50% of patients, it can be documented by physical examination in only about 20% of patients. More typical symptoms include cough, dyspnea, chronic tachypnea and retractions, exercise limitation, and frequent respiratory infections (Figure 6–5). Symptoms tend to be more continuous in ILD and more episodic in asthma, which helps to distinguish between the two conditions.

A search for precipitating factors should include a careful feeding history to rule out potential causes of aspiration, any prior acute or severe respiratory infections, and environmental exposures, especially to birds or molds. Hemoptysis may indicate a pulmonary vascular disorder or hemosiderosis. Joint disease or rash may indicate a systemic process such as connective tissue disease. A family history of relatives or siblings with similar lung conditions may be a clue to genetic or familial lung diseases such as SP-B deficiency.

On physical examination, tachypnea and retractions are often observed, and crackles are commonly heard, particularly at the bases. Severe cases are characterized by cyanosis, clubbing, an increased pulmonic second sound (P_2), and evidence of growth failure (Figure 6–6).

DIAGNOSTIC EVALUATION

A systematic approach to pediatric patients with ILD is essential when confronting a symptom complex with a large and varied differential of rare conditions. Diagnostic studies can be divided into those used to (1) assess the extent and severity of disease, (2) identify disorders that predispose to ILD, and (3) identify the primary ILD (Table 6–4). In adults with ILD, Raghu[149] suggested a diagnostic process that begins with a thorough history and physical examination, continues with noninvasive tests, and finally involves invasive studies that

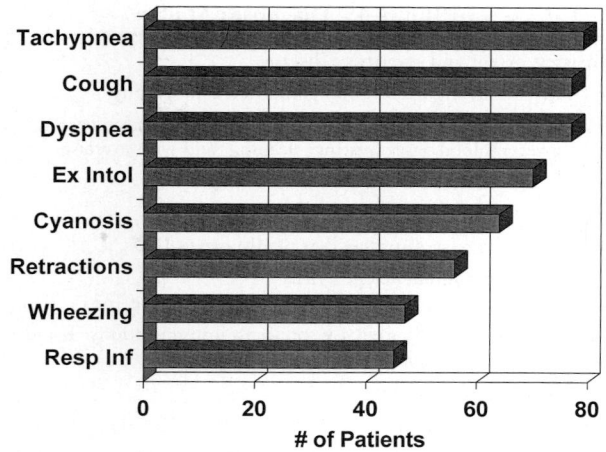

Figure 6–5   Symptoms in 99 children with ILD seen at the University of Colorado from 1980 to 1994. Ex Intol = exercise intolerance; Resp Inf = frequent respiratory infections.

include bronchoalveolar lavage, transbronchial biopsy, and open lung biopsy, if previous less invasive studies have not provided a specific diagnosis. Based on a retrospective chart review of 48 children with ILD,[69] this author and colleagues independently developed an algorithm remarkably similar to the one developed by Raghu and used it prospectively in the evaluation of 51 children presenting with ILD.[39] In this study, a specific diagnosis was established by history and physical examination alone in 1 patient, noninvasive studies alone in 8 others, and invasive studies that included a lung biopsy in another 26. Of the remaining patients, 8 had a suggestive diagnosis, and 8 had no specific diagnosis. This study suggests that a systematic approach to the diagnosis of pediatric ILD is useful, and that lung biopsy is

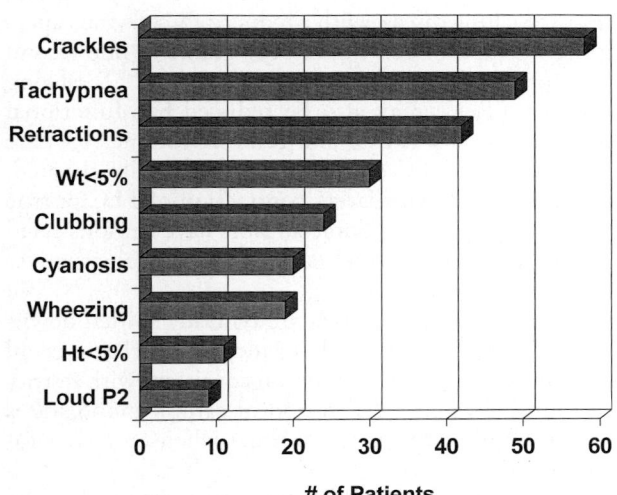

Figure 6–6   Physical findings in the same group as in Figure 6–5. Wt < 5% = weight less than the fifth percentile for age; Ht < 5% = height less than the fifth percentile for age.

TABLE 6–4   Diagnostic Studies

To assess extent and severity of disease

Chest films, high-resolution computed tomography

Pulmonary function studies: spirometry; pulse oximetry and arterial blood gases (resting, sleeping, and with exercise); diffusion, pressure-volume curve, infant studies

Electrocardiogram, echocardiogram

To identify primary disorders that predispose to ILD

Human immunodeficiency virus

Immune studies: immunoglobulins including IgE, skin tests for delayed hypersensitivity, response to immunizations, T and B subsets, complement, others as indicated

Barium swallow, pH probe

To identify primary ILD

Antinuclear antibody

Angiotensin converting enzyme

Antineutrophil cytoplasmic antibody

Antiglomerular basement membrane antibody

Hypersensitivity screen

Infectious disease evaluation: cultures, titers, skin tests

Cardiac catheterization (in selected cases)

Bronchoalveolar lavage and transbronchial biopsy

Transthoracic biopsy

ILD = interstitial lung disease.

not always required for diagnosis. These findings were essentially confirmed in a larger multicenter study, although noninvasive studies alone were slightly less helpful in establishing a diagnosis.[150]

Pulmonary Function Tests

Pulmonary function tests typically show a pattern of restrictive lung disease with a reduced forced vital capacity (FVC) and forced expiratory volume in one second (FEV_1) as well as a normal FEV_1/FVC ratio.[69] Total lung capacity (TLC) may also be reduced but functional residual capacity (FRC) and residual volume (RV) are variable. FRC/TLC and RV/TLC are usually elevated, reflecting a relatively larger contraction of TLC or true hyperinflation.[73,77,151] Some authors have demonstrated airflow limitation, which suggests mixed obstructive/restrictive disease.[4]

Pressure-volume curves are typically shifted downward and to the right with an increase in elastic recoil pressure at maximum inspiration consistent with restrictive lung disease.[73,77] Diffusion of carbon monoxide is low in absolute terms but normal when corrected for alveolar volume.[73,151]

Infant pulmonary function testing can also be used to follow infants with ILD and their response to treatment. In three infants with chronic ILD, respiratory system compliance, measured by multiple occlusion and end-inspiratory techniques, improved following administration of hydroxycholoroquine and/or pulse corticosteroids.[152]

Severity of illness can be graded by oxygen saturation and the development of pulmonary hypertension (Table 6–5).[1,153] Most patients with mild disease are normoxic under all conditions, but they may desaturate with exercise or during sleep as the disease progresses and ventilation-perfusion mismatch ensues. Patients with more advanced disease will be hypoxemic at rest. The development of pulmonary hypertension is often indicative of a poor prognosis (see section on "Outcome"). Children with ILD have increased neural drive either due to hypoxemia or to increased elastic load.[154]

High-Resolution Computed Tomography

As in adults, high-resolution computed tomography (HRCT) has become an important diagnostic tool in the evaluation of children with ILD.[155–157] It combines thin-section computed tomography with a high-frequency resolution algorithm and reduces the field of view to image one lung or a portion of one lung. It is often difficult to obtain optimal studies in infants whose rapid breathing creates motion artifacts, although this problem has been corrected to some degree by helical or spiral computed tomography (scan time: 0.6 seconds) or by the use of ultrafast computed tomography (Imatron) (scan time: 0.17 seconds).

Compared to plain chest radiographs, HRCT provides more precise detail about the extent and distribution of parenchymal disease. This information can then be used to select favorable biopsy sites. In a recent study of 20 children with biopsy-proven ILD, Lynch and colleagues[158] found that 56% of the confident first-choice diagnoses on HRCT were correct. Diseases were classified into five distinct groups based on dominant HRCT features: geographic hyperlucency (BO or bronchocentric granulomatosis), septal thickening (lymphangiomatosis, hemangiomatosis, microlithiasis), ground-glass opacification (DIP, LIP, HP), lung cysts and nodules (histiocytosis), and consolidation (aspiration, bronchiolitis obliterans organizing pneumonia). In this study, HRCT increased the level of diagnostic confidence for the diagnosis of pediatric ILD, improved diagnostic accuracy, and provided a useful classification

TABLE 6–5   Classification of Severity of Illness

1. Asymptomatic

2. Symptomatic, normal room air oxygen saturation under all conditions

3. Symptomatic, normal resting room air saturation but abnormal saturation with sleep or exercise

4. Symptomatic, abnormal resting room air saturation

5. Symptomatic with pulmonary hypertension

system. The diagnostic accuracy of HRCT in pediatric ILD was confirmed in another recent study.[159]

In children, HRCT is a valuable tool in the diagnosis of BO. The characteristic features of this lesion are striking, geographic, low lung density, attenuation of pulmonary vasculature, and central bronchiectasis.[160] In Swyer-James syndrome, these findings are associated with a unilateral, small hyperlucent lung (Figure 6–7). The author's experience suggests that in the absence of unilateral hyperlucency, characteristic HRCT findings may be sensitive but not specific for BO in children.

Bronchoalveolar Lavage

In children, as in adults, the recovery of pulmonary cells and alveolar lining fluid by BAL has been used to diagnose certain pulmonary disorders and to study disease mechanisms.[161–163] The technique can be performed under direct vision with a pediatric flexible fiberoptic bronchoscope or as a blind technique with a catheter placed through an endotracheal tube.[1,164,165]

Recent reports have established normal pediatric BAL indices with which abnormal values can be compared.[166–170] In most of these studies, the normal pediatric values for BAL fluid constituents were similar to those found in adults. The technique is not yet standardized with respect to lavage fluid amount and temperature, dwell time, and inclusion of the first aliquot. Pediatric pulmonologists either correct for size or body weight (eg, 10% FRC or 1 mL/kg/aliquot × 3 aliquots)[1,166–169] or use a fixed amount of lavage fluid regardless of size (eg, 10 mL/aliquot × 2 aliquots).[170] A recent report supports the former approach by demonstrating that a BAL protocol adjusted to body weight will yield constant fractions of epithelial lining fluid in children aged 3 to 15 years, facilitating the comparison of BAL fluid constituents in children of different age groups.[168]

The most common indication for pediatric BAL has been to detect infection in the immunocompromised host.[171–190] The overall diagnostic yield for a specific infectious agent was 47% (117 of 249 patients) in eight studies of immunocompromised children without AIDS.[178–185] The yield was 77% (134 of 174 patients) in five studies of children with AIDS.[186–190]

The usefulness of BAL to detect infection has also been demonstrated in immunocompetent hosts.[191–197] It is, however, often difficult to determine whether recovered organisms represent true infection, colonization, or contamination. In a recent study of healthy children requiring intubation for minor surgery, potentially pathogenic bacteria were recovered from the larynx and trachea in the majority of these children, suggesting that healthy children harbor potential pathogens in their upper airways and that aspirates from the trachea or larynx are of limited value in the diagnosis of bacterial pneumonia.[198] Similarly, BAL in children may be prob-

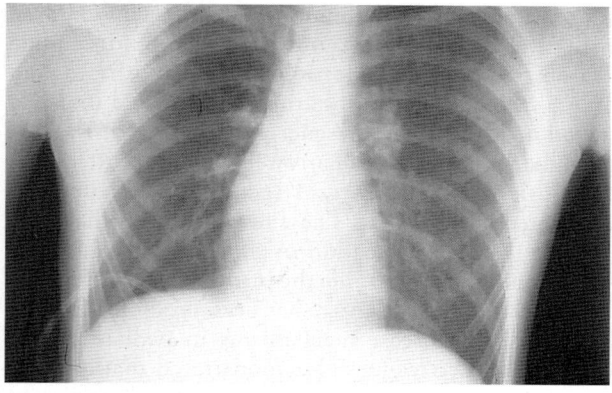

A

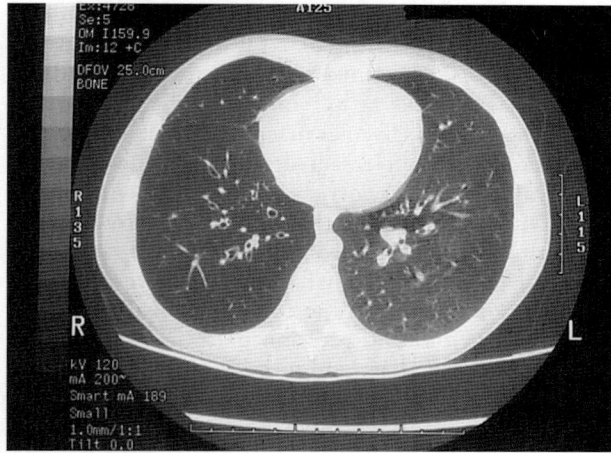

B

Figure 6–7   Swyer-James syndrome in a child. *A*, Chest roentgenogram shows a small right lung with decreased bronchovascular markings. *B*, HRCT scan shows central bronchiectasis, hyperlucency, and vascular attenuation in the right lung, and mild peripheral hyperlucency with vascular attenuation in the left lung.

lematic for detecting bacterial infection due to contamination. In studies that compare nasal or oropharyngeal lavage cultures with BAL cultures, BAL culture was used as the standard by which the upper airway cultures were compared, but the significance of a positive BAL culture was not adequately addressed.[192,197]

Other pediatric conditions identified by BAL include aspiration by the detection of lipid-laden macrophages[17–22] and pulmonary hemorrhage by the detection of hemosiderin-laden macrophages.[122] The presence of lipid- and hemosiderin-laden macrophages in BAL fluid may, however, be sensitive to but not specific for aspiration and alveolar hemorrhage syndromes, respectively.[23] As suggested earlier, the detection of specific milk proteins in alveolar macrophages in BAL fluid may ultimately be more sensitive and specific for aspiration.[25] In addition, BAL has been used to diagnose alveolar proteinosis,[199] lysosomal storage disorders,[200,201] and histiocytosis[202] in children.

As a diagnostic tool in immunocompetent children with ILD, this author found that BAL fluid, studied prospectively, was diagnostic of a primary disorder in only 5 of 29 patients; aspiration was detected in 3 and infection in 2.[23] The presence of lymphocytosis, neutrophilia, or eosinophilia narrowed down the differential diagnosis in 15 patients. A secondary disorder was uncovered in 8 patients. These results suggest that BAL provides useful information in children with ILD, but that its ability to determine the primary cause is limited.

Bronchoalveolar lavage has been used on a limited basis to study disease mechanisms in pediatric ILD. Clement and colleagues[203] demonstrated that alveolar macrophages in children with ILD released more oxygen metabolites, compared with a control group, and this finding correlated with disease activity. Chadelat and colleagues[204] found that BAL fluid from children with sarcoidosis contained more lymphocytes, with an elevated CD4/CD8 ratio, similar to the findings in adults. In addition, alveolar macrophages demonstrated enhanced ability to release hydrogen peroxide, an effect that diminished after corticosteroid treatment. Tessier and colleagues[205] showed that BAL cells from children with sarcoidosis contained varying degrees of IL-1β, TNF-α, IL-6, and transforming growth factor-β expression not found in the control group. They suggested that cytokine expression patterns may help to evaluate disease activity and severity. Chadelat and colleagues[206] found increased expression of insulin-like growth factor binding protein-2 in children with ILD, suggesting that this protein is important in the injury/repair process. In a group of children with chronic diffuse lung disease, Rhonchetti and colleagues[207] reported increased numbers of foamy macrophages and increases in fibronectin, hyaluronic acid, and albumin in the early stages of disease and increased lymphocytes in long-standing disease.

Lung Biopsy

Most diseases are classified in terms of previously described histopathologic patterns, therefore, lung biopsy is the gold standard for the diagnosis of pediatric ILD.[150] Lung tissue adequate for diagnosis has been successfully obtained by transbronchial biopsy (TBB), percutaneous needle biopsy, conventional open lung biopsy (OLB), and video-assisted thoracoscopy (VAT).

Pediatric TBB has been used primarily to monitor for infection or allograft rejection in children with lung or heart/lung transplants.[173,208–210] Transbronchial biopsy also has high diagnostic yield in pediatric sarcoidosis, but it is of limited value in differentiating among other types of ILD.[211–213] Because the operating channel in conventional pediatric flexible bronchoscopes is not sufficiently large to pass standard biopsy forceps, the technique has been limited mainly to older children who can tolerate an adult bronchoscope. Transbronchial biopsy has, however, been performed successfully in younger children using either general anesthesia and a rigid bronchoscope[208–210] or a suction catheter and an ultrathin flexible bronchoscope.[214]

Several recent reports have advocated percutaneous needle biopsy[215] combined with HRCT guidance[216] as a cost effective, acceptable-risk alternative to open lung biopsy. Although this procedure appears to hold promise, its exact role in the diagnosis of pediatric ILD remains to be seen.[217,218]

Transthoracic lung biopsy, either OLB[219–227] or VAT,[228–236] is the most reliable way to obtain adequate tissue for diagnosis. Whatever technique is used, lung biopsy material must be processed in a consistent manner to ensure optimal interpretation. This includes the preparation of imprints from biopsy tissue and the preservation of tissue using several modalities for optimum diagnostic yield. Tissue for light microscopy should be fixed or frozen in expansion by methods previously reported.[1] It is critical that all such biopsies be interpreted by a pathologist with considerable expertise in pediatric lung disease, because the normal lung of an infant differs markedly from that of an older child or adolescent, and any pathologic findings should be interpreted in the light of the normal age-dependent variations of lung architecture.

As in adults, the use of VAT is rapidly becoming the method of choice for lung biopsy in children, and technical modifications have permitted it even in infants.[232,233] In a recent prospective study in a small group of immunocompetent children with ILD, this author found that the diagnostic yield was comparable for OLB (57%) and VAT (54%), but the morbidity from VAT was clearly lower with respect to duration of surgery, chest tube, and hospitalization.[211] Although multiple lobe biopsies directed by HRCT have been advocated for the diagnosis of both adult and pediatric ILD, this study did not show a difference in the diagnostic yield for single-versus multiple-lobe biopsies. Overall, the diagnostic yield from transthoracic lung biopsy (OLB and VAT) was disappointing, due in large part to an extremely low diagnostic yield in children less than two years of age. As this study was done before many of the recently defined diffuse diseases of infants were described, the diagnostic yield in infants is probably higher.

TREATMENT

Supportive care includes adequate nutrition, annual influenza vaccination, aggressive treatment of intercurrent infections, a carefully supervised fitness and exercise program, avoidance of inhalant hazards such as tobacco smoke, selective use of bronchodilators, and administration of oxygen for chronic hypoxemia. Patients with underlying systemic disorders need primary treatment for that disorder (eg, gamma globulin for hypogammaglobulinemia).[237,238] Specific therapy for primary ILD is preferable to less specific treatment, and includes anti-infective therapy for chronic infections, interferon alpha for pulmonary hemangiomatosis,[239,240] and lung lavage[241] and possibly granulocyte-macrophage colony–stimulating factor[242] for alveolar proteinosis. Avoidance is critical when environmental agents such as bird antigens are causative.

Although controlled clinical studies are lacking, corticosteroids have been used to treat UIP,[72–77] DIP,[77–87] LIP,[91,93,101,106] and hypersensitivity pneumonitis.[40,41,43,48,54,55,59,63] On the assumption that suppression of inflammation might be beneficial, corticosteroids are, in general, the treatment of choice for most patients with ILD.[243] In the author's retrospective study, corticosteroids were judged to be effective in 40% (12/30) of treated children with ILD as demonstrated by improved clinical status, decreased oxygen requirements, and improved pulmonary function.[69] Thus, a trial of prednisone or an equivalent corticosteroid, 1 to 2 mg/kg/day, for at least 6 to 8 weeks, is probably warranted. Alternatively, pulse methylprednisolone therapy, 20 to 30 mg/kg given intravenously once a day for 3 days, administered monthly has been anecdotally reported to improve infants with pulmonary fibrosis,[130] and a child with DIP.[244]

Other unproven therapy includes hydroxychloroquine, azathioprine, cyclophosphamide, methotrexate, cyclosporin, and intravenous gammaglobulin. Of these, hydroxychloroquine has probably been used most frequently.[69,77,84,85,101,132,134,152,245,246] Although the precise mechanism of action is unknown, chloroquine and hydroxychloroquine have demonstrated immunosuppressive effects and inhibit both the functional capabilities of monocytes as well as the generation of antibody-forming cells.[247] In one study, seven children with ILD were treated with chloroquine and hydroxychloroquine with generally favorable results.[245] This author's experience[69] has been similar to that of Sharief and colleagues.[77] in that these drugs work well in some patients but not in others. Although used mainly for DIP or nonspecific ILD, chloroquine has been reported to be effective in LIP[69] and pulmonary hemosiderosis.[246] Hydroxychloroquine is preferable to chloroquine because the former is believed to be associated with a lower incidence of retinal toxicity. The recommended dose in children for the treatment of ILD is 10 mg/kg/day.

The existence of so many alternative pharmacologic approaches to ILD implies that conventional therapy is often ineffective. New strategies based on animal models of pulmonary fibrosis and recent advances in the cellular and molecular biology of inflammatory reactions are being developed.[8,9] Such therapies are directed against certain cytokines, oxidants, and growth factors that may be involved in the fibrotic process. The potential to deliver specific inflammatory inhibitors or inhibitors of collagen biosynthesis directly to the lung via aerosolization should make delivery of these agents more efficient than to other internal organs.

More children than in the past are receiving lung transplantation for end-stage ILD.[248–251] For example, from June, 1990, to January, 1996, 105 children received lung or heart-lung transplants at St. Louis Children's Hospital (Mallory and Cohen, personal communication, 1996). Nineteen of these children, ages 1 month to 17 years (mean 6.8 years), had interstitial lung disease, including pulmonary fibrosis (11), SP-B deficiency (3), alveolar proteinosis (2), bronchopulmonary dysplasia (2), and familial chronic interstitial lung disease of infancy (1). To date, the 1- and 3-year survival is 88%, which is higher but not statistically different from the survival of recipients with other conditions. Thus far there has been no evidence of recurrence of underlying disease in the allografts.

OUTCOME

The prognosis for children with ILD is variable. Infants with NEHI generally do well, although they may remain symptomatic and require oxygen for years. At the other end of the spectrum, children with growth failure, pulmonary hypertension, and severe fibrosis do poorly.

In contrast to adult studies, histologic appearance graded on the basis of inflammation versus fibrosis did not correlate with response to treatment or outcome in two studies,[72,77] although the presence of fibrosis on biopsy was associated with a lower specific dynamic lung compliance in another study.[75] Thus, the prognostic significance of inflammation versus fibrosis found on lung biopsy is uncertain in children.

The overall mortality rates for pediatric ILD remain high. In a series of 25 children with fibrosing alveolitis or DIP, Sharief and colleagues[77] reported a poor response to treatment in 9 patients, with 4 deaths. In a review of 28 patients with DIP, Stillwell and colleagues[82] reported that only 17 patients survived. In a series of 17 children with a variety of ILD, including DIP, LIP, pulmonary hemosiderosis, HP, and interstitial fibrosis associated with severe combined immunodeficiency, Diaz and Bowman[4] reported that 50% had a poor quality of life and that 19% died. In a recent series of biopsy-proven ILD, Nicholson and colleagues[70] reported 4 deaths in 17 patients with known outcome.

Fan and Kozinetz recently reviewed the outcome of 99 children with a variety of chronic ILDs seen in Denver, Colorado over a 15-year period (1980 to 1994).[153] There were 15 recorded deaths with a probability that a patient would survive to 24, 48, and 60 months after the onset of symptoms of 83, 72, and 64%, respectively (Table 6–6). Of the clinical features present at the time of initial evaluation, weight < 5%, crackles, clubbing, family history of ILD, and symptom duration were not associated with decreased survival. The simple scoring system for severity of illness, previously shown in Table 6–4, appears to be a useful measure of outcome in children with ILD. An increasing score was associated with a higher probability of decreased survival (Table 6–7).

TABLE 6–6   ILD Diagnoses and Deaths

	# Patients	# Dead
Specific diagnosis	71	
Infection/no bronchiolitis obliterans	10	0
Bronchiolitis obliterans/adenovirus	5	0
Bronchiolitis obliterans/no adenovirus	4	0
Hypersensitivity pneumonitis	7	1
Pulmonary vascular disease	8	5
Lymphocytic interstitial pneumonitis	6	0
Desquamative interstitial pneumonitis	4	4
Usual interstitial pneumonitis	2	0
Aspiration	4	1
Hemosiderosis	5	1
Lymphangiomatosis	4	1
Sarcoidosis	2	0
Connective tissue disease	2	0
Pulmonary infiltrates with eosinophilia	2	0
Miscellaneous (BOOP, IBD, PAP, PM, BCG, Lymphoma)	6	1
Suggestive diagnosis	9	
Hypersensitivity pneumonitis	5	0
Miscellaneous (aspiration, sarcoidosis, EBV, LIP)	4	0
No specific diagnosis	19	1
TOTAL	99	15

BOOP = bronchiolitis obliterans organizing pneumonia; IBD = inflammatory bowel disease; PAP = pulmonary alveolar proteinosis; PM = pulmonary microlithiasis; BCG = bronchocentric granulomatosis; EBV = Epstein-Barr virus; LIP = lymphocytic interstitial pneumonitis. Adapted from Fan LL and Kozinetz CA.[153]

SUMMARY

Pediatric ILD comprises a large, heterogeneous group of mostly rare disorders that are associated with considerable morbidity and mortality and are difficult to diagnose and treat. Although many of these diseases overlap

TABLE 6–7   Probability of Survival by Severity of Illness Score

	Probability of Survival (%)			
Score	24 mo	48 mo	60 mo	p Value
2	100	67	67	—
3, 4, 5	78	71	61	.09
2, 3	100	67	67	—
4, 5	76	69	59	.03
2, 3, 4	93	76	76	—
5	57	57	38	.001

Adapted from Fan LL and Kozinetz CA.[153]

their adult counterparts, many have features unique to children. A systematic approach to diagnosis is valuable to clinicians confronted with so large a differential diagnosis. As in adult ILD, the response to treatment of pediatric ILD is inconsistent. Due to the rarity of each entity in children, multicenter collaboration, already started in Europe,[150] should be encouraged because no single center can see a sufficient number of patients to adequately study these diseases.[252]

REFERENCES

1. Fan LL, Langston C. Chronic interstitial lung disease in children. Pediatr Pulmonol 1993;16:184–96.
2. Fan LL. Evaluation and therapy of chronic interstitial lung pneumonitis in children. Curr Opin Pediatr 1994;6:248–54.
3. Bokulic RE, Hilman BC. Interstitial lung disease in children. Pediatr Clin North Am 1994;41:543–66.
4. Diaz RP, Bowman CM. Childhood interstitial lung disease. Semin Respir Med 1990;11:253–68.
5. Laraya-Cuasay LR, Hughes WT. Interstitial lung disease in children. Boca Raton: CRC Press, 1988.
6. Crouch E. Pathobiology of pulmonary fibrosis. Am J Physiol 1990;259:L159–84.
7. Cherniack RM, Crystal RG, Kalica AR. Current concepts in idiopathic pulmonary fibrosis: a road map for the future. Am Rev Respir Dis 1991;143:680–3.
8. Goldstein RH, Fine A. Potential therapeutic initiatives for fibrogenic lung diseases. Chest 1995;108:848–55.
9. Hunninghake GW, Kalica AR. Approaches to the treatment of pulmonary fibrosis. Am J Respir Crit Care Med 1995;151:915–8.
10. Bauer ML, Figueroa-Colon R, Georgeson K, et al. Chronic pulmonary aspiration in children. South Med J 1993;86:789–95.
11. Colombo JL. Assessment of aspiration syndromes in children. Clin Pulm Med 1998;5:300–6.
12. Wolfson BJ, Allen JL, Panitch HB, et al. Lipid aspiration pneumonia due to gastroesophageal reflux. Pediatr Radiol 1989;19:545–7.
13. Kurlandsky LE, Vaandrager V, Davy CL, et al. Lipoid pneumonia in association with gastroesophageal reflux. Pediatr Pulmonol 1992;13:184–8.
14. Owayed AF, Campbell DM, Wang EEL. Underlying causes of recurrent pneumonia in children. Arch Pediatr Adolesc Med 2000;154:190–4.
15. Fan LL, Graham LM. Lipoid pneumonia from mineral oil aspiration. Arch Pediatr Adolesc Med 1994;148:205–6.
16. Becton DL, Lowe JE, Falletta JM. Lipoid pneumonia in an adolescent girl secondary to use of lip gloss. J Pediatr 1984;105:421–3.
17. Colombo JL, Hallberg TK. Recurrent aspiration in children: lipid-laden alveolar macrophage quantitation. Pediatr Pulmonol 1987;3:86–9.
18. Nussbaum E, Maggi JC, Mathis R, et al. Association of lipid-laden alveolar macrophages and gastroesophageal reflux in children. J Pediatr 1987;110:190–4.
19. Colombo JL, Hallberg TK, Sammut PH. Time course of lipid-laden pulmonary macrophages with acute and recurrent milk aspiration in rabbits. Pediatr Pulmonol 1992;12:95–8.
20. Ahrens P, Noll C, Kitz R, et al. Lipid-laden alveolar macrophages (LLAM): a useful marker of silent aspiration in children. Pediatr Pulmonol 1999;28:83–8.
21. Bauer M, Lyrene RK. Chronic aspiration in children: evaluation of the lipid-laden macrophage index. Pediatr Pulmonol 1999;28:94–100.

22. Sacco O, Fregonese B, Silvestri M, et al. Bronchoalveolar lavage and esophageal pH monitoring data in children with "difficult to treat" respiratory symptoms. Pediatr Pulmonol 2000;30:313–9.

23. Fan LL, Lum Lung MC, Wagener JS. The diagnostic value of bronchoalveolar lavage in immunocompetent children with chronic diffuse pulmonary infiltrates. Pediatr Pulmonol 1997;23:8–13.

24. Knauer-Fischer S, Ratjen F. Lipid-laden macrophages in bronchoalveolar lavage fluid as a marker for pulmonary aspiration. Pediatr Pulmonol 1999;27:419–22.

25. Elidemir O, Fan LL, Colasurdo GN. A novel diagnostic method for pulmonary aspiration in a murine model-immunocytochemical staining of milk proteins in alveolar macrophages. Am J Respir Crit Care Med 2000;161: 622–6.

26. Wohl MEB, Chernick V. Bronchiolitis. Am Rev Respir Dis 1978;118:759–81.

27. Teper AM, Kofman CD, Maffey AF, et al. Lung function in infants with chronic pulmonary disease after severe adenoviral illness. J Pediatr 1999;134:730–3.

28. Laraya-Cuasay LR, DeForest A, Huff D, et al. Chronic pulmonary complications of early influenza virus infection in children. Am Rev Respir Dis 1977;116:617–25.

29. Stokes D, Sigler A, Khouri NF, et al. Unilateral hyperlucent lung (Swyer-James syndrome) after severe *Mycoplasma pneumoniae* infection. Am Rev Respir Dis 1978;117:145–52.

30. Kim CK, Chung CY, Kim JS, et al. Late abnormal findings on high-resolution computed tomography after *Mycoplasma* pneumonia. Pediatrics 2000;105:372–8.

31. Harrison HR, Taussig LM, Fulginiti VA. *Chlamydia trachomatis* and chronic respiratory disease in childhood. Pediatr Infect Dis 1982;1:29–33.

32. Mistchenko AS, Lenzi HL, Thompson FM, et al. Participation of immune complexes in adenovirus infection. Acta Paediatr 1992;81:983–8.

33. Mistchenko AS, Diez RA, Mariani AL, et al. Cytokines in adenoviral disease in children: association of interleukin-6, interleukin-8, and tumor necrosis factor alpha levels with clinical outcome. J Pediatr 1994;124:714–20.

34. Chang AB, Masel JP, Masters B. Post-infectious bronchiolitis obliterans: clinical, radiological and pulmonary function sequelae. Pediatr Radiol 1998;28:23–9.

35. Chan PWK, Muridan R, Debruyne JA. Bronchiolitis obliterans in children: clinical profile and diagnosis. Respirology 2000;5:369–75.

36. Zhang L, Irion K, Kozakewich H, et al. Clinical course of postinfectious bronchiolitis obliterans. Pediatr Pulmonol 2000;29:341–50.

37. Jobe AH, Bancalari E. Bronchopulmonary dysplasia. Am J Respir Crit Care Med 2001;163:1723–9.

38. Bousvaros A, Sundel R, Thorne GM, et al. Parvovirus B19-associated interstitial lung disease, hepatitis, and myositis. Pediatr Pulmonol 1998;26:365–9.

39. Fan LL, Kozinetz CA, Deterding RR, et al. Evaluation of a diagnostic approach to pediatric interstitial lung disease. Pediatrics 1998;101:82–5.

40. Eisenberg JD, Montanero A, Lee RG. Hypersensitivity pneumonitis in an infant. Pediatr Pulmonol 1992;12:186–90.

41. Stiehm ER, Reed CE, Tooley WH. Pigeon breeder's lung in children. Pediatrics 1967;39:904–15.

42. Shannon DC, Andrews JL, Recavarren S, et al. Pigeon breeder's lung disease and interstitial pulmonary fibrosis. Am J Dis Child 1969;117:504–10.

43. Chandra S, Jones HE. Pigeon fancier's lung in children. Arch Dis Child 1972;47:716–8.

44. Reiss JS, Weiss NS, Payette KM, et al. Childhood pigeon breeder's disease. Ann Allergy 1974;32:208–12.

45. Allen DH, Basten A, Williams GV, et al. Familial hypersensitivity pneumonitis. Am J Med 1975;59:505–14.

46. Purtilo DT, Brem J, Ceccaci L, et al. A family study of pigeon breeders' disease. J Pediatr 1975;86:569–71.

47. Miller MM, Patterson R, Fink JN, et al. Chronic hypersensitivity lung disease with recurrent episodes of hypersensitivity pneumonitis due to a contaminated central humidifier. Clin Allergy 1976;6:451–62.

48. Cunningham AS, Fink JN, Schlueter DP. Childhood hypersensitivity pneumonitis due to dove antigens. Pediatrics 1976;58:436–42.

49. Bureau MA, Fecteau C, Patriquin H, et al. Farmer's lung in early childhood. Am Rev Respir Dis 1979;119:671–5.

50. El-Hefny A, Ekladious EM, El-Sharkawy S, et al. Extrinsic allergic bronchiolo-alveolitis in children. Clin Allergy 1980;10:651–8.

51. Saltos N, Saunders NA, Bhagwandeen SB, et al. Hypersensitivity pneumonitis in a mouldy house. Med J Aust 1982;2:244–6.

52. Keith HH, Holsclaw DS, Dunsky EH. Pigeon breeder's disease in children. A family study. Chest 1981;79:107–10.

53. Vergesslich KA, Gotz M, Kraft D. [Bird breeder's lung with conversion to fatal fibrosing alveolitis.] Dtsch Med Wochenschr 1983;108:1238–42.

54. Chiron CC, Gaultier C, Boule M, et al. Lung function in children with hypersensitivity pneumonitis. Eur J Respir Dis 1984;65:79–91.

55. Barker PM, Warner JO. "Atypical pneumonia" due to parakeet sensitivity: bird fancier's lung in a 10-year-old girl. Br J Dis Chest 1984;78:404–7.

56. Park SM, Tremper L. Hypersensitivity pneumonitis in pediatric patients. Immunol Allergy Pract 1987;9:420–3.

57. Wolf SJ, Stillerman A, Weinberger M, Smith W. Chronic interstitial pneumonitis in a 3-year-old child with hypersensitivity to dove antigens. Pediatrics 1987;79:1027–9.

58. Balasubramaniam SK, O'Connell EJ, Yunginger JW, et al. Hypersensitivity pneumonitis due to dove antigens in an adolescent. Clin Pediatr 1987;26:174–6.

59. O'Connell EJ, Zorn JA, Gillespie DN, et al. Childhood hypersensitivity pneumonitis (farmer's lung): four cases in siblings with long-term follow-up. J Pediatr 1989;114:995–7.

60. Yee WFH, Castile RG, Cooper A, et al. Diagnosing bird fancier's disease in children. Pediatrics 1990;85:848–52.

61. Grammer LC, Roberts M, Lerner C, et al. Clinical and serologic follow-up of four children and five adults with bird-fancier's lung. J Allergy Clin Immunol 1990;85:655–60.

62. Swingler GH. Summer-type hypersensitivity pneumonitis in southern Africa. A report of 5 cases in one family. S Afr Med J 1990;77:104–7.

63. Krasnick J, Patterson R, Stillwell PC, et al. Potentially fatal hypersensitivity pneumonitis in a child. Clin Pediatr 1995;34:388–91.

64. Tsai E, Couture D, Hughes DM. A pediatric case of pigeon breeder's disease in Nova Scotia. Can Respir J 1998; 5:507–10.

65. Grech V, Vella C, Lenicker H. Pigeon breeder's lung in childhood: varied clinical picture at presentation. Pediatr Pulmonol 2000;30:145–8.

66. du MSG, Merkus PJ, de Jongste JC. A family with extrinsic allergic alveolitis caused by wild city pigeons: a case report. Pediatrics 2000;105:E62.

67. Cron RQ, Sherry DD, Wallace CA. Methotrexate-induced hypersensitivity pneumonitis in a child with juvenile rheumatoid arthritis. J Pediatr 1998;132:901–2.

68. Liebow AA. Definition and classification of interstitial pneumonias in human pathology. Prog Respir Res 1975;8:1–33.

69. Fan LL, Mullen ALW, Brugman SM, et al. Clinical spectrum of chronic interstitial lung disease in children. J Pediatr 1992;121:867–72.

70. Nicholson AG, Kim H, Corrin B, et al. The value of classifying interstitial pneumonitis in childhood according to defined histological patterns. Histopathology 1998;33:203–11.

71. Katzenstein AL, Myers JL. Idiopathic pulmonary fibrosis: clinical relevance of pathologic classification. Am J Respir Crit Care Med 1998;157:1301–15.

72. Hewitt CJ, Hull D, Keeling JW. Fibrosing alveolitis in infancy and childhood. Arch Dis Child 1977;52:22–37.

73. Zapletal A, Houstek J, Samanek M, et al. Lung function in children and adolescents with idiopathic interstitial pulmonary fibrosis. Pediatr Pulmonol 1985;1:154–66.

74. Chetty A, Bhuyan UN, Mitra DK, et al. Cryptogenic fibrosing alveolitis in children. Ann Allergy 1987;58:336–40.

75. Steinkamp G, Müller KM, Schirg E, et al. Fibrosing alveolitis in childhood. Acta Paediatr Scand 1990;79:823–31.

76. Riedler J, Golser A, Huttegger I. Fibrosing alveolitis in an infant. Eur Respir J 1992;5:359–61.

77. Sharief N, Crawford OF, Dinwiddie R. Fibrosing alveolitis and desquamative interstitial pneumonitis. Pediatr Pulmonol 1994;17:359–65.

78. Rosenow EC, O'Connell EJ, Harrison EG. Desquamative interstitial pneumonia in children. Am J Dis Child 1970;120:344–8.

79. Howatt WF, Heidelberger KP, LeGlovan DP, et al. Desquamative interstitial pneumonia. Am J Dis Child 1973;126:346–8.

80. Barnes SE, Godfrey S, Millward-Sadler GH, et al. Desquamative fibrosing alveolitis unresponsive to steroid or cytoxic therapy. Arch Dis Child 1975;50:324–27.

81. Wigger HJ, Berdon WE, Ores CN. Fatal desquamative interstitial pneumonia in an infant. Arch Pathol Lab Med 1977;101:129–32.

82. Stillwell PC, Norris DG, O'Connel EJ, et al. Desquamative interstitial pneumonitis in children. Chest 1980;77:165–71.

83. Boner A, Wilmott RW, Dinwiddie R, et al. Desquamative interstitial pneumonia and antigen-antibody complexes in two infants with congenital rubella. Pediatrics 1983;72:835–9.

84. Leahy F, Pasterkamp H, Tal A. Desquamative intersitial pneumonia responsive to chloroquine. Clin Pediatr 1985;24:230–2.

85. Springer C, Maayan C, Katzir Z, et al. Chloroquine treatment in desquamative interstitial pneumonia. Arch Dis Child 1987;62:76–7.

86. DiMaio MF, Dische R, Gordon RE, et al. Alveolar brush cells in an infant with desquamative interstitial pneumonia. Pediatr Pulmonol 1988;4:185–91.

87. Buchta RM, Park S, Giammona ST. Desquamative interstitial pneumonia in a 7-week-old infant. Am J Dis Child 1970;120:341–3.

88. Schroten H, Manz S, Köhler H, et al. Fatal desquamative interstitial pneumonia associated with proven CMV infection in an 8-month-old boy. Pediatr Pulmonol 1998;25:345–7.

89. Koss MN. Pulmonary lymphoid disorders. Semin Diagn Pathol 1995;12:158–71.

90. Kradin RL, Mark EJ. Benign lymphoid disorders of the lung, with a theory regarding their development. Hum Pathol 1983;14:857–67.

91. Pitt J. Lymphocytic interstitial pneumonia. Pediatr Clin North Am 1991;38:89–94.

92. Joshi VV, Kauffman S, Oleske JM, et al. Polyclonal polymorphic B-cell lymphoproliferative disorder with prominent pulmonary involvement in children with acquired immune deficiency syndrome. Cancer 1987;59:1455–62.

93. O'Brodovich HM, Moser MM, Lu L. Familial lymphoid interstitial pneumonia: a long-term follow-up. Pediatrics 1980;65:523–8.

94. Rogers BB, Browning I, Rosenblatt H, et al. A familial lymphoproliferative disorder presenting with primary pulmonary manifestations. Am Rev Respir Dis 1992;145:203–8.

95. Franchi LM, Chin TW, Nussbaum E, et al. Familial pulmonary nodular lymphoid hyperplasia. J Pediatr 1992;121:89–92.

96. Lovell D, Lindsley C, Langston C. Lymphoid interstitial pneumonia in juvenile rheumatoid arthritis. J Pediatr 1984;105:947–50.

97. Uziel Y, Hen B, Cordoba M, et al. Lymphocytic interstitial pneumonitis preceding polyarticular juvenile rheumatoid arthritis. Clin Exp Rheumatol 1998;16:617–9.

98. Tangsinmankong N, Wayne AS, Howenstine MS, et al. Lymphocytic interstitial pneumonitis, elevated IgM concentration, and hepatosplenomegaly in ataxia-telangiectasia. J Pediatr 2001;138:939–41.

99. Steele RW. A 13-year-old black male with splenomegaly and interstitial pneumonia. Ann Allergy 1983;51:569–83.

100. Church JA, Isaaca H, Saxon A, et al. Lymphoid interstitial pneumonitis and hypogammaglobulinemia in children. Am Rev Respir Dis 1981;124:491–6.

101. Waters KA, Bale P, Isaacs D, Mellis C. Successful chloroquine therapy in a child with lymphoid interstitial pneumonitis. J Pediatr 1991;119:989–91.

102. Marquis JR, Berman CZ, DiCarlo F, et al. Radiographic patterns of PLH/LIP in HIV positive children. Pediatr Radiol 1993;23:328–30.

103. Campos JMS, Simonetti JP. Treatment of lymphoid interstitial pneumonia with chloroquine. J Pediatr 1993;122:503.

104. Joshi VV, Oleske JM, Minnefor AB, et al. Pathologic pulmonary findings in children with AIDS. Hum Pathol 1985;16:241–6.

105. Scott GB, Hutto C, Makuch R, et al. Survival in children with perinatally acquired human immunodeficiency virus type 1 infection. N Engl J Med 1989;321:1791–6.

106. Rubinstein A, Bernstein LJ, Charytan M, et al. Corticosteroid treatment for pulmonary lymphoid hyperplasia in chidren with acquired immune deficiency syndrome. Pediatr Pulmonol 1988;4:13–7.

107. Rubinstein A, Morecki R, Goldman H. Pulmonary disease in infants and children. Clin Chest Med 1988;9:507–17.

108. Rubinstein A, Morecki R, Silverman B, et al. Pulmonary disease in children with acquired immune deficiency syndrome and AIDS-related complex. J Pediatr 1986;108:498–503.

109. Wilson H, Robinson C, Fan LL. Probable EB viral lung disease in a 2-year-old with AIDS-related complex. Pediatr Pathol 1986;5:121.

110. Fackler JC, Nagel JE, Adler WH, et al. Epstein-Barr virus infection in a child with acquired immunodeficiency syndrome. Am J Dis Child 1985;139:1000–4.

111. Katz BZ, Berkman AB, Shapiro ED. Serologic evidence of active Epstein-Barr virus infection in Epstein-Barr virus-associated lymphoproliferative disorders of children with acquired immunodeficiency syndrome. J Pediatr 1992;120:228–32.

112. Andiman WA, Martin K, Rubinstein A, et al. Opportunistic lymphoproliferations associated with Epstein-Barr viral DNA in infants and children with AIDS. Lancet 1985;ii:1390–3.

113. Malamou-Mitsi V, Tsai MM, Gal AA, et al. Lymphoid interstitial pneumonia not associated with HIV infection: role of Epstein-Barr virus. Mod Pathol 1992;5:487–91.

114. Deterding RR, Hay TC, Langston C, et al. Persistent tachypnea of infancy. Am J Respir Crit Care Med 1997;155:A715.

115. Pye C, Fan LL, Langston C. Pulmonary neuroendocrine cell hyperplasia in persistent tachypnea in infancy. Mod Pathol 1998;11:4P.

116. Kinane BT, Mansell AL, Zwerdling RG, et al. Follicular bronchitis in the pediatric population. Chest 1993;104:1183–6.

117. Hull J, Chow CF, Robertson CF. Chronic idiopathic bronchiolitis of infancy. Arch Dis Child 1997;77:512–5.

118. Schroeder SA, Shannon DC, Mark EJ. Cellular interstitial pneumonitis in infants—a clinicopathologic study. Chest 1992;101:1065–9.

119. Case records of the Massachusetts General Hospital. Case 40-1999. N Engl J Med 1999;341:2075–83.

120. Montana E, Etzel RA, Allan T, et al. Environmental risk fac-

tors associated with pediatric idiopathic pulmonary hemorrhage and hemosiderosis in a Cleveland community. Pediatrics 1997;99:1–8.

121. Pappas MD, Sarnaik AP, Meert KL, et al. Idiopathic pulmonary hemorrhage in infancy—clinical features and management with high frequency ventilation. Chest 1996;110:553–5.

122. Sherman JM, Winnie G, Thomassen MJ, et al. Time course of hemosiderin production and clearance of human pulmonary macrophages. Chest 1984;86:409–11.

123. Etzel RA, Montana E, Sorenson WG, et al. Acute pulmonary hemorrhage in infants associated with exposure to *Stachybotrys atra* and other fungi. Arch Pediatr Adolesc Med 1998;152:757–62.

124. Elidemir O, Colarsurdo GN, Rossman SN, et al. Isolation of *Stachybotrys* from the lung of a child with pulmonary hemosiderosis. Pediatrics 1999;104:964–6.

125. Office of the Director, Centers for Disease Control and Prevention. Update: pulmonary hemorrhage/hemosiderosis among infants-Cleveland Ohio, 1993–1996. MMWR 2000;49:180–4.

126. Vesper SJ, Dearborn DG, Elidemir O, et al. Quantification of siderophore and hemolysin from *Stachybotrys chartarum* strains, including a strain isolated from the lung of a child with pulmonary hemorrhage and hemosiderosis. Appl Environ Microbiol 2000;66:2678–81.

127. Katzenstein AL, Gordon LP, Oliphant M, et al. Chronic pneumonitis of infancy—a unique form of interstitial lung disease occurring in early childhood. Am J Surg Pathol 1995;19:439–47.

128. Fisher M, Roggli V, Merten D, et al. Coexisting endogenous lipoid pneumonia, cholesterol granulomas, and pulmonary alveolar proteinosis in a pediataric population: a clinical, radiographic, and pathologic correlation. Pediatr Pathol 1992;12:365–83.

129. Osika E, Muller MH, Boccon-Gibod L, et al. Idiopathic pulmonary fibrosis in infants. Pediatr Pulmonol 1997;23:49–54.

130. Desmarquest P, Tamalet A, Fauroux B, et al. Chronic interstitial lung disease: response to high-dose intravenous methylprednisolone pulses. Pediatr Pulmonol 1998;26:332–8.

131. Hacking D, Smyth R, Shaw N, et al. Idiopathic pulmonary fibrosis in infants: good prognosis with conservative management. Arch Dis Child 2000;83:152–7.

132. Tal A, Maor E, Bar-Ziv J, et al. Fatal desquamative interstitial pneumonia in three infant siblings. J Pediatr 1984;104:873–6.

133. Buchino JJ, Keenan WJ, Algren JT, et al. Familial desquamative interstitial pneumonitis occurring in infants. Am J Med Genet Suppl 1987;3:285–91.

134. Balasubramanyan N, Murphy A, O'Sullivan J, et al. Familial interstitial lung disease in children: response to chloroquine treatment in one sibling with desquamative interstitial pneumonitis. Pediatr Pulmonol 1997;23:55–61.

135. Nogee LM, deMello DE, Dehner LP, et al. Brief report: deficiency of pulmonary surfactant protein B in congenital alveolar proteinosis. N Engl J Med 1993;328:406–10.

136. Hamvas A, Nogee LM, Mallory GB, et al. Lung transplantation for treatment of infants with surfactant protein B deficiency. J Pediatr 1997;130:231–9.

137. Nogee LM, Gamier G, Dietz HC, et al. A mutation in the surfactant protein B gene responsible for fatal neonatal respiratory disease in multiple kindreds. J Clin Invest 1994;93:1860–3.

138. deMello DE, Nogee LM, Heyman S, et al. Molecular and phenotypic variability in the congenital alveolar proteinosis syndrome associated with inherited surfactant protein B deficiency. J Pediatr 1994;125:43–50.

139. Hamvas A, Cole S, deMello DE, et al. Surfactant protein B deficiency: antenatal diagnosis and prospective treatment with surfactant replacement. J Pediatr 1994;125:356–61.

140. Cutz E, Wert SE, Nogee LM, et al. Deficiency of lamellar bodies in alveolar type II cells associated with fatal respiratory disease in a full-term infant. Am J Respir Crit Care Med 2000;161:608–14.

141. Nogee LM, Dunbar AE, Wert SE, et al. A mutation in the surfactant protein C gene associated with familial interstitial lung disease. New Engl J Med 2001;344:573–9.

142. Amin RS, Wert SE, Baughman RP, et al. Surfactant protein deficiency in familial interstitial lung disease. J Pediatr 2001;139:85–92.

143. Abdallah HI, Karmazin N, Marks LA. Late presentation of misalignment of lung vessels with alveolar capillary dysplasia. Crit Care Med 1993;21:628–30.

144. Boggs S, Harris MC, Hoffman DJ, et al. Misalignment of pulmonary veins with alveolar capillary dysplasia: affected siblings and variable phenotypic expression. J Pediatr 1994;124:125–8.

145. Steinhorn RH, Cox PN, Fineman JR, et al. Inhaled nitric oxide enhances oxygenation but not survival in infants with alveolar capillary dysplasia. J Pediatr 1997;130:417–22.

146. Shapiro JL, Stillwell PC, Levien MG, et al. Diffuse pulmonary arteriovenous malformations (angiodysplasia) with unusual histologic features: case report and review of the literature. Pediatr Pulmonol 1996;21:255–61.

147. Justo RN, Dare AJ, Whight CM, et al. Pulmonary veno-occlusive disease: diagnosis during life in four patients. Arch Dis Child 1993;68:97–100.

148. Sondheimer HM, Lum Lung MC, Brugman SM, et al. Pulmonary vascular disorders masquerading as interstitial lung disease. Pediatr Pulmonol 1995;20:284–8.

149. Raghu G. Interstitial lung disease: a diagnostic approach. Are CT scan and lung biopsy indicated in every patient? Am J Respir Crit Care Med 1995;151:909–14.

150. Barbato A, Panizzolo C, Cracco A, et al. Interstitial lung disease: a multicentre survey on diagnostic approach. Eur Respir J 2000;16:509–13.

151. Gaultier CI, Chaussain M, Boulé M, et al. Lung function in interstitial lung diseases in children. Bull Eur Physiopathol Respir 1980;16:57–66.

152. Kerem E, Bentur L, England S, et al. Sequential pulmonary function measurements during treatment of infantile chronic interstitial pneumonitis. J Pediatr 1990;116:61–7.

153. Fan LL, Kozinetz CA. Factors influencing survival in children with chronic interstitial lung disease. Am J Respir Crit Care Med 1997;156:939–42.

154. Gaultier CI, Perret L, Boule M, et al. Control of breathing in children with interstitial lung disease. Pediatr Res 1982;16:779–83.

155. Lynch DA, Brasch RC, Hardy KA, et al. Pediatric pulmonary disease: assessment with high-resolution ultrafast CT. Radiology 1990;176:243–8.

156. Kuhn JP. High-resolution computed tomography of pediatric pulmonary parenchymal disorders. Radiol Clin North Am 1993;31:533–51.

157. Koh DM, Hansell DM. Computed tomography of diffuse interstitial lung disease in children. Clin Radiol 2000;55:659–67.

158. Lynch DA, Hay T, Newell JD, et al. Pediatric diffuse lung disease: diagnosis and classification using high-resolution CT. AJR Am J Radiol 1999;173:713–8.

159. Copley SJ, Coren M, Nicholson AG, et al. Diagnostic accuracy of thin-section CT and chest radiography of pediatric interstitial lung disease. AJR Am J Radiol 2000;174:549–54.

160. Carlson BA, Swensen SJ, Edell ES, et al. High-resolution computed tomography for obliterative bronchiolitis. Mayo Clin Proc 1993;68:307–8.

161. Henderson AJW. Bronchoalveolar lavage. Arch Dis Child 1994;70:167–9.

162. Boat TF, Tepper R, Stecenko A, et al. Assessment of lung function and dysfunction in studies in infants and children. Am Rev Respir Dis 1993;148:1105–8.

163. ERS Task Force on bronchoalveolar lavage in children. Bronchoalveolar lavage in children. Eur Respir J 2000;15:217–31.

164. Alpert BE, O'Sullivan BP, Panitch HB. Nonbronchoscopic approach to bronchoalveolar lavage in children with artificial airways. Pediatr Pulmonol 1991;13:38–41.

165. Koumbourlis AC, Kurland G. Nonbronchoscopic bronchoalveolar lavage in mechanically ventilated infants: technique, efficacy, and applications. Pediatr Pulmonol 1993;15:257–62.

166. Ratjen F, Bredendiek M, Brendel M, et al. Differential cytology of bronchoalveolar lavage fluid in normal children. Eur Respir J 1994;7:1865–70.

167. Ratjen F, Bredendiek M, Zheng L, et al. Lymphocyte subsets in bronchoalveolar lavage fluid of children without bronchopulmonary disease. Am J Respir Crit Care Med 1995;152:174–8.

168. Ratjen F, Bruch J. Adjustment of bronchoalveolar lavage volume to body weight in children. Pediatr Pulmonol 1996;21:184–8.

169. Riedler J, Grigg J, Stone C, et al. Bronchoalveolar lavage cellularity in healthy children. Am J Respir Crit Care Med 1995;152:163–8.

170. Midulla F, Villani A, Merolla R, et al. Bronchoalveolar lavage studies in children without parenchymal lung disease: cellular constituents and protein levels. Pediatr Pulmonol 1995;20:112–8.

171. Abernathy-Carver KJ, Fan LL, Bognuniewicz M, et al. *Legionella* and *Pneumocystis* pneumonias in asthmatic children on high doses of systemic steroids. Pediatr Pulmonol 1994;18:135–8.

172. Mauch RJ, Bratton S, Myers T, et al. Influenza B virus infection in pediatric solid organ transplant recipients. Pediatrics 1994;94:225–9.

173. Kurland G, Noyes BE, Jaffe R, et al. Bronchoalveolar lavage and transbronchial biopsy in children following heart-lung and lung transplantation. Chest 1993;104:1043–8.

174. Parham DM, Bozeman P, Killian C, et al. Cytologic diagnosis of respiratory syncytial virus infection in a bronchoalveolar lavage specimen from a bone marrow transplant recipient. Am J Clin Pathol 1993;99:588–92.

175. Wood RE, Leigh MW, Retsch-Bogart G. Diagnosis of pneumonia in immunocompromised patients [letter]. J Pediatr 1990;116:836–7.

176. McCray PB, Wagener JS, Howe CWS. Bronchoscopic diagnosis of cytomegalovirus pneumonia following pediatric bone marrow transplantation. Am J Pediatr Hematol Oncol 1986;8:338–41.

177. Leigh MW, Henshaw NG, Wood RE. Diagnosis of *Pneumocystis carinii* pneumonia in pediatric patients using bronchoscopic bronchoalveolar lavage. Pediatr Infect Dis J 1985;4:408–10.

178. McCubbin MM, Trigg ME, Hendricker CM, et al. Bronchoscopy with bronchoalveolar lavage in the evaluation of pulmonary complications of bone marrow transplantation in children. Pediatr Pulmonol 1992;12:43–7.

179. Snyder CL, Ramsay NK, McGlave PB, et al. Diagnostic open-lung biopsy after bone marrow transplantation. J Pediatr Surg 1990;25:871–7.

180. Winthrop AL, Waddell T, Superina RA. The diagnosis of pneumonia in the immunocompromised child: use of bronchoalveolar lavage. J Pediatr Surg 1990;25:878–80.

181. Breuer R, Lossos IS, Lafair JS, et al. Utility of bronchoalveolar lavage in the assessment of diffuse pulmonary infiltrates in the nonAIDS immunocompromised patients. Respir Med 1990;84:313–6.

182. Allen KA, Markin RS, Rennard SI, et al. Bronchoalveolar lavage in liver transplant patients. Acta Cytol 1989;33:539–43.

183. Stokes DC, Shenep JL, Parham D, et al. Role of flexible bronchoscopy in the diagnosis of pulmonary infiltrates in pediatric patients with cancer. J Pediatr 1989;115:561–7.

184. Pattishall EN, Noyes BE, Orenstein DM. Use of bronchoalveolar lavage in immunocompromised children with pneumonia. Pediatr Pulmonol 1988;5:1–5.

185. Frankel LR, Smith DW, Lewiston NJ. Bronchoalveolar lavage for diagnosis of pneumonia in the immunocompromised child. Pediatrics 1988;81:785–8.

186. Abadco DL, Amaro-Galvez R, Rao M, et al. Experience with flexible fiberoptic bronchoscopy with bronchoalveolar lavage as a diagnostic tool in children with AIDS. Am J Dis Child 1992;146:1056–9.

187. Mattey JE, Fitzpatrick SB, Josephs SH, et al. Bronchoalveolar lavage for *Pneumocystis* pneumonia in HIV-infected children. Ann Allergy 1990;64:393–7.

188. de Blic J, Blanche S, Danel C, et al. Bronchoalveolar lavage in HIV infected patients with interstitial pneumonia. Arch Dis Child 1989;64:1246–50.

189. Sculerati N, Ambrosino MM, Avni-Singer AJ, et al. Diagnostic flexible bronchoscopy in human immunodefiency virus (HIV)-positive children. Int J Pediatr Otorhinolaryngol 1989;18:119–27.

190. Birriel JA, Adams JA, Saldana MA, et al. Role of flexible bronchoscopy and bronchoalveolar lavage in the diagnosis of pediatric acquired immunodeficiency syndrome-related pulmonary disease. Pediatrics 1991;87:897–9.

191. Chan S, Abadco DL, Steiner P. Role of flexible fiberoptic bronchoscopy in the diagnosis of childhood endobronchial tuberculosis. Pediatr Infect Dis J 1994;13:506–9.

192. Wang D, Clement P, Lauwers S. Comparison of bacterial culture results in bronchoalveolar lavage and nasal lavage fluid in children with pulmonary infection. Int J Pediatr Otorhinolaryngol 1994;28:149–55.

193. Grigg J, van den Borre C, Malfroot A, et al. Bilateral fiberoptic bronchoalveolar lavage in acute unilateral lobar pneumonia. J Pediatr 1993;122:606–8.

194. Derish MT, Kulhanjian JA, Frankel LR, et al. Value of bronchoalveolar lavage in diagnosing severe respiratory syncytial virus in infants. J Pediatr 1991;119:761–3.

195. Wheeler WB, Kurachek SC, Lobas JG, Einzig MJ. Acute hypoxemic respiratory failure caused by *Chlamydia trachomatis* and diagnosed by flexible bronchoscopy. Am Rev Respir Dis 1990;142:471–3.

196. Rock MJ. The diagnostic utility of bronchoalveolar lavage in immunocompetent children with unexplained infiltrates on chest radiograph. Pediatrics 1995;95:373–7.

197. Avital A, Uwyyed K, Picard E, et al. Sensitivity and specificity of oropharyngeal suction versus bronchoalveolar lavage in identifying respiratory tract pathogens in children with chronic pulmonary infection. Pediatr Pulmonol 1995;20:40–3.

198. Hjuler IM, Hansen MB, Olsen B, et al. Bacterial colonization of the larynx and trachea in healthy children. Acta Paediatr 1995;84:566–8.

199. Mahut B, Delacourt C, Scheinmann P, et al. Pulmonary alveolar proteinosis: experience with eight pediatric cases and a review. Pediatrics 1996;97:117–22.

200. Niggermann B, Rebien W, Rahn W, et al. Asymptomatic pulmonary involvement in 2 children with Niemann-Pick disease type B. Respiration 1994;61:55–7.

201. Carson KF, Williams CA, Rosenthal DL, et al. Bronchoalveolar lavage in a girl with Gaucher's disease—a case report. Acta Cytol 1994;38:597–600.

202. Refabert L, Rambaud C, Mamou-Mani T, et al. Cd1a-positive cells in bronchoalveolar lavage samples from children with Langerhans' cell histiocytosis. J Pediatr 1996;129:913–5.

203. Clement A, Chadelat K, Masliah J, et al. A controlled study of oxygen metabolite release by alveolar macrophages from children with interstitial lung disease. Am Rev Respir Dis 1987;136:1424–8.

204. Chadelat K, Baculard A, Grimfeld A, et al. Pulmonary sarcoidosis in children: serial evaluation of bronchoalveolar lavage cells during corticosteroid treatment. Pediatr Pulmonol 1993;16:41–7.

205. Tessier V, Chadelat K, Baculard A, et al. BAL in children—a controlled study of different cytology and cytokine expresson profiles by alveolar cells in pediatric sarcoidosis. Chest 1996;109:1430–8.

206. Chadelat K, Boule M, Corroyer S, et al. Expression of insulin-like growth factors and their binding proteins by bronchoalveolar lavage cells from children with and without interstitial lung disease. Eur Respir J 1998;11:1329–36.

207. Ronchetti R, Midulla F, Sandstrom T, et al. Bronchoavleolar lavage in children with chronic diffuse parenchymal lung disease. Pediatr Pulmonol 1999;27:395–402.

208. Scott JP, Higenbottam TW, Smyth RL, et al. Transbronchial biopsies in children after heart-lung transplantation. Pediatrics 1990;86:698–702.

209. Whitehead B, Scott JP, Helms P, et al. Technique and use of transbronchial biopsy in children and adolescents. Pediatr Pulmonol 1992;12:240–6.

210. Muntz HR, Wallace M, Lusk RP. Pediatric transbronchial lung biopsy. Ann Otol Rhinol Laryngol 1992;101:135–7.

211. Fan LL, Kozinetz CA, Wojtczak HA, et al. The diagnostic value of transbronchial, thoracoscopic, and open lung biopsy in immunocompetent children with chronic interstitial lung disease. J Pediatr 1997;131:565–9.

212. Fitzpatrick SB, Stokes DC, Marsh B, Wang K. Transbronchial lung biopsy in pediatric and adolescent patients. Am J Dis Child 1985;1239:46–9.

213. Treitman P, Herskowitz JL, Bass HN. Churg-Strauss syndrome in a 14-year-old boy diagnosed by transbronchial lung biopsy. Clin Pediatr 1991;30:502–5.

214. Mullins D, Livne M, Mallory GB, et al. A new technique for transbronchial biopsy in infants and small children. Pediatr Pulmonol 1995;20:253–7.

215. Smyth RL, Carty H, Thomas H, et al. Diagnosis of interstitial lung disease by a percutaneous lung biopsy sample. Arch Dis Child 1994;70:143–4.

216. Spencer AD, Alton HM, Raafat F, et al. Combined percutaneous lung biopsy and high-resolution computed tomography in the diagnosis and management of lung disease in children. Pediatr Pulmonol 1996;22:11–6.

217. Bush A. Diagnosis of interstitial lung disease. Pediatr Pulmonol 1996;2:81–2.

218. Flake AW. Is a CT guided needle better than a knife? Pediatr Pulmonol 1996;22:83–4.

219. Coren ME, Nicholson AG, Goldstraw P, et al. Open lung biopsy for diffuse interstitial disease in children. Eur Respir J 1999;14:817–21.

220. Early GL, Williams TE, Kilman JW. Open lung biopsy. Its effects on therapy in the pediatric patient. Chest 1985;87:467–9.

221. Prober CG, Whyte H, Smith CR. Open lung biopsy in immunocompromised children with pulmonary infiltrates. Am J Dis Child 1984;138:60–3.

222. Adeyemi SD, Ein SH, Simpson JS, et al. The value of emergency open lung biopsy in infants and children. J Pediatr Surg 1979;14:426–7.

223. Hewitt CJ, Hull D, Keeling JW. Open lung biopsy in children with diffuse lung disease. Arch Dis Child 1974;49:27–35.

224. Leijala M, Louhimo I, Lindfors EL. Open lung biopsy in children with diffuse pulmonary lesions. Acta Paediatr Scand 1982;71:717–20.

225. Stillwell PC, Cooney DR, Telander RL, et al. Limited thoracotomy in the pediatric patient. Mayo Clin Proc 1981;56:673–7.

226. Folglia RP, Shilyansky J, Fonkalsrud EW. Emergency lung biopsy in immunocompromised pediatric patients. Ann Surg 1989;210:90–2.

227. Doolin EJ, Luck SR, Sherman JO, et al. Emergency lung biopsy: friend or foe of the immunosuppressed child. J Pediatr Surg 1986;21:485–7.

228. Janik JS, Nagaraj HS, Groff DB. Thoracoscopic evaluation of intrathoracic lesions in children. J Thorac Cardiovasc Surg 1982;83:408–13.

229. de Campos JRM, Filho LOA, Werebe EC, et al. Thoracoscopy in children and adolescents. Chest 1997;111:494–7.

230. Rodgers BM, Moazam F, Talbort JL. Thoracoscopy in children. Ann Surg 1979;169:176–80.

231. Schropp KP. Thoracoscopy. Pediatr Ann 1993;22:686–96.

232. Rothenberg SS. Thoracoscopy in infants and children. Semin Pediatr Surg 1994;3:277–82.

233. Rothenberg SS, Wagener JS, Chang JHT, et al. The safety and efficacy of thoracoscopic lung biopsy for diagnosis and treatment of infants and children. J Pediatr Surg 1996;31:100–4.

234. Bullard KM, Adzick NS. Pediatric thoracoscopy: a new vista. Pediatr Pulmonol 1996;22:129–35.

235. Wood RE. Pediatric thoracoscopy. Pediatr Pulmonol 1996;22:79.

236. de Campos JRM, Filho LOA, Werebe EC, et al. Thoracoscopy in children and adolescents. Chest 1997;111:494–7.

237. Sweinberg SK, Wodell RA, Grodofsky MP. Retrospective analysis of the incidence of pulmonary disease in hypogammaglobulinemia. J Allergy Clin Immunol 1991;88:96–104.

238. Sotomayor JL, Douglas SD, Wilmott RW. Pulmonary manifestations of immune deficiency disease. Pediatr Pulmonol 1989;6:275–92.

239. White CW, Sondheimer HM, Crouch EC, et al. Treatment of pulmonary hemangiomatosis with recombinant interferon alfa-2a. N Engl J Med 1989;320:1197–200.

240. White CW, Wolf SJ, Korones D, et al. Treatment of childhood angiomatous diseases with recombinant interferon alfa-2a. J Pediatr 1991;118:59–66.

241. Hurrion EM, Pearson GA, Firmin RK. Childhood pulmonary alveolar proteinosis—extracorporeal membrane oxygenation with total cardiopulmonary support during bronchoalveolar lavage. Chest 1994;106:638–40.

242. Barraclough RM, Gillies AJ. Pulmonary alveolar proteinosis: a complete response to GM-CSF therapy. Thorax 2001;56:664–5.

243. de Benedictis FM, Canny GJ, Levison H. The role of corticosteroids in respiratory disease in children. Pediatr Pulmonol 1996;22:44–57.

244. Paul K, Klettke U, Moldenhauer J, et al. Increasing dose of methylprednisolone pulse therapy treats desquamative interstitial pneumonia in a child. Eur Respir J 1999;14:1429–32.

245. Avital A, Godfrey S, Maayan C, et al. Chloroquine treatment of interstitial lung disease in children. Pediatr Pulmonol 1994;18:356–60.

246. Bush A, Sheppard MN, Warner JO. Chloroquine in idiopathic pulmonary hemosiderosis. Arch Dis Child 1992;67:625–7.

247. Salmeron G, Lipsky PE. Immunosuppressive potential of antimalarials. Am J Med 1983;75:S19–24.

248. Mallory GB. The special challenges of pediatric lung transplantation. J Respir Dis Pediatr 2001;3:105–14.

249. Bellon G, Ninet J, Louis D, et al. Heart-lung transplantation in a 16-month-old infant. Chest 1992;102:299–300.

250. Bridges ND, Mallory GB, Huddleston CB, et al. Lung transplantation in infancy and early childhood. J Heart Lung Transplant 1996;15:895–902.

251. Noyes BE, Kurland G, Orenstein DM. Lung and heart-lung transplantion in children. Pediatr Pulmonol 1997;23:39–48.

252. Hilman BC. Diagnosis and treatment of ILD. Pediatr Pulmonol 1997;23:1–7.

7

GENETIC BASIS OF INTERSTITIAL LUNG DISEASE

FRANCIS X. MCCORMACK

Interstitial lung disease (ILD) is thought to result from dysfunction or disruption in pathways that regulate pulmonary inflammation, repair, and/or epithelial-mesenchymal interactions. Pulmonary fibrosis is the final common pathway for a variety of insults, and experimental reconstruction of the complex course of cellular and molecular events that lead to its development has proven to be a difficult, if not impossible, task. Recent advances in molecular genetics provide the opportunity to approach ILD pathogenesis from the vantage point of a primary molecular defect. The power of genetic analyses to focus attention on critical intracellular pathways and therapeutic targets is exemplified by the scientific trajectory in the pulmonary vascular and airway biology fields since the discovery of mutations in the cystic fibrosis transmembrane regulator gene in patients with cystic fibrosis, the α_1-antitrypsin gene in patients with inherited emphysema, and the bone morphogenetic protein receptor II (BMPRII) gene in patients with primary and sporadic pulmonary hypertension. Over the past 5 years, our understanding of the genetic basis of ILD has increased significantly. Investigators have identified the genes and gene products that are required for the maintenance of lysosomal pathways in Gaucher's disease, Hermansky-Pudlak syndrome, and Niemann-Pick disease; for surfactant homeostasis in pulmonary alveolar proteinosis; and for control of cellular growth and differentiation in lymphangioleiomyomatosis (LAM). Dissection of the fibrogenic pathways in these disease processes promises to shed light on the mechanisms of fibrosis in more common diseases such as idiopathic pulmonary fibrosis (IPF), sarcoidosis, and hypersensitivity pneumonitis.

Important principles of fibrogenesis have already begun to emerge from genetic ILD studies in mice and humans. The finding that ILD develops in patients with cytotoxic mutations in surfactant protein C (SP-C), a gene expressed only in alveolar type II cells, has underscored the importance of the integrity of the alveolar epithelium in the pathogenesis of alveolar fibrosis. Genetic modifier effects and environmental influences are clearly determinants of disease expression in SP-C-related ILD, because family members with inherited SP-C mutations can be unaffected or can present at any time from the first through the sixth decade of life with histopathologic manifestations that vary from nonspecific interstitial pneumonitis (NSIP) to usual interstitial pneumonitis (UIP). Gene-targeted mice with a deficiency of SP-C develop ILD on some backgrounds. The important role that cytokines and growth factors play in alveolar remodeling and synthetic function has been elucidated by genetic analysis of the granulocyte macrophage colony-stimulating factor (GM-CSF) pathway. Murine models of GM-CSF deficiency developed for the study of hematopoiesis were unexpectedly found to develop alveolar lipoprotein accumulation consistent with alveolar proteinosis. Subsequent studies in humans have revealed that familial alveolar proteinosis can result from mutations in genes for GM-CSF receptors and that sporadic alveolar proteinosis can occur in patients with circulating neutralizing antibodies to GM-CSF. The serendipitous discovery of the molecular basis of some forms of alveolar proteinosis attests to the power of genetic murine models to yield groundbreaking insights into human disease.

This chapter will focus primarily on the cellular and molecular basis of genetic ILD resulting from mutations in tumor suppressor genes, genes required for metabolic homeostasis, the SP-C gene, connective tissue genes, and other loci. The attention devoted to each disease reflects the state of scientific knowledge about the genetic basis of the illness and the frequency of ILD in the populations being discussed. The rationale for the latter criterion is that diseases associated with a very high penetrance of pulmonary fibrosis, such as Hermansky-Pudlak syndrome and tuberous sclerosis, are more likely to reveal causal links between genetic defects and the fibrosis, whereas genetic mutations associated with a low incidence of ILD may indicate that fibrosis occurs through secondary mechanisms. The potential of minor degrees of familial clustering in the more prevalent forms of ILD such as sarcoidosis, hypersensitivity pneumonitis, and IPF to yield insights into the pathogenesis of ILD will also be discussed, but the multicenter cooperative studies necessary for definitive conclusions are just being formed. Reports of candidate ILD loci and ILD-associated polymorphisms have been largely inconclusive and are often misleading; will only be mentioned briefly.

Murine models of ILD will be reviewed, including those with naturally occurring and experimentally induced genetic mutations that result in spontaneous ILD or altered susceptibility to ILD.

TUMOR SUPPRESSOR SYNDROMES

Patients with inherited cancer syndromes and phakomatoses resulting from tumor suppressor gene mutations are at risk of developing benign or malignant tumors, and in some cases are also susceptible to ILD (Table 7–1).[1] Tumor suppressor genes produce proteins that regulate orderly cell growth and differentiation by sensing the surrounding environment, transmitting signals from the membrane or cytoplasmic compartments to the nucleus, or directly influencing deoxyribonucleic acid (DNA) synthesis and cell division. In general, one copy of a tumor suppressor gene is adequate to maintain homeostasis, but functional inactivation of both copies results in a growth advantage relative to cells with normal tumor suppressor gene function. Affected individuals are typically born heterozygous for a loss-of-function mutation in one copy of an allele (ie, a germline mutation) but do not exhibit disease manifestations until an additional mutational event inactivates the wild-type copy of the allele (ie, a somatic mutation). The most common mechanism of loss of heterozygosity is deletion of a segment of DNA containing the normal gene; a deletion which can be identified by methods to detect the loss of genetic markers in the region of the gene. In some cases, disease may also result from two somatic mutational events in a tumor suppressor gene. Fibrotic pulmonary diseases are associated with mutations in the genes responsible for tuberous sclerosis complex (TSC) and neurofibromatosis (NF). The mechanisms by which tumor suppressor gene mutations result in LAM and multifocal micronodular pneumocyte hyperplasia (MMPH) in TSC and in

emphysema, pulmonary hypertension, and pulmonary fibrosis in NF are not fully understood.

Tuberous Sclerosis Complex

LAM and MMPH

TSC is an autosomal dominant tumor suppressor syndrome that is associated with hamartomas and dysplasias in multiple organs including angiofibromas of the skin, retinal hamartomas, abdominal angiomyolipomas (AMLs) of the kidney, liver, or spleen, and subependymal nodules, giant cell astrocytomas, and cortical tubers of the central nervous system.[2] TSC is known to result from mutations in either of two genes: the hamartin gene (*TSC1*) on chromosome 9 (9q34) or the tuberin gene (*TSC2*) on chromosome 16 (16p13.3).[3–5] Although familial TSC results from inheritance of germline mutations, de novo mutations arising during embryogenesis account for two-thirds of TSC cases. Rarely, TSC may be transmitted to offspring from parents who do not themselves have TSC, as a result of germline mosaicism (TSC mutations occurring only in germ cells and not in somatic cells).

Lung Involvement in TSC

There are two major lung manifestations of TSC: LAM (TSC-LAM) and MMPH. LAM is an uncommon progressive cystic lung disease that is characterized by diffuse infiltration of the pulmonary parenchyma with histologically benign smooth muscle-like cells.[6] Although LAM occurs almost exclusively in women, radiographic cystic changes consistent with LAM and biopsy-confirmed disease have also been reported in men with TSC.[7,8] LAM also occurs in women who do not have TSC. Like TSC-LAM patients, these 'sporadic' LAM (S-LAM) patients

TABLE 7–1   Genetic Basis of Tumor Suppressor Syndromes Associated With ILD

	Inheritance	Chromosome Locus	Locus Name	Protein	Pulmonary Disease	Pathologic ILD Pattern	Murine Model
Tuberous sclerosis	AD	9q34	*TSC1*	Hamartin	LAM MMPH	Smooth muscle infiltration Cystic change	TSC1 (+/–)[47]
	AD	16p13.3	*TSC2*	Tuberin	LAM MMPH	Nodular proliferation of alveolar type II cells	TSC2 (+/–)[48]
Sporadic LAM	Not inheritable	16p13.3	*TSC2*	Tuberin	LAM	Smooth muscle infiltration & cystic change	None
NF	AD	17q11.2	*NF1*	Neurofibromin	Bullae, ILD, PAH	UIP	NF1 (–/–)[94]
	AD	22q12.2	*NF2*	Merlin	None	None	NF2 (+/–)[96]

AD = autosomal dominant; ILD = interstitial lung disease; LAM = lymphangioleiomyomatosis; MMPH = multifocal micronodular pneumocyte hyperplasia; NF = neurofibromatosis; PAH = pulmonary arterial hypertension; TSC = tuberous sclerosis complex; UIP = usual interstitial pneumonia.

may also have intra- or extrarenal AMLs, lymphangiomyomas, and axial lymphadenopathy in the abdomen or thorax, but they do not exhibit manifestations of TSC in the skin, eye, central nervous system, or other organs, and they do not transmit LAM or TSC to their children. In both TSC-LAM and S-LAM, some smooth muscle cells of the LAM lesion are positive for staining with HMB-45, an antibody originally raised against melanoma cells. MMPH, which was first described by Popper and colleagues in 1991,[9,10] presents with multiple diffuse pulmonary nodules on chest radiograph or high-resolution computed tomography (HRCT) scan, as a result of nodular proliferation of alveolar type II cells.[11] MMPH has been reported in males and females with and without TSC, in males and females with TSC and LAM, and in women with S-LAM.[11,12] LAM and MMPH frequently coexist in patients with TSC, but they may also occur separately. Fewer than 20 cases of biopsy-confirmed MMPH have been published in the literature, and the physiological and prognostic consequences of MMPH are not known. Clear cell tumor of the lung is a very rare, HMB-45-positive neoplasm associated with TSC.[13,14]

Epidemiology of TSC-LAM and S-LAM

The results of registry-based efforts to locate LAM patients in the United States, France, and the United Kingdom have suggested a value for minimum prevalence of 2 to 6 cases per million women.[15–17] Given a world population of approximately 3 billion women, these figures predict a total of approximately 15,000 LAM patients worldwide. However, recent studies in patients with TSC suggest that the actual number of LAM-affected women may be much higher. The incidence of LAM in TSC patients was initially estimated to be 0.1 to 1% in a review of cases in the literature through 1971 and 2.3% of TSC patients that presented to the Mayo Clinic over a 43-year period.[18] A recent retrospective analysis of lung images from TSC patients, which were captured on abdominal and chest computed tomography (CT) scans, suggested that LAM may affect up to 26% of women with TSC,[19] and two recent prospective series have indicated that up to 34 to 39% of women with TSC have cystic changes consistent with LAM.[12,20] The estimated incidence of TSC is 1 per 6,000 to 11,000 births, and the estimated North American and worldwide prevalence of TSC is 40,000 and 1,000,000 cases, respectively.[21] Based on these data and the equal gender distribution of TSC, there may be as many as 10,000 patients with TSC-LAM in North America and over 100,000 TSC-LAM patients on earth.

Because of its protean presentation and lack of markers for early detection, the true prevalence of S-LAM is much more difficult to estimate. Although S-LAM may be more common than present available data suggest, it is likely that it is considerably less common that TSC-LAM. Paradoxically, most of the LAM patients than are reported in clinical series who present to pulmonologists who treat adults have S-LAM rather than TSC-LAM. Indeed, TSC-LAM was represented only 10, 8, and 4% of the LAM patients in United States, United Kingdom, and French registry series, respectively.[15–17] The underrepresentation of TSC-LAM in these populations indicates that it may be underdiagnosed, that TSC-LAM may be a milder disease than S-LAM, or that TSC comorbidities may prevent TSC-LAM from becoming a health priority for TSC patients.

Genetic Basis of LAM

Over 600 mutations have been identified in *TSC1* and *TSC2*, including protein-truncating mutations, missense (*TSC2* only) and nonsense mutations, splice mutations, and small and large deletions and insertions.[22–24] Overall, the clinical presentation of patients with TSC1 and TSC2 disease are quite similar, although a recent detailed study has suggested that *TSC1* mutations may produce somewhat milder TSC manifestations in general.[22] TSC-LAM has been reported in patients with mutations in either *TSC1* or *TSC2*, but *TSC2*-related LAM appears to be much more common.[24] Franz and colleagues reported that mutations identified in a group of TSC patients with pulmonary cystic changes were distributed throughout *TSC2*.[12] *TSC2* mutations were found in all cyst-positive patients from whom DNA samples were available, suggesting that *TSC2* mutations are more commonly associated with pulmonary cystic change than are mutations in *TSC1*. However, *TSC2* mutations account for about five times as many TSC cases as *TSC1* mutations, in general.[22–24] Three particularly interesting mutations were found at the 3' end of the *TSC2* gene in the cyst-positive group only. A missense mutation and small deletion in exon 38 were located in the region of homology to Rap1GAP, encoded by exons 34 to 38, which had previously been identified as a minor hotspot for *TSC2* mutations.[4,25] The missense mutation in exon 39 was located in a region that may interact with the Rab-5 adaptor, Rabaptin-5, encoded by exons 38 to 41.[26] TSC mutation information is available from 14 additional TSC patients with clinical LAM, and there are also 3 TSC-LAM patients with missense mutations or small deletions in exons 40 and 41.[24,27–30] Collectively, these data suggest that LAM can be caused by any of the diverse mutations that inactivate the *TSC1* or *TSC2* genes and cause TSC.

Great strides in our understanding of the genetic basis of LAM have been made in the past few years. Clinicians had long suspected, based on nearly identical histopathologic presentations, that the cystic lung disease familiar to neurologists who follow patients with TSC and S-LAM seen by adult pulmonary physicians might have a common genetic basis.[31,32] The presence of TSC genetic abnormalities in S-LAM patients was independently identified and jointly reported by Smolarek and Henske in 1998.[33]

They found loss of heterozygosity for *TSC2* in AMLs and lymph nodes from patients with S-LAM, but TSC mutations were not found in the circulating blood cells from S-LAM patients.[33,34] Carsillo and colleagues subsequently demonstrated the presence of missense and protein-truncating *TSC2* mutations associated with loss of heterozygosity in the lesional lung and kidney tissue of patients with S-LAM.[35] Interestingly, the circulating lymphocytes and perilesional normal lung and kidney tissue in S-LAM patients were free from detectable *TSC2* mutations. These data suggest that S-LAM may arise through two somatic mutations rather than the more typical tumor suppressor mechanism, which involves a combination of an inherited or developmental germline mutation and a somatic mutation. The lack of any documented cases of mother-to-daughter transmission of S-LAM, which has been reported in TSC-LAM, is also consistent with a somatic origin for bi-allelic mutations in patients with S-LAM.[36] Until recently, only *TSC2* mutations had been reported to cause S-LAM, but a single case, which was classified as S-LAM on clinical grounds, was recently found to be due to a germline *TSC1* mutation.[37] The patient in that study had cystic lung disease but no other TSC manifestations on skin examination, eye examination, or head CT scan.

Additional genetic and clinical evidence led Carsillo and colleagues to postulate that the smooth muscle cell infiltration and cystic degeneration of lung tissue in LAM may be a consequence of seeding of the lung with 'benign' angiomyolipoma cells.[35] This hypothesis was based on the finding of matching sets of *TSC2* mutations in the kidney and lung lesions of four LAM patients. The data were felt to be consistent with either a subdetectable level of mosaicism for *TSC2* mutations, a common extrarenal and extrapulmonary source that seeded both organs, or with a benign metastasis of tumor-forming cells from the kidney to the lung (or lung to kidney). The recurrence of LAM in the donor lungs of LAM patients who underwent transplantation is also consistent with the metastatic theory, although in two studies, the proliferating lesional cells appeared to be of donor origin.[38–40] In a small prospective study of female TSC-LAM patients, lung cysts were frequently associated with large or problematic angiomyolipomas, raising the possibility that more extensive kidney tumors may more readily seed the lung and cause cyst formation.[12] In several other respects, however, LAM bears little resemblance to hematogenous lung diseases. The intravascular histopathologic lesions and preferential dependent lung zone involvement that are characteristic of metastatic cancers, tumor emboli, and benign metastasizing leiomyoma are not typical presentations for LAM. The fact that only about 50% of S-LAM patients have radiographically apparent angiomyolipomas implies that the spread of LAM cells from the kidney to the lung could not apply to all cases.[41] It is possible, however, that the LAM cells that are deposited in the lung could originate from other sources, such as subdetectable (by CT scan) AMLs, axial lymph nodes, and/or lymphangiomyoma, which are frequent extrapulmonary manifestations in LAM patients.[42] The metastatic theory of LAM pathogenesis is provocative and controversial, and, if validated, may provide new opportunities for early intervention in LAM.

Function of Tuberin and Hamartin

The mechanisms by which hamartin and tuberin regulate cellular proliferation are not known, but co-immunoprecipitation experiments demonstrating that the two proteins interact intraceullularly indicate that their molecular pathways converge. Tuberin is a 180-kD protein that contains a Rap1GAP homology domain near its C-terminal and has been shown to have Rap1GAP activity as well as Rab5GAP activity.[4,25,26] Tuberin has also been reported to bind to calmodulin via a specific C-terminal domain and to be involved in cell cycle control and transcriptional events.[43,44] Recently, tuberin was found to regulate cellular growth of human LAM cells through rapamycin-reversible activation of the p70S6 kinase (p70S6K) pathway and phosphorylation of the cell cycle control protein, ribosomal S6.[45] Hamartin is a 130-kD protein that may play a role in cellular adhesion events and Rho-dependent signaling in actin stress fiber formation through interactions with ezrin-radixin-moesin (ERM) proteins.[46]

Animal Models of TSC

Gene-targeting experiments in mice have demonstrated that homozygous null mutations in *TSC1* or *TSC2* are embryonic lethal due to hypoplasia of the liver and other organs.[47,48] Heterozygous null *TSC1* and *TSC2* animals ([+/–], or one normal gene and one null disrupted allele) develop renal cystadenomas, which exhibit time-dependent malignant transformation, as well as hepatic hemangiomas. Interestingly, TSC1 (+/–) animals die from bleeding into smooth muscle-rich hepatic hemangiomas, beginning at about 1 year of age, at a rate that is three to four times higher in females than in males.[47] Although neither the TSC1 (+/–) or TSC2 (+/–) murine models develop cystic lung disease or pulmonary smooth muscle cell infiltration, the histopathologic features and gender predilection of the liver disease in these animals suggest that TSC1 (+/–) mice may be a reasonable model for LAM. TSC1 (–/–) murine embryonic fibroblasts (MEFs) exhibit constitutive activation of the PI3K-mTOR-S6K pathway, which regulates cell proliferation, including rapamycin-inhibitable hyperphosphorylation of p70S6K and its substrate, S6K.[49] The site of intersection between the hamartin pathway and the PI3K pathway is not clear but appears to occur distal to the kinase Akt, which is not activated in the TSC1 (–/–) MEFs. The PI3K pathway has also been implicated in the defect in cell size regulation in *Drosophila* harboring mutations in *dTSC1* and *dTSC2*.[50–52]

Molecular Basis of LAM Cell Accumulation and Pulmonary Cyst Formation

The source of LAM cells, the mechanism of accumulation of LAM cells in the lung, and the relationship between smooth muscle cell infiltration and cystic change are unknown. There are at least two cellular morphologies that characterize the LAM lesion: an HMB-45-positive, proliferating cell nuclear antigen (PCNA)-negative (nonproliferating) epithelioid cell that has been described in other neoplasms[53] and a spindle-shaped PCNA-positive cell.[54] A smooth muscle origin for LAM cells is suggested by their expression of α-actin and desmin.[53,55] LAM cells also express vimentin, which is not a characteristic of mature smooth muscle cells; this suggests to some investigators that LAM cells are immature myocytes or myofibroblasts.[56–58] A vascular origin has been proposed, based on coexpression of smooth muscle α-actin, desmin, and vimentin, a phenotype that has been demonstrated in smooth muscle cells from arterial walls.[59,60] An endothelial origin for LAM cells is unlikely, because they do not express Factor VIII, and lymphatics do not normally contain smooth muscle or pericytes.[55] The data are inconclusive and can be misleading, because the phenotypic markers expressed on LAM cells may reflect dysregulated gene expression rather than cell lineage. Whether LAM cells arise from pulmonary vascular, interstitial, or bronchial compartments or even from extrapulmonary sites, the mechanism of accumulation in the lung may also include a persistent proliferative stimulus, which may be extrinsic or intrinsic, or a failure of apoptosis. Two reports that the proliferating cells in recurrent LAM lesions posttransplant are donor derived suggest a circulating mitogenic stimulus.[38–40] Recent data indicate that tuberin- and hamartin-deficient mesenchymal cells derived from angiofibromas secrete 'growth factors' that stimulate the proliferation of tuberin- and hamartin-sufficient endothelial cells.[61] In another study, LAM cells exhibited robust expression of Bcl-2, an antiapoptotic cell surface molecule, possibly contributing to an imbalance between proliferation and cell death in LAM.[62] It is also possible that proliferating LAM cells are 'bystanders' that repopulate damaged lung matrix in a reactive response to an unknown lung injury. The finding that some early LAM lesions have pronounced cystic changes in the presence of only trivial smooth muscle cell infiltration is possibly consistent with this notion. The link between LAM cell accumulation and cystic destruction is not understood. One hypothesis is that LAM cells express matrix metalloproteinases (MMPs) and other matrix-degrading enzymes that produce cystic changes.[63] Hayashi and colleagues described increased expression of MMP-2, MMP-9, and MMP-1 without an associated increase in immunostaining for tissue inhibitors of metalloproteinases (TIMPs).[64] The authors speculated that elastin degradation may play a role in cyst formation in LAM through an increase in MMP-2 and MMP-9 that is unbalanced by an increase in TIMPs.

Clinical Presentation and Differential Diagnosis of LAM

Symptomatic patients with LAM may be identified very early or very late in their disease course, depending on the disease manifestations that bring them to medical attention. Acute or subacute shortness of breath or chest pain due to pneumothorax or chylous pleural effusion may be the presenting features of patients with a wide range of pulmonary involvement, including those with very few pulmonary cysts (Figure 7–1). Conceptually, therapeutic intervention in these early-presenting patients may have the greatest potential impact. The most common presentation, however, is progressive breathlessness.[16,17,65–67] Patients with LAM with chronic progressive dyspnea on exertion usually have advanced cystic changes on chest radiograph or HRCT scans of the chest (Figure 7–2). Additional atypical presentations of LAM include an isolated abdominal mass due to lymphangiomyomas or lymphadenopathy, flank pain due to hemorrhage into an AML, and ascites, chyloptysis, chyluria, hemoptysis, or chylopericardium (Figure 7–3). The differential of the thin-walled cystic lung disease of the type that is seen in LAM includes lymphangiomatosis,[68–71] lymphangiectasis,[68] benign metastasizing lymphangioma with cystic change,[72] emphysema, or pulmonary Langerhans cell histiocytosis, also known as pulmonary histiocytosis X or eosinophilic granuloma.[73] Centrilobular emphysema and pulmonary histiocytosis X are very uncommon in nonsmoking patients, but genetic emphysema that results from α_1-antitrypsin deficiency must be excluded, regardless of the tobacco use history. In the nonsmoking female with normal α_1-antitrypsin levels, the diagnosis of pulmonary LAM can be made on clinical grounds on the basis of typical diffuse thin-walled cystic changes on

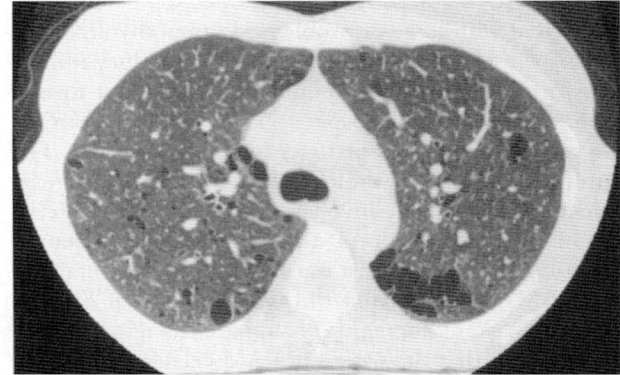

Figure 7–1 High-resolution computed tomography (HRCT) screening of this asymptomatic woman with tuberous sclerosis identified early cystic changes (TSC-LAM) that were not visible on chest radiograph. Reproduced with permission from the LAM Foundation.

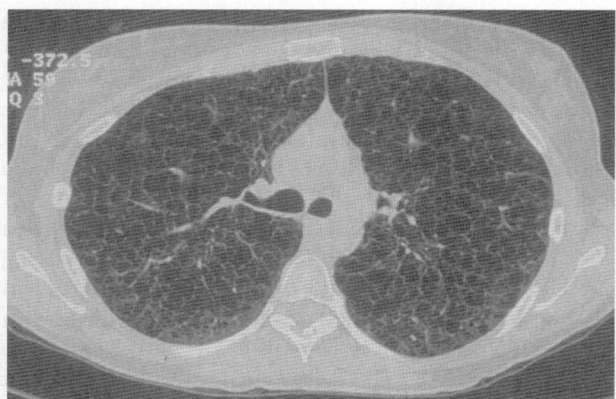

Figure 7–2   Advanced cystic changes in a patient who presented short of breath with sporadic lymphangioleiomyomatosis (S-LAM):

HRCT scans of the chest and at least one other associated feature, including known TSC, renal or lymphatic masses containing fat density on CT or ultrasound scanning of the abdomen, chylous ascites, chylous pleural effusion, or other chylous collection. Recurrent pneumothoraces in a young nonsmoking female are suggestive of LAM, but even in the face of consistent cystic changes on HRCT scan are not generally sufficiently specific to obviate the need for tissue confirmation in the absence of the associated features mentioned above.

The clinical course of patients with LAM varies widely, from relatively stable disease over decades to relentlessly progressive dyspnea on exertion, recurrent pneumothoraces, and chylous pleural effusions. In a survey of 330 patients registered with the LAM Foundation, the first symptom or manifestation of LAM was dyspnea in 51%, spontaneous pneumothorax in 40%, cough in 6%, hemoptysis in 5%, and chest pain in 5%. The most troubling current symptom or manifestation in 395 patients surveyed was dyspnea in 78%, spontaneous pneumothorax in 6%, chest pain in 5%, cough in 2%, and hemoptysis in 1%. More than 90% of patients had a pneumothorax at some point in their disease course. The average age of diagnosis of LAM in the Foundation database and in the literature is approximately 35 years, and the mean survival is frequently reported to be less than 10 years.[16,17,65–67] Recent data, however, suggest a more optimistic prognosis.[74–76] LAM is often radiographically undetectable in the early stages, and the clinical presentation mimics that of asthma. For these reasons, the diagnosis is delayed for an average of 3 to 5 years or more, and most patients seen in practice and studied in clinical series have advanced disease.[16,17,65–67,77] It is difficult to directly compare disease manifestations in S-LAM and TSC-LAM because there are few series of patients with TSC-LAM in the literature.[7,18] Costello and colleagues reported that 7 of 9 patients with TSC-LAM had presenting pulmonary complaints of dyspnea or pneumothorax, and all of those had severe obstructive physiology and advanced cystic changes on HRCT scans

of the chest.[7,19] Although 8 of 9 had renal AMLs, none had chylous complications.[19] In contrast, Franz and colleagues screened 23 female patients with TSC with HRCT and reported that only 3 of 9 of the cyst-positive patients with TSC-LAM had a remote history of pneumothorax, and none had chronic dyspnea. Most of the patients had mild to moderate cystic changes on HRCT scan of the chest, and there were no chylous complications.[12] Clearly, the screening of female TSC patients for lung cysts identifies a LAM population with far fewer disease manifestations than are seen in the patient population with S-LAM. Although definitive conclusions must await a properly designed study, it seems likely that LAM manifestations will prove to be similar in TSC and non-TSC patients who present with breathlessness, with the possible exception of a reduced incidence of chylous effusions in patients with TSC-LAM.[19]

Treatment

LAM is empirically managed with anti-estrogen therapies, based largely on the observed gender restriction and reports that birth control pills and pregnancy can worsen the disease, but there is no convincing evidence that these strategies are effective.[78,79] There have been no prospective randomized trials of hormonal therapy, and the available literature is limited to isolated case reports, meta-analyses of compiled case reports, and retrospective case series that are inconclusive. The state of the science is such that, at the time of this writing, "no pharmacologic treatment" for pulmonary LAM manifestations is generally accepted as a completely reasonable alternative for patients with LAM at all disease stages.

Progesterone has been used as an empiric therapy for LAM for decades. Four early case studies have suggested that progesterone may stabilize disease progression in some patients, especially those with chylous effusions and ascites.[16,67,77,80] The latter conclusion may

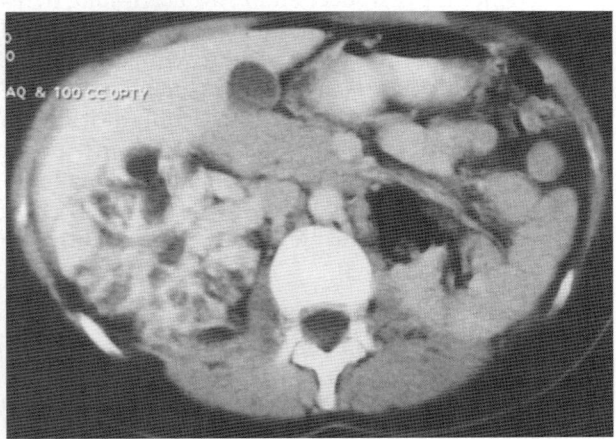

Figure 7–3   Large angiomyolipoma involving the right kidney. Note areas of fat density scattered throughout the mass.

contain inherent bias, because effusions are perhaps the most measurable manifestation of LAM and can spontaneously remit. Improvement, based on outcomes of dyspnea or an increase in forced expiratory volume in 1 second (FEV$_1$), are uncommon but consistently reported in all four series. A retrospective study from the United Kingdom suggested that progesterone reduced the rate of decline in FEV$_1$ in premenopausal patients with LAM from −170 to −47 mL/yr, although the effect did not quite reach statistical significance (p = .06). Progesterone treatment did slow the decline in diffusing capacity for carbon monoxide (DL$_{CO}$), from −2.15 to −0.19 mL/min/mm Hg per year (p < .05).[81] Although the available data concerning the clinical efficacy of progesterone are flawed by retrospective design, concomitant use of multiple treatments, and heterogeneity in patient populations, the anecdotal reports of benefit, the reasonable safety profile, and the lack of any acceptable alternative will likely continue to perpetuate the use of progesterone for symptomatic LAM until a definitive clinical trial is performed or a more promising therapy emerges. Gonadotropin releasing hormone (GnRH) agonists have also been used for LAM but there are no data available that addresses their efficiency.

Reversible airflow obstruction is present in up to 25% of patients with LAM, and a trial of bronchodilators should be considered.[66] Patients with LAM should be treated with supplemental oxygen to maintain saturations greater than 90% with rest, exercise, and sleep. Bone densitometry should be routinely obtained at baseline and as part of routine follow-up, and bone loss should be aggressively treated. Patients with LAM on anti-estrogen therapies are at increased risk for atherosclerotic cardiovascular disease and should be screened for hyperlipidemia and counseled regarding appropriate dietary modifications and exercise.

Lung Transplantation in LAM

There have been well over 100 lung transplants in LAM patients since the first successful LAM heart–lung transplant performed in 1983 and the first single-lung LAM transplant in 1988.[82,83] A retrospective analysis of the outcome of lung transplantation for patients with LAM reported that, despite excess LAM complications of intraoperative hemorrhage due to adhesions, pneumothorax in the native lung following single-lung transplant, and recurrence of LAM in the allograft, lung transplantation is a valuable therapy for patients with end-stage LAM.[84]

Recurrence of LAM in Lung Allografts

There have been three case reports of recurrent LAM in the donor allografts of patients with LAM who have undergone lung transplantion.[38–40] The transplant recipients in studies from Munich, St. Louis, and Pittsburgh were females aged 34 to 45 years, and each received a lung from a male donor. All three women succumbed to infection or acute respiratory failure 20 to 30 months posttransplant. The pathology of the LAM lesion in all three patients revealed multifocal involvement of the walls of blood vessels and bronchioles by proliferation of spindle cells that generally mirrored the lymphatic investment of the structures. In two cases, in situ hybridization with a Y-chromosome probe suggested that the proliferating cells in the LAM lesion were of male (donor) origin, and in the only case tested, the lesional cells stained with HMB-45. These data suggested that a circulating factor, rather than a metastatic cell, was responsible for development of the LAM lesion in the donor allograft. Candidate sites for the origin of the mitogenic stimulus or a mutostatic source may have been the AML that was present in one patient, the lymphadenopathy that was present in the remaining two patients, or the LAM lesions in the native lung in all three patients.

Summary

LAM should be considered in any female with TSC, recurrent pneumothoraces, unexplained chylous effusions in the abdomen or chest, or renal AML. The Tuberous Sclerosis Alliance recommends that all women with TSC should be screened for LAM at least once upon reaching maturity.[85] The clinical diagnosis of LAM is based on radiographic evidence of cystic lung disease in combination with TSC, an AML, and/or chylous effusions. An open lung biopsy may be required to differentiate LAM from emphysema or eosinophilic granuloma in cases where cystic lung disease is present without these associated features. Patients with LAM should be counseled that birth control pills and pregnancy have been associated with disease exacerbations.[16,78,79,86] The current therapeutic options for patients with LAM include watchful observation, progestin therapy at suprapharmacologic or conventional doses, or gonadotropin-releasing hormone (GnRH) agonist therapy. Oophorectomy is rarely recommended. Given the bone and cardiovascular risks of anti-estrogen therapies and the uncertain benefits of currently available surgical and medical treatment modalities, many clinicians avoid treatment of asymptomatic patients. Either progestins (usually at a low dose) or no therapy at all are often considered for patients who have had an initial pneumothorax or chylothorax or who have stable symptomatic disease; progestins (high- or low-dose) or GnRH agonists are frequently recommended for patients who wish to try therapy for progressive disease, recurrent pneumothoraces, or chylothoraces.

Neurofibromatosis

Neurofibromatosis 1 (NF1) and neurofibromatosis 2 (NF 2) are genetically and clinically distinct autosomal dominant tumor suppressor syndromes. Both diseases are inheritable, although sporadic mutations account for 50% of cases. The penetrance of NF is almost 100%, but expressivity is variable. Both disorders can result in the development of benign or malignant tumors, especially of the peripheral and central nervous systems. There is no known sex or racial predominance. Disease severity is greater and age of onset is lower in maternally inherited cases than in paternally inherited cases for both NF1 and NF2, a phenomenon known as genetic imprinting.[87] Pulmonary disease is occasionally associated with NF, but it usually does not become apparent until adulthood and is typically associated with NF1 rather than NF2.

NF1

NF1, the most common cancer predisposition syndrome affecting the nervous system, occurs with a frequency of approximately 1 of 2,500 to 3,300 and has a prevalence of 1 of 5,000. About 25% of patients with NF1 develop disabling disease. NF1 typically presents with cutaneous neurofibromas and pigmentary disorders of the skin, including café-au-lait macules and skin freckling of the intertriginous area of the axilla or groin. Neurofibromas are discrete sessile or papular benign tumors of the dermis, composed of Schwann cells, neurons, perineural fibroblasts, and infiltrating mast cells, that occur in more that 95% of patients and can number in the thousands. Areolar neurofibromas occur in at least 85% of women and tend to appear at the time of puberty.[88] Neurofibromas of the skin (and elsewhere) increase in size and number at puberty in both sexes and also during pregnancy.[89,90] Lisch nodules of the iris, which are true hamartomas, are also present in more than 90% of patients. Less common manifestations include scoliosis, pseudoarthrosis of the tibia, mental retardation, hypertension, and hypoglycemia. Although NF1 has been called peripheral NF, it has also been associated with tumors of the central nervous system. Children with NF1 can present with low-grade glial tumors involving the optic pathway, whereas in adolescents and adults, benign tumors composed of Schwann cells and fibroblasts, pheochromocytomas, and leukemias are more common. Aggressive Schwann cell tumors also occur but are rare.

Molecular Basis of NF1.   The NF1 tumor suppressor protein is a Ras-specific guanosine triphosphatase-activating (RasGTPase) protein that controls cellular proliferation by negative regulation of p21Ras signaling.[49,91] The *NF1* gene was localized to chromosome 17q11.2 by linkage analysis. The gene spans 350 kb with 59 exons and encodes a protein of 2,818 amino acids called neurofibromin, which is widely expressed in a variety of tissues.[92] Neurofibromin has a central Ras-GTPase-activating domain, but no other informative homologies are present.[93] Neurofibromin deficiency has been shown to correlate with elevated Ras activity in a variety of NF1-associated tumors and to down-regulate

Ras-related cellular proliferation in NF (–/–) hematopoetic stem cells. Over 80% of germline mutations predict truncation of neurofibromin. Based on homology between the NF1 protein product and members of the GTPase-activating family, the name NF1GAP-related protein was suggested. The Knudson two-hit hypothesis for tumor formation in NF1 has been validated for most tumor types in NF1 disease. Interestingly, in benign neurofibromas, loss of heterozygosity only occurs in the Schwann cell, which likely recruits other cell types to the lesion.

Animal Models of NF1.   Mice that are heterozygous for inactivating mutations in NF1 are tumor prone and develop pheochromocytomas and myeloid leukemia, but do not develop neurofibromas or nerve sheath tumors. However, it is not uncommon for the phenotypes of mice carrying individual mutations in tumor suppressor genes to fail to closely mimic their cognate human diseases. NF1 (–/–) mice die because of failure of cardiac development, but chimeric mice that are composed in part of NF (–/–) cells develop multiple neurofibromas, demonstrating that loss of the wild-type allele is rate limiting in tumor formation.[94] NF1-deficient mice do not develop pulmonary disease, at least not on the background strains that have been tested to date.

NF2

The birth incidence of NF2 lies between 1 of 33,000 and 1 of 40,000, with a prevalence of approximately 1 of 200,000.[87] Bilateral vestibular schwannomas are the defining feature of NF2 disease. Patients usually present with bilateral hearing loss at a mean age of 24 years. Other tumors that may develop include meningiomas, gliomas, and ependymomas. Most patients do not have café-au-lait spots or peripheral neurofibromata. Most of the literature regarding pulmonary disease in NF is quite dated and does not distinguish between NF1 and NF2 disease, but pulmonary disease is not thought to be associated with *NF2* mutations.

Molecular Basis of NF2.   The *NF2* gene was localized to chromosome 22q12.1 by positional cloning. It spans 100 kb and encodes a 587-amino acid cytoskeletal protein known as merlin, which bears striking sequence homology to a family of proteins that link the actin cytoskeleton to the cell surface ERM proteins.[95] Although the molecular basis of merlin's growth-suppressive function is unknown, recent evidence suggests that merlin may control the localization and trafficking of signaling molecules through its effects on actin cytoskeletal organization.

Animal Models of NF2.   Mice that are hemizygous for *NF2* do not develop schwannomas, but rather develop osteosarcomas, fibrosarcomas, and hepatocellular carcinomas.[96] All three tumor types readily metastasize, an unusual feature of endogenous murine tumors. This observation suggests an important role for merlin in tumor cell migration and invasion, the most poorly understood and lethal consequence of malignant transformation. Conditional homozygous NF (–/–) mice develop schwannomas, cataracts, and osseous metaplasia, but lung disease is not known to occur in any NF2 animal models.

Pulmonary Presentation of NF

The true prevalence of pulmonary disease in patients with NF is not known, but most studies report values from 5 to 10% to as high as 20% of patients with NF.[97–100] Thoracic diseases associated with NF include interstitial fibrosis, pneumocyte hyperplasia, intrapulmonary neurofibromas, emphysema, bullous changes, pulmonary hypertension, bronchiectasis, intrathoracic schwannomas, and scoliosis. Papillary adenomas of type II pneumocytes, reminiscent of the micronodular pneumocyte hyperplasia (MMPH) that has been described in patients with LAM, has been reported in a 13-year-old boy with NF.[101] Pulmonary hypertension in the presence[98,102] and absence of pulmonary fibrosis have been described.[103] Bronchiectasis was reported in 2 of 70 NF patients by Webb and Goodman.[99] Chest wall involvement may also occur, including notching of the ribs due to rib erosion by intercostal fibromas or to a primary defect in bone formation. Twisted rib deformities and severe restrictive lung disease have been described in patients with severe skeletal NF disease. Recently, bilateral diaphragmatic paralysis due to phrenic nerve involvement in NF has been reported.[104]

Davies and coworkers first recognized the association between NF1 and pulmonary fibrosis found in 20 of 76 patients with NF seen at Veterans Administration hospitals.[105] Webb and Goodman reviewed 70 consecutive cases of NF and found interstitial fibrosis or bullae in 10% of all patients and 20% of subjects over the age of 30 years.[99] Transmission of pulmonary fibrosis due to NF from mother to son has been reported.[106]

Pulmonary symptoms and exercise limitation may be mild to severe, in some cases leading to respiratory failure and death in patients with NF-ILD.[106] Pulmonary function tests may reveal a restrictive or obstructive pattern, and the DL_{CO} is frequently reduced.[98] The chest radiograph shows diffuse irregular nodular shadows or honeycombing, typically in the lung bases. In patients observed over a period of years, radiographic progression of interstitial disease from nodular to mottled densities to coarse linear streaking has been seen.[106] Bullous changes are usually associated with fibrotic changes and occur predominantly in the upper lobes, although bullae in the absence of fibrosis[107] or isolated to the lower zones have been reported.[98,108]

The histologic appearance of the lung fibrosis in NF is similar to that of UIP, with a peripheral and subpleural predominance. In the early stages, the alveolar septa become expanded with a cellular infiltrate and excess connective tissue matrix. Later, the cellular response is replaced by fibrosis, destruction of the alveolar wall, bullae formation, and obliteration of blood vessels. Lumenal infiltration by alveolar macrophages is common and can be sufficiently robust to suggest a diagnosis of desquamative interstitial pneumonitis.[109]

Summary

Pulmonary complications can occur in patients with NF because of NF1 mutations, but they are rarely the presenting or the most troubling manifestation. The true prevalence of lung disease has not been carefully defined. The most common pulmonary problems that have been identified in NF are emphysema, pneumothorax, pulmonary fibrosis, pulmonary hypertension, neurogenic thoracic tumors, thoracic and skeletal bony abnormalities, and bronchiectasis. Physicians should be vigilant in looking for pulmonary symptoms in patients with NF and consider imaging and functional studies to define airway, vascular, and interstitial lung disease.

SURFACTANT PROTEIN-C MUTATIONS

Idiopathic Interstitial Pneumonias and Misprocessing of SP-C

Pulmonary surfactant is composed of phospholipids (PLs) and surfactant proteins A, B, C, and D, which are secreted into the alveolar space by alveolar type II cells of the pulmonary epithelium. By reducing surface tension at the air-liquid interface, surfactant makes the lungs compliant and respiration almost effortless. Hyperplasia of alveolar type II cells is a consistent finding in all forms of ILD, but whether injury to the alveolar epithelium is the cause or the result of interstitial fibrosis remains unclear. The finding that cytotoxic mutations in SP-C, which is expressed only in alveolar type II cells, can result in ILD suggests that the pulmonary epithelium can play a primary role in fibrogenesis (Table 7–2).[110] Ongoing microinjury to the alveolar epithelium produced by misprocessing of SP-C may disrupt epithelial-mesenchymal growth and differentiation signals that regulate the synthetic and proliferative functions of fibroblasts and myofibroblasts in the interstitium.[111]

Structure and Function of SP-C

SP-C is an extremely hydrophobic integral membrane protein that is expressed only in alveolar type II cells of the lung. It was first identified in the organic extract of lamellar bodies and in the bronchoalveolar lavage (BAL) fluid of patients with alveolar proteinosis by Phizackerley and colleagues.[112] Glasser and colleagues used a nucleotide probe based on the valine-rich N-terminal of SP-C to isolate a cDNA and genomic DNA encoding the human pro-

TABLE 7–2   Genetic Basis of SP-C ILD

	Inheritance	Chromosome Locus	Locus Name	Protein	Pulmonary Disease	Pathologic ILD Pattern	Murine Model
SP-C ILD	AD	8p23.1	SFTP2	SP-C	ILD, ARDS	DIP/NSIP/UI	SP-C (–/–)[128]

ARDS = acute respiratory distress syndrome; DAD = diffuse alveolar damage; DIP = desquamative interstitial pneumonitis; NSIP = nonspecific interstitial pneumonitis; SP-C = surfactant protein C.

tein.[113,114] SP-C is encoded by a single gene on the short arm of chromosome 8, centromeric to 8p23.1.[115,116] The locus, referred to as SFTP2, spans only 3.5 kb and contains six exons and five introns.[117] The *SP-C* gene is located in close proximity to the gene for bone morphogenic protein I (BMPI), whose transcription start site is only 706 base pairs (bp) downstream of the SP-C polyadenylation site. The SP-C gene encodes a 0.86-kb messenger ribonucleic acid (mRNA), which directs the synthesis of a 22-kD 191- or 197-amino acid proprotein. After folding of proSP-C in the endoplasmic reticulum and Golgi body of the type II cell, the 24- and 138-amino acid N- and C-terminal propeptides are cleaved in the multivesicular body, liberating an extremely hydrophobic 34- to 35-amino acid mature peptide. The deduced primary sequence of the mature fragment reveals an alpha helical membrane-spanning domain rich in valine, isoleucine, and leucine, and a basic hydrophilic extramembrane region containing two palmitoylated cysteine residues at positions 5 and 6.[118] Mature SP-C intercalates into phospholipid (PL) membranes in the multivesicular body and lamellar body where surfactant is stored inside the type II cell, and, in sufficient forms in the alveolar space. The primary function of SP-C in the alveolar space is most likely to stabilize surfactant films by disrupting PL acyl-chain packing and enhancing PL recruitment to spreading monolayers and multilayers in the alveolar space. Mature SP-C can self-associate to form intracellular aggresomes or extracellular fibrillar structures in patients with alveolar proteinosis.[119,120] Inappropriate self-aggregation of SP-C may produce cellular toxicity and alveolar type II cell dropout.[121]

Genetic Basis of Interstitial Pneumonias in Three Families with Mutations or Deficiency of SP

Nogee and colleagues described mutations in the gene encoding SP-C in an infant with a family history of ILD.[122] The mother had received a diagnosis of desquamative interstitial pneumonia (DIP) at 1 year of age and had been treated with corticosteroids through age 15; the maternal grandfather had died of long-standing ILD of unknown cause. The infant developed tachypnea and cyanosis at 6 weeks of age, associated with hyperinflation and increased interstitial markings on chest radiograph. An open lung biopsy from the infant revealed a cellular or NSIP. There was hyperplasia of alveolar type II cells, filling of alveolar spaces with CD68+ macrophages, and interstitial expansion with mature lymphocytes and occa-

sional myofibroblasts. The mother developed worsening respiratory failure after delivery and died. Her lung biopsy revealed areas of diffuse fibrosis and honeycombing, with patchy areas of mild interstitial lymphocytic infiltration, macrophage accumulation, and areas of superimposed diffuse alveolar damage. Immmunostaining for SP-C revealed deficiency of the protein in the infant and the mother, but the misprocessed SP-C precursor was readily detected in alveolar type II cells of both patients. A heterozygous substitution of A for G was identified at the first base of intron 4 (G1728A), disrupting the normal donor splice site (IVS4+1 G→A) and resulting in a deletion of exon 4. Restriction analysis confirmed the presence of this mutation in the patient and the mother, and reverse transcriptase polymerase chain reaction (RT-PCR) revealed the presence of a truncated ribonucleic acid (RNA) lacking exon 4 in both patients. Subsequent screening of 34 individuals with familial and sporadic chronic lung disease identified 12 with mutations or uncommon polymorphisms of one allele of the *SP-C* gene.[123] One infant had a de novo mutation in the same location as the family described above (G1728T), one had a frameshift mutation, and the remaining ten had nucleotide mutations resulting in substitutions in highly conserved amino acids. These data indicate that *SP-C* mutations are a cause of familial and sporadic ILD.

Amin and colleagues subsequently reported the association of ILD and SP-C deficiency in an 11-year-old girl, her 4-year-old half-sister, and her mother.[124] The children had initially been diagnosed at ages 7 (the 11-year-old) and 3.5 weeks (the half-sister), and the mother had developed respiratory distress and infiltrates associated with the two pregnancies, which responded to treatment with corticosteroids. The histopathology of the lung in the sisters revealed variable interstitial fibrosis, type II cell hyperplasia, and moderately severe interstitial inflammation associated with lymphocytic and plasma cell infiltration. Examination of BAL fluid revealed an absence of SP-C and reduced levels of SP-A and SP-B in all three patients. Immunostaining of the lung revealed markedly reduced proSP-C, but DNA sequence analysis revealed no evidence of mutations in the SP-B or SP-C coding sequences.

A large kindred composed of 32 family members in 5 generations, reported by Thomas and colleagues, had 14 members affected by pulmonary fibrosis.[121] Pathologic data were available for 9 members, including 3 children with NSIP, 5 adults with UIP, and 1 adult with "fibrocystic pulmonary dysplasia." A heterozygous exon

5 + 128 T/A transversion that encoded a leucine to glutamine substitution (L188Q) in the C-terminal region of proSP-C was present in 6 affected family members and 2 unaffected obligate heterozygotes, but not in 4 unaffected family members and 88 controls. This region of SP-C has been shown to be critical for proper folding and processing of proSP-C.[119,125,126] Expression of the mutant SP-C in murine lung epithelial cells resulted in reduced growth and the formation of intracellular inclusions consistent with cytotoxity associated with misfolded protein aggregates. The fact that heterozygotes for SP-C mutations can develop ILD suggest that mutant SP-C can interfere with the function of endogenous SP-C in a dominant-negative fashion. Furthermore, the observation that not all patients who are heterozygous for SP-C mutations within a given family were affected indicates that environmental factors or genetic modifiers play an important role in the pathogenesis of ILD. Interestingly, the same genetic mutation can result in NSIP in children and in UIP, suggesting the possibility that NSIP may be a precursor for UIP. Finally, the fact that patients can present in their sixth decade with UIP suggests that some cases of 'sporadic' IPF may be due to mutations in SP-C.

Animal Models

In mice, lung-specific overexpression of a mutant SP-C cDNA encoding mature SP-C without the N- or C-terminal propeptides arrested lung development and resulted in neonatal death.[127] Targeted disruption of the murine SP-C gene in outbred Swiss Black mice did not appear to affect survival, surfactant PL levels, or lung morphology through 8 weeks of age but resulted in subtle surfactant instability detected by measurements of lung mechanics and surface tension of isolated surfactant.[128] The surfactant defect in the Swiss Black animals was exacerbated by oxygen-induced lung injury and a concomitant deficiency of SP-B.[129] Preliminary evidence that the genetically engineered inbred 129/Sv SP-C-deficient strain develops severe age-dependent IPF similar to the human interstitial pneumonitis was recently presented.[130]

Summary

Collectively, the data indicate that expression of a mutant proSP-C protein or the deletion of the SP-C gene can cause fibrotic lung disease. Cell injury that results from misfolding and misprocessing of the SP-C precursor may result in fibrosis caused by loss of the antifibrogenic function of the epithelium, or, alternatively, SP-C deficiency may result in surfactant dysfunction and altered alveolar surface tension forces that ultimately cause interstitial pneumonia through shear stress at the level of the alveolar epithelium. Although the data clearly indicate that SP-C mutations cause some forms of familial interstitial pneumonia, additional studies will be required to determine if nonfa-

milial idiopathic interstitial pneumonias are associated with deficiency or dysfunction of SP-C. Perhaps most importantly, SP-C-related ILD introduces a new disease paradigm for ILD; that misfolding of alveolar epithelial proteins due to genetic, environmental, or pharmacologic influences may result in pulmonary fibrosis.

METABOLIC PULMONARY DISEASE

Gaucher's Disease

Gaucher's disease, the most prevalent lysosomal storage disease, is an autosomal recessive disorder caused by defective hydrolysis of glucosylceramides.[131,132] The disease results from mutations in the gene for β-glucosidase, the enzyme that catabolizes glucosylceramide.[133] Mutations in the gene encoding for lysosomal hydrolase or glucocerebrosidase can also cause Gaucher's disease. Decreased enzymatic activity leads to the accumulation of periodic acid-Schiff (PAS)-positive tubular ("crumpled tissue paper") inclusions containing glucocerebroside in macrophages of the reticuloendothelial system (Figures 7–4, 7–5). Tissue infiltration with Gaucher's cells results in hepatosplenomegally, anemia, thrombocytopenia, neurologic impairment, skeletal disease, and, less commonly, lung disease.[131] Pulmonary manifestations may include pulmonary hypertension or ILD. The majority of patients with Gaucher's disease are females, and more than 95% are Ashkenazi Jews. The recent development of an efficacious therapy based on a solid understanding of the cellular and genetic basis of the disease makes Gaucher's a model for molecular medicine.

Genetic Basis of Gaucher's Disease

The human β-glucosidase gene and a nonprocessed pseudogene span 32 kb on chromosome 1, in close proximity to the genes for metaxin and thrombospondin. The functional gene is 7,600 bp and contains 11 exons.

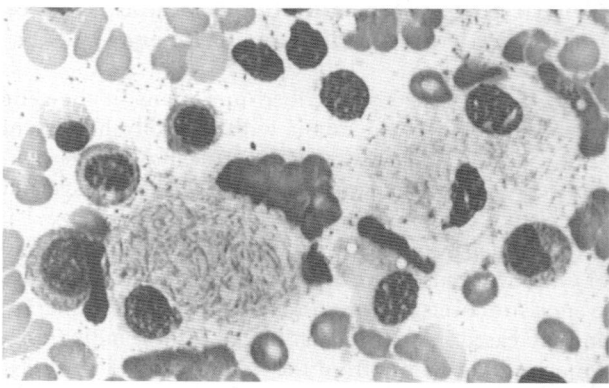

Figure 7–4   Light micrograph of two Gaucher's cells containing characteristic "crumpled tissue paper-like" striated cytoplasmic inclusions. Reproduced with permission from Gregory Grabowski, MD.

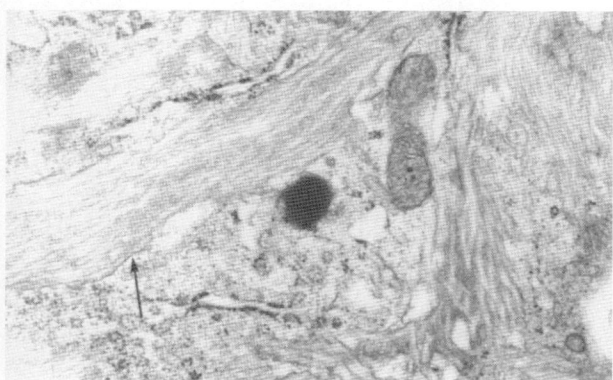

Figure 7–5   High-magnification electron micrograph illustrating the tubular morphology of Gaucher's cell inclusions. Reproduced with permission from Gregory Grabowski, MD.

Most disease alleles in Gaucher's disease lead to nonfunctional or dysfunctional enzymes, but some result in enzyme instability.

Animal Models

Complete disruption of the glucocerebrosidase (*Gba*) gene in mice results in neonatal demise due to altered epithelial barrier function.[134] Introduction of the human Gaucher's-causing mutation L444P into mice results in partial enzyme deficiency and a milder phenotype.[135] With optimal housing conditions, the L444P mice survive for prolonged periods and develop Gaucher's-like manifestations without evidence of classic Gaucher's cells or the typical tissue accumulation of glucosylceramide. The L444P mice exhibit evidence of systemic inflammation, anemia and leukopenia, lymphadenopathy, accumulation of lipofuscin granules in macrophages, and inflammatory infiltrates in the liver and skin. Lung histology reveals expansion of alveolar septa with inflammatory infiltrates consisting of neutrophils, macrophages, and lymphocytes.

Clinical Presentation of Gaucher's Disease

The first case of Gaucher's disease was described by Philippe Charles Ernest Gaucher over a century ago.[136] In published studies, the age at diagnosis ranges from the first week of life to as late as 86 years. Three types of Gaucher's have been described, based on the extent of neurologic, osseous, or visceral involvement. The non-neuronotropic form, type 1, is the most common, found in about 1 of 1,500 Ashkenazi Jews and about 1 of 100,000 of other Whites. Patients typically present at an average age of 21 years with splenomegally as the presenting sign. Other common presenting features include hepatomegally, anemia, and bone disease, including infarcts and necrosis, but there is substantial phenotypic variability. Screening studies of families and populations identify subjects with particularly mild disease. Severely

affected children may die with pancytopenias, liver, and skeletal abnormalities in the first or second decade of life. Type 2 is the rarest (<1 of 500,000 live births) and most severe variant. It is typically apparent in the first year of life and is neuronopathic and relentlessly progressive. Brainstem involvement with cranial nerve signs, mild to moderate hepatosplenomegally, and pulmonary involvement are general features. Death frequently occurs by the age of 3 years. Type 3 occurs in about 1 of 100,000 patients and is less severe, with more variable central nervous system involvement than in type 2. Visceral involvement is common, especially in type 3b disease, which is distinguished by its early onset. Type 3a is characterized by later onset, less visceral involvement, and more severe central nervous system disease. Pulmonary disease eventually occurs in virtually all patients with neuronotropic types 2 and 3b, with grave prognostic consequences, but it is less common in type 1 disease.[137]

Physiological and Radiographic Abnormalities

Although pulmonary involvement in Gaucher's disease is infrequently reported, the true incidence may be more common than is generally appreciated.[133,138,139] In a prospective study from a 95-patient cohort, 68% of patients with Gaucher's disease had some pulmonary function abnormality, occurring, in many cases, in the absence of symptoms.[140] The most common abnormalities included a reduced functional residual capacity in 45% of patients, a reduced diffusion capacity in 42%, and a reduced total lung capacity in 22%. Forced expiratory flows were reduced in 33%, and air trapping was seen in 18%, especially in males. Chest roentgenogram abnormalities were found in 17% of patients but were only severe in 4%. Radiographic manifestations included reticulonodular or miliary changes.[141] Out of 125 of Gaucher's patients followed at the University of Southern California, 5 had pulmonary symptoms. In one patient, the chest radiograph revealed only a calcified granuloma, and the HRCT scan was normal. Chest radiographs were normal in two patients, and HRCT revealed only patchy peripheral thickening of the inter and intralobular septa. In the final two symptomatic patients, the chest radiograph revealed bilateral basilar reticulonodular changes, whereas the HRCT scan revealed bilateral diffuse interstitial changes associated with septal thickening and geographic areas of ground glass. Pulmonary hypertension has been reported in several patients with Gaucher's disease.[142] Gross specimens of the lung reveal patches of scarring and thickened pleura and septal lines (Figure 7–6). Two histopathologic patterns have been described: (1) isolated accumulation of Gaucher's cells in alveolar spaces and (2) Gaucher's cell infiltration of the alveolar, interstitial, and pleural compartments (Figure 7–7).[139,143] Gaucher's cells may be detected in the BAL fluid.[144] Elevated levels of serum angiotensin-converting enzymes have been documented in some patients.[145] Patients may develop hypoxemia due to functional arteriovenous shunts as a result of severe liver involvement.

Treatment of Gaucher's Disease

Gaucher's's disease is a prototype for intracellular enzyme therapy. Modified β-glucosidase is prepared on an industrial scale from human placenta, and recombinant therapies are now available. Several reported trials in over 200 patients have shown the clinical and biochemical efficacy of exogenous β-glucosidase therapy, and over 1,000 patients worldwide are receiving the drug. Liver and spleen sizes routinely decrease by 20 to 40% with drug therapy. Hematologic indexes also improve, often to normal, for red blood cell counts. Platelet counts improve slowly, especially in patients with very large spleens. The enzyme is targeted to macrophages by the presence of α-mannosyl-terminated oligosaccharides on the protein. There have been case reports of improved pulmonary function in patients who receive enzyme replacement therapy.[146–148] However, in most cases it appears that pulmonary and other visceral and bony manifestations of Gaucher's disease are slow to respond to enzyme therapy.[149] The avail-

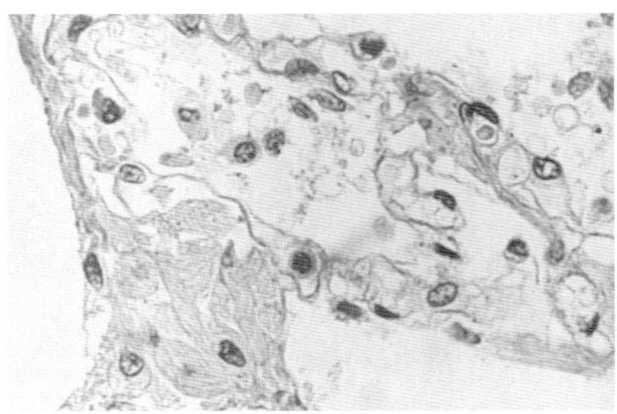

Figure 7–7 Light micrograph of the lung in a patient with Gaucher's disease. Note Gaucher's cells in the alveolar lumen and expanding alveolar septa. Reproduced with permission from Gregory Grabowski, MD.

ability of effective enzyme therapies for Gaucher's make autologous bone marrow transplantation unnecessary in all but unusual cases.

Hermansky-Pudlak Syndrome

Hermansky-Pudlak syndrome (HPS) is an autosomal recessive disorder characterized by tyrosinase-positive oculocutaneous albinism, defective platelet function, and lysosomal accumulation of ceroid lipofuscin in reticuloendothelial cells (Figure 7–8). Clinical manifestations include a variable deficiency of skin and hair pigmentation, reduced visual acuity, congenital nystagmus, and a platelet defect that results in easy bruising of soft tissues and a bleeding diathesis. The sine qua non of the diagnosis of HPS is the absence of platelet-dense granules on electron microscopic analysis of cells from a patient with albinism and easy bruising (Figure 7–9). Lysosomal accumulation of a ceroid lipofuscin in macrophages, a poorly characterized lipid/protein complex, is associated with pulmonary fibrosis and granulomatous colitis.[150] Pulmonary disease, which is very common in HPS, manifests as a restrictive disorder with interstitial infiltrates and can progress to respiratory insufficiency and death by the fourth or fifth decade of life.[151,152]

Genetic and Cellular Basis of HPS

HPS in humans is a heterogenous genetic disorder caused by mutations in at least four separate loci. The existence of over a dozen genetically distinct murine models of HPS suggests that there are several additional HPS loci yet to be discovered in humans.[153] All manifestations of HPS appear to arise from defects in genes involved in the biogenesis of lysosomes, or specialized intracellular organelles that are related to lysosomes, including melanosomes and platelet-dense granules.

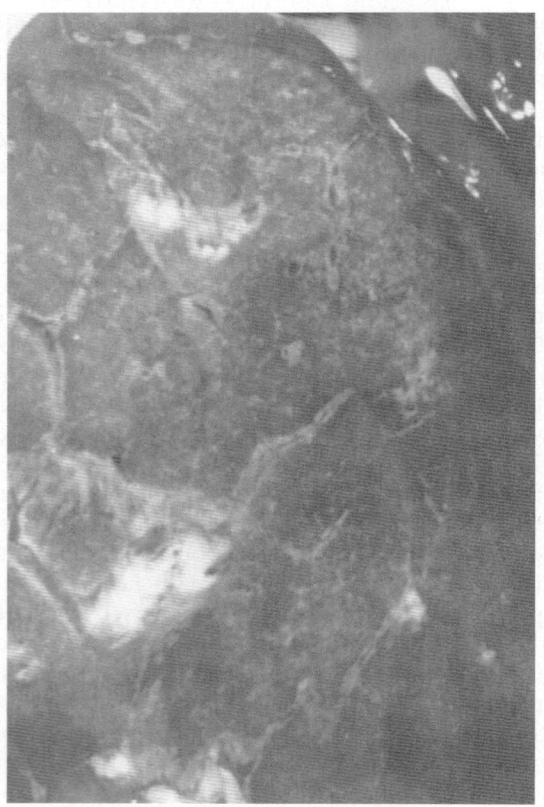

Figure 7–6 Gross appearance of the surface of the lung from a patient with Gaucher's disease. Note reticular appearance due to infiltration of interlobular septa and pleural surfaces with Gaucher's cells. Reproduced with permission from Gregory Grabowski, MD.

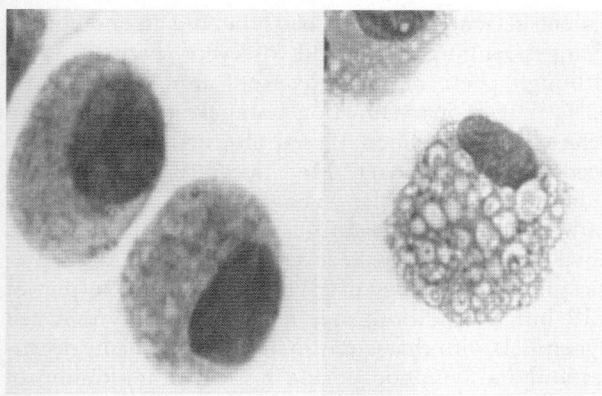

Figure 7–8 Macrophages containing lysosomal inclusions from a patient with Hermansky-Pudlak syndrome (right) are compared to a normal patient (left). Reproduced with permission from Mark Brantly, MD.

HPS may be the most common single genetic disorder in Puerto Rico, where 1 of 20 people carry the gene, and the disease is found in 1 of 1,800 people.[154] Most HPS in Puerto Ricans is caused by mutations in the *HPS1* gene and, less commonly, by mutations in *HPS3*. Outside of Puerto Rico, *HPS1* accounts for only about one half of HPS cases, and *HPS3* mutations are rare.[154–156] *HPS4* has recently been established as an additional HPS locus in humans.[157]

HPS1

HPS1 spans 20 exons on 10q23.1-q23.2 and encodes a ubiquitously expressed 700-amino acid, 79.3-kD protein with no known function or informative homologies

to other proteins. The most common mutation is a 16-bp duplication in exon 15. The protein product of *HPS1* is contained in two distinct high-molecular weight complexes distributed between uncoated vesicles, early stage melanosomes, and the cytosol. The mouse pale ear (*ep*) gene is the murine analogue of *HPS1* in humans.[158,159]

HPS2

The recognition of an HPS-like phenotype in *Drosophila*, including pigment granule defects, led to the identification of the *hypersensitivity pneumonitis2* locus on chromosome 5. The observation that the *Drosophila* pigmentation gene *garnet* encodes the β₃-adaptin subunit of the adaptor complex (AP-3) suggested an association between HPS and mutations in proteins that mediate trafficking of vesicular cargo proteins to cytoplasmic organelles. Dell'Angelica and colleagues subsequently identified mutations in the gene for the β_3-adaptin subunit of the heterotetrameric AP-3 complex in two patients with HPS.[160] The cDNA for the β_3-adaptin subunit predicted a protein composed of 1,094 amino acids and a mass of 140 kD. Fibroblasts from these subjects contained drastically reduced levels of AP-3 due to enhanced degradation of mutant β_3-adaptin. The AP-3 deficiency resulted in increased surface expression of the lysosomal membrane proteins CD63, LAMP-1, and LAMP-2, but not of nonlysosomal proteins, suggesting that the *HPS3* gene product is required at an early stage of melanosome biogenesis and maturation. The authors suggested that AP-3 functions in protein sorting to lysosomes and that HPS provides an example of a human disease in which altered trafficking of integral membrane proteins results from mutations in a component of the

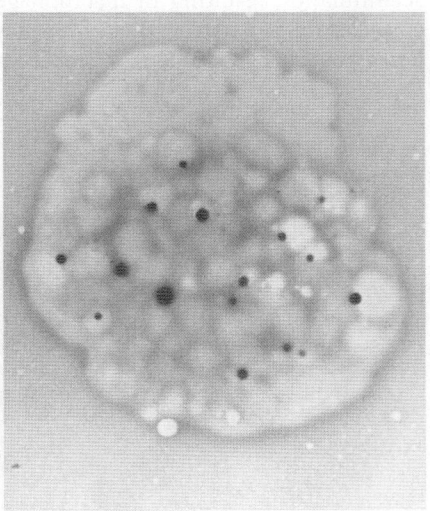

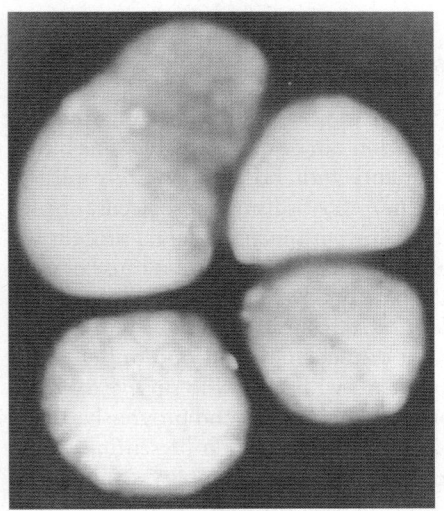

A   B

Figure 7–9 Electron micrograph of platelets from a normal subject (A) and from a patient with Hermansky-Pudlak syndrome (HPS) (B). Note the absence of dense bodies in the HPS patient. Provided by White JG, MD and the Hermansky-Pudlak Syndrome Network.

sorting machinery.[160] The murine models of *HPS2,* the pearl and mocha mice, develop ILD.[161]

HPS3

Aniskter and Oh identified a subset of 13 Puerto Rican HPS patients who did not have the 16-bp duplication characteristic of *HPS1,* and used homozygosity mapping of pooled DNA from their six families to identify a new HPS susceptibility locus on 3q24, called *HPS3.*[156,162] The *HPS3* gene encodes a 114-kD protein that consists of 1,004 amino acids, including a clathrin-binding motif, and that signals for targeting to lysosomal vesicles. The gene mutated in the cocoa (*coa*) mouse is homologous to the human *HPS3* locus.[163]

HPS4

Naturally occurring mutations in mice that result in pigment dilution and platelet dysfunction have revealed an additional HPS gene, *HPS4.*[157] The light-ear mouse was known to have a phenotype that was identical to the pale-ear mouse. The gene responsible for the light-ear phenotype was mapped to a region of the murine chromosome that is syntenic with human chromosome 22q11.2-q12.2. The human gene, termed *HPS4,* encodes a 708-amino acid protein with an apparent molecular mass of 76.9 kD. Of 21 unrelated Puerto Rican HPS patients who lacked the *HPS1* mutation who were screened, 7 were found to have non-sense, frameshift, and in-frame insertion mutations in *HPS4.* Although the function of the *HPS4* gene product is not known, it appears to play a role in the same pathway of membrane biogenesis as the *HPS1* gene product. The light-ear mouse is the rodent counterpart of *HPS4* in humans.[157]

Clinical Presentation of HPS

Albinism in HPS is tyrosinase positive, meaning that the loss of skin pigmentation can be quite variable. The bleeding diathesis in patients with HPS varies from mild to severe and may include easy bruising, nosebleeds, or prolonged or heavy bleeding with menses, dental procedures, and surgery. Fatal hemorrhage is a common cause of early mortality in HPS patients.[164] Some subjects develop a granulomatous colitis that is similar to that seen in Crohn's disease, and renal or cardiac failure may occur.[165,166] ILD develops in most patients with HPS who survive to adulthood.[167-170] A nonproductive cough and progressive dyspnea on exertion are the most common presenting symptoms. The mean age of onset of pulmonary symptoms is about 35 years, and there is no gender predominance. Chest radiograph patterns may vary from normal to fine reticular changes to end-stage honeycombing. Bulla and bronchiectasis have been reported in the upper lung zones. Brantly and colleagues reported that 82% of 38 HPS

patients screened by HRCT had ground-glass and fibrotic changes ranging from mild to severe (Figure 7–10), although chest radiographs were abnormal in only 42%.[171] Pulmonary function tests revealed a restrictive defect, although superimposed obstructive defects have been reported in smokers. More than 50% of patients had reduced FVC and DL_{CO}, and the mean values for the entire group were 71 and 72 % of predicted, respectively. Total lung capacity was reduced to a mean of 72% of predicted. The pathology of HPS is very similar to that of UIP, but, in addition, may reveal alveolar type II cell hyperplasia with characteristic swelling and foamy degeneration, and lymphocytic and histiocytic infiltration of respiratory bronchioles.[172] There is a significant interindividual variability in the severity of pulmonary disease that is not clearly related to age or specific mutations. The variability may derive from environmental factors or may be due to epigenetic phenomena.

Genotype–Phenotype Correlations

The 16-bp duplication in *HPS1* that is prevalent in Puerto Rico is associated with an increased risk of ILD.[166] Gahl and colleagues reported that 9 of 16 HPS patients with the duplication, but none of the 10 HPS patients without it, had a DL_{CO} less than 80% of predicted.[166] HRCT analysis of the patients with the duplication revealed a greater incidence and severity of pulmonary fibrosis than was found in patients with other HPS mutations.

Summary

HPS is strongly associated with ILD that is histologically similar to UIP. The mechanism of lung fibrosis of HPS is unknown, but aberrant lysosomal processing and ceroid accumulation resulting in macrophage and/or alveolar epithelial dysfunction are thought to play a role. The locus heterogeneity of HPS phenotypes in mice suggests that

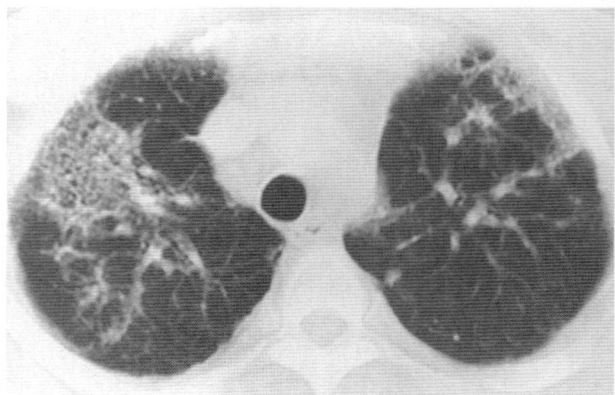

Figure 7–10 High-resolution computed tomography from a patient with Hermansky-Pudlak syndrome demonstrating reticulonodular infiltrates and honeycombing. Reproduced with permission from Mark Brantly, MD.

there may be several additional HPS gene loci to be discovered in humans. All patients with albinism and a bruising or bleeding diathesis should be screened for HPS. All patients with HPS should be screened for pulmonary involvement with pulmonary function tests and chest radiographs. There are currently no treatments available for the pulmonary manifestations of HPS. Vigilance and early treatment for respiratory infections and avoidance of smoking should be encouraged. Bronchoscopy by the oral route should be considered to avoid nasal bleeding.

Niemann-Pick Disease

Niemann-Pick Disease (NPD) is a rare autosomal recessive lipid-storage disease characterized by intracellular accumulation of sphingomyelin and cholesterol.[173,174] NPD is clinically and biochemically heterogeneous, divided into six variant forms designated types A through F. Infiltration of the reticuloendothelial system with lipid-laden Pick cells results in hepatosplenomegally and anemia due to bone marrow replacement. Variable degrees of neurologic involvement may occur. For example, type A NPD is associated with severe neurodegeneration leading to death in early childhood, whereas type B NPD patients survive into adulthood without neurologic involvement.

Genetic and Molecular Basis of NPD

The biochemical defect varies, ranging from lysosomal sphingomyelinase deficiency (types A and B) to altered intracellular cholesterol processing.[175] Types A and B NPD are caused by mutations in the *SMPD1* locus at 11p15.4-15.1. Types C1 and D (Nova Scotia) disease result from mutations in the *NPC1* gene for a lysosomally targeted protein of unknown function on 18q11-18q12. Type C2 disease results from mutations in the *NPC2* (*HE1*) gene on 14q24.3, encoding a protein called epididymal secretory protein, which is required for cholesterol esterification.

Murine Models of NPD

Gene-targeted mice that are deficient in acid sphingomyelinase, but not those that are deficient in neutral sphingomyelinase, accumulate sphingomyelin in the brain, the lung, and the reticuloendothelial system of liver, spleen, and bone marrow.[176] In addition, the ganglionic cell layer of Purkinje's cells of the cerebellum degenerates, leading to impairment of neuromotor coordination.[177,178] A naturally occurring murine model of type C disease also develops organomegally and neurologic dysfunction.[179]

Clinical, Radiographic, and Pathologic Presentation of NPD

Significant respiratory problems including pulmonary infiltration and fibrosis, occur in NPD, although the true incidence and association with NPD subtypes is difficult to ascertain from the literature, which is composed of approximately 40 case reports.[174] In general, pulmonary disease is more common in infantile and neuronotropic forms of the disease and rarer in adult forms. The most common physiological abnormality in NPD is a reduction in DL_{CO}, but exercise desaturation and restrictive changes may also occur.[180–186] Chest radiographs may reveal reticulonodular infiltrates, which are usually most prominent in the lung bases.[187,188] HRCT scans typically reveal areas of nodular, centrilobular ground-glass opacification in the upper lung zones, presumably due to infiltration with Pick's cells, and thickening of interlobular septa in the lower lung zones.[182] Axial lymph nodes may be enlarged, and cavitary changes in the pulmonary parenchyma may occur rarely, but pleural disease has not been reported.[174] Lung histopathology reveals an accumulation of NP cells in the alveoli and interstitium, associated with variable degrees of alveolar septal expansion with excess connective tissue matrix. Histiocytes, which stain intensely with May-Grunwald-Giemsa stain, known as "sea blue histiocytes," are typical of NPD but are not pathognomonic because they have been seen in other settings.[181,185,186] There is no specific treatment for NPD, but successful whole lung lavage for life-threatening hypoxia resulting from lipoid pneumonia in a patient with NPD disease was recently reported .[189]

GM₁ Gangliosidosis

GM$_1$ gangliosidosis, also known as Morquio's syndrome, type B or mucopolysaccharidosis type IVB, is a rare storage disorder caused by a deficiency of β-galactosidase. The disease is associated with severe cerebral degeneration, which usually leads to death within the first years of life; hepatosplenomegaly; accumulation of GM$_1$ ganglioside in reticuloendothelial cells, neurons, and renal epithelium; and skeletal deformities. Miliary shadows and reticulonodular changes have been observed on chest radiographs, and respiratory insufficiency may occur. Infiltration of alveolar structures with foamy macrophages has been described.[190,191] The disease-causing gene encoding β-galactosidase has been mapped to 13p21.33. Gene-targeted β-galactosidase-deficient mice develop cerebral degeneration, ataxia, and tremor due to neuronal accumulation of GM$_1$ ganglioside, but lung histology has not been reported in those animals.[192]

Pulmonary Alveolar Proteinosis

Pulmonary alveolar proteinosis (PAP) was first described in 1958, but little progress was made in the understanding of the molecular basis of the disorder until murine models of GM-CSF deficiency were found to exhibit an unexpected pulmonary disorder that mimicked the human disease.[193–195] The revelation that the

GM-CSF pathway was critical to pulmonary homeostasis led to the discovery of autoantibodies to GM-CSF in most patients with primary PAP and the identification of PAP families with mutations in the GM-CSF receptor. These and other studies have revealed a critical, nonredundant role for GM-CSF in the regulation of alveolar macrophage differentiation and surfactant metabolism. Novel therapeutic strategies based on these findings are beginning to be implemented. The work with PAP is an excellent example of the potential of transgenic technology to improve the lives of patients with ILD.

Clinical Presentation of PAP

PAP is an uncommon disorder characterized by accumulation of surfactant-enriched material in the distal air spaces.[196] Patients with PAP present with dyspnea on exertion, exercise intolerance, and impaired gas exchange. The onset of the disease is typically quite insidious, and the presentation mimics pneumonia, which can lead to delays in diagnosis. The absence of fever, failure to respond to antibiotic therapy, and the tendency of the disease to remit and relapse are typical. Chest radiographs may show a diffuse or focal ground-glass or consolidated appearance, and CT scan may reveal geographic patterns of density and lucency termed 'crazy paving.'[197] Sampling of the distal airways by alveolar lavage yields a flocculent creamy protein- and PL-rich sediment, which has a biochemical composition similar to that of pulmonary surfactant.[198] Furthermore, ultrastructural examination of PAP sediment reveals typical surfactant aggregate forms, including tubular myelin, membranous vesicles, and lamellated structures resembling lamellar bodies. Lung histology reveals amorphous eosinophilic PAS-positive material in the alveolar spaces and foamy alveolar macrophages. The alveolar septa and pulmonary interstitial spaces are usually normal but may be thickened and fibrotic, especially in chronic relapsing disease.

PAP can occur in the absence of associated disorders (primary PAP), or it can be associated with underlying hematologic malignancies, lymphoma, immunosuppression, connective tissue disease, thymic aplasia, or environmental exposures including silica dust, aluminum powder, fiberglass, and nitrogen or silicon dioxide (secondary PAP).[199–203] PAP is also associated with pulmonary infection, including *Nocardia,*[204] *Aspergillus, Cryptococcus,*[205] *Mycobacterium tuberculosis*[206] and nontuberculous mycobacteria, *Pneumocystis carinii,*[207] and *Histoplasma capsulatum.*[208] Although some investigators have postulated that these organisms may cause PAP, it is more likely that pulmonary infection in PAP is due to defective microbial clearance and the favorable growth environment for microbes. The disease usually occurs between the ages of 20 and 50 years, although young children and newborns are also affected. There is a male predominance.[209]

Animal Models of PAP

The molecular basis of surfactant accumulation in naturally occurring animal models of PAP, including the beige mouse and the severe combined immunodeficient (SCID) mouse, and in experimental rat models of silica and quartz exposure are not known.[210–213] In mice, targeted disruption in the genes that encode GM-CSF or its receptor had no discernable effects on hematopoiesis but resulted in a time-dependent accumulation of surfactant components resembling PAP in humans.[194,195,214] Alveolar and tissue levels of the signature surfactant lipid, saturated phosphatidylcholine, increased 10-fold and 2- to 4 fold, respectively, in 7- to 9-week old GM-CSF-deficient mice. Although there was a slight increase in surfactant PL synthesis in the animals, surfactant protein transcription was not altered, and the major abnormality in the GM-CSF-deficient mice was a marked catabolic defect for surfactant lipids and proteins.[215] Lung histology revealed air space accumulation of eosinophilic proteinaceous material and foamy alveolar macrophages associated with perivascular and peribronchiolar mononuclear cell infiltrates. Overexpression of GM-CSF in the pulmonary epithelium or airway administration of aerosolized GM-CSF corrected PAP in GM-CSF-deficient mice, but systemic administration did not.[216] An unexpected finding from mice that overexpressed GM-CSF in either the GM-CSF null or wild-type background was exuberant type II cell hyperplasia, alveolar macrophage accumulation in the distal air spaces, and a 30 to 40% increase in the size of the lungs compared to mice without the GM-CSF transgene.[217]

The correction of PAP in GM-CSF receptor-deficient mice with the use of bone marrow transplantation from wild-type mice suggests that the predominant target for GM-CSF in regulating pulmonary homeostasis in the lung is the alveolar macrophage rather than the alveolar type II cell.[196] GM-CSF is known to play an important role in promoting the growth, differentiation, and activation of monocytic and granulocytic precursor cells.[218] Alveolar macrophages isolated from GM-CSF-deficient mice exhibit marked defects in the catabolism of SP-A and PLs.[219] The defect in surfactant catabolism in GM-CSF-deficient mice appeared to result from arrested macrophage differentiation and was associated with marked down-regulation of the transcription factor PU.1.[220] Overexpression GM-CSF in the pulmonary epithelium of GM-CSF (–/–) mice restored PU.1 expression, and retrovirus-mediated expression of PU.1 in macrophages from GM-CSF (–/–) mice corrected the defect in surfactant catabolism.[220] Other differentiated functions that were found to be down-regulated in alveolar macrophages isolated from GM-CSF (–/–) mice included lipopolysaccharide-induced tumor necrosis factor (TNF)-α expression; Toll receptor pathway expression of TLR2, TLR4, and CD14; mannose receptor expression; phagocytosis; and intracellular killing.

GM-CSF/Interleukin-3/Interleukin-5 Receptor Common β-Chain Defects

The unexpected PAP phenotype of the genetically engineered murine models led to several important discoveries in patients with PAP. Failure to express the GM-CSF/interleukin (IL)-3/IL-5 receptor common β-chain was identified in a number of pediatric PAP patients and a single adult PAP patient.[221] In one patient, the causative mutation was found to be a proline to threonine substitution in codon 602 of the β-chain of the receptor. Genetically engineered mice with a deficiency of the common β-chain develop alveolar proteinosis.[214,222]

Circulating Anti-GM-CSF Autoantibody

In 1999, Kitamura and colleagues discovered that most cases of primary PAP are caused by a circulating, neutralizing antibody of the IgG isotype against GM-CSF in lavage fluid.[223–225] The antibody was found to be present in all specimens of BAL fluid and sera obtained from 11 primary PAP patients but not in samples from 2 secondary PAP patients, 53 normal subjects, or 14 patients with other lung diseases.

The conventional treatment for symptomatic PAP is therapeutic whole lung lavage. This intervention typically alleviates symptoms, improves gas exchange and pulmonary function, and reduces radiographic infiltrates, but it requires hospital admission and general anesthesia. Novel therapies based on an improved understanding of the molecular basis of PAP are beginning to emerge. Treatment of PAP patients with parenteral recombinant GM-CSF has produced a response rate of 43% in patients with neutralizing GM-CSF antibody, including an average 23.3 mm Hg increase in the alveolar–arteriolar gradient for oxygen P(A-a)O$_2$.[226,227] GM-CSF therapy is well tolerated, and responses have lasted for a mean of 39 weeks. A latex agglutination test using recombinant GM-CSF-coated beads was developed and can be used for the serological identification of PAP with a sensitivity of 100% and specificity of 98%.[224] Several therapeutic strategies to increase GM-CSF activity by inhibiting immune responses that result in generation of the antibody or by direct removal of the antibody are under investigation.

Lysinuric Protein Intolerance

Lysinuric protein intolerance (LPI) is a rare autosomal recessive disorder of cationic amino acid transport at the basolateral epithelial membrane in the kidney and small intestine.[228] Predominant disease manifestations include mental retardation, delayed physical development, intestinal malabsorption, vomiting, failure to thrive, and increased urinary excretion of lysine, ornithine, and arginine. The disease is usually diagnosed in childhood, at an average age of 5 to 6 years. The only reported life-threatening manifestation of LPI is respiratory insufficiency that results from progressive pulmonary alveolar proteinosis and alveolar hemorrhage.

The transport of arginine and ornithine across the basolateral cellular membrane produces a deficiency of substrate for the urea cycle enzyme, ornathine decarboxylase, and results in hyperammonemia with usual amounts of dietary protein. LPI families have been reported in Finland, Italy, and Japan. It is caused by mutations in the heterotrimeric amino acid transporter (HAT) gene *SLC7A7*, which was initially assigned to chromosome 14q11.2 by linkage analysis and later identified by candidate positional cloning.[229] HATs are composed of heavy subunits that bear sequence homology to β-glucosidases and contain a single transmembrane domain linked by an interchain disulfide bond to a 'light' subunit containing 12 membrane-spanning domains.[228]

Patients with LPI can develop pulmonary hemorrhage and alveolar proteinosis.[230–232] Parto and colleagues reported that of 38 patients with LPI diagnosed in Finland between 1964 and 1994, 4 patients had died, all with pulmonary insufficiency. Three of the cases were found to have typical alveolar proteinosis at autopsy, and all four were found to have evidence of pulmonary hemorrhage. Asymptomatic patients with LPI who were screened with HRCT were found to have acinar nodules, inter- and/or intralobular thickening of the interstitial septa, and subpleural cysts.[233] Of 25 symptom-free LPI patients studied in Finland, one-third (8 of 25) had signs suggestive of pulmonary fibrosis on chest radiograph and two-thirds (8 of 14) had evidence of ILD on HRCT scan.[230] The mechanism of surfactant accumulation in LPI is unknown.

SP-B Mutations

Hereditary deficiency of SP-B is an autosomal recessive disorder that results in lethal respiratory distress in morphologically normal infants and is associated with accumulation of surfactant lipids and proteins reminiscent of what occurs in PAP.[234] Full-term infants develop respiratory distress within the first 12 to 24 hours of life and usually succumb within 1 to 6 months. The mechanisms responsible for accumulation of surfactant in SP-B-deficient infants are not known, but surfactant metabolism is clearly deranged, because lamellar bodies are dysmorphic or absent, and the processing of SP-C is abnormal.

The *SP-B* gene spans 10 kb on chromosome 2 and has 11 exons, of which only the first 10 are translated. The 2-kb transcript directs the synthesis of a 381-amino acid proprotein, which is glycosylated and proteolytically cleaved to liberate an 8-kD mature protein encoded by exons 6 and 7. *SP-B* is composed of four amphipathic helices and is intimately associated with surfactant PLs in the alveolar space. Affected infants in the initial kindred were homozygous for mutations that involved small deletions and insertions in codon 121 of exon 4 of the *SP-B* gene, which resulted in a frameshift and premature termination.[235] Incompletely processed proSP-C accumulates intracellularly in SP-B-deficient infants with congenital alveolar proteinosis.[236] Gene-targeted mice that are deficient in SP-B develop respiratory distress and die at birth.

Summary

PAP is a clinically and biochemically heterogeneous disorder that may result from environmental exposures, diseases associated with monocyte/macrophage dysfunction, abnormalities in the pathways for GM-CSF signaling, and amino acid transport or surfactant protein production. Currently available therapies for PAP include therapeutic lavage and exogenously administered GM-CSF. Pulmonary fibrosis may result from long-standing or recurrent PAP.

DISORDERS OF THE PULMONARY MATRIX

Discovery of the genetic basis of hereditary disorders of the pulmonary connective tissue matrix, including Marfan syndrome, Ehlers-Danlos syndrome, cutis laxa, and pseudoxanthoma elasticum, has elucidated the molecular mechanisms that can result in emphysema and formation of bullae. Of these, however, only Marfan syndrome has been associated with the development of pulmonary fibrosis.

Marfan Syndrome

Marfan syndrome is an uncommon hereditary connective tissue abnormality characterized by tall stature, excessively long limbs, a high arched palate with crowded teeth, an anterior chest deformity, joint laxity, subluxation of the lens of the eye, and scoliosis. Cardiovascular manifestations include aortic aneurysms, dissection of the thoracic aorta, aortic and mitral regurgitation, and annuloaortic ectasia. The most common pulmonary manifestation of Marfan syndrome is spontaneous pneumothorax, but diffuse emphysema, bronchiectasis, and upper lobe-predominant fibrosis have also been reported.[237–239]

Identification of the Gene

The discovery of the fibrillin gene began with a morphological observation. Patients with Marfan were known to have structural abnormalities of the ciliary zonule, a ligamentous structure in the eye. Fibrillin was localized to the ciliary zonule of skin and fibroblasts of Marfan patients by immmunohistochemistry, and pulse-chase experiments demonstrated abnormal synthesis, secretion, or extracellular matrix deposition from cultured fibroblasts of Marfan patients.[240–242] Linkage studies mapped the Marfan gene to the same region of chromosome 15 that contained the fibrillin gene (*FBN1*), and linkage between the Marfan phenotype and the fibrillin gene was demonstrated. The *FBN1* gene contains 65 exons and spans 110 kb on chromosome 15q21.1.[243] Identification of fibrillin as a Marfan gene was confirmed by the identification of point mutations in the fibrillin gene in patients with Marfan syndrome.[244–246] Many more mutations have been identified, but there are no clear genotype–phenotype correlations except a clustering of mutations between exons 24 and 32 in neonatal Marfan syndrome.[247]

Biochemical Basis of Marfan Syndrome

Marfan can present as an autosomal recessive disorder with variable penetrance or as an autosomal dominant disorder, but in all known cases, the disease is due to a mutation in *FBN1* (Table 7–3). Characterization of the cDNA for fibrillin was reported by Maslan and coworkers.[248] The profibrillin sequence encodes a 350-kD 2,871-amino acid protein that is highly repetitive and contains multiple domains, including a stretch of basic amino acids at the N-terminus, a proline-rich region, and 46 epidermal growth factor (EGF)-like repeats.[249,250] The EGF-repeats contain cysteine-rich domains, and 43 of 46 contain a consensus sequence for calcium binding, which may play important roles in protein–protein interactions. The tandem repetition of EGF repeats is interrupted by eight cysteine-containing motifs that bear homology to the TB domains of transforming growth factor (TGF)-β_1-binding protein. Fibrillin is a large glycoprotein, expressed in multiple tissues, that complexes with elastin to form elastic fibers and is also a major component of microfibrils. Fibrillins form the structural framework that endows connective tissues with long-range elasticity.

The tight-skinned mouse, which contains a duplication in the murine homologue of the fibrillin gene, has abnormal bone development, vascular abnormalities, stiff skin, and pulmonary emphysema.[251,252] The mutation results in the production of mutant murine fibrillin (418 kD), which has a mass that is almost 20% greater than that of the wild-type protein (350 kD). The lung and bone abnormalities in the mice appear to be caused by copolymerization of mutant and wild-type molecules into functionally defective microfibrils.[252] Gene targeting of the *FBN1* gene in mice that results in fibrillen deficiency recapitulates the Marfan phenotype, however.[253]

OTHER GENETIC ILDS

Other familial disorders that result in ILD are listed in Table 7–4 and discussed below.

TABLE 7–3   Genetic Basis of Metabolic Disorders Associated with ILD

	MOI	Type	Chromosome Locus	Locus Name	Protein	Pulmonary Disease	Pathologic ILD Pattern	Murine Model
Fabry's	XL		Xq22	GLA	α-galactosidase	Obstructive lung disease	Airway infiltration and epithelial inclusions	α-GalA (−/−)[367]
Gaucher's	AR AR AR	Type 1 infantile Type 2 visceral Type 3 adult	1q21 1q21 1q21	GBA GBA GBA	β-glucosidase, acid-β	PAH, ILD, pleural disease	Gaucher's cell infiltration, fibrosis	Gba (−/−)[135]
Niemann-Pick	AR	Type A and B	11p15.4-p15.1	SMPD1	Sphingomyelinase, phosphodiesterase-1	Respiratory insufficiency	Alveolar Pick cell infiltration	Smpd1 (−/−)[178]
	AR	Type C1 and D	18q11-q12	NPC1	Unknown function	Reticulonodular infiltrates		NPC1 (−/−)[368]
	AR	Type C2	14q24	NPC2	Epididymal secretory protein			None
Hermansky-Pudlak	AR	HPS-1	10q23.1-q23.3	HPS1	Unknown function	Occurs in most long-lived HPS patients; worse in HPS-1	UIP-like lesion with foamy macrophages and type II cells	Pale-ear (ep)[158]
	AR	HPS-2	Chromosome 5	HPS2	Unknown function			Pearl[161]
	AR	HPS-3	3q24	HPS3	AP-3			Cocoa[163]
	AR	HPS-4	22q11.2-q12.2	HPS4	Unknown function			Light-ear[157]
Alveolar proteinosis	?	IL-3/GM-CSF receptor mutations	22q12.2	CSF2RB	GM-CSF receptor	PAP	Lipoproteinaceous debris and macrophage accumulation in alveoli	βc (−/−) & βc (−/−), GM-CSF (−/−)[222]
	AR	Congenital SP-B deficiency	2q12.2-p11.2	SFTPB	Surfactant protein B	Respiratory failure, PAP		SP-B (−/−)[369]
	AR	Lysinuric protein intolerance	14q	SLC7A7	Cationic amino acid transporter	PAP, hemoptysis		None
GM$_1$ gangliosidosis	?	Infantile and adult	13p21.33	GLB1	β-galactosidase	Respiratory insufficiency & miliary shadows	Infiltration of alveolar septa and lumen with foamy macrophages	β-Gal (−/−)[192]

AR = autosomal recessive; GM-CSF = granulocyte macrophage colony-stimulating factor; HPS = Hermansky-Pudlak syndrome; MOI, mode of inheritance; PAP = pulmonary alveolar proteinosis; SP-B = surfactant protein B; XL = X linked.

Familial Hypocalciuric Hypercalcemia

Familial hypocalciuric hypercalcemia (FHH) was first described by Foley and colleagues as a cause of hypercalcemia and hypermagnesemia associated with low urinary calcium secretion.[254] An association between pulmonary fibrosis and FHH was first reported by Auwerx and coworkers.[255,256] Manifestations of pulmonary fibrosis, including reticulonodular radiographic infiltrates, reduced DL_{CO}, and restrictive pulmonary physiology, typically become apparent by the fourth decade of life and may progress to end-stage disease with honeycomb changes. FHH is also associated with recurrent infections resulting from low myeloperoxidase levels and granulocyte dysfunction.[257] Examination of BAL fluid reveals elevated cell counts, multinucleated giant cells, macrophages containing dark cytoplasmic inclusions, and increased neutrophils that are suggestive of alveolitis. Tissue specimens from lung biopsies exhibit interstitial inflammatory infiltrates and conchoid-body aggregates surrounded by multinucleated giant cells and loosely formed granulomas.

Cellular and Genetic Basis of FHH

The genetic basis of FHH has recently been elucidated. From a study of 25 families with primary parathyroid hyperplasia, two autosomal dominant disorders were discovered, including type I multiple endocrine adenomatosis (MEA) and familial hypocalciuric hypercalcemia.[258,259] Although the prevalence of hypercalcemia and hypermagnesemia approached 50%, unlike the MEA patients, the FHH was not associated with hypercalciuria, nephrolithiasis, or peptic ulcer. FHH results from heterozygous loss-of-function mutations, whereas heterozygous gain-of-function mutations cause autosomal dominant and sporadic hypoparathyroidism. Homozygous loss-of-function mutations result in lethal neonatal hyperparathyroidism (LNH). FHH and LNH result from mutations in the calcium-sensing receptor (*CaR*) gene on chromosome 3, a seven-transmembrane G protein-coupled receptor that appears to set the extracellular calcium level.[260–262] In the kidney, activation of *CaR* decreases calcium resorption, and in the parathyroid, activation of *CaR* regulates secretion of parathyroid hormone. A second locus for FHH, termed *HHC3*, has been mapped to 19q13.[263]

Murine Models of FHH

A murine model of FHH was developed by gene targeting of the *CaR* locus. Like patients with FHH, *CaR* (+/–) mice had hypocalciuria and modest elevations of serum calcium, magnesium, and parathyroid hormone levels.[264] In contrast, *CaR* (–/–) mice, like patients with severe LNH, had markedly elevated serum calcium and parathyroid hormone levels, parathyroid hyperplasia, bone abnormalities, retarded growth, and premature death.

TABLE 7–4   Genetic Basis of Miscellaneous Disorders

	MOI	Type	Chromosome Locus	Locus Name	Protein	Pulmonary Disease	ILD Pathologic Pattern	Murine Model
Marfan	AR or AD		15q21.1	FBN1	Fibrillin	Upper lobe fibrosis; bullae, PAH	UIP-like	FBN1 (−/−)[253]
Familial hypocalciuria hypercalcemia	AD	I	3q13.3-q21	CASR or HHC1	Calcium-sensing receptor	Fibrosis, recurrent infections	Loose granulomas, foamy macrophages, conchoid body inclusions	Casr (+/−)[264]
	AD	III	19q13	HHC3	?			None
Pulmonary alveolar microlithiasis	AR		?	?	?	Respiratory insufficiency, fibrosis, micronodular radiographic pattern	Fibrosis & microliths	nackt[279]
Lipid proteinosis	AR		1q21	ECM1	ECM1	Fibrosis, laryngeal lesions	Alveolar septal expansion	None
X-linked dyskeratosis congenita	X-linked & AD		Xq28 &3q	DKC1 & TERC	Dyskerin & RNA telomerase	Fibrosis	UIP-like	None mTR (−/−)[370]

MOI = mode of inheritance; ECM1 = extracellular matrix protein 1; FHH = familial hypocalciuric hypercalcemia; PAM = pulmonary alveolar microlithiasis; UIP = usual interpneumonitis.

Summary

FHH is an autosomal dominant disorder caused by mutations in genes that regulate calcium homeostasis. The role of the CaR receptor in the pathogensis of lung fibrosis is not known, but the CaR family appears to play a role in potentiating the effects of a number of profibrotic mediators, including thrombin and angiotensin II.[265]

Pulmonary Alveolar Microlithiasis

Pulmonary alveolar microlithiasis (PAM) is a rare progressive lung disorder that can result in pulmonary fibrosis, respiratory insufficiency, and death. Approximately 300 cases have been reported in the literature, in patients ranging in age from premature infants (twins) to an 80-year-old woman.[266–268] PAM is characterized by the presence of innumerable pulmonary alveolar calcifications, causing a sandlike micronodular radiographic pattern that is readily distinguished from other pulmonary disorders associated with calcification.[269] About half of the reported cases in large series are inherited, and many have been associated with consanguinity.[270,271] Most familial cases have occurred in siblings, suggesting a possible environmental component. Data suggesting that PAM is more common in females have been challenged.[266,272] A disproportionate number of the reported cases in the literature have been from Spain and Turkey. PAM occurs most commonly as an isolated pulmonary disorder, typically with normal serum calcium levels, but some cases have been associated with pleural calcification, urolithiasis, cholelithiasis, azoospermia, and multiple skeletal exostoses.[273,274] The most common symptom is dyspnea on exertion, followed by nonproductive cough and hemoptysis (rare). Late stages of the disease may be associated with clubbing, pulmonary hypertension, and respiratory failure. The characteristic radiographic pattern of very fine micronodularity may require increased exposure time to clearly delineate. The radiographic findings are often striking and out of proportion to the symptomatology of the patient. In fact, changes consistent with PAM may be apparent on radiographs from decades before and on those of asymptomatic relatives. HRCT reveals a calcified reticular pattern and thickening of the interlobular septa, especially along perilobular regions and along bronchovascular bundles, with a predominantly basal and peripheral lung distribution.[275] Subpleural air cysts and paraseptal emphysema may also be present. Sarcoidosis can occasionally produce a calcified micronodular pattern that mimics PAM.[276] Bronchoscopy may reveal characteristic calcospherites in the recovered BAL fluid, and transbronchial biopsy can reveal calcified foci.[266] Reduced residual volumes, elevated arterial–alveolar gradients, and mild reductions in lung volumes have been reported. Open lung biopsy, while rarely indicated, reveals a fine granular appearance due to filling of the alveolar spaces with 250 to 750 μM calcium phosphate microliths

having PAS-positive cores. Interstitial fibrosis of alveolar walls associated with giant cell formation is apparent in some cases. There are no known effective therapies for PAM, although single-lung transplantation has been performed successfully.[277] Improvement in the profusion of radiographic infiltrates was noted after 1 year of treatment with sodium etidronate in one patient.[278] The genetic basis for PAM is not known. Mice that are homozygous for mutations in nackt (nkt) develop diffuse alopecia, a marked CD4 T-cell peripheral deficiency in the thymus and lymph nodes, and multiple 30- to −100-μm rounded to oval PAS-positive alveolar septal concretions that resemble those which occur in patients with PAM.[279,280] The causative mutation is a 1,180-bp deletion in the cathepsin L gene, which is required for the degradation of the invariant chain, a critical chaperone for class II major histocompatibility complex (MHC) molecules.[281]

Lipoid Proteinosis

Lipoid proteinosis, also known as hyalinosis cutis et mucosae or Urback-Wiethe disease, is a rare autosomal recessive disorder associated with abnormal protein and lipid deposition in several tissues including the lung. It has been described in over 250 case reports from around the world, but it is especially prevalent in certain areas such as the Northern Cape province of South Africa, where it occurs in a population of mixed Khoisan and European origin. Clinical manifestations include hoarseness due to laryngeal infiltration, beaded or warty papules on the skin and eyelid margins, thickening of the tongue and frenulum, alopecia, epilepsy, and neuropsychiatric abnormalities.[282] Lung manifestations are rare but may include reticulonodular changes consistent with diffuse interstitial fibrosis on the chest radiograph.[283,284] On pathologic examination, alveolar septa are expanded by amorphous eosinophilic material.[284] The gene for lipoid proteinosis has been mapped to 1q21 with the use of DNA from a consanguineous Saudi Arabian family.[285] Six different homozygous mutations in extracellular matrix (ECM) protein 1 (ECM1) have been found with the use of a candidate gene approach. ECM is a glycoprotein of unknown function, which has been implicated in the regulation of endochondral bone formation, keratinocyte differentiation, and angiogenesis.[286–288] ECM is expressed as two alternatively spliced transcripts: ECM1, which is predominantly present in the heart, lung, and the gastrointestinal and genitourinary tracts, and ECM1b, which is found in the skin and tonsils.[289]

Fabry's Disease

Fabry's disease is an inherited X-linked disorder that results in accumulation of the glycosphingolipid ceramide trihexoside in blood vessels and epithelial cells from multiple tissues, including the skin, the kidneys, and the heart. It is caused by deficiency of α-galactosidase A, the enzyme responsible for metabolizing ceramide trihexoside. The most characteristic presentation of Fabry's is the appearance of red spots on the skin, followed by renal and myocardial failure within a decade. Pulmonary manifestations of Fabry's disease include dyspnea, wheezing, hemoptysis, pneumothorax, frequent respiratory infections, pulmonary vascular infiltration, and fixed airflow obstruction, which is presumed to be secondary to glycolipid accumulation in airway walls.[290] Lung histology reveals lamellar inclusions in bronchial epithelial cells and infiltration of small airways. The gene for α-galactosidase is found at Xq22, and dozens of loss-of-function mutations have been described.[291]

X-linked Dyskeratosis Congenita

Dyskeratosis congenita is a rare multisystem disorder associated with epiphora, lesions of the skin and appendages, early dental loss, urinary tract abnormalities, frequent bone marrow failure, and a predisposition to gastrointestinal malignancies. Pulmonary fibrosis with pathology that is consistent with UIP has been reported in four patients but is probably underestimated.[292-295] The X-linked form of the disease is caused by mutations in the *DKC1* gene on Xq28, which encodes dyskerin,[296,297] whereas the autosomal dominant form of the disease is caused by a deletion of 3q, which removes the 74 bases of RNA telomerase.[298]

FAMILIAL CLUSTERING IN IPF, CONNECTIVE TISSUE-RELATED ILD, SARCOIDOSIS, AND HYPERSENSITIVITY PNEUMONITIS

Minor degrees of familial clustering have been described in several ILDs, suggesting important genetic influences on the development of the disease. Although most IPF and sarcoidosis is not inherited, it is clear that multiple genes influence the response to environmental challenges and the complex interactions between inflammatory and repair pathways that result in fibrosis.

Familial Sarcoidosis

Sarcoidosis is an idiopathic systemic granulomatous disorder that often involves the lung. Familial clustering and associations with genetic polymorphisms and with the major histocompatibility locus on chromosome 6p suggest that genetic factors play an important role in the disease. The prevalence of familial sarcoidosis varies between populations; it is reported to be 3.6% in Finnish patients,[299] 4.3% in Japanese patients,[299] 9.6% in Irish patients,[300] 6.9% in Swedish patients,[300] and 19% in black patients.[302] The prevalence of sarcoidosis in first-degree relatives of 80 black patients was 1.5% in one study[303] and was 2.5% of 488 parents and siblings of 179 black sarcoidosis cases in another.[304] In a primarily white population, McGrath and coworkers reported a sibling relative risk for sarcoidosis between 3.6 and 7.3.[305] The familial relative risk in 10,862 first-degree and 17,047 second-degree relatives of 706 age-, sex-, and geographically matched cases who participated in the multicenter ACCESS (A Case-Controlled Etiology Study of Sarcoidosis) trial was 4.7.[306] Cases in white patients revealed a markedly higher familial risk than did black cases (OR = 18 vs 2.8; *p* = .098). Siblings had the highest relative OR (5.8) followed by avuncular relatives (5.7), grandparents (5.2), and then parents (3.8).

Familial IPF

Familial IPF, which has been reported in dozens of case studies, is transmitted as an autosomal dominant trait with reduced penetrance.[307-320] Unaffected family members of patients with inherited IPF may have evidence of subclinical alveolitis, based on increased neutrophils, activated macrophages, and increased levels of fibroblast growth factors in BAL fluid.[320] Forty-three IPF families had been reported in the literature through 1997. Marshall and colleagues reviewed the clinical and epidemiologic findings in 67 patients from 25 families with IPF from the United Kingdom and concluded that familial cases occur in younger patients and account for 0.5 to 2.2% of all cases of IPF.[311] The ratio of men to women was 1.75:1. Patients with connective tissue-related ILD and sarcoidosis were excluded, and lung biopsies were available in approximately one-third of cases. The mean age at presentation to a respiratory physician was 55 years, most commonly with complaints of shortness of breath and cough. About one-half of the patients had a previous history of smoking, with a median pack-years smoked of 28.3. HRCT data were available in 93% of cases and revealed changes that were typical for IPF. Restrictive physiology and reduced DL_{CO} were present. A screening study of all 29 pulmonary clinics in Finland revealed a frequency for IPF of 16 to 18 per 100,000 people and an incidence of familial IPF cases involving 2 to 5 family members of 5.9 per million. The familial form accounted for 3.3 to 3.7% of all IPF in the country.[321] Familial lung disease resembling desquamative interstitial pneumonitis was described in several sets of siblings, their parents, and second-degree relatives.[322-326]

ILD-ASSOCIATED GENETIC POLYMORPHISMS

Genetic polymorphisms are variations in the DNA sequence that occur in more than 1% of the population and which can be useful in defining pathophysiological mechanisms and predicting susceptibility to disease, disease progression, and/or pharmacologic responses to treatment.[327] Polymorphisms may affect disease expression when they encode for amino acid substitutions in the protein product of a gene or when they regulate the level of expression of a gene by affecting promoter function or mRNA stability. Polymorphisms that occur in DNA regions that are not involved in gene transcription do not affect the level or function of proteins but may be useful markers for disease susceptibility or for linkage analysis. Unfortunately, most polymorphism studies in ILD populations are uninformative because of inadequate statistical power or poor design. Well-executed studies define patient populations and disease phenotypes carefully, contain adequate sample sizes, account for environmental influences, and employ appropriate controls.[327] Definitive polymorphism dissociation studies for most ILDs will require cooperative multicenter studies.

IPF

The selection of candidate genes for polymorphism studies in IPF usually focuses on cytokines, inflammatory mediators, and human leukocyte antigen (HLA) loci. Many studies are plagued by small sample size and failure to discriminate between IPF and connective tissue disease-related ILD, which causes them to yield confusing and often conflicting results. Pantelidis and colleagues found no association between IPF and polymorphisms in TNF, lymphotoxin-α, TNF receptor 2, or IL-6 when compared with a matched control population, with the exception of an overrepresentation of a particular TNF haplotype in the female IPF population.[328] Polymorphisms in the genes encoding IL-1 receptor antagonists, TNF immunoglobulin phenotypes, and the angiotensin-converting enzyme have been reported in patients with IPF.[310,329,330] Reported associations between HLA antigens and IPF include HLA-B15, HLA-Dw6, HLA-DR2, HLA-B12, and HLA-DR2.[331,332] Available data on the association of IPF and α_1-antitrypsin Z and S alleles are conflicting.[333,334] Genetic studies of the candidate region near the HLA region of chromosome 6 in familial IPF/UIP and in sporadic IPF have been inconclusive. Familial IPF has been linked to the HLA loci B8, B15, Dw6, DR2, and B12.[331,332,335,336]

Connective Tissue Disease-Related ILD

An apparent association between abnormal α_1-antitrypsin genes and rheumatoid arthritis related ILD (RA-ILD) was not confirmed in a subsequent larger study.[333,337] A strong association between pulmonary fibrosis in patients with systemic sclerosis and HLA-DR3 and/or -DRw52a has been reported.[338]

Granulomatous ILD

Individuals with the HLA polymorphism HLA-DPB1 Glu69, which encodes glutamic acid at position 69 of the DPβ-chain, have a 10-fold higher risk of developing chronic beryllium disease on appropriate exposure.[339] Functional studies confirm the importance of the HLA-DPβ1 glutamate 69 polymorphism in the responsiveness of T-cell clones derived from patients.[340] However, there was no association between the glutamate 69 polymorphism and sarcoidosis despite histologic and phenotypic similarities between the diseases.[341] An association between sarcoidosis and HLA-B8 and -DR5 has also been reported.[342–345]

HLA-DR7 has been associated with hypersensitivity pneumonitis in 48 patients with pigeon breeder's lung.[346] Selman and colleagues examined polymorphisms of the MHC class II alleles and TNF-α promoter in 44 patients with pigeon breeder's lung, 99 healthy unrelated controls, and 50 exposed but asymptomatic patients.[347] The alleles HLA-DRB1*1305 and HLA-DQB1*0501 were overrepresented in the patients with pigeon breeder's lung, and HLA-DRB1*0802 was underrepresented compared with both control groups ($p < .05$). Haplotype analysis revealed an increase of DRB1*1305-DQB1*0301 and a decrease of DRB1*0802-DQB1*0402. The TNF-2(-)(308) allele was also associated with hypersensitivity pneumonitis and with younger age and more active alveolitis based on BAL fluid lymphocyte counts. These results suggest that genetic factors located in the MHC region contribute to the development of pigeon breeder's lung. Patients with the TNF-2(-)(308) allele develop more robust TNF responses to antigen challenge than do patients without this allele.[348]

MURINE MODELS OF PULMONARY FIBROSIS

Animal models are invaluable tools for dissecting the molecular pathways that lead to pulmonary fibrosis. Genetic murine models of ILD can be divided into three categories: those with naturally occurring mutations that result in fibrosis, such as the moth-eaten mouse; those in which overexpression or ablation of a specific gene results in pulmonary fibrosis (Table 7–5); and those in which overexpression or ablation of a specific gene results in altered susceptibility to a fibrogenic agent (Table 7–6).

Naturally Occurring Murine Models of Interstitial Lung Disease

Moth-eaten mice are one of only a very few murine models of naturally occurring ILD that have been identified. Moth-eaten mice develop lethal hemorrhagic pneumonitis at 8 to 10 weeks of age due to expansion and dysfunction of cells of the myelomonocytic lineage. The lung pathology progresses through three distinct stages, including focal intra-alveolar hemorrhage with accumulations of alveolar macrophages and neutrophils in the lower respiratory tract, alveolitis and reparative processes associated with abundant mitotic fibroblasts and alveolar type II alveolar cells, and marked derangement and fibrosis of the alveolar walls.[349] The deficiency of Src homology 2 domain-containing cytosolic phosphatase 1 (*SHP1*), responsible for the moth-eaten phenotype, is complete in the moth-eaten (*me/me*) strains and partial (20%) in the moth-eaten viable (*me^v^/me^v^*) strains.[350] Loss of SHP-1 results in dysregulated or persistent phosphorylation of receptor tyrosine kinases, cytokine receptors, and cytosolic signaling effectors, which causes derangements in myelomonocytic cell function, including increased oxidant production and expression of CD18, as well as markedly diminished chemotaxis.[351] The importance of myelomonocytic cells in the pathogenesis of lung injury in moth-eaten mice is underscored by the attenuation of lung inflammation in moth-eaten mice treated with the macrophage depleting autobody, anti-Mac-1.[352]

Genetic Manipulations That Result in Lung Inflammation and Fibrosis

Transgenic or adenoviral-mediated overexpression of several proinflammatory cytokines results in lung inflammation and/or pulmonary fibrosis, including platelet-derived growth factor, IL-13, IL-1β, TGF-α, GM-CSF, and TNF-α.[353–355] In several of these models, intense leukocyte infiltration followed by alveolar septal expansion with excess connective tissue reaffirms an important role for inflammation in lung remodeling in some forms of pulmonary fibrosis. Albation of presenilin-2 and caveolin-1 also resulted in interstitial changes in the lung through mechanisms that are unclear.[356]

Genetic Manipulations That Alter Susceptibility to Lung Inflammation and Fibrosis

Genetically engineered animal models have been used to elucidate the molecular pathways that contribute to pulmonary fibrosis that occurs in response to toxic agents, such as bleomycin. Not surprisingly, the deficiency of proinflammatory (eg, interferon-γ) and profibrotic (eg, TGF-β) mediators and receptors (eg, TNFR) generally confers protection from bleomycin-induced lung injury.[357,358] Deficiency of phospholipase A2 and lipoxygenase, enzymes involved in membrane degradation and the generation of proinflammatory lipid signaling molecules, also protects mice from bleomycin-induced pulmonary fibrosis.[359,360] The importance of cellular adhesion molecules, integrins, and components of the lung extracellular matrix in the lung's response to fibrogenic agents has also been tested in animal models.[361–363] Genetic ablation of the clotting pathway molecule plasminogen activator inhibitor protein 1 was associated with protection from bleomycin-induced pulmonary fibrosis, whereas a deficiency of fibrinogen α- or γ-chains had no effect.[364–366]

SUMMARY AND FUTURE DIRECTIONS

Our understanding of the genetic basis of ILD has advanced tremendously since the last edition of this textbook was published. Several of the genes and mutations responsible for lung disease-causing disorders, including LAM, NF, HPS, Gaucher's disease, Niemann-Pick disease, and PAP, are now known. In many of these cases, however, our ability to identify the genetic loci associated with lung disease has outstripped our ability to determine the function of the proteins encoded by ILD genes or the mechanisms that lead to fibrosis. These problems will most likely be solved by using genetically engineered animal models that recapitulate human ILD or elucidate the pathways that determine susceptibility to fibrogenic agents.

For many investigators, the ultimate objective is to gain insight into the pathogenesis of the more common, predominantly nonfamilial, interstitial lung diseases: IPF, sarcoidosis, and hypersensitivity pneumonitis. Complex

---

TABLE 7–5   Genetic Manipulations in Mice Resulting in Pulmonary Fibrosis

Protein	Locus	Genetic Manipulation	Inflammation	Other Effects of Genetic Manipulation
PDGF[353]	PDGF	Transgenic overexpression	Increased	Patchy fibrosis, emphysema
IL-13[354]	IL-13	Transgenic overexpression	Increased	Associated with increased activity of TGF-β₁
IL-1β[371]	IL-1β	Adenovirus expression	Increased	Profound inflammation and remodeling
TGF-α	TGF-α	Transgenic overexpression	Increased	Fibrosis also associated with emphysema, increased compliance, and airflow obstruction. Can be reversed by expression of dominant-negative mutant TGF-α receptor.[372]
TNF-α	TNF-α	Adenovirus expression Transgenic overexpression	Increased	Myofibroblast accumulation associated with increased TGF-β₁ production. Fujita reported fibrosis very minor[373]
Presenilin-2	PS2	Ablation	NA	Transmembrane protein involved in apoptosis and processing of amyloid precursor protein
Calveoli[356]	Caveolin 1	Ablation	NA	Endothelial cell hyperplasia, expanded alveolar septa
GM-CSF[355]	GM-CSF	Adenovirus expression	Increased	Myofibroblast accumulation associated with increased TGF-β₁ production

IL = interleukin; PDGF = platelet-derived growth factor; TGF = transforming growth factor; TNF = tumor necrosis factor.

TABLE 7–6   Genetic Manipulations in Mice and Susceptibility to Lung Fibrosis

Protein/Class	Locus	Genetic Manipulation	Fibrogenic Stimulus	Inflammation	Fibrosis	Other Effects of Genetic Manipulation
Cytoplasmic phospholipase[359]	$cPLA_2$	Ablation	Bleomycin	Decreased	Decreased	Decreased thromboxanes and leukotrienes in $cPLA_2$ (–/–) mice
Adhesion molecule[361]	ICAM	Ablation	Radiation	Decreased	Decreased	Improved pulmonary compliance in ICAM-1 (–/–) mice
PAI[364]	PAI-1	Ablation	Bleomycin	NA	Decreased	Enhanced fibrinolysis, improved survival in PAI-1 (–/–) mice
Fibrinogen[365]	α-chain Fg	Ablation	Bleomycin	Unchanged	Unchanged	Hydroxyproline unchanged in Fg (–/–) mice
Fibrinogen[366]	γ-chain Fg	Ablation	Bleomycin	Decreased	Unchanged	Hydroxyproline unchanged in Fg (–/–)
TGF-β transcription factor[374]	SMAD7	Adenovirus expression	Bleomycin	Decreased	Decreased	Reduced hydroxyproline content and Smad2 phosphorylation
TNFR[357,358]	TNFR	Receptor ablation	Bleomycin; silica; asbestos	Decreased	Decreased	TNFR (–/–) mice protected from fibrosis despite up-regulation of TNF expression
IFN[375]	IFN-γ	Ablation	Bleomycin	Decreased	Decreased	Decreased weight loss, mortality, hydroxyproline accumulation
Matrix molecule[363]	Decorin	Adenovirus expression	Adenovirus expression of TGF-β	NA	Decreased	Decreased hydroxyproline, TGF-β
Bleomycin hydrolase[376]	Bh	Ablation	Bleomycin	NA	Increased	Neonatal and postbleomycin survival of Bh (–/–) mice reduced
$\alpha_v\beta_6$-Integrin (–/–)[362]	$\alpha_v\beta_6$ (–/–)	Ablation	Bleomycin	Increased	Decreased	$\alpha_v\beta_6$ (–/–) mice accumulate less hydroxyproline
TGF-β transcription factor[377]	SMAD3	Ablation	Bleomycin	Decreased	Decreased	SMAD3 (–/–) mice have reduced procollagen mRNA and hydroxyproline in lung
T cell stimulatory molecule[378]	CD28	Ablation	Bleomycin	Decreased	Decreased	Bleomycin-induced lung fibrosis restored by adoptive transfer of CD28-sufficient cells
GM-CSF[379]	GM-CSF	Ablation	Bleomycin	Unchanged	Increased	Decreased macrophage PGE2 synthesis in GM-CSF (–/–) mice
IL-12p40[380]	IL-12p40	Ablation	Bleomycin	Decreased	Increased	IL-12p40 (–/–) mice had higher levels of hydroxyproline and IL-6 but lower levels of IP-10, RANTES, and eotaxin
Monocyte chemotactic protein[381]	CCR2	Ablation	Bleomycin; FITC instillation	Decreased	Decreased	CCR (–/–) mice have increased GM-CSF and reduced TGF-α; CCR5 (–/–) mice not protected from fibrosis
Lipoxygenase[360]	5-LO	Ablation	Bleomycin	Decreased	Decreased	Decreased cysteinyl LTs; decreased collagen and hydroxyproline, elevated IFN-γ and PGE₂

ICAM = intercellular adhesion molecule; IFN = interferon; NA = not available; PAI-1 = plasminogen activator inhibitor protein; PGE_2 = prostaglandin E_2; PLA_2 = phospholipase A_2; RANTES = regulated upon activation normal T-cell expressed and secreted; TNFR = tumor necrosis factor receptor.

multigene disorders such as these are inherently difficult to study, but there is reason for optimism. The identification of the genetic loci responsible for familial IPF and familial sarcoidosis are now being examined with the use of multicenter genome-wide screening techniques. The data from these studies will greatly enhance the power of polymorphism studies to elucidate the interaction between genes that results in fibrosis. It is likely that key observations made in rare fibrotic disorders associated with high penetrance and UIP-like pathology, including Hermansky-Pudlak syndrome and SP-C-related ILD, will shed light on disease mechanisms in IPF. One of the lessons learned from the genetic analysis of pulmonary hypertension is that mutations that cause rare familial forms of disease may also be a cause of common sporadic forms, even those that present relatively late in life. The finding that sporadic LAM is caused by genetic mutations in tuberous sclerosis genes demonstrates that ILD can have a genetic basis without being inheritable. Serendipitous discoveries made in animal models produced for other purposes, such as the appearance of PAP in GM-CSF-null mice generated for the study of hematopoiesis, lead to powerful and unexpected advances, such as the revelation that an anti-GM-CSF antibody is responsible for most cases of primary PAP.

A more complete understanding of the genetic basis of ILD will permit us to identify patients at risk, to define the natural history, and to study fibrogenic pathways in the forward direction, beginning with the molecular defect.

REFERENCES

1. Gutmann DH. The neurofibromatoses: when less is more. Hum Mol Genet 2001;10(7)747–55.

2. Lie JT. Pulmonary tuberous sclerosis in tuberous sclerosis complex. In: Gomez MR, Sampson JR, Whittemore VH, editors. Oxford: Oxford University Press; 1999. p. 207–17.

3. van Slegtenhorst M, de Hoogt R, Hermans C, et al. Identification of the tuberous sclerosis gene *TSC1* on chromosome 9q34. Science 1997;277:805–8.

4. The European Chromosome 16 Tuberous Sclerosis Consortium. Identification and characterization of the tuberous sclerosis gene on chromosome 16. Cell 1993;75(7):1305–15.

5. Povey S, Burley MW, Attwood J, et al. Two loci for tuberous sclerosis: one on 9q34 and one on 16p13. Ann Hum Genet 1994;58:107–27.

6. Sullivan EJ. Lymphangioleiomyomatosis. A review. Chest 1998;114:1689–703.

7. Dwyer JM, Hickie JB, Garvan J. Pulmonary tuberous sclerosis. Report of three patients and a review of the literature. QJM 1971;40:115–25.

8. Aubry MC, Myers JL, Ryu JH, et al. Pulmonary lymphangioleiomyomatosis in a man. Am J Respir Crit Care Med 2000;162(2):749–52.

9. Popper HH, Juettner-Smolle FM, Pongratz MG. Micronodular hyperplasia of type II pneumocytes—a new lung lesion associated with tuberous sclerosis. Histopathology 1991; 18(4):347–54.

10. Myers JL. Micronodular pneumocyte hyperplasia. The versatile type 2 pneumocyte all dressed up in yet another brand new suit! Adv Anat Pathol 1999;6:49–55.

11. Muir TE, Leslie KO, Popper H, et al. Micronodular pneumocyte hyperplasia. Am J Surg Pathol 1998;22:465–72.

12. Franz DN, Brody A, Meyer C, et al. Mutational and radiographic analysis of pulmonary disease consistent with lymphangioleiomyomatosis and micronodular pneumocyte hyperplasia in women with tuberous sclerosis. Am J Respir Crit Care Med 2001;164(4):661–8.

13. Flieder DB, Travis WD. Clear cell "sugar" tumor of the lung association with lymphangioleiomyomatosis and multifocal micronodular pneumocyte hyperplasia in a patient with tuberous sclerosis. Am J Surg Pathol 1997;21(10):1242–7.

14. Hironaka M, Fukayama M. Regional proliferation of HMB-45-positive clear cells of the lung with lymphangioleiomyomatosislike distribution, replacing the lobes with multiple cysts and a nodule. Am J Surg Pathol 1999;23(10):1288–93.

15. Foundation L. LAM Foundation database. 2000 http://lam.uc.edu.

16. Urban T, Lazor R, Lacronique J, et al. Pulmonary lymphangioleiomyomatosis. A study of 69 patients. Groupe d'Etudes et de Recherche sur les Maladies "Orphelines" Pulmonaires (GERM"O"P). Medicine (Baltimore) 1999;78(5):321–37.

17. Johnson S. Rare diseases. 1. Lymphangioleiomyomatosis: clinical features, management and basic mechanisms. Thorax 1999;54(3):254–64.

18. Castro M, Shepherd CW, Gomez MR, et al. Pulmonary tuberous sclerosis. Chest 1995;107:189–95.

19. Costello LC, Hartman TE, Ryu JH. High frequency of pulmonary lymphangioleiomyomatosis in women with tuberous sclerosis complex. Mayo Clin Proc 2000;75(6):591–4.

20. Moss J, Avila NA, Barnes PM, et al. Prevalence and clinical characteristics of lymphangioleiomyomatosis (LAM) in patients with tuberous sclerosis complex. Am J Respir Crit Care Med 2001;164(4):669–71.

21. O'Callaghan FJ, Shiell AW, Osborne JP, et al. Prevalence of tuberous sclerosis estimated by capture-recapture analysis. Lancet 1998;351:1490.

22. Dabora SL, Jozwiak S, Franz DN, et al. Mutational analysis in a cohort of 224 tuberous sclerosis patients indicates increased severity of TSC2, compared with TSC1, disease in multiple organs. Am J Hum Genet 2001;68(1):64–80.

23. Cheadle JP, Reeve MP, Sampson JR, et al. Molecular genetic advances in tuberous sclerosis. Hum Genet 2000;107(2): 97–114.

24. Jones AC, Shyamsundar MM, Thomas MW, et al. Comprehensive mutation analysis of TSC1 and TSC2 and phenotypic correlations in 150 families with tuberous sclerosis. Am J Hum Genet 1999;64(5):1305–15.

25. Wienecke R, Konig A, DeClue JE. Identification of tuberin, the tuberous sclerosis-2 product. Tuberin possesses specific Rap1GAP activity. J Biol Chem 1995;270(27): 16409–14.

26. Xiao GH, Shoarinejad F, Jin F, et al. The tuberous sclerosis 2 gene product, tuberin, functions as a Rab5 GTPase activating protein (GAP) in modulating endocytosis. J Biol Chem 1997;272(10):6097–100.

27. Beauchamp RL, Banwell A, McNamara P, et al. Exon scanning of the entire TSC2 gene for germline mutations in 40 unrelated patients with tuberous sclerosis. Hum Mutat 1998;12(6):408–16.

28. Niida Y, Lawrence-Smith N, Banwell A, et al. Analysis of both TSC1 and TSC2 for germline mutations in 126 unrelated patients with tuberous sclerosis. Hum Mutat 1999;14(5): 412–22.

29. Zhang H, Yamamoto T, Nanba E, et al. Novel TSC2 mutation in a patient with pulmonary tuberous sclerosis. Lack of loss of heterozygosity in a lung cyst. Am J Med Genet 1999; 82(5):368–70.

30. Strizheva GD, Carsillo T, Kruger WD, et al. The spectrum of mutations in TSC1 and TSC2 in women with tuberous sclerosis and lymphangiomyomatosis. Am J Respir Crit Care Med 2001;163(1):253–8.

31. Bonetti F, Chiodera P. Lymphangioleiomyomatosis and tuberous sclerosis: where is the border [editorial]? Eur Respir J 1996;9(3):399–401.

32. Lana R, Sanchez-Alarcos JM, Martinez-Cruz R, et al. [Lymphangioleiomyomatosis and tuberous sclerosis. A casual association or a causative one?] Arch Bronconeumol 1998; 34(9):463–5.

33. Smolarek TA, Wessner LL, McCormack FX, et al. Evidence that lymphangiomyomatosis is caused by TSC2 mutations. Chromosome 16p13 loss of heterozygosity in angiomyolipomas and lymph nodes from women with lymphangiomyomatosis. Am J Hum Genet 1998;62(4):810–5.

34. Astrinidis A, Khare L, Carsillo T, et al. Mutational analysis of the tuberous sclerosis gene TSC2 in patients with pulmonary lymphangioleiomyomatosis. J Med Genet 2000; 37(1):55–7.

35. Carsillo T, Astrinidis A, Henske EP. Mutations in the tuberous sclerosis complex gene TSC2 are a cause of sporadic pulmonary lymphangioleiomyomatosis. Proc Natl Acad Sci U S A 2000;97(11):6085–90.

36. Slingerland JM, Grossman RF, Chamberlain D, et al. Pulmonary manifestations of tuberous sclerosis in first-degree relatives. Thorax 1989;44(3):212–4.

37. Sato T, Seyama K, Fujii H, et al. Mutation analysis of the TSC1 and TSC2 genes in Japanese patients with pul-

monary lymphangioleiomyomatosis. J Hum Genet 2002; 47(1):20–8.

38. Bittmann I, Dose TB, Muller C, et al. Lymphangioleiomyomatosis. Recurrence after single lung transplantation. Hum Pathol 1997;28(12):1420–3.

39. Nine JS, Yousem SA, Paradis IL, et al. Lymphangioleiomyomatosis. Recurrence after lung transplantation. J Heart Lung Trans 1994;13:714–9.

40. O'Brien JD, Lium JH, Parosa JF, et al. Lymphangioleiomyomatosis recurrence in the allograft after single lung transplantation. Am J Respir Crit Care 1995;151:2033–6.

41. Bernstein SM, Newell JD Jr, Adamczyk D, et al. How common are renal angiomyolipomas in patients with pulmonary lymphangiomyomatosis? Am J Respir Crit Care Med 1995;152:2138–43.

42. Avila NA, Bechtle J, Dwyer AJ, et al. Lymphangioleiomyomatosis. CT of diurnal variation of lymphangioleiomyomas. Radiology 2001;221(2):415–21.

43. Henry KW, Yuan X, Koszewski NJ, et al. Tuberous sclerosis gene 2 product modulates transcription mediated by steroid hormone receptor family members. J Biol Chem 1998;273(32):20535–9.

44. Tsuchiya H, Orimoto K, Kobayashi K, et al. Presence of potent transcriptional activation domains in the predisposing tuberous sclerosis (Tsc2) gene product of the Eker rat model. Cancer Res 1996;56(3):429–33.

45. Goncharova EA, Goncharov DA, Eszterhas A, et al. Tuberin regulates p70 S6 kinase activation and ribosomal protein S6 phosphorylation. a role for the TSC2 tumor suppressor gene in pulmonary lymphangioleiomyomatosis (LAM). J Biol Chem 2002;3:3.

46. Lamb RF, Roy C, Diefenbach TJ, et al. The TSC1 tumour suppressor hamartin regulates cell adhesion through ERM proteins and the GTPase Rho. Nat Cell Biol 2000;2(5):281–7.

47. Kwiatkowski DJ, Zhang H, Bandura JL, et al. A mouse model of TSC1 reveals sex-dependent lethality from liver hemangiomas, and up-regulation of p70S6 kinase activity in Tsc1 null cells. Hum Mol Genet 2002;11(5):525–34.

48. Onda H, Lueck A, Marks PW, et al. Tsc2(+/–) mice develop tumors in multiple sites that express gelsolin and are influenced by genetic background. J Clin Invest 1999;104(6): 687–95.

49. Ammit AJ, Panettieri RA Jr. The circle of life. Cell cycle regulation in airway smooth muscle. J Appl Physiol 2001; 91(3):1431–7

50. Tapon N, Ito N, Dickson BJ, et al. The *Drosophila* tuberous sclerosis complex gene homologs restrict cell growth and cell proliferation. Cell 2001;105(3):345–55.

51. Potter CJ, Huang H, Xu T. *Drosophila* Tsc1 functions with Tsc2 to antagonize insulin signaling in regulating cell growth, cell proliferation, and organ size. Cell 2001;105(3):357–68.

52. Gao X, Pan D. TSC1 and TSC2 tumor suppressors antagonize insulin signaling in cell growth. Genes Dev 2001;15(11): 1383–92.

53. Vang R, Kempson RL. Perivascular epithelioid cell tumor ('PEComa') of the uterus. A subset of HMB-45-positive epithelioid mesenchymal neoplasms with an uncertain relationship to pure smooth muscle tumors. Am J Surg Pathol 2002;26(1):1–13.

54. Matsui R, Brody JS, Yu Q. FGF-2 induces surfactant protein gene expression in foetal rat lung epithelial cells through a MAPK-independent pathway. Cell Signal 1999;11(3): 221–8.

55. Peyrol S, Gindre D, Cordier JF, et al. Characterization of the smooth muscle cell infiltrate and associated connective matrix of lymphangiomyomatosis. Immunohistochemical and ultrastructural study of two cases. J Pathol 1992;168(4):387–95.

56. Basset F, Soler P, Marsac J, et al. Pulmonary lymphangiomyomatosis: three new cases studied with electron microscopy. Cancer 1976;38(6):2357–66.

57. Vazquez JJ, Fernandez-Cuervo L, Fidalgo B. Lymphangiomyomatosis: morphogenetic study and ultrastructural confirmation of the histogenesis of the lung lesion. Cancer 1976;37(5):2321–8.

58. Corrin B, Liebow AA, Friedman PJ. Pulmonary lymphangiomyomatosis. A review. Am J Pathol 1975;79(2):348–82.

59. Schmid E, Osborn M, Rungger-Brandle E, et al. Distribution of vimentin and desmin filaments in smooth muscle tissue of mammalian and avian aorta. Exp Cell Res 1982;137(2): 329–40.

60. Gabbiani G, Schmid E, Winter S, et al. Vascular smooth muscle cells differ from other smooth muscle cells. Predominance of vimentin filaments and a specific alpha-type actin. Proc Natl Acad Sci U S A 1981;78(1):298–302.

61. Nguyen-Vu PA, Fackler I, Rust A, et al. Loss of tuberin, the tuberous-sclerosis-complex-2 gene product is associated with angiogenesis. J Cutan Pathol 2001;28(9):470–5.

62. Usuki J, Horiba K, Chu SC, et al. Immunohistochemical analysis of proteins of the Bcl-2 family in pulmonary lymphangioleiomyomatosis. Association of Bcl-2 expression with hormone receptor status. Arch Pathol Lab Med 1998;122(10):895–902.

63. Matsui K, Takeda K, Yu ZX, et al. Role for activation of matrix metalloproteinases in the pathogenesis of pulmonary lymphangioleiomyomatosis. Arch Pathol Lab Med 2000; 124(2):267–75.

64. Hayashi T, Fleming MV, Stetler-Stevenson WG, et al. Immunohistochemical study of matrix metalloproteinases (MMPs) and their tissue inhibitors (TIMPs) in pulmonary lymphangioleiomyomatosis (LAM). Hum Pathol 1997;28(9): 1071–8.

65. Oh YM, Mo EK, Jang SH, et al. Pulmonary lymphangioleiomyomatosis in Korea. Thorax 1999;54(7):618–21.

66. Chu SC, Horiba K, Usuki J, et al. Comprehensive evaluation of 35 patients with lymphangioleiomyomatosis. Chest 1999;115(4):1041–52.

67. Kitaichi M, Nishimura K, Itoh H, et al. Pulmonary lymphangioleiomyomatosis. A report of 46 patients including a clinicopathologic study of prognostic factors. Am J Respir Crit Care Med 1995;151:527–33.

68. Faul JL, Berry GJ, Colby TV, et al. Thoracic lymphangiomas, lymphangiectasis, lymphangiomatosis, and lymphatic dysplasia syndrome. Am J Respir Crit Care Med 2000;161(3 Pt 1):1037–46.

69. Swensen SJ, Hartman TE, Mayo JR, et al. Diffuse pulmonary lymphangiomatosis: CT findings. J Comput Assist Tomogr 1995;19(3):348–52.

70. Tazelaar HD, Kerr D, Yousem SA, et al. Diffuse pulmonary lymphangiomatosis. Hum Pathol 1993;24(12):1313–22.

71. Swank DW, Hepper NG, Folkert KE, et al. Intrathoracic lymphangiomatosis mimicking lymphangioleiomyomatosis in a young woman. Mayo Clin Proc 1989;64(10):1264–8.

72. Shin MS, Fulmer JD, Ho KJ. Unusual computed tomographic manifestations of benign metastasizing leiomyomas as cavitary nodular lesions or interstitial lung disease. Clin Imaging 1996;20(1):45–9.

73. Vassallo R, Ryu JH, Colby TV, et al. Pulmonary Langerhans' cell histiocytosis. N Engl J Med 2000;342(26):1969–78.

74. Avila NA, Chen CC, Chu SC, et al. Pulmonary lymphangioleiomyomatosis: correlation of ventilation-perfusion scintigraphy, chest radiography, and CT with pulmonary function tests. Radiology 2000;214(2):441–6.

75. Taveira-DaSilva AM, Hedin C, Stylianou MP, et al. Reversible airflow obstruction, proliferation of abnormal smooth muscle cells, and impairment of gas exchange as predictors of outcome in lymphangioleiomyomatosis. Am J Respir Crit Care Med 2001;164(6):1072–6.

76. Matsui K, Beasley MB, Nelson WK, et al. Prognostic significance of pulmonary lymphangioleiomyomatosis histologic score. Am J Surg Pathol 2001;25(4):479–84.

77. Taylor JR, Ryu J, Colby TV, et al. Lymphangioleiomyomatosis. Clinical course in 32 patients. N Engl J Med 1990; 323(18):1254–60.

78. Shen A, Iseman MD, Waldron JA, et al. Exacerbation of pul-

monary lymphangioleiomyomatosis by exogenous estrogens. Chest 1987;91(5):782–5.

79. Warren SE, Lee D, Martin V, et al. Pulmonary lymphangiomyomatosis causing bilateral pneumothorax during pregnancy. Ann Thorac Surg 1993;55(4):998–1000.

80. Eliasson AH, Phillips YY, Tenholder MF. Treatment of lymphangioleiomyomatosis. A meta-analysis. Chest 1989; 96(6):1352–5.

81. Johnson SR, Tattersfield AE. Decline in lung function in lymphangioleiomyomatosis. Relation to menopause and progesterone treatment. Am J Respir Crit Care Med 1999; 160(2):628–33.

82. Wellens F, Estenne M, de Francquen P, et al. Combined heart-lung transplantation for terminal pulmonary lymphangioleiomyomatosis. J Thorac Cardiovasc Surg 1985;89(6): 872–6.

83. Estenne M, de Francquen P, Wellens F, et al. Combined heart-and-lung transplantation for lymphangioleiomyomatosis [letter]. Lancet 1984;i:275.

84. Boehler A, Speich R, Russi EW, et al. Lung transplantation for lymphangioleiomyomatosis. N Engl J Med 1996;335: 1275–80.

85. Roach ES, DiMario FJ, Kandt RS, et al. Tuberous Sclerosis Consensus Conference. Recommendations for diagnostic evaluation. National Tuberous Sclerosis Association. J Child Neurol 1999;14(6):401–7.

86. Brunelli A, Catalini G, Fianchini A. Pregnancy exacerbating unsuspected mediastinal lymphangioleiomyomatosis and chylothorax [letter]. Int J Gynaecol Obstet 1996;52(3): 289–90.

87. Evans DG, Huson SM, Donnai D, et al. A genetic study of type 2 neurofibromatosis in the United Kingdom. I. Prevalence, mutation rate, fitness, and confirmation of maternal transmission effect on severity. J Med Genet 1992; 29(12):841–6.

88. Riccardi VM. Pathophysiology of neurofibromatosis. IV. Dermatologic insights into heterogeneity and pathogenesis. J Am Acad Dermatol 1980;3(2):157–66.

89. Jarvis GJ, Crompton AC. Neurofibromatosis and pregnancy. Br J Obstet Gynaecol 1978;85(11):844–6.

90. Ansari AH, Nagamani M. Pregnancy and neurofibromatosis (von Recklinghausen's disease). Obstet Gynecol 1976; 47(1):25S–9S.

91. Martin GA, Viskochil D, Bollag G, et al. The GAP-related domain of the neurofibromatosis type 1 gene product interacts with ras p21. Cell 1990;63(4):843–9.

92. Gutmann DH, Wood DL, Collins FS. Identification of the neurofibromatosis type 1 gene product. Proc Natl Acad Sci U S A 1991;88(21):9658–62.

93. Xu GF, Lin B, Tanaka K, et al. The catalytic domain of the neurofibromatosis type 1 gene product stimulates ras GTPase and complements ira mutants of S. cerevisiae. Cell 1990;63(4):835–41.

94. Cichowski K, Shih TS, Schmitt E, et al. Mouse models of tumor development in neurofibromatosis type 1. Science 1999;286:2172–6.

95. den Bakker MA, Tascilar M, Riegman PH, et al. Neurofibromatosis type 2 protein co-localizes with elements of the cytoskeleton. Am J Pathol 1995;147(5):1339–49.

96. McClatchey AI, Saotome I, Mercer K, et al. Mice heterozygous for a mutation at the Nf2 tumor suppressor locus develop a range of highly metastatic tumors. Genes Dev 1998; 12(8):1121–33.

97. Burkhalter JL, Morano JU, McCay MB. Diffuse interstitial lung disease in neurofibromatosis. South Med J 1986; 79(8):944–6.

98. Massaro D, Katz S. Fibrosing alveolitis: its occurrence, roentgenographic, and pathologic features in von Recklinghausen's neurofibromatosis. Am Rev Respir Dis 1966;93(6):934–42.

99. Webb WR, Goodman PC. Fibrosing alveolitis in patients with neurofibromatosis. Radiology 1977;122(2):289–93.

100. Sagel SS, Forrest JV, Askin FB. Interstitial lung disease in neurofibromatosis. South Med J 1975;68(5):647–9.

101. Kurotaki H, Kamata Y, Kimura M, et al. Multiple papillary adenomas of type II pneumocytes found in a 13-year-old boy with von Recklinghausen's disease. Virchows Arch A Pathol Anat Histopathol 1993;423(4):319–22.

102. Porterfield JK, Pyeritz RE, Traill TA. Pulmonary hypertension and interstitial fibrosis in von Recklinghausen neurofibromatosis. Am J Med Genet 1986;25(3):531–5.

103. Aoki Y, Kodama M, Mezaki T, et al. von Recklinghausen disease complicated by pulmonary hypertension. Chest 2001;119(5):1606–8.

104. Hassoun PM, Celli BR. Bilateral diaphragm paralysis secondary to central von Recklinghausen's disease. Chest 2000;117(4):1196–200.

105. Davies PDB. Diffuse pulmonary involvement in neurofibromatosis. Thorax 1963;19:198.

106. Israel-Asselain MR, Chebat J, Sors C, et al. Diffuse interstitial pulmonary fibrosis in a mother and son with von Recklinghausen's disease. Thorax 1965;20:153–7.

107. Webb WR, Goodman PC. Fibrosing alveolitis in patients with neurofibromatosis. Radiology 1966;122:289–93.

108. Klatte EC, Franken EA, Smith JA. The radiographic spectrum in neurofibromatosis. Semin Roentgenol 1976;11(1):17–33.

109. De Scheerder I, Elinck W, Van Renterghem D, et al. Desquamative interstitial pneumonia and scar cancer of the lung complicating generalised neurofibromatosis. Eur J Respir Dis 1984;65(8):623–6.

110. Nogee LM. Abnormal expression of surfactant protein C and lung disease. Am J Respir Cell Mol Biol 2002;26(6):641–4.

111. Selman M, King TE, Pardo A. Idiopathic pulmonary fibrosis. Prevailing and evolving hypotheses about its pathogenesis and implications for therapy. Ann Intern Med 2001; 134(2):136–51.

112. Phizackerley PJ, Town MH, Newman GE. Hydrophobic proteins of lamellated osmiophilic bodies isolated from pig lung. Biochem J 1979;183(3):731–6.

113. Glasser SW, Korfhagen TR, Weaver T, et al. cDNA and deduced amino acid sequence of human pulmonary surfactant—associated proteolipid SPL(Phe). Proc Natl Acad Sci U S A 1987;84(12):4007–11.

114. Glasser SW, Korfhagen TR, Weaver TE, et al. cDNA, deduced polypeptide structure and chromosomal assignment of human pulmonary surfactant proteolipid, SPL (pVal). J Biol Chem 1988;263(1):9–12.

115. Wood S, Yaremko ML, Schertzer M, et al. Mapping of the pulmonary surfactant SP5 (SFTP2) locus to 8p21 and characterization of a microsatellite repeat marker that shows frequent loss of heterozygosity in human carcinomas. Genomics 1994;24(3):597–600.

116. Fisher JH, Emrie PA, Drabkin HA, et al. The gene encoding the hydrophobic surfactant protein SP-C is located on 8p and identifies an EcoRI RFLP. Am J Hum Genet 1988; 43(4):436–41.

117. Glasser SW, Korfhagen TR, Perme CM, et al. Two SP-C genes encoding human pulmonary surfactant proteolipid. J Biol Chem 1988;263(21):10326–31.

118. Curstedt T, Johansson J, Persson P, et al. Hydrophobic surfactant-associated polypeptides. SP-C is a lipopeptide with two palmitoylated cysteine residues, whereas SP-B lacks covalently linked fatty acyl groups. Proc Natl Acad Sci U S A 1990;87(8):2985–9.

119. Kabore AF, Wang WJ, Russo SJ, et al. Biosynthesis of surfactant protein C. Characterization of aggresome formation by EGFP chimeras containing propeptide mutants lacking conserved cysteine residues. J Cell Sci 2001;114(Pt 2): 293–302.

120. Gustafsson M, Thyberg J, Naslund J, et al. Amyloid fibril formation by pulmonary surfactant protein C. FEBS Lett 1999;464(3):138–42.

121. Thomas AQ, Lane K, Phillips J III, et al. Heterozygosity for a surfactant protein C gene mutation associated with usual

interstitial pneumonitis and cellular nonspecific interstitial pneumonitis in one kindred. Am J Respir Crit Care Med 2002;165(9):1322–8.

122. Nogee LM, Dunbar AE III, Wert SE, et al. A mutation in the surfactant protein C gene associated with familial interstitial lung disease. N Engl J Med 2001;344(8):573–9.

123. Nogee LM, Dunbar AE III, Wert S, et al. Mutations in the surfactant protein C gene associated with interstitial lung disease. Chest 2002;121(3 Suppl):20S–1S.

124. Amin RS, Wert SE, Baughman RP, et al. Surfactant protein deficiency in familial interstitial lung disease. J Pediatr 2001;139(1):85–92.

125. Beers MF, Lomax CA, Russo SJ. Synthetic processing of surfactant protein C by alevolar epithelial cells. The COOH terminus of proSP-C is required for post-translational targeting and proteolysis. J Biol Chem 1998;273(24):15287–93.

126. Keller A, Steinhilber W, Schafer KP, et al. The C-terminal domain of the pulmonary surfactant protein C precursor contains signals for intracellular targeting. Am J Respir Cell Mol Biol 1992;6(6):601–8.

127. Conkright JJ, Na CL, Weaver TE. Overexpression of surfactant protein-C mature peptide causes neonatal lethality in transgenic mice. Am J Respir Cell Mol Biol 2002;26(1):85–90.

128. Glasser SW, Burhans MS, Korfhagen TR, et al. Altered stability of pulmonary surfactant in SP-C-deficient mice. Proc Natl Acad Sci U S A 2001;98(11):6366–71.

129. Ikegami M, Weaver TE, Conkright JJ, et al. Deficiency of SP-B reveals protective role of SP-C during oxygen lung injury. J Appl Physiol 2002;92(2):519–26.

130. Glasser SW, Detmer EA, Ikegami M, et al. Emphysema and pulmonary fibrosis in SP-C gene targeted mice [abstract]. Am J Respir Crit Care Med 2002;165:A705.

131. Beutler E. Gaucher's disease. Curr Opin Hematol 1997;4(1):19–23.

132. Grabowski GA, Saal HM, Wenstrup RJ, et al. Gaucher's disease. A prototype for molecular medicine. Crit Rev Oncol Hematol 1996;23(1):25–55.

133. Goitein O, Elstein D, Abrahamov A, et al. Lung involvement and enzyme replacement therapy in Gaucher's disease. QJM 2001;94(8):407–15.

134. Tybulewicz VL, Tremblay ML, LaMarca ME, et al. Animal model of Gaucher's disease from targeted disruption of the mouse glucocerebrosidase gene. Nature 1992;357:407–10.

135. Mizukami H, Mi Y, Wada R, et al. Systemic inflammation in glucocerebrosidase-deficient mice with minimal glucosylceramide storage. J Clin Invest 2002;109(9):1215–21.

136. Gaucher PCE. De l'epithelioma primitif de late rate, hypertrophie idiopathique de late rate sans leucemie; Thesis, Paris 1882.

137. Ross DJ, Spira S, Buchbinder NA. Gaucher's cells in pulmonary-capillary blood in association with pulmonary hypertension. N Engl J Med 1997;336(5):379–81.

138. Lee SY, Mak AW, Huen KF, et al. Gaucher's disease with pulmonary involvement in a 6-year-old girl. Report of resolution of radiographic abnormalities on increasing dose of imiglucerase. J Pediatr 2001;139(6):862–4.

139. Amir G, Ron N. Pulmonary pathology in Gaucher's disease. Hum Pathol 1999;30(6):666–70.

140. Kerem E, Elstein D, Abrahamov A, et al. Pulmonary function abnormalities in type I Gaucher's disease. Eur Respir J 1996;9(2):340–5.

141. Jackson DC, Simon G. Unusual bone and lung changes in a case Gaucher's disease. Br Med J 1965;38:698.

142. Pastores GM, Miller A. Pulmonary hypertension in Gaucher's disease. Lancet 1998;352:580.

143. Lee RE. The pathology of Gaucher's disease. Prog Clin Biol Res 1982;95:177–215.

144. Carson KF, Williams CA, Rosenthal DL, et al. Bronchoalveolar lavage in a girl with Gaucher's disease. A case report. Acta Cytol 1994;38(4):597–600.

145. Lieberman J, Beutler E. Elevation of serum angiotensin-converting enzyme in Gaucher's disease. N Engl J Med 1976;294(26):1442–4.

146. Beutler E, Kay A, Saven A, et al. Enzyme replacement therapy for Gaucher's disease. Blood 1991;78(5):1183–9.

147. Banjar H. Pulmonary involvement of Gaucher's disease in children. A common presentation in Saudi Arabia. Ann Trop Paediatr 1998;18(1):55–9.

148. Pelini M, Boice D, O'Neil K, et al. Glucocerebrosidase treatment of type I Gaucher's disease with severe pulmonary involvement. Ann Intern Med 1994;121(3):196–7.

149. Grabowski GA, Leslie N, Wenstrup R. Enzyme therapy for Gaucher's disease. The first 5 years. Blood Rev 1998;12(2):115–33.

150. Feng L, Novak EK, Hartnell LM, et al. The Hermansky-Pudlak syndrome 1 (HPS1) and HPS2 genes independently contribute to the production and function of platelet dense granules, melanosomes, and lysosomes. Blood 2002;99(5):1651–8.

151. Davies BH, Tuddenham EG. Familial pulmonary fibrosis associated with oculocutaneous albinism and platelet function defect. A new syndrome. QJM 1976;45(178):219–32.

152. DePinho RA, Kaplan KL. The Hermansky-Pudlak syndrome. Report of three cases and review of pathophysiology and management considerations. Medicine (Baltimore) 1985;64(3):192–202.

153. Swank RT, Novak EK, McGarry MP, et al. Mouse models of Hermansky-Pudlak syndrome. A review. Pigment Cell Res 1998;11(2):60–80.

154. Wildenberg SC, Oetting WS, Almodovar C, et al. A gene causing Hermansky-Pudlak syndrome in a Puerto Rican population maps to chromosome 10q2. Am J Hum Genet 1995;57(4):755–65.

155. Fukai K, Oh J, Frenk E, et al. Linkage dysequilibrium mapping of the gene for Hermansky-Pudlak syndrome to chromosome 10q23.1-q23.3. Hum Mol Genet 1995;4(9):1665–9.

156. Oh J, Ho L, Ala-Mello S, et al. Mutation analysis of patients with Hermansky-Pudlak syndrome. A frameshift hot spot in the HPS gene and apparent locus heterogeneity. Am J Hum Genet 1998;62(3):593–8.

157. Suzuki T, Li W, Zhang Q, et al. Hermansky-Pudlak syndrome is caused by mutations in HPS4, the human homolog of the mouse light-ear gene. Nat Genet 2002;30(3):321–4.

158. Gardner JM, Wildenberg SC, Keiper NM, et al. The mouse pale-ear (ep) mutation is the homologue of human Hermansky-Pudlak syndrome. Proc Natl Acad Sci U S A 1997;94(17):9238–43.

159. Feng GH, Bailin T, Oh J, et al. Mouse pale-ear (ep) is homologous to human Hermansky-Pudlak syndrome and contains a rare 'AT-AC' intron. Hum Mol Genet 1997;6(5):793–7.

160. Dell'Angelica EC, Shotelersuk V, Aguilar RC, et al. Altered trafficking of lysosomal proteins in Hermansky-Pudlak syndrome due to mutations in the beta 3A subunit of the AP-3 adaptor. Mol Cell 1999;3(1):11–21.

161. Feng L, Seymour AB, Jiang S, et al. The beta3A subunit gene (Ap3b1) of the AP-3 adaptor complex is altered in the mouse hypopigmentation mutant pearl, a model for Hermansky-Pudlak syndrome and night blindness. Hum Mol Genet 1999;8(2):323–30.

162. Anikster Y, Huizing M, White J, et al. Mutation of a new gene causes a unique form of Hermansky-Pudlak syndrome in a genetic isolate of central Puerto Rico. Nat Genet 2001;28(4):376–80.

163. Suzuki T, Li W, Zhang Q, et al. The gene mutated in cocoa mice, carrying a defect of organelle biogenesis, is a homologue of the human Hermansky-Pudlak syndrome-3 gene. Genomics 2001;78(1-2):30–7.

164. Witkop CJJ, Quevedo WCJ, Kirkpatrick TB, et al. Albinism. In: Scriver R, Beaudet EL, Sly WS, et al., editors. The metabolic basis of inherited disease. Vol 6. New York: McGraw-Hill; 1989. p. 2905–47.

165. Garay SM, Gardella JE, Fazzini EP, et al. Hermansky-Pudlak syndrome. Pulmonary manifestations of a ceroid storage disorder. Am J Med 1979;66(5):737–47.

166. Gahl WA, Brantly M, Kaiser-Kupfer MI, et al. Genetic defects and clinical characteristics of patients with a form of oculocutaneous albinism (Hermansky-Pudlak syndrome). N Engl J Med 1998;338(18):1258–64.

167. Shimizu K, Matsumoto T, Miura G, et al. Hermansky-Pudlak syndrome with diffuse pulmonary fibrosis. Radiologic-pathologic correlation. J Comput Assist Tomogr 1998; 22(2):249–51.

168. Reynolds SP, Davies BH, Gibbs AR. Diffuse pulmonary fibrosis and the Hermansky-Pudlak syndrome. Clinical course and postmortem findings. Thorax 1994;49(6):617–8.

169. Hoste P, Willams J, Devriendt J, et al. Familial diffuse interstitial pulmonary fibrosis associated with oculocutaneous albinism. Report of two cases with a family study. Scand J Respir Dis 1979;60(3):128–34.

170. White DA, Smith GJ, Cooper JA Jr, et al. Hermansky-Pudlak syndrome and interstitial lung disease. Report of a case with lavage findings. Am Rev Respir Dis 1984;130(1):138–41.

171. Brantly M, Avila NA, Shotelersuk V, et al. Pulmonary function and high-resolution CT findings in patients with an inherited form of pulmonary fibrosis, Hermansky-Pudlak syndrome, due to mutations in HPS-1. Chest 2000;117(1): 129–36.

172. Nakatani Y, Nakamura N, Sano J, et al. Interstitial pneumonia in Hermansky-Pudlak syndrome. Significance of florid foamy swelling/degeneration (giant lamellar body degeneration) of type-2 pneumocytes. Virchows Arch 2000; 437(3):304–13.

173. Crocker AC, Farber S. Niemann-Pick disease. A review of 18 patients. Medicine 1958;37:1–98.

174. Minai OA, Sullivan EJ, Stoller JK. Pulmonary involvement in Niemann-Pick disease: case report and literature review. Respir Med 2000;94(12):1241–51.

175. Kolodny EH. Niemann-Pick disease. Curr Opin Hematol 2000;7(1):48–52.

176. Zumbansen M, Stoffel W. Neutral sphingomyelinase 1 deficiency in the mouse causes no lipid storage disease. Mol Cell Biol 2002;22(11):3633–8.

177. Otterbach B, Stoffel W. Acid sphingomyelinase-deficient mice mimic the neurovisceral form of human lysosomal storage disease (Niemann-Pick disease). Cell 1995;81(7):1053–61.

178. Horinouchi K, Erlich S, Perl DP, et al. Acid sphingomyelinase deficient mice. A model of types A and B Niemann-Pick disease. Nat Genet 1995;10(3):288–93.

179. Pentchev PG, Boothe AD, Kruth HS, et al. A genetic storage disorder in BALB/C mice with a metabolic block in esterification of exogenous cholesterol. J Biol Chem 1984; 259(9):5784–91.

180. Niggemann B, Rebien W, Rahn W, et al. Asymptomatic pulmonary involvement in 2 children with Niemann-Pick disease type B. Respiration 1994;61(1):55–7.

181. Long RG, Lake BD, Pettit JE, et al. Adult Niemann-Pick disease. Its relationship to the syndrome of the sea-blue histiocyte. Am J Med 1977;62(4):627–35.

182. Ferretti GR, Lantuejoul S, Brambilla E, et al. Case report. Pulmonary involvement in Niemann-Pick disease subtype B. CT findings. J Comput Assist Tomogr 1996;20(6):990–2.

183. Tabak L, Yilmazbayhan D, Kilicaslan Z, et al. Value of bronchoalveolar lavage in lipidoses with pulmonary involvement. Eur Respir J 1994;7(2):409–11.

184. Lever AM, Ryder JB. Cor pulmonale in an adult secondary to Niemann-Pick disease. Thorax 1983;38(11):873–4.

185. Putterman C, Zelingher J, Shouval D. Liver failure and the sea-blue histiocyte/adult Niemann-Pick disease. Case report and review of the literature. J Clin Gastroenterol 1992;15(2):146–9.

186. Dewhurst N, Besley GT, Finlayson ND, et al. Sea blue histiocytosis in a patient with chronic non-neuropathic Niemann-Pick disease. J Clin Pathol 1979;32(11):1121–7.

187. Duchateau F, Dechambre S, Coche E. Imaging of pulmonary manifestations in subtype B of Niemann-Pick disease. Br J Radiol 2001;74(887):1059–61.

188. Lachman R, Crocker A, Schulman J, et al. Radiological findings in Niemann-Pick disease. Radiology 1973;108(3):659–64.

189. Nicholson AG, Wells AU, Hooper J, et al. Successful treatment of endogenous lipoid pneumonia due to Niemann-Pick Type B disease with whole-lung lavage. Am J Respir Crit Care Med 2002;165(1):128–31.

190. Matsumoto T, Matsumori H, Taki T, et al. Infantile G_{M1}-gangliosidosis with marked manifestation of lungs. Acta Pathol Jpn 1979;29(2):269–76.

191. Semenza GL, Pyeritz RE. Respiratory complications of mucopolysaccharide storage disorders. Medicine (Baltimore) 1988;67(4):209–19.

192. Hahn CN, del Pilar Martin M, Schroder M, et al. Generalized central nervous system disease and massive G_{M1}-ganglioside accumulation in mice defective in lysosomal acid beta-galactosidase. Hum Mol Genet 1997;6(2):205–11.

193. Rosen SG, Castleman B, Liebow AA. Pulmonary alveolar proteinosis. N Engl J Med 1958;258:1123–4.

194. Stanley E, Lieschke GJ, Grail D, et al. Granulocyte/macrophage colony-stimulating factor-deficient mice show no major perturbation of hematopoiesis but develop a characteristic pulmonary pathology. Proc Natl Acad Sci U S A 1994;91(12):5592–6.

195. Dranoff G, Crawford AD, Sadelain M, et al. Involvement of granulocyte-macrophage colony-stimulating factor in pulmonary homeostasis. Science 1994;264:713–6.

196. Trapnell BC, Whitsett JA. GM-CSF regulates pulmonary surfactant homeostasis and alveolar macrophage-mediated innate host defense. Annu Rev Physiol 2002;64:775–802.

197. Holbert JM, Costello P, Li W, et al. CT features of pulmonary alveolar proteinosis. AJR Am J Roentgenol 2001;176(5): 1287–94.

198. Martin RJ, Coalson JJ, Rogers RM, et al. Pulmonary alveolar proteinosis. The diagnosis by segmental lavage. Am Rev Respir Dis 1980;121(5):819–25.

199. Carnovale R, Zornoza J, Goldman AM, et al. Pulmonary alveolar proteinosis. Its association with hematologic malignancy and lymphoma. Radiology 1977;122(2):303–6.

200. Green D, Dighe P, Ali NO, et al. Pulmonary alveolar proteinosis complicating chronic myelogenous leukemia. Cancer 1980;46(8):1763–6.

201. Ruben FL, Talamo TS. Secondary pulmonary alveolar proteinosis occurring in two patients with acquired immune deficiency syndrome. Am J Med 1986;80(6):1187–90.

202. Colon AR Jr, Lawrence RD, Mills SD, et al. Childhood pulmonary alveolar proteinosis (PAP): report of a case and review of the literature. Am J Dis Child 1971;121(6):481–5.

203. Samuels MP, Warner JO. Pulmonary alveolar lipoproteinosis complicating juvenile dermatomyositis. Thorax 1988; 43(11):939–40.

204. Supena R, Karlin D, Strate R, et al. Pulmonary alveolar proteinosis and Nocardia brain abscess. Report of a case. Arch Neurol 1974;30(3):266–8.

205. Sunderland WA, Campbell RA, Edwards MJ. Pulmonary alveolar proteinosis and pulmonary cryptococcosis in an adolescent boy. J Pediatr 1972;80(3):450–6.

206. Witty LA, Tapson VF, Piantadosi CA. Isolation of mycobacteria in patients with pulmonary alveolar proteinosis. Medicine (Baltimore) 1994;73(2):103–9.

207. Tran Van Nhieu J, Vojtek AM, Bernaudin JF, et al. Pulmonary alveolar proteinosis associated with *Pneumocystis carinii*. Ultrastructural identification in bronchoalveolar lavage in AIDS and immunocompromised non-AIDS patients. Chest 1990;98(4):801–5.

208. Hartung M, Salfelder K. Pulmonary alveolar proteinosis and histoplasmosis. Report of three cases. Virchows Arch A Pathol Anat Histopathol 1975;368(4):281–7.

209. Wang BM, Stern EJ, Schmidt RA, et al. Diagnosing pulmonary alveolar proteinosis. A review and an update. Chest 1997;111(2):460–6.

210. Gross NJ, Barnes E, Narine KR. Recycling of surfactant in

black and beige mice. Pool sizes and kinetics. J Appl Physiol 1988;64(5):2017–25.

211. Jennings VM, Dillehay DL, Webb SK, et al. Pulmonary alveolar proteinosis in SCID mice. Am J Respir Cell Mol Biol 1995;13(3):297–306.

212. Dethloff LA, Gilmore LB, Brody AR, et al. Induction of intra- and extra-cellular phospholipids in the lungs of rats exposed to silica. Biochem J 1986;233:111–8.

213. Heppleston AG, Fletcher K, Wyatt I. Abnormalities of lung lipids following inhalation of quartz. Experientia 1972;28(8):938–9.

214. Robb L, Drinkwater CC, Metcalf D, et al. Hematopoietic and lung abnormalities in mice with a null mutation of the common beta subunit of the receptors for granulocyte-macrophage colony-stimulating factor and interleukins 3 and 5. Proc Natl Acad Sci U S A 1995;92(21):9565–9.

215. Ikegami M, Ueda T, Hull W, et al. Surfactant metabolism in transgenic mice after granulocyte macrophage-colony stimulating factor ablation. Am J Physiol 1996;270(4 Pt 1):L650–8.

216. Reed JA, Ikegami M, Cianciolo ER, et al. Aerosolized GM-CSF ameliorates pulmonary alveolar proteinosis in GM-CSF-deficient mice. Am J Physiol 1999;276(4 Pt 1):L556–63.

217. Ikegami M, Jobe AH, Huffman Reed JA, et al. Surfactant metabolic consequences of overexpression of GM-CSF in the epithelium of GM-CSF-deficient mice. Am J Physiol 1997;273(4 Pt 1):L709–14.

218. Hamblin MW, Metcalf MA, McGuffin RW, et al. Molecular cloning and functional characterization of a human 5-HT1B serotonin receptor. A homologue of the rat 5-HT1B receptor with 5-HT1D-like pharmacological specificity. Biochem Biophys Res Commun 1992;184(2):752–9.

219. Yoshida M, Ikegami M, Reed JA, et al. GM-CSF regulates protein and lipid catabolism by alveolar macrophages. Am J Physiol 2001;280(3):L379–86.

220. Shibata Y, Berclaz PY, Chroneos ZC, et al. GM-CSF regulates alveolar macrophage differentiation and innate immunity in the lung through PU.1. Immunity 2001;15(4):557–67.

221. Dirksen U, Nishinakamura R, Groneck P, et al. Human pulmonary alveolar proteinosis associated with a defect in GM-CSF/IL-3/IL-5 receptor common beta chain expression. J Clin Invest 1997;100(9):2211–7.

222. Reed JA, Ikegami M, Robb L, et al. Distinct changes in pulmonary surfactant homeostasis in common β-chain-and GM-CSF-deficient mice. Am J Physiol 2000;278(6):L1164–71.

223. Kitamura T, Tanaka N, Watanabe J, et al. Idiopathic pulmonary alveolar proteinosis as an autoimmune disease with neutralizing antibody against granulocyte/macrophage colony-stimulating factor. J Exp Med 1999;190(6):875–80.

224. Kitamura T, Uchida K, Tanaka N, et al. Serological diagnosis of idiopathic pulmonary alveolar proteinosis. Am J Respir Crit Care Med 2000;162(2 Pt 1):658–62.

225. Thomassen MJ, Yi T, Raychaudhuri B, et al. Pulmonary alveolar proteinosis is a disease of decreased availability of GM-CSF rather than an intrinsic cellular defect. Clin Immunol 2000;95(2):85–92.

226. Seymour JF, Presneill JJ, Schoch OD, et al. Therapeutic efficacy of granulocyte-macrophage colony-stimulating factor in patients with idiopathic acquired alveolar proteinosis. Am J Respir Crit Care Med 2001;163(2):524–31.

227. Kavuru MS, Sullivan EJ, Piccin R, et al. Exogenous granulocyte-macrophage colony-stimulating factor administration for pulmonary alveolar proteinosis. Am J Respir Crit Care Med 2000;161(4 Pt 1):1143–8.

228. Chillaron J, Roca R, Valencia A, et al. Heteromeric amino acid transporters. Biochemistry, genetics, and physiology. Am J Physiol 2001;281(6):F995–1018.

229. Torrents D, Mykkanen J, Pineda M, et al. Identification of SLC7A7, encoding y+LAT-1, as the lysinuric protein intolerance gene. Nat Genet 1999;21(3):293–6.

230. Parto K, Svedstrom E, Majurin ML, et al. Pulmonary manifestations in lysinuric protein intolerance. Chest 1993;104(4):1176–82.

231. Parto K, Maki J, Pelliniemi LJ, et al. Abnormal pulmonary macrophages in lysinuric protein intolerance. Ultrastructural, morphometric, and x-ray microanalytic study. Arch Pathol Lab Med 1994;118(5):536–41.

232. Parto K, Kallajoki M, Aho H, et al. Pulmonary alveolar proteinosis and glomerulonephritis in lysinuric protein intolerance. Case reports and autopsy findings of four pediatric patients. Hum Pathol 1994;25(4):400–7.

233. Santamaria F, Parenti G, Guidi G, et al. Early detection of lung involvement in lysinuric protein intolerance. Role of high-resolution computed tomography and radioisotopic methods. Am J Respir Crit Care Med 1996;153(2):731–5.

234. Nogee LM, de Mello DE, Dehner LP, et al. Brief report. Deficiency of pulmonary surfactant protein B in congenital alveolar proteinosis. N Engl J Med 1993;328(6):406–10.

235. Nogee LM, Garnier G, Dietz HC, et al. A mutation in the surfactant protein B gene responsible for fatal neonatal respiratory disease in multiple kindreds. J Clin Invest 1994;93(4):1860–3.

236. deMello DE, Nogee LM, Heyman S, et al. Molecular and phenotypic variability in the congenital alveolar proteinosis syndrome associated with inherited surfactant protein B deficiency. J Pediatr 1994;125(1):43–50.

237. Wood JR, Bellamy D, Child AH, et al. Pulmonary disease in patients with Marfan syndrome. Thorax 1984;39(10):780–4.

238. Tanoue LT. Pulmonary involvement in collagen vascular disease. A review of the pulmonary manifestations of the Marfan syndrome, ankylosing spondylitis, Sjögren's syndrome, and relapsing polychondritis. J Thorac Imaging 1992;7(2):62–77.

239. Hall JR, Pyeritz RE, Dudgeon DL, et al. Pneumothorax in the Marfan syndrome. Prevalence and therapy. Ann Thorac Surg 1984;37(6):500–4.

240. Sakai LY, Keene DR, Glanville RW, et al. Purification and partial characterization of fibrillin, a cysteine-rich structural component of connective tissue microfibrils. J Biol Chem 1991;266(22):14763–70.

241. Sakai LY, Keene DR, Engvall E. Fibrillin, a new 350-kD glycoprotein, is a component of extracellular microfibrils. J Cell Biol 1986;103(6 Pt 1):2499–509.

242. Milewicz DM, Pyeritz RE, Crawford ES, et al. Marfan syndrome. Defective synthesis, secretion, and extracellular matrix formation of fibrillin by cultured dermal fibroblasts. J Clin Invest 1992;89(1):79–86.

243. Biery NJ, Eldadah ZA, Moore CS, et al. Revised genomic organization of FBN1 and significance for regulated gene expression. Genomics 1999;56(1):70–7.

244. Dietz HC, Cutting GR, Pyeritz RE, et al. Marfan syndrome caused by a recurrent de novo missense mutation in the fibrillin gene. Nature 1991;352(6333):337–9.

245. Dietz HC, Pyeritz RE. Mutations in the human gene for fibrillin-1 (FBN1) in the Marfan syndrome and related disorders. Hum Mol Genet 1995;4:1799–809.

246. Nijbroek G, Sood S, McIntosh I, et al. Fifteen novel FBN1 mutations causing Marfan syndrome detected by heteroduplex analysis of genomic amplicons. Am J Hum Genet 1995;57(1):8–21.

247. Collod-Beroud G, Beroud C, Ades L, et al. Marfan database (third edition): New mutations and new routines for the software. Nucleic Acids Res 1998;26(1):229–3.

248. Maslen CL, Corson GM, Maddox BK, et al. Partial sequence of a candidate gene for the Marfan syndrome. Nature 1991;352:334–7.

249. Corson GM, Chalberg SC, Dietz HC, et al. Fibrillin binds calcium and is coded by cDNAs that reveal a multidomain structure and alternatively spliced exons at the 5' end. Genomics 1993;17(2):476–84.

250. Pereira L, D'Alessio M, Ramirez F, et al. Genomic organization of the sequence coding for fibrillin, the defective gene product in Marfan syndrome. Hum Mol Genet 1993;2(7):961–8.

251. Green MC, Sweet HO, Bunker LE. Tight-skin, a new mutation of the mouse causing excessive growth of connective tissue and skeleton. Am J Pathol 1976;82(3):493–512.

252. Gayraud B, Keene DR, Sakai LY, et al. New insights into the assembly of extracellular microfibrils from the analysis of the fibrillin 1 mutation in the tight skin mouse. J Cell Biol 2000;150(3):667–80.

253. Pereira L, Andrikopoulos K, Tian J, et al. Targetting of the gene encoding fibrillin-1 recapitulates the vascular aspect of Marfan syndrome. Nat Genet 1997;17(2):218–22.

254. Foley TP Jr, Harrison HC, Arnaud CD, et al. Familial benign hypercalcemia. J Pediatr 1972;81(6):1060–7.

255. Auwerx J, Boogaerts M, Ceuppens JL, et al. Defective host defence mechanisms in a family with hypocalciuric hypercalcaemia and coexisting interstitial lung disease. Clin Exp Immunol 1985;62(1):57–64.

256. Tran Van Nhieu J, Valeyre D, Rainfray M, et al. [Idiopathic pulmonary fibrosis and familial benign hypercalcemia syndrome without deficiency in leukocyte myeloperoxidase. A case.] Presse Med 1988;17(13):637–8.

257. Demedts M, Auwerx J, Goddeeris P, et al. The inherited association of interstitial lung disease, hypocalciuric hypercalcemia, and defective granulocyte function. Am Rev Respir Dis 1985;131(3):470–5.

258. Marx SJ, Spiegel AM, Brown EM, et al. Family studies in patients with primary parathyroid hyperplasia. Am J Med 1977;62(5):698–706.

259. Marx SJ, Spiegel AM, Brown EM, et al. Divalent cation metabolism. Familial hypocalciuric hypercalcemia versus typical primary hyperparathyroidism. Am J Med 1978; 65(2):235–42.

260. Pollak MR, Brown EM, Chou YH, et al. Mutations in the human Ca(2+)-sensing receptor gene cause familial hypocalciuric hypercalcemia and neonatal severe hyperparathyroidism. Cell 1993;75(7):1297–303.

261. Chou YH, Pollak MR, Brandi ML, et al. Mutations in the human Ca(2+)-sensing-receptor gene that cause familial hypocalciuric hypercalcemia. Am J Hum Genet 1995; 56(5):1075–9.

262. Brown EM, Pollak M, Chou YH, et al. Cloning and functional characterization of extracellular Ca(2+)-sensing receptors from parathyroid and kidney. Bone 1995;17(2 Suppl): 7S–11S.

263. Lloyd SE, Pannett AA, Dixon PH, et al. Localization of familial benign hypercalcemia, Oklahoma variant (FBHOk), to chromosome 19q13. Am J Hum Genet 1999;64(1): 189–95.

264. Ho C, Conner DA, Pollak MR, et al. A mouse model of human familial hypocalciuric hypercalcemia and neonatal severe hyperparathyroidism. Nat Genet 1995;11(4): 389–94.

265. Brown EM, MacLeod RJ. Extracellular calcium sensing and extracellular calcium signaling. Physiol Rev 2001;81(1): 239–97.

266. Mariotta S, Guidi L, Papale M, et al. Pulmonary alveolar microlithiasis. Review of Italian reports. Eur J Epidemiol 1997;13(5):587–90.

267. Caffrey PR, Altman RS. Pulmonary alveolar microlithiasis occurring in premature twins. J Pediatr 1965;66:758.

268. Sears MR, Chang AR, Taylor AJ. Pulmonary alveolar microlithiasis. Thorax 1971;26(6):704–11.

269. Chan ED, Morales DV, Welsh CH, et al. Calcium deposition with or without bone formation in the lung. Am J Respir Crit Care Med 2002;165(12):1654–69.

270. Ucan ES, Keyf AI, Aydilek R, et al. Pulmonary alveolar microlithiasis. Review of Turkish reports. Thorax 1993; 48(2):171–3.

271. Caffrey PR, Altman RS. Pulmonary alveolar microlithiasis in premature twins. J Pediatr 1965;66:758–63.

272. Senyigit A, Yaramis A, Gurkan F, et al. Pulmonary alveolar microlithiasis. A rare familial inheritance with report of six cases in a family. Contribution of six new cases to the number of case reports in Turkey. Respiration 2001;68(2): 204–9.

273. Pant K, Shah A, Mathur RK, et al. Pulmonary alveolar microlithiasis with pleural calcification and nephrolithiasis. Chest 1990;98(1):245–6.

274. Chatterji R, Gaude GS, Patil PV. Pulmonary alveolar microlithiasis diagnosed by sputum examination and transbronchial biopsy. Indian J Chest Dis Allied Sci 1997; 39(4):263–7.

275. Cluzel P, Grenier P, Bernadac P, et al. Pulmonary alveolar microlithiasis. CT findings. J Comput Assist Tomogr 1991;15(6):938–42.

276. Weinstein DS. Pulmonary sarcoidosis. Calcified micronodular pattern simulating pulmonary alveolar microlithiasis. J Thorac Imaging 1999;14(3):218–20.

277. Jackson KB, Modry DL, Halenar J, et al. Single lung transplantation for pulmonary alveolar microlithiasis. J Heart Lung Transplant 2001;20(2):226.

278. Ozcelik U, Gulsun M, Gocmen A, et al. Treatment and follow-up of pulmonary alveolar microlithiasis with disodium editronate. Radiological demonstration. Pediatr Radiol 2002;32(5):380–3.

279. Starost MF, Benavides F, Conti CJ. A variant of pulmonary alveolar microlithiasis in nackt mice. Vet Pathol 2002; 39(3):390–2.

280. Benavides F, Giordano M, Fiette L, et al. Nackt (nkt), a new hair loss mutation of the mouse with associated CD4 deficiency. Immunogenetics 1999;49(5):413–9.

281. Benavides F, Venables A, Poetschke Klug H, et al. The CD4 T cell-deficient mouse mutation nackt (nkt) involves a deletion in the cathepsin L (CtsI) gene. Immunogenetics 2001;53(3):233–42.

282. Dinakaran S, Desai SP, Palmer IR, et al. Lipoid proteinosis. Clinical features and electron microscopic study. Eye 2001;15(Pt 5):666–8.

283. Weidner WA, Swischuk LE, Wenzi JE. Roentgenographic findings in lipoid proteinosis. A case report. Am J Roentgenol Radium Ther Nucl Med 1970;110(3):457–61.

284. Caplan RM. Visceral involvement in lipoid proteinosis. Arch Dermatol 1967;95:149.

285. Hamada T, McLean WH, Ramsay M, et al. Lipoid proteinosis maps to 1q21 and is caused by mutations in the extracellular matrix protein 1 gene (ECM1). Hum Mol Genet 2002;11(7):833–40.

286. Deckers MM, Smits P, Karperien M, et al. Recombinant human extracellular matrix protein 1 inhibits alkaline phosphatase activity and mineralization of mouse embryonic metatarsals in vitro. Bone 2001;28(1):14–20.

287. Smits P, Poumay Y, Karperien M, et al. Differentiation-dependent alternative splicing and expression of the extracellular matrix protein 1 gene in human keratinocytes. J Invest Dermatol 2000;114(4):718–24.

288. Han Z, Ni J, Smits P, et al. Extracellular matrix protein 1 (ECM1) has angiogenic properties and is expressed by breast tumor cells. FASEB J 2001;15(6):988–94.

289. Smits P, Ni J, Feng P, et al. The human extracellular matrix gene 1 (ECM1): genomic structure, cDNA cloning, expression pattern, and chromosomal localization. Genomics 1997;45(3):487–95.

290. Brown LK, Miller A, Bhuptani A, et al. Pulmonary involvement in Fabry disease. Am J Respir Crit Care Med 1997;155(3):1004–10.

291. Eng CM, Resnick-Silverman LA, Niehaus DJ, et al. Nature and frequency of mutations in the alpha-galactosidase A gene that cause Fabry disease. Am J Hum Genet 1993; 53(6):1186–97.

292. Imokawa S, Sato A, Toyoshima M, et al. Dyskeratosis congenita showing usual interstitial pneumonia. Intern Med 1994;33(4):226–30.

293. Vanbiervliet P, Blockmans D, Bobbaers H. Dyskeratosis congenita and associated interstitial lung disease. A case report. Acta Clin Belg 1998;53(3):198–202.

294. Paul SR, Perez-Atayde A, Williams DA. Interstitial pulmonary disease associated with dyskeratosis congenita. Am J Pediatr Hematol Oncol 1992;14(1):89–92.

295. Safa WF, Lestringant GG, Frossard PM. X-linked dyskeratosis congenita. Restrictive pulmonary disease and a novel mutation. Thorax 2001;56(11):891–4.

296. Luzzatto L, Karadimitris A. Dyskeratosis and ribosomal rebellion. Nat Genet 1998;19(1):6–7.

297. Knight SW, Heiss NS, Vulliamy TJ, et al. X-linked dyskeratosis congenita is predominantly caused by missense mutations in the DKC1 gene. Am J Hum Genet 1999;65(1):50–8.

298. Vulliamy T, Marrone A, Goldman F, et al. The RNA component of telomerase is mutated in autosomal dominant dyskeratosis congenita. Nature 2001;413:432–5.

299. Pietinalho A, Ohmichi M, Hirasawa M, et al. Familial sarcoidosis in Finland and Hokkaido, Japan—a comparative study. Respir Med 1999;93(6):408–12.

300. Brennan NJ, Crean P, Long JP, et al. High prevalence of familial sarcoidosis in an Irish population. Thorax 1984;39(1):14–8.

301. Wiman LG. Familial occurrence of sarcoidosis. Scand J Respir Dis Suppl 1972;80:115–9.

302. Harrington DW, Major M, Rybicki B, et al. Familial analysis of 91 families. Sarcoidosis 1994;11:240–3.

303. Headings VE, Weston D, Young RC Jr, et al. Familial sarcoidosis with multiple occurrences in eleven families. A possible mechanism of inheritance. Ann NY Acad Sci 1976;278:377–85.

304. Rybicki BA, Kirkey KL, Major M, et al. Familial risk ratio of sarcoidosis in African-American sibs and parents. Am J Epidemiol 2001;153(2):188–93.

305. McGrath DS, Daniil Z, Foley P, et al. Epidemiology of familial sarcoidosis in the UK. Thorax 2000;55(9):751–4.

306. Rybicki BA, Iannuzzi MC, Frederick MM, et al. Familial aggregation of sarcoidosis. A case-control etiologic study of sarcoidosis. Am J Respir Crit Care Med 2001;164(11):2085–91.

307. Peabody JW, et al. Idiopathic pulmonary fibrosis. Its occurrence in twin sisters. Dis Chest 1950;18:330–4.

308. McMillan JM. Familial pulmonary fibrosis. Dis Chest 1951;20:426–36.

309. Adelman AG, Chertkow G, Hayton RC. Familial fibrocystic pulmonary dysplasia. A detailed family study. Can Med Assoc J 1966;95(12):603–10.

310. Musk AW, Zilko PJ, Manners P, et al. Genetic studies in familial fibrosing alveolitis. Possible linkage with immunoglobulin allotypes (Gm). Chest 1986;89(2):206–10.

311. Marshall RP, Puddicombe A, Cookson WO, et al. Adult familial cryptogenic fibrosing alveolitis in the United Kingdom. Thorax 2000;55(2):143–6.

312. Stinson JC, Tomkin GH. Familial cryptogenic fibrosing alveolitis. A case report. Ir J Med Sci 1992;161(2):42–3.

313. Barzo P. Familial idiopathic fibrosing alveolitis. Eur J Respir Dis 1985;66(5):350–2.

314. Pazsy A. [Mode of heredity of familial idiopathic fibrosing alveolitis.] Orv Hetil 1982;123(9):569.

315. Barzo P, Szokol M, Czako Z. [Familial idiopathic fibrosing alveolitis.] Orv Hetil 1981;122(47):2907–10.

316. Murphy A, O'Sullivan BJ. Familial fibrosing alveolitis. Ir J Med Sci 1981;150(7):204–9.

317. Javaheri S, Lederer DH, Pella JA, et al. Idiopathic pulmonary fibrosis in monozygotic twins. The importance of genetic predisposition. Chest 1980;78(4):591–4.

318. Thomas H, Costabel U. [Progressive course of idiopathic pulmonary fibrosis in 2 monozygotic twin sisters.] Pneumologie 1996;50(9):679–82.

319. Marshall RP, McAnulty RJ, Laurent GJ. The pathogenesis of pulmonary fibrosis. Is there a fibrosis gene? Int J Biochem Cell Biol 1997;29(1):107–20.

320. Bitterman PB, Rennard SI, Keogh BA, et al. Familial idiopathic pulmonary fibrosis. Evidence of lung inflammation in unaffected family members. N Engl J Med 1986;314(21):1343–7.

321. Hodgson U, Laitinen T, Tukiainen P. Nationwide prevalence of sporadic and familial idiopathic pulmonary fibrosis. Evidence of founder effect among multiplex families in Finland. Thorax 2002;57(4):338–42.

322. Liebow AA, Stees A, Billingsley JC. Desquamative interstitial pneumonitis. Am J Med 1965;39:369–404.

323. Landing BH, Dixon LG. Congenital malformations and genetic disorders of the respiratory tract (larynx, trachea, bronchi, and lungs). Am Rev Respir Dis 1979;120(1):151–85.

324. Farrell PM, Gilbert EF, Zimmerman JJ, et al. Familial lung disease associated with proliferation and desquamation of type II pneumonocytes. Am J Dis Child 1986;140(3):262–6.

325. Buchino JJ, Keenan WJ, Algren JT, et al. Familial desquamative interstitial pneumonitis occurring in infants. Am J Med Genet Suppl 1987;3:285–91.

326. Tsukahara M, Yoshii H, Imamura T, et al. Desquamative interstitial pneumonia in sibs. Am J Med Genet 1995;59(4):431–4.

327. Iannuzzi MC, Maliarik M, Rybicki B. Genetic polymorphisms in lung disease. Bandwagon or breakthrough? Respir Res 2002;3(1):15.

328. Pantelidis P, Fanning GC, Wells AU, et al. Analysis of tumor necrosis factor-alpha, lymphotoxin-alpha, tumor necrosis factor receptor II, and interleukin-6 polymorphisms in patients with idiopathic pulmonary fibrosis. Am J Respir Crit Care Med 2001;163(6):1432–6.

329. Whyte M, Hubbard R, Meliconi R, et al. Increased risk of fibrosing alveolitis associated with interleukin-1 receptor antagonist and tumor necrosis factor-alpha gene polymorphisms. Am J Respir Crit Care Med 2000;162(2 Pt 1):755–8.

330. Morrison CD, Papp AC, Hejmanowski AQ, et al. Increased D allele frequency of the angiotensin-converting enzyme gene in pulmonary fibrosis. Hum Pathol 2001;32(5):521–8.

331. Varpela E, Tiilikainen A, Varpela M, et al. High prevalences of HLA-B15 and HLA-Dw6 in patients with cryptogenic fibrosing alveolitis. Tissue Antigens 1979;14(1):68–71.

332. Libby DM, Gibofsky A, Fotino M, et al. Immunogenetic and clinical findings in idiopathic pulmonary fibrosis. Association with the B-cell alloantigen HLA-DR2. Am Rev Respir Dis 1983;127(5):618–22.

333. Geddes DM, Webley M, Brewerton DA, et al. α$_1$-Antitrypsin phenotypes in fibrosing alveolitis and rheumatoid arthritis. Lancet 1977;ii:1049–51.

334. Michalski JP, McCombs CC, Scopelitis E, et al. α$_1$-Antitrypsin phenotypes, including M subtypes, in pulmonary disease associated with rheumatoid arthritis and systemic sclerosis. Arthritis Rheum 1986;29(5):586–91.

335. Turton CW, Morris LM, Lawler SD, et al. HLA in cryptogenic fibrosing alveolitis. Lancet 1978;i:507–8.

336. Crystal RG, Fulmer JD, Roberts WC, et al. Idiopathic pulmonary fibrosis. Clinical, histologic, radiographic, physiologic, scintigraphic, cytologic, and biochemical aspects. Ann Intern Med 1976;85(6):769–88.

337. Hubbard R, Baoku Y, Kalsheker N, et al. α$_1$-Antitrypsin phenotypes in patients with cryptogenic fibrosing alveolitis. A case-control study. Eur Respir J 1997;10(12):2881–3.

338. Briggs DC, Vaughan RW, Welsh KI, et al. Immunogenetic prediction of pulmonary fibrosis in systemic sclerosis. Lancet 1991;338:661–2.

339. Richeldi L, Sorrentino R, Saltini C. HLA-DPB1 glutamate 69. A genetic marker of beryllium disease. Science 1993;262:242–4.

340. Lombardi G, Germain C, Uren J, et al. HLA-DP allele-specific T cell responses to beryllium account for DP-associated susceptibility to chronic beryllium disease. J Immunol 2001;166(5):3549–55.

341. Maliarik MJ, Chen KM, Major ML, et al. Analysis of HLA-DPB1 polymorphisms in African-Americans with sarcoidosis. Am J Respir Crit Care Med 1998;158(1):111–4.

342. Ishihara M, Ohno S, Ishida T, et al. Molecular genetic studies of HLA class II alleles in sarcoidosis. Tissue Antigens 1994;43(4):238–41.

343. Nowack D, Goebel KM. Genetic aspects of sarcoidosis. Class II histocompatibility antigens and a family study. Arch Intern Med 1987;147:481–3.

344. Olenchock SA, Heise ER, Marx JJ Jr, et al. HLA-B8 in sarcoidosis. Ann Allergy 1981;47(3):151–3.

345. Brewerton DA, Cockburn C, James DC, et al. HLA antigens in sarcoidosis. Clin Exp Immunol 1977;27(2):227–9.

346. Selman M, Teran L, Mendoza A, et al. Increase of HLA-DR7 in pigeon breeder's lung in a Mexican population. Clin Immunol Immunopathol 1987;44(1):63–70.

347. Camarena A, Juarez A, Mejia M, et al. Major histocompatibility complex and tumor necrosis factor-alpha polymorphisms in pigeon breeder's disease. Am J Respir Crit Care Med 2001;163(7):1528–33.

348. Schaaf BM, Seitzer U, Pravica V, et al. Tumor necrosis factor-alpha-308 promoter gene polymorphism and increased tumor necrosis factor serum bioactivity in farmer's lung patients. Am J Respir Crit Care Med 2001;163(2):379–82.

349. Rossi GA, Hunninghake GW, Kawanami O, et al. Motheaten mice—an animal model with an inherited form of interstitial lung disease. Am Rev Respir Dis 1985;131(1):150–8.

350. Kozlowski M, Mlinaric-Rascan I, Feng GS, et al. Expression and catalytic activity of the tyrosine phosphatase PTP1C is severely impaired in motheaten and viable motheaten mice. J Exp Med 1993;178(6):2157–63.

351. Kruger J, Butler JR, Cherapanov V, et al. Deficiency of Src homology 2-containing phosphatase 1 results in abnormalities in murine neutrophil function. Studies in motheaten mice. J Immunol 2000;165(10):5847–59.

352. Koo GC, Manyak CL, Dasch J, et al. Suppressive effects of monocytic cells and transforming growth factor-beta on natural killer cell differentiation in autoimmune viable motheaten mutant mice. J Immunol 1991;147(4):1194–200.

353. Hoyle GW, Li J, Finkelstein JB, et al. Emphysematous lesions, inflammation, and fibrosis in the lungs of transgenic mice overexpressing platelet-derived growth factor. Am J Pathol 1999;154(6):1763–75.

354. Lee CG, Homer RJ, Zhu Z, et al. Interleukin-13 induces tissue fibrosis by selectively stimulating and activating transforming growth factor beta (1). J Exp Med 2001;194(6):809–21.

355. Xing Z, Tremblay GM, Sime PJ, et al. Overexpression of granulocyte-macrophage colony-stimulating factor induces pulmonary granulation tissue formation and fibrosis by induction of transforming growth factor-beta 1 and myofibroblast accumulation. Am J Pathol 1997;150(1):59–66.

356. Drab M, Verkade P, Elger M, et al. Loss of caveolae, vascular dysfunction, and pulmonary defects in caveolin-1 gene-disrupted mice. Science 2001;293:2449–52.

357. Ortiz LA, Lasky J, Lungarella G, et al. Upregulation of the p75 but not the p55 TNF-alpha receptor mRNA after silica and bleomycin exposure and protection from lung injury in double receptor knockout mice. Am J Respir Cell Mol Biol 1999;20(4):825–33.

358. Liu JY, Brass DM, Hoyle GW, et al. TNF-alpha receptor knockout mice are protected from the fibroproliferative effects of inhaled asbestos fibers. Am J Pathol 1998;153(6):1839–47.

359. Nagase T, Uozumi N, Ishii S, et al. A pivotal role of cytosolic phospholipase A(2) in bleomycin-induced pulmonary fibrosis. Nat Med 2002;8(5):480–4.

360. Peters-Golden M, Bailie M, Marshall T, et al. Protection from pulmonary fibrosis in leukotriene-deficient mice. Am J Respir Crit Care Med 2002;165(2):229–35.

361. Hallahan DE, Geng L, Shyr Y. Effects of intercellular adhesion molecule 1 (ICAM-1) null mutation on radiation-induced pulmonary fibrosis and respiratory insufficiency in mice. J Natl Cancer Inst 2002;94(10):733–41.

362. Munger JS, Huang X, Kawakatsu H, et al. The integrin alpha v beta 6 binds and activates latent TGF beta 1. A mechanism for regulating pulmonary inflammation and fibrosis. Cell 1999;96(3):319–28.

363. Kolb M, Margetts PJ, Galt T, et al. Transient transgene expression of decorin in the lung reduces the fibrotic response to bleomycin. Am J Respir Crit Care Med 2001;163(3 Pt 1):770–7.

364. Eitzman DT, McCoy RD, Zheng X, et al. Bleomycin-induced pulmonary fibrosis in transgenic mice that either lack or overexpress the murine plasminogen activator inhibitor–1 gene. J Clin Invest 1996;97(1):232–7.

365. Hattori N, Degen JL, Sisson TH, et al. Bleomycin-induced pulmonary fibrosis in fibrinogen-null mice. J Clin Invest 2000;106(11):1341–50.

366. Wilberding JA, Ploplis VA, McLennan L, et al. Development of pulmonary fibrosis in fibrinogen-deficient mice. Ann NY Acad Sci 2001;936:542–8.

367. Ohshima T, Murray GJ, Swaim WD, et al. α-Galactosidase A-deficient mice. A model of Fabry disease. Proc Natl Acad Sci U S A 1997;94(6):2540–4.

368. Loftus SK, Morris JA, Carstea ED, et al. Murine model of Niemann-Pick C disease. Mutation in a cholesterol homeostasis gene. Science 1997;277:232–5.

369. Clark JC, Wert SE, Bachurski CJ, et al. Targeted disruption of the surfactant protein B gene disrupts surfactant homeostasis, causing respiratory failure in newborn mice. Proc Natl Acad Sci U S A 1995;92(17):7794–8.

370. Rudolph KL, Chang S, Lee HW, et al. Longevity, stress response, and cancer in aging telomerase-deficient mice. Cell 1999;96(5):701–12.

371. Kolb M, Margetts PJ, Anthony DC, et al. Transient expression of IL-1beta induces acute lung injury and chronic repair leading to pulmonary fibrosis. J Clin Invest 2001;107(12):1529–36.

372. Hardie WD, Kerlakian CB, Bruno MD, et al. Reversal of lung lesions in transgenic transforming growth factor alpha mice by expression of mutant epidermal growth factor receptor. Am J Respir Cell Mol Biol 1996;15(4):499–508.

373. Fujita M, Shannon JM, Irvin CG, et al. Overexpression of tumor necrosis factor-alpha produces an increase in lung volumes and pulmonary hypertension. Am J Physiol 2001;280(1):L39–49.

374. Nakao A, Fujii M, Matsumura R, et al. Transient gene transfer and expression of Smad7 prevents bleomycin-induced lung fibrosis in mice. J Clin Invest 1999;104(1):5–11.

375. Chen ES, Greenlee BM, Wills-Karp M, et al. Attenuation of lung inflammation and fibrosis in interferon-gamma-deficient mice after intratracheal bleomycin. Am J Respir Cell Mol Biol 2001;24(5):545–55.

376. Schwartz DR, Homanics GE, Hoyt DG, et al. The neutral cysteine protease bleomycin hydrolase is essential for epidermal integrity and bleomycin resistance. Proc Natl Acad Sci U S A 1999;96(8):4680–5.

377. Zhao J, Shi W, Wang YL, et al. Smad3 deficiency attenuates bleomycin-induced pulmonary fibrosis in mice. Am J Physiol 2002;282(3):L585–93.

378. Okazaki T, Nakao A, Nakano H, et al. Impairment of bleomycin-induced lung fibrosis in CD28-deficient mice. J Immunol 2001;167(4):1977–81.

379. Moore BB, Coffey MJ, Christensen P, et al. GM-CSF regulates bleomycin-induced pulmonary fibrosis via a prostaglandin-dependent mechanism. J Immunol 2000;165(7):4032–9.

380. Sakamoto H, Zhao LH, Jain F, et al. IL-12p40(–/–) mice treated with intratracheal bleomycin exhibit decreased pulmonary inflammation and increased fibrosis. Exp Mol Pathol 2002;72(1):1–9.

381. Moore BB, Paine R III, Christensen PJ, et al. Protection from pulmonary fibrosis in the absence of CCR2 signaling. J Immunol 2001;167(8):4368–77.

8

INFLAMMATION IN THE PATHOGENESIS OF INTERSTITIAL LUNG DISEASES

DAVID W.H. RICHES
G. SCOTT WORTHEN
ANDREI AUGUSTIN
RAZVAN LAPADAT
EDWARD D. CHAN

The interstitial lung diseases are a heterogeneous group of disorders of the lower respiratory tract that are characterized by both acute and chronic inflammation and a generally irreversible and relentless process of fibrosis within the interstitium and alveolar spaces. Idiopathic pulmonary fibrosis (IPF), also known as cryptogenic fibrosing alveolitis, exhibits the pathologic lesions of usual intersititial pneumonitis characterized by intra-alveolar and interstitial accumulations of inflammatory cells, principally neutrophils and macrophages, and less frequently immune cells, especially B cells, $\alpha\beta$ and $\gamma\delta$ T cells, and immunoglobulin-secreting plasma cells. As can be seen in Figure 8–1, the alveolar epithelium becomes damaged and denuded, frequently progressing to damage or destruction of the underlying basement membrane in association with the activation of inflammatory and immune effector cells. In addition, matrix components such as hyaluronan are released in a soluble form from the interstitium and accumulate in the alveolar spaces. As opposed to the injury caused by a single event, these continuous inflammatory events ultimately lead to the collapse and fusion of alveolar units and to an exuberant fibrotic response, orchestrated in part by macrophages, that results in increased collagen synthesis by interstitial and intra-alveolar fibroblasts and myofibroblasts and ultimately leads to loss of function of the gas exchange units.

The events leading to scarring in the lungs in IPF in some respects resemble the process of wound repair, as occurs in the skin following injury. In the skin, the general sequence of events that are initiated in response to injury is comprised of (1) the activation of the coagulation system leading to a cessation of blood flow and the formation of a provisional matrix, (2) the local generation of a variety of chemotactic factors formed both from preformed plasma proteins and locally secreted

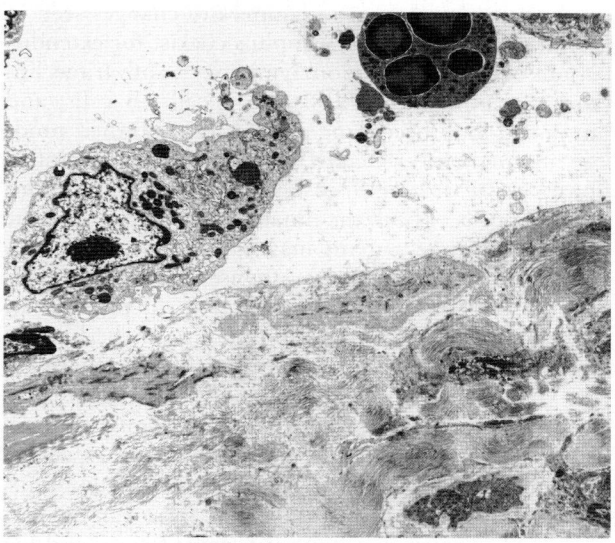

Figure 8–1 Electron micrograph of a lung biopsy specimen from a patient with IPF showing some of the hallmarks of the disease. These include a macrophage and neutrophil as well as cellular and proteinaceous debris in the air space and a basal lamina that is denuded of epithelial cells. In addition, excessive deposition of collagen bundles is seen within the interstitium together with both intact and damaged smooth muscle cells and fibroblasts (×5,600 original magnification). The electron micrograph was generously provided by Jan Henson.

chemokines that attract inflammatory cells to the site of injury, (3) the sequential influx of neutrophils and monocytes, (4) the débridement of damaged connective tissue matrix, (5) the initiation of neovascularization, and (6) the stimulation of mesenchymal cell proliferation and connective tissue matrix remodeling. However, although scarring in adult skin repair is associated with a good functional outcome as a result of abundant collagen synthesis by fibroblasts that proliferate and differentiate into myofibroblasts within the provisional matrix, such an outcome within the alveolus and interstitium is devastating and ultimately results in a fatal loss of the gas exchange properties of the lung. Thus, understanding what distinguishes the processes leading to (1) the resolution and restoration of function or (2) fibrosis resulting in the loss of function, may allow treatment strategies to be developed to ameliorate interstitial and alveolar fibrosis in susceptible individuals.

In both the lung and the skin, the inflammatory response is initiated within minutes of the initiation of injury. Neutrophils are the first blood leukocytes to be attracted and demobilized at the site of injury and their numbers steadily increase before peaking after 24 to 48 hours. Shortly thereafter, the number of monocytes and macrophages begin to increase. In the self-resolving inflammatory responses seen in the skin and in acute lung injury as occurs, for example, in response to the intratracheal instillation of neutrophil chemotactic fragments, neutrophil numbers decline rapidly leaving macrophages as the principal professional phagocyte. In contrast, in the chronic inflammatory changes seen in IPF, macrophages and neutrophils coexist for extended periods of time. In addition, lymphocytes of various lineages, including $\alpha\beta$ T cells, $\gamma\delta$ T cells, B cells, and immunoglobulin-secreting plasma cells and their products are frequently detected in IPF and other noninfectious interstitial lung diseases.[1-3] Thus, one must consider that cells of both the innate inflammatory and the adaptive immune systems may contribute to the hallmark chronic inflammatory response that is seen in IPF.

The objective of this chapter is to provide an overview of the inflammatory response in the lung in interstitial lung diseases with a particular emphasis on IPF. We will discuss the principal cell types that are present and play a role in interstitial and alveolar fibrosis, namely (1) the polymorphonuclear leukocytes, especially the neutrophil, but also the eosinophil, (2) the mononuclear phagocyte, with an emphasis on its role in the regulation of collagen synthesis and degradation, and (3) the role of the adaptive immune system in regulating tissue inflammation and fibrosis. This discussion will form the basis of a review of animal models of pulmonary fibrosis and the concepts of disease progression that have emerged from such studies, including early pathogenic processes that are frequently absent at the time of patient presentation. Finally, we will present a summary of possible interactions between the various elements of the host inflammatory and immune systems that appear to play a role in the pathogenesis of IPF.

INFLAMMATORY AND IMMUNE CELLS IMPLICATED IN ALVEOLAR AND INTERSTITIAL FIBROSIS

Leukocytes emigrate into the alveolus through the walls of the pulmonary capillaries, which necessitates movement across the endothelium, the capillary basement membrane, the alveolar interstitium, the epithelial basement membrane, and junctions between the alveolar epithelial cells.[4-6] This site of migration in the pulmonary circulation contrasts with the postcapillary venule migratory route in the systemic microvascular bed.[7,8] We have suggested that the unique localization of leukocyte interaction within the lung may relate to the peculiar properties of the pulmonary circulation as a low pressure system with pulsatile flow that leads to transient conditions of low shear force in the capillaries rather than in the venules as in other systems.[9-12] These conditions place the capillary and alveolar walls at considerable risk for injury. Futhermore, migration appears largely to occur through the thick side of the alveolar wall rather than directly through the fused basement membrane of the thin side. Whatever the reason for this, the route clearly places the pulmonary interstitium in the path of potential injury.

Inflammation, however, does not always cause lung injury. Leukocyte influx into the alveolar walls and air spaces can occur without leading to a significant increase in vascular permeability and without inducing vascular endothelial cell[13-15] or alveolar epithelial cell damage.[16,17] The injurious potential of leukocytes is not manifested simply by their migration into the interstitium and alveolar space but rather is inherent in other aspects of their function including multiple synergistically interacting stimuli or changes in the overall environment that are encountered during their emigration into the lung.

Illustrated in Figure 8–2 is a broad scheme showing the multiple components involved in leukocyte migration into the airspaces. Leukocyte sequestration in the pulmonary microvasculature is a key early event in leukocyte recruitment to the lung and seems to serve as a point of control for the intensity and perhaps persistence of the inflammatory response. The accumulation of leukocytes is regulated first by mechanisms that control their delivery to, and retention by, the microvasculature. Delivery to the lung is dependent on the kinetics of leukocyte release from the bone marrow, on leukocyte mobilization from organs in which they are marginated (the lung itself, liver, and spleen,[18-20]) and on the distribution of the blood supply to the lung.

Because leukocyte diameter (7.5 to 8 μm)[21,22] is greater than the mean diameter of the capillary segments of the lung (5.5 μm),[23] leukocytes must deform in order to traverse this vascular network. An independent or concurrent alteration in endothelial cell deformability may also influence leukocyte passage through the pulmonary capillaries. In the low-pressure system of the pulmonary circulation, this suggests one reason for the capillary localization. Leukocyte deformability is largely determined by the degree of actin organization[24,25] and by cytoplasmic viscosity[26] which is also regulated by the state of the cytoskeletal assembly.[27] Inflammatory mediators induce a net assembly and/or redistribution of actin in the leukocytes, which increases their stiffness as

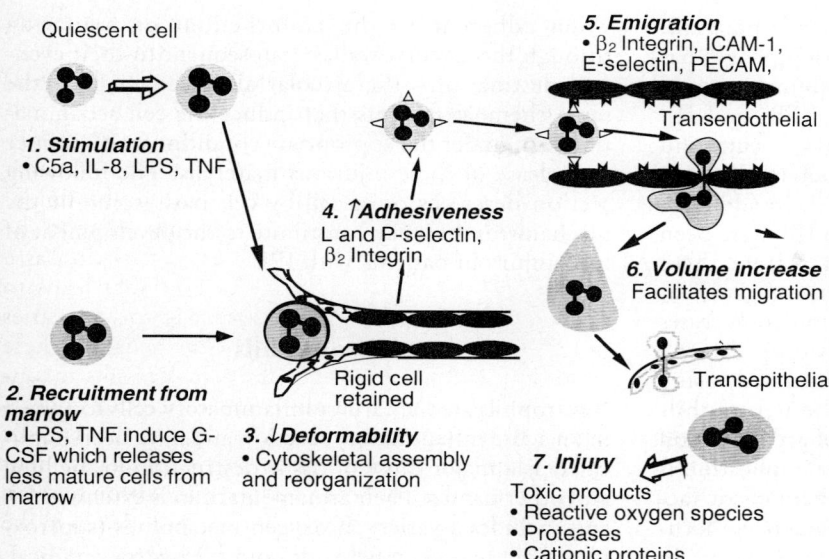

Quiescent cell

1. Stimulation
• C5a, IL-8, LPS, TNF

2. Recruitment from marrow
• LPS, TNF induce G-CSF which releases less mature cells from marrow

3. ↓Deformability
• Cytoskeletal assembly and reorganization

Rigid cell retained

4. ↑Adhesiveness
L and P-selectin, β_2 Integrin

5. Emigration
• β_2 Integrin, ICAM-1, E-selectin, PECAM,

Transendothelial

6. Volume increase
Facilitates migration

Transepithelial

7. Injury
Toxic products
• Reactive oxygen species
• Proteases
• Cationic proteins

Figure 8–2   Scheme illustrating the role of adherence, deformability, transendothelial migration, and cytoplasmic volume changes in neutrophil attraction to the air spaces. C5a = the complement C5-derived anaphylatoxin; IL-8 = interleukin-8; LPS = lipoplysaccharide; TNF = tumor necrosis factor; G-CSF = granulocyte-colony stimulating factor; ICAM-1 = intercellular adhesion molecule 1; PECAM = platelet-endothelial cell adhesion molecule.

well as induces changes in their geometric shape and viscoelastic properties.[16,18,25,28] In vivo, these events would be expected to promote leukocyte sequestration in the microvasculature. In keeping with this suggestion, prevention of actin assembly by pretreatment with cytochalasin D reduced the retention of leukocytes in artifical pores in vitro and localization of these cells in the lung during inflammatory reactions in vivo.[25,28]

An additional or alternative mechanism thought to contribute to leukocyte retention in the microvasculature (and thus to pulmonary tissue injury) is adhesion. Inflammatory mediators induce the upregulation, activation, and/or reorganization of leukocyte and vascular endothelial cell adhesion molecules (CD11/CD18, intercellular adhesion molecules [ICAMs], E-selectin also known as endothelial leukocyte adhesion molecules [ELAM][29–32] which together function to regulate leukocyte-endothelial cell adhesion and disadhesion mechanisms. Such molecules are likely important in contributing to the interaction of leukocytes with the capillary wall and the venular endothelial surface.[29–34] For example, antibodies directed against CD18 have variously been reported to reduce leukocyte retention and injury. In one study, neutrophil retention and injury in the gut were reduced with only minimal effects in the lung.[35,36] By contrast, other studies have demonstrated a significant reduction in neutrophil retention and partial attenuation of pulmonary vascular lung injury in a rabbit ischemia-reperfusion system[37] and decreased plasma leakage into an inflammatory skin site.[38] Our own data suggest that treatment of rabbits in vivo with these antibodies has a greater effect on monocyte than neutrophil accumulation in the pulmonary microvasculature in response to endotoxemia.[28] The observation that such inhibition is incomplete, or in some studies absent, supports the presence of alternative and additional adherence mechanisms or nonadherent processes (eg, those associated with cell deformability). In

contrast, the lung appears to use mechanisms for the initiation of sequestration and then integrin-based mechanisms for the maintenance of retention in tissues supplied by the systems vasculature. The initial slowing (rolling) is mediated by L-selectin on the neutrophil and P-selectin on the endothelial cell, conditions that allow integrin-dependent mechanisms to induce more firm interactions. Since the length of time an activated leukocyte is in contact with a potential target is likely to dictate the degree of injury it sustains,[17] this combination would become a critical determinant of the injurious potential of leukocyte accumulation in the lung.

In order for these retained leukocytes to gain access to the lung parenchyma or alveolar space, the cells must migrate through the alveolar wall. Several specific and nonspecific chemoattractants that lead to this type of accumulation have been described. They include leukotriene B_4 (LTB_4) and interleukin-8 (IL-8) for the neutrophil; C5a the complement anaphylatoxin, fibronectin fragments containing the RGD cell-binding domain, and monocyte chemotactic peptide-1 (MCP-1) for the monocyte; IL-1 in the case of lymphocytes; and mast-cell-derived eosinophilic chemotactic factor, LTB_4, C5a, eotaxin, and IL-5 for the eosinophils. Recent in vivo studies suggest that during migration through the endothelium there is a coexpression/upregulation of the endothelial cell adhesion molecules E-selectin and ICAM[39–42] as well as in the overall system, the presence of chemoattractants. The transmigration process involves intimate contact of the leukocyte with the endothelium, interstitial cells and connective tissue, and the alveolar epithelium. This level of contact provides ample opportunity for damage by any of the toxic products or metalloproteinases released or expressed during the migration process.

There are many potential sources for the chemoattractants and the leukocyte and endothelial stimuli that seem to be involved in acute and chronic inflammation. Activation of alveolar and interstitial macrophages has been shown to lead to the generation of numerous neutrophil chemotactic agents, including LTB_4 and IL-8,[43–47] which could induce several cycles of neutrophil influx into areas of inflammation and potentially contribute to the persistence of these stimuli. In addition, alveolar macrophages from patients with IPF have been shown to spontaneously express and secrete these chemoattractants.[45,48] It is of interest in this regard that in the joint[49] and lung,[50] neutrophil accumulation ceases only when the chemotactic factor levels drop below a critical level. Since we have also demonstrated, using ^{111}In-tagged cells, that the number of neutrophils detected by lavage closely reflects rates of accumulation of such cells in these patients,[51] the clear implication is that there is a persistent production of chemotactic factors that leads to persistent low levels of leukocyte accumulation, over a time frame that has to be measured in years. Macrophages are not the only potential sources of IL-8, however, lymphocytes[52,53] epithelial cells and endothelial cells[54] are also capable of IL-8 transcription and translation. Similarly, it would be naive to suggest that IL-8 is the only chemoattractant for neutrophils that might be involved. Lung epithelial cells express the cysteine-x-cysteine (CXC) chemokine ENA-78, which is also a potent chemoattractant for neutrophils. This issue is also discussed in Chapter 10, "Cytokine Biology and the Pathogenesis of Interstitial Lung Disease."

Digestion of interstitial collagen,[55] elastin,[56] and fibronectin[57] by the leukocyte enzymes elastase[58] and collagenase can lead to the generation of fragments that have been shown in vitro to exhibit monocyte-specific chemotactic activity. In the case of the fibronectin fragment, this property appears to be dependent on a unique cryptic domain that includes the cell-binding RGDS site.[57] Instillation of this monocyte chemotactic fibronectin fragment into rabbit lungs initiated neutrophil-independent accumulation of monocytes into the air spaces.[59] Since we had shown monocyte accumulation in a C5a-mediated inflammatory reaction in rabbit lung to be neutrophil-dependent,[19] a neutrophil-dependent generation of fibronectin fragments containing the RGDS cell-binding domain seemed likely to be a mechanism regulating this monocyte accumulation. This hypothesis was supported by showing that monocyte accumulation was inhibited by antifibronectin antibodies.[59] Here again, however, it is likely that a myriad of potential attractants are involved in the specific cell accumulation and subsequent tissue injury. Furthermore, in the case of interstitial mononuclear phagocytes, a local proliferation of resident or emigrated inflammatory monocytes/macrophages or mononuclear cell precursors may also contribute to the lung content of these cells.[60–63]

As indicated, these inflammatory cells have the potential to synthesize and/or release a variety of materials that are capable of inducing lung injury either when adherent to the endothelium or migrating through the alveolar wall, or subsequent to their eventual destination—the alveolar air space. In fact, the same chemoattractants that induce the cell accumulation can, under the appropriate conditions, also induce the release of these injurious materials. The following section describes on a cell-by-cell basis some of the mechanisms that may contribute to the development of lung injury in patients with IPF.

Neutrophils

Neutrophils are the earliest inflammatory cells to appear in an acute inflammatory reaction and have been implicated as a major cause of tissue destruction in the lung and other tissues. Their armamentarium is extensive[64–66] and includes a variety of oxygen metabolites (superoxide anion, hydrogen peroxide, and the hydroxyl radical, hypochlorous acid) and proteases (elastase, cathepsin G, collagenase, gelatinase). Whereas these are felt to be the most potent and destructive,[67] constituents such as cationic proteins, peptides, and polyamines may also be directly toxic to lung parenchymal cells and hence contribute to the tissue injury.[65]

Each of these groups of agents can be released from neutrophils under the influence of appropriate stimulation. However, as previously mentioned, the mere accumulation of neutrophils in the lung does not of itself necessarily cause significant injury. Chemotaxis alone, therefore, does not seem to be a sufficient stimulus for the release of enough of the toxic agents or, alternately, does not allow the degree of contact with the target necessary to cause the injury. By contrast, phagocytosis of particles by neutrophils does result in a significant release of toxic constituents, which cause injury to pulmonary epithelial cells in vitro.[68] Nathan[69] has shown that, in comparison to cells in suspension, hydrogen peroxide secretion from neutrophils was enhanced and prolonged if these leukocytes were adherent to a variety of surfaces including plastic, laminin, fibronectin, vitronectin, and human umbilical vein endothelial cell monolayers. These data suggest that the adherence of neutrophils to surfaces in the lung (endothelial or epithelial cells or interstitial matrix materials) may lead to a more pronounced effect not only because the toxic materials are directly applied to the targets but because the degree of leukocyte stimulation is enhanced.

Neutrophils, eosinophils, monocytes, and macrophages can be raised to a heightened state of responsiveness by prior exposure to a priming stimulus that in itself does not initiate the function in question. Lipopolysaccharide (LPS) priming for superoxide production was one of the first such stimuli to be described,[70,71] but the process extends to the release of other constituents as well.[72] Since then, a long list of priming stimuli has been described for neutrophils that includes platelet-activating factor (PAF), tumor necrosis factor-α (TNF-α),[73] granulocyte-macrophage colony–stimulating factor (GM-CSF),[74] and IL-1.[75] It has even been suggested that complete neutrophil activation *requires* the combination of both a priming and stimulating agent(s)[76] so that a single stimulus that appears to initiate the responses by itself, might in reality, exhibit the property of initiating (directly or indirectly) both priming and triggering steps.

If leukocytes can migrate to the lung in response to chemotactic stimuli alone (ie, in the absence of priming), it is conceivable that they would not secrete sufficient toxic materials to damage the surrounding tissues. In the presence of priming stimuli, then, increased secretion could result in increased injury. In support of this suggestion, exposure of endothelial cells in culture to neutrophils stimulated with chemoattractants resulted in damage to the endothelial monolayer only when appropriate priming agents were included.[77] Similar combinations of priming and triggering stimuli (LPS and chemotactic factors, respectively) were required to induce pulmonary vascular injury in vivo.[15] In these systems, LPS probably acts directly on the leukocyte to induce priming[15,28,34,72] but could also enhance the reaction by stimulating the production of cytokines such as TNF and/or IL-1, which are reported to act as neutrophil priming agents.[75,78–82] Thus, prolonged residence of the inflammatory cell could result in additional priming and triggering by the plethora of mediators accumulating in the inflammatory reaction, resulting in increased damage.

Neutrophil-derived oxygen metabolites have been shown to injure normal tissues in vivo[83–85] and cell cultures in vitro.[69,86–88] Antioxidants and oxygen metabolite scavengers including catalase, azide, and methionine can prevent lung injury induced by these agents.[67,84]

Proteases, such as elastase and cathepsin G, are released from neutrophil granules and have been implicated in damage not only to connective tissue substrates but to cells of the lung including the endothelium.[65,89–91] These proteases are, however, susceptible to inhibition by several of the antiproteases normally present in the lung (eg, alpha$_1$-proteinase inhibitor, alpha$_2$-macroglobulin, and secretory leukoproteinase inhibitor). It is presumed that the enzymes can avoid the effects of the inhibitors when the leukocyte is closely applied to the matrix or cellular target, another reason for the close connection between adherence and injury. This issue is also pertinent to the mechanisms of macrophage involvement in débridement as described in the section on macrophages. Indeed, this phenomenon has been demonstrated in vitro where leukocytes adherent to connective tissue substrates can mediate their digestion in the presence of antiproteases by excluding access of the inhibitors to the matrix immediately under the cell.[92,93]

Alpha$_1$-antitrypsin (AAT) is the most abundant serine protease inhibitor in humans with normal serum concentrations of 1 to 3 mg/mL but rising fourfold above basal levels in states of inflammation. The poly-morphic AAT gene locus is designated *Pi* and the wild-type nonmutated gene is designated *PiM*. *PiM* encodes a 52 kDa glycoprotein with a serum half-life of 4 to 5 days. An array of mutations identified by isoelectric focusing include Z and S designations. In addition to inhibiting lung neutrophil elastase, AAT has been shown to have anti-inflammatory effects, including inhibition of TNF-α secretion.[94,95] Although frank deficiency of AAT is known to produce emphysema, AAT may also be protective against the development of lung injury and fibrosis. One plausible mechanism is that relative or absolute AAT deficiency may predispose to unopposed elastase-mediated lung injury with subsequent disrepair that results in fibrosis, and, as discussed later, intraperitoneal AAT administration is protective against the development of bleomycin-induced pulmonary fibrosis.[96]

Some clinical epidemiologic data would lend support to this hypothesis. Geddes and colleagues[97] performed *Pi* phenotyping in five groups of individuals: 200 healthy controls, 55 patients with rheumatoid arthritis (RA) with no evidence of chest disease, 33 patients with RA with obstructive disease or recurrent chest infections, 22 patients with RA and interstitial pulmonary fibrosis, and 49 patients with pulmonary fibrosis but without RA. In the normal controls, there was a 14% incidence of the non-MM phenotype (10% MS, 3% MZ, 1% other). There was no significant difference in the frequency of the non-MM phenotype between RA patients without chest disease or RA patients with airflow limitation compared with controls. In contrast, there was a significant increase in the frequency of the non-MM phenotype in patients with pulmonary fibrosis with or without RA (28.6% and 50% non-MM prevalence, respectively). One possible explanation for this association may be a genetic linkage between a putative susceptibility gene to interstitial pulmonary fibrosis and the AAT gene. Another possibility is that *PiMS* and *PiMZ* individuals, with a relative deficiency of AAT, may be predisposed to pulmonary fibrosis because AAT is a broad-spectrum antiserine protease, inhibiting the actions of trypsin, elastase, collagenase, and lysosomal proteases released during inflammation. Although pulmonary fibrosis associated with RA is relatively rare, subclinical pulmonary parenchymal disease is relatively common. Perhaps the reduced tryptic inhibitory capacity of *PiMS* or *PiMZ* patients may provide an impetus to progression to clinical fibrosis. Recently, mice with a genetic disruption of secretory leukocyte protease inhibitor (Slpi–/–), another serine protease inhibitor, were found to exibit impaired cutaneous wound healing with increased inflammation and elastase activity.[98] Interestingly, these Slpi–/– mice also had enhanced transforming growth factor-β (TGF-β) expression.

Neither reactive oxygen species nor proteases produced by neutrophils are likely to act alone. Thus, it has been proposed that because oxidants are short-lived and proteases are held in check by antiproteases or by their own latency, a cooperative effort between both systems is required for neutrophil-induced tissue injury.[67] Further, oxidants may alter the structure of target proteins to render them more susceptible to proteolytic attack and may inactivate the aforementioned antiproteases.[99] Cations released from leukocytes[65,91] are also significantly toxic in cells, and, indeed, some of the damaging effects of the proteases may result from their own highly positive charge.

Eosinophils

Eosinophils, another leukocyte frequently observed in the lung tissue of IPF patients, are a major source of many agents that in themselves or in conjunction with oxidants or halides may potentially induce tissue injury. They are particularly rich in cationic proteins such as major basic protein, eosinophilic cationic protein, eosinophilic derived neurotoxin, and eosinophilic peroxidase. Like neutrophils, however, they also contain cathepsin G, gelatinase[100] and collagenases, which have been shown to degrade connective tissue components present in the parenchyma of the lung, including type I and type III collagens.[101] Little is known regarding the mechanisms by which these cells contribute to the injury of the lung during inflammation. Several cytokines, including IL-3, IL-5, and GM-CSF, increase bone marrow production of eosinophils and thus delivery to the lung, prolong their survival in vitro, increase their leukotriene production, and enhance their cytotoxicity and degranulation, and are thus major candidates for the regulation of eosinophil contributions to inflammation and injury. Eosinophils respond to many of the same chemoattractants as neutrophils, so the mechanisms underlying accumulation of these cells in eosinophil rich interstitial pulmonary disease remains unclear. Thus, although PAF has been reported to be a relatively selective eosinophil chemotactic agent[102–106] that also promotes eosinophil adherence to endothelial cells,[107–109] it also acts on neutrophils and may not provide a ready explanation of selective eosinophil accumulation.

Macrophages

For many years, macrophages were viewed as scavenger cells involved principally in the removal and degradation of injured and/or infected tissue debris, in preparation for repair. However, studies first reported by Leibovitch and Ross in 1975[110] changed that view with the demonstration that depletion of both circulating blood monocytes and local tissue macrophages in guinea pigs resulted not only in a severe retardation of tissue débridement but also in a marked delay in fibroblast proliferation and subsequent wound repair. These data suggested that macrophages play a vital role in the orchestration

and execution of both the degradative and reparative phases of the inflammatory response. The mechanisms involved in tissue degradation and the important role of matrix degrading metalloproteinases and their inhibitors are now beginning to be resolved. In addition, macrophages serve as an important source of growth factors that stimulate the proliferation of fibroblasts, smooth muscle cells, and endothelial cells. The reduced oxygen tension within the inflammatory site is thought to stimulate macrophages to secrete angiogenic cytokines thereby initiating neovascularization of the inflammatory site. Finally, in response to a variety of stimuli pertinent to the fibrotic response, macrophages play a critical role as a source of growth factors and cytokines that control the synthesis of connective tissue proteins, especially collagen, by other cell types. Clearly the breadth of macrophage involvement in the inflammatory and fibrotic response is immense and also includes the critical role of this cell in the production of proinflammatory and profibrotic chemokines and cytokines as well as in the response to these important mediators and modulators. However, covering such a topic is beyond the scope of this chapter and the reader is referred to a recent review of lung macrophages[111] as well as to Chapter 10, "Cytokine Biology and the Pathogenesis of Interstitial Lung Disease." The main objective of this section is to discuss the involvement of macrophages in tissue remodeling through their actions on collagen degradation and as a source of growth factors that regulate and control the fibrotic response in the lung.

As discussed earlier, what distinguishes the self-resolving inflammatory response from the fibrotic response seen in IPF is a dramatic displacement of collagen synthesis in favor of net collagen accumulation mainly associated with increases in collagen types I and III. Thus, consideration must be given to the mechanisms that mediate this imbalance. Based on work conducted in Geoffrey Laurent's laboratory,[112,113] three intuitive mechanisms have been suggested to underlie the increase in total lung collagen in IPF, namely: (1) a failure of matrix-degrading enzymes to control collagen accumulation, (2) an increase in net collagen and matrix synthesis, and (3) a combination of both mechanisms. As we will discuss, ample data now suggest that interstitial and alveolar fibrosis in IPF represents dysregulation of both collagen synthesis and degradation and in the following sections, we will review the broad mechanisms involved.

Collagen Degradation

In a purely reductionist sense, the extracellular connective tissue matrix consists of a framework of cross-linked collagen fibrils to provide tensile strength, a network of elastin fibers to provide the tissue with elastic properties, and a collection of proteoglycans and other glycoproteins such as fibronectin and laminin that facilitate cell-matrix interactions and other functions. Successful breakdown of the extracellular connective tissue matrix requires enzymes that are capable of degrading these major constituents. Macrophages synthesize and secrete several neutral and acid pH-optimum proteases and glycosidases including a number of metalloproteinases that play instrumental roles in this degradative process. In addition, the fibroblast is also an important source of matrix metalloproteinases. Collectively, these different matrix degrading enzymes initiate matrix degradation extracellularly, such that macrophages can endocytose material and complete the process of matrix degradation intracellularly.[114-116]

Monocytes express a heterogeneous group of tissue degrading enzymes whose activities significantly overlap with those of neutrophils, macrophages, and fibroblasts. Consisting mainly of metalloproteinases, serine and cysteine proteases, and acid hydrolases, these enzymes can, under certain circumstances, be active both intracellularly and extracellularly. Of principal importance to collagen degradation are a group of metalloproteinases that hydrolyse either (1) intact collagen (collagenases) or (2) partially-denatured collagen (gelatinases). Collagen degradation by monocytes appears to be mainly mediated by matrix metalloproteinase-1 (MMP-1).[117] However, the levels of MMP-1 secreted by monocytes are low by comparison with that of macrophages, even when the cells are stimulated with LPS or phorbol diesters.[117] Monocytes and the promonocytic cell line U937 also secrete MMP-9, a 92 kDa gelatinase[118] that functions to support further degradation of cleaved native collagen and hence is important in the degradation of damaged or partially degraded collagen found at sites of injury. As will be discussed further in the context of IPF, the activities of both MMP-1 and MMP-9 are opposed by tissue inhibitors of metalloproteinases (TIMPs), of which TIMP-1 is constitutively secreted in abundant levels by monocytes.[117] TIMP activity may therefore serve to limit the activity of secreted metalloproteinases, particularly those released from damaged or dead cells or have diffused away from the cells from which they were secreted.

The precise role of monocytes in extracellular connective tissue matrix breakdown is obviously difficult to define with any precision. Because the monocyte does not appear to secrete MMP-3 (stromelysin),[119] a metalloproteinase that is required to activate MMP-1, alternative mechanisms would be required for MMP-1 to become activated. In addition, the level of synthesis of MMP-1 is small in comparison with that of macrophages and fibroblasts. However, monocytes do secrete at least one gelatinase (MMP-9) that can degrade damaged or cleaved collagen.

Macrophages synthesize and secrete a similar number of metalloproteinases as monocytes with a couple of notable exceptions. Hibbs and colleagues[120] observed that human alveolar macrophages secrete MMP-9 on culture in vitro that is identical to human neutrophil gelatinase.

In a study of human macrophage metalloproteinases, Welgus and colleagues[118] showed that human alveolar macrophages also secrete MMP-1 and MMP-3 although the mechanisms underlying their expression appear distinct. MMP-3 was secreted only in response to stimulation of alveolar macrophages with LPS, but, as pointed out earlier, MMP-3 is capable of activating MMP-1 thereby further stimulating collagen degradation. Thus, in comparison with monocytes, macrophages secrete a broader spectrum of metalloproteinases and in greater quantities as the cells become more differentiated.[118]

Fibroblasts also play a critical role in collagen breakdown under both physiologic and pathologic conditions. The secretion of metalloproteinases by fibroblasts is induced and is tightly controlled by cytokines secreted by macrophages and other cell types. Macrophage regulation of fibroblast collagenase secretion was first reported by Huybrechts-Godin and colleagues,[121] who observed that co-incubation of macrophages and fibroblasts on a ^{14}C-labeled collagen film led to a more rapid and extensive degradation of the collagen matrix, when compared with either fibroblasts or macrophages alone. Later investigations focused on the identity of factors responsible for the induction of fibroblast collagenase synthesis[122] and showed the macrophage factors to include the profibrogenic cytokines IL-1β platelet-derived growth factor (PDGF),[123] and TNF-α.[124,125] Thus collectively, macrophages, neutrophils, and fibroblasts contribute to collagen breakdown, and macrophages appear to play an important role in regulating this process. However, as will be discussed in the following section, the ability of cells present within the lung to degrade the excessive amounts of collagen deposited in IPF is overwhelmed, thereby contributing to net collagen accumulation in this disease.

Dysregulation of Collagen Degradation in Idiopathic Pulmonary Fibrosis

There is now clear evidence to suggest that the accumulation of collagen in the alveolus and interstitium in IPF arises in part from a failure to degrade or remodel collagen. Selman and colleagues[126] studied net collagen synthesis and degradation in homogenized biopsy specimens in 11 patients with IPF and 6 control subjects. As has been shown by a number of groups in both humans as well as in animal models of pulmonary fibrosis,[113,126-128] total lung collagen levels are significantly increased compared with controls. By quantifying the incorporation of ^{3}H-proline into hydroxyproline, no significant differences in collagen synthesis between the two groups were detected, although these measurements are complicated by technical and interpretational issues. Importantly, however, measurements of total collagenolytic activity indicated a marked reduction in the activity in lung homogenates from IPF patients compared with controls. Furthermore, the decrease in collagenolytic activity was detected both spontaneously and in response to activation of latent collagenases with aminophenylmercuric acetate. Arden and Adamson[127] have studied the synthesis and degradation of types I and III collagen in rat lung during the development of interstitial fibrosis following instillation of crocidolite asbestos fibers, and have also concluded that reduced degradation of collagen contributes to the fibrotic process in this animal model. In addition, Pardo and colleagues[129] studied collagenase secretion by fibroblast cell lines established from patients with IPF and controls and reported decreased spontaneous collagenase secretion in a number of fibroblast lines obtained from IPF patients. Unfortunately, none of these studies addressed the question of which metalloproteinases were involved in collagen degradation in either the normal or the fibrotic lung, although recent work by Hayashi and colleagues[130] has suggested that MMP-2 may be associated with type IV collagen in epithelial basement membranes, although its signficance is unclear.

These findings raise the question of the mechanism(s) that culminate in reduced collagen degradation in IPF. Metalloproteinase activity is regulated at a number of levels including the level of expression of the appropriate metalloproteinases, the activation of the proenzyme, and interactions between the various TIMPs. Four TIMPs have been described, and they show overlapping functions. TIMP-1 binds to all known metalloproteinases as well as to the proenzyme form of MMP-9, whereas TIMP-2 has been shown to interact with the proenzyme form of MMP-2.[131–133] Several groups have shown increased levels of TIMPs in IPF. For example, Pardo and colleagues[129] have quantified the secretion of TIMP by fibroblast cell lines from IPF patients compared with controls and suggested that the molar ratio of TIMP to collagenase was markedly increased in IPF. Similarly, Montano and colleagues[134] have shown the level of total TIMP in homogenized lung samples to be increased approximately fifteenfold in IPF over control values. Using immunocytochemistry and confocal microscopy, the increased amount of TIMP-1 in IPF appeared to be localized to epithelial cells with only minimal increases in reactivity being detected in macrophages, although other studies, discussed earlier, have suggested that macrophages express TIMP constitutively. TIMP-4 was originally shown to be mainly expressed in the heart and absent from the lung.[135] However, a recent study combining reverse transcriptase polymerase chain reaction (RT-PCR) analysis, in situ hybridization, and immnocytochemistry has confirmed the absence of TIMP-4 from normal lung tissue but has provided strong evidence to indicate its presence in epithelial cells, and particularly, in interstitial macrophages and plasma cells, in patients with IPF.[136] In addition, there is some evidence to suggest that cytokines both produced by and acting on macrophages, including TGF-β, can markedly augment TIMP production.[137] Thus, as illustrated schematically in Figure 8–3, although many mechanisms may con-

tribute to the decreased ability of the fibrotic lung to degrade collagen, increased expression of TIMP may be an important factor.

Collagen Synthesis

There is now clear evidence from the analysis of both human lung biopsy specimens and from the study of animal models of pulmonary fibrosis that collagen synthesis is increased in the lung in IPF.[138] Recent studies using in situ hybridization and/or Northern blot analysis to investigate the extent of types I and III collagen gene expression have shown that both types of collagen are expressed in increased amounts in response to the induction of pulmonary fibrosis following the instillation of bleomycin, asbestos, or silica. There are also data to indicate that col-

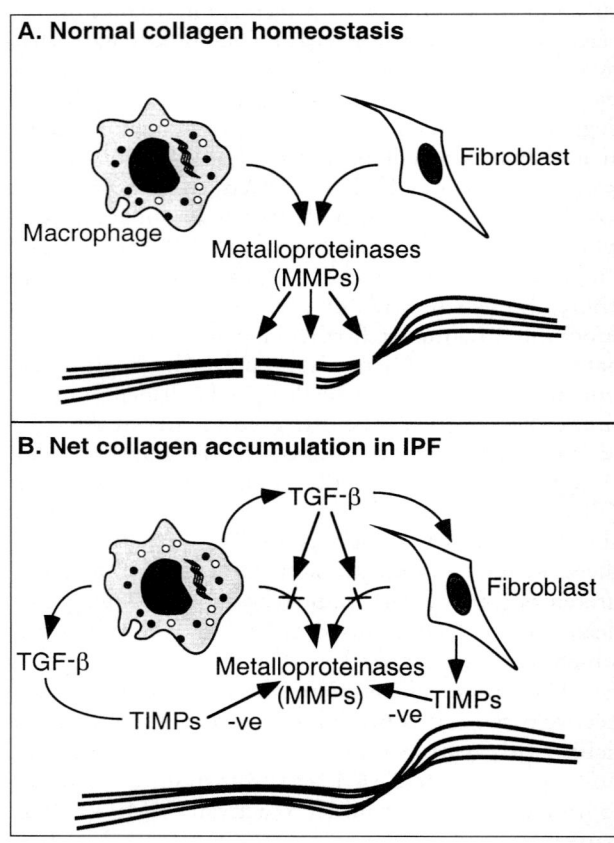

Figure 8–3   Illustration of the role of collagen-degrading matrix metalloproteinases (MMPs) and tissue inhibitors of metalloproteinases (TIMPs) in collagen accumulation in IPF. *A*, Collagen turnover in the normal lung results in a controlled degradation of collagen by metalloproteinases derived from both macrophages and fibroblasts. In this situation, collagen is simply replaced and does not accumulate. *B*, In contrast, in IPF, the action of metalloproteinases is suppressed both as a result of decreased synthesis of metalloproteinases and inhibition by the markedly increased levels of tissue inhibitors of metalloproteinases (TIMPs). Transforming growth factor-β (TGF-β) plays a central role by both suppressing synthesis of metalloproteinases and increasing the synthesis of TIMPs.

lagen type IV expression colocalizes with collagen types I and III in IPF, although in bronchiolitis obliterans organizing pneumonia (BOOP), colocalization is principally with type III collagen.[139] Although collagen is expressed almost exclusively by fibroblasts and myofibroblasts whose numbers are dramatically increased in alveolar and interstitial fibrosis, attention has been directed toward the macrophage and its role in controlling the proliferation of, and collagen expression by, fibroblasts.

A large number of macrophage-derived growth factors and cytokines have been shown to stimulate fibroblast proliferation and/or the synthesis of collagen and other components of the extracellular connective tissue matrix and hence are of significance to the development of alveolar and interstitial fibrosis. Of these pleiotropic factors, five currently stand out as being particularly important, namely TGF-β, PDGF, insulin-like growth factor (IGF-I), fibroblast growth factor (FGF), and TGF-α. All of these growth factors have been shown to be expressed by macrophages during the inflammatory response. In addition, there exists a large body of literature that documents their expression both by alveolar macrophages, as studied by bronchoalveolar lavage, and by interstitial macrophages as have been generally studied by in situ hybridization or immunocytochemistry. In the following sections, we will review each of these growth factors in terms of their biologic activities and the role that they play in the fibrotic response of the lung.

Transforming Growth Factor-β. TGF-β is a group of related proteins that currently comprises five members, namely TGF-β1, TGF-β2, TGF-β3, TGF-β4, and TGF-β5.[140] With the exception of TGF-β4, which comprises 304 amino acids, each family member is synthesized as a latent precursor protein with a molecular weight of approximately 50 kDa and consists of 380 to 412 amino acids. Following dimerization, the precursor protein is cleaved in the COOH terminus to yield the mature 25 kDa dimeric TGF-β protein, which remains noncovalently associated with the larger NH$_2$-terminal portion of the precursor (74 kDa). This complex is, in turn, covalently bound to a 135 kDa TGF-β1 binding protein.[141] While in this state, TGF-β remains functionally inactive. Release of active TGF-β from the latent protein complex can be stimulated by acidification to pH 1.5 or by proteolysis by a number of enzymes including cathepsin D and plasmin.[142] Because both the TGF-β1 binding protein and the 74 kDa precursor contain N-linked oligosaccharides, hydrolysis with endo-F or sialidase has been reported to induce release of active dimeric TGF-β from the latent complex.[143]

Only recently have studies begun to identify stimuli capable of initiating the release of active and latent TGF-β by macrophages. The expression of TGF-β is stringently regulated at both the transcriptional and translational level. In unstimulated macrophages, TGF-β mRNA is constitutively expressed but translationally repressed.[144–146] Work first reported by Assoian and colleagues[144] showed that incubation of human alveolar macrophages with concanavalin A or human monocytes with LPS stimulated the synthesis and release of latent TGF-β from these cells. Since that time, a number of other stimuli have been shown to induce the release of latent and/or active TGF-β from macrophages. These include the inflammatory particulate stimulus, β 1,3-glucan,[146] the human immunodeficiency virus (HIV) tat protein,[147] and obligate and facultative intracellular parasites such as *Toxoplasma gondii*[148] and *Mycobacterium avium-intracellulare*[149] that use macrophages derived TGF-β to inactivate macrophage killing mechanisms thereby allowing the survival of the organisms. Other recent studies have shown that the phagocytosis of apoptotic cells by macrophages also stimulates the production of active TGF-β,[150] an event that suppressed the production of proinflammtory cytokines and chemokines. In addition, studies using adenoviral-mediated gene transfer of GM-CSF to airway and alveolar epithelial cells and macrophages have been shown to initiate an intense fibrotic response.[151] Importantly, the response to GM-CSF did not result in the production of detectable levels of TNF-α but did result in a marked influx of mononuclear phagocytes and the accumulation of large amounts of TGF-β, which has been shown to be derived, at least in part, from newly recruited macrophages. Thus, in vivo, the phagocytosis of apoptotic cells or locally produced GM-CSF may be important inducers of TGF-β expression in the lung.

Studies in experimental animal models have revealed TGF-β to be critically important in the fibrotic response. As will be discussed in more detail in "Animal Models of Interstitial and Alveolar Fibrosis," in the bleomycin model of pulmonary fibrosis, Phan and Kunkel[152] have shown an increase in total lung TGF-β mRNA prior to the induction of increased collagen synthesis while at the protein level, Khalil and colleagues[153] showed that total lung TGF-β protein was increased roughly 30-fold over control animals in response to intratracheal instillation of bleomycin. Immunohistochemical staining of TGF-β in lung sections revealed intense staining of macrophages in the alveolar interstitium during the early stages of development of the fibrotic response, while at later time points, TGF-β was localized extracellularly. Using a similar approach to study TGF-β expression in biopsy specimens from patients with idiopathic pulmonary fibrosis, Khalil and colleagues[154] also showed an increased abundance of TGF-β in macrophages and epithelial cells compared with patients without fibrosis.

Transforming growth factor-β is a potent stimulant of collagen synthesis in vivo and in vitro. Roberts and colleagues[155] initially showed that subcutaneous injection of TGF-β into 1-day-old mice led to the formation of granulation tissue characterized by the presence of neutrophils, fibroblasts, endothelial cells, and macrophages surrounded by a newly formed collagenous capsule. Interestingly, the effect of TGF-β was reversible and self-resolving suggesting that the availability of TGF-β was an important determinant of the duration of the fibrotic response. The ability of TGF-β to stimulate the synthesis of collagen by fibroblasts has also been confirmed in vitro. For example, fibroblasts obtained from skin and lung exposed to TGF-β have been shown to stimulate the expression and secretion of a variety of collagen genes including collagen types I and III,[156–159] the major collagen isoforms deposited in the lung in IPF. The increased expression of collagen genes appears to be mediated in part by increased transcription of collagen mRNAs through effects of TGF-β on NF1 and Sp1 binding sites in the collagen promoter[160,161] as well as by increased stability of the procollagen mRNA.[159] TGF-β has also been shown to increase the level of fibronectin in healing wounds and since fibronectin appears to be one avenue for fibroblast migration and proliferation in the provisional matrix, TGF-β coordinately upregulates several mechanisms for fibroblast proliferation and matrix synthesis.

As might be expected for a pleiotropic growth factor, the effects of TGF-β in fibrosis are not restricted to stimulating collagen synthesis. For example, as illustrated earlier in Figure 8–3, TGF-β inhibits the expression of MMP-1 and MMP-2 by fibroblasts,[162–164] a response stimulated by many agents including the growth factors PDGF[165] and IL-1β.[166,167] In addition, as discussed earlier, the activities of MMP-1, MMP-3, and other connective tissue degrading metalloproteinases are kept in check by a number of inhibitors including TIMPs. In vitro studies reported by Wright and colleagues[137] have shown that TGF-β acts to stimulate the synthesis and secretion of TIMP by IL-1β–stimulated human rheumatoid synovial fibroblasts. Thus, in addition to stimulating collagen synthesis, TGF-β also may attenuate collagen degradation by blocking the synthesis of collagen-degrading enzymes and by increasing the synthesis of TIMPs thus promoting an imbalance between collagen synthesis and its degradation.

Platelet-Derived Growth Factor.   PDGF exists in either homodimeric or heterodimeric complexes as PDGF-AA, PDGF-BB, and PDGF-AB and acts as a mesenchymal competence type growth factor. Studies of bronchoalveolar lavage fluid in IPF and other pulmonary disorders characterized by intra-alveolar or interstitial fibrosis initially showed the levels of PDGF-like bioactivity and, in particular, the PDGF-B chain to be markedly elevated compared with normal healthy controls and that alveolar macrophages were an important source. Martinet and colleagues[168] showed that when alveolar macrophages from patients with IPF or cells from normal controls were cultured in vitro, macrophages obtained from IPF patients secreted approximately four times the amount of PDGF than control macrophages. Furthermore, when PDGF-A and B-chain mRNA expression by alveolar macrophages was quantified, Nagaoka and colleagues[169] found an approximately 10-fold increase in PDGF-B expression by alveolar macrophages compared with normal healthy volunteers with a marked skewing of production toward PDGF-B in that only about one-tenth the level of expression of PDGF-A was detected compared with PDGF-B. The mature PDGF dimer exhibits a molecular mass of ~30 to 34 kDa by sodium dodecyl sulfate–polyacrylamide gel electrophoresis (SDS-PAGE). However, studies of bronchoalveolar lavage fluid (BALF) from patients with acute lung injury, as well as supernatants obtained from asbestos and carbonyl iron–stimulated rat alveolar macrophages, have revealed both higher- and lower-molecular-weight PDGF isoforms.[170,171] It is not clear how these different isoforms may arise, although they appear to contain both PDGF-BB and PDGF-AB but not PDGF-AA–like activity and do not represent single chains. It has been suggested that the low molecular weight 14 to 18 kDa isoforms may arise by proteolytic cleavage or by de novo synthesis.[170,171]

Within the lung parenchyma, studies using immunocytochemistry and in situ hybridization have shed a significant amount of light on the cell types that express PDGF in human fibrotic lung disorders and their animal models. Antoniades and colleagues[172] employed in situ hybridization to explore the cell types responsible for PDGF expression in IPF and showed that both alveolar macrophages and epithelial cells were significant sources of PDGF. Similarly, Homma and colleagues[173] have shown that in early IPF, PDGF was localized to a number of different cell types including macrophages, fibroblasts, type II alveolar epithelial cells, and vascular endothelial cells while in late stage IPF, PDGF expression was exclusively localized to alveolar macrophages. In a similar study, Vignaud and colleagues[174] showed that interstitial macrophages were also a significant source of PDGF and that the number of PDGF-positive interstitial macrophages increased by threefold in biopsy specimens from patients with IPF compared with controls.

The stimuli responsible for inducing PDGF expression and secretion by macrophages have not been systematically investigated, although a number of autocrine- and paracrine-acting cytokines, including IL-1β[175] and interferon-γ (IFN-γ),[176] have been shown to induce PDGF expression. In addition, certain phagocytic stimuli such as β 1,3-glucan and, as discussed above, asbestos fibers and iron particles are also capable of inducing PDGF expression.[146,170]

Insulin-Like Growth Factor-I.   IGF-I is a progression type growth factor, which, in conjunction with a competence-type growth factor, such as PDGF or fibronectin, allows receptor-bearing cell types to progress though the G_1 phase of the cell cycle and to synthesize DNA. Although produced predominantly by the liver and circulating in the plasma in combination with IGF-I binding proteins, there is now extensive evidence that IGF-I can also be expressed at increased levels at extrahepatic sites, especially in the lung. IGF-I protein and/or growth-promoting activity has been found in elevated levels in the BALF of patients with pulmonary fibrosis arising in coal workers' pneumoconiosis, asbestosis, silicosis, and in IPF.[177–180] In addition, alveolar macrophages from patients with these fibrotic disorders secrete elevated amounts of this growth factor.[181] Similarly, in the bleomycin-induced pulmonary fibrotic response in mice, alveolar macrophages have been shown to express up to sixfold higher levels of IGF-I mRNA as detected by RT-PCR analysis.[182] Other studies also have shown that IGF-I can stimulate collagen synthesis by lung fibroblasts in vitro[183,184] thus implying that IGF-I may serve to regulate both fibroblast proliferation and fibroblast collagen synthesis. At the ultrastructural level, we have localized IGF-I expression to alveolar macrophages and airway and alveolar epithelium in normal and IPF subjects, whereas in IPF patients, IGF-I expression appears to be increased in interstitial macrophages.[185] Importantly, the degree of expression of IGF-I by interstitial macrophages in patients with IPF was found to correlate with the degree of disease severity suggesting that localized expression of this growth and survival factor in the pulmonary interstitium may be important in the pathogenesis and/or progression of fibrosis.[185]

Seeking to further understand the mechanism controlling IGF-I expression by macrophages, we[186] investigated the hypothesis that components of the extracellular matrix might stimulate the expression of fibrogenic growth factors, especially IGF-I. In pulmonary fibrosis and asthma, several matrix components have been detected in cell-free BALF, including hyaluronic acid.[187,188] Importantly, the increased abundance of hyaluronic acid in BALF is thought to precede tissue fibrosis.[188] This suggested that hyaluronic acid may regulate IGF-I expression by macrophages. In vitro exposure of mouse bone marrow–derived macrophages to hyaluronic acid stimulated a two to fourfold increase in the synthesis of IGF-I protein with maximal stimulation being observed approximately 18 to 24 hours after stimulation, an effect not seen with other glycosaminoglycans including chondroitin sulfate A or heparan sulfate.[186] The interaction between hyaluronic acid and macrophages was shown to be mediated by the cell surface receptor CD44. In addition to stimulating the synthesis of IGF-I, hyaluronic acid stimulated the expression of TNF-α and IL-1β with a time course that preceded the expression of IGF-I. To address the possible involvement of these cytokines in the regulation of IGF-I expression, macrophages were exposed to hyaluronic acid in the presence of antibodies directed against either TNF-α or IL-1β. Antibodies directed against TNF-α but not against IL-1β inhibited the stimulation of IGF-I synthesis in response to hyaluronic acid. Furthermore, purified recombinant TNF-α was found to directly stimulate the expression of IGF-I. Taken together, these data suggest that hyaluronic acid stimulates IGF-I synthesis in a TNF-α–dependent fashion,[186] thus providing a potential linkage between TNF-α and fibrogenic growth factors.

Fibroblast Growth Factors. The fibroblast growth factor family now includes 22 members with molecular weights that range from 17 to 34 kDa.[189] Members of the FGF family play critical and divergent roles during embryonic development and in adults. Genetic disruption of FGF genes in mice has provided compelling data to show that FGF-10 is essential for lung development[190]; whereas FGF-7 is required for hair growth.[191] In the context of repair, most studies have focused on FGF-1 (previously known as acidic FGF) and, in particular, FGF-2 (also known as basic FGF). Although always suspected as being important in wound repair responses, studies in FGF-2–deficient mice have now clearly established that FGF-2 plays an important role in skin wound repair.[192] Constitutive expression of FGF-2 by mouse peritoneal exudate macrophages was first reported by Baird and colleagues[193] who detected the growth factor by immunocytochemistry. Analyses of FGF expression in animal models of injury and repair have revealed infiltrating macrophages to be a major cellular source of FGF-2. Rappolee and colleagues[194] detected FGF-2 mRNA in macrophages isolated from subepidermally implanted wound cylinders, although expression of the FGF-2 protein was not investigated.

In the context of lung injury and the fibrotic response that occurs in a subset of patients recovering from this disorder, Henke and colleagues[195] showed that FGF-2 mRNA and protein were expressed during the fibroproliferative phase following acute lung injury in humans. PCR and Northern blot analysis of RNA isolated from alveolar macrophages revealed the presence of two species of FGF-2 mRNA, and biosynthetic labeling with ^{35}S-methionine followed by immunoprecipitation with anti-FGF-2 antibody revealed the presence of the 18 kDa protein. Importantly, immunocytochemical staining of lung tissue obtained postmortem revealed the presence of numerous FGF-2–staining macrophages in alveoli containing variable degrees of fibroplasia. In addition, using a combination of approaches including immunocytochemistry, Inoue and colleagues have reported that mast cells are also an important source of FGF-2 in IPF as well as in areas of fibroproliferation in patients with chronic beryllium disease.[196] Furthermore, FGF-2 levels were markedly increased in BALF and sera from patients with severe interstitial and alveolar fibrosis. Thus, alveolar macrophages and mast cells appear to be an important source of FGF-2 in the induction of alveolar fibrosis following lung injury.

Although it is generally thought that the expression of FGF-1 is restricted to the brain and neuronal tissue, recent work has also suggested that macrophages may, under certain conditions, express FGF-1. In a study of FGF expression in atheromatous and nonatheromatous human arteries, Brogi and colleagues[197] detected marked expression of FGF-1 in atheromatous but not in control arteries. Expression of FGF-1 was greatest in areas of neovascularization and in macrophage-rich regions of plaque. Moreover, the expression of FGF-1 by macrophages was extended by showing that the human monocytic cell line THP-1 expressed FGF-1 mRNA following stimulation with the phorbol ester, phorbol myristate acetate (PMA). Thus, these collective data indicate that human macrophages are capable of expressing FGF-1 and suggest that plaque macrophages may contribute to the neovascularization seen in human atheroma. In the context of pulmonary fibrosis, Barrios and colleagues[198] have documented a pronounced increase in FGF-1 mRNA and protein expression by macrophages and epithelial cells in the lungs of rats in which fibrosis was induced with paraquat and hyperoxia (see "Animal Models of Interstitial and Alveolar Fibrosis" for more information about this model). Additional studies, however, are clearly needed to establish if additional FGFs, especially those involved in normal lung development, are also involved in the fibrotic response given the notion that repair and fibrosis may in some way recapitulate normal embryonic and neonatal lung development.

Once released from cells, FGF is strongly bound by elements of the extracellular connective tissue matrix and while in this state appears to be incapable of stimulating cell proliferation. However, work reported by Falcone and colleagues have suggested that macrophages may play an important role in releasing FGF-2 from matrix components thereby rendering the growth factor available for growth stimulation.[199,200] The enzyme responsible appeared to be a membrane-associated urokinaselike plasminogen activator since the release of FGF-2 from cell-derived matrices was enhanced by plasminogen. Importantly, this property was not restricted to FGF-2 since matrix bound TGF-β was also released under the same conditions. Furthermore, purified soluble TGF-β, although not FGF-2, TNF-α, or IL-1β, stimulated the activity of the macrophage urokinaselike plasminogen activator indicating that TGF-β may be capable of amplifying the release of growth factors and/or cytokines from the extracellular tissue matrix.[199] Thus, macrophages may play a key role in maintaining the bioavailability of a number of fibrogenic growth factors including those that are known to regulate the fibrotic response.

Transforming Growth Factor-α. Transforming growth factor-α is a comparatively small macrophage-derived growth factor with a molecular weight of approximately 5 to 6 kDa. Sequence analysis has revealed that TGF-α shares almost 40% homology with epidermal growth factor (EGF) and interacts with responsive cells via the EGF-receptor. TGF-α stimulates the growth of endothelial cells, epithelial cells, and fibroblasts and has been found to stimulate angiogenesis in vivo. TGF-α is secreted by alveolar macrophages stimulated in vitro with endotoxin[201] and crysotile asbestos fibers.[202] Work conducted in the promyelocytic cell line HL-60 has shown that differentiation along the monocytic pathway in response to PMA results in an induction of TGF-α expression leading to both secretion

and intracellular retention of the newly synthesized protein.[203] Evidence was presented to suggest that proteases mediate the release of TGF-α from the cells, because in the presence of protease inhibitors, the secretion of TGF-α was decreased whereas intracellular levels increased.

In the lung, TGF-α also appears to be intimately involved in the initiation of a fibrotic response. Korfhagen and colleagues[204] have shown that overexpression of the human TGF-α gene under the influence of the surfactant protein-C (SP-C) promoter in transgenic mice led to the development of patchy hypercellular fibrotic lesions in the interstitium especially near pulmonary vessels and bronchioles. The fibrotic lesions were comprised principally of fibroblastoid interstitial cells and also were associated with thickening of the pleural surfaces. Interestingly, although macrophages were, in general, more abundant in the transgenic mice, neutrophils were not present. TGF-α protein has also been detected at distinct locations in the lungs of rats in which fibrosis had been induced by inhalation of aerosolized chrysotile asbestos fibers.[202] Specifically, TGF-α protein expression was up-regulated within 24 hours of asbestos exposure in regions of the bronchiolar-alveolar ducts in which asbestos fibers had lodged. Furthermore, although the animals were only given a single exposure to asbestos, the increased staining for TGF-α persisted for up to 2 weeks. In a similar study, Madtes and colleagues[201] showed that levels of TGF-α protein and mRNA increased in rats in response to instillation of bleomycin and that TGF-α protein was localized within macrophages, alveolar septal cells, and epithelial cells in regions of apparent fibroproliferation. These collective lines of evidence suggest that TGF-α may play a significant role in stimulating cell proliferation during the fibrotic response.

Lymphocytes

Perhaps the cell lineage that is most often overlooked as playing a role in the control of the fibrotic response is the lymphoid lineage, although it is well known that the fibrotic process is often preceded and/or accompanied by an intra-alveolar and interstitial inflammatory infiltration that contains activated lymphocytes.[205] The initial phase may not always be detected among patients, but it is thought to precede the fibrotic process. Usual interstitial pneumonitis is associated with diseases of largely unknown etiology but is associated with various factors, ranging from environmental chemical substances to infectious agents. In all these cases, the participation of lymphocytes in the evolution of the disease is intriguing because their presence suggests the possibility of an antigen-specific reaction as a part of the pathogenesis of pulmonary fibrosis. Although not formally demonstrated, an antigen-specific immune reaction has been suggested from experimental data and is supported by the latest notions on the special properties of resident pulmonary lymphocytes. To discuss the role of immune reactivity during the development of lung fibrosis, we must first expose some basic data concerning resident pulmonary lymphocytes (RPL). These lymphocytes have been identified as independent entities only recently, and their discovery was connected to the study of pulmonary γδ T cells in the lung.

γδ *Resident Pulmonary Lymphocytes*

γδ Resident pulmonary lymphocytes reside in murine lungs and readily respond to aerosol immunization with mycobacterial antigens as well as to self-heat-shocked cells.[206,207] Subsequently, T-cell hybrids with such reactivity were established and it appeared that they expressed a monomorphic Vγ6Vδ1 T-cell receptor (TCR). It was also shown that a homogeneous population of γδ T cells that express this receptor constitutes the first set of T cells to colonize the lung, beginning right before birth.[208] γδ T cells that express this receptor share a similar pattern of reactivity with the predominant mycobacterial antigen-specific Vγ9Vδ2 γδ T-cell population found in man. Both sets of γδ T cells react to sonicated mycobacteria but not to recombinant heat shock protein (HSP)-65 antigen.[209] In humans, however, there is little tissue specific restriction of TCR Vγ gene expression, as has been observed for mice. Nonetheless, it has been reported that in some patients suffering from sarcoidosis, there is an oligoclonal expansion of some Vγ9Vδ2 T cells in the lesions.[210,211] Very recently, a nonpeptide family of pyrophosphate compounds have been shown to stimulate the human Vγ9Vδ2 T cells.[212] These compounds are also able to stimulate the murine Vγ6Vδ1 T cells. This extensive similarity between the murine pulmonary γδ T cells and their human equivalent suggests the relevance of the murine experimental system to human lung pathology. To study the functions of these cells in detail, transgenic mice were generated that express various levels of this TCR.[209] With the help of such transgenic mice, the striking analogies between the reactivities of some murine and human γδ T cells were further analyzed. Thus, human Vγ9Vδ2 T cells and the Vγ6Vδ1 murine T cells share not only this specific reactivity to mycobacteria but also reactivity to plasmodial antigens and to some pyrophosphate compounds such as farnesyl pyrophosphate.[212] When stimulated, γδ RPL are able to produce IL-2 and IL-4 for only a short period of time (24 h), but they exhibit a sustained production of IFN-γ.

Extrathymic Selection of Pulmonary γδ T cells by Polymorphic Self-Ligands. In analyzing the γδ RPL repertoire, we have characterized, in the mouse, two additional predominant γδ clonotypes: (1) BALB/c-invariant delta (BID), which is distinguished by an invariant Vδ5 TCR[213] and (2) GxYS a VJ junctional amino acid coding sequence, which consists of a family of Vγ4 chains differing from each other only at one specific amino acid.[214] Both clonotypes are subjected to strain-dependent positive

selection in the periphery but their selective expansion is independent of classic H-2 or the presence of the thymus. This pattern of γδ T-cell selection in the periphery has subsequently been reported in humans.[215] The role of the thymus is mainly oriented towards "supervising" a programmed Vγ and Vδ gene rearrangement and not toward positive selection of clonotypes, as is the case for αβ T cells.[216] It is interesting to note that the "driving force" responsible for peripheral expansion of lung γδ T cells was postulated to be controlled by gene products whose expression can be amplified under special conditions such as local inflammatory stress, which might appear in the induction phase of lung fibrosis. This is exactly the case in at least one circumstance, where an endogenous retrovirus (Mpmv-30) drives the peripheral expansion of γδ T cells.[217] The increased expression of endogenous retroviral gene products in cells under stress could lead to a boost of the local γδ T-cell population, as a secondary phenomenon, in the course of lung fibrosis.

Proliferating Vγ6Vδ1 Murine T Cells Produce Keratinocyte Growth Factor. Keratinocyte growth factor (KGF) has recently been identified as a factor that can promote the regeneration of epithelial cells in vivo. However, it is not yet clear which cell types are the main producers of this growth factor. It now appears that γδ T cells that reside in various epithelia can produce substantial amounts of KGF when activated. It has been reported recently that when stimulated to proliferate, both dendritic epithelial γδ T cells of the skin (DEC) and intestinal intraepithelial γδ T lymphocytes (iIEL) produce significant amounts of KGF mRNA.[218] We have tested various populations of cells of pulmonary origin for KGF production and concluded that (1) Vγ6Vδ1 T cells are KGF producers when activated and that this activity is present in both transgenic and normal RPL; (2) systemic lymphocytes do not produce KGF on activation, in agreement with the previous report; (3) transgenic Vγ6Vδ1 T cells, even when homed to lymphoid organs, are still good KGF producers, an observation that indicates that KGF production is constitutive to the cell type and is not environmentally instructed; and (4) KGF expression by γδ thymocytes is high during fetal life and is a property of early γδ T cells produced by day-15 thymocytes when γδ cells are the only lineage well represented in the thymus, whereas in the postnatal period, KGF production by thymocytes decreases. Thus, the activity and secretory properties of γδ RPLs may serve to help epithelial regrowth following injury through the production of KGF, while the secretion of IFN-γ may, as discussed both earlier and in following sections, serve to limit collagen production and fibroblast growth during the fibrotic response.

Double Negative (CD4⁻CD8⁻) αβ+ T Cells. Double negative (CD4⁻CD8⁻) αβ+ T cells constitute about 20% of all αβ+ T cells in murine lungs and are another variety of resident lymphocytes in the lung. We found that in BALB/c mice, 60% of the double negative αβ+ pulmonary T cells express receptors of the Vβ8 family whereas only 33% of single positive (CD4+ and CD8+) pulmonary T cells express Vβ8. However, in C57BL/6 mice, equal frequencies (25%) of double negative and single positive αβ+ pulmonary T cells express Vβ8. The high frequency of double negative Vβ8+ pulmonary T cells is dominantly inherited in (C57BL/6 × BALB/c) F1 offspring, and is not due to positive selection events involving classic major histocompatibility complex (MHC) region gene products. On exposure to mycobacterial antigens, double negative αβ+ pulmonary T cells are coenriched in vitro in parallel with γδ+ T cells, suggesting functional similarities between these two T-cell subsets. This interesting parallel selection and antigen reactivity between γδ RPL and double negative (CD4−CD8−) αβ+ pulmonary T cells is probably not a coincidence. One should thus consider the possibility that during the fibrotic process, these two types of cells may synergize.[219]

Colonization and Selection of γδ T Cells in the Murine Lung: Thymic and Extrathymic Origins of Resident Pulmonary Lymphocytes. How well individualized is the population of resident pulmonary lymphocytes? Is their typical pattern of gene expression an indication of a different pathway of differentiation or simply of lung specific homing? The answer to these questions may be especially relevant if one designs experiments in which the function of RPLs is investigated during a specific pathologic process, as in pulmonary fibrosis. We investigated the kinetics of colonization of the lung by resident pulmonary γδ T cells with the idea that it would indicate whether the localization of certain γδ T cells in the lung is due to preferential homing or whether it is the product of site-specific proliferation. We found that at birth, T lymphocytes that colonize the lung are mainly of the γδ subset, whereas αβ T cells predominate in the spleen.[208] Thus, the lung is a preferred site for the homing of γδ T cells in the perinatal period. However, after birth, the pattern of Vγ gene usage among RPLs changes with age, from a predominance of Vγ6 at birth to a predominance of Vγ4 in older mice. These data indicate that pulmonary T lymphocytes are derived from both migrants of thymic origin and from precursors that have undergone differentiation and selection in the lung. The population that is generated in situ and that has not been selected in the thymus may include cells that are typical for the pulmonary environment. Thus, it appears that the resident pulmonary T-cell population consists of cells that are generated and selected locally, as well as of cells that are generated in the thymus but may be further selected and expanded in the pulmonary environment.[208]

Recirculating Lymphocytes

CD4+ and CD8+ αβ T Cells. CD4+ and CD8+ αβ T cells constitute a heterogeneous population in terms of T-cell receptor usage and to date there is no clear indication that such cells might be strictly resident in the lung. They probably belong to the recirculating pool and can be activated locally in various conditions of antigen triggering. Among CD4+ T cells, two subsets of lymphocytes have been distinguished based on their ability to produce specific lymphokines on induction: (1) Th$_1$ (which mainly secretes IL-2 and IFN-γ) and (2) Th$_2$ (producing IL-4, IL-5 , IL-6, and IL-10). Both Th$_1$ cells, which are responsible for the production of delayed-type hypersensitivity reactions, and Th$_2$ cells, which are responsible for helping B cells during a humoral response, have been detected in IPF.[1] As we shall see, this observation is in agreement with the data obtained from the study of experimental fibrosis in mice.

B Cells. Although rare in normal lung tissue, B cells are frequently found in the interstitium of IPF patients. Such B lymphocytes usually form aggregates in the vicinity of an air space displaying bronchial metaplasia or hyperplasia of type II epithelial cells.[2] Moreover, in some cases, lymphocytes are organized in germinal centers. In many of these structures, T lymphocytes also were detected and the presence on their surface of the CD45RO+ marker suggests that they belong to the memory T cell pool.[2] These observations suggest the development of an antigen specific immune response during lung fibrosis. Indeed, in 80% of patients with IPF, autoantibodies directed against lung-specific proteins were detected in the peripheral blood.[3] It still remains to be determined whether such a response is a primary event directly related to the course of fibrosis or only a secondary immune phenomenon in response to a profound alteration of the lung architecture seen in IPF. Interestingly, lymphocyte aggregates (which contain predominantly B cells) have been detected both in the areas with active interstitial pneumonitis as well as in the areas displaying end-stage fibrosis. The regulation of the immunoglobulin class secreted by pulmonary plasma cells in the fibrotic lung has not been extensively studied yet. However, in the induction of fibrosing alveolitis by tracheal instillation of cellulose in rats, an increased production of IgA has been detected in the bronchoalveolar lavage fluid.[220]

Lymphocytes in Animal Models of Pulmonary Fibrosis: a Case for Active Involvement in Human Disease

Studies in animal models have contributed significantly to our understanding of the molecular mechanisms underlying the disease process and they are extensively discussed in "Animal Models of Interstitial and Alveolar Fibrosis." A commonly employed experimental system is the induction of pulmonary interstitial fibrosis by the intratracheal instillation of bleomycin. The role of cytokines in the evolution of the fibrotic response has been extensively addressed. A large body of experimental data indicate that cytokine networks mediate the response to bleomycin. In particular, two regulatory cytokines, TNF-α and IFN-γ, have been shown to have important and opposing effects on the development of pulmonary fibrosis in mice.[221-223] In bleomycin induced pulmonary fibrosis, IFN-γ reduces the degree of collagen accumulation and fibroblast proliferation.[221] On the other hand, TNF-α has been shown to promote or at least enhance fibrosis.[224] Fibrosis can be prevented by treatment with anti-TNF-α antibody and aggravated by the infusion of mouse recombinant TNF-α. Although it is well established that IFN-γ is the product of activated T lymphocytes and TNF-α is produced by monocytes and macrophages, the production of TNF-α is dependent on T-cell activities. In vivo depletion of T cells abolishes the production of TNF-α. These data imply that T cells could be the key players in influencing the evolution of pulmonary fibrosis. Prior to that, it was reported that the *nude* mutation protects against bleomycin-induced pulmonary fibrosis. The lesions associated with bleomycin-induced pulmonary fibrosis in athymic nude mice were significantly diminished, compared to euthymic mice, suggesting that the participation of the cellular immune system contributed to the development of fibrosis in normal mice.[225] Although the elimination of T cells can prevent bleomycin-induced fibrosis[223] it is not clear whether T-cell participation is required in the initiation or maintenance phase of the disease, or both. Moreover, the observed inhibitory effects of IFN-γ on collagen accumulation and fibroblast proliferation in bleomycin-induced fibrosis suggest that T cells could also play a role in the resolution of fibrosis.[221] This point of view is further supported by clinical data showing that among patients with fibrosing lung diseases, those with the highest levels of circulating IFN-γ responded best to corticosteroids. This has been taken as an indication that in the high IFN-γ producers, the stage of their disease is in a "less fibrotically inclined" phase, because their immune system is still capable of producing IFN-γ.[226] This could be further corroborated with the observation that untreated patients with impaired IFN-γ production exhibit a greater tendency toward spontaneous deterioration of their conditions.

If T cells are responsible for the initiation and maintenance of fibrosis, how can they participate in its resolution? This apparent contradiction can easily be resolved if one considers that T cells are actually divided into many functionally distinct subsets, apart from the long-recognized category of cytotoxic and helper T cells. Even phenotypically identical subsets that bear the same type of T-cell receptor can be separated into functionally distinct subpopulations.[227] A well-known example is the Th$_1$/Th$_2$ division among the CD4$^+$ T cells discussed earlier in "CD4$^+$ and CD8$^+$ $\alpha\beta$ T Cells." These cells are indistinguishable if one divides the lymphoid population according to their TCR expression. However, they can be easily distinguished functionally by their ability to secrete either IFN-γ or IL-4, following activation. Moreover, there are two different lineages of T cells: those that express

the $\alpha\beta$ T-cell receptor and those that express the $\gamma\delta$ T-cell receptor. These two types of T cells are known to exhibit different kinetics of activation in immune responses to pathogens.[228-230] It is therefore conceivable that T cells that participate in the initiation and maintenance of fibrosis are functionally distinct and differ from those that enhance the process of resolution. Despite this dichotomous paradigm, it is important to emphasize that the same naive T-helper cell (Th$_0$) can functionally differentiate into either the Th$_1$ or Th$_2$ T cell depending on the type of cytokine present in the microenvironment in which it is functionally activated.[231,232] Therefore, some T cells may recognize the same antigen in the context of the same MHC molecule but produce different functional consequences.

An interesting experimental model in which a T-cell mediated immune response to a nominal antigen causes pulmonary interstitial fibrosis has been developed by Hu and Stein-Streilein.[233] In this hapten-immune mouse model, mice were first immunized by painting trinitrophenyl (TNP) onto their shaven abdomen. Subsequent challenge by an intratracheal dose of the same antigen resulted in the induction of lung fibrosis. Subset depletion by in vivo treatment with anti-CD4 and/or anti-CD8 antibodies revealed that both CD4 and CD8 T cells contribute to this process. The authors suggested that skin priming drove antigen-specific cytotoxic T-cell (CTL) precursors into differentiation. CTL effector cells were generated and ready to do damage to the lung tissue on delivery of the antigen to the pulmonary microenvironment, and that T-cell mediated assaults on antigen-derivatized lung cells induced the fibrosing process. This system provides evidence in support of the idea that antigen-specific T cells can be the initiating factor in the development of pulmonary fibrosis. Another potentially interesting animal model for studying the cells participating in lung fibrosis has been constructed by intratracheal instillation with fluorescein isothiocyanate (FITC). This molecule is both a potent T-cell immunogen that forms a covalent bond with tissue protein and a fluorescent substance so that its distribution in the lung tissue can be tracked easily.[234] A long-lasting T-cell reaction, in the vicinity of the fluorescent lung areas, accompanies pulmonary fibrosis. Interestingly, however, recent studies by Christensen and colleagues have suggested that the induction of pulmonary fibrosis in this model is T-cell independent.[235]

A Paradigm for the Role of T cells in Augmenting and Preventing Pulmonary Fibrosis

T-cell activation is an intrinsic part of a normal immune response. Given that T-cell activities appear crucial to the process of pulmonary fibrosis as discussed above, it is possible that over a certain period of time, otherwise "normal" immune responses can influence the development of pulmonary fibrosis. This hypothesis deserves closer examination. One way in which this process can occur is through the generation of a sufficient number of memory cells of various specificities, some of which might be reactive to self-antigens. These memory cells are more readily triggered than naive T cells and can, therefore, be more easily mobilized by stimuli. It was observed in the past,[236] that in an immune response, in addition to the antigen-specific component, there is a "bystander" effect whereby cells that are not specific to the immunizing antigens are "trans-stimulated" and expanded. Today, we know that the cohort of cytokines secreted by various cell types during an antigen-initiated immune response is responsible for the recruitment and expansion of these bystander T cells. It follows that the more frequent an immune reaction takes place in a particular microenvironment, the higher the frequency and variety of memory cells.

If T cells can participate in different phases of the development of fibrosis, the existence of a larger reservoir of memory cells would imply a greater probability that some T cells would become activated in the face of a challenge by an unknown environmental antigen. In line with the theme developed above, it would be important to determine whether a normal immune response (elicited by a well-defined antigen targeting and activating a specific T cell population) could still be elicited at different phases in the course of the evolution of pulmonary interstitial fibrosis.

The major health hazard associated with pulmonary fibrosis is the replacement of pulmonary epithelial tissues by fibroblasts in the repair process following tissue injury, which results in a loss of functional gas exchange units. A growth factor that can potentially counteract fibrosis by promoting the regeneration of the epithelial layer is keratinocyte growth factor.[237,238] As shown above, it was demonstrated that resident pulmonary γδ T cells can secrete KGF when activated. Thus the production of KGF appears to be a conserved feature of epithelial tissue associated γδ T cells. The tendency of γδ T cells to be localized in various epithelial tissues has long been postulated to be a reflection of their role in the preservation of epithelial integrity. The ability of activated but not resting γδ T cells of epithelial origin to secrete KGF suggests that these cells have the capacity to nurse injured epithelia. Thus, they could exert a positive influence in minimizing epithelial damage and diminishing the magnitude of lung fibrosis. The striking similarities between the murine pulmonary γδ T cells and their human equivalents suggest the relevance of the murine experimental system to human lung pathology. Apart from the production of KGF, γδ T cells can also secrete IFN-γ, a cytokine that appears to attenuate the development of fibrosis. Given their ability to produce KGF and IFN-γ, γδ T cells have the potential to contribute positively toward a better reconstruction of the epithelial layer in the repair process and minimize the formation of fibrous tissue.

In summary, recent data indicate that the lung is the site of development, differentiation, and reactivity of several lymphocyte subsets. Their ability to secrete lymphokines, which could affect directly or indirectly the fibrotic process, is now documented. In particular, the pulmonary γδ T cells, which on stimulation produce KGF and IFN-γ, are interesting candidates for modulating this process. On the other hand, the involvement of αβ T cells in experimental lung fibrosis induced in mice and rats suggests that these cells are directly involved in the chain of phenomena leading ultimately to fibrosis. There is, however, no clear and unified view on the modality in which such cells are activated and on their precise effector function during the course of the disease. Thus, a specific therapeutic intervention aimed at modulating lymphocyte reactivity during lung fibrosis should wait for a definite answer to these questions. In the following section, we will discuss further how animal models of pulmonary fibrosis have been helpful in more fully defining the role of the inflammatory and immune systems in disease initiation and progression.

ANIMAL MODELS OF INTERSTITIAL AND ALVEOLAR FIBROSIS

Although pathologic studies on biopsy specimens from patients with pulmonary fibrosis have afforded insights into the mechanisms contributing to the inflammatory and fibrotic processes,[239] the limitation of this approach is that biopsy specimens represent single points in time and do not make it possible for the investigator to dissect early events in disease pathogenesis. In contrast, experimental animal models allow morphologic observation and mechanistic dissection of the early stages of the initial injury and inflammation and the latter stages of dysregulation leading to fibrosis.[240,241] These models can also be sampled at various stages of the injury and repair processes, and can be manipulated, for example, by the administration of experimental agents that may either inhibit or potentiate/ induce fibrosis. Such studies would be difficult or impossible in humans. However, animal models often do not completely mimic the disease in humans. For example, in many animal models, there is often an acute lung injury in response to the inciting stimulus, followed by a slower, but still relatively rapid, phase of fibrosis that differs from the chronic and insidious nature of clinical pulmonary fibrosis in humans. Nevertheless, an array of experimental approaches have been used in an attempt to develop an accurate animal model of human pulmonary fibrosis. These models include the adminstration of intravenous and intratracheal bleomycin,[242] intraperitoneal cyclophosphamide,[243] subcutaneous Freund's adjuvant,[244] subcutaneous paraquat,[245] intravenous oleic acid,[246] intratracheal cadmium chloride,[247] intratracheal silica,[248] and intratracheal asbestos.[249] In the following section, we will discuss current models of pulmonary fibrosis, and reiterate their helpfulness in understanding the pathogenesis and progression of this disorder.

Bleomycin Model

Among the many different animal models of interstitial lung diseases, bleomycin-induced pulmonary fibrosis is the most well studied, paralleled with the fact that bleomycin pulmonary toxicity is one of the most common and significant drug-induced lung diseases in the clinical setting, with an overall incidence of clinically apparent pulmonary toxicity of 10% and a mortality rate of 1%.[250,251] Although bleomycin-induced lung injury is a long-standing model for pulmonary fibrosis, Borzone and coworkers[252] recently showed that the chronic histologic and physiologic changes in rats challenged with intratracheal bleomycin were quite distinct from that seen in IPF. One-hundred and twenty days after bleomycin administration, the main features were normal lung compliance and focal peribronchiolar inflammation and fibrosis associated with paracicatricial emphysematous changes. However, it is possible that the route of bleomycin administration may dictate the different pathologic changes. For example, in beagle dogs given multiple *intravenous* injections of bleomycin over a few weeks, the characteristic pulmonary findings were an interstitial pneumonitis with fibrosis that had a predilection for the subpleural surfaces,[242] a pattern of fibrosis similar to that seen in IPF. Other notable features in this model of bleomycin-induced lung injury included marked hyperplasia and metaplasia of type II pneumocytes and a pleiomorphic inflammatory infiltrate in the interstitial and alveolar spaces composed of histiocytes, lymphocytes, plasma cells, neutrophils, and mast cells.[242] Occasionally, the alveolar inflammation was organized into polypoid projections covered by metaplastic type II epithelial cells. This study revealed that alveolar inflammation is a major component of the initial inflammatory process in interstitial lung diseases; importantly, the thickened interstitium that results is due, in large part, to re-epithelialization of the organized alveolar infiltrate.[253] However, others have shown that in rats repeatedly administered intratracheal bleomycin, alveolitis and interstitial fibrosis were diffusely distributed throughout the lungs.[254] Such descriptive analysis of the injurious and inflammatory phases of fibrosis is one of the major advantages of studying animal models. In the following sections, we will outline the pertinent mechanisms reported in the literature by which (1) bleomycin induces lung injury, (2) discuss how it mediates fibrosis, and (3) summarize investigations examining various agents that may ameliorate bleomycin-induced fibrosis and be potentially useful in formulating strategies to combat pulmonary fibrosis.

Mechanisms of Injury in the Bleomycin Model

There have been a number of studies examining the mechanisms by which bleomycin induces lung injury in experimental models. These include nonspecific injury such as that mediated by reactive oxygen species and immune-mediated injury. In addition, some of these mechanisms may not be mutually exclusive. Adamson and Bowden[255] induced pulmonary fibrosis in mice by the intravenous administration of bleomycin, and using electron microscopy, they showed that the earliest changes were endothelial damage in the pulmonary arterioles and venules, followed by a perivascular edema with a lymphoplasmacytic infiltrate. Even when administered intratracheally, bleomycin resulted in an increase in lung vascular permeability,[256] which may, in part, explain the increase in the influx of macrophages into the alveolar spaces.[257] Subsequent to the initiating event, there was focal necrosis of type I epithelial cells, accumulation of alveolar macrophages and fibrin in the alveolar spaces, proliferation of type II cells, and progressive fibrosis.[256] Although the lymphoplasmacytic infiltrate suggested an immune mechanism, possibly due to immune complex deposition, there was no evidence of electron-dense deposits in the capillary basement membranes.

It has been suggested that reactive oxygen species mediate lung injury caused by bleomycin.[258–261] Compared to control animals, superoxide (O_2^-) production by alveolar macrophages from bleomycin-treated rats was significantly increased on stimulation with either phorbol myristate acetate or opsonized zymosan.[262] The concomitant administration of bleomycin and hyperoxia to hamsters results in a synergistic development of pulmonary injury characterized by diffuse alveolar damage and interstitial fibrosis.[261] In hamsters made iron deficient, there was less bleomycin-induced pulmonary fibrosis and less lipid peroxidation, suggesting that iron-catalyzed oxygen radicals may be responsible for the initial injury.[263] Administration of manganese superoxide dismutase inhibited bleomycin-induced fibrosis,[264] further implicating reactive oxygen species in mediating bleomycin-induced lung injury. Platelet-activating factor has also been implicated in complement-neutrophil–mediated injury,[265] and thus is a candidate mediator in bleomycin-induced lung injury. In lung homogenates of bleomycin-treated hamsters, the density of PAF receptors is significantly upregulated.[266] More importantly, the functional activities of PAF receptors in alveolar macrophages, measured by an increase in cytosolic Ca^{2+}, is significantly greater in bleomycin-treated animals compared with controls. Thus, it is possible that the numeric and functional upregulation of PAF receptors may contribute to the initial injury in the bleomycin-induced model. In ICR strain mice intratracheally instilled with bleomycin, Fas and Fas ligand (FasL) mRNA expression were upregulated in alveolar epithelial cells and infiltrating lymphocytes, respectively.[267] This finding correlated with the apoptosis of bronchial and alveolar epithelial cells and the progression to fibrosis. Corticosteroids ameliorated the upregulation of Fas/FasL apoptosis and fibrosis.[268]

The adaptive immune system has also been implicated in mediating bleomycin-induced lung injury. Cultured BALF cells and blood lymphocytes from control and bleomycin-treated rabbits both exhibited spontaneous proliferation and cytolytic activity under basal conditions. However, in the presence of IL-2, both proliferation and concanavalin A–dependent cell mediated cytotoxicity were significantly increased in the cells exposed to bleomycin, suggesting that T cells were primed in the bleomycin-treated animals.[269]

Mechanisms of Fibrosis in the Bleomycin Model

The presence and severity of fibrosis likely depend on the severity and protraction of the initial lung injury induced by bleomycin.[270] One major determinant of fibrosis is the degree of accumulation of fibrin in the alveolar spaces. Fibrin has recently been demonstrated in the alveolar lining of IPF patients, in diffuse alveolar damage, and in BOOP; it is considered to be a necessary substratum for fibroblasts invading the alveolar spaces from the vascular and interstitial compartments.[239] Fibrin may not only serve to attract fibroblasts and neutrophils but may also stimulate angiogenesis. In bleomycin-treated rats, vascular casts of fibrotic lungs revealed marked neovascularization in the fibrotic areas, with the neoformed vessels arising from bronchial arteries.[271] Recently, it was demonstrated in bleomycin-treated mice that an imbalance existed between the activities of (1) procoagulant molecules such as tissue factor (TF) and type 1 plasminogen activator inhibitor (PAI-1) and (2) fibrinolytic mediators such as urokinase or type 1 plasminogen activator. Procoagulant activity predominated in the drug-injured lungs, resulting in the accumulation of extracellular fibrin in the alveolar spaces.[272] Although urokinase mRNA was also upregulated in the fibrous lesions, the accumulation of PAI-1 served to inhibit the former's fibrinolytic activity, resulting in a localized hypofibrinolytic state and the formation of the fibrin network.

The major cell that appears to be directly linked to the actual fibrosis is the myofibroblast, characterized by the expression of alpha-smooth muscle actin, desmin, and procollagen mRNA.[273] These proliferating fibroblasts appear to be derived initially from a population of cells located in the adventia of bronchioles, terminal bronchioles, and adjacent blood vessels.[273] Immunohistochemical staining has revealed that myofibroblasts are principally localized to the fibrotic regions of the lungs and are likely responsible for the majority of the morphologic findings and mechanical properties observed with bleomycin-induced lung fibrosis.[274] In a study examining the cellular constituents responsible for the increased elasticity in the experimental fibrotic lung, the contractility of strips of lung parenchyma from control and bleomycin-treated rats was measured in response to various stimuli. As expected, there was an increase in the contractile force generated by the bleomycin-treated lung; however, this increase in elasticity was not due to an increase in smooth muscle cells but rather to an increase in the number of myofibroblasts in the interstitium.[275] Another important mediator in the fibrotic process is fibronectin, a fibrin-bound glycoprotein that functions as an adhesive molecule for other extracellular matrix components such as collagen and is a chemoattractant and a competence-type growth factor for lung fibroblasts.[276]

At a subcellular level, the concentration of cyclic adenosine monophosphate (cAMP) may be an important regulator of collagen expression by fibroblasts, with an inverse relation between intracellular cAMP levels and collagen production. The lungs of bleomycin-treated hamsters have decreased stimulation of adenylate cyclase by various stimuli compared with untreated animals.[277] Thus, decreased cAMP formation in bleomycin-treated animals may be a mechanism by which collagen deposition is increased. Moreover, these investigators also showed that β-adrenergic receptors, which may augment the activity of membrane-bound adenylate cyclase and thus augment cAMP, were decreased in the lungs of bleomycin-treated animals compared with controls. In rats, intratracheal bleomycin also increases the activity of lysyl hydroxylase, the enzyme catalyzing the conversion of collagen-bound lysine to hydroxylysine, resulting in increased collagen cross-linking and fibrous scar formation.[278,279]

In a rat bleomycin model, an increase in lung TGF-β levels preceded the maximum collagen synthesis.[153] The major source of TGF-β was found to be interstitial macrophages. In the later stages of fibrosis, TGF-β was associated with the extracellular matrix and collagen. In vitro treatment of rat lung fibroblasts with bleomycin demonstrated that these cells were also a source of TGF-β.[280] The mRNA of two other fibroblast growth factors, PDGF-A and IGF-I, are increased in the BAL cells of bleomycin-treated mice compared with controls.[182] Another profibrotic cytokine shown to be activated by bleomycin in responder CBA strain mice, but not in nonresponder BALB/c mice, is TNF-α, peaking 7 days after bleomycin administration and preceding the increase in the transcription of collagen types I and III.[152] As discussed earlier, others have also shown the importance of TNF-α in the pathogenesis of bleomycin-induced pulmonary fibrosis.[223] In vitro, TNF-α is also a stimulus for IGF-I expression in mouse macrophages.[186] More recently, a transgenic mouse was developed, which overexpressed the murine TNF-α gene driven by the human surfactant protein SP-C promoter. Many of these mice died perinatally from severe pulmonary inflammation. The surviving mice transmitted a pulmonary disease to their offspring, characterized initially by a lymphocytic (T-cell) alveolitis, followed by progressive interstitial fibrosis.[281]

In normal wound repair, accumulation of hyaluronic acid and other glycosaminoglycans occurs prior to collagen deposition. In IPF, BALF contains an increased amount of hyaluronic acid,[187] and this has been confirmed in the bleomycin model with the accumulation of hyaluronic acid in the interstitium and in BALF.[188] In normal lung fibroblast cultures, the production of hyaluronic acid was enhanced by the addition of either BALF or alveolar macrophage-conditioned media obtained from bleomycin-treated rats.[282] Using neutralizing antibodies to various fibrogenic growth factors, it was further shown that the stimulatory activity in the BALF of bleomycin-treated rats was due to TGF-β. A positive feedback mechanism for inflammation and fibrosis may be operative because (1) hyaluronic acid synthesis may be stimulated by a number of fibrogenic growth factors such as PDGF, TGF-β, and IGF-1, (2) TNF-α may induce the synthesis of these same growth factors,[186,283] and (3) hyaluronic acid, by binding to CD44 present on macrophage cell surfaces, may induce the expression of TNF-α. In the C57BL/6 bleomycin-sensitive mice, repeated administration of bleomycin resulted in increased expression of gelatinase A, macrophage metalloelastase, and TIMP-1.[284] This finding is consistent with the prevailing thought that both tissue matrix degradation and deposition are operative in pulmonary inflammation leading to fibrosis, but that an imbalance results in a net gain of pulmonary fibrosis.

In contrast to the profibrotic profile that is typically demonstrated with bleomycin, in vitro studies with supernatants from alveolar macrophages obtained from bleomycin-treated rats revealed an activity, identified as IL-1, that inhibited fibroblast proliferation.[285] However, maximal production of IL-1 occurred early, within 6 to 12 hours after drug challenge and was undetectable by 7 days. Pretreatment of mice with rhIL-1β also attenuated the bleomycin-induced pneumonitis.[286] Interestingly, a hepatocyte-stimulating factor, shown in humans to be identical to IL-6, peaked 28 days after bleomycin.[285] How these cytokines retard the fibrotic process and the significance of this antagonism in the in vivo model is not known. It is possible that such counter-regulatory cytokine expression is not uncommon, but that in those animals that proceed to the fibrotic stage, there is an overwhelming profibrotic phenotypic expression.

Ameliorating the Fibrosis in the Bleomycin Model

A number of studies have evaluated the role of various molecules or reagents in ameliorating the inflammatory and fibrotic response in the bleomycin model of lung fibrosis. These studies not only have potential therapeutic ramifications but, by disrupting key cellular events, are also important in helping to elucidate the myriad components of the inflammatory and fibrotic process in the bleomycin model. Among the endogenous cytokines known to have antifibrotic effects, the interferons appear most promising and best studied. Consistent with the observation that a paucity of IFN-γ is present in IPF lungs,[287] either IFN-γ[288] or the IFN-α/β inducers polyinosinic-polycytidylic acid (poly I:C)[289] or bropirimine[290] has been shown to reduce the bleomycin-induced pulmonary fibrosis seen in mice and hamsters. Although bropirimine had no significant effect on bleomycin-induced lung injury, it reduced both hydroxyproline content and lung prolyl hydroxylase activity that were normally enhanced by bleomycin.[290] In the mouse model, concurrent administration of intratracheal bleomycin and intramuscular IFN-γ was shown to decrease the expression of TGF-β and procollagen α$_1$ (I) and α$_2$ (III) mRNA levels with no effect on the level of β-actin.[291] In addition, IFN-γ treatment also reduced the bleomycin-induced increase in hydroxyproline content.[288] Similarly, in rats given poly (I)-poly (C$_{12}$U) intraperitoneally, there was a reduction in the lung hydroxyproline content and prolyl hydroxylase activity compared with the treatment using bleomycin alone.[292] The mechanism by which IFNs or poly I:C ameliorate the fibrotic process is not well established in the bleomycin model. One study observed that in hamsters, which had been prophylactically treated with poly I:C prior to challenge with bleomycin, there was a reduction in the number of neutrophils in the BALF compared with animals not treated with poly I:C.[289] This study suggested that by limiting the number of neutrophils in the initial inflammatory process and thus limiting the injury, the later fibrotic process could be controlled; however, other studies have shown that exuberant fibrosis may occur despite neutrophil depletion.[293,294] In vitro, IFN-γ, -α$_A$, -α$_D$, and -β have all been shown to inhibit the growth of normal human lung fibroblasts[295] and to inhibit fibroblast proliferation in the bleomycin model of pulmonary fibrosis.[221] Another mechanism by which interferons may have antifibrotic activity is their ability to alter phenotypic differentiation in macrophages. We have shown[296] that in mouse macrophages, the presence of IFN-8 or -β inhibits the induction of IGF-I, a stimulus for fibroblast growth and collagen synthesis. The IFNγ-inducible protein-10 (IP-10), an angiostatic molecule. Systemic administration of IP-10 significantly reduced bleomycin-induced pulmonary fibrosis; furthermore, IP-10 had no direct effect on isolated pulmonary fibroblasts.[297] A molecular basis for the antifibrotic effect of IFN-γ may be the antagonism of TGF-β–induced JunD homodimerization by IFN-γ-induced Stat1α.[298] Because the JunD isoform of AP-1 transcription factor is an essential mediator of TGF-β–induced effects on lung fibroblasts, IFN-γ may serve to directly antagonize TGF-β signaling. IFN-γ also reduced the bleomycin-induced increases in TGF-β mRNA, and type I and type III procollagen mRNAs.[291,299] IFN-γ may also upregulate hepatocyte growth factor (HGF) receptor expression; HGF is a potent mitogen for alveolar epithelial cells and may repress the fibrotic process.[300] In contrast to these findings suggesting that IFN-γ may ameliorate bleomycin-induced pulmonary fibrosis, Chen and coworkers[301] recently found that IFN-γ–deficient mice (IFN-γ–/–) had significantly lower amounts of early inflammation and mortality and reduced pulmonary fibrosis at 3 weeks after bleomycin exposure. This finding is supported by the observation that fibrosis-prone C57BL/6J and A/J mice have elevated expression of IFN-γ protein in BALF after bleomycin challenge.[301,302] Furthermore, alveolar macrophages from both normal controls and interstitial lung disease patients showed increased PDGF-B mRNA production after IFN-γ stimulation.[176] Thus, it remains possible that IFN-γ exerts different effects at different times during the pathogenesis and progression of pulmonary fibrosis. These contradictory findings also emphasize the need to be cautious in the interpretation and extrapolation of findings in different models.

The class of compounds collectively known as the nonsteroidal anti-inflammatory drugs (NSAIDs), which have the ability to inhibit the cyclo-oxygenase pathway in prostaglandin synthesis, have been shown to have both profibrotic and antifibrotic properties in the bleomycin model. Indomethacin has been used to determine its in vivo effect on bleomycin-induced pulmonary fibrosis in rats.[256] In animals that received indomethacin subcutaneously, there was a decrease in the amount of extractable lung collagen, a decrease in the vascular permeability associated with bleomycin, a decrease in pulmonary fibrosis, and a decrease in the peripheral eosinophilia seen with bleomycin treatment. The mechanism by which indomethacin inhibited the fibrosis is not known although these findings suggest that prostaglandins (PG) somehow exhibit or support a profibrotic effect. In support of this notion, we[303] showed in vitro that PGE$_2$ augmented macrophage expression of the fibroblast growth factor IGF-I. However, prostaglandins have also been shown to have anti-inflammatory and potentially antifibrotic properties in the bleomycin model.[304] Prostaglandin E$_2$ metabolism is also decreased in bleomycin-treated hamsters, but the significance is not known.[305] In a hamster bleomycin model, not only did ibuprofen not have any effect on the lung hydroxyproline content but there was an increase in the severity of lung damage and mortality in ibuprofen-treated animals challenged with bleomycin compared with the bleomycin-alone group.[306] Thus, a consistent paradigm for the role of prostaglandins in pulmonary fibrosis is not well established.

High-dose prednisolone administered intraperitoneally and concomitantly with intratracheal bleomycin to rats had no suppressive effect on hyaluronic acid concentration in lung tissue or in BALF.[307] Unexpectedly, systemic corticosteroids also did not have any suppressive effect on the number or type of inflammatory cells in the lavage fluid. The effects of corticosteroids on the compliance of bleomycin-injured lungs were measured in rats.[308] It was dexamethasone and not methylprednisolone that significantly inhibited the decrease in compliance associated with bleomycin although both corticosteroids inhibited the inflammatory response to bleomycin.

Relaxin, a human cytokine implicated in structural remodeling of the interpubic ligament and cervix preceding childbirth, inhibited both the alveolar thickening and the increase in lung hydroxyproline content induced by intravenous bleomycin.[309] Subcutaneous relaxin was intentionally given 7 days after bleomycin administration in order to determine its effect on the fibrotic phase. In vitro, relaxin inhibited the TGF-β stimulation of fibronectin and collagen types I and III in a dose-dependent fashion and augmented the expression of matrix metalloproteinase-1 in human lung fibroblasts. Thus, the antifibrotic properties of relaxin are its ability to decrease collagen expression and increase collagen degradation.

Niacin[310–312] and nicotinamide[312] have been found to attenuate the fibrosis induced by bleomycin. The mechanism by which these agents protect against bleomycin-induced fibrosis is not known but is not considered to be due to any inhibitory effect on the initial lung injury, inflammation, or oxygen radical scavenging.[312] It was speculated that niacin may inhibit the fibrosis by maintaining nicotinamide-adenine dinucleotide (NAD) levels, thus maintaining local adenosine triphosphate (ATP) levels required for repair of the damaged epithelial cells; however, the direct inhibitory effects of niacin on collagen synthesis and cross-linking can not be excluded.[313]

In an intratracheal bleomycin-model of pulmonary fibrosis, hamsters treated intraperitoneally with AAT at 6 mg 1 day before bleomycin and then once weekly for a month showed a significant decrease in the amount of lung injury (day 7) and pulmonary fibrosis (day 30) compared with bleomycin-alone animals.[96] In addition, BAL analysis revealed that in AAT plus bleomycin-treated animals, early and late cellular infiltration in the lungs were decreased compared with bleomycin-treated hamsters. However, these findings occurred despite any difference in elastase activity, chemotaxis, or superoxide generation in neutrophils between the animals with or without AAT administration. Other AAT functions that may account for these salutary effects include inhibitory effects on fibroblast proliferation, inhibition of adherence of neutrophils to endothelial cells, and inhibition of kallikrein activity.

A nontoxic bleomycin resistance protein (BRP), which binds bleomycin and prevents DNA strand breakage, has been shown to protect against bleomycin-induced lung toxicity. BRP is encoded by a *Streptoalloteichus hindustanus* (Sh) *ble* gene. In a series of elegant experiments, prevention of bleomycin-induced lung fibrosis was shown in either transgenic mice overexpressing the Sh *ble* bleomycin-resistance gene[314] or in adenovirus-mediated transfer of Sh *ble* in C57BL/6 mice.[315] Other measures reported to ameliorate bleomycin-induce interstitial fibrosis in experimental animals include anti-CD11 antibodies,[316] antibodies to TGF-β,[317] IL-12,[318] soluble TNF-α receptors,[319] and inhibition of apoptosis by a caspase inhibitor.[320] Unexpectedly, the monoclonal antibody to IL-12 attenuated bleomycin-induced pneumopathy in mice.[321] Because IL-12 stimulates IFN-γ production, one hypothesis of this effect is that the monoclonal antibody neutralizes the IL-12 p40 subunit preferentially, which normally antagonizes the biologic activity of IL-12 p70 via competition for its receptor and thus suppresses Th$_1$-mediated responses. In IFN-γ–receptor deficient mice, where there is a defect in IFN-γ signaling, infection with murine gammaherpesvirus-68 resulted in widespread organ fibrosis, including the lung, compared to wild-type mice.[322]

Paraquat Model

Pulmonary fibrosis can be induced in animals challenged with the herbicide paraquat. However, there is often an acute lung injury with significant edema and high mortality within the first few days of administration.[323] In an attempt to further correlate clinical and experimental pulmonary fibrosis, Thurlbeck and Thurlbeck[324] demonstrated in both human paraquat poisoning and experimental paraquat-induced pulmonary toxicity in rats the occurrence of two distinct patterns of pulmonary fibrosis. One form was characterized by interstitial fibrosis and a honeycomb pattern after epithelial necrosis of the alveolar walls. The other pattern of fibrosis was characterized by fibrous organization of protein-rich edema fluid in the alveolar spaces due to damaged epithelial cells but with a preserved alveolar architecture. Repeated subcutaneous injections of paraquat are necessary to induce pulmonary interstitial fibrosis, possibly suggesting an immunologic mechanism.[245] However, the simultaneous administration of complete Freund's adjuvant (CFA), which was expected to enhance the inflammation, actually reduced the interstitial inflammation and fibrosis. It was speculated that the paraquat may have acted as a haptan in CFA-treated animals with subsequent induction of a blocking antibody that reduced the degree of ligand binding to lung tissues.

Paraquat pulmonary toxicity is considered to be mediated by reactive oxygen species[44] and is enhanced by the simultaneous administration of a high concentration of oxygen.[325] In a detailed chronologic study of paraquat-induced fibrosis, the sequence of morphologic findings was very similar to other models of experimental fibrosis.[95] Early lesions consisted of endothelial and type I epithelial cell damage, followed by a neutrophilic and a mononuclear cell inflammation, and then progressive fibrosis with proliferation of fibroblasts and mast cells. The intense inflammatory phase has been associated with elastin degradation due to the release of elastase from the inflammatory cells.[326] Such degeneration of elastic fibers in the alveolar walls may lead to the alveolar dilatation that often accompanies the fibrosis. Increased expression of ICAM-1 and of various integrins by macrophages in the early inflammatory phase and by macrophages, epithelial cells, and fibroblasts in

the fibrotic phase in rats exposed to both paraquat and hyperoxia may enhance cellular interactions during the pathogenic process.[327]

Silica and Asbestos Models

One of the major issues with many animal model studies is that, clinically, the primary insult in IPF and in fibrosing pneumoconiosis is considered to be initiated by an inhaled antigen. Although the silica animal model would appear ideal because there is a parallel fibrotic lung disease in humans due to inhalation of silica, species variability in animals and type of silica administered often affect the variable responses that have been described in experimental silicosis.[328] Experimentally, the dose of inhaled silica[329] and the formation of reactive oxygen species[330] have been implicated in silica-induced pulmonary injury. It was hypothesized that when the alveolar clearance mechanism is overwhelmed, there is an induction of a T-cell inflammatory response leading to fibrosis.[329] An immune mechanism is suggested in silica-induced injury because mice injected intratracheally with latex beads have significantly less cellular inflammation and collagen deposition than those treated with silica.[331] Halme and colleagues[248] were able to show that in rats injected intratracheally with silica, an increase in proline hydroxylase activity occurred in the early phase of the fibrotic process, preceding any obvious signs of fibrosis measured histologically or by hydroxyproline content. Similar to the bleomycin model, TNF-α[332] and TGF-β[333] have been implicated in silica-induced experimental pulmonary fibrosis. In transgenic mice overexpressing IL-9, there was significantly less pulmonary fibrosis after an inhalational silica challenge.[334]

Asbestosis is a chronic fibrosing lung disease that may occur many years after inhalational exposure to asbestos fibers. In vitro, various asbestos fiber types are known to increase the expression of TNF-α and IL-1β, which, in turn, may increase collagen types I and III and fibronectin gene expression.[335] Although an animal model of asbestos lung injury can be useful in studying the effects of the asbestos fibers in the lung, its correlation to the classic forms of pulmonary fibrosis is limited because of significant airway fibrosis and airflow limitation that develops in addition to the interstitial fibrosis.[93,249,331,336] To determine if reactive oxygen intermediates are involved in the pathogenesis of inflammation and subsequent fibrosis in an inhalational asbestosis model in rats, a novel study was performed in which the animals were given chronic administration of an antioxidant, catalase conjugated to polyethylene glycol, via an osmotic pump.[337] In those animals receiving the systemic antioxidant, there was less cellular and biochemical inflammation in the BALF and a decrease in lung fibrosis as measured by hydroxyproline levels and by histopathology.

Immune-Mediated Models

An immune model of interstitial lung fibrosis would appear to be an attractive model considering the high incidence of interstitial lung disease in various autoimmune diseases and the putative association between immune complex deposition and IPF.[43] Furthermore, as discussed in the section on lymphocytes Wallace and coworkers[1] showed by in situ hybridization and immunochemistry that lungs from IPF patients have a greater dominance of Th_2 cytokines such as IL-4 and IL-5 than the Th_1 cytokine IFN-γ. They speculated that because IL-4 and IFN-γ may be important regulatory factors for pulmonary fibroblasts, the relative paucity of IFN-γ may contribute to the excessive fibroblast activation and collagen deposition. Brentjens and colleagues[338] showed that immune complex deposition, due to repeated challenges with bovine serum albumin in rabbits, resulted in interstitial pneumonitis and fibrosis. However, others have shown that soluble and particulate antigens given into the lungs by aerosolization resulted in an alveolitis but failed to produce chronic interstitial fibrosis.[339] Because chronic intravenous challenges with bacille Calmette-Guérin (BCG) were able to cause a chronic fibrosis, it was hypothesized that effective clearance by alveolar macrophages protected the nonsusceptible animals from the inhaled antigen. A hapten-immune model of pulmonary interstitial fibrosis was described in hamsters that were initially skin painted with trinitrophenol and then challenged intratracheally with the immunizing hapten.[340] The response was specific because animals challenged with an unrelated hapten did not develop fibrosis. The inflammatory and fibrotic responses to trinitrophenol could be adoptively transferred with immune lymphocytes; furthermore, administration of anti-CD4 or anti-CD8 monoclonal antibodies to sensitized mice suppressed the inflammation and lung collagen deposition.[233] Inducing tolerance to trinitrophenol in the mouse model prevented the development of delayed type hypersensitivity and interstitial pulmonary fibrosis.[107] Thus, the hapten-immune model shows that a specific T-cell–mediated immune response can result in the induction of pulmonary fibrosis. The requirement of the delayed-type hypersensitivity response along with the increased expression of IL-2 and TNF-β suggests that the immune response may be deviated toward a Th_1 phenotype. In autoimmune MRL/lpr mice, there was a correlation in the age-associated increase in antinuclear antibodies and immune complexes and the development of interstitial pneumonitis.[341] In another hapten-induced model of lung inflammation and fibrosis, FITC was used as a hapten as well as marker for its sites of deposition due to its fluorescent nature.[234] When instilled into the trachea of mice, FITC induced an acute granulocytic response, followed by a predominantly T-lymphocyte infiltrate that progressed over several months to an interstitial pulmonary fibrosis. However, Christensen and colleagues[235]

recently showed, using T-cell–deficient animals, that FITC-induced pulmonary fibrosis is not dependent on an intact T-cell immunity. Similar to other types of experimental models of pulmonary fibrosis, TGF-β is an important fibrogenic growth factor in immune-mediated fibrosis. In a heat-killed BCG model of pulmonary fibrosis, the simultaneous intraperitoneal injection of a monoclonal antibody to TGF-β significantly decreased the histologic and biochemical markers of fibrosis.[342] Interestingly, the anti-TGF-β antibody also decreased the inflammatory cytokines IL-1β and TNF-α, suggesting that TGF-β, in addition to its fibrotic properties, may also have proinflammatory activity.

Other Models of Pulmonary Fibrosis

Amiodarone, a highly effective antiarrhythmic, has many potential side effects, the most serious being the development of life-threatening pulmonary fibrosis.[343] One characteristic finding in patients who have been exposed to amiodarone is the presence of intra-alveolar foam cells, which are composed of both macrophages and desquamated type II pneumocytes filled with amiodarone-phospholipid complexes. Amiodarone also has a tendency to cause an accumulation of phospholipids within lysosomes in the lungs and other tissues, due to the inhibition of phospholipase A.[343] Amiodarone has been shown to stimulate fibroblast proliferation in vitro.[344] The best available data suggest that either a direct toxic or an indirect immunologic effect may occur from amiodarone exposure.[345] An indirect mechanism that is well documented in amiodarone pulmonary toxicity is a hypersensitivity pneumonitis with features of CD8$^{(+)}$ T-cell lymphocytosis in the lungs.[346] Potential mechanisms for a more direct toxic effect of amiodarone include (1) the accumulation of cellular drug-phospholipid complexes, which interferes with normal cellular metabolic pathways leading to direct cell injury and death; (2) the disruption of the phospholipid bilayer of the cellular and organelle membrane function, and (3) the generation of toxic oxygen species by amiodarone.[345] Amiodarone[347] and its metabolite desethylamiodarone[348] have been used to induce pulmonary fibrosis after intratracheal instillation in experimental animals.

Cellulose has also been used as a noxious stimulus for the induction of experimental fibrosis in the rat, and produces a pattern of granulomatous inflammation and fibrosis identical to that seen clinically in plant dust–induced (Scadding's) fibrosing alveolitis.[349] The initiating injury is suggested to be due to the generation of reactive oxygen intermediates. Intratracheal instillation of cadmium chloride ($CdCl_2$) may also serve as a model of interstitial pulmonary fibrosis.[247] The pathologic findings in rat lungs exposed to $CdCl_2$ were similar to other animal models of fibrosis, and typically consist of alveolitis and damage to type I epithelial cells. Interestingly, fibroblasts were observed to pass through gaps in the denuded alveolar basement membranes into the alveolar spaces. However, significant small airway findings were also observed, including intraluminal fibrosis, intra-bronchiolar budding, and obliterative changes. Other challenges used for induction of pulmonary fibrosis include butylated hydroxytoluene-oxygen. Interestingly, in this model, electron microscopic studies demonstrated intimate associations between the regenerating alveolar lining cells and cells located in the interstitium. The presence of cytoplasmic processes extending from the lining cells into the interstitium suggests that communication between the regenerating epithelium and the underlying interstitium is part of the reparative process.[350] Monocrotaline, a plant alkaloid, is best known for inducing pulmonary hypertension in animals and man. However, it has also been shown to induce pulmonary fibrosis in laboratory animals.[351] In rats that were fed monocrotaline daily for 6 weeks, endothelial dysfunction (as evidenced by decreased activities of angiotensin converting enzyme [ACE] and plasminogen activator [PLA]), pulmonary hypertension, and interstitial fibrosis were all evident in the lungs. Interestingly, the ACE inhibitor captopril ameliorated the pulmonary fibrosis as evinced by the reduced lung hydroxyproline content.[351]

Approaches in Transgenic and Knockout Mice

Studies with mice that are genetically altered by a particular gene being overexpressed (transgenics) or deleted (knockouts) have a great potential in identifying the role of specific gene products in the inflammatory and fibrotic process in the lung. In addition to the SPC promoter TNF-α transgenics, in which a T-cell alveolitis and progressive fibrosis in the offspring occur, there have been other genomically altered models of pulmonary fibrosis. As discussed in the section on "Transforming growth factor-α" in a similar transgenic model in which the animals were expressing TGF-α under the control of the SPC promoter, adult mice expressing this transgene developed severe pulmonary fibrosis.[204] The motheaten mice also represent an inheritable model of interstitial lung fibrosis.[352] The motheaten gene is a single recessive mutation in the *PTPIC* gene, and thus homozygosity is required for full expression of interstitial lung disease. Typically, the affected mice have intra-alveolar hemorrhage; alveolitis with infiltration of macrophages, neutrophils, and lymphocytes; type II cell and fibroblast proliferation; and organization and fibrosis. Except for the initial intra-alveolar hemorrhage, the findings are similar to other animal models of pulmonary fibrosis due to noxious stimulation.

In summary, animal studies have been invaluable in dissecting the mechanisms involved in pulmonary injury leading to chronic inflammation and fibrosis. Such key findings include (1) the presence of endothelial injury that occurs in the early injurious phase of inflammation and that may potentiate the inflammatory process and subsequent fibrosis; (2) the prerequisite of type I epithelial cell apoptotic damage that precipitates alveolar and interstitial fibrosis; (3) the occurrence of significant alveolar fibrosis and re-epithelialization that comprises a major part of the thickened fibrotic interstitium; and (4) the presence of a dichotomous expression of cytokines and growth factors that are either profibrotic (TNF-α, TGF-β, IGF-I, PDGF) or antifibrotic (IFN-γ, IL-1β).

MECHANISM UNDERLYING THE DEVELOPMENT OF PULMONARY FIBROSIS

There is an immense wealth of data contributing to our understanding of the basic mechanisms behind the development of pulmonary fibrosis. Although this is encouraging in terms of building a fuller picture of the disease process and its mechanism of control, some fundamental questions still remain. For example, it is known that the innate inflammatory and adaptive immune system are activated, but it is not clear if all the components of each system play a detrimental or beneficial role and whether this occurs some or all of the time. Furthermore, whereas epithelial damage and/or derangement have been generally thought to be key factors in the initiation of the scarring process, other elements such as microvascular or endothelial damage have received scant attention and may or may not induce or contribute to scarring. In addition, it is clear that certain forms of lung injury are associated with an intense inflammatory response and yet fully resolve to normal or near-normal structure and function, but there are other forms of lung injury that result in scarring and loss of function. In this final section, we will briefly attempt to address some of these fundamental, yet difficult, questions and provide an integrated view of the major features of the disease process.

Idiopathic pulmonary fibrosis is by definition a disease of unknown origin. However, many other interstitial lung diseases in which the inciting stimulus can be defined can also go on to end-stage fibrosis. Examples include asbestosis, silicosis, and radiation-induced fibrosis of which uranium exposure is the best studied. In addition, many of the systemic autoimmune collagen vascular diseases, such as rheumatoid arthritis and progressive systemic sclerosis, are also accompanied by the development of pulmonary interstitial fibrosis. Thus, no single stimulus appears to be the cause of all forms of pulmonary fibrosis. Therefore, the development of the fibrotic response is likely to represent a final common pathway that is induced by many mechanisms, such as the immune system and the inflammatory system. This obviously raises the questions: What events are common, and where and when within the common pathway do different stimuli act?

It is obvious that not all inflammatory lung diseases lead to fibrosis. For example, pneumoccocal pneumonia

Figure 8–4 Contrasting features of disrepair leading to fibrosis in IPF or normal repair and resolution of function of the alveolar-capillary units. Injury to the epithelium leading to, or arising from, the activation of the inflammatory system is viewed to be a common feature of a variety of inflammatory lung diseases including IPF and ARDS. It is suggested that what distinguishes the two outcomes of (1) normal repair and restoration of function or (2) disrepair and loss of function is the ability in a timely fashion to repair and re-epithelialize the basal lamina. A failure to repair in a timely fashion is suggested to result in the activation of a scarring process as seen in IPF. In contrast, once the integrity of the basal lamina has been restored, re-epithelialization with type I and type II cells leads to varying degrees of function in the gas exchange units. ROI = reactive oxygen intermediates; TNF-α = tumor necrosis factor-α; IL = interlukin; LTB$_4$ = leukotriene B$_4$; PDGF = platelet-derived growth factor; IGDF-I = insulin-like growth factor-I.

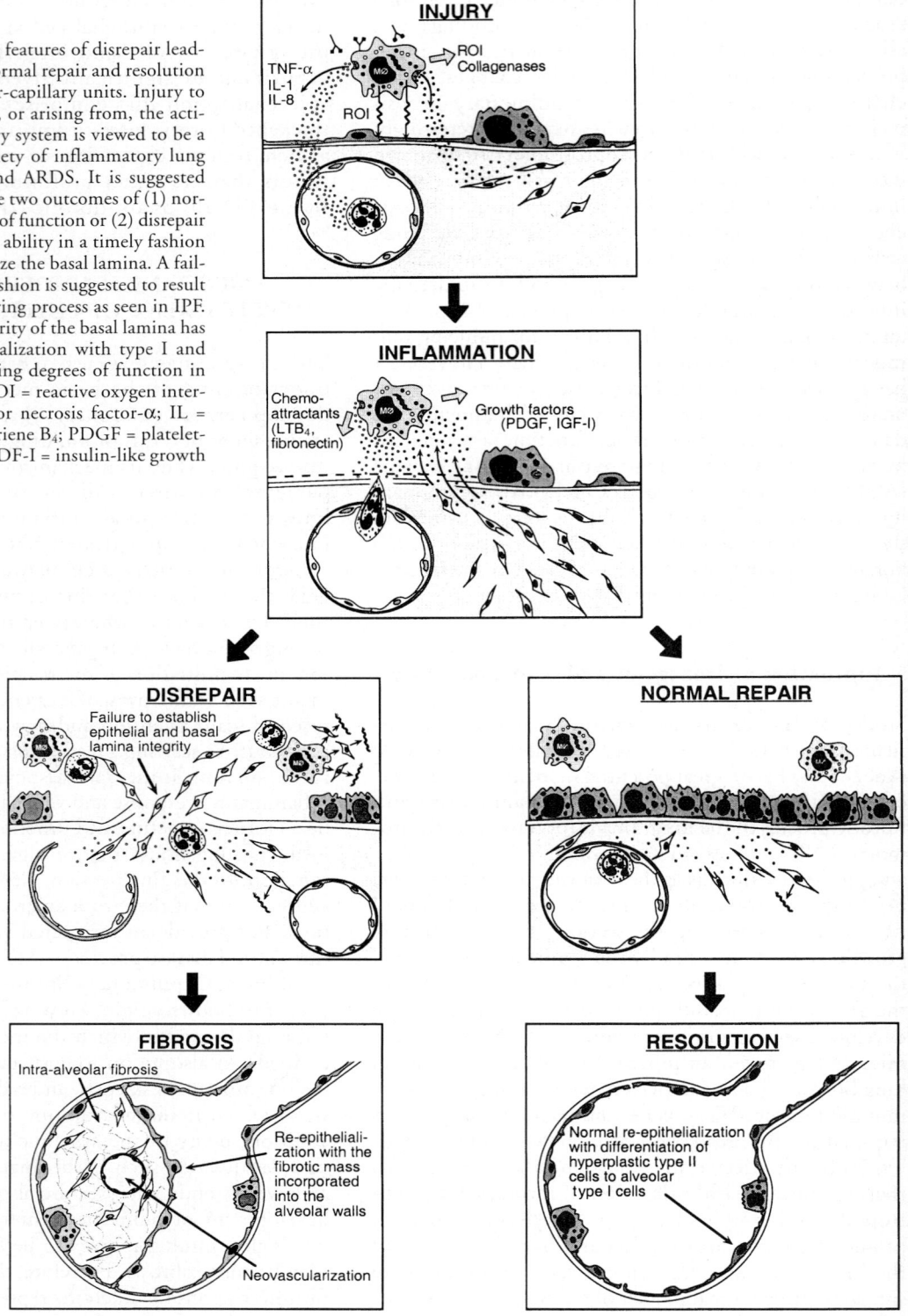

is associated with an acute inflammatory alveolitis with marked neutrophilic infiltration of the alveolar space in response to the microorganism. During the intense inflammation, fibrin and red blood cells accumulate in the alveolar space, obscuring the alveolar architecture. However, unlike the alveolitis that is seen with experimental and clinical models of pulmonary fibrosis, the alveolar septae in typical pneumococcal pneumonia are preserved. In the latter stages of resolution, which may be accelerated by the administration of antibiotics, the consolidated exudate within the alveolar spaces undergoes progressive enzymatic digestion and clearing via the mucociliary escalator. Thus, the architecture of the lung essentially reverts back to its previous normal state. In survivors of such pneumonia, there is usually little or no parenchymal sequelae such as pulmonary fibrosis. Thus, an acute inflammatory response per se, in which the epithelium and alveolar septae are generally preserved, is not sufficient to induce a fibrotic response. In contrast, in the acute respiratory distress syndrome (ARDS), the epithelium is often severely damaged as is the basal lamina. In this situation, a number of individuals are capable of adequately repairing the damage and re-establishing epithelial integrity and thus restoring the functions of the alveolar-capillary units. However, other patients fail to accomplish this and initiate a scarring response. What distinguishes these two outcomes? In Figure 8–4, we have highlighted some of the key events that distinguish the injury leading to fibrosis and the injury leading to repair, with the objective of defining mechanisms that lead to fibrosis.

Injury to the epithelium leading to exposure of the basal lamina can occur in many ways, such as alveolar deposition of bleomycin, activation of the immune system, aspiration of acid or other nonspecifically acting agents, or as a result of ARDS. Several mechanisms have been proposed to explain how epithelial injury may occur. Recent studies in mouse models have suggested that excessive epithelial cell apoptosis may be mediated, at least in part, by Fas/FasL interaction.[267,268,353,354] These experimental studies have been supported by findings of increased Fas and FasL expression in T lymphocytes and epithelial cells in biopsy specimens from patients with IPF.[355] In addition, elevated levels of soluble FasL have been found in the BALF of patients with IPF and interstitial pneumonitis associated with collagen vascular disease.[356] Others, however, have been unable to confirm a role of Fas/FasL in the induction of bleomycin-induced pulmonary fibrosis in mice.[357] Furthermore, the Fas and FasL-deficient mice that were used in the initial studies that supported a role of Fas/FasL interactions in the development of pulmonary fibrosis also spontaneously develop interstitial pneumonitis. In addition some of the mutant mice were on an MLR strain background which itself exhibits abnormalities in wound repair. Hence these issue may cloud interpretations regarding the role of Fas/FasL interaction in the induction of fibrosis. As illustrated schematically in Figure 8–4, perhaps what distinguishes these two outcomes are (1) a deficiency, possibly genetically based, in the ability of patients prone to fibrosis to adequately repair and re-epithelialize their denuded basement membranes in a timely fashion; or (2) a difference in the acute and chronic response to the inciting stimulus. In this latter situation, a persistent stimulus, for example, an autoantigen, would likely never be cleared

and thus would behave as a chronic immune and inflammatory stimulus, whereas a foreign protein antigen or hapten might ultimately be cleared, thus eliminating the stimulus.

Another potential mechanism for a fibrotic phenotype is the chronicity of the antigenic stimulus. In contrast to the overwhelming but short-lived antigenic stimulus that is characteristic of pneumococcal pneumonia, the chronic interstitial lung diseases may be characterized by a low but chronic stimulation with an antigen. This hypothesis is supported by pneumoconioses such as silicosis and asbestosis, in which failure of the host to eliminate the silica or asbestos fibers may increase the susceptibility to a fibrotic phenotype. Another related factor that may lead to the fibrotic phenotype following acute pulmonary inflammation is the cytokine profile that is initiated and sustained. For example, the IFNs that are activated by host defense cells in response to microorganisms also have potent anti-inflammatory and antifibrotic properties. Thus it is plausible that a localized Th_2 response by the host may lead to excessive fibrosis, whereas a predominantly Th_1 response may protect the host from an exuberant fibrotic response. There are emerging data to support the notion that the activation of a Th_2 response may be detrimental to the host and favor the development of a fibrotic response. In addition, the Th_1 cytokine IFN-γ has been shown to attenuate the formation of collagen in animal models of pulmonary fibrosis and work reported by Prior and Haslam[358] has suggested that patients with higher levels of IFN-γ have a better response to corticosteroid therapy and have reduced degrees of fibrosis compared with patients with lower IFN-γ levels. Thus, therapeutic intervention with IFN-γ may be beneficial in reducing fibrosis especially when treated early. Indeed, in a preliminary study comparing the treatment of IPF patients with IFN-γ and low-dose prednisolone showed striking improvement in lung function compared with the control group that received prednisolone alone.[359] Furthermore, IFN-γ treatment decreased the amount of TGF-β mRNA expressed in the IPF lungs compared with before treatment. Clearly, while much has been learned about the role of inflammatory cells in the induction of pulmonary fibrosis, many questions still remain to be addressed.

REFERENCES

1. Wallace WA, Ramage EA, Lamb E, Howie SE. A type 2 (Th2-like) pattern of immune response predominates in the pulmonary interstitium of patients with cryptogenic fibrosing alveolitis (CFA). Clin Exp Immunol 1995;101:436.
2. Wallace WAH, Howie SEM, Krajewski AS, Lamb D. The immunological architecture of B-lymphocyte aggregates in cryptogenic fibrosing alveolitis. J Pathol 1996:178:323.
3. Wallace WAH, Roberts SN, Caldwell H, et al. Circulating antibodies to lung protein(s) in patients with cryptogenic fibrosing alveolitis. Thorax 1994;49:218.
4. Shaw JO. Leukocytes in chemotactic-fragment-induced lung

inflammation: vascular emigration and alveolar surface migration. Am J Pathol 1980;101:283.

5. Lipsomb MF, Onofrio JM, Nash J. A morphologic study of the role of phagocytes in the clearance of *Staphylococcus aureus* from the lung. J Reticuloendothel Soc 1983;33:429.

6. Lien DC, Capen RL, Hanson WL. The acute inflammatory response in the canine lung: direct observation of neutrophil behavior in response to C5 fragments. 1991. [Submitted]

7. Allison F Jr, Smith MR, Wood WB. Studies on the pathogenesis of acute inflammation. I. The inflammatory reaction to thermal injury as observed in the rabbit ear chamber. J Exp Med 1955;102:669.

8. Bjork J, Hugli TE, Smedegard G. Microvascular effects of anaphylatoxins C3a and C5a. J Immunol 1985;134:1115.

9. Lien DC, Worthen GS, Capen RL. Neutrophil kinetics in the pulmonary microcirculation: effects of pressure and flow in the dependent lung. Am Rev Respir Dis 1990;141:953.

10. Martin BA, Wright JL, Thommasen H, Hogg JC. Effect of pulmonary blood flow on the exchange between the circulating and marginating pool of polymorphonuclear leukocytes in dog lungs. J Clin Invest 1982;69:1277.

11. Mayrovitz HN, Wiedeman MP, Tuman RF. Factors influencing leukocyte adherence in microvessels. Thromb Haemost 1977;38:823.

12. Schmid-Schonbein GW, Fung YC, Zeifach BW. Vascular endothelium-leukocyte interaction: striking shear force in venules. Circ Res 1975;36:173.

13. Libbey P, Wyler DJ, Janicka MW, Dinarello CA. Differential effects of human interleukin 1 on growth of human fibroblasts and vascular smooth muscle cells. Atherosclerosis 1985;5:186.

14. Meyrick B, Hoffman LH, Brighma KL. Chemotaxis of granulocytes across bovine pulmonary artery intimal explants without endothelial cell injury. Tissue Cell 1984;16:1.

15. Worthen GS, Haslett C, Rees AJ. Neutrophil mediated pulmonary vascular injury: synergistic effect of trace amounts of lipopolysaccharide and neutrophil stimuli on vascular permeability and neutrophil sequestration in the lung. Am Rev Respir Dis 1987;136:19.

16. Milks LC, Brontoli MJ, Cramer EB. Epithelial permeability and the transepithelial migration of human neutrophils. J Cell Biol 1983;96:1241.

17. Parsons PE, Sugahara K, Cott GK. The effect of neutrophil migration and prolonged neutrophil contact on epithelial permeability. Am J Pathol 1987;129:302.

18. Doerschuk CM, Winn RK, Coxson HO, Harlan JM. CD18-dependent and independent mechanisms of neutrophil emigration in the pulmonary and systemic microcirculation of rabbits. J Immunol 1990;144:2327.

19. Doherty DE, Downey G, Worthen GS. Monocyte retention and migration in pulmonary inflammation: requirement for neutrophils. Lab Invest 1988;59:200.

20. Haslett C, Shen AS, Feldsien DC. ᴵᴵᴵIndium-labeled neutrophil migration into the lungs of bleomycin-treated rabbits assessed noninvasively by external scintigraphy. Am Rev Respir Dis 1989;140:756.

21. Downey G, Doherty DE, Schwab B III. Retention of leukocytes in capillaries: role of cell size and deformability. J Appl Physiol 1990;69:1767.

22. Schmidt-Schonbein GW, Shih YY, Chien S. Morphometry of human leukocytes. Blood 1985;56:866.

23. Guntheroth WG, Lachter DL, Kawabori I. Pulmonary microcirculation: tubules rather than sheet and post. J Appl Physiol 1982;53:510.

24. Downey GP, Gumbay RS, Doherty DE. Enhancement of pulmonary inflammation by prostagladin E: evidence for a vasodilator effect. J Appl Physiol 1988;54:728.

25. Worthen GS, Schwab B, Elson EL, Downey GP. Mechanics of stimulated neutrophils: cell stiffening retention in capillaries. Science 1989;245:183.

26. Chien S, Schmid-Schonbein GW, Sung KL, et al. Viscoelastic properties of leukocytes. Kroc Found Ser 1984;16:19.

27. Howard TH, Casella J, Lin S. Correlation of the biological effects and binding of cytochalasins to human polymorphonuclear leukocytes. Blood 1981;57:399.

28. Doherty DE, Worthen GS. Lipopolysaccharide-induced monocyte lung retention in the rabbit: the role of the CD11/CD18 leukocyte adhesion complex and cell stiffness. Am Rev Respir Dis 1991;143:A583.

29. Rosen SD. An emerging family of cell-cell adhesion receptors based upon carbohydrate recognition. Am J Respir Cell Mol Biol 1990;3:397.

30. Osborn L. Leukocyte adhesion to endothelium in inflammation. Cell 1990;62:3.

31. Kishimoto TK. A dynamic model for neutrophil localization to inflammatory sites. Journal of NIH Research 1991;3:75.

32. Harlan JM, Killen PD, Senecal FM. The role of neutrophil membrane glycoprotein GP-150 in neutrophil adherence to endothelium in vitro. Blood 1985;66:167.

33. Doherty DE, Haslett C, Tonneson MG, Henson PM. Human monocyte adherence: a primary effect of chemotactic factors on the monocyte to stimulate adherence to human endothelium. J Immunol 1987;138:1762.

34. Doherty DE, Zagarella L, Henson PM, Worthen GS. Lipopolysaccharide stimulates monocyte adherence by effects on both the monocyte and the endothelial cell. J Immunol 1989;143:3673.

35. Doerschuk CM, Downey GP, Doherty DE. Leukocyte and platelet migration within the microvasculature of rabbit lungs. J Appl Phys 1990;68:1956.

36. Vedder NB, Winn RK, Rice CL. A monoclonal antibody to the adherence-promoting leukocyte glycoprotein, CD18, reduces organ injury and improves survival from hemorrhagic shock and resuscitation in rabbits. J Clin Invest 1988;81:939.

37. Horgan MJ, Wright SD, Malik AB. Antibody against leukocyte integrin (CD18) prevents reperfusion-induced lung vascular injury. Am J Physiol 1990;259:L315.

38. Arfors K-E, Lundberg C, Lindbom L. A monoclonal antibody to the membrane glycoprotein complex CD18 inhibits polymorphonuclear leukocyte accumulation and plasma leakage in vivo. Blood 1987;69:338.

39. Luscinskas FW, Mark DE, Brunkhorst B. The role of transmembrane cationic gradients in immune complex stimulation of human polymorphonuclear leukocytes. J Cell Physiol 1988;134:211.

40. Luscinskas FW, Brock AF, Aarnaout MA, Gimbrone MA Jr. Endothelial-leukocyte adhesion molecule-1 dependent and leukocyte (CD11/CD18)-dependent mechanisms contribute to polymorphonuclear leukocyte adhesion to cytokine-activated human vascular endothelium. J Immunol 1989;142:2257.

41. Luscinskas FW, Cybulsky MI, Kiely JM. Cytokine-activated human endothelial monolayers support enhanced neutrophil transmigration via a mechanism involving both endothelial-leukocyte adhesion molecule-1 and intercellular adhesion molecule-1. J Immunol 1991;146:1617.

42. Bochner BS, Luscinskas FW, Gimbrone MA Jr. Adhesion of human basophils, eosinophils, and neutrophils to interleukin 1-activated human vascular endothelial cells: contributions of endothelial cell adhesion molecules. J Exp Med 1991;173:1553.

43. Hunninghake GW, Gallin JI, Fauci AS. Immunologic reactivity of the lung: the in vivo and in vitro generation of a neutrophil chemotactic factor by alveolar macrophages. Am Rev Respir Dis 1978;117:15.

44. Kunkel SL, Standiford T, Kasahara K, Strieter RM. Stimulus specific induction of monocyte chemotactic protein-1 (MCP-1) gene expression. Adv Exp Med Biol 1991;305:65.

45. Carre PC, Mortensen RL, King TE Jr, et al. Increased expression of the interleukin-8 gene by alveolar macrophages in idiopathic pulmonary fibrosis. A potential mechanism for the recruitment and activation of neutrophils in lung fibrosis. J Clin Invest 1991;88:1802.

46. Pennington JE, Rossing TH, Boerth LW, Lee TH. Isolation and partial characterization of a human alveolar macrophage-derived neutrophil activating factor. J Clin Invest 1985;75:1230.

47. Robbins RA, Justice JM, Rasmussen JK. Role of chemotactic factor inactivator in modulating alveolar macrophage-derived neutrophil chemotactic activity. J Lab Clin Med 1987;109:164.

48. Carre PC, King TE Jr, Mortensen R, Riches DWH. Cryptogenic organizing pneumonia: increased expression of interleukin-8 and fibronectin genes by alveolar macrophages. Am J Respir Cell Mol Biol 1994;10:100.

49. Haslett C, Jose PJ, Giclas PC. Cessation of neutrophil influx in C5a-induced acute experimental arthritis is associated with loss of chemoattractant activity from the joint space. J Immunol 1989;142:3510.

50. Haslett C, Downey GP, Doherty DE, Henson PM. Early cessation of neutrophil migration after intrapulmonary instillation of C5f des arg (C5f) in rabbits. Am Rev Respir Dis 1988;137:A44.

51. Worthen GS, Downey GP, Young SK. Neutrophil interaction with the lung in human beings: studies in normals and patients with inflammatory lung disorders. Am Rev Respir Dis 1988;137:42A.

52. Smyth MJ, Zachariae COC, Norihisa Y. IL-8 gene expression and production in human peripheral blood lymphocyte subsets. J Immunol 1991;146:3815.

53. Blanchard DK, Michelini-Norris MB, Djeu J. Production of granulocyte-macrophage colony-stimulating factor by large granular lymphocytes stimulated with *Candida albicans*: role in activation of human neutrophil function. Blood 1991;77:2259.

54. Hebert CA, Luscinskas FW, Kiely J-M. Endothelial and leukocyte forms of IL-8: conversion by thrombin and interactions with neutrophils. J Immunol 1990;145:3033.

55. Postlethwaite AE, Kang AH. Collagen-and collagen peptide-induced chemotaxis of human blood monocytes. J Exp Med 1976;143:1299.

56. Senior RM, Griffin GL, Mecham RP. Chemotactic activity of elastin-derived peptides. J Clin Invest 1980;66:859.

57. Clark RAF, Wickner NE, Doherty DE, Norris DA. Cryptic chemotactic activity of fibronectin for human monocytes resides in the 120k Da fibroblastic cell-binding fragment. J Biol Chem 1988;263:12115.

58. McDonald JA, Kelley DG. Degradation of fibronectin by human leukocyte elastase. J Biol Chem 1980;255:8848.

59. Doherty DE, Henson PM, Clark RAF. Fibronectin fragments containing the RGDS cell-binding domain mediate monocyte migration into the rabbit lung: a potential mechanism for C5 fragment-induced monocyte lung accumulation. J Clin Invest 1990;86:1065.

60. Shellito J, Esparza C, Armstrong C. Maintenance of the normal rat alveolar macrophage cell population. Am Rev Respir Dis 1987;135:78.

61. Sawyer RT, Strausbauch PH, Volkman A. Resident macrophage proliferation in mice depleted of blood monocytes by strontium-89. Lab Invest 1982;46:165.

62. Coggle JE, Tarling JD. The proliferation kinetics of pulmonary alveolar macrophages. J Leukoc Biol 1984;35:317.

63. Tarling JD, Coggle JE. Evidence for the pulmonary origin of alveolar macrophages. Cell Tissue Kinetics 1982;15:577.

64. Malech HL, Gallin JI. Neutrophils in human diseases. N Engl J Med 1987;317:687.

65. Henson PM, Johnston RB Jr. Tissue injury in inflammation: oxidants, proteinases, and cationic proteins. J Clin Invest 1987;79:669.

66. Lehrer RI, Ganz T, Selsted ME. Neutrophils and host defense. Ann Intern Med 1988;109:127.

67. Weiss SJ. Tissue destruction by neutrophils. N Engl J Med 1989;320:365.

68. Hunt TK, Knighton DR, Thakral KK, et al. Studies on inflammation and wound healing: angiogenesis and collagen synthesis stimulated *in vivo* by resident and activated wound macrophages. Surgery 1984;96:48.

69. Nathan CJ. Neutrophil activation on biological surfaces: massive secretion of hydrogen peroxide in response to products of macrophages and lymphocytes. J Clin Invest 1987;80:1550.

70. Guthrie LA, McPhail LC, Henson PM, Johnston RB Jr. The priming of neutrophils for enhanced release of superoxide anion and hydrogen peroxide by bacterial lipopolysaccharide: evidence for increased activity of the superoxide-producing enzyme. J Exp Med 1984;160:1656.

71. Pabst MJ, Aida Y. Effect of adherence on triggering and priming of the respiratory burst. J Immunol 1991;146:1271.

72. Haslett C, Guthrie LA, Kopaniack MM. Modulation of multiple neutrophil functions by preparative methods and trace amounts of bacterial lipopolysaccharide. Am J Pathol 1985;119:101.

73. Berkow RL, Wang D, Larrick JW. Enhancement of neutrophil superoxide production by preincubation with recombinant human tumor necrosis factor. J Immunol 1987;139:3783.

74. DiPersio JF, Billing P, Williams R, Gasson JC. Human granulocyte-macrophage colony stimulating factor and other cytokines prime human neutrophils for enhanced arachidonic acid release and leukotriene B_4 synthesis. J Immunol 1988;140:4315.

75. Kharazmi A, Nielsen H, Bendtzen K. Recombinant interleukin-1 alpha and beta prime human monocyte superoxide production but have no effect on chemotasis and oxidative burst response of neutrophils. Immunobiology 1988;177:32.

76. Dewald B, Thelen M, Baggiolini M. Two transduction sequences are necessary for neutrophil activation receptor agonists. J Biol Chem 1988;263:16179.

77. Smedly LA, Tonnesen MG, Sandhaus RA. Neutrophil-mediated injury to endothelial cells: enhancement by endotoxin and essential role of neutrophil elastase. J Clin Invest 1986;77:1233.

78. Crouch E. Pathobiology of pulmonary fibrosis. Am J Physiol 1990;259:L159.

79. Bauldry SA, Bass DA, Cousart SL, McCall CE. Tumor necrosis factor alpha priming of phospholipase D in human neutrophils: correlation between phosphatidic acid production and superoxide generation. J Biol Chem 1991;266:4173.

80. Rabinovici R, Esser KM, Lysko PG. Priming by platelet-activating factor of endotoxin-induced lung injury and cardiovascular shock. Circ Res 1991;69:12.

81. Wewers MD, Rinehart JJ, She ZW. Tumor necrosis factor infusions in humans prime neutrophils for hypochlorous acid production. Am J Physiol 1990;259:L276.

82. Schopf RE, Keller R, Rehder M. TNF alpha primes polymorphonuclear leukocytes for an enhanced respiratory burst to a similar extent as bacterial lipopolysaccharide. J Invest Dermatol 1990;95:216S.

83. Fantone JC. Role of oxygen-derived free radicals and metabolites in leukocyte-dependent inflammatory reactions. Am J Pathol 1982;107:397.

84. Till GO, Johnson KS, Kunkel R, Ward PA. Intravascular activation of complement and acute lung injury: dependency on neutrophils and toxic oxygen metabolites. J Clin Invest 1982;69:1125.

85. Johnson KJ, Fantone JC III, Kaplan J, Ward PA. In vivo damage of rat lungs by oxygen metabolites. J Clin Invest 1981;67:983.

86. Hellewell PG, Henson PM, Downey GP, Worthen GS. Control of local blood flow in pulmonary inflammation: role for neutrophils, PAF, and thromboxane. J Appl Physiol 1991;70:1184.

87. Weiss SJ, Young J, LoBuglio AF. Role of hydrogen peroxide in neutrophil-mediated destruction of cultured endothelial cells. J Clin Invest 1981;68:714.

88. Cross CE, Halliwell B, Borish ET. Oxygen radicals and human disease. Ann Intern Med 1987;107:526.

89. Chen CR, Voelkel NF, Chang SW. PAF potentiates protamine-induced lung edema: role of pulmonary venoconstriction. J Appl Physiol 1990;686:1059.

90. Ginsburg I. Cationic polyelectrolytes: potent opsonic agents which activate the respiratory burst in leukocytes. Free Radic Res Commun 1989;8:11.

91. Rochat T, Casale J, Hunninghake GW, Peterson MW. Neutrophil cathepsin G increases permeability of cultured type II pneumocytes. Am J Phyisol 1988;255:C603.

92. Campbell EJ, Senior RM, McDonald JA, Cox DL. Proteolysis by neutrophils: relative importance of cell substrate contact and oxidative inactivation of protease inhibitors in vivo. J Clin Invest 1982;70:845.

93. Campbell EJ, Campbell MA. Pericellular proteolysis by neutrophils in the presence of proteinase inhibitors: effects of substrate opsonization. J Cell Biol 1988;106:667.

94. Scuderi P. Suppression of human leukocyte tumor necrosis factor secretion by the serine protease inhibitor p-toluenesulfonyl-L-arginine methyl ester (TAME). J Immunol 1989;143:168.

95. Scuderi P, Dorr RT, Liddil JD, et al. Alpha-globulins suppress human leukocyte tumor necrosis factor secretion. Eur J Immunol 1989;19:939.

96. Nagai A, Aoshiba K, Ishihara Y, et al. Administration of α1-proteinase inhibitor ameliorates bleomycin-induced pulmonary fibrosis in hamsters. Am Rev Respir Dis 1992;145:651.

97. Geddes DM, Webley M, Brewerton DA, et al. Alpha 1-antitrypsin phenotypes in fibrosing alveolitis and rheumatoid arthritis. Lancet 1977;ii:1049.

98. Ashcroft GS, Lei K, Jin W, et al. Secretory leukocyte protease inhibitor mediates non-redundant functions necessary for normal wound healing. Nature Med 2000;6:1147.

99. McGowan SE, Murray JJ. Direct effects of neutrophil oxidants on elastase-induced extracellular matrix proteolysis. Am Rev Respir Dis 1987;135:1286.

100. Gleich GJ, Adolphson CR. The eosinophilic leukocyte: structure and function. Adv Immunol 1986;39:177.

101. Davis WB, Fells GA, Sun X. Eosinophil-mediated injury to lung parenchymal cells and interstitial matrix. J Clin Invest 1984;74:269.

102. Little MM, Casale TB. Comparison of platelet-activating factor-induced chemotaxis of normodense and hypodense eosinophils. J Allergy Clin Immunol 1991;88:187.

103. Silva PM, Martins MA, Faria-Neto HC. Generation of an eosinophilic activity in the pleural cavity of platelet-activating factor-injected rats. J Pharmacol Exp Ther 1991;257:1039.

104. Martins MA, Etienne A, Soulard C. Chemotactic effect of PAF-acether on peritoneal eosinophils from normal rats. Braz J Med Biol Res 1989;22:1151.

105. Morita E, Schroder JM, Christophers E. Differential sensitivities of purified human eosinophils and neutrophils to defined chemotaxins. Scand J Immunol 1989;29:709.

106. Sigal CE, Valone FH, Holtzman MJ, Goetzl EJ. Preferential human eosinophil chemotactic activity of the platelet-activating factor (PAF): 1-0-hexadecyl-2-acetyl-sn-glyceryl-3-phosphocholine (AGEPC). J Clin Immunol 1987;7:179.

107. Kimura R, Hu H, Stein-Streilein J. Tolerance to hapten prevents specific delayed type hypersensitivity and pulmonary interstitial fibrosis in the mouse model. Chest 1993;103:122S.

108. Dobrina A, Menegazzi R, Carlos TM. Mechanisms of eosinophil adherence to cultured vascular endothelial cells: eosinophils bind to the cytokine-induced glad vascular cell adhesion molecule-1 via the very late activation antigen-4 integrin receptor. J Clin Invest 1991;88:20.

109. Lamas AM, Mulroney CM, Schleimer RP. Studies on the adhesive interaction between purified human eosinophils and cultured vascular endothelial cells. J Immunol 1988;140:1500.

110. Leibovitch SJ, Ross R. The role of the macrophage in wound repair. A study with hydrocortisone and antimacrophage serum. Am J Pathol 1975;78:71.

111. Riches DWH. Monocytes, macrophages and dendritic cells of the lung. In: Murray JF, Nadel JA, Mason RJ, Bouchay HA, editors. Textbook of respiratory medicine. Philadelphia: WB Saunders Company; 200. p. 385.

112. Laurent GJ. Lung collagen: more than scaffolding. Thorax 1986;41:418.

113. Kirk JME, Da Costa PE, Laurent GJ, et al. Biochemical evidence for an increased and progressive deposition of collagen in lungs of patients with pulmonary fibrosis. Clin Sci 1986;70:39.

114. Etherington DJ. Proteinases in connective tissue breakdown. Ciba Found Symp 1979;75:87.

115. Etherington DJ, Pugh D, Silver IA. Collagen degradation in an experimental inflammatory lesion: studies on the role of the macrophage. Acta Biol Med Ger 1981;40:1625.

116. Etherington DJ, Taylor MA, Henderson B. Elevation of cathepsin L levels in the synovial lining of rabbits with antigen-induced arthritis. Br J Exp Pathol 1988;69:281.

117. Campbell EJ, Cury JD, Lazarus CJ, Wegus HG. Monocyte procollagenase and tissue inhibitor of metalloproteinases. Identification, chacterization, and regulation of secretion. J Biol Chem 1987;262:15862.

118. Welgus HG, Campbell EJ, Cury JD, et al. Neutral metalloproteinases produced by human mononuclear phagocytes. Enzyme profile, regulation, and expression during cellular development. J Clin Invest 1990;86:1496.

119. Campbell EJ, Cury JD, Shapiro SD, et al. Neutral proteinases of human mononuclear phagocytes. Cellular differentiation markedly alters cell phenotype for serine proteinases, metalloproteinases, and tissue inhibitor of metalloproteinases. J Immunol 1991;146:1286.

120. Hibbs MS, Hoidal JR, Kang AH. Expression of a metalloproteinase that degrades native type V collagen and denatured collagens by cultured human alveolar macrophages. J Clin Invest 1987;80:1644.

121. Huybrechts-Godin G, Hauser P, Vaes G. Macrophage-fibroblast interaction in collagenase production and cartilage degradation. Biochem J 1979;184:643.

122. Huybrechts-Godin G, Peeters-Joris C, Vaes G. Partial characterization of the macrophage factor that stimulates fibroblasts to produce collagenase and to degrade collagen. Biochim Biophys Acta 1985;846:51.

123. Hiraoka K, Sasaguri Y, Komiya S, et al. Cell proliferation-related production of matrix matalloproteinases 1 (tissue collagenase) and 3 (stromelysin) by cultured human rheumatoid synovial fibroblasts. Biochem Int 1992;27:1083.

124. Chua CA, Chua BH. Tumor necrosis factor-alpha induces mRNA for collagenase and TIMP in human skin fibroblasts. Connect Tissue Res 1990;25:161.

125. Ito A, Sato T, Iga T, Mori Y. Tumor necrosis factor bifunctionally regulates matrix metalloproteinases and tissue inhibitor of metalloproteinases (TIMP) production by human fibroblasts. FEBS Lett 1990;269:93.

126. Selman M, Montano M, Ramos C, Chapela R. Concentration, biosynthesis and degradation of collagen in idiopathic pulmonary fibrosis. Thorax 1986;41:355.

127. Arden MG, Adamson IYR. Collagen synthesis and degradation during the development of asbsestos-induced pulmonary fibrosis. Exp Lung Res 1992;18:9.

128. Shahzeidi S, Mulier B, de Crombrugghe B, et al. Enhanced type III collagen gene expression during bleomycin induced lung fibrosis. Thorax 1993;48:622.

129. Pardo A, Selman M, Ramirez R, et al. Production of collagenase and tissue inhibitor of metalloproteinases by fibroblasts derived from normal and fibrotic human lungs. Chest 1992;102:1085.

130. Hayashi T, Stetler-Stevenson WG, Fleming MV, et al. Immunochemical study of metalloproteinases and their tissue inhibitors in the lungs of patients with diffuse alveolar damage and idiopathic pulmonary fibrosis. Am J Pathol 1996;149:1241.

131. Carmichael DF, Sommer A, Thompson RC, et al. Primary structure and cDNA cloning of human fibroblast collagenase inhibitor. Proc Natl Acad Sci U S A 1986;83:2407.

132. Goldberg GI, Marmer BL, Grant GA, et al. Human 72-kilodalton type IV collagenase forms a complex with a tissue inhibitor of metalloproteinases designated TIMP-2. Proc Natl Acad Sci U S A 1989;86:8207.

133. Stetler-Stevenson WG, Krutzsch HC, Liotta LA. Tissue inhibitor of metalloproteinase (TIMP-2): a new member of the metalloproteinase inhibitor family. J Biol Chem 1989;264:17374.

134. Montano M, Ramos C, Gonzalez G, et al. Lung collagenase inhibitors and spontaneous and latent collagenase activity in idiopathic pulmonary fibrosis and hypersensitivity pneumonitis. Chest 1989;96:1115.

135. Greene J, Wang M, Liu YE, et al. Molecular cloning and characterization of human tissue inhibitor of metalloproteinase 4. J Biol Chem 1996;271:30375.

136. Selman M, Ruiz V, Cabrera S, et al. TIMP-1, -2, -3, and -4 in idiopathic pulmonary fibrosis. A prevailing nondegradative lung microenvironment? Am J Physiol 2000;279:L562.

137. Wright JK, Cawston TE, Hazleman BL. Transforming growth factor beta stimulates the production of the tissue inhibitor of metalloproteinases (TIMP) by human synovial and skin fibroblasts. Biochim Biophys Acta 1991;1094:207.

138. Coalson JJ. The ultrastructure of human fibrosing alveolitis. Virchows Arch 1982;395:181.

139. Specks U, Nerlich A, Colby TV, et al. Increased expression of type IV collagen in lung fibrosis. Am J Respir Crit Care Med 1995;151:1956.

140. Roberts AB, Sporn MB. The transforming growth factor-bs. In: Sporn IMB, Roberts AB, editors. Peptide growth factors and their receptors. New York: Springer-Verlag; 1991. p. 419.

141. Wakefield LM, Smith DM, Flanders KC, Sporn MB. Latent transforming growth factor-b from human platelets. J Biol Chem 1988;263:7646.

142. Lyons RM, Keski-Oja J, Moses HL. Proteolytic activation of latent transforming growth factor-b from fibroblast conditioned medium. J Cell Biol 1988;106:1659.

143. Miyazono K, Heldin C-H. Interaction between TGF-b1 and carbohydrate structures in its precursor renders TGF-b1 latent. Nature 1989;338:158.

144. Assoian RK, Fleurdelys BE, Stevenson HC, et al. Expression and secretion of type beta transforming growth factor by activated human macrophages. Proc Nat Acad Sci U S A 1987;84:6020.

145. Laszlo DJ, Henson PM, Weinstein L, et al. Development of functional diversity in mouse macrophages. Mutual exclusion of two phenotypic states. Am J Pathol 1993;143:587.

146. Noble PW, Henson PM, Carre PC, Riches DWH. TGFß primes macrophages to express inflammatory gene products in response to particulate stimuli by an autocrine/paracrine mechanism. J Immunol 1993;151:979.

147. Zauli G, Davis BR, Re MC, et al. tat protein stimulates production of transforming growth factor-beta 1 by marrow macrophages: a potential mechanism for human immunodeficiency virus-1-induced hematopoietic suppression. Blood 1992;80:3036.

148. Bermudez LE, Covaro G, Remington J. Infection of murine macrophages with Toxoplasma gondii is associated with release of transforming growth factor beta and downregulation of expression of tumor necrosis factor receptors. Infect Immun 1993;61:4126.

149. Bermudez LE. Production of transforming growth factor-beta by Mycobacterium avium-infected human macrophages is associated with unresponsiveness to IFN-gamma. J Immunol 1993;150:1838.

150. Fadok VA, Bratton DL, Konowal A, et al. Macrophages that have ingested apoptotic cells in vitro inhibit proinflammatory cytokine production through autocrine/paracrine mechanisms involving TGF-beta, PGE2, and PAF. J Clin Invest 1998;101:890.

151. Xing Z, Tremblay GM, Sime PJ, Gauldie J. Overexpression of granulocyte-macrophage colony-stimulating factor induces pulmonary granulation tissue formation and fibrosis by induction of transforming growth factor-β1 and myofibroblast accumulation. Am J Pathol 1997;150:59.

152. Phan SH, Kunkel SL. Lung cytokine production in bleomycin-induced pulmonary fibrosis. Exp Lung Res 1992;18:29.

153. Khalil N, Bereznay O, Sporn M, Greenberg AH. Macrophage production of transforming growth factor beta and fibroblast collagen synthesis in chronic pulmonary inflammation. J Exp Med 1989;170:727.

154. Khalil N, O'Connor RN, Unruh HW, et al. Increased production and immunohistochemical localization of transforming growth factor-beta in idiopathic pulmonary fibrosis. Am J Respir Cell Mol Biol 1991;5:155.

155. Roberts AB, Sporn MB, Assoian RK, et al. Tranforming growth factor b: rapid induction of fibrosis and angiogenesis in vivo and stimulation of collagen formation in vitro. Proc Natl Acad Sci U S A 1986;83:4167.

156. Appling WD, O'Brien WR, Johnston DA, Duvic M. Synergistic enhancement of type I and III collagen production in cultured fibroblasts by transforming growth factor-beta and ascorbate. FEBS Lett 1989;250:541.

157. Fine A, Goldstein RW. The effect of transforming factor-beta on cell proliferation and collagen formation by lung fibroblasts. J Biol Chem 1987;262:3897.

158. Fine A, Poliks CF, Smith BD, Goldstein RH. The accumulation of type I collagen mRNAs in human embryonic lung fibroblasts stimulated by transforming growth factor-beta. Connect Tissue Res 1990;24:237.

159. Raghow R, Postlethwaite AE, Keski OJ, et al. Transforming growth factor-beta increases steady state levels of type I procollagen and fibronectin messenger RNAs posttranscriptionally in cultured human dermal fibroblasts. J Clin Invest 1987;79:1285.

160. Inagaki Y, Truter S, Ramirez F. Transforming growth factor-beta stimulates alpha 2(I) collagen gene expression through a cis-acting element that contains an Sp1-binding site. J Biol Chem 1994;269:14828.

161. Rossi P, Karsenty G, Roberts AB, et al. A nuclear factor 1 binding site mediates the transcriptional activation of a type I collagen promoter by transforming growth factor-beta. Cell 1988;52:405.

162. Overall CM, Wrana JL, Sodek J. Independent regulation of collagenase, 72-kDa progelatinase, and metalloendoproteinase inhibitor expression in human fibroblasts by transforming growth factor-beta. J Biol Chem 1989;264:1860.

163. Overall CM, Wrana JL, Sodek J. Transforming growth factor-beta regulation of collagenase, 72 kDa-progelatinase, TIMP and PAI-1 expression in rat bone cell populations and human fibroblasts. Connect Tissue Res 1989;20:289.

164. Overall CM, Wrana JL, Sodek J. Transcriptional and posttranscriptional regulation of 72-kDa gelatinase/type IV collagenase by transforming growth factor-beta 1 in human fibroblasts. Comparisons with collagenase and tissue inhibitor of matrix metalloproteinase gene expression. J Biol Chem 1991;266:14064.

165. Circolo A, Welgus HG, Pierce GF, et al. Differential regulation of the expression of proteinases/antiproteinases in fibroblasts. Effects of interleukin-1 and platelet-derived growth factor. J Biol Chem 1991;266:12283.

166. Ito A, Goshowaki H, Sato T, et al. Human recombinant interleukin-1 alpha-mediated stimulation of procollagenase production and suppression of biosynthesis of tissue inhibitor of metalloproteinases in rabbit uterine cervical fibroblasts. FEBS Lett 1988;234:326.

167. Unemori EN, Ehsani N, Wang M, et al. Interleukin-1 and transforming growth factor-alpha: synergistic stimulation of metalloproteinases, PGE2, and proliferation in human fibroblasts. Exp Cell Res 1994;210:166.

168. Martinet Y, Rom WN, Grotendorst GR, et al. Exaggerated spontaneous release of platelet-derived growth factor by alveolar macrophage from patients with idiopathic pulmonary fibrosis. N Engl J Med 1987;317:202.

169. Nagaoka I, Trapnell BC, Crystal RG. Upregulation of platelet-derived growth factor-A and -B gene expression in alveolar macrophages of individuals with idiopathic pulmonary fibrosis. J Clin Invest 1990;85:2023.

170. Bonner JC, Osornio AR, Badgett A, Brody AR. Differential proliferation of rat lung fibroblasts induced by the platelet-derived growth factor-AA, -AB, and -BB isoforms secreted by rat alveolar macrophages. Am J Respir Cell Mol Biol 1991;5:539.

171. Snyder LS, Hertz MI, Peterson MS, et al. Acute lung injury. Pathogenesis of intraalveolar fibrosis. J Clin Invest 1991;88:663.

172. Antoniades HN, Bravo MA, Avila RE, et al. Platelet-derived growth factor in idiopathic pulmonary fibrosis. J Clin Invest 1990;86:1055.

173. Homma S, Nagaoka I, Abe H, et al. Localization of platelet-derived growth factor and insulin-like growth factor-I in the fibrotic lung. Am J Respir Crit Care Med 1995;152:2084.

174. Vignaud J-M, Allam M, Martinet N, et al. Presence of platelet-derived growth factor in normal and fibrotic lung is specifically associated with interstitial macrophages, while both interstitial macrophages and alveolar epithelial cells express the c-sis proto-oncogene. Am J Respir Cell Mol Biol 1991;5:531.

175. Raines EW, Dower SK, Ross R. Interleukin-1 mitogenic activity for fibroblasts and smooth muscle cells is due to PDGF-AA. Science 1989;243:393.

176. Shaw RJ, Benedict SH, Clark RAF, King TE Jr. Pathogenesis of pulmonary fibrosis in interstitial lung disease: alveolar macrophage PDGF(B) gene activation an up-regulation by interferon gamma. Am Rev Respir Dis 1991;143:167.

177. Chen F, Deng HY, Ding GF, et al. Excessive production of insulin-like growth factor-I by silicotic rat alveolar macrophages. APMIS 1994;102:581.

178. McAnulty RJ, Guerreiro D, Cambrey AD, Laurent GJ. Growth factor activity in the lung during compensatory growth after pneumonectomy: evidence of a role for IGF-1. Eur Respir J 1992;5:739.

179. Melloni B, Lesur O, Bouhadiba T, et al. Partial characterization of the proliferative activity for fetal lung epithelial cells produced by silica-exposed alveolar macrophages. J Leukoc Biol 1994;55:574.

180. Vanhee D, Gosset P, Wallaert B, et al. Mechanisms of fibrosis in coal workers' pneumoconiosis. Increased production of platelet-derived growth factor, insulin-like growth factor type I, and transforming growth factor beta and relationship to disease severity. Am J Respir Crit Care Med 1994;150:1049.

181. Rom WN, Basset P, Fells GA, et al. Alveolar macrophages release an insulin-like growth factor-1-type molecule. J Clin Invest 1989;82:1685.

182. Maeda A, Hiyama K, Yamakido H, et al. Increased expression of platelet-derived growth factor A and insulin-like growth factor-I in BAL cells during the development of bleomycin-induced pulmonary fibrosis in mice. Chest 1996;109:780.

183. Goldstein RM, Poliks CF, Pilch PF, et al. Stimulation of collagen formation by insulin and insulin-like growth factor I in cultures of human lung fibroblast. Endocrinology 1989;124:964.

184. Gillery P, Leperre A, Maquart FX, Borel JP. Insulin-like growth factor-I (IGF-I) stimulates protein synthesis and collagen gene expression in monolayer and lattice cultures of fibroblasts. J Cell Physiol 1992;152:389.

185. Uh ST, Inoue Y, King TE Jr, et al. Morphometric analysis of insulin-like growth factor-I localization in lung tissues of patients with idiopathic pulmonary fibrosis. Am J Respir Crit Care Med 1998;158:1626.

186. Noble PW, Lake FR, Henson PM, Riches DWH. Hyaluronate activation of CD44 induces insulin-like growth factor-1 expression by a tumor necrosis factor-alpha-dependent mechanism in murine macrophages. J Clin Invest 1993;91:2368.

187. Bjermer L, Lundgren R, Hallgen R. Hyaluron and type III procollagen peptide concentrations in bronchoalveolar lavage fluid in idiopathic pulmonary fibrosis. Thorax 1989;44:126.

188. Nettelbladt O, Hallgren R. Hyaluronan (hyaluronic acid) in bronchoalveolar lavage fluid during the development of bleomycin-induced alveolitis in the rat. Am Rev Respir Dis 1989;140:1028.

189. Ornitz DM, Itoh N. Fibroblast growth factors. Genome Biol 2001;2:3005.

190. Min H, Danilenko DM, Scully SA, et al. Fgf-10 is required for both limb and lung development and exhibits striking functional similarity to Drosophila branchless. Genes Dev 1998;12:3156.

191. Guo L, Degenstein L, Fuchs E. Keratinocyte growth factor is required for hair development but not for wound healing. Genes Dev 1996;10:165.

192. Ortega S, Ittmann M, Tsang SH, et al. Neuronal defects and delayed wound healing in mice lacking fibroblast growth factor 2. Proc Natl Acad Sci U S A 1998;95:5672.

193. Baird A, Mormede P, Böhlen P. Immunoreactive fibroblast growth factor in cells of peritoneal exudate suggests its identity with macrophage-derived growth factor. Biochem Biophys Res Commun 1985;126:358.

194. Rappolee DA, Mark D, Banda MJ, Werb Z. Wound macrophages express TGF-alpha and other growth factors in vivo: analysis by mRNA phenotyping. Science 1988;241:708.

195. Henke C, Marineili W, Jessurun J, et al. Macrophage production of basic fibroblast growth factor in the fibroproliferative disorder of alveolar fibrosis after lung injury. Am J Pathol 1993;143:1189.

196. Inoue Y, King TE Jr, Tinkle SS, et al. Human mast cell basic fibroblast growth factor in fibrotic disorders. Am J Pathol 1996;149:2037.

197. Brogi E, Winkles JA, Underwood R, et al. Distinct patterns of expression of fibroblast growth factors and their receptors in human atheroma and nonatherosclerotic arteries. Association of acidic FGF with plaque microvessels and macrophages. J Clin Invest 1993;92:2408.

198. Barrios R, Pardo A, Ramos C, et al. Upregulation of acidic fibroblast growth factor during development of experimental lung fibrosis. Am J Physiol 1997;273:L451.

199. Falcone DJ, McCaffrey TA, Haimovitz FA, Garcia M. Transforming growth factor-beta 1 stimulates macrophage urokinase expression and release of matrix-bound basic fibroblast growth factor. J Cell Physiol 1993;155:595.

200. Falcone DJ, McCaffrey TA, Haimovitz FA, et al. Macrophage and foam cell release of matrix-bound growth factors. Role of plasminogen activation. J Biol Chem 1993;268:11951.

201. Madtes DK, Busky HK, Standjord TP, Clark JG. Expression of transforming growth factor-α and epidermal growth factor receptor is increased following bleomycin-induced lung injury in rats. Am J Respir Cell Mol Biol 1994;11:540.

202. Liu J-Y, Morris GF, Lei W-H, et al. Up-regulated expression of transforming growth factor-α in the bronchiolar-alveolar duct regions of asbestos-exposed rats. Am J Pathol 1996;149:205.

203. Davies D, Farmer S, Alexander P. Synthesis and release of TGF alpha from the myeloid leukemia cells hl60 treated with phorbol ester [meeting abstract]. Br J Cancer 1990;62:490.

204. Korfhagen TR, Swantz RJ, Wert SE, et al. Respiratory epithelial cell expresssion of human transforming growth factor-α induces lung fibrosis in transgenic mice. J Clin Invest 1994;93:1691.

205. Weissler JC. Idiopathic pulmonary fibrosis: cellular and molecular pathogenesis. Am J Med Sci 1989;297:91.

206. Augustin A, Kubo RT, Sim GK. Resident pulmonary lymphocytes expressing the gamma/delta T-cell receptor. Nature 1989;340(6230):239.

207. Rajasekar R, Sim GK, Augustin A. Self heat shock and γδ T cell reactivity. Proc Natl Acad Sci U S A 1990;87:1767.

208. Sim GK, Rajaserkar R, Dessing M, Augustin A. Homing and in situ differentiation of pulmonary lymphocytes. Int Immunol 1994;6:1287.

209. Sim GK, Olsson C, Augustin A. Commitment and maintainance of the αβ and γδ T cell lineages. J Immunol 1995;154:5821.

210. Balbi B, Moller DR, Kirby M, et al. Increased numbers of T lymphocytes with γδ-positive antigen receptors in a subgroup of individuals with pulmonary sarcoidosis. J Clin Invest 1990;85:1353.

211. Tamura N, Holroyd KJ, Banks T, et al. Diversity in junctional sequences associated with the common human V gamma 9 and V delta 2 gene segments in normal blood and lung compared with the limited diversity in a granulomatous disease. J Exp Med 1990;172:169.

212. Tanaka Y, Morita CT, Tanaka Y, et al. Natural and synthetic non-peptide antigens recognized by human gamma delta T cells. Nature 1995;375:155.

213. Sim GK, Augustin A. Dominantly inherited expression of BID, an invariant undiversified T cell receptor δ chain. Cell 1990;61:397.

214. Sim GK, Augustin A. Extrathymic positive selection of γδ T cells: Vg4Jg1 rearrangements with GxYS junctions. J Immunol 1991;146:2439.

215. Parker CM, Groh V, Band H. Evidence for extrathymic changes in the T cell receptor γδ repertoire. J Exp Med 1990;171:1597.

216. Asarnow DM, Cado D, Raulet D. Selection is not required to produce invariant T cell receptor γ gene junctional sequences. Nature 1993;362:158.

217. Sim GK, Augustin A. The presence of an endogenous murine leukemia virus sequence correlates with the peripheral expansion of gamma delta T cells bearing the BALB invariant delta (BID) T cell receptor delta. J Exp Med 1993;178:1819.

218. Boismenu R, Havran WL. Modulation of epithelial cell growth by intraepithelial gamma delta T cells. Science 1994;266:1253.

219. Rajasekar R, Augustin A. Selection of CD4–CD8– ab+ T cells expressing Vb8 TCR. Am J Respir Cell Mol Biol 1994;10:79.

220. Tatrai E, Brozik M, Adamis Z, et al. In vivo pulmonary toxicity of cellulose in rats. J Appl Toxicol 1996;16:129.

221. Hyde DM, Henderson TS, Giri SN, et al. Effect of murine gamma interferon on the cellular responses to bleomycin in mice. Exp Lung Res 1988;14:687.

222. Hyde DM, Giri SN. Polyinosinic-polycytidylic acid, an interferon inducer, ameliorates bleomycin-induced lung fibrosis in mice. Exp Lung Res 1990;16:533.

223. Piguet PF, Collart MA, Grau GE, et al. Tumor necrosis factor/cachectin plays a key role in bleomycin-induced pneumopathy and fibrosis. J Exp Med 1989;170:655.

224. Piguet PF, Collart MA, Grau GE, et al. Requirement of tumour necrosis factor for development of silica-induced pulmonary fibrosis. Nature 1990;344:245.

225. Schrier DJ, Phan SH, McGarry BM. The effects of the nude (nu/nu) mutation on bleomycin-induced pulmonary fibrosis. A biochemical evaluation. Am Rev Respir Dis 1983;127:614.

226. Prior C, Haslam PL. In vivo levels and in vitro production of interferon-gamma in fibrosing interstitial lung diseases. Clin Exp Immunol 1992;88:280.

227. Sher A, Coffman RL. Regulation of immunity to parasites by T cells and T cell-derived cytokines. Ann Rev Immunol 1992;10:385.

228. Carding SR, Allan W, Kyes S, et al. Late dominance of the inflammatory process in murine influenza by gamma/delta + T cells. J Exp Med 1990;172:1225.

229. Mombaerts P, Arnoldi J, Russ F, et al. Different roles of alpha beta and gamma delta T cells in immunity against an intracellular bacterial pathogen. Nature 1993;365:53.

230. Ohga S, Yoshikai Y, Takeda Y, et al. Sequential appearance of gamma/delta- and alpha/beta-bearing T cells in the peritoneal cavity during an i.p. infection with Listeria monocytogenes. Eur J Immunol 1990;20:533.

231. Hsieh CS, Heimberger AB, Gold JS, et al. Differential regulation of T helper phenotype development by interleukins 4 and 10 in an alpha beta T-cell-receptor transgenic system. Proc Natl Acad Sci U S A 1992;89:6065.

232. Hsieh CS, Macatonia SE, Tripp CS, et al. Development of TH1 CD4+ T cells through IL-12 produced by Listeria-induced macrophages [see comments]. Science 1993;260:547.

233. Hu H, Stein-Streilein J. Hapten-immune pulmonary interstitial fibrosis (HIPIF) in mice requires both CD4+ and CD8+ T lymphocytes. J Leukocyte Biol 1993;54:414.

234. Roberts SN, Howie SEM, Wallace WAH, et al. A novel model for human interstitial lung disease: hapten-driven lung fibrosis in rodents. J Pathol 1995;176:309.

235. Christensen PJ, Goodman RE, Pastoriza L, et al. Induction of lung fibrosis in the mouse by intratracheal instillation of fluorescein isothiocyanate is not T-cell-dependent. Am J Pathol 1999;155:1773.

236. Augustin AA, Julius MH, Cosenza H. Antigen-specific stimulation and trans-stimulation of T cells in long-term culture. Eur J Immunol 1979;9:665.

237. Ulich TR, Yi ES, Longmuir K. Keratinocyte growth factor is a growth factor for type II pneumocytes in vivo. J Clin Invest 1994;93:1298.

238. Panos RJ, Rubin JS, Csaky KG, et al. Keratinocyte growth factor and hepatocyte growth factor/scatter factor are heparin-binding growth factors for alveolar type II cells in fibroblast-conditioned medium. J Clin Invest 1993;92:969.

239. Kuhn CI, Boldt J, King TE Jr, et al. An immunohistochemical study of architectural remodeling and connective tissue synthesis in pulmonary fibrosis. Am Rev Respir Dis 1989;140:1693.

240. Reid LM. Needs for animal models of human diseases of the respiratory system. Am J Pathol 1980;101(3 Suppl):S89.

241. Snider GL. Interstitial pulmonary fibrosis. Chest 1986;89 (3 Suppl):115S.

242. Fleischman RW, Baker JR, Thompson GR, et al. Bleomycin-induced interstitial pneumonia in dogs. Thorax 1971;26:675.

243. Gould VE, Miller J. Sclerosing alveolitis induced by cyclophosphamide. Am J Pathol 1975;81:513.

244. von Wichert P, Morgenroth K. Comparison between pathological and biochemical investigations on an experimental model of fibrosing alveolitis. Respiration 1976;33:36.

245. Butler C. Pulmonary interstitial fibrosis from paraquat in the hamster. Arch Pathol 1975;99:503.

246. Derks CM, Jacobovitz-Derks D. Embolic pneumopathy induced by oleic acid. Am J Pathol 1977;87:143.

247. Damiano VV, Cherian PV, Frankel FR, et al. Intraluminal fibrosis induced unilaterally by lobar instillation of CdCl$_2$ into the rat lung. Am J Pathol 1990;137:883.

248. Halme J, Uitto J, Kahanpaa K, et al. Protocollagen proline hydroxylase activity in experimental pulmonary fibrosis of rats. J Lab Clin Med 1970;75:535.

249. Glassroth JL, Bernardo J, Lucey EC, et al. Interstitial pulmonary fibrosis induced in hamsters by intratracheally administered chrysotile asbestos. Histology, lung mechanics, and inflammatory events. Am Rev Respir Dis 1984; 130:242.

250. Jules-Elysee K, White DA. Bleomycin-induced pulmonary toxicity. Clin Chest Med 1990;11:1.

251. Muggia FM, Louie AC, Sikic BI. Pulmonary toxicity of antitumor agents. Cancer Treat Rep 1983;10:221.

252. Borzone G, Moreno R, Urrea R, et al. Bleomycin-induced chronic lung damage does not resemble human idiopathic pulmonary fibrosis. Am J Respir Crit Care Med 2001;163: 1648.

253. Basset F, Ferrans VS, Soler P, et al. Intraluminal fibrosis in interstitial lung disorders. Am J Pathol 1986;122:443.

254. Brown RF, Drawbaugh RB, Marrs TC. An investigation of possible models for the production of progressive pulmonary fibrosis in the rat. The effects of repeated intra-tracheal instillation of bleomycin. Toxicology 1988;51:101.

255. Adamson IYR, Bowden DH. The pathogenesis of bleomycin-induced pulmonary fibrosis in mice. Am J Pathol 1974; 77:185.

256. Thrall RS, McCormick JR, Jack RM, et al. Bleomycin-induced pulmonary fibrosis in the rat: inhibition by indomethacin. Am J Pathol 1979;95:117.

257. Tryka AF, Godleski JJ, Brain JD. Alterations in alveolar macrophages in hamsters developing pulmonary fibrosis. Exp Lung Research 1984;7:41.

258. Hakkinen PJ, Whiteley JW, Witschi HR. Hyperoxia, but not thoracic X-irradiation, potentiates bleomycin- and cyclophosphamide-induced lung damage in mice. Am Rev Respir Dis 1982;126:281.

259. Rinaldo J, Goldstein RH, Snider JL. Modification of oxygen toxicity after lung injury by bleomycin in hamsters. Am Rev Respir Dis 1982;126:1030.

260. Tryka AF, Skornik WA, Godleski JJ, Brain JD. Potentiation of bleomycin-induced lung injury by exposure to 70% oxygen; morphologic assessment. Am Rev Respir Dis 1982;126:1074.

261. Tryka AF, Godleski JJ, Skornik WA, Brain JD. Progressive pulmonary fibrosis in hamsters. Exp Lung Res 1983;5:155.

262. Slosman DO, Costabella PM, Roth M, et al. Bleomycin primes monocytes-macrophages for superoxide production. Eur Respir J 1990;3:772.

263. Chandler DB, Barton JC, Briggs DD, et al. Effect of iron deficiency on bleomycin-induced lung fibrosis in the hamster. Am Rev Respir Dis 1988;137:85.

264. Parizada B, Werber MM, Nimrod A. Protective effect of human recombinant MnSOD in adjuvant arthritis and bleomycin-induced lung fibrosis. Free Radic Res Commun 1991;15:297.

265. Chang SW, Feddersen CO, Henson PM, Voelkel NF. Platelet activating factor mediates hemodynamic changes and lung injury in endotoxin treated rats. J Clin Invest 1987;79: 1498.

266. Chen J, Ziboh V, Giri SN. Up-regulation of platelet-activating factor receptors in lung and alveolar macrophages in the bleomycin-hamster model of pulmonary fibrosis. J Pharmacol Exp Ther 1997;280:1219.

267. Hagimoto N, Kuwano K, Miyazaki H, et al. Induction of apoptosis and pulmonary fibrosis in mice in response to ligation of Fas antigen. Am J Respir Cell Mol Biol 1997; 17:272.

268. Hagimoto N, Kuwano K, Nomoto Y, et al. Apoptosis and

269. Karpel JP, Aldrich TK, Mitsudo S, Norin AJ. Lung lymphocytes in bleomycin-induced pulmonary disease. Lung 1989;167:163.

270. Shen AS, Haslett C, Feldsin DC, et al. The intensity of chronic lung inflammation and fibrosis after bleomycin is directly related to the severity of acute injury. Am Rev Respir Dis 1988;137:564.

271. Peao MN, Aguas AP, de Sa CM, Grande NR. Neoformation of blood vessels in association with rat lung fibrosis induced by bleomycin. Anatomic Rec 1994;238:57.

272. Olman MA, Mackman N, Gladson CL, et al. Changes in procoagulant and fibrinolytic gene expression during bleomycin-induced lung injury in the mouse. J Clin Invest 1995;96:1621.

273. Zhang K, Gharaee-Kermani M, McGarry B, Phan SH. In situ hybridization analysis of rat lung alpha 1 (I) and alpha 2 (I) collagen gene expression in pulmonary fibrosis induced by endotracheal bleomycin injection. Lab Invest 1994; 70:192.

274. Mitchell J, Woodcock-Mitchell J, Reynolds S, et al. Alpha-smooth muscle actin in parenchymal cells of bleomycin-injured rat lung. Lab Invest 1989;60:643.

275. Evans JN, Kelley J, Low RB, Adler KB. Increased contractility of isolated lung parenchyma in an animal model of pulmonary fibrosis induced by bleomycin. Am Rev Resp Dis 1982;125:89.

276. Limper AH, Roman J. Fibronectin: a versatile matrix protein with roles in thoracic development, repair and infection. Chest 1992;101:1663.

277. Giri SN, Sanford DAJ, Robison TW, Tyler NK. Impairment in coupled beta-adrenergic receptor and adenylate cyclase system during bleomycin-induced lung fibrosis in hamsters. Exp Lung Res 1987;13:401.

278. Last JA, Gerriets JE, Armstrong LC, et al. Hydroxylation of collagen by lungs of rats administered bleomycin. Am J Respir Cell Mol Biol 1990;2:543.

279. Last JA, King TE, Nerlich AG, Reiser KM. Collagen cross-linking in adult patients with acute and chronic fibrotic lung disease. Am Rev Respir Dis 1990;141:307.

280. Breen E, Shull S, Burne S, et al. Bleomycin regulation of transforming growth factor-b mRNA in rat lung fibroblasts. Am J Respir Cell Mol Biol 1992;6:146.

281. Miyazaki Y, Araki K, Vesin C, et al. Expression of a tumor necrosis factor-alpha transgene in murine lung causes lymphocytic and fibrosing alveolitis. A mouse model of progressive pulmonary fibrosis. J Clin Invest 1995;96:250.

282. Teder P, Nettelbladt O, Heldin P. Characterization of the mechanism involved in bleomycin-induced increased hyaluronan production in rat lung. Am J Respir Cell Mol Biol 1995;12:181.

283. Lake FR, Noble PW, Henson PM, Riches DWH. Functional switching of macrophage responses to TNFα by interferons. Implications for the pleiotropic activities of TNFα. J Clin Invest 1994;93:1661.

284. Swiderski RE, Dencoff JE, Floerchinger CS, et al. Differential expression of extracellular matrix remodeling genes in a murine model of bleomycin-induced pulmonary fibrosis. Am J Pathol 1998;152:821.

285. Jordana M, Richards C, Irving LB, Gauldie J. Spontaneous in vitro release of alveolar-macrophage cytokines after the intratracheal instillation of bleomycin in rats. Am Rev Respir Dis 1988;137:1135.

286. Yasui W, Ji ZQ, Kuniyasu H, et al. Expression of transforming growth factor alpha in human tissues: immunohistochemical study and Northern blot analysis. Virchows Arch A Pathol Anat Histopathol 1992;421:513.

287. Wallace WA, Howie SE. Immunoreactive interleulin 4 and

interferon-gamma expression by type II alveolar epithelial cells in interstitial lung disease. J Pathol 1999;187:475.

288. Giri SN, Hyde DM, Marafino BJ. Ameliorating effect of murine interferon gamma on bleomycin-induced lung collagen fibrosis in mice. Biochem Med Metab Biol 1986; 36:194.

289. Giri SN, Hyde DM. Ameliorating effect of an interferon inducer polyinosinic-polycytidylic acid on bleomycin-induced lung fibrosis in hamsters; morphologic and biochemical evidence. Am J Pathol 1988;133:525.

290. Zia S, Hyde DM, Giri SN. Effects of an interferon inducer bropirimine on bleomycin-induced lung fibrosis in hamsters. Pharmacol Toxicol 1992;71:11.

291. Gurujeyalakshmi G, Giri SN. Molecular mechanisms of antifibrotic effect of interferon gamma in bleomycin-mouse model of lung fibrosis: downregulation of TGF-beta and procollagen I and III gene expression. Exp Lung Res 1995;21:791.

292. Wild JS, Hyde DM, Hubbell HR, Giri SN. Dose-related effects of Ampligen (poly (I).poly (C12U)), a mismatched double-stranded RNA, in a bleomycin-mouse model of pulmonary fibrosis. Exp Lung Res 1996;22:375.

293. Thrall RS, Phan SH, McCormick JR, Ward PA. The development of bleomycin-induced pulmonary fibrosis in neutrophil-depleted and complement-depleted rats. Am J Pathol 1981;105:76.

294. Clark JG, Kuhn C. Bleomycin-induced pulmonary fibrosis in hamsters: effect of neutrophil depletion on lung collagen synthesis. Am Rev Respir Dis 1982;126:737.

295. Elias JA, Jimenez SA, Freundlich B. Recombinant gamma, alpha, and beta interferon regulation of human lung fibroblast proliferation. Am Rev Respir Dis 1987;135:62.

296. Lake FR, Dempsey EC, Spahn JD, Riches DWH. Involvement of protein kinase C in macrophage activation by poly (I:C). Am J Physiol 1994;266:C134.

297. Keane MP, Belperio JA, Arenberg DA, et al. IFN-gamma-inducible protein-10 attenuates bleomycin-induced pulmonary fibrosis via inhibition of angiogenesis. J Immunol 1999;163:5686.

298. Eickelberg O, Pansky A, Koehler E, et al. Molecular mechanisms of TGF-(beta) antagonism by interferon (gamma) and cyclosporine A in lung fibroblasts. FASEB J 2001;15:797.

299. Okada T, Sugie I, Aisaka K. Effects of gamma-interferon on collagen and histamine content in bleomycin-induced lung fibrosis in rats. Lymphokine Cytokine Res 1993;12:87.

300. Nagahori T, Dohi M, Matsumoto K, et al. Interferon-gamma upregulates the c-Met/hepatocyte growth factor receptor expression in alveolar epithelial cells. Am J Respir Cell Mol Biol 1999;21:490.

301. Chen ES, Greenlee BM, Wills-Karp M, Moller DR. Attenuation of lung inflammation and fibrosis in interferon-γ-deficient mice after intratracheal bleomycin. Am J Respir Cell Mol Biol 2001;24:545.

302. Gur I, Or R, Segel MJ, et al. Lymphokines in bleomycin-induced lung injury in bleomycin-sensitive C57BL/6 and -resistant BALB/c mice. Exp Lung Res 2000;26:521.

303. Fournier T, Riches DWH, Winston BW, et al. Divergence in macrophage insulin-like growth factor-I (IGF-I) synthesis induced by TNF-α and prostaglandin E2. J Immunol 1995;155:2123.

304. Clark J, Kostal KM, Marino BA. Bleomycin induced pulmonary fibrosis in hamsters: an alveolar macrophage product that increases fibroblast prostaglandin E2 and cyclic adenosine monophosphate and suppresses fibroblast proliferation and collagen production. J Clin Invest 1983; 72:2082.

305. Chandler DB, Jackson RM, Briggs AD, et al. The effect of bleomycin on lung metabolism of prostaglandin E2 in hamsters. Prostaglandins Leukot Med 1985;19:139.

306. Giri SN, Hyde DM. Increases in severity of lung damage and

mortality by treatment with cyclo and lipoxygenase inhibitors in bleomycin and hyperoxia model of lung injury in hamsters. Pathology 1987;19:150.

307. Nettelbladt O, Tengblad A, Hallgren R. High-dose corticosteroids during bleomycin-induced alveolitis in the rat do not suppress the accumulation of hyaluronan (hyaluronic acid) in lung tissue. Eur Resp J 1990;3:421.

308. Grunze MF, Parkinson D, Sulavik SB, Thrall RS. Effect of corticosteroids on lung volume-pressure curves in bleomycin-induced lung injury in the rat. Exp Lung Res 1988;14:183.

309. Unemori EN, Pickford LB, Salles AL, et al. Relaxin induces an extracellular matrix-degrading phenotype in human lung fibroblasts in vitro and inhibits lung fibrosis in a murine model in vivo. J Clin Invest 1996;98:2739.

310. Wang Q, Giri SN, Hyde DM, et al. Niacin attenuates bleomycin-induced lung fibrosis in the hamster. J Biochem Toxicol 1990;5:13.

311. Wang Q, Giri SN, Hyde DM, Congfen L. Amelioration of bleomycin-induced pulmonary fibrosis in hamsters by combined treatment with taurine and niacin. Biochem Pharmacol 1991;42:1115.

312. Nagai A, Matsumiya H, Hayashi M, et al. Effects of nicotinamide and niacin on bleomycin-induced acute injury and subsequent fibrosis in hamster lungs. Exp Lung Res 1994; 20:263.

313. Blaisdell RJ, Schiedt MJ, Giri SN. Dietary supplementation with taurine and niacin prevents the increase in lung collagen cross-links in the multidose bleomycin hamster model of pulmonary fibrosis. J Biochem Toxicol 1994;9:79.

314. Weinbach J, Camus A, Bara J, et al. Transgenic mice expressing the Sh *ble* bleomycin-resistance gene are protected against bleomycin-induced pulmonary fibrosis. Cancer Res 1996;56:5659.

315. Tran PL, Weinbach J, Opolon P, et al. Prevention of bleomycin-induced pulmonary fibrosis after adenovirus-mediated transfer of the bacterial bleomycin resistance gene. J Clin Invest 1997;99:608.

316. Piguet PF, Vesin C, Grau GE, Thompson RC. Interleukin 1 receptor antagonist (IL-1ra) prevents or cures pulmonary fibrosis elicited in mice by bleomycin or silica. Cytokine 1993;5:57.

317. Giri SN, Hyde DM, Hollinger MA. Effect of antibody to transforming growth factor-β on bleomycin induced accumulation of lung collagen in mice. Thorax 1993;48:959.

318. Keane MP, Belperio JA, Burdick MD, Strieter RM. IL-12 attenuates bleomycin-induced pulmonary fibrosis. Am J Physiol Lung Cell Mol Physiol 2001;281:L92.

319. Piguet PF, Vesin C. Treatment of human recombinant soluble TNF receptor of pulmonary fibrosis induced by bleomycin or silica in mice. Eur Respir J 1994;7:515.

320. Kuwano K, Kunitake R, Maeyama T, et al. Attenuation of bleomycin-induced pneumopathy in mice by a caspase inhibitor. Am J Physiol Lung Cell Mol Physiol 2001; 280:L316.

321. Maeyama T, Kuwano K, Kawasaki M, et al. Attenuation of bleomycin-induced pneumopathy in mice by monoclonal antibody to interleukin-12. Am J Physiol Lung Cell Mol Physiol 2001;280:L1128.

322. Ebrahimi B, Dutia BM, Brownstein DG, Nash AA. Murine gammaherpesvirus-68 infection causes multi-organ fibrosis and alters leukocyte trafficking in interferon-gamma receptor knockout mice. Am J Pathol 2001;158:117.

323. Griffin M, Smith LL, Wynne J. Changes in transglutaminase activity in an experimental model of pulmonary fibrosis induced by paraquat. Br J Exp Pathol 1979;60:653.

324. Thurlbeck WM, Thurlbeck SM. Pulmonary effects of paraquat poisoning. Chest 1976;69:276.

325. Selman M, Montano M, Montfort I, Perez-Tamayo R. A new model of diffuse interstitial pulmonary fibrosis in the rat. Exp Mol Pathol 1985;43:375.

326. Fukuda Y, Ferrans VJ. Pulmonary elastic fiber degradation in paraquat toxicity. An electron microscopic immunohistochemical study. J Submicrosc Cytol Pathol 1988;20:15.

327. Barquin N, Chou P, Ramos C, et al. Increased expression of intercellular adhesion molecule 1, CD11/CD18 cell surface adhesion glycoproteins and alpha 4 beta 1 integrin in a art model of chronic interstitial lung fibrosis. Pathobiology 1996;64:187.

328. Reiser KM, Last JA. Silicosis and fibrogenesis: fact and artifact. Toxicology 1979;13:51.

329. Velan GM, Kumar RK, Cohen DD. Pulmonary inflammation and fibrosis following subacute inhalational exposure to silica: determinants of progression. Pathology 1993;25:282.

330. Yamano Y, Kagawa J, Hanaoka T, et al. Oxidative DNA damage induced by silica in vivo. Environ Res 1995;69:102.

331. Callis AH, Sohnle PG, Mandel GS, et al. Kinetics of inflammatory and fibrotic pulmonary changes in a murine model of silicosis. J Lab Clin Med 1985;105:547.

332. Bissonnette E, Rola-Pleszczynski M. Pulmonary inflammation and fibrosis in a murine model of asbestosis and silicosis. Possible role of tumor necrosis factor. Inflammation 1989;13:329.

333. Mariani TJ, Roby JD, Mecham RP, et al. Localization of type I procollagen gene expression in silica-induced granulomatous lung disease and implication of transforming growth factor-beta as a mediator of fibrosis. Am J Pathol 1996;148:151.

334. Arras M, Huaux F, Vink A, et al. Interleukin-9 reduced lung fibrosis and type 2 immune polarization induced by silica particles in a murine model. Am J Respir Cell Mol Biol 2001;24:368.

335. Zhang Y, Lee TC, Guillemin B, et al. Enhanced IL-1β and tumor necrosis factor-α release and messenger RNA expression in macrophages from idiopathic pulmonary fibrosis or after asbestos exposure. J Immunol 1993;150:4188.

336. Filipenko D, Wright JL, Churg A. Pathologic changes in the small airways of the guinea pig after amosite asbestos exposure. Am J Pathol 1985;119:273.

337. Mossman BT, Marsh JP, Sesko A, et al. Inhibition of lung injury, inflammation, and interstitial pulmonary fibrosis by polyethylene glycol-conjugated catalase in a rapid inhalation model of asbestosis. Am Rev Respir Dis 1990;145:1266.

338. Brentjens JR, O'Connell DW, Pawlowski IB, et al. Experimental immune complex disease of the lung: the pathogenesis of a laboratory model resembling certain human interstitial lung diseases. J Exp Med 1974;140:105.

339. Richerson HB, Seidenfeld JJ, Ratajczak HV, Richards DW. Chronic experimental interstitial pneumonitis in the rabbit. Am Rev Respir Dis 1978;117:5.

340. Stein-Streilein J, Lipscomb MF, Fisch H, Whitney PL. Pulmonary interstitial fibrosis induced in hapten-immune hamsters. Am Rev Respir Dis 1987;136:119.

341. Okudaira H, Ogita T, Miyamoto T, et al. Interstitial pneumonitis in autoimmune MRL/lpr mice and its treatment with cyclosporin A. Clin Immunol Immunopathol 1986;38:47.

342. Denis M. Neutralization of transforming growth factor-beta 1 in a mouse model of immune-induced lung fibrosis. Immunology 1994;82:584.

343. Mason JW. Amiodarone. N Engl J Med 1987;316:455.

344. Antony VB, Hadley KJ. Mechanism of amiodarone-induced pulmonary fibrosis: amiodarone stimulates proliferation in vitro [abstract]. Clin Res 1988;36:502A.

345. Martin WJ, Rosenow EC. Amiodarone pulmonary toxicity. Recognition and pathogenesis (Part 2). Chest 1988;93:1242.

346. Akoun GM, Gauthier-Rahman S, Milleron BJ, et al. Amiodarone-induced hypersensitivity pneumonitis: evidence of an immunological cell-mediated mechanism. Chest 1984;85:133.

347. Reinhart PG, Lai YL, Gairola CG. Amiodarone-induced pulmonary fibrosis in Fischer 344 rats. Toxicology 1996;110:95.

348. Daniels JM, Brien JF, Massey TE. Pulmonary fibrosis induced in the hamster by amiodarone and desethylamiodarone. Toxicol Appl Pharmacol 1989;100:350.

349. Tatrai E, Adamis Z, Bohm U, et al. Role of cellulose in wood dust-induced fibrosing alveo-bronchiolitis in rat. J Appl Toxicol 1995;15:45.

350. Brody AR, Soler P, Basset F, et al. Epithelial-mesenchymal associations of cells in human pulmonary fibrosis and in BHT-oxygen-induced fibrosis in mice. Exp Lung Res 1981;2:207.

351. Molteni A, Ward WF, Ts'ao C-H, et al. Monocrotaline-induced pulmonary fibrosis in rats: amelioration by captopril and penicillamine. Proc Soc Exp Biol Med 1985;180:112.

352. Rossi GA, Hunninghake GW, Kawanami O, et al. Motheaten mice—an animal model with an inherited form of interstitial lung disease. Am Rev Respir Dis 1985;131:150.

353. Kuwano K, Miyazaki H, Hagimoto N, et al. The involvement of Fas-Fas ligand pathway in fibrosing lung diseases. Am J Respir Cell Mol Biol 1999;20:53.

354. Kuwano K, Hagimoto N, Kawasaki M, et al. Essential role of the Fas-Fas ligand pathway in the development of pulmonary fibrosis. J Clin Invest 1999;104:13.

355. Kuwano K, Kaneko Y, Hagimoto N, et al. Expression of B7-1, B7-2, and interleukin-12 in anti-Fas antibody-induced pulmonary fibrosis in mice. Int Arch Allergy Immunol 1999;119:112.

356. Kuwano K, Kawasaki M, Maeyama T, et al. Soluble form of Fas and Fas ligand in BAL fluid from patients with pulmonary fibrosis and bronchiolitis obliterans organizing pneumonia. Chest 2000;118:451.

357. Aoshiba K, Yasui S, Tamaoki J, Nagai A. The Fas/Fas-ligand system is not required for bleomycin-induced pulmonary fibrosis in mice. Am J Respir Crit Care Med 2000;162:695.

358. Prior C, Haslam PL. Increased levels of serum interferon-gamma in pulmonary sarcoidosis and relationship with the response to corticosteroid therapy. Am Rev Respir Dis 1991;143:53.

359. Ziesche R, Hofbauer E, Wittmann K, et al. A preliminary study of long-term treatment with interferon gamma-1b and low-dose prednisolone in patients with idiopathic pulmonary fibrosis. N Engl J Med 1999;341:1264.

9

ROLE OF THE ALVEOLAR EPITHELIUM IN THE PATHOGENESIS OF PULMONARY FIBROSIS

FRANCIS X. MCCORMACK
JOHN M. SHANNON

The interstitial lung diseases (ILDs) are a heterogenous group of more than 100 disorders that are characterized by inflammation and fibrosis in the lung.[1] One of the most consistent findings in lung biopsy specimens from patients with ILD is pathologic evidence of injury to the alveolar epithelium. It has been known for several decades that alveolar type II cells have the capacity to restore the alveolar epithelium after injury through proliferation, coordinated movement, and terminal differentiation into type I cells. An expanding body of evidence suggests that the alveolar epithelium also actively participates in the modulation of the fibroproliferative process and that repeated epithelial injury and aberrant epithelial repair may even be a primary pathogenic mechanism of fibrosis in idiopathic pulmonary fibrosis (IPF).[2] In this chapter, IPF will be used as a paradigm within which to review the role of the alveolar epithelium, especially alveolar type II cells, in the remodeling and repair of the lung. Parallels between lung repair and lung development will be explored, and the recently proposed role of circulating stem cells in the repopulation of the lung epithelium will be introduced. Several concepts are central to this discussion: (1) There is a shift in the synthetic repertoire of the alveolar epithelium after lung injury, resulting in the appearance of membrane receptors and soluble factors that are critical for lung repair and remodeling; (2) Alveolar epithelial cells and mesenchymal cells within the interstitium and the air space direct the response to injury and the reparative process through reciprocal interactions mediated by cell-matrix contact, cell-cell contact, and the release of paracrine mediators; (3) Extensive or repeated epithelial injury, impediments to reepithelialization, and loss of the integrity of the connective tissue scaffolding promote scarring in the lung; (4) Surfactant produced by the epithelium is abnormal in IPF, and surfactant dysfunction may contribute to several

of the characteristic features of the disease, including the restrictive physiologic defect, impaired gas exchange, and even the propensity of the lung to scar. The important roles that inflammatory cells, proinflammatory cytokines, and the lung matrix play in lung repair are discussed in Chapter 8, "Inflammation in the Pathogenesis of Interstitial Lung Diseases," Chapter 11 "Extracellular Matrix in the Pathogenesis of Lung Injury and Repair" and Chapter 12, "Immunologic Events in the Development of Interstitial Lung Disease: The Paradigm of Sarcoidosis," of this book and will only be mentioned here in the context of alveolar epithelial functions.

NORMAL ALVEOLAR EPITHELIUM

The alveolar wall is a three-layered structure consisting of (1) capillary endothelial cells; (2) basement membrane and extracellular matrix containing elastin, collagen (types I and IV), and fibronectin; and (3) alveolar epithelial cells (types I and II). Type I cells are thin, flat cells that make up less than 40% of all cells in the alveolar unit but line more than 90% of the alveolar surface area.[3] The attenuated cytoplasm of the type I cell provides for close approximation of the alveolar lumen and the bloodstream, which facilitates the diffusion of the respiratory gases oxygen and carbon dioxide. The type I cell is thought to be terminally differentiated and metabolically quiescent, based on the relative paucity of mitochondria, endoplasmic reticulum, and other organelles compared with synthetically active cells.[4] Type II pneumocytes are multifunctional cells that are predominantly found at the septal intersections and oblique angles of the alveoli. They are cuboidal in shape and make up about 15% of all cells in the lung. As the progenitor cells of the alveolus, type II cells regenerate the alveolar epithelium by proliferation and differentiation into type I cells.[5,6] Type II cells are also the site of synthesis, storage, and secretion of surfactant, a heterogeneous mixture of proteins and phospholipids that lines the alveolar epithelium and reduces the natural surface tension forces that promote alveolar collapse. Water and ion transport channels on the surface of type I cells[7,8] and type II cells[7,9] have been described by several laboratories, and clearance of fluid from the alveolar space may be mediated by both cell types of the alveolar epithelium.[10,11] Interestingly, class II major histocompatibility antigens are expressed on type II cells of patients with IPF, suggesting that type II cells may be capable of antigen presentation (Figure 9–1).[12,13] Type II cells also express components of complement.[14] Thus, loss of epithelial integrity with lung injury has multiple potential consequences, including markedly increased alveolar permeability, loss of water and ion transport, diminished surfactant production, and loss of epithelial modulation of the fibrogenic process.

OVERVIEW OF ALVEOLAR EPITHELIAL REPAIR

Epithelial injury triggers a patterned series of responses, including inflammation, angiogenesis, fibroplasia, matrix accumulation, apoptosis, and matrix degradation, that depend on complex interactions between multiple cell lineages. In IPF, although the source of the injury is obscure, there is microscopic evidence of ongoing epithelial injury and repair coexisting with end-stage fibrosis at all stages of the disease.[15,16] The molecular events that occur in wound healing after epithelial injury to the skin have been intensively studied and can serve as a framework to model the less well-characterized process of lung repair (Figure 9–2).[17]

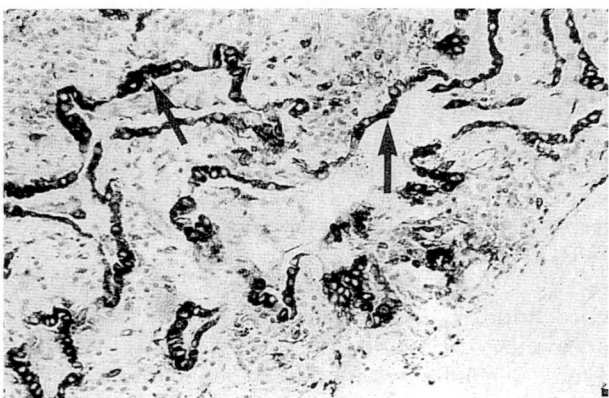

Figure 9–1   Epithelial expression of HLA-DR in IPF. Immunostaining with the anti-HLA-DR antibody LN-3 (ICN Immunobiologicals, Costa Mesa, CA) is positive in epithelial cells, macrophages, and some interstitial cells. Reproduced with permission from Mason and McCormack.[297]

Type I cells are uniquely susceptible in most forms of diffuse lung injury, probably because of their limited synthetic and reparative capacity and their large surface area. Morphologic signs of damage to type I cells include bleb formation, vacuolization, necrosis, and detachment from the basement membrane.[18] Type II cells, although more resilient than type I cells, can also manifest signs of injury, including derangement in the size, number, and morphology of lamellar bodies.[19,20] The loss of type I cells exposes the underlying connective tissue matrix. Exudative material that seeps into the alveolar space through the defect in the epithelium clots to provide hemostasis and a provisional matrix for initiation of the repair process. Components of the coagulation cascade tightly regulate the amount of fibrin in the wound to prevent exuberant clot formation and contraction that might compromise alveolar integrity and gas exchange. Fibroblasts are recruited to the wound and adjacent interstitium by factors that are released, or that fail to be released, from damaged or apoptotic epithelial cells through defects in the basement membrane induced by injury and protease digestion.[2] Various stimuli, including transforming growth factor (TGF)-β, transform fibroblasts into myofibroblasts, which contract the wound and secrete new extracellular matrix. A relatively recent histopathologic observation in IPF is that myofibroblast foci, areas of dense interstitial and air space fibroblast and myofibroblast infiltration invested by hypertrophic alveolar type II cells, are often enriched at the advancing edge of fibrosis. New blood vessel formation, which is stimulated by the release of angiogenic factors, including vascular endothelial growth factor, is generally not apparent in the myofibroblast foci but can be found in adjacent, more densely scarred tissue and is particularly abundant in the more reversible fibromyxoid air space lesions of cryptogenic organizing pneumonia.[21] Hyperplastic and hypertrophic type II cells are a conspicuous feature in lung biopsy specimens from all patients with IPF and are thought to represent the proliferating population that will ultimately restore that epithelium by replacing type I cells (Figure 9–3).[5] There appear to be more hypertrophic type II cells in injured lung than are necessary to perform regenerative functions,[20,22] however, and some investigators have suggested that phenotypic heterogeneity indicates different roles for these cells (Table 9–1).[23] Some type II cells may replace type I cells, others may function as stem cells to replenish the type II cell population,[24] and others may be removed by apoptosis.[25–26] The type II epithelial cells at the edge of the wound are stimulated to proliferate by local factors, which, by analogy with factors implicated in skin regeneration, may include loss of contact inhibition from type I cell dropout, exposure of basement membrane components and gain or loss of soluble agonists or antagonists of growth respectively.[17] Cell kinetic studies in injured lungs have suggested that alveolar type II cells have the capacity to restore high numbers of damaged type I cells within only a few hours[27] and to completely turn over within 3 days, compared to a steady-state turnover rate in uninjured lungs of 4 to 5 weeks.[6,29,30] In IPF, increased or inappropriate epithelial apoptosis, both in normal alveoli and in myofibroblast foci, may deter reepithelialization and promote fibrosis.[30–33] Type II cells up-regulate cell surface adhesion molecule expression and facilitate the adherence and migration on exposed matrix components.[34] Migration and healing may be enhanced by the property of alveolar type II cells to produce their own matrix components, including fibronectin, type IV collagen, and proteoglycan.[34–38] The fibrinous exudate at the leading epithelial edge is probably dissolved by proteases (and indirectly through protease activators) secreted by advancing type II cells,[39] as well as mesenchymal cells including macrophages and fibroblasts.[40] Water and ion channels that are up-regulated by lung injury may assist in the clearance of excess fluid from the alveolar space.[7,41] Once the wound has been reepithelialized, signals to arrest proliferation and stimulate differentiation of type II cells into type I cells are activated. Contact inhibition and matrix interactions likely play an important role in these poorly understood processes.

Recent studies challenge the dogma that alveolar type II cells serve as the sole progenitor cells for the restoration of the alveolar epithelial barrier after

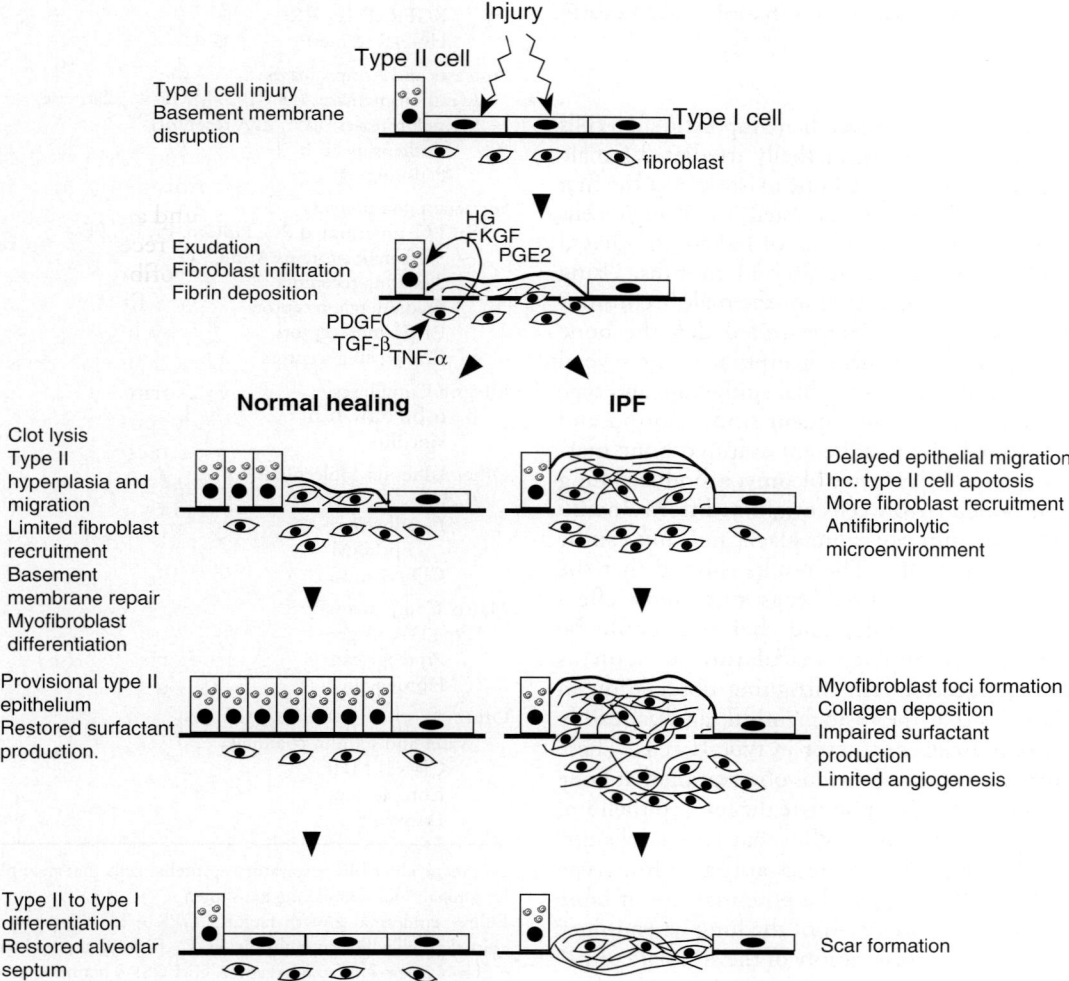

Figure 9–2   Hypothetical model of alveolar repair. Injury to the alveolar epithelium results in type I cell dropout and fragmentation of the basement membrane. Fibrin clot formation provides a provisional matrix, and fibroblasts are recruited by signals from the mesenchymal and epithelial compartments. In normal healing, hyperplastic type II cells close the epithelial defect and secrete factors that limit further myofibroblast differentiation and fibroblast accumulation. Restoration of the basement membrane, protease-dependent matrix degradation, and cellular clearance through apoptosis results in complete structural and functional recovery. In IPF, type II cell dysfunction may inhibit hyperplasia and epithelial migration, which are necessary for closure of the epithelial defect. Myofibroblast differentiation and fibroblast recruitment continues unabated, resulting in further matrix deposition and scarring. Adapted from Selman et al.[2]

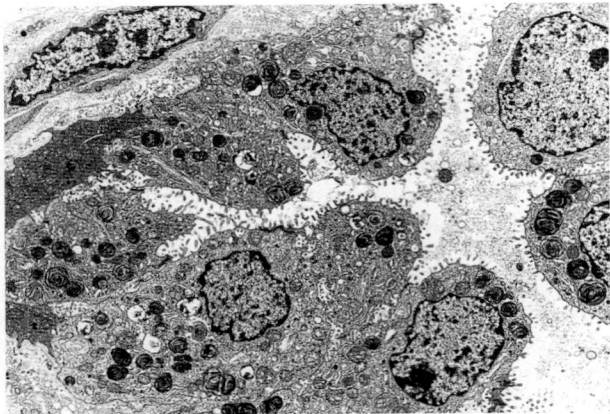

Figure 9–3   Electron micrograph of hyperplastic type II cells in an idiopathic pulmonary fibrosis (IPF) patient (×4,900 original magnification). Reproduced with permission from Robert L. Mason, MD and Jan Henson, MD, National Jewish Medical and Research Center, Denver, CO.

injury.[28,29] Bone marrow-derived hematopoietic stem cells from male mice injected into lethally irradiated female mice homed to the spleen and bone marrow over the first 48 hours.[42] The cells were reharvested, then single cells were re-injected into a second set of lethally irradiated females, which were sacrificed after 11 months. Using fluorescent in situ hybridization for the male Y chromosome, these investigators demonstrated that the bone marrow-derived stem cells were incorporated into several cell lineages, including the bronchial epithelium and type II cells of the lung. In a subsequent study, Kotton and colleagues injected plastic-adherent cultured bone marrow cells into mice 5 days after bleomycin-induced lung injury.[43] The bone marrow cells originated from Rosa26 mice, which constitutively express lacZ and thus can be identified histochemically. The results showed that the injected cells engrafted injured lungs much more effectively than uninjured lungs and that cells could be detected in the pulmonary vasculature as soon as 24 hours after injection. An intriguing observation in these studies was that the histochemical tag was readily detected in type I cells but never in type II cells. These data therefore confirm the previous observation that bone marrow-derived cells can repopulate the lung epithelium, but add the provocative possibility that type I cells differentiating after injury do not necessarily arise from type II cells. Both studies suggest the potential use of bone marrow cells to effect the repair of the lung when injury is so severe that the intrinsic ability of the alveolar epithelium to repair itself is compromised. Collectively, these data suggest that cells outside the lung could function as progenitors for repair of the lung epithelium.

The relative paucity of inflammatory infiltrates found in biopsy specimens of patients with IPF, the lack of association between fibrogenic foci and inflammation, and the failure of anti-inflammatory therapy to improve the outcome of IPF patients have reduced

TABLE 9–1   Factors that May Play Roles in Lung Repair and Remodeling

Growth Factors and Cytokines
   EGF
   TGF-β
   HB-EGF
   acidic FGF
   basic FGF
   FGF-10
   IGFs
   PDGF
   TGF-βs
   TNF-α
   MCP-1
   IL-1, -6, -8, -10, -11
   GM-CSF

Growth Factor Receptors
   EGFR
     FGFR
     KGFR (FGF- IIR)
     HGF-R (c-met)

Proteases and Antiproteases
   Metalloproteinases (MMP-2, MMP-9, gelatinase)
   Serine proteases (uPA, uPA receptor)
     Cathepsins H, E
     Pepsinogen II

Surfactant components
   Sat PC, unsaturated PC, PtdGro, PI, PS, PE
     Surfactant proteins A, B,C, D
     Signaling receptors
     β-adrenergic receptors
     P1 purinoreceptors
     P2Y purinoreceptors

Integrin Complexes
   β₁, α₂β₁, αᵥβ₃, αᵥβ₁
     vinculin

Other Adhesion Molecules
   ICAM
     E-cadherin
       Ep-CAM
     CD44s and v

Matrix Components
   Type IV collagen
     Proteoglycan
     Fibronectin

Other
   Water and sodium channels
     Class II MHC
     Complement
     Lysozyme

Factors produced by respiratory epithelial cells that may play a part in lung repair and remodeling are shown.
EGF = epidermal growth factor; EGFR = EGF receptor; EpCAM = epithelial cell adhesion molecule; FGF = fibroblast growth factor; FGFR = fibroblast growth factor receptor; GM-CSF = granulocyte-macrophage colony-stimulating factor; HB-EGF = heparin-binding EGF; ICAM = intercellular adhesion molecule; IGF = insulin-like growth factor; KGF = keratinocyte growth factor; KGFR = KGF receptor; MCP = monocyte chemoattractant protein; MHC = major histocompatibility complex; MMP = matrix metalloproteinase; PDGF = platelet-derived growth factor; PE = phosphatidylethanolamine; PtdGro = phosphatidylglycerol; PI = phosphatidylinositol; PS = phosphatidylserine; Sat PC = saturated phosphatidylcholine; TGF = transforming growth factor; TNF = tumor necrosis factor; uPa = urokinase plasminogen activator.

enthusiasm for the theory that scarring in IPF results from unrelenting inflammation. Recently, Selman and King have proposed the alternative hypothesis that IPF results from abnormal wound healing in response to poorly understood multifocal alveolar epithelial cell injury.[2] In this model, dysregulation of the processes of cellular migration, proliferation, and differentiation described above may promote fibrosis by delaying reepithelialization.[27] Release of fibrogenic mediators leads to recruitment and proliferation of fibrogenic cells and reduced myofibroblast apoptosis, producing fibroblast–myofibroblast foci that persist and coalesce into areas of mature fibrosis.[44] Further epithelial cell dropout, resulting from the secretion of proapoptotic factors such as angiotensinogen by fibroblasts and myofibroblasts, perpetuates the cycle of epithelial injury and fibrosis.[30,33] Imbalances between metalloproteinases and their inhibitors may contribute to fibrosis, both by facilitating remodeling and by independent effects on myofibroblast proliferation and apoptosis. Future therapeutic strategies in IPF will likely target pathways that result in epithelial injury and aberrant repair rather than inflammation. Drugs that promote fibroblast apoptosis (eg, lovastatin) block endogenous growth factor release or action (eg, pirfenidone), promote or inhibit angiogenesis (eg, imatinib [STI-571]), block collagen synthesis (D-penicillamine), or stimulate type II cell hyperplasia (keratinocyte growth factor) are among the candidates that may be considered.[2]

EPITHELIAL–MESENCHYMAL INTERACTIONS THAT MEDIATE LUNG DEVELOPMENT AND REPAIR

Advances in our understanding of the molecular mechanisms controlling lung development has led to the hypothesis that the processes of repair and remodeling in the lung may be similarly regulated by reciprocal interactions between the mesenchymal and epithelial compartments of the distal air spaces.[45] Although supported by only limited data at the present time, the hypothesis that lung repair recapitulates ontogeny is attractive because, like the developing lung, the repair of the epithelium after injury requires proliferative expansion of a relatively undifferentiated cell population followed by differentiation into highly-specialized cell types. Thus the growth factors, cytokines, cell–matrix interactions, and direct cell–cell contact that are involved in normal lung development may also play important roles in the inflammatory, cytokinetic, and proliferative processes that are critical to effective wound healing.

Overview of Lung Development

The lung is a complex organ with simple beginnings, arising from the seventh pair of pharyngeal pouches in the foregut endoderm. In humans, the nascent lung is first detected as the laryngotracheal groove, which subsequently bifurcates caudally to form the primary bronchi and rudimentary lung buds. A series of dichotomous and lateral branchings of the epithelial rudiments gives rise to the pulmonary tree, a process that is classically referred to as branching morphogenesis. Alveolization begins towards the end of gestation and continues postnatally. Development of the pulmonary epithelium is accompanied by the parallel development of the pulmonary vasculature; recent studies in rodents have shown that vascular precursors are closely associated with the lung epithelium as soon as it evaginates from the endoderm.[46] Concomitant with the elaborate patterning of the lung is the specification in both the epithelium and the mesenchymal compartments of highly specialized cell types that will constitute the mature functioning lung.

Pattern formation and the spatially correct differentiation of the plethora of cell types in the developing lung require the tightly coordinated expression of multiple genes in the correct spatial and temporal contexts. Recent identification of a number of the genes that have an impact on lung development has provided new insights into how lung morphogenesis and differentiation are controlled, but much about how these genes exert their effects or interact with other genes remains unknown. One tenet of lung development that has emerged from classic embryological studies has remained unchallenged: that lung specifies epithelial morphogenesis and cytodifferentiation by means of a short-range induction.

The first report of a mesenchymal requirement for lung morphogenesis was made nearly 70 years ago by Rudnick, who showed that chick lung development in ovo ceased when the mesenchyme was removed.[47] The development of methods for in vitro culture of embryonic lungs, along with techniques of tissue separation and recombination, extended these observations to show not only that the developing lung epithelium required association with mesenchyme but also that only lung mesenchyme could serve as the inducer.[48,49] Further experiments with transfilter cultures showed that the molecules responsible for the induction and maintenance of lung epithelial branching and cytodifferentiation were diffusible over a short distance. An important additional observation in these experiments was that this induction was reciprocal: differentiated cell types also did not arise in the lung mesenchyme when it was separated from lung epithelium.[48]

Autocrine- and Paracrine-Soluble Factors that Mediate Epithelial–Mesenchymal Interactions in the Lung

The molecular characterization of growth factor molecules has progressed substantially in the past two decades, primarily from investigations of wound repair in the skin and liver.[17,50] Most of these proteins are synthesized as inactive polypeptides, which are cleaved to an active form by specific proteases. Many growth factors contain structural domains that mediate binding to components of the extracellular matrix, forming a reservoir that releases growth factors in response to injury or early proliferative events. The fully processed proteins are recognized by their target cells through specific high-affinity plasma membrane receptors. The effects of receptor binding include, but are not limited to, growth, proliferation, differentiation, migration, and induction of synthesis of adhesion molecules and exudate-clearing proteases (Table 9–2). In recent years, a number of lung growth factors and receptors have been shown to appear at sites of lung injury in temporal patterns that are consistent with a role in the fibroproliferative process. Several laboratories are exploring the physiological importance of each of these factors in the complex and redundant circuitry of lung development and wound repair. Four families of growth factors of ligands and receptors will be considered in this discussion: (1) the fibroblast growth factor (FGF) family, (2) the epithelial growth factor (EGF) family, (3) hepatocyte growth factor (HGF), and (4) tumor necrosis factor (TNF)-α. The FGF family will be reviewed in detail because it illustrates the molecular complexity of growth factor-induced differentiation and proliferation and because genetic deletion of FGF receptors and ligands has the most compelling effects on lung development (Table 9–3). For a more complete review of cytokine and growth factor networks in ILD, the reader is referred to Chapter 12, "Immunologic Events in the Development of Interstitial Lung Disease: The Paradigm of Sarcoidosis."

The FGF Family

The first FGF was described over 25 years ago by Gospodarowicz, who discovered that basic FGF was a potent mitogen for 3T3 cells.[51] Subsequent studies have revealed that this FGF is but one member of a family of at least 23 related ligands. All of the known members of the FGF family share significant protein sequence identity within a core of approximately 120 amino acids responsible for the ability of these proteins to bind heparin.[52] Acidic and basic FGF (hereafter FGF1 and FGF2, respectively) were the first FGF family members to be identified, and they differ from the other FGFs in that they do not contain a signal peptide for classic protein secretion. The high-affinity receptors for FGF1 and FGF2 are expressed on cell surfaces, however, suggesting that these ligands act extracellularly.

FGF Receptors.   Four high affinity FGF receptors (FGFRs), which are members of the tyrosine kinase family of receptors, have been described. The four FGFRs, which are encoded by separate genes, are all found in the lung and share a common general structure.[53] A secretory signal sequence at the N-terminal is followed by two or three immunoglobulin (Ig)-like disulfide loops that constitute the extracellular domain. A transmembrane domain anchors the receptors to the plasma membrane, thus defining the FGFRs as cell surface receptors. The intracellular portion of the FGFR consists of two tyrosine kinase domains that are divided by a short interkinase domain. The complexity of the FGFR family is significantly increased by alternate RNA splicing. At least 20 different splice variations occurring at single sites have been found, the majority of which have been described in FGFR1 and FGFR2.[52] These variations occur in virtually every functional domain of the FGFRs. A functionally important variant occurs in the C-terminal portion of the third Ig-like loop, which affects ligand specificity and affinity. Alternative splicing of 49 amino acids in the C-terminal half of the third Ig-like loop in FGFR2 results in what have been termed the IIIb and IIIc splice variants of this receptor. This single variation has a profound effect on receptor function. The IIIb variant binds FGF1, FGF3, FGF7, and FGF10 with high affinity and FGF2 with lower affinity, whereas the IIIc variant binds FGF1, FGF2, FGF4, FGF6, and FGF9.[54]

The binding of FGFs to the FGFRs initiates a signaling cascade, the first step of which is the formation of receptor homo- or heterodimers. Dimerization of FGFRs

TABLE 9–2   Epithelial Growth Factors and Receptors Known to be Expressed in Injured Lung

	Type II Mitogen	Expressed in Type II	Other Source	Other Functions
EGF	+	+	Mesenchyme	Differentiation, migration, matrix deposition
TGF-β	+	+	Mesenchyme	Fluid resorption
HB-EGF	+	+	Macrophages, eosinophils	
EGFR	NA	+	Mesenchyme	
Acidic FGF	+	+*	Macrophages, septa	
Basic FGF	+	+	Basement membrane	
KGF	+++	−	Mesenchyme	KGF may induce fluid resorption via IL-1 and IL-6 prophylactic against injury, type II differentiation type II migration, uPa expression
FGFR	NA	+*	Macrophages, fibroblasts	
HGF	++	−	Mesenchyme	Prophylactic against injury
HGFR	+	+	None	

*Not detectable in normal lung.
NA = not applicable.

TABLE 9–3 Fibroblast Growth Factor Family Members in Lung Development

	Epithelial or Mesenchymal Expression	Receptor	Mitogen	Differential Factor	Overexpression	Deletion
FGF1	Epithelial and mesenchymal	All FGFRs	Epithelium fibroblasts	Dependent on source	–	No lung phenotype
FGF2	Epithelial and mesenchymal	All FGFRs	Epithelium fibroblasts	Epithelial	–	No lung phenotype
FGF7	Tracheal and distal airway mesenchyme	FGFR2IIIb	Epithelium	Epithelial	Cystadenoma; Type II hyperplasia; Increased surfactant	No lung phenotype
FGF9	Epithelial early, later mesenchymal only	FGFR2IIIc	Fibroblasts	Probably	–	Hypoplasia
FGF10	Distal airway mesenchyme	FGFR2IIIb, FGFR1IIIb	Fibroblasts; Epithelium	Probably not	Tumorlike type II hyperplasia	Aplasia below trachea
FGF18	Mesenchyme	?	Chondrocytes, ?	Probably not	Tracheal cartilage defect	No phenotype

stabilizes interactions between their cytoplasmic domains and is followed by transphosphorylation of one receptor by the other. The requirement for dimerization of FGFRs has allowed the use of dominant-negative strategies that have provided important information about the role of FGFs in lung development. The relevant interaction of FGFs with heparin occurs through their low-affinity binding of the related molecule, heparan sulfate. Heparan sulfate is found on cell surfaces and in the extracellular matrix in the form of heparan sulfate proteoglycan (HSPG). It is currently believed that HSPGs bind FGFs and induce or stabilize formation of FGF dimers or a ternary complex composed of ligand plus high- and low-affinity receptors. Beyond acting as co-receptors for FGFs on the cell surface, the HSPG that exists in the extracellular matrix can bind FGFs and thus may act as a reservoir for FGFs in the extracellular space.[55]

FGFs as Mediators of Tissue Interactions in the Developing Lung.   Evidence from many systems has shown that FGFs play a critical role in the development of organs, affecting cells from all three germ layers. FGF family members cause changes in cell proliferation, morphology, differentiation, and migration during organogenesis. All of these responses effected by FGFs have been demonstrated in the developing lung. The most compelling data suggesting a primary role of FGFs in lung development have come from studies in which FGF signaling pathways have been disrupted by the alteration or elimination of FGF receptors. Using the surfactant protein (SP) -C promoter to target overexpression of a dominant-negative FGFR2IIIb to the surface of lung epithelial cells, Peters demonstrated that lung development did not progress beyond the generation of the trachea and two unbranched bronchi.[56] Celli and colleagues used the metallothionein promoter to express a soluble dominant-negative FGFR2IIIb throughout the entire developing embryo and also observed lung bud initiation but no branching morphogenesis.[57] Targeted deletion of the FGFR2 gene resulted in embryonic lethality shortly after implantation due to trophectoderm defects.[58] When

these defects were circumvented with the use of tetraploid fusion chimeras, FGFR2-null mice showed no development of the respiratory tree below the trachea.[59] Using the Cre-loxP recombination system, De Moerlooze and colleagues showed that pulmonary agenesis occurred when just the DNA coding for the IIIb exon was deleted, suggesting a critical role for those FGF ligands that bind FGFR2IIIb in early lung development.[60] FGFR2 is not the only FGF receptor signaling system used in the developing lung, however. Although mice null for FGFR3 or FGFR4 have no abnormal lung phenotype, mice null for both FGFR3 and FGFR4 show defective alveolar septation and abnormally elevated elastin. The role of FGFR1-mediated signaling in lung development is at present unknown, because animals null for FGFR1 die early in development.[61]

FGF1, FGF2, FGF7, FGF9, FGF10, and FGF18 have all been localized to the developing lung.[54,62–70] Information on some of these ligands is sketchy; others have been investigated in much greater detail. FGF18 is the most recent FGF to be described and is found in mesenchymal cells adjacent to epithelial ducts, suggesting a role for FGF18 in mediating epithelial–mesenchymal interactions. However, the FGF receptor to which FGF18 binds and its cellular distribution have not yet been determined; thus the role of FGF18 in lung development remains unknown.

FGF9, which binds the mesenchyme-associated FGFR2IIIc, is expressed in the mouse lung endoderm and pleura on embryonic day 10.5 (day e10.5). Expression in the endoderm is extinguished on day e12.5 but persists in the pleura.[66] Despite its limited distribution in the lung, targeted deletion of FGF9 results in pulmonary hypoplasia and death shortly after birth due to hypoxia. It has been suggested that FGF9 affects lung size by stimulating mesenchymal proliferation and the expression of FGF10.

FGF7 (keratinocyte growth factor [KGF]) has no demonstrated effects on fibroblasts but is, instead, a potent mitogen and differentiation factor for epithelial cells. FGF7 will only bind and activate FGFR2IIIb. FGF7 mRNA has been demonstrated in mesenchymal cells of day e14.5 mouse lung by in situ hybridization and is continuously expressed until adulthood.[67,68] By reverse transcriptase-polymerase chain reaction (RT-PCR), FGF7 has been detected in the developing rat lung as early as day e12, again only in the mesenchyme.[71] Because the FGFR2IIIb splice variant is only found in epithelial cells in the lung, FGF7 is a prime candidate molecular mediator of epithelial–mesenchymal interactions.[72] FGF7 has potent effects on both the prenatal and postnatal lung. Targeted overexpression of FGF7 to the developing lung epithelium with the use of the SP-C promoter resulted in abnormal development that resembled pulmonary cystadenomatoid malformation.[73] Similarly, increasing FGF7 levels in the postnatal lung, either by instillation or by conditional targeted overexpression, led to epithelial hyperplasia.[74,75] FGF7 also has potent effects in vitro. Lung explants treated with FGF7 show epithelial hyperplasia and dilation.[76,77] In mesenchyme-free culture, FGF7 by itself induced cystic dilation of embryonic mouse lung epithelium and patchy expression of SP-C.[78] FGF7 also stimulated extensive proliferation and widespread expression of SP-C in embryonic rat lung epithelial rudiments when given with other competence factors.[79] The importance of competence factors to the FGF7 response cannot be overstated: when embryonic rat tracheal epithelium was treated with FGF7 alone, there was no response. In the presence of serum and elevated cyclic AMP, however, FGF7 induced the transdifferentiation of tracheal epithelium to an alveolar type II cell phenotype. Because the competence factors by themselves were unable to elicit this response, it was concluded that FGF7 was necessary, but not sufficient, to induce lung epithelial differentiation.[80] The fact that cultured adult alveolar type II cells show increased synthesis of surfactant proteins and phospholipids in response to FGF7 suggests that the effects of FGF7 on epithelial differentiation continue into adulthood.[81,82] Furthermore, pretreatment with FGF7 appears to protect the adult lung in a number of injury models.[83,84] The mechanism of protection is not clear, but presumably the expansion of the type II cell population by FGF7 enhances the restoration of epithelial continuity and/or promotes the release of factors (such as surfactant or cytokines) that attenuate lung injury.[84] After injury to the skin, the mRNA for FGF7, but not the other FGFs, is markedly up-regulated (>100-fold). Interleukin (IL)-1 is a potent inducer of FGF7 expression in injured lung and skin fibroblasts, suggesting one potential mechanism for FGF7 up-regulation in states of inflammation.[85,86] FGF7 may also play a role in modulating ion and fluid transport in the lung by stimulating epithelial migration and enhancing expression of plasminogen activator.[87–89] Importantly, however, mice with a targeted deletion of FGF7 exhibit no apparent pre- or postnatal lung abnormalities, suggesting functional compensation by another FGF ligand(s).[90]

FGF10 has been found in the lungs of humans and rodents.[91–93] Like FGF7, expression of FGF10 mRNA has been localized to mesenchymal cells around distal epithelial tips of the developing lung.[67,94] FGF7 is found in both lung and tracheal mesenchyme, however, whereas FGF10 is found only in mesenchymal cells associated with distal lung epithelium. Like FGF7, FGF10 binds the FGFR2IIIb with high affinity, but unlike FGF7, FGF10 also binds FGFR1IIIb.[95] FGF10 appears to be the evolutionarily conserved homologue of the *Drosophila* gene branchless, which guides tracheal epithelial buds to specific sites within the larva, thereby playing a primary role in patterning the *Drosophila* respiratory system.[96] Similarly, FGF10-soaked beads induced dramatic chemotaxis of embryonic lung epithelium, supporting the role of FGF10 in determining the spatial coordinates of the early lung.[94,97] The importance of FGF10 to lung development was most strikingly demonstrated in FGF10-null mice, which had no lung development below the trachea; this phenotype is identical to that seen in mice in which FGFR2IIIb was deleted.[98,99] This indicates that FGF10 plays a unique role in the induction of lung patterning that cannot be compensated for by other FGF ligands. Conditionally overexpressed FGF10 in the adult lung results in tumorlike epithelial growth that is morphologically distinguishable from the malformations seen with FGF7 overexpression.[100] These data present a paradox, because FGF7 and FGF10 both bind the same receptor (FGFR2IIIb) in the lung epithelium. Thus the effects of FGFs on morphogenetic patterning and cellular differentiation may be separable processes in the lung. Although a primary role for FGF10 in lung patterning is apparent, its role in specification of epithelial phenotype is unclear. In vitro, FGF10 caused budding of embryonic lung epithelium in mesenchyme-free culture; the ability of FGF10 to sustain expression of SP-C by itself, however, was not determined.[67,68,94] Furthermore, unlike FGF7, FGF10 could not reprogram embryonic rat tracheal epithelium to express an alveolar type II cell phenotype.[80]

FGF1 mRNA was not detected in the mouse lung on day e11.5 but was found in both the epithelium and mesenchyme on day e13.5.[68] A role for FGF1 in lung development was suggested by the observation that FGF1 elicited growth and budding of day e11 mouse lung epithelium in mesenchyme-free culture; FGF1 by itself, however, was unable to sustain expression of the distal lung epithelial marker SP-C.[78,101] In a more complex medium containing other competence factors, Deterding and Shannon demonstrated that bovine brain FGF1 could sustain growth and SP-C expression in day e13 rat lung epithelium.[102] The ability of FGF1 to effect transdifferentiation of embryonic rat tracheal epithelium to a lung phenotype, however, was less impressive.[80] Importantly, mice null for FGF1 exhibited no abnormalities in lung development.[103] FGF1 has been shown to stimulate the proliferation of fetal rat pulmonary epithelial cells[105] and adult rat alveolar type II cells.[105,106] FGF1 is undetectable in normal adult rodent lung but is up-regulated after experimental lung injury with paraquat and hyperoxia.[107] Immunohistochemical staining of the injured lungs localized both FGF1 and FGFR staining to alveolar epithelial cells and macrophages. FGF1 also stimulates the proliferation of fibroblasts and down-regulates collagen gene expression in the skin, but it is not clear if it has the same effects in the lung.[108]

Localization of FGF2 in the developing lung by immunohistochemistry has given variable results, with some investigators finding expression in the epithelium,[63] whereas others do not.[63] The developing human lung epithelium, however, contains FGF2 mRNA.[109] At high concentrations (1,000 ng/mL), FGF2 induced modest growth and numerous small buds in day e11 mouse lung epithelium in mesenchyme-free culture.[101] FGF2 has also been shown to affect lung epithelial cell differentiation, inducing significant increases in expression of SP-A, SP-B, and SP-C in midgestation fetal rat lung epithelial cells.[110] These data suggest a potential autocrine role for FGF2, but confirmation of this awaits a detailed description of FGF2 expression in the developing lung. How these FGF2 effects on the lung epithelium are mediated is unclear, because high-affinity receptors for FGF2 are located in the lung mesenchyme; it should be noted, however, that FGF2 has been shown to bind FGFR2IIIb but at much lower affinity than FGF7 or FGF10.[111] If FGF2 plays a role in lung development, it can be compensated for by other FGFs, because mice with a targeted deletion for FGF2 or null for both FGF1 and FGF2 have completely normal lungs.[103,112] FGF2 is also a type II cell mitogen, and type II cells have been shown to be at least one source of the growth factor.[113,114] FGF2 is particularly enriched in the alveolar basement membrane, and, in rats, hyperoxia increases the intensity of immunostaining within the alveolar extracellular matrix. The activity of FGF2 and other growth factors bound to HSPG and other matrix components appears to be influenced by the level of sulfation of the extracellular matrix.[114,115] Proteolytic activity associated with injury and early proliferative events may release FGF2, thereby increasing its biological activity. FGF2 expression is up-regulated in ILD and is especially enriched in the fibromyxoid connective tissue lesions of bronchiolitis obliterans organizing pneumonia compared to the less reversible lesions of usual interstitial pneumonia.[116] The role of FGF2 in the proliferative response of type II cells and lung scarring in ILD is unclear, however.

The EGF Family

The EGF family comprises at least five members, of which three have been characterized in the lung, including EGF itself, TGF-α, and heparin-binding EGF (HB-EGF). The EGFs are synthesized as transmembrane precursors that are cleaved by an elastase-like protease to yield active soluble peptides.[117] A common structural motif of three intramolecular disulfide loops in the liberated fragments, called the EGF domain, is critical for receptor binding.[118] The EGF receptor (EGFR) is a 170-kD homodimer with an extracellular cysteine-rich binding region and a cytoplasmic tyrosine kinase domain. Binding of the EGFs to the EGFR results in autophosphorylation of cytoplasmic tyrosine residues and intracellular signaling through Janus kinase (JAK)-, signal transducer and activator of transcription (STAT)-, and mitogen-activated protein kinase-dependent pathways.[119,120] EGF ligands can interact with the receptor in their soluble forms, resulting in autocrine (when arising from the same cell) or paracrine (when arising from another cell) stimulation or can bind in their membrane-associated forms through direct cell–cell contact, resulting in so called "juxtacrine" stimulation.

EGF and TGF-α are type II cell mitogens and therefore may play an important role in lung development and repair.[106,113,121,122] The distribution of the EGFs in developing, adult, and injured lungs has been explored with the techniques of in situ hybridization and immunohistochemistry. EGF mRNA is primarily found in the mesenchymal cells of the developing mouse lung, but EGF protein has been detected in both epithelial and mesenchymal cells from adult animals, as well as in the extracellular matrix.[123] Abrogation of signaling through the EGFR in the developing lung results in decreased branching morphogenesis and neonatal lethality due to pulmonary insufficiency.[124,125] Both EGF and EGFR are expressed by alveolar type II cells, suggesting that EGF may act as an autocrine regulator of type II cell function.[126] TGF-α, EGF, and EGFR are all expressed in injured human lungs (Figure 9–4), and TGF-α and EGFR are expressed in the airway and septal epithelial cells after bleomycin-and asbestos-induced fibrosis in rats.[127–130] TGF-α is detectable at biologically relevant levels in the pulmonary edema fluid of patients with acute lung injury.[131] Transgenic mice that overexpress TGF-α under the control of the human SP-C promoter

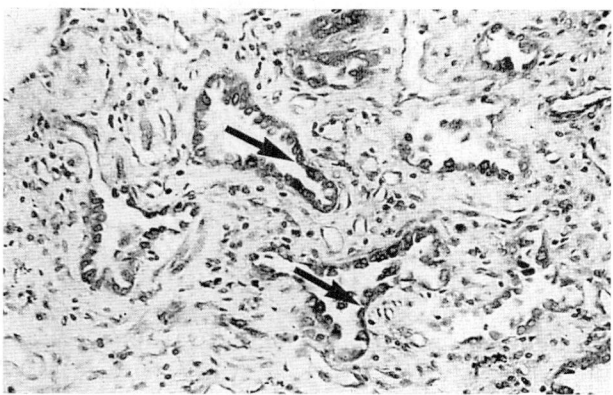

Figure 9–4 Epithelial expression of transforming growth factor (TGF)-β in IPF. Lung biopsy specimens of some but not all patients with IPF demonstrate epithelial staining for TGF-β. Reproduced with permission from Mason and McCormack.[297]

develop peribronchiolar fibrosis and fibrotic pleural lesions associated with marked dilation of the distal airspaces.[132] The severity of the observed emphysematous changes was related to the extent to which TGF-α was overexpressed and was independent of pulmonary inflammation.[133] The introduction of a dominant-negative form of the EGFR to the respiratory epithelial cells of the TGF-α mice reversed the pulmonary fibrosis and significantly improved the abnormal air space dilation.[133] The latter observation supports the concept that the distal respiratory epithelium plays a central role in the development of fibrosis in the TGF-α mice through an autocrine or paracrine mechanism. HB-EGF is the most recent EGF family member to be described in the lung.[134] HB-EGF is produced by macrophages, eosinophils, and type II cells and has been shown to be mitogenic for rat alveolar type II cells.[135] Hyperoxia greatly increases HB-EGF expression, mostly due to the presence of HB-EGF in eosinophils that infiltrate the lung.[136] Although expression of HB-EGF mRNA in human lung is much higher than in the rat, HB-EGF mRNA expression in alveolar macrophages from patients with ILD was not different from that in normal subjects.[135]

In addition to stimulation of type II cell proliferation, the EGFs may play important roles in other aspects of wound repair. The crawling process of cellular migration involves lamellipodial extension and the assembly of focal adhesion complexes, both of which are influenced by the EGFs through activation of the guanosine triphosphatase Rac.[137–139] EGF and TGF-α, may be important for lung remodeling by stimulating the production of matrix-degrading metalloproteinases during development and from airway epithelial cells during repair.[140,141] TGF-α has also been implicated in the clearance of alveolar liquid through a tyrosine kinase-dependent mechanism.[142] Finally, in utero treatment of fetal monkey lungs with EGF results in accelerated type II cell differentiation, DNA synthesis, and surfactant production, suggesting the EGFs may play a role in the modulation of the alveolar type II cell phenotype during development.[143,144]

HGF

HGF, also known as scatter factor (SF), is a mesenchyme-derived, pleiotropic, heparin-binding growth factor that was first identified in the serum of partially hepatectomized rats.[145] The gene for HGF encodes a 728-amino acid, functionally inactive polypeptide that is proteolytically processed into an active disulfide-linked heterodimer. The subunits of the mature protein include a 69-kD α-chain containing four kringle domains and a 34-kD β-chain that contains sequence homology to the serine protease family.[146] The receptor for HGF (HGFR) is expressed on a variety of epithelial cells and has been shown to be identical to the c-met proto-oncogene.[147] Binding of the HGF/SF ligand

results in autophosphorylation of the tyrosine residues of the HGFR and intracellular signaling that stimulates proliferation of hepatocytes and other cell lines, enhances cell motility and tissue invasion, and induces epithelial tubulogenesis.[148,149] Increasing evidence suggests that HGF/SF is involved in tissue repair and remodeling in the liver, but the role of HGF/SF in lung injury and repair is just beginning to be explored.[150]

HGF mRNA is present in the mesenchymal cells in the developing lungs of rodents and humans, whereas c-met mRNA is expressed in the epithelium, thus suggesting a role for HGF in mediating epithelial–mesenchymal interactions. Mice with a targeted deletion of HGF died between day e13 and day e16 of gestation, but their lungs at this stage were identical to those of controls. Therefore, if HGF plays a role in lung development, it occurs later than the glandular stage.

Expression of HGF is associated with protection or repair in several models of lung injury. HGF levels are up-regulated in rat airways after acid instillation.[151] In the bleomycin model of lung injury, HGF expression is greatly increased in whole lung tissue shortly after epithelial necrosis[152]; furthermore, HGF given either simultaneously with or after bleomycin repressed fibrotic changes in the lung.[153,154] HGF levels also rise in response to the administration of asbestos[155] and ischemia-reperfusion injury in the lung.[156]

Remote injury in other organs, including the liver and kidney, has also been shown to induce HGF mRNA in macrophages and endothelial cells of the lung by an unknown mechanism.[157] Recent studies with reporter genes linked to promoters for HGF and HGFR suggest that IL-1 and IL-6 may be involved.[158–160] HGF is both motogenic and mitogenic for alveolar type II cells.[161] Intratracheal instillation of HGF into rats results in type II cell proliferation of a magnitude that is roughly twice the peak proliferation seen on day 2 of recovery from hyperoxia, a rather modest effect.[162] In the liver, the minimal periportal hepatocyte proliferation seen after instillation of HGF into the portal vein is markedly enhanced by preinjection with a small amount of collagenase, suggesting that the cells may need to be primed to respond to the HGF stimulus.[163–165] It may be that cells in the lung also need to be primed to elicit the maximal response to HGF and other growth factors. Protease activators secreted by alveolar type II cells, including urokinase plasminogen activator (uPA), may activate matrix-degrading metalloproteinases and release HGF and other growth factors bound to matrix molecules in the interstitium.[50,166,167] Furthermore, uPA can directly cleave HGF into its active two-chain form.[168,169] A significant proportion of the mitogenic activity present in the salt extracts of normal human lung is attributable to HGF, and HGF expression is up-regulated in inflammatory and fibrotic lung disease.[170] Levels of HGF found in the bronchoalveolar lavage (BAL) fluid of patients with IPF, rheumatoid lung disease, and sarcoidosis are increased compared to levels in normal controls, and the hyperplastic alveolar type II epithelial cells and alveolar macrophages of IPF lungs are strongly stained with anti-HGF.[171] Elevated levels of both HGF and FGF7 are also seen in the pulmonary edema fluid of patients with acute lung injury.[172]

TNF-α

TNF-α mediates a number of inflammatory processes, including induction of cellular adhesion, migration, and coagulation, and has been implicated in several systemic responses such as fever, septic shock, and cachexia.[44] TNF-α is synthesized as a 26-kD precursor composed of 236 amino acids, which is cleaved to a 17-kD, 157-amino acid mature form.[173] Membrane-associated TNF-α can give rise to a biologically active soluble form by cleavage of the transmembrane domain. Although TNF-α is commonly referred to as a mononuclear phagocyte and T-lymphocyte-derived cytokine, alveolar epithelial cells are a primary source of TNF-α in the lung.[174] Overexpression of TNF-α in the alveolar type II cells of mice results in histopathologic and physiological evidence of emphysema associated with limited peribrochiolar, subpleural, and perivascular pulmonary fibrosis, whereas deficiency of TNF-α in gene-targeted mice enhances resistance to bleomycin-induced pulmonary fibrosis.[175] Recently, TNF-α receptor polymorphisms have been shown to be associated with the risk of IPF.[176] TNF-α may promote fibrosis through induction of matrix-degrading metalloproteinases, fibroblast proliferation, and enhancing TGF-β1- and platelet-derived growth factor (PDGF)-dependent collagen production.[177]

Other Cytokines and Growth Factors Secreted by Type II Cells

Monocyte chemoattractant protein (MCP)-1 is the predominant monocyte chemoattractant secreted by a variety of different cell types in culture. Antoniades and colleagues demonstrated that lung epithelial cells from patients with IPF, but not control lung tissue, strongly expressed MCP-1 RNA and protein.[178] MCP-1 expression is induced by the cytokines IL-1 and TNF-α, and secretion is directed toward the apical compartment, consistent with a role in the recruitment of alveolar macrophages.[179] Type II cells have also been reported to express IL-6,[180] IL-8,[181] IL-11,[182] granulocyte macrophage colony-stimulating factor (GM-CSF),[183] and nitric oxide.[184]

Factors Produced by Epithelium that Directly Affect Fibroblast Growth and Matrix Deposition

The growth factors KGF and HGF are excellent examples of paracrine signaling molecules, which arise from the mesenchymal compartment and directly affect alveolar type II cell function. The reciprocal interaction, epithelial modulation of mesenchymal function, is exemplified by two cytokines, TGF-β and PDGF and by the eicosanoid prostaglandin (PG) E_2.

The TGF-β Family

The TGFs, comprised of isoforms denoted β1, β2, β3, and β4, were originally named for their ability to morphologically transform fibroblasts to an anchorage-independent phenotype.[185] They are synthesized as single-chain precursor polypeptides that are cleaved at conserved tetrabasic sites and assembled into a biologically active disulfide-linked homodimers.[186] TGF-β-stimulated growth inhibition and transcriptional activation are mediated by a family of TGF-β-specific cell surface receptors that are autophosphorylated in Serine/Threonine (Ser/Thr)-specific kinase domains of the protein upon binding of the TGF-β ligands.[187] Although all members of TGF have similar biological functions, only TGF-β1 is consistently identified in fibrotic foci.[188] TGF-β1 stimulates collagen deposition by fibroblasts, by enhancing transcription and inhibiting proteolytic degradation. TGF-β1 is also a chemoattractant for fibroblasts and can inhibit or promote fibroblast proliferation via PDGF-dependent pathways. Macrophages, monocytes, platelets, and fibroblasts are generally considered to be sources of TGF-β in the lung, but recently lung epithelial cells have also been shown to synthesize the cytokine, and especially hyperplastic type II cells, in areas of honeycombing and myofibroblast foci.[189–192] TGF-β receptors are present on fibroblasts, macrophages, lymphocytes, and type II cells. Mink lung epithelial cells in culture have been shown to express all known TGF-β receptor subtypes, including I, II, III, and V.[187] TGF-β are important for the modulation of lymphocyte proliferation and differentiated function and for the regulation of extracellular matrix deposition and fibroblast proliferation in many tissues, including the lung. TGF-β is also a potent inhibitor of epithelial cell proliferation,[192] but under certain conditions it can stimulate proliferation, depending on the cellular microenvironment.[186] Inhibitory and stimulatory influences of TGF-β are probably modulated by differential interaction of the peptides with distinct TGF-β receptors present in target tissues. In addition to its effects on cell growth, TGF-β induces bronchial epithelial cell differentiation and modulates the phenotype of alveolar type II cells, upregulating the expression of fibronectin, chondroitin sulfate/dermatan sulfate proteoglycan, and decreasing SP-C expression.[35,36] Recently, animal models of TGF-β have confirmed a central role for the cytokine in pulmonary fibrosis. Intratracheal delivery of adenoviral vectors that express an active form of TGF-β induce a severe progressive pulmonary fibrosis in rats.[194] TGF-β produced by type II cells also appears to play an important role in fibrogenesis in the rat silicosis model. With immunohistochemical staining, the TGF-β1/latency-associated peptide was localized to type II cells adjacent to silicotic granulomas, identifying the site of synthesis of the proprotein precursor for TGF-β. Mature TGF-β protein was localized to fibroblasts and the collagenous stroma.[189] TGF-β is also believed to be a critical mediator in the development of bleomycin-induced interstitial fibrosis, but myofibroblasts, fibroblasts, and eosinophils appear to be the major sources of the cytokine in that model.[195] Gene-targeted mice deficient in $\alpha_v\beta_6$-integrin, which binds and activates TGF-β1, were protected from pulmonary fibrosis despite exuberant inflammation.[196] In the biopsy specimens of patients with IPF, TGF-β is present in macrophages and the extracellular matrix near foci of activated fibroblasts expressing fibronectin, procollagen, and smooth muscle actin, as well as in hyperplastic type II pneumocytes.[192,197] Systemic administration of an anti-TGF antibody reduced the fibrosis induced by intratracheal administration of bleomycin.[198] Thus, TGF-β produced by fibroblasts and alveolar type II cells is markedly up-regulated in the injured lung and may play a role in enhancing matrix production, limiting proliferation, and modulating the phenotypes of both cell types. Pirfenidone inhibits TGF-β mediated collagen synthesis and appears to have a beneficial effect in patients with IPF.[199]

PDGF Family

PDGF is a potent fibroblast mitogen and chemoattractant. PDGF is a 32-kD heterodimeric polypeptide that acts as a competence factor for fibroblast proliferation and is a potent chemoattractant for smooth muscle cells and fibroblasts in vitro.[200] PDGF consists of three species that are disulfide-bridged: AA, AB, and BB heterodimers of the closely related A and B polypeptide chains derived from separate genes. The B-chain is nearly identical to p28sis, the transforming protein of simian sarcoma virus.[201] The PDGF receptor is composed of α- and β-receptor subunits, which dimerize upon binding the ligand, leading to the assembly of αα, αβ, and ββ receptor subtypes. Autophosphorylation by the receptor kinase domain leads to intracellular signaling through tightly regulated pathways that result in potent mitogenic and chemotactic effects on mesenchymal cells.[202,203] The AA isoform binds only to the αα receptor, the AB isoform to the αβ and ββ receptors, and the BB isoform to all three receptors, providing one plausible explanation for the differential effects of PDGF species on different target tissues.[204] Although originally purified from platelets, it has been found that PDGF is produced by many cell types, including endothelial cells, vascular smooth muscle cells, activated macrophages and monocytes, and epithelial cells. In a rat model of fibroproliferative lung disease, PDGF-A and -B mRNAs and protein are found in macrophages and bronchoalveolar cells following a short exposure to crysolite asbestos fiber.[205] Exogenous administration of PDGF or adenoviral expression of PDGF in rat lungs results in a fibrotic response.[206] In lung tissue of patients with IPF, the production of PDGF is much greater in type II epithelial cells than in macrophages.[207–209] Thus, local production of PDGF from the lung epithelium may contribute to the recruitment of fibroblasts and the local accumulation of collagen in the lung parenchyma of patients with IPF. Suppression of PDGF synthesis with the antifibrotic agent pirfenidone correlates with protection from bleomycin-induced fibrosis in the hamster.[210]

Eicosanoid-Dependent Factors

Recent in vitro studies indicate that alveolar type II cells can influence fibroblast proliferation through eicosanoid-dependent pathways.[211] Coculturing of human or rat lung fibroblasts with well-differentiated adult rat type II cells result in inhibition of fibroblast proliferation. This inhibition was mediated by PGE_2 that was produced by the fibroblasts themselves, but this only occurred in the presence of type II cells. Furthermore, addition of FGF7 to the medium enhanced the inhibitory effect. Therefore, differentiated type II cells are producing some factor(s), possibly IL-1α and/or IL-1β, that, in turn, stimulates PGE_2 production by fibroblasts, which then acts as an autocrine inhibitor of proliferation. Treatment with the inhibitor of prostaglandin synthesis indomethacin, worsens bleomycin-induced pulmonary fibrosis in wild-type mice.[212] GM-CSF-null mice develop greater degrees of bleomycin-induced pulmonary fibrosis, through PGE_2-dependent pathways, than do control mice.[213] The mechanism of fibrosis in these animals may also involve the alveolar epithelium, because GM-CSF is known to be a potent mitogen for type II cells in vivo.[212] Importantly, cultured lung fibroblasts from patients with IPF have a diminished capacity to secrete PGE_2.[214] These results support the hypothesis that the alveolar epithelium limits the fibrotic response. Other peptide and nonpeptide factors that may have important anti-proliferative effects in the lung include IL-10, interferon-β, and other prostaglandins.

Direct Contact between Epithelial and Mesenchymal Cells

Another mechanism by which signaling may occur during fibrogenesis is through intercellular contact.[217–219] In the airway, a subpopulation of flat stellate fibroblasts is found closely apposed to the lamina reticularis of the basement membrane, where they make numerous contacts with the lamina densa.[220] This layer of fibroblasts, referred to as the attenuated fibroblast sheath, may mediate responses between the epithelium, extracellular matrix, neural tissues, and migratory cells during fibrogenesis.[221] Although most intensively studied in airway remodeling in asthma, the sheath probably terminates as scattered interstitial fibroblasts in alveolar septa and may play a role in pulmonary fibrosis involving terminal airways.[222] In the alveolus, foot process of alveolar type II cells penetrate the epithelial basement membrane and make contact with cells in the mesenchymal compartment, especially fibroblasts. Intercellular contacts between type II cells and fibroblasts have been described in normal and fibrotic adult lung, as well as in animal models of lung injury.[223] In rats exposed to high oxygen tensions, the incidence of cell–cell contacts decreased during the period of maximal type II cell division, and then increased. Adamson and colleagues suggested that type II cells may inhibit fibroblast growth by this direct physical interaction and that fibroblast proliferation may occur when the epithelial injury interferes with cell contact.[223] The characterization of molecules with known function that are clustered in type II cell foot process, such as CD44 adhesion complexes, may provide important clues regarding the modulatory effects of cell contact in the lung.[27]

EPITHELIAL FUNCTIONS IN WOUND HEALING AND REMODELING

Adhesion Molecule Expression and Type II Cell Migration

Integrins are a large family of heterodimeric transmembrane glycoproteins that were initially identified as receptors for mediating cell adhesion to components of the extracellular matrix.[224] Integrins also play important roles in cellular migration, spreading, and proliferation that are critical for wound repair.[225–227] After injury, epithelial cells at the wound edge up-regulate the expression of integrins that are necessary for binding to molecular components of the exposed connective tissue matrix. Signals that result in the adjustment of the type II cell integrin repertoire probably include loss of contact inhibition and the local elaboration of growth factors and cytokines.[228] The cytoplasmic domains of the β-integrin subunits are linked to actin through the coupling molecules talin and vinculin.[229–231] Cell movement occurs by contraction of actinomyosin filaments of the type II cell cytoskeleton that insert into the membrane-associated adhesion complexes.[232] Many cells predominantly use the $\alpha_v\beta_1$-integrin for binding to fibronectin, the $\alpha_v\beta_3$-integrin for binding to fibronectin and fibrinogen and the $\alpha_v\beta_1$-integrin for binding to collagens. Human type II cells and freshly isolated rat type II cells have both been shown to express integrin subunits.[232,233] Isolated alveolar type II cells adhere to the matrix proteins fibronectin, vitronectin, fibrinogen, and fibrin via β_1-and $\alpha_v\beta_3$-integrins and migrate more

effectively on fibronectin than on type I collagen. The migration on collagen is mediated primarily by the $\alpha_2\beta_1$-integrin, whereas the $\alpha_v\beta_3$-and β_1-integrins partially mediate migration on fibronectin.[234] Antibodies against $\alpha_v\beta_1$-integrin and vinculin strongly stain areas of intra-alveolar fibrosis in biopsies of patients with diffuse alveolar damage.[235] The $\alpha_4\beta_6$-integrin is expressed in fibrotic, but not in normal, epithelium.[236] Thus, it is clear that lung injury causes an up-regulation in the expression of integrins that mediate binding to connective tissue elements that are exposed or accumulating in the wound. Very little is known about the regulation of other adhesion molecules in fibrotic lung disease. E-cadherin is a calcium-dependent 120-kD transmembrane glycoprotein found at the adherens junctions between alveolar epithelial cells and mediates homotypic (type I-type I, type II-type II) and heterotypic (type I-type II) cellular adhesion. The predominantly basolateral expression of E-cadherin is transformed to a cytoplasmic pattern after lung injury in human and rat lungs.[237,238] The functional consequences of the redistribution of E-cadherin in injury are not known. In the healthy lung, intercellular adhesion molecule (ICAM)-1, the adhesion molecule responsible for the attachment and recruitment of neutrophils, is expressed only on type I cells. In the injured lung, ICAM-1 expression also occurs on type II cells.[239,240]

Expression of Proteolytic Enzymes

The complex network of proteins and proteoglycans that makes up the pulmonary extracellular matrix is extensively remodeled in the fibrosing lung diseases.[241,242] The local elaboration of proteolytic enzymes is responsible for the degradation of collagen, elastin, and fibronectin, which precedes the deposition of new matrix components. The major families of proteases are defined by the critical amino acids or ions of the active site, which mediate peptide cleavage. In many cases the enzymes are secreted in an inactive form that requires proteolytic processing for activation. The matrix metalloproteinases (MMPs) are a family of tightly regulated zinc peptidases that includes collagenases, gelatinases, stromolysins, and macrophage metalloelastases. In normal lung, MMP-2 (72-kD type IV collagenase) and MMP-9 (92-kD type IV collagenase), as well as their tissue inhibitors, were found in type II cells, macrophages, ciliated cells, endothelial cells, and smooth muscle cells.[241] Immunoreactivity was increased for each protein in the epithelial cells and myofibroblasts of patients with IPF, and MMP-2 colocalized in areas of disrupted basement membranes, indicating the activation of collagenolysis. This notion was supported by a study that demonstrated that collagenase and tissue inhibitors of metalloproteinases (TIMPs) are increased in fibrotic lung homogenates.[243] Recent data suggest that, in fibrotic lungs, there is a relative excess of TIMPs when compared to collagenases, indicating that there is a nondegrading fibrillar collagen microenvironment in patients with IPF that may contribute to incomplete resolution of the wound.[244] Dunsmore and colleagues reported that collagenase-1, stomelysin-1, and 92-kD gelatinase were not produced in normal or injured lung epithelium but that matrilysin was expressed in migrating airway cells of injured lungs, suggesting a possible role in reepithelialization.[245] Increased procoagulant activity has been described in fibrotic lung disorders.[246–249] The serine protease family includes uPA, plasmin, and neutrophil elastase. Alveolar type II pneumocytes express uPA and its receptor, suggesting an important role for uPA in the regulation of cellular interaction and migration during tissue repair.[250,251] Transgenic mice that overexpressed uPA-1 were more susceptible to bleomycin-induced injury than littermate controls. Neutrophil elastase has been most clearly implicated in an inherited form of human emphysema, α_1-proteinase deficiency but may also be one of many proteases involved in the development of pulmonary fibrosis. In the hamster, administration of a truncated form of the neutrophil elastase inhibitor secretory leukoprotease inhibitor or α_1-antiproteinase ameliorated pulmonary fibrosis resulting from intratracheal administration of bleomycin.[252] Two aspartic proteases, pepsinogen II and cathepsin E, were localized immunohistochemically to alveolar type II cells and bronchiolar Clara cells, and epithelial hyperplasia in the lungs of patients with ILD was associated with enhanced expression of each.[253]

Much of the lung scarring in IPF results from fibrosis within the alveolar space rather than within the interstitium.[254] The exudate that forms the provisional matrix for early fibrogenesis is composed of serum proteins that gain access to the alveolar lumen through the permeablized alveolar basement membrane and epithelial lining; inflammatory cells are recruited through a host of signals from the injured lung (Figure 9–5) (see Chapter 8, "Inflammation in the Pathogenesis of Interstitial Lung Diseases"). The alveolar epithelium performs several functions that suggest it may play an important role in the clearance of the alveolar exudate. Fluid and ion resorption from the air space may occur through water and ion channels that are up-regulated on type I and II cells after lung injury.[7,8,41] Fibrinolytic proteases dissolve clotted proteins in the alveolar space. One of the major proteases that may be involved is plasmin, which is derived from plasminogen within the intra-alveolar exudate. Activation of plasmin is mediated by tissue plasminogen activator or uPA expressed by alveolar epithelial cells and can be inhibited by plasminogen activator inhibitor (PAI)-1.[250] Complexes of uPA and PAI-1 are removed by endocytosis upon binding to the scavenger family molecule GP-330 on the surface of type II cells.[255,256] Clearance of sloughed alveolar epithelial cells and mesenchymal cells within the alveolar space and walls may occur through apoptosis (see below). Apoptotic cells express markers on their surface, which leads to rapid recognition and clearance by phagocytes with little associated inflammation.

Collapse Induration

One hypothesis for the tendency of the lung to scar in IPF is that alveolar walls become irreversibly fused through "collapse induration."[257] In this model, extensive epithelial injury, which leads to near complete denudation of the alveolar membrane, results in flooding of the alveolar space with serum proteins. Monomeric fibrin, fibrin peptides, and other proteins contaminate surfactant and interfere with its function, causing alveolar surface tension to rise.[258,259] The mechanism of inhibition is not clear but may be due to interference with lipoprotein complexes in the alveolar subphase or competition for occupancy of sites within the monolayer.[259] Surfactant dysfunction is compounded by a relative deficiency of specific surfactant components, probably a result of the impaired synthetic capacity of injured type II cells.[260,261] In particular, deficiency of SP-A may render surfactant more vulnerable to inactivation. SP-A has been shown to protect the surface activity of surfactant monolayers from protein inhibition both in vitro and in vivo.[262,263] Elevation of surface tension promotes further alveolar flooding and, ultimately, collapse of the alveolar space. If the reepithelialization of the alveolar membrane is impeded, denuded basement membranes become tightly apposed, and fibrotic fusion of the structures may result in irreversible architectural distortion. Myers and Katsenstein observed ultrastructural evidence of epithelial necrosis and alveolar collapse in a patient with usual interstitial pneumonia.[264] These findings generally support the concept that alveolar collapse following epithelial necrosis plays a role in lung remodeling in ILD.

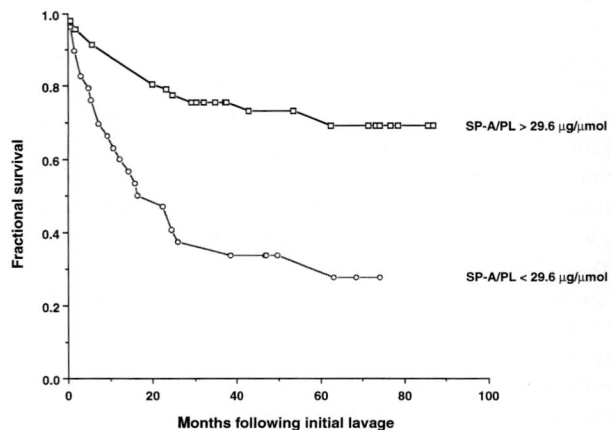

Figure 9–5 Survival of patients with IPF correlates with the level of surfactant protein (SP) A isolated by bronchoalveolar lavage (BAL). SP-A was measured in the BAL fluid of patients with IPF and normalized to total BAL fluid phospholipid (PL) (SP-A:PL) as an index of alveolar sampling. Patients were assigned to two groups based on the relationship of their SP-A:PL value to the median of 29.6 µg/µmol. The 5-year survival of patients with an SP-A:PL above the median was 68%, whereas patients below the median had a 5-year survival of 30% (p = .007). Reproduced with permission from McCormack et al.[290]

AN INTACT EPITHELIAL LAYER IS ESSENTIAL FOR EFFECTIVE WOUND HEALING

Animal models have helped elucidate several characteristics of epithelial injury and repair that are associated with lung scarring rather than effective healing.[265] It is intuitively obvious that a severe epithelial insult is associated with a more pronounced fibrotic response, but there is surprisingly limited experimental evidence to support this notion. Shen and colleagues observed that there was a correlation between the severity of the initial injury and the ultimate degree of fibrosis in rabbits after intratracheal instillation of bleomycin.[266] The extent and localization of the injury to the epithelium was inferred, however, based on the measurement of PO_2 and the route of administration of the drug, respectively. Adamson and colleagues reported that lung explants taken from animals exposed to hyperoxia for prolonged periods (6 days) were more likely to exhibit an enhanced fibrotic response than explants from less severely damaged lungs.[20] If the injury destroys the connective tissue scaffolding, coordinated migration of type II cells is disrupted, and the normal lung architecture is lost or replaced with disorganized connective tissue elements.[265] Repeated injury also increases the tendency of the lung to scar after injury. Hamsters who were challenged with an intratracheal oxidant-generating cocktail of glucose, glucose oxidase, and lactoperoxidase developed a neutrophilic alveolitis that did not progress to fibrosis after a single instillation. Repeated instillations resulted in fibrotic, consolidated parenchyma and polypoid plugs covered by hyperplastic, undifferentiated epithelium within the distal airspaces.[267] These data indicate that repeated or continuous epithelial injury, such as that which is histologically evident throughout the course of IPF, may contribute to the development of pulmonary fibrosis.

The presence of an intact pulmonary epithelial layer suppresses fibroblast proliferation and matrix deposition. This property of the epithelium has been confirmed in vivo and ex vivo with several animal models, which demonstrates that delayed alveolar epithelialization after lung injury leads to an enhanced fibrotic response.[268] Terzaghi and colleagues demonstrated the importance of airway epithelium in limiting fibrosis with the use of tracheal grafts.[269] Grafts that were denuded of and then repopulated with epithelial cells did not scar, but those that were not reepithelialized developed gradual and complete obliteration of the lumen by fibrotic tissue. In another study, mice given intraperitoneal injections of butylated hydroxytoluene (BHT) developed diffuse alveolar damage, characterized by widespread necrosis of the alveolar epithelium and the capillary bed.[270] The damaged lung parenchyma healed without fibrosis when the repair process was allowed to proceed unimpeded. However, when the mice were treated with BHT and then exposed to hyperoxia or radiation during the epithelial repair phase, they invariably developed diffuse interstitial pulmonary fibrosis.[271,272] If oxygen exposure was delayed until epithelial recovery was completed, no fibrotic changes developed.[268] The same conclusion was reached in a study of acute lung injury in which alveolar epithelialization was delayed with cytotoxic agents.[268] Recently, Hagimoto and colleagues observed that stimulation of pulmonary epithelial apoptosis in mice by repeated inhalation of anti-Fas antibody resulted in the development of pulmonary fibrosis over a 4-week period, associated with early expression of TNF-α and mid- to late-course expression of TGF-β.[26] These observations suggest that the epithelial cells may secrete one or more inhibitory mediators that modulate the fibroblast response (such as PGE_2) and that loss of the epithelial layer shifts the balance toward fibroblast migration and activation. Alternatively, apoptotic type II cells may release proinflammatory mediators. Damage to the DNA of alveolar type II cells, and the resultant apoptosis, is thought to play an important role in the development of bleomycin-induced lung fibrosis and even in the markedly delayed pulmonary fibrosis seen in children given carmustine.[26,273–275] It remains to be determined whether the altered replicative or reparative potential of damaged type II cells plays a role in the scarring process in IPF.

Ultrastructural and in situ labeling studies suggest that inappropriate or premature apoptosis may play an important role in the epithelial cell dropout that is a consistent histopathologic feature in IPF biopsy specimens.[31,33] Enrichment in apoptosis adjacent to fibroblastic foci suggests that programed cell death may be induced by signals or factors arising from the mesenchymal compartment. In support of this notion, fibroblasts isolated from injured rodent lungs have been shown to induce apoptosis in alveolar epithelial cells in vitro.[30] Recent evidence suggests that autocrine control of epithelial apoptosis may be mediated by angiotensinogen and angiotensin II or through Fas-dependent pathways.[31,276] Fas antigen is a type 1 membrane receptor protein and member of the TNF superfamily that induces apoptosis upon binding of another cell surface molecule called Fas ligand. Fas and Fas ligand are critical for the process of negative selection that removes autoreactive lymphocytes, but expression has also been described in epithelial progenitor cells in the liver, skin, ovary, and lung.[277] Fas expression has also been reported to be up-regulated in IPF lungs as has Fas death domain protein and the apoptosis-associated proteases caspase-1 and caspase-3.[276,278] Fas expression is restricted to a subpopulation of type II cells in the lungs of mice and apoptosis can be induced by intratracheal administration of an anti-Fas antibody that mimics the Fas ligand.[25] In mice with bleomycin-induced pulmonary fibrosis, Fas mRNA was up-regulated in alveolar epithelial cells, and Fas ligand mRNA was increased in lung lymphocytes.[26] TNF-α and TGF-β up-regulate apoptotic cofactors in hyperplastic type II cells, which are required for Fas-dependent cell death.[279] The evidence regarding whether Fas/Fas ligand-mediated apoptosis is required for pulmonary fibrosis is conflicting, however.[276,280] Collectively, the available data suggest that increased apoptosis in IPF may play an important role in the loss of the antifibrogenic effects of an intact pulmonary epithelium and in tissue remodeling after injury. Inhibition of alveolar epithelial apoptosis with captopril is a strategy for limiting pulmonary fibrosis that is currently being explored in clinical trials in Mexico.[2]

SURFACTANT COMPONENTS AS EPITHELIAL MARKERS OF DISEASE ACTIVITY AND PROGRESSION

One of the major functions of the alveolar epithelium is the production of pulmonary surfactant. Surfactant secreted by alveolar type II cells forms a monolayer at the air–liquid interface of the lung that resists compression and reduces surface tension. The major surfactant phospholipids are dipalmitoylphosphatidylcholine (DPPC), which accounts for most of the surface tension-lowering activity of surfactant, and unsaturated phosphatidylcholine (PC), phosphatidylglycerol (PtdGro), and phosphatidylinositol (PI). The major protein components of surfactant are the surfactant proteins A, B, C, and D. SP-B and SP-C are hydrophobic proteins that assist in the adsorption and spreading of phospholipids at the air–liquid interface of the lung. SP-A and SP-D are hydrophilic glycoproteins that may play a role in surfactant function, but increasing evidence suggests that their principal roles may be as host defense proteins.[281] SP-D may also be important for maintaining alveolar structure and surfactant homeostasis.

Surfactant deficiency and dysfunction in the infant and acute respiratory distress syndromes result in physiological abnormalities that are also characteristic of the ILDs, including reduced lung compliance, increased work of breathing, and impaired gas exchange. Surfactant components also have been shown to be abnormal in several of the ILDs including IPF. In rats with bleomycin-induced pulmonary fibrosis, elastic recoil of the lung is increased and part of the loss in compliance is clearly due to abnormalities in the physical properties of surfactant.[282,283] In patients with ILD, however, the expansion of the interstitium of the lung with inflammatory cells and excess connective tissue matrix causes restrictive and gas exchange abnormalities that confound attempts to characterize the impact of surfactant abnormalities in ILD with physiological measurements. Very recent evidence that mutations in the surfactant protein C gene can result in pulmonary fibrosis highlights the importance of surfactant component in the pathogenesis of ILD (see Chapter 7, "Genetic Basis of Interstitial Lung Disease"). However, the extent to which surfactant dysfunction contributes to the altered physiology of ILD remains unclear.

However, the levels of several surfactant components in the lung may be useful as markers of disease activity and outcome. Multiple laboratories have confirmed that surfactant recovered by BAL is abnormal in both quantity and composition in patients with IPF.[260,284] Consistent findings include a reduction in total phospholipid (PL) and PtdGro and an increase in PI. Changes in DPPC, PtdGro, and PI in BAL fluids have also been described in a number of animal models of rapidly developing pulmonary fibrosis.[285–288] In one study of 32 patients with IPF, the reduction in PtdGro did not correlate with clinical outcome, but an early and persistent increase in the percentage of PtdGro following therapy was associated with clinical improvement.[289] Robinson and colleagues found that patients with more normal pretreatment total PL recoveries were more likely to respond to therapy, but there was no correlation between clinical outcome and the PtdGro to PI ratio. However, patients with histologically advanced, acellular fibrotic lesions had lower initial PtdGro to PI ratios than patients with more normal ratios who had more reversible alveolar septal inflammatory infiltrates. We also observed that total PL recovered by BAL was reduced in patients with IPF, to levels approximately 60% of those in normal volunteers, but the percentage of total PC that was saturated was not altered.[261] The content of SP-A in lavage was reduced, even when normalized for the total PL recovered. The SP-A to PL ratio at initial lavage correlated both with the course of disease over a 6-month interval, as estimated with the multifarious clinical-radiologic-physiologic (CRP) score and with mortality. The 5-year survival of patients with a ratio of SP-A:PL above the median value was more than twice that of patients below the median (see Figure 9–5).[290] The ratio of SP-A:PL improved upon prediction of survival modeled by most routine physiologic variables, with the exception of percent predicted total lung capacity (TLC) and CRP score. Given the small but not insignificant risk associated with BAL in IPF patients and that simple physiological assessments are as useful for prognostication; the measurement of surfactant components in lavage fluid is not recommended for the routine management of IPF.

Recent data suggest that the ectopic appearance of surfactant components in serum may prove to be more accessible markers for disease progression in IPF than BAL fluid markers. In the serum of healthy subjects, SP-A and SP-D are present at very low levels. Surfactant proteins A and D have recently been shown to be elevated in the serum of patients with a variety of interstitial and infectious lung diseases and in patients with IPF.[291,292] The mechanisms by which SP-A and SP-D gain access to the serum in IPF are not known but may include altered alveolar membrane permeability or alveolar epithelial polarity for secretion. Early studies suggested that the serum surfactant protein levels correlated with disease activity in a small number of patients.[291–293] Takahashi and colleagues subsequently reported that serum levels of SP-A and SP-D correlated with the extent of alveolitis and 3-year mortality but not with the extent of fibrosis.[294,295] Serum SP-D was also predictive of a decline in pulmonary function. In another study, serum SP-D detected computed tomography-documented ILD in scleroderma patients with normal chest radiographs, and normal serum SP-A and SP-D levels were quite specific for excluding ILD in this patient population.[295] Greene and colleagues have recently reported that serum SP-D levels correlate with radiographic abnormalities and that both serum SP-A and SP-D correlate with survival in patients with IPF.[296] The data suggest the SP-A and SP-D may be useful biomarkers in patients with IPF.

SUMMARY

Injury to the alveolar epithelium is a consistent finding in the ILDs. The alveolar type II cell plays an important role in the closure of the epithelial defect, the resorption of excess alveolar fluid, the dissolution of unwanted connective tissue matrix, and the modulation of fibroblast proliferation and matrix production. Each of these functions requires a shift in the synthetic repertoire of the type II cell after injury and the elaboration of specialized cell surface proteins and soluble factors. Many of the signals for adjustment in the type II cell phenotype arise from the extracellular matrix and cells within the mesenchymal compartment. Continuous, repeated, or extensive damage to the epithelium is associated with fibrosis, but when reepithelialization is allowed to progress unimpeded, healing can lead to perfect functional and structural recovery of the injured lung.

Accumulating evidence suggests that in the injured lung the alveolar epithelium is not simply reacting to injury and taking instructions from the environment, but is actually directing the process of repair. Fibrosis in IPF may be due to the failure of the type II cell to coordinate and organize the healing functions of fibroblasts, myofibroblasts, and inflammatory cells at sites of alveolar epithelial damage.

REFERENCES

1. Crystal RG, Bitterman PB, Rennard SI, et al. Interstitial lung diseases of unknown cause: disorders characterized by chronic inflammation of the lower respiratory tract. N Engl J Med 1984;310:154–66.
2. Selman M, King TE, Pardo A. Idiopathic pulmonary fibrosis and evolving hypotheses about its pathogenesis and implications for therapy. Ann Intern Med 2001;134(2):136–51.
3. Mason RJ, Shannon JM. Alveolar type II cells. In: Crystal RG, editor. The lung: scientific foundations. Philadelphia: Lippincot-Raven; 1997.
4. Voelker DR, Mason RJ. Alveolar type II epithelial cells. In: Massaro D, editor. Lung cell biology. New York: Marcel Dekker; 1989. p. 487–538.
5. Witschi H. Proliferation of type II alveolar cells: a review of common responses in toxic lung injury. Toxicology 1976;5:267–77.
6. Bowden DH. Alveolar response to injury. Thorax 1981;2:357–75.
7. King LS, Nielsen S, Agre P. Aquaporin-1 water channel protein in lung: ontogeny, steroid-induced expression and distribution in rat. J Clin Invest 1996;97:2183–91.
8. Lee MD, King LS, Nielsen S, et al. Genomic organization and developmental expression of aquaporin-5 in lung. Chest 1997;111:111S–113S.
9. Cott GR, Sugahara K, Mason RJ. Stimulation of net active ion transport across alveolar type II cell monolayers. Am J Physiol 1986;250:C222–C227.
10. Haskell JF, Yue G, Benos DJ, et al. Upregulation of sodium-conductive pathways in alveolar type II cells in sublethal hyperoxia. Am J Physiol 1994;266:L30–L37.
11. Olivera W, Ridge K, Wood LD, et al. Active sodium transport and alveolar epithelial Na-K-ATPase increase during subacute hyperoxia in rats. Am J Physiol 1994;266:L577–84.
12. Kallenberg CG, Schilizzi BM, Beaumont F, et al. Expression of class II MHC antigens on alveolar epithelium in fibrosing alveolitis. Clin Exp Immunol 1987;67:182–90.
13. Kallenberg CG, Schilizzi BM, Beaumont F, et al. Expression of class II major histocompatibility complex antigens on alveolar epithelium in interstitial lung disease: relevance to the pathogenesis of idiopathic pulmonary fibrosis. J Clin Pathol 1987;40:725–33.
14. Strunk RC, Eidlen DM, Mason RJ. Pulmonary alveolar type II epithelial cells synthesize and secrete proteins of the classical and alternative complement pathways. J Clin Invest 1988;81:1419–26.
15. Coalson JJ. The ultrastructure of human fibrosing alveolitis. Virchows Arch 1982;395:181–99.
16. Corrin B, Dewar A, Rodriquez-Roison R, et al. Fine structural changes in cryptogenic fibrosing alveolitis. J Pathol 1985;147:107–19.
17. Martin P. Wound healing–aiming for perfect skin regeneration. Science 1997;276:75–80.
18. Kuhn C. The pathogenesis of pulmonary fibrosis. Monogr Pathol 1993;36:78–92.
19. Chretien J, Jaubert F, Basset F. Type II pneumocyte injury in human respiratory diseases. Curr Probl Clin Biochem 1983;13:56–72.
20. Adamson IYR, Young L, Bowden DH. Relationship of alveolar epithelial injury and repair to the induction of pulmonary fibrosis. Am J Pathol 1988;130:377–83.
21. Keane MP, Belperio JA, Burdick MD, et al. IL-12 attenuates bleomycin-induced pulmonary fibrosis. Am J Physiol 2001;281(1):L92–7.
22. Bitterman PB, Polunovsky VA, Ingbar DH. Repair after acute lung injury. Chest 1994;105:118S–21S.
23. Suwabe A, Panos RJ, Voelker DR. Alveolar type II cells isolated after silica-induced lung injury in rats have increased surfactant protein A (SP-A) receptor activity. Am J Respir Cell Mol Biol 1991;4:264–72.
24. Mason RJ, Williams MC, Moses HL, et al. Stem cells in lung development, disease, and therapy. Am J Respir Cell Mol Biol 1997;16:355–63.
25. Fine A, Anderson NL, Rothstein TL, et al. Fas expression in pulmonary alveolar type II cells. Am J Physiol 1997;273:L64–71.
26. Hagimoto N, Kuwano K, Nomoto Y, et al. Apotosis and expression of Fas/Fas ligand mRNA in bleomycin-induced pulmonary fibrosis in mice. Am J Respir Cell Mol Biol 1997;16:91–101.
27. Kasper M, Haroske G. Alterations in the alveolar epithelium after injury in pulmonary fibrosis. Histol Histopathol 1996;11:463–83.
28. Adamson IYR, Bowden DH. The type 2 cell as progenitor of alveolar epithelial regeneration. Lab Invest 1974;30:35–42.
29. Evans MJ, Cabral LJ, Stephens RJ, et al. Transformation of alveolar type II cells to type I cells following exposure to nitrogen dioxide. Exp Mol Pathol 1975;22:145–50.
30. Uhal BD, Joshi I, True AL, et al. Fibroblasts isolated after fibrotic lung injury induce apoptosis of alveolar epithelial cells in vitro. Am J Physiol 1995;269(6 Pt 1):L819–28.

31. Wang R, Ramos C, Joshi I, et al. Human lung myofibroblast-derived inducers of alveolar epithelial apoptosis identified as angiotensin peptides. Am J Physiol 1999;277(6 Pt 1): L1158–64.

32. Barbas-Filho JV, Ferreira MA, Sesso A, et al. Evidence of type II pneumocyte apoptosis in the pathogenesis of idiopathic pulmonary fibrosis (IFP)/usual interstitial pneumonia (UIP). J Clin Pathol 2001;54(2):132–8.

33. Uhal BD, Joshi I, Hughes WF, et al. Alveolar epithelial cell death adjacent to underlying myofibroblasts in advanced fibrotic human lung. Am J Physiol 1998;275(6 Pt 1): L1192–9.

34. Clark RAF, Mason RJ, Folkvord JM, et al. Fibronectin mediates adherence of rat alveolar type II epithelial cells via the fibroblastic cell-attachment domain. J Clin Invest 1986; 77:1831–40.

35. Maniscalco WM, Sinkin RA, Watkins RH, et al. Transforming growth factor-β modulates type II cell fibronectin and surfactant protein C expression. Am J Physiol 1994;267: L569–77.

36. Maniscalco WM, Campbell MH. Transforming growth factor-β induces a chondroitin sulfate/dermatan sulfate proteoglycan in alveolar type II cells. Am J Physiol 1994;266: L672–80.

37. Simon RH, Scott MJ, Reza MM, et al. Type IV collagen production by rat pulmonary alveolar epithelial cells. Am J Respir Cell Mol Biol 1993;8:640–6.

38. Sage H, Farin FM, Striker GE, et al. Granular pneumocytes in primary culture secrete several major components of the extracellular matrix. Biochemistry 1983;22:2148–55.

39. Simon RH, Gross TJ, Edwards JA, et al. Fibrin degradation by rat pulmonary alveolar epithelial cells. Am J Physiol 1992; 262:L482–8.

40. Gronski TJ Jr, Martin RL, Kobayashi DK, et al. Hydrolysis of a broad spectrum of extracellular matrix proteins by human macrophage elastase. J Biol Chem 1997;272:12189–94.

41. Borok Z, Lubman RL, Danto SI, et al. Keratinocyte growth factor modulates alveolar epithelial cell phenotype in vitro [abstract]. Am J Respir Crit Care Med 1997;155:A829.

42. Krause DS, Theise ND, Collector MI, et al. Multi-organ, multi-lineage engraftment by a single bone marrow-derived stem cell. Cell 2001;105(3):369–77.

43. Kotton DN, Ma BY, Cardoso WV, et al. Bone marrow-derived cells as progenitors of lung alveolar epithelium. Development 2001;128(24):5181–8.

44. Allen JT, Spiteri MA. Growth factors in idiopathic pulmonary fibrosis: relative roles. Respir Res 2002;3(1):13.

45. Warburton D, Tefft D, Mailleux A, et al. Do lung remodeling, repair, and regeneration recapitulate respiratory ontogeny? Am J Respir Crit Care Med 2001;164(10 Pt 2):S59–S62.

46. Gebb SA, Shannon JM. Tissue interactions mediate early events in pulmonary vasculogenesis. Dev Dyn 2000; 217(2):159–69.

47. Rudnick D. Developmental capacities of the chick lung in chorioallantoic grafts. J Exp Zool 1933;66:125–54.

48. Taderera JT. Control of lung differentiation in vitro. Dev Biol 1967;16:489–512.

49. Ball WD. Development of the rat salivary glands. III. Mesenchymal specificity in the morphogenesis of the embryonic submaxillary and sublingual glands of the rat. J Exp Zool 1974;188:277–88.

50. Michalopoulos GK, DeFrances MC. Liver regeneration. Science 1997;276:60–6.

51. Gospodarowicz D, Ferrara N, Schweigerer L, et al. Structural characterization and biological functions of fibroblast growth factor. Endocrinol Rev 1987;8:95–114.

52. McKeehan WL, Wang F, Kan M. The heparan sulfate-fibroblast growth factor family: diversity of structure and function. Prog Nucleic Acid Res Mol Biol 1998;59:135–76.

53. Weinstein M, Xu X, Ohyama K, et al. FGFR-3 and FGFR-4 function cooperatively to direct alveogenesis in the murine lung. Development 1998;125(18):3615–23.

54. Ornitz DM, Xu J, Colvin JS, et al. Receptor specificity of the fibroblast growth factor family. J Biol Chem 1996;271(25): 15292–7.

55. Mason IJ, Fuller-Pace F, Smith R, et al. FGF-7 (keratinocyte growth factor) expression during mouse development suggests roles in myogenesis, forebrain regionalization and epithelial-mesenchymal interactions. Mech Dev 1994;45: 15–30.

56. Peters K, Werner S, Liao X, et al. Targeted expression of a dominant negative FGF receptor blocks branching morphogenesis and epithelial differentiation of the mouse lung. EMBO J 1994;13:3296–301.

57. Celli G, LaRochelle WJ, Mackem S, et al. Soluble dominant-negative receptor uncovers essential roles for fibroblast growth factors in multi-organ induction and patterning. EMBO J 1998;17(6):1642–55.

58. Arman E, Haffner-Krausz R, Chen Y, et al. Targeted disruption of fibroblast growth factor (FGF) receptor 2 suggests a role for FGF signaling in pregastrulation mammalian development. Proc Natl Acad Sci U S A 1998;95(9):5082–7.

59. Arman E, Haffner-Krausz R, Gorivodsky M, et al. FGFR2 is required for limb outgrowth and lung-branching morphogenesis. Proc Natl Acad Sci U S A 1999;96(21):11895–9.

60. De Moerlooze L, Spencer-Dene B, Revest J, et al. An important role for the IIIb isoform of fibroblast growth factor receptor 2 (FGFR2) in mesenchymal-epithelial signalling during mouse organogenesis. Development 2000;127(3):483–92.

61. Ciruna BG, Schwartz L, Harpal K, et al. Chimeric analysis of fibroblast growth factor receptor-1 (FGFR1) function: a role for FGFR1 in morphogenetic movement through the primitive streak. Development 1997;124(14):2829–41.

62. Fu YM, Spirito P, Yu ZX, et al. Acidic fibroblast growth factor in the developing rat embryo. J Cell Biol 1991;114(6): 1261–73.

63. Han RNN, Liu J, Tanswell AK, et al. Expression of basic fibroblast growth factor and receptor: immunolocalization studies in developing rat fetal lung. Pediatr Res 1992;31:435–40.

64. Gonzalez A-M, Buscaglia M, Ong M, et al. Distribution of basic fibroblast growth factor in the 18-day rat fetus: localization in the basement membranes of diverse tissues. J Cell Biol 1990;110:753–65.

65. Finch PW, Cunha GR, Rubin JS, et al. Pattern of keratinocyte growth factor and keratinocyte growth factor receptor expression during mouse fetal development suggests a role in mediating morphogenetic mesenchymal-epithelial interactions. Dev Dyn 1995;203:223–40.

66. Colvin JS, Feldman B, Nadeau JH, et al. Genomic organization and embryonic expression of the mouse fibroblast growth factor 9 gene. Dev Dyn 1999;216(1):72–88.

67. Bellusci S, Grindley J, Emoto H, et al. Fibroblast growth factor 10 (FGF10) and branching morphogenesis in the embryonic mouse lung. Development 1997;124(23):4867–78.

68. Bellusci S, Furuta Y, Rush MG, et al. Involvement of sonic hedgehog (Shh) in mouse embryonic lung growth and morphogenesis. Development 1997;124:53–63.

69. Hu MC, Qiu WR, Wang YP, et al. FGF-18, a novel member of the fibroblast growth factor family, stimulates hepatic and intestinal proliferation. Mol Cell Biol 1998;18(10):6063–74.

70. Ohbayashi N, Hoshikawa M, Kimura S, et al. Structure and expression of the mRNA encoding a novel fibroblast growth factor, FGF-18. J Biol Chem 1998;273(29):18161–4.

71. Post M, Souza P, Liu J, et al. Keratinocyte growth factor and its receptor are involved in regulating early lung branching. Development 1996;122(10):3107–15.

72. Orr-Urtreger A, Bedford MT, Burakova T, et al. Developmental localization of the splicing alternatives of fibroblast growth factor receptor-2 (FGFR2). Dev Biol 1993;158(2):475–86.

73. Simonet WS, DeRose ML, Bucay N, et al. Pulmonary malformation in transgenic mice expressing human keratinocyte growth factor in the lung. Proc Natl Acad Sci U S A 1995;92:12461–5.

74. Ulich TR, Yi ES, Longmuir K, et al. Keratinocyte growth factor is a growth factor for type II pneumocytes in vivo. J Clin Invest 1994;93:1298–306.

75. Tichelaar JW, Lu W, Whitsett JA. Conditional expression of fibroblast growth factor-7 in the developing and mature lung. J Biol Chem 2000;275(16):11858–64.

76. Shiratori M, Oshika E, Ung LP, et al. Keratinocyte growth factor and embryonic rat lung morphogenesis. Am J Respir Cell Mol Biol 1996;15(3):328–38.

77. Zhou L, Graeff RW, McCray PB Jr, et al. Keratinocyte growth factor stimulates CFTR-independent fluid secretion in the fetal lung in vitro. Am J Physiol 1996;271(6 Pt 1):L987–94.

78. Cardoso WV, Itoh A, Nogawa H, et al. FGF-1 and FGF-7 induce distinct patterns of growth and differentiation in embryonic lung epithelium. Dev Dyn 1997;208:398–405.

79. Deterding RR, Jacoby CR, Shannon JM. Acidic fibroblast growth factor and keratinocyte growth factor stimulate fetal rat pulmonary epithelial growth. Am J Physiol 1996;271(4 Pt 1):L495–505.

80. Shannon JM, Gebb SA, Nielsen LD. Induction of alveolar type II cell differentiation in embryonic tracheal epithelium in mesenchyme-free culture. Development 1999;126(8):1675–88.

81. Sugahara K, Rubin JS, Mason RJ, et al. Keratinocyte growth factor increases mRNAs for SP-A and SP-B in rat alveolar type II cells in culture. Am J Physiol 1995;269:L344–50.

82. Shannon JM, Pan T, Nielsen LD, et al. Lung fibroblasts improve differentiation of rat type II cells in primary culture. Am J Respir Cell Mol Biol 2001;24(3):235–44.

83. Deterding RR, Havill AM, Yano T, et al. Prevention of bleomycin-induced lung injury in rats by keratinocyte growth factor. Proc Assoc Am Physicians 1997;109(3):254–68.

84. Panos RJ, Bak PM, Simonet WS, et al. Intratracheal instillation of keratinocyte growth factor decreases hyperoxia induced mortality in rats. J Clin Invest 1995;96:2026–33.

85. Brauchle M, Angermeyer K, Hubner G, et al. Large induction of keratinocyte growth factor expression by serum growth factors and pro-inflammatory cytokines in cultured fibroblasts. Oncogene 1994;9:3199–204.

86. Chedid M, Rubin JS, Csaky KG, et al. Regulation of keratinocyte growth factor expression by interleukin 1. J Biol Chem 1994;269:10753–7.

87. Simonet WS, DeRose ML, Buay N, et al. Pulmonary malformation in transgenic mice expressing keratinocyte growth factor in the lung. Proc Natl Acad Sci U S A 1995;92:12461–5.

88. Zhou L, Graeff RW, McCray PBJ, et al. Keratinocyte growth factor stimulates CFTR-independent fluid secretion in the fetal lung in vitro. Am J Physiol 1996;271:L987–94.

89. Tsuboi R, Sato C, Kurite Y, et al. Keratinocyte growth factor (FGF-7) stimulates migration and plasminogen activator activity of normal human keratinocytes. J Invest Dermatol 1993;101:49–53.

90. Guo L, Degenstein L, Fuchs E. Keratinocyte growth factor is required for hair development but not for wound healing. Genes Dev 1996;10:165–75.

91. Emoto H, Tagashira S, Mattei MG, et al. Structure and expression of human fibroblast growth factor-10. J Biol Chem 1997;272:23191–4.

92. Yamasaki M, Miyake A, Tagashira S, et al. Structure and expression of the rat mRNA encoding a novel member of the fibroblast growth factor family. J Biol Chem 1996;271:15918–21.

93. Tagashira S, Harada H, Katsumata T, et al. Cloning of mouse FGF10 and up-regulation of its gene expression during wound healing. Gene 1997;197(1–2):399–404.

94. Park WY, Miranda B, Lebeche D, et al. FGF-10 is a chemotactic factor for distal epithelial buds during lung development. Dev Biol 1998;201(2):125–34.

95. Lu W, Luo Y, Kan M, et al. Fibroblast growth factor-10. A second candidate stromal to epithelial cell andromedin in prostate [published erratum appears in J Biol Chem 1999;274(39):28058]. J Biol Chem 1999;274(18):12827–34.

96. Sutherland D, Samakovlis C, Krasnow MA. Branchless encodes a *Drosophila* FGF homolog that controls tracheal cell migration and the pattern of branching. Cell 1996;87(6):1091–101.

97. Weaver M, Dunn NR, Hogan BL. BMP4 and FGF10 play opposing roles during lung bud morphogenesis. Development 2000;127(12):2695–704.

98. Min H, Danilenko DM, Scully et al. FGF-10 is required for both limb and lung development and exhibits striking functional similarity to *Drosophila* branchless. Genes Dev 1998;12(20):3156–61.

99. Sekine K, Ohuchi H, Fujiwara M, et al. FGF10 is essential for limb and lung formation. Nat Genet 1999;21(1):138–41.

100. Clark JC, Tichelaar JW, Wert SE, et al. FGF-10 disrupts lung morphogenesis and causes pulmonary adenomas in vivo. Am J Physiol 2001;280(4):L705–15.

101. Nogawa H, Ito T. Branching morphogenesis of embryonic mouse lung epithelium in mesenchyme-free culture. Development 1995;121:1015–22.

102. Deterding RR, Shannon JM. Proliferation and differentiation of fetal rat pulmonary epithelium in the absence of mesenchyme. J Clin Invest 1995;95:2963–72.

103. Miller DL, Ortega S, Bashayan O, et al. Compensation by fibroblast growth factor 1 (FGF1) does not account for the mild phenotypic defects observed in FGF2-null mice [published erratum appears in Mol Cell Biol 2000;20(10):3752]. Mol Cell Biol 2000;20(6):2260–8.

104. Deterding RR, Jacoby CR, Shannon JM. Acidic fibroblast growth factor and keratinocyte growth factor stimulate fetal rat pulmonary epithelial growth. Am J Physiol 1996;271:L495–L505.

105. Leslie CC, McCormick-Shannon K, Mason RJ, et al. Proliferation of rat alveolar epithelial cells in low density primary culture. Am J Respir Cell Mol Biol 1993;9:64–72.

106. Leslie CC, McCormick-Shannon K, Robinson PC, et al. Stimulation of DNA synthesis in cultured rat alveolar type II cells. Exp Lung Res 1985;8:53–66.

107. Barrios R, Pardo A, Ramos C, et al. Upregulation of acidic fibroblast growth factor during the development of lung fibrosis. Am J Physiol 1997;17:L451–8.

108. Tan EML, Rouda S, Greenbaum SS, et al. Acidic and basic fibroblast growth factors down-regulate collagen gene expression in keloid fibroblasts. Am J Pathol 1993;142:463–70.

109. Gonzalez AM, Hill DJ, Logan A, et al. Distribution of fibroblast growth factor (FGF)-2 and FGF receptor-1 messenger RNA expression and protein presence in the midtrimester human fetus. Pediatr Res 1996;39(3):375–85.

110. Matsui R, Brody JS, Yu Q. FGF-2 induces surfactant protein gene expression in foetal rat lung epithelial cells through a MAPK-independent pathway. Cell Signal 1999;11(3):221–8.

111. Wang F, Kan M, Xu J, et al. Ligand-specific structural domains in the fibroblast growth factor receptor. J Biol Chem 1995;270(17):10222–30.

112. Ortega S, Ittmann M, Tsang SH, et al. Neuronal defects and delayed wound healing in mice lacking fibroblast growth factor 2. Proc Natl Acad Sci U S A 1998;95(10):5672–7.

113. Leslie CC, McCormick-Shannon K, Mason RJ. Heparin-binding growth factors stimulate DNA synthesis in rat alveolar type II cells. Am J Respir Cell Mol Biol 1990;2:99–106.

114. Sannes PL, Khosla J, Johnson S, et al. Basic fibroblast growth factor in fibrosing alveolitis induced by oxygen stress. Chest 1996;109:445–55.

115 Sannes PL, Burch KK, Khosla J. The immunohistochemical localization of epidermal growth factor and acidic and basic fibroblast growth factor in post natal developing and adult rat lungs. Am J Respir Cell Mol Biol 1992;7:230–7.

116. Lappi-Blanco E, Soini Y, Kinnula V, et al. VEGF and bFGF are highly expressed in intraluminal fibromyxoid lesions in bronchiolitis obliterans organizing pneumonia. J Pathol 2002;196(2):220–7.

117. Boonstra J, Rijken P, Humbel B, et al. The epidermal growth factor. Cell Biol Int 1995;19:413–30.

118. Massague J. Transforming growth factor-β. J Biol Chem 1990;265:21393–6.

119. Kumar V, Bustin SA, McKay IA. Transforming growth factor-α. Cell Biol Int 1995;19:373–88.

120. Ullrich A, Schelssinger J. Signal transduction by receptors with tyrosine kinase activity. Cell 1990;61:203–12.

121. Shiratori M, Michalopoulos R, Shinozuka H, et al. Hepatocyte growth factor stimulates DNA synthesis in alveolar epithelial type II cells in vitro. Am J Respir Cell Mol Biol 1995;12:171–80.

122. Ryan RM, Mineo-Kuhn MM, Kramer CM, et al. Growth factors alter neonatal type II alveolar epithelial cell proliferation. Am J Physiol 1994;266:L17–22.

123. Warburton D, Seth R, Shum L, et al. Epigenetic role of epidermal growth factor expression and signalling in embryonic mouse lung morphogenesis. Dev Biol 1992;149:123–33.

124. Miettinen PJ, Berger JE, Meneses J, et al. Epithelial immaturity and multiorgan failure in mice lacking epidermal growth factor receptor. Nature 1995;376:337–41.

125. Sibilia M, Wagner EF. Strain-dependent epithelial defects in mice lacking the EGF receptor. Science 1995;269:234–8.

126. Raaberg L, Nexo E, Buckley S, et al. Epidermal growth factor transcription, translation and signal transduction by rat type II pneumocytes in culture. Am J Respir Cell Mol Biol 1992;6:44–9.

127. Strandjord TP, Clark JC, Guralnick DE, et al. Immunolocalization of transforming growth factor-α, epidermal growth factor (EGF) and EGF-receptor in normal and injured developing human lung. Pediatr Res 1995;38:851–5.

128. Madtes DK, Busby TP, Strandjord TP, et al. Expression of transforming growth factor-α and epidermal growth factor is increased following bleomycin-induced lung injury in rats. Am J Respir Cell Mol Biol 1994;11:540–51.

129. Liu JY, Morris GF, Lei WH, et al. Upregulated expression of transforming growth factor-α in the bronchiolar-alveolar duct regions of asbestos-exposed rats. Am J Pathol 1996;149:205–17.

130. Vivekananda J, Lin A, Coalson JJ, et al. Acute inflammatory injury in the lung precipitated by oxidant stress induces fibroblasts to synthesize and release transforming growth factor-α. J Biol Chem 1994;269:25057–61.

131. Chesnutt AN, Kheradmand F, Folkesson HG, et al. Soluble transforming growth factor-α is present in the pulmonary edema fluid of patients with acute lung injury. Chest 1997;111:652–6.

132. Korfhagen TR, Swantz RJ, Wert SE, et al. Respiratory epithelial cell expression of human transforming growth factor-α induces lung fibrosis in transgenic mice. J Clin Invest 1994;93:1691–9.

133. Hardie WD, Kerlakian CB, Bruno MD, et al. Reversal of lung lesions in transgenic transforming growth factor-α mice by expression of mutant epidermal growth factor receptor. Am J Respir Cell Mol Biol 1996;15:499–508.

134. Abraham JA, Damm D, Bajardi J, et al. Heparin-binding EGF-like growth factor: characterization of rat and mouse cDNA clones, protein domain conservation across species, and transcript expression in tissues. Biochem Biophys Res Commun1993;190:125–33.

135. Leslie CC, McCormick-Shannon K, Shannon J, et al. Heparin-binding EGF-like growth factor is a mitogen for rat alveolar type II cells. Am J Resp Cell Mol Biol 1997;16:379–87.

136. Powell PP, Klagsbrun M, Abraham JA, et al. Eosinophils expression heparin-binding growth factor mRNA localize around lung microvessels in pulmonary hypertension. Am J Pathol 1993;143:784–93.

137. Nobes CD, Hall A. Rho, rac, ad cdc42 GTPases regulate the assembly of focal complexes associated with actin stress fibers, lamellipodia and filopodia. Cell 1995;81:53–62.

138. Ridley AJ, Hall A. The small GTP-binding protein rho regulates the assembly of focal adhesions and actin stress fibers in response to growth factors. Cell 1992;70:389–99.

139. Ridley AJ, Comoglio PM, Hall A. Regulation of scatter factor/hepatocyte growth factor responses by ras, rac, and rho in MDCK cells. Mol Cell Biol 1995;15:1110–22.

140. Ganser GL, Stricklin GP, Matrisian L. EGF and TGF-α influence in vitro lung development by the induction of matrix-degrading metalloproteinases. Int J Dev Biol 1991;35:453–61.

141. Buisson AC, Zahm JM, Polette M, et al. Gelatinase B is involved in the in vitro wound repair of human respiratory epithelium. J Cell Physiol 1996;166:413–26.

142. Folkesson HG, Pittet JF, Nitenberg G, et al. Transforming growth factor-α increases alveolar liquid clearance in anesthetized ventilated rats. Am J Physiol 1996;271:L236–44.

143. Plopper CG, St. George JA, Read LC, et al. Acceleration of alveolar type II cell differentiation in fetal rhesus monkey lung by administration of EGF. Am J Physiol 1992;262:L313–21.

144. Goetzman BW, Read LC, Plopper CG, et al. Prenatal exposure to epidermal growth factor attenuates respiratory distress syndrome in rhesus infants. Pediatr Res 1994;35:30–6.

145. Nakamura T, Nishizawa T, Hagiya M, et al. Molecular cloning and expression of human hepatocyte growth factor. Nature 1989;342:440–3.

146. Nakamura T. Structure and function of hepatocyte growth factor. Prog Growth Factor Res 1991;3:67–85.

147. Bottaro DP, Rubin JS, Faletto DL, et al. Identification of the hepatocyte growth factor receptor as the c-met-proto-oncogene product. Science 1991;251:802–4.

148. Naldini L, Weidner KM, Vigna E, et al. Scatter factor and hepatocyte growth factor are indistinguishable ligands for the MET receptor. EMBO J 1991;10:2867–78.

149. Weidner KM, Hartmann G, Sachs M, et al. Properties and functions of scatter factor/hepatocyte growth factor. Am J Respir Cell Mol Biol 1993;8:229–37.

150. Gohda E, Tsubouchi H, Nakayama H, et al. Purification and partial characterization of hepatocyte growth factor from plasma of a patient with fulminant hepatic failure. J Clin Invest 1988;81:414–9.

151. Yanagita K, Matsumoto K, Sekiguchi K, et al. Hepatocyte growth factor may act as a pulmotropic factor on lung regeneration after acute lung injury. J Biol Chem 1993;268:21212–7.

152. Adamson IY, Bakowska J. Relationship of keratinocyte growth factor and hepatocyte growth factor levels in rat lung lavage fluid to epithelial cell regeneration after bleomycin. Am J Pathol 1999;155(3):949–54.

153. Yaekashiwa M, Nakayama S, Ohnuma K, et al. Simultaneous or delayed administration of hepatocyte growth factor equally represses the fibrotic changes in murine lung injury induced by bleomycin. A morphologic study. Am J Respir Crit Care Med 1997;156(6):1937–44.

154. Dohi M, Hasegawa T, Yamamoto K, et al. Hepatocyte growth factor attenuates collagen accumulation in a murine model of pulmonary fibrosis. Am J Respir Crit Care Med 2000;162(6):2302–7.

155. Adamson IY, Bakowska J. KGF and HGF are growth factors for mesothelial cells in pleural lavage fluid after intratracheal asbestos. Exp Lung Res 2001;27(7):605–16.

156. Yamada T, Hisanaga M, Nakajima Y, et al. Enhanced expression of hepatocyte growth factor by pulmonary ischemia-reperfusion injury in the rat. Am J Respir Crit Care Med 2000;162(2 Pt 1):707–15.

157. Yanagita K, Nagaike M, Ishibashi H, et al. Lung may have an endocrine function producing hepatocyte growth factor in response to injury of distal organs. Biochem Biophys Res Commun 1992;182:802–9.

158. Kitamura N, Miyazawa K, Uehara Y, et al. Gene expression and regulation of HGF-SF. EXS 1993;65:49–65.

159. Moghul A, Lin L, Beedle A, et al. Modulation of c-Met proto-oncogene (HGF receptor) mRNA abundance by cytokines and hormones: evidence for rapid decay of the 8-kb c-Met transcript. Oncogene 1994;9:2045–52.

160. Matsumoto K, Okazaki H, Nakamura T. Up-regulation of hepatocyte growth factor gene expression by interleukin-1 in human skin fibroblasts. Biochem Biophys Res Comm 1992;188:235–43.

161. Rubin JS, Chan AM-L, Bottaro DP, et al. A broad spectrum human fibroblast derived mitogen is a variant of hepatocyte growth factor. Proc Natl Acad Sci U S A 1991;88:415–9.

162. Panos RJ, Patel R, Bak PM. Intratracheal administration of hepatocyte growth factor/scatter factor stimulates rat alveolar type II cell proliferation in vivo. Am J Respir Cell Mol Biol 1996;15:574–81.

163. Liu M-L, Mars WM, Zarnegar R, et al. Collagenase pretreatment and the mitogenic effects of hepatocyte growth factor and transforming growth factor-α in adult rat liver. Hepatology 1994;19:1521–7.

164. Roos F, Ryan AM, Chamow SM, et al. Induction of liver growth in normal mice by infusion of hepatocyte growth factor/scatter factor. Am J Physiol 1995;268:G380–6.

165. Webber EM, Godowski PJ, Fausto N. In vivo response of hepatocytes to growth factors requires and initial priming stimulus. Hepatology 1994;19:489–97.

166. Rifkin DB. Plasminogen activator expression and matrix degradation. Matrix Suppl 1992;1:20–2.

167. Blasi F. Urokinase and urokinase receptor:a paracrine/autocrine system in regulating cell migration. Bioessays 1993;15:105–11.

168. Naldini L, Vigna E, Bardelli A, et al. Biological activation of pro-HGF (hepatocyte growth factor) by urokinase is controlled by a stoichiometric reaction. J Biol Chem 1995;270:603–11.

169. Mars WM, Zarnegar R, Michalopoulos GK. Activation of hepatocyte growth factor by the plasminogen activators uPA and tPA. Am J Pathol 1993;143(3):949–58.

170. Mason RJ, McCormick-Shannon K, Rubin JS, et al. Hepatocyte growth factor is a mitogen for alveolar type II cells in rat lavage fluid. Am J Physiol 1996;271:L46–53.

171. Sakai T, Satoh K, Matsushima K, et al. Hepatocyte growth factor in bronchoalveolar lavage fluids and cells in patients with inflammatory diseases of the lower respiratory tract:detection by RIA and in situ hybridization. Am J Respir Cell Mol Biol 1997;16:388–97.

172. Verghese GM, McCormick-Shannon K, Mason RJ, et al. Hepatocyte growth factor and keratinocyte growth factor in the pulmonary edema fluid of patients with acute lung injury. Biologic and clinical significance. Am J Respir Crit Care Med 1998;158(2):386–94.

173. Pennica D, Nedwin GE, Hayflick JS, et al. Human tumour necrosis factor:precursor structure, expression and homology to lymphotoxin. Nature 1984;312(5996):724–9.

174. Piguet PF, Ribaux C, Karpuz V, et al. Expression and localization of tumor necrosis factor-α and its mRNA in idiopathic pulmonary fibrosis. Am J Pathol 1993;143(3):651–5.

175. Fujita M, Shannon JM, Irvin CG, et al. Overexpression of

176. Whyte M, Hubbard R, Meliconi R, et al. Increased risk of fibrosing alveolitis associated with interleukin-1 receptor antagonist and tumor necrosis factor-α gene polymorphisms. Am J Respir Crit Care Med 2000;162(2 Pt 1):755–8.

177. Kapanci Y, Desmouliere A, Pache JC, et al. Cytoskeletal protein modulation in pulmonary alveolar myofibroblasts during idiopathic pulmonary fibrosis. Possible role of transforming growth factor-β and tumor necrosis factor-α. Am J Respir Crit Care Med 1995;152(6 Pt 1):2163–9.

178. Antoniades HN, Neville-Golden J, Galanopoulos T, et al. Expression of monocyte chemoattractant protein 1 mRNA in human idiopathic pulmonary fibrosis. Proc Natl Acad Sci U S A 1992;89:5371–5.

179. Paine Rr, Rolfe MW, Standiford TJ, et al. MCP-1 expression by rat type II alveolar cells in primary culture. J Immunol 1993;150:4561–70.

180. Crestani B, Cornillet P, Dehoux M, et al. Alveolar type II epithelial cells produce interleukin-6 in vitro and in vivo. Regulation by alveolar macrophage secretory products. J Clin Invest 1994;94:731–40.

181. Kunkel SL, Standiford T, Kasahara K, et al. Interleukin-8 is the major neutrophil chemotactic factor in the lung. Exp Lung Res 1991;17:17–23.

182. Elias JA, Zheng T, Einarsson O, et al. Epithelial interleukin 11. Regulation by cytokines, respiratory syncytial virus, and retinoic acid. J Biol Chem 1994;269:22261–8.

183. Blau HS, Riklis V, Kravstov V, et al. Secretion of cytokines by rat alveolar epithelial cells:possible regulatory role for SP-A. Am J Physiol 1994;266:L148–55.

184. Blau H, Riklis S, Minc-Golomb D, et al. Nitric oxide production in vitro by rat alveolar macrophages can be modulated in vitro by surfactant protein A. Am J Physiol 1997;272:L1198–204.

185. De Larco JE, Todaro GJ. Growth factors from murine sarcoma virus transformed cells. Proc Natl Acad Sci U S A 1978;75:4001–5.

186. Roberts AB, Sporn MB. In: Sporn MB, Roberts AB, editors. Peptide growth factors and their receptors. New York: Springer; 1990.

187. Liu Q, Huang SS, Huang JS. Function of the type V transforming growth factor-β receptor in transforming growth factor-β-induced growth inhibition of mink lung epithelial cells. J Biol Chem 1997;272:18891–5.

188. Lasky JA, Brody AR. Interstitial fibrosis and growth factors. Environ Health Perspect 2000;108 Suppl 4:751–62. http://62lasky/abstract.html.

189. Williams AO, Flanders KC, Saffioti U. Immunohistochemical localization of transforming growth factor-β1 in rats with experimental silicosis and alveolar type II epithelial hyperplasia and lung cancer. Am J Physiol 1993;142:L1831–40.

190. Corrin B, Butcher D, McAnulty BJ, et al. Immunohistochemical localization of transforming growth factor-β1 in the lungs of patients with systemic sclerosis, cryptogenic fibrosing alveolitis, and other lung disorders. Histopathology 1994;24:145–50.

191. Khalil N, O'Connor R, Unruh H, et al. Increased production and immunocytochemical localization of transforming growth factor-β (TGF-β) in idiopathic pulmonary fibrosis (IPF). Am J Respir Cell Mol Biol 1991;5:155–62.

192. Khalil N, O'Connor RN, Unruh HW, et al. Increased production and immunohistochemical localization of transforming growth factor-β in idiopathic pulmonary fibrosis. Am J Respir Cell Mol Biol 1991;5:155–62.

193. Moses HL, Yang EY, Pietenpol JA. TGF-β stimulation and inhibition of cell proliferation: new mechanistic insights. Cell 1990;63:245–9.

tumor necrosis factor-α produces an increase in lung volumes and pulmonary hypertension. Am J Physiol 2001;280(1):L39–L49.

194. Sime PJ, Xing Z, Graham FL, et al. Adenovector-mediated gene transfer of active transforming growth factor-β1 induces prolonged severe fibrosis in rat lung. J Clin Invest 1997;100(4):768–76.

195. Zhang K, Flanders KC, Phan SH. Cellular localization of transforming growth factor-β expression in bleomycin-induced pulmonary fibrosis. Am J Pathol 1995;147:352–61.

196. Munger JS, Huang X, Kawakatsu H, et al. The integrin $\alpha_v\beta_6$ binds and activates latent TGF-β1: a mechanism for regulating pulmonary inflammation and fibrosis. Cell 1999; 96(3):319–28.

197. Broekelmann TJ, Limper AH, Colby TV, et al. Transforming growth factor β is present at sites of extracellular matrix gene expression in human pulmonary fibrosis. Proc Natl Acad Sci U S A 1991;88:6642–6.

198. Giri SN, Hyde DM, Hollinger MA. Effect of antibody to transforming growth factor-β on bleomycin-induced accumulation of lung collagen in mice. Thorax 1993;48:959–66.

199. Raghu G, Johnson WC, Lockhart D, et al. Treatment of idiopathic pulmonary fibrosis with a new antifibrotic agent, pirfenidone:results of a prospective, open-label Phase II study. Am J Respir Crit Care Med 1999;159(4 Pt 1):1061–9.

200. Marinelli WA, Polunovsky VA, Harmon KR, et al. Role of platelet-derived growth factor in pulmonary fibrosis. Am J Respir Cell Mol Biol 1991;5:503–4.

201. Waterfield MD, Scrace GT, Whittle N, et al. Platelet-derived growth factor is structurally related to the putative transforming p28sis of simian sarcoma virus. Nature 1983;304:35–9.

202. Ross RJA, Glomset B, Kariya B, et al. A platelet-dependent serum factor that stimulates the proliferation of arterial smooth muscle cells in vitro. Proc Natl Acad Sci U S A 1974;71:1207–10.

203. Claesson-Welsh L. Signal transduction by the PDGF receptors. Progr Growth Factor Res 1994;5:37–54.

204. Meyer-Ingold W, Eichner W. Platelet-derived growth factor. Cell Biol Int 1995;19:389–98.

205. Liu J-Y, Morris GF, Lei W-H, et al. Rapid activation of PDGF-A and -B expression at sites of lung injury in asbestos-exposed rats. Am J Respir Cell Mol Biol 1997;17:129–40.

206. Yoshida M, Sakuma J, Hayashi S, et al. A histologically distinctive interstitial pneumonia induced by overexpression of the interleukin 6, transforming growth factor-β1, or platelet-derived growth factor B gene. Proc Natl Acad Sci U S A 1995;92(21):9570–4.

207. Vignaud JM, Allam M, Martinet N, et al. Presence of platelet-derived growth factor in normal and fibrotic lung is specifically associated with interstitial macrophages, while both interstitial macrophages and alveolar epithelial cells express the c-sis proto-oncogene. Am J Respir Cell Mol Biol 1991;5:155–62.

208. Antoniades HN, Bravo MA, Avila RE, et al. Platelet-derived growth factor in idiopathic pulmonary fibrosis. J Clin Invest 1990;86:1055–64.

209. Homma S, Nagaoka I, Abe H, et al. Localization of platelet-derived growth factor and insulin-like growth factor I in the fibrotic lung. Am J Respir Crit Care Med 1995;152(6 Pt 1):2084–9.

210. Gurujeyalakshmi G, Hollinger MA, Giri SN. Pirfenidone inhibits PDGF isoforms in bleomycin hamster model of lung fibrosis at the translational level. Am J Physiol 1999;276(2 Pt 1):L311–8.

211. Pan T, Mason RJ, Westcott JY, et al. Rat alveolar type II cells inhibit lung fibroblast proliferation in vitro. Am J Respir Cell Mol Biol 2001;25(3):353–61.

212. Huffman Reed JA, Rice WR, Zsengeller ZK, et al. GM-CSF enhances lung growth and causes alveolar type II epithelial cell hyperplasia in transgenic mice. Am J Physiol 1997;273(4 Pt 1):L715–25.

213. Moore BB, Coffey MJ, Christensen P, et al. GM-CSF regulates bleomycin-induced pulmonary fibrosis via a prostaglandin-dependent mechanism. J Immunol 2000;165(7):4032–9.

214. Wilborn J, Crofford LJ, Burdick MD, et al. Cultured lung fibroblasts isolated from patients with idiopathic pulmonary fibrosis have a diminished capacity to synthesize prostaglandin E2 and to express cyclooxygenase-2. J Clin Invest 1995;95(4):1861–8.

215. Moore KW, O'Garra R, deWaal Malfut R, et al. Interleukin 10. Annu Rev Immunol 1993;11:165–90.

216. Badgett AJ, Bonner JC, Brody AR. Interferon γ modulates lung macrophage production of PDGF-BB and fibroblast growth. J Lipid Mediat Cell Signal 1996;13:89–97.

217. Young L, Adamson IY. Epithelial-fibroblast interactions in bleomycin-induced lung injury and repair. Environ Health Perspect 1993;101:56–61.

218. Adamson IY, Young L, King GM. Reciprocal epithelial-fibroblast interactions in the control of fetal and adult rat lung cells in culture. Exp Lung Res 1991;17:821–35.

219. Bowden DH, Young L, Adamson IY. Fibroblast inhibition does not promote normal lung repair after hyperoxia. Exp Lung Res 1994;20:251–62.

220. Evans MJ, Van Winkle LS, Fanucchi MV, et al. The attenuated fibroblast sheath of the respiratory tract epithelial-mesenchymal trophic unit. Am J Respir Cell Mol Biol 1999;21(6):655–7.

221. Brewster CE, Howarth PH, Djukanovic R, et al. Myofibroblasts and subepithelial fibrosis in bronchial asthma. Am J Respir Cell Mol Biol 1990;3(5):507–11.

222. Roche WR. Inflammatory and structural changes in the small airways in bronchial asthma. Am J Respir Crit Care Med 1998;157(5 Pt 2):S191–4.

223. Adamson IYR, Hedgecock C, Bowden DH. Epithelial cell-fibroblast interactions in lung injury and repair. Am J Pathol 1990;137:385–92.

224. Sheppard D. Epithelial integrins. Bioessays 1996;18:655–60.

225. Ruoslahti E, Reed JC. Anchorage dependence, integrins, and apotosis. Cell 1994;77:477–8.

226. Juliano RL, Haskill S. Signal transduction from the extracellular matrix. J Cell Biol 1993;120:577–85.

227. Hynes RO. Integrins: versatility, modulation, and signaling in cell adhesion. Cell 1992;69:11–25.

228. Kumar NM, Sigurdson SL, Sheppard D, et al. Differential modulation of integrin receptors and extracellular matrix laminin by transforming growth factor-β1 in rat alveolar epithelial cells. Exp Cell Res 1995;221:385–94.

229. Chen JD, Kim JP, Zhang K, et al. Epidermal growth factor (EGF) promotes human keratinocyte locomotion on collagen by increasing the α_2-integrin subunit. Exp Cell Res 1993;209:26602–5.

230. Bartfield NS, Pasquale EB, Geltosky JE, et al. The $\alpha_v\beta_3$-integrin associates with a 190-kDa protein that is phosphorylated on tyrosine in response to platelet-derived growth factor. J Biol Chem 1993;268:17270–6.

231. Bellas RE, Bendori R, Farmer SR. Epidermal growth factor activation of vinculin and β1-integrin gene transcription in quiescent Swiss 3T3 cells. Regulation through a protein kinase C-independent pathway. J Biol Chem 1991;266:12008–14.

232. Kim HJ, Ingbar DH, Henke CA. Integrin mediation of type II cell adherence to provisional matrix proteins. Am J Physiol 1996;271:L277–86.

233. Guzman J, Izumi T, Nagai S, et al. ICAM-1 and integrin expression on isolated human alveolar type II cells. Eur Respir J 1994;7:736–9.

234. Kim HJ, Henke CA, Savik SK, et al. Integrin mediation of alveolar epithelial cell migration on fibronectin and type I collagen. Am J Physiol 1997;273:L134–41.

235. Fukuda Y, Basset F, Ferrans VJ, et al. Significance of early intraalveolar fibrotic lesions and integrin expression in lung biopsy specimens from patients with idiopathic pulmonary fibrosis. Human Pathol 1995;26:53–61.

236. Wu F, Buckley S, Bui KC, et al. Differential expression of cyclin D2 and cdc2 genes in proliferating and nonproliferating alveolar epithelial cells. Am J Respir Cell Mol Biol 1995;12:95–103.

237. Kasper M, Huber O, Grobmann H, et al. Immunocytochemical distribution of E-cadherin in normal and injured lung tissue of the rat. Cell Biol 1995;104:383–90.

238. Kasper M, Behrens J, Schuh D, et al. Distribution of E-cadherin and EpCAM in the human lung during development and after injury. Histochemistry 1995;103:281–6.

239. Burns AR, Takei F, Doerschuk CM. Quantitation of ICAM-1 expression in mouse lung during pneumonia. J Immunol 1994;153:3189–98.

240. Kang BH, Crapo JD, Wegner CD, et al. Intercellular adhesion molecule-1 expression on the alveolar epithelium and its modification by hyperoxia. Am J Respir Cell Mol Biol 1993;9:350–5.

241. Hayashi T, Stetler-Stevenson WG, Fleming MV, et al. Immunohistochemical study of metalloproteinases and their inhibitors in the lungs of patients with diffuse alveolar damage and idiopathic pulmonary fibrosis. Am J Pathol 1996;149:1241–56.

242. Matrisian LM. Metalloproteinases and their inhibitors in connective tissue remodelling. Trends Genet 1990;6:121–5.

243. Pardo A, Selman M, Ramirez R, et al. Alveolar epithelial cells constituitively produce several members of the matrix metalloproteinase family [abstract]. Am J Respir Crit Care Med 1992;651:802A.

244. Selman M, Ruiz V, Cabrera S, et al. TIMP-1, -2, -3, and -4 in idiopathic pulmonary fibrosis: a prevailing nondegradative lung microenvironment? Am J Physiol 2000;279(3):L562–74.

245. Dunsmore SE, Saarialho-Kere UK, Roby JD, et al. Matrilysin expression and function in airway epithelium. J Clin Invest 1998;102(7):1321–31.

246. Kotani I, Sato A, Hayakawa H, et al. Increased procoagulant and antifibrinolytic activities in the lungs with idiopathic pulmonary fibrosis. Thromb Res 1995;77(6):493–504.

247. Imokawa S, Sato A, Hayakawa H, et al. Tissue factor expression and fibrin deposition in the lungs of patients with idiopathic pulmonary fibrosis and systemic sclerosis. Am J Respir Crit Care Med 1997;156(2 Pt 1):631–6.

248. Chapman HA, Allen CL, Stone OL. Abnormalities in pathways of alveolar fibrin turnover among patients with interstitial lung disease. Am Rev Respir Dis 1986;133(3):437–43.

249. Chapman HA, Bertozzi P, Reilly JJ. Role of enzymes mediating thrombosis and thrombolysis in lung disease. Chest 1988;93:1256–63.

250. Gross TJ, Simon RH, Kelly CJ, et al. Rat alveolar epithelial cells concomitantly express plasminogen activator inhibitor-1 and urokinase. Am J Physiol 1991;260:L286–95.

251. Gross TJ, Simon RH, Sitrin RG. Expression of urokinase-type plasminogen activator by rat pulmonary alveolar epithelial cells. Am J Respir Cell Mol Biol 1990;3:449–56.

252. Mitsuhashi H, Asano S, Nonaka T, et al. Administration of truncated secretory leukoprotease inhibitor ameliorates bleomycin-induced pulmonary fibrosis in hamsters. Am J Respir Crit Care Med 1996;153:369–74.

253. Bosi F, Silini E, Luisetti M, et al. Aspartic proteases in normal lung and intersitital pulmonary diseases. Am J Respir Cell Mol Biol 1993;8:626–32.

254. Kuhn IC, Boldt J, King TE Jr, et al. An immunohistochemical study of architectural remodeling and connective tissue synthesis in pulmonary fibrosis. Am Rev Respir Dis 1989;140:1693–703.

255. Steffanson S, Kounnas MZ, Henkin J, et al. GP330 on type II pneumocytes mediates endocytosis leading to degradation of pro-urokinase, plasminogen activator inhibitor-1 and urokinase-plasminogen activator inhibitor-1 complex. J Cell Sci 1995;108:2361–8.

256. Moestrup SK, Nielsen S, Andreasen P, et al. Epithelial glycoprotein-330 mediates endocytosis of plasminogen activator inhibitor type 1 complexes. J Biol Chem 1993;268:16564–70.

257. Burkhardt A. Alveolitis and collapse in the pathogenesis of pulmonary fibrosis. Am Rev Respir Dis 1989;140:513–24.

258. Holm BA. Surfactant inactivation in the adult respiratory distress syndrome. In: Robertson B, van Golde LMG, Batenburg JJ, editors. Pulmonary surfactant: from molecular biology to clinical practice. Amsterdam: Elsevier; 1992.

259. Holm BA, Enhorning G, Notter RH. A biophysical mechanism by which plasma proteins inhibit lung surfactant activity. Chem Phys Lipids 1988;49:49–55.

260. Robinson PC, Watters LC, King TE, et al. Idiopathic pulmonary fibrosis. Abnormalities in bronchoalveolar lavage fluid phospholipids. Am Rev Respir Dis 1988;137:585–91.

261. McCormack FX, King Jr TE, Voelker DR, et al. Idiopathic pulmonary fibrosis. Abnormalities in the bronchoalveolar lavage content of surfactant protein A. Am Rev Respir Dis 1991;144:160–6.

262. Cockshutt AM, Weitz J, Possmayer F. Pulmonary surfactant protein A enhances the surface activity of lipid extract surfactant and reverses inhibition by blood proteins in vitro. Biochemistry 1990;29:8424–9.

263. Yukitake K, Brown CL, Schlueter MA, et al. Surfactant apoprotein A modifies the inhibitory effect of plasma proteins on surfactant activity in vivo. Pediatr Res 1994;37:21–5.

264. Myers JL, Katzenstein AA. Epithelial necrosis and alveolar collapse in the pathogenesis of usual interstitial pneumonia. Chest 1988;94:1309–11.

265. Crouch E. The pathobiology of pulmonary fibrosis. Am J Physiol 1990;259:L159–84.

266. Shen AS, Haslett C, Feldsien DC, et al. The intensity of chronic lung inflammation and fibrosis after bleomycin is directly related to the severity of acute injury. Am Rev Respir Dis 1988;137:564–71.

267. Nakashima JM, Levin JR, Hyde DM, et al. Repeated exposures to enzyme-generated oxidants cause alveolitis, epithelial hyperplasia, and fibrosis in hamsters. Am J Pathol 1991;139:1485–99.

268. Haschek WM, Witschi H. Pulmonary fibrosis–a possible mechanism. Toxicol Appl Pharm 1979;51:475–87.

269. Terzaghi M, Nettesheim P, Williams ML. Repopulation of denuded tracheal grafts with normal, preneoplastic and neoplastic epithelial cell populations. Cancer Res 1978;38:4546–53.

270. Hirai K-I, Witschi H, Côté MG. Electron microscopy of butylated hydroxytoluene-induced lung damage in mice. Exp Mol Pathol 1977;27:295–308.

271. Haschek WM, Meyer KR, Ulrich RL, et al. Potentiation of chemically induced lung fibrosis by thorax irradiation. Int J Radiat Oncol Biol Phys 1980;6:449–55.

272. Adamson IY, Bowden DH, Côté MG, et al. Lung injury induced by butylated hydroxytoluene: cytodynamic and biochemical studies in mice. Lab Invest 1977;36:26–32.

273. Watanabe-Fukunaga R, Brannan CI, Copeland NG, et al. Lymphoproliferation disorder in mice explained by defects in Fas antigen that mediates apotosis. Nature 1992;356:314–7.

274. Omar T, Gerladine P, Belehradek J Jr, et al. Bleomycin, an apotosis-mimetic drug that induces two types of cell death depending on the number of molecules internalized. Cancer Res 1993;53:5462–9.

275. O'Driscoll BR, Kalra S, Gattamaneni HR, et al. Late carmustine lung fibrosis. Age at treatment may influence severity and survival. Chest 1995;107:1355–7.

276. Kuwano K, Hagimoto N, Kawasaki M, et al. Essential roles of the Fas-Fas ligand pathway in the development of pulmonary fibrosis. J Clin Invest 1999;104(1):13–9.

277. Watanabe-Fukunga R, Brannan CI, Itoh N, et al. The cDNA structure, expression and chromosomal assignment of mouse Fas ligand. J Immunol 1997;148:1274–9.

278. Maeyama T, Kuwano K, Kawasaki M, et al. Upregulation of Fas-signalling molecules in lung epithelial cells from patients with idiopathic pulmonary fibrosis. Eur Respir J 2001;17(2):180–9.

279. Chapman HA. A Fas pathway to pulmonary fibrosis. J Clin Invest 1999;104(1):1–2.

280. Aoshiba K, Yasui S, Tamaoki J, et al. The Fas/Fas-ligand system is not required for bleomycin-induced pulmonary fibrosis in mice. Am J Respir Crit Care Med 2000;162(2 Pt 1):695–700.

281. Persson A, Chang D, Rust K, et al. Purification and biochemical characterization of CP4 (SP-D), a collagenous surfactant-associated protein. Biochemistry 1989;28:6361–7.

282. Horiuchi T, Ikegami M, Cherniak RM, et al. Increased surface tension of the lung and surfactant in bleomycin-induced pulmonary fibrosis in rats. Am J Respir Crit Care Med 1996;154:1002–5.

283. Horiuchi T, Mason RJ, Kuroki Y, et al. Surface and tissue forces, surfactant protein A, and the phospholipid components of pulmonary surfactant in bleomycin-induced pulmonary fibrosis in the rat. Am Rev Respir Dis 1990;141:1006–13.

284. Honda Y, Tsunematsu K, Suzuki A, et al. Changes in phospholipids in bronchoalveolar lavage fluid of patients with interstitial lung diseases. Lung 1988;166:293–301.

285. Thrall RS, Swendsen CL, Shannon TH, et al. Correlation of changes in pulmonary surfactant phospholipids with compliance in bleomycin-induced pulmonary fibrosis in the rat. Am Rev Respir Dis 1987;136:113–8.

286. Baker G, Duck-Chong C, Cleland K, et al. The surfactant system as an intrinsic monitor of acute interstitial lung disease. Chest 1986;89:126S–7S.

287. Low RB, Adler KB, Woodcock-Mitchell J, et al. Bronchoalveolar lavage lipids during development of bleomycin-induced fibrosis in rats. Relationship to altered epithelial cell morphology. Am Rev Respir Dis 1988;138:709–13.

288. Crapo JD, Barry BE, Foscue HA, et al. Structural and biochemical changes in rat lungs occurring during exposures to lethal and adaptive doses of oxygen. Am Rev Respir Dis 1980;122:123–43.

289. Hughes DA, Haslam PL. Changes in phosphatidylglycerol in bronchoalveolar lavage fluids from patients with cryptogenic fibrosing alveolitis. Chest 1989;95:82–9.

290. McCormack FX, King TEJ, Bucher BL, et al. Surfactant protein A predicts survival in idiopathic pulmonary fibrosis. Am J Respir Crit Care Med 1995;152:751–9.

291. Honda Y, Kuroki Y, Matsuura E, et al. Pulmonary surfactant protein D in sera and bronchoalveolar lavage fluids. Am J Respir Crit Care Med 1995;152:1860–6.

292. Honda Y, Kuroki Y, Shijubo N, et al. Aberrant appearance of lung surfactant protein A in sera of patients with idiopathic pulmonary fibrosis and its clinical significance. Respiration 1995;62:64–9.

293. Kuroki Y, Tsutahara S, Shijubo N, et al. Elevated levels of lung surfactant protein A in sera from patients with idiopathic pulmonary fibrosis and pulmonary alveolar proteinosis. Am Rev Respir Dis 1993;147:723–9.

294. Takahashi H, Kuroki Y, Tanaka H, et al. Serum levels of surfactant proteins A and D are useful biomarkers for interstitial lung disease in patients with progressive systemic sclerosis. Am J Respir Crit Care Med 2000;162(1):258–63.

295. Takahashi H, Fujishima T, Koba H, et al. Serum surfactant proteins A and D as prognostic factors in idiopathic pulmonary fibrosis and their relationship to disease extent. Am J Respir Crit Care Med 2000;162(3 Pt 1):1109–14.

296. Greene KE, King TE Jr, Kuroki Y, et al. Serum surfactant proteins A and D as biomarkers in idiopathic pulmonary fibrosis. Eur Respir J 2002;19(3):439–46.

297. Mason RJ, McCormack FX. Alveolar type II cells in pathologic states. In: Muller B, Wichert PV, editors. Lung surfactant: basic research in the pathogenesis of lung disorders, Prog Respir Res. Vol 27. Basel, Switzerland: Karger; 1994. p. 195–200.

10

CYTOKINE BIOLOGY AND THE PATHOGENESIS OF INTERSTITIAL LUNG DISEASE

MICHAEL P. KEANE
JOHN A. BELPERIO
ROBERT M. STRIETER

Resolution of acute lung injury results in rapid restoration of tissue integrity and function following a variety of insults, including trauma, immunologically mediated lung inflammation, and infection. Although repair is a complex interplay between humoral, cellular, and extracellular matrix networks, this process occurs in a sequential, yet overlapping, manner. Following tissue injury, the reparative process immediately begins with hemorrhage and extravasation of plasma into tissue. This results in activation of the intrinsic and extrinsic coagulation pathways, leading to fibrin deposition and the establishment of a provisional matrix.[1-3] Platelet activation and degranulation also occur during coagulation leading to the release of a number of cytokines into the provisional matrix.[1-3] These cytokines are either important growth factors or chemotaxins that incite leukocyte, endothelial cell, fibroblast, and epithelial cell activation.[1-3]

The elicitation of leukocytes into the lung is dependent on a dynamic and complex series of events. The steps that lead to leukocyte recruitment include endothelial cell activation and expression of endothelial cell–derived adhesion molecules, leukocyte activation and expression of leukocyte-derived adhesion molecules, leukocyte-endothelial cell adhesion, leukocyte diapedesis, and directional leukocyte migration beyond the vascular compartment via chemotactic gradients.[4-6] Adhesion between leukocytes (L-selectin, and β_1 and β_2 integrin adhesion molecules) and endothelial cells (P-selectin, E-selectin, intercellular adhesion molecule 1 [ICAM-1], and vascular cell adhesion molecule [VCAM-1] adhesion molecules) is a prerequisite interaction for successful leukocyte extravasation at sites of inflammation, however, the subsequent steps leading to diapedesis and migration beyond the vascular compartment are dependent on both the continued expression of β_1 and β_2 integrins and the movement along a leukocyte-specific chemokine gradient.[4-6] Neutrophils are usually the first leukocytes to arrive at the site of tissue injury; their primary function is to phagocytose debris. However, these leukocytes have the capacity to produce a number of cytokines that are instrumental in orchestrating the progression of tissue repair.[7-10] While neutrophils are important for initial host defense in response to pulmonary injury, the second wave of leukocytes consists of mononuclear cells, with the mononuclear phagocyte representing a pivotal leukocyte in the progression of lung repair. This leukocyte has the ability to generate a number of inflammatory mediators that are important in transforming the provisional matrix to mature granulation tissue.[1,7,11]

The transition of tissue repair from acute inflammation to granulation tissue is an essential event as granulation tissue consists of a variety of mediators, appropriate extracellular matrix constituents, fibroblasts, endothelial cells, and leukocytes that form either the connective tissue foundation or act as the stimulus for angiogenesis. The process of neovascularization is paramount, as this process sustains a continual supply of oxygen and nutrients to the cellular constituents of tissue. During the early phases of granulation tissue formation, the immature connective tissue resembles undifferentiated mesenchyme with the presence of fibrin, an embryonic form of fibronectin, a predominance of collagen type III as compared to type I collagen, and a highly vascularized capillary bed.[1,2,12-14] This phase is followed by a transformation to mature granulation tissue that is associated with the increased deposition of collagen type I, fibronectin, and protease-dependent remodeling of the extracellular matrix.[15] This granulation tissue provides the foundation for the initiation of re-epithelialization. This response is followed by epithelial cell regeneration and the production of basement membrane extracellular constituents (fibronectin, type IV and VII collagen, heparin sulfate proteoglycans, and laminin) that re-establish the integrity of the epithelium.[1]

The pathogenesis of interstitial lung disease (ILD) leading to the loss of type I epithelial cells and endothelial cells, proliferation of type II cells, recruitment and proliferation of endothelial cells and fibroblasts, and deposition of extracellular matrix leading to end-stage alveolar fibrosis, involves the complex and dynamic interplay between diverse immune effector cells and cellular constituents of the alveolar-capillary membrane and interstitium of the lung.[16–19] Interaction of these diverse cell populations and the mediators that they produce culminate in lung injury, persistent extracellular matrix deposition, and ultimately, end-stage fibrosis. However, the initial stimulus for inflammatory cell recruitment and the mechanisms responsible for the perpetuation and evolution of chronic inflammation, granulation tissue formation, and end-stage fibrosis have not been fully elucidated. Inhaled antigens, viruses, or toxins may induce an exaggerated immune response leading to the extravasation of activated leukocytes resulting in lung injury.[16–19] Aberrant expression of class II major histocompatibility complex (MHC) molecules on alveolar epithelial cells, endothelial cells, and alveolar macrophages may promote exuberant antigen presentation and immune cell activation, which leads to the perpetuation of chronic inflammation in ILD.[16–19] The development of local chemotactic gradients may result in marked expansion of diverse populations of leukocytes within the air spaces and interstitium of the lung. Although the cellular mechanisms by which leukocytes are recruited in ILD have not been fully characterized, cellular constituents of the alveolar-capillary membrane and interstitium probably are central to recruiting activated leukocytes that further amplify the immune/inflammatory process within the lung.[16–19]

As chronic inflammation proceeds, there is a dramatic increase in the number of fibroblasts within the interstitium of the lung (alveolar, perivascular, and peribronchiolar spaces) that is due to both the local release of fibroblast chemoattractants and enhanced fibroblast proliferation.[16–19] Additionally, net accumulation of granulation tissue occurs within the alveolar space and interstitium of the lung due to enhanced synthesis and reduced extracellular matrix degradation.[16–19] A marked increase in type III interstitial collagen is seen early in the disease, whereas, a predominance of type I interstitial collagen is found in the later stages of ILD.[16–19]

It has recently been suggested that inflammation plays little or no role in the pathogenesis of idiopathic pulmonary fibrosis (IPF).[20,21] This notion is based largely on observational studies of single biopsy specimens and the poor response to conventional anti-inflammatory therapy.[22–24] Unfortunately most patients present late in the pathogenesis of ILD, especially IPF. Their biopsy specimens actually represent established disease with evidence of end-stage fibrosis. Unfortunately, we have no data that adequately reflects the natural history or pathogenesis of end-stage ILD such as IPF. Based on single biopsy specimens there is no way of excluding preceding inflammation as the stimulus for ongoing fibroblast proliferation and deposition of extracellular matrix. Indeed, all animal models of fibrosis start with a brisk inflammatory response that precedes the fibrotic response.[25,26] The exceptions to this are models where a proinflammatory cytokine such as transforming growth factor-β (TGF-β) is artificially overexpressed using an adenovirus thereby bypassing the initial inflammatory stimulus for TGF-β production.[27] Indeed transient overexpression of interleukin (IL)-1β leads to the local production of proinflammatory cytokines and a vigorous inflammatory response that subsequently leads to the sustained production of TGF-β and the development of fibrosis.[21] This suggests that inflammation is important in the initiation of the fibrotic response but is not necessary to sustain the process once it has been initiated. Furthermore, transient but prolonged (7 to 10 days) overexpression of tumor necrosis factor-α (TNF-α) in rat lung using an adenoviral vector leads to severe pulmonary inflammation and patchy interstitial fibrogenesis with the subsequent prolonged induction of TGF-β, activation of myofibroblasts, and development of fibrosis.[28] Transgenic expression of TNF-α in the murine lung under the control of the surfactant protein (SP)-C promoter leads to a lymphocytic alveolitis in the first 2 months of life followed by the subsequent development of fibrosis that bears many of the pathologic features of human IPF.[29]

Similarly, the lack of response to corticosteroids cannot be taken as evidence that inflammation is not important. Asthma is a classic pulmonary inflammatory disorder and yet up to 25% of severe asthmatics demonstrate some level of unresponsiveness to corticosteroids.[30] Obliterative bronchiolitis (OB) associated with lung transplantation is a chronic fibrotic disease of the small airways that is characterized by peribronchiolar leukocyte infiltration with the subsequent fibrotic obliteration of the airway.[31] The major risk factor for the development of OB is repeated episodes of acute rejection underscoring the critical role of inflammation in this fibrotic process.[32] Further support for the notion of a continuum of inflammation to fibrosis is seen in the study by Flaherty and colleagues.[33] They describe histologic variability in surgical biopsies taken from multiple lobes in the same patient.[33] They found differing diagnoses between lobes in 26% of patients. Patients concordant for usual interstitial pneumonia (UIP) in all lobes were older than those discordant for UIP who, in turn, were older than those with nonspecific interstitial pneumonia (NSIP) in all lobes, supporting the concept of an evolving process.[33] Rather than trying to separate inflammation and fibrosis, we feel that emphasis should be placed on the importance of both mechanisms as a continuum, with the initial inflammation representing a necessary event that ultimately leads to self-perpetuating fibrosis. Once the fibrotic phase predominates, inflammation is no longer necessary to sustain the response. This is not withstanding the likely importance of the macrophage, which by definition is a chronic inflammatory cell that persists in the interstitium and likely plays an important role in the fibrotic response. The inability to deplete these cells in animal models has deflected attention from their importance. The purpose of this chapter will be to review some of the cytokines that are present in ILD and to discuss their potential role in perpetuating chronic inflammation and deposition of extracellular matrix in the lung (Figure 10–1).

CYTOKINES

Early Response Proinflammatory Cytokines

Interleukin-1 Family of Cytokines

The interleukin-1 family of cytokines consists of two agonists, interleukin-1 alpha (IL-1α) and interleukin-1 beta (IL-1β), and one antagonist, interleukin-1 receptor antagonist (IL-1ra).[34,35] The interleukin-1 agonists are pleiotropic cytokines that exist as two distinct genes with protein isoforms with two isoelectric points (pI), pI 5.0 and pI 7.0, for IL-1α and IL-1β, respectively.[34,35] These two forms of IL-1 are also distinguished by whether they are found predominantly membrane associated (IL-1α) or secreted (IL-1β).[34,35] The cDNAs for IL-1α and IL-1β encode a 23 kD and 33 kD protein, respectively, that lack a typical hydrophobic signal sequence.[34,35] The 33 kD pro-IL-1β protein represents a precursor molecule for the secreted form of IL-1β with a molecular mass of 17 kD.[34,35] Both isoforms of IL-1 are produced by a variety of cells and bind to the type I IL-1 receptor on target cells with similar biologic function.[34–37] Alpha and beta forms of IL-1 only share approximately 26% amino acid sequence homology,[34,35] however site-directed mutagenesis studies of IL-1α and IL-1β have determined that they contain two specific binding sites for the type I receptor.[36,37]

Interleukin-1 ligand binding to the IL-1 type I receptor and the IL-1 receptor–associated protein recruits an intracellular adapter molecule, MyD88, which in turn recruits IL-1 receptor–associated kinase (IRAK). IRAK recruits the adapter molecule, tumor necrosis factor receptor–associated factor 6 (TRAF6), which recruits the nuclear factor-kappa B (NF-κB)–inducing kinase (NIK). NIK activates the I kappa B (IκB) kinase complex (IKK), which phosphorylates IκBα leading to ubiquitination and release of NF-κB for translocation to the nucleus and subsequent transactivation of a number of genes (ie, cyclooxygenase, adhesion molecules, cytokines, nitric oxide [NO] synthase, acute phase proteins, cytokines, and chemokines).[38,39] Although IL-1 signaling can occur through other distinct pathways (ie, p38/MAP kinase pathway and C-Jun-N-terminal kinase [JNK] pathways), the effects are often to synergize with those of NF-κB activation.[40] Interestingly, the signal coupling of IL-1 and the IL-1 type I receptor is identical to the signaling coupling of lipopolysaccharide (LPS) on toll like receptor (TLR4).[40–45] These two divergent ligand-receptor pairs

ultimately signal through the same cytoplasmic pathway leading to NF-κB activation, nuclear translocation, and transactivation of several genes critical to the amplification of the inflammatory and innate host response. This exemplifies that an exogenous factor such as LPS may be the initial triggering event on specific cells that express the complex of CD14/TLR4/MD-2, however, host endogenous ligands, such as IL-1 can further amplify this response. The presence of IL-1 receptors on essentially all immune and nonimmune cells affords the ability of IL-1 to bind to the IL-1 type I receptor, activate, and engage all of these cells as participants of the inflammatory/innate host response. In addition to the IL-1 type I receptor, IL-1 also binds to an IL-1 type II or decoy receptor that does not signal.[46,47] Binding of IL-1 to the IL-1 type II receptor may be a mechanism to sequester IL-1 from interacting with the IL-1 type I receptor.[46,47]

In contrast to the two IL-1 agonists, IL-1ra is the only known naturally occurring cytokine with specific antagonistic activity. The discovery of the IL-1ra has led to an appreciation of a dynamic balance between IL-1 agonists and IL-1ra in the maintenance of IL-1–dependent homeostasis and inflammation and has necessitated investigations into the role of IL-1ra in disease.[34,35] Two structural variants of IL-1ra have previously been described, a 17 kD protein that is secreted by monocytes, macrophages, and neutrophils as a variably glycosolated protein (sIL-1ra), and a second intracellular 18 kD protein that remains in the cytoplasm of monocytes, epithelial cells, and keratinocytes (icIL-1ra).[48] In addition, a smaller isoform of intracellular IL-1ra has been described.[49] A variety of cell populations, including monocytes, polymorphonuclear cells, alveolar macrophages, fibroblasts, keratinocytes, and also tumor cells have been demonstrated to elaborate IL-1ra.[34] IL-1ra is produced in response to a variety of agents, the most potent being adherent immunoglobulin G (IgG), LPS, granulocyte-macrophage colony–stimulating factor (GM-CSF), and IL-4.[48] Investigations have demonstrated that IL-1ra acts as a pure antagonist of either IL-1α or IL-1β and, when present in sufficient quantities, can attenuate a variety of IL-1 actions in both in vitro and in vivo model systems.[34] The ability of IL-1ra to both bind to the type I IL-1 receptor without signal coupling and competitively inhibit either IL-1α or IL-1β is related to its ability to bind to only one, as compared with two sites on the receptor.[36,37] These studies have led to an appreciation that IL-1ra normally modulates IL-1–dependent activity and speculation that it may play a role in the resolution of the pulmonary inflammatory cascade necessary for the lung to return to homeostasis.

The role of the IL-1 family of cytokines in the regulation of fibrosis in ILD is interesting, as these cytokines may have dual and opposing functions (Table 10–1). Both IL-1α and IL-1β induce the expression of procollagen type I and type III mRNA from fibroblasts, type IV collagen mRNA from epithelial cells, and stimulate the production of glycosaminoglycans and

**TABLE 10–1   The Role of
Interleukin-1 Family of Cytokines in Fibrosis**

Promotion of fibrosis

    Induce expression of adhesion molecules for leukocyte
      trafficking

    Induces fibroblast expression of procollagen type I and
      type III mRNA

    Stimulates fibroblast production of glycosaminoglycans and
      fibronectin

    Induces epithelial cell expression of type IV collagen mRNA

    Induces fibroblast expression of PDGF and indirectly mediates
      fibroblast proliferation

    Induces fibroblast expression of other cytokines, such as IL-6,
      CXC, and CC chemokines

Inhibition of fibrosis

    Induces fibroblast production of tissue collagenase (matrix
      metalloproteinase-1 [MMP-1]) and gelatinase

    Induces fibroblast production of prostaglandin E_2

    Induces fibroblast production of plasminogen activator

Bottom line

    Transient expression of IL-1β leads to progressive fibrosis with
      a sustained increase in levels of TGF-β_1

    Exogenous IL-1ra inhibits bleomycin- or silica-induced
      pulmonary fibrosis

PDGF = platelet-derived growth factor; IL = interleukin; TGF = transforming growth factor.

fibronectin by fibroblasts.[50] In addition, these cytokines can behave as indirect mitogens for fibroblast proliferation via the expression of the ligand platelet-derived growth factor (PDGF; homodimer, PDGF-AA) and the PDGF alpha receptor on fibroblasts (see below).[51] Furthermore, IL-1α and IL-1β can serve as proximal mediators of chronic inflammation that may promote fibrosis by inducing fibroblasts to produce a variety of cytokines that include additional IL-1, IL-6, and both CXC and CC chemokines.[52,53] In contrast, both IL-1s mediate the production of tissue collagenase (matrix metalloproteinase-1 [MMP-1]), gelatinase, prostaglandin E_2 (PGE$_2$), and plasminogen activator, which are important in enhancing extracellular matrix degradation.[50] Moreover, both IL-1s can inhibit fibroblast proliferation via the production of PGE$_2$.[54] These studies together with the ability of IL-1ra to modulate the biologic function of IL-1, suggest that IL-1 biology in regulating pulmonary fibrosis is extremely complex.

In order to effectively assess the relevance of a cytokine during the pathogenesis of pulmonary fibrosis in vivo, it is necessary to use an animal model of fibrotic lung disease. Bleomycin sulfate has been used in rodents to initiate fibrotic lung lesions that have many of the histologic components of IPF.[25,55] Bleomycin administration results in a route-, dose-, and strain-dependent pulmonary inflammatory response characterized by increases in leukocyte accumulation, especially mononu-

clear phagocytes, fibroblast proliferation, and enhanced deposition of extracellular matrix.[25,55–59] In addition, the lungs of these animals typically exhibit necrosis of type I pneumocytes within the first 24 hours postchallenge, acute alveolitis 2 to 3 days postchallenge, and intense interstitial inflammation 4 to 12 days postchallenge.[25,60–63] Moreover, fibroblast proliferation and extracellular matrix synthesis are initiated 4 to 14 days postbleomycin challenge with collagen content elevated approximately twofold, 3 weeks postchallenge.[25,55–63] Although these pathologic changes occur in a more rapid fashion than human IPF, the rodent pulmonary inflammatory response to intratracheal bleomycin challenge constitutes a representative model of human pulmonary fibrosis.

Specifically, Piguet and associates determined that exogenous IL-1ra can inhibit bleomycin- or silica-induced pulmonary fibrosis.[64] Infusion of IL-1ra via an intraperitoneal osmotic minipump significantly attenuated lung hydroxyproline deposition and histologic evidence of fibrosis. No significant change was noted in the cellularity of the bronchoalveolar lavage fluid (BALF) of the IL-1ra–treated animals that received either bleomycin or silica.[64] The specific mechanism for the decline in collagen deposition, either decreased collagen production, increased collagen degradation, or both, was not examined in this study. Moreover, these experiments did not determine the magnitude of the presence of endogenous IL-1ra, nor whether depleting endogenous IL-1ra enhanced bleomycin- or silica-induced pulmonary fibrosis. Increased IL-1ra mRNA expression has been found in an immune complex model of lung inflammation, and neutralization of IL-1ra led to augmented inflammation.[65] Recently, it has been demonstrated that transient expression of IL-1β using an adenoviral vector can lead to progressive fibrosis long after the IL-1β levels have declined and the acute inflammatory response has resolved.[66] There was an early increase in levels of the proinflammatory cytokines IL-6 and TNF and the profibrotic cytokine PDGF, followed by a sustained increase in levels of TGF-β1.[66] This study demonstrates that IL-1β has an important role in promoting the initial injury that leads to a self-perpetuating fibrotic response related to the persistent expression of TGF-β.[66] Interestingly, TGF-β can attenuate IL-1 activity by inhibiting IL-1–receptor expression and by inducing the elaboration of IL-1ra.[67] This concept is important as persistent inflammation may attenuate the deposition of extracellular matrix via the elaboration of proteinases that are important in the removal of extracellular matrix. At the same time, the self-perpetuating fibrosis required the initial trigger of inflammation; therefore, we cannot look at these events in isolation.

Our laboratory has previously demonstrated that patients with either sarcoidosis or IPF have elevated levels of IL-1ra protein in cell-free BALF that was tenfold higher than levels of IL-1β.[68,69] This stoichiometric relationship of IL-1ra:IL-1β in the cell-free BALF is inhibitory of IL-1β–dependent biology.[34] To extend these studies, lung tissue homogenates were assayed for IL-1ra, IL-1β, TNF-α, and TGF-β and normalized to total protein.[69] IL-1ra was significantly increased in IPF, as compared with "normal" tissue obtained from patients undergoing thoracic surgery for reasons other than ILD. In contrast, interstitial levels of IL-1β were significantly depressed in IPF patients, as compared with controls. Overall, the ratio of IL-1ra:IL-1β was 19:1 for IPF as compared with 1.3:1 for controls. Immunolocalization and in situ hybridization demonstrated little expression of IL-1ra and IL-1β protein and mRNA in normal lung tissue. In contrast, lung tissue from IPF patients demonstrated marked qualitative increases in both IL-1ra protein and mRNA that was localized primarily to hyperplastic type II pneumocytes lining the alveoli, macrophages, and fibroblasts scattered throughout the extracellular matrix. IPF lung tissue demonstrated only scattered, but focal, areas of detectable IL-1β within the extracellular matrix. In a parallel fashion to IL-1ra, TGF-β protein levels were tenfold higher in IPF lung tissue as compared with control lung tissue as measured by specific enzyme-linked immunosorbent assay (ELISA), whereas no change was seen in TNF-α levels.[69]

Although IL-1α was not measured in these studies, these findings suggested that IL-1ra levels in IPF were stoichiometrically appropriate to inhibit IL-1β–dependent biology. The chronic imbalance between IL-1β and IL-1ra may result in the propagation of an overexuberant reparative and fibrotic phase, with a failure to return the interstitium of the lung to homeostasis. However, unlike previous investigations, which examined the in vitro cytokine production by cell populations isolated by BALF from IPF patients,[70,71] cytokine content of the recovered fluid was directly examined as a reflection of in vivo activity. Lavage fluid from patients with IPF contained a threefold increase in antigenic IL-1ra, as compared with healthy, nonsmoking volunteers. This increase in IL-1ra in the alveolar space was accompanied by an associated, but much less proportional, increase in IL-1β content. These findings demonstrate that the cytokine environment within the alveoli of patients with established IPF is not, as previously speculated, more proinflammatory than normals as defined by IL-1 biology. In contrast, the slightly increased ratio of IL-1ra:IL-1β in the BALF of IPF patients when fibrosis is established may even suggest a less inflammatory milieu, through the local attenuation IL-1β–dependent activity within the alveolar space. Interestingly, we have found that IL-ra levels measured by ELISA from lung tissue homogenates of patients with IPF may directly correlate with mortality.[72]

These findings suggest that chronic end-stage fibrotic changes of IPF, and possibly other interstitial lung diseases associated with increased deposition of extracellular matrix, may result from an overexuberant "fibrotic" phase, which may be partially mediated by excessive IL-1ra production by nonimmune cells. TGF-β is also present in greater quantities in IPF and likely plays a significant role in the pathogenesis of this disorder.[73] Interestingly, in addition to directly stimulating matrix synthesis and inhibiting matrix degradation, TGF-β may also attenuate IL-1 activity by inhibiting IL-1–receptor expression and by inducing the elaboration of IL-1ra.[67] The consequence of these events may be reflected in the type II cell hyperplasia and the excessive aberrant fibroblast collagen synthesis and deposition, which ultimately result in the obliteration of normal structures in IPF. Simultaneously, the inhibition of normal "fibrolytic" activity mediated by IL-1–dependent collagenases may be evident in both the lack of resorption of excessive collagen, and the failure to repair and resculpture the matrix into functional lung tissue. IL-1 has been shown to both directly and indirectly, through the induction of PDGF, initiate fibroblast proliferation and affect fibroblast synthetic behavior.[74] Collagen synthesis is also altered by IL-1, and, as demonstrated in the synovium, there is enhanced synthesis of type I and III collagen and inhibition of type II collagen formation.[75] Importantly, the production of both PGE_2 and various collagenases is also induced by IL-1.[76] Although these factors are responsible for acute, local tissue inflammation, they are also required for normal tissue remodeling during resolution and tissue repair. Thus, the pathology of IPF may demonstrate the loss of coordination between these two processes and the resulting failed orchestration of normal tissue remodeling necessary for the return to homeostasis.

Epidemiologic data, the presence of immune complexes and autoantibodies in IPF patients, and the association of similar interstitial lung disease in patients with collagen-vascular disorders all strongly suggest that autoimmune phenomena are a common, and perhaps causative, component in the pathophysiology of IPF and other interstitial lung disease. Dysregulation of the immune response, resulting from either an intrinsic defect in communication between immune cells or from the deleterious effects of aberrant cytokine production by nonimmune cells, may have important consequences in IPF. It is increasingly apparent that the primary pathologic feature in IPF is the failure to complete the cycle from local inflammation, regardless of the specific initiating event, through the resolution of proinflammatory events, on through an appropriate degree of tissue repair and remodeling, and then finally back to a normal steady-state homeostasis. Further studies will be needed to definitively establish the pathogenic role of IL-1 cytokines in IPF and identify potential targets to modulate these adverse effects through novel therapeutic strategies.

Tumor Necrosis Factor-Alpha

Tumor necrosis factor is a mononuclear phagocyte–derived cytokine, which has been increasingly recognized for its pleiotropic effects on numerous inflammatory and immunologic responses (Table 10–2). It is one of 10 known members of a family of ligands that activate a corresponding family of receptors.[77] TNF is produced primarily by monocytes/macrophages, and has many overlapping biologic activities with IL-1. In solution, TNF is a homotrimer and binds to two different cell surface receptors, p55 and p75.[77,78] The TNF-receptor family consists of transmembrane proteins with an extracellular domain that contains a recurring cysteine-rich motif and an intracellular domain that demonstrates more variability than the extracellular domain.[77] The p55 receptor and the Fas receptor contain a 60 amino-acid domain known as the "death domain," which is essential for signal transduction of an apoptotic signal.[77]

Elevated levels of TNF have been implicated in the pathogenesis of a number of disease states, including septic shock/sepsis syndrome,[78] acute respiratory distress syndrome (ARDS),[79] hepatic ischemia/reperfusion injury,[80] acquired immunodeficiency syndrome (AIDS)-related cachexia,[81] chronic parasitic infections,[82] graft-versus-host disease,[83] and heart, kidney, liver, and lung allograft rejection.[84] Furthermore, it has been suggested that autoimmune disorders are a result of mutations in the receptors for TNF and its related ligands, which are important in mediating apoptosis.[85] The resultant defect

may lead to a compensatory increase in the relevant ligand with subsequent inflammatory damage typical of complex autoimmune disorders such as rheumatoid arthritis and Crohn's disease.[85] Specifically, mutations in the Fas receptor gene leads to a lymphoproliferative disorder with splenomegaly and signs of autoimmunity at an early age.[86,87] Moreover, anti-TNF therapies are known to ameliorate both rheumatoid arthritis and Crohn's disease.[88,89]

TNF exhibits a variety of inflammatory effects, including the induction of neutrophil– and mononuclear cell–endothelial cell adhesion and transendothelial migration via the expression of adhesion molecules and chemokines; enhancement of a procoagulant environment by upregulating the expression of tissue factor and plasminogen activator inhibitor and suppressing the protein C pathway; and acting as an early response cytokine in the promotion of a proinflammatory/fibrotic cytokine cascade.[6,78,90–93] Although TNF may be a significant mediator of proximal nonspecific inflammation, this cytokine may have a role in mediating specific immune inflammatory events in the lung. Studies have demonstrated immunoregulatory functions of TNF that include regulation of B-lymphocyte differentiation[94] and enhanced cytolytic activity of human natural killer (NK) cells.[95] Resting T lymphocytes do not specifically bind TNF, however, Scheurich and associates[96] have identified that anti-CD3 antibody-activated T lymphocytes express specific TNF receptors in a kinetic fashion similar to the expression of IL-2 receptors. These TNF receptors have a biologic function, as TNF enhances the expression of MHC class II antigens, induces the expression of high-affinity IL-2 receptors, and synergizes with IL-2 to stimulate T-lymphocyte proliferation and production of interferon gamma (IFN-γ). In addition, TNF has been shown to stimulate T-lymphocyte colony formation, which may be mediated through the TNF-induced production of IL-1,[97] and to enhance antigen and mitogen-induced T-lymphocyte proliferation.[98]

TNF has a diverse effect on the biology of fibroblasts. TNF induces the proliferation of fibroblasts via the autocrine and paracrine production of fibroblast PDGF.[99] In addition, TNF enhances the production of fibroblast-derived prostaglandin E_2,[100] collagenase (MMP-1) and gelatinase,[101,102] glycosaminoglycans,[101,103] CXC and CC chemokines,[104,105] granulocyte-monocyte–colony stimulating factor,[106] and interleukin-1 and -6.[92] Moreover, TNF has been found to reduce TGF-β-induced production of type I procollagen from fibroblasts at the level of transcription that is independent of PGE_2 production.[107,108] These findings suggest that TNF plays an important role as a cytokine that bridges inflammation, reparative responses, fibrosis and may be involved in extracellular matrix remodeling.

TNF has been found to be significantly elevated in bleomycin-induced pulmonary fibrosis.[18,63] TNF mRNA peaks from days 4 to 15 postbleomycin instillation and subsequently returns to control levels.[18] Interestingly,

---

TABLE 10–2   The Role of Tumor Necrosis Factor-Alpha in Fibrosis

Promotion of fibrosis

   Induces expression of adhesion molecules for leukocyte trafficking

   Orchestrates the innate and adaptive immune responses via cytokine networks

   Induces fibroblast expression of glycosaminoglycans, procollagen type I and type III mRNA

   Induces the proliferation of fibroblasts via the autocrine and paracrine production of platelet-derived growth factor (PDGF)

   Induces the expression of fibroblast-derived cytokines
     IL-1
     IL-6
     CXC and CC chemokines
     GM-CSF

Inhibition of fibrosis

   Enhances the production of fibroblast collagenase (MMP-1) and gelatinase

   Enhances the production of fibroblast-derived prostaglandin E_2

   Inhibits TGF-β-induced fibroblast production of type I and III procollagens

Bottom line

   TNF transgenic (SP-C promoter) mice display increased fibrosis

   Antagonists of TNF inhibit fibrosis
     Neutralizing antibodies
     Soluble TNF receptors

IL = interleukin; GM-CSF = granulocyte-macrophage colony–stimulating factor; MMP = matrix metalloproteinase; TGF = transforming growth factor; TNF = tumor necrosis factor.

these levels are paralleled by the increase in the gene expression of TGF-β.[18] In addition, maximal levels of steady-state mRNA for TNF and TGF-β proceed the gene expression of both types I and III procollagen.[18,63] When bleomycin-treated animals are passively immunized with neutralizing antibodies to TNF, depletion of TNF results in an attenuation of the cellularity of the parenchyma of the lung, reduces alveolar septal thickening, and decreases the disruption of the alveolar architecture, as compared with the control antibody-treated group.[63] These findings are accompanied by a reduction in total lung hydroxyproline content.[63] These studies have been further substantiated with the use of a recombinant soluble TNF receptor (rsTNFR) that impairs binding of TNF to cellular TNF receptors.[109] In this investigation, bleomycin-treated animals either received rsTNFR at the time of bleomycin instillation or after a delay of 25 days postbleomycin challenge. The inhibition of the biologic effect of TNF using these strategies resulted in a marked reduction of early as well as established pulmonary fibrosis, as measured by total lung hydroxyproline at both 15 days and 25 days postbleomycin.[109] Further support for a role of TNF in mediating pulmonary fibrosis has come from a study that examined the overexpression of localized TNF.[29] The murine gene for TNF was expressed under the control of the human surfactant protein SP-C promoter in transgenic mice.[29] In the TNF transgenic mice, TNF mRNA was detected in the type II pneumocytes.[29] In the first two months of life, these transgenic mice exhibited a predominant lymphocytic alveolitis with evidence of elevated expression of the endothelial cell adhesion molecule, VCAM-1.[29] However, in the TNF transgenic animals, the pathology of the lung demonstrated a continuum of inflammation to fibrosis demonstrating that the lung parenchyma developed thickened alveolar septa, progressive accumulation of desmin-containing fibroblasts, augmented collagen deposition, and persistence of interstitial lymphocytes.[29] The loss of alveolar architecture was associated with an increase in the presence of hyperplastic type II pneumocytes.[29] Although the early histopathology of the TNF transgenic mice was similar to changes that are associated with the subacute phases of acute respiratory distress syndrome, the histopathology associated with prolonged tonic exposure to TNF resembled those related to IPF. Interestingly, the TNF transgenic animals in these studies did not have elevated levels of TGF-β or PDGF.[29] However, despite these findings, there is evidence for TNF-mediated TGF-β expression. Inhibition of TNF inhibits the expression of TGF-β, IL-5, and eosinophil infiltration in bleomycin-induced pulmonary fibrosis.[110] Similarly, transient but prolonged (7 to 10 days) overexpression of TNF in rat lung using an adenoviral vector leads to severe pulmonary inflammation and patchy interstitial fibrogenesis with induction of TGF-β and activation of myofibroblasts.[28] The fibrosis associated with this exposure persisted beyond 64 days.[28] Furthermore these stud-

ies support the notion that TNF may be an important cytokine in the pathogenesis of fibrosing alveolitis.

These studies demonstrate an important role for TNF in fibrosis and suggest that therapy with anti-TNF antibodies might be beneficial, however, there are several potential limitations to this approach. First, anti-TNF antibodies do not prevent lymphotoxin from signaling the TNF receptors. Second, formation of immune complexes may lead to the activation of complement with potentially harmful effects. Third, murine monoclonal antibodies, and even humanized monoclonal antibodies, are antigenic, which may preclude long-term therapy. Attempts to overcome these obstacles have led to the development of chimeric inhibitor molecules. These molecules contain the extracellular domain of the TNF receptor joined to an immunoglobulin heavy chain fragment and are minimally antigenic.[77] They are highly specific and neutralize all ligands for the TNF receptor including lymphotoxin-α.[111] The two molecules available to target TNF activity are a chimeric IgG$_1$ antibody, infliximab, and a 75 kD fusion, protein etanercept.[112] These chimeric inhibitors have demonstrated efficacy in the treatment of rheumatoid arthritis, ankylosing spondylitis, Crohn's disease, and psoriatic arthritis.[112–115] These beneficial effects however may be at the expense of increased risk for infectious complications. An increased incidence of tuberculosis has been reported in a large cohort of patients that were treated with anti-TNF therapy (infliximab).[116]

The Type 1/Type 2 (Th$_1$/Th$_2$) Paradigm and Pulmonary Fibrosis

Type 1 and type 2 cytokine patterns in mice were originally identified from a panel of T helper (Th) cell clones and include IFN-γ and IL-2 versus IL-4, IL-5, and IL-10, respectively.[117] The realization that Th type 1 and Th type 2 cytokines are expressed by a variety of immune and nonimmune cells and the function of these cytokines are different, suggest that an imbalance in the expression of type 1/type 2 cytokines may be important in dictating different immunopathologic responses.[118] For example, type 1 cytokines appear to be involved in cell-mediated immunity associated with autoimmune disorders and allograft rejection; whereas, type 2 cytokines are predominately involved in mediating allergic inflammation and chronic fibroproliferative disorders, such as asthma, atopic dermatitis, IPF, and systemic sclerosis.[118] Thus, it is more appropriate to define certain diseases in terms of the predominate cytokine profile (ie, type 1 or type 2 cytokine type) rather than the predominate T helper cell subset. The strict definition of type 1 and type 2 responses may break down in a scenario where the initial inciting agent triggers an unsuccessful type 1 response. The subsequent host reaction to the antigen or the chronicity of the disorder may induce a switch to a response dominated by type 2 cytokines.

The manifestation of this latter response is the scenario of stromal cell/fibroblast proliferation and deposition of extracellular matrix and ultimately fibrosis. Thus, the cytokine pattern in particular diseases is often predictable and appropriate; whereas, severe pathologic consequences may result if an inappropriate cytokine phenotype is expressed. This latter situation may play a role in certain chronic inflammatory diseases, such as ILD, where unknown etiologies lead to dysregulated repair with exaggerated chronic inflammation, subsequent fibroblast proliferation, deposition of extracellular matrix, angiogenesis, and finally fibrosis that accompanies end-stage pulmonary fibrosis.

There is evidence suggesting that a cytokine profile of the natural immune/inflammatory response determines the disease phenotype responsible for either resolution or progression to end-stage fibrosis. Supporting evidence is derived from studies demonstrating that interferons, especially IFN-γ, have profound suppressive effects on the production of extracellular matrix proteins, such as collagen and fibronectin.[101,119] Investigations have demonstrated that IFN-γ can inhibit both fibroblast and chondrocyte collagen production in vitro, as well as decrease the expression of steady-state type I and III procollagen mRNA.[120–122] IFN-γ reduces PDGF-induced lung fibroblast growth but stimulates PDGF production by alveolar macrophages.[123] IFN-γ up-regulates the major matrix-degrading metalloproteinase, stromelysin-1 gene expression by fibroblasts.[124] IFN-γ differentially regulates ICAM-1 and VCAM-1 expression on fibroblasts.[125] The administration of IFN-γ in vivo can cause a reduction of extracellular matrix in animal models of fibrosis.[101,119,126] Furthermore we have recently shown that IL-12 attenuates bleomycin-induced pulmonary fibrosis in an IFN-γ–dependant manner.[127] Moreover, IFN-γ treatment of patients with either systemic sclerosis or IPF for one year demonstrated improved pulmonary function.[128,129] This information supports the concept that IFN-γ is one of the major type 1 cytokines that possesses profound regulatory activity for collagen deposition during chronic inflammation.

The opposing effects of type 1 and type 2 cytokines in fibrosis are supported by a number of recent investigations demonstrating that IL-4 is an important mediator of fibroblast activation.[130] In contrast to the type 1 cytokine IFN-γ, IL-4 is a major type 2 cytokine that promotes the production of fibroblast-derived extracellular matrix, including type I and III procollagens and fibronectin.[130] IL-4 treatment of fibroblasts leads to increases in steady-state levels of extracellular matrix mRNA and protein. IL-4 has been identified as a chemotactic factor for fibroblasts.[131] IL-4 can induce fibroblast proliferation and cytokine production. The intensity of IL-4–induced fibroblast collagen synthesis is on the same order of magnitude as that induced by equivalent amounts of TGF-β. Additional studies have demonstrated that fibroblasts possess both membrane bound and soluble forms of the IL-4 receptor. The sol-

uble IL-4 receptor is derived from a truncation of the membrane form and may serve as either an IL-4 binding protein with antagonist activity or as a carrier of IL-4 with its biologic properties intact.[132] Interestingly, pulmonary expression of IL-4 in transgenic mice leads to little or no fibrosis, suggesting a disparity between the in vitro and in vivo effects.[133] Similarly, IL-4 depletion studies and studies with IL-4 –/– mice fail to demonstrate an indispensable role for IL-4 in models of type 2–mediated inflammation and fibrosis.[134–136]

Recent work has shown that fibroblast cell lines express IL-4 receptor alpha (Rα), IL-13Rα1, and IL-13Rα2, but not the IL-2 common γ chain necessary for specific IL-4 signaling. This suggests that many of the fibroblast activation properties of IL-4 are shared by IL-13. As a type 2 cytokine, IL-13 has similar biologic properties to IL-4, and has been implicated in the pathogenesis of fibroproliferative disorders.[137] IL-13 induces the expression of fibroblast-derived type I and III procollagens in a similar magnitude as IL-4 and TGF-β.[137] IL-13 inhibits IL-1–induced MMP-1 and MMP-3 production and enhances tissue inhibitor of metalloproteinase (TIMP)-1 generation from fibroblasts.[137] Recently, IL-13 was selectively expressed in the lungs using a Clara cell promoter.[138] The phenotype of the transgenic mice expressing IL-13 demonstrated airway epithelial cell hypertrophy, mucus cell metaplasia, the hyperproduction of neutral and acidic mucus, and subepithelial airway fibrosis.[138] Similarly IL-13 has been shown to induce fibrosis by selectively stimulating the production and activation of TGF-β.[139] These data demonstrate both the profibrotic effects of IL-13 on collagen homeostasis and the potential differential regulation of collagen homeostasis in fibroblast subtypes.

The similarities and overlapping functions of IL-4 and IL-13 have led to an interest in the IL-13–receptor (IL-13R) complex and its relationship to the IL-4–receptor (IL-4R) complex.[140] The IL-4R complex is composed of at least two subunits, IL-4Rα and the IL-2Rγ (common γ chain).[141] The IL-13 receptor complex is composed of various combinations of IL-4Rα, IL-13Rα1, IL-13Rα2, and IL-2Rγ.[142,143] IL-4Rα appears to be an essential component of both the IL-4 and IL-13 receptors although it can not by itself bind IL-13.[143,144] Studies of chronic leishmaniasis using both IL-4 –/– mice and IL-4Rα –/– mice have demonstrated that the IL-4 –/– deficient mice are able to clear the infection but the IL-4Rα –/– mice developed progressive infection and death.[144] This indicates an important and independent role for IL-13 receptor signaling in this model system. In addition, this concept is further supported by a schistosomiasis model of hepatic fibrosis. There was a greater reduction in hepatic fibrosis by inhibition of IL-13 using soluble IL-13Rα2-Fc, than was seen in IL-4 –/– mice.

While animal models of pulmonary fibrosis have provided insight into a role for type 2 cytokines in the mediation of pulmonary fibrosis, recent studies have confirmed this profile in IPF. Lung tissue of patients with IPF have been examined for the presence of a type 1 versus a type 2 pattern of cytokine expression by in situ hybridization and immunolocalization of cytokine protein.[145] Although there is a pattern for the existence of both type 1 (characterized by the expression of IFN-γ) and type 2 (characterized by the expression of IL-4 and IL-5) cytokines in IPF lung tissue, the presence of type 2 cytokines predominated over the expression of IFN-γ.[145] This pattern of cytokine expression may be related to the potential role for the humoral response in the pathogenesis of IPF or be related to the inability of IFN-γ to tilt the balance away from an IL-4/IL-13–dependent profibrotic environment. In further support of an imbalance of the presence of type 2 cytokines as compared to IFN-γ, is the finding that IFN-γ levels are inversely related to the levels of type III procollagen in the BALF of IPF patients.[146] The levels of IFN-γ were especially correlated with patients that demonstrate progression of their pulmonary fibrosis by evidence of further deterioration of their pulmonary function.[146] These findings have been further substantiated by the recent suggestion that in IPF patients who had failed to respond to glucocorticoids, treatment with IFN-γ may be beneficial.[129] These findings suggest that the persistent imbalance in the expression of type 1 and type 2 cytokines in the lung may be a mechanism for the progression of diffuse pulmonary fibrosis.

IL-10 is a type 2 cytokine that inhibits a variety of innate and adaptive immune activities. IL-10 inhibits a number of proinflammatory cytokines that include IFN-γ, IL-1, TNF, IL-12, and CXC and CC chemokines.[147,148] The exogenous administration of IL-10 may protect the lung from injury in response to either LPS or immune-complex deposition,[149–151] however, IL-10 can be detrimental to the host under conditions of microorganism invasion.[152] The role of IL-10 in pulmonary fibrosis is controversial. Interestingly, patients with chronic hepatitis C who fail to respond to interferon have been treated with IL-10 with improved histology and decreased liver fibrosis.[153] Paradoxically, it has been shown that patients with hepatitis C that are genetically predisposed to high levels of IL-10 production, as determined by genetic analysis of the IL-10 locus, have a poor response to IFN-α.[154] Exogenous administration of IL-10 using a liposomal vector significantly inhibited bleomycin-induced pulmonary fibrosis in a murine model.[155] IL-10 down-regulates quartz-induced pulmonary inflammation and cell activation in a rat model.[156] In contrast silica induces fibrosis in NMRI mice who display decreased TNF activity and protracted overproduction of IL-10.[157] Similarly in IL-10 –/– mice that have been exposed to silica there is increased inflammation but decreased fibrosis suggesting that IL-10 has both anti-inflammatory and profibrotic activity.[158] With increasing evidence of a type 2 profile in IPF, the possibility of IL-10 exacerbating the disease can not be excluded. It is likely that there are significant variations in response depending on the dose of IL-10 that is used.

Interestingly IL-9, which is another type 2 cytokine that has been implicated in the pathogenesis of asthma, has been shown to attenuate silica-induced pulmonary fibrosis in a murine model.[159] This was demonstrated both in transgenic mice that systemically overexpressed IL-9 and also in wild-type mice that received systemic IL-9 by intraperitoneal injection.[159] Of particular interest was the fact that the overexpression of IL-9 was paradoxically associated with a reduced shift toward a type 2 response.[159] One possible explanation for this may be the difference between the response to the artificial overexpression of IL-9 as compared with its expression during a natural type 2 response.[160]

Growth Factors

Platelet-Derived Growth Factors

The PDGFs, first isolated from human platelets, have since been found to be produced by a variety of cell types including macrophages and endothelial cells.[161,162] PDGFs are a cationic, 31 kD family of mitogenic dimeric glycoproteins that are also chemotaxins for fibroblasts, myofibroblasts, and smooth muscle cells (Table 10–3).[161,162] As mitogens, the PDGFs are competence factors that mediate the transition of resting cells in G_0, to enter G_1 of the cell cycle.[16] The dimers of PDGF are derived from two separate genes and consist of two chains that may be assembled as homodimers, AA or BB, or as a heterodimer, AB. These chains are 60% homologous on an amino acid level.[16] The ligands interact with two receptors, alpha and beta receptors. The AA, AB, and BB dimers bind with high affinity to alpha receptor. In contrast, only the BB dimer binds with high affinity to the beta receptor. The AB heterodimer binds to the beta receptor with tenfold lower affinity than the BB homodimer. Ligand binding and receptor dimerization of both receptors lead to mitogenic activity, whereas, ligand binding to the beta receptor results in a chemotactic signal on appropriate cells.[163] Macrophages secrete primarily PDGF-AB and PDGF-BB whereas mesenchymal cells produce PDGF-AA. Alveolar macrophages recovered by bronchoalveolar lavage from patients with idiopathic pulmonary fibrosis have markedly greater spontaneous release of PDGF-like activity than alveolar macrophages isolated from normal subjects.[164,165] Both PDGF and

TABLE 10–3   The Role of Platelet-Derived Growth Factor in Fibrosis

Competence factor mediating transition from G_0 to G_1

Chemotactic for fibroblasts, myofibroblasts, and smooth muscle cells

Present in bronchoalveolar fluid of animal models of pulmonary fibrosis

PDGF receptor-α induced in rat myofibroblasts during fibrogenesis

IGF-1 have been found in bronchoalveolar lavage (BAL) during the development of animal models of bleomycin-induced pulmonary fibrosis.[166] Suppression of PDGF synthesis with pirfenidone, attenuated bleomycin-induced pulmonary fibrosis.[167] Overexpression of PDGF-BB in rat lung by means of an adenoviral vector leads to pulmonary fibrosis.[168] Furthermore, the PDGF receptor-α has been shown to be induced in rat myofibroblasts during fibrogenesis using a vanadium pentoxide model of lung injury.[169] Inhibition of autophosphorylation of the PDGF-R is 90% effective in preventing fibrosis in response to vanadium pentoxide in a rat model suggesting an important role for PDGF in this model of pulmonary fibrosis.[170] Taken together, these findings suggest an important role for PDGF in the development of pulmonary fibrosis.

Insulin-Like Growth Factor-1

Insulin-like growth factor-1 (IGF-1) or somatomedin C is a 25 kD polypeptide, formerly known as alveolar macrophage–derived growth factor (AMDGF).[171–173] IGF-1 is a progression factor that allows cells to proceed from G_1 through the remainder of the cell cycle.[16] A competence factor is necessary for an optimal concentration of a progression factor to induce cellular proliferation. In fact, IGF-1 acts synergistically with PDGF to promote fibroblast proliferation (Table 10–4).[173] Tissue-type macrophage-derived IGF-1 is substantially larger than serum IGF-1, which is only 6 to 7 kD.[173] The IGF-1 receptor is a cell surface tetrameric glycoprotein with significant homology to the insulin receptor.[174] The receptor consists of two alpha and two beta subunits with an intracellular cytoplasmic tyrosine kinase domain.[174] IGF-1 causes fibroblast proliferation after priming with a competence factor (serum).[171–173] Enhanced expression and release of IGF-1 have been shown in IPF.[175] IGF-1 bioavailability is dependent on high-affinity IGF-binding proteins that act as an extracellular sink to maintain IGF-1 levels.[176] There is evidence that post-translational modification of IGF-1 by insulin-like growth factor binding proteins (IGFBPs) leads to enhanced fibrogenesis in sarcoidosis and thus potentially other interstitial lung diseases.[177] Furthermore, there is evidence that IGFBPs may have some IGF independent actions themselves.[178] In bleomycin-induced pulmonary fibrosis, both PDGF and IGF-1 mRNAs from BAL cells are significantly elevated and parallel the deposition of extracellular matrix.[166] In IPF lung tissue, it has been shown that IGF-1 immunolocalizes to alveolar macrophages, interstitial macrophages, alveolar epithelial cells, and ciliated columnar epithelium.[179] The degree of clinical impairment and collagen deposition in the interstitium correlated with the degree of staining of CD68+ interstitial macrophages.[179] These findings support a role for interstitial macrophages as a source of IGF-1 in IPF. It has also been reported that in early IPF, in association with a more inflammatory phase, PDGF and IGF are predominantly localized in alveolar macrophages, monocytes, fibroblasts, type II pneumocytes, vascular endothelial cells, and smooth muscle cells.[164] In contrast, in later IPF, in association with a more fibrotic phase, PDGF and IGF-1 are exclusively localized to alveolar macrophages.[164] These findings suggest that the early expression of PDGF and IGF-1 from a number of pulmonary cells may contribute to the proliferation of mesenchymal cells and progression of lung fibrosis.

Basic Fibroblast Growth Factor

Basic fibroblast growth factor (bFGF or FGF-2) belongs to a large family of polypeptides (FGF-1 through FGF-22).[180] Similar to the effects of PDGF, bFGF is a competence factor in regulating the cell cycle of fibroblasts and other mesenchymal cells. The gene for bFGF is located on human chromosome 4 and does not encode a typical signal sequence for secreted proteins. The mature form of bFGF has a pI of 9.6, is 18 kD in mass, and is 55% homologous with acidic FGF (aFGF or FGF-1).[181] Basic FGF is produced in a variety of cells, including endothelial cells, fibroblasts, neuronal cells, mast cells and macrophages, and type II epithelial cells.[181–185] The bFGF receptor consists of three extracellular immunoglobulin-like domains and belongs to the family of transmembrane receptor tyrosine kinases.[181] Similar to PDGF receptors, ligand binding and dimerization of the receptor leads to signal coupling.[181] In addition, bFGF can induce the proliferation and differentiation of a number of cells, including fibroblasts, smooth muscle cells, and endothelial cells (Table 10–5).[181] This latter effect and the ability of bFGF to stimulate endothelial cell migration support its role in regulating angiogenesis. Although the role of bFGF has not been well defined during the pathogenesis of pulmonary fibrosis, it has been shown to be elevated both in serum and BAL of patients with IPF, which correlated with BAL cellularity and gas exchange abnormalities.[183] The mast cell was found to be the predominant cellular source of bFGF.[183] This was confirmed in another study, which found that bFGF is localized to the majority of mast cells from normal skin and lung and in tissue samples characterized by fibrosis and hyperplasia.[184] Studies have demonstrated altered immunohistochemical local-

---

**TABLE 10–4 The role of
Insulin-Like Growth Factor-1 in Fibrosis**

Competence factor mediating transition from G_0 to G_1

Synergistic with platelet-derived growth factor in promoting fibroblast proliferation

Elevated in idiopathic pulmonary fibrosis (IPF) lung tissue and animal models of fibrosis

Predominantly expressed by macrophages in IPF

**TABLE 10–5   The Role of
Basic Fibroblast Growth Factor in Fibrosis**

Competence factor for fibroblasts and other mesenchymal cells

Induces proliferation of fibroblasts, smooth muscle cells, and
endothelial cells

Elevated in serum and bronchoalveolar lavage fluid of patients
with idiopathic pulmonary fibrosis

TGF-β_1 induces marked increase in bFGF from type II cells

TGF = transforming growth factor; bFGF = basic fibroblast growth factor.

ization of bFGF after bleomycin-induced lung injury.[186]
Bleomycin-induced lung fibrosis is associated with the
presence of immunoreactive bFGF in the extracellular
matrix that colocalizes with evidence of cellular proliferation.[186] The predominant cellular source of bFGF
is the tissue mast cell.[186] Furthermore, macrophages
have been shown to be a major source of bFGF during the development of intra-alveolar fibrosis associated with ARDS.[182] It has recently been demonstrated
that TGF-β1 leads to a marked increase in bFGF from
type II cells suggesting that bFGF has an important role
in the fibrotic response.[185] In addition to the direct effects
on fibroblast proliferation, lung fibroplasia, and extracellular matrix deposition, bFGF is associated with neo-
vascular changes, and the presence of this potent angiogenic factor may play a role in the pathogenesis of
pulmonary fibrosis.[187,188]

Connective Tissue Growth Factor

Connective tissue growth factor (CTGF) was first
described as a polypeptide growth factor secreted by
endothelial cells and that stimulated DNA synthesis and
chemotaxis in fibroblasts.[189] It is now recognized as a
member of the structurally related CCN (*ctgf/cyr61/
nov*) gene family that contains six genes: *CTGF, cyr61,
nov, elm1, cop1, WISP-3*.[190] CTGF I is produced by vascular smooth muscle cells, fibroblasts, endothelial cells,
and epithelial cells and is activated by a number of factors, particularly TGF-β.[190] CTGF has in vitro activities
that include fibroblast proliferation, fibroplasia, and
extracellular matrix production (Table 10–6).[178,190,191]
Furthermore, its presence has been documented in skin
lesions of systemic sclerosis, keloids, scar tissue, and
eosinophilic fasciitis and in BALF from patients with
IPF and sarcoidosis.[178,190,191] Decreases in levels of CTGF
have been shown to correlate with objective clinical
response to IFN-γ treatment after 6 months in patients
with IPF.[129] The mechanism of action of CTGF has not
been fully elucidated. It is not clear what the cellular
receptor is although CTGF has heparin-binding properties and has been shown to interact with $\alpha_V\beta_3$ integrins
on endothelial cells.[190] However, this interaction has not
been shown to lead to intracellular signaling.[190] CTGF

may be responsible for many of the downstream actions
of TGF-β and is a potential therapeutic target for the
treatment of interstitial lung disease.

Fibrotic Cytokines

Transforming Growth Factor-Beta

Mammalian TGF-β belongs to a superfamily of genes
and exists as three closely homologous (72 to 80%)
dimeric isoforms, TGF-β_1, TGF-β_2, and TGF-β_3.[192,193]
The three isoforms of TGF-β are initially translated as a
prepropolypeptide that contains the hydrophobic signal
sequence, a latency-associated peptide, and the mature
form of the monomeric TGF-β.[194] TGF-β undergoes
initial NH_2-terminal cleavage with the removal of a 29
amino acid signal peptide, followed by dimerization and
secretion as an inactive latent-TGF-β complex.[194] Desta-
bilization of the latent-TGF-β complex and release of
the active 25 kD cytokine occurs with either proteolytic
activation or alterations in the ionic environment (eg, an
acidic pH).[192–195] Although the three isoforms of TGF-β
appear to have overlapping biologic activity, the predominant isoform of TGF-β is TGF-β_1.[192,193] There are
two TGF-β receptors designated TGF-β_1 type I receptor
(TβR-1) and TGF-β_1 type II receptor (TβR-2), which
are structurally similar and possess intrinsic serine/thre-
onine kinase activity.[196] Signaling occurs through het-
erodimerization of TβR-1 and TβR-2.[197,198] Binding of
ligand leads to a conformational change that causes activation of TβR-1 by the constitutively active TβR-2. Signal transduction to the nucleus is via the Smad group of
proteins.[197] Smad 1, 2, 3, 4, 5, 8 and 9 are activating signals, whereas, Smad 6 and 7 are inhibitory signals of
TGF-β_1 signaling.[197] IL-7 down-regulates TGF-β production in an IFN-γ–dependent manner,[199] and we have
shown that it is mediated via Smad 7 signaling [unpub-
lished observation].

TGF-β is produced by a variety of cells, including
platelets, neutrophils, eosinophils, mononuclear leukocytes, fibroblasts, and endothelial cells.[192,193,200,201] TGF-β
is a pleiotropic cytokine that can modulate inflamma-
tory and immune responses and orchestrate fibrosis and
tissue repair (Table 10–7). For example, TGF-β can

**TABLE 10–6   The Role of
Connective Tissue Growth Factor in Fibrosis**

Produced by vascular smooth muscle cells, fibroblasts, and
endothelial cells

Induces fibroblast proliferation, fibroplasia, and extracellular
matrix production

Present in bronchoalveolar lavage fluid from patients with
idiopathic pulmonary fibrosis and sarcoidosis

Present in a variety of fibrotic skin processes

Activated by transforming growth factor (TGF)-β

directly and indirectly, via regulation of IL-6, induce the production of acute phase proteins.[202] TGF-β can suppress macrophage respiratory burst, which results in significant attenuation of the generation of macrophage-derived H_2O_2.[203] TGF-β is a potent chemoattractant for monocytes and macrophages,[204] and can activate these cells to express IL-1, TNF, PDGF, and itself (TGF-$β_1$).[204,205] TGF-β can inhibit IgE synthesis in B cells stimulated with IL-4 and suppress other immunoglobulin (Ig) isotype production by inhibiting their synthesis and the switch from the membrane form to the secreted form of Ig mRNA.[206] TGF-β is a potent immunosuppressive agent that inhibits IL-1–dependent lymphocyte proliferation via down regulation of IL-2 receptors.[207]

In the context of fibrosis and tissue repair, TGF-β is chemotactic for fibroblasts and can indirectly induce their proliferation via the expression and autocrine and paracrine activity of PDGF B chain.[208,209] TGF-β is perhaps the most potent and efficacious promoter of extra-

cellular matrix production. TGF-β induces the gene expression and protein production of the following extracellular matrix constituents: fibronectin, osteopontin, tenascin, elastin, hyaluronic acid, chondroitin/dermatan sulfate proteoglycans, osteonectin, thrombospondin, and collagens I, III, IV, and V.[192,210] TGF-β promotes the production of connective tissue, however, it is equally efficacious for reducing the degradation of extracellular matrix by both inhibiting the generation of serine proteases (plasminogen activator), metalloproteinases, collagenases, elastases, and transin, and augmenting the expression of TIMP and plasminogen activator inhibitor.[192,210] In addition, although TGF-β inhibits endothelial proliferation in vitro, it is a potent stimulator of angiogenesis in vivo.[211] This in vivo angiogenic activity is due to the ability of this cytokine to indirectly stimulate angiogenesis by recruiting angiogenic macrophages.[204,212] The net result of increased production and decreased degradation of the connective tissue and promotion of angiogenesis is amplified deposition and persistence of new extracellular matrix. This suggests that TGF-β is a pivotal mediator of fibrosis in the lung.

In support of this contention is a number of studies that have clearly demonstrated that TGF-β is a cytokine involved in the promotion of pulmonary fibrosis. In bleomycin responsive (C57Bl/6) and -resistant (BALB/c) strains of mice, the lung content of $α_2$I procollagen, $α_1$III procollagen, and fibronectin mRNA is significantly increased in the bleomycin-responsive but not-resistant strains of mice.[18,213] The augmented gene expression for constituents of the extracellular matrix was paralleled by the gene expression and bioactivity of TGF-β.[18,213] These findings were also corroborated in hamster lungs after bleomycin-induced pulmonary fibrosis.[214] In addition, the gene expression of TGF-β has been associated with expression of small proteoglycans, such as biglycan, decorin, and fibromodulin during bleomycin-induced pulmonary fibrosis.[215] Although TGF-$β_1$, TGF-$β_2$, and TGF-$β_3$ can stimulate fibroblast procollagen production in vitro, these TGF-βs are differentially expressed during bleomycin-induced lung fibrosis.[216] In normal mouse lung, TGF-$β_1$ and TGF-$β_3$ mRNA transcripts are abundant in bronchiolar epithelium; however, in bleomycin-induced pulmonary fibrosis maximal expression of TGF-$β_1$ is predominately found and is primarily produced by macrophages along with its expression localized in lung mesenchymal cells that include endothelial cells and mesothelial cells.[216] In contrast, TGF-$β_3$ expression is unchanged, as compared with controls, and TGF-$β_2$ is not detected during bleomycin-induced pulmonary fibrosis.[216] These findings suggest that various isoforms of TGF-β are differentially regulated during bleomycin-induced pulmonary fibrosis, and TGF-$β_1$ is the predominate isoform expressed during the pathogenesis of fibrosis. Further evidence for the role of TGF-$β_1$ in pulmonary fibrosis is seen in the study by Sime and colleagues, who demonstrated that transient overexpression of active, but not

TABLE 10–7   The Role of Transforming Growth Factor-β in Fibrosis

Promotion of fibrosis
    Chemoattractant for mononuclear phagocytes
    Activates mononuclear phagocytes to express:
        IL-1
        TNF
        PDGF
        TGF-$β_1$

Chemotactic factor for fibroblasts

Indirectly induces fibroblast proliferation via the expression of PDGF

Promotes extracellular matrix production
    Fibronectin
    Osteopontin
    Tenascin
    Elastin
    Hyaluronic acid
    Chondroitin/dermatan sulfate proteoglycans
    Osteonectin
    Thrombospondin
    Collagens I, III, IV, V

Reduces the degradation of extracellular matrix, inhibits the generation of:
    Serine proteases (ie, plasminogen activators)
    Metalloproteinases
    Collagenases
    Elastases

Induces the expression of:
    Tissue inhibitor of metalloproteinases (TIMP)
    Plasminogen activator inhibitor

Inhibition of fibrosis
    Potent immunosuppressive factor that inhibits IL-1–dependent lymphocyte proliferation via down-regulation of IL-2 receptors

Bottom line
    Transient overexpression of active TGF-$β_1$ results in prolonged and severe interstitial and pleural fibrosis

IL = interleukin; TNF = tumor necrosis factor; PDGF = platelet-derived growth factor; TGF = transforming growth factor.

latent, TGF-β_1 resulted in prolonged and severe interstitial and pleural fibrosis characterized by extensive deposition of the extracellular matrix (ECM) proteins: collagen, fibronectin, and elastin.[27] The same authors have shown that transfer of TNF-α to rat lung induces severe pulmonary inflammation and patchy interstitial fibrogenesis that is due, in part, to the induction of TGF-β_1 with associated myofibroblasts.[28] In another study, it was shown that transfer of the *GM-CSF* gene to rat lung induces fibrosis.[217] Subsequent studies demonstrated that this effect was mediated through the induction of TGF-β_1 from alveolar macrophages.[218] Similarly, it has been demonstrated that the transient expression of IL-1β using an adenoviral vector can lead to progressive fibrosis long after the IL-1β levels have declined and the acute inflammatory response has resolved. The development of fibrosis under these conditions was associated with a sustained increase in levels of TGF-β1.[66] These results illustrate the role of TGF-β_1 and the importance of its activation in potentially sustaining the profibrotic environment in pulmonary fibrosis, and suggest that targeting active TGF-β_1 and steps involved in TGF-β_1 activation and signal transduction are likely to be valuable antifibrogenic therapeutic strategies.

The activation of TGF-β has been shown to be pivotal to the development of the fibrotic process. The integrin $\alpha v \beta 6$ has been shown to have an important role in the binding and activation of latent TGF-β1.[219] Mice that are deficient in $\alpha v \beta 6$ develop exaggerated inflammation but are protected from the development of fibrosis in response to bleomycin.[219] This illustrates the importance of TGF-β both in the promotion of fibrosis and as a potent anti-inflammatory cytokine. The fact that inflammation and fibrosis can be separated in this and other transgenic models should not be mistaken as evidence that the processes are separate and isolated events. Inflammation is a potent inducer of integrins, which can subsequently activate TGF-β; similarly, there are proteolytic pathways for the activation of TGF-β_1.[220] Furthermore it has recently been described that IL-13 is a potent inducer and activator of TGF-β_1 via protease-dependent mechanisms.[139] Macrophages were the major source of TGF-β_1 production.[139] IL-13 is classically associated with type 2–mediated inflammation and is further evidence for the importance of initial inflammation in the subsequent activation of TGF-β_1 and development of fibrosis. Once TGF-β_1 has been activated there is a positive feedback loop whereby TGF-β_1 itself induces $\beta 6$ integrin subunit expression thereby amplifying the anti-inflammatory and profibrotic cycle.[221]

In other studies, the passive immunization of bleomycin-treated mice with both neutralizing antibodies to TGF-β_1 and TGF-β_2 results in a significant reduction in total lung collagen content, as measured by the level of hydroxyproline.[222] This has been verified in another animal model of pulmonary fibrosis. Studies using heat-killed bacille Calmette-Guérin (BCG) to induce lung fibrosis followed by passive immunization

with neutralizing TGF-β_1 antibodies resulted in a marked decline in the presence of collagen deposition, as determined by morphometric analysis of Masson trichrome stain of lung sections and total lung hydroxyproline levels.[223] These studies support the contention that TGF-β may be an important mediator of pulmonary fibrosis in humans. In IPF, increased expression of TGF-β has been found by immunohistochemistry and is localized to bronchiolar epithelial cells, epithelial cells of honeycomb cysts, and hyperplastic type II pneumocytes. In addition, TGF-β has been found in IPF in association with constituents of the extracellular matrix.[224] The predominate isoform of TGF-β in IPF, similar to what has been found in bleomycin-induced pulmonary fibrosis, is TGF-β_1.[225] Our laboratory found that TGF-β protein levels, as measured by specific ELISA of lung tissue homogenates, were elevenfold higher in patients with IPF, as compared with normal control lung.[69] Interestingly, we found no significant difference in the levels of TGF-β from patients with IPF that exhibited a predominant histopathologic pattern of desquamative interstitial pneumonitis (DIP) versus UIP.[69] However, our ELISA did not specifically differentiate between active and latent forms of TGF-β. Furthermore, we have found that levels of TGF-β in BAL from patients with IPF may directly correlate with mortality.[72] These findings suggest that TGF-β is a critical cytokine for the promotion of pulmonary fibrosis.

Chemotactic Cytokines

Chemokines

Although not all inflammatory disorders result in fibrosis, fibrotic responses are always preceded and potentially perpetuated by chronic inflammation, especially mononuclear phagocyte infiltration. The salient feature of chronic inflammation is the association of leukocyte infiltration. These recruited leukocytes, and in particular macrophages, contribute to the pathogenesis of chronic inflammation and promote fibrosis via the elaboration of a variety of cytokines. The maintenance of leukocyte recruitment during inflammation requires intercellular communication between infiltrating leukocytes and the endothelium, resident stroma, and parenchymal cells. These events are mediated via the generation of early response cytokines (eg, IL-1 and TNF), the expression of cell-surface adhesion molecules, and the production of chemotactic molecules, such as chemokines.

The human CXC, CC, C, and CXXXC chemokine families of chemotactic cytokines are four closely related polypeptide families that behave, in general, as potent chemotactic factors for neutrophils, eosinophils, basophils, monocytes, mast cells, dendritic cells, NK cells, and T and B lymphocytes (Table 10–8). These cytokines in their monomeric form range from 7 to

10 kD and are characteristically basic heparin-binding proteins. The chemokines display highly conserved cysteine amino acid residues. The CXC chemokine family has the first two NH_2-terminal cysteines separated by one nonconserved amino acid residue, the CXC cysteine motif. The CC chemokine family has the first two NH_2-terminal cysteines in juxtaposition, the CC cysteine motif. The C chemokine has one lone NH_2-terminal cysteine amino acid, the C cysteine motif; the CXXXC chemokine has the first two NH_2-terminal cysteines separated by three nonconserved amino acid residues. Interestingly, CXC chemokines are, in general, clustered on human chromosome 4 and exhibit between 20 to 50% homology on the amino acid level;

TABLE 10–8   The Human C, CC, CXC, and CXXXC Chemokine Families of Chemotactic Cytokines

C Chemokines
XCL1	Lymphotactin
XCL2	SCM-1β

CC Chemokines
CCL1	I-309
CCL2	Monocyte chemotactic protein-1 (MCP-1)
CCL3	Macrophage inflammatory protein-1 alpha (MIP-1α)
CCL4	Macrophage inflammatory protein-1 beta (MIP-1β)
CCL5	Regulated on activation normal T-cell expressed and secreted (RANTES)
CCL7	Monocyte chemotactic protein-3 (MCP-3)
CCL8	Monocyte chemotactic protein-2 (MCP-2)
CCL9	Macrophage inflammatory protein-1 delta (MIP-1δ)
CCL11	Eotaxin
CCL13	Monocyte chemotactic protein-4 (MCP-4)
CCL14	HCC-1
CCL15	HCC-2
CCL16	HCC-4
CCL17	Thymus and activation-regulated chemokine (TARC)
CCL18	DC-CK-1
CCL19	Macrophage inflammatory protein-3 beta (MIP-3β)
CCL20	Macrophage inflammatory protein-3 alpha (MIP-3α)
CCL21	6Ckine
CCL22	MDC
CCL23	MPIF-1
CCL24	MPIF-2
CCL25	TECK
CCL26	Eotaxin-3
CCL27	CTACK

CXC Chemokines
CXCL1	Growth-related oncogene alpha (GRO-α)
CXCL2	Growth-related oncogene beta (GRO-β)
CXCL3	Growth-related oncogene gamma (GRO-γ)
CXCL4	Platelet factor-4 (PF4)
CXCL5	Epithelial neutrophil activating protein-78 (ENA-78)
CXCL6	Granulocyte chemotactic protein-2 (GCP-2)
CXCL7	Neutrophil activating protein-2 (NAP-2)
CXCL8	Interleukin-8 (IL-8)
CXCL9	Monokine induced by interferon- γ (MIG)
CXCL10	Interferon-γ-inducible protein (IP-10)
CXCL11	Interferon inducible T cell alpha chemoattractant (ITAC)
CXCL12	Stromal cell derived factor-1 (SDF-1)
CXCL13	B cell-attracting chemokine-1 (BCA-1)

CXXXC Chemokines
CXC3CL1	Fractalkine

CC chemokines are, in general, clustered on human chromosome 17 and exhibit between 28 to 45% homology on the amino acid level. The one C chemokine, lymphotactin, is located on human chromosome 1, and the one CXXXC, fractalkine, is located on human chromosome 16. There is approximately 20 to 40% homology between the members of the four chemokine families.

The murine homologues of the human CXC chemokines, KC/CXCL1, macrophage inflammatory protein-2 (MIP-2)/CXCL2, IP-10/CXCL10, MIG/CXCL9, and SDF-1/CXCL12 are structurally homologous to human GRO-α/CXCL1, GRO-β/GRO-γ (CXCL2/CXCL3), IP-10/CXCL10, MIG/CXCL9, and SDF-1/CXCL12, respectively.[226,227] No murine or rat structural homologue exists for human IL-8.[226,227] The murine CC and C chemokines, in general, are known by the same names as their human counterparts.[6,226–228] The CXXXC chemokine, fractalkine/CX3CL1, was initially described on nonhematopoietic cells, and it can exist as either a membrane-anchored or shed glycoprotein, which act as a potent adhesion molecule or chemoattractant, respectively, for T cells and monocytes.[229,230]

Chemokines have been found to be produced by an array of cells including monocytes, alveolar macrophages, neutrophils, platelets, eosinophils, mast cells, T and B lymphocytes, NK cells, keratinocytes, mesangial cells, epithelial cells, hepatocytes, fibroblasts, smooth muscle cells, mesothelial cells, and endothelial cells. These cells can produce chemokines in response to a variety of factors, including viruses, bacterial products, IL-1, TNF, C5a, LTB_4, and IFNs. The production of chemokines by both immune and nonimmune cells supports the contention that these cytokines may play a pivotal role in orchestrating chronic inflammation. We will focus our discussion on the role of the CXC and CC chemokine families in the context of pulmonary fibrosis.

CXC Chemokines

The CXC chemokines can be further divided into two groups on the basis of a structure/function domain consisting of the presence or absence of three amino acid residues (Glu-Leu-Arg; "ELR" motif) that precedes the first cysteine amino acid residue in the primary structure of these cytokines.[6,226,228,231–234] The ELR⁺ CXC chemokines are chemoattractants for neutrophils and act as potent angiogenic factors.[235–237] In contrast, the ELR⁻ CXC chemokines are chemoattractants for mononuclear cells and are potent inhibitors of angiogenesis (Table 10–9).[237,238]

Based on the structural/functional difference, the members of the CXC chemokine family are unique cytokines in their ability to behave in a disparate manner in the regulation of angiogenesis. The angiogenic members include IL-8/CXCL8, epithelial neutrophil activating protein-78 (ENA-78)/CXCL5, growth-related genes (GRO-α, -β, and -γ)/CXCL1, 2 and 3, granulocyte chemotactic protein-2 (GCP-2)/CXCL6, and NH_2-terminal truncated forms of platelet basic protein (PBP), which are generated by proteolytic cleavage with monocyte-derived proteases and include connective tissue activating protein-III (CTAP-III), beta-thromboglobulin (β-TG), and neutrophil activating protein-2 (NAP-2). GRO-α, -β, and -γ are closely related CXC chemokines, with GRO-α/CXCL1 originally described for its melanoma growth stimulatory activity (see Table 10–9). IL-8/CXCL8, ENA-78/CXCL5, and GCP-2/CXCL6 were all initially identified on the basis of neutrophil activation and chemotaxis.

The angiostatic (ELR⁻) members of the CXC chemokine family include platelet factor 4 (PF4)/CXCL4, which was originally described for its ability to bind heparin and inactivate heparin's anticoagulation function. Other angiostatic ELR⁻ CXC chemokines include MIG/CXCL9 and IP-10/CXCL10 (see Table 10–9). Stromal cell–derived factor (SDF-1)/CXCL12 gained notoriety when it was shown that SDF-1/CXCL12 induces lymphocyte migration and prevents infection of T cells by lymphotropic strains of human immunodeficiency virus (HIV)-1. Although SDF-1/CXCL12 is another ELR⁻ CXC chemokine, it remains unclear whether it inhibits angiogenesis. SDF-1/CXCL12 was found to induce in vitro migration of human umbilical vein endothelial cells, whereas, in another study, SDF-1/CXCL12 was found to attenuate the in vivo angiogenic activity of either ELR⁺ CXC chemokines, bFGF, or vascular endothelial growth factor (VEGF) using the rat cornea micropocket assay of neovascularization.[239]

Of particular interest is the fact that IP-10/CXCL10 and MIG/CXCL9 are highly induced by interferons. IP-10/CXCL10 can be induced by all three interferons (IFN-α, -β, and -γ). MIG/CXCL9 is unique in that it is only induced by IFN-γ. In addition, IL-12 and IL-18, via the induction of IFN-γ, have been found to induce the expression of IP-10/CXCL10 and MIG/CXCL9.[240]

While interferons induce the production of the angiostatic CXC chemokines, IP-10/CXCL10 and MIG/CXCL9, they attenuate the expression of the angiogenic CXC chemokines IL-8/CXCL8, GRO-α/CXCL1, and ENA-78/CXCL5. This differential regulation of angiostatic versus angiogenic CXC chemokines by interferons is likely to account for their previously documented inhibitory effect on angiogenesis.

Interesting information on chemokine function can be obtained from transgenic animal models. Transgenic mice that overexpress IL-8/CXCL8 on a liver-specific promoter do not develop neutrophil infiltrates in their liver.[241] They have high circulating IL-8/CXCL8 levels that are associated with L-selectin shedding from the neutrophils and lack the ability to induce neutrophil accumulation in response to local stimuli.[241] Similarly, intravenous administration of IL-8/CXCL8 in rabbits prevents local neutrophil accumulation, although L-selectin shedding was not observed.[242,243] Furthermore, mice that express KC (murine homologue of GRO-α/CXCL1) on a lung cc10 promoter have demonstrated that chronic unregulated expression of KC/CXCL1 is associated with attenuated recruitment of neutrophils over time.[244] Similar findings have been reported in the thymus.[245] Furthermore, the neutrophil accumulation that was seen early in the lungs of KC/CXCL1 transgenic mice is not associated with tissue injury or evidence for the development of fibrosis or emphysema.[244] Similarly, mice that express MCP-1/CCL2 under the control of the insulin promoter develop a monocytic insulitis without tissue damage or diabetes.[246] These studies demonstrate that chemokines exert their attractant effects only when expressed locally at low levels and that chemoattraction is not always associated with leukocyte activation. Furthermore, this may explain the relative lack of neutrophils in chronic inflammatory/fibroproliferative disorders associated with significant levels of IL-8/CXCL8 or other ELR⁺ CXC chemokines, whereas these chemokines are acting as angiogenic factors.[247–250]

CXC Chemokine Receptors

Chemokine activities are mediated through G protein–coupled receptors. Six CXC chemokine receptors have been identified (Table 10–10).[251,252] The ELR⁺ chemokines bind to CXCR1 and CXCR2 receptors that are found on neutrophils, T lymphocytes, monocytes, basophils, keratinocytes, mast cells, and endothelial cells.[253,254] The CXCR1 and CXCR2 receptor genes are found on human chromosome 2(q34-q35) and may have arisen from duplication of a common ancestral gene. Whereas the transmembrane and the second and third intracellular/cytoplasmic domains of these receptors are well conserved, the NH_2- and COOH-terminal ends of these receptors are variable. The intracellular COOH-terminus of these receptors is rich in serine and threonine amino acid residues that may be important in phospho-

TABLE 10–9   The CXC Chemokines that Display Disparate Angiogenic Activity

Angiogenic CXC chemokines containing the ELR motif

CXCL1	Growth-related oncogene alpha (GRO-α)
CXCL2	Growth-related oncogene beta (GRO-β)
CXCL3	Growth-related oncogene gamma (GRO-γ)
CXCL5	Epithelial neutrophil activating protein-78 (ENA-78)
CXCL6	Granulocyte chemotactic protein-2 (GCP-2)
CXCL7	Neutrophil activating protein-2 (NAP-2)
CXCL8	Interleukin-8 (IL-8)

Angiostatic CXC chemokines that lack the ELR motif

CXCL4	Platelet factor-4 (PF4)
CXCL9	Monokine induced by interferon-γ (MIG)
CXCL10	Interferon-γ-inducible protein (IP-10)
CXCL11	Interferon inducible T cell alpha chemoattractant (ITAC)
CXCL12	Stromal cell derived factor-1 (SDF-1)

TABLE 10–10   The CXC Chemokine Receptors

Receptor	Ligand
CXCR1	CXCL6, CXCL8
CXCR2	CXCL1, CXCL2, CXCL3, CXCL5, CXCL6, CXCL7, CXCL8
CXCR3	CXCL9,CXCL10, CXCL11
CXCR4	CXCL12
CXCR5	CXCL13

rylation and signal coupling via G proteins.[255–257] In general, these receptors are coupled to $G_{\alpha i}$ proteins that are inhibited in response to pertussis toxin.[252,258–262]

Members of the herpesvirus family have been demonstrated to encode genes that mimic the chemokine receptors.[263] Both herpesvirus saimiri (HVS) and Kaposi's sarcoma–associated herpesvirus (KSHV) have the genes, *ECRF3* and *ORF74*, respectively, that encode a G protein–coupled receptor, with significant homology to CXCR2.[264,265] These receptors are functional and specific receptors for the CXC chemokines. Similarly, human CMV can encode four G protein–coupled receptors, UL33, US27, US28, and UL78.[263] US28 binds CC chemokines and has homology with CX_3CR1 and binds fractalkine.[263] Human herpesvirus 6 encodes a functional chemokine receptor homologue designated US12, which binds CC chemokines.[263] Moreover, the expression of these receptors suggests a potential role for chemokines in mediating the pathogenesis associated with the infection of these viruses. For example, *ORF74* expression on the cell surface is associated with constitutive activity that can induce cellular proliferation, cell transformation, and tumorigenicity.[266,267] In addition, ELR$^+$ CXC chemokine ligands, such as IL-8 and GRO-α, can bind to this receptor and further augment signal transduction of this receptor.[268] Furthermore the non-ELR CXC chemokine, IP-10, has been found to inhibit signaling of this receptor.[268]

The receptor for IP-10 and MIG, CXCR3, is expressed on activated T lymphocytes in the presence of IL-2; however, it is not significantly present on resting T and B lymphocytes, monocytes, or neutrophils.[269] CXCR4 is the specific receptor for SDF-1 and is the cofactor for lymphotropic HIV-1, and SDF-1 is a potent inhibitor of HIV entry into T lymphocytes.[252,270,271] In contrast to CXCR3, CXCR4 appears to be expressed on resting T lymphocytes.[252,270,271] These findings suggest that ELR$^-$ CXC chemokines and their receptors are important in regulating mononuclear cell function. CXCR1, CXCR2, and CXCR4 are expressed on human umbilical vein endothelial cells (HUVEC) and the spontaneously transformed HUVEC cell line, ECV304.[272] We have found that CXCR2 is expressed on human microvascular endothelial cells (HMVEC) and that it mediates the angiogenic effects of ELR$^+$ chemokines.[253] Recent evidence suggests that the expression of CXCR3 on HUMVEC is cell cycle dependant.[273]

CXCR5 is the receptor for B-cell-attracting chemokine-1 (BCA-1).[274] It was originally described on Burkitt's lymphoma cells and B lymphocytes and was noticed to have many structural similarities to other chemokine receptors.[275] BCA-1 and CXCR5 are necessary for the homing of B lymphocytes and proper development of the B-cell-rich regions of lymphoid organs.[276] CXCR6 is a receptor for the recently described CXCL16, which differs from other CXC chemokines in that its sequence predicts that it is membrane bound and suspended by a mucin stalk in a similar fashion to fractalkine/CX3C.[277] CXCR6 was initially described as an orphan receptor that could serve as a coreceptor for HIV.[261,278] CXCR6 is predominantly expressed on type 1 polarized T cells suggesting it may have a role in type 1–mediated processes.[279]

Although the CXCRs have been demonstrated to have functional activity with ligand binding, another chemokine receptor has been identified that apparently binds chemokines without a subsequent signal-coupling event. This receptor demonstrates promiscuity in that it binds both CXC and CC chemokines without apparent signal coupling.[252,255–257] This receptor was originally found on human erythrocytes and felt to represent a "sink" for chemokines.[257] In addition to binding of the chemokine family, this receptor has been found to be shared by the malarial parasites, *Plasmodium vivax* and *P. knowlesi*, and may allow their invasion into erythrocytes.[257] This receptor has been cloned and found to be identical to the Duffy blood group antigen and is now referred to as the Duffy antigen receptor for chemokines (DARC). Its structure demonstrates a seven transmembrane spanning receptor motif similar to other chemokine receptors.[252,257] Further studies are required to examine the functional nature of this receptor.

The Role of CXC Chemokines in Pulmonary Fibrosis

Idiopathic pulmonary fibrosis is a disease of unknown etiology that is characterized by the accumulation of neutrophils within the air space and mononuclear cells within the interstitium, followed by the progressive deposition of collagen within the interstitium and subsequent destruction of lung tissue.[16,17] Further support for the notion of a continuum of inflammation to fibrosis is seen in the study by Flaherty and colleagues who found differing diagnoses between lobes in 26% of patients undergoing surgical biopsy for ILD.[33] Patients concordant for UIP in all lobes were older than those discordant for UIP who, in turn, were older than those with NSIP in all lobes, supporting the concept of an evolving process.[33] Whereas the mechanisms of cellular injury and the role of classic inflammatory cells remain unclear, activated alveolar macrophages, interstitial macrophages, and neutrophils undoubtedly play a significant role in the pathogenesis of the inflammatory lung lesion of IPF.[16,17,20]

Increases in neutrophils in BALF and in lung tissue have been demonstrated from patients with IPF. Although the number or proportion of neutrophils in BALF does not correlate with the activity of alveolitis and has limited prognostic value, declines in BALF neutrophils typically occur among patients exhibiting favorable responses to therapy.[280] Neutrophilic alveolitis has been described in humans with IPF, collagen vascular diseases with associated ILD, as well as diverse animal models of pulmonary fibrosis. The neutrophil represents a potent immune effector cell and has the capacity to release oxygen radicals, complement fragments, arachidonic acid metabolites, proteolytic enzymes, and various cytokines, which may inflict lung injury and mitigate the transition from innate to adaptive immunity.[16,17] Recent work in rabbit lungs suggests that pulmonary fibrosis in response to a variety of fibrogenic substances correlates with the duration of tissue neutrophil activation.[281] The signals responsible for the recruitment of neutrophils to the lung and the perpetuation of neutrophilic alveolitis are not known. Our laboratory and others have found that IL-8/CXCL8 is significantly elevated in IPF, as compared to either normal or sarcoidosis patients, and correlates with the BALF presence of neutrophils.[282,283] Several of these studies have identified the alveolar macrophage to be an important cellular source of IL-8/CXCL8 in IPF.[282,283] In addition, these studies have suggested that levels of IL-8/CXCL8 in IPF may correlate with a worse prognosis.[284]

Although studies have suggested an importance for IL-8/CXCL8 in mediating neutrophil recruitment, CXC chemokines have been found to exert disparate effects in regulating angiogenesis.[237] This latter issue is relevant to IPF, as the pathology of IPF demonstrates features of dysregulated and abnormal repair with exaggerated angiogenesis, fibroproliferation, and deposition of extracellular matrix, leading to progressive fibrosis and loss of lung function. The existence of neovascularization in IPF was originally identified by Turner-Warwick who examined the lungs of patients with IPF and demonstrated neovascularization leading to anastomoses between the systemic and pulmonary microvasculature.[188] Further evidence of neovascularization during the pathogenesis of pulmonary fibrosis has been demonstrated in bleomycin-induced pulmonary fibrosis following the perfusion of the vascular tree of rat lungs with methacrylate resin at a time of maximal bleomycin-induced pulmonary fibrosis.[187] Using scanning electron microscopy, these investigators demonstrated major vascular modifications that included neovascularization of an elaborate network of microvasculature located in the peribronchial regions of the lungs and distortion of the architecture of the alveolar capillaries. The location of neovascularization was closely associated with regions of pulmonary fibrosis, similar to the findings for human lungs,[188] and this neovascularization appeared to lead to the formation of systemic-pulmonary anastomoses.[187] Recently, angiogenesis has been shown to develop in the mouse lung within 6 days in response to ischemia, with

the new vessels arising entirely from vessels between the parietal and visceral pleura and accounting for 15% of the normal pulmonary blood flow.[285] Although these studies supported the presence of angiogenesis, there have been limited investigations to delineate factors that may be involved in the regulation of this angiogenic activity during pulmonary fibrosis.

Our laboratory has demonstrated that in IPF lung tissue there is an imbalance in the presence of CXC chemokines that behave as either promoters of angiogenesis (IL-8/CXCL8) or inhibitors of angiogenesis (IP-10/CXCL10).[247] This imbalance favors augmented net angiogenic activity.[247] Lung tissue from IPF patients have elevated levels of IL-8/CXCL8, as compared with control lung tissue and demonstrate in vivo angiogenic activity that can be significantly attributed to IL-8/CXCL8.[247] Immunolocalization of IL-8 demonstrated that the pulmonary fibroblast was the predominant interstitial cellular source of this chemokine, and areas of IL-8/CXCL8 expression were essentially devoid of neutrophil infiltration.[247] This would seem to be discordant with the previous observations of augmented BALF IL-8/CXCL8 in IPF, in association with BALF neutrophilia.[283] However, this disparity may be explained by the different compartments analyzed in these studies (ie, BALF versus lung interstitium); moreover, BALF neutrophilia may simply be a marker of disease without neutrophils actually contributing to the pathogenesis of IPF. In further support of IL-8/CXCL8's role as an angiogenic factor is its association with the regulation of angiogenic activity in psoriasis, coronary artery atherosclerosis, rheumatoid arthritis, non–small cell lung cancer, and melanoma.[250,286–292] This supports an alternative biologic role for IL-8/CXCL8 or other ELR+ CXC chemokines in the interstitium of IPF lung tissue.

In contrast to the increased angiogenic activity attributable to IL-8/CXCL8, we found a deficiency in the production of the angiostatic factor IP-10/CXCL10 in IPF, as compared with controls.[247] Interestingly, IFN-γ, a major inducer of IP-10/CXCL10 from a number of cells, is a known inhibitor of wound repair, in part, due to its angiostatic properties, and has been shown to attenuate fibrosis in bleomycin-induced pulmonary fibrosis.[126] This supports the notion that a distal mediator of the affect of IFN-γ is IP-10/CXCL10, and an imbalance in the expression of this angiostatic CXC chemokine is found in IPF. These results suggest that attenuation of the angiogenic (IL-8/CXCL8) or augmentation of the angiostatic (IP-10/CXCL10) CXC chemokines may represent a viable therapeutic option for the treatment of IPF.

The pulmonary fibroblast is the predominant cellular source of IL-8/CXCL8 in the interstitium of IPF, supporting the notion that the pulmonary fibroblast has a pivotal role in mediating the angiogenic activity during the pathogenesis of IPF.[247] Indeed the pulmonary fibroblast has received increasing attention as a pivotal cell in the pathogenesis of IPF.[20] Relative levels of IL-8/CXCL8 and IP-10/CXCL10 from IPF pulmonary fibroblast–conditioned media demonstrated a significant imbalance favoring IL-8/CXCL8–induced angiogenic activity. In contrast, normal pulmonary fibroblasts had greater levels of bioactive IP-10/CXCL10 that favored a net inhibition of angiogenesis.[247] The difference in expression of IL-8/CXCL8 and IP-10/CXCL10 between IPF and control pulmonary fibroblasts lends further support to the notion of a phenotypic difference between IPF and normal pulmonary fibroblasts, which has been well described.[293]

We have recently shown that ENA-78/CXCL5 is an additional important regulator of angiogenic activity in IPF.[294] We found that lung tissue from patients with IPF expressed greater levels of ENA-78/CXCL5 as compared with normal control lung tissue. These higher levels of ENA-78/CXCL5 were associated with increased angiogenic activity as assessed by the corneal micropocket assay that was significantly attributable to ENA-78/CXCL5. The predominant cellular sources of ENA-78/CXCL5 were hyperplastic type II cells and macrophages. These hyperplastic type II cells are associated with areas of active inflammation and are often found in proximity to fibroblastic foci. This is in contrast to our previous findings that pulmonary fibroblasts were the predominant cellular source of IL-8/CXCL8 and suggests that the expression of chemokines with similar biologic functions does not necessarily indicate redundancy.[247] Furthermore, it is further support for the role of nonimmune cells in the pathogenesis of IPF and may explain the failure of conventional immunosuppressive agents in this disease.

The finding that both IL-8/CXCL8 and ENA-78/CXCL5 have important roles in the pathogenesis of IPF raises the question of the relative roles of IL-8/CXCL8 and ENA-78/CXCL5 in promoting angiogenesis in IPF. In our corneal micropocket model, we have previously shown that neutralizing antibodies to IL-8/CXCL8 significantly inhibit the angiogenic activity of IPF samples, and we have now also shown that anti–ENA-78/CXCL5 antibodies significantly inhibit the angiogenic activity of IPF samples. This is similar to previous findings in rheumatoid arthritis.[289] As IL-8/CXCL8 and ENA-78/CXCL5 share the same receptor (CXCR2), one possible explanation is heterologous desensitization of the receptor, whereby neutralization of ENA-78/CXCL5 may overexpose the receptor to IL-8/CXCL8 (and vice versa), thereby resulting in desensitization of the receptor as is seen in chemotaxis assays at high concentrations of the ligand.[295] Our results do not show that either ENA-78/CXCL5 or IL-8/CXCL8 is more important but merely that they both play an important role in angiogenic activity in IPF. Furthermore we cannot exclude that other angiogenic factors might be involved. Our laboratory has recently described CXCR2 as the receptor that mediates the angiogenic activity of the ELR+ CXC chemokines.[253] As both IL-8/CXCL8 and ENA-78/CXCL5 bind to CXCR2, this may represent an attractive therapeutic target with respect to the inhibition of angiogenesis, thereby inhibiting or retarding the progression of IPF.

To determine whether the imbalance in the expression of these CXC chemokines is relevant to the pathogenesis of pulmonary fibrosis, the expression and biologic activity of murine MIP-2 (MIP-2/CXCL2; an angiogenic ELR+ CXC chemokine homologous to human GRO-β/γ/CXCL2/3) and the angiostatic CXC chemokine, IP-10/CXCL10, were correlated with the extent of fibrosis during bleomycin-induced pulmonary fibrosis in a murine model system.[296,297] MIP-2/CXCL2 and IP-10/CXCL10 were temporally measured during bleomycin-induced pulmonary fibrosis from whole lung tissues and were found to be directly and inversely correlated, respectively, using total lung hydroxyproline levels, a measure of lung collagen deposition.[296,297] Moreover, if either endogenous MIP-2/CXCL2 was depleted by passive immunization with neutralizing antibodies, or exogenous IP-10/CXCL10 was administered to the animals during bleomycin exposure, both treatment strategies resulted in marked attenuation of pulmonary fibrosis that was entirely attributable to a reduction in angiogenesis in the lung.[296,297] These findings support the notion that angiogenesis is a critical biologic event that supports fibroplasia and deposition of ECM in the lung during pulmonary fibrosis, and that angiogenic and angiostatic factors, such as CXC chemokines, play an important role in the pathogenesis of this process.

We have recently shown that IL-12 attenuates bleomycin-induced pulmonary fibrosis via the induction of IFN-γ.[127] Moreover, the beneficial effects of IL-12 can be inhibited by simultaneous administration of anti–IFN-γ antibodies.[127] These findings provide further support for IFN-γ, and thereby the interferon-inducible chemokines, IP-10/CXCL10 and MIG/CCL9, as inhibitors of fibrosis. In contrast, an antibody to IL-12 was found to attenuate bleomycin-induced pulmonary fibrosis.[298] Although these findings appear contradictory, they can be explained by the fact that during bleomycin-induced fibrosis the IL-12 p40 subunit is preferentially expressed over IL-12 p70.[298] This is relevant due to the fact that IL-12 p40 antagonizes the effect of IL-12 p70 thereby suppressing type 1 mediated responses.[298] Furthermore, there was no change in levels of IFN-γ protein in this study.[298] Interestingly, bleomycin-induced pulmonary fibrosis was shown to be attenuated in IFN-γ –/– mice.[299] This would appear to contradict previous studies that have shown that IFN-γ inhibits wound repair[300] and attenuates fibrosis in bleomycin-induced pulmonary fibrosis.[301,302] The difference may be related to timing, IFN-γ may be necessary to initiate the inflammatory response, which was diminished in the IFN-γ –/– mice and only exerts antifibrotic effects once the fibrotic process has been initiated. With the recent demonstration of the efficacy of the IFN-γ treatment of IPF patients,[129] the above studies substantiate that the IFN-γ treatment of IPF may mediate its effect, in part, by shifting the imbalance of the expression of ELR[+] and ELR[−] CXC chemokines to favor an angiostatic environment. This leads to inhibition of dysregulated neovascularization/vascular remodeling, fibroproliferation, and deposition of the extracellular matrix in IPF patients.

CC Chemokines

The CC chemokines (see Table 10–9) are chemoattractants for monocytes, T and B lymphocytes, NK cells, dendritic cells, basophils, mast cells, and eosinophils.[226,2000#401,227] The genes for CC chemokines are, in general, clustered on human chromosome 17 (q11.2-q12).[226,2000#401,227] In general, the CC chemokine genes have three exons and two introns. The first and second introns of all the genes of this chemokine family are highly conserved.[6,226,228] The splice junctions between the second and third exons in all CC chemokine genes occur at precisely the same position, suggesting that the CXC and CC chemokine superfamily may have diverged from a common ancestral gene.[6,226,228]

The CC chemokines have been found to be produced by an array of cells including monocytes, alveolar macrophages, neutrophils, platelets, eosinophils, mast cells, T cells, B cells, NK cells, keratinocytes, mesangial cells, epithelial cells, hepatocytes, fibroblasts, smooth muscle cells, mesothelial cells, and endothelial cells.[6,226,228] These cells can produce CC chemokines in response to a variety of factors, including viruses, bacterial products, IL-1, TNF, C5a, LTB$_4$, and IFNs and appear to be significantly susceptible to suppression by IL-10.[6,226,228]

The primary structure of members of the CC chemokine family is similar to MCP-1/CCL2.[6,226,228,303] There is a 29 to 71% sequence homology on the amino acid level of the other CC chemokines with MCP-1/CCL2. The CC and CXC chemokines are similar in size and in primary structures and form two intrachain disulfide bonds; whereas, I-309 and 6Ckine have six cysteine amino acid residues and form three intrachain disulfide bonds. The CC chemokines lack a conserved NH$_2$-terminal sequence analogous to the ELR motif of the CXC chemokine family.[6,226,228,303] MCP-1/CCL2 has also been found in two isoforms from the same gene product, that are 13 kD and 9 kD in size and can be distinguished by lectin binding.[304] The 13 kD isoform of MCP-1 contains the disaccharide galactose-beta 1-3D-N-acetyl galactosamine, whereas, the 9 kD isoform lacks this glycosylation. However, the glycosylation of the 13 kD isoform appears to not alter its ability to mediate migration of monocytes.[304]

NH$_2$-terminal processing of CC chemokines also influences their activity in the recruitment of mononuclear cells. CD26/dipeptidyl peptidase IV, a lymphocyte membrane–associated peptidase, selectively cleaves peptides with proline or alanine at the second position and cleaves dipeptides at the NH$_2$-terminus.[305] Whereas NH$_2$-terminal truncation of the CXC chemokine GCP-2 (GCP-2/CXCL6[227]) by CD26 does not alter neutrophil chemotactic activity,[305,306] NH$_2$-terminal truncation of regulated on activation normal T-cell expressed and secreted RANTES/CCL5, eotaxin/CCL11, and macrophage-derived chemokine (MDC/CCL22) by CD26 markedly impaired chemotactic activity.[305,306] While NH$_2$-terminal truncation of RANTES/CCL5 by CD26 reduced activation of CCR1 and CCR3 receptors, binding to CCR5 is preserved after proteolysis.[306] Thus, proteolytic modification of RANTES/CCL5 by CD26 increased receptor selectivity and responses during innate and adaptive immune responses. In contrast, NH$_2$-terminal processing of LD78beta (CCL3[227]), an isoform of macrophage inflammatory peptide-1α (MIP-1α/CCL3),[227] by CD26 increased its chemotactic activity,[307] an effect mediated by the chemokine receptors CCR1 and CCR5.[307] Thus, extracellular processing of leukocyte chemoattractants modifies their ability to recruit leukocytes and influence subsequent inflammatory responses.

CC Chemokine Receptors

CC chemokine activities are mediated by seven-transmembrane-domain, G protein–coupled receptors. The CC chemokine receptors are structurally homologous. Whereas the transmembrane and the second and third intracellular/cytoplasmic domains of these receptors are well conserved, the NH$_2$- and COOH-terminal ends of these receptors are highly variable. This suggests that the conserved domains are involved in G protein signal coupling, and the variable domains are involved in specific ligand interaction and unique cellular signaling. Currently, at least ten cellular CC chemokine receptors have been cloned, expressed, and identified to have specific ligand-binding profiles (Table 10–11).[252,260–262,308–310]

The expression of specific CCRs may be restricted to a state of cellular activation (ie, resting or activated) and differentiation. Mononuclear phagocytes stimulated with IL-2 express CCR2; whereas, MCP-1/CCL2 has no effect in regulating expression of CCR2 on these cells.[311] In addition to CC chemokine ligand-receptor interaction leading to chemoattraction of mononuclear phagocytes, IL-2 induces the expression of CCR1 and CCR2 on CD45RO[+] T cells, the primary receptors for RANTES/CCL5 and MCP-1/CCL2, respectively.[312] The expression of CCR1 and CCR2 was directly correlated to their migration in response to RANTES/CCL5 and MCP-1/CCL2, respectively.[312] Moreover, the ability of these cells to express CCRs and respond to CC chemokine ligands was dependent on continued IL-2 exposure.[312] This response was mimicked by IL-12 but not in the presence of other cytokines.[312] Combined activation of the TCR/CD3 complex with CD28 antigen caused rapid down-regulation of

TABLE 10–11   The CC Chemokine Receptors

Receptor	Ligand
CCR1	CCL3, CCL5, CCL7, CCL14, CCL15, CCL16, CCL23
CCR2	CCL2, CCL7, CCL13,
CCR3	CCL5, CCL7, CCL11, CCL11, CCL15, CCL26
CCR4	CCL17, CCL22
CCR5	CCL3, CCL4, CCL5
CCR6	CCL20
CCR7	CCL19
CCR8	CCL1
CCR9	CCL25
CCR10	CCL27

CCR1 and CCR2 expression. This effect was paralleled by a decline in chemotactic response to either RANTES/CCL5 or MCP-1/CCL2, even in the presence of IL-2.[312] These findings support the notion that IL-2, by induction of specific CCRs, in conjunction with specific CC chemokine ligand production can have a significant impact on the recruitment of mononuclear cells.

Type 1 T helper cells and type 2 T helper cells can be differentially recruited to promote different types of inflammatory reactions. It has become increasingly recognized that chemokine receptors are differentially expressed on T cells depending on their antigenic experience and type of polarization.[313] Chemokines and their receptors are essential components of type 1– and type 2–mediated responses.[313] Naive T cells express CXCR4 and CCR7 and migrate in response to SDF-1 and MIP-3β.[314] CXCR3 is present on most peripheral blood memory cells and is expressed at higher levels on type 1 cells than type 2.[313] CCR5 is mainly expressed on type 1 cells whereas CCR3, CCR4, and CCR8 are more characteristic of type 2 cells.[313,314] CXCR6 is predominantly expressed on type 1 polarized T cells.[279] Furthermore, polarized type 1/type 2 cells differentially respond to the appropriate ligand for these receptors including IP-10 and MIP-1β for type 1 cells and MDC, I309, and eotaxin for type 2 cells.[314] These findings demonstrate that chemokines are important in the amplification of polarization of T cells. There is increasing evidence that pulmonary fibrosis is predominantly a type 2 mediated process.

The use of CC chemokine receptor knockout mice has provided additional insight into the biology of chemokines and their receptors in animal models of inflammation. Mice genes targeted to lack CCR2 develop normally and have no hematopoietic abnormalities, yet they have profound defects in their ability to recruit mononuclear cells in response to intraperitoneal thioglycollate or to mount a delayed-type hypersensitivity (DTH) response in the context of granuloma formation.[315–317] In addition, CCR2 –/– mice were found to have lower levels of IFN-γ as compared with CCR +/+ mice. Furthermore CCR2 –/– mice have less tracheal obliteration with extracellular matrix and improved graft

survival in a murine model of obliterative bronchiolitis.[31] The beneficial effects were directly related to the absence of CCR2-expressing macrophages demonstrating the importance of a specific population of macrophages in the development of fibrosis.[31] CCR1 –/– mice, as compared with littermate controls, have a reduced ability to form granulomas, which were associated with defects in the production of type 1 and type 2 cytokines, and have improved graft survival in a cardiac transplant model.[318,319] These studies support the notion that understanding the biology of CC chemokine ligands and their receptors will provide important insight into mechanisms of leukocyte trafficking during inflammation and the evolution of chronic fibrosis.

The Role of CC Chemokines in Pulmonary Fibrosis

Animal models, such as bleomycin-induced pulmonary fibrosis have demonstrated the presence and contribution of CC chemokines to the pathogenesis of fibrosis. Time-dependent expression of MCP-1/CCL2 has been reported in response to bleomycin challenge in rodents.[320,321] MCP-1/CCL2 mRNA levels were significantly elevated from BALF cells at 24 hours postbleomycin challenge; however, MCP-1/CCL2 mRNA in lung tissue was maximally elevated at 7 days, correlating with eosinophil and mononuclear cell infiltration,[320] MIP-1α/CCL3 protein and mRNA expression in lung tissue homogenates also has been found to be elevated postbleomycin challenge with detectable levels of MIP-1α/CCL3 protein peaking at 2 and 16 days.[60,61] In contrast to MCP-1/CCL2, the kinetics of whole-lung MIP-1α/CCL3 expression is similar to MIP-1α/CCL3 expression in BALF.[60,61] The kinetics of expression of both MIP-1α/CCL3 and MCP-1/CCL2 during the first week postbleomycin challenge temporally correlates with accumulation of lung mononuclear cells.[60,61] In the second week postbleomycin challenge, increased MIP-1α expression coincided with increases in macrophages, while elevated MCP-1/CCL2 is not observed.[60,61] The predominate cellular source of both MCP-1/CCL2 or MIP-1α/CCL3 is the alveolar macrophage.[60,61] In addition, eosinophils, epithelial cells, and interstitial macrophages are also significant cellular sources of MCP-1/CCL2 and MIP-1α/CCL3, respectively.[60,61,320] Passive immunization of mice with either neutralizing antibodies to murine MCP-1/CCL2 or MIP-1α/CCL3 resulted in a reduction of infiltrating cells into the lungs of bleomycin-treated animals by 30 and 35%, respectively.[60,61] Depletion of MCP-1/CCL2 had the greatest effect on mononuclear cells, whereas neutralization of MIP-1α/CCL3 reduced B lymphocyte, macrophage, and neutrophil infiltration.[60,61]

To determine the contribution that these CC chemokines have in mediating pulmonary fibrosis, bleomycin-challenged mice that were passively immunized with neutralizing anti-MIP-1α/CCL3 antibodies demonstrated a 49% decrease in total lung collagen, as measured by lung hydroxyproline content.[60,61] Depletion of MIP-1α/CCL3 did not completely abrogate either the inflammatory or fibrotic response to bleomycin. This suggests the existence of other mediators with similar or overlapping activities. Certainly, other CC chemokines have been shown to have activities similar to MIP-1α/CCL3 and may be concomitantly expressed and induce the observed leukocyte recruitment that supports a profibrotic environment.

In addition to the ability of CC chemokines to modulate leukocyte recruitment in the lung during the pathogenesis of pulmonary fibrosis, MCP-1/CCL2 has been found to be an important cofactor for the stimulation of fibroblast collagen production and the induction of the expression of TGF-β_1.[322] MCP-1/CCL2 treatment of rat lung fibroblasts results in both a dose- and time-dependent gene expression of type I procollagen.[322] However, the expression of procollagen by these cells was found to be delayed by 24 hours, suggesting an alternative means for MCP-1/CCL2 induction of gene expression of type I procollagen. Subsequent studies demonstrated that the delay was due to the initial induction of endogenous TGF-β_1. MCP-1/CCL2 stimulation of pulmonary fibroblasts induced the gene expression of TGF-β_1 that preceded gene expression of type I procollagen. Moreover, a strategy using an antisense to TGF-β_1 attenuated all of the effect of MCP-1/CCL2–induced procollagen gene expression.[322] These findings support the notion that MCP-1/CCL2 stimulation of pulmonary fibroblasts is an important event leading to gene expression of endogenous TGF-β_1 and subsequent gene expression of type I procollagen.

Several studies have demonstrated the presence of CC chemokines in ILD.[323–325] MIP-1α/CCL3 has been found in BALF of patients with ILD.[324] MIP-1α/CCL3 was found in equivalent levels in the BALF of 22 out of 23 patients with sarcoidosis and 9 out of 9 patients with IPF, whereas, detectable MIP-1α/CCL3 was found in only 1 out of 7 healthy subjects. In addition, these levels correlated with increased monocyte chemotactic activity in the BALF obtained from patients with sarcoidosis and IPF, respectively, as compared with healthy subjects.[324] The monocyte chemotactic activity was reduced by approximately 22 when BALF from sarcoidosis and IPF patients was preincubated with rabbit antihuman–MIP-1α/CCL3 antibodies.[324] The predominant cellular sources of MIP-1α/CCL3 within the lung of these patients, by immunolocalization, were both alveolar and interstitial macrophages and pulmonary fibroblasts.[324] Minimal to no detectable MIP-1α/CCL3 was expressed in normal subjects. Furthermore, pulmonary fibroblasts isolated from patients with IPF produced greater amounts of MIP-1α/CCL3 after challenge with IL-1β than did similarly treated pulmonary fibroblasts recovered from patients without fibrotic lung disease. Similar to the findings for MIP-1α/CCL3,

MCP-1/CCL2 has been found to be significantly elevated in ILD.[323] MCP-1/CCL2 mRNA and protein has been detected in pulmonary epithelial cells, mononuclear phagocytes, fibroblasts, endothelial cells, and vascular smooth muscle cells.[323,325] In addition, MCP-1/CCL2 was produced to a greater extent in the presence of either TNF or IL-1β from isolated pulmonary fibroblasts of patients with IPF, as compared with normal controls.[325] Moreover, pulmonary fibroblasts from IPF patients demonstrated a reduced ability to down-modulate their MCP-1/CCL2 expression in the presence of either PGE$_2$ or the glucocorticoid, dexamethasone.[325] These findings suggested that both MIP-1α/CCL3 and MCP-1/CCL2 are expressed in increased amounts within the air space and interstitium of patients with ILD, and that these chemokines may be important mediators of the mononuclear cell recruitment that characterizes and perpetuates these diseases.

Furthermore, it has been shown that MCP-1/CCL2 can stimulate IL-4 production, and its overexpression is associated with defects in cell-mediated immunity, indicating that it might be involved in type 2 polarization.[326] Furthermore, neutralization of MCP-1/CCL2 using polyclonal serum leads to a reduction in IL-4 and an augmentation in IFN-γ production by CD4+ lymphocytes when cocultured with fibroblasts.[327] These findings suggest that endogenous MCP-1/CCL2 has an important role in the modulation of CD4+ T-cell activation during cell-cell interactions with lung fibroblasts and that these interactions may dictate the cytokine profile associated with an inflammatory response.[327] MCP-1/CCL2–deficient mice are unable to mount type 2 responses. Lymph node cells from immunized MCP-1/CCL2 –/– mice synthesize extremely low levels of IL-4, IL-5, and IL-10, but normal amounts of IFN-γ and IL-2.[326] Thus, MCP-1/CCL2 may have both a direct role in the pathogenesis of pulmonary fibrosis through effects on monocytes and an indirect role through control of T helper cell polarization. Similarly, the murine CC chemokine, C10/CCL6, is differentially regulated by type 1 and type 2 cytokines.[328] Bone marrow–derived macrophages produce C10/CCL6 in response to IL-4, IL-10, and IL-13 in a dose-dependent manner.[328] In contrast, IFN-γ inhibits IL-3– and GM-CSF–induced expression of C10/CCL6.[328] Furthermore, the type 2 cytokine, IL-13, has been shown to stimulate eotaxin/CCL11 production from airway epithelial cells.[329] This is further evidence for the interaction of CC chemokines and type 2 cytokines and suggests that chemokines may have an important role in the switch toward a profibrotic type 2 phenotype.

CCR1 has been shown to play an important role in the pathogenesis of bleomycin-induced pulmonary fibrosis.[330] Following the administration of bleomycin, the expression of CCR1 mRNA peaked at 7 days. This paralleled the expression of RANTES/CCL5 and MIP-1α/CCL3, the major ligands for CCR1. Treatment with antibodies to CCR1 leads to a reduction in both

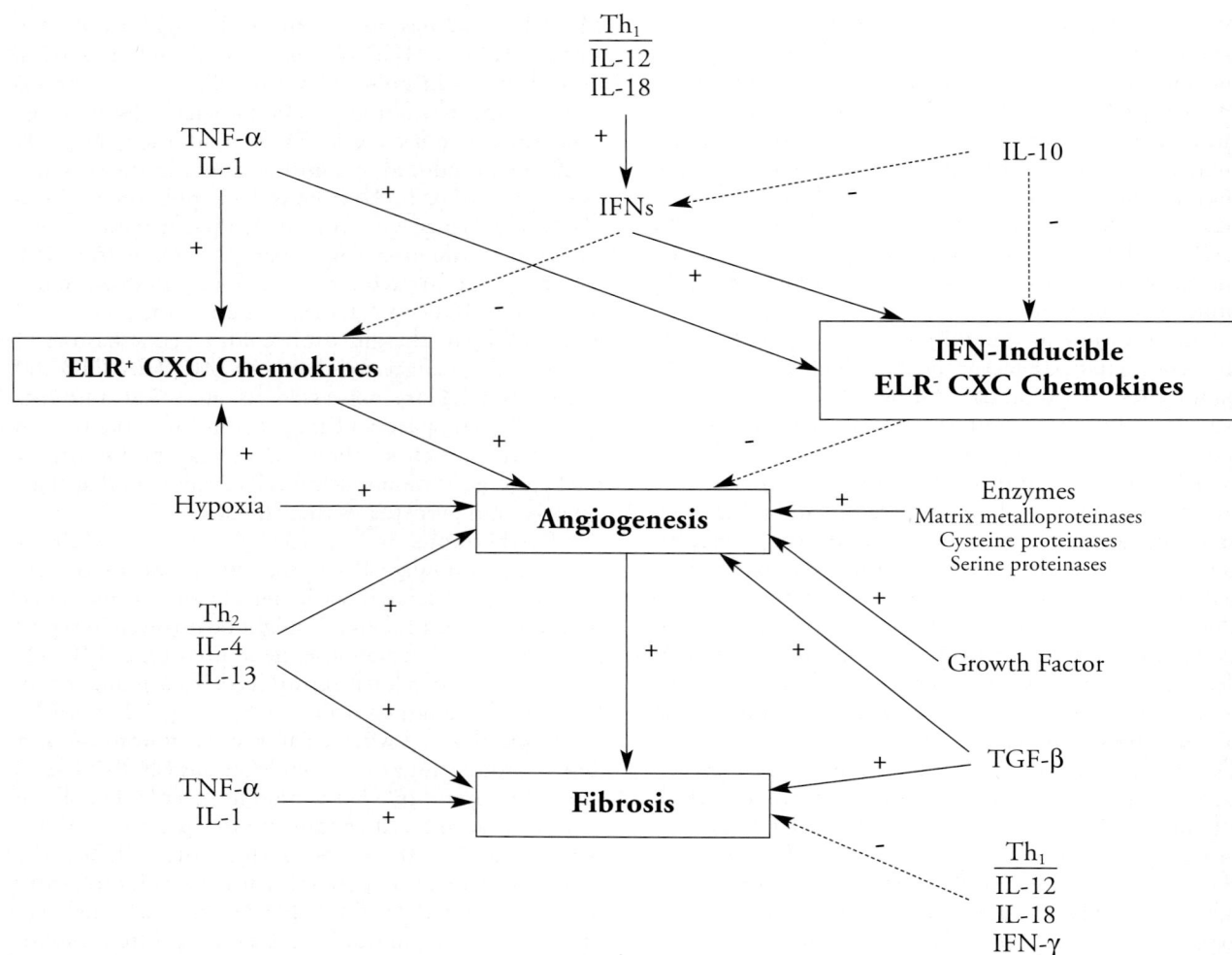

Figure 10–1   Cytokine networks involved in pulmonary fibrosis. TNF = tumor necrosis factor; IL = interleukin; IFN = interferon; TGF = transforming growth factor; ELR = glutamic acid (E) - leucine (L) -arginine (R) motif; Th = T helper.

inflammatory cell infiltrates and the development of fibrosis.[330] Similarly CCR2 –/– mice are protected from pulmonary fibrosis in response to bleomycin.[331] Similar effects have been seen in murine model of obliterative bronchiolitis where the fibrotic response associated with this disorder was attenuated in CCR2 –/– mice.[31] This suggests that targeting chemokine receptors may be an efficient way to inhibit pulmonary fibrosis.

Recently, the importance of receptor polymorphisms in various disease states has been demonstrated. CCR5 is the major receptor for MIP-1α/CCL3, MIP-1β/CCL4, and RANTES/CCL5. Homozygosity for the CCR5Δ32 mutation has been shown to predict prolonged renal allograft survival (90% at 20 years), reduced risk of asthma, and decreased severity of rheumatoid arthritis.[332,333] In contrast, there was an increased frequency of the CCR5Δ32 allele in patients with sarcoidosis that was associated with more apparent disease and an increased need for corticosteroids.[334] This suggests that CCR5Δ32 is associated with altered susceptibility to immmunolog-

ically mediated diseases, and that the balance between chemokines and their appropriately expressed receptor is necessary for the full manifestation of various diseases. Similarly, polymorphisms in the CXCR2 gene have been described in patients with systemic sclerosis both with and without evidence of interstitial lug disease, suggesting that CXCR2 may have a role in the fibrotic process.[335]

CONCLUSIONS

In this chapter, we have examined the role of a variety of cytokines that may contribute to pulmonary fibrosis. We have emphasized the role of chemokines in ILD. Interestingly, many of these proteins are detectable in the BALF of patients with ILD and may eventually serve as useful laboratory markers of disease activity. Although there are many complex interactions involving cytokine networks and cascades in pulmonary fibrosis, attempts to eliminate a single cytokine in clinical trials may be difficult. Given the limited efficacy of the therapeutic armamentarium currently used to treat patients with ILD/IPF, it seems prudent to consider alternative therapeutic regimens, such as the ablation of multiple cytokines or switching the "cytokine profile" in order to prevent pulmonary fibrosis and the associated pathophysiology. Future directions in cytokine research may include systemic or local intrapulmonary cytokine gene therapy, that may either attenuate or augment the expression of specific cytokines or groups of cytokines. Hopefully, the study of cytokines and their networks will lead to specific immunomodulatory therapies that will benefit patients with ILD and prevent end-stage pulmonary fibrosis leading to reduced morbidity and mortality.

REFERENCES

1. Davidson JM. Wound repair. In: Gallin JI, Goldstein IM, Snyderman R, editors. Inflammation: basic principles and clinical correlates. New York: Raven Press, Ltd; 1992.

2. Clark RA. Basics of cutaneous wound repair. J Dermatol Surg Oncol 1993;19:693–706.

3. Clark RA, Lanigan JM, Dellapelle P, et al. Fibronectin and fibrin provide a provisional matrix for epidermal cell migration during wound re-epithelialization. J Invest Dermatol 1982;79:264–9.

4. Butcher EC. Leukocyte-endothelial cell recognition: three (or more) steps to specificity and diversity. Cell 1991;67:1033–5.

5. Springer TA. Adhesion receptors of the immune system. Nature 1990;346:425–34.

6. Strieter RM, Lukacs NW, Standiford TJ, Kunkel SL. Cytokines and lung inflammation. Thorax 1993;48:765–9.

7. Grotendorst GR, Smale G, Pencev D. Production of transforming growth factor beta by human peripheral blood monocytes and neutrophils. J Cell Physiol 1989;140:396–402.

8. Wertheim WA, Kunkel SL, Standiford TJ, et al. Regulation of neutrophil-derived IL-8: the role of prostaglandin E_2, dexamethasone, and IL-4. J Immunol 1993;151:2166–75.

9. Kasama T, Strieter RM, Standiford TJ, et al. Expression and regulation of human neutrophil-derived macrophage inflammatory protein-1 alpha. J Exp Med 1993;178:63–72.

10. Kasama T, Strieter RM, Lukacs NW, et al. Regulation of neutrophil-derived chemokine expression by IL-10. J Immunol 1994;152:3559–69.

11. Sibille Y, Reynolds HY. Macrophages and polymorphonuclear neutrophils in lung defense and injury. Am Rev Respir Dis 1990;141:471–501.

12. French-Constant C, Van DWL, Dvorak HF, Hynes RO. Reappearance of an embryonic pattern of fibronectin splicing during wound healing in the adult rat. J Cell Biol 1989;109:903–14.

13. Kurkinen M, Vaheri A, Roberts PJ, Stenan S. Sequential appearance of fibronectin and collagen in experimental granulation tissue. Lab Invest 1980;43:47–51.

14. Epstein EHJ. [a1(III)3] human skin collagen: release by pepsin digestion and preponderance in fetal life. J Biol Chem 1974;249:3225–31.

15. Donoff RB, McLennan JE, Grillo HC. Preparation and properties of collagenases from epithelium and mesenchyme of healing mammalian wounds. Biochem Biophys Acta 1971;227:639–53.

16. Vaillant P, Menard O, Vignaud J-M, et al. The role of cytokines in human lung fibrosis. Monaldi. Arch Chest Dis 1996;51:145–52.

17. Phan SH. New strategies for treatment of pulmonary fibrosis. Thorax 1995;50:415–21.

18. Phan SH, Kunkel SL. Lung cytokine production in bleomycin-induced pulmonary fibrosis. Exp Lung Res 1992;18:29–43.

19. Gauldie J, Jordana M, Cox G. Cytokines and pulmonary fibrosis. Thorax 1993;48:931–5.

20. Sheppard D. Pulmonary fibrosis: a cellular overreaction or a failure of communication? J Clin Invest 2001;107:1501–2.

21. Kolb M, Margetts PJ, Anthony DC, et al. Transient expression of IL-1beta induces acute lung injury and chronic repair leading to pulmonary fibrosis. J Clin Invest 2001;107:1529–36.

22. King TE Jr, Schwarz MI, Brown K, et al. Idiopathic pulmonary fibrosis: relationship between histopathologic features and mortality. Am J Respir Crit Care Med 2001;164:1025–32.

23. Collard HR, King TE Jr. Treatment of idiopathic pulmonary fibrosis: the rise and fall of corticosteroids. Am J Med 2001;110:326–8.

24. Selman M, King TE, Pardo A. Idiopathic pulmonary fibrosis: prevailing and evolving hypotheses about its pathogenesis and implications for therapy. Ann Intern Med 2001;134:136–51.

25. Chandler DB. Possible mechanisms of bleomycin-induced fibrosis. Clin Chest Med 1990;11:21–30.

26. Christensen PJ, Goodman RE, Pastoriza L, et al. Induction of lung fibrosis in the mouse by intratracheal instillation of fluorescein isothiocyanate is not T-cell-dependent. Am J Pathol 1999;155:1773–9.

27. Sime PJ, Xing Z, Graham FL, et al. Adenovector-mediated gene transfer of active transforming growth factor-beta1 induces prolonged severe fibrosis in rat lung. J Clin Invest 1997;100:768–76.

28. Sime PJ, Marr RA, Gauldie D, et al. Transfer of tumor necrosis factor-alpha to rat lung induces severe pulmonary inflammation and patchy interstitial fibrogenesis with induction of transforming growth factor-beta1 and myofibroblasts [in process citation]. Am J Pathol 1998;153:825–32.

29. Miyazaki Y, Araki K, Vesin C, et al. Expression of a tumor necrosis factor-alpha transgene in murine lung causes lymphocytic and fibrosing alveolitis. A mouse model of progressive pulmonary fibrosis. J Clin Invest 1995;96:250–9.

30. Leung DY, de Castro M, Szefler SJ, Chrousos GP. Mechanisms of glucocorticoid-resistant asthma. Ann N Y Acad Sci 1998;840:735–46.

31. Belperio JA, Keane MP, Burdick MD, et al. Critical role for the chemokine MCP-1/CCR2 in the pathogenesis of bronchiolitis obliterans syndrome. J Clin Invest 2001;108:547–56.

32. Trulock EP. Lung transplantation. Am J Respir Crit Care Med 1997;155:789–818.

33. Flaherty KR, Travis WD, Colby TV, et al. Histopathologic variability in usual and nonspecific interstitial pneumonias. Am J Respir Crit Care Med 2001;164:1722–7.

34. Dinarello CA. Biologic basis for interleukin-1 in disease. Blood 1996;87:2095–147.

35. Dinarello CA. Interleukin-1 and interleukin-1 antagonism. Blood 1991;77:1627–35.

36. Vigers GPA, Anderson LJ, Caffes P, Brandhuber BJ. Crystal structure of the type-I interleukin-1 receptor complexed with interleukin-1b. Nature 1997;386:190–4.

37. Schreuder H, Tardif C, Trump-Kallmeyer S, et al. A new cytokine-receptor binding mode revealed by the crystal structure of the IL-1 receptor with an antagonist. Nature 1997;386:194–200.

38. Murphy JE, Robert C, Kupper TS. Interleukin-1 and cutaneous inflammation: a crucial link between innate and acquired immunity. J Invest Dermatol 2000;114:602–8.

39. Ghosh S, May MJ, Kopp EB. NF-kappa B and Rel proteins:

evolutionarily conserved mediators of immune responses. Annu Rev Immunol 1998;16:225–60.

40. Saklatvala J, Dean J, Finch A. Protein kinase cascades in intracellular signalling by interleukin-I and tumour necrosis factor. Biochem Soc Symp 1999;64:63–77.

41. Medzhitov R, Janeway C Jr. Innate immunity. N Engl J Med 2000;343:338–44.

42. Medzhitov R, Janeway C Jr. Innate immune recognition: mechanisms and pathways. Immunol Rev 2000;173:89–97.

43. Medzhitov R, Preston-Hurlburt P, Janeway CA Jr. A human homologue of the *Drosophila* Toll protein signals activation of adaptive immunity [see comments]. Nature 1997;388:394–7.

44. Brightbill HD, Modlin RL. Toll-like receptors: molecular mechanisms of the mammalian immune response. Immunology 2000;101:1–10.

45. Brightbill HD, Libraty DH, Krutzik SR, et al. Host defense mechanisms triggered by microbial lipoproteins through toll-like receptors. Science 1999;285:732–6.

46. Mantovani A, Muzio M, Ghezzi P, et al. Regulation of inhibitory pathways of the interleukin-1 system. Ann N Y Acad Sci 1998;840:338–51.

47. Dinarello CA. Interleukin-1 beta, interleukin-18, and the interleukin-1 beta converting enzyme. Ann N Y Acad Sci 1998;856:1–11.

48. Arend WP, Malyak M, Guthridge CJ, Gabay C. Interleukin-1 receptor antagonist: role in biology. Annu Rev Immunol 1998;16:27–55.

49. Malyak M, Guthridge JM, Hance KR, et al. Characterization of a low molecular weight isoform of IL-1 receptor antagonist. J Immunol 1998;161:1997–2003.

50. Bienkowski RS, Gotkin MG. Control of collagen deposition in mammalian lung. Proc Soc Exp Biol Med 1995;209:118–40.

51. Lindroos PM, Coin PG, Osornio-Vargas AR, Bonner JC. Interleukin 1 beta (IL-1b) and the IL-1 beta-alpha2-macroglobulin complex upregulate the platelet-derived growth factor alpha-receptor on rat pulmonary fibroblasts. Am J Respir Cell Mol Biol 1995;13:455–65.

52. Koch AE, Kunkel SL, Harlow LA, et al. Macrophage inflammatory protein-1 alpha. A novel chemotactic cytokine for macrophages in rheumatoid arthritis. J Clin Invest 1994;93:921–8.

53. Koch AE, Kunkel SL, Harlow LA, et al. Enhanced production of monocyte chemoattractant protein-1 in rheumatoid arthritis. J Clin Invest 1992;90:772–9.

54. Jordana M, Newhouse MT, Gauldie J. Alveolar macrophage/peripheral blood monocyte-derived factors modulate proliferation of primary lines of human lung fibroblasts. J Leukoc Biol 1987;42:51–60.

55. Adamson IY, Bowden DH. The pathogenesis of bleomycin-induced pulmonary fibrosis in mice. Am J Pathol 1974;77:185–97.

56. Bowden DH. Unraveling pulmonary fibrosis: the bleomycin model. Lab Invest 1984;50:487–8.

57. Bedrossian CMW, Grennberg SD, Yawn DH, O'Neil RM. Experimentally induced bleomycin sulfate pulmonary toxicity. Arch Pathol Lab Med 1977;101:248–54.

58. Aso Y, Yoneda Y. Morphological and biochemical study of pulmonary changes induced by bleomycin in mice. Lab Invest 1976;35:558–68.

59. Schrier DJ, Kunkel RG, Phan SH. The role of strain variation in murine bleomycin-induced pulmonary fibrosis. Am Rev Respir Dis 1983;127:63–6.

60. Smith RE, Strieter RM, Phan SH, et al. Production and function of murine macrophage inflammatory protein-1 alpha in bleomycin-induced lung injury. J Immunol 1994;153:4704–12.

61. Smith RE, Strieter RM, Phan SH, Kunkel SL. CC chemokines: novel mediators of the profibrotic inflammatory response to bleomycin challenge. Am J Respir Cell Mol Biol 1996;15:693–702.

62. Chandler DB, Hyde DM, Gin SN. Morphometric estimates of infiltrative cellular changes during the development of bleomycin-induced pulmonary fibrosis in hamsters. Am J Pathol 1983;112:170–7.

63. Piguet PF, Collart MA, Grau GE, et al. Tumor necrosis factor/cachectin plays a key role in bleomycin-induced pneumopathy. J Exp Med 1989;170:655–63.

64. Piguet P, Vesin C, Grau G, Thompson RC. Interleukin 1 receptor anatgonist (IL-1ra) prevents or cures pulmonary fibrosis elicited in mice by bleomycin or silica. Cytokine 1993;5:57–61.

65. Shanley TP, Peters JL, Jones ML, et al. Regulatory effects of endogenous interleukin-1 receptor antagonist protein in immunoglobulin G immune complex-induced lung injury. J Clin Invest 1996;97:963–70.

66. Kolb M, Margetts PJ, Anthony DC, et al. Transient expression of IL-1beta induces acute lung injury and chronic repair leading to pulmonary fibrosis. J Clin Invest 2001;107:1529–36.

67. Wahl SM, Allen JB, Wong HL, et al. Antagonistic and agonistic effects of transforming growth factor-beta and IL-1 in rheumatoid synovium. J Immunol 1990;145:2514–9.

68. Rolfe MW, Standiford TJ, Kunkel SL, et al. Interleukin-1 receptor antagonist expression in sarcoidosis. Am Rev Respir Dis 1993;148:1378–84.

69. Smith DR, Kunkel SL, Standiford TJ, et al. Increased interleukin-1 receptor antagonist in idiopathic pulmonary fibrosis. A compartmental analysis. Am J Respir Crit Care Med 1995;151:1965–73.

70. Kline JN, Schwartz DA, Monick MM, et al. Relative release of interleukin-1beta and interleukin-1 receptor antagonist by alveolar macrophages. Chest 1993;104:47–53.

71. Janson RW, King TEJ, Hance KR, Arend WP. Enhanced production of IL-1 receptor antagonist by alveolar macrophages from patients with interstitial lung diseases. Am Rev Respir Dis 1993;148:495–503.

72. DiGiovine B, Lynch III JP, Martinez FJ, et al. The presence of pro-fibrotic cytokines correlate with outcome in patients with idiopathic pulmonary fibrosis. Chest 1996;110:37S.

73. Broekelmann TJ, Limper AH, Colby TV, McDonald JA. Transforming growth factor beta-1 is present at sites of extracellular matrix gene expression in human pulmonary fibrosis. Proc Natl Acad Sci U S A 1991;88:6642–51.

74. Raines EW, Dower SK, Ross R. Interleukin-1 mitogenic activity for fibroblasts and smooth muscle cells is due to PDGF-AA. Science 1989;243:393–6.

75. Goldring MB, Krane SM. Modulation by recombinant interleukin-1 of synthesis of types I and III collagens and associated procollagen mRNA levels in cultured human cells. J Biol Chem 1987;262:16724–34.

76. Dayer J-M, Rochemonteix BD, Burrus B, et al. Human recombinant interleukin I stimulates collagenase and prostaglandin E_2 production by human synovial cells. J Clin Invest 1986;77:645–8.

77. Bazzoni F, Beutler B. The tumor necrosis factor ligand and receptor families. N Engl J Med 1996;334:1717–25.

78. Strieter RM, Kunkel SL, Bone RC. Role of tumor necrosis factor-alpha in disease states and inflammation. Crit Care Med 1993;21:S447–63.

79. Millar AB, Foley NM, Singer M, et al. TNF in bronchopulmonary secretions of patients with adult respiratory distress syndrome. Lancet 1989;ii:712–4.

80. Colletti LM, Remick DG, Burtch GD, et al. Role of tumor necrosis factor-alpha in the pathophysiologic alterations after hepatic ischemia/reperfusion injury in the rat. J Clin Invest 1990;85:1936–43.

81. Lahdevirta J, Maury CPJ, Teppo AM, Reppo H. Elevated

levels of circulating cachectin/tumor necrosis factor in patients with acquired immunodeficiency syndrome. Am J Med 1988;85:289–91.

82. Scuderi P, Lam KS, Ryan KJ, et al. Raised serum levels of tumour necrosis factor in parasitic infections. Lancet 1986;ii:1364–5.

83. Piguet P-F, Grau GE, Allet B, Vassalli P. Tumor necrosis factor/cachectin is an effector of skin and gut lesions of the acute phase of graft-vs-host disease. J Exp Med 1987;166:1280–9.

84. DeMeester SR, Rolfe MW, Kunkel SL, et al. The bimodal expression of tumor necrosis factor–α in association with rat lung reimplantation and allograft rejection. J Immunol 1993;150:2494–505.

85. Beutler B, Bazzoni F. TNF, apoptosis and autoimmunity: a common thread? Blood Cells Mol Dis 1998;24:216–30.

86. Watanabe-Fukunaga R, Brannan CI, Copeland NG, et al. Lymphoproliferation disorder in mice explained by defects in Fas antigen that mediates apoptosis. Nature 1992;356:314–7.

87. Adachi M, Watanabe-Fukunaga R, Nagata S. Aberrant transcription caused by the insertion of an early transposable element in an intron of the Fas antigen gene of lpr mice. Proc Natl Acad Sci U S A 1993;90:1756–60.

88. Feldmann M, Brennan FM, Elliott M, et al. TNF alpha as a therapeutic target in rheumatoid arthritis. Circ Shock 1994;43:179–84.

89. van Dullemen HM, van Deventer SJ, Hommes DW, et al. Treatment of Crohn's disease with anti-tumor necrosis factor chimeric monoclonal antibody (cA2). Gastroenterology 1995;109:129–35.

90. Beutler B, Cerami A. Cachectin and tumor necrosis factor as two sides of the same biological coin. Nature 1986;320:584–8.

91. Beutler B, Cerami A. The biology of cachectin/TNF-A primary mediator of the host response. Annu Rev Immunol 1989;7:625–50.

92. Le J, Vilcek J. Tumor necrosis factor and interleukin 1: cytokines with multiple overlapping biological activities. Lab Invest 1987;56:234–48.

93. Sherry B, Cerami A. Cachectin/tumor necrosis factor exerts endocrine, paracrine, and autocrine control of the inflammatory responses. J Cell Biol 1988;107:1269–77.

94. Kashiwa H, Wright SC, Bonavida B. Regulation of B cell maturation and differentiation: I. suppression of pokeweed mitogen-induced B cell differentiation by tumor necrosis factor (TNF). J Immunol 1987;138:1383–90.

95. Ostensen ME, Thiele DL, Lipsky PE. Tumor necrosis factor-alpha enhances cytolytic activity of human natural killer cells. J Immunol 1987;138:4185–91.

96. Scheurich P, Thoma B, Ucer U, Pfizenmaier K. Immunoregulatory activity of recombinant human tumor necrosis factor (TNF)-α: induction of the TNF receptors on human T cells and TNF-α-mediated enhancement of T cell responses. J Immunol 1987;138:1786–90.

97. Zucali JR, Elfenbein GJ, Barth KC, Dinarello CA. Effects of human interleukin 1 and human tumor necrosis factor on human T lymphocyte colony formation. J Clin Invest 1987;80:772–7.

98. Yokota S, Geppert TD, Lipsky PE. Enhancement of antigen- and mitogen-induced human T lymphocyte proliferation by tumor necrosis factor-α. J Immunol 1988;140:531–6.

99. Paulsson Y, Austgulen R, Hofsli E, al el. Tumor necrosis factor-induced expression of platelet-derived growth factor A-chain messenger RNA in fibroblasts. Exp Cell Res 1989;180:490–6.

100. Elias JA, Gustilo K, Baeder W, Freundlich B. Synergistic stimulation of fibroblast prostaglandin production by recombinant interleukin 1 and tumor necrosis factor. J Immunol 1987;138:3812–6.

101. Duncan MR, Berman B. Differential regulation of collagen, glycosaminoglycan, fibronectin, and collagenase activity production in cultured human adult dermal fibroblasts by interleukin-1-alpha and beta and tumor necrosis factor-alpha and beta. J Invest Dermatol 1989;92:699–706.

102. Nakagawa H, Kitagawa H, Aikawa Y. Tumor necrosis factor stimulates gelatinase and collagenase production by granulation tissue in culture. Biochem Biophys Res Commun 1982;142:791–7.

103. Elias JA, Krol RC, Freundlich B, Sampson PM. Regulation of human lung fibroblast glycosaminoglycan production by recombinant interferons, tumor necrosis factor and lymphotoxin. J Clin Invest 1988;81:325–33.

104. Rolfe MW, Kunkel SL, Standiford TJ, et al. Pulmonary fibroblast expression of interleukin-8: a model for alveolar macrophage-derived cytokine networking. Am J Respir Cell Mol Biol 1991;5:493–501.

105. Rolfe MR, Kunkel SL, Standiford TJ, et al. Expression and regulation of human pulmonary fibroblast-derived monocyte chemotactic peptide-1. Am J Physiol 1992;263:L536–45.

106. Munker R, Gasson J, Ogawa M, Koeffler MP. Recombinant TNF induces production of granulocyte-monocyte colony-stimulating factor. Nature 1986;323:79–82.

107. Solis Herruzo JA, Brenner DA, Chojkier M. Tumor necrosis factor alpha inhibits collagen gene transcription and collagen synthesis in cultured human fibroblasts. J Biol Chem 1988;263:5841–5.

108. Kahari VM, Chen YQ, Su MW, et al. Tumor necrosis factor-alpha and interferon-gamma suppress the activation of human type I collagen gene expression by transforming growth factor-beta 1. Evidence for two distinct mechanisms of inhibition at the transcriptional and post-transcriptional levels. J Clin Invest 1990;86:1489–95.

109. Piguet PF, Vesin C. Treatment by human recombinant soluble TNF receptor of pulmonary fibrosis induced by bleomycin or silca in mice. Eur Respir J 1994;7:515–8.

110. Zhang K, Gharaee-Kermani M, McGarry B, et al. TNF-alpha-mediated lung cytokine networking and eosinophil recruitment in pulmonary fibrosis. J Immunol 1997;158:954–9.

111. Peppel K, Crawford D, Beutler B. A tumor necrosis factor (TNF) receptor-IgG heavy chain chimeric protein as a bivalent antagonist of TNF activity. J Exp Med 1991;174:1483–9.

112. Braun J, de Keyser F, Brandt J, et al. New treatment options in spondyloarthropathies: increasing evidence for significant efficacy of anti-tumor necrosis factor therapy. Curr Opin Rheumatol 2001;13:245–9.

113. Maini R, St Clair EW, Breedveld F, et al. Infliximab (chimeric anti-tumour necrosis factor alpha monoclonal antibody) versus placebo in rheumatoid arthritis patients receiving concomitant methotrexate: a randomised phase III trial. ATTRACT Study Group. Lancet 1999;354:1932–9.

114. Mease PJ, Goffe BS, Metz J, et al. Etanercept in the treatment of psoriatic arthritis and psoriasis: a randomised trial. Lancet 2000;356:385–90.

115. Brandt J, Haibel H, Cornely D, et al. Successful treatment of active ankylosing spondylitis with the anti-tumor necrosis factor alpha monoclonal antibody infliximab. Arthritis Rheum 2000;43:1346–52.

116. Keane J, Gershon S, Wise RP, et al. Tuberculosis associated with infliximab, a tumor necrosis factor alpha-neutralizing agent. N Engl J Med 2001;345:1098–104.

117. Mosmann TR, Cherwinski H, Bond MW. Two types of murine helper T cell clones. I. Definition according to profiles of lymphokine activities and secreted proteins. J Immunol 1986;136:2348–57.

118. Romagnani S. Th1/Th2 cells. Inflamm Bowel Dis 1999;5:285–94.

119. Giri SN, Hyde DM, Marafino BJ. Ameliorating effect of murine interferon gamma on bleomycin-induced lung

collagen fibrosis in mice. Biochem Med Metab Biol 1986; 36:194–7.

120. Chizzolini C, Rezzonico R, Ribbens C, et al. Inhibition of type I collagen production by dermal fibroblasts upon contact with activated T cells: different sensitivity to inhibition between systemic sclerosis and control fibroblasts. Arthritis Rheum 1998;41:2039–47.

121. Cornelissen AM, Von den Hoff JW, Maltha JC, Kuijpers-Jagtman AM. Effects of interferons on proliferation and collagen synthesis of rat palatal wound fibroblasts. Arch Oral Biol 1999;44:541–7.

122. Jaffe HA, Gao Z, Mori Y, et al. Selective inhibition of collagen gene expression in fibroblasts by an interferon-gamma transgene. Exp Lung Res 1999;25:199–215.

123. Brody AR, Bonner JC, Badgett A. Recombinant interferon-gamma reduces PDGF-induced lung fibroblast growth but stimulates PDGF production by alveolar macrophages in vitro. Chest 1993;103(2 Suppl):121S–2S.

124. Lewis M, Amento EP, Unemori EN. Transcriptional inhibition of stromelysin by interferon-gamma in normal human fibroblasts is mediated by the AP-1 domain. J Cell Biochem 1999;72:373–86.

125. Spoelstra FM, Postma DS, Hovenga H, et al. Interferon-gamma and interleukin-4 differentially regulate ICAM-1 and VCAM-1 expression on human lung fibroblasts. Eur Respir J 1999;14:759–66.

126. Hyde DM, Henderson TS, Giri SN, et al. Effect of murine gamma interferon on the cellular responses to bleomycin in mice. Exp Lung Res 1988;14:687–95.

127. Keane MP, Belperio JA, Burdick MD, Strieter RM. IL-12 attenuates bleomycin-induced pulmonary fibrosis. Am J Physiol Lung Cell Mol Physiol 2001;281:L92–7.

128. Hein R, Behr J, Hundgen M, et al. Treatment of systemic sclerosis with gamma–interferon. Br J Dermatol 1992;126: 496–501.

129. Ziesche R, Hofbauer E, Wittmann K, et al. A preliminary study of long-term treatment with interferon gamma-1b and low-dose prednisolone in patients with idiopathic pulmonary fibrosis [see comments]. N Engl J Med 1999; 341:1264–9.

130. Postlethwaite AE, Holness MA, Katai H, Raghow R. Human fibroblasts synthesize elevated levels of extracellular matrix proteins in response to interleukin-4. J Clin Invest 1992; 90:1479–85.

131. Postlethwaite AE, Seyer JM. Fibroblast chemotaxis induction by human recombinant interleukin-4. Identification by synthetic peptide analysis of two chemotactic domains residing in amino acid sequences 70-88 and 89-122. J Clin Invest 1991;87:2147–52.

132. Sempowski GD, Beckmann MP, Derdak S, Phipps RP. Subsets of murine lung fibroblasts express membrane-bound and soluble IL-4 receptors. J Immunol 1994;152:3606–14.

133. Rankin JA, Picarella DE, Geba GP, et al. Phenotypic and physiologic characterization of transgenic mice expressing interleukin 4 in the lung: lymphocytic and eosinophilic inflammation without airway hyperreactivity. Proc Natl Acad Sci U S A 1996;93:7821–5.

134. Chensue SW, Warmington K, Ruth JH, et al. Mycobacterial and schistosomal antigen-elicited granuloma formation in IFN-gamma and IL-4 knockout mice: analysis of local and regional cytokine and chemokine networks [published erratum appears in J Immunol 1999;162:3106]. J Immunol 1997;159:3565–73.

135. Metwali A, Elliott D, Blum AM, et al. The granulomatous response in murine schistosomiasis mansoni does not switch to Th1 in IL-4-deficient C57BL/6 mice. J Immunol 1996;157:4546–53.

136. Pearce EJ, Cheever A, Leonard S, et al. *Schistosoma mansoni* in IL-4-deficient mice. Int Immunol 1996;8:435–44.

137. Oriente A, Fedarko NS, Pacocha SE, et al. Interleukin-13

modulates collagen homeostasis in human skin and keloid fibroblasts. J Pharmacol Exp Ther 2000;292:988–94.

138. Zhu Z, Homer RJ, Wang Z, et al. Pulmonary expression of interleukin-13 causes inflammation, mucus hypersecretion, subepithelial fibrosis, physiologic abnormalities, and eotaxin production. J Clin Invest 1999;103:779–88.

139. Lee CG, Homer RJ, Zhu Z, et al. Interleukin-13 induces tissue fibrosis by selectively stimulating and activating transforming growth factor beta(1). J Exp Med 2001;194:809–21.

140. Callard RE, Matthews DJ, Hibbert L. IL-4 and IL-13 receptors: are they one and the same? Immunol Today 1996;17:108–10.

141. Hilton DJ, Zhang JG, Metcalf D, et al. Cloning and characterization of a binding subunit of the interleukin 13 receptor that is also a component of the interleukin 4 receptor. Proc Natl Acad Sci U S A 1996;93:497–501.

142. Donaldson DD, Whitters MJ, Fitz LJ, et al. The murine IL-13 receptor alpha 2: molecular cloning, characterization, and comparison with murine IL-13 receptor alpha 1. J Immunol 1998;161:2317–24.

143. Jensen PL. The interleukin 13 receptor complex. Stem Cells 2000;18:61–2.

144. Mohrs M, Ledermann B, Kohler G, et al. Differences between IL-4- and IL-4 receptor alpha-deficient mice in chronic leishmaniasis reveal a protective role for IL-13 receptor signaling. J Immunol 1999;162:7302–8.

145. Wallace WAH, Ramage EA, Lamb D, Howie EM. A type 2 (Th2-like) pattern of immune response predominates in the pulmonary interstitium of patients with crytogenic fibrosingalveolitis (CFA). Clin Exp Immunol 1995;101:436–41.

146. Kuroki S, Ohta A, Sueoka N, et al. Determination of various cytokines and type III procollagen aminopeptide levels in bronchoalveolar lavage fluid of the patients with pulmonary fibrosis: inverse correlation between type III procollagen aminopeptide and interferon-γ in progressive fibrosis. Br J Rheum 1995;34:31–6.

147. de Waal Malefyt R, Yssel H, Roncarolo MG, et al. Interleukin-10. Curr Opin Immunol 1992;4:314–20.

148. Moore KW, O'Garra A, de Waal Malefyt R, et al. Interleukin-10. Annu Rev Immunol 1993;11:165–90.

149. Mulligan MS, Jones ML, Vaporciyan AA, et al. Protective effects of IL-4 and IL-10 against immune complex-induced lung injury. J Immunol 1993;151:5666–74.

150. Howard M, Muchamuel T, Andrade S, Menon S. Interleukin 10 protects mice from lethal endotoxemia. J Exp Med 1993;177:1205–8.

151. Standiford TJ, Strieter RM, Lukacs NW, Kunkel SL. Neutralization of IL-10 increases lethality in endotoxemia. Cooperative effects of macrophage inflammatory protein-2 and tumor necrosis factor. J Immunol 1995;155:2222–9.

152. Greenberger MJ, Strieter RM, Kunkel SL, et al. Neutralization of IL-10 increases survival in a murine model of *Klebsiella pneumonia*. J Immunol 1995;155:722–9.

153. Nelson DR, Lauwers GY, Lau JY, Davis GL. Interleukin-10 treatment reduces fibrosis in patients with chronic hepatitis C: a pilot trial of interferon nonresponders. Gastroenterology 2000;118:655–60.

154. Edwards-Smith CJ, Jonsson JR, Purdie DM, et al. Interleukin-10 promoter polymorphism predicts initial response of chronic hepatitis C to interferon alfa. Hepatology 1999;30:526–30.

155. Arai T, Abe K, Matsuoka H, et al. Introduction of the interleukin-10 gene into mice inhibited bleomycin-induced lung injury in vivo. Am J Physiol Lung Cell Mol Physiol 2000;278:L914–22.

156. Driscoll KE, Carter JM, Howard BW, et al. Interleukin-10 regulates quartz-induced pulmonary inflammation in rats. Am J Physiol 1998;275(5 Pt 1):L887–94.

157. Huaux F, Lardot C, Arras M, et al. Lung fibrosis induced by silica particles in NMRI mice is associated with an upregula-

tion of the p40 subunit of interleukin-12 and Th-2 manifestations. Am J Respir Cell Mol Biol 1999;20:561–72.

158. Huaux F, Louahed J, Hudspith B, et al. Role of interleukin-10 in the lung response to silica in mice. Am J Respir Cell Mol Biol 1998;18:51–9.

159. `Arras M, Huaux F, Vink A, et al. Interleukin-9 reduces lung fibrosis and type 2 immune polarization induced by silica particles in a murine model. Am J Respir Cell Mol Biol 2001;24:368–75.

160. Hoyle GW, Brody AR. IL-9 and lung fibrosis: a Th2 good guy? Am J Respir Cell Mol Biol 2001;24:365–7.

161. Raines EW, Bowen-Pope DF, Ross R. Platelet-derived growth factor. In: Sporn MB, Roberts AB, editors. Peptide growth factors and their receptors. Handbook of experimental pharmacology. Heidelberg, Germany: Springer-Verlag; 1990. p. 173–262.

162. Remmers EF, Sano H, Wilder RL. Platelet-derived growth factors and heparin-binding (fibroblast) growth factors in the synovial tissue pathology of rheumatoid arthritis. Semin Arthritis Rheum 1991;21:191–9.

163. Eriksson A, Siegbahn A, Westermark B, et al. Platelet-derived growth factor alpha- and beta-receptors activate unique and common signal transduction pathways. EMBO J 1992;11:543–50.

164. Homma S, Nagaoka I, Abe H, et al. Localization of platelet-derived growth factor and insulin-like growth factor in the fibrotic lung. Am J Respir Crit Care Med 1995;152:2084–9.

165. Antoniades HN, Bravo MA, Avila RE, et al. Platelet-derived growth factor in idiopathic pulmonary fibrosis. J Clin Invest 1990;86:1055–64.

166. Maeda A, Hiyama K, Yamakido H, et al. Increased expression of platelet-derived growth factor A and insulin-like growth factor-1 in BAL cells during the development of bleomycin-induced pulmonary fibrosis in mice. Chest 1996;109:780–6.

167. Gurujeyalakshmi G, Hollinger MA, Giri SN. Pirfenidone inhibits PDGF isoforms in bleomycin hamster model of lung fibrosis at the translational level. Am J Physiol 1999;276(2 Pt 1):L311–8.

168. Yoshida M, Sakuma J, Hayashi S, et al. A histologically distinctive interstitial pneumonia induced by overexpression of the interleukin 6, transforming growth factor beta 1, or platelet-derived growth factor B gene. Proc Natl Acad Sci U S A 1995;92:9570–4.

169. Bonner JC, Lindroos PM, Rice AB, et al. Induction of PDGF receptor-alpha in rat myofibroblasts during pulmonary fibrogenesis in vivo. Am J Physiol 1998;274(1 Pt 1):L72–80.

170. Lindroos PM, Wang YZ, Rice AB, Bonner JC. Regulation of PDGFR-alpha in rat pulmonary myofibroblasts by staurosporine. Am J Physiol Lung Cell Mol Physiol 2001;280:L354–62.

171. Bitterman PB, Adelberg S, Crystal RG. Mechanisms of pulmonary fibrosis. Spontaneous release of the alveolar macrophage-derived growth factor in the interstitial lung disorders. J Clin Invest 1983;72:1801–13.

172. Bitterman PB, Rennard SI, Hunninghake GW, Crystal RG. Human alveolar macrophage growth factor for fibroblasts. Regulation and partial characterization. J Clin Invest 1982;70:806–22.

173. Rom WN, Bassette P, Fells GA, et al. Alveolar macrophages release insulin-like growth factor-I-type molecule. J Clin Invest 1988;82:1658–93.

174. Rechler MM, Nissley SP. The nature and regulation of the receptors for insulin-like growth factors. Annu Rev Physiol 1986;47:425–42.

175. Aston C, Jagirdar J, Lee TC, et al. Enhanced insulin-like growth factor molecules in idiopathic pulmonary fibrosis. Am J Respir Crit Care Med 1995;151:1597–603.

176. Jones JL, Clemmons DR. Insulin-like growth factors and their binding proteins. Endocr Rev 1995;16:3–34.

177. Allen JT, Bloor CA, Knight RA, Spiteri MA. Expression of insulin-like growth factor binding proteins in bronchoalveolar lavage fluid of patients with pulmonary sarcoidosis. Am J Respir Cell Mol Biol 1998;19:250–8.

178. Allen JT, Spiteri MA. Growth factors in idiopathic pulmonary fibrosis. Respir Res 2001;3:13–21.

179. Uh ST, Inoue Y, King TE Jr, et al. Morphometric analysis of insulin-like growth factor-I localization in lung tissues of patients with idiopathic pulmonary fibrosis. Am J Respir Crit Care Med 1998;158(5 Pt 1):1626–35.

180. Nakatake Y, Hoshikawa M, Asaki T, et al. Identification of a novel fibroblast growth factor, FGF-22, preferentially expressed in the inner root sheath of the hair follicle. Biochim Biophys Acta 2001;1517:460–3.

181. Mason IJ. The ins and outs of fibroblast growth factors. Cell 1994;78:547–52.

182. Henke C, Marineili W, Jessurun J, et al. Macrophage production of basic fibroblast growth factor in the fibroproliferative disorder of alveolar fibrosis after lung injury. Am J Pathol 1993;143:1189–99.

183. Inoue Y, King TE Jr, Tinkle SS, et al. Human mast cell basic fibroblast growth factor in pulmonary fibrotic disorders. Am J Pathol 1996;149:2037–54.

184. Qu Z, Liebler JM, Powers MR, et al. Mast cells are a major source of basic fibroblast growth factor in chronic inflammation and cutaneous hemangioma. Am J Pathol 1995;147:564–73.

185. Li CM, Khosla J, Pagan I, et al. TGF-beta1 and fibroblast growth factor-1 modify fibroblast growth factor-2 production in type II cells. Am J Physiol Lung Cell Mol Physiol 2000;279:L1038–46.

186. Liebler JM, Picou MA, Powers MR, Rosenbaum JT. Altered immunohistochemical localization of basic fibroblast growth factor after bleomycin-induced lung injury. Growth Factors 1997;14:25–38.

187. Peao MND, Aguas AP, DeSa CM, Grande NR. Neoformation of blood vessels in association with rat lung fibrosis induced by bleomycin. Anat Rec 1994;238:57–67.

188. Turner-Warwick M. Precapillary systemic-pulmonary anastomoses. Thorax 1963;18:225–37.

189. Bradham DM, Igarashi A, Potter RL, Grotendorst GR. Connective tissue growth factor: a cysteine-rich mitogen secreted by human vascular endothelial cells is related to the SRC-induced immediate early gene product CEF-10. J Cell Biol 1991;114:1285–94.

190. Moussad EE, Brigstock DR. Connective tissue growth factor: what's in a name? Mol Genet Metab 2000;71:276–92.

191. Brigstock DR. The connective tissue growth factor/cysteine-rich 61/nephroblastoma overexpressed (CCN) family. Endocr Rev 1999;20:189–206.

192. Roberts AB, Sporn MB. The transforming growth factor-betas. In: Sporn MB, Roberts AB, editors. Peptide growth factors and their receptors. Handbook of experimental pharmacology. Berlin, Germany: Springer-Verlag; 1990. p. 419–72.

193. Laiho M, Keski-Oja J. Transforming growth factors-beta as regulators of cellular growth and phenotype. Crit Rev Oncog 1992;3:1–26.

194. Derynck R, Jarrett JA, Cehn EY, Goeddel DV. The murine transforming growth factor-b precursor. J Biol Chem 1986;261:4377–9.

195. Lyons RM, Keski-Oja J, Moses HL. Proteolytic activation of latent transforming growth factor-β from fibroblast-conditioned medium. J Cell Biol 1985;106:1659–65.

196. Heldin CH, Miyazono K, ten Dijke P. TGF-beta signalling from cell membrane to nucleus through SMAD proteins. Nature 1997;390:465–71.

197. Derynck R, Zhang Y, Feng XH. Smads: transcriptional activators of TGF-beta responses. Cell 1998;95:737–40.

198. Monteleone G, Kumberova A, Croft NM, et al. Blocking Smad7 restores TGF-beta1 signaling in chronic inflammatory bowel disease. J Clin Invest 2001;108:601–9.

199. Dubinett SM, Huang M, Dhanani S, et al. Down-regulation of macrophage transforming growth factor-beta messenger RNA expression by IL-7. J Immunol 1993;151:6670–80.

200. Zhang K, Flanders KC, Phan SH. Cellular localization of transforming growth factor-β expression in bleomycin-induced pulmonary fibrosis. Am J Pathol 1995;147:352–61.

201. Phan SH, Gharaee-Kermani M, Wolber F, Ryan US. Stimulation of rat endothelial cell transforming growth factor-β production by bleomycin. J Clin Invest 1991;87:148–54.

202. Mackiewicz A, Ganapathi MK, Schultz D, et al. Transforming growth factor-β1 regulates production of acute-phase proteins. Proc Natl Acad Sci U S A 1990;87:1491–5.

203. Tsunawaki S, Sporn M, Nathan C. Comparison of transforming growth factor-beta and a macrophage-deactivating polypeptide from tumor cells: differences in antigenicity and mechanism of action. J Immunol 1989;142:3462–8.

204. Wahl S, Hunt DA, Wakefield LM, et al. Transforming growth factor type-β induces monocyte chemotaxis and growth factor production. Proc Natl Acad Sci U S A 1987;84:5788–2.

205. McCartney-Francis N, Mizel D, Wong H, et al. TGF-β regulates production of growth factors and TGF-β by human peripheral blood monocytes. Growth Factors 1990;4:27–35.

206. Kehrl JH, Thevenin C, Rieckmann P, Fauci AS. Transforming growth factor-β suppresses human B lymphocyte Ig production by inhibiting synthesis and switch from the membrane form to the secreted form of Ig mRNA. J Immunol 1991;146:4016–22.

207. Wahl SM, Hunt DA, Wong HL, et al. TGF-β is a potent immunosuppressive agent that inhibits IL-1 dependent lymphocyte proliferation. J Immunol 1988;140:3026–32.

208. Postlethwaite AE, Keski-Oja J, Moses HL, Kang AH. Stimulation of the chemotactic migration of human fibroblasts by transforming growth factor beta. J Exp Med 1987;165:251–6.

209. Leof EB, Proper JA, Goustin AS, et al. Induction of c-*sis* mRNA and activity similar to platelet-derived growth factor by transforming growth factor β: a proposed model for indirect mitogenesis involving autocrine activity. Proc Natl Acad Sci U S A 1986;83:2453–7.

210. Bruijn JA, Roos A, deGues B, deHeer E. Transforming growth factor-β and the glomerular extracellular matrix in renal pathology. J Lab Clin Med 1994;123:34–47.

211. Klagsbrun M, D'Amore PA. Regulators of angiogenesis. Annu Rev Physiol 1991;53:217–39.

212. Wiseman DM, Polverini PJ, Kamp DW, Leibovich SI. Transforming growth factor-beta (TGF-β) is chemotactic for human monocytes and induces their expression of angiogenic activity. Biochem Biophys Res Commun 1988;157:793–800.

213. Hoyt DG, Lazo JS. Alterations in pulmonary mRNA encoding procollagens, fibronectin, and transforming growth factor-β precede bleomycin-induced pulmonary fibrosis. J Pharmacol Exp Ther 1988;246:765–71.

214. Raghow R, Irish P, Kang AH. Coordinate regulation of transforming growth factor β gene expression and cell proliferation in hamster lungs undergoing bleomycin-induced pulmonary fibrosis. J Clin Invest 1989;84:1836–42.

215. Westergren-Thorsson G, Hernnas J, Sarnstrand B, et al. Altered expression of small proteoglycans, collagen, and transforming growth factor-β1 in developing bleomycin-induced pulmonary fibrosis in rats. J Clin Invest 1993;92:632–7.

216. Laurent CRK, Shahzeidl S, Lympany PA, et al. Transforming growth factors-beta 1, -beta 2, -beta 3 stimulate fibroblast procollagen production in vitro but are differentially expressed during bleomycin-induced lung fibrosis. Am J Pathol 1997;150:981–91.

217. Xing Z, Ohkawara Y, Jordana M, et al. Transfer of granulocyte-macrophage colony-stimulating factor gene to rat lung induces eosinophilia, monocytosis, and fibrotic reactions. J Clin Invest 1996;97:1102–10.

218. Xing Z, Tremblay GM, Sime PJ, Gauldie J. Overexpression of granulocyte-macrophage colony-stimulating factor induces pulmonary granulation tissue formation and fibrosis by induction of transforming growth factor-beta 1 and myofibroblast accumulation. Am J Pathol 1997;150:59–66.

219. Munger JS, Huang X, Kawakatsu H, et al. The integrin alpha v beta 6 binds and activates latent TGF beta 1: a mechanism for regulating pulmonary inflammation and fibrosis. Cell 1999;96:319–28.

220. Schultz-Cherry S, Chen H, Mosher DF, et al. Regulation of transforming growth factor-beta activation by discrete sequences of thrombospondin 1. J Biol Chem 1995;270:7304–10.

221. Wang A, Yokosaki Y, Ferrando R, et al. Differential regulation of airway epithelial integrins by growth factors. Am J Respir Cell Mol Biol 1996;15:664–72.

222. Gira SN, Hyde DM, Hollinger MA. Effect of antibody to transforming growth factor β on bleomycin induced accumulation of lung collagen in mice. Thorax 1993;48:959–66.

223. Denis M. Neutralization of transforming growth factor-β1 in a mouse model of immune-induced lung fibrosis. Immunology 1994;82:584–90.

224. Khalil N, O'Connor N, Unruh HW, et al. Increased production and immunohistochemical localization of transforming growth factor-β in idiopathic pulmonary fibrosis. Am J Respir Cell Mol Biol 1991;5:155–62.

225. Khalil N, O'Connor RN, Flanders KC, Unruh H. TGF-beta 1, but not TGF-beta 2 or TGF-beta 3, is differentially present in epithelial cells of advanced pulmonary fibrosis: and immunohistochemical study. Am J Respir Cell Mol Biol 1996;14:131–8.

226. Strieter RM, Kunkel SL. Chemokines in the lung. In: Crystal R, West J, Weibel E, Barnes P, editors. Lung: scientific foundations. 2nd ed. New York: Raven Press; 1997. p. 155–86.

227. Zlotnik A, Yoshie O. Chemokines: a new classification system and their role in immunity. Immunity 2000;12:121–7.

228. Koch AE, Strieter RM. Chemokines in disease. Austin (TX): RG Landes, Co., Biomedical Publishers; 1996.

229. Rossi D, Hardiman G, Copeland NG, et al. Cloning and characterization of a new type of mouse chemokine. Genomics 1998;47:163–70.

230. Bazan JF, Bacon KB, Hardiman G, et al. A new class of membrane-bound chemokine with a CX3C motif. Nature 1997;385:640–4.

231. Farber JM. HuMIG: a new member of the chemokine family of cytokines. Biochem Biophys Res Commun 1993;192:223–30.

232. Taub DD, Oppenheim JJ. Chemokines, inflammation and immune system. Therapeutic Immunol 1994;1:229–46.

233. Proost P, Wolf-Peeters CD, Conings R, et al. Identification of a novel granulocyte chemotactic protein (GCP-1) from human tumor cells: in vitro and in vivo comparison with natural forms of GROa, IP-10, and IL-8. J Immunol 1993;l150:1000–10.

234. Walz A, Burgener R, Car B, et al. Structure and neutrophil-activating properties of a novel inflammatory peptide (ENA-78) with homology to interleukin-8. J Exp Med 1991;174:1355–62.

235. Clark-Lewis I, Dewald B, Geiser T, et al. Platelet factor 4 binds to interleukin 8 receptors and activates neutrophils when its N terminus is modified with Glu-Leu-Arg. Proc Natl Acad Sci U S A 1993;90:3574–7.

236. Hebert CA, Vitangcol RV, Baker JB. Scanning mutagenesis of interleukin-8 identifies a cluster of residues required for receptor binding. J Biol Chem 1991;266:18989–94.

237. Strieter RM, Polverini PJ, Kunkel SL, et al. The functional role of the "ELR" motif in CXC chemokine-mediated angiogenesis. J Biol Chem 1995;270:27348–57.

238. Luster AD, Greenberg SM, Leder P. The IP-10 chemokine binds to a specific cell surface heparan sulfate shared with platelet factor 4 and inhibits endothelial cell proliferation. J Exp Med 1995;182:219–32.

239. Arenberg DA, Polverini PJ, Kunkel SL, et al. In vitro and in vivo systems to assess role of CXC chemokines in regulation of angiogenesis. Methods Enzymol 1997;288:190–220.

240. Coughlin CM, Salhany KE, Wysocka M, et al. Interleukin-12 and interleukin-18 synergistically induce murine tumor regression which involves inhibition of angiogenesis. J Clin Invest 1998;101:1441–52.

241. Simonet WS, Hughes TM, Nguyen HQ, et al. Long-term impaired neutrophil migration in mice overexpressing human interleukin-8. J Clin Invest 1994;94:1310–9.

242. Hechtman DH, Cybulsky MI, Fuchs HJ, et al. Intravascular IL-8. Inhibitor of polymorphonuclear leukocyte accumulation at sites of acute inflammation. J Immunol 1991; 147:883–92.

243. Ley K, Baker JB, Cybulsky MI, et al. Intravenous interleukin-8 inhibits granulocyte emigration from rabbit mesenteric venules without altering L-selectin expression or leukocyte rolling. J Immunol 1993;151:6347–57.

244. Lira SA, Fuentes ME, Strieter RM, Durham SK. Transgenic methods to study chemokine function in lung and central nervous system. Methods Enzymol 1997;287:304–18.

245. Lira SA, Zalamea P, Heinrich JN, et al. Expression of the chemokine N51/KC in the thymus and epidermis of transgenic mice results in marked infiltration of a single class of inflammatory cells. J Exp Med 1994;180:2039–48.

246. Grewal IS, Rutledge BJ, Fiorillo JA, et al. Transgenic monocyte chemoattractant protein-1 (MCP-1) in pancreatic islets produces monocyte-rich insulitis without diabetes: abrogation by a second transgene expressing systemic MCP-1. J Immunol 1997;159:401–8.

247. Keane MP, Arenberg DA, Lynch III JP, et al. The CXC chemokines, IL-8 and IP-10, regulate angiogenic activity in idiopathic pulmonary fibrosis. J Immunol 1997;159: 1437–43.

248. Koch AE, Leibovich SJ, Polverini PJ. Stimulation of neovascularization by human rheumatoid synovial tissue macrophages. Arthritis Rheum 1989;29(4):471–9.

249. Koch AE, Polverini PJ, Kunkel SL, et al. Interleukin-8 (IL-8) as a macrophage-derived mediator of angiogenesis. Science 1992;258:1798–801.

250. Nickoloff BJ, Mitra RS, Varani J, et al. Aberrant production of interleukin-8 and thrombospondin-1 by psoriatic keratinocytes mediates angiogenesis. Am J Pathol 1994; 144:820–8.

251. Broxmeyer HE, Kim CH. Regulation of hematopoiesis in a sea of chemokine family members with a plethora of redundant activities. Exp Hematol 1999;27:1113–23.

252. Premack BA, Schall TJ. Chemokine receptors: gateways to inflammation and infection. Nat Med 1996;2:1174–8.

253. Addison CL, Daniel TO, Burdick MD, et al. The CXC chemokine receptor 2, CXCR2, is the putative receptor for ELR(+) CXC chemokine-induced angiogenic activity [in process citation]. J Immunol 2000;165:5269–77.

254. Lippert U, Artuc M, Grutzkau A, et al. Expression and functional activity of the IL-8 receptor type CXCR1 and CXCR2 on human mast cells. J Immunol 1998;161:2600–8.

255. Ahuja SK, Gao JL, Murphy PM. Chemokine receptors and molecular mimicry. Immunol Today 1994;15:281–7.

256. Murphy PM. The molecular biology of leukocyte chemoattractant receptors. Ann Rev Immunol 1994;12:593–633.

257. Horuk R. Molecular properties of the chemokine receptor family. Trends Pharmacol Sci 1994;15:159–65.

258. Rollins BJ. Chemokines. Blood 1997;90:909–28.

259. Luster AD. Chemokines—chemotactic cytokines that mediate inflammation. N Engl J Med 1998;338:436–45.

260. Imai T, Chantry D, Raport CJ, et al. Macrophage-derived

261. Liao F, Alkhatib G, Peden KW, et al. STRL33, a novel chemokine receptor-like protein, functions as a fusion cofactor for both macrophage-tropic and T cell line-tropic HIV-1. J Exp Med 1997;185:2015–23.

262. Liao F, Alderson R, Su J, et al. STRL22 is a receptor for the CC chemokine MIP-3alpha. Biochem Biophys Res Commun 1997;236:212–7.

263. Stine JT, Chantry D, Gray P. Virally encoded chemokines and chemokine receptors: genetic embezzlement of host DNA. In: Mantovani A, editor. Chemokines. Basel: Karger; 1999. p. 161–80.

264. Ahuja SK, Murphy PM. Molecular piracy of mammalian interleukin-8 receptor type B by herpesvirus saimiri. J Biol Chem 1993;268:20691–4.

265. Arvanitakis L, Geras-Raaka E, Varma A, et al. Human herpesvirus KSHV encodes a constitutively active G-protein-coupled receptor linked to cell proliferation. Nature 1997;385:347–9.

266. Bais C, Santomasso B, Coso O, et al. G-protein-coupled receptor of Kaposi's sarcoma-associated herpesvirus is a viral oncogene and angiogenesis activator [see comments] [published erratum appears in Nature 1998;392:210]. Nature 1998;391:86–9.

267. Geras-Raaka E, Varma A, Ho H, et al. Human interferon-gamma-inducible protein 10 (IP-10) inhibits constitutive signaling of Kaposi's sarcoma-associated herpesvirus G protein-coupled receptor. J Exp Med 1998;188:405–8.

268. Rosenkilde MM, Kledal TN, Brauner-Osborne H, Schwartz TW. Agonists and inverse agonists for the herpesvirus 8-encoded constitutively active seven-transmembrane oncogene product, ORF-74. J Biol Chem 1999;274:956–61.

269. Loetscher M, Gerber B, Loetscher P, et al. Chemokine receptor specific for IP10 and mig: structure, function, and expression in activated T-lymphocytes. J Exp Med 1996;184:963–9.

270. Oberlin E, Amara A, Bachelerie F, et al. The CXC chemokine SDF-1 is the ligand for LESTR/fusin and prevents infection by T-cell-line-adapted HIV-1. Nature 1996;382:833–5.

271. Bleul CC, Farzan M, Choe H, et al. The lymphocyte chemoattractant SDF-1 is a ligand for LESTR/fusin and blocks HIV-1 entry. Nature 1996;382:829–3.

272. Murdoch C, Monk PN, Finn A. CXC chemokine receptor expression on human endothelial cells. Cytokine 1999;11: 704–12.

273. Romagnani P, Annunziato F, Lasagni L, et al. Cell cycle-dependent expression of CXC chemokine receptor 3 by endothelial cells mediates angiostatic activity. J Clin Invest 2001;107:53–63.

274. Legler DF, Loetscher M, Roos RS, et al. B cell-attracting chemokine 1, a human CXC chemokine expressed in lymphoid tissues, selectively attracts B lymphocytes via BLR1/CXCR5. J Exp Med 1998;187:655–60.

275. Dobner T, Wolf I, Emrich T, Lipp M. Differentiation-specific expression of a novel G protein-coupled receptor from Burkitt's lymphoma. Eur J Immunol 1992;22:2795–9.

276. Forster R, Mattis AE, Kremmer E, et al. A putative chemokine receptor, BLR1, directs B cell migration to defined lymphoid organs and specific anatomic compartments of the spleen. Cell 1996;87:1037–47.

277. Wilbanks A, Zondlo SC, Murphy K, et al. Expression cloning of the STRL33/BONZO/TYMSTR ligand reveals elements of CC, CXC, and CX3C chemokines. J Immunol 2001;166:5145–54.

278. Deng HK, Unutmaz D, KewalRamani VN, Littman DR. Expression cloning of new receptors used by simian and human immunodeficiency viruses. Nature 1997;388: 296–300.

279. Kim CH, Kunkel EJ, Boisvert J, et al. Bonzo/CXCR6 expression

defines type 1-polarized T-cell subsets with extralymphoid tissue homing potential. J Clin Invest 2001;107:595–601.

280. Turner-Warwick M, Haslam PL. The value of serial bronchoalveolar lavages in assessing the clinical progress of patients with cryptogenic fibrosing alveolitis. Am Rev Respir Dis 1987;135:26–34.

281. Jones HA, Schofield JB, Krauss T, et al. Pulmonary fibrosis correlates with the duration of tissue neutrophil activation. Am J Respir Crit Care 1998;158:620–8.

282. Carre PC, Mortenson RL, King TE Jr, et al. Increased expression of the interleukin-8 gene by alveolar macrophages in idiopathic pulmonary fibrosis. A potential mechanism for the recruitment and activation of neutrophils in lung fibrosis. J Clin Invest 1991;88:1802–10.

283. Lynch III JP, Standiford TJ, Kunkel SL, et al. Neutrophilic alveolitis in idiopathic pulmonary fibrosis: the role of interleukin-8. Am Rev Respir Dis 1992;145:1433–8.

284. Southcott AM, Jones KP, Li D, et al. Interleukin-8, differential expression in lone fibrosing alveolitis and systemic sclerosis. Am J Respir Crit Care 1995;151:1604–12.

285. Mitzner W, Lee W, Georgakopoulos D, Wagner E. Angiogenesis in the mouse lung. Am J Pathol 2000;157:93–101.

286. Koch AE, Leibovich SJ, Polverini PJ. Stimulation of neovascularization by human rheumatoid synovial tissue macrophages. Arthritis Rheum 1986;29:471–9.

287. Smith DR, Polverini PJ, Kunkel SL, et al. IL-8 mediated angiogenesis in human bronchogenic carcinoma. J Exp Med 1994;179:1409–15.

288. Arenberg DA, Kunkel SL, Polverini PJ, et al. Inhibition of interleukin-8 reduces tumorigenesis of human non-small cell lung cancer in SCID mice. J Clin Invest 1996;97:2792–802.

289. Koch AE, Volin MV, Woods JM, et al. Regulation of angiogenesis by the C-X-C chemokines interleukin-8 and epithelial neutrophil activating peptide 78 in the rheumatoid joint. Arthritis Rheum 2001;44:31–40.

290. Simonini A, Moscucci M, Muller DW, et al. IL-8 is an angiogenic factor in human coronary atherectomy tissue. Circulation 2000;101:1519–26.

291. Yuan A, Yang PC, Yu CJ, et al. Interleukin-8 messenger ribonucleic acid expression correlates with tumor progression, tumor angiogenesis, patient survival, and timing of relapse in non-small-cell lung cancer. Am J Respir Crit Care Med 2000;162:1957–63.

292. Haghnegahdar H, Du J, Wang D, et al. The tumorigenic and angiogenic effects of MGSA/GRO proteins in melanoma. J Leukoc Biol 2000;67:53–62.

293. Jordana M, Schulman J, McSharry C, et al. Heterogeneous proliferative characteristics of human adult lung fibroblast lines and clonally derived fibroblasts from control and fibrotic tissue. Am Rev Respir Dis 1988;137:579–84.

294. Keane MP, Belperio JA, Burdick M, et al. ENA-78 is an important angiogenic factor in idiopathic pulmonary fibrosis. Am J Respir Crit Care Med 2001. [In press].

295. Ben-Baruch A, Michiel DF, Oppenheim JJ. Signals and receptors involved in recruitment of inflammatory cells. J Biol Chem 1995;270:11703–6.

296. Keane MP, Belperio JA, Moore TA, et al. Neutralization of the CXC chemokine, macrophage inflammatory protein-2, attenuates bleomycin-induced pulmonary fibrosis. J Immunol 1999;162:5511–8.

297. Keane MP, Belperio JA, Arenberg DA, et al. IFN-gamma-inducible protein-10 attenuates bleomycin-induced pulmonary fibrosis via inhibition of angiogenesis [in process citation]. J Immunol 1999;163:5686–92.

298. Maeyama T, Kuwano K, Kawasaki M, et al. Attenuation of bleomycin-induced pneumopathy in mice by monoclonal antibody to interleukin-12. Am J Physiol Lung Cell Mol Physiol 2001;280:L1128–37.

299. Chen ES, Greenlee BM, Wills-Karp M, Moller DR. Attenuation of lung inflammation and fibrosis in interferon-

300. Stout AJ, Gresser I, Thompson D. Inhibition of wound healing in mice by local interferon alpha/beta injection. Int J Exp Pathol 1993;74:79–85.

301. Hyde DM, Henderson TS, Giri SN, et al. Effect of murine gamma interferon on the cellular responses to bleomycin in mice. Exp Lung Res 1988;14:687–704.

302. Gurujeyalakshmi G, Giri SN. Molecular mechanisms of antifibrotic effect of interferon gamma in bleomycin-mouse model of lung fibrosis: downregulation of TGF-beta and procollagen I and III gene expression. Exp Lung Res 1995;21:791–808.

303. Schall TJ. Biology of the RANTES/SIS cytokine family. Cytokine 1991;3:165–83.

304. Jiang Y, Tabak LA, Valente AJ, Graves DT. Initial characterization of the carbohydrate structure of MCP-1. Biochem Biophys Res Commun 1991;178:1400–4.

305. De Meester I, Korom S, Van Damme J, Scharpe S. CD26, let it cut or cut it down. Immunol Today 1999;20:367–75.

306. Proost P, De Meester I, Schols D, et al. Amino-terminal truncation of chemokines by CD26/dipeptidyl-peptidase IV. Conversion of RANTES into a potent inhibitor of monocyte chemotaxis and HIV-1-infection. J Biol Chem 1998;273:7222–7.

307. Proost P, Menten P, Struyf S, et al. Cleavage by CD26/dipeptidyl peptidase IV converts the chemokine LD78beta into a most efficient monocyte attractant and CCR1 agonist. Blood 2000;96:1674–80.

308. Nibbs RJB, Wylie SM, Pragnell IB, Graham GJ. Cloning and characterization of a novel murine beta chemokine receptor, D6. Comparison to three other related macrophage inflammatory protein-1alpha receptors, CCR-1, CCR-3, and CCR-5. J Biol Chem 1997;272:12495–504.

309. Nibbs RJ, Wylie SM, Yang J, et al. Cloning and characterization of a novel promiscuous human beta-chemokine receptor D6. J Biol Chem 1997;272:32078–83.

310. Rossi D, Zlotnik A. The biology of chemokines and their receptors. Annu Rev Immunol 2000;18:217–42.

311. Sica A, Saccani A, Borsatti A, et al. Bacterial lipopolysaccharide rapidly inhibits expression of C-C chemokine receptors in human monocytes. J Exp Med 1997;185:969–74.

312. Loetscher P, Seitz M, Baggiolini M, Moser B. Interleukin-2 regulates CC chemokine receptor expression and chemotactic responsiveness in T lymphocytes [see comments]. J Exp Med 1996;184:569–77.

313. Sallusto F, Lanzavecchia A, Mackay CR. Chemokines and chemokine receptors in T-cell priming and Th1/Th2-mediated responses. Immunol Today 1998;19:568–74.

314. Allavena P, Luini W, Bonecchi R, et al. Chemokines and chemokine receptors in the regulation of dendritic cell trafficking. In: Mantovani A, editor. Chemical immunology; chemokines. Basel: Karger; 1999. p. 69–85.

315. Boring L, Gosling J, Chensue SW, et al. Impaired monocyte migration and reduced type 1 (Th1) cytokine responses in C-C chemokine receptor 2 knockout mice. J Clin Invest 1997;100:2552–61.

316. Kuziel WA, Morgan SJ, Dawson TC, et al. Severe reduction in leukocyte adhesion and monocyte extravasation in mice deficient in CC chemokine receptor 2. Proc Natl Acad Sci U S A 1997;94:12053–8.

317. Kurihara T, Warr G, Loy J, Bravo R. Defects in macrophage recruitment and host defense in mice lacking the CCR2 chemokine receptor. J Exp Med 1997;186:1757–62.

318. Gao W, Topham PS, King JA, et al. Targeting of the chemokine receptor CCR1 suppresses development of acute and chronic cardiac allograft rejection. J Clin Invest 2000;105:35–44.

319. Gao JL, Wynn TA, Chang Y, et al. Impaired host defense, hematopoiesis, granulomatous inflammation and type 1-

gamma-deficient mice after intratracheal bleomycin. Am J Respir Cell Mol Biol 2001;24:545–55.

type 2 cytokine balance in mice lacking CC chemokine receptor 1. J Exp Med 1997;185:1959–68.

320. Zhang K, Gharaee-Kermani M, Jones ML, et al. Lung monocyte chemoattractant protein-1 gene expression in bleomycin-induced pulmonary fibrosis. J Immunol 1994; 153:4733–41.

321. Brieland JK, Jones ML, Flory CM, et al. Expression of monocyte chemoattractant protein-1 (MCP-1) by rat alveolar macrophages during chronic lung injury. Am J Respir Cell Mol Biol 1993;9:300–5.

322. Gharaee-Kermani M, Denholm EM, Phan SH. Costimulation of fibroblast collagen and transforming growth factor beta1 gene expression by monocyte chemoattractant protein-1 via specific receptors. J Biol Chem 1996;271: 17779–84.

323. Antoniades HN, Neville-Golden J, Galanopoulos T, et al. Expression of monocyte chemoattractant protein-1 mRNA in human idiopathic pulmonary fibrosis. Proc Natl Acad Sci U S A 1992;89:5371–5.

324. Standiford TJ, Rolfe MW, Kunkel SL, et al. Macrophage inflammatory protein-1α expression in interstitial lung disease. J Immunol 1993;151:2852–63.

325. Standiford T, Rolfe M, Kunkel S, et al. Altered production and regulation of monocyte chemoattractant protein-1 from pulmonary fibroblasts isolated from patients with idiopathic pulmonary fibrosis. Chest 1993;103:121S.

326. Gu L, Tseng S, Horner RM, et al. Control of TH2 polarization by the chemokine monocyte chemoattractant protein-1. Nature 2000;404:407–11.

327. Hogaboam CM, Lukacs NW, Chensue SW, et al. Monocyte chemoattractant protein-1 synthesis by murine lung fibroblasts modulates CD4+ T cell activation. J Immunol 1998;160:4606–14.

328. Orlofsky A, Wu Y, Prystowsky MB. Divergent regulation of the murine CC chemokine C10 by Th(1) and Th(2) cytokines. Cytokine 2000;12:220–8.

329. Matsukura S, Stellato C, Georas SN, et al. Interleukin-13 upregulates eotaxin expression in airway epithelial cells by a STAT6-dependent mechanism. Am J Respir Cell Mol Biol 2001;24:755–61.

330. Tokuda A, Itakura M, Onai N, et al. Pivotal role of CCR1-positive leukocytes in bleomycin-induced lung fibrosis in mice. J Immunol 2000;164:2745–51.

331. Moore BB, Paine R 3rd, Christensen PJ, et al. Protection from pulmonary fibrosis in the absence of ccr2 signaling. J Immunol 2001;167:4368–77.

332. Fischereder M, Luckow B, Hocher B, et al. CC chemokine receptor 5 and renal-transplant survival. Lancet 2001;357: 1758–61.

333. Strieter RM, Belperio JA. Chemokine receptor polymorphism in transplantation immunology: no longer just important in AIDS. Lancet 2001;357:1725–6.

334. Petrek M, Drabek J, Kolek V, et al. CC chemokine receptor gene polymorphisms in Czech patients with pulmonary sarcoidosis. Am J Respir Crit Care Med 2000;162(3 Pt 1): 1000–3.

335. Renzoni E, Lympany P, Sestini P, et al. Distribution of novel polymorphisms of the interleukin-8 and CXC receptor 1 and 2 genes in systemic sclerosis and cryptogenic fibrosing alveolitis. Arthritis Rheum 2000;43:1633–40.

11 EXTRACELLULAR MATRIX IN THE PATHOGENESIS OF LUNG INJURY AND REPAIR

JESSE ROMAN

The interstitial lung diseases (ILDs) are a diverse group of disorders characterized by dramatic alterations in lung structure and function. Over the past two decades, the cellular events triggered by acute and chronic forms of lung injury and the molecules and mechanisms potentially involved in the development of ILD have become increasingly clear. The use of animal models of lung injury induced by agents capable of producing architectural changes in the lung that resemble the human condition (eg, bleomycin) has helped to improve our understanding of the pathologic changes associated with ILD. Advances in other fields of research, as diverse as growth factors and lung cell biology, and the development of novel and sophisticated cellular and molecular biologic techniques have also contributed. These advances notwithstanding, we still lack a clear understanding of the fundamental processes by which normal human lung tissue becomes nonfunctional in patients with ILD. These gaps in knowledge represent the major obstacle to the development of sensitive tests for the early detection of disease and safe and efficient therapies to halt or reverse disease and its consequences. An observation that may provide clues to the pathogenesis of ILD is that independent of the inciting agent(s) or the initiating factors involved, uncontrolled deposition and turnover of fibrous connective tissue is a common pathway in the development of ILD. This chapter will focus on the aberrant deposition of fibrous connective tissue in the lungs of patients with acute and chronic forms of lung injury and its potential effect on inflammatory and repair processes within the lung.

Virtually all studies that have examined the lungs of patients with ILD show evidence of abnormal lung tissue remodeling that is characterized by aberrant extracellular matrix deposition and degradation. The extent of the fibrous connective tissue affected during this process and the compartments involved (ie, airways, vessels, interstitium) dictate the physiologic alterations seen in any given patient with ILD. For example, excessive fibrous connective tissue deposition in the lung interstitium leads to lung "stiffness" and the obliteration of gas exchange units

in diseases such as idiopathic pulmonary fibrosis (IPF), whereas, deposition of fibrous tissue within small airways leads to airflow limitation in obliterative bronchiolitis. However, the consequences of fibrous connective tissue deposition in ILD appear to surpass the architectural effects that lead to ILD-associated physiologic abnormalities. Mounting evidence suggests that in contrast to normal lungs (where the connective tissue is considered mainly responsible for structural support), after injury, cells and extracellular matrix (ECM) molecules newly deposited within the airway walls and interstitium may become major players in the control of inflammatory and tissue repair responses. These observations suggest that the development and progression of ILD after exposure to an injurious agent are highly dependent on the ability of the host to control the tissue remodeling response and to clear the fibrous connective tissue deposited by the injured lung in an attempt to heal the wound (Figure 11–1).

In view of the potential significance of tissue remodeling and regulation of ECM synthesis, deposition, and degradation in the pathogenesis of ILD, this chapter will summarize our current understanding of these processes. First, it describes the various molecules that combine to form the lung ECM and reviews the difference in content and distribution between normal and diseased states. Second, it discusses data generated in animal models of lung injury and explains the relevance of these data to the human condition. Third, it explores the cellular origin of ECMs and the factors that control ECM expression following injury to the mammalian lung. Fourth, it examines the mechanisms of ECM degradation in the lung, since the total amount of ECM deposited in any tissue is greatly dependent on the balance between factors involved in ECM deposition and those responsible for its degradation. Fifth, it summarizes the evidence that implicates ECMs in regulation of the inflammatory and repair responses that play prominent roles in acute and chronic forms of lung injury and the mechanisms by which ECMs exert their biologic effects. The information summarized herein indicates that the activation of tissue remodeling in the lung, with the consequent changes in

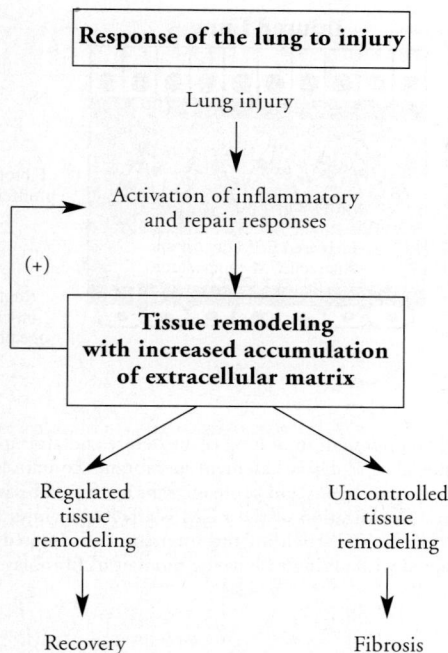

Response of the lung to injury

Lung injury

↓

Activation of inflammatory
and repair responses

↓

(+)

**Tissue remodeling
with increased accumulation
of extracellular matrix**

Regulated   Uncontrolled
tissue   tissue
remodeling   remodeling

↓   ↓

Recovery   Fibrosis

Figure 11–1   Mechanisms of lung injury and repair. This scheme summarizes the events triggered after lung injury. Lung injury appears to trigger an early inflammatory response that is followed by tissue remodeling. Extracellular matrix deposition during remodeling not only affects lung architecture but may amplify the inflammatory process. Thus, recovery from injury depends on control of excessive extracellular matrix deposition during remodeling.

extracellular matrix expression, deposition, and degradation, is a key event that is triggered early after diverse forms of acute and chronic lung injury, which has profound effects on lung architecture as well as on cellular functions. This process must be appropriately controlled by the activation of counter regulatory mechanisms directed at allowing wound healing while preventing excessive ECM deposition, destruction of the original architecture, and loss of lung function due to scarring.

EXTRACELLULAR MATRIX IN HEALTHY AND DISEASED HUMAN LUNGS

Extracellular Matrices in Healthy Adult Lungs

Connective tissue comprises approximately 25% of the total normal human adult lung mass[1,2] and is composed of collagens, elastin, proteoglycans, and noncollagenous glycoproteins such as laminin and fibronectin. Of these ECM molecules, *elastin* constitutes more than 30% of the dry weight of the normal adult lung. This polymeric molecule is predominant in the pleura, alveolar septae, and walls of blood vessels and airways; it is primarily responsible for the elastic properties of the lung. *Collagens* also constitute over 20% of the dry weight of the lung. Of the three categories of collagens (fibrillar, non-

fibrillar, and the low-molecular-weight collagens), the fibrillar collagens (eg, collagens type I, II, and III) constitute over 65% of all lung collagens. Fibrillar collagens are considered critical to the maintenance of structural support, since they associate laterally to form thick cables that provide strength to the lung connective tissue. *Proteoglycans* are high-molecular-weight molecules that consist of a protein core linked to polysaccharide chains of chondroitin, dermatan, keratan, and heparan sulfates. Proteoglycans are integral membrane components of cells and are present within the insoluble ECM. *Fibronectins* are glycoproteins present in plasma and connective tissue matrices. Fibronectins produced by hepatocytes and secreted into the plasma are termed "plasma" fibronectins, whereas "cellular" fibronectins are produced within tissues only by certain cell types such as fibroblasts and epithelial cells in response to injury. Increased expression of these and other ECMs in lung tissue is often considered an early marker of lung injury.[3]

Some ECM components organize into basement membranes, which are specialized structures that serve as interfaces between epithelia, peripheral nerves, or muscle cells and their surrounding tissue microenvironments.[4–6] *Laminin*, the most abundant glycoprotein found in basement membranes, associates with other ECMs such as collagen type IV, entactin, and heparan- and chondroitin-sulfate proteoglycans. Basement membranes not only help compartmentalize cells but also serve as semipermeable barriers and regulators of cell function. Furthermore, basement membranes delineate the normal architecture of the lung and, in doing so, are believed to serve as roadmaps for re-epithelialization after epithelial cell denudation during injury. It is felt that in the absence of such maps, due to basement membrane disruption, the return to the original tissue architecture after injury is unlikely.

Extracellular matrix components interact with one another covalently and noncovalently to form insoluble, heterogeneous connective tissue matrices. In the lung, the connective tissue is organized into the axial and peripheral connecting fiber networks that make up the lung "fiber skeleton."[7] This structure supports the airways and alveoli and also transmits stresses imposed at the alveolar wall to adjacent alveoli, to loose connective tissue in the lobules, and to visceral pleura. In addition to interacting with one another, ECMs interact with cells by binding to specific cell-surface receptors capable of signal transduction.[8] Thus, by interacting with one another and with cells, ECMs create a complex network that provides structural integrity and can modulate lung cell function. This well-organized tissue is disturbed during injury (Figure 11–2).

Extracellular Matrices are Increased in Interstitial Lung Disease

In contrast to healthy adult lungs, injured lungs undergo tissue changes in the process of eliminating noxious sub-

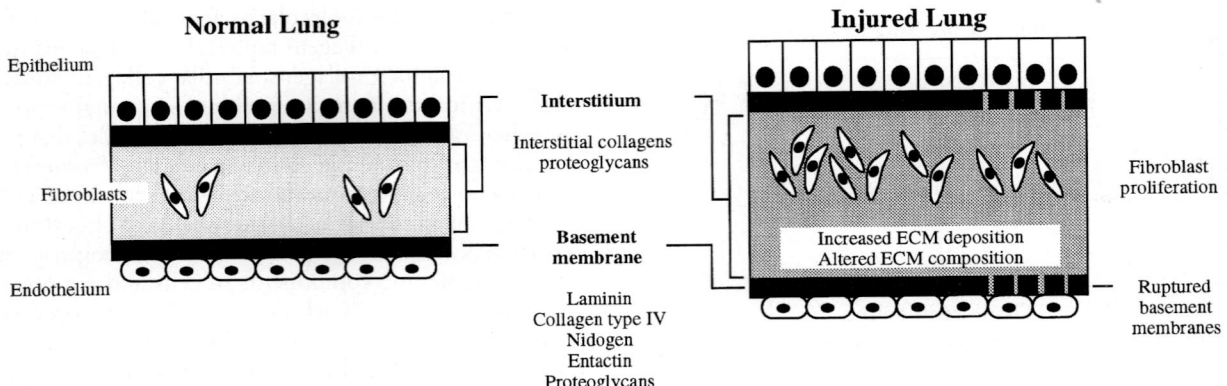

Figure 11–2 Extracellular matrix in normal and diseased lungs. This is a schematic representation of lung tissue before and after injury. In normal lungs, basement membranes help to compartmentalize epithelial and endothelial cells. These basement membranes contain laminin, collagen type IV, and nidogen, as well as other extracellular matrices (ECMs). Interstitial collagens and proteoglycans are found between the basement membranes of the lung epithelium and endothelium. The distribution and organization of the ECM is affected in injured lungs (eg, when basement membranes are disrupted and the amount and composition of the ECM within the interstitium is altered). More fibronectin and fibrin are deposited at the site of injury. These alterations are associated with an increase in the number of fibroblasts.

stances and healing the wounds they cause.[9] Early after injury, the lung increases in weight mainly due to edema caused by increased vascular permeability and by the influx of immune cells such as neutrophils. This early stage is termed the *acute* or *inflammatory* phase of lung injury and precedes a *reparative* phase, which is characterized by monocytic cell infiltration and tissue reorganization in the interstitium and alveolar spaces. Tissue reorganization during the reparative phase of lung injury is mainly due to the deposition of ECMs in basement membranes and lung parenchyma. This scheme is fairly stereotypical for most forms of acute lung injury such as that observed in the acute respiratory distress syndrome (ARDS).[10] The mechanisms involved in the architectural reorganization observed in chronic forms of lung injury (eg, IPF), however, are less well defined but are believed to be similar to those described above. The differences between acute (eg, ARDS) and chronic (eg, idiopathic pulmonary fibrosis) forms of lung injury lie in the intensity of the inciting event and the slower pace of disease progression after injury.

Altered expression and deposition of ECMs is common to both acute and chronic forms of lung injury as demonstrated in studies that examine the distribution of fibronectin and interstitial collagens showing dysregulation during injury.[3] Plasma fibronectin is readily detected in normal adult lungs where it localizes in alveolar capillary and epithelial basal lamina and is associated with interstitial collagens.[11] In contrast, cellular fibronectin is poorly detected in normal adult lung parenchyma, suggesting that most fibronectin detected in the adult lung is of plasma origin.[12] In injured lungs, however, cellular fibronectins can be readily detected. In one study in which lung tissue sections obtained from patients with acute and chronic forms of lung injury were examined, there were striking alterations in the distribution of these ECM

molecules.[12] For example, in patients with ARDS, focal discontinuities in the alveolar basal lamina were consistent with disruption of the basement membranes. The air spaces contained an infiltrate composed of fibroblastic cells and organizing ECM. Fibroblasts within the alveolar spaces and interstitium stained positively with an antiprocollagen antibody. This finding correlates well with new synthesis of collagen type I. Intense staining for cellular fibronectin and collagen type III also was observed. When the biopsy samples of 22 patients with chronic pulmonary fibrosis were examined, only 13 cases showed positive staining for procollagen, supporting the idea that differences in tissue responses depend on the host. When present, the staining was most prominent in fibroblasts that formed subepithelial clusters near the air-tissue interface. These fibrogenic foci stained diffusely with polyclonal antifibronectin antibodies; the staining for cellular fibronectin, which indicates new synthesis, corresponded to the location of the collagen-synthesizing fibroblasts. In patients with bronchiolitis obliterans and organizing pneumonia (BOOP), staining for collagen type III, plasma fibronectin, and cellular fibronectin was detected within the matrix of polypoid buds of fibroblasts known as Masson bodies and in ECMs projecting into the lumens of respiratory bronchioles. The fibroblasts within these bodies stained intensely for procollagen type I.

Similar alterations in fibronectin, collagen, and other ECM components (eg, proteoglycans, tenascin) have been demonstrated in other types of lung disease (see Table 11–1). Figure 11–3 demonstrates an example of increased accumulation of collagen and fibronectin in the lungs of a patient with BOOP. Of particular interest are the ILDs characterized by lung granulomatous inflammation. Elevated concentrations of the matrix components vitronectin, hyaluronan, and fibronectin have been found in the bronchoalveolar lavage (BAL)

TABLE 11–1   Examples of Altered Extracellular Matrix in Human Lung Disease

Lung Disease	ECM
Acute lung injury	
ARDS	HA[208,209]
	VER, Coll, Dec[52]
Bronchopulmonary dysplasia	FN[210,211]
Chronic lung injury	
Idiopathic pulmonary fibrosis	FN, Coll[43,212,213,224]
	Coll[12,42]
	TN, Thr, SPARC[214]
	VER[52]
Bronchiolitis obliterans	[215]
	Coll type VI[216]
	VER[52]
	TN, Thr, SPARC[214]
Farmer's lung	HA, Coll[217]
	Lam[218]
Alveolar proteinosis	HA[219]
Asbestos exposure	FN, Coll[32]
Chronic injury (children)	
Chronic inflammation	FN[220,223]
Cystic fibrosis	[221]
Granulomatous inflammation	
Sarcoidosis	FN, Coll[14,222]
	Dec[87]
	VN, FN, HA[13]
	HA[225]
	Lam[219]
Airways inflammation	
Asthma	FN, Coll[206,207]

HA = hyaluronic acid; VER = versican; FN = fibronectin; TN = tenascin; Dec = decorin; Coll = collagen; Lam = laminin; VN = vitronectin; Thr = thrombospondin; SPARC = secreted protein, acidic, and rich in cysteine.

fluid of patients with sarcoidosis.[13] Immunohistochemical studies of lung sections of patients with sarcoidosis revealed prominent staining for collagen type I at the periphery of sarcoid granulomas, whereas fibronectin staining was present in cells and stroma within and surrounding the granulomas.[14] Examination of the tissues with antibodies to procollagen and cellular fibronectin indicated that the increased deposition of collagen type I and fibronectin was mainly due to production in situ.

Overall, these studies reveal that alterations in ECM expression and deposition occur in most, if not all, acute and chronic forms of lung injury examined to date, independent of the elapsed time between the insult and specimen collection.

EXTRACELLULAR MATRIX EXPRESSION IN ANIMAL MODELS OF LUNG INJURY

Since dysregulation of ECM expression and deposition is one of the most important determinants of disease progression, it is critical to identify the mechanisms involved in ECM production in human lung. However, due to the complexity of human diseases, investigators have turned to various animal models to study ECM expression in lung injury. Using these models, investigators have demonstrated increased levels of messenger ribonucleic acid (mRNA) encoding for matrix components as well as chemically and immunohistochemically detectable ECM protein accumulation after lung injury.[3] This has been demonstrated in animal models of lung injury induced by exposure to bleomycin,[15,16] paraquat,[17,18] and hyperoxia,[19] among other potentially injurious substances (Table 11–2).

Of these models, the one considered most similar to human pulmonary fibrosis is that of bleomycin-induced lung injury. Bleomycin, a complex of water-soluble peptides extracted from *Streptomyces verticillus*, is a cytotoxic antimicrobial drug currently used to treat a variety of tumors; it causes interstitial pulmonary disease in humans.[20] In rodents, a single intratracheal injection, multiple subcutaneous injections, or administration via a continuous infusion pump causes an early diffuse hemorrhagic interstitial pneumonia that is consistently followed by lung fibrosis characterized by intra-alveolar buds, mural incorporation, and obliterative changes. All of these changes are morphologic alterations typically seen in human fibrotic lung diseases.[21,22] Furthermore, these morphologic alterations are accompanied by significant changes in lung mechanics.[23] Early studies performed almost two decades ago revealed marked alterations in ECM synthesis and deposition in the lungs of rodents exposed to bleomycin.[21,22,24–26] In mice, alterations in ECM protein accumulation after bleomycin administration follow overexpression of genes encoding for fibronectin and procollagens type I and III.[15,26] In mice receiving bleomycin by subcutaneous injection, increases in these mRNAs were detected as early as 1 to 2 weeks after initiation of bleomycin treatment, with peaks at 3 weeks.[27]

Altered expression of ECM components has also been demonstrated in animal models of granulomatous inflammation.[28] Trehalose-6,6'-dimycolate (TDM), a glycolipid found in the cell walls of mycobacteria and a major component of mycobacterial cord factor, induces the formation of granuloma-like lesions.[14] The lesions are characterized by edema and the accumulation of mononuclear cells at discrete foci within the lung interstitium (Figure 11–4). The number of these granuloma-like lesions peaks 3 to 5 days after the injection of the glycolipid. Over the next two weeks, the lesion slowly resolves, with total return of the normal lung architecture. New fibronectin and collagen type I deposition can be detected within and surrounding the granuloma-like lesions.[14] The early expression and deposition of fibronectin and collagen type I in this model overlap with the spatial and temporal kinetics of the mononuclear cell response. In other words, fibronectin and type I collagen are located within the granuloma-like lesions

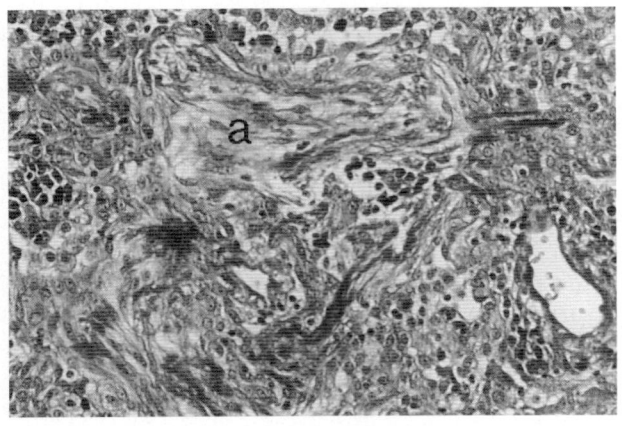

A

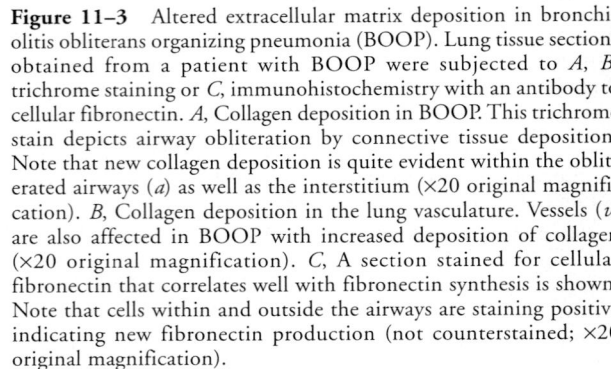

Figure 11–3 Altered extracellular matrix deposition in bronchiolitis obliterans organizing pneumonia (BOOP). Lung tissue sections obtained from a patient with BOOP were subjected to *A*, *B*, trichrome staining or *C*, immunohistochemistry with an antibody to cellular fibronectin. *A*, Collagen deposition in BOOP. This trichrome stain depicts airway obliteration by connective tissue deposition. Note that new collagen deposition is quite evident within the obliterated airways (*a*) as well as the interstitium (×20 original magnification). *B*, Collagen deposition in the lung vasculature. Vessels (*v*) are also affected in BOOP with increased deposition of collagen (×20 original magnification). *C*, A section stained for cellular fibronectin that correlates well with fibronectin synthesis is shown. Note that cells within and outside the airways are staining positive indicating new fibronectin production (not counterstained; ×20 original magnification).

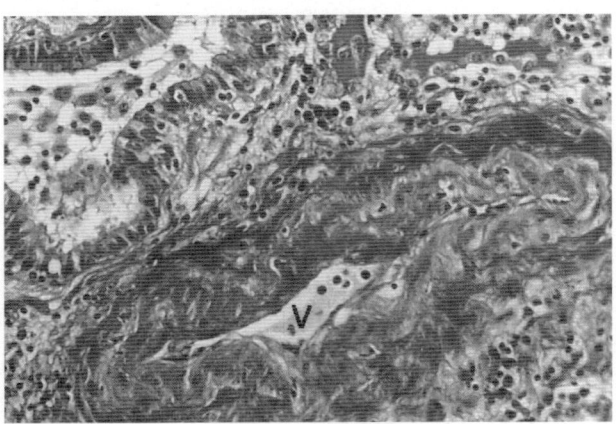

B

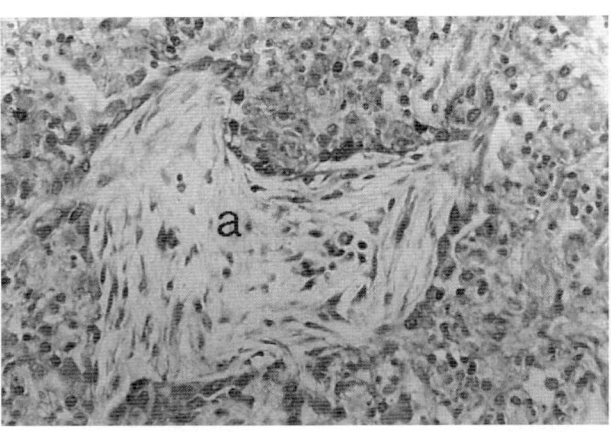

C

TABLE 11–2   Examples of Altered Extracellular Matrix in Animal Models of Lung Injury

Agent	Species	ECM
Paraquat	Monkey	Coll[143]
	Rat	FN, Coll[17,226]
Bleomycin	Hamster	FN, Coll, Elastin[15]
	Rat	FN, HA, Coll[26,227]
	Mouse	Elastin, Coll[228,229]
Hyperoxia	Rat	FN, Coll[19]
Heavy metal	Rabbit	FN[35]
Radiation	Rat	FN[230]
Cadmium chloride	Rat	Coll, Elastin[231]
Crocidolite	Mouse	Coll[232]
	Sheep	FN, Coll[32]
Ozone	Rat	FN, Coll[233]
CCL$_4$	Rat	Coll[234]
ROFA	Rat	FN[235]
Shistosome	Mouse	FN, Coll[28]
TDM	Mouse	FN, Coll[14]

HA = hyaluronic acid; FN = fibronectin; Coll = collagen; ECM = extracellular matrix; CCL$_4$ = carbon tetrachloride; ROFA = residual oil fly ash; TDM = trehalose-6,6'-dimycolate.

when they appear, and they disappear as the lesions resolve. Of significance is that these alterations in matrix deposition were observed prior to the evidence of fibrosis on light microscopy.

The above studies focus on ECM glycoproteins (eg, fibronectin) and collagens; however, evidence for the increased expression of proteoglycans and elastin is also available.[21] Elastin, for example, is increased in the lungs of animals after the administration of silica, and this is associated with alterations in lung elastase and airway resistance.[29]

The observations above underscore several important points. They show that many and diverse types of agents (eg, bleomycin, ozone, TDM) induce similar responses that lead to lung tissue remodeling characterized by excessive ECM synthesis and deposition. They reveal that the excessive ECM deposition observed in animals after lung injury is similar to that seen in humans, suggesting that mechanisms of wound healing are similar across mammalian species. They show that the increase in ECM deposition observed after injury is due largely to altered expression of ECM molecules by many cell types, including cells within the lung vasculature. This does not negate the contribution of leaked plasma proteins (eg, fibrinogen and fibronectin), but demonstrates that a major source of ECMs in the lung after injury is the lung itself. Most importantly, these studies suggest that events characteristic of both the inflammatory response (eg, edema and neutrophilic infiltration) and the tissue remodeling response (eg, increased ECM expression/deposition and degradation) occur very early after injury and often simultaneously. This suggests that both the initiation and maintenance of the inflammatory and tis-

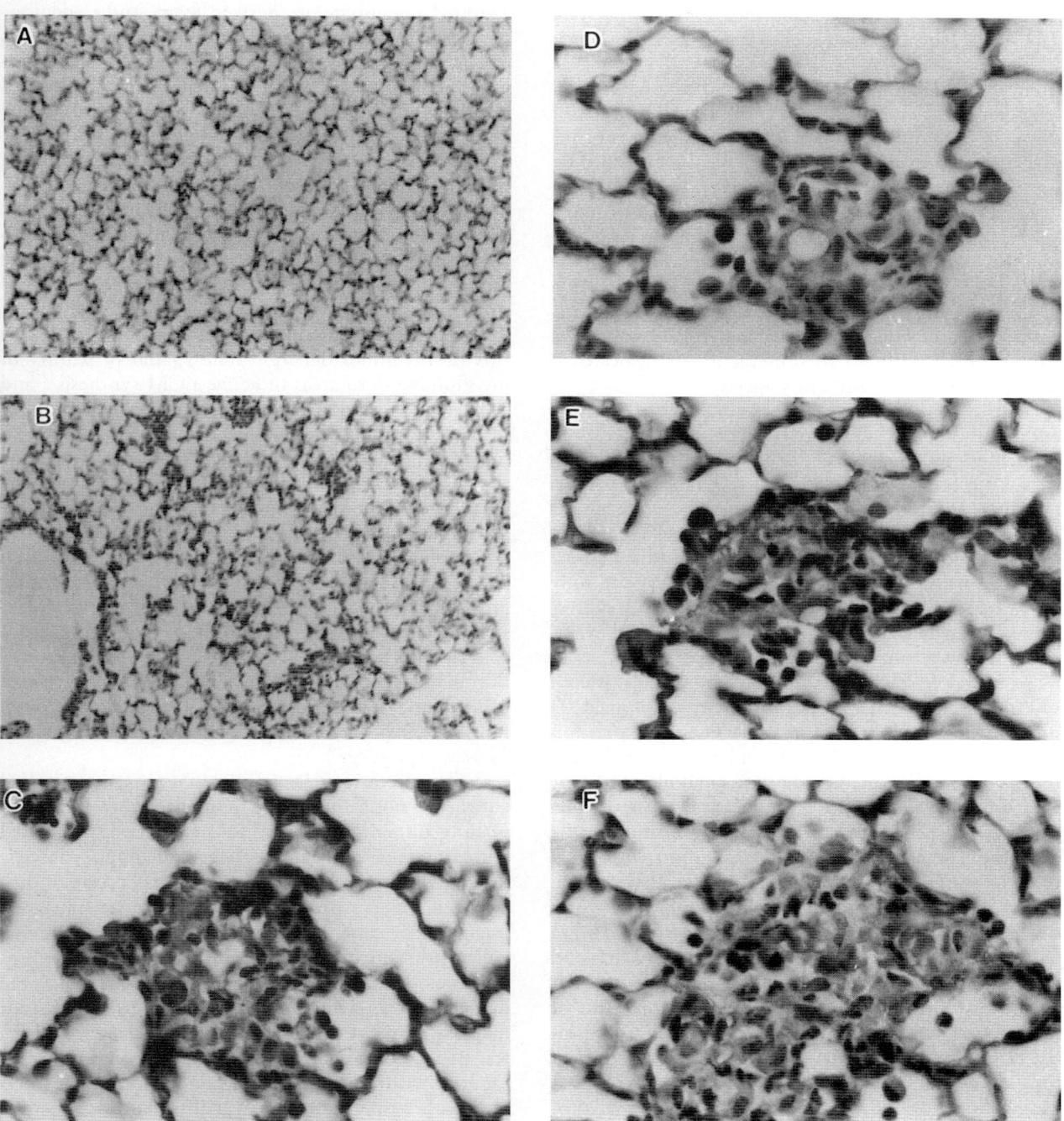

Figure 11–4   Distribution of extracellular matrices, matrix receptors, and transforming growth factor-β_1 in a murine model of trehalose-6,6'-dimycolate lung injury. Mice (C57BL) were injected with trehalose-6,6'-dimycolate (TDM) and the animals euthanized after three days. *B*, Note the accumulation of immune cells in TDM-treated animals as compared with *A*, controls (×10 original magnification). When examined by immunohistochemistry, the granuloma-like lesions contained *C*, procollagen type I as well as *D*, fibronectin (×40 original magnification). *E*, Cells within and outside the lesions expressed the fibronectin integrin receptor $\alpha_5\beta_1$ (×40 original magnification). *F*, These lesions also contained transforming growth factor-β_1 (×400 original magnification).

sue remodeling phases of lung injury may depend on common factors and mechanisms of action.

MECHANISMS OF EXTRACELLULAR MATRIX EXPRESSION IN INTERSTITIAL LUNG DISEASE

Cellular Origin of Extracellular Matrices in Lung

Many lung cells can produce ECM components after lung injury. For example, the increased concentration of fibronectin found in the BAL fluid obtained from clinical and experimentally injured lungs are derived mostly from the alveolar macrophage. Increased production of fibronectin has been demonstrated in alveolar macrophages obtained from human subjects with scleroderma-associated lung disease,[30] rheumatoid arthritis,[31] asbestos exposure,[32] and a variety of other ILD-associated diseases.[33] Similarly, the exaggerated production of ECMs has been demonstrated in alveolar macrophages obtained from animals exposed to mineral dust,[34] asbestos,[32] metal,[35] hyperoxia,[36] and other agents.

Other sources of ECM components include endothelial cells,[37] alveolar type II epithelial cells,[38] bronchial epithelial cells,[39] and lung fibroblasts.[40] Of these, the lung fibroblast is the cell type most commonly associated with ILD. Zhang and colleagues[41] investigated the expression of collagen using in situ hybridization in rats with bleomycin-induced pulmonary fibrosis. Early after bleomycin treatment, only a few scattered fibroblasts were found with weak expression of the alpha 1 (I) procollagen gene localized exclusively in the adventitia of many bronchi as well as in major blood vessels. After three days, however, scattered interstitial cells with significantly increased alpha 1 (I) procollagen and alpha 2 (I) procollagen gene expression were seen in the adventitia of respiratory bronchioles, terminal bronchioles, and adjacent small blood vessels. In 7 to 14 days, many interstitial cells expressed alpha 1 (I) procollagen. This was followed by a drop in gene expression by days 21 and 28. The authors concluded that, in this model, increased numbers of interstitial cells with high expression of procollagen type I genes are derived primarily from the fibroblasts in the adventitia of bronchioles, terminal bronchioles, and adjacent blood vessels, as well as the submesothelial region.[41] Broekelmann and colleagues[42] demonstrated expression of mRNAs for procollagen type I and fibronectin in fibroblasts within intra-alveolar organizing foci in a study of lung tissue obtained from subjects with IPF. Using a monoclonal antibody to detect new synthesis of procollagen type I in fibrotic lungs, McDonald and colleagues[43] and Kuhn and colleagues[12] found a striking increase in new collagen synthesis in some lung fibroblasts but not others. These data suggested the presence of an altered collagen-synthesizing fibroblast phenotype typical of fibrotic lung lesions.

To date, it is unclear whether the alterations observed in fibroblast production of ECMs in injured lungs are due to acquired phenotypic alterations that turn on a cellular program characterized by matrix production and proliferation or to the expansion of a pre-existing subpopulation of fibroblasts with exaggerated matrix production capabilities. Data favoring an acquired phenotype are derived from studies demonstrating that soluble mediators produced in injured lungs can act as mitogens for lung fibroblasts.[44-46] These soluble mediators may also be responsible for enhanced matrix production.[47] The idea of an acquired altered fibroblast phenotype in fibrotic lung lesions is further supported by the appearance of *myofibroblasts* in fibrotic lesions in ILD. Myofibroblasts get their name from their morphologic fibroblastic features and from the fact that they show increased expression of cytoskeletal components such as α-smooth muscle actin.[48] The emergence of myofibroblasts in lung injury also has been confirmed in animal models of pulmonary fibrosis.[49,50] They appear to originate from the adventitial fibroblast, although this is still under debate.[51] The spatial proximity of myofibroblasts to areas of active ECM synthesis[52] and the demonstration in vitro that myofibroblasts produce increased amounts of collagen when compared with fibroblasts,[53] suggest that they are actively involved in the tissue remodeling that accompanies ILD. The factors that promote the appearance of myofibroblasts are considered important targets for investigation because they are potentially relevant to the development of ILD. Treatment of cultured fibroblasts with transforming growth factor-beta (TGF-β) induces the expression of α-smooth muscle actin in these cells,[54,55] which suggests a role for this mediator in the generation of an altered fibroblast phenotype in ILD.[56] This is one of the pieces of evidence that implicates TGF-β as a key factor in lung fibrotic processes (see "Cytokines and Extracellular Matrix Expression").

The alterations in cellular phenotype described above may not be limited to lung fibroblasts. Induction of lung inflammation by TDM in mice is associated with the detection of procollagen in monocytic cells located within the lung lesions.[14] The detection of procollagen in cells of monocytic/phagocytic lineage is intriguing because these cells are not usually considered collagen-producing cells. However, the factors that trigger development of ILD or the conditions created by the disease may somehow lead these cells to switch to a matrix-producing phenotype. Others have reported the transformation of human leukocyte antigen (HLA)-DR monocytes into neofibroblasts under conditions associated with tissue remodeling, as in osteomyelosclerosis and tumor encapsulation.[57,58] This transformation appears to depend on the presence of T lymphocytes and is associated with the production of collagen.[58]

Another explanation for the appearance of myofibroblasts in certain patients with ILD is that the agent that induces the disease (or the conditions created in the lung by the disease) may induce the expansion of a pre-existent population of matrix-producing fibroblasts. The apparent heterogeneity of fibroblasts derived from the lungs of human and experimental animals with fibrosis that can be sustained in culture favors this "clonal expansion hypothesis."[59] For example, faster growth characteristics have been demonstrated in fibroblast lines that originate in lung tissue obtained from patients with ILD.[59,60] It appears that the mitogenic response of fibroblasts to various agents may be altered in ILD when compared with fibroblasts obtained from patients with limited lung disease.[61] Thus, the detection of this "semistable" fibroblast phenotype during cell culture suggests that, as seen in lymphocytes, lung fibroblasts also consist of subpopulations with different phenotypes and functions.[62]

Cytokines and Extracellular Matrix Expression

A number of soluble mediators with matrix-inducing capacity have been demonstrated in both humans and other animals at sites of active fibrosis.[63] These mediators can be expressed by inflammatory cells such as macrophages and eosinophils as well as by epithelial cells and fibroblasts. Mediators potentially involved in ILD include TGF-β, interleukins, tumor necrosis factor-α (TNF-α), platelet-derived growth factor (PDGF), fibroblast growth factor (FGF), and transforming growth factor-α (TGF-α). The actions of these mediators in vitro, and their detection in the lungs of patients with ILD, have implicated them in the modulation of inflammation and tissue repair responses that follow lung injury. Their ability to induce ECM expression in many cell types is most relevant to this discussion. For example, both protein release and messenger RNA expression for interleukin (IL)-1β and TNF-α, which are known to induce fibronectin and collagen expression in diploid lung fibroblasts, are enhanced in macrophages obtained from subjects with IPF or in macrophages exposed to asbestos.[64] Studies showing that bleomycin-induced lung injury and silica-induced pulmonary fibrosis can be greatly ameliorated by interventions that affect

cytokine production or function (eg, TNF-α,[65,66] IL-12,[67] interferons,[68] osteopontin[69]) suggest an important role for these molecules in ILD. The protective effects associated with deficiencies in certain cytokines further support this role.[70] However, the activity of these interventions has been generally ascribed to their anti-inflammatory properties rather than to their ability to affect tissue remodeling.

Members of the TGF-β family have received the most attention in the genesis of fibrotic lung diseases. Their potential role in tissue fibrosis is supported by in vitro studies demonstrating the ability of these factors (in particular TGF-β1) to increase the expression of ECM components by bronchial epithelial cells,[39,71] alveolar type II cells,[72] macrophages,[73,74] and fibroblasts[47] among other cell types. In lung fibroblasts, the stimulatory effects of TGF-β1 appear to be mediated via both TGF-β1 type I and type II serine/threonine kinase receptors,[75] and its activation appears dependent on specific integrin receptors.[76] In addition, TGF-β can directly decrease the expression of matrix-degrading enzymes or indirectly inhibit their function by stimulating inhibitors of their activity.[77,78] Thus, by stimulating ECM expression while decreasing matrix degradation, TGF-β may disrupt the ECM deposition/degradation balance and favor ECM accumulation (Figure 11–5).

The observation that production of TGF-β correlates with the development of fibrosis in animal models of lung injury induced by bleomycin,[79] thoracic irradiation,[80] and silicosis[81] further supports a role for TGF-β1 in the control of tissue remodeling in the lung. Studies demonstrating the ability of inhibitors of TGF-β to affect progression of lung fibrosis in animals or humans are scarce in spite of overwhelming data supporting a role for TGF-β in fibrotic lung diseases and the demonstrated beneficial effect of preventing TGF-β function in other injured organs.[77,82] One example is the work of Giri and colleagues[83] who showed that inhibition of TGF-β function by intravenous injection of anti-TGF-β2 and anti-TGF-β1 antibodies reduced the bleomycin-induced accumulation of lung collagen when lungs were examined 14 days after bleomycin administration. This

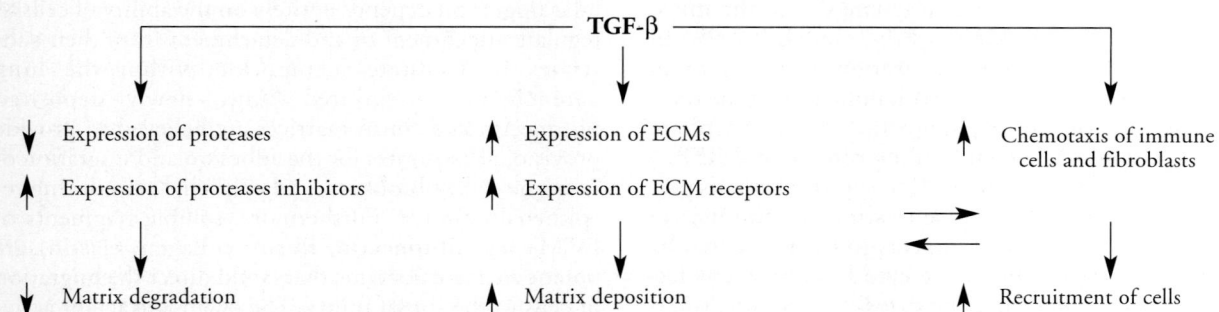

Figure 11–5   Diagrammatic representation of the potential effects of transforming growth factor (TGF)-β1 during lung injury. TGF-β1 induces the expression of extracellular matrix (ECM) while decreasing the expression and activity of matrix-degrading enzymes. In this fashion, TGF-β1 may, if uncontrolled, promote excessive ECM deposition. This effect may be amplified by the influx and activation of cells in injured lungs.

type of manipulation could ultimately prove useful in the clinical setting.

Immunohistochemistry and in situ hybridization have been used to examine the distribution and cellular origin of TGF-β in human lungs with IPF.[42] The TGF-β$_1$ mRNA expression was highest in alveolar macrophages in these diseases, although some TGF-β$_1$ was detected in fibrogenic foci codistributing with active collagen expression. Others have reported increased expression of TGF-β$_1$ in epithelial cells and macrophages in lung sections that show advanced fibrosis and honeycombing, which were obtained from patients with IPF, asbestosis, hypersensitivity pneumonitis, and other ILDs.[84,85] This is in contrast to the observations made in normal lungs where TGF-β$_1$ was not found in alveolar macrophages, epithelial cells, or extracellularly. Abundant TGF-β$_1$ has also been demonstrated in lung biopsy samples obtained from patients with eosinophilic granuloma[86] as well as in the epithelioid histiocytes within the non-necrotizing granulomas of lungs of patients with sarcoidosis.[14,87]

In addition to its effects on ECM and integrin expression, TGF-β might have indirect effects related to tissue remodeling. For example, TGF-β$_1$ can negatively affect the metabolism of glutathione in the lung thereby increasing its susceptibility to oxidant injury.[88] The resulting increase in oxidant stress can stimulate ECM expression.[89] This pathway has recently been implicated in the development of ARDS and in the increased susceptibility to ARDS observed in chronic alcoholics.[90] TGF-β$_1$ may also induce other profibrotic mediators such as the connective tissue growth factor (CTGF), which is a peptide that is mitogenic for fibroblasts and that induces fibronectin and collagen expression.[91] Conversely, other factors may work via the induction of TGF-β. This was demonstrated for the chemokine monocyte chemoattractant protein-1 (MCP-1) that induces collagen expression in lung fibroblasts in part by stimulating TGF-β$_1$.[92]

With the exception of the few studies that delineate the promoter elements present in genes encoding for ECM molecules,[93,94] information about the signaling and transcriptional mechanisms involved in the regulation of cytokine-induced ECM gene expression is very limited. Several studies suggest a role for specific protein kinases including protein kinase C and the mitogen-activated protein kinases Erk-1 and Erk-2.[95,96] In the case of fibronectin, the activation of these protein kinase pathways is associated with induction of the transcription factor cyclic adenosine monophosphate (cAMP)-response element binding protein or CREB.[95] This factor interacts with cAMP response elements present in the 5' end of the gene to stimulate fibronectin expression.[95] This process appears to be modulated by the organizational state of the cytoskeleton.[95] The latter is not surprising since the cytoskeleton, in particular the microtubular system, is considered to be a "retention receptor for protein kinases or kinase activators."[97] In the case of collagen, TGF-β has been shown to interact with specific "TGF-β–activating elements" present within the alpha 1(I) collagen promoter thereby stimulating its expression.[93]

Overall, the aforementioned studies emphasize the potential role of cytokines and other soluble mediators in the control of ECM expression after lung injury. Less is known about the mechanisms by which these mediators induce the expression of ECMs. Regardless of the mechanisms involved in their expression, newly deposited ECMs are likely to affect many cellular functions necessary to repair the injured lung.

BIOLOGIC EFFECTS OF EXTRACELLULAR MATRICES

Effects of Extracellular Matrices on Cell Function

The exact role of ECMs in normal and diseased lungs remains unclear despite advances in molecular biology and genetics. One significant hindrance to our understanding of ECM function in the lung is that knockout mutations of many ECM genes (eg, fibronectin and its integrin receptor $\alpha_5\beta_1$) are embryonic lethal and, therefore, are difficult to study.[98,99] Nevertheless, histological and physiologic analyses of tissues show that the exaggerated deposition of ECMs in injured lungs has dramatic effects on lung structure and function. In addition, mounting evidence suggests that newly deposited ECMs are not inert and that they affect many processes at the cellular level that modulate lung inflammatory and tissue repair responses even after ECM expression has subsided (Figure 11–6). This is possible because cells express surface receptors that can transmit intracellular signals after binding to the matrix. In this way, incoming and resident cells are likely to be affected by the alterations in ECM composition observed in ILD. The role(s) these cell-matrix interactions play in vivo are unclear; however, they can be inferred from in vitro data that suggest roles in the regulation of cell adhesion, migration, proliferation, differentiation, and activation.[8]

During the early stage of lung injury, inflammation is characterized by the activation and migration of immune and nonimmune cells to the site of injury. Cellular migration depends entirely on the ability of cells to regulate attachment to and detachment from their substrates to facilitate locomotion within the lung parenchyma. In injured lungs, newly deposited fibronectin and fibrin matrices are believed to provide provisional substrates for the adhesion and migration of immune cells, fibroblasts, and epithelial cells during re-epithelialization.[100] Furthermore, soluble fragments of ECMs (eg, fibronectin, fibrin, collagen, elastin) are potent chemoattractants that could direct the migration of cells to the site of injury. The chemoattractant activity of ECM fragments has been demonstrated for epithelial and endothelial cells, fibroblasts, neutrophils, monocytes, and alveolar macrophages.[101–107] In addition,

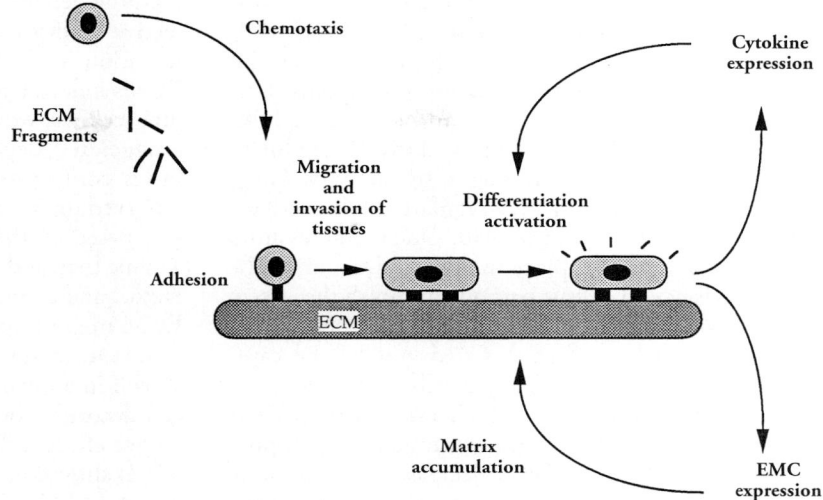

Figure 11–6 Effects of extracellular matrices (ECMs) on cellular function. ECMs enhance the adhesion and migration of immune and nonimmune cells. In addition, the fragments of certain ECM components are chemotactic to many cell types. These fragments can be released during tissue destruction after injury. ECMs may also alter the proliferation and differentiation of cells. Most relevant to lung injury, ECMs may activate immune cells to express cytokines and procoagulant factors that further enhance inflammation and fibrosis.

insoluble matrices are also believed to affect the directional migration of cells. This effect is known as *haptotaxis*, a form of chemotaxis elicited by an insoluble gradient (rather than a soluble one) that is created by the differential deposition of certain ECM components. In other words, cells are considered capable of detecting differences in insoluble matrix content, which leads their migration from sites of poor ECM deposition (distal to the injury site) to the injury site where new ECM deposition is greatest. On arrival, the very high concentrations of ECM at the injury site may enhance cell adhesion to the point of preventing further migration, thereby retaining the cell at the wound site.[108] Therefore, ECMs may influence the directional movement of immune and other cell types during inflammation by inducing chemotaxis and by providing a substrate for cell adhesion and migration during haptotaxis. The retention of immune cells in the lung might perpetuate injury, whereas the retention of fibroblasts in interstitial and alveolar spaces might promote further ECM deposition with subsequent thickening of the interstitium and "carnification" of the alveolar spaces.

Although the recruitment of blood-borne cells is considered a major mechanism for the observed accumulation of immune cells at the injury site, increased proliferation of incoming and resident cells is also contributory. Newly deposited ECMs are believed to affect this process as well. Fibronectin, for example, is a competence factor for lung fibroblast proliferation in vitro that promotes cytokinesis in serum-free defined medium.[109] This mechanism may be particularly relevant to the pathogenesis of pulmonary fibrosis in which increased fibroblast proliferation is seen.[59,60] Not only can ECM components affect proliferation directly, but they may serve as reservoirs or as carriers for growth factors that may be released during matrix degradation. Moreover, the growth-promoting effects of these factors may be synergized by their binding to ECMs.[110,111]

Alterations in matrix as well as in matrix-receptor expression that coincide with the differentiation of monocyte/macrophages and other cell types have implicated ECMs in cell differentiation.[112-114] In monocytic cells, differentiation induced by treatment with phorbol esters is associated with increased expression of cell-surface receptors for some matrix ligands but not for others.[115]

Extracellular matrix–derived signals capable of regulating cell proliferation and terminal differentiation may also be involved in the induction of apoptosis (programmed cell death).[116] In general, most studies indicate that attachment of a cell to its substrate may prevent or delay apoptosis. However, this protective effect appears highly dependent on the type of ECM molecules present in the substrate.[117] Work by Polunovsky and colleagues[118] has demonstrated the potential relevance of this phenomenon in lung injury and the development of ILD. These authors showed that exposure of fibroblasts and endothelial cells to BAL fluid obtained from patients with lung injury results in death of these cells by apoptosis. They also detected apoptotic cells within the air space granulation tissue in lungs obtained from patients with acute lung injury. These findings suggest that apoptosis may be yet another mechanism involved in tissue remodeling after lung injury, and that ECMs deposited in injured lungs may modulate this process.

Finally, ECMs can activate immune cells and stimulate their production of proinflammatory factors such as prostaglandins,[119] superoxide anions,[107,119] the cytokine IL-1β,[120–122] TNF-α,[123] and IL-6,[124] among others. In turn, as mentioned above, these molecules can affect leukocyte function and promote further deposition of ECMs by fibroblasts. The mechanisms responsible for induction of cytokine expression in immune cells exposed to ECMs are of great interest since they represent potential targets for the modulation of inflammation. The exposure of monocytic cells to fibronectin and type I collagen in vitro results in the expression of IL-1β mRNA and synthesis and secretion of both the precursor and active forms of IL-1β.[120,121] Both fibronectin and type I collagen also induce the expression of the interleukin-1 receptor antagonist (IL-1ra), a member of the IL-1 family produced by mononuclear cells.[121,125] Like interleukins, IL-1ra binds to IL-1 receptors, but without agonistic activity. Thus, this competitive inhibitor may regulate the bioactivity of IL-1β both in vitro and in vivo. One would assume that if these events take place in vivo, induction of IL-1ra by ECMs would at least partially diminish the effects of matrix-induced IL-1β in injured lungs. However, recent studies suggest that this may not be the case. Exposure of human mononuclear cells to collagen and fibronectin simultaneously, which mimics the mixed composition of the ECM in vivo, stimulates IL-1β production but results in a relative decrease in the amount of IL-1ra produced.[121,126] Exposure of human monocytes to fibrin produces the same effect.[122] Since these are the very same ECM components typically found in injured lungs, it is postulated that ECMs might enhance the bioactivity of IL-1β thereby boosting inflammation by inducing IL-1β (and other cytokines) while decreasing its inhibitor (ie, IL-1ra).

Additional evidence of the ability of ECMs to stimulate cell activation relates to the increase in procoagulant activity demonstrated in cultured human monocytic cells exposed to fibronectin, type I collagen, and fibrin [Roman and colleagues, unpublished observations, 1993]. This is relevant to the understanding of ILD since many studies have demonstrated that coagulation is enhanced and fibrinolysis depressed in the interstitial and alveolar spaces of the lung in diffuse acute and chronic interstitial lung diseases and in animals with experimental lung injury.[12,127–138] The importance of disturbances in coagulation in lung injury is best depicted in studies demonstrating that interventions designed to alter the balance between coagulation and fibrinolysis favoring the latter (eg, anticoagulation, transgenic animals deficient in plasminogen activator inhibitor-1), reduce inflammation and tissue remodeling.[137,139] By binding to specific cell-surface receptors on alveolar macrophages[140] and other immune cells, certain ECMs could stimulate the expression of procoagulants such as tissue factor,[141] which, in turn, promotes the crosslinkage of fibrinogen monomers extravasated from the vasculature into insoluble fibrin matrices. Once deposited in the extravascular spaces of the lung, fibrin serves as a scaffold for the accumulation of other ECM components and provides a provisional matrix for the migration, activation, and organization of fibroblasts and other cells.[100,142] This mechanism may be particularly relevant to the process of acute lung injury since ultrastructural studies of injured lungs show intra-alveolar fibrin deposits intermingled with fibronectin and associated with intra-alveolar fibroblasts.[143] In sarcoidosis, extensive deposition of fibrin occurs in the core of the granulomas.[122] In animals, alterations in fibrinolysis related to inhibition of

plasminogen activator inhibitor-1 were found to be protective against bleomycin-induced hydroxyproline accumulation in the lung.[144] If further studies confirm that ECMs indeed regulate the expression of procoagulants in lung cells, it would be reasonable to postulate that the exaggerated deposition of ECMs observed in injured lungs contribute greatly to the increased coagulation observed under these circumstances.

Based on the information presented above, one can assume that, as demonstrated in the case of certain growth factors and cytokines, interventions designed to alter the ECM might impact the progression of lung disease after acute and chronic forms of lung injury. This has been shown in animals that transiently express the proteoglycan decorin. The expression of this molecule had a protective effect against bleomycin-induced lung fibrosis.[145]

It should be emphasized that not all of the biologic effects of ECMs are detrimental. In fact, the activation of tissue remodeling in injured lungs is likely to be adaptive in nature. For example, the ability of ECMs and their fragments to stimulate the recruitment and activation of immune cells into the lung after injury and to serve as nonimmune opsonins[146] are clearly protective mechanisms relevant during infection. Also, the ability of ECMs to promote coagulation is very important during bleeding. The many connections between ECMs and cells serve as a "glue" to maintain tissue integrity after injury. Moreover, ECMs have been shown to promote vasculogenesis and angiogenesis in vitro and therefore are likely to play roles in the revascularization of ischemic lung tissue.[147] With regard to the vasculature, ECMs, in particular fibronectin, have been implicated in the regulation of vascular permeability in lung injury associated with sepsis.[148] Therefore, in patients with ILD, the excessive and unopposed activation of tissue remodeling might represent an adaptive response turned maladaptive.

EXTRACELLULAR MATRIX RECEPTORS

Extracellular matrices are able to affect cellular processes during normal states and tissue injury because cells express surface receptors that not only bind ECMs but are also capable of transmitting intracellular signals that affect gene expression. Many types of molecules mediate cell-matrix interactions.[149] The discussion will be limited to the *integrins*, a ubiquitous and highly conserved receptor family that mediates both cell-cell and cell-matrix interactions.[150] Blood-borne leukocytes, fibroblasts, tissue macrophages, bronchial and alveolar epithelial cells, and endothelial cells express integrins and, consequently, are capable of interacting with ECMs. Integrins are heterodimeric transmembrane receptors composed of two noncovalently linked glycoprotein α and β subunits (Figure 11–7). Distinct α subunits help confer ligand-binding specificity, whereas the β subunit may be common to other integrins. These αβ

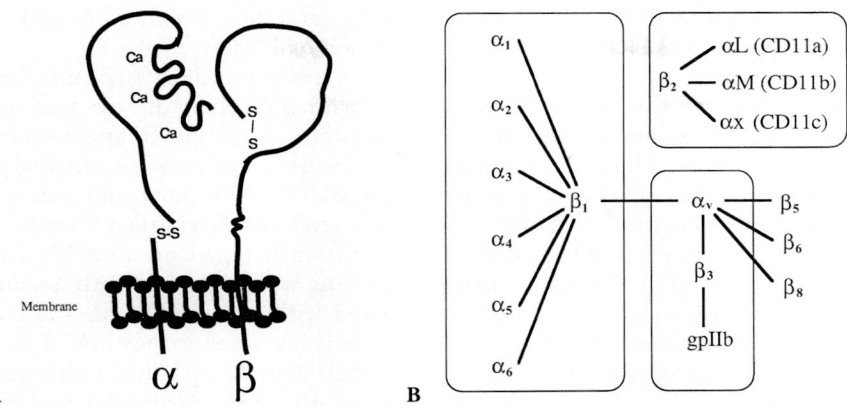

Figure 11–7   The integrin receptor family. *A*, Schematic representation of an integrin receptor. Integrins are heterodimeric glycoproteins expressed by diverse cell types including fibroblasts and leukocytes and consist of transmembrane α and β subunits. The α subunit contains several divalent cation binding sites, which are considered important for ligand binding. In general, the β subunits contain conserved cysteines that are arranged in four repeating units. *B*, Integrin subunit associations. Integrin α subunits associate with different β subunits. The identity of each subunit in any given heterodimer determines ligand-binding specificity. For example, the association of α_5 and β_1 subunits results in a receptor for fibronectin ($\alpha_5\beta_1$), whereas the association of α_2 and β_1 subunits results in a receptor for collagen and laminin ($\alpha_2\beta_1$). Initially, integrins were divided into three subfamilies according to their β subunit (ie, β_1, β_2, β_3), but newly discovered integrin subunits and their associations have limited the usefulness of this classification scheme.

complexes are classified into subfamilies, depending on their β subunit. To date, over 8 β and 30 α subunits have been identified, but the functions (their in vivo ligands) have not been determined for many of them.

The signaling pathways elicited by ligand binding to integrins have not been entirely characterized.[151] In general, ligand binding is followed by the clustering of integrins at the focal adhesion complex, a membrane structure that serves as a scaffold for the assembly and organization of integrins and intracellular proteins such as the cytoskeletal components talin, α-actinin, vinculin, and actin(Figure 11–8).[152] These interactions between integrins and the cytoskeleton allow for induction of cell shape changes, which could, in and of themselves, induce signal transduction.[153] In addition, integrin binding triggers the activation of intracellular secondary messengers,[154] including protein phosphorylation, transmembrane calcium ion fluxes, alterations in intracellular pH, altered levels of cAMP, breakdown of membrane phosphatidylinositols, and activation of protein kinases.[155] This occurs as a result of the spatial proximity of integrins and these signaling molecules at the focal adhesion complex. These signaling events have been implicated in many cellular processes that range from cell adhesion and migration to activation and cytokine expression. Many of these signals can be triggered by a single stimulus, converging to generate their effects. For example, in human monocytic cells, fibronectin induces the secretion of IL-1β protein by engaging the integrin $\alpha_5\beta_1$. The activation of $\alpha_5\beta_1$ is followed by the activation of serine/threonine protein kinase C and the induction of the transcription factor activator protein-1 (AP-1) that, after translocation into the nucleus, acts on the IL-1β promoter to induce gene transcription and, ulti-

mately, protein synthesis. This cascade of signaling events appears to be modulated by the state of organization of the cytoskeleton and the coactivation of mitogen-activated protein kinases.[156–158]

More recently, attention has been directed to the transcription factors induced by ECMs. Two transcription factors known to be induced after cell adhesion to fibronectin are AP-1 and nuclear factor-kb (NF-kb).[95,157] These factors are known to bind to promoter regions of genes that encode for proinflammatory mediators such as the cytokines IL-1β and TNF-α,[123,126] and adhesion molecules.[159] The activation of potent transcription factors known to modulate the expression of proinflammatory genes further highlights the reciprocal interaction that exists between inflammatory and tissue remodeling processes in injured lungs.

Studies demonstrating a role for various integrins in leukocyte recruitment during lung inflammation have highlighted the importance of these molecules in lung injury and repair. However, for the most part, most of these studies have focused on β_2 integrins, which are known for their ability to mediate cell-cell interactions.[150] As an example, Piguet and colleagues demonstrated that the pretreatment of animals with anti-integrin antibodies specific for a member of the β_2 integrin subfamily (ie, CD11b/CD18) prevented bleomycin- and silica-induced lung fibrosis.[160,161] Much less is known about the in vivo function of matrix-binding integrins. Nevertheless, in view of their ability to mediate the communication of cells with their surrounding ECM, the matrix-binding integrins are potential candidates for the development of therapeutic agents that could prove useful in the treatment of lung injury and ILD.

DESTRUCTION OF
EXTRACELLULAR MATRICES

Although lung injury can lead to tissue fibrosis in many instances, patients with acute lung injury do not always progress to overwhelming fibrosis. Thus, it is assumed that the human lung is protected by defense mechanisms that prevent excessive deposition of ECMs and that disturbances of these mechanisms could be involved in the pathogenesis of ILD. One of these mechanisms is the expression of matrix-degrading proteases capable of degrading newly deposited fibrous connective tissue. Of these, the family of matrix metalloproteinases (MMP) has received much attention (Table 11–3). The MMPs are zinc- and calcium-dependent endopeptidases that can degrade connective tissue components such as collagens, elastin, laminins, and fibronectin.[162,163] The MMPs differ from other matrix-degrading enzymes (eg, serine proteases) in at least two respects. First, these molecules are secreted as inactive zymogens and require extracellular activation after production. Second, many tissues produce specific inhibitors of MMPs termed TIMPs (for tissue inhibitors of MMPs). Consequently, the activity of MMPs in tissues depends on their expression, extracellular activation, and the relative concentration of TIMPs.

Members of the MMP family have been implicated in many pulmonary diseases including cystic fibrosis,[164] bronchiectasis,[165] and idiopathic interstitial pneumonias such as IPF, nonspecific interstitial pneumonia (NSIP), and BOOP.[166] Montano and colleagues[167] demonstrated high levels of collagenase inhibitory activity in lung samples from five patients with IPF and six samples from patients with hypersensitivity pneumonitis when compared with controls. Ricou and colleagues[168] demonstrated increased expression of the 92 kD gelatinase (MMP-9) in the BAL fluid rather than plasma of patients with early ARDS. Although its corresponding TIMP also was elevated, the MMP-9/TIMP ratio remained elevated throughout the late phases of prolonged ARDS. In sarcoidosis, O'Connor and colleagues[169] found latent collagenase activity in the BAL fluid of 16 of 43 patients with sarcoidosis but not in any patient in the control group. On follow-up, 62% of patients with BAL collagenase required treatment, whereas only 23% without activity required treatment. A consistent correlation between the amount of MMPs (or their activity) and the clinical presentation and progression of disease has not been estab-

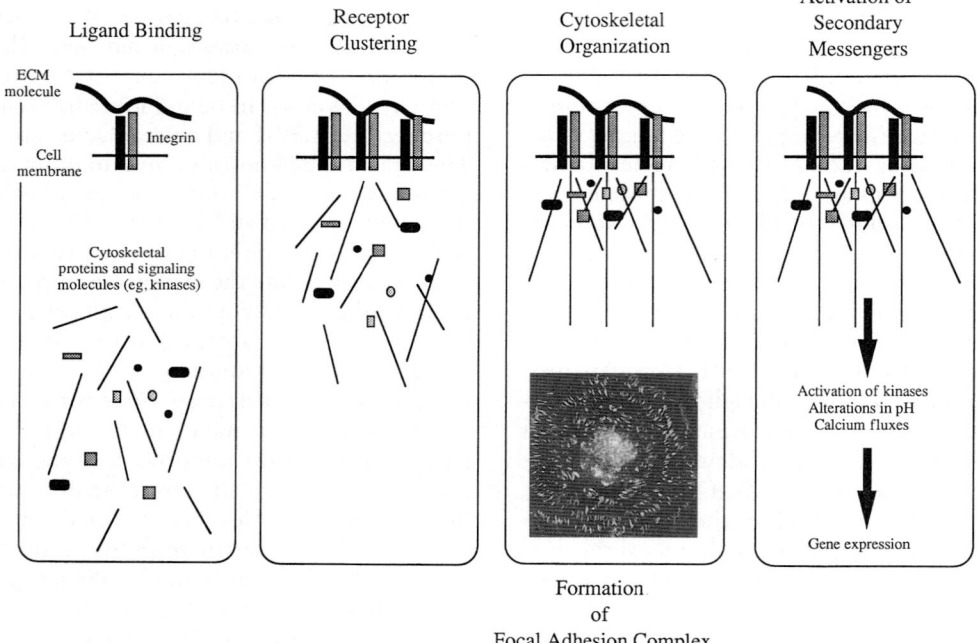

Figure 11–8   Signal transduction via integrins. Adhesion of cells to the extracellular matrix results in signal transduction via integrin receptors. The events involved in signaling via integrins are believed to occur in the following sequence. First, *ligand binding* occurs. This depends on the state of activation of the receptor and on the presence of divalent cations. Second, ligand binding triggers *receptor clustering*. Third, receptor clustering is associated with the *organization* of cytoskeletal proteins such as talin, vinculin, and α-actinin at the cell surface. The membrane structure that contains the extracellular ligand, the integrin, and the intracellular cytoskeletal proteins mentioned above are called the *focal adhesion complex* or *FAC*. FACs in association with integrins are believed to provide a scaffold for the assembly of signaling molecules at the cell surface. Interactions between integrins, cytoskeletal proteins, and signaling proteins present at the FAC result in the *activation* of intracellular secondary messengers and the transduction of signals that ultimately affect gene expression. *Insert*, immunofluorescence staining of fibronectin receptors adherent to fibronectin in human lung fibroblasts. Note the needle-eye shape of the clustered receptors at the cell surface. These structures show the localization of FACs.

TABLE 11–3 The Family of the Matrix Melloproteinases

Subgroup	Name	MMP Number	Substrate	Native Inhibitor
Collagenases	Interstitial collagenase	1	Collagen types I, II, III, VII, X; gelatin, proteoglycans	TIMP-1 and -2
	Neutrophil collagenase	8	Collagen types I, II, III; proteoglycans	TIMP-1 and -2
Gelatinases	Gelatinase A	2	Collagen types IV, V, VII, X; gelatin	TIMP-1 and -2
	Gelatinase B	9	Collagen types IV, V, VII, X	TIMP-1 and -2
Stromelysins	Stromelysin 1	3	Collagen types III, IV, V, IX; laminin, fibronectin, elastin, gelatin, proteoglycans, progelatinase B, procollagenase	TIMP-1 and -2
	Stromelysin 2	10	Same as for stromelysin 1	TIMP-1 and -2
	Stromelysin 3	11	Gelatin, fibronectin, proteoglycan	TIMP-1 and -2
	PUMP-1	7	Gelatin, fibronectin, laminin, collagen type IV, procollagenase, proteoglycan core protein	TIMP-1 and -2
Metalloelastases		12	Elastin	TIMP-1 and -2
Membrane-type MMP	MT-MMP	—	Collagen type IV, gelatin, progelatinase A	TIMP-1 and -2

MT-MMP = membrane type-metalloproteinase; TIMP = tissue inhibitor of metalloproteinase; PUMP-1 = matrilysin; MMP = matrix metalloproteinase.

lished. However, a recently published short report described a small but significant inverse correlation between levels of gelatinolytic activity in the bronchoalveolar lavage fluid of subjects with sarcoidosis and lung function tests including forced expiratory volume in one second and forced vital capacity.[170] Of note, the subgroup with the highest gelatinolytic activity also had the worst pulmonary function and this association persisted over time indicating a role for MMPs in the pathogenesis of chronic lung disease related to sarcoidosis.

Similar derangements in MMP expression and activity have been demonstrated in animal models of lung injury. Hyperoxia, for example, is known to induce type I and IV collagenase mRNA expression and to increase type I and IV collagenolytic activity in the lungs of newborn rats.[171] The MMP and elastase activities were examined in cultured alveolar macrophages and polymorphonuclear neutrophils obtained from the BAL fluid of a guinea pig model of acute lung injury induced by intratracheal instillation of a lipopolysaccharide.[172] Increased free and total gelatinase activity was detected. Pardo and colleagues[173] found that exposure of adult rats to 100% oxygen induces an increase in gelatinolytic and collagenolytic activities. This correlated with increased type IV collagenases as well as interstitial collagenase mRNA as determined by in situ hybridization. Increased MMP activity has also been detected in the lungs of animal models of infectious disease typically associated with lung destruction such as tuberculosis.[174]

The cells responsible for and the mechanisms involved in altered MMP expression in injured lungs are beginning to be discovered. At least three types of lung cells are considered capable of producing collagenolytic enzymes in the lower respiratory tract: fibroblasts, macrophages, and neutrophils.[175] In these cells, expression of MMPs can be upregulated by polypeptide growth factors and cytokines. For example, IL-1 induces collagenase synthesis[176] and stromelysin gene expression.[177] Tumor necrosis factor-α also induces collagenase production.[178] The ECM itself may affect MMP expression. Collagen types I and III, for example, stimulate collagenase expression.[179] Matrigel, which contains mainly basement membrane components such as laminin and type IV collagen, induces fibroblasts to produce collagenase.[175] Fibronectin induces collagenase and stromelysin.[154] Fibroblasts produced MMP-1 when cultured in collagen sponges and collagen-glycosaminoglycan sponges.[175] Fibroblasts cultured on granuloma matrix complexes isolated from tissues obtained from subjects with sarcoidosis are stimulated to produce MMP-1 as well.[175] The effects of ECMs on MMP expression are mediated via specific integrins.[154,180]

The above studies implicate MMPs in the remodeling of the lung during injury, but few studies have carefully delineated the alterations in MMP function under these circumstances by examining in detail the expression and activity of MMPs and that of their inhibitors simultaneously. Nevertheless, the data available to date suggest that the alterations in MMP expression and activity observed after lung injury parallel those observed in ECM expression. It should be mentioned, however, that several reports have demonstrated a decrease, rather than an increase, in matrix-degrading activity after lung injury. For example, lung collagenase activity decreased significantly in rats after 12-hour exposure to normobaric hyperoxia.[181] Intratracheal instillation of quartz DQ-12 resulted in a significant decrease in tissue collagenolytic activity in a well known model of silicosis.[182] Pardo and colleagues[183] set out to study this discrepancy, and they tested the production of matrix-degrading enzymes in fibroblastic cells obtained from human normal lung specimens and lungs from patients with IPF. They observed that although fibroblasts from both types of hosts were capable of producing the enzymes, fibroblasts from patients with IPF secreted about half of the amount produced by the others. They concluded that certain subpopulations of lung fibroblasts could have different potentials for producing collagenase activity and TIMP in vivo. In view of these latter observations, it has been postulated that certain injurious agents could cause lung fibrosis by restraining matrix-degrading activity.[184] It is clear that further work is needed to delineate the exact timing of their expression as well as the role matrix-degrading enzymes might play during different periods after lung injury. Nevertheless, it appears that a tight balance between ECM deposition and degradation in injured lungs is necessary to preserve lung function. Alterations in this balance favoring matrix deposition may lead to tissue fibrosis, whereas excessive expression/function of matrix-degrading enzymes may lead to destruction of bronchial walls and alveolar septae. The latter supposition is supported by the work of D'Armiento and colleagues who demonstrated that overexpression of collagenase in mice results in alterations in lung architecture consistent with emphysema.[185] Strategies designed to regulate the exaggerated expression and function of MMPs might prove beneficial in the treatment of interstitial lung disease. In a recent report, investigators showed that an MMP inhibitor termed batimastat ameliorated bleomycin-induced lung fibrosis.[186]

It should be emphasized that MMPs are not the only family of proteases involved in lung connective tissue degradation. As described above, a deficiency in plasminogen activator inhibitor-1 is protective in bleomycin-induced lung fibrosis.[144] However, these associations appear to be more complex than previously anticipated since fibrinogen-null mice were not protected against bleomycin-induced lung injury.[187] In other work, it has been demonstrated that targeted alterations in the coagulation cascade induced by the administration of activated protein C inhibited bleomycin-induced lung fibrosis.[188]

CLINICAL IMPLICATIONS

Studies in humans and animals with acute and chronic forms of lung injury invariably show that increased expression and deposition of ECM components is part of the stereotypical response of the lung to injury. The origins of this response are unclear, but the response may have evolved to combat parasitic infections.[189] Under these circumstances, deposition of connective tissue around the parasite could wall off the invading organism and contain its spread. This wound-healing response may have also prevented death due to massive bleeding after trauma. Regardless of its origin, it has become increasingly clear that this response, when uncontrolled, becomes maladaptive and leads to excessive connective tissue deposition with destruction of the original lung architecture, loss of lung function, and, in many cases, respiratory failure and death. Thus, it has been proposed that ECM deposition during tissue remodeling plays a key role in the repair responses that follow lung injury. How tissue remodeling occurs and affects the overall progression of lung disease in acute and chronic forms of lung injury is not entirely clear. The following is an attempt to reconcile the latest information about ECMs with our current understanding of lung injury in general and interstitial lung disease in particular.

As discussed earlier, descriptive studies performed in clinical and experimental lung specimens have revealed that lung injury elicits a wound-healing response characterized by inflammatory and tissue remodeling responses. Independent of the triggering factors and the mechanisms of action, these types of studies also suggest that recovery or progression to loss of lung function is highly dependent on the intensity of the elicited responses (Figure 11–9A). In the current scheme of thought, the inflammatory and tissue remodeling responses are triggered in tandem. In this view of lung injury and wound healing, the elicited inflammatory and tissue remodeling responses are regulated by distinct factors that exert their effects via different mechanisms of action. Several observations have dramatically shaped this view. One observation is that newly deposited ECMs can modulate many inflammatory processes in vitro and thus are likely to have similar effects in vivo. ECMs could amplify and perhaps perpetuate inflammation, thereby leading to abnormal wound healing and progression to fibrosis. Another observation is that some of the same soluble polypeptide growth factors found in injured lungs during the inflammatory phase of lung injury are also found during the repair phase. In vitro, these polypeptides can affect both inflammatory and tissue remodeling processes. A third observation comes from the evaluation of data generated in animal models of lung injury. In essentially all animal models studied, the inflammatory and tissue remodeling responses elicited by lung injury overlap temporally and are often triggered simultaneously, suggesting similar modes of regulation. These three pieces of information imply that the so-called early inflammatory and late repair responses of lung injury are manifestations of the same wound-healing response. In other words, lung injury simultaneously triggers both inflammation and tissue remodeling (Figure 11–9B). Most importantly, there appears to be a recriprocal interaction between inflammation and tissue remodeling such that the intensity of one of these responses has important effects on the other. To some, this statement may seem to contradict observations made in clinical and experimental lung injury where "cellular" or inflammatory changes usually do not coexist with "fibrotic" changes. However, this is not surprising during the early stages of lung injury when edema and inflammation are readily detected by light microscopy, but ECM expression, deposition, and degradation are not. It is only when light microscopy is used in conjunction with immunohistochemistry or in situ hybridization that new matrix expression and deposition can be detected before fibrosis is evident. Studies in which these techniques are used clearly demonstrate that ECM expression is altered very early after lung injury, much earlier than anybody would have anticipated years ago. The same cannot be said about the late stages of lung injury, when fibrosis can be detected with little evidence of inflammation. This suggests that even though inflammation and tissue remodeling can be triggered simultaneously, the two responses can be dissociated. Furthermore, it supports the idea that the factors sustaining some of the processes that take place during the early stage of lung injury (eg, edema, recruitment of immune cells) can be established independently of those factors involved in matrix production and tissue remodeling.

Although the foregoing statements are related more to acute forms of lung injury, similar processes could be postulated for chronic forms as well. In the latter, the inflammatory response is likely characterized by less dramatic physiologic alterations that do not lead to symptoms during the early stages of the disease (Figure 11–9C). Under those circumstances, symptoms become apparent only after significant tissue remodeling has occurred and fibrosis is overwhelming. Thus, even though both inflammation and tissue remodeling are triggered early in acute and chronic forms of lung injury, the higher intensity of the response in acute lung injury is responsible for its early detection before fibrosis is evident by light microscopy, whereas in chronic forms of lung injury, late detection occurs when fibrosis is the most obvious component.

Assuming the above hypothesis is correct, strategies directed toward the treatment of ILD should exert their effects on both inflammatory and tissue remodeling aspects of the wound-healing response at a very early stage. Current therapeutic strategies (ie, immunosuppressants) are directed mainly toward the reduction of inflammation but appear to be ineffective against aberrant tissue remodeling, which explains our unsuccessful attempts at curtailing the progression of these diseases. It is now apparent that effective options for the treatment of fibrotic lung diseases may become available only with a better understanding of the mechanisms that control ECM expression/deposition and degradation in the lung and after the mechanisms of fibrous connective tissue replacement by functional tissue have been clarified.

The task of identifying potential therapeutic agents for ILD is particularly difficult because the etiology of many ILDs such as IPF and sarcoidosis remains unknown. In other instances, the inciting agents are known (eg, asbestos, silica), but the cellular events that lead to fibrosis in response to these agents are unclear. Meanwhile, new and old therapeutic agents should be tested for their effect on ECM turnover both in vitro and in vivo. Certain agents such as prostaglandin E, which

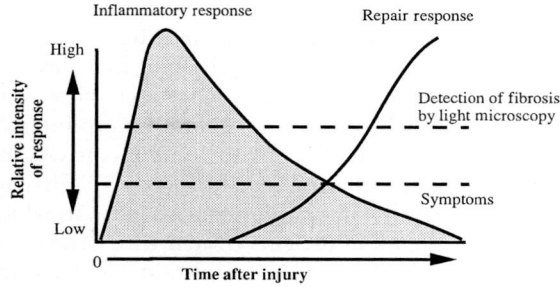

A

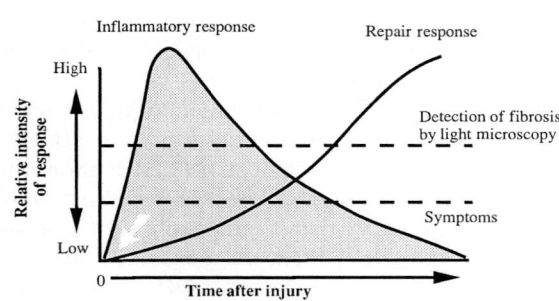

B

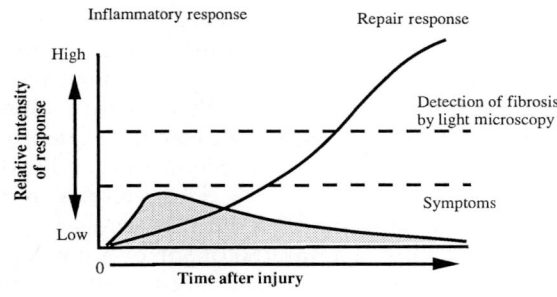

C

Figure 10–9 Schematic representation of the events triggered by lung injury. *A,* Lung injury triggers inflammatory and repair responses. This image represents our current understanding of the events triggered by acute lung injury. Note that, in general, it is believed that lung injury triggers an early inflammatory response that precedes the repair response by as much as several days. Under these circumstances, symptoms are evident very early, and the morphologic alterations that characterize inflammation are readily noted by light microscopy. Only later can the fibrotic response be detected by the same means. *B,* Schematic representation of proposed sequence of events triggered by lung injury. Based on studies described in the text, one can propose that lung injury triggers inflammation and tissue remodeling simultaneously (compare beginning of repair response in A and B). Lung biopsies obtained early in the disease demonstrate inflammation, but fibrosis will not be detected until later unless light microscopy is used in conjunction with other techniques such as in situ hybridization. *C,* Schematic representation of proposed sequence of events triggered after chronic lung injury. Chronic lung injury such as IPF is detected late in the course of the disease when fibrosis is evident by light microscopy. It is assumed that the early inflammatory reaction was insufficient to induce symptoms, thereby explaining the delay in detection. However, it is possible that repair responses with increased ECM deposition may be totally dissociated from inflammation in certain kinds of chronic lung injury. In other words, injury could induce fibrosis in the absence of an early inflammatory process.

has a uniformly negative effect on net collagen accumulation, have already been shown to affect ECM accumulation.[190] The alkaloid, colchicine, has both anti-inflammatory and antifibrotic properties in vitro, which include its ability to diminish fibronectin production in alveolar macrophages[191] and to inhibit conversion of procollagen to collagen in fibroblasts.[192] This may explain the results of a published case series in which a benefit was shown in patients treated with colchicine as compared with those who received steroids alone.[193] Unfortunately, further studies failed to reveal significant improvements with this agent. Another agent with antifibrotic properties is pirfenidone, which has been shown in a limited number of patients with IPF to slow the progression of disease.[194]

Despite these promising observations, it appears that single agents with unique targets of action are unlikely to be effective against ILD. It is more likely that "cocktails" of drugs will be more effective, considering the redundancy that is innate to proinflammatory and profibrotic mechanisms in the lung. Thus, agents capable of inhibiting ECM accumulation are likely to be most useful when coupled with strategies directed at diminishing cell injury (eg, antioxidants), inhibiting growth factor and proinflammatory cytokine activity, modulating proteases, and reducing fibroblast proliferation.[194] The polypeptide relaxin, a growth factor present in serum particularly during pregnancy, recently has been observed to decrease the synthesis and secretion of interstitial collagens, increase the expression of collagenase, and decrease the production of TIMP in human dermal fibroblasts.[195] These effects may be related to its ability to inhibit the matrix-inducing activity of TGF-β.[196] The pretreatment of animals with relaxin inhibits bleomycin-induced lung fibrosis in mice, a protective effect that is probably related to its impact on various processes involved in tissue remodeling.[196] An intriguing concept highlighted by these and other studies is that inflammation might be diminished by controlling the fibrotic response. If one subscribes to the above hypothesis that both inflammatory and repair responses are manifestations of the same wound-healing response and thus can be controlled by similar, and sometimes identical, factors, then this is within the realm of possibility.

In evaluating approaches to treatment of ILD, clinicians should bear in mind that many patients with these disorders are identified late in the course of the disease, and that chronicity is one of the most important determinants of a poor response to therapy. This problem is compounded by the difficulty in detecting disease in many chronic forms of lung injury (eg, IPF) prior to the development of symptoms and in the identification of patients who have "active" rather than "dormant" disease. This is an area in which tools capable of identifying ECM products in serum and BAL fluid might be useful. Peters and colleagues[197] reported increased levels of intact cellular fibronectin in the plasma of patients

with collagen vascular disorders. However, the source of these ECM components remains unclear. The collagen metabolite procollagen-III-peptide can be detected in the BAL fluid of patients with hypersensitivity pneumonitis but not in normal controls. Its levels correlated well with that of vitronectin and fibronectin as measured by enzyme-linked immunosorbent assay (ELISA).[198,199] Vincent and colleagues[200] examined the release of total fibronectin and cellular fibronectin into the plasma-free perfusate of isolated perfused rabbit lung after oxidant challenge. In this model, continuous infusion of H_2O_2 caused an increase in lung weight over 60 minutes and endothelial protein permeability after 20 minutes. Fibronectin antigen was detected in the perfusate as early as 15 minutes after the oxidant injury. This occurred in the presence of inhibitors of protein synthesis and suggests mainly degradation and remodeling. Recent data suggest that the determination of MMP activity in bronchoalveolar lavage fluid might prove useful in the evaluation of disease activity in sarcoidosis.[170] Taken together, these observations suggest that detection of ECM products in serum and BAL fluid in patients suspected of or diagnosed with ILD may provide a convenient means by which disease activity can be measured. Further studies will be required to determine whether there is a correlation between levels of ECM products in body fluids and abnormalities in lung physiology, and ultimately, between progression of disease and survival.

If the disease is not detected early, fibrosis, which is considered an irreversible event, ensues. The fact that some patients with ARDS, sarcoidosis, and BOOP, in which excessive connective tissue deposition is evident, experience recovery of lung function suggests cure is possible at least in some patients. To date, it is unclear as to what extent fibrous connective tissue can be remodeled and replaced by functional tissue. In some subjects, tissue remodeling is due to alveolar collapse and "carnification" of airway and alveolar spaces with little destruction of basement membranes.[10] Based on our discussion, intact basement membranes may help maintain the underlying architecture of the lung; in these cases, a significant degree of recovery may occur with appropriate treatment.

SUMMARY AND RESEARCH NEEDS

The development and progression of acute and chronic forms of lung injury are heavily influenced by the extent of matrix accumulation with excessive ECM deposition that leads to fibrosis and excessive ECM degradation that leads to tissue destruction. Factors that control the balance between fibrogenic and antifibrogenic forces during tissue remodeling, in large part, determine the outcome. The data available to date suggest that this tissue remodeling response is triggered early after injury, often simultaneously with inflammation, and that it might modulate the inflammatory process. Thus, interventions directed at controlling tissue remodeling should be instituted very early after lung injury to prevent irreversible tissue damage. Such interventions, however, are not available. It is expected that further understanding of the pathophysiologic processes involved in lung tissue remodeling will help in the development of agents that can reverse fibrosis and return some, if not all, of the lost pulmonary function (Figure 11–10). It is evident that much work in the area of tissue remodeling still needs to be done to achieve these goals. Research is urgently needed in the area of control of ECM accumulation in the lung, including regulation of transcription and translation of genes coding for ECM molecules, post-translational modifications of ECM proteins, and secretion and fibril organization and cross-linking into an insoluble matrix, all involving tightly regulated complex mechanisms that determine ECM assembly.[201] Research in the area of extracellular degradation of ECM molecules and their potential role in the control of tissue remodeling is also needed. The evaluation of old and new potential therapeutic agents should include a careful examination of their effects on matrix production. The immunologic responses that promote ECM accumulation should also be evaluated, as should the mechanisms for regulation of the immune response by newly deposited matrices. The mechanisms of expression and functional regulation of profibrotic growth factors require further attention.[202] Animal models that closely resemble chronic forms of lung injury will help to better address questions regarding such illnesses. Further clinical and epidemiologic studies that examine the potential interaction between matrix turnover and disease development and progression should be conducted, and questions regarding the potential determinants of susceptibility to ILD and the effects of environmental factors (eg, cigarette smoking, ethanol, FDA-approved drugs, alternative medicines) on matrix accumulation should be addressed. Studies directed at evaluating the role of mechanical ventilation on tissue remodeling,[203] the role of tissue remodeling in lung rejection after transplantation, and the role of chronic hypoxia on the regulation of lung tissue remodeling[204] are just a few of those areas of investigation that are not only likely to have an impact upon the understanding and treatment of ILD but are likely to affect the management of other diseases where alterations in ECM accumulation have been recently recognized as important (eg, obstructive airway diseases, primary pulmonary hypertension).[205–207] Information obtained from such studies may suggest new approaches in which inflammation and tissue remodeling are considered together in an attempt to prevent the devastating effects of ILD.

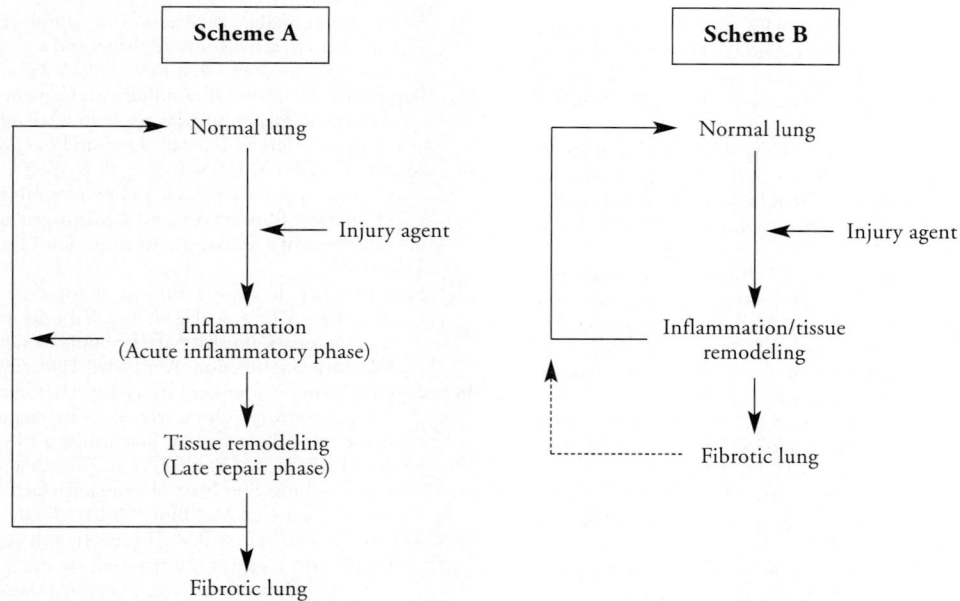

Figure 11–10   Role of tissue remodeling in lung injury and repair. *A*, Current understanding of lung injury. In general, lung injury is believed to trigger an acute inflammatory response followed by tissue remodeling and extracellular matrix deposition. Tissue remodeling may lead to irreversible fibrosis if uncontrolled. As depicted here, inflammation and tissue remodeling involve separate mechanisms of action, which are regulated independently. *B*, Proposed scheme for lung injury and repair. Experimental evidence suggests that lung injury may simultaneously trigger inflammation and tissue remodeling. Furthermore, both inflammation and tissue remodeling may be two manifestations of the same wound healing response. If so, interventions that affect both responses should be considered early after injury to avoid irreversible tissue fibrosis. One can also propose that not all fibrotic lung may be irreversibly damaged. Because deposited matrices can be degraded by various enzymes, interventions directed at regulating these enzymes may prove beneficial in the recovery of functional tissue.

REFERENCES

1. Clark JG, Kuhn C, McDonald JA, Mecham P. Lung connective tissue. Annu Rev Conn Tissue Res 1983;10:249–331.

2. Hance AJ, Crystal RC. The connective tissue of lung. Am Rev Respir Dis 1975;112:657–711.

3. Roman J, McDonald JA. Fibronectins and fibronectin receptors in lung development, injury and repair. In: Crystal RG, West JB, Barnes P, Cherniack NS, Weibel ER, editors. The lung: scientific foundations. Philadelphia: Lippincott-Raven Publishers; 1996. p. 737–55.

4. Sannes PL, Wang J. Basement membranes and pulmonary development. Exp Lung Res 1997;23:101–8.

5. Paulsson M. Basement membrane proteins: structure, assembly, and cellular interactions. Crit Rev Biochem Mol Biol 1992;27:93–127.

6. Yurchenco PD, Schittny C. Molecular architecture of basement membranes. FASEB J 1990;4:1577–90.

7. Weibel ER. Looking into the lung: what can it tell us? AJR Am J Roentgenol 1979;133:1021–31.

8. Roman J. Extracellular matrices and lung inflammation. Immunol Res 1996;15:163–78.

9. Roman J, McDonald JA. Cellular processes in lung repair. Chest 1991;100:245–8.

10. Burkhardt A. Alveolitis and collapse in the pathogenesis of pulmonary fibrosis. Am Rev Respir Dis 1989;140:513–24.

11. Torikata C, Villiger B, Kuhn C, McDonald JA. Ultrastructural distribution of fibronectin in normal and fibrotic human lung. Lab Invest 1985;52:399–408.

12. Kuhn C, Boldt J, King TE, et al. An immunohistochemical study of architectural remodeling and connective tissue synthesis in pulmonary fibrosis. Am Rev Respir Dis 1989; 140:1693–703.

13. Eklund AG, Sigurdardottir O, Ohrn M. Vitronectin and its relationship to other extracellular matrix components in bronchoalveolar lavage fluid in sarcoidosis. Am Rev Respir Dis 1992;145:646–50.

14. Roman J, Jeon Y-J, Gal A, Perez RL. Distribution of extracellular matrices, matrix receptors, and transforming growth factor beta-1 in human and experimental lung granulomatous inflammation. Am J Med Sci 1995;309:124–33.

15. Raghow R, Lurie S, Seyer JM, Kang AH. Profiles of steady state levels of messenger RNAs coding for type 1 procollagen, elastin, and fibronectin in hamster lungs undergoing bleomycin-induced interstitial pulmonary fibrosis. J Clin Invest 1985;76:1733–9.

16. Kelley J, Newman RA, Evans JN. Bleomycin-induced pulmonary fibrosis in the rat: prevention with an inhibitor of collagen synthesis. J Lab Clin Med 1980;96:954–64.

17. Dubaybo BA, Thet LA. Changes in lung tissue and lavage fibronectin after paraquat injury in rats. Res Commun Chem Pathol Pharmacol 1986;51:211–20.

18. Shirai M, Fujise H, Masaoka T, et al. Histometric changes in connective fibers of the lung following paraquat administration in rats. J Toxicol Sci 1993;18:167–70.

19. Durr RA, Dubaybo BA, Thet LA. Repair of chronic hyperoxic lung injury: changes in lung ultrastructure and matrix. Exp Mol Pathol 1987;47:219–40.

20. Luna MA, Bedrossian CWM, Lichtiger EA. Interstitial pneumonitis associated with bleomycin therapy. Am J Clin Pathol 1972;58:501–10.

21. Adamson IYR, Bowden DH. The pathogenesis of bleomycin-induced pulmonary fibrosis in mice. Am J Pathol 1974;77:185–98.

22. Harrison JH, Lazo JS. High dose continuous infusion of bleomycin in mice: a new model for drug-induced pulmonary fibrosis. J Pharmacol Exp Ther 1987;243:1185–93.

23. Ebihara T, Venkatesan N, Tanak R, Ludwig MS. Changes in extracellular matrix and tissue viscoelasticity in bleomycin-induced lung fibrosis. Temporal aspects. Am J Respir Crit Care Med 2000;162:1569–76.

24. Clark JG, Overton JE, Marino BA, et al. Collagen biosynthesis in bleomycin-induced pulmonary fibrosis in hamsters. J Lab Clin Med 1980;96:943–9.

25. Schrier DJ, Phan SH, McGarry BM. The effects of the nude (nu/nu) mutation on bleomycin-induced pulmonary fibrosis. Am Rev Respir Dis 1983;127:614–7.

26. Kelley J, Chrin L, Shull S, et al. Bleomycin selectively elevates mRNA levels for procollagen and fibronectin following acute lung injury. Biochem Biophys Res Commun 1985; 131:836–43.

27. Hoyt DG, Lazo JS. Alterations in pulmonary mRNA encoding procollagens, fibronectin, and transforming growth factor-β precede bleomycin-induced pulmonary fibrosis in mice. J Pharmacol Exp Ther 1988;246:765–71.

28. Adnani MSA. Concomitant immunohistochemistry localization of fibronectin and collagen in schistosome granulomata. J Pathol 1985;147:77–85.

29. Faffe DS, Silva GH, Kurtz PM, et al. Lung tissue mechanics and extracellular matrix composition in a murine model of silicosis. J Applied Physiol 2001;90:1400–6.

30. Kinsella MB, Smith EA, Miller KS, et al. Spontaneous production of fibronectin by alveolar macrophages in patients with scleroderma. Arthritis Rheum 1989;32:577–83.

31. Perez T, Farre JM, Gosset P, et al. Subclinical alveolar inflammation in rheumatoid arthritis: superoxide anion, neutrophil chemotactic activity, and fibronectin generation by alveolar macrophages. Eur Respir J 1989;2:7–13.

32. Begin R, Mertel M, Desmarais Y, et al. Fibronectin and procollagen 3 levels in bronchoalveolar lavage of asbestos-exposed human subjects and sheep. Chest 1986;89:237–43.

33. Rennard SI, Hunninghake GW, Bitterman PB, Crystal RG. Production of fibronectin by the human alveolar macrophage: mechanism for the recruitment of fibroblasts to sites of tissue injury in interstitial lung diseases. Proc Natl Acad Sci U S A 1981;78:7147–51.

34. Davies R, Erdogdn G. Secretion of fibronectin by mineral dust-derived alveolar macrophages and activated peritoneal macrophages. Exp Lung Res 1989;15:285–7.

35. Berghem L, Hansson M, Lundborg M, Camner P. Fibronectin concentrations in lung lavage fluid after inhalation exposure to low levels of metals. Environ Res 1987;43:179–85.

36. Kradin RL, Zhu Y, Hales CA, et al. Response of pulmonary macrophages to hyperoxic pulmonary injury. Acquisition of surface fibronectin and fibrin/ogen and enhanced expression of a fibronectin receptor. Am J Pathol 1986;125:349–57.

37. Saba TM, Jaffe E. Plasma fibronectin (opsonic glycoprotein): its synthesis by vascular endothelial cells and role in cardiopulmonary integrity after trauma as related to reticuloendothelial function. Am J Med 1980;68:577–94.

38. Sage H, Farin FM, Striker GE, Fisher AB. Granular pneumocytes in primary culture secrete several major components of the extracellular matrix. Biochemistry 1983;22:2148–55.

39. Shoji S, Rickard KA, Ertl RF, et al. Bronchial epithelial cells produce lung fibroblast chemotactic factor: fibronectin. Am J Respir Cell Mol Biol 1989;1:13–20.

40. Roman J, LaChance RM, Broekelmann TJ, et al. The fibronectin receptor is organized by extracellular matrix fibronectin: implications for oncogenic transformation and for cell recognition of fibronectin matrices. J Cell Biol 1989;108:2529–43.

41. Zhang K, Gharaee-Kermani M, McGarry B, Phan SH. In situ hybridization analysis of rat lung alpha 1 (I) and alpha 2 (I) collagen gene expression in pulmonary fibrosis induced by endotracheal bleomycin injection. Lab Invest 1994;70:192–202.

42. Broekelmann TJ, Limper AH, Colby TV, McDonald JA. Transforming growth factor β1 is present at sites of extra-

cellular matrix gene expression in human pulmonary fibrosis. Proc Natl Acad Sci U S A 1991;88:6642–6.

43. McDonald JA, Broekelmann TJ, Matheke ML, et al. A monoclonal antibody to the carboxyterminal domain of procollagen type I visualizes collagen-synthesizing fibroblast detection of an altered fibroblast phenotype in lungs of patients with pulmonary fibrosis. J Clin Invest 1986;78:1237–44.

44. Bitterman PB, Rennard SI, Hunninghake GW, Crystal RG. Human alveolar macrophage growth factor for fibroblasts: regulation and partial characterization. J Clin Invest 1982;70:806–22.

45. Bitterman PB, Rennard S, Adelberg S, Crystal RG. Role of fibronectin in fibrotic lung disease: a growth factor for human lung fibroblasts. Chest 1983;83:96S.

46. Jordana M, Newhouse MT, Gauldie J. Alveolar macrophage/peripheral blood monocyte-derived factors modulate proliferation of primary lines of human lung fibroblasts. J Leukoc Biol 1987;42:51–60.

47. Roberts CJ, Birkenmeier TM, McQuillan JJ, et al. Transforming growth factor-β stimulates the expression of fibronectin and of both subunits of the human fibronectin receptor by cultured human lung fibroblasts. J Biol Chem 1988;263:4586–92.

48. Kuhn C, McDonald JA. The roles of the myofibroblast in idiopathic pulmonary fibrosis. Am J Pathol 1991;138:1257–65.

49. Mitchell J, Woodcock-Mitchell J, Reynolds S, et al. Alpha-smooth muscle actin in parenchymal cells of bleomycin-injured rat lung. Lab Invest 1989;60:643–50.

50. Zhang K, Rekhter MD, Gordon D, Phan SH. Myofibroblasts and their role in lung collagen gene expression during pulmonary fibrosis: a combined immunohistochemical and in situ hybridization study. Am J Pathol 1994;145:114–25.

51. Phan SH. Role of the myofibroblast in pulmonary fibrosis. Kidney Int 1996;49:S46–8.

52. Bensadoun ES, Burke AK, Hogg JC, Roberts CR. Proteoglycan deposition in pulmonary fibrosis. Am J Respir Crit Care Med 1996;154:1819–28.

53. Majno G, Gabbiani G, Hirschel BJ, et al. Contraction of granulation tissue in vitro: similarity to smooth muscle. Science 1971;173:548–50.

54. Roy SG, Nozaki Y, Phan SH. Regulation of alpha-smooth muscle actin gene expression in myofibroblast differentiation from rat lung fibroblasts. Int J Biochem Cell Biol 2001:723–34.

55. Hashimoto S, Gon Y, Takeshita I, et al. Transforming growth factor-beta1 induces phenotypic modulation of human lung fibroblasts to myofibroblast through a c-Jun-NH$_2$-terminal kinase-dependent pathway. Am J Respir Crit Care Med 2001;163:152–7.

56. Desmouliere A, Geinoz A, Gabbiani F, Gabbiani G. Transforming growth factor-β1 induces α-smooth muscle actin expression in granulation tissue myofibroblasts and in quiescent and growing cultured fibroblasts. J Cell Biol 1993;122:103–11.

57. Labat ML, Bringuier AF, Seebold C, et al. Monocytic origin of fibroblasts: spontaneous transformation of blood monocytes into neo-fibroblastic structures in osteomyelosclerosis and Engelmann's disease. Biomed Pharmacother 1991;45:289–99.

58. Bringuier AF, Seebold-Choqueux C, Moricard Y, et al. T-lymphocytes control of HLA-DR monocytes, involving not only collagen but also uromodulin, amyloid-beta peptide, alpha-fetoprotein and carcinoembryonic antigen. Biomed Pharmacother 1992;46:91–108.

59. Jordana M, Schulma J, MeSharry C, et al. Heterogeneous proliferative characteristics of human adult lung fibroblast lines and clonally derived fibroblasts from control and fibrotic tissue. Am Rev Respir Dis 1988;137:579–84.

60. Raghu G, Chen Y, Rush V, Rabinovitch PS. Differential proliferation of fibroblasts cultured from normal and fibrotic human lungs. Am Rev Respir Dis 1988;138:703–8.

61. Mio T, Nagai S, Kitaichi M, et al. Proliferative characteristics of fibroblast lines derived from open lung biopsy specimens of patients with IPF (UIP). Chest 1992;102:832–7.

62. Fries KM, Blieden T, Looney RJ, et al. Evidence of fibroblast heterogeneity and the role of fibroblast subpopulations in fibrosis. Clin Immunol Immunopathol 1994;72:283–92.

63. Lasky JA, Brody AR. Interstitial fibrosis and growth factors. Environ Health Perspect 2000;108:751–62.

64. Zhang Y, Lee TC, Guillemin B, et al. Enhanced IL-1 beta and tumor necrosis factor-alpha release and messenger RNA expression in macrophages from idiopathic pulmonary fibrosis or after asbestos exposure. J Immunol 1993;150:4188–96.

65. Piguet PF, Collart MA, Grau GE, et al. Tumor necrosis factor/cachectin plays a key role in bleomycin-induced pneumopathy and fibrosis. J Exp Med 1989;170:655–63.

66. Piguet PF, Collart MA, Grau GE, et al. Requirement for tumour necrosis factor for development of silica-induced pulmonary fibrosis. Nature 1990;344:245–7.

67. Keane MP, Belperio JA, Burdick MD, Strieter RM. IL-12 attenuates bleomycin-induced pulmonary fibrosis. Am J Physiol 2001;281:L92–7.

68. Berkman N, Kremer S, Or R, et al. Human recombinant interferon-alpha2a and interferon-alpha A/D have different effects on bleomycin-induced lung injury. Respiration 2001;68:169–77.

69. Takahashi F, Takahashi K, Okazaki T, et al. Role of osteopontin in the pathogenesis of bleomycin-induced pulmonary fibrosis. Am J Respir Crit Care Med 2001;24:264–71.

70. Chen ES, Greenlee BM, Wills-Karp M, Moller DR. Attenuation of lung inflammation and fibrosis in interferon-gamma-deficient mice after intratracheal bleomycin. Am J Respir Crit Care Med 2001;24:545–55.

71. Romberger DJ, Beckmann JD, Claassen L, et al. Modulation of fibronectin production of bovine bronchial epithelial cells by transforming growth factor-β. Am J Respir Cell Mol Biol 1992;7:149–55.

72. Maniscalco WM, Campbell MH. Transforming growth factor-beta induces a chondroitin sulfate/dermatan sulfate proteoglycan in alveolar type II cells. Am J Physiol 1994;266:L672–80.

73. Khalil N, Bereznay O, Sporn M, Greenberg A. Macrophage production of transforming growth factor-ß and fibroblast collagen synthesis in chronic pulmonary inflammation. J Exp Med 1989;170:727–37.

74. Assoian RK, Fleurdelys BE, Stevenson HC, et al. Expression and secretion of type β transforming growth factor by activated human macrophages. Proc Natl Acad Sci U S A 1987;84:6020–4.

75. Zhao Y. Transforming growth factor-beta (TGF-beta) type I and type II receptors are both required for TGF-beta-mediated extracellular matrix production in lung fibroblasts. Mol Cell Endocrinol 1999;150:91–7.

76. Munger JS, Huang X, Kawakatsu H, et al. The integrin alpha v beta 6 binds and activates latent TGF beta 1: a mechanism for regulating pulmonary inflammation and fibrosis. Cell 1999;96:319–28.

77. Grande JP. Role of transforming growth factor-β in tissue injury and repair. Proc Soc Exp Biol Med 1997;214:27–40.

78. Eickelberg O, Kohler E, Reichenberger F, Bertschin S, et al. Extracellular matrix deposition by primary human lung fibroblasts in response to TGF-beta1 and TGF-beta3. Am J Physiol 1999;276:L814–24.

79. Santana A, Saxena B, Noble NA, et al. Increased expression of transforming growth factor-β isoforms (β1, β2, β3) in bleomycin-induced pulmonary fibrosis. Am J Respir Cell Mol Biol 1995;13:34–44.

80. Finkelstein JN, Johnston CJ, Baggs R, Rubin P. Early alterations in extracellular matrix and transforming growth factor-beta

gene expression in mouse lung indicative of late radiation fibrosis. Int J Radiat Oncol Biol Phys 1994;28:621–31.

81. Williams AO, Flanders KC, Saffiotti U. Immunohistochemical localization of transforming growth factor-beta 1 in rats with experimental silicosis, alveolar type II hyperplasia, and lung cancer. Am J Pathol 1993;142:1831–40.

82. Border WA, Okuda S, Languino LR, et al. Suppression of experimental glomerulonephritis by antiserum against transforming growth factor-β1. Nature 1992;346:371–4.

83. Giri SN, Hyde DM, Hollinger MA. Effect of antibody to transforming growth factor-beta on bleomycin induced accumulation of lung collagen in mice. Thorax 1993;48:959–66.

84. Khalil N, O'Connor RN, Unruh HW, et al. Increased production and immunohistochemical localization of transforming growth factor-β in idiopathic pulmonary fibrosis. Am J Respir Cell Mol Biol 1991;5:155–62.

85. Khalil N, O'Connor RN, Flanders KC, Unruh H. TGB-beta 1, but not TGF-beta 2 or TGF-beta 3, is differentially present in epithelial cells of advanced pulmonary fibrosis: an immunohistochemical study. Am J Respir Cell Mol Biol 1996;14:131–8.

86. Asakura S, Colby TV, Limper AH. Tissue localization of transforming growth factor-beta 1 in pulmonary eosinophilic granuloma. Am J Respir Crit Care Med 1996;154:1525–30.

87. Limper AH, Colby TV, Sanders MS, et al. Immunohistochemical localization of transforming growth factor-β in the nonnecrotizing granulomas of pulmonary sarcoidosis. Am J Respir Crit Care Med 1994;149:197–204.

88. Pittet JF, Griffiths MJ, Geiser T, et al. TGF-β is a critical mediator of acute lung injury. J Clin Invest 2001;107:1537–44.

89. Peters JH, Ginsberg MH, Bohl BP, et al. Intravascular release of intact cellular fibronectin during oxidant-induced injury of the in vitro perfused rabbit lung. J Clin Invest 1986;78:1596–603.

90. Holguin F, Moss I, Brown LA, Guidot DM. Chronic ethanol ingestion impairs alveolar type II cell glutathione homeostasis and function and predisposes to endotoxin-mediated acute edematous lung injury in rats. J Clin Invest 1998;101:761–8.

91. Frazier K, Williams S, Kothapalli D, et al. Stimulation of fibroblast cell growth, matrix production, and granulation tissue formation by connective tissue growth factor. J Invest Dermatol 1996;107:404–11.

92. Gharaee-Kermani M, Denholm EM, Phan SH. Costimulation of fibroblast collagen and transforming growth factor-beta gene expression by monocyte chemoattractant protein-1 via specific receptors. J Biol Chem 1996;271:17779–84.

93. Ritzenthaler JD, Goldstein RH, Fine A, Smith SD. Regulation of the alpha 1(I) collagen promoter via a transforming growth factor-beta activation element. J Biol Chem 1993;268:13625–31.

94. Dean DC. Expression of the fibronectin gene. Am J Respir Cell Mol Biol 1989;1:5–10.

95. Roman J, Ritzenthaler JD, Fenton M. Transcriptional regulation of the human IL-1β gene by fibronectin: role of protein kinase C and AP-1. Cytokine 2000;12:1581–96.

96. Force T, Bonventre JV. Growth factors and MAP kinases. Hypertension 1998;31:152–61.

97. Manie S, Schmid-Alliana A, Kubar J, et al. Disruption of microtubule network in human monocytes induces expression of interleukin-1 but not that of interleukin-6 nor tumor necrosis factor-α. J Biol Chem 1993;268:13675–81.

98. Sheppard D. In vivo functions of integrins: lessons from null mutations in mice. Matrix Biology 2000;19:203–9.

99. Yan JT, Hynes RO. Fibronectin receptor functions in embryonic cells deficient in α5β1 integrin can be replaced by αv integrins. Mol Biol Cell 1996;7:1737–48.

100. Clark RAF, Lanigan JM, DellaPelle P, et al. Fibronectin and fibrin provide a provisional matrix for epidermal cell migration during wound reepithelialization. J Invest Dermatol 1982;79:264–9.

101. Parekh T, Saxena B, Reibman J, et al. Neutrophil chemotaxis in response to TGF-beta isoforms (TGF-beta 1, TGF-beta 2, TGF-beta 3) is mediated by fibronectin. J Immunol 1994;152:2456–66.

102. Clark RAF, Wikner NE, Doherty DE, Norris DA. Cryptic chemotactic activity of fibronectin for human monocytes resides in the 120-kDa fibroblastic cell-binding fragment. J Biol Chem 1988;263:12115–23.

103. Denholm EM, Wolber FM, Phan SH. Secretion of monocyte chemotactic activity by alveolar macrophages. Am J Pathol 1989;135:571–80.

104. Bowersox JC, Sorgente N. Chemotaxis of aortic endothelial cells in response to fibronectin. Cancer Res 1982;42:2547–51.

105. Postlethwaite AE, Kang AH. Collagen- and collagen-peptide-induced chemotaxis of human blood monocytes. J Exp Med 1976;143:1299–307.

106. Postlethwaite AE, Keski-Oja J, Balian G. Induction of fibroblast chemotaxis by fibronectin. J Exp Med 1981;153:494–9.

107. Laskin DL, Soltys RA, Berg RA, Riley DJ. Activation of alveolar macrophages by native and synthetic collagen-like polypeptides. Am J Respir Cell Mol Biol 1994;10:58–64.

108. Akiyama SK, Yamada SS, Chen WY, Yamada KM. Analysis of fibronectin receptor function with monoclonal antibodies: roles in cell adhesion, migration, matrix assembly, and cytoskeletal organization. J Cell Biol 1989;109:863–75.

109. Bitterman PD, Rennard SI, Adelberg S, Crystal RG. Role of fibronectin as a growth factor for fibroblasts. J Cell Biol 1983;97:1925–32.

110. Roy F, DeBlois C, Doillon CJ. Extracellular matrix analogs as carriers for growth factors: in vitro fibroblast behavior. J Biomed Mater Res 1993;27:389–97.

111. End P, Engel J. Multidomain proteins of the extracellular matrix and cellular growth. In: McDonald JA, Mecham RP, editors. Receptors for extracellular matrices. San Diego: Academic Press; 1991. p. 79–129.

112. Vachon PH, Simoneau A, Herring-Gillam FE, Beaulieu JF. Cellular fibronectin expression is down-regulated at the mRNA level in differentiating human intestinal epithelial cells. Exp Cell Res 1995;216:30–4.

113. Cardarelli PM, Pierschbache MD. T-lymphocyte differentiation and the extracellular matrix: identification of a thymocyte subset that attaches specifically to fibronectin. Proc Natl Acad Sci U S A 1986;83:2647–51.

114. Prieto J, Eklund A, Patarroyo M. Regulated expression of integrins and other adhesion molecules during differentiation of monocytes into macrophages. Cell Immunol 1994;156:191–211.

115. Ferreira OC, Valinsky JE, Sheridan K, et al. Phorbol ester-induced differentiation of U937 cells enhances attachment to fibronectin and distinctly modulates the α5β1 and α4β1 fibronectin receptors. Exp Cell Res 1991;193:20–6.

116. Ruoslahti E, Reed JC. Anchorage dependence, integrins and apoptosis. Cell 1994;77:477–8.

117. Boudreau N, Sympson CJ, Werb Z, Bissell MB. Supression of ICE and apoptosis in mammary epithelial cells by extracellular matrix. Science 1995;267:891–3.

118. Polunovsky VA, Chen B, Henke C, et al. Role of mesenchymal cell death in lung remodeling after injury. J Clin Invest 1993;92:388–97.

119. Gudewicz PW, Frewin MB, Heinel LA, Minnear FL. Priming of human monocyte superoxide production and arachidonic acid metabolism by adherence to collagen- and basement membrane-coated surfaces. J Leukoc Biol 1994;55:423–9.

120. Pacifici R, Basilico C, Roman J, et al. Collagen-induced release of interleukin-1 from human blood mononuclear cells. Potentiation by fibronectin binding to the α5β1 integrin. J Clin Invest 1992;89:61–7.

121. Graves KL, Roman J. Fibronectin modulates the expression of

interleukin-1β and its receptor antagonist in human mononuclear cells. Am J Physiol 1996;271:L61–9.

122. Perez RL, Roman J. Fibrin matrices enhance the expression of interleukin-1β by human peripheral blood mononuclear cells. Implications for lung granulomatous inflammation. J Immunol 1995;154:1879–87.

123. Chang ZL, Beezhold DH, Personius CD, Shen ZL. Fibronectin cell-binding domain triggered transmembrane signal transduction in human monocytes. J Leukoc Biol 1993;53:79–85.

124. Xing Z, Jordana M, Gauldie J. IL-1 beta and IL-6 gene expression in alveolar macrophages: modulation by extracellular matrices. Am J Physiol 1992;262:L600–5.

125. Arend WP. Interleukin-1 receptor antagonist: a new member of the interleukin family. J Clin Invest 1991;88:1445–51.

126. Juliano RL, Haskill S. Signal transduction from the extracellular matrix. J Cell Biol 1993;120:577–85.

127. Chapman HA, Allen CL, Stone OL. Abnormalities in pathways of alveolar fibrin turnover among patients with interstitial lung disease. Am Rev Respir Dis 1986;133:437–43.

128. Bertozzi P, Astedt B, Zenzius L, et al. Depressed bronchoalveolar urokinase activity in patients with adult respiratory distress syndrome. N Engl J Med 1990;322:890–7.

129. Idell S, Kumar A, Koenig KB, Coalson JJ. Pathways of fibrin turnover in lavage of premature baboons with hyperoxic lung injury. Am J Respir Crit Care Med 1994;149:767–75.

130. Idell S, Peterson BT, Gonzalez K, et al. Local abnormalities of coagulation and fibrinolysis and alveolar fibrin deposition in sheep with oleic acid-induced lung injury. Am Rev Respir Dis 1988;138:1282–94.

131. Kalifat SR, Bouteille M, Delarue J. Changes in connective tissue in sarcoid granuloma: hyalin, paraamyloid, and fibrinoid. Electron microscopic study of 11 cases. Virchows Arch 1969;3:348–58.

132. Idell S, Gonzalez K, Bradford H, et al. Procoagulant activity in bronchoalveolar lavage in the adult respiratory distress syndrome. Contribution of tissue factor associated with factor VII. Am Rev Respir Dis 1987;136:1466–74.

133. Idell S, Gonzalez K, MacArthur CK, et al. Bronchoalveolar lavage procoagulant activity in bleomycin-induced lung injury in marmosets. Characterization and relationship to fibrin deposition and fibrosis. Am Rev Respir Dis 1987;136:124–33.

134. Hasday JD, Bachwich PR, Lynch JP, Sitrin RG. Procoagulant and plasminogen activator activities of bronchoalveolar fluid in patients with pulmonary sarcoidosis. Exp Lung Res 1988;14:261–78.

135. Nakstad B, Lyberg T, Skjonsberg OH, Boye NP. Local activation of the coagulation and fibrinolysis systems in lung disease. Thromb Res 1990;57:827–38.

136. Perez RL, Duncan A, Hunter RL, Staton GW. Elevated D dimer in the lungs and blood of patients with sarcoidosis. Chest 1993;103:1100–6.

137. Perez RL, Roman J, Staton GW, Hunter RL. Extravascular coagulation and fibrinolysis in murine lung granulomatous inflammation induced by the mycobacterial cord factor trehalose-6,6'-dimycolate. Am J Respir Crit Care Med 1992;149:510–8.

138. Olman MA, Mackman N, Gladson CL, et al. Changes in procoagulant and fibrinolytic gene expression during bleomycin-induced lung injury in the mouse. J Clin Invest 1995;96:1621–30.

139. Eltzman DT, McCoy RD, Zheng X, et al. Bleomycin-induced pulmonary fibrosis in transgenic mice that either lack or overexpress the murine plasminogen activator inhibitor-1 gene. J Clin Invest 1996;97:232–7.

140. Lyberg T, Nakstad B, Hetland O, Boye NP. Procoagulant (thromboplastin) activity in human bronchoalveolar lavage fluids is derived from alveolar macrophages. Eur Respir J 1990;3:61–7.

141. Fan S-T, Mackman N, Cui M-Z, Edgington TS. Integrin regulation of an inflammatory effector gene. Direct induction

of the tissue factor promoter by engagement of β1 or α4 integrin chains. J Immunol 1995;154:3266–74.

142. Ciano PS, Colvin RB, Dvorak AM, et al. Macrophage migration in fibrin gel matrices. Lab Invest 1986;54:62–70.

143. Fukuda V, Ferrans VJ, Schoenberger CI, et al. Patterns of pulmonary structural remodeling after experimental paraquat toxicity: the morphogenesis of intraalveolar fibrosis. Am J Pathol 1985;118:452–75.

144. Eitzman DT, McCoy RD, Zheng X, et al. Bleomycin-induced pulmonary fibrosis in transgenic mice that either lack or overexpress the murine plasminogen activator inhibitor-1 gene. J Clin Invest 1996;97:232–7.

145. Kolb M, Margetts PJ, Galt T, et al. Transient transgene expression of decorin in the lung reduces the fibrotic response to bleomycin. Am J Respir Crit Care Med 2001;163:770–7.

146. Limper AH, Roman J. Fibronectin: a versatile matrix protein with roles in pulmonary development, repair, and infection. Chest 1992;101:1663–73.

147. Ingber DE, Folkman J. Mechanochemical switching between growth and differentiation during fibroblasts growth factor-stimulated angiogenesis in vitro: role of extracellular matrix. J Cell Biol 1989;109:317–30.

148. Resnikoff M, Brien T, Vincent PA, et al. Lung matrix incorporation of plasma fibronectin reduces vascular permeability in postsurgical bacteremia. Am J Physiol 1999;277:L749–59.

149. Albelda SM, Smith CW, Ward PA. Adhesion molecules and inflammatory injury. FASEB J 1994;8:504–12.

150. Hynes RO. Integrins: versatility, modulation, and signaling in cell adhesion. Cell 1992;69:11–25.

151. Giancotti FG, Ruoslahti E. Integrin signaling. Science 1999;285:1028–32.

152. Burridge K, Faith K, Kelly T, et al. Focal adhesions: transmembrane junctions between the extracellular matrix and the cytoskeleton. Ann Rev Cell Biol 1988;4:487–525.

153. McDonald JA. Extracellular matrix effects on cell shape and gene expression. Curr Opin Cell Biol 1989;1:995–9.

154. Werb Z, Tremble PM, Behrendtsen O, et al. Signal transduction through the fibronectin receptor induces collagenase and stromelysin gene expression. J Cell Biol 1989;109:877–89.

155. Clark EA, Brugge JS. Integrins and signal transduction: the road taken. Science 1995;268:233–9.

156. Lee B, Park R, Choi J, et al. Stimulation of fibronectin synthesis through protein kinase C signaling pathway in normal and transformed human lung fibroblasts. Biochem Mol Biol Int 1996;39:895–904.

157. Roman J, Ritzenthaler J, Perez RL, Roser S. Differential modes of regulation of interleukin-1β expression by extracellular matrices. Immunology 1999;98:228–37.

158. Ritzenthaler JD, Roman J. Interleukin-1β gene transcription in U937 cells is modulated by type I collagen and cytoskeletal integrity via distinct signaling pathways. J Interferon Cytokine Res 2000;21:105–16.

159. Quinlan KL, Naik SM, Cannon G, et al. Substance P activates coincident NF-AT- and NF-kappa B-dependent adhesion molecule gene expression in microvascular endothelial cells through intracellular calcium mobilization. J Immunol 1999;163:5656–65.

160. Piguet PF, Rosen H, Vesin C, Grau GE. Effective treatment of the pulmonary fibrosis elicited in mice by bleomycin or silica with anti-CD/11 antibodies. Am Rev Respir Dis 1993;147:435–41.

161. Piguet PF, Tacchini-Cottier F, Vesin C. Administration of anti-TNF-α or anti-CD11a antibodies to normal adult mice decreases lung and bone collagen content: evidence for an effect of platelet consumption. Am J Respir Cell Mol Biol 1995;12:227–31.

162. Murphy G, Docherty AJP. The matrix metalloproteinases and their inhibitors. Am J Respir Cell Mol Biol 1992;7:120–5.

163. Nagase H, Woessner JF. Matrix metalloproteinases. J Biol Chem 1999;274:21491–4.

164. Delacourt C, Bourgeois ML, D'Ortho MP, et al. Imbalance between 95 kDa type IV collagenase and tissue inhibitor of metalloproteinases in sputum of patients with cystic fibrosis. Am J Respir Crit Care Med 1995;152:765–74.

165. Sepper R, Konttinen YT, Sorsa T, Koski H. Gelatinolytic and type IV collagenolytic activity in bronchiectasis. Chest 1994;106:1129–33.

166. Suga M, Iyonaga K, Okamoto T, et al. Characteristic elevation of matrix metalloproteinase activity in idiopathic interstitial pneumonias. Am J Respir Crit Care Med 2000;162:1949–56.

167. Montano M, Ramos C, Gonzalez G, et al. Lung collagenase inhibitors and spontaneous and latent collagenase activity in idiopathic pulmonary fibrosis and hypersensitivity pneumonitis. Chest 1988;106:1115–9.

168. Ricou B, Nicod L, Lacraz S, et al. Matrix metalloproteinases and TIMP in acute respiratory distress syndrome. Am J Respir Crit Care Med 1996;154:346–52.

169. O'Connor CM, Power C, Vanbreda A, et al. Fibronectin and collagenase in bronchoalveolar lavage (BAL) fluid from patients with sarcoidosis. Thorax 1986;41:230–1.

170. Roman J, Silverboard H, Perez RL, Aguayo SM. Gelatinolytic activity in the BAL fluid of patients with sarcoidosis. Chest 2001;120:43S.

171. Devaskar UP, Taylor W, Govindrajan R, et al. Hyperoxia induces interstitial (type I) and increases type IV collagenase mRNA expression and increases type I and IV collagenolytic activity in newborn rat lung. Biol Neonate 1994;66:76–85.

172. D'Ortho MP, Jarreau PH, Delacourt C, et al. Matrix metalloproteinase and elastase activities in LPS-induced lung injury in guinea pigs. Am J Physiol 1994;266:L209–16.

173. Pardo A, Selman M, Ridge K, et al. Increased expression of gelatinases and collagenases in rat lungs exposed to 100% oxygen. Am J Respir Crit Care Med 1996;154:1067–75.

174. Rivera-Marrero C, Schuyler W, Roman J. Induction of MMP-9 mediated gelatinolytic activity in human monocytic cells by cell wall components of *M. tuberculosis*. Microbial Pathogenesis 2000;29:231–44.

175. Emonard H, Takiya C, Dreze S, et al. Interstitial collagenase (MMP-1), gelatinase (MMP-2) and stromelysin (MMP-3) released by human fibroblasts cultured on acellular sarcoid granulomas (sarcoid matrix complex, SMC). Matrix Biol 1989;9:382–8.

176. Mizel SB, Dayer JM, Krane SM, Mergenhagen SE. Stimulation of rheumatoid synovial cell collagenase and prostaglandin production by partially purified lymphocyte-activating factor (interleukin-1). Proc Natl Acad Sci U S A 1981;78:2474–7.

177. Saus J, Quinones S, Otani Y, et al. The complete primary structure of human matrix metalloproteinases-3. Identity with stromelysin. J Biol Chem 1988;263:6742–5.

178. Dayer JM, Beutler B, Cerami A. Cachectin/tumor necrosis factor stimulates collagenase and prostaglandin E2 production by human synovial cells and dermal fibroblasts. J Exp Med 1985;162:2163–8.

179. Biswas C, Dayer JM. Stimulation of collagenase production by collagen in mammalian cell cultures. Cell 1979;18:1035–41.

180. Langholz O, Rockel D, Mauch C, et al. Collagen and collagenase gene expression in three-dimensional collagen lattices are differentially regulated by alpha 1 beta 1 and alpha 2 beta 1 integrins. J Cell Biol 1995;131:1903–15.

181. Ledwozyw A, Borowicz B. The influence of normobaric hyperoxia on hydroxyproline content and collagenase and elastase activities in rat lung. Arch Vet Pol 1993;33:117–22.

182. Montano M, Ramos C, Pardo A, Selman M. Comparison between lung parenchyma and bronchoalveolar lavage collagenolytic activity. Lung 1993;171:87–93.

183. Pardo A, Selman M, Ramirez R, et al. Production of collagenase and tissue inhibitor of metalloproteinases by fibro-

184. Ledwozyw A, Rucinski T, Synowiec R. The influence of endotracheally administered bleomycin on hydroxyproline content and collagenase and elastase activity in rat lungs. Arch Vet Pol 1992;32:49–55.

185. D'Armiento J, Dalal SS, Okada Y, et al. Collagenase expression of the lungs of transgenic mice causes pulmonary emphysema. Cell 1992;71:955–61.

186. Corbel M, Caulet-Maugendre S, Germain N, et al. Inhibition of bleomycin-induced pulmonary fibrosis in mice by the matrix metalloproteinase inhibitor batimastat. J Pathol 2001;193:538–45.

187. Hattori N, Degen JL, Sisson TH, et al. Bleomycin-induced pulmonary fibrosis in fibrinogen-null mice. J Clin Invest 2000;106:1441–3.

188. Yasui H, Gabazza EC, Tamaki S, et al. Intratracheal administration of activated protein C inhibits bleomycin-induced lung fibrosis in the mouse. Am J Respir Crit Care Med 2001;163:1660–8.

189. Polednak AP. Connective tissue responses in Blacks in relation to disease: further observations. Am J Phys Anthropol 1987;74:357–71.

190. Bienkowski RS, Gotkin MG. Control of collagen deposition in mammalian lung. Proc Soc Exp Biol Med 1995;209:118–40.

191. Rennard SI, Bitterman PB, Ozaki T, et al. Colchicine suppresses the release of fibroblast growth factors for alveolar macrophages *in vitro*. Am Rev Respir Dis 1988;137:181–5.

192. Ehrlich HP, Bornstein P. Microtubules in transcellular movement of procollagen. Nature 1972;238:257–60.

193. Douglas WW, Ryu JH, Bjoraker JA, et al. Colchicine versus prednisone as treatment of usual interstitial pneumonia. Mayo Clin Proc 1997;72:201–9.

194. Hunninghake GW, Kalica AR. Approaches to the treatment of pulmonary fibrosis. Am J Respir Crit Care Med 1995;151:915–8.

195. Unemori EN, Amento EP. Relaxin modulates synthesis and secretion of procollagenase and collagen by human dermal fibroblasts. J Biol Chem 1990;265:10681–5.

196. Unemori EN, Pickford LB, Salles AL, et al. Relaxin induces an extracellular matrix-degrading phenotype in human lung fibroblasts in vitro and inhibits lung fibrosis in a murine model in vivo. J Clin Invest 1996;98:2739–45.

197. Peters JH, Maunder RJ, Woolf AD, et al. Elevated plasma levels of ED1+ (cellular)fibronectin in patients with vascular injury. J Lab Clin Med 1989;113:586–97.

198. Teschler H, Thompson AB, Pohl WR, et al. Bronchoalveolar lavage procollagen-III-peptide in recent onset hypersensitivity pneumonitis: correlation with extracellular matrix components. Eur Respir J 1993;6:709–14.

199. Teschler H, Pohl WR, Thompson AB, et al. Elevated levels of bronchoalveolar lavage vitronectin in hypersensitivity pneumonitis. Am Rev Respir Dis 1993;147:332–7.

200. Vincent PA, Rebres RA, Lewis EP, et al. Release of ED1 fibronectin from matrix of perfused lungs after vascular injury is independent of protein synthesis. Am J Physiol 1993;265:L485–92.

201. McDonald JA. Extracellular matrix assembly. Methods Enzymol 1994;245:518–31.

202. Gupta SK, Reinhart PG, Bhalla DK. Enhancement of fibronectin expression in rat lung by ozone and an inflammatory stimulus. Am J Physiol 1998;275:L330–5.

203. Berg JT, FU X, Breen EC, et al. High lung inflation increases mRNA levels of ECM components and growth factors in lung parenchyma. J Appl Physiol 1997;83:120–8.

204. Berg JT, Breen EC, Fu Z, et al. Alveolar hypoxia increases gene expression of extracellular matrix proteins and platelet-derived growth factor-B in lung parenchyma. Am J Respir Crit Care Med 1998;158:1920–8.

205. Kazuyoski K, Bosken CH, Pare PD, et al. Small airway dimen-

blasts derived from normal and fibrotic human lungs. Chest 1992;102:1085–9.

sions in asthma and chronic obstructive pulmonary disease. Am Rev Respir Dis 1983;148:1220–5.

206. Roche WR, Beasley R, Williams J, Holgate ST. Subepithelial fibrosis in the bronchi of asthmatics. Lancet 1989;i:520–4.

207. Brewster CEP, Howarth PG, Djukanovic R, et al. Myofibroblasts and subepithelial fibrosis in bronchial asthma. Am Rev Respir Cell Mol Biol 1990;3:507–11.

208. Snow RL, Davies P, Pontoppidan H, et al. Pulmonary vascular remodeling in adult respiratory distress syndrome. Am Rev Respir Dis 1982;126:887–92.

209. Hallgren R, Samuelsson T, Laurent TC, Modig J. Accumulation of hyaluronan in the lung in adult respiratory distress syndrome. Am J Respir Dis 1989;139:682–7.

210. Watts CL, Bruce MC. Effect of dexamethasone therapy on fibronectin and albumin levels in lung secretions of infants with bronchopulmonary dysplasia. J Pediatr 1992;121:597–607.

211. Watts CL, Fanaroff AA, Bruce MC. Elevation of fibronectin levels in lung secretions of infants with respiratory distress syndrome and development of bronchopulmonary dysplasia. J Pediatr 1992;120:614–20.

212. Rennard SI, Crystal RG. Fibronectin in human bronchopulmonary lavage fluid: evaluation in patients with interstitial lung disease. J Clin Invest 1982;69:113–22.

213. Kirk J, Heard BE, Kerr I, et al. Quantitation of types I and III collagen in biopsy lung samples from patients with cryptogenic fibrosing alveolitis. Coll Relat Res 1984;4:169–82.

214. Kuhn C, Mason RJ. Immunolocalization of SPARC, tenascin, and thrombospondin in pulmonary fibrosis. Am J Pathol 1995;147:1759–69.

215. Cordier JF, Loire R, Peyrol S. Bronchiolitis obliterans organizing pneumonia (BOOP). Characteristics and boundaries of an anatomo-clinical entity. Rev Mal Respir 1991;8:139–52.

216. Specks U, Nerlich A, Colby TV, et al. Increased expression of type VI collagen in lung fibrosis. Am J Respir Crit Care Med 1995;151:1956–64.

217. Bjermer L, Engstrom-Laurent A, Lundgren R, et al. Hyaluronate and type III procollagen peptide concentrations in bronchoalveolar lavage fluid as markers of disease activity in farmer's lung. BMJ 1987;295:803–6.

218. Perez-Arellano JL, Pedraz MJ, Fuertes A, et al. Laminin fragment P1 is increased in the lower respiratory tract of patients with diffuse interstitial lung diseases. Chest 1993;104:1163–9.

219. Sahu S, Lynn WS. Hyaluronic acid in the pulmonary secretions of patients with alveolar proteinosis. Inflammation 1978;3:149–58.

220. Nagy B, Katona E, Erdei J, et al. Fibronectin in bronchoalveolar lavage fluid and plasma from children with chronic inflammation of lungs. Acta Paediatr Scand 1988;77:727–33.

221. Valletta EA, Rigo A, Bonazzi L, et al. Modification of some markers of inflammation during treatment for acute respiratory exacerbation in cystic fibrosis. Acta Paediatr 1992;81:227–30.

222. Peyrol S, Takiya C, Cordier J-F, Grimaud J-A. Organization of the connective matrix of the sarcoid granuloma. Evolution and cell-matrix interactions. Ann N Y Acad Sci 1986;465:268–85.

223. Roman J, McDonald JA. Expression of fibronectin, the integrin VLA-5 and α-smooth muscle actin in lung and heart development. Am J Respir Cell Mol Biol 1992;6:472–80.

224. Limper AH, Broekelmann TJ, Colby TV, et al. Analysis of local mRNA expression for extracellular matrix proteins and growth factors using in situ hybridization in fibroproliferative lung disorders. Chest 1991;99:55S–56S.

225. Hallgren R, Eklund A, Engstrom-Laurent A, Schmekei B. Hyaluronate in bronchoalveolar lavage fluid: a new marker in sarcoidosis reflecting pulmonary disease. BMJ 1985;290:1778–81.

226. Dubaybo BA, Durr RA, Thet LA. Unilateral paraquat-induced lung fibrosis: evolution of changes in lung fibronectin and collagen after graded degrees of lung injury. J Toxicol Environ Health 1987;22:439–57.

227. Hernnas J, Nettelbladt O, Bjermer L, et al. Alveolar accumulation of fibronectin and hyaluronan precedes bleomycin-induced pulmonary fibrosis in the rat. Eur Respir J 1992;5:404–10.

228. Lucey EC, Ngo HQ, Agarwal A, et al. Differential expression of elastin and alpha 1 (I) collagen mRNA in mice with bleomycin-induced pulmonary fibrosis. Lab Invest 1996;74:12–20.

229. Swiderski RE, Dencoff JE, Floerchinger CS, et al. Differential expression of extracellular matrix remodeling genes in a murine model of bleomycin-induced pulmonary fibrosis. Am J Pathol 1998;152:821–8.

230. Lafuma C, Wegrowski J, Labat-Robert J, et al. Parallel increase of plasma fibronectin and perchlorosoluble serum glycoproteins in radiation-induced lung damage. Clin Physiol Biochem 1987;5:61–9.

231. Kobrle V, Mirejovska E, Holusa R, Hurych J. Changes in pulmonary connective tissue proteins after a single intratracheal instillation of cadmium chloride in the rat. Environ Res 1986;40:3–14.

232. Bowden DH, Adamson IY. Bronchiolar and alveolar lesions in the pathogenesis of crocidolite-induced pulmonary fibrosis in mice. J Pathol 1985;147:257–67.

233. Choi AM, Elbon CL, Bruce SA, et al. Messenger RNA levels of lung extracellular matrix proteins during ozone exposure. Lung 1994;172:15–30.

234. Paakko P, Anttila S, Sormunen R, et al. Biochemical and morphological characterization of carbon tetrachloride-induced lung fibrosis in rats. Arch Toxicol 1996;70:540–52.

235. Su WY, Kodavanti UP, Jaskot RH, et al. Temporal expression of cellular distribution of pulmonary fibronectin gene induction following exposure to an emission source particle. J Environ Pathol Toxicol Oncol 1995;14:215–25.

12

IMMUNOLOGIC EVENTS IN THE DEVELOPMENT OF INTERSTITIAL LUNG DISEASE: THE PARADIGM OF SARCOIDOSIS

GIANPIETRO SEMENZATO
CARLO AGOSTINI

Complex multistep processes have been claimed to interpret the large spectrum of events involved in inducing and maintaining inflammatory responses in the pulmonary microenvironment of patients with interstitial lung disease (ILD). During the 1980s, most research efforts were focused on the relevance of immunocompetent cells in the pathogenesis of ILD. Taking advantage of two- and three-color flow cytometry, pulmonary cells of patients with ILD were extensively investigated using a variety of monoclonal antibodies (mAbs), which provided information directly related to the differentiation and activation state of lung immune cells. In addition, mAbs recognizing relevant epitopes were successfully applied to cryostat and paraffin embedded lung tissue specimens to study the in situ distribution of T, B, and natural killer (NK) cell subsets at sites of pulmonary inflammation.

In the 1990s, understanding the role of cytokines in pulmonary immune responses, however, marked the beginning of a new era. Taking advantage of the cloning of cytokine genes, in situ hybridization methods and cytokine receptor characterization, it was possible to shed some light on the complex network of interactions between cells and biologic response modifiers that control the state of activation of the pulmonary immune system.[1-4] The definition of the importance of cytokine patterns in inflammation also had a powerful impact on the field of ILD. In fact, it is well established that the release of a cascade of interacting extracellular signaling proteins orchestrates the trafficking of immune cells during ILD. Through their binding to relevant receptors on neighboring cells, cytokines regulate the expression of adhesion molecules on the lung vascular endothelium within and around the site of inflammation. This in turn favors the entrance and activation of inflammatory effector cells and modulates local survival and proliferation of different types of immune cells (see Chapter 10). If the inciting antigen(s) that locally initiates the ILD is removed, the inflammatory response generally resolves. However, there are ILDs that are associated with the persistence of the etiologic agents and/or an imbalance of mechanisms for the removal of inflammatory cells and their by-products, ultimately leading to an ongoing inflammatory response. As a result, cytokines with proinflammatory, destructive biologic functions are locally produced; overall, these cytokines set the stage for the development of irreversible remodeling of the lung tissue, the evolution toward pulmonary granuloma formation, and, in some individuals, the development of fibrosis.

This chapter reviews the available knowledge concerning cell-to-cell communications leading to the early accumulation of immunoinflammatory cells at sites of ongoing inflammation during ILD. It will also provide a detailed description of cellular interactions that govern the dynamics of hypersensitivity granuloma and diffuse fibrosis in ILD. As a paradigm for our discussion we will focus on sarcoidosis (ie, the most frequently observed granulomatous ILD in which the immune processes have been most intensively studied).[5] Conceptually, sarcoidosis can be considered the archetype of immune granulomatous disorders, because there is good circumstantial evidence that several immunoregulatory mechanisms that are important in the development of sarcoid granuloma also modulate the pathogenetic events taking place in the interstitium and air spaces of other ILDs.[6-8]

The aim of this chapter is to provide readers with an overview of the biologic effects by which a granulomatous process is initiated, sustained, and clinically presented, with the ultimate hope of relating immunologic phenomena to a management rationale (Table 12–1). From a clinical point of view, we will comment on the

TABLE 12–1   A Summary of Immunologic Abnormalities Observed in Patients with Sarcoidosis

- Alveolar and interstitial accumulation of CD4+ cells showing a Th_1 cytokine profile. As a consequence, a marked increase of CD4/CD8 ratio in the lung and other involved tissues may be observed. A Th_1/Th_2 shift may occur in patients evolving toward fibrosis.
- B-cell hyperactivity and spontaneous in situ production of immunoglobulins
- Expansion of T cells bearing a restricted Vβ and Vα TCR repertoire in involved tissues. This pattern is consistent with a TCR oligoclonality. Expansion of the γδ TCR cell pool in the lung of a subset of patients
- Increased expression of members of TNF-ligand and TNF-receptor superfamilies by sarcoid T cells
- Increased spontaneous rate of proliferation of lung immunocompetent cells
- Accumulation of macrophages expressing a monocyte-like phenotype (CD14), increased levels of activation markers (HLA-DR, HLA-DQ, CD71) and adhesion molecules (CD49a, CD54, CD102)
- Increased antigen presenting cell capacity by alveolar macrophages
- Increased production of macrophage-derived cytokines (IL-1, IL-6, IL-8, IL-15, IL-18, TNF-α, and GM-CSF)
- Increased production of chemokines (CXCL10/IP-10, CCL2/MCP-1, CCL3/MIP-1α, CCL5/RANTES, and other chemokines), which favor the development of alveolitis and granuloma accretion
- Increased production of macrophage-derived fibrogenetic cytokines (TGF-β and related cytokines, PDGF, and IGF-I), favoring evolution toward fibrosis
- BAL neutrophilia, which correlates with IL-8/CXCL8 production in patients with fibrosis

Th_1 = T helper Type 1; TCR = T-cell receptor; TNF = tumor necrosis factor; IL = interleukin; GM-CSF = granulocyte-macrophage colony–stimuling factor; TGF = transforming growth factor; PDGF = growth factor; IGF = insulin-like growth factor.

role of the immunologic evaluations in the management of patients with sarcoidosis and how new and old immunosuppressants have their place in the setting of sarcoidosis, as a paradigm of ILD.

ANTIGENIC AND GENETIC FACTORS INVOLVED IN SARCOID INFLAMMATION

Morphologically, sarcoid granuloma represents a typical delayed-type hypersensitivity granuloma. The central core is made up of a number of monocyte/macrophages and epithelioid cells, which are derived from mononuclear phagocytes; it also contains giant multinucleated cells that derive from the aggregation of macrophage cells. Epithelioid cell foci are surrounded by a mantle of CD4+ T lymphocytes and, to a far lesser extent, B cells and plasma cells.

Granulomatous disorders may be due to a wide variety of etiologic agents. In the past, advances in molecular diagnostic techniques were responsible for the identification of microorganisms involved in granulomatous disorders that previously were of unknown etiology.[9] Furthermore, immunologic studies using a beryllium-induced delayed-type hypersensitivity model have contributed to the understanding that chronic exposure to an antigen (beryllium) may cause a granulomatous disorder.[10] Although the etiology of sarcoidosis is still unknown, the combination of the characteristic morphologic and immunohistologic aspects of the granuloma suggest that sarcoid granuloma is the result of an exaggerated immunologic response against an undefined antigen that has persisted at the sites of disease involvement, perhaps because of its low solubility and degradability.

Relationship Between Sarcoidosis and Infections

Despite intensive research in recent years, all attempts to discover an infectious microorganism as the causative agent of sarcoidosis have failed.[11,12] Several pathogens, including *Yersinia enterocolitica*, *Borellia burgdorferi*, *Aspergillus*, and *Nocardia*, have been cultured from the serum, skin lesions or lymph nodes of patients with sarcoidosis; however, their presence seems to be largely coincidental rather than causal. In addition, numerous chemicals have been claimed to be inciting agents, but none is yet universally accepted. More convincing data have recently been provided by several groups attempting to detect mycobacterial deoxyribonucleic acid (DNA) by polymerase chain reaction (PCR) in samples from patients with sarcoidosis. Most of the studies have reported at least a few specimens that are positive for *Mycobacterium tuberculosis*, and the findings are sufficiently persuasive to suggest that at least some of the patients diagnosed as having sarcoidosis have a disease that is initiated by a mycobacterial infection.[13] By molecular techniques, *Propionibacterium acnes* has been identified also in sarcoid granulomas, and a link to the etiology of sarcoidosis has been claimed.[14]

High titers of antibodies against lymphotropic viruses (Epstein-Barr virus, cytomegalovirus, herpes simplex virus, human herpesvirus type 6) and other human viruses (rubella viruses, parainfluenza viruses) have been anecdotally described in patients with sarcoidosis. Nevertheless, the many efforts have been unsuccessful in isolating a virus from cultures of sarcoid tissues,[15] suggesting that the presence of virus-specific serum antibodies may reflect a hyperactivity of the B-cell system rather than a direct causal relationship with sarcoidosis. Retroviruses also have been causatively linked with sarcoidosis. In fact, preliminary data have demonstrated the presence of retrovirus-like particles in the sera and bronchoalveolar lavage (BAL) fluid of patients with sarcoidosis and in the membrane fraction of Kveim-Siltzbach suspensions obtained from spleen with sarcoidosis. Furthermore, alveolar macrophages (AMs) of a subgroup of patients with sarcoidosis can produce an endogenous retrovirus-related protein, HERV-E 4-1 Env protein,[16] suggesting a role for a retrovirus as an etiologic agent of sarcoidosis; these data need appropriate confirmation.

The Kveim-Siltzbach Test and Other Experimental Models

The Kveim-Siltzbach (KS) skin test has been widely used to confirm the diagnosis of sarcoidosis. The technique consists of the intradermal injection of a heat-sterilized suspension usually obtained from splenic tissues with sarcoidosis. The cutaneous reaction mimics the immunologic events seen in the naturally occurring sarcoid granuloma. After injection, a subcutaneous lymphocytic infiltrate develops, which is predominantly sustained by CD4+ helper-related cells, and within 3 weeks a granuloma is formed. The granuloma shows morphologic and immunologic features of a sarcoid nodule: the central area contains particulate KS material and aggregates of monocyte-macrophages and is surrounded by a number of CD4+ cells and plasma cells, whereas rare CD8+ cells are confined to the periphery of the structure.[17]

The sequence of events leading to the formation and organization of the granuloma would per se suggest that the KS reaction could be an ideal in vivo model for studying the nature of the causative agent of sarcoidosis. Unfortunately, this assumption has not been subsequently confirmed because any attempt to identify putative transmissible or infectious agents from KS material has remained unsuccessful to date. Neither viral nor bacterial products have been identified in the several different KS batches examined nor did any individual develop sarcoidosis following injection of KS suspensions. More recently, the KS reaction has been used to obtain information on the diversity of the T-cell receptor (TCR) repertoire in granulomatous response.[18] The sequence analysis of paired KS biopsies and blood specimens in individuals with sarcoidosis revealed that CD4+ T cells surrounding the KS reaction are oligoclonal, suggesting that they respond to a single antigen or to a limited number of antigens.

During the past few years, a number of other models of granuloma formation have been taken into account to study the evolution of sarcoid granuloma.[19] When administered by intradermal injection, several factors produce sarcoid-like lesions both in humans and animals. Granulomas resembling those obtained with KS extracts have been reproduced by using chemicals; bacterial, fungal, and viral products; and autologous lung cells and neoplastic cells.[20–24] Animal models have been successfully used to study experimental pulmonary fibrosis. These models have undoubtedly improved our understanding of the mechanisms of granuloma formation and the development of sarcoidosis-associated fibrosis but have not been useful in definitively identifing the etiology of sarcoidosis, which still remains a mystery.

Genetic Factors

Differences in the occurrence and course of sarcoidosis have been reported by several epidemiologic studies.[25] The disease is more frequent in developed countries and in some ethnic groups. Furthermore, the possibility of family clustering has been generally accepted by several investigators.[26] A shared determinant (either genetic or environmental) seems to be operating in familial sarcoidosis, and it has been suggested that this determinant is similar for all ethnic groups.[27]

Many polymorphic genes have been suggested to contribute to the genetic susceptibility to sarcoidosis. Genes encoding human leukocyte antigen (HLA) products (classic and nonclassic), chemokine receptors, angiotensin converting enzyme (ACE), vitamin D3 hydroxylase, TCR genes, and the immunoglobulins Gm and Km have been involved in the genetic predisposition to sarcoidosis. As far as the association between HLA genes and the disease is concerned, class I major histocompatibility complex (MHC) HLA-A1, -B8, -B13, -B27, -Cw7, class II MHC HLA-DR3, -DR5, and HLA-DPB1 are the determinants that have been associated with susceptibility to sarcoidosis, even if in most cases the associations are weak.[28–32] A highly significant reduction in the frequency of individuals carrying HLA-DR alleles with a hydrophobic residue at position 11 has been observed in sarcoidosis cases, suggesting that this HLA-DR residue is an important protective marker in sarcoidosis.[33]

Epidemiologic studies have also demonstrated the positive association between MHC alleles and some aspects of the disease. There is a relationship between B13 and B35 expression and an early onset of disease while A30, B8, DR3, and DR4 alleles are associated with late onset. Cases of pulmonary sarcoidosis associated with B27 expression and HLA-DR3 patients commonly have a favorable outcome. Likely, HLA molecules are also important for controlling the susceptibility to cardiac sarcoidosis.[34] Thus, although the expression of MHC molecules depends to a large extent on the selection of the patients who belong to different racial groups, data on HLA expression may help in establishing a molecular basis that explains the clinical heterogeneity of sarcoidosis and, in particular, the differences in the degree of extrapulmonary involvement among patients coming from different areas of the world.

Other genes could, in theory, contribute to the genetic susceptibility to sarcoidosis and/or to clinical manifestations of the disease. There is a correlation between 25-hydroxyvitamin D3 1 alpha-hydroxylase gene expression in alveolar macrophages with the activity of sarcoidosis and its associated disturbances in calcium metabolism[35]; by contrast, polymorphism of the vitamin D receptor (VDR) is not a risk factor for hypercalcemia in sarcoidosis.[36] Although ACE is involved in the pathogenesis of sarcoidosis, there are data indicating that ACE polymorphism is not an inherited main cause of the disease, but rather that the ACE I/D genotype DD might be a promoter of the clinical manifestation of the disease.[37] Concerning the regulation of genes encoding for B- and T-cell receptors, the evaluation of the frequency of serologic polymorphism of the immunoglobulin G heavy chain (Gm) and kappa (K) light chain (Km) markers have shown the "protective" effect of the Gm (3 5*) phenotype in the sarcoid group and a reduced frequency of Gm (3 23 5*) in patients with an advanced chest radiographic stage.[28] Furthermore, the predominant TCR V alpha 2.3 gene usage in compartmentalized CD4+ BAL T lymphocytes has been linked to the HLA-DR3(w17), DQw2 haplotype in Swedish patients.[38]

A genetic regulation for the production of chemokines and cytokines seems to take place at sites of disease activity during sarcoidosis. Genes for chemokine receptors, which are characterized by polymorphisms resulting in expression of a nonfunctional receptor, have been implicated in the susceptibility to sarcoidosis: there are data indicating that CCR5Delta32 allelic frequency is increased in sarcoidosis and associated with clinically more apparent disease[39]; furthermore, the presence of the CCR2-64I allele confers a lower risk for the development of sarcoidosis.[39,40] Predisposition for tumor necrosis factor (TNF)-α production seems to be genetically regulated[41]; however, the TNF-α gene controls the genetic susceptibility to cardiac sarcoidosis,[42] and the genotyping of -308 TNF-α promoter polymorphism and HLA-DR may be of prognostic value for monitoring the course of the disease.[43–45] Interleukin (IL)-1 levels are elevated in sarcoidosis and the allelic distribution of IL-1 alpha*137 is strongly associated with sarcoidosis.[46] For TGF-β and IL-10, statistical comparisons of the allele and genotype frequencies between the clinically defined sarcoidosis groups and healthy blood donors do not reveal significant differences.[47]

Taken together, these data implicate a role for these polymorphisms in disease susceptibility, suggesting that genetic factors could be considered a background terrain in which other still unknown, provocative factors lead to the clinical development of the disease.

HOST FACTORS INVOLVED IN THE INITIATION AND MAINTENANCE OF INFLAMMATORY RESPONSES IN INTERSTITIAL LUNG DISEASE

Much of the present knowledge of the network of interactions that set the stage for the pathogenesis of ILD and sarcoidosis has been acquired from the evaluation of cell populations retrieved from BAL fluid and from immunohistologic analysis of tissue involved by the disease. As in other hypersensitivity reactions, the first manifestation of the disease is an accumulation in involved organs of mononuclear inflammatory cells, mostly helper T cells and monocyte-macrophages. The inflammatory process is followed by the formation of sarcoid granulomas, a compact structure made by a central aggregate of mononuclear phagocytes and their progeny (epithelioid and multinucleated cells) surrounded by a rim of T cells, consisting mostly of CD4+ T cells but also containing rare CD8+ T cells and B cells (see "Pulmonary Lymphocytes").

Before discussing advances in the pathophysiology of sarcoidosis, we will summarize the pattern of functional activities shown by cellular and soluble products of the mononuclear inflammatory cells that participate in the sarcoidosis process. The description of cells and cytokines is proposed in the context of their relevance in the pathogensis of sarcoidosis and other ILDs.

Pulmonary Lymphocytes

According to their specific properties and discrete functions, lung lymphocytes are functionally compartmentalized into primary, secondary, and tertiary lymphoid organs.[48] The great majority of organized lymphoid tissue is represented by the so-called bronchus-associated lymphoid tissue (BALT) and lymph nodes that receive drainage from the nose or lung. Lymphoid follicles are located throughout the bronchial tree as far down as the small bronchioles and are constituted by B-cell germinal centers surrounded by T cells, macrophages, and dendritic cells (DC).[3,49] In general, AMs, DCs, and T cells expressing discrete surface molecules and secreting peculiar molecules determine the type and direct the magnitude of the immune response at sites of pulmonary inflammation. As shown in Chapter 8, the recruitment of immunoinflammatory cells is the result of the binding of primed lymphocytes to ligands expressed by the endothelium and whose expression is induced by soluble mediators that are locally released following antigenic challenge.[4,50]

Although lung parenchyma normally contains only a few lymphoid elements, the lymphocyte populations are strikingly compartmentalized in sarcoidosis air spaces and interstitium. In a normal nonsmoking individual, more than 90% of the cells retrieved from the BAL are macrophages, whereas lymphocytes account for 5 to 10% of the entire BAL cell population. Less than 1×10^6 lymphocytes are usually recovered from a normal BAL; they are CD45R0 T "memory" cells[51,52] that coexpress the αβ TCR although few lung T cells (about 5%) stain with the mAb TCRδ1 that recognizes γδ TCR cells. Both CD4+ and CD8+ T cells are present in approximately the same proportions as in the peripheral blood (pulmonary ratio CD4/CD8 around 2).

In patients with pulmonary sarcoidosis, T lymphocytes dramatically increase both in percentage and in absolute number. The equivalent of 25×10^6 T cells can be recovered from the BAL fluid of most patients with active disease. The lung lymphocytes are predominantly CD4+ T cells, the ratio of CD4+ to CD8+ T cells being 5 to 15:1. In common with their normal counterparts, sarcoidosis lung T cells are CD45R0 T memory cells that coexpress the $\alpha\beta$ T-cell receptor. Interestingly, in a subset of patients, pulmonary $\gamma\delta$ TCR cells may increase,[53,54] but the precise mechanism by which $\gamma\delta$ cells contribute to the sarcoid immune response still remains to be established. The marked accumulation of CD4+ lymphocytes can be observed at all sites of disease activity, including lymph nodes, spleen, conjunctiva, skin, and other tissues affected by the sarcoidosis immunoinflammatory process.[3] At all sites of granuloma formation, the CD4/CD8 ratio is extremely high (usually greater than 10) and is secondary to the local increase in the CD4 population. In other words, an infiltrate of CD4+ activated T cells represents the immunologic hallmark of sarcoidosis.

Networks of interacting cytokines are responsible for controlling the characteristc hypersensitivity reaction taking place in the lung during sarcoidosis. The following section will focus on the pattern of lymphokine production within the respiratory tract during ILDs, including sarcoidosis.

Interleukin-2

Actively released by pulmonary T cells, the role of IL-2 in the pulmonary immune system, as in other organs, is to expand activated T-cell populations via the binding with its receptor, which is formed by 3 different chains: α (CD25), β (CD122), and γ (CD132). IL-2 can act as a local growth factor for T lymphocytes infiltrating the lung tissues of patients with sarcoidosis.[55–57] Inasmuch as some AMs normally express the $\beta\gamma$ IL-2R at low density and considering the fact that the addition of IL-2 to activated AMs increases granulocyte-macrophage colony–stimulating factor (GM-CSF) expression, it is likely that IL-2 could also be involved in the activation of some functional capabilities of sarcoidosis AMs. The presence of binding sites for IL-2 may also be demonstrated on human lung fibroblasts. The addition of IL-2 to fibroblasts leads to an enhanced expression of the gene coding for monocyte chemoattractant protein-1 (MCP-1/CCL2), a chemokine that is involved in fibrosis through the regulation of profibrotic cytokine generation and matrix. IL-2 may thus serve to integrate fibroblasts and sarcoidosis macrophages into a coordinated response of the connective tissue initiated by T-helper (Th)$_1$ lymphocytes at sites of disease activity.

Interleukin-4

This lymphokine, released by Th$_2$ cells, is a cofactor for the proliferation of multiple cell lineages, including fibroblasts. Inducing the expression of class II MHC antigens on the surface membrane of accessory cells, it acts in synergism with IL-2 in stimulating the growth of T cells. The production of IL-4 during pulmonary inflammation has been related to the development of pulmonary fibrosis in ILD, including sarcoidosis.[19,58,59] The IL-4/IL-13 axis is involved in the triggering and maintaining of the recruitment, homing, and activation of inflammatory cells during the remodeling process of the airways.[60] However, IL-4 induces the release of chemokines from human bronchial epithelial cells, including IL-8/CXCL8. This effect is thought to be of particular importance in attracting neutrophils and monocytes to sites of inflammation.

Interleukin-9

Interleukin-9 is a multifunctional cytokine produced by activated Th$_2$ cells in vitro and during Th$_2$-like T-cell responses in vivo. Lung expression of IL-9 in transgenic mice causes massive airway inflammation, epithelial cell hypertrophy associated with accumulation of mucus-like material within nonciliated cells, and increased subepithelial deposition of collagen. Because human fibroblasts express the IL-9 receptor, it is believed that this cytokine might be involved in fibroproliferative responses.

Interleukin-10

Activated Th$_2$ cells may represent a source for this molecule in the pulmonary microenvironment. IL-10 has anti-inflammatory and immunoregulatory properties: it inhibits proinflammatory cytokine and chemokine production in addition to blocking T-cell responses to specific antigens. It acts primarily through the inhibition of costimulatory properties of macrophages. There are data on its involvement in the regulation of the pathophysiology of lung fibrosis.[59] IL-10 shows inhibitory activity on the release of interferon (IFN)γ and IL-2 by Th$_1$ cells, stimulates mast cell growth, and regulates the accessory function of antigen presenting cells. It has been proposed that increased local secretion of IL-10 may represent a downmodulating mechanism involved in the spontaneous resolution of alveolitis in sarcoidosis.[61]

Interleukin-13

Interleukin-13 is expressed in activated Th$_0$ cells, Th$_1$-like cells, Th$_2$-like cells, and T cells expressing CD8.[62] This molecule strongly inhibits cytokine secretion induced by lipopolysaccharides (LPS) in monocyte-macrophages, including IL-1, IL-6, TNF-α, and IL-8. IL-13 also is a monocyte chemoattractant and has effects on fibrogenesis. It increases adhesion molecule and inflammatory cytokine expression in human lung fibroblasts and is critical for the recruitment of inflammatory cells. It is debated whether this cytokine is important in the pathophysiology of lung fibrosis.[63,64]

Interleukin-17

This cytokine is produced by CD4 T cells and is able to induce cytokine expression, including IL-6 and IL-8, on target cells. It enhances the surface expression of intercellular adhesion molecule (ICAM)-1 on fibroblasts. Recent evidence also indicates that IL-17 can link the activation of certain T lymphocytes to the recruitment and activation of airway neutrophils.[65] The IL-17–induced neutrophil recruitment is mediated via induced CXC chemokine release through steroid-sensitive mechanisms and is modulated by the release of endogenous tachykinins. These effects of IL-17 are potentiated by other proinflammatory cytokines such as IL-1β and TNF-α. Taken together, these findings suggest the potential role of this cytokine in T-cell driven lung fibrosis.[65,66]

Interferon-γ

This Th₁ cytokine is a key factor in the events that favor local immune responses in sarcoid lung. IFN-γ enhances the accessory function of AMs, increases the cytotoxic function of lung macrophages and lymphocytes, and regulates the secretion of an array of lymphokines, cytokines, and chemokines into the surrounding microenvironment. IFN-γ is typically expressed by T cells infiltrating the lung during most ILDs, including sarcoidosis, hypersensitivity pneumonitis, tuberculosis, and human immunodeficiency virus (HIV) infection.[67–70] There are data suggesting that monocyte/macrophages may represent a cell source of IFN-γ in the lungs, but the data are debated.

Through its pleiotropic effects on cytokine production, IFN-γ modulates mucosal immune responses in ILD.[71] IFN-γ upregulates the expression of the costimulatory molecules on pulmonary accessory cells, including CD80 and CD86.[72] It influences cell-mediated mechanisms of cytotoxicity and modulates T-cell growth and functional differentiation. However, by inducing non-ERL chemokines (MIG/CXCL9, IP-10/CXCL10, ITAC/CXCL11), the cytokine plays a major role in the recruitment of activated CXCR3+ T cells into inflamed tissues of patients with ILD (see Chemokines). IFN-γ also has crucial antifibrotic effects, because it inhibits the proliferation of endothelial cells and the synthesis of collagens by fibroblasts.

The Th₁/Th₂ Model

The pattern of Th₁ and Th₂ cytokine production in sarcoid lung can be summarized in the context of the Th₁/Th₂ paradigm.[73] As better specified below, the clinical story of diffuse lung disease may in fact be influenced by the Th₁/Th₂ pattern of cytokine production. Th₁ cells producing IFN-γ or IL-2 are responsible for initiating the alveolitis in the lung of patients with sarcoidosis. A Th₁ CD4 or Tc1 T-cell profile predominates during the formation of the typical T-cell–mediated alveolitis. The net effect of the Th₁ response is the development of a hypersensitivity reaction, such as in sarcoidosis, or an antigen-specific immune response, as in the case of hypersensitivity pneumonitis. In general terms, an inhibition of fibrogenetic processes may be observed in this phase. However, depending on the host susceptibility, a switch to Th₂ cells may occur in patients evolving toward lung fibrosis with the concomitant release of cytokines, including IL-4, which stimulate the production of extracellular matrix proteins and chemoattractants for fibroblasts.

Alveolar Macrophages

The representatives of the mononuclear phagocyte system in the lung arise from circulating monocytes that migrate through the alveolar walls into the lungs.[74,75] The daily contribution rate of the monocyte traffic in the homeostatic maintenance of the AM population is relatively low in healthy individuals (1.25% per day), but it notably increases in the lung of patients with sarcoidosis and other ILDs. As better specified in the following sections, local epithelial regulatory factors with the potential to regulate leukocyte homing[76] and the production of chemoattractant monokines cooperate in this phenomenon.[77–80] Furthermore, the local release of macrophage growth factors may also increase the self-renewal of the resident macrophage pool.[81,82] This multistep process results in a macrophagic alveolitis, which can be demonstrated in the BAL of the majority of individuals with active sarcoidosis.

Surface phenotypic analysis reveals that AMs are quite heterogeneous both in healthy subjects and in patients with ILD. In their steady state, AMs express class II MHC-related determinants and show high-affinity receptors for the Fc portion of immunoglobulin (Ig)G (CD64), IgE (CD23), and complement (CD11b).[83,84] Unlike peripheral blood monocytes, they either do not bear or bear at low levels the CD14 determinant (LPS-binding protein) and express low levels of molecules involved in cell-to-cell, cell-to-endothelium, or cell-to-matrix contact.[83,84] For these reasons, under normal conditions AMs are poor antigen-presenting cells. Mature AMs show a suppressive action on local T-cell immune responses, which is directly proportional to the local TGF-β secretion and lack of expression of counter-receptors that are needed to provide costimulatory signaling to lung T cells, including CD80.[85,86]

In contrast, in patients with sarcoidosis a massive monocyte influx takes place. This may explain why in sarcoidosis and other ILDs pulmonary macrophages act as professional antigen-presenting cells (APCs) for local immune responses. Freshly recruited monocytes are able to produce cytokines that may influence the functional and proliferative activities of lung T cells. Acting as accessory cells, AMs express costimulatory molecules including CD80/CD86 and CD72.[72] AMs release an array of biologic mediators of the immune response, such as IL-1, IL-6, IL-8, INF-γ, and GM-CSF, which favor the expansion of T-cell, AM, and neutrophil pools as well as the enhancement of local effector cell functions.[87] Furthermore, GM-CSF delays the differentiation of AM precursors into immunosuppressive mature AMs.

The interaction between IFN-γ and its receptor triggers AMs to become "primed" in sarcoidosis. This activation state of AMs is indicated by increased metabolic activity and by enhanced secretion of immunomodulatory molecules, such as the proinflammatory cytokines, chemokines, and other cytokines that are specified in the following paragraphs.

Interleukin-1

Alveolar macrophages in sarcoidosis are capable of producing detectable amounts of IL-1. The role of IL-1 in the lung is to provide accessory growth-factor activity for T cells. Promoting the adhesion of neutrophils, monocytes, and T cells by enhancing the expression of adhesion molecules such as ICAM-1/CD54 and CD62E/ELAM (endothelial leukocyte adhesion molecule), IL-1 regulates the development of the alveolar inflammation (alveolitis). Moreover, IL-1 may per se stimulate granuloma formation and fibrosis development by inducing fibroblast proliferation and increasing collagen production.

Interleukin-6

This factor, which stimulates B-cell growth and T-cell proliferation, is produced by lung T cells, AMs, endothelial cells, and fibroblasts. It causes fever and the active synthesis of acute-phase proteins and has weak antiviral IFN-like effects. Dysregulated production of IL-6 was suggested to be involved in a variety of chronic pulmonary inflammatory diseases, including sarcoidosis, tuberculosis, berylliosis, HIV infection, and ILD associated with autoimmune disorders. Furthermore, IL-6 is also involved in the control of the in situ proliferation of sarcoid fibroblasts.

Interleukin-12

Interleukin-12 is involved in Th₁ immune responses and stimulates the proliferation and the lytic activity of activated lung T cells. Specifically, IL-12 induces the Th₀ versus Th₁ shift and stimulates the proliferation and the

lytic activity of activated T cells and NK cells. In synergy with IL-15, IL-12 favors contact between activated T cells and APCs. The cytokine acts by interacting with specific receptors (IL-12Rβ) expressed by lymphocytes accumulating in the lung during most Th₁-driven diffuse lung diseases.[88] However, its involvement in the development of lung granulomas, including sarcoidosis, has been recently demonstrated.[70,89–91]

Interleukin-15

This pleiotropic lymphokine shares biologic activities and components of its receptor with IL-2 (βγ IL-2r). In the lung, IL-15 is mainly produced by macrophages and dendritic cells. IL-15 is produced by alveolar macrophages and supports the growth and chemotaxis of T cells, favoring the development of T-cell alveolitis.[92,93] It also behaves as a costimulatory factor for the production of other cytokines and chemokines (IL-17, CXCL8/IL-8, CCL2/MCP-1, GM-CSF, IFN-γ, and TNF-α) and for the expression of molecules involved in the antigen-presenting capability of resident accessory cells (CD80/CD86). Furthermore, the finding that IL-15 down-modulates the apoptosis rate of lung T cells introduces IL-15 as a possible inhibitor of death-inducing effects of physiologic apoptotic stimuli. In addition, IL-15 may regulate neutrophil functions in the lung. In fact, it induces cytoskeletal rearrangements, enhances phagocytosis, and delays apoptosis of neutrophils.[94] Moreover, IL-15 has been found to elicit other functional responses in neutrophils, such as chemokine production, that may influence pulmonary host defense mechanisms.

Interleukin-18

Previously known as IFN-γ–inducing factor (IGIF), IL-18 has activity roughly similar to, though distinct from, that of IL-1.[95] Mainly produced by monocytes and macrophages, it induces expression of IFN-γ and granulocyte colony–stimulating factor (G-CSF), while it inhibits production of IL-10. Interestingly, IL-18 and IL-12 act on Th₁ cells synergistically to induce IFN-γ, pointing to the possibility that both cytokines cooperate in the development of Th₁-type immune response in sarcoid lung.[69,96–98] In particular, it is thought that IL-18, via the activation of AP1 and NF-kappaB, leads to enhanced IL-2 gene expression and IL-2 protein production and concomitant T-cell activation in sarcoid lung.[96]

Colony Stimulating Factors

Granulocyte-macrophage colony–stimulating factor, G-CSF, monocyte-CSF (M-CSF), and IL-3 are able to induce the growth and differentiation of myeloid progenitors in bone marrow, facilitating the accumulation of macrophages in the lung of patients with sarcoidosis.[81,99] Furthermore, GM-CSF modulates cytokine production and enhances the antigen-presenting capacity and the growth of sarcoid AMs.[82]

Transforming Growth Factor-β and Related Cytokines

Transforming growth factor-β (TGF-β) and the family of TGF-related cytokines are secreted by monocyte-macrophages and activated lymphocytes, including pulmonary lymphocytes. TGF-β is a potent immunosuppressive molecule that exerts chemotactic activity on monocytes and modulates the synthesis and the effect of several other molecules, including IL-1, IL-2, IL-3, GM-CSF, IFN-γ, and TNF-α. TGF-β, which is constitutively released in the respiratory tract, has been involved in the development of fibrotic processes.[100]

Tumor Necrosis Factor and Other Molecules Belonging to the TNF-Ligand Superfamily

Tumor necrosis factor-α is a pleiotropic factor predominantly produced by activated cells belonging to the monocyte-macrophage lineage. TNF-α activates both neutrophils and macrophages leading to protease release, stimulation of the respiratory burst, and the induction of vascular adhesion molecule expression, which are essential for cell recruitment at sites of inflammation. TNF-α is actively produced by pulmonary macrophages. It plays a critical role in pulmonary injury and in the regulation of fibroblast growth via the induction of IL-6. Furthermore, TNF-α stimulates and regulates the synthesis and release of other lymphokines (IL-1, GM-CSF, platelet activating factor, and IL-6) and increases prostaglandin (PGE$_2$) production.

TNF-α is a member of an emerging family of soluble molecules with several and complex immunoregulatory properties that interact with specific receptors (TNF-R). TNF-α and other ligands of the TNF superfamily (TNF-L) has a role in modulating apoptotic mechanisms at sites of inflammation. There are data suggesting that the chronic overexpression of TNF-α and IFN-γ and the dysregulation of TNF-R/TNF-L set the stage for the persistence and the progression of inflammatory events during some ILDs.[68,101–103] In some circumstances, the alteration of the TNF-R/TNF-L balance leads to the chronic recruitment of inflammatory cells, which, once in the inflamed tissue, assemble granulomatous structures. On the other hand, it has been shown that TNF-α is induced in inflammatory cells during the resolution phase of granulomatous processes, rather suggesting a role for the cytokine in the recovery from the inflammation. Both phenomena are likely to take place in the lung. TNF-α may be essential or have little impact on the control of apoptotic mechanisms

depending on a combination of genetic factors, previous environmental exposure, and local alterations of immunocompetence.

Other Macrophage-Derived Factors

Fibrosing processes taking place in the lung result in the generation of other macrophage-derived molecules, including platelet-derived growth factor (PDGF) and insulin-like growth factor I (IGF-I). These growth factors for fibroblasts and epithelial cells and their receptors are abundantly expressed in fibrotic lung. They cooperate with the TGF family in promoting fibroblast growth and deposition of collagen fibrils.

Another group of mediators whose role in the evolution of fibrosis has recently been investigated are the 5-lypoxygenase metabolites of arachidonic acid (LTB$_4$ and LTC$_4$). AMs of patients with lung fibrosis elaborate significant amounts of leukotrienes. In addition, lung fibroblasts isolated from these subjects show a striking defect in their capacity to synthesize the anti-inflammatory and anti-fibrogenic molecules PGE$_2$ and phospholipase A2. In view of the fact that LTB$_4$ and LTC$_4$ stimulate fibroblast proliferation and chemotaxis and favor collagen deposition, their hyperproduction and the defect in PGE synthesis could be relevant in the pathogenesis of lung fibrosis.

Polymorphonuclear Cells

Although in normal nonsmokers BAL polymorphonuclear neutrophils (PMNs) are rare (less than 5%),[104] they can be found in excess in the BAL fluid of patients with sarcoidosis and other ILDs who show radiographic evidence of fibrosis. Compartmentalization of PMNs in ILD-associated fibrosis involves the interaction of homing receptors on the surface of rolling neutrophils (CD62, CD11a/CD18 complex, and CD49 antigens) with organ-specific molecules expressed by cytokine-stimulated endothelial cells of the pulmonary tissue (CD54, CD62P, and CD106). The migration of PMNs to the sites of fibrosis can be initiated and driven by AMs, which release chemotactic factors for granulocytes.[105] For instance, it has been shown that IL-1, TNF-α, and leukotriene B$_4$ are potent chemotactic factors for granulocytes. Furthermore, a recently discovered phagocyte-derived lymphokine, called IL-8/CXCL8, has been implicated in the mechanisms that control the neutrophil recruitment.

Interestingly, activated neutrophils can be induced to express a number of genes whose products lie at the core of the sarcoid inflammatory response, including cytokines (TNF-α, IL-1, vascular endothelial growth factor, IL-12) and a number of chemokines further amplifying local inflammatory responses. Neutrophils are also equipped with lysosomal granules containing a large repertoire of enzymes, including lactoferrin, cathepsin

G, elastase, myeloperoxidase, hydrolase, and bacterial permeability-inducing proteins.[104] Furthermore, migrating PMNs are capable of releasing a wide variety of oxygen intermediates, such as hydrogen peroxide, superoxide, and hydroxyl radicals capable of degrading many components of the extracellular matrix. Increased concentrations of neutrophil granule enzymes can be found in the BAL fluid of patients with sarcoidosis with fibrotic changes. It is therefore widely believed that these cells participate in the oxidant or protease-mediated damage to lung cells and extracellular matrix. This sequence of events explains the pathogenesis of the lung damage in sarcoidosis, which has long been known to be associated with a persistent neutrophilic alveolitis. Details in mechanisms by which parenchymal cells (mesenchymal cells, fibroblasts, smooth muscle cells) re-establish normal alveolar structures with consequent derangement of the normal architecture of the lung parenchyma are discussed in the following sections.

Chemokines and Other Chemotactic Molecules

A number of data have recently pointed out the role of chemokines in the development of the sarcoid inflammatory process. The superfamily of chemokines consists of an array of chemoattractant proteins that can be divided into four branches (C, CC, CXC, CXXXC), according to variations in a shared cysteine. The current roster approaches 50 related proteins.[106] Structural variations of chemokines have been demonstrated to be associated with differences in their ability to regulate the trafficking of immune cells during sarcoid inflammation.

CC Chemokines

Most molecules of this chemokine branch are highly expressed in the lung during inflammatory responses, including sarcoidosis. Monocyte chemoattractant protein 1 (MCP-1/CCL2), monocyte inflammatory protein-1α (MIP-1α/CCL3), MIP-1β/CCL4, regulated on activation normal T cell expressed and secreted (RANTES)/CCL5, and eotaxin/CCL11 cooperate to immobilize several leukocyte subpopulations in perivascular foci of inflammation.[107] MCP-1/CCL2 and RANTES/CCL5 interacting with CCR1/CCR2 or CCR1/CCR3/CCR5, respectively, may be chemoattractant for different cell targets that characterize the different phases of the sarcoid inflammatory process, including macrophages, T lymphocytes, and neutrophils.

CXC Chemokines

Three lymphocyte-specific CXC chemokines, which are produced in response to IFN-γ (ie, CXCL10, Mig/CXCL9, and I-TAC/CXCL11),[71] play an impor-

tant role in the recruitment of activated T cells into the pulmonary micoenvironment during sarcoidosis. Signaling mediated by these non-ERL CXC chemokines (CXC chemokines without the Glu-Leu-Arg [ERL] motif before the CXC motif) is mostly directed toward pulmonary activated T lymphocytes. AMs are the main cell source for these molecules; they release high amounts of CXCL10 and CXCL9 that, by interacting with specific receptors expressed by Th_1 and Tc_1 cells (CXCR3), allow for the accumulation of pulmonary T lymphocytes and contribute to granuloma formation.[87] Activated bronchial epithelium is another important source of CXCL9, CXCL10, and CXCL11.

IL-8/CXCL8, a chemokine that favors T cell and neutrophil recruitment,[107] is actively released in the airways during different ILDs associated with lung damage. Usually, elevated BAL neutrophil percentage as well as levels of the granulocyte activation markers, myeloperoxidase and eosinophil cationic protein, correlate with BAL levels of this chemokine. Immunolocalization of IL-8 demonstrated that the pulmonary fibroblast is the predominant cellular source of IL-8, even if there are data suggesting that macrophages may release this chemokine. Interestingly, pulmonary fibrosis may be associated with an increased release of IL-8/CXCL8 and a dysregulation of CXCL10 production, suggesting that the balance in chemokine production is an important factor in the regulation of local angiogenesis and fibrogenesis. CXC chemokines, like CXCL12/SDF-1, are also able to favor DC recruitment and activation.

Chemokines and Lung Th_1/Th_2 Cells

Chemokines are also believed to regulate Th_1 and Th_2 cells, which in turn may influence chemokine release.[108] For instance, MCP-1/CCL2 favors the formation of the eosinophil-rich type-2 granuloma and also appears to have a broader role in the regulation of Th differentiation and expression at sites of granuloma formation. Two other possible candidates involved in regulating the Th pattern are (1) IL-10, which promotes the Th_2-type immune response via the inhibition of Th_1-type reactions and (2) IL-12, which has proinflammatory properties, induces the Th_0 versus Th_1 shift, and stimulates the proliferation and lytic activity of activated T cells. In synergy with IL-15, IL-12 also favors the contact between activated T cells and APC. The balance between IL-10 and IL-12 may thus dictate the outcome of pulmonary inflammation. On the other hand, the release of Th_1 or Th_2 cytokines in lung tissue can polarize lung fibroblasts to produce either RANTES/CCL5 or eotaxin/CCL11 as major eosinophil attractants.[59]

Other Chemotactic Molecules

Interleukin-16 is a proinflammatory cytokine produced by CD8 T cells, CD4 T cells, eosinophils, mast cells, and bronchial epithelial cells.[109] This cytokine induces the migratory response of CD4 cells, increases intracellular calcium and inositol 1,4,5-triphosphate levels, and induces the production of proinflammatory cytokines. This cytokine is involved in the pathogenesis of hypersensitivity reactions even at the pulmonary level and plays a role in directing lymphocyte migration from the circulation into sites of inflammation and tissue injury. IL-16 shares chemoattractant activity for eosinophils and CD4 T cells, and high amounts of IL-16 can be detected in the lung at sites where a perivascular accumulation of lymphocytes may be demonstrated.

IL-15 is also able to favor the chemotaxis of T cells.[110] It induces migration of lung T cells, bearing an effective IL-15 receptor formed by three chains (ie, IL-15Rα, IL-15Rβ, and IL-15Rγ), during inflammatory diseases of the lung that are associated with a T-cell alveolitis. Collectively, these data emphasize the role of chemokines and chemotactic molecules in the development of sarcoid inflammation. It is also likely that cell-to-cell and cell-to-matrix interactions modulate the local chemokine expression, contributing to the pathologic progression toward fibrosis of inflammatory lesions.

THE ACCUMULATION OF INFLAMMATORY CELLS SETS THE STAGE FOR GRANULOMA FORMATION

Sarcoid granuloma formation can be arbitrarily divided into a series of immune events consisting of (1) the triggering of CD4+ Th1 cells by local antigen presenting cells, (2) the release of cytokines with multiple and overlapping functions, and (3) the accumulation of immunocompetent cells at sites of disease activity.[6,87,111] All of them ultimately lead to the organization of the local inflammatory process, which leads to granuloma formation. Although closely linked, these events will be discussed independently in the following section. The accumulation of immunoinflammatory cells at sites of ongoing inflammation represents the first step leading to granuloma formation (Figure 12–1). From a pathogenetic point of view, two mechanisms account for the increased number of inflammatory cells in affected organs (ie, a cellular redistribution from the peripheral blood to the lung and an in situ proliferation).[7]

Mechanisms Leading to T-Cell Compartmentalization

Suggestions for the concept of T-cell subset redistribution come from the comparison of the results obtained from the lymphocytic pattern in peripheral blood and at sites of disease activity. In patients with sarcoidosis a peripheral CD4 lymphopenia is associated with a dramatic increase in CD4 memory T cells in the lung, lymph nodes, liver, spleen, conjunctiva, skin, and other tissues where the sarcoid inflammatory process takes place.[112,113] These cells mainly produce IFN-γ or IL-2 and belong to the Th1 cell subset. This finding substantiates the concept of a Th1 T-cell compartmentalization, because it is presumable that the marked increase of Th1 CD4+ T cells at sites of involvement might lead to the consequent decrease in peripheral T lymphocytes.

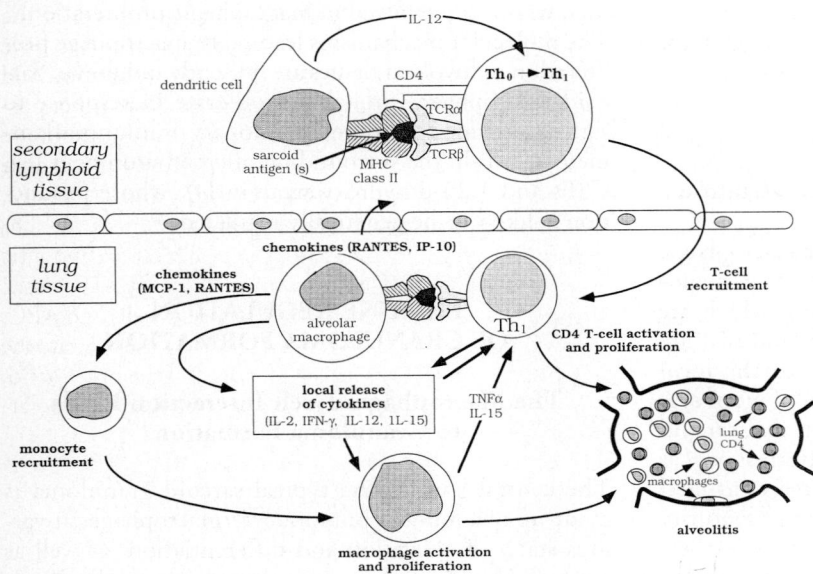

Figure 12–1 Schematic events leading to alveolitis in patients with sarcoidosis. Two mechanisms account for the increased number of CD4+ Th1 T cells in the lung (ie, a cellular redistribution from the secondary lymphoid tissues and peripheral blood to the lung and an in situ proliferation). Chemoattractant cytokines (IL-8, IL-15, CXCL10, RANTES, MCP-1) are likely to favor the expansion of the intra-alveolar pool of CD4+ T cells and monocytes within the inflamed area. Other cytokines that cooperate with IL-2 in T-cell proliferation (IL-15 and TNF-α) and molecules involved in macrophagic proliferation (GM-CSF) aid in the accumulation and activation of inflammatory cells releasing proinflammatory cytokines within the lung. IL = interleukin; IFN = interferon; TNF = tumor necrosis factor; AM = alveolar macrophage; DC = dendritic cell; CSFs = colony-stimulation factors; TGF = transforming growth factor; PDGF = platelet-derived growth factor; IGF = insulin-like growth factor; Th1 = T helper type 1.

As extensively reported in the section dedicated to the role of cytokines and chemokines in sarcoid lung, a possible scenario is that AMs or mucosal and intra-alveolar cells (dendritic, epithelial, and endothelial cells) could favor lymphocyte-endothelium adhesion at sites of sarcoid inflammation through cytokine and chemokine release.[7,111,114] In fact, it is known that macrophage-derived cytokines (such as IL-1, IL-15, IFN-γ, and TNF-α) can up-regulate the expression of messenger ribonucleic acid (mRNA) for adhesion molecules on endothelial cells. Furthermore, recent data suggest that chemoattractant cytokines are likely to cooperate in the expansion of the intra-alveolar pool of CD4 T cells within the inflamed areas.[72,79,92,93,115,116] High levels of CXCL10 and IL-16 can be found in the BAL fluid of some patients with sarcoidosis and a direct relationship between CXCL10 levels in BAL fluid and the degree of T-cell alveolitis has been demonstrated.[116] MCP-1/CCL2, another chemokine that is actively released in sarcoid lung, is significantly related to the degree of alveolitis.[79] CD13/aminopeptidase N, a molecule up-regulated by IFN-γ and expressed by sarcoid AMs, is also able to induce the in vitro chemotactic migration of T lymphocytes, suggesting its role in the pathogenesis of alveolitis.[117]

A second mechanism responsible for the accumulation of Th₁ cells is the in situ proliferation of these cells (see Figure 12–1). Various studies have shown that IL-2 and IL-15 act as local growth factors for T lymphocytes infiltrating lung tissues of sarcoid patients.[55,57,68,92,118] A number of sarcoid lymphocytes are CD25⁺ (the p55 chain of the IL-2 receptor) and express the p75 (CD122) and p64 (CD132) subunits of the IL-2 receptor.[92,119] Sarcoid BAL lymphocytes are also able to proliferate in vitro in response to IL-2 and IL-15 and constitutively synthesize and secrete IL-2. Furthermore, the discovery that an increased number of BAL T cells of sarcoid patients express the cell-cycle related Ki67 antigen indicates that sarcoid T cells can proliferate in situ.[120]

Mechanisms Leading to Monocyte-Macrophage Compartmentalization

The cellular redistribution also involves the macrophagic component of the alveolitis (see Figure 12–1). Chemotactic and activating factors for leukocytes, which are secreted in the lung of patients with sarcoidosis, are capable of recruiting blood monocytes to the local milieu.[77,78,105] Proof supporting the concept of monocyte redistribution comes from the observation that sarcoid AMs show a monocyte-like phenotype pattern as well as reduced or missing activity of tartrate-resistant acid phosphatase, which is regarded as a marker of maturity for cells of the monocyte-macrophage lineage. Furthermore, macrophages in early granulomatous lesions and around blood vessels in the intergranulomatous areas express the calcium binding protein calgranulin Mac387

(an antigen shared by granulocytes and circulating monocytes but only by a minimal proportion of tissue macrophages), thus confirming that the recruitment of adherent cells drives the development of the core of the granuloma.

Most events responsible for the recruitment of sarcoid monocytes from the bloodstream to sites of inflammation have been identified. High levels of monocyte chemoattractants, including CCL2/MCP-1, CCL3/MIP-1α, and CCL5/RANTES, have been demonstrated both in BAL fluid and the lung of patients with sarcoidosis. Once attracted by relevant chemotactic stimuli, monocytes acquire the ability to release type IV collagenase, an enzyme that is capable of binding and degrading the major structural component of the basement membrane of vessel walls (ie, type IV collagen).[74] By modifying the macromolecular organization of the basement membrane, this proteinase causes discontinuities through which circulating monocytes may enter the sarcoid tissues. Following the secretion of this enzyme, a heightened number of circulating monocytes enters the interstitium and under the influx of macrophage-derived cytokines (M-CSF and GM-CSF), mature AMs are generated, thus favoring the accumulation of mononuclear inflammatory cells releasing proinflammatory cytokines within the lung.

AMs are also able to proliferate in sarcoid lung[121] (see Figure 12–1). Sarcoid AMs show an increased mitotic activity and form colonies when placed in soft agar and incubated in vitro. They also actively synthesize DNA, as demonstrated by the enhanced incorporation of 3H-thymidine. From a phenotypic point of view, AMs from patients with active sarcoidosis are equipped with the CD71 antigen, which is related to proliferating cells following stimulation by growth factors. In addition, a high proportion of sarcoid macrophages show enhanced expression of the M-CSF and GM-CSF receptors, which are involved in macrophagic proliferation.[81] The molecular mechanisms leading to macrophage proliferation in involved tissues are presently unknown. Sarcoid macrophages probably proliferate in response to signals provided by other pulmonary immunoinflammatory cells in the surrounding microenvironment (eg, CSFs and 1,25-dihydroxy vitamin D), whose production is likely to be genetically regulated.[36]

IMMUNE REGULATION OF GRANULOMA FORMATION

The Macrophage–T-cell Interaction Leads to Granuloma Formation

The central core of the typical sarcoid granuloma is made up of a number of monocyte/macrophages at various states of activation and differentiation, as well as epithelioid cells and multinucleated giant cells. Typically, when the macrophage cells aggregate into more mature components of the granuloma, they lose expression of the calgranulin Mac387 antigen and their mitotic activity. In fact, in granulomatous mononuclear cell inflammation, proliferating cells are restricted to T lymphocytes. Using double-marker analysis with mAbs recognizing cycle-related markers (Ki67 and proliferating cell nuclear antigen [PCNA]) on sarcoid lymph nodes, it is possible to demonstrate that in granuloma areas only T lymphocytes exhibiting the CD4/CD45R0 helper-memory phenotype actively proliferate.[120]

Immunohistochemical analysis used mAbs recognizing adhesion molecules (CD11a, CD11c, CD54/ICAM-1, CD56/N-CAM, and CD36) to investigate the membrane interactions occurring among different subsets of macrophages within granulomas. Epithelioid cells forming sarcoid granulomas exhibit a very high expression of CD11a and CD11c as well as the leukocyte function-associated antigen (LFA)-1 specific ligand CD54/ICAM-1 but completely lack other adhesion molecules such as the receptor for thrombospondin (CD36), the collagen/laminin receptor VLA-1, and CD56/N-CAM. This pattern suggests that the reciprocal recognition of CD11a/LFA-1 and CD54/ICAM-1 molecules is a major mechanism involved in homotypic adhesion of inflammatory macrophages recruited from the peripheral blood and activated at sites of ongoing inflammation.[2] Epithelioid and giant cells probably arise from the aggregation and coalescence of the mononuclear phagocytes. In this regard, it is thought that GM-CSF contributes to the development of the macrophage core of the granuloma, since there is a relationship between AM proliferation and fusion and the subsequent formation of granuloma.[122,123]

A number of CD4 lymphocytes and plasma cells surround the central core of the granuloma; in contrast, a few CD8 cells are confined to the borders of the lesion. Histopathologic data also have demonstrated the presence of interdigitating HLA-DR cells in the T-cell areas and that mature macrophages and epithelioid cells immunoreact with IL-1 and class II MHC determinants.[124] This characteristic pattern clearly indicates that CD4+ cells together with macrophages participate in processing a persistent unknown antigenic stimulus. Acting as accessory cells, AMs play a role in antigen presentation and account for T-cell recruitment and activation as well as for the release of cytokines, which ultimately lead to the accumulation of immunocompetent cells.[125] The expression of cytokine genes inside granulomas was recently investigated in sarcoid lymph nodes by in situ hybridization techniques and immunohistologic studies. IL-1β, IFN-γ, and CXCL10 are preferentially expressed by cells located inside the granuloma whereas cells containing TNF-α, IL-1α, IL-6, and IL-2 mRNA are scattered and randomly distributed. These findings suggest that cells producing IL-1β (ie, macrophages) and IFN-γ (ie, Th$_1$ cells) are involved in the local recruitment and activation of immunocompetent cells. Once inside the sites of involvement, these freshly recruited cells contribute to the development of the new granuloma.

Molecules with chemotactic properties and inhibitors of monocytic mobility also cooperate to immobilize monocytes in perivascular foci of inflammation, thus contributing to the perpetuation of the granuloma. In particular, the in situ production of RANTES/CCL5, in lymph nodes presenting typical delayed-type hypersensitivity (DTH) lesions related to sarcoidosis, has been recently evaluated.[115] A positive signal has been detected in sarcoid lesions, whereas very few positive cells could be detected in the normal residual lymphoid tissue surrounding them or in reactive lymph nodes involved in a B lymphocyte response. Other chemotactic molecules, (ie, IP-10/CXCL10, Mig/CXCL9, and IL-16)[102] also have been involved in the formation of sarcoid granulomas. Immunochemistry performed with an anti-CXCL10 antibody in lymph nodes displaying abundant sarcoid granulomas showed that cells bearing CXCL10 are mainly located inside granulomas. In particular, epithelioid cells and CD68+ macrophages are stained, indicating that these cells produce CXCL10; in contrast, scattered positive cells are present in the perigranulomatous inflammatory reaction area. Furthermore, IL-16 is expressed in areas where there is perivascular accumulation of lymphocytes. Osteopontin and IL-16 represent other molecules that have chemotactic activity in sarcoidosis and whose expression correlates with granuloma maturity.[126,127] In particular, osteopontin induces T-cell chemotaxis, supports T-cell adhesion (an effect enhanced by thrombin cleavage of osteopontin), and costimulates T-cell proliferation, indicating a mechanism by which osteopontin and thrombin modulate the formation of sarcoid granuloma.

The compartmentalization of different regulatory T cells is likely to provide distinct effects on the evolution of the granuloma. In fact, at least in animal models, helper T cells facilitate and suppressor T cells downmodulate the growth of the granulomatous process.[20] Furthermore, CD4 positive cells predominate in the inner area of sarcoid granulomas whereas the few CD8 cells that are present predominate in the outer margin of the lymphocyte rim. It has been suggested, therefore, that suppressor cells may limit the exaggerated immunologic response against the antigen causing sarcoidosis, thus exerting a suppressive effect on the formation of the sarcoid granuloma. It remains to be established whether a defective recruitment of CD8 cells might lead to an ineffective control of the expansion of CD4 cells. In fact, the possibility cannot be excluded that in a subset of patients who progress toward advanced disease, the equilibrium between helper and suppressor signals may be lost, favoring the persistence of antigenic pressure, the maintenance of the inflammatory response, and the evolution of the granulomatous process.

However, the different pattern of cytokine production by T cells and, in particular, alteration of the Th$_1$/Th$_2$ balance may also influence the evolution of granulomatous lung inflammation (Figure 12–2). It is assumed that T cells isolated from patients with active sarcoidosis show a dominant Th₁ cytokine expression, with elevated mRNA and protein levels of IFN-γ and IL-2, but not IL-4. More specifically, at the site of granuloma formation, an accumulation of Th₁ cells as well as of intermediate (between Th₁ and Th₀) cell types occurs, whereas in the alveolar lumen, large numbers of Th₁ and Th₂ cells with a simultaneous decrease in Th₀ cells can be observed.[128] Furthermore, AMs are major regulators of Th₁ response because they produce large amounts of IL-12,[69,70,89] a cytokine that is known to stimulate IFN-γ production and is involved in the differentiation of Th₀ cells into Th₁ cells. When these data are reviewed together, it is conceivable that AMs favor the development of the characteristic Th₁ granulomatous response at sites of disease activity.

Local Proliferation of a Limited Number of Activated T-cell Clones Favors the Development of Sarcoid Granuloma

In human peripheral blood, two variable types of antigen receptors are independently expressed on T cells, the αβ and the γδ TCR. Just as for immunoglobulins on B cells, the antigen specificity and diversity of the TCR arise through the rearrangement of the large repertoire of V, D, J, and C gene segments during T-cell ontogeny. The use of mAbs for the α, β, γ, and δ chains of the TCR that have specificity for defined V regions together with DNA molecular analysis of the αβ or the γδ TCR genes, can verify whether the cell population being dealt with is composed of cells consistently possessing an identical TCR rearrangement (monoclonal expansion), by cells belonging to a limited number of clones (oligoclonal expansion), or by a multitude of cells that are different from each other (polyclonal expansion).

Taking advantage of these molecular biology procedures, the repertoire of the TCR of lavage and blood T lymphocytes from sarcoid patients has been evaluated.[18,38,129–137] Analysis of the use of β-chain constant region segments (Cβ1 versus Cβ2) and variable elements (Vβ) by BAL T cells has suggested that the TCR repertoire may be restricted in sarcoid lung, confirming a growth pattern in the lung that is consistent with TCR oligoclonality. Interestingly, there are data that indicate that the alveolitis in sarcoidosis results from two different processes, a local clonal expansion of T cells and a heterogeneous and presumably nonspecific accumulation of T cells with an extremely diverse Vβ repertoire. The relative contribution of these two processes is likely to vary in different patients and over time in the same individual.

Parallel evaluation of the Vα frequencies has shown that a strong compartmentalization of Vα2.3 CD4 cells may also occur in sarcoidosis. The increase of Vα2.3 CD4 cells may be so consistent that in some patients with active sarcoidosis these cells may represent more than 30% of BAL T cells. This data clearly indicates a role for this T-cell subset in the clinical manifestations of the active granulomatous disease. Interestingly, the preferential Vα2.3 usage is significantly linked to a discrete haplotype and to the course of the disease, because a 100% positive correlation between TCR Vα2.3⁺ CD4⁺ lung T-cell expansions and the expression of the HLA-DR3(17),DQ2 haplotype can be found. Furthermore,

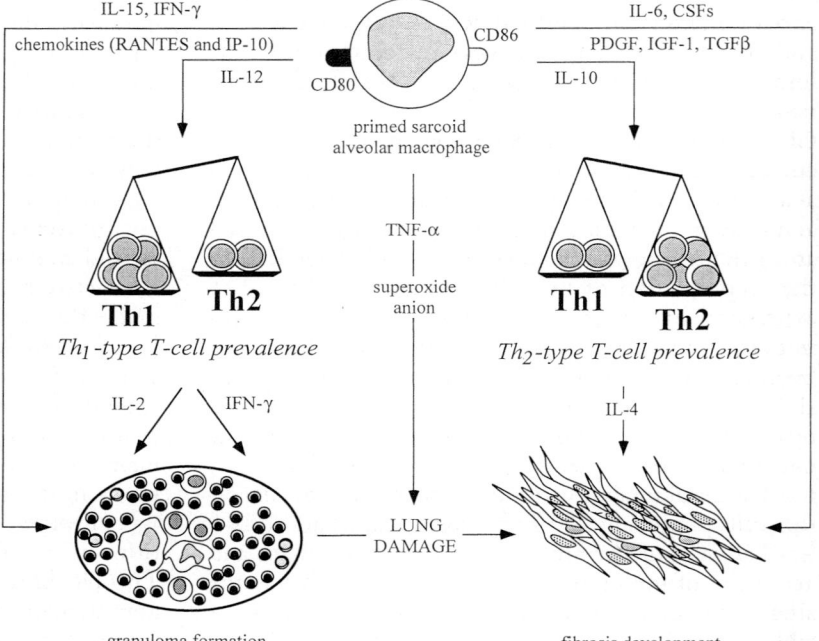

Figure 12–2 Different cytokine profiles drive granuloma formation or the development of pulmonary fibrosis. The prevalence of Th₁-type T cells favors the T-cell compartmentalization, and the net effect of this phenomenon is the development of the sarcoid granuloma and an inhibition of the fibrogenetic processes. However, depending on host susceptibility, a switch to Th₂ cells may occur in patients evolving toward lung fibrosis with a concomitant release of cytokines, including IL-4, which stimulate the production of extracellular matrix proteins and/or are chemoattractants for fibroblasts. IL = interleukin; IFN = interferon; AM = alveolar macrophages; Th₁ = T helper type 1; IP-10 = interferon γ-inducible protein-10.

there is an association between the BAL/peripheral blood TCR Vα2.3+ CD4+ T-cell ratio, clinical signs of disease activity and response to therapy.

Different mechanisms could account for the limited usage of the TCR repertoire in the lung of patients with sarcoidosis. One hypothesis is that the putative antigen(s) drives an oligoclonal expansion of T cells using particular Vα or Vβ regions. Alternately, the antigenic or superantigenic stimulation of T cells might induce a preferential growth of cells with a limited TCR leading to an oligoclonal proliferation. In addition, the in situ release of cytokines likely plays a role in this phenomenon. After in vitro growth in IL-2–supplemented media, BAL T cells from sarcoid patients show a selective expansion of particular Vβ-expressing subsets. Junctional region sequencing indicates that the IL-2 stimulated T cells are strikingly oligoclonal and derive from T-cell clones already selectively expanded in vivo.

A third possibility could be that the preferential expression of particular V region segments may be due to the accumulation of T cells that acquire a peculiar tropism for the pulmonary tract in that they express certain V genes of the TCR. Although there are no indications of HLA sharing between patients with sarcoidosis it is also possible that a local entity behaving as a "superantigen" leads to the development of the sarcoid granulomatous damage.

In synthesis, it is thought that the antigen(s) involved in granulomatous lesions favors the massive proliferation of a limited number of T-cell clones and an up-regulation of the physiologic activation state of tissue T lymphocytes. When a sufficient amount of pulmonary tissues is involved by inflammatory T cells, clinical signs of disease activity appear and are sensed by the individual as dyspnea.

Are Alterations of Programed Cell Death Mechanisms Involved in the Pathophysiology of Granuloma?

Although the granuloma structure is aimed at containing the dissemination of inciting agents in hypersensitivity reactions, it is to be expected that the inflammatory response will spontaneously clear once the etiologic factors are isolated. This paradigm is not supported in the case of progressive sarcoidosis. In about 60% of patients with sarcoidosis the course of the disease is self-limiting with spontaneous resolution of the granuloma, whereas patients with progressive sarcoidosis show a massive development of granulomas and do not recover even if strong immunosuppressive therapy is used. The uncontrolled development of granulomas results in fibrosis.

Possibly, in subjects with refractory sarcoidosis, the persistent, exaggerated T-cell growth and the consequent continuous formation of immune granulomas are a reflection of the dysregulation of mechanisms controlling T-cell homeostasis. This is strictly controlled by soluble factors and membrane receptors that activate proliferative and apoptotic processes. In particular, activation-induced T-cell death or apoptosis is characterized by specific morphologic and biochemical events. Schematically, the process can be divided in three functionally distinct steps: (1) the initiation phase, which is induced by heterogeneous death-inducing signals, lack of obligatory survival factors, shortage of metabolic supply, binding of death-signal-transmitting receptors (eg, members of the TNF-R superfamily), and subnecrotic damage by toxins, heat, or irradiation; (2) a complex pattern of metabolic events that lead to the degradation phase; and (3) the degradation phase, characterized by the typical morphologic and biochemical features of apoptosis (eg, DNA fragmentation, massive protein degradation, chromatin condensation). T cells, as well as other immune cells, may undergo this three-step sequence of events during negative intrathymic selection of the TCR repertoire. In the post-thymic phase, death of responsive T cells on specific activation of the TCR/CD3 complex assures rapid disappearance of the immune response on antigenic clearance, avoiding the metabolic costs involved in sustaining a large number of effector cells in inflamed tissues. Furthermore, programmed cell death of antigen-specific T cells prevents putative immune responses against related self-antigens.

A number of data suggest that the binding of death-signal-transmitting receptors or modulators of T-cell apoptosis may have undesirable, pathogenetic effects in subjects with progressive sarcoidosis. TNF-α may have a conflicting role in modulating apoptotic mechanisms at sites of inflammation. There are data suggesting that the chronic overexpression of TNF-α and IFN-γ sets the stage for the persistence and the progression of inflammatory events in patients with chronic sarcoidosis; in some circumstances, alteration of the TNF-R/TNF-L balance leads to the chronic recruitment of inflammatory cells, which, once in the inflamed tissue, assemble new granulomatous structures. On the other hand, it has been shown that TNF-α is induced in inflammatory cells during the resolution phase of the granulomatous process, suggesting a role for the cytokine in recovery from the disease. Both phenomena are likely to be possible. TNF-α may be essential or have little impact on the control of apoptotic mechanisms within the granulomatous structure depending on a combination of genetic factors, previous environmental exposure, and local alterations of the immunocompetence.

IL-15 is another cytokine belonging to the Th$_1$ system that is involved in the formation of the granulomatous process and may in theory influence granuloma maintenance. IL-15 also antagonizes the clearance of T cells from sites of chronic inflammation via an inhibition of T-cell apoptosis due to cytokine deprivation; this effect seems to be mediated by the up-regulation of BCL2 expression.[138] These data introduce IL-15 as a possible inhibitor of the death-inducing effects of physiologic apoptosis stimuli during chronic hypersensitivity reactions, including sarcoidosis. As a matter of fact, alveolar macrophages of patients with sarcoidosis over-produce IL-15, which supports the growth and survival of sarcoid T cells, favoring granuloma growth.[92]

Another system that is involved in the regulation of the T-cell inflammatory processes is the Fas/Fas-L system. Fas protein, which is expressed at high levels by chronically stimulated T cells, limits the expansion of antigen-reactive T cells after ligation with a specific ligand belonging to the TNF-L superfamily (Fas-L), thus preventing excessive accumulation of antigen-activated lymphocytes.[139] Both these systems have been evaluated in sarcoidosis.[140] Fas molecules are expressed at higher levels on sarcoid T lymphocytes than in normal T-cell subpopulations,[101] setting the stage for the development of irreversible remodeling of the lung tissue and, as discussed in the following section, the evolution toward fibrosis. Programmed T-cell death is also inhibited by oncogene products. The *BCL2* oncogene in particular belongs to a family of apoptosis-regulatory products that may either be death antagonists or agonists. Overexpression of some family members (eg, *BCL2* and *BCLX_L*) protects lymphoid cells from programed cell death when certain growth factors, such as IL-2, are withdrawn, whereas overexpression of others (eg, *BAD, BAX,* and *BID*) overrides the incoming signals from the cytokine-receptor and induces apoptosis. Like Fas, *BCL2* is highly expressed by T lymphocytes surrounding granulomatous lesions of patients with sarcoidosis.[141] Applying high-density human gene-chip probe-arrays for RNA expression profiling, it has been shown that a number of apoptosis-related gene products, including growth factors and the *BCL2* family of genes, are up-regulated in patients with sarcoidosis, consistent with a prosurvival profile.[142] Furthermore, patients with progressive disease show an up-regulation of NFκB and a lack of down-regulation of inhibitors of apoptosis.[142] It has also been shown that interaction with fibroblasts can inhibit the apoptosis of cytokine-deprived activated T cells by a selective effect on *BCLX_L*: this phenomenon is probably mediated by a soluble factor released by fibroblasts that up-regulates glutathione synthesis and maintains high *BCLX_L* levels and may help maintain the granulomatous process. Therefore, it is possible that overexpression of this inhibitor of apoptosis may prevent the clearance of activated T cells, favoring the formation of new granulomatous lesions in multisystemic granulomatous disorders.

MECHANISMS LEADING TO PULMONARY FIBROSIS

Although normal inflammatory reactions in the lung generally resolve, in patients with sarcoidosis, the rapidity and efficiency with which inflammatory constituents are removed from alveolar air spaces are altered. The loss of balance between events that mediate resolution or perpetuation of inflammatory responses sets the stage for the irreversible development of pulmonary fibrosis.[7,143,144]

Immune Activation Involvement in Lung Injury

The alveolitis and invasion of host tissues by granuloma may alter the permeability of type I cells, causing alveolar and interstitial edema and derangement of alveolar structures of the lung. These phenomena lead to physiologic repair reactions by parenchymal cells, which try to restore and re-establish normal alveolar structures. The repair processes lead to an exaggerated production of collagen associated with fibroblast migration and proliferation and an abnormal increase in the extracellular matrix with derangement of alveolar structures and resultant fibrosis. Given the above, it clearly appears that the severity of the lung injury and the extension of the tissue involvement by granulomatous areas represent the limiting factors in determining the degree of permanent structural alterations of the respiratory tract. With continued activity of the inflammatory cells, fibrosis becomes more widespread and involves the vasculature.

Immunologic mechanisms that drive pulmonary fibrosis in sarcoidosis show many features in common with other ILDs. Apart from the earliest, reversible phases of the sarcoid process in which Th$_1$ lymphocytes act as mediators of the initial alveolar injury, the fibrotic changes that follow are modulated by an increased number of activated macrophages, neutrophils, eosinophils, and mast cells overlying or interspersed in the alveoli; in the fibrotic phase, lymphocytes are not usually increased. The BAL fluid of individuals evolving toward fibrosis contains myeloperoxidase, elastase, proteases and other products of neutrophil granules, eosinophil cation protein, and secretory products of mast cells that may be directly toxic to epithelial lung cells.[145,146] Furthermore, an overproduction of superoxide anion and oxygen radicals by neutrophils and macrophages can cause local injury, disruption of the epithelial basement membrane, and alteration of epithelial permeability with a consequent derangement of the normal architecture of lung parenchyma.

Enzymes and oxidant radicals can be found in the BAL fluid[146] of patients with sarcoidosis because PMNs degranulate. Macrophage mediators can also operate in two directions at the sites of fibrosis. First, by releasing TNF-α, IL-1, superoxide anions, and type IV collagenase, sarcoid AMs contribute to injury. In particular, the derangement of collagen aggregates (which are important for epithelial basement membrane integrity) favors alveolar collapse. AM-derived cytokines can induce injury both directly (TNF-α) and via the recruitment and activation of neutrophils. Furthermore, AM-derived cytokines (including IL-1, IL-6, IFN-γ, TNF-α, GM-CSF) and IgG immune complexes may up-regulate the expression of the inducible form of nitric oxide synthetase (iNOS) and NO production in granuloma cells,[147] thus contributing to the injury.

Other cell components of the granuloma, such as epithelioid cells, giant cells, and dendritic cells can initiate the pathogenesis of fibrosis. It is thought that epithelioid cells, by releasing biologic response modifiers, favor the recruitment of inflammatory leukocytes and fibroblasts as well as alter the metabolism of lung connective tissue. However, since human fibroblasts appear to be an important source of IL-16 and of other mediators that are responsible for monocyte chemokinetic activity, fibroblasts may per se have key roles in the perpetuation of sarcoid inflammatory responses.[148,149] Deposition of immunocomplexes and the activation of the complement pathway with complement-mediated recruitment of neutrophils probably represent additional events that contribute to the development of tissue damage.

Cytokines Involved in the Recruitment of Fibroblasts

With the continued activity of macrophages and neutrophils, a fibrotic process develops that is strictly correlated to the recruitment of fibroblasts and the increased production of matrix macromolecules. In particular, migration of fibroblasts and epithelial cells from the interstitium to the alveolar spaces and adhesive interactions of fibroblasts with the surrounding interstitial matrix are the major factors that contribute to the development of fibrosis. Fibroblasts derived from fibrotic areas show an enhanced migratory capability,[150] and a typical fibroblast migration can be observed through discontinuities in the basement membrane of epithelia.[151] The migratory process reflects the local release of a variety of molecules that can act as chemoattractant factors for fibroblasts, such as chemokines, products of coagulation and the fibrinolytic cascade, matrix proteins (collagen peptides, laminin, fibronectins, elastin-derived peptides), and cytokines such as IL-4 and IL-13.[151–154]

TNF and its superfamily of TNF-like molecules are considered of crucial importance in the regulation of the accumulation of fibroblasts.[155] As for granuloma formation, dysregulation of the physiologic cell-death mechanisms (under the control of TNF-like molecules) may alter inflammatory and mesenchymal cell functions leading to a perpetuation of inflammation and/or lung injury. Furthermore, alteration of the apoptotic index can alter the destruction rate of alveolar walls. In fact, fibroblasts derived from fibrotic lung injury are able to release soluble factors that induce epithelial cell death and disruption of the basement membrane.[156] Due to their contribution to alveolar collapse, apoptotic factors are reasonably expected to dictate the extension of lung injury, the deposition of collagen, and, ultimately, the fibrotic changes.

Adhesion molecules and other integrins capable of interacting with specific receptors on the surface membrane of fibroblasts represent other molecules that permit interactions of fibroblasts with the surrounding environment. Recent findings point to the so-called antiadhesive proteins as mediators of fibroblast migration and adhesion (ie, osteonectin or secreted protein, acidic and rich in cysteine [SPARC], tenascin-C, and thrombospondin-1). These extracellular proteins, that do not have a structural role in normal lung, are selectively localized in fibrotic lesions. In particular, SPARC and tenascin are abundant in fibroblast foci, a pattern that is consistent with their role in the migration of fibroblasts to sites of lung injury as well as in epithelial adhesion and migration. Furthermore, it is now clear that the thickness and staining intensity of tenascin around granulomas appear in some way related to the duration of the lesion.[157] Thin fibrillary deposits of tenascin are common around young sarcoid granulomas characterized by a large number of monocyte-like macrophages and a rich CD4+ T-cell perigranulomatous cuff, whereas very thick tenascin fibrous bands are common in lymphocyte-depleted fibrotic lesions.[157] On the basis of these findings it is likely that the proportion and position of tenascin can be relevant in modulating the adhesive and repulsive attitude of sarcoid immune cells and fibroblasts with respect to the extracellular matrix.

Changes in the local expression of adhesion molecules that are involved in epithelial cell–extracellular matrix or epithelial cell–fibroblast interactions represent a second pathway that can accelerate fibroblast migration. As a matter of fact, pathologic alterations in pulmonary fibrosis are accompanied by a disruption of the histoarchitecture, cytoplasmic hyaladherin deposition in the damaged epithelium, and loss of expression of molecules that mediate homing via hyaluronate binding.[158] Likely, expression of integrins by epithelial and mesenchymal cells in areas of intra-alveolar fibrosis might render these cells actively adherent to fibronectin, favoring progressive fibrosis throughout the affected lung.

Cytokines Involved in Fibroblast Proliferation

Several soluble effector molecules secreted by sarcoid inflammatory cells prime fibroblasts to enter the G_1 phase of the growth cycle to proliferate. AMs have been shown to play a key role in these steps by releasing mediators that evoke a generalized proliferative response. Accumulated macrophagic cells express IL-1, IL-6, IFN-γ, PDGF, TGF-β, IGF-1, fibronectin, IL-3, and CSFs. Eosinophils are also able to act as direct modulatory cells in fibroblast proliferation and collagen synthesis, in part, through TGF-β.[159] These factors lead to a generalized proliferative response by cells present in the area of tissue damage, including fibroblasts, endothelial, and epithelial cells.[160–162] As a matter of fact, an increased proportion of fibroblasts isolated from patients with pulmonary fibrosis demonstrate an unexpected growth capability and a higher rate of cell division than fibroblasts isolated from normal lung.

Other cellular components and soluble products are involved in fibroblast changes. Endothelial cells, epithelial cells, and smooth-muscle cells can proliferate, leading to structural modification of the air space. It is thought that epithelial cells also may directly drive the fibroblast growth via the in situ release of members of the TGF family, which are involved in the pathogenesis of fibrosis.[163] In normal tissues, cytokine binding proteins (which include α-macroglobulins, extracellular matrix proteins, monospecific cytokine binding proteins, and secreted extracellular domains of cytokine receptors) are critical avenues for the clearance of fibrogenetic cytokines during physiologic repair processes. Abnormal expression of these proteins can be related to the abnormal fibroblast proliferation, because alteration of these clearance mechanisms might lead to the local overexpression of TGF and PDGF.

Cytokines Involved in the Synthesis of Matrix Components

Newly recruited and proliferating fibroblasts, which adhere to connective tissue at sites of fibrosis, undergo cellular activation. In fact, they show morphologic evidence of an increased secretory activity of matrix components. Furthermore, immunohistochemistry has revealed that the evolution from the granulomatous response to irreversible and unchangeable fibrosis is influenced by a number of components present in the lung tissue of these patients, including fibronectin, collagen, integrin receptors, and TGF.[22] In particular, it has been shown that TGF-β_1 staining assessed by immunohistochemistry is intense in epithelioid histiocytes comprising non-necrotizing granuloma and in bronchiolar epithelial cells, in hyperplastic type II pneumocytes, and occasionally in AMs, and, interestingly, overproduction of TGF-β_1 is associated with functional impairment in patients with pulmonary sarcoidosis.[164] Type-I collagen can be found in the border of sarcoid granulomas sometimes extending between cells toward the center. Fibronectin occurs in both the periphery and the center of granulomas, whereas procollagen type-I is mainly central.

The mechanisms accounting for the increased production of fibronectin and collagen components by these cells are under investigation. Local production of the profibrogenic molecule IGF-1 is subject to post-translational regulation by IGF-binding proteases that enhance fibrogenesis in patients with sarcoidosis with evidence of progression or fibrosis.[165] However, evidence suggests that the in vitro treatment of lung macrophages and fibroblasts with cytokines (IFN-γ, TGF-β, and PDGF) is associated with an abnormal synthesis of matrix components and expression of matrix receptors. Thus, alterations in the cytokine network may contribute to mural accretion of the alveoli and to the consequent development of air space fibrosis. The local shifts of the Th$_1$/Th$_2$ regulatory networks may also drive the development of fibrotic lesions via the deposition of matrix components.

As specified above, it is postulated that in the early phases, sarcoid T cells produce Th$_1$ cytokines that favor the accretion of the granuloma (ie, IL-2) or have suppressive effects on the production of extracellular proteins (ie, IFN-γ). The net effect of the Th$_1$ response is the development of the sarcoid granuloma and an inhibition of fibrogenetic processes (see Figure 12–2). However, depending on host susceptibility, a switch to Th$_2$ cells may occur in patients evolving toward lung fibrosis with concomitant release of cytokines, including IL-4, which stimulate the production of extracellular matrix proteins and/or are chemoattractants for fibroblasts.[166] Thus, the Th$_2$ shift might be involved in the expansion of the mesenchymal cell population, with increased deposition of extracellular matrix components in the surrounding environment.

MOLECULAR TARGETS FOR IMMUNOSUPPRESSIVE DRUGS IN SARCOIDOSIS

There is no question that corticosteroids represent the therapy of choice for sarcoidosis.[167–169] In spite of their widespread use to treat sarcoidosis, the exact mechanisms by which these drugs suppress the activity of the disease are still under investigation. In general terms, steroids are able to down-modulate the expression of IL-2r on target cells and the production of IL-2 by relevant cells, mainly CD4$^+$ lymphocytes equipped with high-affinity receptors for glucocorticoids. Furthermore, they induce apoptosis in target cells and inhibit various macrophagic activities, including TNF-α and IL-1 release, accessory function, and tumoricidal activity.

In patients with sarcoidosis, steroid therapy leads to a reduction in the number and activity of BAL T cells probably via the induction of programed cell death of lung T cells. Furthermore, they favor a diminished expression of the IL-2 gene by pulmonary T cells. Steroids also modify the phenotypic profile of the macrophagic component of alveolitis reverting the monocyte-like pattern of alveolitis to a more mature, AM-like phenotype. Corticosteroids also influence monocyte-macrophage functions, influencing the release of molecules, such as hydrogen peroxide, TNF-α, MIP-1α, and RANTES, which are known to be strictly associated with the immunopathogenesis of the disease.[170,171]

Methotrexate is another effective immunosuppressive agent for long-term therapy in sarcoidosis.[172] The drug is particularly helpful in the treatment of chronic skin lesions, including lupus pernio. The treatment with this antimetabolite affects both macrophagic and lymphocytic components of the sarcoid inflammatory process. It causes a drop in the number of pulmonary CD4 cells and a consequent decrease in the CD4/CD8 ratio: in addition, it leads to a significative fall in the amounts of TNF-α and hydrogen peroxide released by sarcoid AMs.[173] Similarly to steroids, methotrexate favors a decrease in B lymphocytes; furthermore, it inhibits various neutrophil functions, including the release of proinflammatory molecules and neutrophil adherence.

The drug also antagonizes the proinflammatory effects of IL-1 and inhibits fibroblast proliferation. Thus, although methotrexate does not directly affect the T-helper number and function in vitro, it has potent effects on lung CD4 in vivo, entirely superimposable to those displayed by steroid therapy.

Alternate forms of treatments may be warranted when a particular organ is involved or when the disease is refractory to conventional treatment and evolves toward fibrosis. Thus, many steroid-resistant patients are treated with cytotoxic agents like azathioprine.[174–176] Cyclosporin A (CyA), a fungal-derived drug, is the prototype of the immunosuppressive agents that interfere with cytokine synthesis. It binds to cytosolic binding proteins (immunophilins), and the CyA/immunophilin complex blocks early events in the activation of T cells, including Ca^{2+}-dependent IL-2 gene transcription and, in particular, the nuclear site for the nuclear factor of activated T cells (NFAT). Surprisingly, this drug, which, in theory, could inhibit the production of IL-2 in sarcoid $CD4^+$ T cells, has no apparent benefits in sarcoidosis.[177,178] Even if the drug suppresses the spontaneous release of IL-2 by pulmonary T cells in vitro and inhibits their spontaneously exaggerated replication, the oral administration of conventional doses of CyA is ineffective in controlling lung T-cell activation and does not alter the clinical course of the disease. Two hypotheses can be proposed to explain the paradoxical ineffectiveness of CyA in a disease that is characterized by an accumulation of CD4 T cells actively secreting IL-2. One possibility lies in the fact that the drug does not reach therapeutic levels at sites of disease activity. Alternately, CyA might not be able to overcome the specific action of the inciting stimuli that are putatively present at sites of disease activity. A third comprehensive explanation for the ineffectiveness of CyA in controlling lung T-cell proliferation in patients with sarcoidosis could be related to the fact that only drugs that are capable of controlling the number and the activation state of the macrophagic component of alveolitis represent effective agents in this disorder.

Research on immunosuppressive drugs is progressing rapidly. Several drugs that exhibit different inhibitory effects on cells of the immune system offer considerable promise as adjunctive therapeutic immunosuppressive agents for patients with sarcoidosis who do not respond to steroids or have severe corticosteroid-induced side effects. New immunosuppressants with inhibitor activity on cytokine synthesis and action (ie, tacrolimus and sirolimus), have been developed. In particular, rapamycin is an interesting drug that affects IL-2 signal transduction pathways, inhibits expression of the Th_2 cytokines, and suppresses the production of other proinflammatory cytokines. Mycophenolate mofetil is another immunosuppressant that shows selective antiproliferative effects on lymphocytes. Leflunomide (Arava) is an isoxazole that inhibits pyrimidine synthesis. Its mode of action is similar to methotrexate. Recently, the combination of methotrexate and leflunomide has begun to be used for ocular sarcoidosis to avoid the possible increased risk for malignancy due to multicombination chemotherapy with azathioprine.[179]

A combination of these new immunosuppressants could be used in the future with the objective of controlling sarcoidosis in patients who do not improve with glucocorticoids. For instance, 15-deoxyspergualin could represent an alternative for controlling the first phase of the cell-mediated immune response of the sarcoid inflammatory process (ie, the T lymphocyte/macrophage interaction). This semisynthetic polyamine inhibits monocyte/macrophage function, affecting oxidative metabolism, IL-1 synthesis, and cell-surface expression of accessory molecules that are involved in cell-to-cell interactions. Furthermore, the antiproliferative mycophenolate mofetil could be used alone or with IL-2 inhibitors to decrease the accumulation of lymphocytes into sites of ongoing sarcoid inflammation. In fact, this drug, in clinically attainable doses, is able to control the recruitment of lymphocytes and monocytes, inhibits the glycosylation of adhesion molecules, and limits the proliferation of smooth muscle cells.

As previously reported, cytokines set the stage for pathogenetic mechanisms involved in granuloma formation and fibrosis development. Advances in clinical management of sarcoidosis will depend on the ability to develop anticytokine approaches at sites of disease activity. Currently, most interest in soluble cytokine receptors, natural cytokine inhibitors, genetically engineered antagonists, and single or combinations of anti-inflammatory cytokines has focused on the possibility that they may become standard pharmacologic agents for controlling and modulating the complex network of cytokines interrupting the sequel of immunologic events that lead to granuloma formation and fibrosis development.[102] In particular, there are data that raise the possibility for the therapeutic use of anti-TNF agents in sarcoidosis, including the chimeric IgG_1 monoclonal antibody infliximab and the fusion protein etanercept. Infliximab is a chimerized monoclonal antibody that is able to recognize the cytokine bound to TNF-receptors expressed by activated macrophages and T cells; it has also been suggested that the IgG_1 Fc fragment of the mAb triggers the activation of complement-pathway components, leading to the neutralization of cells that are involved in tissue injury and inflammation. Etanercept is a fusion peptide comprised of two separate molecules: the p75 TNF-α receptor is joined to the Fc portion of a human IgG_1. It binds to soluble TNF-α and prevents its interaction with the cell-surface TNF-α receptor. Etanercept has the advantage that with its clearance from circulation, TNF-α is again available and biologically active, which is important in the event that TNF-α is needed for an intercurrent problem such as an infection. Not unexpectedly, there are data suggesting that infliximab has beneficial effects in reducing clinical signs and symptoms in patients with sarcoidosis who are unresponsive to conventional therapy (steroids).[180,181]

These data are preliminary and should promote further clinical trials to confirm both the efficacy and tolerability of anticytokine agents when used in patients with sarcoidosis and other interstitial lung diseases that are characterized by an up-regulation of cytokine and chemokine expression in the pulmonary milieu.

CONCLUSION

The paradigm of sarcoidosis has furnished an enormous amount of detailed molecular and cellular information on the immunopathogenesis of ILD and granulomatous disorders. It is now recognized that several cytokines that are secreted in the pulmonary environment during the sarcoid inflammatory process potentially participate in the pathogenesis of several ILDs. As detailed above, high-affinity receptors for immunomodulatory cytokines participating in granuloma and fibrosis development have been recently cloned. There is clearly much more to be learned. More research is required to define on a molecular basis the actions of cytokines on granuloma formation, pulmonary tissue injury, and collagen metabolism. Furthermore, it is easy to anticipate that the development of potential immunosuppressive strategies to inhibit cytokine activity will be a major challenge to researchers involved in the clinical management of ILD. The selection of the immunotherapy of choice for those mechanisms, to measure the efficacy of our therapeutic intervention, and then to prevent the spontaneous exacerbations of the disease will represent the actual endpoints of this task. We are still a long way from these goals, but it is likely that they are achievable using sarcoidosis as a model for studying the host granulomatous inflammatory response against persistent antigens. Hope in this regard comes from the current revolution in the areas of clinical immunology and molecular biology as well as from the development of new immune techniques, which could improve our knowledge of this area of medicine.

ACKNOWLEDGMENT

We wish to thank Mr. Martin Donach for his help in the preparation of this manuscript.

REFERENCES

1. Lipscomb MF, Bice DE, Lyons CR, et al. The regulation of pulmonary immunity. Adv Immunol 1995;59:369–455.
2. Lukacs NW, Ward PA. Inflammatory mediators, cytokines, and adhesion molecules in pulmonary inflammation and injury. Adv Immunol 1996;62:257–304.
3. Semenzato G, Bortolin M, Facco M, et al. Lung lymphocytes: origin, biological functions, and laboratory techniques for their study in immune-mediated pulmonary disorders. Crit Rev Clin Lab Sci 1996;33:423–55.
4. Zhang P, Summer WR, Bagby GJ, Nelson S. Innate immunity and pulmonary host defense. Immunol Rev 2000;173: 39–51.
5. Newman LS, Rose CS, Maier LA. Sarcoidosis. N Engl J Med 1997;336:1224–34.
6. Newman LS. Immunologic mechanisms in granulomatous lung disease. Immunopharmacology 2000;48:329–31.
7. Semenzato G, Adami F, Maschio N, Agostini C. Immune mechanisms in interstitial lung diseases. Allergy 2000;55: 1103–20.
8. Vourlekis JS, Sawyer RT, Newman LS. Sarcoidosis: developments in etiology, immunology, and therapeutics. Adv Intern Med 2000;45:209–57.
9. Zumla A, James DG. Granulomatous infections: etiology and classification. Clin Infect Dis 1996;23:146–58.
10. Saltini C, Amicosante M. Beryllium disease. Am J Med Sci 2001;321:89–98.
11. Agostini C, Semenzato G, James DG. Immunological, clinical and molecular aspects of sarcoidosis. Mol Aspects Med 1997;18:91–165.
12. Popper HH, Klemen H, Hoefler G, Winter E. Presence of mycobacterial DNA in sarcoidosis. Hum Pathol 1997;28: 796–800.
13. Grosser M, Luther T, Muller J, et al. Detection of *M. tuberculosis* DNA in sarcoidosis: correlation with T-cell response. Lab Invest 1999;79:775–84.
14. Ishige I, Usui Y, Takemura T, Eishi Y. Quantitative PCR of mycobacterial and propionibacterial DNA in lymph nodes of Japanese patients with sarcoidosis. Lancet 1999;354: 20–3.
15. Maeda H, Niimi T, Sato S, et al. Human herpesvirus 8 is not associated with sarcoidosis in Japanese patients. Chest 2000;118:923–7.
16. Tamura N, Iwase A, Suzuki K, et al. Alveolar macrophages produce the Env protein of a human endogenous retrovirus, HERV-E 4-1, in a subgroup of interstitial lung diseases. Am J Respir Cell Mol Biol 1997;16:429–37.
17. Mishra BB, Poulter LW, Janossy G, James DG. The distribution of lymphoid and macrophage like cell subsets of sarcoid and Kveim granulomata: possible mechanism of negative PPD reaction in sarcoidosis. Clin Exp Immunol 1983;54:705–15.
18. Klein JT, Horn TD, Forman JD, et al. Selection of oligoclonal V beta-specific T cells in the intradermal response to Kveim-Siltzbach reagent in individuals with sarcoidosis. J Immunol 1995;154:1450–60.
19. Moller DR. Cells and cytokines involved in the pathogenesis of sarcoidosis. Sarcoidosis Vasc Diffuse Lung Dis 1999; 16:24–31.
20. Chensue SW, Wellhausen SR, Boros DL. Modulation of granulomatous hypersensitivity. II. Participation of Ly 1+ and Ly 2+ T lymphocytes in the suppression of granuloma formation and lymphokine production in *Schistosoma mansoni*-infected mice. J Immunol 1981;127:363–7.
21. Pfeifer S, Bartlett R, Strausz J, et al. Beryllium-induced disturbances of the murine immune system reflect some phenomena observed in sarcoidosis. Int Arch Allergy Immunol 1994 104:332–9.
22. Roman J, Jeon YJ, Gal A, Perez RL. Distribution of extracellular matrices, matrix receptors, and transforming growth factor-beta 1 in human and experimental lung granulomatous inflammation. Am J Med Sci 1995;309:124–33.
23. Huang H, Meyer KC, Kubai L, Auerbach R. An immune model of beryllium-induced pulmonary granulomata in mice. Histopathology, immune reactivity, and flow-cytometric analysis of bronchoalveolar lavage-derived cells. Lab Invest 1992;67:138–46.
24. Holter JF, Park HK, Sjoerdsma KW, Kataria YP. Nonviable autologous bronchoalveolar lavage cell preparations induce intradermal epithelioid cell granulomas in sarcoidosis patients. Am Rev Respir Dis 1992;145:864–71.

25. Luisetti M, Beretta A, Casali L. Genetic aspects in sarcoidosis. Eur Respir J 2000;16:768–80.

26. Elford J, Fitch P, Kaminski E, et al. Five cases of sarcoidosis in one family: a new immunological link? Thorax 2000;55:343–4.

27. McGrath DS, Daniil Z, Foley P, et al. Epidemiology of familial sarcoidosis in the UK. Thorax 2000;55:751–4.

28. Martinetti M, Dugoujon JM, Tinelli C, et al. HLA-Gm/kappam interaction in sarcoidosis. Suggestions for a complex genetic structure. Eur Respir J 2000;16:74–80.

29. Luisetti M, Martinetti M, Cuccia M, et al. HLA Class I, II and III polymorphisms in sarcoidosis. Sarcoidosis 1993;10:151–3.

30. Martinetti M, Tinelli C, Kolek V, et al. "The sarcoidosis map": a joint survey of clinical and immunogenetic findings in two European countries. Am J Respir Crit Care Med 1995;152:557–64.

31. Schurmann M, Lympany PA, Reichel P, et al. Familial sarcoidosis is linked to the major histocompatibility complex region. Am J Respir Crit Care Med 2000;162:861–4.

32. Arbustini E, Grasso M, Leo G, et al. Polymorphism of angiotensin-converting enzyme gene in sarcoidosis. Am J Respir Crit Care Med 1996;153:851–4.

33. Foley PJ, McGrath DS, Puscinska E, et al. Human leukocyte antigen-DRB1 position 11 residues are a common protective marker for sarcoidosis. Am J Respir Cell Mol Biol 2001;25:272–7.

34. Naruse TK, Matsuzawa Y, Ota M, et al. HLA-DQB1*0601 is primarily associated with the susceptibility to cardiac sarcoidosis. Tissue Antigens 2000;56:52–7.

35. Inui N, Murayama A, Sasaki S, et al. Correlation between 25-hydroxyvitamin D3 1 alpha-hydroxylase gene expression in alveolar macrophages and the activity of sarcoidosis. Am J Med 2001;110:687–93.

36. Niimi T, Tomita H, Sato S, et al. Vitamin D receptor gene polymorphism and calcium metabolism in sarcoidosis patients. Sarcoidosis Vasc Diffuse Lung Dis 2000;17:266–9.

37. Schurmann M, Reichel P, Muller-Myhsok B, et al. Angiotensin-converting enzyme (ACE) gene polymorphisms and familial occurrence of sarcoidosis. J Intern Med 2001;249:77–83.

38. Grunewald J, Janson CH, Eklund A, et al. Restricted V alpha 2.3 gene usage by CD4+ T lymphocytes in bronchoalveolar lavage fluid from sarcoidosis patients correlates with HLA-DR3. Eur J Immunol 1992;22:129–35.

39. Petrek M, Drabek J, Kolek V, et al. CC chemokine receptor gene polymorphisms in Czech patients with pulmonary sarcoidosis. Am J Respir Crit Care Med 2000;162:1000–3.

40. Hizawa N, Yamaguchi E, Furuya K, et al. The role of the C-C chemokine receptor 2 gene polymorphism V64I (CCR2-64I) in sarcoidosis in a Japanese population. Am J Respir Crit Care Med 1999;159:2021–3.

41. Seitzer U, Swider C, Stuber F, et al. Tumour necrosis factor alpha promoter gene polymorphism in sarcoidosis. Cytokine 1997;9:787–90.

42. Takashige N, Naruse TK, Matsumori A, et al. Genetic polymorphisms at the tumour necrosis factor loci (TNFA and TNFB) in cardiac sarcoidosis. Tissue Antigens 1999;54:191–3.

43. Swider C, Schnittger L, Bogunia-Kubik K, et al. TNF-alpha and HLA-DR genotyping as potential prognostic markers in pulmonary sarcoidosis. Eur Cytokine Netw 1999;10:143–6.

44. Foley PJ, Lympany PA, Puscinska E, et al. Analysis of MHC encoded antigen-processing genes TAP1 and TAP2 polymorphisms in sarcoidosis. Am J Respir Crit Care Med 1999;160:1009–14.

45. Seitzer U, Gerdes J, Muller-Quernheim J. Evidence for disease phenotype associated haplotypes (DR.TNF) in sarcoidosis. Sarcoidosis Vasc Diffuse Lung Dis 2001;18:279–83.

46. Rybicki BA, Maliarik MJ, Malvitz E, et al. The influence of T cell receptor and cytokine genes on sarcoidosis susceptibility in African Americans. Hum Immunol 1999;60:867–74.

47. Murakozy G, Gaede KI, Zissel G, et al. Analysis of gene polymorphisms in interleukin-10 and transforming growth factor-beta 1 in sarcoidosis. Sarcoidosis Vasc Diffuse Lung Dis 2001;18:165–9.

48. Pabst R, Schuster M, Tschernig T. Lymphocyte dynamics in the pulmonary microenvironment: implications for the pathophysiology of pulmonary sarcoidosis. Sarcoidosis Vasc Diffuse Lung Dis 1999;16:197–202.

49. Tschernig T, Pabst R. Bronchus-associated lymphoid tissue (BALT) is not present in the normal adult lung but in different diseases. Pathobiology 2000;68:1–8.

50. Mulligan MS, Vaporciyan AA, Warner RL, et al. Compartmentalized roles for leukocytic adhesion molecules in lung inflammatory injury. J Immunol 1995;154:1350–63.

51. Saltini C, Kirby M, Trapnell BC, et al. Biased accumulation of T lymphocytes with "memory"-type CD45 leukocyte common antigen gene expression on the epithelial surface of the human lung. J Exp Med 1990;171:1123–40.

52. Fazel SB, Howie SE, Krajewski AS, Lamb D. Increased CD45RO expression on T lymphocytes in mediastinal lymph node and pulmonary lesions of patients with pulmonary sarcoidosis. Clin Exp Immunol 1994;95:509–13.

53. Forrester JM, Newman LS, Wang Y, et al. Clonal expansion of lung V delta 1+ T cells in pulmonary sarcoidosis. J Clin Invest 1993;91:292–300.

54. Balbi B, Moller DR, Kirby M, et al. Increased numbers of T lymphocytes with gamma delta–positive antigen receptors in a subgroup of individuals with pulmonary sarcoidosis. J Clin Invest 1990;85:1353–61.

55. Hunninghake GW, Bedell GN, Zavala DC, et al. Role of interleukin-2 release by lung T-cells in active pulmonary sarcoidosis. Am Rev Respir Dis 1983;128:634–8.

56. Pinkston P, Bitterman PB, Crystal RG. Spontaneous release of interleukin-2 by lung T lymphocytes in active pulmonary sarcoidosis. N Engl J Med 1983;308:793–800.

57. Muller-Quernheim J, Pfeifer S, Kienast K, Zissel G. Spontaneous interleukin 2 release of bronchoalveolar lavage cells in sarcoidosis is a codeterminator of prognosis. Lung 1996;174:243–53.

58. Wallace WA, Howie SE. Immunoreactive interleukin 4 and interferon-gamma expression by type II alveolar epithelial cells in interstitial lung disease. J Pathol 1999;187:475–80.

59. Lukacs NW, Hogaboam C, Chensue SW, et al. Type 1/type 2 cytokine paradigm and the progression of pulmonary fibrosis. Chest 2001;120:5S–8S.

60. Striz I, Mio T, Adachi Y, et al. IL-4 and IL-13 stimulate human bronchial epithelial cells to release IL-8. Inflammation 1999;23:545–55.

61. Bingisser R, Speich R, Zollinger A, et al. Interleukin-10 secretion by alveolar macrophages and monocytes in sarcoidosis. Respiration 2000;67:280–6.

62. Brubaker JO, Montaner LJ. Role of interleukin-13 in innate and adaptive immunity. Cell Mol Biol (Noisy-le-grand) 2001;47:637–51.

63. Hancock A, Armstrong L, Gama R, Millar A. Production of interleukin 13 by alveolar macrophages from normal and fibrotic lung. Am J Respir Cell Mol Biol 1998;18:60–5.

64. Zhu Z, Homer RJ, Wang Z, et al. Pulmonary expression of interleukin-13 causes inflammation, mucus hypersecretion, subepithelial fibrosis, physiologic abnormalities, and eotaxin production. J Clin Invest 1999;103:779–88.

65. Linden A, Hoshino H, Laan M. Airway neutrophils and interleukin-17. Eur Respir J 2000;15:973–7.

66. Laan M, Cui ZH, Hoshino H, et al. Neutrophil recruitment by human IL-17 via C-X-C chemokine release in the airways. J Immunol 1999;162:2347–52.

67. Robinson BW, McLemore TL, Crystal RG. Gamma interferon is spontaneously released by alveolar macrophages and lung

T lymphocytes in patients with pulmonary sarcoidosis. J Clin Invest 1985;75:1488–95.

68. Wahlstrom J, Katchar K, Wigzell H, et al. Analysis of intracellular cytokines in CD4+ and CD8+ lung and blood T cells in sarcoidosis. Am J Respir Crit Care Med 2001;163: 115–21.

69. Shigehara K, Shijubo N, Ohmichi M, et al. IL-12 and IL-18 are increased and stimulate IFN-gamma production in sarcoid lungs. J Immunol 2001;166:642–9.

70. Moller DR, Forman JD, Liu MC, et al. Enhanced expression of IL-12 associated with Th1 cytokine profiles in active pulmonary sarcoidosis. J Immunol 1996;156:4952–60.

71. Farber JM. Mig and IP-10: CXC chemokines that target lymphocytes. J Leukoc Biol 1997;61:246–57.

72. Agostini C, Trentin L, Perin A, et al. Regulation of alveolar macrophage-T cell interactions during Th1-type sarcoid inflammatory process. Am J Physiol 1999;277:L240–50.

73. Romagnani S. The Th1/Th2 paradigm. Immunol Today 1997;18:263–6.

74. Agostini C, Garbisa S, Trentin L, et al. Pulmonary alveolar macrophages from patients with active sarcoidosis express type IV collagenolytic proteinase. An enzymatic mechanism for influx of mononuclear phagocytes at sites of disease activity. J Clin Invest 1989;84:605–12.

75. Lohmann-Matthes ML, Steinmuller C, Franke-Ullmann G. Pulmonary macrophages. Eur Respir J 1994;7:1678–89.

76. Thompson AB, Robbins RA, Romberger DJ, et al. Immunological functions of the pulmonary epithelium. Eur Respir J 1995;8:127–49.

77. Iyonaga K, Suga M, Ichiyasu H, et al. Measurement of serum monocyte chemoattractant protein-1 and its clinical application for estimating the activity of granuloma formation in sarcoidosis. Sarcoidosis Vasc Diffuse Lung Dis 1998;15: 165–72.

78. Hashimoto S, Nakayama T, Gon Y, et al. Correlation of plasma monocyte chemoattractant protein-1 (MCP-1) and monocyte inflammatory protein-1alpha (MIP-1alpha) levels with disease activity and clinical course of sarcoidosis. Clin Exp Immunol 1998;111:604–10.

79. Sugiyama Y, Kasahara T, Mukaida N, et al. Chemokines in the bronchoalveolar lavage fluid of patients with sarcoidosis. Ann Intern Med 1997;36:856–60.

80. Smith RE, Strieter RM, Zhang K, et al. A role for C-C chemokines in fibrotic lung disease. J Leukoc Biol 1995; 57:782–7.

81. Kreipe H, Radzun HJ, Heidorn K, et al. Proliferation, macrophage colony-stimulating factor, and macrophage colony-stimulating factor-receptor expression of alveolar macrophages in active sarcoidosis. Lab Invest 1990;62: 697–703.

82. Enthammer C, Zambello R, Trentin L, et al. Synthesis and release of granulocyte-macrophage colony–stimulating factor by alveolar macrophages of patients with sarcoidosis. Sarcoidosis 1993;10:147–8.

83. Agostini C, Trentin L, Zambello R, et al. Pulmonary alveolar macrophages in patients with sarcoidosis and hypersensitivity pneumonitis: characterization by monoclonal antibodies. J Clin Immunol 1987;7:64–70.

84. Krombach F, Gerlach JT, Padovan C, et al. Characterization and quantification of alveolar monocyte-like cells in human chronic inflammatory lung disease. Eur Respir J 1996;9:984–91.

85. Toossi Z, Hirsch CS, Hamilton BD, et al. Decreased production of TGF-beta 1 by human alveolar macrophages compared with blood monocytes. J Immunol 1996;156:3461–8.

86. Chelen CJ, Fang Y, Freeman GJ, et al. Human alveolar macrophages present antigen ineffectively due to defective expression of B7 costimulatory cell surface molecules. J Clin Invest 1995;95:1415–21.

87. Agostini C, Adami F, Semenzato G. New pathogenetic insights

into the sarcoid granuloma. Curr Opin Rheumatol 2000; 12:71–6.

88. Rogge L, Papi A, Presky DH, et al. Antibodies to the IL-12 receptor beta 2 chain mark human Th1 but not Th2 cells in vitro and in vivo. J Immunol 1999;162:3926–32.

89. Shigehara K, Shijubo N, Ohmichi M, et al. Enhanced mRNA expression of Th1 cytokines and IL-12 in active pulmonary sarcoidosis. Sarcoidosis Vasc Diffuse Lung Dis 2000;17: 151–7.

90. Minshall EM, Tsicopoulos A, Yasruel Z, et al. Cytokine mRNA gene expression in active and nonactive pulmonary sarcoidosis. Eur Respir J 1997;10:2034–9.

91. Taha RA, Minshall EM, Olivenstein R, et al. Increased expression of IL-12 receptor mRNA in active pulmonary tuberculosis and sarcoidosis. Am J Respir Crit Care Med 1999;160:1119–23.

92. Agostini C, Trentin L, Facco M, et al. Role of IL-15, IL-2, and their receptors in the development of T cell alveolitis in pulmonary sarcoidosis. J Immunol 1996;157:910–8.

93. Zissel G, Baumer I, Schlaak M, Muller-Quernheim J. In vitro release of interleukin-15 by broncho-alveolar lavage cells and peripheral blood mononuclear cells from patients with different lung diseases. Eur Cytokine Netw 2000;11:105–12.

94. Cassatella MA, McDonald PP. Interleukin-15 and its impact on neutrophil function. Curr Opin Hematol 2000;7:174–7.

95. Dinarello CA. Interleukin-18, a proinflammatory cytokine. Eur Cytokine Netw 2000;11:483–6.

96. Greene CM, Meachery G, Taggart CC, et al. Role of IL-18 in CD4+ T lymphocyte activation in sarcoidosis. J Immunol 2000;165:4718–24.

97. Fukami T, Miyazaki E, Matsumoto T, et al. Elevated expression of interleukin-18 in the granulomatous lesions of muscular sarcoidosis. Clin Immunol 2001;101:12–20.

98. Shigehara K, Shijubo N, Ohmichi M, et al. Increased levels of interleukin-18 in patients with pulmonary sarcoidosis. Am J Respir Crit Care Med 2000;162:1979–82.

99. Itoh A, Yamaguchi E, Kuzumaki N, et al. Expression of granulocyte-macrophage colony-stimulating factor mRNA by inflammatory cells in the sarcoid lung. Am J Respir Cell Mol Biol 1990;3:245–9.

100. Zissel G, Homolka J, Schlaak J, et al. Anti-inflammatory cytokine release by alveolar macrophages in pulmonary sarcoidosis. Am J Respir Crit Care Med 1996;154:713–9.

101. Agostini C, Zambello R, Sancetta R, et al. Expression of tumor necrosis factor-receptor superfamily members by lung T lymphocytes in interstitial lung disease. Am J Respir Crit Care Med 1996;153:1359–67.

102. Agostini C. Cytokine and chemokine blockade as immunointervention strategy for the treatment of diffuse lung diseases. Sarcoidosis Vasc Diffuse Lung Dis 2001;18:18–22.

103. Baughman RP, Strohofer SA, Buchsbaum J, Lower EE. Release of tumor necrosis factor by alveolar macrophages of patients with sarcoidosis. J Lab Clin Med 1990;115:36–42.

104. Sibille Y, Marchandise FX. Pulmonary immune cells in health and disease: polymorphonuclear neutrophils. Eur Respir J 1993;6:1529–43.

105. Car BD, Meloni F, Luisetti M, et al. Elevated IL-8 and MCP-1 in the bronchoalveolar lavage fluid of patients with idiopathic pulmonary fibrosis and pulmonary sarcoidosis. Am J Respir Crit Care Med 1994;149:655–9.

106. Murphy PM, Baggiolini M, Charo IF, et al. International union of pharmacology. XXII. Nomenclature for chemokine receptors. Pharmacol Rev 2000;52:145–76.

107. Zlotnik A, Morales J, Hedrick JA. Recent advances in chemokines and chemokine receptors. Crit Rev Immunol 1999;19:1–47.

108. Kunkel SL, Lukacs NW, Strieter RM, Chensue SW. Th1 and Th2 responses regulate experimental lung granuloma development. Sarcoidosis Vasc Diffuse Lung Dis 1996; 13:120–8.

109. Yoshimoto T, Wang CR, Yoneto T, et al. Role of IL-16 in delayed-type hypersensitivity reaction. Blood 2000;95: 2869–74.

110. Waldmann T, Tagaya Y, Bamford R. Interleukin-2, interleukin-15, and their receptors. Int Rev Immunol 1998;16:205–26.

111. Agostini C, Basso U, Semenzato G. Cells and molecules involved in the development of sarcoid granuloma. J Clin Immunol 1998;18:184–92.

112. Hunninghake GW, Crystal RG. Pulmonary sarcoidosis: a disorder mediated by excess helper T- lymphocyte activity at sites of disease activity. N Engl J Med 1981;305:429–34.

113. Semenzato G, Pezzutto A, Chilosi M, Pizzolo G. Redistribution of T lymphocytes in the lymph nodes of patients with sarcoidosis. N Engl J Med 1982;306:48–9.

114. Nicod LP, Cochand L, Dreher D. Antigen presentation in the lung: dendritic cells and macrophages. Sarcoidosis Vasc Diffuse Lung Dis 2000;17:246–55.

115. Devergne O, Marfaing-Koka A, Schall TJ, et al. Production of the RANTES chemokine in delayed-type hypersensitivity reactions: involvement of macrophages and endothelial cells. J Exp Med 1994;179:1689–94.

116. Agostini C, Cassatella M, Zambello R, et al. Involvement of the IP-10 chemokine in sarcoid granulomatous reactions. J Immunol 1998;161:6413–20.

117. Tani K, Ogushi F, Huang L, et al. CD13/aminopeptidase N, a novel chemoattractant for T lymphocytes in pulmonary sarcoidosis. Am J Respir Crit Care Med 2000;161:1636–42.

118. Konishi K, Moller DR, Saltini C, et al. Spontaneous expression of the interleukin 2 receptor gene and presence of functional interleukin 2 receptors on T lymphocytes in the blood of individuals with active pulmonary sarcoidosis. J Clin Invest 1988;82:775–81.

119. Semenzato G, Agostini C, Trentin L, et al. Evidence of cells bearing interleukin-2 receptor at sites of disease activity in sarcoid patients. Clin Exp Immunol 1984;57:331–7.

120. Chilosi M, Menestrina F, Capelli P, et al. Immunohistochemical analysis of sarcoid granulomas. Evaluation of Ki67+ and interleukin-1+ cells. Am J Pathol 1988;131:191–8.

121. Bitterman PB, Saltzman LE, Adelberg S, et al. Alveolar macrophage replication. One mechanism for the expansion of the mononuclear phagocyte population in the chronically inflamed lung. J Clin Invest 1984;74:460–9.

122. Xing Z, Braciak T, Ohkawara Y, et al. Gene transfer for cytokine functional studies in the lung: the multifunctional role of GM-CSF in pulmonary inflammation. J Leukoc Biol 1996;59:481–8.

123. Prieditis H, Adamson IY. Alveolar macrophage kinetics and multinucleated giant cell formation after lung injury. J Leukoc Biol 1996;59:534–8.

124. Menestrina F, Lestani M, Mombello A, et al. Transbronchial biopsy in sarcoidosis: the role of immunohistochemical analysis for granuloma detection. Sarcoidosis 1992;9:95–100.

125. Lem VM, Lipscomb MF, Weissler JC, et al. Bronchoalveolar cells from sarcoid patients demonstrate enhanced antigen presentation. J Immunol 1985;135:1766–71.

126. Center DM, Kornfeld H, Cruikshank WW. Interleukin 16 and its function as a CD4 ligand. Immunol Today 1996; 17:476–81.

127. O'Regan AW, Chupp GL, Lowry JA, et al. Osteopontin is associated with T cells in sarcoid granulomas and has T cell adhesive and cytokine-like properties in vitro. J Immunol 1999;162:1024–31.

128. Baumer I, Zissel G, Schlaak M, Muller-Quernheim J. Th1/Th2 cell distribution in pulmonary sarcoidosis. Am J Respir Cell Mol Biol 1997;16:171–7.

129. Usui Y, Kohsaka H, Eishi Y, et al. Shared amino acid motifs in T-cell receptor beta junctional regions of bronchoalveolar T cells in patients with pulmonary sarcoidosis. Am J Respir Crit Care Med 1996;154:50–6.

130. Trentin L, Zambello R, Facco M, et al. Selection of T lymphocytes bearing limited TCR-Vbeta regions in the lung of hypersensitivity pneumonitis and sarcoidosis. Am J Respir Crit Care Med 1997;155:587–96.

131. Jones CM, Lake RA, Wijeyekoon JB, et al. Oligoclonal V gene usage by T lymphocytes in bronchoalveolar lavage fluid from sarcoidosis patients. Am J Respir Cell Mol Biol 1996;14:470–7.

132. Grunewald J, Berlin M, Olerup O, Eklund A. Lung T-helper cells expressing T-cell receptor AV2S3 associate with clinical features of pulmonary sarcoidosis. Am J Respir Crit Care Med 2000;161:814–8.

133. Grunewald J, Olerup O, Persson U, et al. T-cell receptor variable region gene usage by CD4+ and CD8+ T cells in bronchoalveolar lavage fluid and peripheral blood of sarcoidosis patients. Proc Natl Acad Sci U S A 1994;91:4965–9.

134. Forrester JM, Wang Y, Ricalton N, et al. TCR expression of activated T cell clones in the lungs of patients with pulmonary sarcoidosis. J Immunol 1994;153:4291–302.

135. Forman JD, Klein JT, Silver RF, et al. Selective activation and accumulation of oligoclonal V beta-specific T cells in active pulmonary sarcoidosis. J Clin Invest 1994;94:1533–42.

136. Du Bois RM, Kirby M, Balbi B, et al. T-lymphocytes that accumulate in the lung in sarcoidosis have evidence of recent stimulation of the T-cell antigen receptor. Am Rev Respir Dis 1992;145:1205–11.

137. Cerutti A, Trentin L, Zambello R, et al. Selection of Valpha 2.3 cells in the lung of patients with sarcoidosis. Sarcoidosis 1993;10:165–6.

138. Bulfone-Paus S, Ungureanu D, Pohl T, et al. Interleukin-15 protects from lethal apoptosis in vivo. Nat Med 1997;3: 1124–8.

139. Alderson MR, Tough TW, Davis-Smith T, et al. Fas ligand mediates activation-induced cell death in human T lymphocytes. J Exp Med 1995;181:71–7.

140. Kunitake R, Kuwano K, Miyazaki H, et al. Apoptosis in the course of granulomatous inflammation in pulmonary sarcoidosis. Eur Respir J 1999;13:1329–37.

141. Agostini C, Perin A, Semenzato G. Cell apoptosis and granulomatous lung diseases. Curr Opin Pulm Med 1998;4:261–6.

142. Rutherford RM, Kehren J, Staedtler F, et al. Functional genomics in sarcoidosis—reduced or increased apoptosis? Swiss Med Wkly 2001;131:459–70.

143. Agostini C, Semenzato G. Immunology of idiopathic pulmonary fibrosis. Curr Opin Pulm Med 1996;2:364–9.

144. Crouch E. Pathobiology of pulmonary fibrosis. Am J Physiol 1990;259:L159–84.

145. Cassatella MA, Berton G, Agostini C, et al. Generation of superoxide anion by alveolar macrophages in sarcoidosis: evidence for the activation of the oxygen metabolism in patients with high-intensity alveolitis. Immunology 1989;66:451–8.

146. Lenz AG, Costabel U, Maier KL. Oxidized BAL fluid proteins in patients with interstitial lung diseases. Eur Respir J 1996;9:307–12.

147. Facchetti F, Vermi W, Fiorentini S, et al. Expression of inducible nitric oxide synthase in human granulomas and histiocytic reactions. Am J Pathol 1999;154:145–52.

148. Sciaky D, Brazer W, Center DM, et al. Cultured human fibroblasts express constitutive IL-16 mRNA: cytokine induction of active IL-16 protein synthesis through a caspase-3-dependent mechanism. J Immunol 2000;164:3806–14.

149. Koyama S, Sato E, Masubuchi T, et al. Human lung fibroblasts release chemokinetic activity for monocytes constitutively. Am J Physiol 1998;275:L223–30.

150. Suganuma H, Sato A, Tamura R, Chida K. Enhanced migration of fibroblasts derived from lungs with fibrotic lesions. Thorax 1995;50:984–9.

151. Rennard SI, Hunninghake GW, Bitterman PB, Crystal RG. Production of fibronectin by the human alveolar macrophage: mechanism for the recruitment of fibroblasts

to sites of tissue injury in interstitial lung diseases. Proc Natl Acad Sci U S A 1981;78:7147–51.

152. Homma S, Nagaoka I, Abe H, et al. Localization of platelet-derived growth factor and insulin-like growth factor I in the fibrotic lung. Am J Respir Crit Care Med 1995;152:2084–9.

153. Gray AJ, Bishop JE, Reeves JT, et al. Partially degraded fibrin(ogen) stimulates fibroblast proliferation in vitro. Am J Respir Cell Mol Biol 1995;12:684–90.

154. Doucet C, Brouty-Boye D, Pottin-Clemenceau C, et al. IL-4 and IL-13 specifically increase adhesion molecule and inflammatory cytokine expression in human lung fibroblasts. Int Immunol 1998;10:1421–33.

155. Miyazaki Y, Araki K, Vesin C, et al. Expression of a tumor necrosis factor-alpha transgene in murine lung causes lymphocytic and fibrosing alveolitis. A mouse model of progressive pulmonary fibrosis. J Clin Invest 1995;96:250–9.

156. Uhal BD, Joshi I, True AL, et al. Fibroblasts isolated after fibrotic lung injury induce apoptosis of alveolar epithelial cells in vitro. Am J Physiol 1995;269:L819–28.

157. Chilosi M, Lestani M, Benedetti A, et al. Constitutive expression of tenascin in T-dependent zones of human lymphoid tissues. Am J Pathol 1993;143:1348–55.

158. Kasper M, Gunthert U, Dall P, et al. Distinct expression patterns of CD44 isoforms during human lung development and in pulmonary fibrosis. Am J Respir Cell Mol Biol 1995;13:648–56.

159. Levi-Schaffer F, Garbuzenko E, Rubin A, et al. Human eosinophils regulate human lung- and skin-derived fibroblast properties in vitro: a role for transforming growth factor beta (TGF-beta). Proc Natl Acad Sci U S A 1999;96:9660–5.

160. Limper AH, Colby TV, Sanders MS, et al. Immunohistochemical localization of transforming growth factor-beta 1 in the nonnecrotizing granulomas of pulmonary sarcoidosis. Am J Respir Crit Care Med 1994;149:197–204.

161. Shahar I, Fireman E, Topilsky M, et al. Effect of IL-6 on alveolar fibroblast proliferation in interstitial lung diseases. Clin Immunol Immunopathol 1996;79:244–51.

162. Vignaud JM, Allam M, Martinet N, et al. Presence of platelet-derived growth factor in normal and fibrotic lung is specifically associated with interstitial macrophages, while both interstitial macrophages and alveolar epithelial cells express the c-sis proto-oncogene. Am J Respir Cell Mol Biol 1991;5:531–8.

163. Korfhagen TR, Swantz RJ, Wert SE, et al. Respiratory epithelial cell expression of human transforming growth factor-alpha induces lung fibrosis in transgenic mice. J Clin Invest 1994;93:1691–9.

164. Salez F, Gosset P, Copin MC, et al. Transforming growth factor-beta1 in sarcoidosis. Eur Respir J 1998;12:913–9.

165. Allen JT, Bloor CA, Knight RA, Spiteri MA. Expression of insulin-like growth factor binding proteins in bronchoalveolar lavage fluid of patients with pulmonary sarcoidosis. Am J Respir Cell Mol Biol 1998;19:250–8.

166. Agostini C, Siviero M, Semenzato G. Immune effector cells in idiopathic pulmonary fibrosis. Curr Opin Pulm Med 1997;3:348–55.

167. Hunninghake GW, Gilbert S, Pueringer R, et al. Outcome of the treatment for sarcoidosis. Am J Respir Crit Care Med 1994;149:893–8.

168. Gibson GJ, Prescott RJ, Muers MF, et al. British Thoracic Society Sarcoidosis study: effects of long term corticosteroid treatment. Thorax 1996;51:238–47.

169. Paramothayan NS, Jones PW. Corticosteroids for pulmonary sarcoidosis. Cochrane Database Syst Rev 2000;2,CD0011/4.

170. Berkman N, Jose PJ, Williams TJ, et al. Corticosteroid inhibition of macrophage inflammatory protein-1 alpha in human monocytes and alveolar macrophages. Am J Physiol 1995;269:L443–52.

171. Kwon OJ, Jose PJ, Robbins RA, et al. Glucocorticoid inhibition of RANTES expression in human lung epithelial cells. Am J Respir Cell Mol Biol 1995;12:488–96.

172. Baughman RP, Winget DB, Lower EE. Methotrexate is steroid sparing in acute sarcoidosis: results of a double blind, randomized trial. Sarcoidosis Vasc Diffuse Lung Dis 2000;17:60–6.

173. Baughman RP, Lower EE. The effect of corticosteroid or methotrexate therapy on lung lymphocytes and macrophages in sarcoidosis. Am Rev Respir Dis 1990;142:1268–71.

174. Lynch JP 3rd, McCune WJ. Immunosuppressive and cytotoxic pharmacotherapy for pulmonary disorders. Am J Respir Crit Care Med 1997;155:395–420.

175. Lewis SJ, Ainslie GM, Bateman ED. Efficacy of azathioprine as second-line treatment in pulmonary sarcoidosis. Sarcoidosis Vasc Diffuse Lung Dis 1999;16:87–92.

176. Muller-Quernheim J, Kienast K, Held M, et al. Treatment of chronic sarcoidosis with an azathioprine/prednisolone regimen. Eur Respir J 1999;14:1117–22.

177. Martinet Y, Pinkston P, Saltini C, et al. Evaluation of the in vitro and in vivo effects of cyclosporine on the lung T-lymphocyte alveolitis of active pulmonary sarcoidosis. Am Rev Respir Dis 1988;138:1242–8.

178. Wyser CP, van Schalkwyk EM, Alheit B, et al. Treatment of progressive pulmonary sarcoidosis with cyclosporin A. A randomized controlled trial. Am J Respir Crit Care Med 1997;156:1371–6.

179. Baughman RP, Ohmichi M, Lower EE. Combination therapy for sarcoidosis. Sarcoidosis Vasc Diffuse Lung Dis 2001;18:133–7.

180. Baughman RP, Lower EE. Infliximab for refractory sarcoidosis. Sarcoidosis Vasc Diffuse Lung Dis 2001;18:70–4.

181. Yee AM, Pochapin MB. Treatment of complicated sarcoidosis with infliximab anti-tumor necrosis factor-alpha therapy. Ann Intern Med 2001;135:27–31.

13 THE FUTURE OF MEDICAL THERAPY FOR LUNG FIBROSIS

MARVIN I. SCHWARZ
KEVIN K. BROWN

There are several important considerations regarding the development of new approaches for treatment of the fibrotic lung disorders. In idiopathic pulmonary fibrosis (IPF), for example, because the inciting injury(s) is unknown, advice regarding avoidance, as is the case for hypersensitivity pneumonitis, the pneumoconioses, and drug-induced pneumonitis, is not possible. Except for a small number of patients with familial IPF, we are unaware of genetic mutations that place an individual at risk for developing IPF. Although our understanding of pathobiology has increased in the past 20 years because of the development of animal models of lung fibrosis, and in particular the relationship between inflammation, fibrosis, and cytokine function, none of these models are representative of IPF. For most patients with IPF, the initial contact with a pulmonologist occurs at a stage of advanced disease. To date, we do not have reproducible screening biomarkers for this group of diseases. All patients over the age of 60 cannot get screening high-resolution computed tomography (HRCT). Moreover, primary care physicians often discount radiographic abnormalities if symptoms are absent or minimal or if routine physiological testing (office spirometry) shows minimal or no abnormalities. In many cases, particularly those with normal or minimal change on chest radiographs, months to years are lost because inaccurate diagnoses such as reactive airway disease, chronic obstructive lung disease, or congestive failure are made. It is the general rule that interstitial lung diseases, (ILDs) regardless of the etiology, will progress, albeit at different rates, in individual patients. If effective therapy for IPF is developed, it is likely that therapeutic success will be realized if patients are diagnosed during the earlier stages of disease.

CURRENT TREATMENT PROBLEMS

There is no effective therapy for several of the idiopathic interstitial pneumonias (IIPs), including usual interstitial pneumonia (UIP), acute interstitial pneumonia (AIP), and the fibrotic forms of nonspecific interstitial pneumonia (NSIP). The traditional concept that injury evokes inflammation, which in turn signals fibroproliferation, does not hold up in some of these IIPs. Although corticosteroid therapy with or without additional immunosuppression is still recommended for IPF, it is clear that for the great majority of patients, it does not alter the outcome.[1–3] Why then is this still the recommendation? First, no other proven treatments are currently available. Second, this treatment has been shown to be efficacious in other ILDs, and in the absence of a definitive diagnosis, a short trial of several months seems reasonable. Hypersensitivity pneumonia, eosinophilic pneumonia, organizing pneumonia, the more cellular forms of NSIP, and desquamative interstitial pneumonia clearly are responsive. Before the stricter histologic definition of IPF that requires underlying UIP, other IIPs were considered to be earlier, more cellular forms of IPF, and the older literature implies that 10 to 30% of patients will respond to treatment. Third, there are some patients with IPF in whom prolonged survival (5 to 10 years) is possible; these patients are often active or former smokers, are usually younger at the time of diagnosis, and they often show less physiological deterioration when first seen.[4–6] Whether corticosteroid or immunosuppressive treatment contributes to this longer than expected survival is unknown because controlled trials using these therapies have never been carried out. It is clear that a progressive course, which eventually leads to death in under 5 years, is the expected outcome in more than 80% of patients with IPF.

ETIOLOGY OF FIBROSIS AND FUTURE TREATMENT OPTIONS

Three conferences sponsored by the National Heart, Lung and Blood Institute have concluded that new directions in the treatment of IPF must be developed.[7–9] There have been multiple publications by leaders in the field disagreeing with the concept that acute inflammation secondary to some unknown stimulus leads to fibrosis.[10–12] It is now the consensus that fibroproliferation in response to an injury, possibly to the alveolar epithelium, should be the new target for drug development.[7–12]

Two facts remain, however. The first is that the inflammatory milieu as measured in the bronchoalveolar lavage (BAL) fluid of IPF patients is characterized by increases in neutrophils and eosinophils. It is now apparent that these cells are washed from cystic honeycomb spaces in which there is mucostasis and that, possibly due to low-grade clinical infection, acute inflammatory cells accumulate (Figure 13–1). This BAL fluid finding indicates advanced UIP with cystic honeycomb change and represents a secondary rather than a primary event.

It is not known what the inciting injury is for IPF/UIP or NSIP. However, the less fibrotic forms of NSIP have improved survival rates with the standard recommended therapies.[13,14] Could these two histologic patterns represent different responses to the same inciting injury? In patients with a connective tissue disease such as rheumatoid arthritis, the underlying lung disease may be UIP, NSIP, AIP, organizing pneumonia, pulmonary capillaritis, or bronchiolitis obliterans, and presumably results from a common initiating injury. In several cases of familial pulmonary fibrosis, there was an association with a surfactant protein C point mutation, but dissimilar histologic patterns (UIP, NSIP) were found in first-degree relatives.[15] Moreover, there is evidence that demonstrates that both NSIP and UIP can be present in different lung samples from the same patient.[16] The clinical course in these individuals follows that of IPF/UIP.

Fibroproliferation, which characterizes IPF/UIP, represents a dysregulated attempt at repair in response to injury. This is driven by profibrotic cytokines and results in the excessive and persistent accumulation of extracellular matrix. Studies of human lung tissue indicate that there is an up-regulation of a number of profibrotic cytokines, possibly derived from injured epithelial cells, lymphocytes, or the fibroblasts themselves.[9–12]

A key feature of the UIP lesion is the structure known as the fibroblastic focus (Figure 13–2). It is located with the interstitium (alveolar walls) and is subepithelial in location. Its contents are the extracellular matrix elements such as proteoglycans, fibrillar collagen, decorin, and fibronectin, as well as focal aggregates of proliferating fibroblasts and myofibroblasts.[17–19] These foci are often found at the interface between normal and abnormal lung as well as in areas of established fibrosis (Figure 13–3). UIP is a temporally heterogeneous lesion consisting of active early fibroblastic proliferation within the fibroblastic foci, mature dense interstitial collagen, and end-stage cystic honeycomb change. These changes are interspersed in and adjacent to the normal remaining lung. The fibroblastic focus is sometimes the only, and therefore the first, recognizable abnormality seen within the interstitium (Figure 13–4). It is not unreasonable to suggest that, regardless of the initiating injury, potential new therapies for IPF/UIP should be directed toward control of the proliferation of fibroblastic foci and, thereby the inhibition of the dysregulated fibroproliferative response that is driven by proliferating fibroblasts and myofibroblasts.

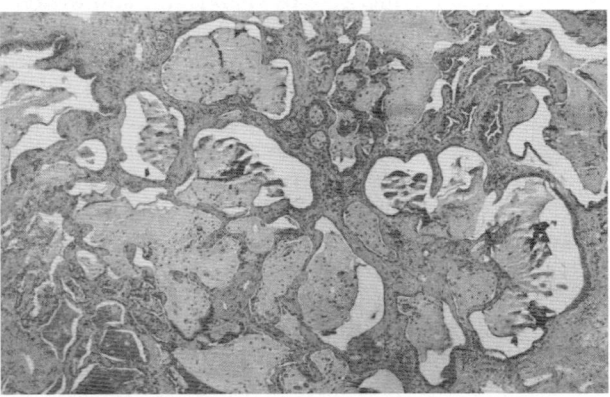

A

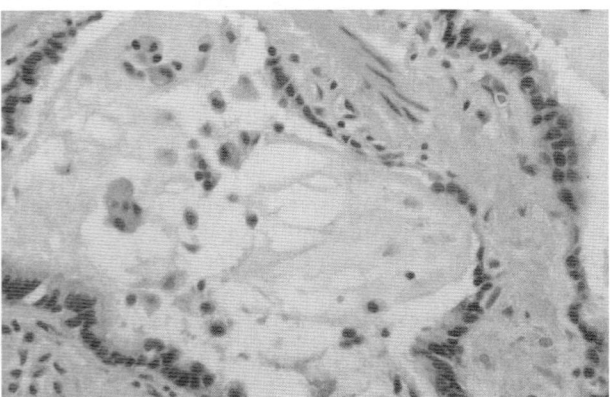

B

Figure 13–1   Usual interstitial pneumonia (UIP) with honeycomb change (hematoxylin and eosin; ×20 original magnification). Note the mucostasis within these cystic structures (A). High-power view (×40 original magnification) of mucus within cyst. Note the type 2 cell hyperplasia lining the cyst and the neutrophils and eosinophils within the cyst lumens (B).

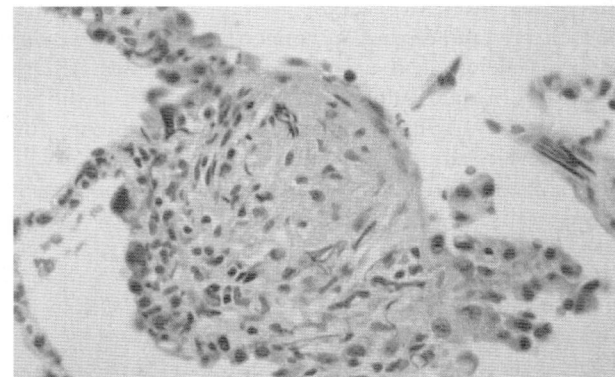

Figure 13–2   Fibroblastic focus in UIP (pentachrome stain; ×40 original magnification). The fibroblastic focus is subepithelial within the lung interstitium.

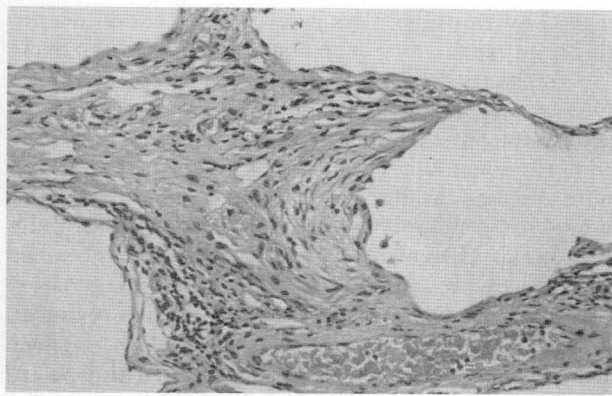

Figure 13–3 Fibroblastic focus in UIP (hematoxylin and eosin; ×20 original magnification). This fibroblastic focus is at the interface between collagenized and normal lung.

The majority of fibroblasts in IPF-affected lung are found within the fibroblastic focus, and in fibrotic collagenized lung are myofibroblasts (Figure 13–5).[19–23] Myofibroblasts are also abundant in granulating skin wounds and are found in areas of active fibrosis in lung models of fibrosis, as well as in human glomerulosclerosis and cirrhosis.[24,25] In the lung, the interstitial myofibroblast is probably derived from an adventitial myofibroblast or results from a phenotypic switch of the interstitial fibroblast, which can be induced by a number of profibrotic cytokines, including transforming growth factor (TGF)-β1 and platelet-derived growth factor (PDGF), which are overexpressed in IPF/UIP.[26–29]

Myofibroblasts can also support fibroproliferation because they are important sources of TGF-β1 and monocyte chemoattractant protein-1.[30] Reestablishment of the overlying epithelium is required to switch off proliferating myofibroblasts and induce myofibroblast apoptosis and is therefore critical for regulated repair. The proliferating subepithelial myofibroblast has

also been shown to induce apoptosis of the overlying epithelium, thereby preventing the return of an intact epithelial layer.[31]

It has recently been demonstrated that the number of fibroblastic foci is the histologic feature that best predicts survival in IPF/UIP.[5,25] The presence of increasing numbers of fibroblastic foci in the initial surgical lung biopsy specimen portends a poorer outcome. The Masson body, which characterizes organizing pneumonia, also consists of proliferating myofibroblasts in a loose connective tissue disease stroma (Figure 13–5). In contrast to an interstitial subepithelial location, as is the case for fibroblastic foci, Masson bodies are found within the lumens of the distal air spaces. Another differentiating feature between the Masson bodies and fibroblastic foci is the excellent therapeutic response and outcome of organizing pneumonia following corticosteroid treatment. Why is there this difference? The terminal deoxynucleotidyltransferase-mediated dUTP nick-end labeling (TUNEL) assay demonstrates apoptosis of myofibroblasts in Masson bodies but no or very little apoptosis in the fibroblastic foci of IPF/UIP.[32] Moreover, there is also decreased vascularity in the fibroblastic focus compared to the Masson body.[11] Future therapies for lung fibrosis (Table 13–1) should be developed to interfere with inducers of collagen production and the deposition of mature collagen.

Role of TGF-β1

All lung and inflammatory cells produce TGF-β1 and have its receptor on their cell surfaces. The profibrotic properties of TGF-β1, which is considered to be the central cytokine in organ fibrosis and wound healing, are summarized in Table 13–2. TGF-β1 is abundant in fibroblastic foci and in collagenized areas in IPF/UIP.[26] In IPF lung it is also expressed in epithelial cells, alveolar macrophages, and in hyperplastic type 2 cells.[33–35]

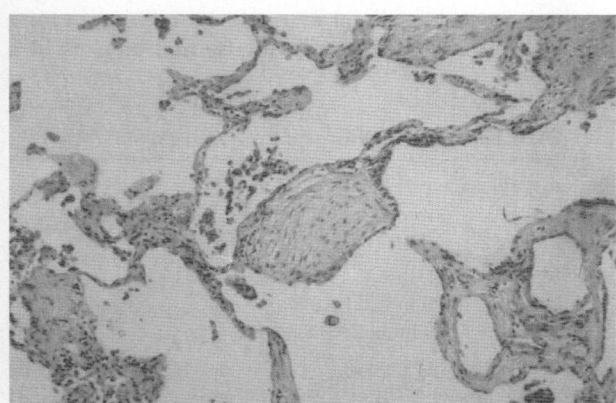

Figure 13–4 Fibroblastic focus in UIP (hematoxylin and eosin ×15 original magnification). The lone fibroblastic focus is expanding an otherwise normal-appearing interstitium.

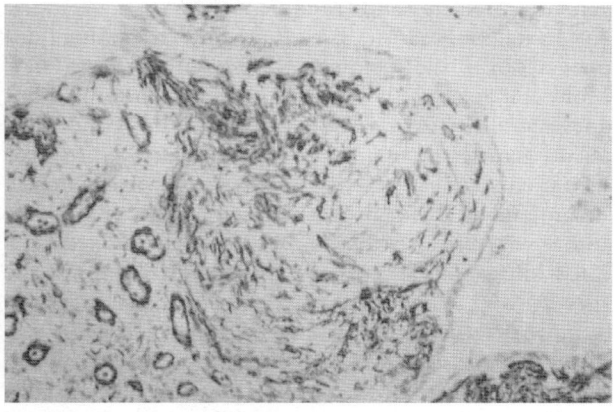

Figure 13–5 Fibroblastic focus in UIP (hematoxylin and eosin; ×40 original magnification). This is an α-smooth muscle actin stain showing myofibroblasts within the fibroblastic focus.

TABLE 13–1   Future Therapies for Lung Fibrosis

Directed against TGF-β_1
  IFN-γ
  Soluble TGF-β_1 receptors
  Human TGF-β_1 antibodies
  Decorin
  SMAD-7
  IL-7
  Pirfenidone
  Human antibodies to connective tissue growth factor
  Taurine/niacin
Directed against myofibroblast induction and survival
  Anti-TGF-β_1 therapies
  ET-1 receptor antagonists
  Anti-TNF-α therapies
    Soluble TNF-α fusion protein
    Chimeric monoclonal antibody
  ACE inhibitor
  Statin agents
Directed against collagen synthesis
  Halfuginone
  Collagen enzyme synthesis inhibitors
  Proline analogues

ACE = angiotensin-converting enzyme; ET-1 = endothelin 1; IFN = interferon; TGF = transforming growth factor; TNF = tumor necrosis factor.

Possible Anti-TGF-β_1 Therapies

Interferon (IFN)-γ is a T helper (Th)$_1$ cytokine produced by lymphocytes and neutral killer cells. It has a suppressive regulatory function affecting the accumulation of extracellular matrix. Its actions are in direct opposition to TGF-β_1. It down-regulates collagen and fibronectin synthesis and diminishes fibroblastic chemotaxis, thereby reducing myofibroblast numbers.[36–38] Importantly, it induces myofibroblast apoptosis via regulation of caspase expression and up-regulates angiostatic chemokines.[39–42] IFN-γ suppresses the Th$_2$ phenotype, reducing the production of interleukin (IL)-4 and IL-13, both profibrotic cytokines.[43] In a bleomycin model, IFN-γ reduced fibrosis, and this was reflected in a reduction in TGF-β_1 levels and decreases in procollagen and collagen I and III expression.[44,45]

In the lung, serum, BAL fluid, and circulating lymphocytes of IPF/UIP patients, IFN-γ is undetectable.[46–49] Molecular assessment of UIP lungs reveals no IFN-γ but does reveal increased levels of TGF-β_1 and connective tissue growth factor. A 12-month phase II trial of 18 patients with IPF/UIP, 9 of whom were treated with subcutaneous IFN-γ 3 times per week plus prednisone and 9 who were treated with prednisone alone, indicated improved gas exchange and lung volumes in the IFN-γ group.[49] The results of a phase III controlled trial of more than 300 patients showed no inhibitor of physiologic progression; however there was some evidence to suggest a survival advantage after 48 weeks versus controls ($p = .8$) (personal communication). Nevertheless, in those patients whose forced vital capacity (FVC) exceeded 33%, there was a significant survival advan-

tage. This however was not a primary endpoint, but rather an explanatory or retrospective look at the data.

Are there other potential anti-TGF-β_1 therapies? One animal model of pulmonary fibrosis involves the gene transfer of TGF-β_1 via an adenoviral vector; decorin, which is a naturally occurring extracellular matrix protein, inhibits the fibrosis induced by TGF-β_1 in this model.[50,51] One potential problem with global inhibition of TGF-β_1 as occasioned by decorin is the unwanted side effects, such as the loss of the anti-inflammatory properties of TGF-β_1. The possibility of trials of human monoclonal antibodies directed against TGF-β_1, which are now being tested in scleroderma, have exciting potential for the treatment of IPF/UIP.[52] TGF-β_1 antibodies have been shown to prevent fibrosis in a bleomycin model of lung fibrosis.[53–55] Connective tissue growth factor, a cytokine that mediates TGF-β_1 induction of collagen synthesis, may also be considered for monoclonal antibody therapy.[56] There is an available chimeric soluble receptor for TGF-β_1, which combines with TGF-β_1 before its attachment to its cellular receptor, that has reduced lung fibrosis in a bleomycin hamster model.[57] Like other cytokines, once TGF-β_1 attaches to its cellular receptor, its signal must be translocated to the nucleus where it effects specific target genes. To accomplish this, cytoplasmic transcription factors (intracellular signaling molecules) are activated. There is a naturally occurring inhibitory molecule (SMAD-7), which, if up-regulated, blocks the signal transmission of TGF-β_1 from the cell surface to the nucleus.[58] Another antifibrotic effect of IFN-γ is the up-regulation of SMAD-7.[57] Moreover, adenoviral transfer of SMAD-7 diminishes fibrosis in a bleomycin model by down-regulation of the TGF-β_1 signal.[58] Recent data demonstrate that IL-7, a Th$_1$ cytokine, inhibits TGF-β_1 production and signaling in fibroblasts in in vitro and in vivo systems.[59] This effect is associated with increases in SMAD-7 and is independent of IFN-γ. Retinoic acid inhibits TGF-β_1 collagen synthesis by inhibiting collagen gene transcription.[60]

Pirfenidone (5-methyl-1-phenyl-2(1H)-pyridone) is a compound that, in vitro, blocks TGF-β_1 collagen synthesis and extracellular matrix accumulation in lung fibroblasts obtained from fibrotic human lungs.[61] In a

TABLE 13–2   Profibrotic Properties of TGF-β_1

Fibroblast chemotaxis
Fibroblast and myofibroblast proliferation
Promotion of extracellular matrix components
Inhibition of the MMPs
Enhances the expression of TIMPs
Transformation of a fibroblast to a myofibroblast
Inhibition of angiogenesis
Up-regulation of connective tissue growth factor
Inhibition of myofibroblast apoptosis

*See references 43, 50, 62–69. MMP = matrix metalloproteinase; TIMP = tissue inhibitor of metalloproteinase.

single-center open label trial of pirfenidone in IPF, results were promising, demonstrating improved survival at 1 and 2 years when compared to historic controls.[70] This type of open label study is inherently difficult to interpret, even though the patients in this study had previously demonstrated progressive disease in spite of corticosteroid and immunosuppressive therapy. Side effects are common with pirfenidone, but only a few subjects in this study had to discontinue treatment. The results of a controlled trial with pirfenidone recently carried out in Japan are being evaluated.

Possible Treatments Directed Against Other Profibrotic Cytokines

Endothelin (ET)-1 is a potent vasoactive cytokine in the pulmonary circulation. It also has significant mitogenic effects on smooth muscle cells and fibroblasts.[71] Under normal conditions, the lung contains the greatest amount of ET-1 of all organs. Moreover, it enhances the transition of the fibroblast to the myofibroblast.[72] In patients with IPF, increased plasma levels of ET-1 and increased expression of this cytokine in lung tissue have been shown.[73] The synthesis of ET-1 is also enhanced by other profibrotic cytokines (TGF-β_1, tumor necrosis factor [TNF]-α, IL-1) as well as by hypoxia.[74–76] An ET-1 receptor antagonist (bosentan) reduced fibrosis induced by bleomycin in an animal model.[77] In humans with IPF, there is increased ET-1 mRNA expression and immunoreactivity in airway epithelial cells, proliferating type II pneumocytes, endothelial cells, and inflammatory cells.[78,79] Bosentan, which has been approved for the treatment of primary or connective tissue disease-associated pulmonary hypertension, is being considered for the treatment of fibrotic lung disorders, including IPF and the pulmonary fibrosis that occurs with scleroderma.

TNF-α

TNF-α is an important mediator of inflammation that causes the activation and margination of neutrophils, activation of the coagulation cascade, and activation of catabolism. Its major sources in the lung are the alveolar epithelium, the alveolar macrophage, and lymphocytes.[80–81] Its effects on fibroblasts are bidirectional. On one hand, it results in fibroblast/myofibroblast proliferation via the production of PDGF from the fibroblast itself, and on the other, it stimulates the fibroblast to release prostaglandin E_2, some metalloproteinases, and glycosaminoglycans, all of which are involved in extracellular matrix remodeling and the down-regulation of the fibroblastic response.[82–83] At the post-transcriptional level, it diminishes the production of fibroblast procollagen I, which is induced by TGF-β_1 stimulation.[84]

In experimental bleomycin models, fibrosis decreases after pretreatment with either antibodies against TNF-α or a recombinant TNF-α-soluble receptor.[85,86] Overexpression of the TNF-α gene induced with the use of a human surfactant protein C promoter in transgenic mice resulted in extensive fibrosis.[87] Compared to control lungs, in IPF lungs, TNF-α is found in proliferating alveolar epithelium and alveolar macrophages.[81] There is a commercially available soluble TNF-α receptor fusion protein that binds with and thereby inactivates the cytokine, as well as a commercially available chimeric monoclonal antibody that binds with circulating TNF-α. One or the other of these agents have shown beneficial clinical effects in rheumatoid arthritis, ankylosing spondylitis, Crohn's disease, and Wegener's granulomatosis.[88] Thalidomide inhibits intracellular processing of TNF-α and has shown efficacy in Crohn's disease.[89] Similar studies are unavailable in pulmonary fibrosis.

Although there are definite concerns about TNF-α blockade for IPF, the bulk of the available data support the profibrotic rather than the antifibrotic properties of this cytokine.

Other Possible Antifibrotic Therapies

Angiotensin-Converting Enzyme Inhibitors

Angiotensin II, which is derived from angiotensin I via proteolytic cleavage by angiotensin-converting enzyme (ACE), has a well-defined role in control of systemic blood pressure and intravascular volume. A less familiar aspect of angiotensin II is its profibrotic properties, more specifically, myofibroblast proliferation, which can be attenuated by ACE inhibitors in animal models of cardiac and renal fibrosis.[90–91] ACE levels are also elevated in the BAL fluid of patients with IPF, as well as in other potentially fibrotic lung diseases, such as sarcoidosis, the acute respiratory distress syndrome, and some pneumoconioses.[92,93] ACE inhibitors were successful in preventing the fibrosis associated with a radiation lung model.[94]

Angiotensin II is mitogenic for human lung fibroblasts in vitro, and this involves an autocrine effect of TGF-β_1. Anti-TGF-β_1 antibodies, but not antibodies to PDGF, inhibited this effect.[95] One human study indicated that there was a lack of protection against radiation-induced pneumonitis in patients receiving ACE inhibitors.[96] There are, however, very clear differences between the pathobiology and histology of radiation pneumonitis and those of IPF.

Statins

One of the key issues in IPF/UIP is the persistence of myofibroblasts in the lungs of IPF patients. There appears to be diminished apoptosis of these cell lines, which contributes to their longevity.[32] Agents that enhance fibroblast/myofibroblast apoptosis could have a role in the treatment of IPF.

The statins (3-hydroxy-3-methylglutaryl coenzyme A [HMG-CoA] reductase inhibitors) have proapoptotic properties in several malignant cell lines. One study of cultured fibroblasts from lungs with IPF indicated that in clinically available concentrations, lovastatin induced fibroblast apoptosis.[97] There are no clinical studies available in fibrotic lung disorders.

Relaxin

Relaxin is a polypeptide growth factor belonging to the insulin growth factor family that is necessary for restructuring the interuterine ligament and cervix during parturition by causing a loosening of collagen bundles or a decrease in their numbers.[98] Relaxin inhibits TGF-β_1-induced collagen and fibronectin production by cultured human lung fibroblasts. It also increases the expression of the proteolytic matrix metalloproteinases and decreases the production of the tissue inhibitors of metalloproteinases, resulting in breakdown or proteolysis of the extracellular matrix.[99] In vivo pretreatment with relaxin inhibited pulmonary fibrosis in two animal models.[100] Human relaxin also reduced interstitial fibrosis in an animal model of renal fibrosis.[101] Recombinant human relaxin has shown some promise in the treatment of diffuse scleroderma; however, the response of the pulmonary component, if present, was not commented on in that study.[102]

N-Acetylcysteine

There is evidence that links oxidative stress and diminished antioxidative activity in IPF.[103] Excessive numbers of reactive oxygen species have been identified in the lower respiratory tract of IPF patients. It has also been shown that glutathione, a major antioxidant in human lung tissue, regulates oxidant-induced cellular damage. Glutathione levels are reduced in the lungs of IPF patients.[104] It has been further suggested that this imbalance leads to oxidative injury to alveolar epithelial cells and tissue injury as a result of the oxidation of proteins and lipids. They also inactivate protease inhibitors and activate lipid mediators (leukotrienes). N-acetylcysteine (NAC) is a known precursor for glutathione synthesis. Aerosolized administration of NAC given 3 days prior to bleomycin attenuated fibrosis in an animal model.[105] However, it appears that this effect resulted from the amelioration of acute inflammation rather than a direct effect on fibroblast proliferation.

One small human study (20 patients) indicated that the oral administration of NAC (600 mg 3 times/day) increased glutathione levels in the BAL fluid. This was accompanied by improvements in pulmonary function.[106] A large-scale phase III trial in Europe is coming to a close. It is not inconceivable that oral NAC may be employed as an adjuvant to other antifibrotic therapy.

Taurine-Niacin

Taurine and niacin have been shown to protect against oxidative tissue damage in in vivo and in vitro models of inflammation and oxidative stress.[107,108] In a bleomycin model of lung fibrosis, this combination reduced collagen accumulation. This was associated with a decrease in types I and III procollagen.[109–111] This reduction in collagen was due in part to a decrease in TGF-β_1 mRNA levels resulting from reduced gene transcription.[111] There have been no human trials with taurine-niacin.

Halfuginone

Halfuginone is an antiparasitic plant alkaloid used in veterinary medicine that inhibits collagen type I synthesis at the transcriptional level.[112] This agent has been shown to prevent fibrosis in graft-versus-host disease in mice and in a bleomycin model of lung fibrosis.[112,113] A phase II trial that makes use of an ointment for the skin fibrosis of scleroderma is in progress.

Interference with Collagen Synthesis

One interesting approach for the treatment of fibrotic disorders is the development of inhibitors of the enzymes involved in the synthesis of collagen. One possibility is an inhibitor to the enzyme prolyl hydroxylase. Inhibition of its enzymatic functions has prevented scarring in models of skin and cardiac fibrosis.[114] This is a posttranslational enzyme, and others include c-proteinase and lysyl oxidase.[115]

Proline analogues are in vivo antifibrotic agents. They become incorporated into developing collagen in place of proline and impair the folding of procollagen, producing a defective product that undergoes degradation. Because these analogues are quickly degraded and potentially toxic, a slowly reduced polymer of a proline analogue was developed (cis-4-hydroxy-L-proline), which demonstrated sustained reduction of collagen in a bleomycin model of lung fibrosis.[116]

Organ-Specific Therapy

The novel therapies discussed require some form of systemic application, thereby increasing the possibility of unwanted side effects. Direct application (organ-specific therapy) via the inhaled route, using delivery systems capable of producing droplet sizes (< 5 µg) that deposit in the small airways and gas exchange units of the lung, could be the wave of the future for the treatment of the diffuse parenchymal lung diseases. The delivery of a protein such as insulin via a handheld nebulizer indicates the metabolic efficacy of this form of therapy. In this case, there is the desired systemic absorption, indicating the passage of protein from the airway to the circulation.[117] Preliminary data regarding aerosol delivery of IFN-γ indicate both biologic activity and a lack of systemic side effects.[118]

REFERENCES

1. International Consensus Statement. Idiopathic pulmonary fibrosis: diagnosis and treatment. Am J Respir Crit Care Med 2000;161:646–64.

2. Douglas WW, Ryu JH, Schroeder DR. Idiopathic pulmonary fibrosis: impact of oxygen and colchicine, prednisone or no therapy in survival. Am J Respir Crit Care Med 2000; 161:1172–8.

3. Gay SE, Kazerooni EA, Towes GB, et al. Idiopathic pulmonary fibrosis: predicting response to therapy and survival. Am J Respir Crit Care Med 1998;157:1063–72.

4. Zisman DA, Lynch JP III, Towes G, et al. Cyclophosphamide in the treatment of idiopathic pulmonary fibrosis: a prospective study in patient who failed to respond to corticosteroids. Chest 2000;117:1619–26.

5. King TE, Schwarz MI, Brown KK, et al. Idiopathic pulmonary fibrosis: relationship between histopathologic features and mortality. Am J Respir Crit Care Med 2001;164:1025–32.

6. King TE, Tooze JA, Schwarz MI, et al. Predicting survival in idiopathic pulmonary fibrosis: scoring system and survival model. Am J Respir Crit Care Med 2001;164:1171–81.

7. Hunninghake GW, Kalica AR. Approaches to the treatment of pulmonary fibrosis. Am J Respir Crit Care Med 1995;151: 915–8.

8. Mason RJ, Schwarz MI, Hunninghake GW, Musson RA. Pharmacological therapy for idiopathic pulmonary fibrosis; past, present, and future. Am J Respir Crit Care Med 1999;160:1771–7.

9. Crystal RG, Bitterman PB, Mossman B, Schwarz MI, et al. Future research directions in idiopathic pulmonary fibrosis. Am J Respir Crit Care Med 2002;166:236–46.

10. Gross TJ, Hunninghake GW. Idiopathic pulmonary fibrosis. N Engl J Med 2001;345:517–25.

11. Selman M, King TE Jr, Pardo A. Idiopathic pulmonary fibrosis: prevailing and evolving hypothesis about its pathogenesis and implications for therapy. Ann Intern Med 2001;134:136–51.

12. Gauldie J. Pro: Inflammatory mechanisms are a minor component of the pathogenesis of idiopathic pulmonary fibrosis. Am J Respir Crit Care Med 2002;165:1205–8.

13. Travis WD, Matsui K, Moss J, Ferrans VJ. Idiopathic non-specific interstitial pneumonia: prognostic significance of cellular and fibrosing patterns: survival comparison with usual interstitial pneumonia and desquamative interstitial pneumonia. Am J Surg Pathol 2000;24:19–33.

14. Nicholson AG, Colby TV, DuBois RM, et al. The prognostic significance of the histologic pattern of interstitial pneumonia in patients presenting with the clinical entity of cryptogenic fibrosing alveolitis. Am J Respir Crit Care Med 2000;162: 2213–7.

15. Thomas AQ, Lane K, Phillips J, et al. Heterozygosity for a surfactant protein C gene mutation associated with usual interstitial pneumonitis and cellular non-specific interstitial pneumonitis in one kindred. Am J Respir Crit Care Med 2002;165:1322–8.

16. Flaherty KR, Travis WD, Colby TV, et al. Histopathologic variability in usual and non-specific interstitial pneumonias. Am J Respir Crit Care Med 2001;164:1722–7.

17. Katzenstein AL, Myers JL. Idiopathic pulmonary fibrosis: clinical relevance of pathologic classification. Am J Respir Crit Care Med 1998;157:1301–15.

18. Basset F, Ferrans VJ, Soler P, et al. Intraluminal fibrosis in interstitial lung disorders. Am J Pathol 1986;122(3):443–61.

19. Kuhn C, McDonald JA. The roles of the myofibroblast in idiopathic pulmonary fibrosis. Ultrastructural and immunohistochemical features of sites of active extracellular matrix synthesis. Am J Pathol 1991;138(5):1257–65.

20. Kuhn CD, Boldt J, King TE Jr, et al. An immunohistochemical study of architectural remodeling and connective tissue synthesis in pulmonary fibrosis. Am Rev Respir Dis 1989;140(6):1693–703.

21. Fukada Y, Basset F, Ferrans VJ, et al. Significance of early intraalveolar fibrotic lesions and integrin expression in lung biopsy specimens from patients with idiopathic pulmonary fibrosis. Hum Pathol 1995;26(1):53–61.

22. Leslie KO, Mitchell J, Low R. Lung myofibroblasts. Cell Motil Cytoskeleton 1992;22(2):92–8.

23. Zhang K, Rekhter MD, Gordon D, et al. Myofibroblasts and their role in lung collagen gene expression during pulmonary fibrosis. A combined immunohistochemical and in situ hybridization study. Am J Pathol 1994;145:114–25.

24. Schuppan D, Cho JJ, Jia JD, et al. Interplay of matrix and myofibroblasts during hepatic fibrogenesis. Curr Top Pathol 1999;93:205–18.

25. el Nahas N, Muchaneta-Kubara EC, Tamimi N, et al. Glomerulosclerosis: the role of interstitial myofibroblasts in its progression. Curr Top Pathol 1999;93:167–71.

26. Broekelmann TJ, Limper AH, Colby TV, et al. Transforming growth factor-β1 is present at sites of extracellular matrix gene expression in human pulmonary fibrosis. Proc Natl Acad Sci U S A 1991;88:6642–6.

27. Phan SH. Role of the myofibroblast in pulmonary fibrosis. Kidney Int Suppl 1996;54:S46–8.

28. Serini G, Gabbiani G. Mechanisms of myofibroblast activity and phenotypic modulation. Exp Cell Res 1999;250: 273–83.

29. Coker RK, Laurent FJ. Anticytokine approaches in pulmonary fibrosis: bringing factors into focus. Thorax 1997;52:294–6.

30. Zhang K, Gharaee-Kermani M, McGarry B, et al. In situ hybridization analysis of rat lung alpha 1 (I) and alpha 2 (I) collagen gene expression in pulmonary fibrosis induced by endotracheal bleomycin injection. Lab Invest 1994; 70:192–202.

31. Wang R, Ramos C, Joshi I, et al. Human lung myofibroblast-derived inducers of alveolar epithelial apoptosis identified as angiotensin peptides. Am J Physiol 1999;277:L1158–64.

32. Lappi-Blanco E, Soini Y, Paakko P. Apoptotic activity is increased in the newly formed fibromyxoid connective tissue in bronchiolitis obliterans organizing pneumonia. Lung 1999;177:367–76.

33. Khalil N, O'Connor RN, Unruh HW, et al. Increased production and immunohistochemical localization of transforming growth factor-β in idiopathic pulmonary fibrosis. Am J Respir Cell Mol Biol 1991;5:155–62.

34. Khan TZ, Wagener JS, Bost T, et al. Early pulmonary inflammation in infants with cystic fibrosis. Am J Respir Crit Care Med 1995;151:1075–82.

35. Corrin B, Butcher D, McAnulty BJ, et al. Immunohistochemical localization of transforming growth factor-β1 in the lungs of patients with systemic sclerosis, cryptogenic fibrosing alveolitis and other lung disorders. Histopathology 1994;24:145–50.

36. Duncan MR, Berman B. Gamma interferon is the lymphokine and beta interferon the monokine responsible for inhibition of fibroblast collagen production and late, but not early fibroblast proliferation. J Exp Med 1985;162:516–27.

37. Jimenez SA, Freundlich B, Rosenbloom J. Selective inhibition of human diploid fibroblast collagen synthesis by interferons. J Clin Invest 1984;74:1112–6.

38. Duncan MR, Berman B. Differential regulation of collagen, glycosaminoglycan, fibronectin and collagenase activity production in cultured human adult dermal fibroblasts by interleukin a alpha and beta and tumor necrosis factor alpha and beta. Invest Dermatol 1989;92:699–706.

39. Chin YE, Katagawa M, Kuida K, et al. Activation of the STAT

signaling pathway can cause expression of caspase 1 and apoptosis. Mol Cell Biol 1997;17:5328–37.

40. Kalvakolanu DV. Interferons and cell growth control. Histol Histopathol 2000;15:523–37.

41. Adelmann-Grill BC, Hein R, Wach F, et al. Inhibition of fibroblast chemotaxis by recombinant human interferon-γ and interferon-α. J Cell Physiol 1987;130:270–5.

42. Elias JA, Freundlich B Kern JA, et al. Cytokine networks in the regulation of inflammation and fibrosis of the lung. Chest 1990;97:1439–45.

43. Leof EB, Proper JA, Goustin AS, et al. Induction of c-sis mRNA and activity similar to platelet-derived growth factor by transforming growth factor -β: a proposed model of indirect mitogenesis involvement. Autocrine activity. Proc Natl Acad Sci U S A 1986;83:2453–7.

44. Okada T, Sugie I, Aisaka K. Effects of gamma interferon on collagen and histamine content in bleomycin-induced lung fibrosis in rats. Lymphokine Cytokine Res 1993;12:87–91.

45. Granstein RD, Flotte TJ, Amento EP. Interferons and collagen production. J Invest Dermatol 1990;95:75S–80S.

46. Ziesche R, Hofbauer E, Wittmann K, et al. A preliminary study of long-term treatment with interferon-γ1b and low-dose prednisolone in patients with idiopathic pulmonary fibrosis. N Engl J Med 1999;341:1264–9.

47. Prior C, Haslam PL. Increased levels of serum interferon-γ in pulmonary sarcoidosis and relationship with response to corticosteroid therapy. Am Rev Respir Dis 1991;143:53–60.

48. Robinson WB, McLemore TL, Crystal RG. Gamma interferon is spontaneously released by alveolar macrophages and lung T lymphocytes in patients with pulmonary sarcoidosis. J Clin Invest 1985;75:1488–95.

49. Prior C, Haslam PL. In vivo levels and in vitro production of interferon-γ in fibrosing interstitial lung diseases. Clin Exp Immunol 1992;88:280–7.

50. Gauldie J, Sime PJ, Xing Z, et al. Transforming growth factor-β gene transfer to the lung induces myofibroblast presence and pulmonary fibrosis. Curr Top Pathol 1999;93:35–45.

51. Zhao J, Sime PJ, Bringas P, et al. Adenovirus-mediated decorin gene transfer prevents TGF-β-induced inhbition of lung morphogenesis. Am J Physiol 1999;277:L412–22.

52. Herrick AL. Development of agents for the treatment of systemic sclerosis. Expert Opin Invest Drugs 2001;10:1255–64.

53. Giri SN, Hyde DM, Hollinger MA. Effect of antibody to transforming growth factor-β on bleomycin-induced accumulation of lung collagen in mice. Thorax 1993;48: 959–66.

54. Lauren GJ, Coker RK, McAnulty RJ. TGF-β antibodies: a novel treatment for pulmonary fibrosis? Thorax 1993;48:953–4.

55. Asakura S, Kato, H, Fujino S, et al. Role of transforming growth factor-β1 and decorin in development of central fibrosis in pulmonary adenocarcinoma. Human Pathol 1999;30:195–8.

56. Duncan MR, Frazer KS, Abramson S, et al. Connective tissue growth factor mediates transforming growth factor-β-induced collagen synthesis: downregulation by cAMP. FASEB J 1999;13:1774–86.

57. Wang O, Wang Y, Hyde DM, et al. Reduction of bleomycin-induced lung fibrosis by transforming growth factor-β-soluble receptor in hamsters. Thorax 1999;34:805–12.

58. Nakao A, Fujii M, Matsumura R, et al. Transient gene transfer and expression of Smad7 prevents bleomycin-induced lung fibrosis in mice. J Clin Invest 1999;104:5–11.

59. Huang M, Sharma S, Zhu LX, et al. IL-7 inhibits fibroblast TGF-β production and signaling in pulmonary fibrosis. J Clin Invest 2002;109:931–7.

60. Redlich CA, Delisser HM. Elias JA. Retinoic acid inhibition of transforming growth factor-β-induced collagen production by human lung fibroblasts. Am J Respir Cell Mol Biol 1995;12:287–95.

61. Iyer SN, Gurujeyalakshmi G, Giri SN. Effect of pirfenidone on transforming growth factor gene expression at the tran-

scriptional level in a bleomycin model of lung fibrosis. J Pharmacol Exp Ther 1999;291:367–73.

62. Blobe GC, Schiemann WP, Lodish HF. Role of transforming growth factor-β in human disease. N Engl J Med 2000; 243:1350–8.

63. Postlethwaite AE. Stimulation of the chemotactic migration of human fibroblasts by transforming growth factor-β. J Exp Med 1987;165:251–6.

64. Roberts A, Sporn MG. Handbook of experimental pharmacology. Peptide growth factors and their receptors. Berlin, Germany: Springer-Verlag; 1990.

65. Bruijn JA, Roos A, de Geus B, et al. Transforming growth factor-β and the glomerular extracellular matrix in renal pathology. J Lab Clin Med 1994;123:34–47.

66. Klagsburn M, D'Amore PA. Regulators of angiogenesis. Annu Rev Physiol 1991;53:217–39.

67. Xing Z, Tremblay GM, Sime PJ, et al. Overexpression of granulocyte-macrophage colony stimulating factor induces pulmonary granulation tissue formation and fibrosis by induction of transforming growth factor-β1 and myofibroblast accumulation. Am J Pathol 1997;150:59–66.

68. Andreutti D, Gabbiani G, Neuville P. Early granulocyte-macrophage colony-stimulating factor expression by alveolar inflammatory cells during bleomycin-induced rat lung fibrosis. Lab Invest 1998;78:1493–502.

69. Sime PJ, Xing Z, Graham FL, et al. Adenovector-mediated gene transfer of active transforming growth factor-β1 induces prolonged severe fibrosis in rat lung. J Clin Invest 1997;100:768–76.

70. Raghu G, Johnson WC. Lockhardt D, et al. Treatment of idiopathic pulmonary fibrosis with a new antifibrotic agent, perfenidone: results of a prospective open label phase II study. Am J Respir Crit Care Med 1999;139:1061–9.

71. Hocher B, Schwarz A, Fagan K, et al. Pulmonary fibrosis and chronic lung inflammation in ET-1 transgenic mice. Am J Respir Cell Mol Biol 2000;23:7–10.

72. Shahar I, Fireman E, Topkisky M, et al. Effect of endothelin-1 on α-smooth muscle actin expression and in alveolar fibroblasts proliferation in interstitial lung diseases. Int J Immunopharmacol 1999;21:759–75.

73. Uguccioni M, Pulsatelli L, Grigolo B, et al. Endothelin-1 in idiopathic pulmonary fibrosis. J Clin Pathol 1995;48:330–4.

74. Kurihawa H, Yoshizumi M, Sugiyana T, et al. Transforming growth factor-β stimulates the expression of endothelin mRNA by vascular endothelial cells. Biochem Biophys Res Commun 1989;159:1435–40.

75. Orisio S, Morigi M, Zoja C, et al. Tumor necrosis factor stimulates endothelin-1 gene expression in cultured bovine endothelial cells. Mediators Inflamm 1992;1:263–6.

76. Kourembarras S, Mardsen PA, McQuinllan LP, et al. Hypoxia induces endothelin gene expression and secretion in cultured human endothelium. J Clin Invest 1991;88:1054–7.

77. Park SH, Saleh D, Giaid A, Michel RP. Increased endothelin-1 in bleomycin-induced pulmonary fibrosis and the affect of an endothelin receptor antagonists. Am J Respir Crit Care Med 1997;156:600–8.

78. Giaid A, Michel RR, Stewart M, et al. Expression of endothelin-1 in lungs of patients with cryptogenic fibrosing alveolitis. Lancet 1993;341:1550–4.

79. Salch D, Furukawa MS, Tsau A, et al. Elevated expression of endothelin-1 and endothelin-1 converting enzyme idiopathic pulmonary fibrosis: possible involvement of proinflammatory cytokines. Am J Respir Cell Mol Biol 1997;16:187–93.

80. Streiter RM, Remick RG, Lynch JP, et al. IL-2-induced TNF expression in human alveolar macrophages and blood monocytes. Am Rev Respir Dis 1989;139:335–42.

81. Piquet PF, Ribaux C, Karpuz J, et al. Expression and localization of tumor necrosis factor-α and its mRNA in idiopathic pulmonary fibrosis. Am J Pathol 1993;143:651–5.

82. Paulsen Y, Austgulen R, Hofsli E, et al. Tumor necrosis factor-induced expression of platelet-derived growth factor A-

chain messenger RNA in fibroblasts. Exp Cell Res 1989;180:490–6.

83. Elias J, Gustilo K, Baeder W, Freundlich B. Synergistic stimulation of fibroblast prostaglandin production by recombinant interleukin 1 and tumor necrosis factor. J Immunol 1987;138:3812–6.

84. Solis-Herruzo JA, Brenner DA, Chojkier M. Tumor necrosis factor-α inhibits collagen gene transcription and collagen synthesis in human lung fibroblasts. J Biol Chem 1988; 263:5841–5.

85. Piquet PF, Collart MA, Grau GE, et al. Tumor necrosis factor/cachetin plays a key role in bleomycin-induced pneumonopathy. J Exp Med 1989;170:655–63.

86. Piquet PF, Vesin C. Treatment by human recombinant soluble TNF receptor of pulmonary fibrosis induced by bleomycin or silica. Eur Respir J 1994;7:515–8.

87. Miyazaki YK, Araki C, Vesin I, et al. Expression of a TNF-α transgene in murine lung causes lymphocytic and fibrosing alveolitis in a mouse model of progressive pulmonary fibrosis. J Clin Invest 1995;96:250–9.

88. Dayer JM, Krane SM. Anti-TNF-α therapy for ankylosing spondylitis—a specific or non-specific treatment? N Engl J Med 2002;346:1399–400.

89. Ehrenpries ED, Kane SV, Cohen, et al. Thalidomide therapy for patients with refractory Crohn's disease: an open-label trial. Gastroenterology 1999;117:1271–7.

90. Linz W, Scholkens BA, Ganten D. Converting enzyme inhibition specifically prevents cardiac hypertrophy in rats. Clin Exp Hypertens 1989;11:1325–50.

91. Cohen EP, Molteni A, Hill P, et al. Captopril preserves function and ultrastructure in experimental radiation nephropathy. Lab Invest 1996;75:349–60.

92. Specks U, Martin WN, Rohrbach MS. Bronchoalveolar lavage fluid angiotensin-converting enzyme in interstitial lung disease. Am Rev Respir Dis 1990;141:117–23.

93. Idell S, Keuppers F, Lippman H, et al. Angiotensin-converting enzyme in bronchoalveolar lavage in ARDS. Chest 1987;91:52–6.

94. Molteni A, Moulder JE, Cohen EF, et al. Control of radiation-induced pneumopathy and lung fibrosis by angiotensin-converting enzyme inhibitors and an angiotensin II receptor blocker. J Radiat Biol 2000;76:523–32.

95. Marshall RP, McAnulty RJ, Laurent GJ. Angiotensin II is mitogenic for human lung fibroblasts via activation of the type I receptor. Am J Respir Crit Care Med 2000;161:1999–2004.

96. Wang LW, Fu XL, Clough R, et al. Can angiotensin-converting enzyme inhibitors protect against symptomatic radiation pneumonitis? Radiat Res 2000;153:405–10.

97. Tan A, Levry H, Dahm C, et al. Lovastatin induces fibroblast apoptosis in vitro and in vivo: a possible therapy for fibroproliferative disorders. Am J Respir Crit Care Med 1999; 159:220–7.

98. Bell JRJ, Eddie LW, Lester AR, et al. Relaxin in human pregnancy serum measured with a homologous radioimmunoassay. Obstet Gynecol 1987;69:585–9.

99. Unimori EN, Pickford LB, Salles AL, et al. Relaxin induces an extracellular matrix-degrading phenotype in human lung fibroblasts in vitro and inhibits lung fibrosis in a murine model in vivo. J Clin Invest 1966;98:2739–45.

100. Unemori EN, Beck LS, Lee WP, et al. Human relaxin decreases collagen accumulation in vivo in two rodent models of fibrosis. J Invest Dermatol 1993;101:280–5.

101. Garvber SL, Mirochnik V, Brecklin CS, et al. Relaxin decrease renal interstitial fibrosis and slows progression of renal diseases. Kidney Int 2001;59:876–82.

102. Seibold JR, Korn JH, Simms R, et al. Recombinant human relaxin in the treatment of scleroderma. A randomized, double-blind, placebo-controlled trial. Ann Intern Med 2000;132:871–9.

103. Cantin AM, North SL, Fells GA, et al. Oxidant-mediated epithelial cell injury in idiopathic pulmonary fibrosis. J Clin Invest 1989;79:1165–73.

104. Cantin AM, Hubbard AC, Crystal RG. Glutathione deficiency in the epithelial lining fluid of the lower respiratory trace in idiopathic pulmonary fibrosis. Am Rev Respir Dis 1989;139:370–2.

105. Hagawara SI, Ishii Y, Kitamura S. Aerosolized administration of N-acetylcysteine attenuates lung fibrosis induced by bleomycin in mice. Am J Respir Crit Care Med 2000;162: 225–31.

106. Behr J, Maier K, Degenkolb B, et al. Antioxidative and clinical effects of high dose N-acetylcysteine in fibrosing alveolitis: adjuvant therapy to maintenance immunosuppression. Am J Respir Crit Care Med 1997;156:1897–901.

107. Wang OA, Hollister MA, Giri SN. Attenuation of amiodarone-induced pulmonary fibrosis and phospholipidosis in hamsters of taurine and/or niacin. J Pharmacol Exp Ther 1992;262:127–32.

108. Brown DR, Heitcamp M, Jong CS. Niacin reduces paraquat toxicity in rats. Science 1981;212:1510–2.

109. Wang O, Giri SN, Hyde DM, Li C. Amelioration of bleomycin-induced pulmonary fibrosis in hamsters by combined treatment with taurine and niacin. Biochem Pharmacol 1991;42:1115–22.

110. Gurufeyalakshmi G, Giri SN. Molecular mechanisms of antifibrotic effect of interferon gamma in a bleomycin mouse model of lung fibroses; down regulation of TGF-β and procollagen I and III gene expression. Exp Lung Res 1986; 21:791.

111. Gurufeyalakshmi G, Hollinger MA, Giri SN. Regulation of transforming growth factor-β1 mRNA expression by taurine and niacin in the bleomycin hamster model of lung fibrosis. Am J Respir Cell Mol Biol 1996;18:334–42.

112. Nagler A, Pines M. Topical treatment of cutaneous graft versus host disease with halfuginone: a novel inhibitor of type I collagen synthesis. Transplantation 1999;68:1806–9.

113. Nagler A, Firman N, Feferman R, et al. Reduction in pulmonary fibrosis in vivo by halfuginone. Am J Respir Crit Care Med 1996;154:1082–6.

114. Franklin TJ, Morris WP, Edwards PN, et al. Inhibition of prolyl-4-hydroxylase in vitro and in vivo by members of a novel series of phenanthrolinones. Biochem J 2001;353:333–8.

115. Prockop DJ, Kivirikko KI. Collagens: molecular biology, diseases and potentials for therapy. Annu Rev Biochem 1995;64:403–34.

116. Greco NJ, Kemnitzer JE, Fox JD, et al. Polymer of proline analogue with sustained antifibrotic activity in lung fibrosis. Am J Respir Crit Care Med 1997;155:1391–7.

117. Cefalu WT, Skyler JS, Kourdies IA, et al. Inhaled human insulin treatment in patients with type Z diabetes mellitus. Ann Intern Med 2001;134:203–7.

118. Jaffee HA, Buhl R, Mastrangelia A, Holroyd KJ, et al. Organ-specific cytokine therapy: local activation of mononuclear phagocytes by delivery of an aerosol of recombinant interferon gamma to the human lung. J Clin Invest 1991; 88:297–302.

14

SARCOIDOSIS

GLEN P. WESTALL
R. G. STIRLING
PAUL CULLINAN
ROLAND M. DU BOIS

Sarcoidosis is a chronic, multiorgan inflammatory disorder of unknown etiology. It is characterized by tissue infiltration by mononuclear phagocytes and lymphocytes and noncaseating granulomas that primarily affect the lungs and the lymphatics.[1-3] Since the first cutaneous description in 1877 by Hutchinson,[4] sarcoidosis has been recognized as a systemic disorder with protean clinical presentations, affecting virtually every organ system. The diagnosis is "established when the clinicoradiological findings are supported by histological evidence of noncaseating epithelioid granulomas. Granulomas of known causes and local sarcoid reactions must be excluded."[5] Despite over a century of clinical observation, the cause of the disorder remains unknown. However, over the past twenty years the development of sophisticated new molecular and cellular probes has led to a greater understanding of the immunologic and pathologic basis of this disease. The consensus view is that sarcoidosis results from exposure of genetically susceptible hosts to specific environmental agents that trigger a Th_1-type cellular immune response with granuloma formation.

The clinical presentation of sarcoidosis has important implications for prognosis, with an acute onset often associated with a self-limited course and resolution, whereas a more insidious onset is often followed by a more chronic course, characterized by pulmonary fibrosis. These differing disease phenotypes and dichotomy in prognosis may well reflect differing immunologic pathways. At present, treatment protocols continue to be refined. In expediting a full understanding of the immune mechanisms, coupled with accurate descriptions of the differing clinical presentation and subsequent disease course, better-targeted therapies will hopefully be achieved. Prognosis is generally good, with the majority of patients recovering spontaneously. Some features of sarcoidosis such as lupus pernio, neurologic involvement, bone cysts, and pulmonary fibrosis predict a more chronic course, with a low rate of remission. In all, approximately one-third of patients suffer a more persis-

tent and progressive disease requiring prolonged treatment with corticosteroids and occasionally with one or more second-line drugs such as azathioprine, methotrexate, hydroxychloroquine, or cyclophosphamide.

MILESTONES

Sarcoidosis was first described more than 100 years ago, and initially the disease was thought to be limited to the skin. In 1877, the English physician, Jonathon Hutchinson described multiple raised purplish cutaneous patches. He ascribed these lesions as atypical gout, but subsequently published further cases that he felt represented a new dermatologic entity.[6] Besnier in 1889 described lupus pernio,[7] and 3 years later the histology on a similar case confirmed the presence of granulomata.[8] In 1899, Caesar Boeck used the phrase "multiple benign sarkoid of the skin," feeling that the skin lesions resembled a benign form of sarcoma.[9] In a subsequent paper, in 1905, he presented a series of five cases. Some of these patients complained of chronic cough and were later shown to have granulomatous nasal disease.[10]

Sarcoid bone cysts were first described in 1904.[11] Over the next few years, Boeck,[10] Heerfordt,[12] and Jungling[13] all described separate eponymous syndromes, before Schaumann in 1934 recognizing a common thread, used the term "lymphogranuloma benigna" to emphasize the systemic nature of the disease.[14] In 1946, Sven Löfgren described a syndrome[15] consisting of fever, hilar lymphadenopathy, polyarthritis, and erythema nodosum; such patients have been shown to have a relatively good prognosis.

The Kveim-Siltzbach test was developed in the 1940s and 1950s. Ansgar Kveim initially observed that a papular eruption arose in 12 of 13 sarcoid patients following intradermal inoculation of sarcoid lymph node tissue.[16] Subsequently Louis Siltzbach refined the test using a splenic suspension and developed a specific and validated antigen that became universally used.[17]

PATHOGENESIS

Etiology

There is abundant evidence to support the concept that sarcoid granulomas are formed in response to a persistent, poorly degradable antigenic stimulus. First, immune granulomas are known to form in response to persistent antigenic epitopes present after infection with organisms such as Schistosoma or mycobacterial infection.[18–22] Second, infectious agents, inorganic agents, and organic particulates may initiate pulmonary immune granulomas; the factor common to all is their low biodegradability and/or persistence, often within macrophages.[23]

Noninfective agents have been suggested as etiologic agents: pine pollen because of an association with the pine forests in the southeastern states of the USA, but this was not confirmed after further epidemiologic studies,[24,25] clay soil,[26] talc,[27] beryllium,[28] and zirconium.[29] None of these theories has endured.

More traditional suggestions of etiology point to infective agents. Support for the concept of a transmissible agent is provided by the finding of granulomas in the lungs of heart and bone marrow transplants from donors not suspected of having sarcoidosis.[30,31] Other infective agents incriminated in the pathogenesis of sarcoidosis are listed in Table 14–1. These include bacteria, viruses, Nocardia, and cell-wall-deficient mycoplasma.[32–41]

Most studies of a possible causal organism have, however, focused on mycobacteria. It is noteworthy that the coexistence of sarcoidosis and tuberculosis has been recognized for some time.[42]

An infective or transmissible cause for sarcoidosis has been supported by animal experiments, particularly the passage experiments of Mitchell and colleagues,[43–45] which showed that a granulomatous response could be produced by passaging pooled, filtered homogenates or supernatants of mouse granulomatous tissue into other mice. Notably, acid-fast organisms were also found in some of these tissues, and mycobacteria having the characteristics of *Mycobacterium tuberculosis* were grown in Löwenstein-Jensen medium from some of these homogenates. There remains some uncertainty about the causative role of mycobacteria because of the difficulty in repeating the passage experiments. However, the findings of Almenoff and colleagues,[46] in identifying cell-wall-deficient forms in patients with sarcoidosis using an antibody raised against *M. tuberculosis* whole-cell antigen (HR37RV), may partly explain the difficulties in isolating cell-wall-deficient organisms that require a specialized culture medium to grow. A number of studies have detected higher levels of antibodies to mycobacteria in patients with sarcoidosis compared with normal controls.[47,48] However, most of these studies fail to detect mycobacterial deoxyribonucleic acid (DNA) in cells or tissue from disease sites

The application of molecular biology techniques has further fueled the mycobacteria debate but has not resolved it. Using mycobacteria-specific primers and the polymerase chain reaction, mycobacterial DNA molecules were identified in granulomatous tissue (lung, skin, or lymph node) in 1 study in 7 out of 16 instances compared with 1 out of 16 normal controls but in only 2 out of 4 tuberculosis controls.[49] A second study by a different group reported contradictory findings: tissue or cell samples from 16 patients with sarcoidosis were compared with 13 control tissue samples, 4 normal bronchoalveolar lavage samples, and 11 normal volunteer lavage samples. Most of the sarcoidosis samples were negative using *Mycobacterium hominis*–specific primers and a technique sensitive enough to detect two mycobacterial genomes— the equivalent of 15 organisms per 106 human cells.[50] These newer technologies, however, have in common with those previously used to detect mycobacteria, the limitations of imperfect sensitivity and specificity, and failure to detect mycobacterium may reflect insensitive tools, whereas positive results may reflect contamination.[51] Thus mycobacterial DNA fingerprints are seen in some patients with sarcoidosis, but they are not seen in all, and although these studies suggest a microbiologic link between mycobacterial infection and the development of sarcoidosis, the clinical correlates are lacking. Over the past century, while there has been a marked reduction in the incidence of tuberculosis, this is not paralleled by changes in new cases of sarcoidosis. Further, involvement of the heart and salivary glands is peculiar to sarcoidosis and is not commonly described with mycobacterial infections. A definitive conclusion on this issue will require more extensive investigations.

TABLE 14–1   Agents Cited as Causes of Sarcoidosis

Nonmycobacterial infective agents
  Bacterial
  Viral
  Mycoplasma
  Nocardia
Mycobacterial infective agents
  Mycobacerium tuberculosis
  Other mycobacteria
  Cell-wall deficient mycobacteria
  Virus/mycobacteria co-infection
Noninfective agents
  Pine pollen
  Clay soil
  Talc
  Zirconium
  Other metals

Epidemiology

Despite almost 100 years of clinical observation, little is known about the distribution of sarcoidosis. Consequently its etiology has remained very largely a mystery. This, in part, reflects a relative lack of interest from epidemiologists; most descriptions of the disease are based on cases seen in specialist clinics, and studies based on whole populations are few. The clinical features of the disease are variable (Table 14–2), and patients present to different hospital specialties. Valid denominators for such case series are difficult to define; the experience of the general population may not be a suitable point of reference. Proof of sarcoidosis in the general population is thus difficult, and the difficulty is compounded by the proportion of cases whose disease is clinically silent. Case series of sarcoidosis report disease that was asymptomatic at presentation in 31 to 68% of cases (Table 14–3); these estimates are inevitably influenced by the method of case collection but, taken together, show that in an important proportion of cases, the disease may go undetected unless (radiographic) screening is undertaken. The lack of enthusiasm for such screening, both in the general population and occupational groups over the past 30 years, is probably responsible for the dearth of new information about the distribution of the disease during that period.

Disease Frequency

Sarcoidosis is often a chronic disease lasting many years; alternately, it may be short-lived and self-limiting. As a result the relationship between its prevalence (the number of cases at a defined time point) and incidence (the number of new cases over a defined time period) may be difficult to delineate. Measures of both prevalence and (more rarely) incidence have been derived from the findings of mass radiographic screening campaigns carried out for the control of tuberculosis in a number of developed countries and for employment purposes and from surveys of presentations to specialist medical services. These alternate techniques have particular, and to some extent mutually exclusive, weaknesses: the first detects only disease that is apparent on chest radiography and depends on the assiduousness with which "suspicious cases" are investigated. On the other hand, mass radiographic surveys have the potential to detect asymptomatic sarcoidosis, much of which is probably missed in surveys based on clinical experience. If appropriately targeted, clinic registers will include cases of nonthoracic sarcoidosis and, arguably, will rely on a more consistent case definition.

Available measures of prevalence suggest that sarcoidosis is not a common disease. Mass surveys from the United Kingdom in the 1950s and 1960s disclosed radiographic abnormalities consistent with sarcoidosis in 9[52] to 36[53] per 100,000 of those screened. Similar studies in Scandinavia, carried out over the same decades, revealed a combined prevalence of 28 per 100,000 examined persons.[54] In 1964, Bauer and Löfgren[55] summarized the findings from 29 surveys (in ten cases nationwide) carried out in 24 countries; the results varied widely from 0.2 per 100,000 (in Portugal, Brazil, and Uruguay) to the highest figure of 64 per 100,000 in Sweden. It is noteworthy that in the city of Malmo in Sweden, autopsies conducted during 1957 to 1962 on 6,707 individuals comprising 60% of all deaths, found evidence for sarcoidosis in 43, only 3 of whom were known to have sarcoidosis in life, a prevalence of 671 per 100,000, about 10 times higher than detected by mass screening. The wide variation in these estimates presumably reflects differences in diagnostic labeling and in the age, gender, and morbid distributions of the screened populations. Milman and Selroos[54] have emphasized the need to express the frequencies measured in this way as a proportion of those undergoing radiography rather than of the whole population.

Incidence rates based on mass radiography also vary considerably, and probably for the same reasons. In Scandinavia, estimates derived from nationwide screening programs range from 14 per 100,000 [56,57] to 42 per 100,000.[58] Sutherland and colleagues[59] reported annual incidence rates of sarcoidosis of between 8.0 and 12.7 per 100,000 among young men and women participating in a trial of bacille Calmette-Guérin (BCG) for tuberculosis. Among the United States male naval personnel, subjected to regular chest radiography, Sartwell and Edwards[60] reported annual, age-adjusted incidence rates of sarcoidosis that ranged between 7.6 per 100,000 (in white men) to 81.8 per 100,000 (in African American men). In Japanese railway workers undergoing annual chest radiography examination, however, the incidence was much lower at 1.5 per 100,000.[61]

TABLE 14–2   Patient Symptoms as Percentage of Patient Population at Disease Presentation

	Caucasian n = 111	Blacks n = 90	Asian n = 44	Overall N = 1,609
Abnormal routine chest radiograph	23	7	10	34
Constitutional symptoms	46	57	55	—
Respiratory symptoms	38	57	55	18
Skin lesions	2	9	7	7
Erythema nodosum	41	9	17	16
Superficial lymphadenopathy	3	34	17	—
Ocular symptoms	12	12	3	9

Adapted from Edmondstone WM et al[70] and Siltzbach LE et al.[595]

TABLE 14–3   Proportion of Cases Asymptomatic at Presentation—Selected Surveys

Lead Author	Country	Method of Case Detection	Proportion of Cases Asymptomatic at Presentation (%)
Sutherland[59]	United Kingdom	Radiographic screening	56
BTTA[63]	United Kingdom	Hospital patients	31
Hillerdal[411]	Sweden	Population health screening	68
Hennessy[77]	United States	Hospital patients	52
Milman[54*]	Scandinavia	Radiographic screening/hospital patients	35–58

BTTA = British Thoracic and Tuberculosis Association.
*Review of several surveys.

Surveys of persons presenting to specialist medical services have also been used to derive measures of disease incidence, although it is often unclear what proportion of reported cases are in fact prevalent at the start of the study. The results of such surveys are heavily dependent on their scope and on the enthusiasm with which cases are sought. In the Isle of Man, for example, the incidence measured following a prospective survey in which "special efforts" were made to detect all cases presenting over a 6-year period was 14.7 per 100,000—significantly higher than the figure of 3.5 per 100,000 derived from a retrospective survey of clinical records.[62] This lower figure approximates to that reported in a survey of cases presenting to chest physicians, dermatologists, or ophthalmologists in four areas of the United Kingdom[63] but is a little lower than that from a similar study in the United States—6.1 per 100,000.[64] Following a "general health" screening program (including annual chest radiography) in Uppsala, Sweden, with a take-up rate of 64%, an annual incidence of 19 per 100,000—or 24 per 100,000 of those screened—was reported.[65] In Japan, where nationwide surveys of sarcoidosis took place in hospitals between 1972 and 1984, the annual incidence rates were lower (1.3 per 100,000).

Taken together, these figures suggest that the annual incidence of sarcoidosis across the whole population in Western Europe and the United States lie around 10 per 100,000; its prevalence, reflecting the chronic nature of sarcoidosis, is somewhat higher. Figures from Japan, and possibly South America, may be much lower. Applying cumulative incidence estimates, the lifetime risk of sarcoidosis is 2.4% for African Americans and 0.85% for American Whites.[66] Geographic and temporal differences between estimates are influenced to an unknown extent by differences in diagnostic ascertainment and population base. For the same reasons, data on temporal trends in the frequency of sarcoidosis are difficult to interpret but do not indicate any important changes in incidence over the relatively brief time periods examined. Incidence rates reported by Yamaguchi and colleagues[67] in Japan as a result of occupational screening between 1960 and 1988, and East Germany following case notification between 1970 and 1985, did not show any systematic changes.

Age and Gender

A consistent finding in the epidemiology of sarcoidosis has been the observation that the peak age of incidence is in young adulthood. Most Scandinavian incidence surveys, based on detection after mass radiography, have reported the majority of new cases in persons aged less than 35 years.[54] Among (male) naval personnel in the United States, the incidence was highest in those aged 24 to 35 years.[60] In the United Kingdom, findings from an inclusive, clinic-based series[63] confirmed these observations, with the highest incidence rates in both genders between the ages of 25 and 34 years. Similarly, in the Rochester, Minnesota, USA series, the peak age of incidence for both genders combined was between 30 and 39 years.[64] A number of observers have described a small difference in the age of presentation between the genders. In the Isle of Man, the peak age of presentation among women was 30 to 39 years, five years higher than among men[62]; the findings mirror those in Rochester, Minnesota, USA. In Uppsala, Sweden a second age peak at 45 to 65 years was observed among women but not among men.[65] The disease is sometimes found among children but appears to be very rare. No cases under the age of 15 years were reported from surveys in the Isle of Man,[62] United States,[64] or mainland United Kingdom[63]—in the last instance, possibly because cases were collected from only adult hospital clinics. In a Japanese series of 2,079 cases,[68] 48% of which arose from mass radiographic screening, 29 (1.4%) were in children under ten years of age.

Similarly, the evidence has been consistent concerning gender distribution; most studies report a higher incidence of the disease in women. In the United Kingdom, for example, the incidence of sarcoidosis presenting to specialist clinics was 40% higher among women than men,[63] a figure mirrored in the mass radiographic surveys from Scandinavia.[54] Interestingly, the difference in incidence between the genders was more than threefold in the study reported by Sutherland and colleagues[59]; a possible explanation is that the higher female incidence among very young adults (the study was confined to those aged less than 25 years) seems difficult to sustain in the light of the findings described earlier. This study aside, it should be noted that the differences in gender distribution, when they are found at all, are generally small.

The possibility of differential access to medical services whereby women would have a higher probability of diagnostic ascertainment should be included among potential explanations for observed differences between the genders. Experience from the Uppsala screening program would, however, suggest that this is not the case. In that setting, women presented with symptoms more frequently than men, rather than had their sarcoidosis detected "by chance."[65]

Race

Sarcoidosis may affect subjects of any nationality or ethnic group of either gender at any age, although the main incidence is in the age group 20 to 40 years (Table 14–4). In Great Britain, it is more frequent among the Irish, British, and West Indian than among the Asian population. In a study of four contrasted areas by the British Thoracic and Tuberculosis Association, 1961 to 1966, the range of annual incidence for men was approximately 2.1 per 100,000 in the most northerly area to 4.1 in the most southerly, whereas in women it was 3.5 to 4.5.[63] Because of the protean nature of the manifestations of sarcoidosis and the few studies to which uniform standards have been applied and because of the rapid changes in population trends in recent years, we have no true appreciation of the incidence at the present time.

Sartwell and Edwards[60] reported that the incidence of sarcoidosis among African American naval personnel was 10.7 times higher (81.8/100,000) than among their white counterparts (7.6/100,000). A similar distribution has been reported in a case series from London,

United Kingdom [69,70] and in South Africa.[71] In one of the London surveys, among patients attending a chest clinic, the prevalence of disease in those of Asian origin was as high as among patients of African origin, the incidence in both being 12 times greater than in the white population. These observations made from clinical practice depend crucially on a clear understanding of the (racial) denominators involved. Assuming these observations to be valid, it is not clear whether they can be attributed to genetic, socioeconomic, geographic, or environmental factors, or indeed to differential access to diagnostic services.

Extrathoracic manifestations of sarcoidosis are reported more frequently in people of African origin than in white patients; as a corollary, "widespread" disease is more common among the former and "asymptomatic" disease among the latter.[72] These differences could be attributed in part, but probably not wholly, to earlier access to medical or screening services available to white patients. Certain populations are characterized by particular disease presentations: erythema nodosum is common in Europeans and less so in Blacks and Japanese,[73] with chronic uveitis and lupus pernio commonly seen in Blacks, and Puerto Ricans, respectively. In Japan, mortality usually relates to myocardial involvement.[74]

Gideon and Mannino[75] showed that mortality from sarcoidosis varied by region, gender, and race. Age-adjusted mortality rates were higher in the African American population as compared with the white population in a nationwide study of mortality in the United States from 1979 to 1991. During this period, 5,791 people died from sarcoidosis or its complications, and age-adjusted mortality rates increased from 1.3 per one million in 1979 to 1.6 per one million in 1991 among men and 1.9 per one million in 1979 to 2.5 per one million in 1991 among women.

TABLE 14–4   Frequency of Organ Involvement in White, Blacks, and Asian Patients

	Caucasian	Blacks	Asian
Hilar nodes	85	90	76
Lungs	50	71	51
Lymph nodes	9	34	17
Liver	3	25	27
Spleen	15	15	10
Skin	9	32	10
Eyes	12	30	17
Kidneys	2	5	—
Salivary glands	3	10	11
Bone	0	5	—
Heart	2	3	3
Central nervous system	3	8	—
> 2 extrathoracic organs	9	48	41

Adapted from Edmondstone WM et al.[70]

Geography

Comparisons of the frequency of sarcoidosis between different geographic areas or countries depend critically on the quality of ascertainment. The apparent rarity of the disease in, for example, rural Africa reflects to an unknown degree under-recognition and the difficulty of distinguishing the disease from tuberculosis, which is endemic in that region. Among countries with more or less equal access to sophisticated diagnostic techniques and with broadly similar views on what constitutes a case of sarcoidosis, the prevalence of the disease follows a rough north-south gradient. Bauer and Löfgren,[55] in their review of mass radiographic studies, reported prevalence rates from 28 countries in Europe, North and South America, Israel, and Japan. These are plotted against the latitude of the country's capital city and a line of least squares drawn, as shown in Figure 14–1. Within-country comparisons, where diagnosis is presumably more uniform, have been less convincing. The highest

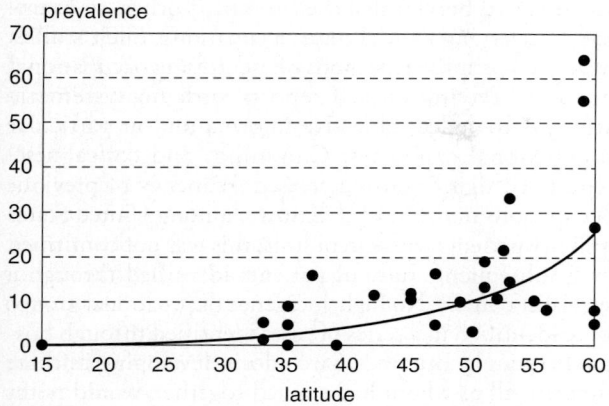

Figure 14–1 Comparison of prevalence rates (per 10^5) by latitude of capital city in 28 countries suggests increasing prevalence with distance from the equator.

incidence in the British case series[63] was in the southernmost of the four study areas with a steady decrease northward, although admittedly over a distance of only 600 miles. Studies within the United States, collated by Bresnitz and Strom,[76] show an increased frequency among patients currently living in southern and eastern States; this appears to be a consistent finding although risk estimates vary widely (from 1.1 to 13.3). Stratified analyses in many of these surveys suggested an interaction between race and geography, whereby the risks for African Americans living in these areas were consistently higher than for Whites. This difference in geographic prevalence lends weight to the argument that sarcoidosis might be caused by environmental exposure to an infectious agent.

There appear to be no classic migrant studies of sarcoidosis. A potential difficulty in conducting such a study was highlighted by Hennessy and colleagues.[77] In their population-based case series from Rochester, Minnesota, USA, immigrants who had been resident in the community for less than 5 years were more likely to present with asymptomatic disease as a result of routine general health medical screening. Thus, disease rates in this group may appear artificially high.

Clustering

Interest in temporal or spatial clusters of sarcoidosis arises from the possibility that the disease is the result of a transmissible agent. An unusually detailed analysis of cases detected on the Isle of Man was reported by Hills and colleagues.[78] Using a method developed by Pike and Smith[79] and selecting controls at random from pathology and radiology records, they reported a highly significant increase in links between cases whose places of residence, during an "infective period" of 5 years before and 2 years after diagnosis, were separated by distances

of less than 100 meters. No excess of residential links within 500 meters or of school or recreational links was found; the significant increase in workplace links probably reflected the fact that 13 (9%) cases were health workers in the island's single hospital. The question of an increase in ascertainment among this latter group remains unexplored. An increase in case pairs diagnosed within 1 year of each other provided some evidence for temporal clustering within the same population.

Other reports of "clusters" depend on small case series of patients in "contact" with one another[70,80]; these are generally uncontrolled and difficult to interpret. Hosoda and colleagues[68] were unable to find any evidence of temporal-spatial clustering in two areas of Japan.

Several authors have described the frequency of sarcoidosis among the immediate family of patients; these reports differ in the assiduousness with which relatives were investigated. The highest frequency was found in an Irish population of 114 patients identified through a specialist clinic[81]; 11 (9.6%) of these were found, largely through questionnaires, to have one or more siblings with the same disease. Although it is likely that the chances of a diagnosis of sarcoidosis are intrinsically higher among the relatives of cases, approximately 2.5% of the sibling pool in this population were thus diagnosed as having the disease, a prevalence almost certainly higher than in the general population. These findings are very similar to those from a study of African American patients in whom a sibling disease frequency of 10% was reported.[82] Other studies, in which the methods were different in some important respects, have reported much lower frequencies ranging between 0.7[83] and 4.6%.[84] A more recent questionnaire study sent to 406 patients with sarcoidosis in the United Kingdom reported that 5.9% of index cases had relatives with biopsy-proven sarcoidosis. A λ_S (relative risk of disease in a sibling compared to population disease prevalence) value of 36 to 73 indicated significant familial clustering.[85] Studies of affected families suggest that the mode of inheritance is polygenic, with the major histocompatibility complex (MHC) contributing to the susceptibility.[86]

Seasonal clustering has been described in several settings. Clearly, the date of diagnosis may bear little relationship to the date of disease onset; most authors have attempted to account for this by restricting analysis to patients with supposedly recent-onset disease. In Greece, following mass radiography of almost 85,000 adults between 1980 and 1989, no diagnoses of asymptomatic stage I sarcoidosis were made between the months of July and November.[87] Forty (70%) cases were identified between the months of March and May in each year. Similarly, in a Spanish population of patients with erythema nodosum and bilateral hilar lymphadenopathy, almost half had a diagnosis made in April, May, or June.[88] Japanese patients with bilateral hilar lymphadenopathy, identified through a nationwide casefinding exercise, were most frequently detected during the months June and July[68]; this pattern was present among those identified by mass radiography as well as those presenting with symptomatic disease. A May "outbreak" of eight cases of acute sarcoidosis, accompanied by arthropathy, was reported in Norfolk, England, in 1988[89]; any family or other spatial contacts between the cases were not described.

Smoking

Several authors have examined the frequency of cigarette smoking among patients with sarcoidosis and have compared it with the frequency among a referent group of the general population. A selection of such studies is presented in Table 14–5. Most have observed a reduced prevalence of smoking among sarcoidosis patients. In some studies, notably those reported by Bresnitz and colleagues[90] and Douglas and colleagues,[91] an exposure-response relationship has been observed, with decreasing risk estimates for those with heavier smoking habits. A variety of biologic mechanisms has been postulated to be responsible for this pattern and it is notable that a similar, inverse relationship has been reported in extrinsic allergic alveolitis,[92] another granulomatous pulmonary disease. Such relationships need, however, to be interpreted with care. Bresnitz and colleagues,[90] for example, reported but did not describe a conflicting relationship in their population between cigarette smoking and socioeconomic status as measured by family income; following multivariate regression, including both these indices, the association between smoking and sarcoidosis was not statistically significant. A possible explanation for this finding, aside from the power of this relatively small study, is an increase in ascertainment of sarcoidosis among high-income groups in whom cigarette smoking is less frequent.

Occupation

An increase in the diagnosis of sarcoidosis in women working in fluorescent light factories in Salem, Massachusetts in the 1940s, led to the recognition that beryllium could cause granulomatous disease, which became known as "Salem sarcoid." The similarities between sarcoidosis and berylliosis have prompted others to examine associations with certain occupations. Such studies have used primitive methods of identifying occupational histories, relying on self-reports with no systematic attempts to collect objective information on particular occupational exposures. Cummings and colleagues[93] reported a significantly increased frequency of previous occupations in the lumber industry among United States military patients with sarcoidosis; this was not confirmed by a subsequent study of patients identified through a specialist clinic.[26] No high-incidence occupational groups were identified in a series of cases identified through hospital clinics in Britain.[63] Sarcoidosis developing in three firemen, all of whom had trained together, would point toward exposure to a common environmental antigen.[94] Such findings have led to the hypothesis that the handling or burning of woods may lead to the development of sarcoidosis, thus explaining the increased incidence of sarcoidosis seen in studies looking at firefighters[95] and those individuals living in rural settings.[96]

An increased frequency of sarcoidosis in particular (often high-income) occupational groups has also been reported in Rochester, Minnesota, USA,[77] where health professionals (14 physicians and 10 nurses) were included among the 129 identified cases. This proportion (19% of all cases) is probably higher than that in the general population (estimated at 6%). Edmonstone[97] reported that 24 (15%) of 156 cases identified through specialist hospital services were hospital workers, and 16 (10%) were nurses; none of the latter group had presented through employment screening services and all had "substantial symptoms." Nonetheless, with findings such as these, it is difficult to dissociate the effects of better access to diagnostic services.

It is clear that a novel approach is required to explain many of the epidemiologic features of the disease, including its rarity in childhood and the difficulty of detecting spatial clustering. Among such explanations, and by analogy with multiple sclerosis with which sarcoidosis shares many distributive features, mycobacterial infection at an unusual age might be included, perhaps in the second decade of life. This explanation would be consistent with the fact that the disease presents in early adulthood, is more common in northern latitudes where, through common behavioral patterns,

---

TABLE 14–5   Risk Estimates for Smoking in Sarcoidosis—Selected Case-Referent Studies

| Lead Author | Country | Comparison Population | Sarcoidosis | | Odds Ratio |
			N	Smoking (%)	
Terris[596]	United States	Medical outpatients	240	53*	0.80
Douglas[91]	United Kingdom	General population	183	22	0.36
Harf[597]	France	Healthy volunteers	101	25	0.26
Bresnitz[90]	United States	Medical outpatients	51	55*	0.70

*Includes exsmokers.

infections common in childhood elsewhere may be delayed. Future epidemiologic studies would profit by concentrating on determining distributive features consistent with such a hypothesis.

Genetic Factors

Sarcoidosis is believed to arise as a result of environmental exposure to an, as yet, unidentified antigen, in genetically predisposed individuals. The evidence for genetic contributions is suggested by racial variations in its epidemiology and familial clustering. Although there is good circumstantial evidence, particularly from beryllium workers, that an exuberant granulomatous response to organic and inorganic stimuli requires some form of host predisposition, the mechanisms of this are not clear. Many studies have explored the class I and II major histocompatibility loci, but different messages emerge from studies that look at small samples of patients with different ethnic backgrounds and at different stages of disease. There is an urgent need for large-scale studies recruiting better-defined patient populations with clear disease phenotypes.

Candidate genes that may account for a genetic predisposition have been identified in pathogenic processes that lead to granuloma formation, namely, in loci that influence T-cell function, antigen recognition and processing, matrix deposition, and lung fibrosis. Genetic factors that may also account for disease phenotype, progression, and subsequent prognosis include angiotensin converting enzyme genes and chemokine/cytokine genes. The human leukocyte antigen (HLA) complex plays a central role in presenting antigens for T-cell recognition. In other immune-based disorders, the pattern of HLA class II allele presentation confers both resistance and susceptibility to disease presentation. Analyzing disease presentation globally, no distinct HLA class II allele has been shown to be absolutely associated with the development of sarcoidosis in all populations although common themes are now emerging.

In a study of 122 Scandinavian patients, HLA-DR14 and -DR15 were associated with chronic disease and -DR17 predicted a good prognosis.[98] There appears to be good evidence that the HLA-B8 allele is associated with erythema nodosum and both HLA-B8 and HLA-DR3 with spontaneous resolution.[99,100] Two detailed Japanese studies have been reported. In one, increased frequencies of HLA-1, -Bw46, -Cx46, -DRw8, -DRw9, and -DR52 were identified by comparison with 478 healthy subjects. Patients with HLA-DR52 were the most common, but there were no differences in clinical features between individuals with or without this allele. HLA-DR5 was associated with a better outcome.[101] In the second study,[102] increases in HLA-B51, -DR4, -DR5, -DRw9, -DR52, and -DR53 were found. These two studies have found different HLA frequencies, even within populations of patients from the same country.

These differences may reflect a heterogeneous group in terms of disease stage or organ involvement. Furthermore, although patients in a good prognostic group were defined, the subset of patients likely to deteriorate was not identified.

Two hundred and thirty-three patients were enrolled in a study in which data was obtained from two European populations (Italian and Czech).[103] There was remarkable agreement between the two populations studied. A positive association with the HLA-1, -B8, and -DR3 haplotype was found. HLA-DR3 and -DR4 were more common among females and -DR5 among males. The B27 allele was found in patients with pure pulmonary sarcoidosis. The study also confirmed the association of HLA-DR3 with a good outcome. Foley and colleagues[104] studied HLA-DR and -DQ allele frequency in case-control samples from three European populations. They demonstrated that across the three population groups, patients with sarcoidosis had a significant reduction in the frequency in the HLA-DR alleles (*HLA-DRB*01* and *-*04*) that contain a hydrophobic residue at position 11. This was confirmed in three other studies suggesting that there may be a common genetic determinant that protects from disease that is independent of ethnic origin.[98,101,103] Other more variable HLA-DR alleles conferred susceptibility and this is consistent with the studies of Schurman and colleagues[86] who identified the MHC class II region to be highly relevant to the genetic predisposition to sarcoidosis in a cohort of German families.

Other studies have demonstrated organ-specific genetic association. Ishihara et al.[105] showed that there was association with *DRB3*0101* in sarcoidosis, and that this allele was in linkage dysequilibrium with DR5- and DR6-associated alleles. In patients with retinal perivasculitis and other ocular lesions, there were significant decreases in DR3, -5, -6, and -8 allele frequencies. Naruse and colleagues[106] described an association of cardiac sarcoidosis with *DQB1*0601*.

In chronic beryllium disease, a disorder with histopathologic appearances identical to sarcoidosis but caused by a hypersensitivity to beryllium salts, an excess of HLA-DP alleles with a glutamine residue at position 69 of the B1 chain was observed by Richeldi and colleagues[107] Lympany and colleagues[108] observed a similar but not so striking association but in sarcoidosis this was not confirmed in subsequent studies.

Serum angiotensin converting enzyme (SACE) has been implicated in the pathophysiology of sarcoidosis and reflects disease activity. SACE levels in normal and sarcoidosis patients are influenced by an insertion (I)/deletion (D) polymorphism in the SACE gene. A number of studies have investigated the significance of SACE gene insertion/deletion (I/D) polymorphism on disease severity and prognosis. SACE genotype corresponds to SACE levels and may influence the development of autoimmune manifestations[109] and bronchial hyperresponsiveness.[110] It remains unclear whether

SACE genotype is a prognostic marker in sarcoidosis. One study suggested that SACE genotype may influence disease presentation in African Americans but not in Whites,[111] but our own group looking at 118 UK and 56 Czech white patients with sarcoidosis found no association between SACE I/D polymorphism and pulmonary disease severity, fibrosis, and progression.[112]

Genetic polymorphisms of the cytokine, tumour necrosis factor (TNF) have been the focus of a number of recent studies. Previous studies have shown high levels of TNF in patients with sarcoidosis and its release from alveolar macrophages is pivotal in granuloma formation. The relative importance of polymorphisms of both the TNF-α and TNF-β gene, despite studies by a number of different groups, awaits clarification. Somoskovi and colleagues[113] analyzed bronchoalveolar lavage fluid (BAL) and showed that TNF-α and TNF-β polymorphisms did not determine the level of TNF-α release of mononuclear cells activated during the course of sarcoid inflammation. A number of studies have suggested that polymorphisms of both the TNF-α and TNF-β genes are linked to prognosis in sarcoidosis.[114–116] The interpretation of these results is made difficult in a number of ways. First, these studies come from different groups studying patients with differing phenotypes from different racial backgrounds. Second, the interpretation of associations of TNF-α and TNF-β polymorphisms is made difficult due to linkage dysequilibrium with other HLA class I and II alleles. Despite these qualifications, TNF polymorphisms, perhaps as part of an extended haplotype with HLA loci, are likely to be relevant to disease manifestation and severity.

Polymorphisms for the genes of the chemokine receptors CCR5 and CCR2 exist and result in nonfunctional receptor expression. In Czech patients with sarcoidosis, the presence of CCR5Δ32 and CCR2-64I are associated with disease susceptibility and protection, respectively.[117]

There is no doubt that genetic predisposition plays a role in sarcoidosis. This predisposition is likely to lie in part in the class I and class II MHC region of the genome, but polymorphisms of other candidate genes probably play a role. These candidate genes will likely include the antigen processing genes, *TAP1*, *TAP2*, *DMA*, *DMB*, and *LMP* and polymorphisms within crucial granuloma-inducing cytokines such as TNF-α, interferon (IFN)-γ, and interleukin (IL)-2.[118,119]

Immune Processes

There are good data to support the concept that sarcoidosis is a T-cell-driven immunologic response. Several distinct immunologic mechanisms are involved in the process: antigen recognition, T-cell proliferation, T-cell recruitment to disease sites, mononuclear cell recruitment to disease sites, granuloma formation, and repair processes.

Models of immune granuloma formation demonstrate that the first phase in granuloma formation is the recruitment of tissue macrophages to the disease site; these macrophages attempt to ingest the partially or completely degraded foreign material.[120] The degraded antigenic material is expressed on the surface of the macrophage or other antigen-presenting cell as small peptide fragments complexed in the groove of class II MHC molecules. This step is essential for T-cell recognition by T-cell antigen receptors.[121,122] Class II MHC molecules are crucial for antigen presentation to CD4+ T cells and are, thus, necessary for the subsequent development of a cell-mediated immune response.[123–127]

In sarcoidosis, there is evidence that alveolar macrophages have a greater capacity to present antigens than do normal macrophages. Alveolar macrophages from patients with sarcoidosis are capable of increased presentation of nonrelevant antigens, such as tetanus toxoid to lymphocytes,[128,129] in comparison with those from normal individuals. They express higher concentrations of HLA-DR molecules on the surface.[130] They express accessory molecules such as the macrophage-adhesion molecules (intercellular adhesion molecule 1 [ICAM-1]. They also express lymphocyte function–associated antigen 3 [LFA-3]), which probably plays a role during antigen presentation in the cell-surface-triggered events leading to lymphocyte activation.[131,132] Sarcoid lung lymphocytes express an increased surface density of CD2 (the sheep erythrocyte receptor), the natural receptor for LFA-3 believed to be an important accessory receptor in T-cell activation and LFA-1 and the ligand for ICAM-1.[133]

T-Cell Antigen Receptors

T lymphocytes predominantly use the $\alpha\beta$ heterodimer form of T-cell (antigen) receptors (TCRs) on their surface to recognize MHC/oligopeptide complexes. Analysis of TCR expression on the surfaces of T cells and levels of messenger ribonucleic acid (mRNA) in the cytoplasm provide further evidence that lung macrophages are presenting antigens to T cells in sarcoidosis. The consequence of TCR triggering is the down-regulation of surface TCR molecules and the up-regulation of TCR mRNA transcript numbers.[134,135] If TCR triggering occurs in sarcoidosis, it would be expected that T cells from active disease sites would exhibit the appropriate surface and mRNA changes, which is the case. Compared with blood T cells, sarcoid lung T lymphocytes exhibit a decrease in density of surface TCR molecules, and they express increased numbers of TCR β-chain mRNA transcripts.[136] This down-regulation of TCRs may explain the reduced proliferative response of lung T cells to recall antigens compared with lung cells obtained from normal individuals.[137]

Studies of the repertoire of TCRs present on T cells at disease sites further support the concept that sarcoidosis is the result of the presence of a specific antigen. The enormous diversity of T cells for specific antigens is created by rearrangement of germline variable (V), diversity (D), junctional (J), and constant (C) region elements of the two types ($\alpha\beta$ and $\gamma\delta$) of TCRs. The number of $\alpha\beta$ TCRs is much higher than $\gamma\delta$. Theoretically, analysis of the relative use of these elements in TCRs should yield evidence as to whether the T cells accumulate in a biased fashion with exaggerated use of specific TCR elements, as would be expected if sarcoidosis resulted from persistent, specific antigen(s) in association with enhanced antigen presentation/T-cell triggering.

The evidence from analysis of TCRs in sarcoidosis points to the persistent antigen hypothesis. Sophisticated molecular biologic studies have shown that particular families of TCR molecules (α chain or β chain) may exhibit individual bias in the expression of specific V beta, V alpha, or gamma/delta + T-cell receptor genes in T-cell subsets from patients who have sarcoidosis. Table 14–6 summarizes studies that have demonstrated the overexpression of particular variable regions of the α- and β-chains of the TCR.[138–147] Further evidence for oligoclonality comes from the studies of MHC and TCR in the same population.[140] A striking association of an excess number of lymphocytes bearing the TCR α chain determinant AV2S3 and a class II MHC haplotype that includes the DR3 (17) allele was demonstrated (ie, that a particular molecule required for antigen presentation, together with an as yet unidentified antigen, is recognized by a TCR that includes a specific α chain variant).[140] More recently, this group demonstrated bias in α chain J region use in this population.[148] Although nucleotide sequences varied in cyclic deoxyribonucleic acid (cDNA) clones from AV2S3 CD4+ cells, the amino acids encoded were identical. In active sarcoidosis, this group have phenotypically characterized the AV2S3 lung T cells, detecting expression of the activation markers CD26, CD28, and CD69 on the T-cell surface. These results suggest ongoing and selective stimulation of AV2S3 T cells by a specific antigen,[149] and have further correlated this with a shorter disease course characterized by an earlier relapse, suggesting that the AV2S3 (+) T cells may have a protective role against a presumed "sarcoid" antigen.[150] Finally, there is evidence of compartmentalization of cells, with Vβ8+ CD4+ cells to the lung (the site of granulomas) and Vβ8+ CD8+ T cells to the blood.

All of these studies support the concept that T-cell activation is driven through the TCR mechanism by an antigen-specific process, leading to a specific oligoclonal response on the background of a generalized polyclonal expansion of T cells. On a cautionary note, the vast variations in TCR V gene use that have been reported from different groups may be influenced by either the heterogeneity in onset of disease (ie, acute versus chronic) or differences in the ethnicity of study populations, thus larger studies need to confirm these findings. It may also be that some of the T-cell clonal expansion is caused by contamination by exogenous antigens that are not involved directly in the development of sarcoidosis.[151]

A bias in TCR use in sarcoidosis is also seen in studies that have analyzed the T cell $\gamma\delta$ TCR. Theoretically, the $\gamma\delta$ TCR is of particular relevance to sarcoidosis because at least some $\gamma\delta$ T cells in normal individuals respond to *M. tuberculosis*, an agent known to evoke a granulomatous response[152] and now suspected as the etiologic factor in sarcoidosis. In normal individuals, less than 10% of blood and lung T cells use this TCR, but there is a marked expansion in the numbers of T cells, particularly in blood but also in lung,[153] in a subgroup of individuals with sarcoidosis. Furthermore, in some individuals a large proportion of these T cells use the same γ chains and the same δ chains, suggesting that they were amplified as a result of a specific, persistent antigenic stimulus.[154] Together, these data are compatible with the concept that sarcoidosis is caused by persistent, specific antigens (exogenous and/or self) that induce a cell-mediated immune response.

Consequences of T-Cell Triggering

A number of results of the initial direct macrophage to T-cell interaction are of importance in the development of the granuloma. These involve the expression of a number of cell-surface molecules on macrophages and lymphocytes and the lymphocytes' release of key cytokines.

Lymphocytes

Cell Surface Markers. Studies of the lymphocyte populations obtained by lavage and from tissue samples support suggestions of an immune basis to the disease. Sarcoidosis is a systemic disorder, but the lymphocyte populations are strikingly compartmentalized. At sites of disease activity such as the lung, there is a marked expansion in lymphocyte numbers, whereas there is a lymphopenia in the blood.[155] Within the lung there is further compartmentalization, with different lymphocyte subsets being distributed in the pulmonary vascular bed, epithelium, interstitium, and the bronchus-associated lymphoid tissue.[156] The distribution of the different lymphocyte subpopulations will reflect the underlying disease state. In sarcoidosis, lymphocyte numbers are increased in the bronchoalveolar space. The lung lymphocytes are predominantly CD4+ T cells, with the ratio

TABLE 14–6   T Cell Receptor Overexpression at Disease Sites in Sarcoidosis

Vα2.3 (AV2S3)
Vβ2,3,5,6,8,14,15,16,18,19
Vγ9
Vδ1

of CD4+ to CD8+ populations being 3 to 10:1. In normal lung the CD4+ to CD8+ ratio is 2:1, approximately 1 to 1.5:1 in sarcoid blood, and 1.5 to 3:1 in normal blood.[155] Occasionally CD8+ cells outnumber CD4+ cells in sarcoidosis. Agostini and colleagues[157] showed this in 15 of 394 patients.

The mechanism of T-cell activation remains unclear, but involves expression of various activation markers including interleukin 2 receptor (IL-2R), HLA-DR class II MHC molecules, and the very-late antigen (VLA)-1 marker of late activation.[158–161] Koura and colleagues[162] studied the distribution of the IL-2R inducer, thioredoxin, and hypothesized its role in the induction of IL-2R expression on T cells, given its coexistence with the IL-2R in the granulomas of sarcoid patients. The expression of these cell-surface markers of activation are also increased on macrophages/monocytes and correlate with the percentage of BAL lymphocytes.[163]

Most T cells are CD45RO+ (in common with normal lung T cells), which denotes that they are of the "antigen-primed" subset of T cells and are leu-8-.[157,164,165] Furthermore, they can express the epitopes identified by the antibodies Ki67 and proliferating cell nuclear antigen (PCNA), which indicate that the cells are proliferating.[166,167] This is consistent with the observation of spontaneous proliferation ex vivo in cells lavaged from patients with active disease.[158] In contrast with those in the lung, blood T cells in active pulmonary sarcoidosis appear relatively quiescent with no evidence of lymphokine release.[168] Mollers and colleagues[169] also demonstrated compartmentalization of naive and memory lymphocytes with significantly higher CD45RO:CD45RA ratios seen in BAL fluid compared with blood. Although some blood T cells do express activation markers such as IL-2R and class II MHC molecules, these cells possibly represent T cells activated in tissues such as the lung that have migrated to the blood.[168]

The accessory function of antigen-presenting cells, such as alveolar macrophages, to facilitate antigen-induced T-cell proliferation, requires presentation of the antigen in association with B7 costimulating molecules.[170] Alveolar macrophages from patients with sarcoidosis with CD4+ T-cell alveolitis demonstrate up-regulated expression of the costimulatory cell surface markers CD80, CD86, and CD72 and high levels of IL-15, suggesting that these molecules may play a role in the regulation of the sarcoid T-cell response. Agostini and colleagues[171] hypothesized that locally released cytokines interact with the alveolar macrophages leading to the development of sarcoid T-cell alveolitis.

There is evidence of B-cell activation in pulmonary sarcoidosis. Levels of immunoglobulins in the blood and lung are often elevated, and immune complexes are found in both the blood and epithelial lining fluid of some patients.[172,173] Immunoglobulin-secreting B cells are likely to be present in the lung parenchyma, rather than on the pulmonary epithelial surface,[174,175] and there appears to be a nonspecific polyclonal activation of these cells by T helper cells in the local microenvironment.[172] Interestingly, anti-T-lymphocyte antibodies are observed in sarcoidosis in blood and lung.[176] These antibodies are predominantly IgM and are mostly directed toward CD8+ T cells; their function is unknown. A more recent study of lung and lymph node biopsies has emphasized the presence of increased numbers of B cells between the granulomas, which may explain the source of the polyclonal increase in immunoglobulins and possibly the immune complexes in the peripheral blood and epithelial lining fluid.[177]

Mononuclear Phagocytes

Cell Surface Markers. Bronchoalveolar lavage studies in sarcoid patients show an increase in the number of alveolar macrophages compared with normal controls.[178] Studies of lung macrophages using monoclonal antibodies have demonstrated that the cells bear the phenotype of young, recently recruited monocytes,[179,180] suggesting migration of cells from the periphery. Granulocyte-macrophage colony–stimulating factor (GM-CSF), a cytokine present in granulomas, can also drive local proliferation of macrophages.[181] Thus the increase in macrophage numbers most likely reflects both local proliferation and recruitment of peripheral blood monocytes. The pulmonary mononuclear phagocyte population in sarcoidosis is also proliferating at a rate that is two to three times higher than normal.[182] Alveolar macrophages are usually poor accessory cells. In patients with sarcoidosis, however, their accessory function can be up-regulated, possibly in response to IFN-γ produced by T cells.[183] As a result of the activation of lung mononuclear phagocytes, the surface density of all categories of class II MHC molecules is increased on these cells.[130,184] Given that pulmonary T cells in sarcoidosis are releasing IFN-γ and because IFN-γ augments class II MHC molecule surface density on alveolar macrophages, it is likely that the T cells participate at least in part in the lung macrophage activation process. The Clara cell 10 kD protein (CC10), a product of nonciliated bronchiolar epithelial cells, has inhibitory effects on IFN-γ and thus may be a regulator of the inflammatory process in sarcoidosis. A putative role is suggested by studies by Shijubo and colleagues[185] demonstrating that patients with sarcoidosis whose disease is in regression have higher levels of CC10 in sera and BAL fluid compared with patients with progressive disease. The importance of IFN-γ in granuloma formation is further highlighted by the lack of granuloma formation that occurs in IFN-γ gene knockout mice after exposure to thermophilic bacteria.[186]

Other macrophage cell-surface molecules that are differentially expressed in sarcoidosis include the D series of antibodies first reported by Poulter and colleagues.[187] Increased numbers of RFD1 (interdigitating cell marker), RFD7 (mature tissue macrophages), and RFD9 (epithelioid cells) are present in sarcoidosis; the dual expression of RFD1/RFD7, a combination not observed in normal tissues, is present on approximately 40% of sarcoid macrophages.[188] This population can downregulate the autologous mixed lymphocyte reaction, suggesting a regulatory role for this subset of cells.[189] Furthermore, this subset is present in higher numbers in active and more advanced (type III) disease.[188]

Macrophages and peripheral blood mononuclear cells have also been shown to have an enhanced expression of surface adhesion molecules that are necessary for close cell-to-cell contact, a necessary prerequisite to antigen presentation. The binding of CD2 (lymphocyte) to LFA-3 (macrophage) has been described above. Other mechanisms involve the beta-2 integrins and the immunoglobulin supergenes. The density of CD11/CD18 was increased on sarcoid blood cells from 21 patients in one study,[190] and the percentage of CD11b+ and ICAM-11 alveolar macrophages was found to be higher in "active" sarcoidosis than in "inactive" sarcoidosis and in normal controls in another.[191] In other studies, more macrophages were found to be CD11a+ in sarcoidosis than controls,[192] and an increased number of macrophages expressing CD11a, b, and c was found by Schaberg and colleagues.[193] Other macrophage surface receptors of interest include CD14.[194] Compared with controls, patients with sarcoidosis had a higher percentage of CD14 positive alveolar macrophages obtained by BAL (34% compared with 22%). Furthermore, the antigen density was higher on the macrophages from patients with sarcoidosis; surface shedding of the receptor was reflected by increased amounts of soluble CD14 present in the serum of patients with sarcoidosis as compared with controls.

All these studies emphasize that the surface-receptor repertoire of macrophages reflects their activation status at disease sites in sarcoidosis, and also that the expression of these molecules will be of functional consequence in terms of cell adhesion and ligand reception.

Cytokines

Monokines. Macrophage mediators implicated in granuloma formation include IL-1 (T-cell chemoattractant and activation cofactor after antigen presentation; adhesion molecule up-regulation), TNF-α (adhesion molecule up-regulation and up-regulator of IL-6 by connective tissue matrix cells), granulocyte colony–stimulating factor (G-CSF; granulocyte differentiation in bone marrow),[195] and arachidonic acid metabolites, which may play a regulatory role by their effects on class II molecule expression. Prostaglandin E (PGE) down-regulates class II molecule expression on macrophages compromising granulomas, whereas prostaglandin F2α up-regulates the expression of these molecules.[196,197]

Evidence that the local microenvironment stimulates newly recruited macrophages was provided by Pantelidis and colleagues.[198] They showed that BAL fluid obtained from patients with sarcoidosis but not from those with other diffuse lung diseases stimulated mononuclear cells to release lysozyme in vitro using a single-cell hemolytic plaque assay.

Although the data are conflicting, the "early" proinflammatory cytokines, TNF-α and IL-1, almost certainly play an important role in granuloma formation. Some studies show no increase, whereas others demonstrate an increase in macrophage IL-1 secretion compared with controls.[199–201] In other studies, evaluation of IL-1 mRNA transcript numbers in sarcoid macrophages showed no difference from controls, and the in vitro IL-1 responses of control and sarcoidosis monocytes and macrophages to lipopolysaccharide were similar, suggesting that there is no difference in the regulation of IL-1 production in sarcoidosis.[201,202] Of the two more recent studies, one has shown that alveolar macrophages from patients with sarcoidosis spontaneously secrete IL-1, TNF-α, and PGE$_2$, but that the amounts secreted from patients with active disease did not differ significantly from patients with inactive disease.[203] By contrast, Muller-Quernheim and colleagues[204] demonstrated that IL-1 and TNF-α were spontaneously released by alveolar macrophages of patients with active sarcoidosis as compared with patients with inactive disease and autologous peripheral blood monocytes.

Alveolar macrophage secretion of TNF-α has been found to be increased in patients with sarcoidosis in some studies [205–207] but not in another.[208] Using a single-cell assay, it has been shown that alveolar macrophages from patients with sarcoidosis spontaneously secrete more TNF-α than normal individuals.[209] When normal macrophages are cultured in the presence of IL-2, a cytokine known to be secreted spontaneously by lymphocytes obtained from the lower respiratory tract of patients with sarcoidosis, increased amounts of TNF-α mRNA transcripts are found.[210] In an in situ hybridization study of granulomas, Myatt and colleagues[211] showed that giant cells and epithelioid cells in the granulomas contained mRNA for TNF-α. In patients with sarcoidosis, soluble TNF receptors (TNF-R) can inhibit TNF-α activity, and furthermore the degree of inhibition may result in a reduced tendency for pulmonary fibrosis. In a study looking at 16 patients with histologically proven sarcoidosis, Armstong and colleagues[212] showed that patients with stage I sarcoidosis had increased inhibition of TNF-α bioactivity by TNF-R, compared with patients with stage II/III disease. They hypothesized that this represents a homeostatic mechanism, which protects the lung from high levels of TNF seen in the chronic inflammatory state. The immediate release of high concentrations of TNF-α and IL-1 from cultured alveolar macrophages suggests that these cells are activated in vivo.

Secretion of the cytokines, IL-12 and IL-15, from activated macrophages appears to be important in driving the Th$_1$ lymphocyte proliferation.[213] Other products released by macrophages from patients with sarcoidosis include G-CSF (inducer of granulopoiesis and neutrophil activation)[214] and the ectoenzyme CD13/aminopeptidase N.[215] The activity of CD13/aminopeptidase N in BAL fluid is higher in patients with sarcoidosis compared with normal controls, and correlates with lymphocyte percentages, the CD4:CD8 ratio, and the degree of parenchymal involvement. CD13/aminopeptidase N induced in vitro chemotactic activity was greater for CD4 T cells compared with CD8 T cells, suggesting a role in lymphocyte recruitment. Anti-inflammatory cytokines such as IL-10, that can deactivate macrophages, may have a role in the spontaneous resolution of alveolitis that is seen in many patients.[216]

These conflicting results suggests that the evaluation of cytokine release in vitro may be confounded by the influence of a number of complex factors, including the effects of adhesion to the culture dishes, the effects of cell-to-cell contact in culture, and the modulating influences of the release of other cytokines and their inhibitors into the culture medium. Recently introduced methods of evaluating the products of single cells in microculture chambers may help to clarify the cytokine profiles of cells from disease sites.[217]

In addition to their secretory capacity, alveolar macrophages have been shown to release increased oxidant species that result in lung injury [218,219] and to produce type IV collagenase that attacks basement membrane collagen.[220]

Lymphokines. Antigen presentation, in association with secondary cytokine signals, stimulates T cells to release a number of lymphokines that activate macrophages and lymphocytes and to provide the building blocks from which granulomas are formed.[2,3,221] The defined lymphokines of most relevance to the generation of granulomas are IL-2 (the T-cell growth factor) and IFN-γ (multiple effects including a potent activator of macrophages). Consistent with this concept, monocytes and alveolar macrophages can be stimulated in vitro by IFN-γ to increase the expression of class II surface antigens, Fc receptors, IL-2 receptors, and transferrin receptors. Furthermore, mononuclear phagocytes form giant cells under the influence of IFN-γ under appropriate circumstances.[222] Prior and Haslam[223] showed that serum levels of IFN-γ were significantly higher in patients with sarcoidosis than in controls but that the levels decreased significantly after administration of corticosteroids. More sustained serum levels often were present in patients who had a better outcome; the higher the pretreatment level, the lower the degree of radiographic abnormality.

Lung lymphocytes express mRNA for GM-CSF (stimulator of granulopoiesis and monopoiesis)[224] and for monocyte colony–stimulating factor (M-CSF; stimulator of monocyte proliferation).[225] The relative contributions of the lymphokines to granuloma formation are not known.

Tissue immunohistochemistry studies have confirmed that lavage cells are representative of those in the lung parenchyma,[226,227] and in situ hybridization supports the roles of cytokines in generating immune granulomas. A detailed study of cytokine expression in lymph nodes has demonstrated the presence of IL-1α and -β, TNF-α, IL-2, IL-6, and IFN-γ in situ and that there is a spatial arrangement of cytokine producing cells. IL-1β, TNF-α, and IFN-γ are restricted to the granuloma itself, whereas the other cytokines are distributed in cells more randomly.[228] The most avidly expressed product was IL-1β, and IFN-γ was 32-fold more abundant than IL-2. These data are consistent with those of Campbell and colleagues[226] and Munro and colleagues[229] who used monoclonal antibodies to identify cell phenotype to define spatial arrangements of cells in immune granulomas.

The common thread that arises from studies performed on cytokine profiles is of a Th$_1$ dominant condition (ie, a predominance of IFN-γ, IL-2, and IL-12) over Th$_2$ cytokines such as IL-4, IL-5, and IL-10. Recent investigations have demonstrated increased expression of IL-12 and IL-18 in BAL fluid from patients with sarcoidosis, cytokines that are known to induce IFN-γ production.[230–232] The prominent shift toward a type Th$_1$ phenotype is predominantly seen in CD4$^+$ T cells[233] but has also been described in CD8$^+$ T cells.[234,235] Th$_2$-type cytokines have also been detected in some patients,[236] and this may reflect compartmentalization of Th$_2$ cytokine-producing T cells into peripheral blood rather than the alveolar compartment.[163] The ratio of Th$_1$/Th$_2$ T cells might explain differences in clinical outcome in pulmonary sarcoidosis; a Th$_1$ cytokine profile leads to granuloma formation and subsequent fibrosis, and a Th$_2$ phenotype favors resolution without chronic sequelae.[237] Factors that influence Th$_0$ differentiation are likely to impact on clinical prognosis in patients with sarcoidosis. It is of interest that HLA-DR17–positive Scandinavian patients who have been shown to have a favorable prognosis,[98] have also been shown to exhibit a less exuberant Th$_1$ response.[234] The Th$_1$ cytokine profile in patients with sarcoidosis is most likely maintained by the ubiquitous Th$_1$ cytokine IFN-γ, given its additional role of suppressing the Th$_2$ lymphocyte response.[238]

As a result of these recent studies, there is now convincing evidence that IL-12 is up-regulated at sites of inflammation in sarcoidosis, which is a result of enhanced expression and dysregulated production by activated alveolar macrophages. Granulomatous models in experimental animals support these observations.[239] As to how a Th$_1$ cytokine–driven immune response could maintain pulmonary fibrosis is less clear, but insights gained from animal models have suggested possible mechanisms. Using the *Schistosoma mansoni* model of immune granuloma, data suggest that pulmonary fibrosis may develop if there is a shift from a Th$_1$ to a Th$_2$ cytokine phenotype with secretion of IL-4, IL-5, IL-6, IL-9, and IL-10. The cytokine profile results in a fibroproliferative response leading to the development of pulmonary fibrosis.[237]

Chemokines

A number of important chemoattractants are relevant to the accumulation of inflammatory cells at lung disease sites. These include the CXC (macrophage inflammatory protein [MIP-1α], monocyte chemotactic protein [MCP-1], and regulated on activation, normal T cell expressed and secreted [RANTES]) and CC (IL-8) chemokine families of cytokines that can be produced by a number of immune cells present in the lung. These cytokines have both chemoattractant and cell-activating properties. Several authors[240–242] have pointed out that MIP-1α is involved in inflammatory cell recruitment in sarcoidosis and that RANTES appears to be a significant factor in both the recruitment of CD45RO+ lymphocytes into the lungs of patients with sarcoidosis[165] and the development of granulomas.[243] Other chemoattractants such as IL-8 and MCP-1 have been shown to be present in increased concentrations in the BAL fluid from patients with sarcoidosis,[244] although Pantelidis and colleagues[245] and Sugiyama and colleagues[246] showed that isolated alveolar macrophages from patients with sarcoidosis secreted no more IL-8 than did control subjects.

Adhesion Molecules. Cells traffic into tissue by initially adhering to endothelial cell-surface adhesion molecules. They then traffic into tissue usually under a chemoattractant gradient. Other adhesion molecules within organs allow close cell-to-cell contact. A selective expression of adhesion molecules is likely to influence recruitment of immune cells to areas of inflammation.[247] Hamblin and colleagues[248] showed high serum levels of circulating ICAM-1, E-selectin, and VCAM-1 in the serum of patients with sarcoidosis, but the most striking increase was in the E-selectin levels. Results by Kaseda and colleagues[249] suggest that L-selectin may be involved in the lymphocytic alveolitis characterized by acute pulmonary fibrosis. The ICAM-1 levels in BAL fluid were found by Shijubo and colleagues[250] to be higher in patients with sarcoidosis than in controls, although serum levels were no different from controls. The expression of ICAM-1 is increased on alveolar macrophages, epithelioid cells, and giant cells in sarcoidosis.[250,251] The soluble components of ICAM-1 (sICAM-1) are shed from the cell surface during binding to ligands, thus its concentration in the serum may reflect the degree of tissue inflammation.[252] The expression of ICAM-1 may be up-regulated by the synthesis and release of 1,25-dihydroxycholecalciferol from alveolar macrophages, that is itself up-regulated in granulomatous disease.[253]

Growth Factors. The accumulation of inflammatory cells and granulomas themselves can cause organ dysfunction, but it is the progression to fibrosis that can result in most of the persistent abnormality. The fibrotic response in the lung is highly variable but can produce significant morbidity. The predisposition to develop marked fibrosis is unclear, and it is not known why the granulomatous infiltrates in some patients resolve completely whereas in others they evolve into a highly fibrotic response. A BAL neutrophilia that is driven by Th$_2$-type cytokines characterize the fibrotic response.

Growth factors have been demonstrated in the lungs of patients with sarcoidosis. Work has concentrated on the role of the anti-inflammatory cytokine, transforming growth factor-beta (TGF-β), but much of this has produced conflicting messages. High levels of TGF-β have been found in the BAL fluid of patients with remitting disease.[254] There is a strong negative correlation between IL-2 and TGF-β levels, suggesting a role in suppressing the Th$_1$ phenotype, given its known inhibitory effect on IL-12 and IFN-γ. Limper and colleagues[255] showed abundant TGF-β localization in the epithelioid cells within the non-necrotizing granulomas of sarcoidosis, which supports a role for growth factors in the healing process. Contrary to this is work by Khalil and colleagues[256] demonstrating increased TGF-β expression leading to extracellular matrix deposition in a number of diffuse lung diseases and that of Salez and colleagues[257] indicating that higher levels of TGF-β were seen in patients with more restricted lung function.

A wealth of different growth factors are produced by alveolar cells and may contribute to the development of fibrosis and include the products TNF-α, IL-1, IFN-γ, TGF-β, GM-CSF, vascular endothelial growth factor (VEGF), insulin-like growth factor (IGF-1), and platelet-derived growth factor (PDGF). Eklund and colleagues[258] found that concentrations of vitronectin, fibronectin, and hyaluronan in the BAL fluid were higher in patients with sarcoidosis than in controls. These connective tissue matrix proteins are important contributors to the repair process. Pohl and colleagues[259] found high levels of serum procollagen III peptide levels in patients with sarcoidosis. This procollagen peptide is cleaved from collagen as it is deposited in tissue and is a surrogate marker for collagen deposition. Furthermore, patients whose chest radiograph features were found to progress had higher levels of serum procollagen III than did patients whose radiographic features were more stable. Luisetti and colleagues[260] also found elevated serum procollagen peptide III in the serum of patients with sarcoidosis but, in contrast with the previous study, demonstrated no relationship to future disease progression or treatment resistance. These data are consistent with those previously reported by O'Connor and colleageus[261] who demonstrated that BAL procollagen peptide levels were higher in patients with sarcoidosis than in controls but found no association between these levels and disease severity or subsequent deterioration.

In sarcoidosis, macrophage secretion of TNF-α leads to an increased fibroblast recruitment, which in concert with the change to a Th$_2$ cytokine profile and the release of a number of different growth factors results in the deposition of collagen matrix products that is typical of the fibrotic response.

PATHOLOGY

Immune (Epithelioid Cell) Granulomas

Granulomas are collections of inflammatory cells at sites of disease or response to foreign invaders. Although central to the pathology of sarcoidosis, they are also a feature of other chronic interstitial lung diseases, including hypersensitivity pneumonitis and berylliosis. "Immune" granulomas result from specific cell-mediated immune mechanisms. The general paradigm of immune granuloma formation suggests a specific, T-cell-mediated response to an antigenic agent that has been processed by macrophages and has then been presented to antigen-specific T lymphocytes. The T cell, in turn, directs the accumulation and differentiation of mononuclear phagocytes in the local microenvironment.[2,3,262]

Immune granulomas are "epithelioid cell granulomas" because the dominant cell is the epithelioid cell, which is derived from the mononuclear phagocyte series of cells.[263,264] These large (20 to 40 μm) polygonal cells contain abundant cytoplasm; pale-staining nuclei are located at the center of the granuloma, surrounded by a mantle of lymphocytes and mature tissue macrophages. Immune granulomas usually contain giant cells, which are also derived from mononuclear phagocytes and are characterized by multiple nuclei.[264] Small numbers of CD4+ helper-inducer T lymphocytes are interspersed among the epithelioid and giant cells. The cells surrounding the epithelioid cells are mostly CD4+ T cells, some CD8+ cells, and mature macrophages.[21,265,266] Early fibrotic changes, including fibroblasts and collagen, may be seen at the periphery of the granuloma.[267]

Most epithelioid cells appear to be secretory cells that contain abundant rough endoplasmic reticulum (RER), a developed Golgi complex and prominent nucleoli, and a plasma membrane forming an interdigitating boundary that interacts with other inflammatory cells.[263,268]

Concepts of Granuloma Formation

Granulomas result as an immune response to antigenic oligopeptides that in the case of sarcoidosis are unknown. These oligopeptides are phagocytosed by macrophages and persist due to their resistance to enzymatic degradation. The oligopeptide is subsequently presented to T cells invoking an immunologic cellular response. The key stages in granuloma formation are shown in Table 14–7. Cellular analysis of granulomas at different time points reveal that the cellular constituents are in a dynamic equilibrium, balanced by the relative rates of cellular reconstitution and cell death/apoptosis. Each component is controlled by the balance of a number of different cytokines in the local milieu. These cytokines released from macrophages and T cells, as a consequence of close cell-cell interactions, act in both an autocrine and a paracrine fashion.

Programmed cell death (apoptosis) is an active suicide mechanism that is involved in normal tissue turnover. Apoptosis aids in the rapid clearance of immune responses following antigen presentation, and, conversely, breakdown in the normal apoptotic pathways can lead to the persistence of immunologic cells at sites of granulomatous inflammation, as is hypothesized to occur in sarcoidosis. A greater understanding of apoptosis and its control with particular regard to granuloma formation may offer future insights into new and potentially novel treatment strategies.

The balance between granuloma growth and resolution reflects the balance between proinflammatory cytokines and factors affecting the rate of cell apoptosis. In sarcoidosis, apoptosis is governed by a number of different factors that include dysregulation of the TNF superfamily, expression of oncogene products, and the Th_1/Th_2 ratio. The TNF superfamily is expressed by immune cells and is recognized as apoptosis signaling receptors. Agostini and colleagues[269] exploring cell surface molecules of the TNF-R superfamily, reported up-regulation of CD70 and CD95 and down-regulation of CD27 in patients with sarcoidosis. However, the expression of the signaling receptors, Fas and TNF-R1, are increased on the macrophages of patients with sarcoidosis.[270] These observations suggest that induction or down-regulation of intracellular signaling pathways may regulate the development of granulomas by influencing cell apoptosis. Oncogene products, such as the $Bcl2$ oncogene, can also control apoptosis and have been

---

TABLE 14–7   Key Events in Granuloma Formation

- Recognition of MHC class II bound antigen on antigen presenting cells by T cells and subsequent activation of the CD4+ lymphocyte subset via the TCR.

- Release of macrophage-derived cytokines TNF-α, IL-1, IL-6, IL-12, IL-15; chemokines IL-8, regulated on activation, normal T cell expressed and secreted (RANTES), monocyte chemotactic protein (MCP-1), macrophage inflammatory protein (MIP-1), and the colony-stimulating factor GM-CSF

- Oligoclonal proliferation of CD4+ T cells with expression of a Th_1 cytokine profile IL-2 and IFN-γ

- Macrophage/lymphocyte interaction via intercellular signaling and cell contact leading to proliferation, activation, and spontaneous cytokine release by both cell lines at sites of inflammation

- Fibrosis associated with shift to Th_2 T-cell profile, up-regulation of macrophage-derived fibrogenic cytokines (TGF-β, PDGF, and IGF-1), and increased production of neutrophil protease products

- Disturbance of normal programmed cell death (apoptosis) by dysregulation of the TNF-L/TNF-R superfamily, abnormal expression of oncogene products, and change in Th_1/Th_2 ratio

MHC = major histocompatibility complex; TCR = T cell receptor; TNF = tumor necrosis factor; IL = interleukin; GM-CSF = granulocyte-macrophage colony–stimulating factor; IFN = interferon; TGF = transforming growth factor; PDGF = platelet-derived growth factor; IGF = insulin-like growth factor.

shown to be increased in T cells located within sarcoid granulomas.[271] Additionally the Th phenotype can influence apoptosis as a result of the predominant cytokine profile. The Th_1 cytokines, IL-2 and IL-15, inhibit macrophage apoptosis, whereas the Th_2 cytokines, IL-4 and IL-10, have the opposite effect, enhancing apoptosis.[272] Contributions from factors that influence and regulate apoptosis may explain why some patients undergo spontaneous remission and others follow a more protracted and chronic course.

CLINICAL PRESENTATION

Nonspecific Constitutional Symptoms

Symptoms such as fever, weight loss, fatigue, and malaise are seen in roughly 30% of patients with sarcoidosis. Sarcoidosis should, thus, always be in the differential diagnosis of any patient being investigated for fever of unknown origin (FUO). The fever is usually low grade. Weight loss can occur. Constitutional symptoms are more common in Blacks than in Whites or Asian patients.

Pulmonary Involvement

Pulmonary involvement in sarcoidosis is almost universal, with abnormal chest radiographs seen in 90 to 95% of patients through the course of the disease. Chest radiographs will be somewhat atypical in 25 to 30% of patients, and this number rises to 59% in those presenting at 50 years of age or older.[273]

Symptoms related to chest disease include dyspnea on exertion, vague central chest discomfort, and cough, which although usually dry may be productive of small amounts of mucoid sputum. Signs in sarcoidosis are few. Clubbing is rare and is usually associated with chronic, widespread pulmonary fibrosis. Chest auscultation is usually unremarkable but may be associated with minimal fine crepitations in alveolitic disease, whereas advanced fibrosis produces changes consistent with this process.

Pulmonary infiltration is almost always bilateral, with nodular shadowing distributed throughout all lung fields but slightly more pronounced in the midzones. More dense infiltration leads to reticulonodular shadowing, nodular opacities, and to fibrotic change of strandlike linear opacities that may radiate from the hilum and be associated with vascular distortion and upward displacement of the hila and fissures. Imaging is discussed in greater detail in "Investigations." Less common presentations include pneumothorax, chylothorax, pleural thickening, and bullous emphysema.[274,275] The relationship between having sarcoidosis and the subsequent relative risk of developing lung cancer remains uncertain. In a retrospective cohort study looking at 8,925 patients with sarcoidosis in Sweden, the relative risk for developing lung cancer was doubled during the first decade of follow-up.[276] The authors suggest that the presence of chronic inflammation is a putative mediator of this risk.

Sarcoidosis of the Upper Respiratory Tract

Sarcoidosis of the upper respiratory tract (SURT) is a relatively uncommon condition and is seen in up to 6% of patients. However, in one extensive series, 66% of cases had upper respiratory symptoms at initial presentation with minimal or undeclared sarcoidosis elsewhere.[277] Neville and colleagues[278] analyzed 32 cases of SURT and observed intrathoracic disease in 81%, skin disease in 59%, bone involvement in 31%, ocular involvement in 22%, and peripheral lymphadenopathy in 19%. Thus, SURT frequently serves as a marker of extrathoracic and fibrotic lung disease.

Nasal stuffiness or blockage is the most frequent symptom. Other symptoms include nasal crusting; nasal discharge, which may be blood stained, mucoid, or purulent; facial pain; stridor; and anosmia.[277] Nasal septal perforation was observed in 4 of 27 patients, 3 of whom had undergone submucosal resection, which clearly indicates the danger of nasal surgery in these patients. Two more patients had a collapse of the bridge of the nose due to the destruction of septal cartilage. Nasal mucosal changes most commonly presented as raised pale yellowish lesions over the nasal septum and/or inferior turbinates, often associated with mucosal hypertrophy characterized by eroded or crusted mucosa. Destruction of other regions of the oropharynx, such as the palate, may occur (Figure 14–2).

Patients with sarcoidosis can present with symptoms of mucosal dryness, and the sicca manifestations make it difficult to exclude Sjögren's syndrome, although patients with sarcoidosis are less likely to have parotid gland enlargement.[279] Performing a minor salivary gland biopsy, to detect either focal sialadenitis or noncaseating granulomas, may be required to discriminate between Sjögren's syndrome and sarcoidosis.

Laryngeal sarcoidosis affects 19% of those with SURT and most frequently involves the epiglottis, arytenoepiglottic folds, false vocal cords, and ventricles; infrequently it affects the vocal cords.[277] The appearance on indirect laryngoscopy is characteristic, with symmetric diffuse swelling of supraglottic tissues.[280]

Sarcoidosis affecting lymphoid tissue has been described in biopsy specimens following adenoid resection for obstructive sleep apnea (OSA) in one case and in a second case undergoing tonsillectomy for persistent sore throat.[277]

Local treatment of nasal symptoms may include nasal douche with an alkaline solution for relief of retained secretions and crusting, followed by betamethasone nasal drops with the patient lying prone with the

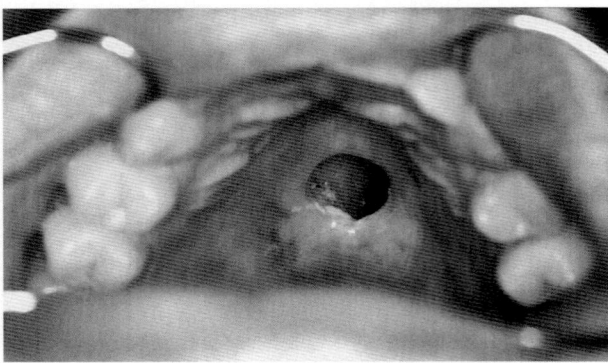

Figure 14–2   Sarcoidosis of the upper respiratory tract may be locally invasive. Shown here is a fistula between the pharynx and nasal cavity through the palate.

head hanging over the side of the bed. Systemic disease dictates the need for systemic steroids. From the Wilson and colleagues[277] series, 22 out of 27 patients required prednisolone in doses of 30 to 60 mg per day for effective symptom relief in all patients, whereas in a subsequent series[281] only one-half of patients required oral corticosteroids.

Typically, SURT is an indolent process but rapid, locally destructive disease that necessitates urgent tracheostomy has been described.[282]

Sarcoidosis is an important consideration in the differential diagnosis of nasopharyngeal granulomatous diseases that include tuberculosis, leprosy, Wegener's granulomatosis, syphilis, and fungal infection.

Skin Involvement

Erythema nodosum (EN) in its earliest description was considered a disease entity in itself. Later, it was recognized as a feature of sarcoidosis and its other systemic associations (Table 14–8). Löfgren[283] defined a syndrome in which bilateral hilar lymphadenopathy (BHL) was associated with EN and fever; patients in this subgroup frequently experienced full remission.

The incidence of EN in sarcoidosis varies between 3 and 34%, appearing more commonly in females and in European, Puerto Rican, and Mexican patients. Erythema nodosum classically presents as an erythematous and exquisitely tender warm raised nodular swelling over the anterior aspects of the lower legs and less frequently upper legs, buttocks, and arms. Initially bright red, the lesion evolves through a dusky red to a bruised appearance. Multiple lesions at different stages of evolution may be present simultaneously. The onset of EN may be preceded by a prodrome of malaise with subsequent troublesome arthralgia, fevers, and hilar lymphadenopathy on chest radiography (CXR). The condition persists between 1 and 6 weeks and regresses spontaneously or with control of the underlying disease process. Seasonal

clustering has been observed with patients typically developing EN in the spring, in both the northern and southern hemispheres, suggesting a common environmental trigger.[284,285]

Histologically, EN is a panniculitis, characterized by a predominant neutrophilic and lymphocytic infiltration of connective tissue septa between the adipose cells in the deep dermis and subcutaneous tissue, with granulomas characteristically absent.

Lupus pernio is the most easily recognizable form of cutaneous sarcoidosis, typically forming purplish papules or plaques that involve the nose, cheeks, lips, ears, eyelids, and occasionally the finger tips (Figure 14–3). Occurring more frequently in women and West Indians, it is commonly a marker of indolent chronically progressive disease.[286] It is associated with intrathoracic disease in up to 74% of patients, SURT in 54%, and bone disease in 43% in addition to having strong associations with renal and ocular disease.[286] Biopsy of these plaques reveals the characteristic noncaseating granuloma.[287] Lesions of the nasal rim are common (Figure 14–4), and appear at the watershed between cutaneous disease and the common association with SURT.[288] Neville and colleagues[278] drew attention to SURT as a strong indicator of chronic fibrotic sarcoidosis and pointed to a high degree of Kveim positivity in this group as a useful test for the differential diagnosis in nasal granulomatous disease.

Cutaneous disease is not uncommon in Caucasians. Veien and colleagues[289] in a review of 189 patients observed infiltrative lesions in 86%, systemic disease in 73%, and solely cutaneous disease in just 26%. The most frequent lesions are those of lupus pernio, granulomatous scar infiltration, and plaque lesions, which tend to exhibit a broad distribution over the face, trunk, and limbs.[290] Cutaneous involvement may also include leukocytoclastic vasculitis, nail dystrophy, maculopapular eruptions, alopecia, and areas of hypo/hyperpigmentation.

TABLE 14–8   Disease Associations with Erythema Nodosum

Inflammatory	Infectious
Sarcoidosis	*Streptococcus* spp.
Crohn's	Coccidioidomycosis
Ulcerative colitis	Histoplasmosis
Polyarteritis nodosa	Blastomycosis
Neoplasia	Leprosy
Leukemia	Tularemia
Lymphoma	Cat scratch disease
Drugs	*Yersinia enterocolitica*
Penicillin	*Trichophyton verrucosum*
Sulfonamides	Epstein-Barr virus
Oral contraceptives	Ornithosis
Bromides	Tuberculosis
Phenacetin	

Corticosteroids, methotrexate, and chloroquine[291] have been effective most frequently in lupus pernio and sarcoid skin disease. A high recurrence rate on cessation of treatment, however, has resulted in a number of other reported treatments. These have been written up as case reports or small trials and include tetracyclines,[292] CO_2 laser therapy,[293] plastic surgery,[294] isotretinoin,[295] clofazimine,[296] allopurinol,[297] and the topical corticosteroid, clobetasol.[298]

The Melkersson-Rosenthal syndrome comprises the triad of orofacial swelling, relapsing facial paralysis, and swelling and fissuring of the tongue associated with a granulomatous histology. A biopsy demonstrating sarcoidlike granulomatosis is required for diagnosis.[299] The syndrome may be mono- or oligosymptomatic. Treatment is with clofazimine and systemic or intralesional corticosteroids, but a significant spontaneous remission rate has also been noted.[300,301]

Neurosarcoidosis

Clinically evident neurosarcoidosis is found in less than 10% of total cases, although postmortem investigation suggests its presence in up to 14% of patients. Black patients appear to have a much higher incidence of involvement than do Whites.[302] In a study of 35 biopsy-proven cases, neurosarcoidosis was the presenting symptom in 31% of patients and the only manifestation in 17%.[303] The diagnosis of neurosarcoidosis is often clear when prompted by the presence of typical thoracic and skin involvement, but it may prove elusive when neurologic signs occur in isolation.

In the series by Chapelon and colleagues,[303] central nervous system (CNS) involvement was noted in 37% of patients, meningitis in 40%, cranial nerve palsies in 37%, peripheral neuropathy in 40%, myopathy in 26%, and multiple neurologic manifestations in 51%.

The use of magnetic resonance imaging (MRI) has greatly facilitated diagnosis in neurosarcoidosis and is now the investigation of choice for CNS disease (Table 14–9). It minimizes artefact, improves resolution, and, with the contrast enhancement provided by gadolinium, improves the resolution of bone, CSF, and especially meningeal disease.[304] Lexa and Grossman,[305] in an MRI study of 24 patients, demonstrated the diversity of neural structures involved and suggested a role for this modality in defining a prognosis. Abnormal contrast enhancement of tissue appeared to identify patients likely to respond to corticosteroid therapy. Nine out of 10 patients with leptomeningeal involvement, 6 out of 6 patients with brain parenchymal masses, 3 out of 3 with cord masses, and 3 out of 3 with periventricular lesions improved with steroid therapy.

Although of limited use in peripheral nerve assessment, MRI has proven effective in evaluation of sar-

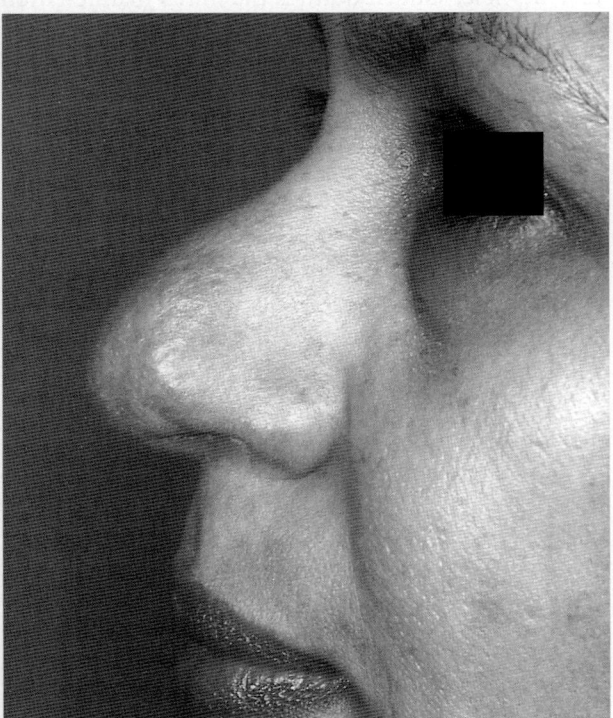

Figure 14–3 Lupus pernio, a violaceous indurating skin lesion affecting chiefly the nose and facial skin, is often a marker of chronic persistent disease.

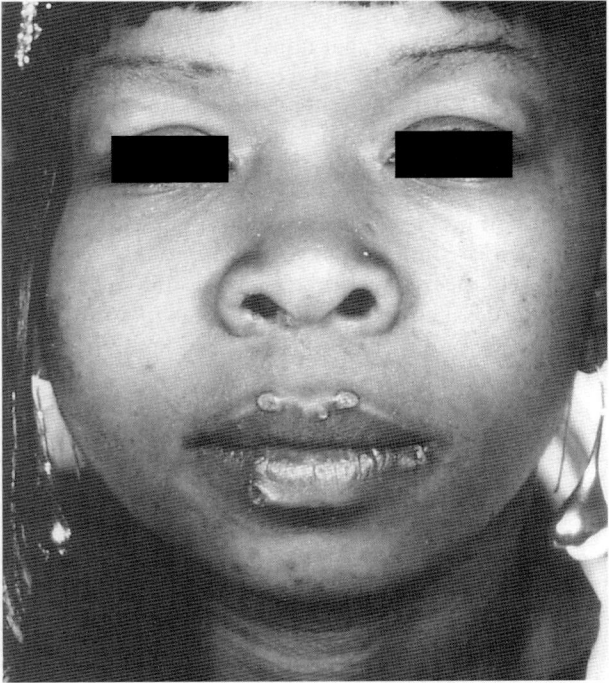

Figure 14–4 Sarcoid plaques are prominent at mucocutaneous junctions of the nose and mouth in this woman with sarcoid nasal septal perforation. Further skin involvement is evident on the right cheek and lacrimal enlargement is seen bilaterally.

coidosis of the orbit and visual pathways. The MR analysis of 15 such patients revealed 8 with optic nerve granulomata, 9 in whom the optic chiasm was affected, 4 with perineural enhancement, 3 with optic nerve enlargement (unenhanced scans), 5 with periventricular white matter changes resembling multiple sclerosis, 3 with orbital masses resembling pseudotumor, and one with diffuse change in the optic radiations.[306] MRI appearances, however, are often nonspecific and may mimic the appearances of multiple sclerosis, cerebral metastases, or meningiomas[307]; thus, definitive histologic diagnosis is often required. The cerebrospinal fluid (CSF) will be abnormal in 80% of patients with neurosarcoidosis, and characteristic findings include lymphocytosis (increased CD4/CD8 ratio), elevated protein, and elevated ACE (50%).[308]

Leptomeningeal involvement is most frequently seen at the base of the brain, where it commonly involves the pituitary gland, the optic chiasm, and cranial nerves II, VII, and VIII. A biopsy study conducted by Cheng and colleagues[309] identified sarcoidosis as the most frequent cause of undiagnosed chronic meningitis (31% of cases), with a higher incidence than metastatic adenocarcinoma (25%). Pituitary dysfunction is not uncommon, and the combination of diabetes insipidus and chiasmal involvement is particularly suggestive of sarcoidosis.[310]

Central nervous system parenchymal disease may take a diffuse infiltrative form (Figure 14–5) or that of coalescent granulomata forming space-occupying lesions (Figure 14–6). Periventricular white matter lesions leading to focal signs and myelopathy have been demonstrated in both the brain and spinal cord. Hydrocephalus has been described with both meningeal disease and mass lesions that impair CSF drainage. Hypothalamic and leptomeningeal involvement with diabetes insipidus and hypernatremia has been observed in two patients presenting with the unusual symptoms of paranoid psychosis.[311]

Sarcoid neuropathy affects cranial and peripheral nerves, commonly presenting as a mononeuropathy or mononeuritis multiplex. The facial nerve is classically involved in the uveoparotid fever syndrome described by Heerfordt.[12] The syndrome comprises parotid gland enlargement, uveitis, fever, and cranial nerve palsies. Symmetric ascending polyneuropathy resembling the Guillain-Barré syndrome has also been described.[312]

Although neurosarcoidosis may initially manifest with psychiatric symptoms, the relationship between sarcoidosis and depression is less clear. Given that sarcoidosis is a chronic multisystem disease it is likely to impact on quality of life and potentially increases the risk of developing depression. Cross-sectional studies, using quality-of-life and depression scales, suggest that the prevalence of depression is 60%, and that female gender, decreased access to medical care, and increased dyspnea predicted depression (odds ratio of 3.33, 11.6, and 2.8, respectively).[313] These studies suggest that attention to psychosocial aspects of the disease is important.

Cardiovascular Involvement

Cardiac involvement in sarcoidosis is not uncommon, but it is frequently not diagnosed until postmortem examination. Sampling bias confounds an accurate estimate of incidence, but clinical involvement is recognized in 5% of patients; autopsy series suggest that it is present in up to 30% of patients.

Of all patients with sarcoidosis, 67% will die of a sarcoid-related complication, and myocardial involvement accounts for half of these deaths. Further, of those with clinically significant myocardial involvement, sudden death is the most common manifestation (65%). In 40% of these, sudden death is the initial manifestation of sarcoidosis.[314–316]

Ventricular arrhythmias occur in 22% of patients[317] and 25% die from progressive congestive cardiac failure (CCF).[318] Other manifestations include conduction disturbances including atrioventricular (AV) nodal block of which complete heart block (CHB) is most common,[319]

TABLE 14–9   Diagnosis and Localization by MRI in 24 Cases of Neurosarcoidosis

Sites of Involvement	Cases
White matter and periventricular changes similar to multiple sclerosis	11
Leptomeningeal disease	11
Parenchymal mass	7
Hydrocephalus	3
Extra-axial mass mimicking meningioma	2
Parenchymal cord mass	3

MRI = magnetic resonance imaging.
Adapted from Lexa FJ, Grossman RI.[305]

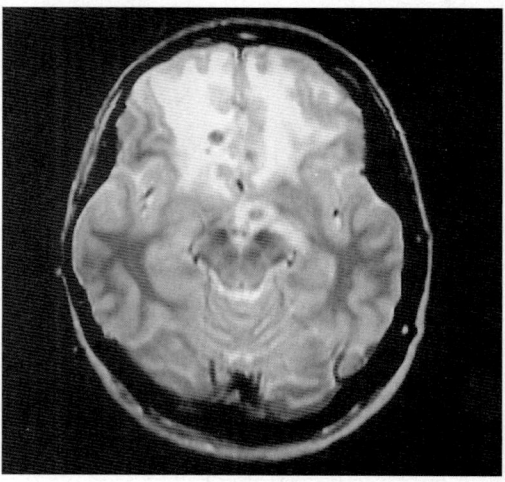

Figure 14–5 Magnetic resonance imaging with gadolinium enhancement is the investigation of choice for suspected neurosarcoidosis. Shown here is diffuse frontal lobe infiltration.

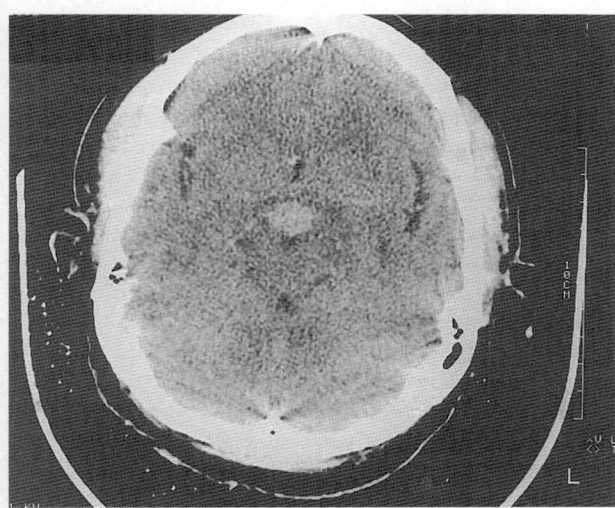

Figure 14–6 Computed tomography scan showing a sarcoid mass lesion infiltrating the pituitary gland.

Analysis of MRI as a diagnostic tool is incomplete, but MRI appears to offer some promise as a noninvasive measure. The histology of myocardial sarcoid is of classic granulomatous infiltration affecting the left ventricular free wall most commonly followed by the interventricular septum.[315] Endomyocardial biopsy provides diagnostic certainty, but sampling problems due to the inhomogeneous distribution of the disease leads to a low yield; thus, a negative result does not exclude the diagnosis.[329]

Steroids are the mainstay of treatment of myocardial sarcoidosis along with diuretics and antiarrhythmics and should be instituted early in the course of the disease.[317,330]

Pacemakers are indicated for CHB and AV-nodal block whereas automatic implantable cardioverting defibrillators have been used for malignant arrhythmias.[331] Cardiac transplantation has proven effective for the treatment of congestive cardiac failure, malignant arrhythmia, and cor pulmonale although a clinically insignificant recurrence of granulomas in the transplanted organ has been noted.[332]

bundle branch block, atrial arrhythmias, papillary muscle dysfunction, ventricular aneurysm, and pericardial effusion.[315] In a study of 81 patients with systemic sarcoidosis but with no overt cardiac disease, mild to moderate pericardial effusions were found in 21% of patients.[320] Of these, 92% had thallium scans that suggested myocardial involvement.

Multiple abnormalities are represented on electrocardiogram (ECG); an abnormal ECG may be seen in up to 50% of those without known myocardial involvement[321] and should prompt consideration of myocardial sarcoidosis. Performing 24-hour Holter monitoring and exercise stress testing increases the diagnostic yield of resting 12-lead electrocardiography.[322]

Although nonspecific, two-dimensional (2D) echocardiography offers useful evaluation of left ventricular systolic and diastolic function, regional wall motion, and assessment of pericardial disease.[323] Diastolic dysfunction with abnormal relaxation, ventricular filling, and prominence of the A wave are features of sarcoid infiltration of the left ventricular wall.[324]

Myocardial scintigraphy with thallium 201 is superior in assessing segmental contraction abnormalities, in contrast to the pattern seen in coronary artery disease, it demonstrates resting perfusion defects that resolve with exercise.[325,326] Lesions are most frequently observed in the interventricular septum. Kinney and Caldwell[327] questioned the sensitivity and specificity of thallium scanning in asymptomatic patients with sarcoidosis by demonstrating that survival correlated solely with age and not with perfusion defects seen on thallium scan. The combined use of ^{67}Ga and ^{201}Tl is effective in diagnosing myocardial sarcoidosis when both tests are positive, but the combination of tests does not improve specificity.[328] The resolution of gallium scan defects with corticosteroid therapy suggests that this may be useful for monitoring steroid therapy.[328]

Musculoskeletal Involvement

Nonspecific arthralgia occurs in 25% of patients, but a deforming arthritis is less common. Acute sarcoid arthritis is a self-limiting disease occurring in 1 to 4% of patients and markedly more frequently in Blacks than in Whites.[71] Some 9% of patients presenting to an Oslo clinic with "acute reactive arthritis" were diagnosed as having sarcoidosis[333]; therefore, it needs to be considered in this differential.

The acute disease manifests as a migratory polyarthropathy typically affecting the ankles but also knees, wrists, and elbows. It is uniformly associated with BHL and often with fever. The triad of arthritis, BHL, and EN occurs in 60 to 88% of cases.[333,334] Complete remission is usual after a mean duration of 11 weeks; although subsequent recurrence has been reported, it rarely occurs.

Joint ultrasonography reveals minor periarticular edema but no erosive changes,[335] and synovial biopsy shows no change or minor mononuclear cell infiltration in a perivascular distribution.[336] Giant cell granulomata have been demonstrated in the synovium in the chronic form,[337] occasionally associated with periarticular bone disease.

The HLA phenotype B8 DR3 is closely linked to a subset of patients at increased risk of acute sarcoid arthritis with hilar adenopathy who do not appear to progress to chronic sarcoid arthritis.[338]

Chronic sarcoid arthritis has a similar joint distribution to the acute form (ie, ankles, knees, wrists, and elbows) but may also affect the metacarpophalangeal and interphalangeal joints. This form is seen more frequently in Black patients and is associated with a greater degree of multiorgan extrathoracic disease.[337] A radiograph shows this to be a nondestructive arthropathy, and synovial biopsy reveals synovitis with hypertrophy of lining cells[339] and occasionally synovial giant cell granulo-mata.[337,339] Granulomatous synovitis may occasionally be associated with periarticular bone disease.

When associated with fever in children this condition may mimic juvenile chronic arthritis with regard to joint features, growth, and pubertal delay.[340]

Tenosynovitis is associated with chronic joint disease and, like this condition, occurs in both early and established disease. It has been confirmed histologically with giant cell granulomata affecting the synovial sheath.[341]

Symptoms of muscle weakness and pain suggest occult sarcoid myositis. Myopathies can occur; they tend to be chronic and are more common in women. A steroid-induced myopathy is the main differential, and muscle biopsies may reveal noncaseating granulomas.

Sarcoid bone disease primarily takes the form of bone cysts and has been described in bones of the hands, feet, nose, skull, vertebrae, and pelvis. These cysts are generally asymptomatic and may be seen in the hands and feet in up to 5% of patients[342]; they are seen more frequently in those with granulomatous skin disease and lupus pernio.[343] These cysts may become symptomatic as a dactylitis in which the finger may become reddened, swollen, and tender over the affected bone or joint (Figure 14–7). Bone scintigraphy aids in the evaluation of these patients.

Osteoporosis

In a computed tomography (CT) study of osteoporosis measuring vertebral cancellous mineral content in untreated sarcoidosis, greater than 50% of patients had significant osteoporosis (ie, Z score < −1). This study considered untreated males and pre- and postmenopausal females with median disease duration of 20 months. Further, the Z score deteriorated with disease duration when comparing early and longstanding untreated sarcoidosis (Z score −1.19 ± 0.24 vs. 0.32 ± 0.39, $p < .001$).[344]

The cause of the osteoporosis is as yet unknown. In one study, the increase in serum 1, 25-dihydroxyvitamin D_3 seemed to be contributory to accelerated bone turnover leading to, in women, reduced bone marrow density.[345] In other studies, serum 1,25-dihydroxyvitamin D_3 levels were elevated in both those with and without osteopenia in sarcoidosis.[346] Malabsorption and putative osteoclastic factors have been postulated as possible contributors to this enhanced bone resorption.

In steroid-treated patients with sarcoidosis, the incidence of osteopenia is approximately 70%.[347] The time course of onset of osteopenia is similar to that seen in other steroid-treated conditions such as asthma and rheumatoid arthritis, and the more severe osteopenia in postmenopausal patients with sarcoidosis suggests synergy between these two conditions. In corticosteroid-treated patients there is a decrease in biochemical markers of bone formation, when compared with untreated patients with sarcoidosis.[348]

Deflazacort, a novel corticosteroid, is reputed to have similar disease-suppressive activity as prednisolone in sarcoidosis but is associated with less osteopenia.[349,350] Nesi and colleagues[350] observed a 15% decrease in lumbar spine bone mineral density over 1 year in prednisolone-treated patients as opposed to 9% in deflazacort-treated patients ($p < .05$). Rizzato and colleagues[344] observed a similar reduction in bone mineral density (−9.81 ± 1.84%) in deflazacort-treated patients but without achieving statistical significance from the prednisolone-treated group (−13.9 ± 2.1%).

Clearly, prevention of bone loss with judicious but appropriate steroid dosing is central to the treatment of osteoporosis. In steroid-treated patients, the concomitant use of the third-generation bisphoshonate, alendronate, has been shown to counteract the increase in markers of bone resorption induced by glucocorticoid therapy. After 12 months of treatment, bone mineral density increased by 0.8% in the alendronate-treated group but decreased

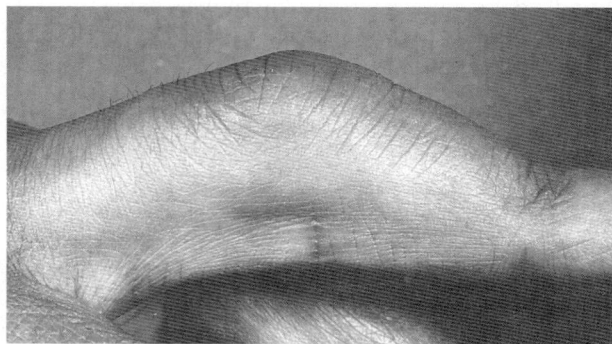

A

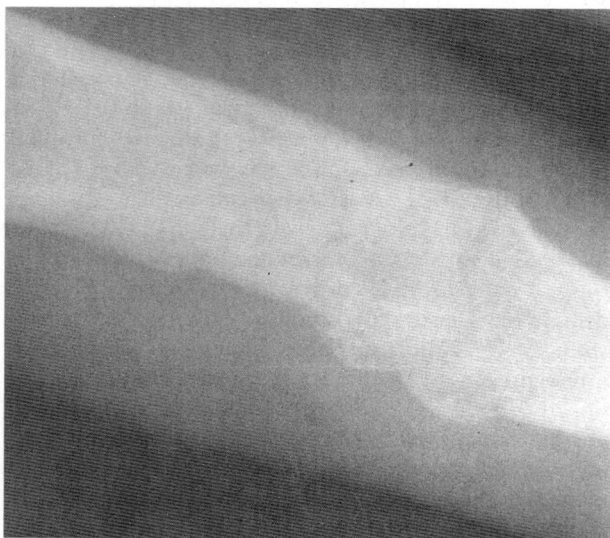

B

Figure 14–7   *A*, A painful dactylitis in chronic sarcoid bone disease presents with a soft tissue swelling. *B*, Overlying cystic bone disease in a periarticular distribution.

by 4.5% in the placebo-treated group ($p < .001$).[348] Salmon calcitonin by intramuscular or nasal routes may offer some protection; in one study, it was associated with a marked reduction in bone mineral loss for treatment over one year when combined with prednisolone therapy (13.9 ± 0.21% compared 2.9 ± 2.9%).[351] Controlled trials on the benefits to bone density of calcium supplementation and hormone replacement therapy in this condition are lacking but should offer some promise.

Eye Disease

Ocular sarcoidosis affects up to 25% of patients at some stage of chronic disease[352,353] and is potentially sight threatening. Manifestations include uveitis, granulomatous conjunctivitis, dryness of the eyes, and pain and diplopia due to orbital granulomata that impinge on orbit and extraocular musculature. Karma[354] reported 23 patients with ocular sarcoidosis and found uveitis in 26%, decreased lacrimal secretion in 78%, and epithelioid cell granulomas in 81% on conjunctival biopsies although only 5 of these patients had manifest ocular complaints.

Uveitis is the most serious presentation but occurs as a primary manifestation of disease only rarely (less than 1.5%).[355] This inflammation may affect all of the uveal tract (iris, ciliary body, and choroid), but most frequently the anterior portion as iridocyclitis, with pain, watering, redness, photophobia, and blurred vision (Figure 14–8). Most commonly bilateral, typical findings include circumcorneal congestion, papillary irregularities, anterior chamber floaters, and sluggish papillary responses. Anterior uveal disease commonly presents as an acute process that may resolve spontaneously or with topical corticosteroid therapy. Edelsten followed 75 patients with sarcoid uveitis for a median of 4 years. At diagnosis, lung involvement was described in 35%, and oral steroids were required in 51%. After 10 years, 54% retained normal visual acuity, although 5% had lost vision to less than 6/36 in both eyes. Further involvement of the central nervous system was seen in 10%.[356]

Chronic uveitis, particularly when associated with posterior synechiae and raised intraocular pressure, has a markedly poorer visual outcome.[353] Thus, regular ophthalmic surveillance is most important in this group.

Posterior uveitis leads to choroidal and retinal changes that are often more difficult to detect. This form of disease is characterized by a retinal periphlebitis and is the cause of the majority of visual morbidity.[352] Fluffy white perivascular cuffing may be seen but is easily missed if peripheral. Vitreous involvement, hemorrhage, and papilledema are also seen, but only rarely.

Lacrimal infiltration, alone or combined with salivary gland infiltration (Mikulicz's syndrome), leads to marked enlargement of these glands. In the chronic phase, this leads to dryness of the eyes. Lacrimal enlargement is also encountered in Heerfordt's syndrome. The lacrimal glands accumulate gallium in up to 75% of acute cases, and ocular uptake is a useful indicator of active eye disease although in the chronic form the gallium scan is frequently negative.[357–359] This ocular uptake is particularly useful diagnostically when presenting with a normal CXR.[358]

Uveitis is a common finding in pediatric sarcoidosis in which the triad of uveitis, arthritis, and skin involvement may result in diagnostic confusion with juvenile chronic arthritis (Still's disease). This triad is common in children under the age of 5 years. In children aged 8 to 15 years, it is associated almost universally with pulmonary involvement and also with liver and spleen infiltration.[360]

Nodular granulomatous involvement of the conjunctivae may be amenable to biopsy and is useful diagnostically; this does not apply to blind conjunctival biopsy.

In a review of 204 cases of biopsy-proven sarcoidosis, Dresner and colleagues[361] found that only 44% of cases had been referred for ophthalmologic review, however, more than half of those examined by an ophthalmologist showed signs of ocular involvement. Sarcoidosis frequently affects the eyes and may lead to serious visual impairment. Ocular disease is often asymptomatic, so close examination is required with early and regular specialist ophthalmologic review.

Renal Disease

The renal system may be affected by sarcoidosis in a number of ways (Table 14–10). Renal involvement is an unusual finding in sarcoidosis but may be histologically confirmed in 20 to 30% of patients as gleaned from biopsy and postmortem studies.[362] A study of renal biopsy in 58 patients with chronic renal failure revealed 4 cases of sarcoidosis (7%) showing granulomatous interstitial nephritis; a diagnosis of sarcoidosis had not previously been made in 2 of these patients.[363] Richmond and colleagues[364] reviewed 75 cases of renal sarcoidosis and found 1 case of membranous glomerulonephritis, 1 case of granulomatous interstitial nephritis, 7 of nephrocalcinosis, and a further 8 that featured abnormal urinary sediment suggesting renal involvement.

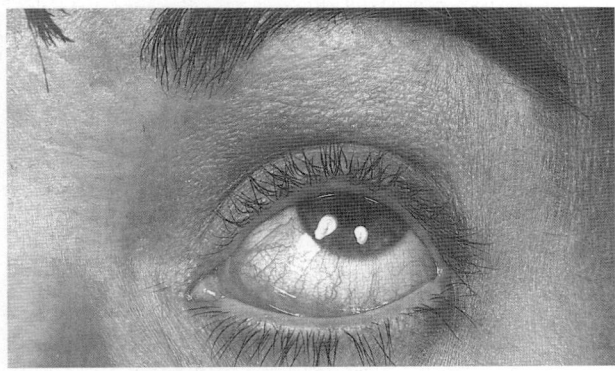

Figure 14–8   Granulomatous conjunctivitis and anterior uveitis may present with a painful red eye.

Granulomatous nephritis is generally thought to be the classic presentation, but biopsies may reveal prominent interstitial nephritis with no evidence of granulomata. It is not clear to what extent sampling bias influences these findings.

Primary glomerular disease is unusual but membranous,[364,365] membranoproliferative,[366] and mesangiocapillary glomerulonephritis[367] have been described.

Renal sarcoidosis is usually asymptomatic and is generally discovered by routine creatinine and calcium estimations. When clinically significant, it presents as chronic renal failure with or without renal stones and hypercalcemia. Urinalysis may reveal minimal proteinuria, few white cells and granular casts, and a fractional excretion of sodium of greater than one. Creatinine clearance is depressed, and the 24-hour calcium excretion is increased leading to hypercalciuria.

Response to corticosteroid therapy is generally prompt and gratifying,[368] although the degree of improvement is related to disease chronicity where interstitial fibrosis, tubular atrophy, and nephrocalcinosis limit treatment response. Relapse occurs on weaning and cessation of treatment but is responsive to the reintroduction of corticosteroids. Maintenance treatment is frequently managed with low-dose prednisolone on a daily or alternate-day basis. When this approach fails, further investigation to exclude alternate causes of renal impairment may be required.

Calcium Metabolism

Hypercalciuria is seen in almost a third of patients with sarcoidosis, and hypercalcemia is seen in approximately 10%. Thus serum calcium should be determined in all patients. Assessment of 24-hour urinary calcium excretion is mandatory in all new presentations of sarcoidosis if urine sediment is abnormal and suggests urinary tract inflammation secondary to nephrocalcinosis. Serum calcium levels in sarcoidosis rise with serum vitamin D levels and with a diet rich in vitamin D; they fluctuate with seasonal sun exposure and prednisolone therapy.[369] This dysregulation of calcium metabolism appears to be modulated through the abnormal synthe-

TABLE 14–10   Renal Involvement in Sarcoidosis

Interstitial nephritis
  Granulomatous
  Nongranulomatous
Glomerulonephritis
  Membranous
  Membranoproliferative
  Mesangiocapillary
Nephrocalcinosis
Urolithiasis
Hypercalcemic renal failure

sis of vitamin D by activated pulmonary macrophages and granulomatous tissue that leads to excessive hydroxylation of 25-monohydroxylated vitamin D precursors.[370] The reason for this apparent up-regulation of vitamin D expression remains obscure, but it could represent an adaptive response to the undefined antigen that causes sarcoidosis. Recent work has recognized that different polymorphisms of the vitamin D gene may have an impact on both bone mineral density and the development of granulomatous disease.[371] In patients with sarcoidosis, although such polymorpisms may affect the serum PTH level, they are not a risk factor for hypercalcaemia.[372]

Hypercalciuria appears to result purely from elevated renal calcium filtration and does not appear to be an independent effect of vitamin D on the kidney.[373] This hypercalciuria leads to renal papillary calcification (or nephrocalcinosis) and urolithiasis. Rizzato and Colombo[374] reported renal stones in 3.6% of 729 consecutive patients at presentation and asymptomatic stones in a further 2.7%, highlighting the high frequency of hypercalciuria in sarcoidosis.

Treatment with corticosteroids leads to rapid normalization of serum and urinary calcium concentrations in the majority of cases, often within 3 to 5 days. In those unresponsive to corticosteroids or intolerant of their side effects, chloroquine,[375] hydroxychloroquine, or ketoconazole offer effective and relatively safe alternatives when used with appropriate supervision. Drug therapy should be linked to dietary modification that reduces intake of vitamin D and calcium-rich foods.

Lymphoreticular Involvement

Small- to moderate-sized rubbery peripheral lymphadenopathy is a very common feature of sarcoidosis and particularly affects the cervical and scalene groups as well as axillary, inguinal, and epitrochlear regions. Peripheral lymphadenopathy may occur in isolation and present years before the onset of multisystem disease.[376]

Abdominal examination by CT shows widespread lymphadenopathy with discernible hepatomegaly in 38% and splenomegaly in 60%. Retroperitoneal lymph nodes are also common. Despite these CT features, palpable hepatosplenomegaly and peritoneal adenopathy are unusual. Computed tomography, however, is a poor tool for the differentiation of sarcoid granulomatous lymphadenopathy from neoplastic lymphadenopathy.[377] To confuse the picture further, sarcoidlike granulomas may occur in association with Hodgkin's lymphoma and non-Hodgkin's lymphoma.

Gastrointestinal And Hepatic Involvement

Clinically significant gastrointestinal sarcoidosis is unusual, but involvement at most levels of the gastrointestinal tract has been described. Disturbed liver function tests (LFTs) with elevated alkaline phosphatase are, however, common, if transient, and are seen in up to 25% of patients.

Lumenal involvement leading to life-threatening hemorrhage,[378] malabsorption,[379,380] protein-losing enteropathy,[381] and obstruction affecting the small and large bowel[382] have been observed, as have appendicitis[383] and cholecystitis.[384] Small bowel disease frequently presents some difficulty in differentiation from small bowel celiac disease, sprue, Whipple's disease, and Crohn's disease. Careful biopsy sampling with culture and periodic acid-Schiff (PAS) staining differentiates granulomatous enterocolitis.[385] Papadopoulos and colleagues,[386] reporting on 89 patients with sarcoidosis, did not demonstrate an increased frequency of the autoimmune diseases, pernicious anemia, or celiac disease but did show a high frequency (40%) of autoimmunity (positive serum autoantibodies in the absence of overt disease).

Devaney and colleagues[387] reviewed 100 patients with sarcoidosis with clinical evidence of liver involvement. All patients had granulomata on biopsy; 58% had cholestatic changes, 41% necroinflammatory changes, and 20% vascular changes. Of those with cholestasis, 19 out of 58 had bile duct pathology similar to primary biliary cirrhosis, and 13 out of 58 had changes similar to primary sclerosing cholangitis. Ductopenia was a common finding in cholestasis and is described elsewhere in a syndrome with fever, loss of weight, anorexia, and marked biochemical cholestasis; it responds symptomatically but not histologically to corticosteroids.[388] Six percent of patients had a dominant mass or sarcoidoma and a further 6% cirrhosis. There are case reports of successful treatment of hepatic sarcoidosis with chloroquine,[389] hormone replacement therapy,[390] and ursodeoxycholic acid.[391]

Portal hypertension and hemorrhage from gastric and esophageal varices have been described. Corticosteroids are of some value as are propranolol and usual therapies.[392,393]

Pancreatic sarcoid masses associated with abdominal pain may mimic adenocarcinoma but have a good prognosis.[394]

Sarcoid-Affected Lymph Nodes In Nonsarcoid Disease

Histopathologic assessment of surgical specimens from a variety of predominantly neoplastic diseases including lymphoproliferative disease,[395] germ cell testicular tumors,[396,397] leiomyosarcoma,[398] renal cell carcinoma,[399] and ovarian mucinous cystadenoma,[400] often return lymph nodes with changes suggestive of sarcoidosis.

Early observations by Brincker[395] suggest an increased incidence of sarcoidosis in patients with malignancy. Fossa and colleagues.[401] noticed the occurrence of sarcoidlike changes in mediastinal and paratracheal lymph nodes that progressed with disease progression and regressed with tumor treatment in germ cell tumor

patients. These coincidences posed several questions that examine the veracity of the initial diagnoses, the prospect of truly coincident disease, and the possibility that malignancy may induce sarcoidlike changes in adjacent lymph nodes if not sarcoidosis itself.

Brincker[395] reviewed 131 cases of coexistent sarcoidosis and malignant disease; the data suggest a higher incidence of sarcoidosis among these patients than among normal patients. There also appeared to be a nonrandom tumor selection, with an approximately threefold increase in the frequency of Hodgkin's disease, acute myeloid leukemia, and lung carcinoma. The chronicity of sarcoidosis and the fact that subclinical sarcoidosis may be uncovered only during tumor investigation as well as a change in the natural history of lymphoproliferative disease by curative treatment make these findings difficult to interpret. More recent studies from Scandinavia could not confirm previous reports of an increased occurrence of malignant neoplasms in patients with sarcoidosis.[401–403]

These observations emphasize the importance of an extremely thorough evaluation of lymphoproliferative disease patients with sarcoidosis to distinguish between benign and malignant mediastinal, gonadal, or other tissue involvement. This cohort also requires particularly vigilant follow-up.

Pregnancy

Unlike other interstitial lung diseases, sarcoidosis has a significant incidence during the reproductive years. Pregnancy, however, appears to have little effect on the long-term course of the disease in the majority of patients. The disease often remits during pregnancy but may relapse postpartum. A poorer prognosis is, however, predicted in those with more severe disease such as fibrotic pulmonary parenchymal change, advanced maternal age, immunosuppressive therapy other than corticosteroids, and extrapulmonary disease.[404,405]

INVESTIGATIONS

Imaging

Chest Radiography

Staging by CXR continues to evolve. Previously, there was general acceptance of the description by James and Thompson[406] of a three-stage disease. Stage I disease displays hilar lymphadenopathy without parenchymal change; stage II shows BHL with parenchymal change; and stage III shows parenchymal mottling without BHL.[407] Some semantic confusion arises over the character of parenchymal change, with some observers using the term "fibrosis" for parenchymal changes in stage III disease.[408] In an attempt to clarify the classification, Scadding and Mitchell[267] added a fourth stage for lung changes radiographically considered fibrotic. DeRemee[409] proposed a useful modification, adding stage 0 disease in which the CXR is interpreted as normal. This modification also made allowance for the inclusion of paratracheal with hilar lymphadenopathy in stage I (Figure 14–9).

Intrathoracic adenopathy most commonly presents a bihilar distribution often more prominent on the right, with rounded, clearly defined nodes distinguishable on CXR. Up to half of the patients exhibit right paratracheal lymph node enlargement but anterior mediastinal nodes are uncommon, which help to differentiate this condition from lymphoma.

Both clinical presentation and the appearance of the plain chest radiograph at the time of diagnosis carry important prognostic information in sarcoidosis.[288,409–413] A major problem in some studies of disease activity markers lies in a failure to account for the important effect of disease presentation on the likelihood of disease progression.[414] Many studies have shown that an acute presentation with fever and EN carries a particularly good outcome, conversely an insidious onset often implies a poor prognosis.[283,288,411–413,415–417] On the other hand, up to 16% of patients presenting with EN, BHL, and acute arthritis, will follow a chronic course.[288] The case mixture in a series (acute presentations vs. chronic disease) influences the sensitivity and specificity of any proposed activity marker. This fact has been mentioned only rarely in published reports.

In stage I disease, 75 to 80% of patients experience complete remission within 5 years and 15% remain unchanged with severe morbidity unusual in this group.[418] Persistence of hilar lymphadenopathy does not indicate ongoing active disease. Half of the patients with stage II disease remit within 5 years, a quarter remain stable, and a quarter progress; in stage III, the spontaneous remission rate is approximately 40%[288]; and 0% of patients with stage IV disease remit (Table 14–11). In patients who have previously improved or remained stable for 2 years, late relapses are uncommon (2 to 8%).[419–424] Failure to improve after 2 years suggests chronicity, and subsequent disease remission is rare.

The chest radiograph must be interpreted within the context of the clinical situation and ancillary tests such as pulmonary function. In patients who become progressively dyspneic, the CXR may show new pulmonary infiltrates but will be unchanged if the cause of dyspnea is due to endobronchial sarcoidosis, pulmonary vascular disease, a steroid myopathy, or cardiac sarcoidosis.

Atypical Pulmonary Involvement. *Pulmonary Nodules.* Coalescent granulomata may lead to larger pulmonary nodules and mimic neoplastic metastatic disease and other granulomatous processes as well as rheumatologic and infective processes. Nodules from 5 mm to greater than 5 cm that are generally bilateral and multiple have been noted. Necrotizing sarcoid granulomatosis (NSG) presents with nodular changes and differs clinically with prominent pleuritic chest pain, frequent pleural involvement, and mediastinal lymphadenopathy.[425] This condition usually responds to corticosteroid therapy.

Pleural Disease. Pleural effusion has been described in 0.16 to 7% of patients[426,427] and is generally associated with granulomatous involvement of the pleura, which may take the form of NSG. Pleural fluid is generally exudative and associated with a relative lymphocytosis.

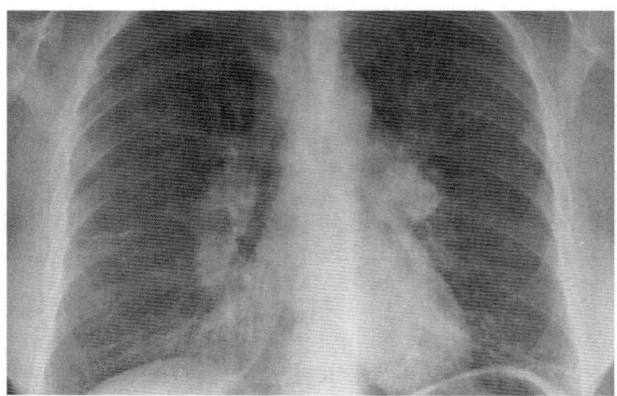

A

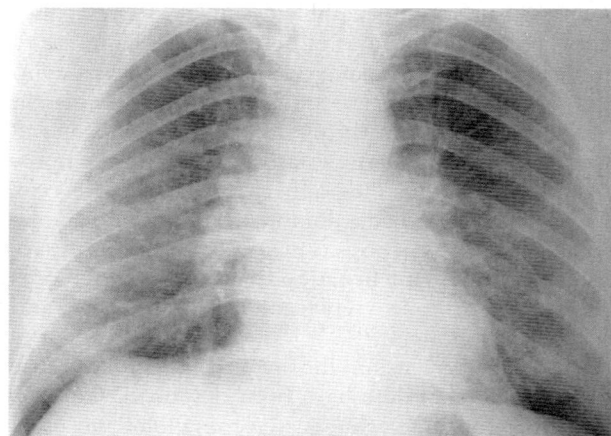

B

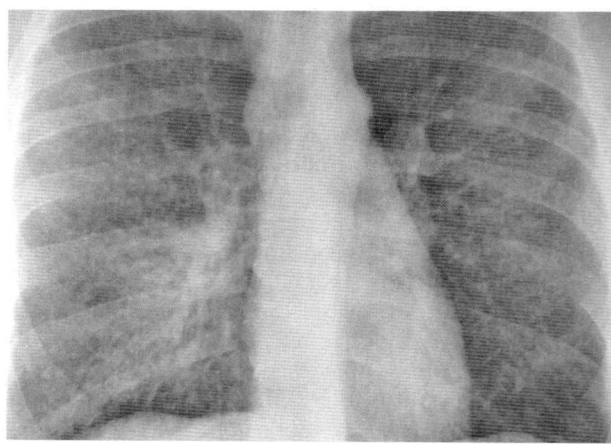

C

Figure 14–9 Chest radiographic staging. *A*, Stage I; bilateral hilar lymphadenopathy (BHL). *B*, Stage II; BHL with pulmonary infiltrates. *C*, Stage III; infiltrates alone.

Most clinicians have found this condition steroid responsive, but its rarity demands complete evaluation to exclude more common causes of this condition.[418] Chronicity of the pleural effusion may lead to pleural thickening that is readily detected by CT.[428]

Cavitation.   Cavitation may follow NSG to produce thick- or thin-walled, single, or multiple cavities.[429] These cavities are unusual, and should be investigated to rule out mycetoma, a recognized complication of this process (Figure 14–10).

Pneumothorax.   Pneumothorax is uncommon but may be associated with NSG due to invasion by subpleural or pleural granulomata. Pneumothoraces may be bilateral and recurrent.[430]

Lymph Node Calcification.   Lymph node calcification, although unusual, becomes more frequent with disease duration. The pattern of calcification is nonspecific and resembles tuberculosis or histoplasmosis and may mimic the eggshell calcification of silicosis.[431]

Atelectasis.   Atelectasis may be seen as a feature of airway collapse, due to either endobronchial sarcoidosis compromising airway patency or due to extrinsic compression by enlarged lymph nodes. The right middle lobe is most frequently involved, probably due to its narrow orifice and the clumping of lymph nodes around its origin. This condition may present with stridor or unilateral rhonchi and has been reported to progress to postobstructive bronchiectasis.[432]

Computed Tomography in Sarcoidosis

The use of high-resolution computed tomography (HRCT) in sarcoidosis is somewhat controversial, given the excellent correlation provided by CXR. However, some 25% of CXR are somewhat atypical including 5 to 10% of HRCT show disease but with a normal CXR. Computed tomography is most useful for these patients (Figure 14–11). Computed tomography has three potential roles in sarcoidosis: diagnosis, assessment of distribution, and assessment of activity.

In a study to assess the diagnostic accuracy in 118 cases of interstitial lung disease, CXR provided a correct diagnosis in 66% of 19 cases of sarcoidosis and CT 77%.[433] This result did not achieve statistical significance and tends to confirm the validity of CXR assessment in diagnostic evaluation in sarcoidosis.

Mahler and colleagues[301] considered the overuse of CT in the initial evaluation of patients with sarcoidosis. Computed tomography was performed in 35 of 100 patients but provided no new clinically significant information when compared to corresponding CXR. In two cases, mediastinal lymph nodes not seen on CXR were noted, and a unilateral pulmonary infiltrate on CXR was noted to be bilateral on CT in a third.

The classic appearance of pulmonary sarcoidosis on lung high HRCT scans are: (1) thickened interlobular septa, (2) widespread small nodules associated with bronchovascular bundles or distributed subpleurally, (3) architectural distortion, (4) interstitial infiltrates, and (5) hilar and mediastinal adenopathy. Other features include reticular changes, septal beading, and consolidation.

Computed tomography is clearly superior to CXR in demonstrating the extent and distribution of disease. The CXR identifies nodules, adenopathy, cystic change, and pleural disease, whereas CT more effectively demonstrates smaller nodules (< 5 mm), bronchovascular, and interlobular septal involvement.[434–436] Both of these techniques, however, can produce negative results with biopsy-proven granulomatous disease, albeit at a low rate.[436]

Computed tomography has not proven particularly effective in the assessment of disease activity. Bergin and colleagues[437] investigated 27 patients with pulmonary sarcoidosis and found that the CT grading of severity of disease correlated well with pulmonary function tests (PFTs) for those groups with a normal CXR, multiple discrete small nodules, and distortion of parenchymal

TABLE 14–11   Chest Radiography Staging at Presentation and Remission Prognosis

Stage	Presentation (%)	Spontaneous Remission (%)
I BHLN	50	75–80
II BHLN + parenchymal infiltrate	25	50
III Parenchymal infiltrate without BHLN	15	40

BHLN = bilateral hilar lymph nodes.
Adapted from Scadding JG, Mitchell DN[267] and Kirtland SH, Winterbauer RH.[418]

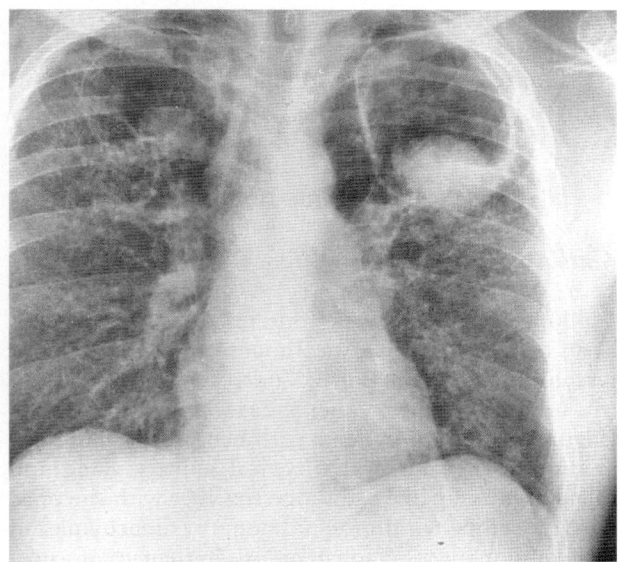

Figure 14–10   Bilateral cavity formation with mycetoma as a complication of chronic pulmonary sarcoidosis.

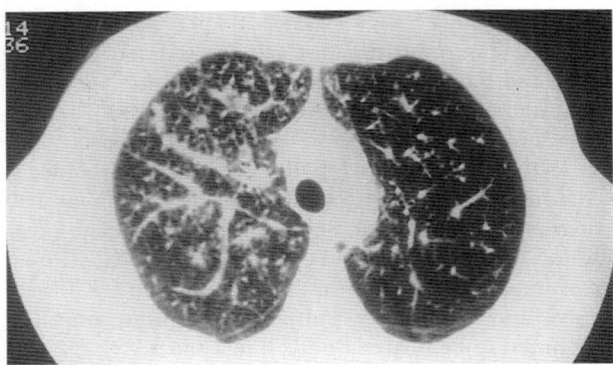

Figure 14–11 High-resolution computed tomography demonstrates the typical bronchovascular bundle distribution of pulmonary involvement creating a "beading" pattern.

structures, whereas patients with segmental alveolar disease and spherical (alveolar) masslike opacities had relatively normal PFTs and thus had no correlation. Further, no correlation was found when gallium scans were compared with CT, PFT, or BAL lymphocyte counts. Lynch and colleagues[438] found an inconsistent correlation between the gallium scan and CT but none nogallium correlation BAL lymphocytosis, whereas Leung and colleagues[439] reported that the presence of nodules and consolidation on the HRCT scan reflected disease activity as measured by ^{67}Ga scan, BAL, and SACE assay. Hansell and colleagues,[440] reporting CT scans in 45 patients with sarcoidosis, described changes compatible with small airways disease in 40 but the presence of decreased attenuation did not correlate with airflow obstruction measured spirometrically. Other studies have, however, found the reverse: lung infiltration on inspiratory HRCT scans and air trapping on expiratory CT correlated with spirometric measures of restrictive and obstructive lung disease, respectively.[441] Overall, CT influences therapeutic decisions in a minority of cases in clinical practice.

Indications for CT scanning in sarcoidosis are summarized in Table 14–12.

Radionuclide Imaging

Gallium Scans

Gallium scans (^{67}Ga) were routinely used in the 1980s as an investigation that was thought to be sensitive for sarcoidosis and of prognostic value.[442–444] The ^{67}Ga scans can be helpful where other indices are not diagnostic (Figure 14–12). In patients with neurologic symptoms and signs, the presence of typical salivary gland and bilateral hilar uptake of isotope together with the presence of isotope within the pulmonary parenchyma can be helpful in identifying sarcoidosis in the face of a normal chest radiograph and lung function tests (Figure 14–13). However, the pulmonary parenchyma may be positive in a wide range of diffuse lung diseases, and in the absence of typical parotid and hilar gland uptake (panda and lambda signs respectively), Gallium 67 scanning cannot be regarded as diagnostic.

Gallium 67 has been assessed as an activity marker in sarcoidosis in several studies.[442,445–451] [67]Ga is predominantly taken up in the lung by macrophages, and there is evidence that ^{67}Ga uptake mainly reflects the presence of granulomata.[445]

Several studies have examined ^{67}Ga scanning in relationship to standard clinical and radiologic measures of disease activity. Line and coworkers[442] found that 65% of their patients with sarcoidosis (n = 41) had increased ^{67}Ga activity in the lungs, but this correlated poorly with clinical, radiologic, and physiologic data. Klech and colleagues[446] found ^{67}Ga scanning to have a 94% sensitivity in detecting active sarcoidosis (defined in terms of clinical symptoms and/or plain chest radiologic deterioration). Negative scans had a poor specificity but a high predictive value for the exclusion of active disease. Gupta and coworkers[452] found abnormal ^{67}Ga scans in 97% of patients with "active" disease (defined in terms of clinical symptoms and abnormal chest radiography) and also in 71% with inactive disease. They concluded that abnormal ^{67}Ga scans were highly sensitive (97%) but had a poor specificity (29%) for clinical disease activity.

Gallium 67 scanning has been used to predict the response to corticosteroid therapy. Baughman and colleagues[448] found a close correlation (r = .95) between initial ^{67}Ga uptake and lung function improvement in 16 patients treated with corticosteroids for clinically active sarcoidosis. Hollinger and colleagues[449] studied 21 patients and found a poor correlation between quantitated ^{67}Ga scans performed before and after steroid treatment and clinical and respiratory function assessment. Turner-Warwick and colleagues[450] rescanned 32 patients with sarcoidosis receiving steroid therapy designed to maximize chest radiographic improvement. Mean follow-up was 19.8 months; during this period, ^{67}Ga scanning information was not used in patient management decisions. Initial ^{67}Ga scanning did not predict treatment response, and scans often remained abnormal despite a normal chest radiograph and lung function. There was a tendency for ^{67}Ga activity to fall with clinical and radiographic improvement.

TABLE 14–12   Guidelines for Computed Tomography in Pulmonary Sarcoidosis

Evaluation of the atypical chest radiograph

Evaluation of the normal chest radiograph with abnormal lung function. Search for covert lymphadenopathy or parenchymal disease

Assessment of unusual symptoms (eg, hemoptysis) and intercurrent chest disease

Localization for diagnostic transbronchial biopsy

Upper respiratory tract disease

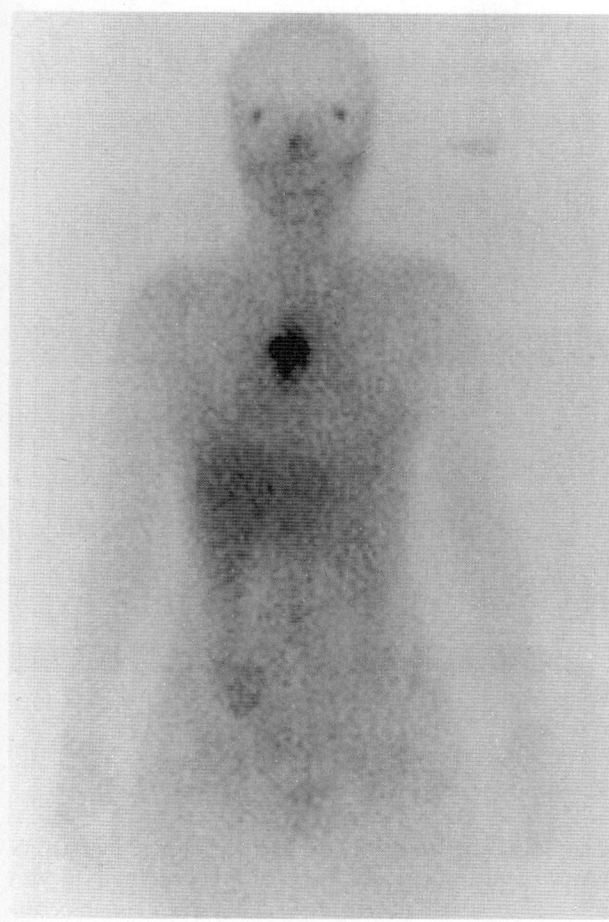

A

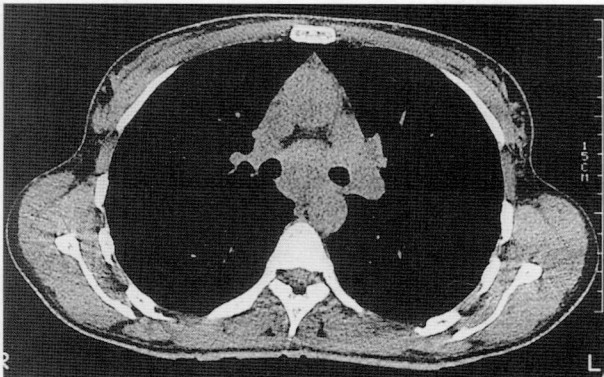

B

Figure 14–12 Computed tomography (CT) is useful in assessing patients with a normal or atypical chest radiograph. *A*, Central thoracic gallium uptake suggests disease and *B*, CT confirms its localization to the subcarinal glands.

Recent work suggests that the use of somatostatin receptor scintigraphy (SRS) may offer better evaluation of organ involvement in patients with sarcoidosis compared to gallium scintigraphy, especially those who have received treatment with steroids.[453]

^{99m}Tc-DTPA Epithelial Permeability Scanning

It is likely that persistent lung inflammation leads to disease progression in sarcoidosis. Technetium 99m diethylenetriamine pentaacetate (DTPA) lung scanning is a measure of epithelial cell permeability and has been evaluated as a marker of disease activity; however, it is not useful for diagnosis. No predictive value was estimated in the majority of reports.

Jacobs and colleagues[454] studied 14 nonsmokers with untreated sarcoidosis and found an increased DTPA clearance in 8; there was no correlation with BAL lymphocyte counts or gallium uptake. Dusser and colleagues[455] measured DTPA clearance in 49 nonsmokers with sarcoidosis and reported an increased value in 12, all of whom showed diffuse lung disease on chest radiography. There was no correlation with BAL lymphocyte counts but some correlation with SACE. The DTPA clearance was decreased when lung function improved, but respiratory function tests were normal in 29% of patients with increased clearance and were abnormal in 24% of patients with normal clearance.

Chinet and colleagues[456] prospectively examined the use of DTPA lung scanning in assessing both the likelihood of disease progression and the treatment response in 37 untreated, nonsmoking patients with sarcoidosis. The DTPA clearance was determined at intervals of 6 or 12 months over a period of 6 to 36 months (mean of 16 months). A 15% or greater deterioration in respiratory function tests occurred in 11 patients, 8 of whom received corticosteroid therapy. In patients who remained stable, regardless of initial values of respiratory function tests, DTPA clearance remained within the normal range; DTPA clearance became abnormal in those who deteriorated. In the 8 treated patients, respiratory function tests improved and DTPA clearance significantly fell. The authors concluded that DTPA clearance can identify those patients who are likely to remain stable (those with normal clearance), and changes in DTPA clearance reflect changes in respiratory function tests in sarcoidosis. Bradvik and colleagues[457] documented that with the introduction of steroids, lung DTPA clearance improved as did the lung ^{67}Ga score and SACE, but changes were not associated with lung function changes. These studies suggest that the technique requires further evaluation with regard to its place in the investigative algorithm for patients with sarcoidosis.

Pulmonary Function

The typical physiologic abnormality is a restrictive ventilatory defect; respiratory function tests, particularly vital capacity (VC) and gas transfer (DL_{CO}), are frequently abnormal in patients with sarcoidosis. Airflow obstruction is seen in extensive endobronchial and fibrotic disease and has been reported as an early abnor-

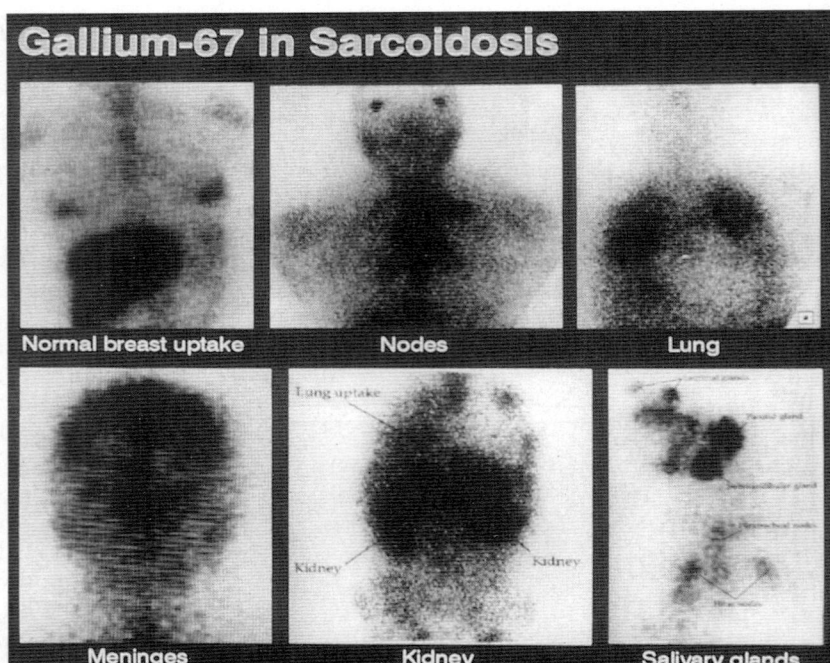

Figure 14–13 Gallium 67 scanning demonstrates regions of granulomatous involvement and is particularly useful in supporting a clinical diagnosis of sarcoidosis if a biopsy site is not available.

mality.[458] Serial respiratory function tests have traditionally been used to monitor disease progression in sarcoidosis and are the only way to evaluate progressive change in organ function.[459] Only 20% of patients with stage I disease will have abnormal lung function tests, compared 40 to 70% of patients with stage II to IV involvement.

Four studies have addressed the correlation between disease extent, which was assessed histologically, and respiratory function.[460–462] All reported some correlation between disease extent and respiratory function. In the largest of these, Huang and colleagues[462] graded 81 open-lung biopsies from patients with sarcoidosis for density of granulomas, degree of interstitial pneumonitis, presence of granulomatous angiitis, and severity of parenchymal fibrosis. Respiratory function tests readily distinguished mild from moderate and severe pathology but did not separate moderate from severe disease; however, it is clear that histologic measures of disease extent and respiratory function are only indirectly related. One group investigated the value of initial respiratory function tests in predicting the likelihood of disease progression[463]; 78 untreated patients with sarcoidosis were divided into two groups based on a VC or DL_{CO} of 65% or less than predicted. During a mean follow-up period of 2 years and 8 months, 26% of the group with a VC above 65% worsened, whereas none of the group (n = 11) with the low VC deteriorated. In the group with the higher DL_{CO} 42% worsened, whereas in the lower DL_{CO} group 25% deteriorated. They concluded that baseline respiratory function tests do not relate to the probability of disease progression.

Bronchoalveolar Lavage

A large number of diffuse lung diseases may be characterized by the presence of excess numbers of lymphocytes in lavage returns, but, typically, a lymphocyte alveolitis is most commonly seen in sarcoidosis, tuberculosis, and extrinsic allergic alveolitis (hypersensitivity pneumonitis).[155,160,464,465] The range of increase in lymphocyte percentages is huge, which makes it difficult to accurately assess the likelihood of sarcoidosis based purely on lavage lymphocyte counts. However, an assessment of CD4:CD8 ratios may help.[464] If the CD4:CD8 ratio is 3.5 or greater, the specificity of diagnosis is 94% with a sensitivity of 52%. With increasing CD4:CD8 ratios, the sensitivity falls and the specificity rises. With a CD4:CD8 ratio as low as 1, sensitivity increases to 90% but with a reduction in specificity to 33%. These data show that CD4:CD8 ratios can be helpful in differential diagnosis but that a considerable number of patients with confirmed sarcoidosis have a lower-than-normal CD4:CD8 ratio. Similarly, in a small percentage of patients, a CD4:CD8 ratio > 3.5% may be observed in diseases other than sarcoidosis. This has been reported in asbestosis, tuberculosis, cryptogenic fibrosing alveolitis, and extrinsic allergic alveolitis. The use of the CD4:CD8 ratio in diagnosis is further undermined by its variability between different patients, with one study reporting that the CD4:CD8 ratio ranged from 0.5 to 37.3 in a population of 86 patients with sarcoidosis.[466] It has been suggested that the sensitivity of the CD4:CD8 ratio in diagnosing sarcoidosis can be improved by assessing the expression of other lymphocyte-addressing molecules. In patients with sarcoidosis, the BAL fluid is characterized by the lack of CD103, which is usually expressed by intraepithelial CD4+ lymphocytes in mucosal areas, and its absence may differentiate sarcoidosis from other lung conditions characterized by CD4 lymphocytosis.[467]

It is probably most helpful to consider a lavage lymphocytosis, particularly with a high CD4:CD8 ratio, as highly suggestive of sarcoidosis in the context of other clinical and investigational indices that are consistent with the diagnosis. Biopsy confirmation remains the gold standard. The 1991 World Association of Sarcoidosis and other Granulomatous Diseases definition of sarcoidosis includes "…supported by histological evidence of noncaseating epithelioid cell granulomas" on histologic assessment.[468]

Initial reports from Crystal and colleagues' group at the National Institutes of Health in the United States suggested that prognosis in sarcoidosis is determined by the degree of BAL lymphocytosis.[444] Nineteen untreated patients with pulmonary disease were serially studied with BAL and ^{67}Ga scans at 6-month intervals for a mean of 10 months. The percentage of lymphocytes in the BAL fluid and the ^{67}Ga scan were used to divide the patients into two groups of low-intensity (less than or equal to 28% lymphocytes and/or ^{67}Ga scan negative) and high-intensity alveolitis (> 28% lymphocytes in the BAL fluid and a positive ^{67}Ga scan). Lung function deteriorated over the next 6 months in 87% of patients with high-intensity alveolitis but in only 8% of patients with a low-intensity alveolitis. Clinical, radiologic, and physiologic tests did not predict deterioration. This study provided a point of departure for many subsequent papers; however, it has been criticized on the small number of patients studied (only 5 patients had high-intensity alveolitis), the relatively short duration of follow-up, and the significantly older age of the patient and longer duration of disease (both known to influence outcome) in the high-intensity group.

Several studies have subsequently investigated the use of alveolitis intensity as a guide to either disease progression or response to treatment. The results have been conflicting, although it appears that the intensity of the alveolitis does not predict outcome.[449,450,469–474] Turner-Warwick and colleagues[450] evaluated serial lavage counts in 32 patients with persistent radiologic and physiologic abnormalities and who had received steroid treatment. Initial lavage lymphocyte counts did not predict a response to therapy, and a good radiographic response occurred in 7 patients whose initial BAL lymphocyte count was normal. However, most patients with a normal lymphocyte count showed persistent radiologic abnormalities. Changes in radiology and respiratory function correlated very poorly with serial lavage data, and several symptom-free patients with normal or stable radiographs remained stable despite persistently abnormal BAL lymphocyte counts. Laviolette and colleagues[475] prospectively studied 98 patients with newly diagnosed sarcoidosis for a mean of 26 months. Twenty-four patients required steroid treatment during this period. Thirty-two percent of the group with an initial BAL lymphocyte percentage of greater than or equal to 30% required steroid therapy compared with 18% of the group with fewer lymphocytes, but this difference was not significant. There was no significant difference between changes in respiratory function tests at follow-up in either the high- or low-intensity alveolitis groups. The authors concluded that BAL lymphocyte counts at the time of diagnosis are not useful predictors of respiratory prognosis in newly diagnosed sarcoidosis.

In some studies, high lymphocytosis is seen in disease that has a high incidence of spontaneous resolution. Foley and colleagues[471] suggested that high-intensity alveolitis is a favorable prognostic factor for lung function. Sixty-seven patients with biopsy-proven sarcoidosis were prospectively followed for 13 to 37 months. Initially, 42 patients with high-intensity alveolitis (BAL lymphocyte count greater than 28%) improved significantly in terms of lung function and chest radiographs, whereas patients with low-intensity alveolitis did not improve. Steroid therapy also caused a greater improvement in patients with high- rather than low-intensity alveolitis. Repeat BAL in 34 patients showed a very weak and not clinically useful correlation between vital capacity response and fall in lymphocyte counts.

The impact of neutrophilia in BAL fluid has been assessed by Drent and colleagues.[476] Twenty-six nonsmoking patients with sarcoidosis were divided into two groups according to the degree of neutrophilia in the BAL fluid. Those patients (n = 11) with > 0.2×10^4 neutrophils per mL had more severe disease as measured by radiographic stage, HRCT, ^{67}Ga scan, and lung function, and these patients were less likely to improve spontaneously when compared with a group (n = 15) with < 0.2×10^4 neutrophils per mL.

Given the invasive technique of obtaining BAL samples there is encouraging work suggesting that equivalent cellular profiles can be obtained by the easier and less invasive technique of induced sputum by inhalation of a hypertonic saline solution.[477] These techniques have been widely used to assess airway inflammation in asthma and chronic obstructive pulmonary disease. The cellular profiles obtained by induced sputum techniques may reflect the more proximal airways disease, rather than the interstitial changes typical of sarcoidosis.

T Lymphocyte CD4:CD8 Ratios

Following the original observations of Hunninghake and Crystal[155] that there is an excess of CD4+ helper/inducer T cells in the lungs of patients with "active sarcoidosis," several groups have suggested that lymphocyte subgroup analysis, based on the ratio of CD4 to CD8 cells, provides a better predictor of outcome and response to treatment than total cell counts alone, but the data in support of this is equivocal.[448,472,478–480] Ceuppens and colleagues[480] analyzed T-cell subsets in 35 patients. The percentage of lymphocytes in the BAL fluid fell in only 6 out of 10 patients who improved clinically, but a fall in the CD4:CD8 ratio accompanied or preceded radiologic and clinical improvement in all cases. In 16 patients assessed before corticosteroid therapy by Baughman and colleagues,[448] there was no correlation between the percentage of lymphocytes in the BAL fluid and changes in vital capacity, but there was a positive correlation (r = .62) between changes in CD4:CD8 ratio and vital capacity. Further support for the predictive power of the CD4:CD8 ratio came from Costabel and colleagues,[478] who serially studied 31 initially untreated patients with sarcoidosis. A normal CD4:CD8 ratio at presentation was highly predictive of a favorable course. Thirteen out of 15 patients with normal ratios remained stable whereas 10 out of 16 with elevated CD4:CD8 ratios deteriorated during follow-up.

Different findings were reported by Verstraeten and colleagues,[472] who followed up 31 patients for 22 to 36 months. Patients who improved radiologically had a higher CD4:CD8 ratio in their initial BAL sample than those who deteriorated or remained unchanged. However, the correlation between the CD4:CD8 ratio and the change in DL_{CO} was only 0.51. In 10 patients in whom BAL was repeated, improvement in chest radiology was accompanied by a decrease in the CD4:CD8 ratio.

The importance of disease duration as a confounding factor in the interpretation of CD4:CD8 ratios was shown by Ward and coworkers.[481] They examined the influence of the type of disease presentation and time of onset of symptoms on lavage lymphocyte counts in 99 patients who were studied at the time of their initial diagnosis. Patients with an acute inflammatory presentation (EN, acute uveitis) almost invariably had a high CD4:CD8 ratio and high BAL lymphocyte counts. They concluded that any series that included a high proportion of patients with an acute onset of illness would not find a high CD4:CD8 ratio or lymphocyte count to be indicative of a poor outcome.

The current role of BAL in sarcoidosis can be summarized as follows. All patients suspected of pulmonary sarcoidosis should undergo BAL to confirm the presence or absence of a lymphocytic alveolitis. The CD4:CD8 analysis can increase the sophistication of differential diagnosis, but there are too many exceptions to recommend this procedure on a routine basis. Setting up a regional BAL processing unit serving a wide area may be the answer rather than expecting all hospitals to provide the service. No additional information is obtained by monitoring BAL lymphocyte counts serially. Well-controlled prospective studies are urgently needed to define more precisely the role of the evaluation of BAL lymphocytes in sarcoidosis. These studies will need to stratify patient entry based on the type of disease at presentation and must have clearly defined end points. Such studies will inevitably need to

be multicentric. An important issue is the duration and stage of disease at the time of BAL analysis. It is likely the differences between these studies are, at least in part, due to different case mixes of individuals with early and late disease.

Biopsy

Biopsy Procedures

Histologic confirmation of the diagnosis should be obtained in all cases, except for Löfgren's syndrome in which the features (and resolution) help make the diagnosis without a reasonable doubt. The site of biopsy sampling is chosen on the basis of organ involvement and most easy access.

Bronchial/Transbronchial Biopsy. Fiberoptic bronchoscopy with endobronchial and transbronchial biopsy (TBB), taking a minimum of four samples, provides a greater than 90% positivity rate (Figure 14–14).[482] Because lung involvement is so common, it is the procedure used most frequently in patients presenting with pulmonary sarcoidosis. In a large series of transbronchial biopsies, Mitchell and colleagues[483] found a close to 80% positive yield in unselected patients. In stage I disease, the yield may be further increased by performing transbronchial needle aspiration in addition.[484] As with other sites of granuloma formation, there are many causes of granulomas in the lung other than sarcoidosis. Thus, a finding of granuloma must be in keeping with a compatible clinical picture.

Mediastinoscopy. Although "blind" TBB will be positive in approximately 60% of patients presenting with BHL with normal lung fields, mediastinoscopy should be performed to exclude malignancy or tuberculosis, particularly if mediastinal lymphadenopathy is not associated with hilar glands or if the hilar lymphadenopathy is not bilateral.[485]

Liver Biopsy. Granulomas within the liver parenchyma or in the periportal region may be found in approximately 70% of patients who present with hilar lymphadenopathy with or without pulmonary infiltration (Figure 14–15).[486] The presence of such granulomas may be associated with an isolated elevation in serum alkaline phosphatase. Ultrasound may show hepatomegaly with a diffuse increase in signal. The percentage of positive results is usually lower among patients who do not have hilar lymphadenopathy. Other causes of liver granuloma must be excluded if no evidence of granuloma is found elsewhere.

Other Biospy Sites. Other organs such as the eye, brain, and heart are relatively less accessible to perform a biopsy and are vulnerable to sampling error, but a biopsy can be confirmatory in some cases (Figure 14–16). Biopsies of areas of erythema nodosum will be unhelpful as they do not contain granulomas.

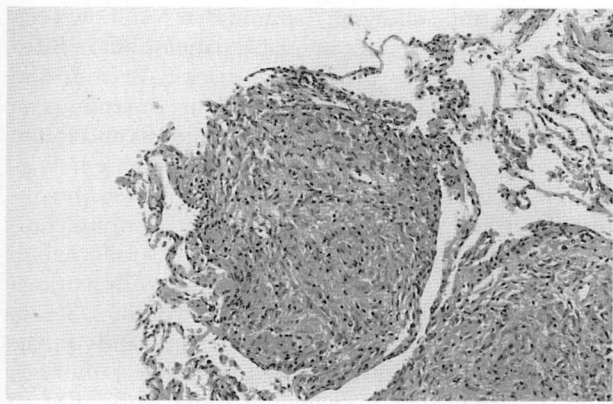

Figure 14-14 Transbronchial lung biopsy (hematoxylin and eosin).

Delayed-Type Hypersensitivity Skin Tests

Delayed skin tests to recall antigens are typically suppressed in patients with sarcoidosis anergy.[487] These include responses to tuberculin, which is helpful in excluding tuberculosis from the differential diagnosis. The exact mechanisms of anergy are not known, but it is possible that the relative lymphopenia, particularly of CD4+ cells, may be a factor. If hydrocortisone is injected with tuberculin, it is possible to restore responsiveness. This suggests the alternate possibility that inhibition of the suppressor mechanism by steroids may be relevant.

Kveim Test

The Kveim test, first described in 1941,[16] although still a potentially useful diagnostic tool today is now unavailable in Europe. The Kveim test acts as an in vivo model of sarcoidosis, wherein the Kveim suspension invokes a tissue response in patients with sarcoidosis that is histologically identical to the sarcoid granuloma that is caused by the disease. Isolation of the causative antigen in the Kveim suspension remains elusive, but an understanding of it may clarify the etiology of sarcoidosis. Given that monoclonal antibodies raised to the Kveim suspension recognize macrophages from sarcoid granulomas and that T cells do not proliferate when exposed to Kveim reagent, it has been postulated that the antigen is situated on the macrophage surface.[488] Transbronchial biopsy now provides a mechanism that permits more rapid diagnosis of lung infiltrates. However, there are frequent instances in which the lungs are normal or the transbronchial approach has failed to provide diagnostic material. Kveim testing would have continued to be a useful diagnostic approach in this situation, particularly in differentiating the cause of multifocal neurologic signs.

The percentage of positive responses depends on the stage of the disease. An acute presentation with fever, EN, arthralgia, and BHL is associated with a positivity of 70 to 90%. In contrast, more extensive stage III disease may yield only 34 to 43% positive responses. Thus, unfortunately, the test is less helpful in exactly those situations in which it is most needed (ie, in disease that is less easy to diagnose). However, it remains the most specific test for sarcoidosis and carries an incidence of false positives in healthy individuals of only 0.7 to 2%, with a similar percentage for patients with other diseases.[16]

Among patients with only extrathoracic manifestations of sarcoidosis, or where granulomas are found unexpectedly in an organ or tissue, a positive test significantly bolsters a tentative diagnosis of sarcoidosis.

Blood Tests

Peripheral blood counts may show a low absolute number of lymphocytes and also neutrophils. Subset analysis has shown that the lymphopenia is due predominantly to a reduction in the numbers of the CD4 subset. In one study, eosinophilia was seen in 41% of patients, but this is unusual and in these patients there was no associated lung tissue eosinophilia.[489] Hemoglobin is rarely affected

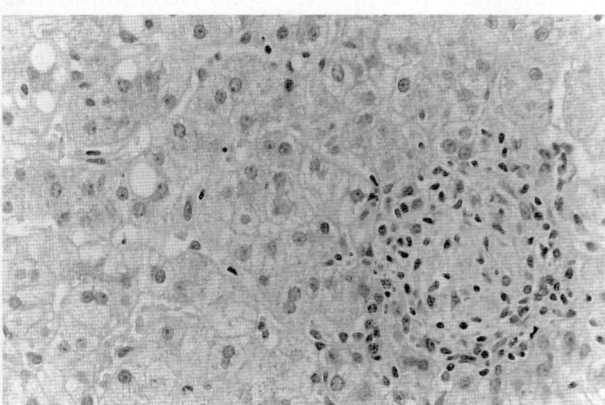

Figure 14-15 Percutaneous liver biopsy (hematoxylin and eosin).

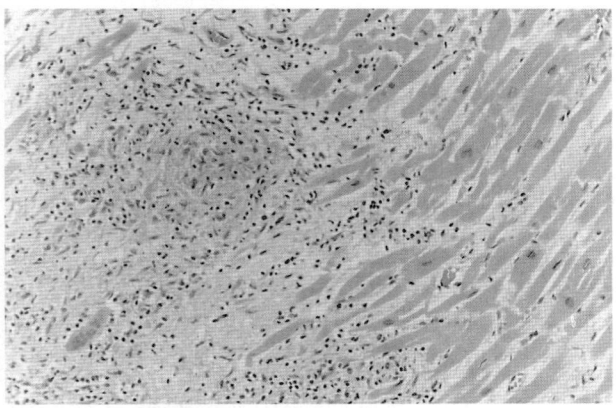

Figure 14-16 Endomyocardial biopsy (hematoxylin and eosin).

but thrombocytopenia may occur. Erythrocyte sedimentation rate may be modestly elevated.

Liver function tests are usually elevated due to granulomatous infiltration, particularly an isolated rise in alkaline phosphatase. Calcium levels may be high in the blood and independently in the urine as a result of vitamin D metabolism in the granulomas, which themselves produce increased amounts of 1,25-dihydroxyvitamin D_3.

Serum angiotensin converting enzyme levels may be elevated, but this is a nonsensitive test for sarcoidosis with better specificity. The SACE level can also be elevated in other granulomatous diseases, such as tuberculosis, leprosy, Gaucher's disease, and hyperthyroidism. A very high level (twice the upper level of normal) is usually associated with sarcoidosis. Since Lieberman's[490] original report, many authors have confirmed the rise in SACE that occurs in sarcoidosis.[446,452,491–495] These series have reported elevated SACE levels in 30 to 100% of patients with sarcoidosis with a mean between 50 and 60%.[496] Studdy and James[497] estimated that SACE has a diagnostic sensitivity of 57% and a specificity of 90.5%.

Serum angiotensin converting enzyme has also been proposed as a marker of disease activity. Two important factors should be considered: (1) SACE is often normal during the first 2 to 3 months of the disease in patients with sarcoidosis presenting acutely with EN.[492,498,499] This is probably explained by its production by granulomata rather than lymphocytes. (2) The SACE levels probably reflect the total granulomatous burden rather than the degree of lung involvement by sarcoidosis. A lack of change in SACE, despite improvements in respiratory function tests, could simply reflect a difference in disease activity in various organs.

The relationship between SACE and disease activity in the lung has been the subject of several studies.[446,491,493–495,500–503] The results of these studies are often contradictory, which may be due to the inclusion of patients with very different disease durations; the lack of a precise definition of disease activity; a difference in activity measures (clinical, radiologic, physiologic, or a combination of these); and a lack of predetermined, regular SACE measurements. It is unclear in some studies whether repeated SACE measurements were made as clinical judgment dictated or as part of a fixed protocol. The discovery of a polymorphism of the SACE gene means that different genotypes will also influence the circulating concentration of SACE and thus its role in diagnosis and subsequent monitoring of patients.[504] Genotype-corrected values may turn out to have greater prognostic value. Finally, corticosteroid treatment may have influenced results. In the majority of studies, some patients received steroids during the follow-up period, and it is often difficult to separate the effect of such treatment on SACE levels. In some studies, the first SACE recordings were not always performed at initial assessment; in one study, they were performed nearly 6 months after the initial visit.

Turton and colleagues[494] found that SACE was elevated in 1 out of 19 clinically stable patients but in 8 out of 13 patients with progressive disease. Selroos and Gronhagen-Riska[491,501] made serial measurements of SACE in patients with untreated sarcoidosis and found some correlation between SACE and worsening radiography or respiratory function. Serum angiotensin converting enzyme also changed significantly during clinically stable periods. Ueda and colleagues[495] followed up 51 patients with sarcoid for at least 1 year with repeated (choice of interval unspecified) SACE recordings. Serum angiotensin converting enzyme fell significantly in the group of patients who achieved complete radiologic remission but did not change in those who failed to remit. In a small group of patients who initially remitted and later relapsed, SACE levels mirrored radiologic change. DeRemee and Rohrback[493] followed up 35 patients for a variable period (up to 640 days) with repeated SACE measurements (intervals not defined). Nine patients were already taking prednisolone at entry, and a further 18 started steroids during the trial. In the 8 who spontaneously resolved, SACE levels fell to normal, and in the 13 who responded to treatment, SACE levels also fell. Weaver and colleagues[500] followed up 18 patients with repeated (time not specified) SACE levels for a median of 11 months (range 1 to 25 months). A weak relationship (r = .35) was found between changes in SACE and gas transfer and between changes in SACE and total lung capacity (r = .58). Klech and coworkers[446] divided 60 patients into active and inactive groups based on clinical and chest radiologic criteria. They found SACE to have a 77% sensitivity and an 88% specificity in assessing disease activity. Ainslie and Benatar[503] measured SACE in 128 patients with sarcoidosis on 303 occasions. Serum angiotensin converting enzyme was significantly higher in patients with stage II or III chest radiographs and was also greater in patients with clinically active disease.

These studies suggest a relationship between disease extent and ACE, as assessed clinically, radiologically, physiologically, and by SACE levels and that SACE can reflect changes in disease extent as assessed radiologically. Unfortunately, there is no large, prospective study that has systematically assessed whether SACE measurements predict outcome; there is insufficient evidence to recommend changes in treatment policy based solely on SACE levels.

Whether SACE predicts a response to corticosteroid treatment has been investigated.[448–450,452,498] Gupta and colleagues[452] noted an inverse correlation between SACE and steroid dose in 80 patients with sarcoidosis. Baughman and colleagues[448] measured SACE before and after corticosteroid treatment in 16 patients with clinically active sarcoidosis. Only a low correlation (r = .37) was found between pretreatment SACE levels and changes in vital capacity. In a similar study, Hollinger and colleagues[449] also recorded SACE before and after steroid therapy in 21 patients. The SACE levels fell with treatment in all patients, but there was no correlation between pretreatment SACE levels and changes in vital capacity. Turner-Warwick and colleagues[450] serially measured SACE in 32 patients given corticosteroids for persistent pulmonary sarcoidosis. Pretreatment SACE levels did not predict outcome in terms of radiologic improvement. Serum angiotensin converting enzyme tended to fall with improvement but some patients had an elevated SACE despite a normal chest radiograph.

Initial SACE levels are a poor guide to predict treatment response, in terms of improvement in chest radiology and respiratory function tests. Serum angiotensin converting enzyme tends to fall with corticosteroid treatment, but the magnitude of change correlates poorly with other measures of improvement.

Urine Tests

It is important to test urine microscopy for evidence of renal tract inflammation. Renal inflammatory and nephrocalcinosis problems may be asymptomatic, and an abnormal sediment may indicate the need for further tests of renal function including 24-hour urine calcium excretion.

Disease Activity and Prognosis

Sarcoidosis runs a variable course, with the disease resolving spontaneously in many patients. In approximately 25 to 30% of instances, however, the disease runs a more protracted course and can result in significant morbidity and death. In this situation, treatment is often instituted, but no studies have confirmed that treatment affects the long-term outcome. At presentation, significant extrapulmonary involvement of the heart or central nervous system is seen in 4 to 7% of cases. Corticosteroids are used in 30 to 50% of cases at presentation, but relapse is common as the dose is reduced. Deaths are usually due to respiratory failure or cardiac and neurologic involvement, and occur in 1 to 5% of patients.[302,314-316] Measures that can predict disease progression (the presence of disease activity) would provide the basis of a rational approach to treatment and trials of treatment. However, the term "activity" has in the past been used loosely and indiscriminately, confusing the central issue. This confusion has been compounded by the quest for a disease activity marker in sarcoidosis that has resulted in often circular logic and self-fulfilling prophecy. Many reported studies have assessed a wide range of clinical, radiologic, and serologic tests as possible activity markers.[410,496,505,506] Despite this enormous research effort, no single test appears satisfactory, and many seem to be of very limited value.

Most clinicians feel intuitively that a definition of disease activity would include disease prognosis and would help make the difficult decision as to which patients should receive treatment. If this definition of disease activity is adopted, it is immediately clear that the only useful validation studies for proposed markers of disease activity will be long-term studies in which repeated measurements of organ function (usually lung) in patients have been made. Studies in which one proposed marker of activity is compared with another would not fulfill the terms of this definition and will not be considered in this review. Furthermore, the ideal marker (or markers) of disease activity would predict subsequent organ dysfunction.

Changes in plain chest radiology and respiratory function tests have traditionally been used as the main indices of change of lung studies and probably remain the best indices of lung dysfunction and failure, although they are not themselves good predictors of disease progression. It is nonetheless appropriate that plain chest radiology, respiratory function, and clinical state continue to remain the standards against which novel putative activity markers are judged.

Other Putative Markers of Disease Activity

A variety of other markers of disease activity have been used in sarcoidosis, but few have been subject to prospective studies, and they add nothing to chest radiography and lung function tests.

Serum lysozyme,[501,507-509] beta$_2$-microglobulin,[496,509] carboxypeptidase,[510] neutral thermolysine-like metal peptidase,[498] and adenosine deaminase [511,512] have all been tested as biochemical markers of disease activity, but none of these tests has proved to be useful clinically.

Markers of connective tissue matrix metabolism have been tested and include collagenase in BAL,[513,514] which is probably the best marker. In one study, patients with collagenase activity had more advanced disease and worse respiratory function tests. During the 12-month follow-up, 55% of the collagenase group required steroid therapy compared with 26% of the collagenase-negative group. The BAL collagenase fell with steroid treatment. In untreated patients, respiratory function tests improved in the collagenase-negative group but worsened in the positive group. Type III procollagen peptide, a cleavage product of type III collagen[259,515,516] is much less specific.

Recent research has also focused on the measurement of cytokines and their receptors as markers of disease activity. Prior and colleagues[517] measured serum IFN-γ and found an association with a better treatment response in terms of radiologic clearing but not in terms of improvements in respiratory function tests. For patients who at presentation do not require treatment with corticosteroids, Ziegenhagen and colleagues[518] demonstrated that high levels of BAL TNF-α or serum soluble interlukin-2 receptor (sIL-2R) predict subsequent disease progression. Hashimoto and colleagues[519] demonstrated that plasma levels of the cytokines, monocyte chemoattractant protein-1alpha and monocyte inflammatory protein-1alpha, reflected disease activity: high levels were seen in active disease with the levels falling as the sarcoidosis went into remission. They postulated that these cytokines played a role in initiating monocyte migration into the tissue. Other studies have suggested roles for the cytokines ICAM-1[252] and KL-6/MUCI.[520]

It is unlikely that any test will be the single measure that defines activity and disease progression in sarcoidosis for all patients. Disease activity remains best defined by disease progression, but the use of other tests of pathophysiology such as DTPA, cytokine levels, or collagenase levels might identify high-risk individuals.

Investigation Algorithm

The diagnostic investigation algorithm in all cases should be tailored to the manner of presentation. Our current approach involves routine screening tests (Table 14–13) at first presentation, supplemented as necessary at a second evaluation by ^{67}Ga scan, and a tissue biopsy as necessary. Further investigation is instituted by the clinical needs.

After achieving a diagnosis, indicators of disease are sought to monitor disease progress and treatment response. The most useful clinical indices beyond clinical examination include SACE, liver function tests, serum calcium, urinary calcium excretion, lung function, and ^{67}Ga scan.

Cardiac and renal involvement is frequently silent, necessitating routine urinary calcium excretion testing and ECG as minimum requirements.

Further cardiac investigation is necessary if there is any ECG abnormality or if there is significant clinical suspicion of involvement. Exercise ECG, and 24-hour ECG monitoring as indirect measures of cardiac function may be supplemented by echocardiography, gallium ± thallium scanning, and potentially MRI scanning in pursuing this important diagnosis.

Renal symptoms, elevated serum creatinine, or hypercalcemia/hypercalciuria necessitate further renal investigation. Renal ultrasound may demonstrate nephrolithiasis and also shows renal size in renal sarcoid involvement. Renal biopsy has proven useful in the diagnosis of renal sarcoidosis as well as to exclude other renal pathologies.

Magnetic resonance imaging is the study of choice in neurosarcoidosis, particularly when meningeal involvement is suspected. Magnetic resonance imaging may also provide important prognostic information.

Specialist ophthalmologic review is recommended for all patients at diagnosis to ensure a thorough visual evaluation and also assessment of sclerae and conjunctivae.

Tissue diagnosis remains the most useful diagnostic test demonstrating noncaseating granulomata in the absence of other causes of granulomatous disease (Table 14–14). The most accessible site for initial biopsy is the skin. Should there be no skin lesions, other tissue can be obtained by transbronchial biopsy or lymph node biopsy. More unusually, deep tissue is sought including liver, kidney, brain, and other viscera as indicated.

TREATMENT

There has been considerable debate over the place of treatment, particularly corticosteroid treatment, in sarcoidosis. There is no dispute that severe symptoms or involvement of vital organs such as the eyes, central nervous system, or the heart require therapy, and that corticosteroids are the most effective treatment option.

However, there is less agreement about the role of corticosteroid treatment in pulmonary sarcoidosis. The main issues revolve around the therapeutic ratio in acute and chronic disease. The natural inclination in these circumstances is to withhold treatment until there are symptoms, but by this stage there may be considerable, irreversible lung injury that treatment will not help, leaving the patient with symptoms. Patients with progressive deterioration in lung function and pulmonary infiltrates should be offered treatment with corticosteroids. With regard to pulmonary sarcoidosis, the early T-cell driven alveolitis and granulomatous inflammation of the acute presentation are likely to be corticosteroid responsive, with the fibrosis of chronic sarcoidosis being less amenable to treatment. Although given that granulomatous inflammation is likely to precede and thus overlap with the development of pulmonary fibrosis, the decision regarding the timing of commencement of treatment with corticosteroids is not so clear-cut. Patients who are likely to require long-term treatment with corticosteroids, or who have progressive disease despite treatment with corticosteroids, should have second-line agents introduced.

Corticosteroids

Corticosteroids have formed the mainstay of treatment in sarcoidosis for over 30 years, and their use in this disease

TABLE 14–13   Routine Screening Tests for Evaluation of New Presentations of Sarcoidosis

Chest radiography

Pulmonary function tests with gas transfer

Full blood count, ESR, serum urea and electrolytes, creatinine, calcium, phosphate, albumin, SACE, liver function tests, random blood glucose

C-reactive protein

Electrocardiogram

Urine 24-hour calcium excretion, creatinine clearance, and protein excretion (if urinary sediment abnormal)

Tuberculin test (Heaf/Mantoux)

ESR = erythrocyte sedimentation rate; SACE = serum angiotensin converting enzyme.

TABLE 14–14   Causes of Granulomatous Lung Disease

Sarcoidosis

Extrinsic allergic alveolitis

Berylliosis

Infection—mycobacterial, bacterial, fungal, protozoal, viral

Foreign body

Wegener's granulomatosis

Churg-Strauss syndrome

Lyphomatoid granulomatosis

Bronchocentric granulomatosis

Langerhans cell histiocytosis

has been critically re-evaluated.[521] While awaiting the identification of the triggering event that initiates granuloma formation, therapies are directed at arresting or limiting the T-cell triggering, activation, and proliferation that incite granuloma formation. Key to this process is the expression of the cytokines IL-2, IFN-γ, IL-1, and IL-2R by T lymphocytes, all of which are suppressed by corticosteroid activity.[522–525] Tumor necrosis factor-α, G-CSF, and GM-CSF[205,524] appear to play an auxiliary role and are also suppressed by corticosteroids.

These findings support the suggestion that corticosteroids are a logical treatment for the control of sarcoidosis. Indeed, short-term oral corticosteroid therapy has proven very effective both in new-onset disease and in late untreated disease providing significant symptomatic relief, improved PFTs, and gas transfer as well as radiographic clearance in the vast majority of treated patients.[419,420,526,527] Hunninghake and colleagues reported a simplified approach to treatment, which was determined by evidence of recent deterioration.[525] If there was no evidence (generally physiologic) of deterioration within the previous 3 months, no corticosteroids were given. The majority of patients not given treatment remained stable, and the authors concluded that change in status should be the determinant of treatment. The patient cohort as a whole had relatively well-preserved lung function, and it is not clear whether those with more severe disease would behave in the same way.

The efficacy of long-term corticosteroids is disputed. There have been few studies that have been designed to address this issue in a prospective trial. In a landmark study, Israel and colleagues[421] used a 3-month period of treatment of 15 mg per day and evaluated the outcome at 5 years. There were no significant differences in objective measures between treated and untreated patients in comparison with the placebo-treated group. These findings were echoed by other studies.[422,423,526] However, the majority of these studies have treated patients for a fixed period only and studied the outcome after a longer untreated period. The study of the British Thoracic Society of sarcoidosis treatment attempted to overcome this design problem by tailoring treatment to response and tapering the dosage of treatment while ensuring that

response was maintained. The study concluded that long-term corticosteroids conferred a functional advantage as assessed by a change in vital capacity.[424] A meta-analysis reviewing the use of corticosteroids in pulmonary sarcoidosis has recently been published by the Cochrane group.[528] With regard to the use of oral corticosteroids, 5 trials involving 516 patients were deemed suitable for inclusion. Outcomes were symptoms, chest radiograph changes, lung function, and global scores (combination of all three outcomes). Their conclusion was "that oral steroids improved the chest x-ray score, and a global score of chest x-ray, symptoms and spirometry over 6-24 months, but there is little evidence of an improvement in lung function. There are no data beyond two years to indicate whether oral corticosteroids have any modifying effect on long-term disease progression. Oral corticosteroids are indicated for patients with Stage II and III disease with moderate-severe or progressive symptoms or CXR changes."

In general, corticosteroids are indicated at presentation as first-line therapy for ocular, cardiac, neurologic, renal disease, hypercalciuria, symptomatic stage II disease, and stage III pulmonary disease.[529–531] An approach to corticosteroid therapy in pulmonary disease is detailed in Table 14–15 and nonpulmonary disease in Table 14–16.

In most cases, a period of observation for 6 to 12 months while monitoring CXR, spirometry, and gas transfer is indicated to allow for spontaneous resolution. In our practice, progressive or unimproved disease is then treated as outlined in Table 14–15. Acute sarcoidosis is often so markedly corticosteroid-sensitive that the benefit is felt within 2 weeks of commencing treatment. A starting dose of 40 mg of prednisolone for 4 weeks is appropriate for most patients. Dosage may be tapered to 10 to 15 mg over 2 months, titrated to improvement in clinical state, CXR, and PFT. The aim is to achieve the lowest effective alternate-day dose possible. Treatment for acute disease is usually necessary for 12 to 18 months, although 6- to 12-month courses of therapy are occasionally effective. There is evidence that disease recurrence is less common if corticosteroid therapy is continued for at least 1 year.[525] Relapse of disease, as evoked by a recurrence of symptoms or the development of new pulmonary infiltrates, is common after stopping corticosteroids, with up to 36% of patients relapsing.[448,532,533] Relapses do not always occur immediately on withdrawal of corticosteroids, with 20% of relapses occurring more than 1 year after cessation of steroid treatment and 10% beyond 2 years.[419]

Alternate-day therapy is as effective as daily therapy and delivers the same weekly dose but may cause fewer corticosteroid-related side effects. Patient selection is important, as this strategy may hinder compliance.[534,535]

Corticosteroid therapy for extrathoracic disease is better defined and is indicated for all disease that impairs or threatens organ function. Doses are typically larger than in pulmonary disease and may be as high as 60 to

80 mg per day; medication is frequently taken for longer periods than in pulmonary disease. Features such as asymptomatic glandular involvement, minor elevation of LFTs, and chronic peripheral neuropathies may not require treatment or may not respond to therapy, and therefore corticosteroid therapy should be avoided. The decision to treat with long-term corticosteroids should be based on the anticipated therapeutic ratio, which may require an initial trial period followed by a concerted effort to achieve the minimum effective dose.

Topical corticosteroids for ocular involvement, intralesional corticosteroids for skin and laryngeal involvement,[536,537] and intravenous pulsed methyl prednisolone[538] have all found some usefulness in chronic disease and may replace the need for oral prednisolone in some patients.

Inhaled Corticosteroids

Given the bronchocentric nature of sarcoidosis, inhalation seems a logical route for corticosteroid delivery. It remains to be seen how effective this route will be in patients with the deformed airway architecture and fibrosis of more chronic sarcoidosis.

Spiteri and colleagues[539] reported clinical improvement in 10 patients treated with budesonide 800 μg nebulized twice daily. All enjoyed symptomatic improvement; 3 had significant radiologic clearing but without significant change in lung function. Hasani and colleagues[540] studied 13 patients with sarcoidosis treated with corticosteroids by various routes and found markedly impaired mucociliary clearance only in the group treated with inhaled corticosteroids, which was not seen in those treated with systemic corticosteroids,

possibly increasing the risk of superinfection in the inhaled treatment group. In a brief study that compared inhaled budesonide with placebo, Erkkila and colleagues[541] observed a significant decrease in SACE levels but no change in lung function or radiography in 19 patients with newly diagnosed sarcoidosis. In one open study,[542] 20 patients were treated with up to 1600 μg of budesonide daily for 3 to 6 months followed by a taper to 400 μg where clinically possible. Treatment continued for 18 months. Disease was assessed at 3- to 6-month intervals. Improvements in symptoms, radiographs, and forced vital capacity were observed, but these did not reach statistical significance. Although these results are encouraging and side effects were minimal (two patients developed hoarse voice), the interpretation of these findings is limited by the lack of a control group and the recruitment strategy that involved a run-in period of only 6 months. Even though progressive disease was noted during this period, it is also possible that spontaneous resolution could have followed.

TABLE 14–16   Treatment Strategies for Nonpulmonary Sarcoidosis

Clinical Features	First Line	Second Line
Fevers Night sweats Arthralgia Löfgren's syndrome	Observation and nonsteroidals	Steroids for severe or recalcitrant symptoms
Ocular	Ophthalmologic assessment	Systemic steroids Topical steroids Immunosuppression Topical cycloplegics
Upper respiratory tract	Nasal alkaline douche	Systemic steroids Topical steroids Hydroxychloroquine Methotrexate
Cardiac	Systemic steroids	Permanent pacemaker Antiarrhythmics Automatic implantable cardiac defibrillator Heart transplant
Skin	Systemic steroids	?CO$_2$ laser Hydroxychloroquine ? Isotretinoin Methotrexate ?Clofazimine ?Clobetasol
Liver and spleen	Systemic steroids	Immunosuppression
Neurosarcoidosis	Systemic steroids	Immunosuppression ? Radiotherapy ? Shunt
Hypercalcemia/ hypercalciuria	Low calcium diet	Ketoconazole Low vitamin D diet Hydroxychloroquine Avoid sunlight Systemic steroids
Renal	Systemic steroids	Immunosuppression Transplantation

? = consider use but not established treatment.

TABLE 14–15   Treatment Strategies for Pulmonary Sarcoidosis

Stage	Treatment
I	Corticosteroids are generally not indicated for stage I disease. NSAIDs are first-line therapy for fever and arthralgia although low-dose, short-course steroids are occasionally used for prominent respiratory symptoms.
II	Asymptomatic patients may be observed off treatment and treatment decision made on change or deterioration in PFT and CXR. Corticosteroids are indicated in symptomatic disease for control of symptoms and titrated to maintain response.
III	No treatment is required for asymptomatic patients with stable, good lung function. Corticosteroid treatment may be of value in control of alveolitis but clinically dependent on change in PFT/CXR parameters. Corticosteroids are indicated for symptomatic disease and are titrated to effect.
IV	Advanced fibrosis is unlikely to be affected by corticosteroid therapy; however, decision to treat must be based on the clinical likelihood of active alveolitis.

NSAIDs = nonsteroidal anti-inflammatory drugs; PFT = pulmonary function tests; CXR = chest radiography.

A double-blind, randomized, controlled trial of high-dose inhaled budesonide in newly diagnosed pulmonary sarcoidosis (within 6 months of diagnosis) demonstrated significant improvement in symptom scores and inspiratory vital capacity but in no other objective indices of lung function or ACE levels.[543] This confirmed a previous study by Milman and colleagues,[544] whose double-blind, placebo-controlled study showed no objective effect of high-dose inhaled corticosteroids in pulmonary sarcoidosis. Other studies have, however, suggested a role for dual therapy with both oral and inhaled corticosteroids. In a double-blind, placebo-controlled study looking at patients with newly diagnosed stage I and stage II pulmonary sarcoidosis, initial treatment with prednisolone followed by long-term inhaled budesonide is more effective than placebo in stage II disease. Study variables included chest radiographs, PFTs, and SACE. Treatment was not needed for stage I disease.[545]

Zych and colleagues,[546] in attempting to evaluate the role of inhaled corticosteroids in maintenance therapy, showed that after an initial 6 weeks of systemic prednisolone, budesonide 1600 μg daily was as effective as prednisolone 10 mg daily as a maintenance treatment for patients with stage II or III pulmonary sarcoidosis. A study by our own group[547] did not show an objective benefit in adding inhaled corticosteroid to patients whose disease is already stable. The previously cited Cochrane review, examined only two studies using inhaled budesonide and concluded that they may have a role in patients whose main symptom is cough.[528]

These studies have demonstrated that inhaled corticosteroids can influence immunopathogenic mechanisms in sarcoidosis but have not clarified their place in the disease. The most likely applications are for early disease, in which these agents may obviate the need for systemic corticosteroid therapy[548] or following reduction of the oral corticosteroid dose for maintenance therapy.[530] These and other indications await fuller evaluation.

Alternate Immunosuppressive Agents

Corticosteroids are clearly beneficial in the short term in sarcoidosis,[267,420–423,450,527,549] but their long-term efficacy has not been proven (see "Corticosteroids" above). These agents are associated with a variety of limiting adverse affects. A wide variety of agents have thus been assessed for their value as potential anti-inflammatory agents or as steroid-sparing agents.

Hydroxychloroquine

The antimalarial chloroquine is recognized as a first line agent in cutaneous sarcoidosis[291] has some suppressive effect on pulmonary disease,[550] and has an adjunctive benefit for the treatment of hypercalcemia.[77]

In 1964, Siltzbach and colleagues[551] demonstrated that 50% of patients with pulmonary or cutaneous sarcoidosis responded to the introduction of chloroquine. Morse and colleagues[552] showed improvement in cutaneous sarcoidosis in all of 7 patients treated with 500 mg of chloroquine daily by mouth, although 4 of these patients relapsed on cessation of the drug. Jones and Callen[553] confirmed these findings with hydroxychloroquine (2 to 3 mg/kg/day), showing regression of cutaneous lesions within 4 to 12 weeks of commencement in 12 out of 17 patients, all of whom were able to discontinue other therapies for their skin disease. Chloroquine in concert with antibiotic and oral corticosteroid therapy also appears beneficial in the treatment of unusual ulcerative cutaneous sarcoidosis. The British Tuberculosis Association[550] had earlier reported the predictability of recurrence on cessation of chloroquine, a feature associated with short-course therapy.

Chloroquine and ketoconazole are effective inhibitors of the pulmonary macrophage-induced hydroxylation of vitamin D precursors, and are thus of some value in the treatment of hypercalcemia.[369,554] Both chloroquine and hydroxychloroquine may have a role in controlling neurologic sarcoidosis in those patients who fail to respond to steroids or in whom their use is limited by adverse events.[555]

The role of chloroquine in pulmonary sarcoidosis has recently been highlighted. In an open, randomized trial, 23 symptomatic patients with biopsy-proven pulmonary sarcoidosis were initially treated for 6 months with chloroquine (750 mg/day). Eighteen patients were then randomized to either maintenance treatment (chloroquine 250mg/day) or to an observation group. Patients who received the maintenance group showed a slower decline in pulmonary function and were less likely to have subsequent relapses.[556] However, it remains unknown whether the antimalarials are more effective than oral corticosteroids, and further studies are required to answer this question.

Patients started on antimalarials require regular ophthalmic assessment, as long-term use may be associated with retinopathy and blindness. Hydroxychloroquine, compared with chloroquine, is less likely to be associated with ocular toxicity, but due to its effect on insulin degradation, may worsen glycemic control if used in diabetics.

Methotrexate

The antimetabolite folate antagonist methotrexate has been used for both pulmonary and extrathoracic disease with both corticosteroid-sparing and primary immunosuppressive intent. It appears thus far to be the most promising alternative to corticosteroids in the treatment of sarcoidosis.

In a small series of 15 cases, Lower and Baughman[557] observed an improvement in lung function

(< 15% increase in forced vital capacity), skin infiltration (50% reduction), and LFTs when treated with low-dose methotrexate. Disease recurrence on the cessation of treatment was seen in five cases, all of whom responded to reinstitution of the drug. In a later study, Lower and Baughman[558] observed the effects of low-dose treatment (10 mg orally per week) over 2 years in 50 patients. More than 60% experienced objective improvement, and 25 out of 30 enjoyed some corticosteroid sparing effect, with 5 patients ceasing steroids after 6 months and 13 after 2 years. A single patient was hospitalized with neutropenia, while other toxicities included mouth sores, nausea, and deranged LFTs. Liver biopsy was performed 41 times in 33 patients and revealed methotrexate-induced changes in 15% of biopsies. No further liver abnormalities were found after discontinuation of the methotrexate. In total, methotrexate was discontinued in 16% of cases due to toxicity (elevated LFTs 6, cough 1, neutropenia 1) with no apparent long-term sequelae.

The same group assessed the role of methotrexate as a steroid-sparing agent during the initial period of treatment of sarcoidosis. Patients (n = 24) with new onset, symptomatic disease were treated with prednisolone according to a standardized regimen, and randomized to receive either methotrexate or placebo for the following year. Although the study was hampered as a result of a large number of dropouts (n = 9), the results demonstrated that patients in the active arm received less prednisolone, suggesting a corticosteroid-sparing role for methotrexate.[559]

Baughman and Lower have recently reviewed their collective experience with methotrexate in patients with chronic sarcoidosis.[560] In their experience, patients should remain on methotrexate for at least 6 months, as the drug effects are often not immediate, and objective improvement can occur until and beyond 6 months. Hypersensitivity pneumonitis can occur in up to 5% of patients treated with methotexate[561]; thus, in patients on methotrexate who develop new pulmonary infiltrates or deteriorating lung function it can be difficult to differentiate between the development of a new hypersensitivity pneumonitis from reactivation of the underlying pulmonary sarcoidosis. The development of hepatotoxicity is the main adverse event associated with long-term use of methotrexate. Guidelines have been established to guide treatment.[562] Liver function tests should be performed prior to starting treatment, and repeated thereafter at 4 to 6 week intervals.

Methotrexate has induced some regression of disfiguring skin lesions when used in treatment of resistant lupus pernio and cutaneous sarcoidosis.[563,564]

A steroid-sparing effect in a small pediatric population has also been observed,[565] with no recorded adverse effects during short-course therapy. Long-term treatment safety is not known. Unfortunately, there is still a dearth of placebo-controlled trials. Thus, long-term and steroid-sparing effects cannot be adequately interpreted given the high spontaneous remission/improvement rate.

Musculoskeletal disease, often viewed as steroid resistant, has been shown by Kaye and colleagues[566] to demonstrate a significant improvement in symptomatology and a 59% reduction in the corticosteroid dose when treated with low-dose (10 mg/week) methotrexate. These benefits appeared to accrue from 8 to 12 weeks and were maintained through 3 years of follow-up.

Methotrexate appears to offer an acceptable alternative to corticosteroids for advanced pulmonary and cutaneous disease. This treatment is not without toxicity and requires regular surveillance of hematologic indices and liver function.

Azathioprine

There is little published data on the use of this agent in sarcoidosis.[567–569] The role of azathioprine as a steroid-sparing agent has been explored by Muller-Quernheim and colleagues[570] who showed in an open study that patients with chronic sarcoidosis could be controlled with a regimen of low-dose prednisolone (0.1 mg/kg) and azathioprine (2 mg/kg) daily.

Elsewhere, azathioprine has been used effectively, albeit in very small numbers of patients, for the treatment of neurosarcoidosis resistant to steroids and in pediatric sarcoidosis.[340] Further studies are required to support optimistic anecdotal results.

Chlorambucil

Chlorambucil is an alkylating cytotoxic agent, widely used in the treatment of chronic lymphocytic leukemia and non-Hodgkin's lymphoma. These agents inhibit DNA synthesis by forming covalent bonds with nucleic acids and by modulating antigen processing.[571] Although recognized as an immunosuppressive agent, its mechanism of action in sarcoidosis is unclear.

Israel and McComb[572] examined the effect of chlorambucil in 31 patients with biopsy-proven sarcoidosis in whom corticosteroids had either failed to control the disease or had caused intolerable side effects. The oral dose was 8 mg daily reduced to 4 mg in those with thrombocytopenia or leukopenia and continued for 3 to 58 months. Six-month courses were repeated in 11 patients, and 1 patient received 3 courses.

Marked symptomatic and objective improvement was seen in 15 cases, and moderate improvement was seen in a further 13 although the objective improvement has not been detailed. Two cases showed no response at all. A high relapse rate on discontinuation of chlorambucil was similar to that noted with corticosteroids. Disease appeared responsive to recommencing treatment.

Kataria[573] reported an anecdotal study of 10 patients with proven corticosteroid-unresponsive disease or marked corticosteroid toxicity. Using daily oral doses between 4 to 12 mg, 8 patients experienced some clinical improvement, 2 with complete remission, and 5 with improvement in their PFTs. In those who improved, improvement occurred within 2 to 3 months of commencing therapy.

Covalent alkylation is mutagenic; however, the long-term effects of this agent on gonadal function is of concern, as are its teratogenesis and the appearance of secondary leukemias. Myelosuppression is the most common toxicity and leads to thrombocytopenia and leukopenia. Long-term experience is required to define the role of chlorambucil as an alternative immunosuppressive agent in sarcoidosis. At present it is not recommended.

Cyclosporin A

Theoretically cyclosporin A remains an attractive agent for use in sarcoidosis due to its potent IL-2 inhibition, suppression of T-lymphocyte proliferation, and reduction of monocyte chemotactic factor expression.[574] Despite apparent in vitro benefit, this did not confer a clear clinical benefit for 8 patients with uncomplicated pulmonary disease. In a larger cohort, 37 patients were randomized in an open-label study to receive either prednisolone alone or prednisolone in combination with cyclosporin A for a total period of 18 months. The use of cyclosporin A did not confer an additional benefit, given that the combination group was characterized by an increase in the number of relapses, infections, and adverse events.[575]

Pia and colleagues[576] observed a complete and lasting remission in 11 patients treated with a combination of methotrexate, cyclosporin, and flucortolone, but the relative role of each agent cannot be determined. Other studies have suggested some benefit in intractable neurosarcoidosis.[577,578]

Ketoconazole

Ketoconazole, the imidazole-derivative antifungal, has significant activity in inhibition of the cytochrome P-450 complex and may inhibit synthesis of 1,25-dihydroxyvitamin D_3 and other steroid hormones in patients with sarcoidosis with both normal and elevated calcium levels.

Adams and colleagues[579] have demonstrated that ketoconazole effectively suppresses the synthesis of vitamin D both in vitro and in vivo and is associated with a rapid decrease in serum calcium levels, purportedly due to the suppression of alveolar macrophage 1α-hydroxylase activity. Ketoconazole has subsequently been shown to be very effective in the treatment of hypercalcemia in oral doses of 600 to 800 mg per day.[579–581] Caveats to the use of ketoconazole include a delayed onset of action of up to 2 days making it inappropriate for the acute control of hypercalcemia, the possibility of significant renal toxicity, and the consequences of generalized inhibition of steroid hormone synthesis with reports of decreased libido secondary to low testosterone.

TNF-α Blockade

New insights clarifying cellular interactions and the role of cytokines in the development of granulomas, have led to speculation that the next generation of drugs will target individual cytokines vital to the granulomatous immune response. Much attention has concentrated on the proinflammatory cytokine, TNF-α. Recently, Zabel and colleagues,[582] postulating a prominent role for TNF-α in granuloma development in sarcoidosis, noted that TNF-α and Th_1 cytokine activity could be more specifically inhibited both in vivo and in vitro with the phosphodiesterase inhibitor, pentoxifylline. A small study of 23 patients with predominantly pulmonary disease demonstrated to be progressive were treated with oral pentoxifylline. None of the patients deteriorated, 11 improved, and 7 remained stable in terms of symptom score, radiology, and PFTs. Three were unable to complete the study due to gastrointestinal side effects. In 3 patients with corticosteroid-dependent disease, the addition of pentoxifylline to the treatment regimen led to rapid and complete regression, suggesting some synergy between the two drugs.

The mechanism of action of pentoxifylline relates to its ability to inhibit the lipopolysaccharide-induced TNF-α production from both peripheral blood monocytes and alveolar macrophages and secondly by also inhibiting the spontaneous TNF-α production of alveolar macrophages.[583] Its importance as a possible target for imunomodulation is further supported by studies exploring the clinical efficacy of the drugs, infliximab and etanercept. Infliximab is a human-mouse chimeric monoclonal antibody that specifically inhibits TNF-α, whereas etanercept is a fusion protein made up of two recombinant p75 TNF receptors fused with the Fc portion of the human IgG_1. In a study limited to 3 patients, 2 with lupus pernio and 1 with restrictive lung disease, all 3 had clinical improvement when started on infliximab, having previously failed to respond to treatment with steroids and immunosuppressive agents.[584] Both drugs, having already been shown to be clinically efficacious in patients with rheumatoid arthritis[585] need to be the subject of further clinical trials in patients with sarcoidosis.

The results of this study offer some hope in the development of more selective agents for the blockade of cytokine-induced inflammation.

Transplantation

Organ transplantation is now a widely available modality for single organ failure but is of limited value in multisystem disorders such as sarcoidosis with multiorgan involvement. Sarcoidosis with a single organ predilection has, however, proved amenable to transplantation.

Yeatman and colleagues[332] reviewed 11 patients with sarcoidosis with end-stage pulmonary fibrosis undergoing heart-lung (5) or lung (6) transplantation. All patients experienced excellent functional recovery. Graft granulomata recurred in 2 of these patients and although 5 deaths were recorded among this group, none were thought to have clinically significant pulmonary sarcoidosis at the time of death.

Johnson and colleagues[586] showed a similar rate of recurrence and observed an increase in the mean grade of rejection during the first 3 months post-transplantation compared with other patients. Similar levels of obliterative bronchiolitis, survival, and pulmonary function were noted. Long-term outcome remains to be elucidated. Conversely, a patient inadvertently transplanted with a sarcoid-affected donor lung showed no histologic, radiologic, or clinical evidence of disease recurrence after 6 months of follow-up.[587]

Cardiac transplantation has been performed for intractable arrhythmia and progressive cardiomyopathy with congestive cardiac failure with some success.[330] Graft granulomata recurrence has been observed with therapeutic response to augmented corticosteroid treatment.[588]

Renal replacement therapy by transplantation is now described for sarcoid-induced granulomatous nephritis and glomerulonephritis.[589–591] Again, graft granulomata recurrence is well recognized and may be treated by augmenting steroid therapy.[592]

Pescovitz and colleagues[593] observed massive retroperitoneal adenopathy in a patient with sarcoidosis 1 year following orthotopic liver transplantation for primary sclerosing cholangitis. In common with other organs transplants, this patient was adequately immunosuppressed under standard transplant protocols, with CD4 suppression suggesting therapeutic effect. Disease recurrence thus occurs independently of transplant immunosuppression but frequently responds to increased corticosteroid treatment.

Radiotherapy

Although radiotherapy has previously been used for various manifestations of sarcoidosis, there is no evidence that it has any beneficial effect. Recently, there have been reports of possible benefit from radiotherapy in the treatment of CNS sarcoidosis, and it is possible that a trial of low-dose radiotherapy to the whole brain or spinal cord may be justified when all conventional measures have failed.

MANAGEMENT STRATEGIES: A SUMMARY

Treatment Algorithm

A summary of the authors' approaches to treatment for the various manifestations of sarcoidosis is shown in Tables 14–15 and 14–16. Fuller reviews are published elsewhere.[1,414,531,594]

Löfgren's Syndrome

This almost always resolves without treatment. Nonsteroidal anti-inflammatory drugs (NSAIDs) may be used for symptomatic relief, which generally occurs over about 3 months, with radiographic resolution generally complete at 9 to 12 months.

Ocular Involvement

Ophthalmologic opinion is crucial if there are any ocular symptoms or if chloroquine therapy is being considered. Routine screening of all patients should be performed. Topical treatment for anterior uveitis is usually all that is needed, but posterior or recalcitrant anterior disease may require oral corticosteroids or immunosuppression.

Bilateral Hilar and/or Paratracheal Lymphadenopathy Alone

This requires no treatment, and the majority resolve spontaneously, but a positive diagnosis should be sought. In a small percentage (< 10%) of patients, the adenopathy is persistent and only rarely gives rise to superior vena cava or bronchial obstruction.

Pulmonary Infiltration

For asymptomatic patients with lung function at least 80% predicted, we give the patients 1 year for spontaneous clearing to occur while carefully monitoring progress. If there has been no improvement at the end of 1 year or if deterioration has occurred during that year, we opt for a trial of oral corticosteroids.

Skin

Corticosteroids or methotrexate (up to 10 to 15 mg/week) or hydroxychloroquine (200 mg/day) are the mainstays of treatment.

Cardiac Involvement

Arrhythmias and cardiac failure are treated as for all other causes. A trial of systemic corticosteroids is justified.

Liver/Gastrointestinal Involvement

Disease is often asymptomatic. Symptomatic disease should be treated with corticosteroids as first-line therapy. Relapse may occur on corticosteroid withdrawal and can be troublesome. Rarely, a grossly enlarged spleen may produce discomfort and hypersplenism; splenectomy may be required.

Hypercalcemia

Initial treatment should be dietary. Uncontrolled hypercalcemia or isolated hypercalciuria may require corticosteroids or second-line agents if steroid reduction causes a relapse.

Neurosarcoidosis

Severe neurosarcoidosis is often refractory to treatment and may require prolonged courses of high-dose oral ± intravenous corticosteroids. Immunosuppression may be necessary if corticosteroid control is suboptimal. Hydrocephalus may require neurosurgical evaluation. Convulsive disorders are treated in the usual manner with due consideration for steroid/anticonvulsant drug interactions.

CONCLUSION

Although many patients experience spontaneous resolution of their disease, a substantial minority require regular ongoing monitoring of both disease and treatment to limit morbidity and mortality. Referral to specialist centers facilitates the creation of management plans for the cooperative care of patients in the community.

REFERENCES

1. Mitchell DN, Scadding JG. Sarcoidosis. Am Rev Respir Dis 1974;110:774–802.
2. Crystal RG, Bitterman PB, Rennard ST, et al. Interstitial lung diseases of unknown cause: disorders characterized by chronic inflammation of the lower respiratory tract. N Engl J Med 1984;310:154–65, 235–44.
3. Thomas PD, Hunninghake GW. Current concepts of the pathogenesis of sarcoidosis. Am Rev Respir Dis 1987;135:747–60.
4. Hutchinson J. Case of livid papillary psoriasis. In: Illustrations of clinical surgery. Vol 1. London: J&A Churchill; 1877. p. 42–3.
5. Statement on Sarcoidosis. Joint statement of the American Thoracic Society (ATS), the European Respiratory Society (ERS) and the World Association of Sarcoidosis and other Granulomatous Disorders (WASOG) adopted by the ATS Board of Directors and by the ERS Executive Committee, February 1999. Am J Respir Crit Care Med 1999;160:736–55.
6. Hutchinson J. On eruptions which occur in connection with gout: case of Mortimer's malady. Arch Surg 1898;9:307–14.
7. Besnier M. Lupus pernio de la face: synovites fungueses (scofula-tuberculeuses) symetriques des extremities superieures. Ann Dermatol Syphiligr 1889;10:333–6.
8. Tenneson M. Lupus pernio (lupus pernio). Bull Soc Fr Dermatol Syphiligr 1892;3:417–9.
9. Boeck C. Multiple benign sarkoid of the skin. J Cutan Genitourinary Dis 1899;17:543–50.
10. Boeck C. Forgesetzle untersuchugen uber des multiple benigne sarkoid [abstract]. Arch Dermatol Syph Wien 1905;73:301–32.
11. Kreibich K. Ueber lupus pernio. Arch Dermatol Syph (Wien) 1904;71:13–6.
12. Heerfordt C. Uber eine Febris uveo-partidea subchronica. Von Graefe's Arch Ophthalmol 1909;70:254–73.
13. Jungling O. Ostitis tuberculosa multiplex cystica. Fortschr Geb Roentgenstr 1920;27:375–83.
14. Schaumann J. Etude anatomo pathologique et histologique sur les localisations viscerales de la lymphogranulomatose benigne. Bull Soc Fr Dermatol Syphiligr 1934;1167–322.
15. Löfgren S. Erythema nodosum: studies on etiology and pathogenesis in 185 adult cases. Acta Med Scand 1946;124:1–197.
16. Kveim A. En ny og spesifikk kutan-reaksjon ved Boecks sarcoid. Nord Med 1941;9:169–72.
17. Stitzbach L. The Kveim test in sarcoidosis: a study of 750 patients. JAMA 1961;178:476–82.
18. Boros DL. Imunoregulation of granuloma formation in murine schistosomiasis mansoni. Ann N Y Acad Sci 1986;465:313–23.
19. Colley DG. Immune responses and immunoregulation in experimental and clinical schistosomiasis. In: Mansfield JM, ed. Parasitic diseases. 1. The immunology. New York: Marcel Dekker; 1985. p. 1–83.
20. Lima MS, Gazzinelli G, Nascimento E, et al. Immune responses during human schistosomiasis mansoni. Evidence for antiidiotypic T lymphocyte responsiveness. J Clin Invest 1988;78:983.
21. Narayanan RB. Immunopathology of leprosy granulomas current status: a review. Lepr Rev 1988;59:75–82.
22. Kaplan G, Laal S, Sheftel G. The nature and kinetics of a delayed immune response to purified protein derivative of tuberculin in the skin of lepromatous leprosy patients. J Exp Med 1988;168:1811–24.
23. Boros DL. Experimental granulomatosis. Clin Dermatol 1986;4:10–21.
24. Cummings MM, Hudgins PC. Chemical constituents of pine pollens and their possible relationship to sarcoidosis. Am J Med Sci 1958;236:311–7.
25. Cummings MM. An evaluation of the possible relationship of pine pollen to sarcoidosis. Acta Med Scand Suppl 1964;425:48–50.
26. Buck AA, Sartwell PE. Epidemiologic investigations of sarcoidosis. I. Introduction; materials and methods [abstract]. Am J Hygiene 1961;74:152–73.
27. Farber HW, Fairman RP, Glauser FL. Talc granulomatosis: laboratory findings similar to sarcoidosis. Am Rev Respir Dis 1982;125:258–61.
28. Williams WJ. Beryllium disease—pathology and diagnosis. Soc Occup Med 1977;27:93–6.
29. Shelley WB, Hurley HL. The allergic origin of zirconium deodorant granulomas. Br J Dermatol 1958;70:75–101.
30. Heyll A, Meckenstock G, Aul C, et al. Possible transmission of sarcoidosis via allogeneic bone marrow transplantation. Bone Marrow Transplant 1994;14:161–4.
31. Burke WM, Keogh A, Maloney PJ, et al. Transmission of sarcoidosis via cardiac transplantation. Lancet 1997;336:1579.
32. Löfgren S, Lundback H. Isolation of virus from 6 cases of sarcoidosis: a preliminary report. Acta Med Scand 1950;138:71–5.
33. Sodja J, Votava L. Isolation of haemabsorptive virus from cases of sarcoidosis. Acta Virol 1966;10:81–4.
34. Fillet AM, Raguin G, Agut H, et al. Evidence of human herpesvirus 6 in Sjögren syndrome and sarcoidosis. Eur J Clin Microbiol Infect Dis 1992;11:564–6.

35. James DG, Neville E. Pathobiology of sarcoidosis. Pathobiol Ann 1977;7:31–61.

36. Manz HJ. Pathobiology of neurosarcoidosis and clinico-pathologic correlation. Can J Neurol Sci 1983;10:50–5.

37. Lipsky BA, Goldberger AC, Tompkins LS, Plorde JJ. Infections caused by nondiphtheria corynebacteria. Rev Infect Dis 1982;4:1220–35.

38. Fick RB, Reynolds HY. *Pseudomonas* respiratory infection in cystic fibrosis: a possible defect in opsonic IgG antibody? Bull Eur Physiopathol Respir 1983;19:151–61.

39. Wirostko E, Johnson L, Wirostko B. Sarcoidosis associated uveitis. Parasitization of vitreous leucocytes by mollicute-like organisms. Acta Ophthalmol 1989;67:415–24.

40. Wirostko E, Johnson LA, Wirostko WJ. Mouse interstitial lung disease and pleuritis induction by human mollicute-like organisms. Br J Exp Pathol 1988;69:891–902.

41. Johnson LA, Edsall JR, Austin JH, Ellis K. Pulmonary sarcoidosis: could mycoplasma-like organisms be a cause? Sarcoidosis Vasc Diffuse Lung Dis 1996;13:38–42.

42. Kent DC, Houk VN, Slliot RC, et al. The definitive evaluation of sarcoidosis. Am Rev Respir Dis 1970;101:721–7.

43. Mitchell DN, Rees RJW, Rees RJ. A transmissable agent from sarcoid tissue. Lancet 1969;ii:81–4.

44. Mitchell DN, Rees RJ. An attempt to demonstrate a transmissible agent from sarcoid material. Postgrad Med J 1970;46:510–4.

45. Mitchell DN, Rees RJ, Goswami KK. Transmissible agents from human sarcoid and Crohn's disease tissues. Lancet 1976;ii:761–5.

46. Almenoff PL, Johnson A, Lesser M, Mattman LH. Growth of acid fast L forms from the blood of patients with sarcoidosis. Thorax 1996;51:530–3.

47. Milman N, Anderson AB. Detection of antibodies in serum against *M. tuberculosis* using Western blot technique: comparison between sarcoidosis patients and healthy subjects. Sarcoidosis 1993;10:29–31.

48. Chapman JS, Speight M. Further studies of mycobacterial antibodies in the sera of sarcoidosis patients. Acta Med Scand Suppl 1964;425:61–7.

49. Fidler HM, Rook GA, Johnson NM, McFadden J. *Mycobacterium tuberculosis* DNA in tissue affected by sarcoidosis. BMJ 1993;306:546–9.

50. Bocart D, Lecossier D, De Lassence A, et al. A search for mycobacterial DNA in granulomatous tissues from patients with sarcoidosis using the polymerase chain reaction. Am Rev Respir Dis 1992;145:1142–8.

51. Mangiapan G, Hance AJ. Mycobacteria and sarcoidosis: an overview and summary of recent molecular biological data. Sarcoidosis 1995;12:20–37.

52. McGregor I. The two year mass radiography campaign in Scotland 1957–1958 [abstract]. Edinburgh: HMSO, 1961.

53. Anderson R, Brett GZ, James DG, Siltzbach LE. The prevalence of intrathoracic sarcoidosis [abstract]. Med Thorac 1963;20:152.

54. Milman N, Selroos O. Pulmonary sarcoidosis in the Nordic countries 1950–1982. Epidemiology and clinical picture. Sarcoidosis 1990;7:50–7.

55. Bauer HJ, Löfgren S. International study of pulmonary sarcoidosis in mass chest radiography [abstract]. Acta Med Scand 1964;176:103–5.

56. Riddervold L. Sarcoidosis in Norway [abstract]. Acta Med Scand 1964;176:111.

57. Fog J, Wilbek E. The epidemiology of sarcoidosis in Denmark [Danish]. Ugeskr Laeger 1974;136:2183–91.

58. Wallgren S. Pulmonary sarcoidosis detected by photofluorographic surveys in Sweden 1950–1957 [abstract]. Nord Med 1958;60:1194–5.

59. Sutherland I, Mitchell DN, D'Arcy Hart P. Incidence of intrathoracic sarcoidosis among young adults participating in a trial of tuberculosis vaccines [abstract]. BMJ 1965;2:497–503.

60. Sartwell PE, Edwards LB. Epidemiology of sarcoidosis in the U.S. Navy. Am J Epidemiol 1974;99:250–7.

61. Hiraga Y, Hosoda Y, Odaka M. Epidemiology of sarcoidosis in a Japanese working group—a ten year study. In: Iwai K, Hosoda Y, editors. Proceedings of the 6th International Conference on Sarcoidosis, Tokyo, Japan. 1974;303–6.

62. Parkes SA, Baker SB, Bourdillon RE, et al. Incidence of sarcoidosis in the Isle of Man. Thorax 1985;40:284–7.

63. Anonymous. Geographical variations in the incidence of sarcoidosis in Great Britain: a comparative study of four areas. A report to the Research Committee of the British Thoracic and Tuberculosis Association. Tubercle 1969;50:211–32.

64. Henke CE, Henke G, Elveback LR, et al. The epidemiology of sarcoidosis in Rochester, Minnesota: a population-based study of incidence and survival. Am J Epidemiol 1986;123:840–5.

65. Hillerdal G, Nou E, Osterman K, Schmekel B. Sarcoidosis: epidemiology and prognosis. A 15-year European study. Am Rev Respir Dis 1984;130:29–32.

66. Rybicki BA, Major M, Popovich Jr J, et al. Racial differences in sarcoidosis incidence: a 5-year study in a health maintenance organization. Am J Epidemiol 1997;145:234–41.

67. Yamaguchi M, Hosoda Y, Sasaki R, Aoki K. Epidemiological study on sarcoidosis in Japan. Recent trends in incidence and prevalence rates and changes in epidemiological features. Sarcoidosis 1989;6:138–46.

68. Hosoda Y, Hiraga Y, Odaka M, et al. A cooperative study of sarcoidosis in Asia and Africa: analytic epidemiology. Ann N Y Acad Sci 1976;278:355–67.

69. Young RC Jr, Hackney RL Jr, Harden KA. Epidemiology of sarcoidosis: ethnic and geographic considerations. J Natl Med Assoc 1974;66:386–8.

70. Edmondstone WM, Wilson AG. Sarcoidosis in Caucasians, Blacks and Asians in London. Br J Dis Chest 1985;79:27–36.

71. Benatar SR. Sarcoidosis in South Africa. A comparative study in Whites, Blacks and Coloureds. S Afr Med J 1977;52:602–6.

72. Israel HL, Washbourne JD. Characteristics of sarcoidosis in black and white patients. In: Jones Williams W, Davies BH, editors. Proceedings of the 8th International Conference on Sarcoidosis. Cardiff: Alpha Omega; 1978:497–507.

73. Pietinalho A, Ohmichi M, Hiraga Y, et al. The mode of presentation of sarcoidosis in Finland and Hokkaido, Japan: a comparative analysis of 571 Finnish and 668 Japanese patients. Sarcoidosis Vasc Diffuse Lung Dis 1996;13:159–66.

74. Iwai K, Sekiguti M, Hosoda R, et al. Racial difference in cardiac sarcoidosis incidence observed at autopsy. Sarcoidosis 1994;11:26–31.

75. Gideon NM, Mannino DM. Sarcoidosis mortality in the United States 1979–1991: an analysis of multiple-cause mortality data. Am J Med 1996;100:423–7.

76. Bresnitz EA, Strom BL. Epidemiology of sarcoidosis. Epidemiol Rev 1983;5:124–56.

77. Hennessy TW, Ballard DJ, DeRemee RA, et al. The influence of diagnostic access bias on the epidemiology of sarcoidosis: a population-based study in Rochester, Minnesota, 1935–1984. J Clin Epidemiol 1988;41:565–70.

78. Hills SE, Parkes SA, de C Backer SB. Epidemiology of sarcoidosis in the Isle of Man—2: evidence for space-time clustering [abstract]. Thorax 1987;42:427–30.

79. Pike MC, Smith PG. Case-control approach to examine diseases for evidence of contagion, including diseases with long latent periods. Biometrics 1974;30:263–79.

80. Stewart IC, Davidson NM. Clustering of sarcoidosis. Thorax 1982;37:398–9.

81. Brennan NJ, Crean P, Long JP, FitzGerald MX. High prevalence of familial sarcoidosis in an Irish population. Thorax 1984;39:14–8.

82. Headings VE, Weston D, Young RC Jr, Hackney RL Jr. Familial sarcoidosis with multiple occurrences in eleven families: a possible mechanism of inheritance. Ann N Y Acad Sci 1976;278:377–85.

83. James DG, Neville E, Piyasena KH, et al. Possible genetic influences in familial sarcoidosis. Postgrad Med J 1974;50:664–70.

84. Sharma OP, Neville E, Walker AN, James DG. Familial sarcoidosis: a possible genetic influence. Ann N Y Acad Sci 1976;278:386–400.

85. McGrath DS, Daniil Z, Foley P, et al. Epidemiology of familial sarcoidosis in the UK. Thorax 2000;55:751–4.

86. Schurmann M, Lympany PA, Reichel P, et al. Familial sarcoidosis is linked to the major histocompatibility complex region. Am J Respir Crit Care Med 2000;162:861–4.

87. Panayeas S, Theodorakopoulos P, Bouras A, Constantopoulos S. Seasonal occurrence of sarcoidosis in Greece. Lancet 1991;338:510–1.

88. Bardinas F, Morera J, Fite E, Plasencia A. Seasonal clustering of sarcoidosis. Lancet 1989;ii:455–6.

89. Jawad ASM, Hamour AA, Wesley WG, Scott DGI. An outbreak of acute sarcoidosis with arthropathy in Norfolk. Br J Rheumatol 1989;28:178.

90. Bresnitz EA, Stolley PD, Israel HL, Soper K. Possible risk factors for sarcoidosis. A case-control study. Ann N Y Acad Sci 1986;465:632–42.

91. Douglas JG, Middleton WG, Gaddie J, et al. Sarcoidosis: a disorder commoner in non-smokers? Thorax 1986;41:787–91.

92. Arima K, Ando M, Ito K, et al. Effect of cigarette smoking on prevalence of summer-type hypersensitivity pneumonitis caused by *Trichosporon cutaneum*. Arch Environ Health 1992;47:274–8.

93. Cummings MM, Dunner E, Williams JH. Epidemiologic and clinical observations in sarcoidosis [abstract]. Ann Intern Med 1959;50:879–90.

94. Kern DG, Neill MA, Wren DS, Varoone JC. Investigation of a unique time-space cluster of sarcoidosis in firefighters. Am Rev Respir Dis 1993;148:974–88.

95. Prezant DJ, Dhala A, Goldstein A, et al. The incidence, prevalence, and severity of sarcoidosis in New York City firefighters. Chest 1999;116:1183–93.

96. Kajdasz DK, Lackland DT, Mohr LC, Judson MA. A current assessment of rurally linked exposures as potential risk factors for sarcoidosis. Ann Epidemiol 2001;11:111–7.

97. Edmondstone WM. Sarcoidosis in nurses: is there an association? Thorax 1988;43:342–3.

98. Berlin MA, Fogdell-Hahn MA, Olerup O, et al. HLA-DR predicts the prognosis in Scandinavian patients with pulmonary sarcoidosis. Am J Respir Crit Care Med 1997;156:1601–5.

99. Neville E, James DG, Brewerton DA, et al. HLA antigens and clinical features of sarcoidosis. In: Jones Williams W, Davies BH, editors. Sarcoidosis. Cardiff: Alpha and Omega Press; 1980. p. 201–5.

100. Smith MJ, Turton CWG, Mitchell DN, et al. Association of HLA-B8 with spontaneous resolution in sarcoidosis. Thorax 1987;36:296–8.

101. Ina Y, Takada K, Yamamoto M, et al. HLA and sarcoidosis in the Japanese. Chest 1989;95:1257–61.

102. Kunikane H, Abe S, Tsuneta Ye. Role of HLA-DR antigens in Japanese patients with sarcoidosis. Am Rev Respir Dis 1987;135:688–91.

103. Martinetti M, Tinelli C, Kolek V, et al. "The sarcoidosis map:" a joint survey of clinical and immunogenetic findings in two European countries. Am J Respir Crit Care Med 1995;152:557–64.

104. Foley PJ, McGrath DS, Puscinska E, et al. Human leukocyte antigen-DRB1 position 11 residues are acommon protective marker for sarcoidosis. Am J Respir Cell Mol Biol 2001;25:272–7.

105. Ishihara M, Ishida T, Mizuki N, et al. Clinical features of sarcoidosis in relation to HLA distribution and HLA-DRB3 genotyping by PCR-RFLP. Br J Ophthalmol 1995;79:322–5.

106. Naruse TK, Matsuzawa Y, Ota M, et al. HLA-DQB1*0601 is primarily associated with the susceptibility to cardiac sarcoidosis. Tissue Antigens 2000;56:52–7.

107. Richeldi L, Sorrentino R, Saltini C. HLA-DPB1 glutamate 69: a genetic marker of beryllium disease. Science 1993;262:242–4.

108. Lympany PA, Petrek M, Southcott AM, et al. HLA-DPB polymorphisms: Glu 69 association with sarcoidosis. Eur J Immunogenet 1996;23:353–9.

109. Papadopoulos KI, Melander O, Orho-Melander M, et al. Angiotensin converting enzyme (ACE) gene polymorphism in sarcoidosis in relation to associated autoimmune diseases. J Intern Med 2000;247:71–7.

110. Niimi T, Tomita H, Sato S, et al. Bronchial responsiveness and angiotensin-converting enzyme gene polymorphism in sarcoidosis patients. Chest 1998;114:495–9.

111. Maliarik MJ, Rybicki BA, Malvitz E, et al. Angiotensin-converting enzyme gene polymorphism and risk of sarcoidosis. Am J Respir Crit Care Med 1998;158:1566–70.

112. McGrath, DS, Foley PJ, Petrek M, et al. ACE gene I/D polymorphism and sarcoidosis pulmonary disease severity. Am J Respir Crit Care Med 2001;164:197–201.

113. Somoskovi A, Zissel G, Seitzer U, et al. Polymorphisms at position –308 in the promoter region of the TNF-α and in the first intron of the TNF-β genes and spontaneous and lipopolysaccharide-induced TNF-alpha release in sarcoidosis. Cytokine 1999;11:882–7.

114. Yamaguchi E, Itoh A, Hizawa N, Kawakami Y. The gene polymorphism of tumour necrosis factor-beta, but not that of tumour necrosis factor-alpha, is associated with the prognosis of sarcoidosis. Chest 2001;119:678–9.

115. Seitzer U, Swider C, Stuber F, et al. Tumour necrosis factor alpha promoter gene polymorphism in sarcoidosis. Cytokine 1997;9:787–90.

116. Takashige N, Naruse TK, Matsumri A, et al. Genetic polymorphisms at the tumour necrosis factor loci (TNFA and TNFB) in cardiac sarcoidosis. Tissue Antigens 1999;54:191–3.

117. Petrek M, Drabek J, Kolek V, et al. CC chemokine receptor gene polymorphisms in Czech patients with pulmonary sarcoidosis. Am J Respir Crit Care Med 2000;162:1000–3.

118. Foley PJ, Lympany PA, Puscinska E, et al. Analysis of MHC encoded antigen-processing genes *TAP1* and *TAP"* polymorphisms in sarcoidosis. Am J Respir Crit Care Med 1999;160:1009–14.

119. Rybicki BA, Maliarik MJ, Malvitz E, et al. The influence of T cell receptor and cytokine genes on sarcoidosis susceptibility in African Americans. Hum Immunol 1999;60:867–74.

120. Dannenberg AMJ. Macrophages in inflammation and infection. N Engl J Med 1975;293:489–93.

121. Berzofsky JA. Structural basis of antigen recognition by T-lymphocytes. Implications for vaccines. J Clin Invest 1988;82:1811–7.

122. Paul WE. The immune system: an introduction. In: Paul WE, editor. Fundamental immunology. New York: Raven Press; 1989. p. 3–19.

123. Mackaness GB. The mechanisms of macrophage activation. In: Mudd S, editor. Infectious agents and host reactions. Philadelphia: W.B. Saunders; 1970. p. 61–75.

124. Unanue ER. Antigen-presenting function of the macrophage. Ann Rev Immunol 1984;2:395–428.

125. Braciale TJ, Morrison LA, Sweetser MT, et al. Antigen presentation pathways to class I and II MHC restricted T lymphocytes. Immunol Rev 1987;98:95–114.

126. Buus S, Sette A, Grey HM. The interaction between protein derived immunogenic peptides and Ia. Immunol Rev 1987;98:115–41.

127. Harding CV, Unanue ER. Antigen processing and intracellu-

lar Ia. Possible roles of endocytosis and protein synthesis in Ia. function. J Immunol 1989;42:12–9.

128. Venet A, Hance AJ, Saltini C, et al. Enhanced alveolar macrophage-mediated antigen-induced T lymphocyte proliferation in sarcoidosis. J Clin Invest 1985;75:293–301.

129. Lem VM, Lipscomb MF, Weissler JC, et al. Bronchoalveolar lavage cells from sarcoid patients demonstrate enhanced antigen presentation. J Immunol 1985;135:1766–71.

130. Campbell DA, du Bois RM, Butcher RG, Poulter LW. The density of HLA-DR antigen expression on alveolar macrophages is increased in pulmonary sarcoidosis. Clin Exp Immunol 1986;65:165–71.

131. Weiss A, Imboden JB. Cell surface molecules and early events involved in human T-lymphocyte activation. Adv Immunol 1987;41:1–38.

132. Sanders ME, Makgoba W, Sharrow SO, et al. Human memory T lymphocytes express increased levels of three cell adhesion molecules (LFA-3, CD2, and LFA-1) and three other molecules (UCHL1, CDw29, and Pgp-1) and have enhanced IFN-gamma production. J Immunol 1988;140:1401–7.

133. Spurzem J, Saltini C, Kirby M, Crystal RG. Compartmentalised expression of adhesion molecules on lung T-lymphocytes. Am Rev Respir Dis 1988;137:A46.

134. Cantrell D, Davies AA, Londel M, et al. Association of phosphorylation of the T3 antigen with immune activation of T-lymphocytes. Nature 1987;325:540–2.

135. Noonan DJ, Isakov N, Theofilopoulos AN, et al. Protein kinase C-activating phorbol esters augment expression of T-cell receptor genes. Eur J Immunol 1987;17:803–7.

136. du Bois RM, Kirby M, Balbi B, et al. T-lymphocytes that accumulate in the lung in sarcoidosis have evidence of recent stimulation of the T-cell antigen receptor. Am Rev Respir Dis 1992;145:1205–11.

137. Lecossier D, Valeyre D, Loiseau A, et al. Antigen-induced proliferative response of lavage and blood T-lymphocytes. Am Rev Respir Dis 1991;144:861–8.

138. Moller DR, Konishi K, Kirby M, et al. Bias toward use of a specific T-cell receptor B-chain variable region in a subgroup of individuals with sarcoidosis. J Clin Invest 1988;82:1183–91.

139. Forman JD, Klein JT, Silver RF, et al. Selective activation and accumulation of oligoclonal V beta-specific T cells in active pulmonary sarcoidosis. J Clin Invest 1994;94:1533–42.

140. Grunewald J, Janson CH, Eklund A, et al. Restricted V alpha 2.3 gene usage by CD41 T lymphocytes in bronchoalveolar lavage fluid from sarcoidosis patients correlates with HLA-DR3. Eur J Immunol 1992;22:129–35.

141. Jones CM, Lake RA, Wijeyekoon JB, et al. Oligoclonal V gene usage by T lymphocytes in bronchoalveolar lavage fluid from sarcoidosis patients. Am J Respir Cell Mol Biol 1996; 14:470–7.

142. Bellocq A, Lecossier D, Pierre-Audigier C, et al. T cell receptor repertoire of T lymphocytes recovered from the lung and blood of patients with sarcoidosis. Am J Respir Crit Care Med 1994;149:646–54.

143. Dohi M, Yamamoto K, Masuko K, et al. Accumulation of multiple T cell clonotypes in lungs of healthy individuals and patients with pulmonary sarcoidosis. J Immunol 1994;152:1983–8.

144. Klein JT, Horn TD, Forman JD, et al. Selection of oligoclonal V beta-specific T cells in the intradermal response to Kveim-Siltzbach reagent in individuals with sarcoidosis. J Immunol 1995;154:1450–60.

145. du Bois RM. Sarcoidosis. In: Walters EH, du Bois RM, editors. Immunology and management of interstitial lung disease. London: Chapman & Hull; 1995. p. 98–102.

146. Muller-Quernheim J. Sarcoidosis: immunopathogenic concepts and their clinical application. Eur Respir J 1998;12:716–38.

147. Moller DR, Forman JD, Liu MC, et al. Enhanced expression of IL-12 associated with Th1 cytokine profiles in active pulmonary sarcoidosis. J Immunol 1996;156:4952–60.

148. Grunewald J, Hultman T, Bucht A, et al. Restricted usage of T cell receptor V alpha/J alpha gene segments with different nucleotide but identical amino acid sequences in HLA-DR31 sarcoidosis patients. Mol Med 1995;1:287–96.

149. Katcher K, Wahlstrom J, Eklund A, Grunewald J. Highly activated T-cell receptor AV2S3(+) CD4(+) lung T-cell expansions in pulmonary sarcoidosis. Am J Respir Crit Care Med 2001;163:1540–5.

150. Grunewald J, Berlin M, Olerup O, Eklund A. Lung T-helper cells expressing T-cell receptor AV2S3 associate with clinical features of pulmonary sarcoidosis. Am J Respir Crit Care Med 2000;161:814–8.

151. Sawabe T, Shiokawa S, Sugisaki K, et al. Accumulation of common clonal T cells in multiple lesions of sarcoidosis. Mol Med 2000;6:793–802.

152. Haregewoin A, Soman G, Hom RC, Finberg RW. Human gamma delta1 T-cells respond to mycobacterial heat shock proteins. Nature 1989;340:309–12.

153. Balbi B, Moller DR, Kirby M, et al. Increased numbers of T-lymphocytes with gamma delta1 antigen receptors in a subgroup of individuals with pulmonary sarcoidosis. J Clin Invest 1990;85:1353–61.

154. Forrester JM, Newman LS, Wang Y, et al. Clonal expansion of lung V delta 11 T cells in pulmonary sarcoidosis. J Clin Invest 1993;91:292–300.

155. Hunninghake GW, Crystal RG. Pulmonary sarcoidosis; a disorder mediated by excess helper T-lymphocyte activity at sites of disease activity. N Engl J Med 1981;305:429–34.

156. Pabst R, Schuster M, Tschernig T. Lymphocyte dynamics in the pulmonary microenvironment: implications for the pathophysiology of pulmonary sarcoidosis. Sarcoidosis Vasc Diffuse Lung Dis 1999;16:197–202.

157. Agostini C, Trentin L, Zambello R, et al. CD8 alveolitis in sarcoidosis: incidence, phenotypic characteristics, and clinical features. Am J Med 1993;95:466–72.

158. Pinkston P, Bitterman PB, Crystal RG. Spontaneous release of interleukin-2 by lung T lymphocytes in active pulmonary sarcoidosis. N Engl J Med 1983;308:793–800.

159. Semenzato G, Agostini C, Trentin L, et al. Evidence of cells bearing interleukin-2 receptor at sites of disease activity in sarcoid patients. Clin Exp Immunol 1984;57:331–7.

160. Costabel U, Bross KJ, Ruhle KH, et al. Ia-like antigens on T-cells and their subpopulations in pulmonary sarcoidosis and in hypersensitivity pneumonitis. Analysis of bronchoalveolar lavage and blood lymphocytes. Am Rev Respir Dis 1985;131:337–42.

161. Saltini C, Hemler ME, Crystal RG. T-lymphocytes compartmentalised on the epithelial surface of the lower respiratory tract express the very late activation antigen complex VLA-1. Clin Immunol Immunopathol 1988;46:221–33.

162. Koura T, Gon Y, Hashimoto S, et al. Expression of thioredoxin in granulomas: possible role in the development of T lymphocyte activation. Thorax 2000;55:755–61.

163. Wahlstrom J, Berlin M, Skold CM, et al. Phenotypic analysis of lymphocytes and monocytes/macrophages in peripheral blood and bronchoalveolar lavage fluid from patients with pulmonary sarcoidosis. Thorax 1999;54:339–46.

164. Fazel SB, Howie SE, Krajewski AS, Lamb D. Increased CD45RO expression on T lymphocytes in mediastinal lymph node and pulmonary lesions of patients with pulmonary sarcoidosis. Clin Exp Immunol 1994;95:509–13.

165. Petrek M, Pantelidis P, Southcott AM, et al. The source and role of RANTES in interstitial lung disease [abstract]. Eur Respir J 1997;10:1207–16.

166. Semenzato G, Chilosi M, Cipriani A, et al. Cells and mediators involved in the mechanisms of granuloma formation in patients with granulomatous disorders. In: Yoshida T, Torisu M, editors. Basic mechanisms of granulomatous inflammation. Amsterdam: Elsevier Science Publishers B.V.; 1989. p. 283–98.

167. Chilosi M, Mombello A, Lestani M, et al. Immunohisto-chemical analysis of cells accounting for granuloma formation. Sarcoidosis 1992;9:199–203.

168. Konishi K, Moller DR, Saltini C, et al. Spontaneous expression of the interleukin-2 receptor gene and presence of functional interleukin-2 receptors on T-lymphocytes in the blood of individuals with active pulmonary sarcoidosis. J Clin Invest 1988;82:775–81.

169. Mollers M, Aries SP, Dromann D, et al. Intracellular cytokine repertoire in different T cell subsets from patients with sarcoidosis. Thorax 2001;56:487–93.

170. Kaneko Y, Kuwano K, Kuntake R, et al. Immunohistochemical localization of B7 costimulating molecules and major histocompatibility complex class II antigen in pulmonary sarcoidosis. Respiration 1999;66:343–8.

171. Agostini C, Trentin L, Perin A, et al. Regulation of alveolar macrophage-T cell interactions during Th$_1$-type sarcoid inflammatory process. Am J Physiol 1999;277:L240–50.

172. Hunninghake GW, Crystal RG. Mechanisms of hypergammaglobulinemia in pulmonary sarcoidosis: site of increased antibody production and role of T-lymphocytes. J Clin Invest 1981;67:86–92.

173. Saint-Remy J, Mitchell DN, Cole PJ. Variation in immunoglobulin levels and circulating immune complexes in sarcoidosis. Correlation and extent of disease and duration of symptoms. Am Rev Respir Dis 1983;127:23–7.

174. Lawrence EC, Martin RR, Blaese RM, et al. Increased bronchoalveolar IgG-screening cells in interstitial lung diseases. N Engl J Med 1980;302:1186–8.

175. Hance AJ, Saltini C, Crystal RG. Does de novo immunoglobulin synthesis occur on the epithelial surface of the human lower respiratory tract? Am Rev Respir Dis 1988;137:17–24.

176. Spurzem JR, Saltini C, Crystal RG. Functional significance of anti-T-lymphocyte antibodies in sarcoidosis. Am Rev Respir Dis 1988;137:600–5.

177. Fazel SB, Howie SE, Krajewski AS, Lamb D. B lymphocyte accumulations in human pulmonary sarcoidosis. Thorax 1992;47:964–7.

178. Pforte A, Gerth C, Voss A, et al. Proliferating alveolar macrophages in BAL and lung function changes in interstitial lung disease. Eur Respir J 1993;6:951–5.

179. Hance AJ, Douches S, Winchester RJ, et al. Characterisation of mononuclear phagocyte subpopulations in the human lung by using monoclonal antibodies: changes in alveolar macrophage phenotype associated with pulmonary sarcoidosis. J Immunol 1985;134:284–92.

180. Campbell DA, Poulter LW, du Bois RM. Phenotypic analysis of alveolar macrophages in normal subjects and in patients with interstitial lung disease. Thorax 1986;41:429–34.

181. Blusse van Oud Albas A, van Furth R. Kinetics and characteristics of alveolar macrophages in the normal steady state. J Exp Med 1979;149:1504–18.

182. Bitterman PB, Saltzman LE, Adelberg J, et al. Alveolar macrophage replication. One mechanism for the expansion of the mononuclear phagocyte population in the chronically inflamed lung. J Clin Invest 1984;72:460–9.

183. Zissel G, Ernst M, Schlaak M, et al. Pharmacological modulation of the IFN-gamma-induced accessory function of alveolar macrophages and peripheral blood monocytes. Inflamm Res 1999;48:662–8.

184. Spurzem JR, Saltini C, Kirby M, et al. Expression of HLA class II genes in alveolar macrophages of patients with sarcoidosis. Am Rev Respir Dis 1989;140:89–94.

185. Shijubo N, Itoh Y, Shigehara K, et al. Association of Clara cell 10-kDa protein, spontaneous regression and sarcoidosis. Eur Respir J 2000;16:414–9.

186. Gudmundsson G, Hunninghake GW. Interferon-γ is necessary for the expression of hypersensitivity pneumonitis. J Clin Invest 1997;99:2386–90.

187. Poulter LW, Campbell DA, Munro C, Janossy G. Discrimina-

188. Ainslie GM, Poulter LW, du Bois RM. Relation between immunocytological features of bronchoalveolar lavage fluid and clinical indices in sarcoidosis. Thorax 1989;44:501–9.

189. Spiteri M, Clarke SW, Poulter LW. Alveolar macrophages that suppress T-cell responses may be crucial to the pathogenetic outcome of pulmonary sarcoidosis. Eur Respir J 1992;5:394–403.

190. Shakoor Z, Hamblin AS. Increased CD11/CD18 expression on peripheral blood leucocytes of patients with sarcoidosis. Clin Exp Immunol 1992;90:99–105.

191. Striz I, Wang YM, Kalaycioglu O, Costabel U. Expression of alveolar macrophage adhesion molecules in pulmonary sarcoidosis. Chest 1992;102:882–6.

192. Melis M, Gjomarkaj M, Pace E, et al. Increased expression of leukocyte function associated antigen-1 (LFA-1) and intercellular adhesion molecule-1 (ICAM-1) by alveolar macrophages of patients with pulmonary sarcoidosis. Chest 1991;100:910–6.

193. Schaberg T, Rau M, Stephan H, Lode H. Increased number of alveolar macrophages expressing surface molecules of the CD11/CD18 family in sarcoidosis and idiopathic pulmonary fibrosis is related to the production of superoxide anions by these cells. Am Rev Respir Dis 1993;147:1507–13.

194. Pforte A, Schiessler A, Gais P, et al. Expression of CD14 correlates with lung function impairment in pulmonary sarcoidosis. Chest 1994;105:349–54.

195. Itoh A, Yamaguchi E, Furuya K, Kawakami Y. Secretion of GM-CSF by inflammatory cells in the lung of patients with sarcoidosis. Respirology 1998;3:247–51.

196. Kunkel SL, Chesnue SW, Plewa M, Higashi GI. Macrophage function in the *Schistosoma mansoni* egg-induced pulmonary granuloma. Role of arachidonic acid metabolites in macrophage Ia antigen expression. Am J Pathol 1984;114:240–49.

197. Chensue SW, Kunkel SL, Ward PA, Higashi GI. Exogenously administered prostaglandins modulate pulmonary granulomas induced by *Schistosoma mansoni* eggs. Am J Pathol 1983;111:78–87.

198. Pantelidis P, Southcott AM, Cambrey AD, et al. Activation of peripheral blood mononuclear cells in bronchoalveolar lavage fluid from patients with sarcoidosis: visualisation of single cell activation products. Thorax 1994;49:1146–51.

199. Hunninghake GW. Release of interleukin-1 by alveolar macrophages of patients with active pulmonary sarcoidosis. Am Rev Respir Dis 1984;129:569–72.

200. Eden E, Turino GM. Interleukin-1 from human alveolar macrophages in lung disease. J Clin Immunol 1986;6:326–33.

201. Wewers MD, Saltini C, Sellers S. Evaluation of alveolar macrophages for the spontaneous expression of the interleukin-1 beta gene. Cell Immunol 1987;107:479–88.

202. Kern JA, Lamb RJ, Reed JC, et al. Interleukin-1-beta gene expression in human monocytes and alveolar macrophages from normal subjects and patients with sarcoidosis. Am Rev Respir Dis 1988;137:1180–4.

203. Pueringer RJ, Schwartz DA, Dayton CS, et al. The relationship between alveolar macrophage TNF, IL-1, and PGE2 release, alveolitis, and disease severity in sarcoidosis. Chest 1993;103:832–8.

204. Muller-Quernheim J, Pfeifer S, Mannel D, et al. Lung-restricted activation of the alveolar macrophage/monocyte system in pulmonary sarcoidosis. Am Rev Respir Dis 1992;145:187–92.

205. Baughman RP, Strohofer SA, Buchsbaum J, Lower EE. Release of tumor necrosis factor by alveolar macrophages of patients with sarcoidosis. J Lab Clin Med 1990;115:36–42.

206. Foley NM, Millar AB, Meager A, et al. Tumour necrosis fac-

tor production by alveolar macrophages in pulmonary sarcoidosis and tuberculosis. Sarcoidosis 1992;9:29–34.

207. Muller-Quernheim J, Pfeifer S, Mannel D, et al. Lung-restricted activation of the alveolar macrophage/monocyte system in pulmonary sarcoidosis. Am Rev Respir Dis 1992;145:187–92.

208. Bachwich PR, Lynch JP, Larrick J, et al. Tumor necrosis factor production by human sarcoid alveolar macrophages. Am J Pathol 1986;125:421–5.

209. Pantelidis P, Southcott AM, Cambrey AD, et al. Activation of peripheral blood mononuclear cells in bronchoalveolar lavage fluid from patients with sarcoidosis: visualisation of single cell activation products. Thorax 1994;49:1146–51.

210. Strieter RM, Remick DG, Lynch JP 3rd, et al. Interleukin-2-induced tumour necrosis factor-alpha (TNF-α) gene expression in human alveolar macrophages and blood monocytes. Am Rev Respir Dis 1989;139:335–42.

211. Myatt N, Coghill G, Morrison K, et al. Detection of tumour necrosis factor alpha in sarcoidosis and tuberculosis granulomas using in situ hybridisation. J Clin Pathol 1994; 47:423–6.

212. Armstrong L, Foley NM, Millar AB. Inter-relationship between tumour necrosis factor-alpha (TNF-alpha) and TNF soluble receptors in pulmonary sarcoidosis. Thorax 1999;54:524–30.

213. Agostini C, Trentin L, Facco M. Role of IL-12 and IL-15 and their receptors in the development of T cell alveolitis in sarcoidosis. J Immunol 1996;156:4952–60.

214. Tazi A, Nioche S, Chastre J, et al. Spontaneous release of granulocyte colony-stimulating factor (G-CSF) by alveolar macrophages in the course of bacterial pneumonia and sarcoidosis: endotoxin-dependent and endotoxin-independent G-CSF release by cells recovered by bronchoalveolar lavage. Am J Respir Cell Mol Biol 1991;4:140–7.

215. Tani K, Ogushi F, Huang L, et al. CD13/aminopeptidase N, a novel chemoattractant for T lymphocytes in pulmonary sarcoidosis. Am J Respir Crit Care Med 2000;161: 1636–42.

216. Bingisser R, Speich R, Zollinger A, et al. Interleukin-10 secretion by alveolar macrophages and monocytes in sarcoidosis. Respiration 2000;67:280–6.

217. Pantelidis P, Southcott AM, du Bois RM. Epithelial lining fluid (ELF) from sarcoid patients activates peripheral blood mononuclear cells (PBM): visualization of single cell activation products [abstract]. Eur Respir J 1992;5:235.

218. Fels AOS, Nathan CF, Cohn ZA. Hydrogen peroxide release by alveolar macrophages from sarcoidosis patients and by alveolar macrophages from normals after exposure to recombinant interferons alphaA, beta, and gamma and 1,25-dihydroxyvitamin D_3. J Clin Invest 1987;80:381–6.

219. Baughman RP, Lower EE, Pierson G, Strohofer S. Spontaneous hydrogen peroxide release from alveolar macrophages of patients with active sarcoidosis: comparison with cigarette smokers. J Lab Clin Med 1988;111:399–404.

220. Poole A, Myllyla R, Davies BH. Activities of enzymes of collagen biosynthesis and levels of type III procollagen peptide in the serum of patients with sarcoidosis. Life Sci 1989;45:319–26.

221. Hunninghake GW, Gadek JE, Young RC, et al. Maintenance of granuloma formation in pulmonary sarcoidosis by T lymphocytes within the lung. N Engl J Med 1980;302:594–8.

222. Nagasawa H, Miyaura C, Abe E, et al. Fusion and activation of human alveolar macrophages induced by recombinant interferon gamma and their suppression by dexamethasone. Am Rev Respir Dis 1987;136:916–21.

223. Prior C, Haslam PL. Increased levels of serum interferon-gamma in pulmonary sarcoidosis and relationship with response to corticosteroid therapy. Am Rev Respir Dis 1991;143:53–60.

224. Ishioka S, Saito T, Hiyama K, et al. Increased expression of tumor necrosis factor-alpha, interleukin-6, platelet-derived growth factor-B, and granulocyte-macrophage colony-stimulating factor mRNA in cells of bronchoalveolar lavage fluids from patients with sarcoidosis. Sarcoidosis Vasc Diffuse Lung Dis 1996;13:139–45.

225. Kreipe H, Radzun HJ, Heidorn K, et al. Proliferation, macrophage colony-stimulating factor and macrophage colony-stimulating factor-receptor expression of alveolar macrophages in active sarcoidosis. Lab Invest 1990;62: 697–703.

226. Campbell DA, Poulter LW, du Bois RM. Immunocompetent cells in bronchoalveolar lavage reflect the cell populations in transbronchial biopsies in pulmonary sarcoidosis. Am Rev Respir Dis 1985;132:1300–6.

227. Semenzato G, Chilosi M, Ossi E. Bronchoalveolar lavage and lung histology. Comparative analysis of inflammatory and immunocompetent cells in patients with sarcoidosis and hypersensitivity pneumonitis. Am Rev Respir Dis 1985; 132:400–4.

228. Devergne O, Emilie D, Peuchmaur M, et al. Production of cytokines in sarcoid lymph nodes: preferential expression of interleukin-1 beta and interferon-gamma genes. Hum Pathol 1992;23:317–23.

229. Munro CS, Campbell DA, du Bois RM, et al. Dendritic cells in cutaneous, lymph node, and pulmonary lesions of sarcoidosis. Scand J Immunol 1987;25:461–7.

230. Shigehara K, Shijubo N, Ohmichi M, et al. IL-12 and IL-18 are increased and stimulate IFN-gamma production in sarcoid lungs. J Immunol 2001;166:642–9.

231. Shigehara K, Shijubo N, Ohmichi M, et al. Enhanced mRNA expression of Th1 cytokines and IL-12 in active pulmonary sarcoidosis. Sarcoidosis Vasc Diffuse Lung Dis 2000;17: 151–7.

232. Shigehara K, Shijubo N, Ohmichi M, et al. Increased levels of interleukin-18 in patients with pulmonary sarcoidosis. Am J Respir Crit Care Med 2000;162:1979–82.

233. Inui N, Chida K, Suda T, Nakamura H. Th1/Th2 and TC1/TC2 profiles in peripheral blood and bronchoalveolar lavage fluid cells in pulmonary sarcoidosis. J Allergy Clin Immunol 2001;107:337–44.

234. Wahlstrom J, Katchar K, Wigzell H, et al. Analysis of intracellular cytokines in CD4(+) and CD8(+) lung and blood T cells in sarcoidosis. Am J Respir Crit Care Med 2001; 163:115–21.

235. Prasse A, Georges CG, Biller H, et al. Th1 cytokine pattern in sarcoidosis is expressed by bronchoalveolar CD4+ and CD8+ T cells. Clin Exp Immunol 2000;122:241–8.

236. Muller-Quernheim J. Sarcoidosis: immunopathogenic concepts and their clinical application. Eur Respir J 1998;12:716–38.

237. Kunkel SL, Lukacs NW, Strieter RM, et al. Th1 and Th2 responses regulate experimental lung granuloma formation. Sarcoidosis Vasc Diffuse Lung Dis 1996;13:120–8.

238. Chensue SW, Warmington K, Ruth JH, et al. Mycobacteria and schistosomal antigen-elicited granuloma formation in IFN-γ and IL-4 knockout mice. J Immunol 1997;159: 356–73.

239. Chensue SW, Otterness IG, Higashi GI, Kunkel SL. Monokine production by hypersensitivity and foreign body type granuloma macrophages. J Immunol 1989;142:1281–6.

240. Driscoll KE. Macrophage inflammatory proteins: biology and role in pulmonary inflammation. Exp Lung Res 1994; 20:473–90.

241. Keane MP, Standiford TJ, Strieter RM. Chemokines are important cytokines in the pathogenesis of interstitial lung disease [abstract]. Eur Respir J 1997;10:1199–1202.

242. Standiford TJ, Rolfe MW, Kunkel SL, et al. Macrophage inflammatory protein-1 alpha expression in interstitial lung disease. J Immunol 1993;151:2852–63.

243. Oshima M, Maeda A, Ishioka S, et al. Expression of C-C

chemokines in bronchoalveolar lavage cells from patients with granulomatous lung diseases. Lung 1999;177:229–40.

244. Car BD, Meloni F, Luisetti M, et al. Elevated IL-8 and MCP-1 in the bronchoalveolar lavage fluid of patients with idiopathic pulmonary fibrosis and pulmonary sarcoidosis. Am J Respir Crit Care Med 1994;149:655–9.

245. Pantelidis P, Southcott AM, Black CM, du Bois RM. Upregulation of IL-8 secretion by alveolar macrophages from patients with fibrosing alveolitis: a subpopulation analysis. Clin Exp Immunol 1997;108:95–104.

246. Sugiyama Y, Kasahara T, Mukaida N, et al. Chemokines in the bronchoalveolar lavage fluid of patients with sarcoidosis. Intern Med 1997;36:856–60.

247. Berlin M, Lundahl J, Skold CM, et al. The lymphocytic alveolitis in sarcoidosis is associated with increased amounts of soluble and cell-bound adhesion molecules in bronchoalveolar lavage fluid and serum. J Intern Med 1998;244:333–40.

248. Hamblin AS, Shakoor Z, Kapahi P, Haskard D. Circulating adhesion molecules in sarcoidosis. Clin Exp Immunol 1994;96:335–8.

249. Kaseda M, Kadota J, Mukae H, et al. Possible role of L-selectin in T lymphocyte alveolitis in patients with active pulmonary sarcoidosis. Clin Exp Immunol 2000;121:146–50.

250. Shijubo N, Imai K, Shigehara K, et al. Soluble intercellular adhesion molecule-1 (ICAM-1) in sera and bronchoalveolar lavage fluid of patients with idiopathic pulmonary fibrosis and pulmonary sarcoidosis. Clin Exp Immunol 1994;95:156–61.

251. Dalhoff K, Bohnet S, Braun J, et al. Intercellular adhesion molecule 1 (ICAM-1) in the pathogenesis of mononuclear cell alveolitis in pulmonary sarcoidosis. Thorax 1993;48:1140–4.

252. Kim DS, Paik SH, Lim CM, et al. Value of ICAM-1 expression and soluble ICAM-1 level as a marker of activity in sarcoidosis. Chest 1999;115:1059–65.

253. Braun J, Dinkelacker C, Bohnet S, et al. 1,25-dihydroxycholecalciferol stimulates ICAM-1 expression of human alveolar macrophages in healthy controls and patients with sarcoidosis. Lung 1999;177:139–49.

254. Zissel G, Homolka J, Schlaak J, et al. Anti-inflammatory cytokine release by alveolar macrophages in pulmonary sarcoidosis. Am J Respir Crit Care Med 1996;154:713–9.

255. Limper AH, Colby TV, Sanders MS, et al. Immunohistochemical localization of transforming growth factor-beta 1 in the nonnecrotizing granulomas of pulmonary sarcoidosis. Am J Respir Crit Care Med 1994;149:197–204.

256. Khalil N, O'Connor RN, Unruh HW, et al. Increased production and localization of TGFβ in idiopathic fibrosis. Am J Respir Cell Mol Biol 1991;5:155–62.

257. Salez F, Gosset P, Copin MC, et al. Transforming growth factor-beta1 in sarcoidosis. Eur Respir J 1998;12:913–9.

258. Eklund AG, Sigurdardottir O, Ohrn M. Vitronectin and its relationship to other extracellular matrix components in bronchoalveolar lavage fluid in sarcoidosis. Am Rev Respir Dis 1992;145:646–50.

259. Pohl WR, Thompson AB, Kohn H, et al. Serum procollagen III peptide levels in subjects with sarcoidosis. A 5-year follow-up study. Am Rev Respir Dis 1992;145:412–7.

260. Luisetti M, Bulgheroni A, Bacchella L, et al. Elevated serum procollagen III aminopeptide levels in sarcoidosis. Chest 1990;98:1414–20.

261. O'Connor C, Ward K, Van Breda A, et al. Type 3 procollagen peptide in bronchoalveolar lavage fluid. Poor indicator of course and prognosis in sarcoidosis. Chest 1989;96:339–44.

262. Daniele RP, Dauber JH, Rossman MD. Immunologic abnormalities in sarcoidosis. Ann Intern Med 1980;92:406–16.

263. Soler P, Basset F, Bernaudin JF, Chretien J. Morphology and distribution of the cells of a sarcoid granuloma: ultrastructural study of serial sections. Ann N Y Acad Sci 1976;278:147–60.

264. Mitchell DN, Scadding JG, Heard BE, Hinson KFW. Sarcoidosis: histopathological definition and clinical diagnosis. J Clin Pathol 1977;30:395–408.

265. Mishra BB, Poulter LW, Janossy G, James GJ. The distribution of lymphoid and macrophage like cell subsets and Kveim granulomata: possible mechanism of negative PPD reaction in sarcoidosis. Clin Exp Immunol 1983;54:705–15.

266. van Maarsseveen AC, Mullink H, Alons CL, Stam J. Distribution of T-lymphocyte subsets in different portions of sarcoid granulomas: immunohistologic analysis with monoclonal antibodies. Hum Pathol 1986;17:493–500.

267. Scadding JG, Mitchell DN. Sarcoidosis. London: Chapman & Hall; 1985.

268. Jones-Williams W, Erasmus DA, James BMV, Davies T. The fine structure of sarcoid and tuberculosis granulomas. Postgrad Med J 1970;46:496–500.

269. Agostini C, Zambello R, Sancetta R, et al. Expression of tumour-necrosis factor-receptor superfamily members by lung T lymphocytes in interstitial lung disease. Am J Respir Crit Care Med 1996;153:1359–67.

270. Dai H, Guzman J, Costabel U. Increased expression of apoptosis signaling receptors by alveolar macrophages in sarcoidosis. Eur Respir J 1999;13:1451–4.

271. Gombert W, Borthwick NJ, Wallace DL, et al. Fibroblasts prevent apoptosis of IL-2 deprived T-cells without inducing proliferation: a selective effect on Bcl-xL expression. Immunology 1996;89:397–404.

272. Estaquier J, Ameisen J. C: a role for Th1 and Th2 cytokines in the regulation of human monocyte apoptosis. Blood 1997;90:153–60.

273. Conant EF, Glickstein MF, Mahar P, Miller WT. Pulmonary sarcoidosis in the older patient: conventional radiographic features. Radiology 1988;169:315–9.

274. Lynch JP III, Kazerooni EA, Gay SA. Pulmonary sarcoidosis. Clin Chest Med 1997;18:755–85.

275. Judson MA, Strange C. Bullous sarcoidosis: a report of three cases. Chest 1998;114:1474–8.

276. Askling J, Gruewald J, Eklund A, et al. Increased risk for cancer following sarcoidosis. Am J Respir Crit Care Med 1999;160:1668–72.

277. Wilson R, Lund V, Sweatman M, et al. Upper respiratory tract involvement in sarcoidosis and its management. Eur Respir J 1988;1:269–72.

278. Neville E, Mills RG, Jash DK, et al. Sarcoidosis of the upper respiratory tract and its association with lupus pernio. Thorax 1976;31:660–4.

279. Drosos AA, Voulgari PV, Psychos DN, et al. Sicca syndrome in patients with sarcoidosis. Rheumatol Int 1999;18:177–80.

280. Benjamin B, Dalton C, Croxson G. Laryngoscopic diagnosis of laryngeal sarcoid. Ann Otol Rhinol Laryngol 1995;104:529–31.

281. James DG, Barter S, Jash D, et al. Sarcoidosis of the upper respiratory tract (SURT). J Laryngol Otol 1982;96:711–8.

282. Levey M. Extensive sarcoidosis involving the upper respiratory tract. Int Surg 1979;64:73–7.

283. Löfgren S. Primary pulmonary sarcoidosis. Acta Med Scand 1953;145:421–31.

284. Wilsher ML. Seasonal clustering of sarcoidosis presenting with erythema nodosum. Eur Respir J 1999;12:1197–9.

285. Mana J, Gomez-Vaquero C, Montera A, et al. Löfgren's syndrome revisited: a study of 186 patients. Am J Med 1999;107:240–5.

286. James DG. Lupus pernio. Lupus 1992;1:129–31.

287. Norton SA, Chesser RS, Fitzpatrick JE. Scar sarcoidosis in pseudofolliculitis barbae. Mil Med 1991;156:369–71.

288. Neville E, Walker AN, James DG. Prognostic factors predicting the outcome of sarcoidosis: an analysis of 818 patients. QJM 1983;205:525–33.

289. Veien NK, Stahl D, Brodthagen H. Cutaneous sarcoidosis in Caucasians. J Am Acad Dermatol 1987;16:534–40.

290. Elgert ML. Cutaneous sarcoidosis: definitions and types of lesions [abstract]. Clin Dermatol 1986;4:35–45.

291. Zic JA, Horowitz DH, Arzubiaga C, King LE Jr. Treatment of cutaneous sarcoidosis with chloroquine. Review of the literature. Arch Dermatol 1991;127:1034–40.

292. Bachelez H, Senet P, Cadranel J, et al. The use of tetracyclines for the treatment of sarcoidosis. Arch Dermatol 2001;137:69–73.

293. Stack BC Jr, Hall PJ, Goodman AL, Perez IR. CO_2 laser excision of lupus pernio of the face. Am J Otolaryngol 1996;17:260–3.

294. Shaw M, Black MM, Davis PK. Disfiguring lupus pernio successfully treated with plastic surgery. Clin Exp Dermatol 1984;9:614–7.

295. Gollnick H. New indications and new retinoids. Dermatologica 1987;175 Suppl 1:182–95.

296. Mackey JP. Clofazimine in dermatology. Int J Dermatol 1976;15:140–1.

297. Voelter-Mahlknecht S, Benez A, Metzger S, Fierlbeck G. Treatment of subcutaneous sarcoidosis with allopurinol. Arch Dermatol 1999;135:1560–1.

298. Khatri KA, Chotzen VA, Burrall BA. Lupus pernio: successful treatment with a potent topical corticosteroid. Arch Dermatol 1995;131:617–8.

299. Daoud MS, Rogers RS 3rd. Melkersson-Rosenthal syndrome. Semin Dermatol 1995;14:135–9.

300. Sussman GL, Yang WH, Steinberg S. Melkersson-Rosenthal syndrome: clinical, pathologic, and therapeutic considerations. Ann Allergy 1992;69:187–94.

301. Mahler VB, Hornstein OP, Boateng BI, Kiesewetter FF. Granulomatous glossitis as an unusual manifestation of Melkersson-Rosenthal syndrome. Cutis 1924;55:244–6.

302. Delaney P. Neurologic manifestations in sarcoidosis: review of the literature, with a report of 23 cases. Ann Intern Med 1977;87:336–45.

303. Chapelon C, Ziza JM, Piette JC, et al. Neurosarcoidosis: signs, course, and treatment in 35 confirmed cases. Medicine 1990;69:261–76.

304. Kadakia JK, Collette PM, Sharma OP. Role of magnetic resonance imaging in neurosarcoidosis. Sarcoidosis 1993;10:98–9.

305. Lexa FJ, Grossman RI. MR of sarcoidosis in the head and spine: spectrum of manifestations and radiographic response to steroid therapy. Am J Neuroradiol 1994;15:973–82.

306. Carmody RF, Mafee MF, Goodwin JA, et al. Orbital and optic pathway sarcoidosis: MR findings. Am J Neuroradiol 1994;15:775–83.

307. Pickuth D, Heywang-Kobrunner SH. Neurosarcoidosis: evaluation with MRI. J Neuroradiol 2000;27:185–8.

308. Lynch JP, Sharma OP, Baughman RP. Extrapulmonary sarcoidosis. Semin Respir Infect 1998;13:229–54.

309. Cheng TM, O'Neill BP, Scheithauer BW, Piepgras DG. Chronic meningitis: the role of meningeal or cortical biopsy. Neurosurgery 1994;34:590–6.

310. Stuart CA, Neelon FA, Lebovitz HE. Hypothalamic insufficiency: the cause of hypopituitarism in sarcoidosis. Ann Intern Med 1978;88:589–94.

311. O'Brien GM, Baughman RP, Broderick JP, et al. Paranoid psychosis due to neurosarcoidosis. Sarcoidosis 1994;11:34–6.

312. Godwin JE, Sahn SA. Sarcoidosis presenting as progressive ascending lower extremity weakness and asymptomatic meningitis with hypoglycorrhachia. Chest 1990;97:1263–5.

313. Chang B, Steimel J, Moller DR, et al. Depression in sarcoidosis. Am J Respir Crit Care Med 2001;163:329–34.

314. Matsui Y, Iwai K, Tachibana T, et al. Clinicopathological study of fatal myocardial sarcoidosis. Ann N Y Acad Sci 1976;278:455–69.

315. Roberts WC, McAllister HA Jr, Ferrans VJ. Sarcoidosis of the heart. A clinicopathologic study of 35 necropsy patients (group 1) and review of 78 previously described necropsy patients (group 11). Am J Med 1977;63:86–108.

316. Fleming HA, Bailey SM. Sarcoid heart disease. J R Coll Phys Lond 1981;15:245–53.

317. Shammas RL, Movahed A. Sarcoidosis of the heart. Clin Cardiol 1993;16:462–72.

318. Perry A, Vuitch F. Causes of death in patients with sarcoidosis. A morphologic study of 38 autopsies with clinicopathologic correlations. Arch Pathol Lab Med 1995;119:167–72.

319. Fleming HA. Cardiac sarcoidosis. Clin Dermatol 1986;4:143–9.

320. Angomachalelis N, Hourzamanis A, Salem N, et al. Pericardial effusion concomitant with specific heart muscle disease in systemic sarcoidosis. Postgrad Med J 1994;70:Suppl 1:S8–12.

321. Stein E, Jackler I, Stimmel B, et al. Asymptomatic electrocardiographic alterations in sarcoidosis. Am Heart J 1973;86:474–7.

322. Gibbons WJ, Levy RD, Nava S, et al. Subclinical cardiac dysfunction in sarcoidosis. Chest 1991;100:44–50.

323. Lewin RF, Mor R, Spitzer S, et al. Echocardiographic evaluation of patients with systemic sarcoidosis. Am Heart J 1985;110:116–22.

324. Tan LB, Dickie S, McKenna WJ. Left ventricular diastolic characteristics of cardiac sarcoidosis. Am J Cardiol 1986;58:1126–7.

325. Tellier P, Paycha F, Antony I, et al. Reversibility by dipyridamole of thallium-201 myocardial scan defects in patients with sarcoidosis. Am J Med 1988;85:189–93.

326. Tellier P, Valeyre D, Nitenberg A, et al. Cardiac sarcoidosis: reversion of myocardial perfusion abnormalities by dipyridamole. Eur J Nucl Med 1985;11:201–4.

327. Kinney EL, Caldwell JW. Do thallium myocardial perfusion scan abnormalities predict survival in sarcoid patients without cardiac symptoms? Angiology 1990;41:573–6.

328. Okayama K, Kurata C, Tawarahara K, et al. Diagnostic and prognostic value of myocardial scintigraphy with thallium-201 and gallium-67 in cardiac sarcoidosis. Chest 1995;107:330–4.

329. Uemura A, Morimoto S, Hiramitsu S, et al. Histologic diagnostic rate of cardiac sarcoidosis: evaluation of endomyocardial biopsies. Am Heart J 1999;138:299–302.

330. Valantine HA, Tazelaar HD, Macoviak J, et al. Cardiac sarcoidosis: response to steroids and transplantation. J Heart Transplant 1987;6:244–50.

331. Watson J, Smith V, Schmidt D, Navratil D. Automatic implantable cardioverter-defibrillator: early experience at Wilford Hall USAF Medical Center. South Med J 1992;85:161–3.

332. Yeatman M, McNeil K, Smith JA, et al. Lung transplantation in patients with systemic diseases: an eleven-year experience at Papworth Hospital. J Heart Lung Transplant 1996;15:144–9.

333. Glennas A, Kvien TK, Melby K, et al. Acute sarcoid arthritis: occurrence, seasonal onset, clinical features and outcome. Br J Rheumatol 1995;34:45–50.

334. Gran JT, Bohmer E. Acute sarcoid arthritis: a favourable outcome? A retrospective survey of 49 patients with review of the literature. Scand J Rheumatol 1996;25:70–3.

335. Mathur A, Kremer JM. Immunopathology, musculoskeletal features, and treatment of sarcoidosis. Curr Opin Rheumatol 1993;5:90–4.

336. Ferguson EH, Paris J. Sarcoidosis: study of 29 cases, with review of splenic, hepatic, mucous membrane, retinal and joint manifestations. Arch Intern Med 1958;101:1065–84.

337. Sokoloff L, Bunim JJ. Clinical and pathological studies of joint involvement in sarcoidosis. N Engl J Med 1959;260:841–7.

338. Kremer JM. Histologic findings in siblings with acute sarcoid arthritis: association with the B8,DR3 phenotype. J Rheumatol 1986;13:593–7.

339. Bianchi FA, Koech MK. Sarcoidosis with arthritis [abstract]. Ann Rheum Dis 1964;23:463–79.

340. Morris KP, Coulthard MG, Smith PJ, Craft AW. Renovascular and growth effects of childhood sarcoid. Arch Dis Child 1996;75:74–5.

341. Larsen TK. Tenosynovitis as initial diagnosis of sarcoidosis. Case report. Scand J Plast Reconstr Surg Hand Surg 1996; 30:157–9.

342. Löfgren S. Primary pulmonary sarcoidosis: early signs and symptoms. Acta Med Scand 1953;145:424–31.

343. Neville E, Carstairs LS, James DG. Sarcoidosis of bone. QJM 1977;46:215–27.

344. Rizzato G, Montemurro L, Fraioli P. Bone mineral content in sarcoidosis. Semin Respir Med 1992;13:411–23.

345. Hamada K, Nagai S, Tsutsumi T, Izumi T. Bone mineral density and vitamin D in patients with sarcoidosis. Sarcoidosis Vasc Diffuse Lung Dis 1999;16:219–23.

346. Meyrier A, Valeyre D, Bouillon R, et al. Different mechanisms of hypercalciuria in sarcoidosis. Correlations with disease extension and activity. Ann N Y Acad Sci 1986;465: 575–86.

347. Montemurro L, Fraioli P, Riboldi A, et al. Bone loss in prednisone treated sarcoidosis: a two-year follow-up. Ann Ital Med Int 1990;5:164–8.

348. Gonnelli S, Rottoli P, Cepollaro C, et al. Prevention of corticosteroid-induced osteoporosis with alendronate in sarcoid patients. Calcif Tissue Int 1997;61:382–5.

349. Rizzato G, Fraioli P, Montemurro L. Long-term therapy with deflazacort in chronic sarcoidosis. Chest 1991;99:301–9.

350. Nesi D, Sestini P, Fusi L, et al. Comparison of deflazacort and prednisolone therapy in pulmonary sarcoidosis [abstract]. Sarcoidosis 1989;6 Suppl:108.

351. Montemurro L, Schiraldi G, Fraioli P, et al. Prevention of corticosteroid-induced osteoporosis with salmon calcitonin in sarcoid patients. Calcif Tissue Int 1991;49:71–6.

352. Silver MR, Messner LV. Sarcoidosis and its ocular manifestations. J Am Optom Assoc 1994;65:321–7.

353. Jabs DA, Johns CJ. Ocular involvement in chronic sarcoidosis. Am J Ophthalmol 1986;102:297–301.

354. Karma A. Diagnostic aspects of ocular sarcoidosis. Sarcoidosis 1994;11:58–60.

355. Rizzato G, Angi M, Fraioli P, et al. Uveitis as a presenting feature of chronic sarcoidosis. Eur Respir J 1996;9:1201–5.

356. Edelsten C, Pearson A, Joynes E, et al. The occular and systemic prognosis of patients presenting with sarcoid uveitis. Eye 1999;13:748–53.

357. Karma A, Poukkula AA, Ruokonen AO. Assessment of activity of ocular sarcoidosis by gallium scanning. Br J Ophthalmol 1987;71:361–7.

358. Israel HL, Albertine KH, Park CH, Patrick H. Whole-body gallium 67 scans. Role in diagnosis of sarcoidosis. Am Rev Respir Dis 1991;144:1182–6.

359. Mochizuki T, Ichijo K, Takehara Y, Nakamura M. Gallium-67-citrate scanning in patients with sarcoid uveitis. J Nucl Med 1992;33:1851–3.

360. Hoover DL, Khan JA, Giangiacomo J. Pediatric ocular sarcoidosis. Surv Ophthalmol 1986;30:215–28.

361. Dresner MS, Brecher R, Henkind P. Ophthalmology consultation in the diagnosis and treatment of sarcoidosis. Arch Intern Med 1986;146:301–4.

362. Hoffbrand BI. Ocular and renal sarcoidosis. J R Soc Med 1996;89:179–80.

363. Restrick LJ, Blomley MJ, Drayson RA, et al. Percutaneous renal biopsy in the district general hospital. J R Coll Phys Lond 1993;27:247–51.

364. Richmond JM, Chambers B, D'Apice AJ, et al. Renal disease and sarcoidosis. Med J Aust 1981;2:36–7.

365. Khan IH, Simpson JG, Catto GR, MacLeod AM. Membranous nephropathy and granulomatous interstitial nephritis in sarcoidosis. Nephron 1994;66:459–61.

366. Molle D, Baumelou A, Beaufils H, et al. Membranoprolifera-

367. Howard RS, Gabriel R. Glomerulonephritis in sarcoidosis: causal relationship unproven. Postgrad Med J 1992;68:206–8.

368. Romer FK. Renal manifestations and abnormal calcium metabolism in sarcoidosis. QJM 1980;49:233–47.

369. Sharma OP. Vitamin D, calcium, and sarcoidosis. Chest 1996;109:535–9.

370. Adams JS, Sharma OP, Gacad MA, Singer FR. Metabolism of 25-hydroxyvitamin D3 by cultured pulmonary alveolar macrophages in sarcoidosis. J Clin Invest 1983;72:1856–60.

371. Niimi T, Tomita H, Sato S, et al. Vitamin D receptor gene polymorphism in patients with sarcoidosis. Am J Respir Crit Care Med 1999;160:1107–9.

372. Niimi T, Tomita H, Sato S, et al. Vitamin D receptor gene polymorphism and calcium metabolism in sarcoidosis patients. Sarcoidosis Vasc Diffuse Lung Dis 2000;17: 266–9.

373. Broulik PD, Votava V, Pacovsky V. The tubular maximum for calcium reabsorption in patients with chronic active thoracic sarcoidosis. Eur Respir J 1990;3:447–9.

374. Rizzato G, Colombo P. Nephrolithiasis as a presenting feature of chronic sarcoidosis: a prospective study. Sarcoidosis Vasc Diffuse Lung Dis 1996;13:167–72.

375. O'Leary TJ, Jones G, Yip A, et al. The effects of chloroquine on serum 1,25-dihydroxyvitamin D and calcium metabolism in sarcoidosis. N Engl J Med 1986;315:727–30.

376. Rizzato G, Montemurro L. The clinical spectrum of the sarcoid peripheral lymph node. Sarcoidosis Vasc Diffuse Lung Dis 2000;17:71–80.

377. Britt AR, Francis IR, Glazer GM, Ellis JH. Sarcoidosis: abdominal manifestations at CT. Radiology 1991;178: 91–4.

378. Munker M, Sharma OP. Fatal gastrointestinal haemorrhage in sarcoidosis: a previously unreported occurrence. Sarcoidosis 1987;4:55–7.

379. Sprague R, Harper P, McClain S, et al. Disseminated gastrointestinal sarcoidosis. Case report and review of the literature. Gastroenterology 1984;87:421–5.

380. MacRury SM, McQuaker G, Morton R, Hume R. Sarcoidosis: association with small bowel disease and folate deficiency. J Clin Pathol 1992;45:823–5.

381. Lindgren A, Engstrom CP, Nilsson O, Abrahamsson H. Protein-losing enteropathy in an unusual form of sarcoidosis. Eur J Gastroenterol Hepatol 1995;7:1005–7.

382. Hilzenrat N, Spanier A, Lamoureux E, et al. Colonic obstruction secondary to sarcoidosis: nonsurgical diagnosis and management. Gastroenterology 1995;108:1556–9.

383. Tinker MA, Viswanathan B, Laufer H, Margolis IB. Acute appendicitis and pernicious anemia as complications of gastrointestinal sarcoidosis. Am J Gastroenterol 1984;79: 868–72.

384. Freed JS, Reiner MH. Acute cholecystitis as a complication of sarcoidosis. Arch Intern Med 1983;143(11):2188–9.

385. Rouillon A, Menkes CJ, Gerster JC, et al. Sarcoid-like forms of Whipple's disease. Report of 2 cases. J Rheumatol 1993;20:1070–2.

386. Papadopoulos KI, Sjoberg K, Lindgren S, Hallengren B. Evidence of gastrointestinal immune reactivity in patients with sarcoidosis. J Intern Med 1999;245:525–31.

387. Devaney K, Goodman ZD, Epstein MS, et al. Hepatic sarcoidosis. Clinicopathologic features in 100 patients. Am J Surg Pathol 1993;17:1272–80.

388. Murphy JR, Sjögren MH, Kikendall JW, et al. Small bile duct abnormalities in sarcoidosis. J Clin Gastroenterol 1990;12: 555–61.

389. Galwankar S, Vyas M, Desai D, Udwadia ZF. Hepatic sarcoidosis responding to chloroquine as steroid-sparing drug. Indian J Gastroenterol 1999;18:177–8.

390. Chida K, Shirai M, Sato M, et al. Successful treatment of

hepatic sarcoidosis with hormone replacement in a post menopausal woman. Respirology 1999;4:259–6.

391. Baratta L, Cascino A, Delfino M, et al. Ursodeoxycholic acid treatment in abdominal sarcoidosis. Dig Dis Sci 2000;45: 1559–62

392. Melissant CF, Smith SJ, Kazzaz BA, Demedts M. Bleeding varices due to portal hypertension in sarcoidosis. Favorable effect of propranolol and prednisone. Chest 1993;103: 628–9.

393. Mullins PD, Youngs GR. Favourable prognosis following variceal haemorrhage complicating hepatic sarcoidosis. Eur J Gastroenterol Hepatol 1995;7:185–6.

394. Garcia C, Kumar V, Sharma OP. Pancreatic sarcoidosis. Sarcoidosis Vasc Diffuse Lung Dis 1996;13:28–32.

395. Brincker H. Coexistence of sarcoidosis and malignant disease: causality or coincidence? Sarcoidosis 1989;6:31–43.

396. Toner GC, Bosl GJ. Sarcoidosis, "Sarcoid-like lymphadeno-pathy," and testicular germ cell tumors. Am J Med 1990; 89:651–6.

397. Leatham EW, Eeles R, Sheppard M, et al. The association of germ cell tumours of the testis with sarcoid-like processes. Clin Oncol (R Coll Radiol) 1992;4:89–95.

398. Nakamura M, Iemura A, Kojiro M, et al. Leiomyosarcoma of the rectum with sarcoid-like reaction—a case report. Kurume Med J 1990;37:171–5.

399. Campbell F, Douglas-Jones AG. Sarcoid-like granulomas in primary renal cell carcinoma. Sarcoidosis 1993;10:128–31.

400. White A, Flaris N, Elmer D, et al. Coexistence of mucinous cystadenoma of the ovary and ovarian sarcoidosis. Am J Obstet Gynecol 1990;162:1284–5.

401. Fossa SD, Abeler V, Marton PF, et al. Sarcoid reaction of hilar and paratracheal lymph nodes in patients treated for testicular cancer. Cancer 1985;56:2212–6.

402. Seersholm N, Vestbo J, Viskum K. Risk of malignant neoplasms in patients with pulmonary sarcoidosis. Thorax 1997;53:892–4.

403. Romer FK, Hommelgaard P, Schou G. Sarcoidosis and cancer revisited: a long-term follow-up study of 555 Danish sarcoidosis patients. Eur Respir J 1999;12:906–12.

404. Haynes de Regt R. Sarcoidosis and pregnancy. Obstet Gynecol 1987;70:369–72.

405. King TE Jr. Restrictive lung disease in pregnancy. Clin Chest Med 1992;13:607–22.

406. James WB, Thompson AD. The course of sarcoidosis and its modification by treatment. Lancet 1959;i:1057–61.

407. James DG, Timmis B, Barter S, Carstairs S. Radiology of sarcoidosis. Sarcoidosis 1989;6:7–14.

408. Citron KM. Intrathoracic sarcoidosis. Postgrad Med J 1958;34:268–73.

409. DeRemee RA. The roentgenographic staging of sarcoidosis: historic and contemporary perspectives. Chest 1983;83:128–32.

410. Thomas PD, Hunninghake GW. State of art. Current concepts of the pathogenesis of sarcoidosis. Am Rev Respir Dis 1987;135:747–60.

411. Hillerdal G, Nou E, Osterman K, Schmekel B. Sarcoidosis: epidemiology and prognosis. A 15 year European study. Am Rev Respir Dis 1984;130:29–32.

412. Honeybourne D. Ethnic differences in the clinical features of sarcoidosis in southeast London. Br J Dis Chest 1980;74:63–9.

413. Reich JM, Johnson RE. Course and prognosis of sarcoidosis in a nonreferral setting: analysis of 86 patients observed for 10 years. Am J Med 1985;78:61–7.

414. Lynch JP, Strieter RM. Sarcoidosis. In: Lynch JP, DeRemee RA, editors. Immunologically mediated pulmonary diseases. Philadelphia: Lippincott; 1991.

415. Johns CJ, MacGregor MI, Zachary JB, Ball WC. Extended experience in the long-term corticosteroid treatment of pulmonary sarcoidosis. Ann N Y Acad Sci 1976;278:722–31.

416. Levinsky L, Commiskey J, Romer FK. Sarcoidosis in Europe: a cooperative study. Ann N Y Acad Sci 1976;278:335–46.

417. Israel HL, Karlin P, Menduke H, DeLisser OG. Factors affecting outcome in sarcoidosis: influence of race, extrathoracic involvement, and initial radiologic lung lesions. Ann N Y Acad Sci 1986;465:609–18.

418. Kirtland SH, Winterbauer RH. Pulmonary sarcoidosis. Semin Respir Med 1993;14:344–52.

419. Gottlieb JE, Israel HL, Steiner RM, et al. Outcome in sarcoidosis. The relationship of relapse to corticosteroid therapy. Chest 1997;111:623–31.

420. Selroos O, Sellergren TL. Corticosteroid therapy of pulmonary sarcoidosis: a prospective evaluation of alternate day and daily dosage in stage II disease. Scand J Respir Dis 1979; 60:215–21.

421. Israel HL, Fouts DW, Beggs RE. A controlled trial of prednisone treatment of sarcoidosis. Am Rev Respir Dis 1973; 107:609–14.

422. Young RL, Harkerload LE, Lordon RE, Weg JG. Pulmonary sarcoidosis: a prospective evaluation of glucocorticoid therapy. Ann Intern Med 1970;73:207–12.

423. Harkerload LE, Young RL, Savage PJ, et al. Pulmonary sarcoidosis: long-term follow-up of the effects of steroid therapy. Chest 1982;82:84–7.

424. Gibson GJ, Prescott RJ, Muers MF, et al. British Thoracic Society Sarcoidosis study: effects of long term corticosteroid treatment. Thorax 1996;51:238–47.

425. Chittock DR, Joseph MG, Paterson NA, McFadden RG. Necrotizing sarcoid granulomatosis with pleural involvement. Clinical and radiographic features. Chest 1994;106:672–6.

426. Tommasini A, Di Vittorio G, Facchinetti F, et al. Pleural effusion in sarcoidosis: a case report. Sarcoidosis 1994;11:138–40.

427. Wilen SB, Rabinowitz JG, Ulreich S, Lyons HA. Pleural involvement in sarcoidosis. Am J Med 1974;57:200–9.

428. Solomon A, Kreel L, McNicol M, Johnson N. Computed tomography in pulmonary sarcoidosis. J Comput Assist Tomogr 1979;3:754–8.

429. Schiffner RO, Sharma OP. Acute pulmonary cavitation in sarcoidosis. West J Med 1977;127:346–9.

430. Ross RJ, Empey DW. Bilateral spontaneous pneumothorax in sarcoidosis. Postgrad Med J 1983;59:106–7.

431. Rockoff SD, Rohatgi PK. Unusual manifestations of thoracic sarcoidosis. AJR Am J Roentgenol 1985;144:513–28.

432. Goldenberg GJ, Greenspan RH. Middle lobe atelectasis due to endobronchial sarcoidosis with hypercalcaemia and renal impairment. N Engl J Med 1960;262:1112–6.

433. Mathieson JR, Mayo JR, Staples CA, Muller NL. Chronic diffuse infiltrative lung disease: comparison of diagnostic accuracy of CT and chest radiography. Radiology 1989; 171:111–6.

434. Dawson WB, Muller NL. High-resolution computed tomography in pulmonary sarcoidosis. Semin Ultrasound CT MR 1990;11:423–9.

435. Kuhlman JE, Fishman EK, Hamper UM, et al. The computed tomographic spectrum of thoracic sarcoidosis. Radiographics 1989;9:449–66.

436. Muller NL, Mawson JB, Mathieson JR, et al. Sarcoidosis: correlation of extent of disease at CT with clinical, functional, and radiographic findings. Radiology 1989;171:613–8.

437. Bergin CJ, Bell DO, Coblentz CL, et al. Sarcoidosis: correlation of pulmonary parenchymal pattern at CT with results of pulmonary function tests. Radiology 1989;171:619–24.

438. Lynch DA, Webb WR, Gamsu G, et al. Computed tomography in pulmonary sarcoidosis. J Comput Assist Tomogr 1989;13:405–10.

439. Leung AN, Brauner MW, Caillat-Vigneron N, et al. Sarcoidosis activity: correlation of HRCT findings with those of 67Ga scanning, bronchoalveolar lavage, and serum angiotensin-converting enzyme assay. J Comput Assist Tomogr 1998;22:229–34.

440. Hansell DM, Milne DG, Wilsher ML, Wells AU. Pulmonary

sarcoidosis: morphologic associations of airflow obstruction at thin-section CT. Radiology 1998;209:697–704.

441. Chung MH, Edinburgh KJ, Webb EM, et al. Mixed infiltrative and obstructive disease on high-resolution CT: differential diagnosis and functional correlates in a consecutive series. J Thorac Imaging 2001;16:69–75.

442. Line BR, Hunninghake GW, Keogh BA, et al. Gallium-67 scanning to stage the alveolitis of sarcoidosis: correlation with clinical studies, pulmonary function studies, and bronchoalveolar lavage. Am Rev Respir Dis 1981;123:440–6.

443. Line BR, Hunninghake GW, Keogh BA, Crystal RG. Gallium-67 scanning as an indicator of the activity of sarcoidosis. In: Fanburg BL, editor. Sarcoidosis and other granulomatous diseases of the lung. New York: Marcel Dekker; 1983. p. 287–22.

444. Crystal RG, Keogh BA, Hunninghake GW, Line BR. The alveolitis of pulmonary sarcoidosis: evaluation of natural history and alveolitis dependent changes in lung function. Am Rev Respir Dis 1983;128:256–65.

445. Abe S, Munakata M, Nishimura M. Gallium-67 scintigraphy, bronchoalveolar lavage, and pathologic changes in patients with pulmonary sarcoidosis. Chest 1984;85:650–5.

446. Klech H, Kohn H, Kummer F, Mostbeck A. Assessment of activity in sarcoidosis. Sensitivity and specificity of 67 gallium scintigraphy, serum ACE levels, chest roentgenography, and blood lymphocyte subpopulations. Chest 1982;82:732–8.

447. Niden AH, Mishkin FS, Salem F, et al. Prognostic significance of gallium lung scans in sarcoidosis. Ann N Y Acad Sci 1986;465:435–43.

448. Baughman RP, Fernandez M, Bosken CH, et al. Comparison of gallium-67 scanning, bronchoalveolar lavage, and serum angiotensin converting enzyme levels in pulmonary sarcoidosis. Predicting response to therapy. Am Rev Respir Dis 1984;129:676–81.

449. Hollinger WM, Staton GW, Fajman WA, et al. Prediction of therapeutic response in steroid-treated pulmonary sarcoidosis: evaluation of clinical parameters, bronchoalveolar lavage, gallium-67 scanning and serum angiotensin converting enzyme levels. Am Rev Respir Dis 1985;132:65–9.

450. Turner-Warwick M, McAllister W, Lawrence R, et al. Corticosteroid treatment in sarcoidosis: do serial lavage lymphocyte counts, serum angiotensin-converting enzyme measurements, and gallium-67 scans help management? Thorax 1986;41:903–13.

451. Beaumont D, Herry JY, Sapene M, et al. Gallium-67 in the evaluation of sarcoidosis: correlations with serum angiotensin converting enzyme and bronchoalveolar lavage. Thorax 1982;37:11–8.

452. Gupta RG, Oparil S, Szidon J, Daise M. Clinical significance of serum angiotensin converting enzyme levels in sarcoidosis. J Lab Clin Med 1979;93:940–9.

453. Lebtahi R, Crestani B, Belmatoug N, et al. Somatostatin receptor scintigraphy and gallium scintigraphy in patients with sarcoidosis. J Nucl Med 2001;42:21–6.

454. Jacobs MP, Baughman RP, Hughes J, Fernandez-Ulloa M. Radioaerosol lung clearance in patients with active pulmonary sarcoidosis. Am Rev Respir Dis 1985;131:687–9.

455. Dusser DJ, Collignon MA, Stanislas-Leguern G, et al. Respiratory clearance of 99mTc-DTPA and pulmonary involvement in sarcoidosis. Am Rev Respir Dis 1986;134:493–7.

456. Chinet T, Dusser D, Labrune S, et al. Lung function declines in patients with pulmonary sarcoidosis and increased respiratory epithelial permeability to 99mTc-DTPA. Am Rev Respir Dis 1990;141:445–9.

457. Bradvick I, Wollmer P, Evander E, et al. One year follow-up of lung clearance of 99Tc-diethylene triamine penta-acetic acid and disease activity in sarcoidosis. Sarcoidosis Vasc Diffuse Lung Dis 2000;17:281–7.

458. Harrison BDW, Shaylor JM, Stokes TC, Wilkes AR. Airflow limitation in sarcoidosis—a study of pulmonary function in 107 patients with newly diagnosed disease. Respir Med 1991;85:59–64.

459. Winterbauer RH, Hutchinson JF. Use of pulmonary function tests in sarcoidosis. Chest 1980;78:640–7.

460. Young RL, Lourden RE, Krumholz RA, et al. Pulmonary sarcoidosis. I. Pathophysiologic correlations. Am Rev Respir Dis 1968;97:997–1008.

461. Carrington CB, Gaensler EA, Mikus JP, et al. Structure and function in sarcoidosis. Seventh International Conference on Sarcoidosis and Other Granulomatous Disorders. Ann N Y Acad Sci 1976;278:265–84.

462. Huang CT, Heurich AE, Rosen Y, et al. Pulmonary sarcoidosis: roentgenographic, functional and pathologic correlations. Respiration 1979;37:337–45.

463. Colp C. Sarcoidosis: course and treatment. Med Clin North Am 1977;61:84–93.

464. Costabel U, Zaiss AW, Guzman J. Sensitivity and specificity of BAL findings in sarcoidosis. In: Izumi T, editor. Proceedings of the 1991 XII World Congress on Sarcoidosis. Milan: Sigilim s.r.l. Edizioni Bongraf; 1992. p. 211–4.

465. Reynolds HY. Bronchoalveolar lavage. Am Rev Respir Dis 1987;135:250–63.

466. Kantrow SP, Meyer KC, Kidd P, Raghu G. The CD4/CD8 ratio in BAL fluid is highly variable in sarcoidosis. Eur Respir J 1997;10:2699–700.

467. Kolopp-Sarda MN, Kohler C, De March AK, et al. Discriminative immunophenotype of bronchoalveolar lavage CD4 lymphocytes in sarcoidosis. Lab Invest 2000;80:1065–9.

468. Yamamoto M, Sharma OP, Hosoda Y. The 1991 descriptive definition of sarcoidosis. In: Izumi T, editor. Proceedings of the 1991 XII World Congress on Sarcoidosis. Milan: Sigilim s.r.l. Edizioni Bongraf; 1992. p. 34.

469. Lawrence EC, Teague RB, Gottlieb MS, et al. Serial changes in markers of disease activity with corticosteroid treatment in sarcoidosis. Am J Med 1983;74:747–56.

470. Bjermer L, Rosenhall L, Angstrom T, Hallgren R. Predictive value of bronchalveolar lavage cell analysis in sarcoidosis. Thorax 1988;43:284–8.

471. Foley MM, Coral AP, Tung K, et al. Bronchoalveolar lavage cell counts as a predictor of short term outcome in pulmonary sarcoidosis. Thorax 1989;44:732–8.

472. Verstraeten A, Demedts M, Verwilghen J, et al. Predictive value of bronchoalveolar lavage in pulmonary sarcoidosis. Chest 1990;98:560–7.

473. Buchalter S, App W, Jackson L, et al. Bronchoalveolar lavage cell analysis in sarcoidosis: a comparison of lymphocyte counts and clinical course. Ann N Y Acad Sci 1986;465:678–84.

474. Israel-Biet D, Venet A, Chretien J. Persistent high alveolar lymphocytosis as a predictive criteria of chronic pulmonary sarcoidosis. Ann N Y Acad Sci 1986;465:395–406.

475. Laviolette M, La Forge J, Tennina S, Boulet LP. Prognostic value of bronchoalveolar lavage lymphocyte count in recently diagnosed pulmonary sarcoidosis. Chest 1991;100:380–4.

476. Drent M, Jacobs JA, de Vries J, et al. Does the cellular bronchoalveolar lavage fluid profile reflect the severity of sarcoidosis? Eur Respir J 1999;13:1338–44.

477. D'Ippolito R, Foresi A, Chetta A, et al. Induced sputum in patients with newly diagnosed sarcoidosis: comparison with bronchial wash and BAL. Chest 1999;115:1611–5.

478. Costabel U, Bross KJ, Guzman J, et al. Predictive value of bronchoalveolar T-cell subsets for the course of pulmonary sarcoidosis. Ann N Y Acad Sci 1986;465:418–26.

479. Bauer W, Gorney MK, Baumann HR, Morell A. T-lymphocyte subsets and immunoglobulin concentrations in bronchoalveolar lavage of patients with sarcoidosis and high and low intensity alveolitis. Am Rev Respir Dis 1985;132:1060–5.

480. Ceuppens JL, Lacquet LM, Marien G, et al. Alveolar T-cell

subsets in pulmonary sarcoidosis: correlation with disease activity and effect of steroid treatment. Am Rev Respir Dis 1984;129:563–8.

481. Ward K, O'Connor C, Odlum C, FitzGerald MX. Prognostic value of bronchoalveolar lavage in sarcoidosis: the critical influence of disease presentation. Thorax 1989;44:6–12.

482. Gilman MJ, Wang KP. Transbronchial lung biopsy in sarcoidosis. Am Rev Respir Dis 1980;122:721–4.

483. Mitchell DM, Mitchell DN, Collins JV, Emerson CJ. Transbronchial lung biopsy through fibreoptic bronchoscope in diagnosis of sarcoidosis. BMJ 1980;280:679–81.

484. Bilaceroglu S, Perim K, Gunel O, et al. Combining transbronchial aspiration with endobronchial and transbronchial biopsy in sarcoidosis. Monaldi Arch Chest Dis 1999;54:217–23.

485. Mikhail JR, Shepherd M, Mitchell DN. Mediastinal lymph node biopsy in sarcoidosis. Endoscopy 1979;11:5–8.

486. Sherlock S. Diseases of the liver and biliary system. Oxford: Blackwell Scientific Publications; 1985. p. 443.

487. Scadding JG. Insensitivity to tuberculin in pulmonary sarcoidosis. Tubercle 1956;37:371–80.

488. Ishioka S, Fujihara M, Takaishi M, et al. Anti-Kveim monoclonal antibody—new monoclonal antibody reacting to epithelioid cells in sarcoid granulomas. Chest 1999;98:1255–8.

489. Renston JP, Goldman ES, Hsu RM, et al. Peripheral blood eosinophilia in association with sarcoidosis. Mayo Clin Proc 2000;75:586–90.

490. Lieberman J. Evaluation of serum angiotensin converting enzyme (ACE) level in sarcoidosis. Am J Med 1975;59:365–72.

491. Selroos O, Gronhagen-Riska C. Angiotensin converting enzyme. III. Changes in serum level as an indicator of disease activity in untreated sarcoidosis. Scand J Respir Dis 1979;60:328–36.

492. Gronhagen-Riska C, Selroos O, Wager G, Fyhrquist F. Angiotensin converting enzyme. II. Serum activity in early and newly diagnosed sarcoidosis. Scand J Respir Dis 1979; 60:94–101.

493. DeRemee RA, Rohrback MS. Serum angiotensin converting enzyme activity in evaluating the clinical course of sarcoidosis. Ann Intern Med 1980;92:361–5.

494. Turton CW, Grundy E, Firth G, et al. Value of measuring serum angiotensin I converting enzyme and serum lysozyme in the management of sarcoidosis. Thorax 1979; 34:57–62.

495. Ueda E, Kawabe T, Tachibana T, Kokuba T. Serum angiotensin converting enzyme activity as an indicator of prognosis in sarcoidosis. Am Rev Respir Dis 1980;121:667–71.

496. Selroos OB. Biochemical markers of sarcoidosis. Crit Rev Clin Lab Sci 1986;24:185–216.

497. Studdy RP, James DG. The specificity and sensitivity of serum angiotensin converting enzyme in sarcoidosis and other disease. Experience in twelve centres in six different countries. In: Chretien J, editor. Sarcoidosis and other granulomatous diseases. Paris: Pergamon Press; 1983.

498. Almanoff J, Skovrow ML, Teirstein AS. Thermolysine-like serum metallo-endopeptidase. A new marker for active sarcoid that complements serum angiotensin converting enzyme. Ann N Y Acad Sci 1986;465:738–43.

499. Valeyre D, Saumon G, Georges R, et al. The relationship between disease duration and noninvasive pulmonary explorations in sarcoidosis with erythema nodosum. Am Rev Respir Dis 1984;129:938–43.

500. Weaver LJ, Solliday NH, Celic L, Cugell D. Serial observations of angiotensin converting enzyme and pulmonary function in sarcoidosis. Arch Intern Med 1981;141:931–4.

501. Gronhagen-Riska C, Selroos O. Angiotensin converting enzyme. IV. Changes in serum activity and in lysozyme concentrations as indicators of the course of untreated sarcoidosis. Scand J Respir Dis 1979;60:337–44.

502. Rohatgi PK, Ryan JW, Lindeman P. Value of serial manage-

503. Ainslie GM, Benatar SR. Serum angiotensin converting enzyme in sarcoidosis: sensitivity and specificity in diagnosis: correlation with disease activity, duration, extrathoracic involvement radiographic type and therapy. QJM 1985;55:253–70.

504. Stokes GS, Monaghan JC, Schrader AP, et al. Influence of angiotensin converting enzyme (ACE) genotype on interpretation of diagnostic tests for serum ACE activity. Aust N Z J Med 1999;29:315–8.

505. Reynolds HY. Pulmonary sarcoidosis: do cellular and immunochemical lung parameters exist that would separate subgroups of patients for prognosis? Sarcoidosis 1989;6:1–4.

506. Pozzi E, Ghio P, Albera C. Sarcoid disease markers. Sarcoidosis 1988;5:162–5.

507. Pascual RS, Gee JBL, Finch SC. Usefulness of serum lysozyme measurement in diagnosis and evaluation of sarcoidosis. N Engl J Med 1973;289:1074–6.

508. Selroos O, Klockars M. Serum lysozyme in sarcoidosis. Evaluation of its usefulness in determination of disease activity. Scand J Respir Dis 1977;58:110–6.

509. Schmekel B, Hallgren R, Stalenheim G, Venge P. Indices of inflammatory cell activity and pulmonary function in different stages of sarcoidosis. Acta Med Scand 1982;211: 393–9.

510. Rohatgi PK, Ryan JW. Serum angiotensin converting enzyme (SACE) and carboxypeptidase N(CPN) activities in sarcoidosis and other chronic lung diseases. Am Rev Respir Dis 1982;125:115.

511. Taylor A. Serum adenosine deaminase activity is increased in sarcoidosis. Clin Chem 1984;30:499–500.

512. Klockars M, Petterson T, Selroos O, Weber T. Activity of serum adenosine deaminase in sarcoidosis. Clin Chem 1985;31:155.

513. Gadek JE, Kelman JA, Fells GA, et al. Collagenase in the lower respiratory tract of patients with idiopathic pulmonary fibrosis. N Engl J Med 1979;301:737–42.

514. Ward K, O'Connor CM, Odlum C, et al. Pulmonary disease progress in sarcoid patients with and without bronchoalveolar lavage collagenase. Am Rev Respir Dis 1990;142:636–41.

515. Blaschke E, Eklund A, Hernbrand R. Extracellular matrix components in bronchoalveolar lavage fluid in sarcoidosis and their relationship to signs of alveolitis. Am Rev Respir Dis 1990;141:1020–5.

516. Low RB, Cutroneo KR, Davies GS, Giancola MS. Lavage type III procollagen N-terminal peptides in human pulmonary fibrosis and sarcoidosis. Lab Invest 1983;48:755–9.

517. Prior C, Barbee RA, Evans PM, et al. Lavage versus serum measurements of lysozyme, angiotensin converting enzyme and other inflammatory markers in pulmonary sarcoidosis. Eur Respir J 1990;3:1146–54.

518. Ziegenhagen MW, Benner UK, Zissel G, et al. Sarcoidosis: TNF-alpha release from alveolar macrophages and serum level of sIL-2R are prognostic markers. Am J Respir Crit Care Med 1997;156:1586–92.

519. Hashimoto S, Nakayama T, Gon Y, et al. Correlation of plasma monocyte chemoattractant protein-1 (MCP-1) and monocyte inflammatory protein-1alpha (MIP-1alpha) levels with disease activity and clinical course of sarcoidosis. Clin Exp Immunol 1998;111:604–10.

520. Kohno N. Serum marker KL-6/MUCI for the diagnosis and management of interstitial pneumonitis. J Med Invest 1999;46:151–8.

521. du Bois RM. Corticosteroids in sarcoidosis: friend or foe? Eur Respir J 1994;7:1203–9.

522. Robinson BWS, McLemore TL, Crystal RG. Gamma interferon is spontaneously released by alveolar macrophages and lung T lymphocytes in patients with pulmonary sarcoidosis. J Clin Invest 1985;75:1488–95.

523. Pinkston P, Saltini C, Muller-Quernheim J, Crystal RG. Corticosteroid therapy suppresses spontaneous interleukin 2 release and spontaneous proliferation of lung T lymphocytes of patients with active pulmonary sarcoidosis. J Immunol 1987;139:755–60.

524. Munck A, Mendel DB, Smith LI, Orti E. Glucocorticoid receptors and actions. Am Rev Respir Dis 1990;141:S2–S10.

525. Hunninghake GW, Gilbert S, Pueringer R, et al. Outcome of the treatment for sarcoidosis. Am J Respir Crit Care Med, 1994;149:893–8.

526. Zaki MH, Lyons HA, Leilop L, Huang CT. Corticosteroid therapy in sarcoidosis. A five year, controlled follow-up study. N Y State J Med 1987;87:496–9.

527. Odlum CM, FitzGerald MX. Evidence that steroids alter the natural history of previously untreated progressive pulmonary sarcoidosis. Sarcoidosis 1986;3:40–6.

528. Paramothayan NS, Jones PW. Corticosteroids for pulmonary sarcoidosis (Cochrane Review). In: The Cochrane Library, 2. Oxford: Update Software; 2001.

529. Sharma OP. Pulmonary sarcoidosis and corticosteroids. Am Rev Respir Dis 1993;147:1598–600.

530. Selroos O. Treatment of sarcoidosis. Sarcoidosis 1994;11:80–3.

531. Newman LS, Rose CS, Maier LA. Sarcoidosis. N Engl J Med 1997;336:1224–34.

532. Johns CJ, Zachary JB, Ball WC Jr. A ten-year study of corticosteroid treatment of pulmonary sarcoidosis. Johns Hopkins Med J 1974;134:271–83.

533. Rizzato G, Montemurro L, Colmbo P. The late follow-up of chronic sarcoid patients previously treated with corticosteroids. Sarcoidosis Vasc Diffuse Lung Dis 1998;15:19–20.

534. Spratling L, Tenholder MF, Underwood GH, et al. Daily vs alternate day prednisone therapy for stage II sarcoidosis. Chest 1985;88:687–90.

535. Selroos O, Sellergren TL. Corticosteroid therapy of pulmonary sarcoidosis. A prospective evaluation of alternate day and daily dosage in stage II disease. Scand J Respir Dis 1979;60:215–21.

536. Bersani TA, Nichols CW. Intralesional triamcinolone for cutaneous palpebral sarcoidosis. Am J Ophthalmol 1985;99: 561–2.

537. Gallivan GJ, Landis JN. Sarcoidosis of the larynx: preserving and restoring airway and professional voice. J Voice 1993;7:81–94.

538. Wallaert B, Ramon P, Fournier EC, et al. High-dose methylprednisolone pulse therapy in sarcoidosis. Eur J Respir Dis 1986;68:256–62.

539. Spiteri MA, Newman SP, Clarke SW, Poulter LW. Inhaled corticosteroids can modulate the immunopathogenesis of pulmonary sarcoidosis. Eur Respir J 1989;2:218–24.

540. Hasani A, Spiteri M, Pavia D, et al. Tracheobronchial clearance in patients with pulmonary sarcoidosis. Chest 1992;101: 1614–8.

541. Erkkila S, Froseth B, Hellstrom PE, et al. Inhaled budesonide influences cellular and biochemical abnormalities in pulmonary sarcoidosis. Sarcoidosis 1988;5:106–10.

542. Selroos OB. Use of budesonide in the treatment of pulmonary sarcoidosis. Ann N Y Acad Sci 1986;465:713–21.

543. Alberts C, van der Mark TW, Jansen HM. Inhaled budesonide in pulmonary sarcoidosis: a double-blind, placebo-controlled study. Dutch Study Group on Pulmonary Sarcoidosis. Eur Respir J 1995;8:682–8.

544. Milman N, Graudal N, Grode G, Munch E. No effect of high-dose inhaled steroids in pulmonary sarcoidosis: a double-blind, placebo-controlled study. J Intern Med 1994;236: 285–90.

545. Pietinalho A, Tukiainen P, Haahtela T, et al. Oral prednisolone followed by inhaled budesonide in newly diagnosed pulmonary sarcoidosis: a double-blind, placebo-controlled multicenter study. Finnish Pulmonary Sarcoidosis Study Group. Chest 1999;116:424–31.

546. Zych D, Pawlicka L, Zielinski J. Inhaled budesonide vs prednisone in the maintenance treatment of pulmonary sarcoidosis. Sarcoidosis 1993;10:56–61.

547. du Bois RM, Greenhalgh PM, Southcott AM, et al. Randomized trial of inhaled fluticasone propionate in chronic stable pulmonary sarcoidosis: a pilot study. Eur Respir J 1999; 13:1345–50.

548. Selroos O. Inhaled corticosteroids and pulmonary sarcoidosis. Sarcoidosis 1988;5:104–5.

549. Baumann MH, Strange C, Sahn SA. Do chest radiographic findings reflect the clinical course of patients with sarcoidosis during corticosteroid withdrawal? AJR Am J Roentgenol 1990;154:481–5.

550. Anonymous. Chloroquine in the treatment of sarcoidosis. A report from the Research Committee of the British Tuberculosis Association. Tubercle 1967;48:257–72.

551. Sitzbach LE, Teirstein AS. Chloroquine therapy in 43 patients with intrathoracic and cutaneous sarcoidosis. Acta Med Scand Suppl 1964;425:302–8.

552. Morse SI, Cohn ZA, Hirsch JG, et al. The treatment of sarcoidosis with chloroquine. Am J Med 1961;30:779–84.

553. Jones E, Callen JP. Hydroxychloroquine is effective therapy for control of cutaneous sarcoidal granulomas. J Am Acad Dermatol 1990;23:487–9.

554. Adams JS, Diz MM, Sharma OP. Effective reduction in the serum 1,25-dihydroxyvitamin D and calcium concentration in sarcoidosis-associated hypercalcemia with short-course chloroquine therapy. Ann Intern Med 1989;111:437–8.

555. Sharma OP. Effectiveness of chloroquine and hydroxychloroquine in treating selected patients with sarcoidosis with neurological involvement. Arch Neurol 1998;55:1248–54.

556. Baltzan M, Mehta S, Kirkham TH, Cosio MG. Randomized trial of prolonged chloroquine therapy in advanced pulmonary sarcoidosis. Am J Respir Crit Care Med 1999;160:192–7.

557. Lower EE, Baughman RP. The use of low dose methotrexate in refractory sarcoidosis. Am J Med Sci 1990;299:153–7.

558. Lower EE, Baughman RP. Prolonged use of methotrexate for sarcoidosis. Arch Intern Med 1995;155:846–51.

559. Baughman RP, Winget DB, Lower EE. Methotrexate is steroid sparing in acute sarcoidosis: results of a double blind, randomized trial. Sarcoidosis Vasc Diffuse Lung Dis 2000; 17:60–6.

560. Baughman RP, Lower EF. A clinical approach to the use of methotrexate for sarcoidosis. Thorax 1999;54:742–6.

561. Hargreaves MR, Mowat AG, Benson MK. Acute pneumonitis associated with low dose methotrexate treatment for rheumatoid arthritis: report of five cases and review of published reports. Thorax 1992;47:628–33.

562. Kremer JM, Alarcon GS, Lightfoot Jr GW, et al. Methotrexate for rheumatoid arthritis. Suggested guidelines for monitoring liver toxicity. American College of Rheumatology. Arthritis Rheum 1994;37:316–28.

563. Webster GF, Razsi LK, Sanchez M, Shupack JL. Weekly low-dose methotrexate therapy for cutaneous sarcoidosis. J Am Acad Dermatol 1991;24:451–4.

564. Veien NK, Brodthagen H. Cutaneous sarcoidosis treated with methotrexate. Br J Dermatol 1977;97:213–6.

565. Gedalia A, Molina JF, Ellis GS Jr, et al. Low-dose methotrexate therapy for childhood sarcoidosis. J Pediatr 1997;130:25–9.

566. Kaye O, Palazzo E, Grossin M, et al. Low-dose methotrexate: an effective corticosteroid-sparing agent in the musculoskeletal manifestations of sarcoidosis. Br J Rheumatol 1995;34:642–4.

567. Sharma O, Hughes D, James D, Naish P. Immunosuppressive therapy with azathioprine in sarcoidosis. In: Levinsky L, Macholoa F, editors. Fifth International Conference on Sarcoidosis and Other granulomatous Disorders. Prague: Universita Karlova; 1971. p. 635–7.

568. Pacheco Y, Marechal C, Marechal F, et al. Azathioprine treat-

ment of chronic pulmonary sarcoidosis. Sarcoidosis 1985;2:107–13.

569. Lewis SJ, Ainslie GM, Bateman ED. Efficacy of azathioprine as second-line treatment in pulmonary sarcoidosis. Sarcoidosis Vasc Diffuse Lung Dis 1999;16:87–92.

570. Muller-Quernheim J, Kienast K, Held M, et al. Treatment of chronic sarcoidosis with an azathioprine/prednisolone regimen. Eur Respir J 1999;14:1000–1.

571. Harding CV, Unanue ER. Cellular mechanisms of antigen processing and the function of class I and II major histocompatibility complex molecules. Cell Regul 1990;1:499–509.

572. Israel HL, McComb BL. Chlorambucil treatment of sarcoidosis. Sarcoidosis 1991;8:35–41.

573. Kataria YP. Chlorambucil in sarcoidosis. Chest 1980;78:36–43.

574. Martinet Y, Pinkston P, Saltini C, et al. Evaluation of the in vitro effects of cyclosporine on the lung T-lymphocyte alveolitis of active pulmonary sarcoidosis. Am Rev Respir Dis 1988;138:1242–8.

575. Wyser CP, van Schalkwyk EM, Alheit B, et al. Treatment of progressive pulmonary sarcoidosis with cyclosporin A. A randomized controlled trial. Am J Respir Crit Med 1997;156:1369–70.

576. Pia G, Pascalis L, Arescu G, et al. Evaluation of the efficacy and toxicity of the Cyclosporin-A-Flucortolone-Methetrexate combination in the treatment of sarcoidosis. Sarcoidosis Vasc Diffuse Lung Dis 1996;13(2):146–52.

577. Cunnah D, Chew S, Wass J. Cyclosporin for central nervous system sarcoidosis. Am J Med 1988;85:580–1.

578. Kavanaugh AF, Andrew SL, Cooper B, et al. Cyclosporine therapy of central nervous system sarcoidosis. Am J Med 1987;82:387.

579. Adams JS, Gacad MA, Diz MM, Nadler JL. A role for endogenous arachidonate metabolites in the regulated expression of the 25-hydroxyvitamin D-1-hydroxylation reaction in cultured alveolar macrophages from patients with sarcoidosis. J Clin Endocrinol Metab 1990;70:595–600.

580. Bia MJ, Insogna K. Treatment of sarcoidosis-associated hypercalcemia with ketoconazole. Am J Kidney Dis 1991;18:702–5.

581. Conron M, Beynon HL. Ketoconazole for the treatment of refractory hypercalcemic sarcoidosis. Sarcoidosis Vasc Diffuse Lung Dis 2000;17:277–80.

582. Zabel P, Entzian P, Dalhoff K, Schlaak M. Pentoxifylline in treatment of sarcoidosis. Am J Respir Crit Care Med 1997;155:1665–9.

583. Marques LJ, Zheng L, Poulakis N, et al. Pentoxifylline inhibits TNF-alpha production from human alveolar macrophages. Am J Respir Crit Care Med 1999;159:508–11.

584. Baughman RP, Lower EE. Infliximab for refractory sarcoidosis. Sarcoidosis Vasc Diffuse Lung Dis 2001;18:70–4.

585. Elliot MJ, Maini RN, Feldmann M, et al. Randomized double-blind comparison of chimeric monoclonal antibody to tumour necrosis factor α (cA2) versus placebo in rheumatoid arthritis. Lancet 1994;344:1105–10.

586. Johnson BA, Duncan SR, Ohori NP, et al. Recurrence of sarcoidosis in pulmonary allograft recipients. Am Rev Respir Dis 1993;148:1373–7.

587. Heatly T, Sekela M, Berger R. Single lung transplantation involving a donor with documented pulmonary sarcoidosis. J Heart Lung Transplant 1994;13:720–3.

588. Oni AA, Hershberger RE, Norman DJ, et al. Recurrence of sarcoidosis in a cardiac allograft: control with augmented corticosteroids. J Heart Lung Transplant 1992;11:367–9.

589. Beaufils H, Gompel A, Gubler MC, et al. Pre- and posttransplant glomerulonephritis in a case of sarcoidosis. Nephron 1983;35:124–9.

590. Hakaim AG, Stilmant MM, Kauffman J, et al. Successful renal transplantation in a patient with systemic sarcoidosis and renal failure due to focal glomerulosclerosis. Am J Kidney Dis 1992;19:493–5.

591. Brown JH, Jos V, Newstead CG, Lawler W. Sarcoid-like granulomata in a renal transplant. Nephrol Dial Transplant 1992;7:173.

592. Shen SY, Hall-Craggs M, Posner JN, Shabazz B. Recurrent sarcoid granulomatous nephritis and reactive tuberculin skin test in a renal transplant recipient. Am J Med 1986;80:699–702.

593. Pescovitz MD, Jones HM, Cummings OW, et al. Diffuse retroperitoneal lymphadenopathy following liver transplantation—a case of recurrent sarcoidosis. Transplantation 1995;60:393–6.

594. Baughman RP, Lower EE, Lynch JP. Treatment modalities for sarcoidosis. Clin Pulm Med 1994;1:223–31.

595. Siltzbach LE, James DG, Neville E, et al. Course and prognosis of sarcoidosis around the world. Am J Med 1974;57:847–52.

596. Terris M, Chaves AD. An epidemiologic study of sarcoidosis. Am Rev Respir Dis 1966;94:50–5.

597. Harf RA, Ethevenaux C, Gleize J, et al. Reduced prevalence of smokers in sarcoidosis. Results of a case-control study. Ann N Y Acad Sci 1986;465:625–31.

15

SILICOSIS

DAVID N. WEISSMAN
DANIEL E. BANKS

Silicosis refers to a spectrum of pulmonary diseases caused by the inhalation of free crystalline silicon dioxide (silica).[1,2] Written documentation of silicosis extends to the ancient Egyptians and Greeks.[3,4] Silicosis can be prevented, but it continues to exist. Recognition of sentinel cases (particularly of acute and accelerated silicosis) has important public health implications. Recognizing and investigating these cases can lead to the identification of unsafe work places and prevention of additional cases.

FORMS OF SILICA

Silicon dioxide or silica is the most abundant mineral on earth.[5] It is formed from the elements silicon and oxygen under conditions of increased heat and pressure. Silica exists in crystalline and amorphous forms. The polymorphs of crystalline silica include quartz, cristobalite, tridymite, coesite, and stishovite. With the exception of stishovite (which has an octahedral structure), crystalline forms are based on a tetrahedral structure in which the central atom is silicon, and the corners are occupied by oxygen. Two adjacent tetrahedrons share two oxygen atoms. The most common form of crystalline silica is quartz, a typical component of rocks. Quartz-containing materials used in industry include granite, slate, and sandstone. Granite contains about 30% free silica, slate about 40%, and sandstone is almost pure silica.[6] Cristobalite and tridymite occur naturally in lava and are formed when quartz or amorphous silica is subjected to very high temperatures. They are also formed in silica bricks used in industrial furnaces.

Amorphous silica is noncrystalline and is relatively nontoxic after inhalation. It occurs as diatomite (skeletons of prehistoric marine organisms) or as vitreous silica (the result of carefully melting and then quickly cooling crystalline silica). Heating diatomite with or without alkali (a process known as calcining) forms cristobalite, a material that is very toxic after inhalation.

"Free" crystalline silica is unbound to other minerals; "combined" forms are bound to other minerals. Combined forms are also known as silicates. Examples of silicates used in industry include asbestos, talc ($Mg_3Si_4O_{10}[OH]_2$), and kaolinite ($Al_2Si_2O_5(OH)_4$), a major component of china clay or kaolin.[7,8]

OCCUPATIONAL EXPOSURE TO SILICA

A wide variety of industries are associated with the generation of particulate aerosols with sufficient crystalline silica content to cause silicosis. Any occupation that disturbs the earth's crust or exposes the worker to the use or processing of silica-containing rock or sand has potential risks.[9] Occupations mentioned here are important but this list is by no means complete and continues to change over time. Silicosis can occur in industries and work settings not previously recognized to be at risk.[9] Thus, a high index of suspicion for silicosis should be maintained when the clinical history indicates a dusty work environment.

Mining has long been associated with silicosis. Hippocrates reported that miners developed dyspnea with exertion. Ramazzini and Agricola recognized the relationship between rock dust exposure and the development of dyspnea in miners.[3] Underground mining for metals often disturbs quartz-rich ores and generates respirable quartz-containing aerosols. Silicosis may occur in gold, tin, iron, copper, nickel, silver, tungsten, and uranium mining. Mining for other types of minerals can also cause silicosis. For example, underground coal mining can be associated with silicosis. Especially risky activities include tunneling through or roof bolting into rock with high silica content or using sand as a friction material on rails. Although dust exposure levels are generally lower in surface or strip mining, silicosis has been reported in workers who operate the large drills that make holes in which explosives are placed to expose coal deposits (Figure 15–1).[10]

Tunneling through rock with high silica content, such as granite or sandstone, can generate very significant aerosol exposures to silica. Tunneling was responsible for the worst outbreak of silicosis in U.S. history, which occurred during the construction of the Gauley Bridge Tunnel in West Virginia in 1930 and 1931. More than 400 of the estimated 2,000 men engaged in rock drilling died, and about 1,500 contracted silicosis and were eventually disabled.[3] Other occupations involving the disruption of the earth's crust, such as quarrying and stone cutting, are also associated with risk of silicosis.[11]

Foundry work is another potentially hazardous occupation.[11] Foundries are where metal castings are made. The castings are produced by making a mold into

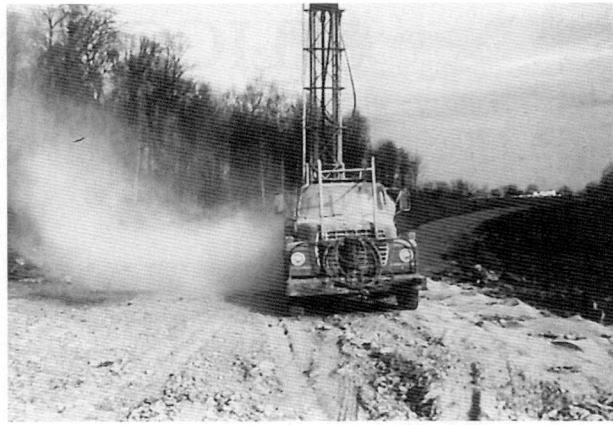

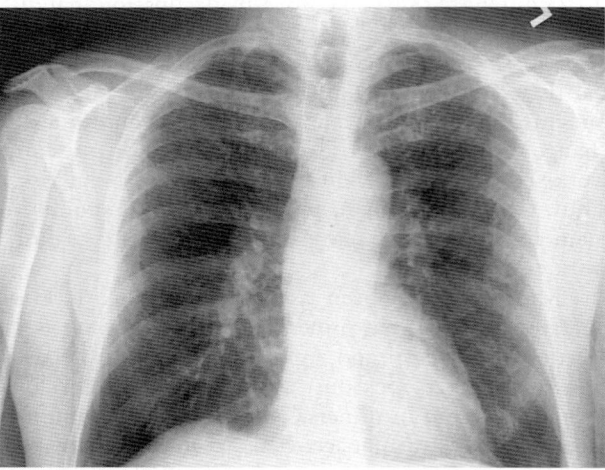

Figure 15–1 *A*, Drilling at a surface coal mine. Note the cloud of dust generated by dry-surface drilling. The operator is exposed to dust as he must be positioned at the back of the truck to monitor drill pressures and change bits as needed. *B*, Simple pneumoconiosis in a bulldozer operator who worked at surface coal mines for 42 years. In the early stages of his career, his bulldozer had an open cab allowing high exposures to dust.

Sandblasting generates respirable aerosols of silica and is associated with great risk for silicosis even when respiratory protection is used.[9,12–14] Sandblasting occurs in ship building, oil rig maintenance, preparing steel for painting, and many other applications where abrasive cleaning of surfaces is required. Sandblasting continues in the U.S. despite the availability of substitutes to sand for abrasive blasting. The United Kingdom has severely restricted the use of abrasives containing silica since 1949, and other European countries abandoned sandblasting in the 1960s. The United States virtually allows the unrestricted use of sand for abrasive blasting, except in the underground mine environment.[15]

Production of silica flour, or finely milled crystalline silica, is associated with the risk of silicosis.[16] This abrasive powder is used in the production of scouring powders, polishes, toothpastes, and sandpaper. It is also used as filler in paints, woods, surfacing materials, rubbers, and plastics.

Production of ceramics has historically been associated with risk of silicosis. Traditionally, a mixture of crushed flint and siliceous clays have been used to form china and earthenware, and the products are polished or fettled prior to glazing. Substitute materials are decreasing the risk of silicosis in this industry.

Diatomaceous earth is amorphous silica and in its native state does not entail a great health hazard. However, if it is calcined, it can be converted into the hazardous crystalline forms cristobalite and tridymite. Exposure to calcined material used in filters, abrasives, insulation materials, and absorbents may cause silicosis in unexpected settings.[11]

Although occupation is the major risk factor for the inhalation of crystalline silica and the development of silicosis, simple silicosis has been reported after environmental exposures in regions where soil silica content is high and dust storms are common.[17]

BIOLOGIC CONSEQUENCES OF SILICA INHALATION

Inhaled crystalline silica particles with favorable characteristics for intrapulmonary deposition are most likely to affect the lungs. The most important characteristic is size. Particles less than 1 μm are believed to be the most pathogenic, and the median diameter of silica particles retained in the human lung range from 0.5 to 0.7 μm.[18] Over time, particle burden within the lung is the result of an equilibrium between dust deposition and dust clearance. Clearance mechanisms include removal in expired air, mucociliary clearance from the upper airways, and phagocytosis by alveolar macrophages with subsequent clearance via either the mucociliary escalator or via pulmonary lymphatics.

The pathogenic mechanisms underlying the induction of inflammation, lung injury, and fibrosis by silicosis are complex.[5] Several processes contribute to the

which molten metal is poured. A core may also be used to produce a hollow casting. After cooling, the solidified casting is then knocked out of the mold. Silica exposure can occur in production of the molds and cores, which are made of quartz sands bonded by clays or resins. However, the greatest risk is associated with knocking out castings and the subsequent cleaning and polishing of the product. Cleaning and polishing is especially dangerous and is known as fettling or dressing. It may be done with hammers, grinding wheels, mills, or abrasive blasting. These activities aerosolize silica, especially the highly toxic cristobalite, which is generated by heating the molds and cores. Foundry workers may also be exposed to inhaled silica when knocking out the linings of furnaces, which often include quartz.

development of disease. First, due to its surface properties, silica is directly cytotoxic to pulmonary target cells. It has been theorized that in the presence of water, the surface of silica becomes hydrated to form silanol groups (-SiOH). These groups may serve as hydrogen donors, with the formation of hydrogen bonds between silica particles and biologic membranes leading to cell damage. In addition, at neutral pH, it is predicted that 1 in 30 -SiOH groups would be negatively charged (–SiO–). Negatively charged silica molecules could react with scavenger receptors on alveolar macrophages, leading to the release of reactive oxygen species and inflammatory cytokines. These, in turn, could cause tissue damage. Finally, silica particles are able to react with water to form hydroxyl radicals. These can react with cell membranes leading to lipid peroxidation and cytotoxicity.[19,20] Of note is that freshly crushed silica forms more hydroxl radicals than similar amounts of aged silica and has been demonstrated to be more cytotoxic, to produce more lipid peroxidation, and to induce alveolar macrophages to produce more superoxide and hydrogen peroxide than does stored or "aged" silica.

Interactions between inhaled silica and target cells such as alveolar macrophages can also generate pulmonary inflammation and fibrosis via a process of cytokine networking between macrophages, lymphocytes, neutrophils, fibroblasts, epithelial cells, and potentially other cell types such as mast cells.[21,22] Alveolar macrophages stimulated in vitro by silica or evaluated ex vivo after in vivo exposure to silica secrete proinflammatory and profibrogenic mediators. For example, enhanced production of interleukin-1β (IL-1β),[23,24] interleukin-6 (IL-6), tumor necrosis factor-α (TNF-α),[25,26] transforming growth factor-β (TGF-β),[27] fibronectin,[28] platelet-derived growth factor (PDGF), and insulin-like growth factor-I (IGF-I)[21] by silica-activated alveolar macrophages have all been demonstrated. Pulmonary stromal cells such as endothelial and smooth muscle cells have the potential to amplify local inflammation by the secretion of chemokines such as IL-8 after stimulation by macrophage-derived IL-1β and TNF-α.[29] Silica may also stimulate chemokine secretion by alveolar epithelial cells by direct action on these cells.[30]

Tumor necrosis factor-α may play a particularly important role in the pathogenesis of silicosis. Increased levels of lung TNF messenger RNA (mRNA) can be demonstrated by in situ hybridization in mice after intratracheal instillation of silica.[25] Deposition of extracellular matrix protein (expressed as an increase in hydroxyproline) can be prevented in this model by pretreatment with anti-TNF antibodies or soluble TNF receptors.[25,31] An inbred strain of TNF-deficient mice shows less inflammation and collagen accumulation in the lungs after instillation of silica when compared with appropriate controls.[32]

The profibrogenic cytokine TGF-β also appears to be important in the pathogenesis of silicosis. It has been demonstrated by immunohistochemical staining in experimental silicosis.[27] In human specimens, TGF-β has been localized in peribronchiolar fibrotic lesions, hyaline centers of nodules, progressive massive fibrosis (PMF) lesions, fibroblasts, and alveolar macrophages of silicotic lungs.[33]

The pathogenesis of acute silicosis is different from that of classic or chronic silicosis. In acute silicosis, the alveoli fill with an amorphous lipoproteinaceous exudate. Animal models of this condition show a dramatic increase in the amounts of intracellular and extracellular phospholipids.[34–36] The composition of lung surfactant is also altered.[37] A distinct population of hypertrophic type II pneumocytes has been observed in experimental acute silicosis. These cells appear to be responsible for the marked increase in the amount of pulmonary surfactant in silica-treated animals.[38,39] In addition to the increased activity of metabolic pathways involved in surfactant production, increased biosynthesis of surfactant protein A (SP-A) and augmented levels of SP-A mRNA have also been shown.[40]

A variety of factors can modify the host response to inhaled silica. The duration and amount of exposure, as well as the content of free crystalline silica, are critical determinants of the progression of silicosis.[9,11,18,41] As previously noted, particle size in the respirable range increases toxicity. Furthermore, freshly fractured silica particles have greater ability to interact with water and generate oxygen radicals and thus may be more toxic than older particles.[19] In the case of mixed dust exposures, the nature of the mixture along with relative silica content is important.

Genetic factors also play a role in modifying the biologic response to inhaled silica. Specific human leukocyte antigen (HLA)-haplotype associations with silicosis have been reported in a Japanese population.[42] In addition, HLA-haplotype associations with coal workers' pneumoconiosis have been reported in a German population.[42] Recent studies have documented relationships between single nucleotide polymorphisms (SNPs) in the genes encoding TNF-α[43] and IL-1 receptor antagonist[43,44] and the development of silicosis.

Previous environmental exposures might also alter the host response to inhaled silica. In one report, experimental exposure to a high concentration of quartz dust produced an alveolar proteinosis response in specific pathogen-free (SPF) rats but resulted in typical granulomatous and fibrotic changes in ordinary stock rats.[45] The only difference seemed to be an inadequately developed lymphatic system in the SPF rats. How previous environmental exposures impact on human responses to silica is unknown. However, differences in responses of smokers and nonsmokers to hard rock mining exposures have been reported.[46]

PATHOLOGY OF SILICOSIS

Detailed reviews of the pathology of silicosis have been published elsewhere.[18,47] Briefly, on gross inspection, the silicotic lung is firm and blacker than normal. The surface is coarse and nodular. The visceral pleura has areas of fibrosis and may be covered by plaquelike lesions. Peribronchial and hilar lymph nodes are typically enlarged. On sectioning, these enlarged nodes show concentrically arranged fibrous tissue. Cutting the lung reveals palpable intrapulmonary nodules, especially in the upper lobes. In simple silicosis, these nodules are usually 2 to 6 mm in diameter. In conglomerate silicosis or progressive massive fibrosis, the lesions are typically 10 to 20 mm in diameter as a result of the coalescence of smaller nodules. Nodules vary in color depending on the presence of other dusts. The extent of nodule calcification is also variable.

The earliest histopathologic lesion in workers with relatively low-dose, chronic exposure to free crystalline silica is a collection of dust-laden macrophages and loose reticulin fibers in the peribronchial, perivascular, and paraseptal or subpleural areas. Later, these lesions become more organized and may appear whorled.

The silicotic nodule is the pathologic hallmark of silicosis (Figure 15–2). Its central zone shows little activity. It is hyalinized and composed of concentrically arranged collagen fibers. The peripheral zone is whorled and becomes less organized toward the edges. It contains macrophages, lymphocytes, and lesser amounts of loosely formed collagen. Under polarized light microscopy, a few weakly birefringent particles may be seen in the center of the nodule, possibly the result of trapped crystalline silica and other dusts. In the periphery of the nodule, the amount of dust and the degree of birefringence differ dramatically. Needle-shaped, strongly birefringent material is intermingled with cells and dust. This is the site of active enlargement of the nodule and of ongoing inflammation. As the disease progresses, the periphery of the silicotic nodule moves farther from the hyalinized center, enmeshing small airways, pleura, and blood and lymphatic vessels in the fibrotic process.

Coalescence of silicotic nodules forms the progressive massive fibrotic lesion, a mass of dense, hyalinized connective tissue with minimal silica content, a small amount of anthracotic pigment, minimal cellular infiltrate, and negligible vascularization. Typically, the centers of these conglomerate lesions cavitate, which is the result of mycobacterial infection or ischemic necrosis when they exceed a certain size.

The histologic pattern of acute silicosis is very different from chronic silicosis. Silicotic nodules are rarely seen and, if identified, are usually poorly developed. The interstitium is thickened with inflammatory cells. There is alveolar filling with proteinaceous material consisting largely of phospholipids or surfactant (or surfactant-like material), which stain with periodic acid–Schiff (PAS) reagent. Because the histologic appearance resembles that of idiopathic alveolar proteinosis, this process occurring in a clinical background of overwhelming silica exposure has also been called silicoproteinosis.[48] On electron microscopic examination,

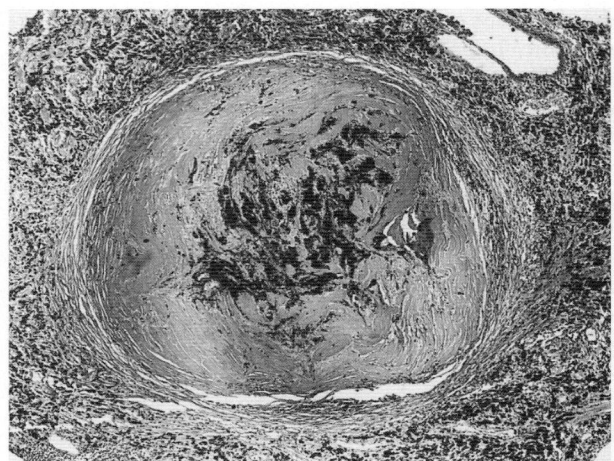

Figure 15–2   Histology section from a patient with silicosis showing a typical silicotic nodule.

the alveoli are lined with prominent epithelial cells, the majority of which are hypertrophic type II pneumocytes.[49] The alveolar exudate is most likely the result of overproduction of phospholipids and surfactant-associated proteins by these hypertrophic type II cells. In addition, desquamated pneumocytes, macrophages, and silica particles are found in the alveolar spaces. Typically, a minimal amount of pulmonary fibrosis is present. Therefore, although the term silicoproteinosis may reflect one of the pathologic changes present, other features of acute alveolar damage syndromes and even of desquamative interstitial pneumonitis are a part of the recognized lung injury.

EPIDEMIOLOGY OF SILICOSIS

The true prevalence of silicosis is difficult to estimate because of the many different occupations involved, the participation of transient workers, and the variability of disease detection methods (eg, autopsy versus compensation or screening data) and reporting practices from place to place. It is common for silicosis to be diagnosed after a worker has left the silica-exposed industry and for it to continue to progress slowly over many decades of life after the exposure has ended. Thus, higher prevalence levels and estimates of exposure risk have been published when studies have included retired workers.[50,51]

In 1956, Trasko obtained estimates of silicosis prevalence by examining records of workers in 20 states who were compensated for silicosis.[52] About 6,000 cases were identified with the largest numbers of cases among metal miners (1,637) and foundry workers (1,645). Autopsy records of 3,365 underground miners submitted to the U.S. National Coal Workers' Autopsy Study between 1971 and 1980 revealed the presence of classic silicotic nodules in 12.5% of the cases.[53] In 1991, it was estimated that 200,000 miners and 1.7 million nonmining workers in the United States had occupational exposures to inhaled silica.[54] Silicosis was identified in 577 workers in the state of Michigan over the period between 1987 and 1995 through a state surveillance system.[55] In the United States between 1987 and 1996, 2,787 deaths were attributed to silicosis.[56]

The prevalence of silicosis increases with increasing silica dust exposure.[41] Conversely, the risk of silicosis can be decreased by appropriate engineering controls to decrease inhalation exposure. The Vermont granite industry is an excellent example of prevention through the control of dust exposure. Workers historically endured heavy silica dust exposures as a result of activities such as granite grinding and chipping. Earlier this century, two studies evaluating this population documented serious dust-induced lung disease and premature death.[57,58] However, beginning in the 1950s, there was evidence that the institution of dust-control measures had produced a safer workplace.[59,60] These data serve as the backbone for current federal regulations for permissible silica exposure. A recent study of Vermont granite workers with initial exposure after 1955 (when exposure limits stabilized at current levels) documented a decreased burden of disease, but 3.5% of these workers still had x-ray film abnormalities consistent with silicosis.[61] Other studies also suggest a continued (even if improved) lifetime risk for silicosis at current exposure levels.[50,51] Continued risk is likely due to both a current permissible exposure level (PEL) that is not completely protective and a lack of compliance with the current PEL.[15]

RADIOGRAPHIC PATTERNS OF SILICOSIS

Specific terminology is used to describe chest radiographic patterns of lung involvement in silicosis. These radiographic patterns together with clinical features such as the duration of clinical exposure to the recognition of disease, define the various clinical types of silicosis.[2]

Two important terms describing the chest radiographic patterns of lung involvement in silicosis are *simple silicosis* and *progressive massive fibrosis*. These two patterns have different radiographic appearances, but are part of a spectrum of illness. Simple silicosis is a profusion of small (less than 10 mm in diameter) opacities (nodules), generally rounded, but sometimes irregular, predominantly in the upper lung zones (Figure 15–3). In some cases, these small opacities gradually enlarge and coalesce to form larger, upper- or midzone opacities of more than 10 mm in diameter. This condition is referred to as conglomerate silicosis or PMF (Figure 15–4). As these opacities progressively enlarge, the hila are retracted upward and the lower zones become hyperinflated. The opacities of PMF often cause concern that a neoplastic process is present, particularly if the opacities are not symmetrical.

Another radiographic presentation occurs more rarely and is referred to as *acute silicosis*.[62–64] This is the result of an overwhelming exposure to respirable crystalline silica over a short time, typically less than several years. The chest radiograph has a basilar alveolar filling pattern (identical to that seen in pulmonary alveolar proteinosis) without rounded opacities or lymph node calcifications (Figure 15–5). This is also termed silicoproteinosis.[48] With time, these features progress from a pattern of lower zone alveolar filling to large masses of coalesced parenchymal tissue, typically bilateral but not always symmetric, in the middle and lower zones.

TYPES OF SILICOSIS

Types of silicosis are defined based on radiographic patterns and clinical features.[2] *Chronic silicosis* develops slowly, usually appearing 10 to 30 years after the first exposure. It is not uncommon for silicosis to first become radiographically apparent many years after cessation of employment in a job associated with exposure.[51] Chronic silicosis most often has a simple radiographic pattern. In a minority of those with simple disease, nodules coalesce to become PMF. *Accelerated silicosis* develops less than 10 years after the first exposure. It has the same radiographic appearance as chronic silicosis and is differentiated only by its more rapid development after the first exposure. Development of silicosis after such a short time signals that the worker is at great risk for immunologic complications of silicosis and for the development of PMF. Finally, *acute silicosis* develops after exposure to high concentrations of respirable crystalline silica and results in symptoms within a few weeks to 4 or 5 years after the initial exposure. As already

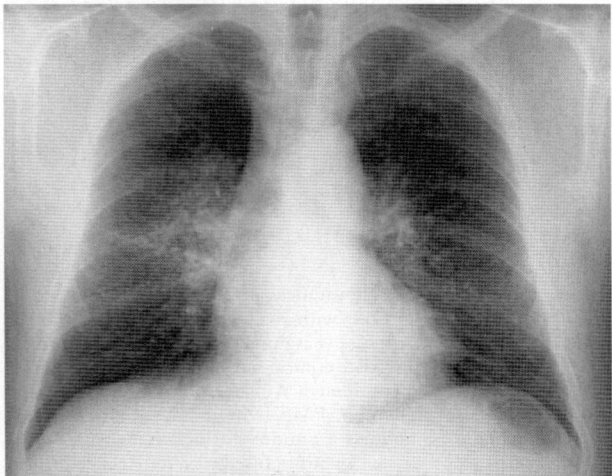

Figure 15–3 Chest radiograph from a patient with simple silicosis. Note the bilateral nodular interstitial process with prominent involvement of the middle and upper zones.

noted, the radiographic pattern of acute silicosis is that of an alveolar-filling process resembling alveolar proteinosis. Symptoms may precede significant radiologic findings. It is not known why some individuals with very high silica exposures develop acute silicosis and others develop accelerated silicosis.

SYMPTOMS AND PHYSICAL FINDINGS OF SILICOSIS

The clinical presentation of chronic or accelerated silicosis is variable. Affected individuals may be asymptomatic and present only with an abnormal chest radiograph. However, chronic cough and dyspnea are common and become more frequent with a worsening radiographic appearance.[65] Physical examination of the chest is usually unremarkable, although coarse adventitious sounds or wheezing may be present.

PMF is, on average, associated with more severe symptoms than simple disease. Over time, progressive coalescence of silicotic nodules leads to progressive respiratory impairment. Physical examination may demonstrate decreased breath sounds due to emphysematous changes associated with PMF. Signs of chronic respiratory failure and cor pulmonale may be present. Crackles do not occur as a result of the interstitial changes but adventitious sounds may be present. PMF is not specifically associated with finger clubbing. If present, another cause should be sought.

Acute silicosis is a grim condition characterized by the rapid onset of symptoms after intense exposures to inhaled silica.[48,64,66,67] Symptoms usually begin 1 to 3 years after exposure, although onset has been reported less than a year after sandblasting. Symptoms include cough, weight loss, fatigue, and sometimes pleuritic pain. On physical examination, crackles are usually present. Patients rapidly develop cyanosis, cor pulmonale, and respiratory failure. Survival after the onset of symptoms is typically less than 4 years, with mycobacterial and fungal infections frequently complicating the clinical course.

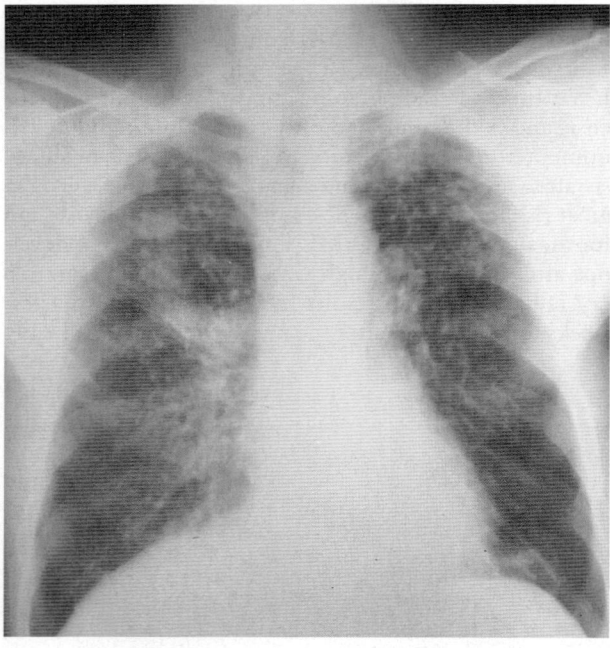

A

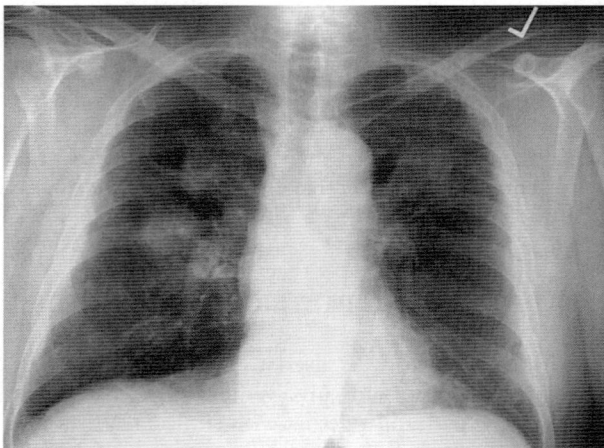

B

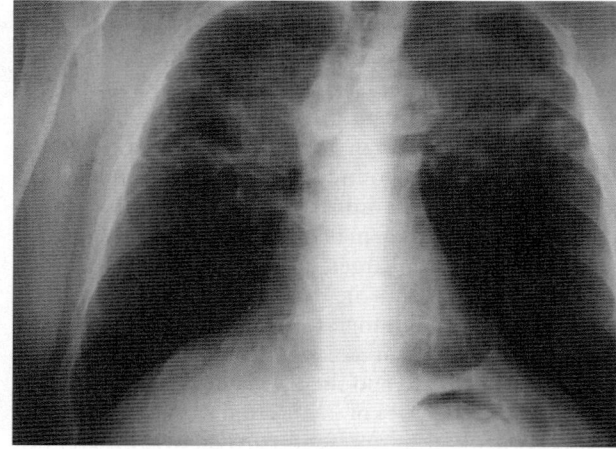

C

Figure 15–4 Different appearances of conglomerate silicosis or PMF. *A*, A soft, fluffy process with coalescence is prominent in the right upper zone. The process is asymmetric as it is far less prominent on the left. In appropriate clinical settings, mycobacterial infection might need to be considered. A background of simple pneumoconiosis is also present. *B*, PMF is more advanced. The large bilateral upper zone nodules are more distinct than in *A*. When asymmetric, such processes can be confused with lung cancer. *C*, Far advanced PMF. Hila and airways are distorted and pulled upward toward the process. Associated severe emphysematous changes are present in the lower zones. This patient had severe airways obstruction and respiratory impairment.

PULMONARY FUNCTION IN SILICOSIS

Recent data suggest that silica exposure, even in the absence of findings on conventional chest radiograph, is associated with excessive decline in spirometric performance. A study of 45,380 Norwegian men aged 30 to 46 years with normal chest radiographs found that the duration of occupational exposure to quartz was an independent predictor for spirometric airflow limitation. Exposure was associated with an excessive decline in forced expiratory volume in 1 second (FEV_1) of 4.3 mL/yr of quartz exposure.[68] The presence of even mild radiographic findings of chronic or accelerated silicosis is associated, on average, with a greater degree of abnormality in pulmonary function. Spirometry shows a mixed picture of obstructive and restrictive ventilatory impairment with decreased FEV_1 and FEV_1/forced vital capacity (FVC) ratio.[65] Pulmonary function, on average, worsens in association with worsening radiographic abnormalities of chronic or accelerated silicosis. PMF is the radiographic appearance associated with the worst pulmonary function abnormalities, including decreased compliance, decreased FEV_1 and FEV_1/FVC ratio, and decreased diffusing capacity.[65,69] Advancing severity of silicosis, in particular PMF, is associated with worsening emphysema detectable by pathology and by computed tomography (CT) scan of the chest.[69–74] In a number of studies using a chest CT scan to evaluate lung parenchyma in chronic or accelerated silicosis, lung function abnormalities have correlated better with the emphysematous changes of silicosis than the nodular changes of silicosis.

INTERNATIONAL LABOUR OFFICE CLASSIFICATION AND CHEST ROENTGENOGRAPHY IN SILICOSIS

As noted above, the chest radiograph plays a key role in the identification and characterization of silicosis. Appropriate and reproducible interpretation of the chest radiograph has therefore been an important concern of epidemiologists as well as clinicians and those involved in the processes of workmen's compensation and litigation. In response to these needs, the International Labour Office (ILO) has developed a series of classification schemes to characterize the chest radiograph in studies of pneumoconiosis.[75] The most recent was developed in 1980 and is described in the ILO publication *Guidelines for the Use of ILO International Classification of Radiographs of Pneumoconioses.*[76] In the United States, the National Institute of Occupational Safety and Health (NIOSH) maintains a training and certification program for physicians seeking to read chest radiographs according to the ILO system. Physicians may qualify as "A" readers (attended training seminars) or "B" readers (passed a comprehensive examination based on 120 roentgenograms read into the ILO classification).

Briefly, in this classification scheme, the reader initially grades film quality and whether or not changes on

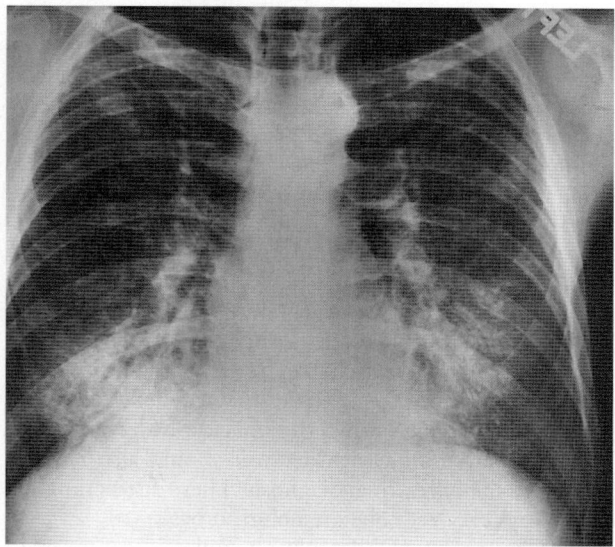

Figure 15–5 Acute silicosis in a surface coal mine driller. Note the bilateral lower zone alveolar filling processes with air bronchograms. Open lung biopsy ruled out the presence of an infectious process and confirmed the diagnosis. Reprinted with permission from Thorax 1983;38:276.

the film might be due to pneumoconiosis. If small opacities are present, they are characterized according to shape and size. Small round opacities are characterized according to size as p (up to 1.5 mm), q (1.5 to 3 mm), or r (3 to 10 mm). Irregular small opacities are classified by width as s, t, or u (same sizes as for small rounded opacities). Level of involvement with small opacities, or profusion, is classified on a 12-point scale between 0/– and 3/+. Next, large opacities are identified. Large opacities are defined as any opacity greater than 1 cm that is present in a film in which there is sufficient evidence to indicate a diagnosis of pneumoconiosis. Large opacities are classified as category A (for one or more large opacities not exceeding a combined diameter of 5 cm), category B (large opacities with combined diameter greater than 5 cm but does not exceed the equivalent of the right upper zone), or category C (bigger than B). Pleural thickening is also assessed with respect to thickness, extent, and degree of calcification. Finally, other abnormal features of the chest radiograph can be commented upon.

The characteristic radiographic pattern of simple silicosis is the presence of rounded opacities. These tend to be of the "q" and "r" types. In the lower profusion categories these opacities are most often in the upper lung zones. In the more advanced stages of the disease, the middle and lower lung zones typically are also involved.

PMF is associated with large opacities exceeding one centimeter. These often occur on a background of small rounded opacities that are recognizable as simple silicosis. The confluence of these nodules begins posteriorly and peripherally and migrates centrally. As with simple silicosis, progressive massive fibrosis develops most prominently in the upper lobes. As these upper lobe fibrous masses progressively enlarge, the hila are retracted upward and the lower zones become hyperinflated and appear as bullous emphysema. As retraction occurs, the large opacities also become associated with subpleural emphysematous changes. The large upper zone opacities often cause concern that neoplastic processes are present, particularly if the opacities are not symmetric. Importantly, progressive massive fibrotic lesions are relatively thin and platelike and are located in the peripheral and posterior aspects of the upper lung zones. These radiographic features are sometimes helpful in differentiating between progressive massive fibrosis and pulmonary malignancy. The large opacities may cavitate. This may be due to ischemia within the opacity; however, tuberculosis or carcinoma with necrosis should also be considered in the differential diagnosis. These distinctions are not always easy to make on a clinical basis.

Enlargement of hilar lymph nodes is common in chronic and accelerated silicosis. In 5 to 10% of cases, the hilar nodes calcify circumferentially, producing the so-called eggshell pattern of calcification (Figure 15–6). This is not pathognomonic of silicosis, as it has also been described in sarcoidosis, postirradiation Hodgkin's disease, blastomycosis, scleroderma, amyloidosis, and histoplasmosis.[77] However, the presence of eggshell hilar calcifications in the setting of typically distributed nodular parenchymal opacities reinforces the clinical impression of silicosis when there is an appropriate exposure history.

In acute silicosis, the chest radiograph typically reveals bibasilar alveolar filling with air bronchograms.[62] The diffuse alveolar filling is best described as a ground-glass appearance. Histologically, small rounded opacities can sometimes be identified, but they are not easily recognized on the chest radiograph. Progression seen on the chest radiograph occurs over a relatively short time. Areas of alveolar filling progress to large masses that are similar to those seen in progressive massive fibrosis but are somewhat larger and often located in the middle compared with upper zones. Tracheal distortion is common and is a result of the parenchymal distortion with stress placed on the trachea. Radiographic demonstration of the process of progression can be accelerated in these workers by superimposed mycobacterial infection. The radiologic differential diagnosis includes pneumonia and other pulmonary infections, pulmonary edema, alveolar hemorrhage, alveolar cell cancer, idiopathic alveolar proteinosis, and other alveolar filling processes. These entities can usually be excluded on a clinical basis.

Several studies have evaluated the performance of the chest radiograph in detecting silicosis as compared to pathologic examination of the lungs at autopsy. In a study of 557 South African gold miners, sensitivities and specificities using ILO profusion classes of 1/0, 1/1, and 1/2 as cutoffs were found to be 50%, 37%, and 25% for sensitivity and 89%, 96%, and 100% for specificity, respectively.[78] A subsequent study by this group of 241 South African gold miners evaluated use of "miniradiographs"

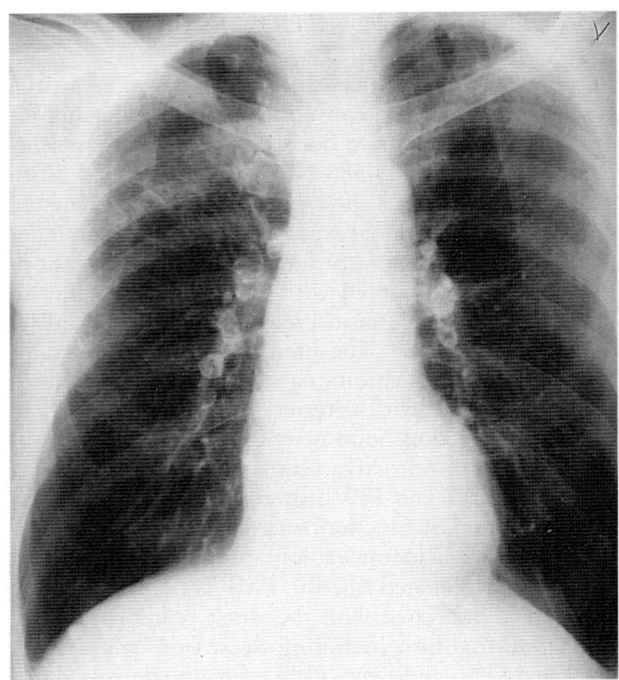

Figure 15–6   A chest radiograph demonstrating enlargement and prominent eggshell calcification of hilar lymph nodes. In addition, there is a minimal background of simple pneumoconiosis and a suggestion of coalescence of nodules in the right upper zone.

with cutoffs at ILO profusion categories 0/1, 1/0, and 1/1. Sensitivities were 89%, 74%, and 71%, respectively and specificities were 73%, 87%, and 96%, respectively.[79] Reasons for the improved performance in the second study were unclear.

Performance of the conventional chest CT scan and high-resolution CT scan of the chest (HRCT) relative to conventional radiography in the diagnosis of silicosis has been somewhat controversial. With regard to diagnosis of early-stage interstitial changes, some have found that chest CT and HRCT have less sensitivity than conventional chest radiography,[72] whereas others have reported improved sensitivity and significantly reduced inter-reader variability for CT/HRCT.[80] In another investigation, HRCT was more reproducible when interpreted by two readers than conventional radiography, but was not felt to be more sensitive.[81] In contrast to the mixed results in the evaluation of early-stage interstitial changes, there is general agreement that CT/HRCT is superior to conventional chest radiography for documentation of PMF lesions and emphysematous changes associated with silicosis (Figure 15–7).

DIAGNOSIS OF SILICOSIS

In general, three elements play a key role in the diagnosis of silicosis. First, a history of silica exposure sufficient to cause this illness. Second, chest imaging (usually a conventional chest radiograph) that shows opacities (ILO category 1/0 or greater) consistent with silicosis. Finally, there are no underlying illnesses more likely to be causing the abnormalities. Diseases capable of mimicking the x-ray appearance of silicosis include infectious processes (such as miliary distribution of a mycobacterial or fungal process), pulmonary malignancy (a consideration when the coalesced lesions of progressive massive fibrosis are unilateral or asymmetric), rheumatoid nodules (referred to as Caplan's syndrome in the presence of pneumoconiosis[82]), or, in rare cases, sarcoidosis.

Determining whether the worker's occupational silica exposure is sufficient to cause silicosis can be difficult. This requires information about the work environment and the worker's exposures. Silicosis occurs in association with industrial processes where silica particles of respirable size are generated and aerosolized. This is the common feature among diverse occupations such as sandblasting, drilling into siliceous rock, or exposure to finely milled silica flour where silicosis is a well-recognized risk.

When the three clinical requirements for the diagnosis of silicosis are met, additional evaluation is not necessary to make the diagnosis. Occasionally, the diagnosis cannot be made clinically. In these instances, biopsy of the lung may be necessary to exclude other diagnoses. The traditional view has been that an open lung biopsy is preferred due to the chance of pneumothorax after transbronchial lung biopsy.[83] The presence of stiff upper zones and emphysematous changes in the lower zones might be predisposing factors for pneumothorax. However, bronchoalveolar lavage and transbronchial lung biopsy have the potential to be informative. In one reported case, bronchoalveolar lavage documented a neutrophilic alveolitis and silica was shown to be present in alveolar macrophages by energy dispersive x-ray analysis despite the absence of birefrin-

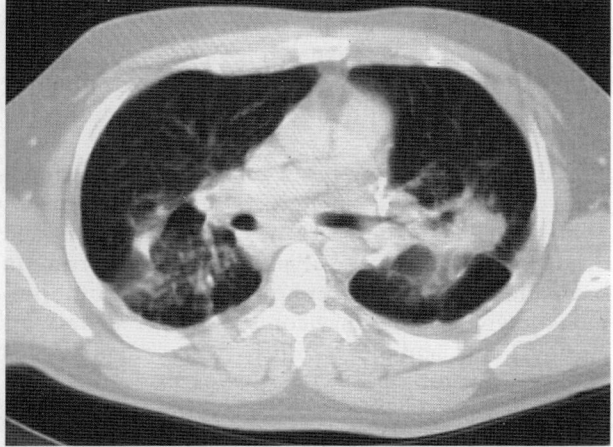

Figure 15–7 A computed tomography scan of the lung demonstrating conglomerate densities in the posterior aspects of both midzones. Note the associated subpleural emphysematous changes.

gent crystal particles. Transbronchial biopsy showed fibrocellular nodules in the parenchyma. Taken together, these findings were deemed consistent with the diagnosis of silicosis.[84]

COMPLICATIONS OF SILICOSIS

Mycobacterial Infections

The association between silicosis and pulmonary tuberculosis (TB) has long been recognized.[9,85] This relationship has been attributed, at least in part, to the impairment of alveolar macrophage function by inhaled crystalline silica.[85] Recent studies have documented that silica exposure alone, even in the absence of radiographic silicosis, is associated with an increased risk of TB.[86–88] The risk of TB is considerably increased in association with radiographic evidence of silicosis; the risk further increases with an increasing profusion of radiographic opacities.[86,88,89] Silicosis is also associated with an increased risk for nontuberculous mycobacterial infection.[90,91] Historically, the incidence of tuberculosis and nontuberculous mycobacterial disease was noted to be especially high in acute and accelerated silicosis.[83]

Mycobacterial infection should always be suspected when a silicotic patient experiences appropriate constitutional symptoms, worsening of respiratory symptoms, or changes in chest radiographs such as cavitation of PMF lesions. It has been recommended that silicotics or those with more that 25 years' exposure to inhaled crystalline silica should have a tuberculin test performed by intradermal injection of 5 tuberculin units (TU) of purified protein derivative (PPD), and that treatment of latent TB infection should be offered to all patients with reactions of greater than 9 mm of induration.[9] Unfortunately, several studies suggest that treatment of latent TB infection may be less effective in the presence of silicosis.[92,93]

Because silicotic changes can make radiographic evaluation for active TB difficult, it is critical to evaluate for active tuberculosis after a positive PPD skin test has been documented. Smear or culture-positive silicotics should be treated with multiple antituberculous drugs. Several studies suggest efficacy for a four-drug regimen including isoniazid, rifampin, pyrazinamide, and streptomycin.[94–96] One of these studies suggests better results when treatment is given for a period of at least eight months.[95]

Immune-Mediated Complications

Silicosis is associated with immune dysfunction, both systemically and in the lung.[97] A major feature of this immune dysfunction is dysregulated and increased immunoglobulin production.[98–102] Increased serum IgG and IgM concentrations have been reported in sandblasters[98]; increased serum IgG and IgA concentrations in silicotic stone masons[99]; increased serum IgG, IgM, and IgA concentrations in slate-pencil workers[100]; increased IgG in quartz crushers[101]; and increased IgG, IgA, and IgE in silicotic miners.[102] Silicosis is also associated with an increased prevalence of serum autoantibodies, such as antinuclear antibody and rheumatoid factor, as well as with an increased prevalence of circulating immune complexes.[18,97–99,101,102] Despite the apparent activation of antibody immunity, silicosis is associated with impaired antimycobacterial defenses, an important cell-mediated immune function (as discussed in "Mycobacterial Infections").

In addition to altered markers of immune function, silicosis also appears to be associated with several autoimmune diseases. A recent statement by the American Thoracic Society noted persuasive evidence relating scleroderma to occupational silica exposures.[9] This observation was first made in Scottish stonemasons in 1914.[103] Subsequent reports have described an increased prevalence of sclerodactyly (acrosclerosis) and progressive systemic sclerosis (PSS) both in patients from dusty trades and in patients with silicosis.[104,105] More recent studies of South African miners have shown an increased incidence of PSS[106] as well as an increased number of PSS cases relative to systemic lupus erythematosis (SLE) cases.[107] A potentially confounding factor in these studies is the induction of acrosclerosis and Raynaud's phenomenon in response to vibration injury to which many workers, including miners who drill rock, are subject.[108] PSS in individuals with silicosis appears clinically identical to PSS occurring in the absence of silicosis.[109]

Current evidence is also highly suggestive of an association between rheumatoid arthritis (RA) and silicosis. A Finnish cohort of 1,026 current and former granite workers had excessive numbers of individuals disabled by or taking medicines for RA compared with age-specific rates in the general population.[110] South African miners with RA were more likely to have silicosis than were miners not exhibiting RA, and their silicosis was more progressive. The study did not assess whether silica exposure increased the risk of RA.[111] Evaluation of a population of silicotics identified by a state surveillance program for silicosis documented a statistically significant 2.73-fold increased risk of RA relative to the general population. PSS and SLE occurred less frequently than RA; the relative risks for these conditions were also increased in silicosis but not to a statistically significant degree.[112] Evaluation of a cohort of 4,626 silica-exposed workers in the industrial sand industry showed a positive dose-response trend for RA on the basis of death certificate data.[113]

Evidence for an association between SLE and mixed connective tissue disorders with silicosis is limited to case reports from populations of sandblasters and workers grinding and handling silica for use in scouring powder.[66,83,114] Current evidence can only support the suspicion of a causal relationship between SLE and silica exposure in the presence of acute or accelerated silicosis.

Lung Cancer

The associations between silica exposure, silicosis, and lung cancer have been an area of controversy. In 1997, the International Agency for Research on Cancer (IARC) reviewed the available literature and concluded in a split vote that inhaled crystalline silica from occupational sources was a definite (group 1) human carcinogen.[115–117] The IARC qualified its decision by noting that the evidence was not entirely consistent and that different forms of silica might have differing potentials for causing lung cancer. A statement by the American Thoracic Society issued in 1997 noted that available data supported the conclusion that silicosis produces an increased risk for bronchogenic carcinoma. The best available evidence of an increased risk was for cigarette smokers, with less information available for never-smokers and for workers exposed to silica but without silicosis.[9] The literature in this area continues to be controversial, especially with regard to the ability of silica exposure, in the absence of silicosis, to cause lung cancer.[116–119]

Chronic Bronchitis and Airflow Obstruction

Silicosis and, to a lesser degree, silica exposure without silicosis are associated with respiratory symptoms and an excessive decline in FEV_1 as was discussed earlier in "Pulmonary Function in Silicosis." A statement by the American Thoracic Society notes that studies from many different work environments suggest that exposure to silica at dust levels not appearing to cause radiographic silicosis, can cause bronchitis symptoms in excess of those expected from smoking alone.[9] A meta-analysis of 13 studies among coal and gold miners confirmed an excess of bronchitic symptoms and obstructive physiology, even among nonsmokers.[120] Pathology studies of such workers exposed to nonasbestos mineral dust have shown pigmentation and fibrosis surrounding small airways, a condition termed "mineral dust small airways disease."[121]

Airways obstruction is a feature of silicosis.[9] In moderate to severe silicosis, nodules occur in close proximity to small and medium airways causing narrowing and distortion of the lumen. Hypertrophy and scarring in bronchial-associated lymphoid tissue and intrapulmonary lymph nodes may compress larger airways. As already noted, radiologic and pathologic emphysema also occurs in association with silicosis, particularly progressive massive fibrosis. In patients with more advanced silicosis, pulmonary function tests usually reflect a mixed pattern of nonreversible airflow obstruction as well as the features of volume restriction and impaired gas exchange expected with diffuse interstitial lung disease.[65,120]

Renal Complications

A relationship between silica exposure and renal disease has been suspected since the 1930s. A report at that time documented a 45% increase in the death rate from chronic nephritis in English and Welsh men with occupations associated with silica exposure relative to age-specific rates in the reference population.[122] More recently, a case-control study of men with end-stage renal disease found elevated odds ratios for "regular occupational exposures to solvents or silica." It stated that other evidence of silica-related renal disease was limited to case reports.[123] In 1997, a retrospective cohort study of 2,412 gold miners found an increased risk for end-stage renal disease (ESRD) relative to the general population. Risk was greatest for "nonsystemic" ESRD caused by glomerulonephritis or interstitial nephritis and among workers with 10 or more years employment underground.[124] In 2001, the same group reported an evaluation of renal disease in a cohort of 4,626 silica-exposed workers in the industrial sand industry. Using death-certificate data, significant excess mortality from acute and chronic renal disease was documented relative to the general population. Using data from the U.S. registry of ESRD, an excess incidence of ESRD, which was highest for glomerulonephritis, was documented. Furthermore, an exposure-response relationship for the incidence of ESRD was documented.[113] In addition to epidemiologic associations between silica exposure and ESRD, case reports also suggest an association between acute silicoproteinosis and glomerular injury.[125,126]

TREATMENT OF SILICOSIS

There is no proven specific therapy for silicosis. Symptomatic therapy includes measures such as treatment of airflow obstruction with bronchodilators, treatment of respiratory tract infection with antibiotics, and use of supplemental oxygen to prevent complications of chronic hypoxemia. As already noted, patients should be screened for TB infection and a high index of suspicion for mycobacterial infection superimposed against the background of silicosis should be maintained.

Corticosteroid therapy has been attempted as a measure to interrupt inflammation and cytokine networking leading to progressive silicosis. In the largest study to date, a 6-month trial of prednisolone was carried out in 34 northern Indian patients with chronic simple and complicated silicosis. Treatment resulted in statistically (although not clinically) significant improvements in lung volumes, diffusing capacity (DL_{CO}), and partial pressure of arterial oxygen (PaO_2). A significant decrease in total cells recovered by bronchoalveolar lavage was also noted.[127] Systemic steroid therapy also has been reported to be beneficial in accelerated and acute silicosis.[128] No large randomized, double-blinded prospective clinical trials have documented the impact of steroid therapy on the long-term outcome of silicosis.

Other experimental treatment measures have been attempted in silicosis. Whole lung lavage (WLL) has been proposed as a therapeutic measure based on its ability to reduce the pulmonary dust burden and remove inflammatory cells from the lung.[129–131] Although current data show the procedure to be safe and technically feasible, its usefulness remains unclear.

Several other agents also have received attention as potential therapies for silicosis, but none of these have achieved usefulness. Modulation of silica-induced toxicity by inhalation of aluminum and inhalational or parenteral administration of a polymer, polyvinyl pyridine N-oxide (PVNO), has been studied in animal models and in humans.[132–135] Tetrandrine, an active component of the Chinese traditional medicine "hanfangii," has been reported in the Chinese literature to inhibit and even reverse pulmonary lesions in experimental silicosis.[136] Tetrandrine appears to function as an anti-inflammatory agent.[137–139] An open clinical trial showed clinical and radiographic improvement in patients with pulmonary fibrosis from silica inhalation,[140] but double-blinded, randomized, prospective studies remain to be conducted. Finally, both anti-TNF-α antibodies and soluble TNF-α receptors have been shown to reduce fibrosis in animal models of silicosis.[25,31] Although both agents are now available for clinical treatment of other diseases, clinical trials for the treatment of silicosis remain to be conducted.

Lung transplantation is a potential option for the treatment of end-stage silicosis and should be seriously considered in appropriate clinical settings. Of note is that one of the earliest reports of unilateral lung transplantation occurred in 1972 and was for acute silicosis in a 23-year-old man.[141]

PREVENTION OF SILICOSIS

Silicosis is a preventable disease. As a consequence of better industrial hygiene practices, silicosis afflicts far fewer people than in the past.[61] As a result of litigation not specifically related to the silica standard, the Occupational Safety and Health Administration has returned to a permissible exposure limit (PEL) for respirable silica at 10 mg/m^3 divided by (%SiO$_2$ + 2) or 250 million particles per cubic foot divided by (%SiO$_2$ + 5), after having enforced an exposure limit of 0.1 mg/m^3 of respirable silica.[142] It has been suggested that this exposure limit is not protective of workers with exposure over an entire working lifetime.[50,51] A recent study of Vermont granite workers concluded that strict adherence to the 0.1 mg/m^3 exposure limit resulted in rare occurrences of radiologic abnormalities but still documented that 3.5% of workers with initial exposure after 1955 (when exposure limits in these stone sheds and quarries stabilized at current levels) had radiographic abnormalities consistent with silicosis.[61] Thus, a lower recommended exposure limit (REL) of 0.05 mg/m³ has been established by the NIOSH.[143]

Achieving protective exposure levels through the use of engineering controls is strongly preferred to the use of personal protective equipment (respirators) as the primary means for limiting inhalation exposures to crystalline silica.[12] Inappropriate respirators or respirator use can lead to significant exposures.[144] Unfortunately, noncompliance with the current PEL appears to be common in construction work, foundry work, mining, sandblasting, and in the cut stone and stone products industries.[61,145]

Although primary prevention through exposure control is the critical component of silicosis prevention, health monitoring of workers with inhalation exposure to crystalline silica using chest radiographs and spirometry may assist in the early identification of people developing disease from their exposures. Efforts at secondary prevention should focus on reducing silica exposure for both the affected workers and others with similar exposures. Many industrialized countries mandate health surveillance for workers at risk of developing silicosis.[146]

A number of NIOSH publications are available addressing such issues as awareness of silica as a workplace hazard, environmental controls, personal protection, and medical monitoring.[12,147,148]

REFERENCES

1. Castranova V, Vallyathan V, Wallace W. Silica and silica-induced lung diseases. Boca Raton: CRC Press, Inc.; 1996.
2. WHO. Concise international chemical assessment document 24. Crystalline silica, quartz. Stuttgart: Wissenschaftliche Verlagsgesellschaft mbH, 2000.
3. Corn J. Historical aspects of industrial hygiene-silicosis. Am Ind Hyg Assoc J 1980;41:125–32.
4. Holt P. Silicosis. In: Holt P, editor. Inhaled dust and disease. New York: John Wiley and Sons; 1987. p. 46–85.
5. Castranova V, Vallyathan V. Silicosis and coal workers' pneumoconiosis. Environ Health Perspect 2000;108(Suppl 4): 675–84.
6. Lapp N. Lung disease secondary to inhalation of nonfibrous minerals. Clin Chest Med 1981;2:219–33.
7. Morgan WKC. Silicates and lung disease. In: Morgan WKC, Seaton A, editors. Occupational lung diseases. Philadelphia: W.B. Saunders Company; 1995. p. 268–307.
8. Gamble JF. Silicate pneumoconiosis. In: Merchant JA, editor. Occupational respiratory diseases. Publication No. DHHS (NIOSH) 86-102. Washington, DC: Government Printing Office, 1986:243–327.
9. Anonymous. American Thoracic Society. Adverse effects of crystalline silica exposure. Am J Respir Crit Care Med 1997;155:761–5.
10. Banks D, Bauer M, Castellan R, et al. Silicosis in surface coalmine drillers. Thorax 1983;38:275–8.
11. Seaton A. Silicosis. In: Morgan WKC, Seaton A, editors. Occupational lung diseases. Philadelphia: W.B. Saunders Company; 1995. p. 222–67.
12. National Institute for Occupational Safety and Health. Request for assistance in preventing silicosis and deaths from sandblasting. Cincinnati: Ref type: report. DHHS(NIOSH); 1992 Publication No. 92-102.
13. Bailey W, Brown M, Buechner H, et al. Silicomycobacterial disease in sandblasters. Am Rev Respir Dis 1974;110:115–25.
14. Glindmeyer HW, Hammad YY. Contributing factors to sandblasters' silicosis: inadequate respiratory protection equipment and standards. J Occup Med 1988;30:917–21.
15. Wagner GR. The inexcusable persistence of silicosis [editoral]. Am J Public Health 1995;85:1346–7.
16. Banks D, Morring K, Boehlecke B, et al. Silicosis in silica flour workers. Am Rev Respir Dis 1981;124:445–50.
17. Norboo T, Angchuk PT, Yahya M, et al. Silicosis in a Himalayan village population: role of environmental dust. Thorax 1991;46:341–3.
18. Anonymous. Silicosis and silicate disease committee. Diseases associated with exposure to silica and nonfibrous silicate minerals. Arch Pathol Lab Med 1988;112:673–720.
19. Vallyathan V, Xianglin S, Dalal N, et al. Generation of free radicals from freshly fractured silica dust. Am Rev Respir Dis 1988;138:1213–9.
20. Ghio AJ, Kennedy TP, Schapira RM, et al. Hypothesis: is lung disease after silicate inhalation caused by oxidant generation? Lancet 1990;336:967–9.
21. Vanhee D, Gosset P, Boitelle A, et al. Cytokines and cytokine network in silicosis and coal workers' pneumoconiosis. Eur Respir J 1995;8:834–42.
22. Hamada H, Vallyathan V, Cool CD, et al. Mast cell basic fibroblast growth factor in silicosis. Am J Respir Crit Care Med 2000;161:2026–34.
23. Schmidt J, Oliver C, Lepe-Zuniga J, et al. Silica-stimulated monocytes release fibroblast proliferation factors identical to interleukin 1. A potential role for interleukin 1 in the pathogenesis of silicosis. J Clin Invest 1984;73:1462–72.
24. Oghiso Y, Kubota Y. Enhanced interleukin 1 production by alveolar macrophages in Ia-positive lung cells in silica-exposed rats. Microbiol Immunol 1986;30:1189–98.
25. Piquet PF, Collart MA, Grau JE, et al. Requirement of tumour necrosis factor for development of silica-induced pulmonary fibrosis. Nature 1990;344:245–7.
26. Mohr C, Gemsa D, Graebner C, et al. Systemic macrophage stimulation in rats with silicosis: enhanced release of tumor necrosis factor-alpha from alveolar and peritoneal macrophages. Am J Respir Cell Mol Biol 1991;5:395–402.
27. Williams AO, Flanders KC, Saffiotti U. Immunohistochemical localization of transforming growth factor-beta 1 in rats with experimental silicosis, alveolar type II hyperplasia, and lung cancer. Am J Pathol 1993;142:1831–40.
28. Rom WN, Bitterman PB, Rennard SI, et al. Characterization of the lower respiratory tract inflammation of nonsmoking individuals with interstitial lung disease associated with chronic inhalation of inorganic dust. Am Rev Respir Dis 1987;136:1429–34.
29. Lukacs NW, Kunkel SL, Allen R, et al. Stimulus and cell-specific expression of C-X-C and C-C chemokines by pulmonary stromal cell populations. Am J Physiol 1995;268: L856–61.
30. Driscoll KE, Howard BW, Carter JM, et al. Alpha-quartz induced chemokine expression by rat lung epithelial cells: effects of in vivo and in vitro particle exposure. Am J Pathol 1996;149:1627–37.
31. Piquet P, Vesin C. Treatment by human recombinant soluble TNF receptor of pulmonary fibrosis induced by bleomycin or silica in mice. Eur Respir J 1994;7:515–8.
32. Davis G, Hill-Eubanks L, Pfeiffer L, et al. Reduced silicosis in C3H/HeJ-LPS^d mice: an implied role for cytokine production deficiency. Am Rev Respir Dis 1992;145: A325.
33. Jagirdar J, Begin R, Dufresne A, et al. Transforming growth factor-β in silicosis. Am J Respir Crit Care Med 1996; 154:1076–81.
34. Heppleston A, Fletcher K, Wyatt I. Changes in the composition of lung lipids and the turnover of dipalmitoyl lecithin

in experimental alveolar lipoproteinosis induced by inhaled quartz. Br J Exp Pathol 1974;55:384–95.

35. Gabor S, Zugravu E, Kovats A, et al. Effects of quartz on lung surfactant. Environ Res 1978;16:443–8.

36. Dethloff L, Gilmore L, Brody A, et al. Induction of intra- and extracellular phospholipids in the lungs of rats exposed to silica. Biochem J 1986;233:111–8.

37. Kawada H, Horiuchi T, Shannon J, et al. Alveolar type II cells, surfactant protein A (SP-A), and the phospholipid components of surfactant in acute silicosis in the rat. Am Rev Respir Dis 1989;140:460–70.

38. Miller B, Dethloff L, Hook G. Silica-induced hypertrophy of type II cells in the lungs of rats. Lab Invest 1986;55:153–63.

39. Miller B, Dethloff L, Gladen B, et al. Progression of type II cell hypertrophy and hyperplasia during silica-induced pulmonary inflammation. Lab Invest 1987;57:546–54.

40. Miller B, Bakewell W, Katyal S, et al. Induction of surfactant protein A (SP-A) biosynthesis and SP-A mRNA in activated type II cells during acute silicosis in rats. Am J Respir Cell Mol Biol 1990;3:217–26.

41. Hughes JM. Radiographic evidence of silicosis in relation to silica exposures. Appl Occup Environ Hyg 1995;10:1064–9.

42. Honda K, Kimura A, Dong R-P, et al. Immunogenetic analysis of silicosis in Japan. Am J Respir Cell Mol Biol 1993;8:106–11.

43. Yucesoy B, Vallyathan V, Landsittel DP, et al. Association of tumor necrosis factor-alpha and interleukin-1 gene polymorphisms with silicosis. Toxicol Appl Pharmacol 2001;172:75–82.

44. Yucesoy B, Vallyathan V, Landsittel DP, et al. Polymorphisms of the IL-1 gene complex in coal miners with silicosis. Am J Ind Med 2001;39:286–91.

45. Eden K, Seebach HV. Atypical dust-induced pneumoconiosis in SPF rats. Virchows Arch (Pathol Anat) 1976;372:1–9.

46. Kreiss K, Greenberg L, Kogut S, et al. Hard-rock mining exposures affect smokers and nonsmokers differently. Am Rev Respir Dis 1989;139:1487–93.

47. Green FHY, Vallyathan V. Pathologic responses to inhaled silica. In: Castranova V, Vallyathan V, Wallace WE, editors. Silica and silica-induced lung diseases. Boca Raton: CRC Press, Inc.; 1996. p. 39–62.

48. Buechner H, Ansari A. Acute silicosis. Dis Chest 1969;55:274–84.

49. Hoffman EO, Lamberty J, Pizzolato P, Coover J. The ultrastructure of acute silicosis. Arch Pathol 1973;96:104–7.

50. Steenland K, Brown D. Silicosis among gold miners: exposure-response analyses and risk assessment. Am J Public Health 1995;85:1372–7.

51. Kreiss K, Zhen B. Risk of silicosis in a Colorado mining community. Am J Ind Med 1996;30:529–39.

52. Trasko V. Some facts on the prevalence of silicosis in the United States. Arch Ind Health 1956;14:379–87.

53. Green F, Althouse R, Weber K. Prevalence of silicosis at death in underground coal miners. Am J Ind Med 1989;16:605–15.

54. National Institute for Occupational Safety and Health. Work-related lung diseases surveillance report. DHHS(NIOSH); 1991 Publication 91-113.

55. Rosenman K, Reilly M, Kalinowsky D. Silicosis in the 1990s. Chest 1997;111:779–86.

56. National Institute for Occupational Safety and Health. Work-related lung disease surveillance report. Cincinnati (OH): DHHS (NIOSH); 1999 Publication No.: 2000-105.

57. Russell AE, Britten RH, Thomson RL, et al. The health of workers in dusty trades. II. Exposure to siliceous dust. Washington (DC): U.S. Treasury Department, Public Health Service; 1929 Public Health Bulletin 187.

58. Russell AE. The health of workers in dusty trades. VII. Restudy of a group of granite workers. Washington (DC): U.S.

Federal Security Agency, Public Health Service; 1941 Public Health Bulletin 269.

59. Hosey AD, Trasko VM, Ashe HB. Control of silicosis in the Vermont granite industry: progress report. Washington (DC): U.S. Department of Health, Education, and Welfare; 1957 Publication 557.

60. Ashe HB, Bergstrom DE. Twenty-six years experience with dust control in the Vermont granite industry. Ind Med Surg 1964;33:73–8.

61. Graham WGB, Vacek PM, Morgan WKC, et al. Radiographic abnormalities in long-tenure Vermont granite workers and the permissable exposure limit for crystalline silica. J Occup Environ Med 2001;43:412–7.

62. Dee P, Suratt P, Winn W. The radiographic findings in acute silicosis. Radiology 1978;126:359–63.

63. Sampson HL. The roentgenogram in so-called "acute" silicosis. Am J Public Health 1933;23:1237–9.

64. Chapman E. Acute silicosis. JAMA 1932;98:1439–41.

65. Wang XR, Christiani DC. Respiratory symptoms and functional status in workers exposed to silica, asbestos, and coal dust mines. J Occup Environ Med 2000;42:1076–84.

66. Suratt P, Winn W, Brody A, et al. Acute silicosis in tombstone sandblasters. Am Rev Respir Dis 1977;115:521–9.

67. Gardner LU. Pathology of so-called "acute" silicosis. Am J Public Health 1933;23:1240–9.

68. Humerfelt S, Eide GE, Gulsvik A. Association of years of occupational quartz exposure with spirometric airflow limitation in Norwegian men aged 30–46 years. Thorax 1998;53:649–55.

69. Begin R, Ostiguy G, Cantin A, et al. Lung function in silica-exposed workers. A relationship to disease severity assessed by CT scan. Chest 1988;94:539–45.

70. Bergin C, Muller N, Vedal S, et al. CT in silicosis: correlation of plain films and pulmonary function tests. AJR Am J Radiol 1986;146:477–83.

71. Kinsella M, Muller N, Vedal S, et al. Emphysema in silicosis. A comparison of smokers with nonsmokers using pulmonary function and computed tomography. Am Rev Respir Dis 1990;141:1497–500.

72. Cowie RL, Hay M, Thomas RG. Association of silicosis, lung dysfunction, and emphysema in gold miners. Thorax 1993;48:429–35.

73. Hnizdo E, Sluis-Cremer GK, Baskind E, et al. Emphysema and airway obstruction in non-smoking South African gold miners with long exposure to silica dust. Occup Environ Med 1994;51:557–63.

74. Gevenois PA, Sergent G, DeMaertelaer V, et al. Micronodules and emphysema in coal mine dust or silica exposure: relation with lung function. Eur Respir J 1998;12:1020–4.

75. Morgan WKC. Epidemiology and occupational lung disease. In: Morgan WKC, Seaton A, editors. Occupational lung diseases. Philadelphia: W.B. Saunders Company; 1995.

76. Guidelines for the use of ILO international classification of radiographs of pneumoconioses. Revised edition. Geneva: International Labour Office; 1980.

77. Gross B, Schneider H, Proto A. Eggshell calcification of lymph nodes: an update. AJR Am J Roentgenol 1980;135:1265–8.

78. Hnizdo E, Murray J, Sluis-Cremer GK, et al. Correlation between radiological and pathological diagnosis of silicosis: an autopsy population based study. Am J Ind Med 1993;24:427–45.

79. Corbett EL, Murray J, Churchyard GJ, et al. Use of miniradiographs to detect silicosis. Comparison of radiological with autopsy findings. Am J Respir Crit Care Med 1999;160:2012–7.

80. Begin R, Ostiguy G, Fillion R, et al. Computed tomography scan in the early detection of silicosis. Am J Respir Crit Care Med 1991;144:697–705.

81. Talini D, Paggiaro PL, Falaschi F, et al. Chest radiography and high resolution computed tomography in the evalua-

tion of workers exposed to silica dust: relation with functional findings. Occup Environ Med 1995;52:262–7.

82. Caplan A. Certain unusual radiographic appearances in the chest of coalminers suffering from rheumatoid arthritis. Thorax 1953;8:29–30.

83. Ziskind M, Jones RM, Weill H. Silicosis. Am Rev Respir Dis 1976;113:643–65.

84. Nugent K, Dodson R, Idell S, et al. The utility of bronchoalveolar lavage and transbronchial lung biopsy combined with energy-dispersive x-ray analysis in the diagnosis of silicosis. Am Rev Respir Dis 1989;140:1438–41.

85. Snider DE. The relationship between tuberculosis and silicosis. Am Rev Respir Dis 1978;118:455–60.

86. Sherson D, Lander F. Morbidity of pulmonary tuberculosis among silicotic and nonsilicotic foundry workers in Denmark. J Occup Environ Med 1990;32:110–3.

87. Chen GX, Burnett CA, Cameron LL, et al. Tuberculosis mortality and silica exposure: a case-control study based on a national mortality database for the years 1983–1992. Int J Occup Environ Health 1997;3:163–70.

88. Hnizdo E, Murray J. Risk of pulmonary tuberculosis relative to silicosis and exposure to silica dust in South African gold miners. Occup Environ Med 1998;55:496–502.

89. Cowie R. The epidemiology of tuberculosis in gold miners with silicosis. Am J Respir Crit Care Med 1994;150:1460–2.

90. Corbett EL, Churchyard GJ, Clayton T, et al. Risk factors for pulmonary mycobacterial disease in South African gold miners. A case-control study. Am J Respir Crit Care Med 1999;159:94–9.

91. Sonnenberg P, Murray J, Glynn JR, et al. Risk factors for pulmonary disease due to culture-positive *M. tuberculosis* or nontuberculous mycobacteria in South African gold miners. Eur Respir J 2000;15:291–6.

92. Hong Kong Chest Service/Tuberculosis Research Centre, Madras/British Medical Research Council. A double-blind placebo-controlled clinical trial of three antituberculosis chemoprophylaxis regimens in patients with silicosis in Hong Kong. Am Rev Respir Dis 1992;145:36–41.

93. Cowie R. Short course chemoprophylaxis with rifampicin, isoniazid and pyrazinamide for tuberculosis evaluated in gold miners with chronic silicosis: a double-blind placebo controlled trial. Tuber Lung Dis 1996;77:239–43.

94. Cowie RL, Langton ME, Becklake MR. Pulmonary tuberculosis in South African gold miners. Am Rev Respir Dis 1989;139:1086–9.

95. Hong Kong Chest Service/Tuberculosis Research Centre, Madras/British Medical Research Council. A controlled clinical comparison of 6 and 8 months of antituberculosis chemotherapy in the treatment of patients with silicotuberculosis in Hong Kong. Am Rev Respir Dis 1991;143:262–7.

96. Cowie R. Silicotuberculosis: long term outcome after short-course chemotherapy. Tuber Lung Dis 1995;76:39–42.

97. Davis GS. Pathogenesis of silicosis: current concepts and hypotheses. Lung 1986;164:139–54.

98. Doll N, Stankus R, Hughes J. Immune complexes and autoantibodies in silicosis. J Allergy Clin Immunol 1981;68:281–5.

99. Autoimmunity phenomena and alterations of humoral immunological responses in silicotic patients. Pittsburgh (PA): DHHS (NIOSH); 1988 90.

100. Karnik AB, Saiyed HN, Nigam SK. Humoral immunologic dysfunction in silicosis. Indian J Med Res 1990;B92:440–2.

101. Nigam SK, Saiyed HN, Malaviya R, et al. Role of circulating immune complexes in the immunopathogenesis of silicosis. Toxicol Lett 1990;51:315–20.

102. Nagaoka T, Tabata M, Kobayashi K, et al. Studies on production of anticollagen antibodies in silicosis. Environ Res 1993;60:12–9.

103. Bramwell B. Diffuse scleroderma: its frequency; its occurrence in stone-masons; its treatment by fibrinolysin: elevations of

104. Erasmus LD. Scleroderma in gold-miners on the Witwatersrand with particular reference to pulmonary manifestations. S Afr J Lab Clin Med 1957;3:209–31.

105. Rodnan G, Benedek R, Medsger T, et al. The association between progressive systemic sclerosis (scleroderma) with coal miners' pneumoconiosis and other forms of silicosis. Ann Intern Med 1967;66:323–34.

106. Cowie RL. Silica-dust-exposed mine workers with scleroderma (systemic sclerosis). Chest 1987;92:260–2.

107. Sluis-Cremer GK, Hessel PA, Hnizdo EH, et al. Silica, silicosis and progressive systemic sclerosis. Br J Ind Med 1985;42:838–43.

108. Pelmear PL, Roos JO, Maehle WM. Occupationally-induced scleroderma. J Occup Med 1992;34:20–5.

109. Haustein UF, Anderegg U. Silica induced scleroderma—clinical and experimental aspects. J Rheumatol 1998;25:1917–26.

110. Klockars M, Koskela RS, Jarvinen E, et al. Silica exposure and rheumatoid arthritis: a follow up study of granite workers 1940–81. BMJ 1987;294:997–1000.

111. Sluis-Cremer G, Hessel P, Hnizdo E, et al. The relationship between silicosis and rheumatoid arthritis. Thorax 1986;41:596–600.

112. Rosenman KD, Moore-Fuller M, Reilly MJ. Connective tissue disease and silicosis. Am J Ind Med 1999;35(4):375–81.

113. Steenland K, Sanderson W, Calvert GM. Kidney disease and arthritis in a cohort study of workers exposed to silica. Epidemiology 2001;12:405–12.

114. Sanchez-Roman J, Wichmann I, Salaberri J, et al. Multiple clinical and biological autoimmune manifestations in 50 workers after occupational exposure to silica. Ann Rheumatol Dis 1993;52:534–8.

115. International Agency for Research on Cancer. Silica, some silicates, coal dust, and para-aramid fibrils. Monograph 68. Evaluation of carcinogenic risks to humans. Ref type: serial (book, monograph). Lyon, France: IARC; 1997.

116. Hessel PA, Gamble JF, Gee JBL, et al. Silica, silicosis, and lung cancer: a response to a recent working group report. J Occup Environ Med 2000;42:704–20.

117. Steenland K, Sanderson W. Lung cancer among industrial sand workers exposed to crystalline silica. Am J Epidemiol 2001;153:695–703.

118. Weill H, McDonald J. Exposure to crystalline silica and risk of lung cancer: the epidemiological evidence. Thorax 1996;51:97–102.

119. Checkoway H, Franblau A. Is silicosis required for silica-associated lung cancer. Am J Ind Med 2000;37:252–9.

120. Oxman AD, Muir DCF, Shannon HS, et al. Occupational dust exposure and chronic pulmonary disease: a systematic overview of the evidence. Am Rev Respir Dis 1993;148:38–48.

121. Churg A. Small airways disease associated with mineral dust exposure. Semin Respir Med 1992;13:140–8.

122. Collis EL, Yule GU. The mortality experience of an occupational group exposed to silica dust, compared with that of the general population and an occupational group exposed to dust not containing silica. J Ind Hyg 1933;15:395–417.

123. Steenland NK, Thun MJ, Ferguson CW, et al. Occupational and other exposures associated with male end-stage renal disease: a case/control study. Am J Public Health 1990;80:153–9.

124. Calvert G, Steenland K, Palu S. End-stage renal disease among silica-exposed gold miners: a new method for assessing incidence among epidemiologic cohorts. JAMA 1997;277:1219–23.

125. Giles RD, Sturgill BC, Suratt PM, et al. Massive proteinuria and acute renal failure in a patient with acute silicoproteinosis. Am J Med 1978;64:336–42.

126. Banks D, Multinovic J, Desnick R, et al. Silicon nephropathy mimicking Fabry's disease. Am J Nephrol 1983;3:279–84.

127. Sharma S, Pande J, Verma K. Effect of prednisolone treatment in chronic silicosis. Am Rev Respir Dis 1991;143:814–21.

128. Lapp N, Goodman G, Castranova V, et al. Acute silicosis responding to corticosteroid therapy. Chest 1990;98:67S.

129. Mason G, Abraham J, Hoffman L, et al. Treatment of mixed-dust pneumoconiosis with whole lung lavage. Am Rev Respir Dis 1982;126:1102–7.

130. Liang Y, Sun U, Chen C, et al. Clinical evaluation of massive whole lung lavage for treatment of coal workers' pneumoconiosis. He Bei Liano Yang (J Hebei Convalescence) 1992;1:1–9.

131. Wilt J, Banks D, Weissman D, et al. Reduction of lung dust burden in penumoconiosis by whole lung lavage. J Occup Environ Med 1996;38:619–24.

132. Kennedy M. Aluminum powder inhalation in the treatment of silicosis. Br J Ind Med 1956;13:85–101.

133. Jinduo Z, Jingde L, Guizhi L. Long-term follow-up observations of the therapeutic effects of PVNO. Zbl Bkt Hyg Abt Orig 1983;B178:259–62.

134. Dubois F, Begin R, Cantin A, et al. Aluminum inhalation reduces silicosis in a sheep model. Am Rev Respir Dis 1988;137:1172–9.

135. Begin R, Masse S, Dufresne A. Further information on aluminum inhalation in silicosis. Occup Environ Med 1995;52:778–80.

136. Yu X, Zou C, Lin M. Observation of the effect of tetrandrine on experimental silicosis in rats. Exotoxicol Environ Saf 1983;7:306–12.

137. Seow W, Ferrante A, Li S-Y, et al. Antiphagocytic and antioxidant properties of plant alkaloid tetrandrine. Int Arch Allergy Appl Immunol 1988;85:404–9.

138. Seow W, Li S-Y, Thong Y. Inhibitory effects of tetrandrine on human neutrophil and monocyte adherence. Immunol Lett 1986;13:83–8.

139. Castranova V, Kang J, Ma J, et al. Effects of bisbenzylisoquinoline alkaloids on alvoelar macrophages: correlation between binding affinity, inhibitory potency, and antifibrotic potential. Toxicol Appl Pharmacol 1991;108:242–52.

140. Li Q, Xu Y, Zhon Z, et al. The therapeutic effect of tetrandrine on silicosis. Chin J Tuber Respir Dis 1981;4:321–4.

141. Vermeire P, Tasson J, F Lamont, et al. Respiratory function after lung homotransplantation with a 10 month survival in man. Am Rev Respir Dis 1972;106:515–27.

142. 29 CFR (United States Code of Federal Regulations) 1910.1000. Washington (DC): Office of the Federal Register, National Archives and Records Administration, U.S. Government Printing Office: 1994.

143. National Institute for Occupational Safety and Health. Criteria for a recommended standard: occupational exposure to crystalline silica. U.S. Department of Health, Education and Welfare, Public Health Service, Center for Disease Control, 1974. HEW Publication Np (NIOSH):75–120.

144. Glindmeyer HW, Hammad YY. Contributing factors to sandblasters' silicosis: inadequate respiratory protection equipment and standards. J Occup Environ Med 1988;30:917–21.

145. Linch KD, Miller WE, Althouse RB, et al. Surveillance of respirable crystalline silica dust using OSHA compliance data (1979–1995). Am J Ind Med 1998;34:547–58.

146. Wagner GR. Screening and surveillance of workers exposed to mineral dusts. Geneva: World Health Organization; 1996.

147. National Institute for Occupational Safety and Health. Request for assistance in preventing silicosis and deaths in rock drillers. Cincinnati: DHHS(NIOSH); 1992 Publication No. 92-107.

148. National Institute for Occupational Safety and Health. Request for assistance in preventing silicosis and deaths in construction workers. Cincinnatti: DHHS(NIOSH); 1996 Publication No. 96-112.

16

COAL WORKERS' PNEUMOCONIOSIS

DANIEL E. BANKS

Coal workers' pneumoconiosis (CWP) is a disease distinct and separate from silicosis. It results from the inhalation and deposition of coal dust in the lungs. Although the coal particle is not nearly as fibrogenic as the silica particle, excessive exposure over a period of time can overwhelm effective clearance mechanisms, stimulate a fibrogenic response, and lead to a spectrum of diseases including industrial bronchitis, simple CWP, and complicated CWP (also known as progressive massive fibrosis [PMF]). In simple CWP, the chest radiograph shows only small rounded opacities (radiographically indistinguishable from the opacities recognized in silicosis). In complicated CWP or PMF, large opacities are present, again radiologically indistinguishable from those seen in silicosis.

Simple CWP is clearly related to the amount of dust deposited within the lungs. PMF most often occurs on a background of simple CWP. In addition to dust deposition, other inadequately defined immunologic and local cellular factors may contribute to the development of PMF.

PMF is clearly associated with alterations in the ventilatory, mechanical, and vascular function of the lungs. These abnormalities in PMF contribute to premature morbidity and mortality. Like silicosis, there is no specific therapy for CWP. Prevention remains the cornerstone of eliminating this disease. Education of workers and employers regarding the hazards of coal dust exposure and measurement and effective control of dust exposure are key elements of disease prevention.

The most recent trends of CWP in the United States, for the years 1985 to 1996, show a continuing decline in the overall number of deaths attributed to this illness. In those over the age of 45 years, mortality rates have significantly declined; however, there has been little change in the age group of 24 to 44 years, implying a continuing high level of exposure in some young adults in mining and mining-related occupations.[1]

HISTORY

The earliest coal mines were outcroppings of coal along river banks. As such, they could be described as surface or "open cast" mines. The drive for coal production on a large scale was associated with the manufacture of iron and derived from the development of the steam engine in the early part of the eighteenth century. It was not until 1762 that a steam engine was used to work a colliery in Scotland. Underground mining grew quickly as effective methods for ventilating fresh air into mines and removing toxic gases and water were developed. As of 1866, in Scotland alone, there were 472 coal mines, 41,000 miners, and 12 million tons of coal produced yearly.

Meiklejohn has extensively reviewed the history of lung disease in miners.[2–4] Lung disease in miners has been referred to as miners' asthma, phthisis, anthracosis, and, in Scotland, miners' black lung. In 1831, the first report of "black lungs" attributed to employment in coal mines was published.[5] A 59-year-old man who had been employed as a miner for 10 or 12 years was hospitalized for generalized anasarca and soon died from progressive heart failure. The lungs were examined and a picture consistent with PMF with cavitation of these large lesions on a background of simple CWP was described.

> At necropsy, the lungs were universally adherent to the chest wall; the pleura was thickened and in places ossified. When cut into, both lungs presented one uniform black carbonaceous color, pervading every part of their substance … The left lung did not appear to contain any cavities, but was condensed and loaded with black serum. Some minute hard points could be felt in various parts of both lungs.

Opinions regarding the explanation for this black pigment included gunpowder, inhalation of lamp-black, or soot from oil lamps of the miners. Marshall, just several years later, concluded that:

> The true explanation of the origin of this disease in colliers seems to be, that it is in consequence of the inhalation of fine coal dust, and its deposition in the substance of the lung. That coal may float through the air in particles sufficiently fine to be inhaled without immediate irritation and that it is thus inhaled is a matter of common observation.[6]

Throughout the nineteenth century, there was considerable controversy and disagreement regarding the impact of coal dust inhalation on the survival of miners. Overall, data showed that the mortality of coal miners only minimally exceeded the mortality of other groups such as farmers or agricultural laborers. The lack of coal dust effect on survival was felt attributable to better mine ventilation and lesser exposures to coal dust. Even at that time, the lesser fibrogenicity of coal dust compared to silica was recognized.[7]

Early in the twentieth century, Collis opined that coal dust did not produce pneumoconiosis (and even served to protect against tuberculosis). He attributed dust disease in miners to silica inhalation and concluded that the disease present was silicosis.[8] It was not until nearly 10 years later when washed coal, free of silica, was recognized to produce dust disease in the lungs in stevedores loading and leveling coal in the holds of ships that CWP was widely accepted as being pathologically distinct from silicosis.[9–11] Later, King and colleagues showed that the radiologic and histologic severity of pneumoconiosis in coal miners was related to the total amount of dust and not the silica content of the coal.[12]

With the development of standardized medical tools necessary to monitor pneumoconiosis in miners such as standardized questionnaires, measurement of lung function, and standardized interpretation of chest radiographs, the emphasis of CWP research from the 1930s to the present time has been on epidemiologic studies. These studies have been critical for developing current dust standards for coal mines, such as those mandated in the United States Federal Coal Mine Health and Safety Acts of 1969 and 1977.[13]

FORMATION AND CHARACTERISTICS OF COAL

Coal is not a pure mineral. It is a mixture of mainly carbon, oxygen, nitrogen, and crystalline silica. Trace elements may include boron, cadmium, nickel, iron, antimony, lead, and zinc. Coal is formed by the accumulation of vegetable matter covered by sedimentary rock (thereby sealing it from air) and subjected to pressure and temperature over the ages. This causes the physical and chemical properties of the matter to change. The matter dries, becomes warmer, and loses oxygen content, while increasing the relative carbon content.[14]

The first step in this conversion of vegetable matter to coal is the formation of peat, a moist spongy material. This transformation of an organic deposit can occur in a stagnant waterbed relatively quickly (at a rate of approximately 1 foot per hundred years). An approximately hundred foot accumulation of peat compresses to form a 1 foot wide coal seam. In the most simple terms, coal is mainly comprised of moisture (which lessens with time, "pure" coal (carbon), and mineral matter.[15]

The process of conversion (coalification) from organic matter follows a sequence from wood to peat, to lignite, to bituminous coal, and finally to anthracite coal. Rank describes the extent of change from vegetation to mineral-free coal; coal is classified primarily by rank. Rank is directly related to the percent of carbon in coal, the completeness of the transformation from vegetation to coal, and the geologic age of the deposit, with new deposits forming above the old. Indeed, Hilt observed that "in a vertical sequence, at any one locality in a coalfield, the rank of the coal seam rises with increasing depth."[16] The type of coal relates to the plant materials that form the coal. The grade refers to the purity of the coal—or the amount of inorganic material (including ash and sulfur) released in the burning of coal. Sulfur is a frequent contaminant of coal and is derived from sulfur in the plants that have formed the coal or from the pooling of water containing sulfur during the formation of coal, or both. In today's world, sulfur released as a by-product of coal burning is an important air pollutant and boiler corrosive, making coal with a high sulfur content less desirable.

Other important descriptive terms include a quantitative measurement of coal moisture (the percentage of water that is contained in coal and released with moderate heat) and the amount of volatile matter (that percentage of substances, mainly gases and coal tar, lost when a sample is well heated). The residue of combusted material remaining after a coal sample is completely burned is ash. The ash content has two sources. The first is the inherent minerals in the decaying organic material and the second is material that was blown or entered the swamp while the peat was being formed.[17]

The composition of coal mine dust varies with the coal steam. Most of the dust is carbon, although in some seams it may only approximate 60% of the dust,[18] with more than 50 different elements and their oxides.[19] Dusts of high rank typically have more silica than dusts of lesser rank. In the case of anthracite coal, seams of this rank of coal often have roofs and floors of quartz, which contaminate the coal during mining.[20]

COAL MINING

Coal mining is inherently dangerous. In addition to its respiratory risks, other serious risks include underground fires and explosions, toxic gas excess, and rock falls. Safety measures must emphasize adequate ventilation (so that methane is removed and the risk of explosion and fire minimized); protect from roof falls; and control dust. Each of the different methods of mining described below presents its own safety challenges.

Coal may be found in outcroppings and in seams that are sometimes just a few feet below the surface. In these deposits, coal can be obtained by scraping away the surface or overburden and extracting the coal with earth-moving equipment (see Chapter 15: Silicosis, Figure 15–1). This is called surface mining, strip mining, or open-cast mining. Dust levels in the air at surface mines are generally considerably lower than in underground mines with a few notable exceptions. In surface miners and coal plant cleaning workers in the anthracite coal mining area of the United States, the mean forced vital capacity (FVC), forced expiratory volume in 1 second (FEV_1), and peak flow rates were not related to the number of years worked in coal-cleaning plants.[21] Yet, there is a group of these workers at special risk for pneumoconiosis. Surface coal mine workers who operate large drills (drillers and driller helpers) to make holes in which explosives are placed in order to remove the overburden, are exposed to silica and are at risk for the development of silicosis rather than CWP.[22–24]

Workers in some exclusively above-ground operations may be exposed to coal dust. These are the workers at tipples where crushing, sizing, washing, and blending of coal is done; at surface coal mine sites away from the drilling operations; and at locations where coal is loaded into ships, railroad cars, or river barges. Although each case needs to be evaluated on an individual basis, the great majority of these exposures are relatively small and unlikely to be sufficient to cause disease.

On hillsides where the coal seam may be many feet below the surface but some outcropping occurs from the side of the hill, a feasible method of mining coal is to bore into the outcropping with an auger. Depending on how far into the hillside the seam extends, this method of mining is a combination of surface and underground mining.

Where coal seams are buried deep, typically greater than 200 feet underground, it is not economically feasible to strip away the overburden. The only practical way of mining the coal is to sink shafts from the surface to the coal seam and then follow the seam with a series of more or less horizontal tunnels. This has been the most prevalent method of mining coal in the past century.

Room and Pillar Mines

Modern underground coal mines are categorized as room and pillar mines or long-wall mines.[25] A room and pillar mine is a series of parallel rooms where mining has occurred separated by pillars of unmined coal. As mining goes on, this looks increasingly like a honeycomb. Two types of mining are performed in room and pillar mining. The first is conventional mining, and it is least mechanized, accounting for less than 10% of US coal mine production.[26] Here, incisions are cut in the sides and bases of the seam and charges inserted through holes drilled in these areas. The roof is first supported, the charges are exploded, and the coal loaded and removed from the face. The cycle is typically performed sequentially in adjacent areas to maximize coal production.

An alternative approach is continuous mining. This approach accounts for approximately half of US coal production. In continuous mining, a machine with a rotating head is used to break coal from the face. The operator advances this machine through the seam, moving the cutting head of the machine up and down to maximize coal breakaway from the face. A conveyor, incorporated into the continuous mining machine, moves the broken coal from the face to waiting underground shuttle cars. The continuous miner may include roof bolter units located just behind the rotating cutter head or have a roof bolting machine nearby. Roof bolting is necessary to provide support of the roof. Workers remain here while mining is conducted. A detailed description of these processes are reported elsewhere.[27]

In this method of mining, a substantial amount of coal remains within the pillars after the rooms are mined. To recover the coal within the pillars, each pillar is mined using timber for temporary roof support. The timber is then removed, causing the roof in that area to collapse. This approach is called retreat mining because after mining of the pillars begins, no attempt is made to go back into the block. The roof caves in and the mine is abandoned.[28]

Long-Wall Mines

Long-wall mining is the most mechanized and the most productive means of underground mining. The number of underground mines employing long-wall mining techniques continues to increase in the United States (and now is used in more than 100 mines). This accounts for more than 40% of US coal production. Long-wall mining may produce up to 40 tons of coal per minute and, in some instances, nearly 4,000 tons per work shift. In this process, the continuous miner cuts out a long wall of coal which may be 600 to 800 feet wide and 5,000 to 12,000 feet long. When the wall is formed, the hydraulically powered roof supports, the cutting machine or shearer (often with built-in water sprays to minimize dust generation), and the conveyors are put into place. The shearer moves across the coal face in a bidirectional manner with a depth of cut of about 2 feet. A conveyor belt, which runs the length of the long wall, captures the newly excavated coal. As each pass is made by the shearer (which requires one or two workers to operate and travels up to 60 ft/min), the roof supports and the conveyor are advanced. As these supports are advanced, the roof behind these supports caves in, another example of retreat mining.[29]

Although it is a very productive way to mine coal, long-wall mining has several disadvantages. First, if the cutting machine or any mechanized aspect necessary for this process fails, production of coal from the entire system stops. Second, a coal face of 600 to 800 feet may have numerous different characteristics. Attempting to mine this extensive block may lead to mining difficulties. Third, developing and setting up a long wall requires considerable time and worker effort. Finally, the large number of roof supports for a long wall are very costly. Using fewer supports would cut costs. This has led operators to combine the roof support system of the long-wall mine with the flexibility of the continuous mining machine. This has been named short-wall mining. With this approach, the face is shortened to about one-third of the length of the long wall, production is increased relative to room and pillar mining, and the miner works under the hydraulic roof support the entire time, thereby lessening the hazards of roof falls.

EPIDEMIOLOGY

Although not all investigators have identified an accelerated decline in lung function among coal miners related to dust exposure,[30] the great number of cross-sectional and longitudinal studies have shown a loss in lung function in miners using parameters that include years of employment, job category, differences in pneumoconiosis prevalence related to different regions of the country, rank of coal mined,[31] and duration and intensity of exposure.[32–34] To further complicate the assessment of the effect of coal dust in workers, there are a number of other potential risk factors that may result in an accelerated decline in FEV_1 independent of coal dust exposure, which might confound the potentially adverse effect of dust on lung function. These include host susceptibility factors,[35] a family history of atopy,[36] cigarette smoking, childhood illnesses,[37] obesity and excessive weight gain,[38] intercurrent chest infections,[39] as well as previous or concurrent environmental exposures.[40] Recent data have suggested that childhood passive exposure to cigarette smoke and possibly indoor smoke exposure due to wood and coal fuels may also be relevant.[41] Not surprisingly, many of the following reports did not or were unable to address these potential influences on lung function.

It should also be recognized that interpretation of longitudinal lung function tests can be difficult and reflect large unexplained rates of decline that appear to occur in members of all populations. For example, a recent retrospective review of lung function separate US coal miners into two serially assessed groups: rapid decliners (> 60 mL decline/year) compared with matched [by age, height, smoking status, and initial FEV_1 to those whose FEV_1 is < 60 mL/year]—no data regarding mine, mining job, or exposure]) versus controls.[42] The mean yearly FEV_1 change was –92 mL/yr versus –5 mL/yr and an FVC decline of –103 mL/yr versus –16 mL/yr in rapid decliners versus controls, respectively. The authors presented this data as reflective of the serious respiratory risk attributable to coal mining. In comparison, steel workers—a healthy population shown to have lung function changes attributable to weight gain, not dust—had serial lung function tests and were separated into rapid decliners versus controls using the same parameters. In this population, the mean FVC changed –96 mL/yr versus +5 mL/yr and FEV_1 changed –95 mL/yr versus + 10 mL/yr in rapid decliners versus controls, respectively, was essentially no different from the coal miners.[43]

Industrial Bronchitis

The most common adverse effect of dust exposure is the development of industrial bronchitis. Miners, as a group, are at considerable risk for this because of their dust exposures in the mine environment.[44–46] Industrial bronchitis is manifest as a productive cough that persists for at least 3 months per year for at least 2 years (chronic bronchitis) associated with workplace dust exposure. The relationship between coal mining and bronchial mucous gland dimensions was presented in an autopsy study by Douglas and colleagues.[47] Coal dust exposure resulted in an increase in the maximal gland-wall ratio independent of smoking, even though no relationship between mucous gland size and lung dust or pneumoconiosis was found. This suggests that pneumoconiosis is related to respirable dust exposure whereas mucous gland enlargement is related to the inhalation of larger (nonrespirable) dust particles that present a chronic burden to the mucociliary escalator and act as irritants to the airway.

Early reports showed that the prevalence of bronchitis in coal miners varied by smoking history, age, and job.[48] In all reports, miners who smoked had bronchitis more frequently than nonsmokers and, when studied, showed that bronchitis increased with age (a surrogate for years of dust exposure in the workplace). Marine and colleagues identified 543 lifetime nonsmokers among 14,888 British coal miners (3.6%) studied between 1953 and 1967 who were less than 65 years of age, who worked at the coal face in most instances and were without PMF, and who participated in three surveys over 10 years. Of these, 17% had bronchitis at the time of the third survey.[49] In a second report of coal miners, 16% had bronchitis.[50]

Dust Exposure and Changes in Lung Function

There is little information on the natural history of chronic bronchitis in nonsmoking miners once they are removed from dust exposure. Bates and colleagues[51] showed no change in the annual rate of lung function decline in miners who retired from mining compared with the rate of decline while mining. Those who were rapid decliners continued at that pace, which was attributed to dust loading of the lung. A repeat analysis of this population, reported approximately 10 years later, showed that smokers continued at an unchanged accelerated rate of FEV_1 decline after leaving mining, while the nonsmokers rate of decline slowed after ceasing mining.[52] Although perhaps not relevant to the mining population, Kauffman and colleagues[53] noted that the rate of lung function decline lessened or returned to normal when Paris factory workers exposed to dust moved to jobs in a nondusty environment.

Among underground miners, those working at the face and exposed to higher concentrations of coal mine dust had a higher prevalence of CWP than surface workers or those who entered the face area intermittently.[54] For example, miners in Pennsylvania anthracite seams had a considerably greater prevalence of CWP than miners in the western plateau of Colorado and Utah who mined a lower rank of coal. In this report, categories of simple pneumoconiosis were not consistently associated with a decline in FEV_1 unless another process (typically bronchitis) was present, whereas complicated pneumoconiosis was generally associated with a significant decline in FEV_1.

In a summary of the results of numerous epidemiologic studies of workers exposed to dust, Becklake[55] observed that "airflow limitation, almost certainly multifactorial in etiology, occurs in those engaged in dusty occupations as well as in those who are not. Among the environmental factors concerned, cigarette smoking is clearly one of the most important, but occupational exposures are increasingly implicated; it is also clear that not all with similar exposures are affected, pointing to the importance of host or personal factors." In this connection, it is natural to consider the variation in responses to dust and why some workers respond to dust exposures by developing clinically evident functional changes whereas others have fewer symptoms.[56]

Yet, it is clear that epidemiologic studies, where no clinical input is available, may not be able to separate the effects of dust from that of other variables. For example, among 203 steel workers who never smoked and had yearly spirometry performed twice or more over the 1980s, 3 of the 203 (1.5%) and 17 of the remaining 200 (8.5%) had final FEV_1 values < 65% or between 65 and 80% predicted, respectively.[57] Of the 3 workers with a FEV_1 < 65% predicted, 1 was morbidly obese (body mass index of 39.6 kg/m²), 1 had a history of trauma with fractured ribs, arm, and pelvis, and a diaphragmatic hernia following a severe crush injury, and 1 had a FEV_1 of 64% and a FVC of 59%, without a clear explanation for this apparent restriction. In the 17 with FEV_1 values between 65 and 80% predicted, 1 chart was unavailable for review, and 14 had either a history of chest trauma, obesity, asthma, hay fever, or a combination of these conditions. Medical conditions that might explain this decline in the remaining 2 workers were not apparent. In this instance attributing the apparent changes in lung function to dust exposures may not be accurate, and reports of this nature illustrate the complexity of straight-forward epidemiologic surveys of workers' health. Furthermore, although a number of studies have suggested a statistically significant association between dust exposure and the loss of lung function, the recognition of these "average effects" provide little indication of the importance of this effect in individual miners.

Population studies of coal miners have been complicated and associated with variable results, although the increasing consensus is that there is a degree of airway obstruction associated with coal dust exposure.

Investigators have identified miners who have suffered severe impairment of lung function. In 31 nonsmoking miners and ex-miners who applied for "black lung" compensation, 6 had a FEV_1 value < 60% pre-

dicted or a FEV_1/FVC ratio < 60%. Of these, 5 had medical conditions that reasonably explained this impairment, yet 1 had unexplained severe obstruction.[58]

Smoking and Dust Exposure

Not surprisingly, when one reviews the estimated annual decline of FEV_1 attributable to smoking and dust exposure in coal mining populations, smoking was constantly a strong predictor for annual decline of FEV_1. In reports by Attfield[59] and Seixas and colleagues,[60] the relationship between dust exposure and lung function was less evident when longitudinal compared with cross-sectional approaches were applied to the same population. Only one of four models in Attfield's report showed a relationship between face work and annual decline of FEV_1 ($p = .01$). In this report, the estimated annual loss of FEV_1 attributed to smoking ranged from 8.5 to 15.5 mL/yr, whereas the decline due to dust exposure was 3.8 to 7.9 mL/yr depending on the level of exposure.

Variations in the rate of FEV_1 decline in longitudinal studies have been found by other investigators. Love and Miller[61] examined the lung function of British coal miners who took part in three surveys. Regression analysis showed that age, height, and smoking each made a strong contribution to explaining the observed loss of FEV_1. After adjustment for these factors, the rate of FEV_1 declined only an additional 3.8 mL/yr with an average observed dust exposure of 117 gram-hours/m³ over approximately 11 years.

A cross-sectional analysis of the relationship between lung function and individual cumulative exposure to respirable coal mine dust was estimated in approximately 4,000 British miners and ex-miners.[62] If those with PMF are excluded, the average loss of FEV_1 due to moderately high dust exposures (a cumulative exposure of 300 gh/m³—approximately 35 years of exposure at twice the current US permissible dust exposure limit) was an excess of 228 mL, which is approximately 6 mL per year. However, in a select group of ex-miners with chronic bronchitis, the estimated effect of this exposure was greater, whereas in 35 ex-smokers (1.6% of the ex-miners), the mean loss was an excess of 940 mL of FEV_1 (approximately a 30 mL additional decline per year resulting in an FEV_1 of about 65% predicted). The authors observed "a third factor, whether intrinsic susceptibility to the effects of dust or an environmental factor not so far identified, must be sought to explain why these men suffered such severe lung damage in response to their exposure to respirable dust."

Marine and colleagues[49] analyzed the results of lung function from 3,380 British miners using a linear logistic model. The average age of the miner was 47 years. The "high" exposure (348 gh/m³) group had an estimated mean dust concentration in the range of 6.1 to 7.2 mg/m³ for a working lifetime. The estimated prevalence of miners who smoke and have a FEV_1 < 65% predicted was 14.2% and 5.0% and in nonsmoking miners was 7.7 and 3.2%, assuming a "high" or "zero" exposure, respectively. This implies that approximately 4% of the nonsmoking miners and 9% of the smoking miners had "clinically significant" obstruction attributable to dust. Regrettably, in attempts to further review this data, no spirometry curves were available for review.

Similarly, Soutar and colleagues[63] showed that in one British colliery where lifetime dust exposures approximated 400 gh/m^3 (35 years of employment at a mean dust exposure of 7 mg/m^3), approximately 20% of the nonsmokers and 45% of the smokers had a "clinically important" deficit in lung function. The authors suggest that these values are greater than those in other reports because miners with PMF were included. In two other collieries, where the exposures were less, such clinically important declines were not shown. This was thought to be due to less dust exposure and possible confounding between dust exposure and age.

Oxman and colleagues[64] reviewed studies on three cohorts of coal miners where dust measurements were available and where the relationship between dust exposure and outcome was determined while controlling for age and smoking. All showed a relationship between lung function and dust exposure. In two other reports,[49,65] data were re-analyzed to show the number of workers by smoking category with clinically significant declines in FEV$_1$. Approximately 1.2% of nonsmoking coal miners (p = .053) and 2.3% of smoking coal miners (p < .001) with a cumulative dust exposure of 122.5 gh/m^3 (35 years of work with a mean dust exposure of 2 mg/m^3) could be expected to have a percent predicted FEV$_1$ < 65%.

The predicted FEV$_1$ versus years of dust exposure were plotted (at a specific mean dust concentration of 4.0 mg/m^3—twice the current US coal dust standard) using regression equations derived from cross-sectional data analyses by Attfield and Hodous.[66] For a nonsmoking White man standardized to age 50, 71 inches tall, and with dust exposures ranging from none to 30 years, the result was an additional maximal 3.6% decline in the FEV$_1$ compared with the predicted FEV$_1$ values of a non-coal miner.[67]

The rate of lung function decline among miners in any given population may not be linear. Longitudinal studies have also suggested that the miner is most susceptible to the dust effect in the early years of mining employment, with the rate of decline plateauing over time. In young Sardinian miners with higher cumulative exposures to dust over a 7-year time period, the later dust exposures had a smaller net effect on the decline in lung function than those early on.[68] Reports on US miners have shown a similar phenomenon, as well as a suggestion that rates of decline, which were accelerated early on, tend to plateau over time.[69]

Petsonk and colleagues[70] have shown that miners employed in the dustiest jobs were less likely to have methacholine hyperresponsiveness than their less-exposed coworkers, suggesting that this "self-selection" may allow them to remain in dusty jobs where others would leave because of respiratory symptoms. When airway responsiveness was measured serially in underground coal miners, those whose hyperresponsiveness lessened over time had a less-accelerated rate of FEV$_1$ decline.[71]

In summary, even though only a few populations have been studied worldwide, there is a statistically significant relationship between mean FEV$_1$ decline and dust exposure. Some workers within a dust-exposed population develop a clinically significant decline. Other illnesses may contribute to this decline. Because of the apparent exaggerated rate of lung function decline among miners in the early years of their employment, it is likely that those with the greatest difficulty in tolerating dust exposure leave the workplace early on.

Incidence and Prevalence of CWP

Institution and enforcement of dust control measures have reduced the attack rate of CWP and may have lessened progression among those with radiographic opacities who continued to work in mines. The US coal dust standard was initiated in 1969 at 3 mg/m^3 and reduced to 2 mg/m^3 in 1972.[72]

The US Public Health Service has performed a series of studies evaluating the prevalence of CWP. Round one of the US coal workers' surveillance program was performed using data collected from 1970 to 1973. The most recent, round five of this same program, was undertaken from 1987 to 1991. Data from these studies have been presented in summary form in a series of reports.[73–75] Mines chosen for evaluation represented different geographic areas, coal seams, and coal mining methods. These studies appear to show a reduction in the prevalence of CWP over time. When comparing studies from the mid-70s to the mid-80s, the number of cases with both simple CWP and PMF declined in all groups with at least 10 years of mining. In one group, miners with a mining tenure of between 15 and 24 years, the prevalence decreased to less than half. Similarly, in those with a lifetime of coal mining, 11% had category 2 simple CWP in round one compared with 2% in round four. An important concern about these data is whether this decline is a true decrease or the effect of self-selection inducing bias. In the years 1970 to 1973, approximately 75% of the nation's 100,000 miners participated in the program. Participation decreased to approximately 15% of the mining work force in the study performed from 1987 to 1991.

In a recent reported study of 43,504 Indian coal miners from the southeastern part of the country, the prevalence of CWP was 3%, with 81% of these being category 1 simple CWP and 18% category 2 simple CWP. Three cases of PMF were detected.[76]

Data from British studies have shown that the attack rate (incidence of new cases) and the probability of progressing to a higher category of simple CWP once the disease is recognized, are related to the mass of respirable dust to which the miner is exposed during his lifetime.[77] As a general rule, once the miner with simple CWP leaves dust exposure, the chest radiograph is not likely to progress. Yet, in an important report regarding progression of CWP described in Scottish underground miners, an accelerated rate of radiologic progression was recognized after some of these miners ceased mining. Investigations into this pattern of progression revealed that these miners had large quartz exposures in the process of mining. Individuals with silicosis are well recognized to progress after ceasing employment.[78]

The same cannot be said for PMF. The rate of progression to PMF appears to be influenced chiefly by the age at which the miner begins to show radiographic changes of CWP. Progression may also be influenced by the presence of a rheumatoid diathesis.[79]

MORTALITY STUDIES

A number of studies have addressed mortality rates in coal miners and CWP. Perhaps the best to summarize the rates of mortality in the first part of the twentieth century was Enterline, who noted that it was not until 1950 that relatively accurate death certificate data, which described an individual's usual occupation, became available.[80] In US Public Health Service data collection from death certificates for the year 1950,[81] there was a gross excess in mortality for all ages for coal miners compared to the general population. For example, in miners aged 45 to 64 years, the standard mortality ratio (SMR = the ratio between the predicted number of deaths and the observed number of deaths) approximated 2.0.

To further emphasize the mortality risk of being a coal miner between the years 1949 and 1963, the Society of Actuaries published SMRs on 44 US occupations using life insurance policy data.[82] Of all of these occupations, coal mining had the highest SMR. The SMR for coal miners was 1.5. The SMR for death attributable to respiratory disease exceeded 40.0 using death certificate data and 11.0 using life insurance policy information. Even when accidents and respiratory disease were eliminated as causes of death, the SMR for coal miners ranged between 1.4 and 1.7 times the death rate for all working men. Even as late as 1979, a coal miner was recognized to have a twofold risk of being killed at work compared to the risk of the average worker.[83]

Studies involving approximately 6,000 miners and ex-miners residing in the Rhondda Fach,[84,85] a mining community in southern Wales, also showed an excess mortality. In the absence of pneumoconiosis, or when simple pneumoconiosis, or even PMF of category A was present, the SMR approximated 1.2. The number of deaths did not vary by pneumoconiosis category unless category B or C large opacities were present. When category B or C large opacities were present, the SMR

nearly doubled that of the comparison group. Chronic bronchitis occurred twice as often as a cause of death among the miners. Additionally, carcinoma of the stomach increased with pneumoconiosis category, a feature frequently reported in other studies. Ortmeyer and colleagues[86] reviewed mortality for compensated Pennsylvania miners by category of opacity on the chest radiograph and recorded similar results.

Stocks was one of the first to present the relationship between mining and gastric cancer, but his report made it clear that it was necessary to compare the mining risks for illness with local controls. He showed that the rate of gastric cancer among miners in the United Kingdom varied, with it being most frequent in south Wales, intermediate in northern England, and least in the Midlands.[87] The relationship between this malignancy and coal dust exposure was also suggested in a study of gastric carcinoma in Utah. Gastric malignancy was increased nearly threefold in residents of two Utah coal mining counties, leading the authors to speculate that swallowed coal particles containing polyaromatic hydrocarbons, such as benzpyrene, increased the gastric cancer risk.[88]

Additional mortality data for US coal miners on the rolls of the United Mine Workers Health and Retirement Fund from 1959 to 1971 were presented by Rockette.[89] Of the 23,232 men enrolled, 7,741 died. The overall SMR for this population was 1.02, a dramatic improvement compared with the above-cited death certificate study by Enterline published in 1994. Yet, the SMRs for several specific categories of illness remained elevated. Specifically, the SMR for nonmalignant respiratory disease was 1.6 and the SMR for accidents was 1.8. Although mortality due to all cancers was not increased, the SMRs for stomach and lung cancer were excessive (1.4 and 1.1, respectively).

In a mortality report of Appalachian coal miners and ex-miners followed from 1963 to 1971, the mortality of current miners was 7% less than expected although the mortality for ex-miners was 24% greater than expected.[90] Simple pneumoconiosis did not affect life expectancy whereas the presence of PMF did.

Meijers and colleagues[91] postulated that coal workers have a greater risk of lung cancer due to their exposure to coal mine dust, a material containing various potentially carcinogenic organic (ie, hydrocarbons) and inorganic (ie, trace elements such as cadmium and chromium) compounds. In support of this hypothesis, crystalline silica, a component of coal dust, had been declared a carcinogen.[92] The cause of death of 334 miners from a cohort of 5,400 miners with CWP employed in 11 Dutch coal mines from 1956 to 1960 was evaluated in 1983. Data showed a higher than expected mortality, primarily attributed to stomach and large and small intestine malignancy, as well as more frequent nonmalignant respiratory diseases.

Exposure data were available for 26,363 coal miners from 20 collieries in England and Wales who first attended medical screening between 1953 and 1958.[93] A chest radiograph, respiratory questionnaire, and coal mining history were recorded and estimates of exposure made. An assessment of the causes of 8,489 deaths was begun in 1980. The general mortality was 13% less on average than in English and Welsh men in the same region. The survival of miners with category A large opacities was less than that of men without pneumoconiosis, yet the mortality rate did not increase with increasing category of simple pneumoconiosis. Mortality due to all causes, as well as that attributable to pneumoconiosis, bronchitis, and emphysema, increased with cumulative dust exposure. Furthermore, in those with greater dust exposures at the start of the evaluation, particularly those of an older age group, a less survival was reported. There was no association between lung cancer and coal mining, but the risk for cancer of the digestive system approached significance. In a later follow-up of this population, survival rates of those with category 1 simple pneumoconiosis were 2% to 3% lower than in miners without radiologic evidence of pneumoconiosis, but there was no consistent increase in mortality with increasing category of pneumoconiosis.[94]

The mortality experience of US coal miners with exposure estimates was reported by Kuempel and colleagues.[95] In this population, the mortality experience of 793 men among a population of 8,878 miners enrolled between 1969 and 1971 and followed until 1979 was evaluated. Overall, the SMR for all causes was 0.85, the SMRs for bronchitis, emphysema, lung cancer, and stomach cancer were not increased. No statistical relationship between deaths due to lung cancer or stomach cancer was reported.

A case-control study compared the risk for lung cancer in smoking and nonsmoking coal miners and showed no evidence of a coal mine dust exposure lung cancer risk and no evidence of an interactive effect between cigarette smoking and coal mine dust exposure.[96]

In summary, a series of mortality reports have not convincingly shown that simple CWP is associated with premature mortality. However, PMF adversely effects survival, especially when category B and C large opacities are present. Although there appears to be no clear difference in the SMR for lung cancer between miners and nonminers,[97] a number of studies show an increase in the SMR for digestive cancer, in general, and stomach cancer, in particular.

PATHOLOGY

As the normal dust clearance mechanisms of the lung are overwhelmed, dust deposition increases. With the initiation and progression of fibrosis, lung lesions increase in size and number. A focal collection of coal dust in pigment-laden macrophages around dilated respiratory bronchioles, which tapers off toward the alveolar duct, is initially apparent.[98] This is the coal macule, the characteristic lesion of CWP (Figure 16–1). A fine network

of reticulin within this collection of cells may be visible early on. Focal emphysema is a specific entity that is an integral part of the simple lesion of simple CWP. The coal macule, the basic pathologic feature of CWP, is associated with enlargement of the air spaces immediately adjacent to this collection of dust, a feature described as centrilobular emphysema.[99]

Emphysema

Ryder and colleagues[100] showed a significant excess of emphysema in coal miners with pneumoconiosis compared to nonminers but did not comment on the prevalence of emphysema in miners without pneumoconiosis. Coal miners in south Wales showed more centrilobular emphysema at autopsy compared to nonminers; however, much of this difference was explained by current smokers over the age of 60 years, a group where PMF was common.[101] Lyons and colleagues[102] reported similar findings.

Centrilobular emphysema was by far the most common type of emphysema encountered in both smokers and nonsmokers; with less decline in FEV_1 in nonsmokers than in smokers. Results from a large autopsy series of miners from 24 British coal mines showed a very strong relationship between smoking and emphysema.[103] As expected, centrilobular emphysema increased with smoking and age. In the absence of pneumoconiosis, there was no detectable effect of dust leading to emphysema. Even though the groups with simple pneumoconiosis and PMF (groups with an increased exposure to coal dust) had an increased chance of centriacinar emphysema, no clear relationship could be demonstrated between the amount of dust in the lung and the extent of emphysema.

Leigh and colleagues[104] noted that the use of the pathologic assessment of the lung to determine the relationship between emphysema and coal dust might

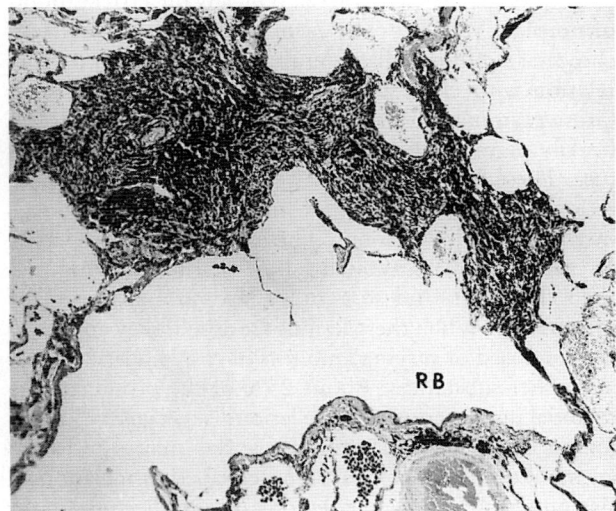

Figure 16–1   Histology section from a patient with coal workers' pneumoconiosis showing a typical coal macule.

induce bias because coal macules might draw attention to emphysematous spaces, resulting in the perspective that emphysema is more common in those with pneumoconiosis. They measured the actual coal content of the lungs and found that in smokers, the emphysema score was driven by the coal content in the lungs, cigarette smoking, and age. In nonsmokers, the coal content and age were most important. Questionnaire data on smoking were reported and correlations among emphysema score, questionnaire, and lung function tests performed during life were attempted. In nonsmokers, the relationship between the decline in FEV_1/FVC and the increase in emphysema score approached significance.

The impact of this pathologic change on lung function has been the subject of considerable discussion. In nonsmoking, nonobstructed miners, Morgan and colleagues[105] showed an increase in the residual volume (RV). In miners without CWP, the RV was 105% of a group of nonminers. This increased to 108% and 114% of controls in miners with category 1 or category 2 and 3 simple CWP, respectively. Although Morgan and colleagues[105] considered that this might be attributable to focal emphysema, they thought that unlikely because pathologic disruption of the bronchioles was absent. Rather, they considered this hyperinflation to be the result of the narrowing of the airways by coal macules located along the airway margins with diminution of the peripheral flow rates and increasing airway resistance.[105]

On gross examination of the lung, larger collections of dust are described as coal nodules, classified as micronodular if they are 7 mm in diameter or less and macronodular if they are larger. These nodules are palpable whereas coal macules are not.

Progressive Massive Fibrosis

PMF is diagnosed when one or more nodules attain a size of 2 cm or greater in diameter, typically on a background of simple CWP.[106,107] The 2 cm diameter is an arbitrary choice of a minimal diameter that has allowed better correlation with clinical and radiographic measurements. Gross examination of the lung in PMF reveals a solid, heavily pigmented lung that is rubbery-to-hard in texture. These features are most apparent in the apical posterior portions of the upper lobes or the superior segments of the lower lobes. These lesions tend to occur asymmetrically, occasionally show first in one lung and then the other, and sometimes lead to a suspicion of malignancy. When these lesions are ashed, they appear to be composed of varying amounts of coal, silica, calcium, and other substances. About 25% of the proteinaceous material in the center of these lesions is collagen.[108] These lesions may also cavitate and the worker may expectorate an inklike fluid (a clinical sign described as melanoptysis), or when these cavitary lesions are cut, they may drain inklike fluid. Airways and vessels adjacent to the lesions are distorted and destroyed within the lesions.

Caplan's Syndrome

Caplan's syndrome is described with coal dust exposure. It is a nodular lung reaction that occurs in dust-exposed individuals who either have rheumatoid arthritis or who develop rheumatoid arthritis within the subsequent 5 to 10 years.[109,110] The nodules vary in diameter from 0.5 to 5.0 cm and are usually multiple, bilateral, and peripherally situated. Grossly, the lesions resemble a giant silicotic nodule. Microscopically the amount of dust in the lesion is small, there is a necrotic area in the center, and there is a surrounding cellular zone infiltrated with lymphocytes and plasma cells. In many nodules there is a peripheral zone of active inflammation with neutrophils and a few macrophages. The natural history of these nodules is unpredictable, as they may increase in size, remain unchanged over time, or resolve.

PATHOGENESIS

Coal workers' pneumoconiosis is the result of coal dust–induced cell damage with activation of the fibrotic process. Lapp and Castranova[111] provided a well-outlined approach to addressing how coal dust causes lung damage and which focuses on the very important role of the alveolar macrophage. Potential mechanisms include the

1. direct cytotoxicity of coal dust;
2. stimulation of alveolar macrophages by coal to release oxidants or enzymes that induce lung damage;
3. stimulation of alveolar macrophages to secrete inflammatory factors that recruit and/or activate neutrophils causing additional damage; and
4. stimulation of alveolar macrophages to secrete factors that induce fibroblast proliferation and stimulate collagen synthesis in the area of coal dust deposition.

Coal dust is much less fibrogenic than silica. A mixture of 10% silica and 90% coal is far more cytotoxic to macrophages than pure coal dust.[112] Although alveolar macrophages in animals are activated after chronic exposure to coal dust, there is little lung damage. Protein and lysosomal enzyme levels in the acellular lavage fluid of these animals are not increased. However, when as little as 2% silica is added, the fibrotic process begins.[113] Castranova and Vallyathan[114] reported on cytotoxicity, activation of oxidants from alveolar macrophages, and dust-induced stimulation of cytokine and chemokine secretion from lung cells exposed to silica and coal dust. Overall, in each of the three categories, silica was more toxic than coal dust. Both silica and coal dusts, when cleaved, show surface radicals by electron spin resonance spectroscopy, a fact which has dramatically changed our understanding of the pathogenesis of these dust diseases.[115] The free radicals generated by crushing anthracite coal are more numerous than those generated by crushing bituminous coal, leading to speculation that this is a way in which anthracite coal dust exposure increases the risk for disease.[116]

Long-term coal dust exposure in animals increases the number of alveolar cells recovered by lung lavage.[117] In addition, an elevation in the number of blood monocytes and an increased rate of mitosis have been recognized in cells from animals undergoing chronic coal dust inhalation.[118] This suggests that recruitment of cells into the lung from the alveolar capillaries and the interstitium of the lung occurs with dust inhalation. Recruited "young" macrophages appear to be more phagocytically active than older macrophages. This may be a mechanism for more effective clearance of particles.

Exposure of alveolar macrophages to particles can result in the release of proteolytic enzymes, reactive oxygen species (ie, hydrogen peroxide, hydroxyl radical, and superoxide anion), and leukotrienes via the breakdown of arachidonic acid in the cell membrane.[119] Again, silica is a much stronger stimulus for the release of these agents than coal dust.[120] Excessive release of these reactive oxygen species has the potential to overwhelm the naturally protective antioxidant system within the lung and begin the process of inflammation and fibrosis.

Activated macrophages secrete a wide variety of mediators that can attract neutrophils into the effected area and then stimulate them to release reactive oxygen species and enzymes.[121] Similarly, the macrophage-derived inflammatory factors can act as chemotactic agents for neutrophils (eg, tumor necrosis factor-alpha, interleukin-8, and leukotrienes) and increase neutrophil adherence and reactive enzyme release (platelet-derived growth factor and platelet activating factor). The presence of these factors escalates the inflammatory process. Finally, secretion of many of the above factors by activated macrophages also enhances fibroblast growth and/or stimulates the production of collagen.

A number of investigators have applied bronchoalveolar lavage (BAL) to evaluate mechanisms of CWP. Lapp and colleagues[122] compared 12 asymptomatic, lifelong nonsmoking coal miners without pneumoconiosis with a mean of 17 years of underground mining exposure using BAL with the results from 18 controls.[122] There was no difference in BAL mean total or differential cell counts, immunoglobulin A (Ig)A or IgG concentration, or spontaneous or stimulated phorbol myristic acetate (PMA)-stimulated alveolar macrophage chemiluminescence in the two groups. BAL total protein levels and particle-stimulated chemiluminescence were decreased in miners. Scanning electron microscopy showed a marked increase in alveolar macrophage cell surface ruffling consistent with activation. Transmission electron microscopy showed particles in macrophages consistent with coal.

Rom and colleagues[123] studied 15 symptomatic, nonsmoking coal miners with simple CWP by BAL. There was no significant difference between miners with CWP and controls in the number of cells recovered, BAL cell differentials, and in the release of superoxide anion or hydrogen peroxide from alveolar macrophages. This contrasted with findings in subjects with asbestosis and silicosis, whose values for the spontaneous release of oxidant superoxide and hydrogen peroxide were significantly greater than controls. BAL levels of fibronectin and alveolar macrophage–derived growth factor (AMDGF) were elevated but not different from the values obtained in subjects with asbestosis and silicosis. Although fibrosis has not been a major part of the pathology of simple CWP, there is evidence of the presence of fibronectin in pneumonoconiotic lesions.[124]

In contrast with other reports, Wallaert and colleagues[125] demonstrated a significantly increased number of total cells in the BAL recovered from miners with simple and complicated CWP. Alveolar cells from miners with simple CWP and PMF spontaneously released significantly more superoxide, as contrasted with the levels generated in the comparison group. However, when these alveolar cells were stimulated with PMA, only cells recovered from miners with PMF showed significantly increased amounts of superoxide release.

As noted, coal dust is much less fibrogenic than silica dust; yet, coal dust is a sufficient stimulus for the secretion and release of macrophage products. These activated macrophages can release enzymes, reactive oxygen species, cytokines, and growth factors that cause fibroblast proliferation.[126] All are important factors in inflammation and the development of CWP.

The chest radiograph in simple CWP correlates with the amount of dust in the lung at autopsy.[127] This is not true of the complicated form of the disease, suggesting that inadequately defined host factors play a role in the development of this lesion. Hypotheses proposed to explain the differences in tissue response to coal dust in those who remain with simple CWP and those who progress to PMF include differing silica contents of inhaled dusts, development of mycobacterial infection, and differences in host immune responses to dust inhalation. None of these appear to be fully satisfactory explanations. PMF has been reported in carbon electrode workers, suggesting that silica exposure is not necessary for PMF. Treatment of miners with simple CWP in Wales with antituberculous drugs did not prevent PMF.[128] Host factors predisposing to the development of PMF have been elusive. If such factors are present, they do not appear to be linked to histocompatibility type.[129]

Relationships between autoantibodies and CWP have been explored extensively. Soutar reported circulating antinuclear factor (ANA) and rheumatoid factor (RF) levels among 109 miners with radiographic evidence of pneumoconiosis. The authors did not identify the region of the country from which the miners came or in which mines they worked. They found positive ANA in 17% and RF in 10% of the miners. The expected prevalence in the male general population of a positive ANA approximate 2 to 3%. The prevalence of ANA was lowest (9%) in simple CWP and 27% in those with category C (PMF). A similar but less striking trend was seen with RF, ranging from 6% in simple CWP to 18% in category C. Combining both ANA and RF resulted in a prevalence of positive results in 13% of the miners with simple CWP and 45% of those with category C PMF.[130]

In 1973, Lippmann and colleagues[131] reported a prevalence study among coal miners in the United States. Sera from 207 coal miners were examined. Of the 196 miners with pneumoconiosis, 9% were positive for RF and 34% had a positive ANA. There were regional variations in ANA that seemed to parallel the prevalence of radiographic changes; namely, a higher prevalence in the anthracite miners and a lower prevalence in bituminous miners.[131] These authors did not find the increased prevalence of RF in miners with PMF compared with simple CWP that Wagner and McCormick[132] reported in Welch miners.

Benedek and colleagues[133] were unable to confirm findings reported by European investigators among miners in the United States. These authors matched 55 pairs of coal miners with rheumatoid arthritis with nonminers with rheumatoid arthritis. The miners and controls did not differ in respect to serum concentrations of IgG or IgA. Elevated levels of IgM were more frequent among the miners but did not reach significance. RF was positive in 82% of miners and only 64% of nonminers ($p < .05$), but there was no correlation with category of pneumoconiosis.

Studies of serum immunoglobulins were also conducted by Hahon and colleagues[134] among 155 US coal miners with chest radiographs demonstrating simple CWP, Caplan's syndrome, and PMF. They found significantly higher serum concentrations of complement (C)3, alpha$_1$-antitrypsin, and IgA and IgG in anthracite miners than in bituminous miners with PMF. There were few differences in these serum proteins among the miners with simple CWP. Compared with normal controls, the miners' C3, alpha$_1$-antitrypsin, and IgG values were elevated. The authors did not find an association between the elevated immunoglobulins and FEV$_1$.

Burrell[135] used an antiglobulin consumption test to identify autoantibodies in the sera of coal miners directed at lung parenchyma and basement membrane. The lung autoantibodies tended to reside in the IgA class. The role of these and other autoantibodies in the pathogenesis of CWP remains unclear.

CLINICAL FEATURES

Three criteria are necessary for the diagnosis of CWP.[77] They include

1. a chest radiograph consistent with the features of CWP;
2. a work history (typically that of underground coal mining) that is sufficient in exposure and latency to result in pneumoconiosis; and
3. the absence of other illnesses that may mimic CWP.

Therefore, the diagnosis of CWP is a clinical and radiologic diagnosis that can be made with confidence and without histologic confirmation. Clinical features such as dyspnea, cough, and sputum production are important in addressing the degree of a miner's overall respiratory impairment but are not a part of the diagnostic criteria.

The radiographic appearance of CWP is indistinguishable from that of silicosis and miners may develop disease from exposure to both dusts (see Chapter 15: Silicosis, Figure 15–1). As is the case of silicosis, the International Labour Office (ILO) classification scheme is used in radiographic interpretation for both compensation assessments and for epidemiologic studies of CWP.[136,137]

Typically, CWP is described as either simple pneumoconiosis or PMF. The chest radiograph has been recognized as the "gold standard" for diagnosing CWP in compensation matters, although it appears that high-resolution computed tomography scans are more sensitive in the detection of small rounded opacities.[138] The chest radiograph in simple pneumoconiosis shows small rounded opacities, ranging in size from a pinhead to 1 cm in diameter. Rounded nodules predominate and tend to appear first in the upper zones and then the rest of the lung as the number of opacities increase. With prolonged excessive exposure these small opacities may coalesce and form larger opacities, recognized as PMF lesions and characterized by one or more large opacities greater than 1 cm in diameter. As the disease progresses, the upper-zone nodules begin to coalesce and distort the lung architecture, a feature that gradually becomes more prominent. This typically presents as deviation of the trachea and major airways to the side of the most prominent area of coalescence, loss of upper-zone lung volume, elevation of the hila, and basilar emphysema (typically of a panacinar type) attributable to traction placed on the lower lung zones by the elevation of the hila.

There are no symptoms or physical signs associated with simple CWP. The not infrequent presence of a chronic cough and sputum production, even in the presence of CWP, is attributable to "industrial bronchitis." Alternately, these same clinical features in a miner who smokes may be partially attributable to bronchitis induced by the inflammatory stimulus of cigarette smoke. Finger clubbing is not a feature of CWP and, if noted, should prompt further investigations.

When PMF is recognized on the chest radiograph, the worker frequently describes dyspnea, cough, and sputum production, although it is well recognized that the degree of impairment or the presence or absence of symptoms does not always correlate well with the extent of chest radiographic abnormalities.

The consultant may be requested to differentiate a primary or metastatic neoplasm from an unusual presentation of PMF. When large opacities of PMF occur bilaterally on a background of simple CWP, one can be reasonably confident that the lesions are not neoplastic disease (see Chapter 4: Imaging of Diffuse Parenchymal Lung Diseases, Figure 4–28). When there is a sparse background of simple CWP or none or there are crops of nodules (as in Caplan's syndrome), the differentiation from a neoplasm may be difficult.

The effect of pneumoconiosis on the heart has been described by several investigators. Lapp and colleagues performed cardiac catheterization during rest and exercise in 47 miners with CWP (23 with airways obstruction and 24 without). In 7 of 12 miners, either chronic obstructive lung disease or PMF appeared to explain the increase in pulmonary artery pressures. The other 5 with increased pressures had the smaller type of pinpoint opacity on their radiograph.[139] It is likely pertinent that the pinpoint type of opacity is associated with diminished diffusion and a diminution of the vascular bed.[140] A later autopsy study of 215 British coal miners (100 with simple CWP or no pneumoconiosis and 115 with PMF) was designed to address the relationship between coal dust exposure and right ventricular hypertrophy (RVH). In this population, the prevalence of RVH was the same in those with simple CWP as in those without pneumoconiosis (approximately 15%) and was related to the extent of airways obstruction. Overall, RV enlargement did not occur unless the coal miner was a smoker with severe airflow obstruction or had developed PMF.[141]

CWP alone does not appear to significantly increase the risk for development of coexisting mycobacterial infection. However, miners often have exposure to silica in drilling (a job typically associated with silica) rather than coal dust exposure. Miners with silica exposure in the workplace may also be at risk for mycobacterial infection. The appearance of a cavity in a PMF lesion or an aggressive and unexplained rate of radiographic progression should prompt examination of the sputum for mycobacteria.

As already noted, CWP is associated with a variety of immunologic abnormalities. An increased prevalence of ANA and RF is present in populations with CWP. Caplan's syndrome can present, often in association with rheumatoid arthritis or subcutaneous nodules. Lesions on the chest radiograph are multiple, peripherally located, and between 0.5 and 5.0 cm in diameter. They usually appear on a background profusion of small opacities of categories 0 or 1 simple CWP, as opposed to PMF in which the background profusion is more advanced. The lesions appear within a short time, often weeks. The lesions can cavitate, develop fluid levels, calcify or even disappear to be followed later by a fresh crop of lesions. Caplan's syndrome can predate rheumatoid arthritis by up to 10 years. Scleroderma may also be a risk of coal mining. In a group of 60 consecutive cases of scleroderma, Rodnan and colleagues[142] described 26 with a history of employment as a coal miner or in an occupation where silica exposure was encountered. Although the course of scleroderma did not vary in the two groups, it appears that chronic fibrogenic dust exposure may be a risk factor for the development of scleroderma.

MANAGEMENT

There is no proven therapy for CWP. The primary prevention of lung disease in miners must include continuing efforts at reducing coal mine dust exposure. Management is best directed at prevention, early recognition, and treatment of complications. The major challenges to the physician are the recognition and management of airflow obstruction, respiratory infection, hypoxemia, respiratory failure, cor pulmonale, arrhythmias, and pneumothorax.

Improved mining methods and lower dust levels appear to be reducing exposures and new cases of both simple and complicated pneumoconiosis in the United States. Medical surveillance programs, using chest radiographs, allow the early recognition of workers with simple pneumoconiosis. Workers with simple pneumoconiosis should be encouraged to transfer from jobs with high dust exposure to jobs with negligible or no dust exposure or to leave the dusty workplace altogether. Any worker with the unexpected finding of PMF should be carefully advised about the hazards of further dust exposures.

Workers presenting with respiratory symptoms should have a careful evaluation. The initial history and examination should be supplemented by a chest radiograph, spirometry with bronchodilators, diffusing capacity, electrocardiogram, and resting arterial blood gas measurement as indicated. A thorough initial data base allows accurate assessment of the worker's respiratory health and serves as a starting point for observing the response to therapy or progression of disease.

Smoking cessation is important regardless of symptoms of respiratory disease, chest radiograph abnormalities, or pulmonary function status. Physician encouragement to stop smoking should be supplemented by psychological support, use of nicotine substitutes or other pharmacologic means to lessen this addiction, and behavior modification techniques.

Coexisting symptomatic reversible airflow obstruction should be treated with inhaled anti-inflammatory and bronchodilator therapy as indicated. Patients with severe obstruction and inadequate improvement from the usual measures should be considered for a trial of glucocorticoids.

Hypoxemia can be a serious complication in those with PMF. As in other interstitial lung disease, it typically first presents during exercise but with advancing illness can occur at rest and during sleep. Chronic hypoxemia can lead to the complications of polycythemia, pulmonary hypertension, cor pulmonale, and cerebral dysfunction. Therapy with low-flow oxygen is indicated when the arterial oxygen tension is less than 55 mm Hg or when clinical evidence of cor pulmonale is present.

Workers with significant airflow obstruction or PMF should receive appropriate immunization with influenza and pneumococcal vaccines. Bacterial and viral episodes of bronchitis or pneumonia should be promptly recognized and appropriately treated. Similarly, miners with concomitant exposure to silica dust (most often roof bolters, drillers, and motormen), deserve special attention with regard to mycobacterial infection as already noted for silicosis. Symptoms of weight loss, fever, sweats, a change in sputum production, or malaise should be promptly investigated with a chest radiograph and examination of respiratory secretions through stain and culture for acid-fast bacilli. Furthermore, a more-rapid-than-expected progression of chest radiographic features of pneumoconiosis suggest mycobacterial infection. Active tuberculosis in this population can be successfully treated with the usual drug regimens provided rifampin is one of the drugs used.[143,144] In coal miners with a significant history of concurrent silica exposure, the treatment for tuberculosis may need to be more aggressive, and long-term follow-up is essential in view of reports of recurrent pulmonary tuberculosis in patients with PMF after completion of apparently adequate therapy.[145]

Pneumothoraces can be particularly troublesome events in miners with pneumoconiosis. Those with bullous disease in the presence of advanced complicated pneumoconiosis appear to be at the greatest risk. Typically, once the lung has collapsed it is difficult to expand, a feature attributable to the decreased compliance associated with interstitial lung disease. Despite this, therapy with one or several chest tubes is often therapeutic. Recurrent pneumothoraces, or a pneumothax that cannot be expanded, may require an open procedure and pleurodesis.

Respiratory failure may complicate advanced PMF as it does in other chronic respiratory diseases. Ventilatory support measures are indicated when the failure is precipitated by a treatable complication. The application of ventilatory support measures should be discussed with the patient before the need arises. In general, miners with advanced pneumoconiosis are poor candidates for long-term mechanical ventilation.

Prevention strategies to decrease the incidence of CWP in miners include education, exposure control, medical surveillance, and research. A series of primary and secondary preventive measures should include the following:

1. Education about the respiratory health hazards from uncontrolled exposures to coal mine dust must be widely available to workers, employers, production managers, government representatives, and health care providers. This information provides the basis for implementing any programs addressing worker health. This is primary prevention.
2. Major efforts must be directed at improving work methods or work practices, including engineering controls, to progressively reduce dust exposures to acceptable levels.
3. Environmental dust surveillance programs should be implemented. Data generated from these programs allow for the critical feedback needed to justify improvement of the ambient air quality and modify work methods if exposures exceed acceptable levels. This is also primary prevention.
4. Medical screening and surveillance programs should be designed to benefit the individual worker and future workers, including feedback to environmental surveillance and work practice evaluations. The recognition of disease provides a strong impetus for changes in environmental surveillance. More important than the identification of a single case is the collection of information that addresses the cumulative burden of disease, or prevalence, in a population. This allows the educators to monitor trends over time and the effectiveness of primary preventive measures. Since case identification represents failures in primary prevention, this is secondary prevention.
5. Research should be encouraged to improve therapy, to improve diagnostic capabilities, and to better understand the pathogenesis of CWP. Critical to the issue of research is the relationship between dust exposure and the development and progression of disease. These research efforts should not displace efforts at achieving effective dust control.

REFERENCES

1. Bang KM, Althouse RB, Kim JH, et al. Recent trends of age-specific pneumoconiosis mortality rates in the United States, 1985–1996: coal workers' pneumoconiosis, asbestosis, and silicosis. Int J Environ Health 1999;5:251–5.
2. Meiklejohn A. History of lung disease of coal miners in Great Britain, part I, 1800–1875. Br J Ind Med 1951;8:127–37.
3. Meiklejohn A. History of lung disease of coal miners in Great Britain, part II, 1875–1920. Br J Ind Med 1952;9:93–8.
4. Meiklejohn A. History of lung disease of coal miners in Great Britain, part III, 1920–1952. Br J Ind Med 1952;9:208–20.
5. Gregory JC. Case of peculiar black infiltration of the lungs resembling melanosis. Edinb Med Surg J 1831;36:389–92.
6. Marshall W. Cases of spurious melanosis of the lungs or phthisis melanotica. Lancet 1983–1834;ii:271–4.
7. Ogle W. Supplement of the 45th annual report of the Registrar General for England and Wales. London: Her Majesty's Stationary Office; 1885.
8. Collis EL. Industrial pneumoconiosis (Milroy lectures, 1915). London: His Majesty's Stationary Office; 1919.
9. Collis EL, Gilchrist JC. Effects of dust upon coal trimmers. J Ind Hyg Toxicol 1928;10:101–9.
10. Gough J. Pneumoconiosis of coal trimmers. J Pathol Bacteriol 1940;51:277–85.
11. Hepplestone AG. The essential lesson of pneumoconiosis in Welch coal workers. J Pathol Bacteriol 1947;59:453–60.
12. King EJ, Maguire BA, Nagelschmidt G. Further studies of the dust in the lungs of coal-miners. Br J Ind Med 1956;13:9–13.
13. Morgan WKC. Epidemiology and occupational lung disease. In: Morgan WKC, Seaton A, editors. Occupational lung diseases. 3rd ed. Philadelphia: WB Saunders Company; 1995.
14. Stahl R. Coal and derivatives. Encyclopedia of occupational health and safety. Geneva: International labour organisation; 1989.
15. Thomas L. Handbook of practical geology. New York (NY): John Wiley & Sons; 1992.
16. Hilt C. Die Beiziehungen zwischen der Zusammensetzung und der technis chen Eigenschaften der Steinkohle. Bezirksvereinigung Ver. Deutsch. Ingenieure Z 1873;17(4):157–69.
17. Haught OL. Coal and coal mining in West Virginia. Morgantown (WV). West Virginia Geological and Economic Survey; 1955.
18. National Institute for Occupational Safety and Health. Criteria for a recommended standard: occupational exposure to respirable coal mine dust. Cincinnati (OH): DHHS; 1995 (NIOSH) publication No.:95–106.

19. Coates DR. Energy and fossil fuels. Environmental geology. New York (NY): John Wiley and Sons; 1981.

20. Wallace WE, Harrison JC, Grayson RI, et al. Aluminosilicate surface contamination of respirable quartz particles from coal mine dusts and from clay works dusts. Ann Occup Hyg 1994;38:439–45.

21. Amandus HE, Petersen MR, Richards TB. Health status of anthracite surface coal miners. Arch Environ Health 1989; 44:75–81.

22. Banks D, Bauer M, Castellan R, Lapp N. Silicosis in surface coalmine drillers. Thorax 1983;38:275–8.

23. Silicosis screening in surface coal miners—Pennsylvania, 1996–1997. MMWR Morb Mortal Wkly Rep 2000;49: 612–5.

24. Love RG, Miller BG, Groat SK, et al. Respiratory health effects of opencast coalmining: a cross sectional study of current workers. Occup Environ Health 1997;54:416–23.

25. Coleman LL. Coal data. Washington (DC): The National Coal Association; 1992.

26. Taylor LD, Thakur PC. Recent developments in coal mining technology and their impact on miners' health. Occupational medicine: state of the art reviews. Philadelphia: Hanley & Belfus, Inc.; 1993. p. 109–26.

27. Parker JE, Banks DE. Lung diseases in coal workers. In: Banks DE, Parker JE, editors. Occupational lung disease: an international perspective. Philadelphia: Lippincott-Raven Publishers; 1998. p. 161–82.

28. Stout KS. Mining methods and equipment. New York (NY): McGraw-Hill, Inc.; 1980.

29. Euler WJ. In: Meyers RA, editor. Coal handbook. New York: Marcel Dekker, Inc.; 1981. p. 75–114.

30. Jain BL, Patrick JM. Ventilatory function in Nigerian coal workers. Br J Ind Med 1981;38:275–80.

31. Lainhart WS, Doyle HM, Enterline PE, et al. Pneumoconiosis in Appalachian bituminous coal miners. Washington (DC): U.S. Government Printing Office; 1969.

32. McBride WW, Pendergrass E, Lieben J. Pneumoconiosis study of Pennsylvania anthracite miners. J Occup Med 1963;5: 376–88.

33. Rogan JM, Attfield MD, Jacobsen M, et al. Role of dust in the working environment in development of chronic bronchitis in British coal miners. Br J Ind Med 1973;30:217–26.

34. Morgan WKC, Handelsman L, Kibelstis J, et al. Ventilatory capacity and lung volumes of U.S. coal miners. Arch Environ Health 1974;282:182–9.

35. Carp H, Miller F, Hoidal JR, et al. Potential mechanism of emphysema: alpha-1-proteinase inhibitor recovered from lungs of cigarette smokers contains oxidized methionine and has decreased elastase inhibitory capacity. Proc Nat Acad Sci U S A 1982;79:2041–5.

36. Mayer AS, Stoller JK, Bartelson BB, et al. Occupational exposure risks in individuals with PI*Z alpha-1-antitrypsin deficiency. Am J Respir Crit Care Med 2000;162:553–8.

37. Myers JE. Differential ethnic standards for lung functions, or one standard for all? S Afr Med J 1984;65:768–72.

38. Wang M-L, McCabhe L, Hankinson JL, et al. Longitudinal and cross sectional analyses of lung function in steel workers. Am J Respir Crit Care Med 1996;153:119–29.

39. Burrows B, Knudson RJ, Lebowitz MD, et al. The relationship of childhood respiratory illness to adult obstructive airway disease. Am Rev Respir Dis 1977;115:751–60.

40. Martinez FD, Antognoni G, Macri F, et al. Parental smoking enhances bronchial responsiveness in nine-year-old children. Am Rev Respir Dis 1988;138:518–23.

41. Wang M-L, Petsonk EL, Beeckman L-A, et al. Clinically important FEV$_1$ declines among coal miners: an exploration of previously unrecognized determinants. Occup Environ Med 1999;56:837–44.

42. Beeckman L-U, Wang M-L, Petsonk EL, et al. Rapid declines in FEV$_1$ and subsequent respiratory symptoms, illnesses

and mortality in coal miners in the US. Am J Respir Crit Care Med 2001;163:633–9.

43. Wang M-L, McCabe L, Petsonk EL, et al. Weight gain and longitudinal changes in lung function in steel workers. Chest 1997;111:1526–32.

44. Rogan JM, Attfield MD, Jacobsen M, et al. Role of dust in the working environment in development of chronic bronchitis in British coal miners. Br J Ind Med 1973;30:217–26.

45. Morgan WKC. Industrial bronchitis. Br J Ind Med 1978;35: 285–91.

46. Attfield MD, Hodgson MJ. Respiratory symptoms and chest illness in underground coal miners. Ann Am Conf Govern Ind Hyg 1986;14:91–100.

47. Douglas AN, Lamb D, Ruckley VA. Bronchial gland dimensions in coalminers: influence of smoking and dust exposure. Thorax 1982;37:760–4.

48. Kibelstis JA, Morgan EJ, Reger R, et al. Prevalence of bronchitis and airway obstruction in American bituminous coal miners. Am Rev Respir Dis 1973;108:886–93.

49. Marine WM, Gurr D, Jacobsen M. Clinically important respiratory effects of dust exposure and smoking in British coal miners. Am Rev Respir Dis 1988;137:106–12.

50. Seixas NS, Robins TG, Attfield MD, et al. Exposure-response relationships for coal mine dust and obstructive lung disease following enactment of the Federal Coal Mine Health and Safety Act of 1969. Am J Ind Med 1992;21:715–34.

51. Bates DV, Pham QT, Chau N, et al. A longitudinal study of pulmonary function in coal miners in Lorraine, France. Am J Ind Med 1985;8:21–32.

52. Dimich-Ward H, Bates DV. Reanalysis of a longitudinal study of pulmonary function in coal miners in Lorraine, France. Am J Ind Med 1994;25:613–23.

53. Kauffmann F, Drouet D, Lellouch J, et al. Occupational exposures and 12-year spirometric changes among Paris area workers. Br J Ind Med 1982;39:221–32.

54. Kibelstis JS, Morgan EJ, Reger R, et al. Prevalence of bronchitis and airways obstruction in American bituminous coal miners. Am Rev Respir Dis 1973;108:886–93.

55. Becklake MR. Chronic airflow limitation: its relationship to work in dusty occupations. Chest 1985;88:608–17.

56. Hurley JF, Soutar CA. Can exposure to coalmine dust cause a severe impairment of lung function? Br J Ind Med 1986; 43:150–7.

57. Banks DE, Shah AA, Lopez M, et al. Chest illnesses and the decline of FEV$_1$ in steel workers. J Occup Environ Med 1999;41:1085–90.

58. Lapp NL, Morgan WKC, Zaldivar G. Airways obstruction, coal mining, and disability. Occup Environ Med 1994;51:234–8.

59. Attfield MD. Longitudinal decline in FEV$_1$ in United States coalminers. Thorax 1985;40:132–7.

60. Seixas NS, Robins TG, Attfield MD, et al. Longitudinal and cross-sectional analysis of exposure to coal mine dust and pulmonary function in new miners. Br J Ind Med 1993; 50:929–37.

61. Love RG, Miller BG. Longitudinal study of lung function in coal-miners. Thorax 1982;37:193–7.

62. Soutar CA, Hurley JF. Relation between dust exposure and lung function in miners and ex-miners. Br J Ind Med 1986; 43:307–20.

63. Soutar C, Campbell S, Gurr D, et al. Important deficits of lung function in three modern colliery populations. Relations with dust exposure. Am Rev Respir Dis 1993;147:797–803.

64. Oxman AD, Muir DCF, Shannon HS, et al. Occupational dust exposure and chronic obstructive pulmonary disease. Am Rev Respir Dis 1993;148:38–48.

65. Hnizdo E, Baskind E, Sluis-Cremer GK. Combined effect of silica dust exposure and tobacco smoking on the prevalence of respiratory impairments among gold miners. Scand J Work Environ Health 1990;16:411–22.

66. Attfield MD, Hodous TK. Pulmonary function of U.S. coal

miners related to dust exposure estimates. Am Rev Respir Dis 1992;14:605–9.

67. Wang M-L, Banks DE. Airways obstruction and occupational inorganic dust exposure. In: Banks DE, Parker JE, editors. Occupational lung disease: an international perspective. Philadelphia: Lippincott-Raven; 1998. p. 69–82.

68. Carta P, Aru G, Barbieri MT, et al. Dust exposure, respiratory symptoms, and longitudinal decline in lung function in young coal miners. Occup Environ Med 1996;53:312–9.

69. Hodous TK, Hankinson JL. Prospective spirometric study of new coal miners. Proceedings of the International Symposium on Pneumoconioses; 1988; Shenyang PRC. Beijing (PRC): Institute of Occupational Medicine, Chinese Academy of Preventive Medicine; p. 206–11.

70. Petsonk EL, Daniloff EM, Mannino DM, et al. Airway responsiveness and job selection: a study in coal miners and non-mining controls. Occup Environ Med 1995;52:745–9.

71. Hodgins P, Henneberger PK, Wang M-L, et al. Bronchial hyperresponsiveness and FEV$_1$ decline: a study in miners and non-miners. Am J Respir Crit Care Med 1998;157:1390–6.

72. US Coal Mine Health and Safety Act. U.S. Pub. L. No. 91-173, Stat. 2917 (1969).

73. Attfield MD, Castellan RM. Epidemiological data on US coal miners' pneumoconiosis, 1960–1968. Am J Public Health 1992;82:964–70.

74. Attfield MD, Althouse RB. Surveillance data on US coal miners' pneumoconiosis, 1970–1986. Am J Public Health 1992;82:971–7.

75. Attfield MD. British data on coal miners' pneumoconiosis and relevance to U.S. conditions. Am J Public Health 1992;82:978–83.

76. Parihar YS, Patnaik JP, Nema PK, et al. Coal workers' pneumoconiosis: a study of prevalence in coal mines of eastern Madhya Pradesh and Orissa states of India. Ind Health 1997;4:467–73.

77. McLintock J, Rae S, Jacobsen M. The attack rate of progressive massive fibrosis in British coal miners. In: Walton WH, editor. Inhaled particles III. Surrey: Unwin Brothers; 1971. p. 933–50.

78. Balaan MR, Weber SL, Banks DE. Clinical aspects of coal workers' pneumoconiosis and silicosis. Occup Med 1993;8:19–24.

79. Davies I, Mann KJ. Ninth International Congress on Industrial Medicine; 1949; Bristol. p. 768.

80. Enterline PE. A review of mortality data for American coal miners. Ann N Y Acad Sci 1972;200:260–72.

81. Enterline PE. Mortality rates among coal miners. Am J Public Health 1964;54:758–68.

82. 1967 Occupational Study. Chicago (IL): Society of Actuaries; 1967.

83. Editorial. Coal mining and mortality. BMJ 1979;2:1168–9.

84. Cochrane AL, Haley TJL, Moore F, et al. The mortality of men in the Rhondda Foch, 1950–1970. Br J Ind Med 1978;36:15–22.

85. Atuhaire LK, Campbell MJ, Cochrane AL, et al. Mortality of men in the Rhondda Fach 1950–1980. Br J Ind Med 1985;42:741–5.

86. Ortmeyer CE, Baier EJ, Crawford GMJ. Life expectancy of Pennsylvania coal miners compensated for disability. Arch Environ Health 1973;27:227–30.

87. Stocks P. On the death rates from cancer of the stomach and respiratory diseases in 1949–1953 among coal miners and other male residents in counties in England and Wales. Br J Cancer 1962;16:592–8.

88. Matolo NA, Klauber MR, Gorishek WM, et al. High incidence of gastric carcinoma in a coal mining region. Cancer 1972;29:733–7.

89. Rockette HE. Cause specific mortality of coal miners. J Occup Med 1977;19:795–801.

90. Ortmeyer CE, Costello J, Morgan WKC, et al. The mortality of Appalachian coal miners. Arch Environ Health 1974;29:67–72.

91. Meijers JMM, Swaen GMH, Slangen JJM, et al. Long-term mortality in miners with coal workers' pneumoconiosis in the Netherlands: a pilot study. Am J Ind Med 1991;19:43–50.

92. IARC. IARC monograph on the evaluation of the carcinogenic risk of chemicals to humans. Silica, some silicates, coal dust, and para-aramid fibrils. Vol. 68. Lyon; International Agency for Research on Cancer: 1997.

93. Jacobsen M, Rae S, Walton WH, Rogan JM. The relation between pneumoconiosis and dust-exposure in British coal mines. In: Walton WH, editor. Inhaled particles III. Surrey: Unwin Brothers; 1971. p. 903–17.

94. Miller BG, Jacobsen M. Dust exposure, pneumoconiosis, and mortality of coal miners. Br J Ind Med 1985;42:723–33.

95. Kuempel ED, Stayner LT, Attfield MD, et al. Exposure-response analysis of mortality among coal miners in the United States. Am J Ind Med 1995;28:167–84.

96. Ames RG, Amandus H, Attfield M, et al. Does coal mine dust present a risk for lung cancer? A case control study of U.S. miners. Arch Environ Health 1983;38:331–3.

97. Vallyathan V, Green FHY, Rodman NF, et al. Lung carcinoma by histologic type in coal miners. Arch Pathol Lab Med 1985;109:419–23.

98. Heppleston AG. The pathogenesis of simple pneumoconiosis in coal workers. J Pathol Bacteriol 1954;67:51–63.

99. Kleinerman J, Green F, Lacquer W, et al. Pathology standards for coal workers' pneumoconiosis. Arch Pathol Lab Med 1979;103:374–432.

100. Ryder RC, Dunnill MS, Anderson JA. A qualitative study of bronchial mucus gland volume, emphysema, and smoking in a necropsy population. J Pathol 1971;104:59–71.

101. Cockcroft A, Wagner JC, Ryder R, et al. Post-mortem study of emphysema in coalworkers and non-coalworkers. Lancet 1982;Sept. 11:600–3.

102. Lyons JP, Ryder RC, Seal EME, et al. Emphysema in smoking and non-smoking coalworkers with pneumoconiosis. Bull Eur Physiopathol Respir 1981;17:75–85.

103. Ruckley VA, Gould SJ, Chapman JS, et al. Emphysema and dust exposure in a group of coalworkers. Am Rev Respir Dis 1984;129:528–32.

104. Leigh J, Dirscoll TR, Cole BD, et al. Quantitative measurement between emphysema and lung mineral content in coalworkers. Occup Environ Med 1994;51:400–7.

105. Morgan WKC, Burgess DB, Lapp NL, et al. Hyperinflation of the lungs in coal miners. Thorax 1971;26:585–90.

106. Hodous TK, Attfield MD. Progressive massive fibrosis developing on a background of minimal simple pneumoconiosis. VIIth International Pneumoconiosis Conference. Pittsburgh (PA): DHHS (NIOSH); 1988. p. 122–6.

107. Shennan DH, Washington JS, Thomas DJ, et al. Factors predisposing to the development of progressive massive fibrosis in British coal miners. Br J Ind Med 1981;38:321–6.

108. Wagner JC. Etiologic factors in complicated coal workers' pneumoconiosis. Ann N Y Acad Sci 1972;200:401–4.

109. Caplan A. Certain unusual radiographic appearances in the chest of coalminers suffering from rheumatoid arthritis. Thorax 1953;8:29–30.

110. Caplan A, Payne RB, Withey JL. A broader concept of Caplan's syndrome related to rheumatoid factors. Thorax 1962;17:205–12.

111. Lapp NL, Castranova V. How silicosis and coal workers' pneumoconiosis develops—a cellular assessment. Banks DE, editor. Occupational medicine: state of the art reviews. Philadelphia: Hanley and Belfus, Inc.; 1993. p. 35–65.

112. Adamis Z, Timlar T. Studies on the effect of quartz, bentonite, and coal dust mixtures on macrophages in vitro. Br J Exp Pathol 1978;59:411–9.

113. Ray SC, King EJ, Harrison CV. The action of small amounts

of quartz and large amounts of coal and graphite on the lungs of rats. Br J Ind Med 1951;8:68–73.

114. Castranova V, Vallyathan V. Silicosis and coal workers' pneumoconiosis. Environ Health Perspect 2000;108 Suppl. 4:674–84.

115. Dalal NS, Jafari B, Petersen M, et al. Presence of stable coal radicals in autopsied coal miners' lungs and its possible correlation to coal workers' pneumoconiosis. Arch Environ Health 1991;46:366–72.

116. Dalal NS, Suryan MM, Vallyathan V, et al. Detection of reactive free radicals in fresh coal mine dusts and their implication for pulmonary injury. Ann Occup Hyg 1989;33:79–84.

117. Castranova V, Bowman L, Reasor M, et al. The response of rat alveolar macrophages to chronic inhalation of coal dust and/or diesel inhalation. Environ Res 1985;36:405–19.

118. Adamson IYR, Bowden DH. Adaptive responses of the pulmonary macrophagic system to carbon. II. Morphologic studies. Lab Invest 1978;38:430–8.

119. Kuhn DC, Stanley CF, el-Ayouby N, et al. Effect of *in vivo* coal dust exposure on arachidonic acid metabolism in the rat alveolar macrophage. J Toxicol Environ Health 1990;29:157–68.

120. Vallyathan V, Xianglin S, Dalal N, et al. Generation of free radicals from freshly fractured silica dust. Am Rev Respir Dis 1988;138:1213–9.

121. Borm PJA, Henderson PT. Symposium on the health effects of occupational exposures to inorganic dusts. Exp Lung Res 1990;16:1–3.

122. Lapp NL, Lewis D, Schwegler-Berry D, et al. Bronchoalveolar lavage in asymptomatic underground coal miners. In: Ramani RV, editor. Proceedings of respiratory dusts in the mineral industry. Society of Mining Engineering; 1991. p. 159–69.

123. Rom WN, Bitterman PB, Rennard SI, et al. Characterization of the lower respiratory tract inflammation of nonsmoking individuals with interstitial lung disease associated with chronic inhalation of inorganic dust. Am Rev Respir Dis 1987;136:1429–34.

124. Wagner JC, Burns J, Munday DE, et al. Presence of fibronectin in pneumoconiotic lesions. Thorax 1982;37:54–6.

125. Wallaert B, Lassalle P, Fortin F, et al. Superoxide anion generation by alveolar inflammatory cells in simple pneumoconiosis and in progressive massive fibrosis of non-smoking coal miners. Am Rev Respir Dis 1990;141:129–33.

126. Vanhee D, Gosset P, Boitelle A, et al. Cytokines and cytokine network in silicosis and coal workers' pneumoconiosis. Eur Respir J 1995;8:834–42.

127. Rivers D, Wise M, King E, et al. Dust content, radiology, and pathology in simple pneumoconiosis of coalworkers. Br J Ind Med 1960;17:87–108.

128. Watson AJ, Black J, Doig AT, et al. Pneumoconiosis in carbon electrode workers. Br J Ind Med 1959;16:274–85.

129. Heise ER, Mentnech MS, Olenchock SA, et al. HLA-A1 and coalworkers' pneumoconiosis. Am Rev Respir Dis 1979;119:903–8.

130. Soutar CA, Turner-Warwick M, Parkes WR. Circulating antinuclear antibody and rheumatoid factor in coal pneumoconiosis. BMJ 1974;3:145–7.

131. Lippmann M, Eckert HL, Hahon N, et al. Circulating antinuclear and rheumatoid factors in United States coal miners. Ann Intern Med 1973;79:807–11.

132. Wagner JC, McCormick JN. Immunological investigations of coalworkers' disease. J R Coll Physicians Lond 1967;2:49–56.

133. Benedek TG, Zwadzki ZA, Medsger TAJ. Serum immunoglobulins, rheumatoid factor and pneumoconiosis in coal miners. Arthritis Rheum 1976;19:731–6.

134. Hahon N, Morgan WKC, Petersen M. Serum immunoglobulin levels in coal workers' pneumoconiosis. Ann Occup Hyg 1980;23:165–74.

135. Burrell R. Immunological aspects of coal workers' pneumoconiosis. Ann N Y Acad Sci 1972;200:94–105.

136. Morgan WKC. Epidemiology and occupational lung disease. In: Morgan WKC, Seaton A, editors. Occupational lung diseases. 3rd ed. Philadelphia: WB Saunders Company; 1995.

137. Guidelines for the use of ILO international classification of radiographs of pneumoconiosis. Revised ed. Geneva: International Labour Office; 1980.

138. Lamers RJ, Schins RP, Wouters EF, et al. High-resolution computed tomography of the lungs in coal miners with a normal chest radiograph. Exp Lung Res 1994;20:411–9.

139. Lapp NL, Seaton A, Kaplan KC, et al. Pulmonary haemodynamics in coal workers' pneumonconiosis. In: Walton WH, editor. Inhaled Particles III. Surrey: Unwin Bros. Ltd; 1971. p. 645–57.

140. Lyons JP, Clarke WG, Hall AM, et al. Transfer factor (diffusing capacity) for the lung in simple pneumoniosis of coal workers. BMJ 1967;4:349–59.

141. Fernie JM, Douglas AN, Lamb D, et al. Right ventricular hypertrophy in a group of coalworkers. Thorax 1983;38:436–42.

142. Rodnan G, Benedek R, Medsger T, et al. The association between progressive systemic sclerosis (scleroderma) with coal miners' pneumoconiosis and other forms of silicosis. Ann Intern Med 1967;66:323–34.

143. Ball JD, Berry G, Clarke WG, et al. A controlled trial of antituberculosis chemotherapy in early complicated pneumoconiosis of coal workers. Thorax 1969;24:399–406.

144. Dubois P, Gyselen A, Prignot J. Rifampicin-combined chemotherapy in coal-workers' pneumoconio-tuberculosis. Am Rev Respir Dis 1977;115:221–8.

145. Morgan E. Silicosis and tuberculosis. Chest 1979;75:202–3.

17

ASBESTOSIS AND ASBESTOS-INDUCED PLEURAL FIBROSIS

MARK P. STEELE
MICHAEL W. PETERSON
DAVID A. SCHWARTZ

Asbestos is a naturally occurring mineral that has several unique physical properties.[1] It is resistant to degradation by both acid and alkaline solutions; it is also resistant to heat and is an excellent, inexpensive insulator. Asbestos degrades throughout its lifetime by splitting longitudinally into ever smaller fibers. This physical characteristic enhances its thermal-insulating properties, but it also increases the fraction of respirable fibers that can be inhaled into the lung and subsequently deposited in the terminal bronchioles.

Between 1940 and 1979, approximately 20 million workers were occupationally exposed to asbestos in the United States.[2] Although these workers were primarily shipbuilders and construction workers, other workers in other industrial sectors such as the automotive and railroad industries were also exposed to relatively high concentrations of asbestos. Morbidity and mortality associated with asbestos exposure in the United States will continue well into this century due to the long latency period between first exposure and the development of asbestos-induced lung disease (15 to 35 years).[3,4] Continued mixing and use of this inexpensive but hazardous form of insulation in the developing countries around the world raises even greater concern.

This discussion will focus on the mineralogy of asbestos and the pathogenic and clinical characteristics of the nonmalignant types of asbestos-induced lung disease (asbestosis and pleural fibrosis). However, asbestos has been associated with the development of two types of lung cancer: bronchogenic (non–small cell and small cell) malignancies and mesothelioma. Both asbestos-induced malignancies may occur independently or may be diagnosed in conjunction with the diagnosis of either asbestosis or asbestos-induced pleural fibrosis. Moreover, bronchogenic malignancies are the most common asbestos-related cause of death among exposed workers. Mesotheliomas are a very aggressive tumor of the chest wall for which there is currently no effective therapy.

CHARACTERISTICS OF ASBESTOS

The aspect ratio (length-to-width ratio) is the distinguishing feature of a particle classifying it as a fiber. By definition, a fiber has an aspect ratio of 3 or greater. Although this definition was not based on aerosol dynamics, the aspect ratio of 3 appears reasonable in light of the effects of fiber surface area and aerodynamic properties on sedimentation and impaction. In fact, the aspect ratio of 3 has been used by the Occupational Safety and Health Administration to define and enforce exposure standards for asbestos. The surface area and the fiber length contribute to patterns of deposition; these fiber characteristics are reportedly important determinants of asbestos-induced lung disease type.[5]

Fiber deposition in the respiratory tract occurs through five aerodynamic mechanisms: impaction, sedimentation, interception, electrostatic precipitation, and diffusion. Whereas impaction and sedimentation are primarily dependent on the aerodynamic diameter of the fiber,[6] interception is governed by fiber length,[5] and electrostatic precipitation is dependent on the electrical charge of the fiber.[5] Processing of asbestos fibers results in aerosols with relatively high levels of electrical charge.[7] Uniform fibers, such as amphibole asbestos, become aligned parallel to the axis of flow and are often deposited in the alveolar ducts.[8] By contrast, fiber aggregates with excess heterogeneity, such as chrysotile asbestos, have a mixed flow pattern and are more frequently deposited at the airway bifurcation.[8]

Fiber mineralogic classification is relevant to the interpretation of basic, clinical, and epidemiologic findings, as well as to the assessment of health risk.[9] Fibers are classified as either asbestos (or asbestiform), other silicates, or man-made mineral fibers (Table 17–1). Asbestos is a naturally occurring family of hydrated mineral silicates derived from either the amphibole (anthophyllite, amosite, or crocidolite) or serpentine (chrysotile) groups.[10]

TABLE 17–1   Mineralogic Classification of Fibers

Asbestos (Asbestiform)	Other Silicates	Man-Made Mineral Fibers
Chrysotile	Attapulgite	Fiberglass (continuous filament)
Crocidolite	Erionite	Insulation wool
Anthophyllite	Sepiolite	Refractory fibers (ceramic)
Amosite	Talc	Special purpose fibers
Tremolite-actinolite	Vermiculite Wollastonite	

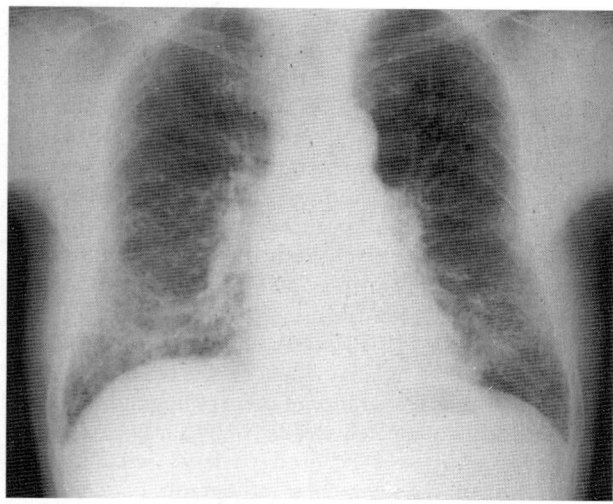

Figure 17–1   A posterior-anterior chest radiograph of an individual with asbestosis. Note the lower lobe and peripheral distribution of the irregular markings.

Amphiboles are rigid and rodlike and consist of double chains of tetrahedral groups linked by cations; they consist primarily of silicon oxide. Serpentine asbestos is pliable and curly and is composed of individual fibrillar subunits that contain silicon oxide sheets arranged in pseudohexagonal arrays. Magnesium is a principal component of serpentine asbestos, which gives it a strongly positive charge. Natural deposits of asbestos are often mixtures of amphibole and serpentine types. Man-made mineral fibers (MMMF) consist of fibrous inorganic material made primarily from rock, clay, slag, or glass filament (glasswool, glass filament, slag wool, rock wool, or ceramic fibers). The MMMF can be manufactured to size specifications that range from 0.1 μm in diameter to over 100 μm in diameter. Unlike asbestos fibers, which fracture along the fiber axis and form smaller fibers, MMMF predominantly break across the fiber axis; aerosols of MMMF are not associated with large numbers of submicron-size fibers.

CLINICAL ASPECTS OF ASBESTOS-INDUCED LUNG DISEASE

Asbestosis

Asbestosis is a diffuse form of interstitial fibrosis affecting both lungs in a symmetric pattern, as can be seen on radiographic examination.[1] There is a latency period of 15 to 20 years from the first exposure to asbestos to the development of asbestosis. Importantly, there is a clear dose-response relationship between exposure to asbestos and the risk of developing asbestosis. Although this relationship exists within several industrial sectors, there appears to be a wide discrepancy in risk between different industrial sectors (ie, mining < construction < textile). This variation in risk is probably due to the different concentrations of respirable fibers in the aerosols that characterize these industries.

Radiographically, asbestosis typically presents as a lower lobe disease with irregular markings in the periphery of the lung (Figure 17–1). In less severe forms of asbestosis, the central and apical portions of the lung are relatively unaffected. The chest radiograph, however, is neither a sensitive nor a specific method for identifying asbestos-induced interstitial fibrosis. In fact, 15 to 20% of individuals with pathologic evidence of asbestosis[11,12] have normal-appearing parenchyma on the chest radiograph.

Several studies[13–15] suggest that the findings on high-resolution computed tomography (HRCT) scan are indicative of histologic evidence of parenchymal inflammation and fibrosis. Whereas conventional CT scans obtain 8 to 10 mm thick slices through the chest, the HRCT scan obtains thinner slices (1 to 3 mm) and uses a different reconstruction algorithm to improve spatial resolution.[16] In idiopathic pulmonary fibrosis, the reticular patchy densities on the HRCT scan correspond to histologic evidence of inflammation and irregular fibrosis.[15] In addition, the cystic (2 to 20 mm) subpleural findings on HRCT appear to represent regions of diffuse fibrosis with honeycombing.[15,17] In asbestosis, the HRCT scan has identified several parenchymal lesions that appear relevant to this interstitial lung disease.[13,14] These abnormalities include short peripheral lines, subpleural curvilinear lines, parenchymal bands, and peripheral cystic lesions (Figure 17–2); these changes are heterogeneously distributed throughout the lung parenchyma (Figure 17–3). Although the short peripheral lines are believed to represent focal thickening of the interalveolar septa, subpleural curvilinear lines may be evidence of extensive collapse and fibrosis of adjacent acinar units. Parenchymal bands are almost always associated with asbestos-induced pleural disease and are believed to represent thickened septal tissue. Cystic lesions in the periphery of the lung appear to represent regions of diffuse fibrosis with honeycombing. These radiographic features are seen in other forms of interstitial lung disease,[18] and histologic confirmation of these abnormalities is only beginning to accumulate.[13,14] Moreover, we have shown[19] that the density of interstitial changes on the HRCT scan is a valid, clinically meaningful, and objective measure of interstitial lung disease that correlates independently with the subjective, physiologic, and inflammatory indices of pulmonary fibrosis. Taken as a group, these studies suggest that the HRCT scan can effectively identify regions of abnormal lung tissue that appear to be associated with pathologic evidence of interstitial fibrosis.

Although the HRCT scan can identify parenchymal abnormalities that are not evident on the plain chest radiograph, the clinical relevance of these radiographic abnormalities is still not entirely clear.[20] We recently have found that among asbestos-exposed patients with normal parenchyma on the plain chest radiograph, patients with pleural disease are more likely to have interstitial abnormalities revealed on the HRCT scan than are those patients with normal pleura.[21] Although these interstitial abnormalities on the HRCT scan are associated with a reduction in lung volume and abnormal gas exchange, these differences were not found to be statistically significant.[21] Staples and colleagues[22] have reported that among asbestos-exposed workers with normal parenchyma on the plain chest radiograph, HRCT scans of approximately one-third of these workers suggest underlying interstitial inflammation, fibrosis, or a combination of the two. Moreover, when compared to HRCT scans of workers with normal parenchyma, those with interstitial changes on the HRCT scan were more dyspneic, had a lower vital capacity, and had diminished gas exchange.[22] Clearly, prospective controlled studies are needed to determine the prognostic significance of these interstitial abnormalities that appear on the HRCT scans of asbestos-exposed workers with and without identifiable interstitial lung disease on the plain chest radiograph.

The diagnosis of asbestosis is based on two simple findings[23-25]: a consistent history of exposure to asbestos and definite evidence of interstitial fibrosis. There must be clear evidence of exposure to asbestos as well as a proper latency period from the first exposure. Exposure is most commonly documented by work history, but it is not available in some situations or the available exposure history may, at times be unreliable. Further documentation of occupational exposure to asbestos can be verified by identifying a sufficient concentration of asbestos fibers or asbestos bodies in the bronchoalveolar lavage (BAL) fluid or in biopsy specimens of lung tissue. The presence of bilateral pleural plaques is virtually pathognomonic for previous exposure to asbestos. In addition to a well-documented exposure history, one must clearly identify interstitial lung disease. Lower lobe interstitial markings in both lung fields are sufficient radiographic evidence of asbestosis. However, because the chest radiograph can demonstrate interstitial lung disease in approximately 85% of patients with asbestosis,[4,5] other tests such as the HRCT scan and pulmonary

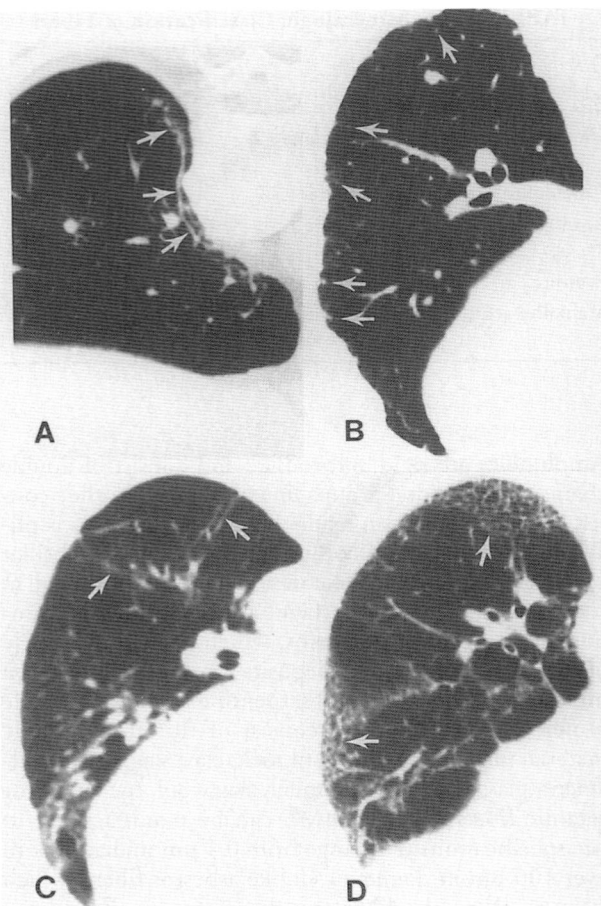

Figure 17–2   Single high-resolution computed tomography sections from four patients with asbestosis with *arrows* demonstrating *A,* curvilinear subpleural lines; *B,* thickened interlobular septal lines; *C,* parenchymal bands; and *D,* honeycombing.

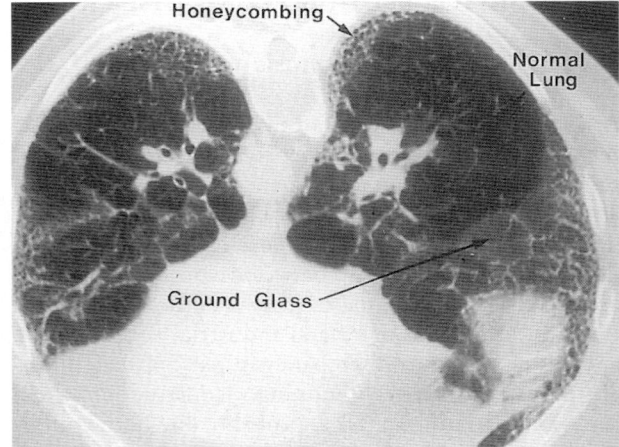

Figure 17–3   This high-resolution computed tomography (HRCT) scan from a patient with severe asbestosis demonstrates both honeycombing and an area of ground-glass infiltrate. This HRCT scan also demonstrates that asbestosis is a heterogeneous disease with radiologically abnormal lung adjacent to normal-appearing lung parenchyma.

function tests may be helpful in pursuing the diagnosis of asbestosis. Although histologic evidence of asbestosis is occasionally required to confirm that the interstitial process is caused by previous exposure to asbestos, this approach is not recommended by either the American Thoracic Society[25] or the American Medical Association[23]; microscopic examination of lung parenchyma is rarely needed to diagnose asbestosis.[26] In well over 90% of the cases of asbestosis, the diagnosis is based on the patient's history, physical examination, and the presence of interstitial fibrosis on the radiograph. Other diseases such as congestive heart failure must be excluded as potential causes of the dyspnea and the interstitial radiographic abnormalities that are present.

Pleural Fibrosis

Asbestos-induced pleural fibrosis is the most common radiographic finding among those exposed to asbestos.[26–28] Circumscribed pleural plaques and diffuse pleural thickening account for more than 90% of asbestos-induced pleural abnormalities[28]; the prevalence of these lesions is expected to increase for at least the next 10 to 15 years.[3,4] The development of pleural fibrosis is dependent on the cumulative dose of asbestos exposure and the elapsed time since initial exposure. These factors taken into account, between 20 and 60% of construction workers exposed to high concentrations of asbestos demonstrate roentgenographic evidence of pleural fibrosis.[29–35]

In 1980, the International Labor Organization (ILO) modified its classification system to incorporate a semiquantitative method of categorizing pleural involvement.[36] However, the definition of circumscribed plaques and diffuse pleural thickening is ambiguous in the ILO 1980 classification. Bourbeau and Ernst[37] found unacceptably low rates of agreement regarding the presence and type of pleural abnormalities between (and within) ILO-trained readers. In fact, in regard to the type of pleural lesion (circumscribed plaque versus diffuse pleural thickening), the intrareader discordance ranged from 17 to 27% and the inter-reader discordance ranged from 19 to 28%. Moreover, autopsy studies and studies using CT scans demonstrate that the chest radiograph is neither a sensitive nor a specific method for identification of asbestos-induced pleural fibrosis. These observations suggest that the 1980 ILO criteria for pleural fibrosis[36] should be modified to improve the overall utility of this classification system. In addition, the specific role of the chest CT scan needs to be further clarified in identifying and defining pleural fibrosis.

Several investigations have found that pleural plaques[30,32,33,38–43] and diffuse pleural thickening[33,44–47] independently contribute to the development of restrictive lung function. After controlling for age, cigarette smoking, and duration of employment, pleural plaques in the absence of interstitial fibrosis were found to be associated with a reduction in vital capacity[30,32,38] as well

as reduction in the diffusing capacity of carbon monoxide.[32,39] Although diffuse pleural thickening has been reported to reduce lung volumes,[33,44–47] concerns about selection of study subjects and potential confounding by factors such as interstitial fibrosis and cigarette smoking have compromised general acceptance of this association. Nonetheless, after controlling for the degree of interstitial fibrosis, Rosenstock and colleagues[33] demonstrated that diffuse pleural thickening was associated with decrements in vital capacity. These studies suggest that asbestos-induced pleural fibrosis is independently associated with restrictive lung function.

To further quantify the physiologic significance of asbestos-induced pleural fibrosis, we evaluated the relationship between roentgenographic evidence of pleural fibrosis and spirometric values in 1,211 sheet metal workers.[34] Of those with pleural fibrosis (N = 334), 260 (78%) had circumscribed plaques and 74 (22%) had diffuse pleural thickening. Among persons with normal-appearing parenchyma and those with interstitial fibrosis, we observed a consistent decline in the percentage-predicted forced vital capacity (FVC) that was significantly associated with the type of pleural fibrosis (Figure 17–4). After controlling for potential confounders (age, years in the trade, pack-years of smoking, and ILO profusion category), linear regression models demonstrated that both circumscribed plaques (140 mL decline; $p = .02$) and diffuse pleural thickening (270 mL decline; $p = .005$) were independently associated with decrements in FVC. Further qualification of the physiologic effect of these pleural lesions using three-dimensional reconstruction techniques demonstrated that the quantitative estimate of pleural fibrosis was inversely related to the total lung capacity.[48] Moreover, regression equations showed a 5 mL decline in total lung capacity for every mL of pleural fibrosis.

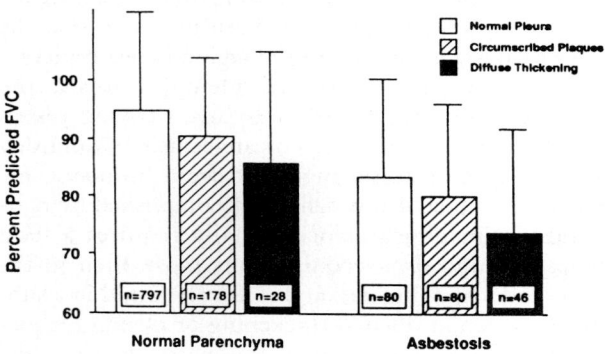

Figure 17–4   The percent predicted forced vital capacity stratified by parenchymal fibrosis (normal = profusion 0/1; asbestosis = profusion ≥ 1/0) and pleural fibrosis (normal pleural circumscribed plaques and diffuse pleural thickening). A significant clinical and statistical decline between categories of pleural fibrosis for those with normal parenchyma (ANOVA F = 8.62; $p = .0002$) and those with asbestosis (ANOVA F = 4.88; $p = .009$) was observed.

Several pieces of evidence suggest that parenchymal inflammation and/or fibrosis are the principal determinants of restrictive lung function in persons with asbestos-induced pleural fibrosis who have normal-appearing parenchyma on the chest radiograph. First, pulmonary function tests indicate that in addition to reduced lung volumes, asbestos-induced pleural fibrosis is associated with lower diffusing capacities for carbon monoxide,[32,41,46] diminished lung compliance,[41] and exercise responses that suggest interstitial lung disease.[49] Second, autopsy studies[50,51] and studies using HRCT scans[2,52] demonstrate that the chest roentgenogram appears to underestimate the presence of parenchymal fibrosis. These studies[2,14,50,52] show that as many as 15% of individuals with anatomically defined interstitial fibrosis have normal routine chest roentgenograms. This implies that asbestos-exposed persons with pleural fibrosis may have interstitial fibrosis that is not readily apparent on the chest roentgenogram but which may be responsible for the development of restrictive lung function. Third, two independent groups[21,53] have shown that individuals with asbestos-induced pleural fibrosis and no evidence of interstitial lung disease on the chest roentgenogram have an elevated percentage of lymphocytes in their BAL fluid when compared with similarly exposed persons with normal chest radiographs. These data suggest that parenchymal inflammation and/or fibrosis not appreciated on the chest radiograph are more likely to be present among persons with pleural fibrosis than similarly exposed individuals with normal pleura and may account for the associated restrictive lung function.

One unique consequence of asbestos-related pleural fibrosis is rounded atelectasis, which was first recognized as a consequence of pleural disease and therapeutic pneumothorax. However, Blesovsky[54] first suggested a relationship between asbestos exposure and rounded atelectasis in 1966, and asbestos exposure is now known to be the most common cause for rounded atelectasis.[55,56] The exact mechanism leading to rounded atelectasis is not known, but it has been proposed that the lung becomes atelectatic in the region beneath pleural thickening. With continued pleural fibrosis, the atelectatic lung is trapped and curls, drawing vessels and bronchi into the area of atelectasis.[55] Rounded atelectasis must be distinguished from bronchogenic carinoma, which can usually be accomplished by radiographic imaging but occasionally requires a lung biopsy. Rounded atelectasis occurs most often in the lower lobes and lingula[55] and is usually found in a subpleural location. Pleural thickening or pleural plaques are often located adjacent to the mass. However, the most useful finding is a "comet tail" or curvilinear shadows that extend toward the hilum.[55] This comet tail is best seen with computerized tomography (Figure 17–5). Asbestos-related rounded atelectasis is usually stable over time and is not associated with an increased risk for bronchogenic carcinoma.

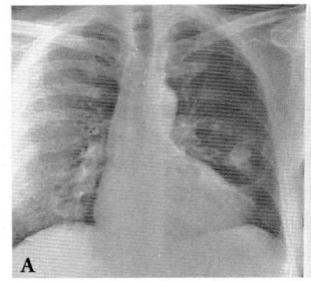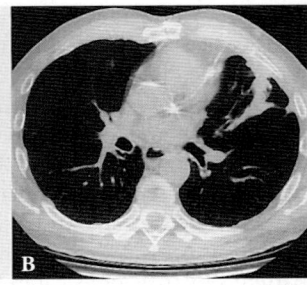

Figure 17–5   *A*, Composite chest radiograph and *B*, selected image from conventional CT scan in an individual with rounded atelectasis. The CT scan shows the classic "comet tail" sign and the underlying pleural-based plaque.

In summary, previous studies indicate that pleural fibrosis is the most common asbestos-induced abnormality, is being underdiagnosed, and is associated with restrictive lung function. Little work has been done to investigate the accuracy of the current criteria for pleural fibrosis established by the ILO, the anatomic and functional validity of these criteria, and the determinants of restrictive lung function in persons with asbestos-induced pleural fibrosis. Further studies are required to advance our understanding of impairment associated with pleural fibrosis. Results from these studies will have clear implications for the clinical assessment and management of workers with asbestos-induced pleural disease.

CELLULAR AND MOLECULAR EFFECTS OF ASBESTOS

Effects of Asbestos on Lung Epithelium

Lung epithelial cells are the first lung cells to contact inhaled asbestos fibers by virtue of their anatomic location lining the airways and alveoli (Figure 17–6). Both animal and human studies demonstrate that the lung epithelium is injured soon after exposure to asbestos. In a rat model of asbestosis, asbestos fibers deposit preferentially at alveolar duct bifurcations[57]; these alveolar duct bifurcations are the site of early fibrotic lesions.[57,58] The impacted asbestos fibers are phagocytosed by both alveolar macrophages and by epithelial cells (Figure 17–7)[57,59] and localize primarily to the perinuclear region in the epithelial cells.[60] In rats, phagocytosis of the fibers is associated with morphometric evidence of subtle lung epithelial injury[61] and increased lung epithelial permeability.[62] This increased permeability is due, at least in part, to direct effects of the fibers because both silica and asbestos directly increase mannitol permeability (a marker of the paracellular pathway) as well as fibrin degradation products permeability across cultured lung epithelial monolayers.[63–65] Subsequent to this injury, rat type II epithelial cell proliferation increases as measured by triturated thymidine uptake.[66,67]

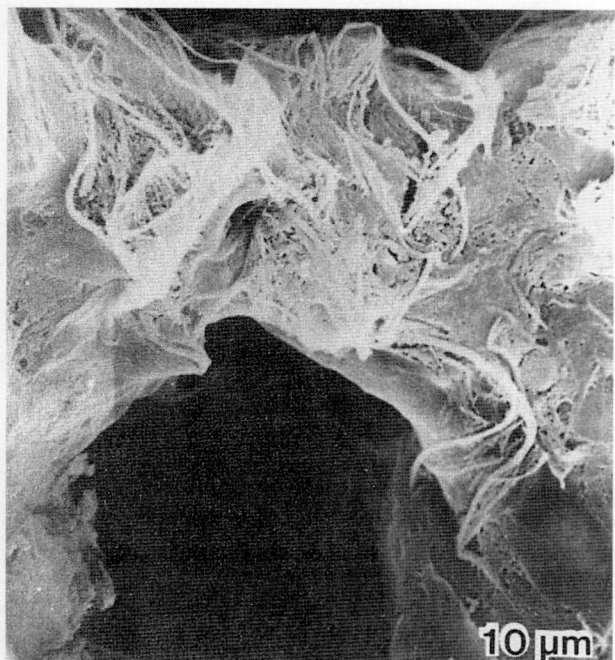

Figure 17–6 Asbestos fibers overlie the first bifurcation of the alveolar duct where they are initially deposited. Reproduced with permission from Brody et al.[212]

Human studies also demonstrate lung epithelial dysfunction soon after asbestos exposure. Using ^{99m}Tc-diethylenetriamine pentaacetate (DTPA) clearance as a marker, lung epithelial permeability is increased in patients with asbestosis.[68,69] This effect is due, at least in part, to the direct effects of asbestos on the epithelial cells; asbestos fibers cause both cytolytic and noncytolytic lung epithelial injury in cultured human bronchial explants and cultured human lung epithelial cells.[63–65,70] These experimental observations are relevant to asbestosis. In asbestosis, lung epithelial injury and increased epithelial permeability can contribute to subsequent fibrosis by creating a microenvironment that leads to collapse-induration in the small airways and alveolar ducts,[71,72] or by increasing the movement of biologically active compounds (platelet-derived growth factor [PDGF], cytokines, and fibrin degradation products) from the air spaces into the lung interstitium.[65]

Asbestos and Reactive Oxygen Species

One proposed mechanism for asbestos-induced lung disease is through reactive oxygen species.[73] Asbestos can increase oxidants in at least two ways. First, depending on the asbestos fiber, they contain varying amounts of iron, either absorbed to the surface as in the case of chrysotile, or incorporated into the mineral structure as in the case of amphiboles. The iron can act to catalyze the Fenton reaction generating •OH from H_2O_2.[74] Alter-

nately, asbestos can increase oxidant generation by stimulating inflammatory cells.[73] Previous experimental systems have provided evidence for and against the hypothesis that asbestos expresses its biologic activity through oxidant production. In support of this hypothesis, using electron spin trapping, asbestos catalyzes hydroxyl radical production (•OH) from H_2O_2 via the Fenton reaction[74]; the iron chelator, deferoxamine, binds to asbestos fibers and blocks this reaction.[75] Oxidants are also generated in vivo after asbestos or silica exposure because •OH is produced in the lungs of animals exposed to asbestos.[76] Further indirect evidence for an oxidant-mediated mechanism is provided by several observations: (1) asbestos exposure increases manganese-superoxide dismutase (MnSOD) antioxidant enzyme levels in cultured tracheal epithelial cells and in type II cells cultured from the lungs of exposed animals[77,78]; (2) lung inflammation following inorganic dust exposure correlates with the amount of iron present in the dust[79]; (3) exogenous polyethylene glycol (PEG)-linked catalase partially protects asbestos-exposed animals from subsequent lung fibrosis in a model of rapid asbestosis[80]; and (4) in A549 cells (a transformed cell line with some alveolar type II cell features), asbestos fibers increase intracellular iron levels, and the pathogenic effects correlate with increases in iron levels and the induction of ferritin expression and intracellular iron storage protein, which functions to limit redox active iron.[81]

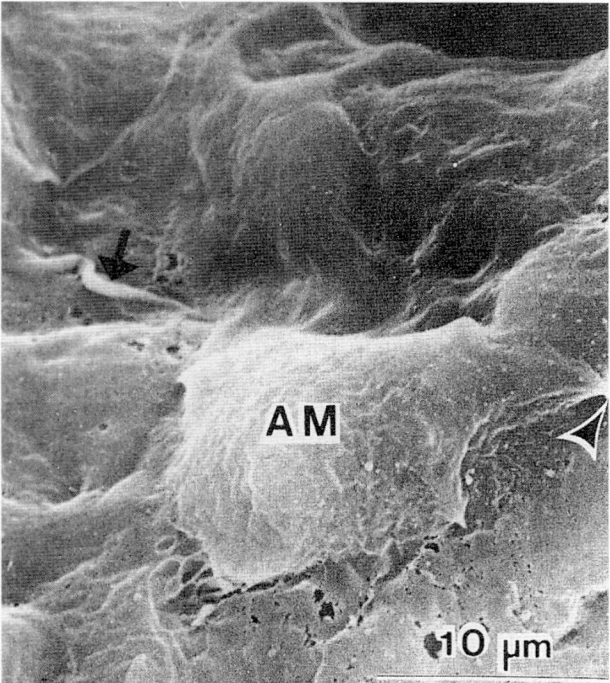

Figure 17–7 Twenty-four hours after exposure, some fibers are seen on alveolar dust surfaces and most fibers are obscured (*arrowheads*) by epithelial cells and alveolar macrophages. Reproduced with permission from Brody et al.[212]

Other experimental observations suggest that asbestos may have biologic effects independent of its ability to generate oxidants. In the animal model of rapid asbestosis, catalase only partially protects the lung from asbestos-induced fibrosis, and it does not prevent increased airway protein as seen in the animal model.[80] Because this increased protein reflects mucosal and vascular permeability, asbestos may affect permeability through nonoxidant pathways. Similarly, evidence for increased oxidant production and asbestos' biologic effects is not always causally linked. Asbestos is toxic for mouse peritoneal macrophages and causes lipid peroxidation. The antioxidant, vitamin E, blocks lipid peroxidation following asbestos exposure, but it does not prevent the cytotoxicity.[82] Similarly, immortalized human mesothelial cells are injured by extracellular oxidants, but are resistant to amosite-asbestos injury even when their antioxidant enzymes are depleted.[83] Finally, the ability of chrysotile asbestos to increase human lung epithelial permeability is not affected by alterations in the iron content by iron loading or by chelating iron with deferoxamine.[64] These observations suggest that asbestos can induce and amplify oxidant production, and that some of the biologic effects of asbestos are linked causally to this mechanism. Asbestos also appears to express biologic effects that are independent of its ability to generate reactive oxygen species.

Asbestos and Reactive Nitrogen Species

More recently, there is increasing evidence that reactive nitrogen species (RNS) might have a role in asbestos-induced lung injury. Nitric oxide, •NO, is produced enzymatically from L-arginine in the presence of O_2• NADPH (the reduced form of nicotinamide-adenine dinucleotide phosphate) and either constitutive or inducible nitric oxide synthase (iNOS). Nitric oxide can interact with •O_2 to form the potent oxidant peroxynitrite (•NOOO). Asbestos fibers induce the activity of iNOS in alveolar macrophages, A549 cells, and mesothelial cells.[84–86] Inhalation of asbestos fibers (crocidolite or chrysotile) increases the formation of reactive nitrogen species and nitrotyrosine, a marker for peroxynitrite formation.[87] The molecular and cellular targets of RNS that cause lung injury are less certain. The proxidant properties of NO may be balanced by antioxidant properties of nitric oxide.[88,89] Given the complex signaling pathways involving nitric oxide, the role of RNS and nitric oxide in asbestos-induced lung injury requires further study.

Asbestos and Cell Signal Transduction Pathways

Asbestos is increasingly recognized to activate signaling pathways in both lung epithelial and mesothelial cells.[90,91] Many cell-membrane-mediated signaling events are mediated by activating phospholipases C or D. Activating these phospholipases can lead to increased intracellular calcium (through inositol, 1,4,5-triphosphate [IP_3] or through phosphatidic acid) and to increased protein kinase C (PKC) activity. Protein kinase C is a ubiquitous calcium-, phosphatidylserine-, and diglyceride-dependent kinase that is usually present in the cell cytoplasm.[92] When activated by increased cell diglycerides, PKC translocates to the cell membrane and phosphorylates its substrate(s). Protein kinase C activation has been implicated in controlling many cell functions including growth, regulation of gene expression, cell shape, and epithelial permeability.[93,94] Crocidolite asbestos exposure at low concentrations can increase both phospholipase C and PKC activity in hamster tracheal epithelial cells.[90] These observations are potentially relevant to asbestos-induced cell injury because asbestos increases ornithine decarboxylase (ODC) gene expression and activity. The ODC is a highly regulated, rate-limiting enzyme in polyamine biosynthesis. Polyamines are organic polycations with multiple roles in cell proliferation.[95] Asbestos-induced ODC activity appears to be linked to phospholipase C activation because both calcium antagonists and PKC inhibitors prevent this increase.[96,97] Because both calcium and PKC affect epithelial permeability, changes in cell calcium and PKC activity are also important to subtle physiologic alterations in lung epithelial function.[93,94,98]

Fibers may also activate tyrosine kinase activity in target cells. Tyrosine kinases are a family of both receptor- and nonreceptor-activated kinases that act by either autophosphorylating tyrosine sites (in the case of receptor-activation) or phosphorylating tyrosine sites on target proteins.[99] Tyrosine kinase activation is involved in cell proliferation and growth factor signal transduction events; it can also alter epithelial cell-to-cell adherence. When epithelial cells are transfected with a temperature-sensitive *src* (a tyrosine kinase) and grown at permissive temperature, cells rapidly lose cell-to-cell contact. This change in morphology is associated with tyrosine phosphorylation of both cell adherence proteins, E-cadherin and β-catenin.[100] The fibrogenic mineral, silica, has recently been reported to increase tyrosine kinase activity in human lung macrophages.[101]

Asbestos exposure can also indirectly alter cell responsiveness by affecting expression of cell surface receptors. Platelet-derived growth factor is secreted by several cells such as alveolar macrophages and is proposed as an important mediator in several fibrotic lung diseases. The PDGF is a potent mitogen and chemoattractant for mesenchymal cells such as fibroblasts. These mesenchymal cells respond to PDGF through cell surface receptors (PDGF-rα which binds PDGF-AA and PDGF-rβ which binds PDGF-BB).[102] Changing these cell surface receptors affects their response to secreted PDGF. Chrysotile asbestos exposure increases PDGF-rα on rat lung fibroblasts and increases their response to PDGF-AA.[103] Changes in these or other receptors could affect the progression of fibrotic lung disease following asbestos exposure.

Asbestos and Signal Transduction and Oncogene Expression

Pathologically, the asbestos-induced lung diseases associated with asbestos exposure are characterized by inflammation, cell proliferation, and cell transformation. These cellular activities can be controlled at the molecular level through the expression of oncogenes. Recent work with asbestos demonstrates that asbestos exposure activates oncogene regulatory pathways. The proto-oncogenes *CFOS* and *CJUN* encode for proteins that form homo- and heterodimeric protein complexes.[104] These complexes are members of the activator protein (AP)-1 transcription factor family and interact with regulatory deoxyribonucleic acid (DNA) sequences known as TPA response elements (TRE). Expression of *CFOS* and *CJUN* is required for transition from the G_1 phase into the S phase in cultured cells.[105] In rat pleural mesothelial cells, both crocidolite and chrysotile asbestos induce persistent elevation in *CFOS* and *CJUN* messenger ribonucleic acid (mRNA).[99] Additionally, in hamster tracheal epithelial cells, asbestos induces *CJUN* expression but not *CFOS* expression[106]; this activation may be oxidant mediated because H_2O_2 similarly increases *CJUN* expression.[107] Increased *CJUN* expression is linked to cell transformation because transfecting hamster tracheal epithelial cells with full length *CJUN* yields cells that grow in soft agar, a marker of cell transformation.[107] Both *CJUN* and *CFOS* code for proteins that bind to AP-1 binding sites on DNA. These proteins appear to be expressed after asbestos exposure because in both cells, asbestos exposure increases protein factors that bind to the AP-1 sites on DNA. Nuclear factor κB (NF-κB) is another transcription factor that regulates genes intrinsic to inflammation and cell proliferation.[108] Crocidolite asbestos exposure causes persistent NF-κB expression in hamster tracheal epithelial cells. This elevated NF-κB expression is associated with increased *CMYC* mRNA expression, a proto-oncogene under NF-κB regulation.[108]

MECHANISMS OF ASBESTOS-INDUCED LUNG DISEASE

Asbestosis

The pathogenesis of asbestosis is unknown. Despite the absence of definitive knowledge regarding the biologic mechanisms that result in pulmonary fibrosis, it is very clear that the chronic inflammatory response is progressive, that the inflammation and fibrosis is heterogeneously distributed throughout the lung, and that the chronic inflammatory process is associated with extensive remodeling and fibrosis of the lower respiratory tract. In the lung parenchyma, this chronic inflammatory process eventually leads to proliferation of mesenchymal cells, intra-alveolar fibrosis, and loss of alveolar capillary units. The mechanisms for asbestos-induced pulmonary fibrosis are complex and probably involve several lung cells and cell mediators (Figure 17–8). Both inflammatory cells—neutrophils and macrophages—and lung epithelial cells are affected by asbestos.

A potential pathway that mediates fibrosis in the lung parenchyma is through chronic alveolitis dominated by alveolar macrophages and neutrophils. Chronically activated alveolar macrophages release several mediators, further amplifying the inflammatory response. Both activated alveolar macrophages and epithelial cells release polypeptide growth factors (transforming growth factor [TGF]-β, PDGF-B, insulin-like growth factor [IGF], and fibronectin) that modulate the growth of mesenchymal cells; they also release cytokines, including tumor necrosis factor (TNF)-α, interleukin (IL)-8, IL-1, and interferon (IFN)-γ, which may amplify the local inflammatory response. The alveolar capillary membrane is injured, and inflammatory cells are activated in pulmonary fibrosis. Thus, inflammatory products may be locally produced and released, contributing to injury of the lung parenchyma. Moreover, it has been proposed that oxidants, cytokines, and growth factors are important mediators of acute and chronic injury and of chronic remodeling of the lower respiratory tract that eventually results in asbestosis.

Several lines of evidence suggest that asbestos contributes to lung fibrosis via oxidant injury to the alveolar structures. As reviewed earlier, asbestos can contribute to oxidant injury by •OH production or by promoting production of reactive oxidants by macrophages and neutrophils. Oxidants can contribute to chronic lung fibrosis. When alveolar cells are recovered from patients with idiopathic pulmonary fibrosis (IPF), a disease of similar clinical expression, they release excess amounts of superoxide anion and hydrogen peroxide.[109,110] Myeloperoxidase, a neutrophil enzyme that converts hydrogen peroxide to a hypohalide radical, is also present in high concentration in BAL fluid in patients with IPF.[111] Glutathione, an antioxidant, is markedly depressed in patients with IPF.[112] Antioxidants appear to play an important protective role in preventing or limiting oxidant-induced lung disease.[113] A patient with partial monosomy 21 who had low superoxide dismutase activity (manganese-superoxide dismutase is on chromosome 21) was found to have an adverse response to supplemental oxygen.[114] Manganese-superoxide dismutase, located near the mitochondrial structures, is a potent antioxidant that converts superoxide anion to hydrogen peroxide. Interestingly, the production of MnSOD is induced in vitro following exposure to TNF-α.[115] Tumor necrosis factor-α has been shown to induce MnSOD mRNA in vivo in several organs in mice.[116] In rats, asbestos inhalation also induces mRNA for MnSOD beginning one day after exposure and persisting for 14 days after cessation of exposure.[117] Tracheal epithelial cell lines transfected with a MnSOD cDNA construct resulting in high levels of SOD activity are protected from crocidolite-induced cytotoxicity.[118] These findings suggest that antioxidants in general and MnSOD in particular may play prominent roles in modulating the lung's response to oxidant injury.

Cytokines are produced by both macrophages and lung epithelial cells and appear to play a prominent role in recruiting inflammatory cells to the site of injury and in promoting and extending the chronic inflammatory process. Both TNF-α and IL-8 illustrate the potential importance of cytokines in the persistent inflammation associated with pulmonary fibrosis. However, other cytokines may prove more important in the pathogenesis of pulmonary fibrosis. Tumor necrosis factor-α has been shown to stimulate fibroblast proliferation[119] as well as fibroblast production of prostaglandin E_2 (PGE_2), collagenase, and collagen.[120,121] Tumor necrosis factor-α has also been shown to activate endothelial cell adhesion molecule expression,[122] stimulate neutrophils to release superoxide anion,[123] and induce epidermal growth factor receptor expression on fibroblasts.[121] Tumor necrosis factor-α can induce target tissues to produce a variety of bioactive molecules such as IL-1,[124] IL-6,[125] granulocyte-macrophage colony–stimulating factor (GM-CSF),[126] monocyte-CSF,[127] and granulocyte-CSF,[126] which may play an important role in modulating the effects of

TNF-α. For example, adding IFN-γ to TNF-α inhibits fibroblast proliferation[128] and collagen production.[129] Asbestos and silica, known to cause pulmonary fibrosis, activate rat alveolar macrophages to release TNF-α in vitro.[130] In mice, bleomycin, another potent fibrogenic agent, has been shown to upregulate the production of mRNA for TNF-α.[131] Importantly, anti-TNF-α antibody prevents bleomycin-induced pulmonary fibrosis.[131] TNF-α receptor knockout mice exposed to asbestos, which have homozygous deletions of both the 55 kD and 75 kD TNF-α receptors, demonstrate decreased proliferative responses assessed by bromodeoxyuridine (bBrdU) incorporation, and decreased mRNA expression of TFG-α and PDGF-A. The TNF-α receptor knockout mice demonstrate in vivo an important role for TNF-α in the fibroproliferative response after asbestos exposure and the importance of other growth factors.[132] Similarly, experimental silicosis is associated with increased pulmonary mRNA for TNF-α; prior treatment with anti-TNF-α antibody appears to prevent pulmonary fibrosis.[133] Macrophages isolated from humans with IPF[134,135] and asbestosis[135] have higher concentrations of mRNA for TNF-α and spontaneously release greater amounts of TNF-α compared with controls. In IPF, mRNA for TNF-α is primarily produced by macrophages and epithelial cells.[134]

Interleukin-8, another chemokine, belongs to a supergene family with potent chemotactic activity for polymorphonuclear leukocytes (PMN).[136] Whereas monocytes and macrophages can produce IL-8, epithe-

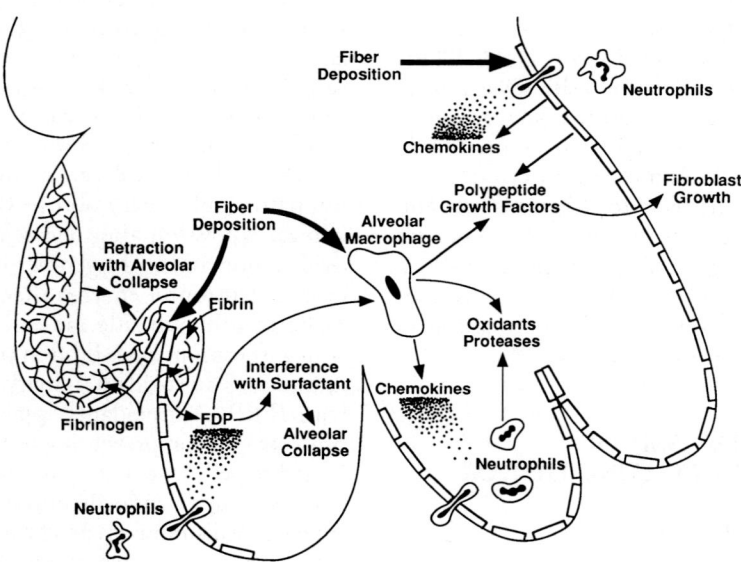

Figure 17–8   The predominant biologic processes involved in the development of fiber-induced pulmonary fibrosis. Fiber deposition stimulates alveolar macrophages, terminal airway, and type I alveolar epithelial cells to release chemotactic factors that attract neutrophils to the alveolar duct. Oxidants, myeloperoxidase, and proteolytic enzymes directly injure the alveolar wall; growth factors enhance mesenchymal proliferation and collagen production; and alveolar injury increases permeability to fibrinogen and other plasma proteins, which ultimately result in induration and collapse of the bronchoalveolar unit. FDP = fibrin degradation products.

lial cells may require a specific host-derived signal (TNF-α or IL-1) for induction of IL-8.[136–141] However, asbestos can directly cause the release of IL-8 by lung epithelial cells.[142] Increased concentrations of IL-8 in BAL fluid have been reported in patients with IPF[143,144] and sarcoidosis.[143] Additional studies indicate that the alveolar macrophage appears to be the primary source of IL-8 in IPF.[144,145] The PMNs are a prominent and expected feature of the inflammatory response in asbestosis.[146] In fact, excess neutrophils in the BAL fluid have been associated with an accelerated decline in gas exchange among individuals exposed to asbestos.[147] Moreover, a decline in BAL neutrophilia was temporally associated with a beneficial response to corticosteroid therapy in patients with IPF.[148] The concentration of IL-8 mRNA extracted from alveolar macrophages is directly related to the concentration of PMNs in the BAL fluid.[145] Taken together, these findings suggest that PMNs play an important role in the pathogenesis of pulmonary fibrosis, and that IL-8 may modulate the concentration of lung PMNs in these chronic forms of interstitial lung disease.

Growth factors released from activated alveolar macrophages promote the mesenchymal proliferation, resulting in enhanced collagen production and re-epithelialization of the alveolar structure, both of which are essential histologic features of pulmonary fibrosis. For the purposes of this discussion, we will highlight only the potential pathogenic effects of PDGF; other growth factors may, however, prove more relevant in the remodeling process. Platelet-derived growth factor-B is a potent mitogen that can trigger early events in the cell cycle (G_0 to G_1 transition) and can induce the synthesis of a number of cell-cycle-related proteins.[149] In models of skin wounding, epithelial cells increase the expression of mRNA for PDGF-B and PDGF-β receptor within the first two days of the lesion; the message levels return to normal following re-epithelialization.[150] In vitro, asbestos fibers enhance the production of PDGF by alveolar macrophages.[150] In patients with interstitial lung disease, alveolar macrophages appear to release significantly higher concentrations of a PDGF-like material than in normal control subjects.[151] Alveolar macrophages from subjects with interstitial lung disease have significantly higher concentrations of PDGF-B mRNA,[152,153] which appears to be specifically up-regulated by IFN-γ.[152] Among patients with pulmonary fibrosis, PDGF-B mRNA is overexpressed in lung biopsy specimens and appears to be localized to alveolar epithelial cells and alveolar macrophages.[154] In individuals with pulmonary fibrosis, the expression of messages for PDGF-B is much more abundant than transcripts for PDGF-A[153,154]; mRNA for PDGF-B colocalizes with the PDGF protein.[154] Interestingly, Hermansky-Pudlak syndrome, a pleiotropic genetic disorder associated with pulmonary fibrosis,[155] is associated with the enhanced release of PDGF-B by alveolar macrophages.[156,157]

Modulation of connective tissue may be a salient component of wound healing and scar resolution/repair. In this context, TGF-β is a family of several similar molecules (β_1, β_2, and β_3) whose genes are highly conserved across species and are believed to modulate the development of fibrosis and other biologic processes.[158] Interestingly, TGF-β may have dual effects in the regulation of fibrotic lung tissue. Transforming growth factor-β_1 (25 kD) is primarily found in alpha granules of platelets but is produced by a variety of cells, including activated T cells, macrophages, and epithelial cells. Transforming growth factor-β_2 is a homodimer consisting of two β_2 subunits, and TGF-β_3 is a heterodimer that contains one β_1 and one β_2 subunit linked by a disulfide bond. Transforming growth factor-β is abundant in the lung, can be demonstrated in BAL fluid, and appears to play a prominent role in modulating inflammation in fibrotic forms of lung disease. Following intratracheal instillation of bleomycin in C57BL/6 mice, TGF-β mRNA in the lung increases five-fold above control levels and is maximally elevated one week following the initial exposure.[159,160] The production of lung collagen following intratracheal instillation of bleomycin is significantly reduced by treatment with antibodies to TGF-β_1 and TGF-β_2.[161] Expression of TGF-β in the extracellular matrix is also a prominent feature in experimental models of radiation injury.[162] In vitro studies using rat lung fibroblasts stimulated with bleomycin demonstrate that increases in TGF-β mRNA precede increases in mRNA for procollagen I and procollagen III.[163] In an experimental model of asbestosis, TGF-β appears to accumulate at the bifurcation of the alveolar duct, the initial site of asbestos deposition and macrophage localization.[164] In pulmonary fibrosis, in situ hybridization studies indicate that macrophages[165,166] and bronchial epithelial cells[166,167] appear to be major sources for TGF-β. Transforming growth factor-β protein appears to localize in the interstitium at the site of fibroblast proliferation.[165,166]

Lung epithelial cells may not only contribute to chronic lung injury by producing cytokines and growth factors, but they may also be targets of injury in fibrotic lung disease. Studies of the histopathology and cell biology of interstitial lung disease provide us with a pathophysiologic model in which lung epithelial injury and dysfunction contribute to the evolution of pulmonary fibrosis. According to this collapse-induration model, the initial injury leads to increased epithelial permeability. Increased permeability results in plasma components entering distal air spaces, contributing to small airway obstruction and distal microatelectasis. Fibrinogen is among the plasma components that enter the air spaces. The distal airways and alveoli are rich in procoagulant tissue factor,[168] which quickly converts fibrinogen to fibrin. The resulting fibrin clot must be lysed and cleared to restore function to the distal air spaces. This fibrinolytic activity must be tightly controlled because both increased and decreased fibrinolysis can contribute to further lung injury. If fibrinolysis is impaired, the fibrin clot will be incompletely resolved, and airway obstruction and/or alveolar atelectasis will persist. This can lead to endoluminal fibrosis with loss of alveolar units.[72] Alternately, increased fibrinolysis can contribute to further lung injury. Plasmin, a serine protease that degrades connective tissue elements in addition to its preferred substrate, fibrin, is the major fibrinolytic enzyme in the lung.[169–171] Degrading basement membrane components such as laminin and fibronectin could contribute directly to lung injury. Plasmin could also contribute to inflammatory injury by activating latent collagenase, growth factors, and cytokines.[169,171] Finally, increased fibrinolytic activity leads to elevated local concentrations of fibrin degradation products (FDP). These FDP injure endothelial cells, activate and recruit inflammatory cells,[172] and interfere with surfactant function, contributing to further alveolar collapse.[173,174] Experimental observations support this mechanism in asbestosis. The FDP are increased in both an animal model of asbestosis and in patients with asbestosis.[175] Some of this increased fibrinolytic activity is due to increased plasmin activation by macrophages, but asbestos also directly increases urokinase production by human lung epithelial cells.[176]

Pleural Fibrosis

Although circumscribed pleural plaques and diffuse pleural thickening are included in the broad category of asbestos-induced pleural fibrosis, these processes are distinct entities that probably involve different clinical pathogenic components. Circumscribed plaques involve the parietal pleura, are often bilateral and symmetric, and occur most commonly between the fifth and eighth ribs in the posterior/lateral portion of the chest while sparing the apices and costophrenic angles.[10,26–28,36,177–180] Diffuse pleural thickening is closely associated with previous pleural effusions,[180,181] primarily involves the visceral pleura, is usually unilateral, and commonly extends into the costophrenic angle.[10,26–28,36,177–181] Although circumscribed pleural plaques remain as discrete lesions of the parietal pleura, diffuse pleural thickening often results in adhesions and fusion of the visceral and parietal pleura.[10,26–28,44,177]

Any hypothesis that addresses the pathogenesis of circumscribed pleural plaques must account for several peculiar characteristics of these lesions. These dense collections of collagenous connective tissue occur primarily in the posterior and lateral aspect of the chest, are usually bilateral and symmetric in shape, are orientated parallel to the ribs, do not have associated pleural adhesions, and spare the apices and costophrenic angle. Although microscopic fragments of asbestos fibers have been observed within the circumscribed pleural plaque,[182–184] it is not certain that these short microfibrils are directly responsible for initiating a localized inflammatory response. Kiviluoto[183] and Meurman[185] have proposed that circumscribed pleural plaques form as a direct result of local inflammation of the parietal pleura from asbestos

fibers that protrude from the visceral pleura. This theory has not gained wide acceptance because supportive pathologic material (such as fibers protruding from the visceral pleura or adhesions between the visceral pleura and circumscribed plaques) has not been reported, and because asbestos fibers are too short to be anchored in the visceral pleura and span the pleural cavity. Animal[186] and human[187] studies have shown that asbestos fibers migrate peripherally in the lung parenchyma; fibers have been demonstrated occasionally in the pleural effusions of asbestos workers.[188] These findings suggest that microfibrils may reach the parietal pleura via a transpleural route.[189] Once in the pleural cavity, asbestos fibers may gain access to the parietal pleura through preformed stomata that connect the pleural cavity to the lymphatics in the parietal pleura.[190] The transpleural migration of fibers might account for the predilection of pleural plaques to form in the gravity-dependent (posterior and basilar) portion of the chest cavity. To date, no studies have confirmed the relationship between inflammation and obliteration of the parietal stomas and the development of pleural plaques. Furthermore, the transpleural route fails to address several salient characteristics of these lesions, such as bilaterality, symmetric shape, orientation parallel to the ribs, and sparing of the apices and costophrenic angle. Since asbestos fibers are cleared by the parenchymal lymphatic plexus and accumulate in the mediastinal lymph nodes,[191] microfibrils probably reach the parietal pleura through retrograde lymphatic drainage involving flow from the mediastinal nodes to the retrosternal and intercostal lymphatics.[192] Given the peculiar characteristics of circumscribed pleural plaques (bilateral, symmetric, and orientated parallel to the ribs), the data presented thus far suggest that microfibrils embolize to the parietal pleura via either the parenchymal lymphatic plexus or via the costal vascular supply. Once present in the parietal pleura, the fiber itself or agents transported by it appear to initiate and promote the inflammatory response. This hypothesis accounts for the finding of fibers in other anatomic sites, but it also raises questions as to why plaques occur in the parietal pleura and not at other sites of fiber deposition.

The pathogenesis of diffuse pleural thickening remains even less well understood. Its location and strong association with interstitial fibrosis suggest that it may be a direct extension of parenchymal fibrosis to the visceral pleura. Both diffuse pleural thickening and parenchymal fibrosis are localized in the lung periphery and result in inflammation and fibrosis of the superficial or pleural lymphatic plexus.[26,182,193,194] This is consistent with the peripheral migration of asbestos fibers that are observed in animal inhalation studies[182,186] and in humans.[187] Moreover, the strong association with interstitial fibrosis[194] suggests that the development of diffuse pleural fibrosis requires exposure to high concentrations of asbestos fibers and may involve pathogenic mechanisms that are similar to asbestos-induced interstitial fibrosis. Alternately, a localized visceral pleural inflammatory reaction to an asbestos-related hemorrhagic pleural effusion may result in diffuse and extensive fibrosis of the visceral pleura.[180,181] This would be analogous to the development of a fibrothorax as a complication of an empyema or a hemothorax.[195] An additional hypothesis that may account for the development of diffuse pleural thickening involves the interaction of specific inflammatory cells and mediators of inflammation within the pleural cavity. Recently, Sahn and Antony[196] have demonstrated that neutrophils and macrophages in the pleural space may help contain and limit the amount of pleural fibrosis that occurs after exposure to asbestos. These findings imply that inflammatory responses to asbestos in the pleural cavity may parallel those observed in the lung parenchyma.

PROGNOSIS AND TREATMENT

Asbestosis and asbestos-induced pleural fibrosis are traditionally believed to be slowly progressive disorders. Radiographic evidence of disease progression appears to be associated with advanced age,[197–199] increased evidence of asbestos-induced lung disease on the chest radiograph,[197,200–203] more extensive occupational exposure to asbestos,[198,201,204–206] and cigarette smoking.[197,203,205] Progressive restrictive physiology has been reported to be associated with cumulative asbestos exposure,[204,207–209] cigarette smoking,[147,207] and either the presence of asbestosis[147,204] or of diffuse pleural thickening[147,200,204] on the chest radiograph. Excess declines in diffusing capacity have been associated with higher concentrations of neutrophils in BAL fluid.[147,210] Risk factors such as advanced age, more extensive occupational exposure to asbestos, cigarette smoking, and specific radiographic abnormalities, which are found to be associated with disease progression, are particularly important when one considers that among those with asbestosis, as much as 20% of the attributable mortality appears to be caused by progressive interstitial fibrosis.[211] Beyond the inherent clinical use of these prognostic factors, specific risk factors may be particularly useful in identifying populations that may benefit from aggressive novel therapeutic trials to diminish the risk of disease progression. To date, clinical trials to determine the efficacy of pharmacologic agents in the presentation or treatment of asbestos-induced interstitial fibrosis have not been conducted. Results from these novel drug trials may prove to be generalizable to other forms of pulmonary fibrosis.

REFERENCES

1. Becklake MR. Asbestos-related diseases of the lung and other organs: their epidemiology and implications for clinical practice. Am Rev Respir Dis 1987;114:187–227.
2. Aberle DR, Gamsu G, Ray CS, Feuerstein IM. Asbestos-related pleural and parenchymal fibrosis: detection with high-resolution CT. Radiology 1988;166:729–34.
3. Nicholson WJ, Perkel G, Selikoff IJ. Occupational exposure to asbestos: population at risk and projected mortality—1980–2030. Am J Ind Med 1982;3:259–311.
4. Walker AM, Loughlin JE, Friedlander ER, et al. Projections of asbestos-related disease 1980–2009. J Occup Environ Med 1983;25:409–25.
5. Lippmann M. Asbestos exposure indices. Environ Res 1988;46:86–106.
6. Timbrell V. An aerosol spectrometer and its applications. In: Mercer T, Morrow PE, Strober W, et al, editors. Assessment of airborne particles. Springfield, IL: Thomas; 1972. p. 290–330.
7. Vincent JH. On the practical significance of electrostatic lung deposition of isometric and fibrous aerosols. J Aerosol Sci 1985;16:511–9.
8. Timbrell V. Deposition and retention of fibers in the human lung. Ann Occup Hyg 1982;26:347–69.
9. Merchant J. Human epidemiology: a review of fiber type and characteristics in the development of malignant and nonmalignant disease. Environ Health Perspect 1990;88:287–93.
10. Craighead JE, Mossman BT. The pathogenesis of asbestos-associated diseases. N Engl J Med 1982;307:1446–55.
11. Epler GR, McCloud TC, Gaensler EA, et al. Normal chest roentgenograms in chronic diffuse infiltrative lung disease. N Engl J Med 1978;298:934–9.
12. Kipen HM, Lilis R, Suzuki Y, et al. Pulmonary fibrosis in asbestos insulation workers with lung cancer: a radiological and histopathological evaluation. Br J Ind Med 1987;44:96–100.
13. Akira M, Yamamoto S, Yokoyama K, et al. Asbestosis: high-resolution CT-pathologic correlation. Radiology 1990;176:389–94.
14. Lynch DA, Gamsu G, Aberle DR. Conventional and high resolution computed tomography in the diagnosis of asbestos-related diseases. Radiographics 1989;9:523–51.
15. Muller NL, Miller RR, Webb WR, et al. Fibrosing alveolitis: CT-pathologic correlation. Radiology 1986;160:585–8.
16. Begin R, Cantin A, Drapeau G, et al. Pulmonary uptake of gallium-67 in asbestos-exposed humans and sheep. Am Rev Respir Dis 1983;127:623–30.
17. Staples CA, Muller NL, Vedal S, et al. Usual interstitial pneumonia: correlation of CT with clinical, functional, and radiologic findings. Radiology 1987;162:377–81.
18. Muller NL, Miller RR. Computed tomography of chronic duffuse infiltrative lung disease: part 1. Am Rev Respir Dis 1990;142:1206–15.
19. Hartley PG, Galvin JR, Hunninghake GW, et al. High-resolution CT-derived measures of lung density are valid indexes of interstitial lung disease. J Appl Physiol 1994;76:271–7.
20. McCloud TC. Asbestos-related pleura and parenchymal fibrosis: detection with high-resolution CT. Invest Radiol 1989;24:636–7.
21. Schwartz DA, Galvin JR, Dayton CS, et al. Determinants of restrictive lung function in asbestos-induced pleural fibrosis. J Appl Physiol 1990;68:1932–7.
22. Staples CA, Gamsu F, Ray CS, Webb WR. High resolution computed tomography and lung function in asbestos-exposed workers with normal chest radiographs. Am Rev Respir Dis 1989;139:1502–8.
23. Affairs COS. A physician's guide to asbestos-related diseases. JAMA 1984;252:2593–7.
24. Jones RN. The diagnosis of asbestosis. Am Rev Respir Dis 1991;144:477–8.
25. Murphy RL, Becklake MR, Brooks SM, et al. The diagnosis of nonmalignant diseases related to asbestos. Am Rev Respir Dis 1986;134:363–8.
26. Craighead JE, Abraham JL, Churg A, et al. The pathology of asbestos-associated diseases of the lungs and the pleural cavities: diagnostic criteria and proposed grading schema. Arch Pathol Lab Med 1982;106:540–96.

27. Hillerdal G. Nonmalignant pleural disease related to asbestos exposure. Clin Chest Med 1985;6:141–52.

28. Rosenstock L, Hudson LD. Nonmalignant asbestos-induced pleural disease. Semin Respir Med 1986;7:197–202.

29. Anderson HA, Selikoff IJ. Pleural reaction to environmental agents. Fed Proc 1978;37:2496–500.

30. Baker EL, Dagg T, Greene RE. Respiratory illness in the construction trades. J Occup Environ Med 1985;27:483–9.

31. Irwig LM, duToit RSJ, Sluis-Cremer GK, et al. Risk of asbestosis in crocidolite and amosite mines in South Africa. Ann N Y Acad Sci 1979;330:35–52.

32. Oliver LC, Eisen EA, Greene R, Sprince NL. Asbestos-related pleural plaques and lung function. Am J Ind Med 1988; 14:649–56.

33. Rosenstock L, Barnhart S, Heyer NJ, et al. The relation among pulmonary function, chest roentgenographic abnormalities, and smoking status in an asbestos-exposed cohort. Am Rev Respir Dis 1988;138:272–7.

34. Schwartz DA, Fuortes LJ, Galvin JR, et al. Asbestos-induced pleural fibrosis and impaired lung function. Am Rev Respir Dis 1990;141:321–6.

35. Selikoff IJ. The occurrence of pleural calcifications among asbestos insulation workers. Ann N Y Acad Sci 1965;132: 351–67.

36. International Labour Office. Guidelines for the use of ILO international classification of radiographs of pneumoconioses. Revised edition. Occupational Safety and Health Series. Vol. 22. Geneva: International Labour Office; 1980. p. 48.

37. Bourbeau J, Ernst P. Between- and within-reader variability in the assessment of pleural abnormality using the ILO 1980 international classification of pneumoconioses. Am J Ind Med 1988;14:537–43.

38. Hjortsberg U, Orbaek P, Arborelius M, et al. Railroad workers with pleural plaques: I. spirometric and nitrogen washout investigation on smoking and nonsmoking asbestos-exposed workers. Am J Ind Med 1988;14:635–41.

39. Hedenstierna G, Alexandersson R, Kolmodin-Hedman B, et al. Pleural plaques and lung function in construction workers exposed to asbestos. Eur J Respir Dis 1981;62: 111–22.

40. Britton MG. Asbestos pleural disease. Br J Dis Chest 1982;76: 1–10.

41. Fridricksson HV, Hedenstrom H, Hillerdal G, Malmberg P. Increased lung stiffness in persons with pleural plaques. Eur J Respir Dis 1981;62:412–24.

42. Jarvholm B, Sanden A. Pleural plaques and respiratory function. Am J Ind Med 1986;10:419–26.

43. Jarvholm B, Larsson S. Do pleural plaques produce symptoms? A brief report. J Occup Environ Med 1988;30:345–7.

44. Miller A, Teirstein AS, Selikoff IJ. Ventilatory failure due to asbestos pleurisy. Am J Med 1983;75:911–9.

45. McGavin CR, Sheers G. Diffuse pleural thickening in asbestos workers: disability and lung function abnormalities. Thorax 1984;39:604–7.

46. Wright PH, Hanson A, Capel LH. Respiratory function changes after asbestos pleurisy. Thorax 1980;35:31–6.

47. Picado C, Laporta D, Grassino A, et al. Mechanisms affecting exercise performance in subjects with asbestos–related pleural fibrosis. Lung 1987;165:45–57.

48. Schwartz DA, Galvin JR, Yagla SJ, et al. Restrictive lung function and asbestos-induced pleural fibrosis: a quantitative approach. J Clin Invest 1993;91:2685–92.

49. Shih J-F, Wilson J, Broderick A, et al. Asbestos-induced pleural fibrosis and impaired exercise physiology. Chest 1994;105: 1370–6.

50. Hillerdal G, Lindgren A. Pleural plaques: correlation of autopsy findings to radiographic findings and occupational history. Eur J Respir Dis 1980;61:315–9.

51. Hourihane DOB, Lessof L, Richardson PC. Hyaline and calcified pleural plaques as an index of exposure to asbestos:

52. a study of radiological and pathological features of 100 cases with a consideration of epidemiology. BMJ 1966;1: 1069–74.

52. Aberle DR, Gamsu G, Ray CS. High-resolution CT of benign asbestos-related diseases: clinical and radiographic correlation. AJR Am J Roentgenol 1988;151:883–91.

53. Wallace JM, Oishi JS, Barbers RG, et al. Bronchoalveolar lavage cell and lymphocyte phenotype profiles in healthy asbestos-exposed shipyard workers. Am Rev Respir Dis 1989;139:33–8.

54. Blesovsky A. The folded lung. Br J Dis Chest 1966;60:19–22.

55. Mintzer RA, Cugell DW. The association of asbestos-induced pleural disease and rounded atelectasis. Chest 1982;81: 457–60.

56. Voisin C, Fisekci F, Voisin-Saltiel S, et al. Asbestos-related rounded atelectasis: radiologic and mineralogic data in 23 cases. Chest 1995;107:477–81.

57. Brody AR, Hill LH, Adkins B, O'Connor RW. Chrysotile asbestos inhalation in rats: deposition pattern and reaction of alveolar epithelium and pulmonary macrophages. Am Rev Respir Dis 1981;123:670–9.

58. Quinlan TR, Berube KA, Marsh JP, et al. Patterns of inflammation, cell proliferation, and related gene expression in lung after inhalation of chrysotile asbestos. Am J Pathol 1995;147:728–39.

59. Haugen A, Schafer PW, Lechner JF, et al. Cellular ingestion, toxic effects, and lesions observed in human bronchial epithelial tissue and cells cultured with asbestos and glass fibers. Int J Cancer 1982;30:265–72.

60. Cole RW, Ault JG, Hayden JH, Rieder CL. Crocidolite asbestos fibers undergo size-dependent microtubule-mediated transport after endocytosis in vertebrate lung epithelial cells. Cancer Res 1991;51:4942–7.

61. Chang L-Y, Overby LH, Brody AR, Crapo JD. Progressive lung cell reactions and extracellular matric production after a brief exposure to asbestos. Am J Pathol 1988;131:156–70.

62. Warheit DB, Hill LH, George G, Brody AR. Time course of chemotactic factor generation and the corresponding macrophage response to asbestos inhalation. Am Rev Respir Dis 1986;134:128–33.

63. Merchant RK, Peterson MW, Hunninghake GW. Silica directly increases permeability of alveolar epithelial cells. J Appl Physiol 1990;68:1354–9.

64. Peterson MW, Walter ME, Gross TJ. Asbestos directly increases lung epithelial permeability. Am J Physiol 1993; 265:L308–18.

65. Gross TJ, Cobb SM, Peterson MW. Asbestos exposure increases paracellular transport of fibrin degradation products across human airway epithelium. Am J Physiol 1994;266:L287–95.

66. McGavran PD, Brody AR. Chrysotile asbestos inhalation induces tritiated thymidine incorporation by epithelial cells of distal bronchioles. Am J Respir Cell Mol Biol 1989;1: 231–5.

67. Brody AR, Overby LH. Incorporation of tritiated thymidine by epithelial and interstitial cells in bronchiolar-alveolar regions of asbestos-exposed rats. Am J Pathol 1989;134:133–9.

68. Gellert AR, Langford JA, Winter RJD, et al. Asbestosis: assessment by bronchoalveolar lavage and measurement of pulmonary epithelial permeability. Thorax 1985;40:508–14.

69. Rinderknecht J, Shapiro L, Krauthammer M, et al. Accelerated clearance of small solutes from the lungs in interstitial lung disease. Am Rev Respir Dis 1980;121:105–17.

70. Kamp DW, Dunne M, Anderson JA, et al. Serum promotes asbestos-induced injury to human pulmonary epithelial cells. J Lab Clin Med 1990;116:289–97.

71. Wright JL, Cagle P, Churge A, et al. Diseases of the small airways. Am Rev Respir Dis 1992;146:240–62.

72. Burkhardt A. Alveolitis and collapse in the pathogenesis of pulmonary fibrosis. Am Rev Respir Dis 1989;140:513–24.

73. Kamp DW, Graceffa P, Pryor WA, Weitzman SA. The role of free radicals in asbestos-induced diseases. Free Radic Biol Med 1992;12:293–315.

74. Lund LG, Aust AE. Iron-catalyzed reactions may be responsible for the biochemical and biological effects of asbestos. Biofactors 1991;3:83–9.

75. Weitzman SA, Chester JF, Graceffa P. Binding of deferoxamine to asbestos fibers in vitro and in vivo. Carcinogenesis 1988;9:1643–5.

76. Shapira RM, Ghio AJ, Effros RM, et al. Hydroxyl radicals are formed in the rat lung after asbestos instillation in vivo. Am J Respir Cell Mol Biol 1994;10:573–9.

77. Janssen YMW, Marsh JP, Absher MP, et al. Expression of antioxidant enzymes in rat lungs after inhalation of asbestos or silica. J Biol Chem 1992;267:10625–30.

78. Holley JA, Janssen YW, Mossman BT, Taatjes DT. Increased manganese superoxide dismutase protein in type II epithelial cells of rat lungs after inhalation of crocidolite asbestos or cristobalite silica. Am J Pathol 1992;141:475–85.

79. Ghio AJ, Kennedy TP, Whorton AR, et al. Role of surface complexed iron in oxidant generation and lung inflammation induced by silicates. Am J Physiol 1992;263:L511–8.

80. Mossman BT, Marsh JP, Sesko A, et al. Inhibition of lung injury, inflammation, and interstitial pulmonary fibrosis by polyethylene glycol-conjugated catalase in a rapid inhalation model of asbestosis. Am Rev Respir Dis 1990;141:1266–71.

81. Fang R, Aust AE. Induction of ferritin synthesis in human lung epithelial cells treated with crocidolite asbestos. Arch Biochem Biophys 1997;340:369–75.

82. Goodglick LA, Peitras LA, Kane AB. Evaluation of the causal relationship between crocidolite asbestos-induced lipid peroxidation and toxicity to macrophages. Am Rev Respir Dis 1989;139:1265–73.

83. Kinnula VL, Aalto K, Raivio KO, et al. Cytotoxicity of oxidants and asbestos fibers in cultured human mesothelial cells. Free Radic Biol Med 1994;16:169–76.

84. Thomas G, Ando T, Verma K, et al. Asbestos fibres and interferon upregulate nitric oxide production in rat alveolar macrophages. Am J Respir Cell Mol Biol 1994;11:707–15.

85. Chao CC, Park SH, Aust AE. Participation of nitric oxide and iron in the oxidation of DNA in asbestos-treated human lung epithelial cells. Arch Biochem Biophys 1996;326:152–7.

86. Choe N, Tanaka S, Kagan E. Asbestos fibres and interleukin-1 upregulate the formation of reactive nitrogen species in rat pleural mesothelial cell. Am J Respir Cell Mol Biol 1998;19:226–36.

87. Tanaka S, Choe N, Hemenway DR, et al. Asbestos inhalation induces reactive nitrogen species and nitrotyrosine formation in the lungs and pleura of the rat. J Clin Invest 1998;102:445–54.

88. Gupta MP, Evanoff V, Hart CM. Nitric oxide attenuates hydrogen peroxide-mediated injury to procine pulmonary artery endothelial cells. Am J Physiol (Lung Cell Mol Physiol 16) 1997;272:L1133–41.

89. Gorbunov NV, Yalowich JC, Gaddam A, et al. Nitric oxide prevents oxidative damage produced by ter-butyl hydroperoxide in erythroleukemia cells via nitrosylation of heme and non-heme iron. J Biol Chem 1997;272:12328–41.

90. Perderiset M, Marsh JP, Mossman BT. Activation of protein kinase C by crocidolite asbestos in hamster tracheal epithelial cells. Carcinogenesis 1991;12:1499–502.

91. Janssen YMW, Heintz NH, Mossman BT. Induction of c-fos and c-jun proto-oncogene expression by asbestos is ameliorated by N-acetyl-L-Cysteine in mesothelial cells. Cancer Res 1995;55:2085–9.

92. Nishizuka Y. The role of protein kinase C in cell surface signal transduction and tumor promotion. Nature 1986;308:693–8.

93. Mullin JM, O'Brien TG. Effects of tumor promoters on LLC-PK1 renal epithelial tight junctions and transepithelial fluxes. Am J Physiol 1986;251:C597–602.

94. Winter M, Wilson JS, Bedell K, Shasby DM. The conductance of cultural epithelial cell monolayers: oxidants, adenosine triphosphate, and phorbol dibutyrate. Am J Respir Cell Mol Biol 1990;2:355–63.

95. Pegg AE. Polyamine metabolism and its importance in neoplastic growth and as a target for chemotherapy. Cancer Res 1988;48:759–74.

96. Marsh JP, Mossman BT. Mechanisms of induction of ornithine decarboxylase activity in tracheal epithelial cells by asbestiform fibers. Cancer Res 1988;48:709–14.

97. Marsh JP, Mossman BT. Role of asbestos and active oxygen species in activation and expression of ornithine decarboxylase in hamster tracheal epithelial cells. Cancer Res 1991;51:167–73.

98. Peterson MW, Gruenhaupt D. A23187 increases permeability of MDCK monolayers independent of phospholipase activation. Am J Physiol 1990;259:C69–76.

99. Marshall CJ. Specificity of receptor tyrosine kinase signaling: transient versus sustained extracellular signal-regulated kinase activation. Cell 1995;80:179–85.

100. Behrens J, Vakaet L, Friis R, et al. Loss of epithelial differentiation and gain of invasiveness correlates with tyrosine phosphorylation of the E-cadherin/B-catenin complex in cells transformed with a temperature-sensitive v-SRC gene. J Cell Biol 1993;120:757–66.

101. Holian A, Kelley K, Hamilton RF. Mechanisms associated with human alveolar macrophage stimulation by particulates. Environ Health Perspect 1994;102:Suppl 10:69–74.

102. Shimokado KE, Raines EW, Madtes DK, et al. A significant part of macrophage-derived growth factor consists of at least two forms of PDGF. Cell 1985;43:277–86.

103. Bonner JC, Goodell AL, Coin PG, Brody AR. Chrysotile asbestos upregulates gene expression and production of α-receptors for platelet-derived growth factor (PDGF-AA) on rat lung fibroblasts. J Clin Invest 1993;92:425–30.

104. Ransone LJ, Verma IM. Nuclear proto-oncogenes fos and jun. Annu Rev Cell Biol 1990;6:539–57.

105. Angel P, Karin M. The role of jun, fos, and the AP-1 complex in cell proliferation and transformation. Biochem Biophys Acta 1991;1072:129–57.

106. Heintz NH, Janssen YM, Mossman BT. Persistent induction of c-fos and c-jun expression by asbestos. Proc Natl Acad Sci U S A 1993;90:3299–303.

107. Timblin CR, Janssen YWM, Mossman BT. Transcriptional activation of the proto-oncogene c-jun by asbestos and H_2O_2 is directly related to increased proliferation and transformation of tracheal epithelial cells. Cancer Res 1995;55:2723–6.

108. Janssen YMW, Barchowsky A, Treadwell M, et al. Asbestos induces nuclear factor κB (NF-κB) DNA-binding activity and NF-κB-dependent gene expression in tracheal epithelial cells. Proc Natl Acad Sci U S A 1995;92:8458–62.

109. Strausz J, Muller-Quernheim J, Steppling H, Ferlinz R. Oxygen radical production by alveolar inflammatory cells in idiopathic pulmonary fibrosis. Am Rev Respir Dis 1990;141:124–8.

110. Cantin A, North SL, Hubbard RC, Crystal RG. Normal alveolar epithelial lining fluid contains high levels of glutathione. J Appl Physiol 1987;63:152–7.

111. Cantin AM, North SL, Fells GA, et al. Oxidant mediated epithelial cell injury in idiopathic pulmonary fibrosis. J Clin Invest 1987;79:1665–75.

112. Cantin AM, Hubbard RC, Crystal RG. Glutathione deficiency in the epithelial lining fluid of the lower respiratory tract in idiopathic pulmonary fibrosis. Am Rev Respir Dis 1989;139:370–2.

113. Sies H. Antioxidant activity in cells and organs. Am Rev Respir Dis 1987;136:478–80.

114. Ackerman AD, Fackler JC, Tuck-Muller CM, et al. Partial monosomy 21, dimished activity of superoxide dismutase and pulmonary oxygen toxicity. N Engl J Med 1988;318:1666–9.

115. Wong GHW, Goeddel DV. Induction of manganous superoxide dismutase by tumor necrosis factor: possible protective mechanism. Science 1988;242:941–4.

116. Heffner JE, Repine JE. Antioxidants and the lung. In: Crystal RG, West JB, editors. The lung: scientific foundations. New York: Raven Press; 1991. p. 1811–20.

117. Quinlan TR, Marsh JP, Janssen YMW, et al. Dose-responsive increases in pulmonary fibrosis after inhalation of asbestos. Am J Respir Crit Care Med 1994;150:200–6.

118. Mossman BT, Sirinrut P, Brinton BT, et al. Transfection of manganese-containing SOD gene into hamster tracheal epithelial cells ameliorate asbestos-mediated cytotoxicity. Free Radic Biol Med 1996;21:125–31.

119. Vilcek J, Palombella VJ, Henriksen-DeStefano D. Fibroblast growth enhancing activity of tumor necrosis factor and its relationship to other polypeptide growth factors. J Exp Med 1986;163:632–43.

120. Dayer J-M, Beutler B, Cerami A. Cachectin/tumor necrosis factor stimulates collagenase and prostaglandin E2 production by human synovial cells and dermal fibroblasts. J Exp Med 1985;162:2163–8.

121. Rochester CL, Elias JA. Cytokines and cytokine networking in the pathogenesis of interstitial and fibrotic lung disorders. Semin Respir Med 1993;14:389–416.

122. Albelda SM, Buck CA. Integrins and other cell adhesion molecules. FASEB J 1990;4:2868–80.

123. Tsujimoto M, Yokota S, Vilcek J, Weissmann G. Tumor necrosis factor provokes superoxide anion generation from neutrophils. Biochem Biophys Res Commun 1986;137:1094–100.

124. Nawroth PP, Bank I, Handley D. Tumor necrosis factor/cachectin interacts with endothelial cell receptors to induce release of interleukin 1. J Exp Med 1986;163:1363–75.

125. Baggiolini M, Walz A, Kunkel SL. Neutrophil-activating peptide-1/interleukin 8, a novel cytokine that activates neutrophils. J Clin Invest 1989;84:1045–9.

126. Leizer T, Cebon J, Layton JE, Hamilton JA. Cytokine regulation of colony stimulating factor production in cultured human synovial fibroblasts. I. Induction of GM-CSF and G-CSF production by interleukin-1 and tumor necrosis factor. Blood 1990;76:1989–96.

127. Akashi M, Saito M, Koeffler HP. Lymphotoxin: stimulation and regulation of colony-stimulating factors in fibroblasts. Blood 1989;74:2383–90.

128. Elias JA. Tumor necrosis factor interacts with interleukin-1 and interferons to inhibit fibroblast proliferation via fibroblast prostaglandin-dependent and independent mechanisms. Am Rev Respir Dis 1988;138:652–8.

129. Kahari V-M, Chen YQ, Su MW. Tumor necrosis factor-α and interferon-γ suppress the activation of human type I collagen gene expression by transforming growth factor-β1. Evidence for two distinct mechanisms of inhibition at the transcriptional and post-transcriptional levels. J Clin Invest 1990;86:1489–95.

130. Lindenschmidt RC, Driscoll KE, Perkins MA, et al. The comparison of a fibrogenic and two nonfibrogenic dusts by bronchoalveolar lavage. Toxicol Appl Pharmacol 1990;102(2):268–81.

131. Piguet PF, Collart MA, Grau GE, et al. Tumor necrosis factor/cachectin plays a key role in bleomycin-induced pneumopathy and fibrosis. J Exp Med 1989;170:655–63.

132. Liu JY, Brass DM, Howle GW, Brody AR. TNF-alpha receptor knockout mice are protected from the fibroproliferative effects of inhaled asbestos fibers. Am J Pathol 1998;153:1839–47.

133. Piguet PF, Collart MA, Grau GE, et al. Requirement of TNF for development of silica-induced pulmonary fibrosis. Nature 1990;344:245–7.

134. Piguet PF, Ribaux C, Karpuz V, et al. Short communication. Expression and localization of tumor necrosis factor-α and its mRNA in idiopathic pulmonary fibrosis. Am J Pathol 1993;143:651–5.

135. Zhang Y, Lee TC, Guillemin B, et al. Enhanced IL-1β and tumor necrosis factor-α release and messenger RNA expression in macrophages from idiopathic pulmonary fibrosis or after asbestos exposure. J Immunol 1993;150:4188–96.

136. Strieter RM, Standiford TJ, Rolfe MW, Kunkel SL. Interleukin-8. In: Kelley J, editor. Cytokines of the lung. New York: Marcel Dekker; 1993. p. 281–305.

137. Beutler B, Milsark IW, Cerami AC. Passive immunization against cachectin/tumor necrosis factor protects mice from lethal effect of endotoxin. Science 1985;229:869–71.

138. Standiford TJ, Kunkel SL, Basha MA, et al. Interleukin-8 gene expression by a pulmonary epithelial cell line: a model for cytokine networks in the lung. J Clin Invest 1990;86:1945–53.

139. Nakamura H. IL-8 gene expression in human bronchial epithelial cells. J Biol Chem 1991;266:19611–7.

140. Massion PP, Inoue H, Richman-Eisenstat J, et al. Novel *Pseudomonas* product stimulates interleukin-8 production in airway epithelial cells in vitro. J Clin Invest 1994;93:26–32.

141. Redl H, Schlag G, Ceska M, et al. Interleukin-8 release in baboon septicemia is partially dependent on tumor necrosis factor. J Infect Dis 1993;167:1464–6.

142. Rosenthal GJ, Germolec DR, Blazka ME, et al. Asbestos stimulates IL-8 production from human lung epithelial cells. J Immunol 1994;153:3237–44.

143. Car BD, Meloni F, Luisetti M, et al. Elevated IL-8 and MCP-1 in the bronchoalveolar lavage fluid of patients with idiopathic pulmonary fibrosis and pulmonary sarcoidosis. Am J Respir Crit Care Med 1994;149:655–9.

144. Carre PC, Mortenson RL, King TE, et al. Increased expression of the interleukin-8 gene by alveolar macophages in idiopathic pulmonary fibrosis. A potential mechanism for the recruitment and activation of neutrophils in lung fibrosis. J Clin Invest 1991;88:1802–10.

145. Lynch JP, Standiford TJ, Rolfe MW, et al. Neutrophilic alveolitis in idiopathic pulmonary fibrosis. The role of interleukin-8. Am Rev Respir Dis 1992;145:1433–9.

146. Crystal RG, Bitterman PB, Rennard SI, et al. Interstitial lung diseases of unknown cause. Disorders characterized by chronic inflammation of the lower respiratory tract. N Engl J Med 1984;310:154–66, 235–44.

147. Schwartz DA, Davis CS, Merchant JA, et al. Longitudinal changes in lung function among asbestos-exposed workers. Am J Respir Crit Care Med 1994;150:1243–9.

148. Turner-Warwick M, Haslam PL. The value of serial bronchoalveolar lavages in assessing the clinical progress of patients with cryptogenic fibrosing alveolitis. Am Rev Respir Dis 1987;135:26–34.

149. Fabisiak JP, Kelley J. Platelet-derived growth factor, In: Kelley J, editor. Cytokines of the lung. New York: Marcel Dekker; 1993. p. 3–39.

150. Antoniades HN, Galanopoulos T, Neville-Golden J, et al. Injury induces in vivo expression of platelet-derived growth factor (PDGF) and PDGF receptor mRNAs in skin epithelial cells and PDGF mRNA in connective tissue fibroblasts. Proc Natl Acad Sci U S A 1991;88:565–9.

151. Bauman MD, Jetten AM, Bonner JC, et al. Secretion of a platelet-derived growth factor homologue by rat alveolar macrophages exposed to particulates in vitro. Eur J Cell Biol 1990;51:327–34.

152. Shaw R, Benedict SH, Clark RAF, King TE. Pathogenesis of pulmonary fibrosis in interstitial lung disease. Alveolar macrophage PDGF(B) gene activation and up-regulation by interferon gamma. Am Rev Respir Dis 1991;143:167–73.

153. Nagaoka I, Trapnell BC, Crystal RG. Upregulation of platelet-

derived growth factor-A and -B gene expression in alveolar macrophages of individuals with idiopathic pulmonary fibrosis. J Clin Invest 1990;85:2023–7.

154. Antoniades HN, Bravo MA, Avila RE, et al. Platelet-derived growth factor in idiopathic pulmonary fibrosis. J Clin Invest 1990;86:1055–64.

155. Depinho RA, Kaplan KL. The Hermansky-Pudlak syndrome: report of three cases and review of pathophysiology and management considerations. Medicine 1985;64:192–202.

156. Witkop C, Townsend D, Bitterman P, Harmon K. The role of ceroid in lung and gastrointestinal disease in Hermansky-Pudlak syndrome. Adv Exp Med Biol 1989;266:283–97.

157. Harmon KR, Witkop CJ, White JG, et al. Pathogenesis of pulmonary fibrosis: platelet-derived growth factor precedes structural alterations in the Hermansky-Pudlak syndrome. J Lab Clin Med 1994;123:617–27.

158. Kelley J. Transforming growth factor-β. In: Kelley J, editor. Cytokines of the lung. New York: Marcel Dekker; 1993. p. 101–31.

159. Hoyt DG, Lazo JS. Alterations in pulmonary mRNA encoding pro-collagens, fibronectin and transforming growth factor-β precede bleomycin-induced pulmonary fibrosis in mice. J Pharmacol Exp Ther 1988;246:765–71.

160. Hoyt DG, Lazo JS. Bleomycin and cyclophosphamide increase pulmonary type IV procollagen mRNA in mice. Am J Physiol 1990;259:L47–52.

161. Giri SN, Hyde DM, Hollinger MA. Effect of antibody to transforming growth factor beta on bleomycin induced accumulation of lung collagen in mice. Thorax 1993;48:959–66.

162. Finkelstein JN, Johnston CJ, Baggs R, Rubin P. Early alteration in extracellular matrix and transforming growth factor beta gene expression in mouse lung indicative of late radiation fibrosis. Int J Radiat Oncol Biol Phys 1994;28:621–31.

163. Phan SH, Gharaee-Kermani M, Wolber F, Ryan US. Stimulation of rat endothelial cell transforming growth factor-beta production by bleomycin. J Clin Invest 1991;87:148–54.

164. Perdue TD, Brody AR. Distribution of transforming growth factor beta-1, fibronectin, and smooth muscle actin in asbestos-induced pulmonary fibrosis in rats. J Histochem Cytochem 1994;42:1061–70.

165. Limper AH, Broekelmann TJ, Colby TV, et al. Analysis of local mRNA expression for extracellular matrix proteins and growth factors using in situ hybridization in fibroproliferative lung disorders. Chest 1991;99:55S–6S.

166. Corrin B, Butcher D, McAnulty BJ, et al. Immunohistochemical localization of transforming growth factor-beta1 in the lungs of patients with systemic sclerosis cryptogenic fibrosing alveolitis and other lung disorders. Histopathology 1994;24:145–50.

167. Khalil N, O'Connor RN, Unruh HW, et al. Increased production and immunohistochemical localization of transforming growth factor-beta in idiopathic pulmonary fibrosis. Am J Respir Cell Mol Biol 1991;5:155–62.

168. Idell S, James KK, Levin EG, et al. Local abnormalities in coagulation and fibrinolytic pathways predispose to alveolar fibrin deposition in the adult respiratory distress syndrome. J Clin Invest 1989;84:695–705.

169. Vassalli J, Sappino A, Belin D. The plasminogen activator/plasmin system. J Clin Invest 1991;88:1067–72.

170. Bertozzi P, Astedt B, Zenzius L, et al. Depressed bronchoalveolar urokinase activity in patients with adult respiratory distress syndrome. N Engl J Med 1990;322:890–7.

171. Henkin J, Marcotte P, Yang H. The plasminogen-plasmin system. Prog Cardiovasc Dis 1991;34:135–64.

172. Leavell KJ, Peterson MW, Gross TJ. The role of fibrin degradation products in neutrophil recruitment to the lung. Am J Respir Cell Mol Biol 1996;14:53–60.

173. Ge M, Ryan TJ, Lum H, Malik AB. Fibrinogen degradation product fragment D increases endothelial monolayer permeability. Am J Physiol 1991;261:L283–9.

174. O'Brodovich H, Weitz J, Possmayer F. Effect of fibrinogen degradation products and lung ground substance on surfactant function. Biol Neonate 1990;57:325–33.

175. Cantin A, Allard C, Begin R. Increased alveolar plasminogen activator in early asbestosis. Am Rev Respir Dis 1989;139:604–9.

176. Gross TJ, Cobb SM, Peterson MW. Asbestos exposure increases human bronchial epithelial cell fibrinolytic activity. Am J Physiol 1993;264:L276–83.

177. Hillerdal G. Pleural plaques in a health survey material: frequency, development and exposure to asbestos. Scand J Respir Dis 1978;59:257–63.

178. Statement A. The diagnosis of nonmalignant disease related to asbestos. Am Rev Respir Dis 1986;134:363–8.

179. Sargent EN, Gordonson J, Jacobson G, et al. Bilateral pleural thickening: a manifestation of asbestos dust exposure. AJR Am J Roentgenol 1978;131:579–85.

180. McLoud TC, Woods BO, Carrington CB, et al. Diffuse pleural thickening in an asbestos-exposed population: prevalence and causes. AJR Am J Roentgenol 1985;144:9–18.

181. Epler GR, McLoud TC, Gaensler EA. Prevalence and incidence of benign asbestos pleural effusion in a working population. JAMA 1982;247:617–22.

182. Lee KP. Lung response to particles with emphasis on asbestos and other fibrous dusts. Crit Rev Toxicol 1985;14:33–86.

183. Kiviluoto R. Pleural calcification as a roentgenologic sign of non-occupational endemic anthophyllite-asbestosis. Acta Radiol 1960;194: Suppl:1–67.

184. Churg A. Asbestos fibers and pleural plaques in a general autopsy population. Am J Pathol 1982;109:88–96.

185. Meurman L. Asbestos bodies and pleural plaques in a Finnish series of autopsy cases. Acta Pathol Microbiol Scand 1966;Suppl 181:1–107.

186. Morgan A, Evans JC, Holmes A. Deposition and clearance of inhaled fibrous minerals in the rat studies using radioactive tracer techniques. Environ Res 1975;10:196–207.

187. Sebastien P, Fondimare A, Bignon J, et al. Topographic distribution of asbestos fibers in human lung in relation to occupational and non-occupational exposure. In: Walton WH, editor. Inhaled particles. Oxford: Pergamon Press; 1977. p. 435–46.

188. Bignon J, Jaurand MC, Sebastien P, Dufour G. Interaction of pleural tissue and cells with mineral fibers. In: Chretien J, Hirsch A, editors. Diseases of the pleura. New York: Masson; 1983. p. 198–207.

189. Hillerdal G. The pathogenesis of pleural plaques and pulmonary asbestosis: possibilities and impossibilities. Eur J Respir Dis 1980;61:129–38.

190. Wang N-S. The preformed stomas connecting the pleural cavity and the lymphatics in the parietal pleura. Am Rev Respir Dis 1975;111:12–20.

191. Bignon J, Sebastien P, Gaudichet A. Measurement of asbestos retention in the human respiratory system related to health effects. In: Gravatt CC, La Fleur PD, Heinrich KFJ, editors. Proceedings of workshop on asbestos: definitions and measurement methods; 1977 July 18–20; National Bureau of Standards, Gaithersburg, Maryland. Washington: Department of Commerce, National Bureau of Standards; 1978. p. 95–119.

192. Taskinen E, Ahlman K, Wiikeri M. A current hypothesis of the lymphatic transport of inspired dust to the parietal pleura. Chest 1973;64:193–6.

193. Lauweryns JM, Baert JH. Alveolar clearance and the role of the pulmonary lymphatics. Am Rev Respir Dis 1977;115:625–83.

194. Stephens M, Gibbs AR, Pooley FD, Wagner JC. Asbestos induced diffuse pleural fibrosis: pathology and mineralogy. Thorax 1987;42:583–8.

195. Sahn SA. The pleura. Am Rev Respir Dis 1988;138:184–234.

196. Sahn SA, Antony VB. Pathogenesis of pleural plaques: rela-

tionship of early cellular response and pathology. Am Rev Respir Dis 1989;139:884–7.

197. Sluis-Cremer GK, Hnizdo E. Progression of irregular opacities in asbestos miners. Br J Ind Med 1989;46:846–52.

198. Liddell D, Eyssen G, Thomas D, McDonald C. Radiological changes over 20 years in relation to chrysotile exposure in Quebec. In: Walton WH, editor. Inhaled particles IV. Proceeding of an International Symposium. The British Occupational Hygiene Society; 1975 September 22–26; Edinburgh, Scotland. Tarrytown, NY: Pergamon Press; 1975. p. 799–813.

199. Cookson W, de Klerk N, Musk AW, et al. The natural history of asbestosis in former crocidolite workers of Wittenoom Gorge. Am Rev Respir Dis 1986;133:994–8.

200. Jones RN, Diem JE, Hughes JM, et al. Progression of asbestos effects: a prospective longitudinal study of chest radiographs and lung function. Br J Ind Med 1989;46:97–105.

201. Rubino GF, Newhouse M, Murray R, et al. Radiologic changes after cessation of exposure among chrysotile asbestos workers in Italy. Ann N Y Acad Sci 1979;330:157–61.

202. McMillan GHG, Rossiter CE. Development of radiological and clinical evidence of parenchymal fibrosis in men with non-malignant asbestos-related pleural lesions. Br J Ind Med 1982;39:54–9.

203. Suorant H, Huuskonen MS, Zitting A, Juntunen J. Radiographic progression of asbestosis. Am J Ind Med 1982; 3:67–74.

204. Jones RN, Diem JE, Glindmeyer H, et al. Progressions of asbestos radiographic abnormalities: relationships to esti-mates of dust exposure and annual decline in lung function. In: Wagner JC, editor. Biological effects of mineral fibres. Lyon: International Agency for Research on Cancer; 1980. p. 537–43.

205. Rossiter CE, Heath JR, Harries PG. Royal naval dockyards asbestosis research project: nine-year follow-up study of men exposed to asbestos in Devonport dockyard. J R Soc Med 1980;72:337–44.

206. Ehrlich R, Lilis R, Chan E, et al. Long term radiological effects of short term exposure to amosite asbestos among factory workers. Br J Ind Med 1992;49:268–75.

207. Ohlson G-G, Bodin L, Rydman T, Hogstedt C. Ventilatory decrements in former asbestos cement workers: a four year follow up. Br J Ind Med 1985;42:612–6.

208. Siracusa A, Cicioni C, Volpi R, et al. Lung function among asbestos cement factory workers: cross sectional and longitudinal study. Am J Ind Med 1984;5:315–25.

209. Enarson DA, Embree V, Maclean L, Grzybowski S. Respiratory health in chrysotile asbestos miners in British Columbia: a longitudinal study. Br J Ind Med 1988;45:459–63.

210. Cullen MR, Merrill WW. Association between neutrophil concentration in bronchoalveolar lavage fluid and recent losses in diffusing capacity in men formerly exposed to asbestos. Chest 1992;102:682–7.

211. Berry G. Mortality of workers certified by pneumoconiosis medical panels as having asbestosis. Br J Ind Med 1981;38:130–7.

212. Brody AR, Hill LH, Warheit DB. Induction of early alveolar injury by inhaled asbestos and silica. Fed Proc 1985;44: 2596–601.

18   BERYLLIUM DISEASE

LEE S. NEWMAN

LISA A. MAIER

Discovered in 1798, the silver-gray metal beryllium has become a favorite material of the 21st century, which is used in many high-technology applications. It is the fourth lightest element, is corrosion resistant, and has a low density, high melting point, and high tensile strength. Unfortunately, although it is a desirable metal in engineering circles, it continues to produce serious and often insidious adverse health effects. Exposure to beryllium occurs during the extraction of the mineral from its ores, beryl and bertrandite, during the processing of beryllium into metal alloys and ceramic products, the machining of near-final parts, and even in the recycling of computers, electronic circuit boards, and other beryllium-containing alloys. Of particular concern is beryllium's ability to cause granulomatous lung disease even after seemingly small exposures to beryllium metal, oxide, alloy dust, or fumes. As indicated in Table 18–1, exposure occurs in a wide variety of industries, including electronics, aerospace, aircraft manufacturing, tool and die, nuclear weapons manufacturing, and dental prosthesis manufacturing. Historically, it was used in the manufacture of fluorescent lamps, although this practice was discontinued more than 30 years ago on recognition of its health hazards. Exposure to beryllium can induce delayed-type hypersensitivity, and pulmonary, dermatologic, and systemic disease, including the granulomatous condition chronic beryllium disease (CBD) (Table 18–2). This chapter will summarize our present knowledge based on epidemiologic workplace studies, basic research on the role of the immune response to beryllium, and clinical research on the diseases that ensue. We will emphasize recent developments in CBD detection and diagnosis since this is now the most common form of beryllium toxicity, which continues to occur in 2 to greater than 20% of exposed workers.

HISTORIC PERSPECTIVE

The toxicity of beryllium was not appreciated until the early part of this century when the industrial processing of beryllium began in earnest. In the 1930s, reports of lung and skin disease in workers in beryllium industries emerged in the European medical literature[1] and in Russia.[2,3] In the early 1940s, investigators described beryllium workers in the United States with an acute chemical pneumonitis or bronchiolitis, although these abnormalities were misattributed initially to other chemicals in the manufacturing process.[4] The link between beryllium and granulomatous lung disease was forged in this country when an outbreak of "sarcoidosis" in fluorescent lamp industry workers in Salem, Massachusetts, was described by Harriet Hardy and Irving Tabershaw.[5] Much of our early understanding of the clinical presentation and course is based on Hardy and colleagues' compilation of many patients with acute and chronic beryllium disease in the US Beryllium Case Registry.[6] In addition to the reports of chronic disease associated with beryllium industry workers, disease was discovered in individuals living in areas surrounding beryllium industries and among household contacts of beryllium industry workers.[7–10] Now CBD is recognized among bystanders, such as secretaries, security guards, laundry workers, and family members.[11] Recently, cases have been reported among office workers whose only exposures came from residual beryllium left in an office building more than 10 years after a machine shop using beryllium alloy was moved out. Thus, those who work directly with beryllium and those with only incidental, secondhand exposures are at risk.

TABLE 18–1   Occupational Exposure: Industries that Use Beryllium

Aerospace
Aircraft manufacture
Alloy manufacturing (aluminum-beryllium, copper-beryllium, nickel-beryllium, magnesium)
Automotive parts
Ceramics
Defense industries
Dental alloy and prosthesis manufacture
Extraction, fabrication, and smelting of beryllium and beryllium alloys
Electronics
Fluorescent lamp manufacture (historic)
Foundries
Metal and metal alloy machining
Nuclear weapons
Plating
Precious metal extraction
Recycling of metal, electronics, and computers
Telecommunications
Tool and die

TABLE 18–2 Diagnostic Criteria for Beryllium Sensitization and Chronic Beryllium Disease

Beryllium sensitization
　Beryllium-specific immune response, usually indicated by one or more of the following:
　　Blood BeLPT
　　Positive skin-patch test using beryllium salts
　　Other tests of specific cellular immune response to beryllium
Beryllium lung disease
　Beryllium-specific immune response, usually indicated by one or more of the following:
　　Blood BeLPT
　　BAL BeLPT
　　Positive skin-patch test using beryllium salts

Histopathology on biopsy or radiographic alterations consistent with beryllium lung disease (granulomas or mononuclear cell interstitial infiltrates)

Clinical findings, if present, may include any of the following:
　Pulmonary signs or symptoms, systemic symptoms
　Compatible abnormalities on chest radiograph or chest computed tomography scan
　Altered pulmonary physiology (see text)

BeLPT = beryllium lymphocyte proliferation test.

Early epidemiologic and exposure assessments in Lorain, Ohio, led Sterner and Eisenbud to observe that CBD occurred at both high (workplace) and low (community) levels of exposure without a clear association between magnitude of exposure and disease incidence.[8] They hypothesized that beryllium disease was immunologically mediated, resulting from a specific response to the antigen beryllium. Knowing that beryllium is retained in the lungs for many years after last exposure, Sterner and Eisenbud speculated that an individual could become "immunologically sensitized" to beryllium long after stopping work, which helped explain the latency of disease development noted in some cases.[8]

A beryllium exposure standard was introduced in the United States in 1949 by the Atomic Energy Commission, setting occupational exposures at a permissible exposure limit of 2 μg/m^3 for an 8-hour time-weighted average and a peak level of 25 μg/m^3. Based in part on a study of neighborhood cases surrounding one beryllium plant, the environmental standard for air around factories was set at 0.01 μg/m^3 averaged over a 30-day period. As a result of these standards, some industrial controls were implemented in the late 1940s and early 1950s, leading to a reduction in the levels emitted by industry. After implementation of this exposure standard, cases of acute beryllium lung disease largely ceased, and the occurrence of neighborhood and household contact cases of CBD diminished, with the exception of sporadic acute cases such as one reported in 1984 in a dental laboratory technician who had been grinding a beryllium alloy for 4 to 6 hours a day for 3 months.[12] Although reduction of beryllium levels in the workplace may have reduced the incidence of acute disease, CBD continues to occur.[13–32] The US Occupational Safety and Health Administration

(OSHA) adopted the old Atomic Energy Commission exposure limits for beryllium and never implemented a full health standard for protecting beryllium workers. Adherence to existing OSHA exposure limits[33,34] does not afford adequate protection from CBD.[16,24–27,30,32,35–38] These standards are now being reexamined by the OSHA, and exposure limits are being voluntarily reduced further by a number of major beryllium users such as the United States Department of Energy.[33,34]

EXPOSURE TO BERYLLIUM

It has been estimated that more than a million individuals in the United States have been exposed to beryllium at some time.[16,39] Other countries, including Canada, the United Kingdom, Sweden, Germany, Belgium, France, Israel, Russia, Kazakhstan, and Japan—with nuclear weapon programs or emerging high-technology industries—have problems with beryllium exposure and have reported cases of CBD. Disease rates for CBD have been estimated at 2 to more than 20% of exposed workers, depending on the group studied.[12,21,24,26,28–32,40,41] Most studies have been cross-sectional and therefore underestimate the true incidence of CBD, missing cases in workers who have already left the workplace or in those who have not yet fulfilled the latency period for disease to occur. Beryllium primarily affects the lungs, lymph nodes, and skin by direct toxicity, its impact on the immune system, or both. Skin lesions, including granulomatous nodules and ulceration, occur following direct inoculation of beryllium splinters into the skin. Cutaneous contact with beryllium salts can induce contact dermatitis.[42–44] Inhalation of fumes and respirable dusts of beryllium salts, metal, oxides, or beryllium-containing metal alloys-mainly copper-beryllium and aluminum-beryllium—results in beryllium-related respiratory disease. Although the definitive study has not been published, exposure to the ore in the form of either beryl or bertrandite has not been shown to cause disease. However, beryllium ore workers have developed sensitization to beryllium.[12] Machining of beryllium and of beryllium alloys generates a high proportion of respirable-size particles,[45] often in the ultrafine (< 1.0 μ) range.[46,47] Once inhaled, the beryllium particles obey the general principles of particle deposition in the lung. Most likely, the chemical properties of the inhaled beryllium particles influence their toxicity. The solubility, particle size, and form of beryllium inhaled influence the development of an immune response and disease.[48] For example, beryllium oxide produced at lower temperatures is less immunogenic than that formed at higher temperatures. Because beryllium machining processes generate very fine particles, the number and surface area of particles that can reach the alveolar space are high.[38,45–47] Wet machining processes do not prevent aerosolization of beryllium particles.[49] Much of the beryllium inhaled is cleared by the lung's mucociliary escalator and alveolar macrophages. Some of the remaining beryllium is moved to the regional lymph nodes and pulmonary interstitium, remaining in the lungs for many years after the last exposure. Species and individual differences also influence the rate of clearance and type of toxicity seen.[41,50,51]

Certain beryllium industrial processes and job tasks increase the risk of developing an immune response to beryllium. For example, machinists have been found to have an increased risk of developing sensitization.[21,22,24,26,29,30,32,52] The exact exposure-response relationship for CBD, still under study, does not appear to be strictly linear. Recent data suggest that both genetic and exposure-related risk factors contribute to CBD risk, as discussed in more detail below.[52] Both dose and duration of beryllium exposure have been associated with increased risk of sensitization and disease. Clearly, this is most evident with acute pneumonitis, which occurs only at high exposures,[5] in the 10 μg/m³ range or greater.[53] On the other hand, CBD also develops in workers with seemingly minimal exposures such as security guards and secretaries,[21,22,30,32,37,38,54–56] and after as short a duration as three months.[29,38,40] Thus, it appears that beryllium's effects may be dose dependent, and that other factors modify the impact of beryllium exposure. In one study, tobacco smoking was found to reduce the risk of sensitization, raising the question of a protective effect from smoking.[24] However, subsequent studies have not confirmed this negative association.

PATHOLOGY

Although CBD is commonly considered to be a granulomatous disorder (Figure 18–1), the pathologic alterations seen in lung biopsy specimens are quite variable. Frieman and Hardy, in a paper reviewing 124 chronic disease cases submitted to the US Beryllium Case Registry, observed that only 69 of the patients (56%) had noncaseating granulomas on biopsy. The remainder of the patients had none or poorly formed granulomas with varying amounts of mononuclear cell interstitial infiltration.[57] Interstitial fibrosis is often found, but to varying extent. Most fibrosis occurs circumferentially around granulomas.[58] When present, the granulomas are composed of epithelioid cells, multinucleated giant cells, numerous CD4+ T lymphocytes, macrophages, and mast cells. Cultures and special stains for acid-fast bacilli and fungi are negative. Inclusions such as conchoid bodies, asteroid bodies, Schaumann's bodies, and cholesterol clefts are often present but are not pathognomonic and do not discriminate CBD from other granulomatous lung diseases. In fact, the histopathologic pattern in CBD can easily be mistaken for pulmonary sarcoidosis.[57,59–61]

Regional lymph nodes may be infiltrated by numerous noncaseating granulomas, indistinguishable from sarcoidosis. Partially or completely hyalinized nodules are also common (40%). Granulomas and these larger nodules may be surrounded by a rim of fibrosis and contain thin-walled vessels and remnants of granulomatous

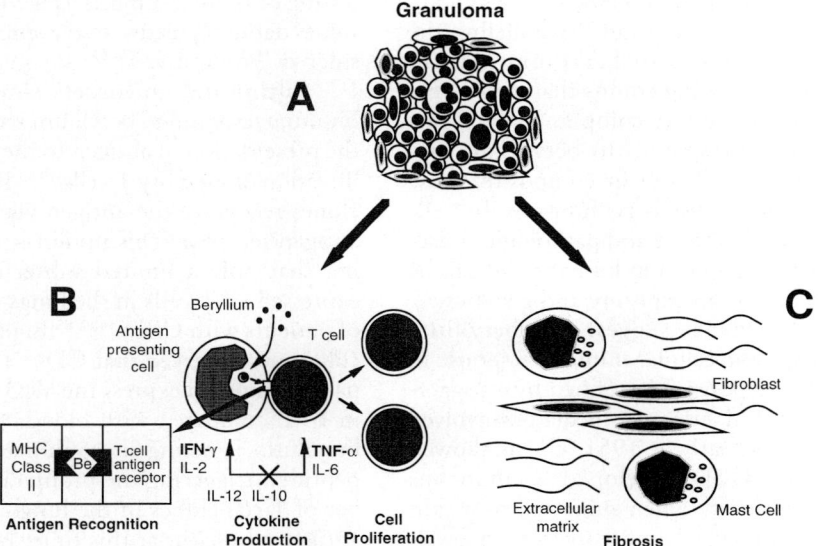

Figure 18–1 Immunopathogenesis of chronic beryllium disease. *A*, The granuloma, which is the hallmark of chronic beryllium disease, is composed of epithelioid cells, multinucleated giant cells, and lymphocytes. The granuloma may be surrounded by a rim of fibrosis and fibroblasts. *B*, After beryllium (Be) is inhaled, a nonspecific inflammatory response probably results. In addition, a beryllium-specific immune response may result when beryllium is internalized and presented to beryllium-specific T cells via major histocompatibility complex (MHC) class II molecules (HLA-DP) on antigen presenting cells. The antigen is recognized by the T-cell antigen receptor (antigen recognition). Following antigen recognition, two key events occur: cytokine production and cellular proliferation. The T cell produces interferon (IFN)-γ and interleukin (IL)-2 while the antigen presenting cells and other inflammatory cells produce tumor necrosis factor (TNF)-α and IL-6. These cytokines, along with others, enhance the inflammatory response and stimulate T-cell proliferation. *C*, Eventually, fibrosis may occur. Mast cells have been shown to produce basic fibroblast growth factor, which may stimulate fibroblasts and promote the production of extracellular matrix in a fibrotic capsule surrounding the granuloma.

organization. Some nodules have areas of necrosis, occasionally with large calcific inclusions. Dermatopathology shows noncaseating granulomas due to beryllium inoculation although in some individuals the appearance is more consistent with chronic atopic dermatitis.

TOXICOLOGY AND IMMUNOPATHOGENESIS

The pulmonary pathologic consequences of beryllium exposure are integrally related to the immune and inflammatory responses to beryllium.[62,63] Inhalation or tracheal instillation of various beryllium moieties produces lung injury ranging from an acute chemical pneumonitis to a mononuclear cellular infiltration and formation of granulomas and/or fibrosis in rats, mice, guinea pigs, dogs, and nonhuman primates.[64-73] In some of the more meticulous animal exposure studies, Haley and colleagues challenged beagle dogs with various forms of beryllium oxide particles and evaluated the pathologic and immune responses longitudinally. Over 1 year, the dogs developed granulomas, fibrosis, and lymphocytic infiltrates in their lungs. A lymphocytic T-helper-predominant alveolitis was observed, along with an in vitro lymphocyte proliferative response to beryllium. Studies using T-cell lines from the beagle lung indicated a beryllium-specific immune response.[68] Mice and nonhuman primates mount a lymphocyte-predominant granulomatous response similar to that in the dog. In one mouse model, in vivo lymphocyte proliferation was demonstrated in granulomas around blood vessels and in areas of white blood cell aggregation,[73] paralleling the lymphoproliferative response to beryllium seen in humans. Mouse and guinea pig strains that differ only in their major histocompatibility complex (MHC) loci mount varying immune responses to beryllium, suggesting genetic regulation. Taken in composite, these animal models suggest that the beryllium-specific cell-mediated[64,65,71] immune response and pathologic consequences are similar to those seen in humans and can be influenced by both beryllium exposure and genetics.

Several lines of evidence suggest that beryllium induces an antigen-specific cellular immune response in humans and that this response is amplified by a triggering of more nonspecific inflammatory mediators involved in innate immunity.[62] As early as 1951, Curtis showed that individuals with CBD developed a cutaneous delayed-type hypersensitivity when subjected to a skin patch test with beryllium salts. Some workers even developed a granulomatous response at the skin patch test site weeks later.[74,75] In vitro studies have confirmed the role of cellular immunity in CBD. When peripheral blood or bronchoalveolar lavage (BAL) cells are cultured in the presence of beryllium salts, lymphocytes that possess "memory" for beryllium are seen to proliferate.[13,14,17,19,20,76–80] These observations form the basis for the beryllium lymphocyte proliferation test (BeLPT) that is now widely used to detect beryllium sensitization and

disease and to distinguish CBD from sarcoidosis.[14,17–22,76,78,81] BAL cells from those with CBD show a marked proliferative response to beryllium salts whereas those from other granulomatous diseases such as sarcoidosis do not (see Figure 18–1 and Table 18–3).[13,17,81] When peripheral blood BeLPT was evaluated as a potential workplace medical screening tool in the 1980s, Kreiss, Newman, and colleagues showed that this immune biomarker enhanced early detection of CBD in many industries.[18,20,21,24,49,76,78] In these studies, some individuals were found to be sensitized to beryllium, as indicated by a positive response in the BeLPT and initiation of the cellular immune response, without evidence of pulmonary disease or granulomas on lung biopsy.[21,22,24,26,49,76,78] Some of these individuals have since developed granulomatous disease in as little as 3 months, indicating that sensitization precedes the inflammatory response in the lung and is a step in the progression from exposure to disease.[21,56,82] The BeLPT and its usefulness in disease surveillance will be discussed in greater depth below. The BeLPT is performed on peripheral blood mononuclear cells or BAL cells in microtiter plates cultured in the absence or presence of beryllium sulfate. Tritiated thymidine is added for the last 24 hours of incubation and the stimulation index (SI) is calculated as the highest uptake of unstimulated cells compared with cells stimulated with any of three concentrations of beryllium sulfate on any day of harvest. An SI of approximately 2.5 to 3 is considered positive, depending on the laboratory-specific cutoff values that are based on the testing of normal subjects' cells. Two or more elevated SI values define a positive test; a single elevated value is considered "borderline."[78,82]

Saltini and coworkers showed that the cellular immune response to beryllium requires class II MHC for the presentation of antigen to the T cells and for the proliferation of memory T cells.[19,83] Beryllium-specific T-cell clones recognize the antigen via their alpha/beta T-cell antigen receptor. This notion is supported by the finding that only a limited subset of T-cell receptors are expressed on T cells in the lungs compared to the blood of patients with CBD.[54,84,85] In particular, Fontenot and colleagues observed that CD4+ T cells from 25% of the patients studied express the Vα3 T-cell antigen receptor in BAL compared with blood.[86] Thus, it is likely that beryllium is acting in conjunction with a hapten (ie, peptide), triggering the proliferation of a limited number of T-cell clones in the lungs. The exact form of the antigen is unclear at this time. Implicit in this hypothesis is that such an antigen or hapten would act in combination with MHC class II molecules on antigen presenting cells. A number of recent studies have confirmed the importance of MHC class II presentation in both beryllium sensitization and CBD, in particular, the role of human leukocyte antigen (HLA)-DP.[87–90] Of the class II molecules, HLA-DPB1 appears to be most important in presenting a beryllium antigen to T cells to induce proliferation. Fontenot and colleagues, for

TABLE 18–3 Comparison of Hypersensitivity Pneumonitis, Chronic Beryllium Disease, and Sarcoidosis

	Hypersensitivity Pneumonitis	Chronic Beryllium Disease	Sarcoidosis
Exposure	Microbials Animal proteins Reactive chemicals	Beryllium salts, alloys, metals, oxides	Unknown
Symptoms	Respiratory and constitutional May fluctuate with exposure	Respiratory and constitutional	Respiratory and constitutional Extrathoracic common, especially eye, skin, lymphatics
Physical examination	Pulmonary	Pulmonary Extrathoracic variably present; skin nodules	Pulmonary Extrathoracic common
Laboratory	Serum precipitins usually present Serum ACE rarely elevated	Beryllium-specific cellular immune response in blood and/or lavage No serum precipitins Serum ACE elevated	No serum precipitins No cellular immune response to beryllium Serum ACE frequently elevated
Pulmonary physiology	Both restrictive and obstructive Gas exchange abnormalities Can be normal	Both restrictive and obstructive (restrictive late in disease) Gas exchange abnormalities are prominent Can be normal	Both restrictive and obstructive Gas exchange abnormalities variably present Can be normal
Chest radiograph	Alveolar and/or interstitial infiltrates Adenopathy unusual Often normal	Interstitial infiltrates Conglomerate masses (late) Pleural thickening in minority Adenopathy common, but rarely large Can be normal	Interstitial infiltrates Adenopathy very common, often large Pleural effusion occasionally present Can be normal
Endobronchial anatomy	Normal or mild bronchitis	Bronchial inflammation often present	Bronchial inflammation often present
Bronchoalveolar lavage	Lymphocytic alveolitis CD4+ or CD8+ (T suppressor) lymphocytes often predominant, but varies with stage Produce T helper 1 cytokines Neutrophils and mast cells present early	Lymphoytic alveolitis CD4+ (T helper) lymphocytes Produce T helper 1 cytokines	Lymphocytic alveolitis CD4+ (T helper) lymphocytes, rarely CD8+ Neutrophils variably but infrequently present Produce T helper 1 cytokines
Histopathology	Inflammation distant from granulomas Peribronchial location of granulomas Granulomas may be small, poorly defined Mononuclear cell infiltrates Fibrosis variable	Inflammation clustered at granulomas or distant Granulomas often perivascular but can be peribronchial Granulomas usually well defined but may be poorly defined Mononuclear cell infiltrates may be prominent Fibrosis variable	Inflammation clustered at granulomas Granulomas often perivascular Well-defined noncaseating granulomas Mononuclear cell infiltrates less prominent Fibrosis variable

example, demonstrated that proliferation of CBD T-cell clones was reconstituted by antigen presenting cell lines possessing an HLA-DPB1 Glu69 variant and could be inhibited by antibody to HLA-DPB1.[89] Lombardi and colleagues[90] confirmed the Fontenot finding of functional significance for HLA-DP molecules that possess a glutamate in position 69—an observation that provides important biologic plausibility for the epidemiologic finding that HLA-DPB1 Glu69 is a genetic susceptibility marker for beryllium sensitization and CBD, as discussed below.

Following antigen presentation and recognition, immune effector cells become activated.[77] When a beryllium-specific T-cell response has been initiated, key inflammatory cytokines, in particular tumor necrosis factor alpha (TNF-α), interleukin (IL)-6,[91] IL-2, and gamma interferon (IFN-α), are produced.[92,93] The response is characteristic of a T helper 1 pattern, with high and sustained IFN-α production and no detectable IL-4 but detectable IL-10. These cytokines enhance the inflammatory and immune response of the lymphocytes, macrophage, and other cells within the lung, while regulating the development of granulomas and the immune response in CBD (see Figure 18–1). This immune response acts in a self-propagating manner that amplifies the inflammatory response in the target organ. In CBD, the beryllium-reactive cells and immune response are largely compartmentalized to the lung.[23,94] Early initiating events probably include a nonspecific inflammatory cascade starting with alveolar epithelial cell injury and increased alveolar-capillary permeability.[95–97] Recent work demonstrating increased production of the mucin-like moiety KL-6 suggests a role for activated alveolar type II epithelium in disease pathogenesis.[95] The epithelial cells and other cells found at sites of granuloma formation may help regulate the inflammatory events in CBD. Recent studies suggest that mast cells accumulate in the circumference of CBD granulomas. They produce the 17.8 kD isoform of the fibrogenic growth factor, basic fibroblast growth factor (bFGF), that may help promote the formation of a fibrotic capsule surrounding the granuloma.[58] The granulomatous and inflammatory response might be sustained because of beryllium's ability to induce macrophage apoptosis.[98] The progression from beryllium exposure to CBD hinges partly on an individual's genetic susceptibility. Both animal and human studies support the importance of genetic susceptibility to beryllium. The finding of familial cases of CBD in identical twins,[99] siblings,[31] and in parents and children[54,55] suggests a genetic predisposition to CBD. Most striking are the results of a study by Richeldi and colleagues who found an increased use of MHC HLA-DPB1 with a glutamate residue at position 69 in patients with CBD compared with exposed individuals.[87,88] Since their original report, a number of other investigators, studying other populations of beryllium-exposed workers, have confirmed and extended this observation, showing that the number of Glu69 variants further increases the CBD risk, and that presence of Glu69 is a risk factor for beryllium sensitization as well as for CBD.[100–102] Other allelic differences have been found in HLA-DRB1, -DRB3, and -DRB5 loci in individuals with CBD but their functional significance and importance as risk markers have been less thoroughly examined.[76] Since HLA class II molecules are involved in the presentation of most antigens to the T-cell antigen receptor, it is hypothesized that genetic differences in the MHC may dictate the ability of a person's cells to mount an immune response to beryllium. It is unlikely that these genetic markers will be clinically useful since a large percentage of the general population has the same CBD-associated allelic substitution[52,87] as do patients with sarcoidosis.[103] The frequency of the Glu69 variant is approximately 85% in beryllium sensitization and CBD compared with approximately 45% of the general population and those with sarcoidosis. Regardless of an individual's genetics, CBD does not occur unless that person has been exposed to beryllium. Recent research in a population of workers in beryllium ceramics demonstrated that genetics and exposure-related risk factors, such as being a machinist with higher dust exposures, contribute independently to the occurrence of CBD.[52]

Two other major groups of potential susceptibility genes have been examined in CBD. The angiotensin converting enzyme (ACE) genotype was assessed both as a CBD susceptibility gene and as a potential marker of disease severity, based on the earlier observation that patients with more severe CBD had elevated serum ACE activity levels.[104] Maier and coworkers found that higher ACE levels were associated with the DD ACE genotype in CBD and suggested that this ACE gene might be more important in rapid progression of CBD, as those patients with the DD genotype developed disease sooner following their first exposure to beryllium.[105] Following the observation that blood and BAL cells from CBD patients express high levels of TNF-α on stimulation with beryllium salts in vitro, Maier and colleagues observed that a polymorphism in the TNF-α promoter region is associated with higher levels of TNF-α production by lung T cells in CBD, which in turn correlates with CBD severity.[106] Further studies will determine whether this and other TNF variants are important in predicting disease outcome. The overall conclusion is that CBD risk is polygenic and exposure dependent. The major HLA-DP marker is predictive of sensitization not CBD. Additional genetic variants are likely to be found that will predict progression from sensitization to disease.

CLINICAL FEATURES

Depending on the amount, form, and route of exposure to beryllium, various diseases may result. Beryllium can cause several forms of lung disease, dermatologic disease, or cancer. Beryllium-related pulmonary manifestations exist on a continuum from acute inhalational injury to acute pneumonitis, beryllium sensitization, and the chronic indolent form of CBD. In fact, a number of early acute beryllium disease survivors eventually developed the chronic form of CBD.[107–109]

Acute Disease

Exposure to elevated concentrations of beryllium produces inflammation of the upper and lower respiratory tract and airways, bronchiolitis, pulmonary edema, and chemical pneumonitis.[107–109] Acute beryllium disease is nonspecific, mimicking other inhalational injuries. The upper airway manifestations include beryllium nasopharyngitis and tracheobronchitis. The former may present with irritation of the nares and pharynx, epistaxis, and a metallic taste. It may imitate a viral upper respiratory infection.[107–109] If left untreated, the nasopharyngitis can lead to fissures, ulcerations, and nasal perforation. Tracheobronchitis may occur rapidly or gradually. It often occurs concomitantly with acute pneumonitis. Nonproductive cough, shortness of breath, substernal chest pain, burning, or tightness are typical, and the airways appear hyperemic. Rales or rhonchi are heard on auscultation. Radiographic evaluation may suggest bronchial wall thickening. Therapy is mainly supportive for acute upper airway disease and should include the person's removal from exposure. The role of such upper airway disease in contributing to beryllium sensitization is not known.

The symptoms of acute beryllium pneumonitis are similar to those of tracheobronchitis. Usually, after an acute high-level inhalation exposure, patients report severe cough, occasionally productive of blood-tinged sputum, chest pain or burning, and dyspnea on exertion that progresses to dyspnea at rest. Systemic symptoms are common and include malaise, anorexia, and low-grade fever. In acute beryllium pneumonitis, individuals usually appear quite ill with cyanosis, tachycardia, tachypnea, and rales. Hypoxemia is often present, and lung volumes show restriction. The chest radiograph may be normal or show diffuse bilateral alveolar infiltrates or even severe bilateral pulmonary edema. Radiographic abnormalities usually develop within a few weeks of the onset of symptoms.[107–109] There are no specific diagnostic criteria or laboratory evaluations available for the acute disease. The history of beryllium exposure with a compatible clinical picture are the principal means of establishing the diagnosis. Pathologically, a nongranulomatous pneumonitis is observed with nonspecific inflammatory infiltrates composed of neutrophils and lymphocytes, bronchiolitis, and intra-alveolar edema. The presence of lymphocytes in the course of this illness and the ability of acute disease to evolve into CBD suggest that acute beryllium pneumonitis is not simply a chemical injury but the beginning of an immunologic process in the context of inflammation.[5,108]

The primary therapeutic intervention for acute beryllium disease is removal from exposure. Corticosteroids, oxygen, bed rest, and even ventilatory support may be required, although no controlled trials of steroids have been reported. The signs and symptoms of the acute chemical pneumonitis may resolve within several weeks to several months. In its most severe form, this acute disease may be fatal. Approximately 17% of acute cases in the US Beryllium Case Registry progressed to CBD.[108] It is unclear whether return to work and further beryllium exposure is safe for individuals who have experienced acute pneumonitis.

Beryllium Sensitization

The use of the blood BeLPT has allowed physicians to define a population of exposed individuals who develop a cell-mediated, antigen-driven immune response to beryllium but in whom there are no pathologic or clinical features of either acute or chronic beryllium disease. These individuals are asymptomatic and have normal pulmonary function, exercise tolerance, chest radiographs, and lung biopsies.[110] Although their blood BeLPT is abnormal, they have not yet developed a clinically detectable inflammatory process in the lung although some display a mild degree of alveolar-capillary leak.[95–97] In published studies, the average rate of beryllium sensitization without disease has ranged from 1 to 5% but varies with time since first exposure.[21,22,24–26,28–30] These cross-sectional studies underestimate the true frequency of sensitization in the worker population. Recent longitudinal studies using serial surveillance with the blood BeLPT have demonstrated that additional beryllium sensization cases are detected by retesting the workforce.[29,30,32] A subset of these individuals eventually develop CBD at a rate of approximately 10% per year.[24,55,56] The risk factors for progression from sensitization to CBD are not known. Thus, sensitized individuals should remain under close medical supervision and be reexamined at intervals for signs of clinical progression. Sensitized individuals should be informed of the risk of future progression to CBD. In some individuals who have borderline or normal blood BeLPT, sensitization can be confirmed using beryllium sulfate patch testing.[75]

Chronic Beryllium Disease

The most common lung manifestation of beryllium exposure today is CBD. Because sensitization to beryllium precedes CBD, the current diagnostic criteria require demonstration of a beryllium-specific cell-mediated immune response, usually with the BeLPT measured in blood or BAL along with evidence of granulomatous or mononuclear cell interstitial inflammation on transbronchial lung biopsy. In order to reduce the need for invasive biopsies, a probable diagnosis of CBD can also be made by relying on evidence of the beryllium-specific immune response plus one or more other indicators of underlying granulomatous lung disease, such as BAL lymphocytosis, abnormal profusion of small opacities on the chest radiograph or chest computed tomography (CT) scan, abnormal lung physiology, or gas exchange abnormalities at rest or with exercise, as discussed in greater detail below. Today, many individuals are evaluated for CBD because they have been found to have one or more abnormal blood BeLPTs, detected as part of workplace medical surveillance programs. Such individuals may be carrying incorrect diagnoses (eg, sarcoidosis, asthma, pulmonary fibrosis) or may be asymptomatic and have normal lung physiology and normal chest imaging studies. Nonetheless, such individuals require clinical evaluation because of the high probability of them being in the early stages of CBD.

Signs and Symptoms

Unlike acute beryllium disease, CBD can develop many years after exposure has ceased and typically has an insidious onset and indolent course. Occasionally, disease occurs after a bout of acute beryllium disease or after a stressor, such as surgery or pregnancy.[59,107–109] Most of the clinical features of CBD are indistinguishable from thoracic involvement with sarcoidosis.[61,107] Misdiagnosis can occur unless more specific immunologic testing for CBD is used. Such testing became clinically available in the 1980s.[13,14,17,18,20,76] The latency from first beryllium exposure to development of clinically obvious disease ranges from a few months to 40 years, averaging 10 years in some series.[18,41,76,107]

Typically, patients report the gradual onset of dyspnea on exertion, cough that can be productive or nonproductive, chest pain, and fatigue. Other systemic symptoms such as anorexia, nonvolitional weight loss, fever, arthralgias, and night sweats also occur. Disease is often limited to the lung parenchyma, with a variable degree of endobronchial granulomatous or lymphocytic infiltration. Disseminated granulomas and/or mononuclear cell interstitial infiltrates can form in other organs, including lymph nodes, liver, spleen, myocardium, skeletal muscle, kidney, salivary glands, and bone. In some advanced cases, the hilar and mediastinal adenopathy can cause compression of the pulmonary arteries, produce chest pain, signs of pulmonary hypertension, and even mimic pulmonary embolism. Skin ulceration and subcutaneous granulomatous infiltration are observed, independent of the pulmonary manifestations, often in response to accidental inoculation with a beryllium splinter or wound contamination. In contrast to sarcoidosis, erythema nodosum and ocular involvement have not been reported in CBD. Chronic beryllium disease can be identified at an early, sometimes asymptomatic, stage through workplace surveillance.[20,76] The majority of these asymptomatic individuals who are detected through the use of the blood BeLPT as a workplace surveillance tool will have one or more abnormality of lung physiology, especially if gas exchange is measured by arterial blood gases at rest and at maximum exercise.

Physical signs of CBD are nonspecific and similar to those observed in other interstitial lung diseases. Bilateral dry rales are often heard. Hepatomegaly occurs in 10% of patients. Signs of cor pulmonale are common in the later stage of the disease. Clubbing occurs in approximately 10% of patients. Palpable lymphadenopathy is rare but may be found on axillary examination. Poorly healed or active ulcerated skin lesions may be seen.

Pulmonary Physiology

The pulmonary function abnormalities noted in CBD are typical of many interstitial lung diseases, especially hypersensitivity pneumonitis and sarcoidosis. Normal lung volumes, often with a mild obstructive pattern, are commonly found early in CBD.[110,111] Restriction occurs in advanced disease. Mixed obstruction and restriction may also be observed.[110,112] The diffusing capacity for carbon monoxide (DL_{CO}) is insensitive, becoming abnormal only in more advanced disease.[110] Exercise tolerance testing is the most sensitive indicator of physiologic impairment, revealing defects in pulmonary physiology even when the lung volumes, spirometry, and DL_{CO} are normal.[110] The most common abnormalities noted on exercise testing include reduced exercise tolerance, decreased oxygen consumption ($\dot{V}O_2$), abnormal

fall in oxygen levels, widened alveolar-arterial gradient, and ventilatory limitations to exercise. Some individuals with histologically-documented CBD may have normal exercise physiology.

DIAGNOSIS OF CHRONIC BERYLLIUM DISEASE

Imaging

Classically, the chest radiographic manifestations of CBD include bilateral, mid-, and upper lobe predominant reticulonodular infiltrates, with mild hilar and mediastinal lymphadenopathy.[15,113,114] Chest radiographic abnormalities range in severity from normal to widespread bilateral interstitial fibrosis and honeycombing in any lung field. Hazy opacification is also commonly observed. Over time, a reduction in lung volumes becomes apparent on serial radiographs, and small nodules coalesce to form larger subpleural nodular opacities (Figure 18–2). The large hilar nodes seen in sarcoidosis are seen infrequently in CBD, although adenopathy is present on chest radiography in approximately one-third of cases.[15,113–116] Pleural abnormalities may be noted in a minority of patients, most often adjacent to areas of greatest parenchymal involvement.[112] The pleural changes correlate histologically with granulomatous and fibrotic pleuritis.

The chest radiograph is an insensitive screening tool.[22] Disease is usually physiologically and symptomatically evident by the time the radiograph appears abnormal. Thin-section CT is more sensitive than the plain radiograph.[18,76] In one study of biopsy-proven CBD cases, abnormalities were noted in 10 of 13 CBD patients with normal chest radiographs and 89% of the 28 patients studied.[115] The most common CT abnormalities are nodules, thickened septal lines, ground-glass opacification, and hilar adenopathy (Figure 18–3). Bronchial wall thickening can be observed even in nonsmokers.[115,117,118] These findings are not specific for CBD but, when combined with specific tests like the blood BeLPT, can confirm the diagnosis, even in the absence of lung biopsy. Notably, even high-resolution chest CT can be completely normal in some cases of biopsy-proven CBD.[115,117]

Bronchoalveolar Lavage

Suspected CBD is a clinical indication for performing BAL, which will demonstrate an increased number of white cells with a lymphocyte predominance.[13,17–19] The lymphocytes are principally CD4+ T cells, similar to those found in sarcoidosis and in some cases of hypersensitivity pneumonitis.[119] Unlike these disorders, BAL cells in CBD proliferate in response to beryllium salts (see Figure 18–1). Tobacco smoke interferes with BAL cell function and increases the macrophage percentage,

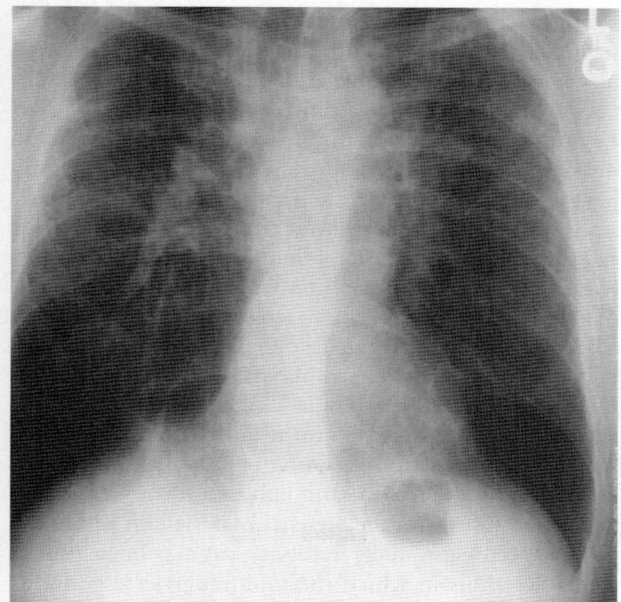

Figure 18–2 A posteroanterior chest radiograph of a patient with advanced chronic beryllium disease reveals changes typical of this lung disease. Upper lobe predominant nodules are evident bilaterally with some coalescence into a conglomerate mass. Hilar adenopathy, volume loss with hilar retraction, and subpleural thickening are also evident.

complicating the interpretation of the BAL cell count and differential in CBD. The extent of BAL cellularity, lymphocytosis, and BeLPT response correlates with disease severity,[23] suggesting that the magnitude of the pulmonary inflammatory and antigenic response may help predict disease progression or response to therapy. The major reason to perform BAL in suspected CBD is to obtain cells for BAL BeLPT testing. This assay is done in only a few laboratories, but samples can be prepared locally and shipped to an experienced laboratory for this test. Because bronchoscopy with BAL is associated with fewer risks than bronchoscopy with transbronchial lung biopsies, in some circumstances BAL may be used in lieu of biopsy to confirm the diagnosis. For example, some individuals with bleeding disorders can undergo BAL and be shown to have a lymphocytosis and an abnormal BAL BeLPT, which confirms CBD without a biopsy. In individuals who were erroneously given a diagnosis of sarcoidosis, granulomas may have already been demonstrated by mediastinal lymph node biopsy or by previous thoracoscopic or transbronchial lung biopsy. In such cases, a BAL might be used to confirm that lung T cells proliferate in response to beryllium salts as a means of confirming the correct diagnosis.

Laboratory Abnormalities

As well as the BeLPT and BAL findings, a number of less specific laboratory abnormalities are noted in some cases

of CBD. These include hyperuricemia,[120] nonspecific elevation of serum immunoglobulins,[121] hypercalcemia, hypercalciuria, and abnormal hepatic enzymes.[107,109] Despite the finding of increased uric acid in 40% of patients, gout has not been noted commonly. Polycythemia is uncommon unless patients have been diagnosed late and have not been appropriately treated with immunosuppressive agents and supplemental oxygen. Changes in the electrocardiogram occur late in the disease, usually with evidence of right atrial enlargement and

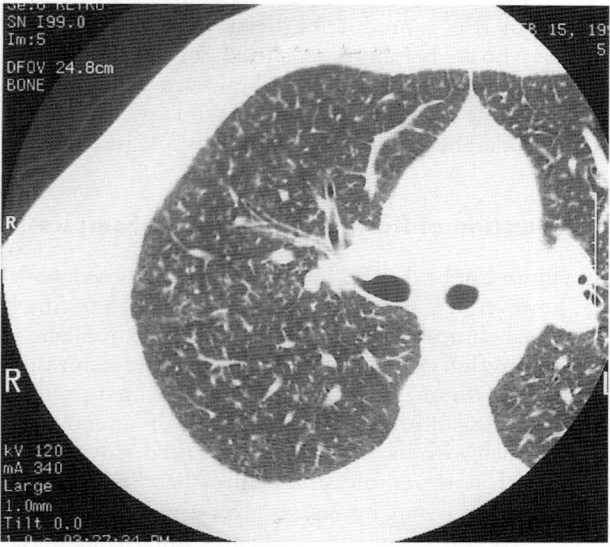

A

B

Figure 18–3 A, Thin-section computed tomography scan reveals diffuse nodules, thickened septal lines, and bronchial wall thickening. B, Ground-glass opacification is another common radiographic manifestation of chronic beryllium disease on thin-section computed tomography.

right ventricular hypertrophy. Occasionally, CBD affects the myocardium and cardiac conducting system, producing heart block and, rarely, sudden death. Elevated serum angiotensin converting enzyme (SACE) levels are frequently found in patients with CBD, analogous to other granulomatous disease such as sarcoidosis.[104,122] Elevated SACE levels correlate with some markers of disease severity, although this test has shown little practical utility in CBD diagnosis or prognostication.[104,122] The SACE level does not differentiate CBD from sarcoidosis. A study of serum neopterin in patients with beryllium sensitization and CBD suggests that this marker of IFN-γ production helps to distinguish individuals who are beryllium sensitized but are without disease from those with CBD.[123] However, as a practical matter, most clinicians rely on physiology, symptoms, and radiography to assess disease activity and progression.

Detection of Beryllium in Biologic Samples

Beryllium can be detected in the urine of exposed workers; however, it is not a marker of disease. Such testing is of no real clinical use, especially because of problems of standardization and quality of the assays used to measure urinary beryllium. Beryllium can be measured in lung, lymph node, and other tissues by one of several techniques, each with its own advantages and disadvantages. In general, however, measurement of beryllium in biologic samples is not necessary, given the availability of BeLPT. As with urine measurements, lung tissue beryllium levels reflect exposure and not disease. The more standard atomic absorption method used can be difficult to interpret because of the significant overlap in the measured amount of beryllium found in normal lungs and in beryllium-diseased lungs.[124] Laser or ion microprobe mass absorption analysis or energy dispersive x-ray microanalysis can identify beryllium within granulomas and "calcific" inclusions that are sometimes seen; however, these techniques require further standardization.[125,126] Nonetheless, in certain cases it may be beneficial to establish the presence of beryllium within the lung tissue as a means of confirming an association between beryllium particles and granulomatous inflammation.

Lung Biopsy

As discussed above, the noncaseating granuloma is the hallmark of CBD (see Figure 18–1) and of some beryllium-related skin lesions but is histologically indistinguishable from the granulomas found in sarcoidosis. Other pathologic abnormalities commonly found include a mononuclear cell interstitial infiltrate and varying degrees of fibrosis.[57,108,109,127] The absence of granulomas on either transbronchial biopsy or thoracoscopic lung biopsy does not fully exclude CBD. The granulomas accumulate primarily in the pulmonary interstitium and bronchial submucosa, often tracking along the bronchovascular bundle, occasionally in the regional lymph nodes, and rarely in the liver, heart, kidney, and in the abdominal and cervical lymph nodes.[128]

In our experience, transbronchial biopsies (8 to 12 samples), taken from the area of greatest radiographic involvement or from random sites throughout one lung, have a very high yield (greater than 90%). On some occasions, it may be necessary to repeat the bronchoscopy if samples are nondiagnostic. High BAL lymphocyte numbers in the face of normal biopsies should raise suspicion of a nondiagnostic procedure and the necessity to pursue a definitive diagnosis. We have found a good correlation between the presence of lymphocytosis in BAL and positive transbronchial biopsies in CBD. On rare occasions, it may be necessary to perform video-assisted thoracoscopic lung biopsy or open-lung biopsy. As always, samples should be examined and cultured for mycobacteria and fungi. Testing for the presence of beryllium within the biopsy specimen is rarely necessary but may be helpful in some situations in which the immunologic response to beryllium cannot be confirmed. Given the high specificity of the BeLPT and the beryllium sulfate patch test, a strong presumptive diagnosis can be made even in the absence of lung biopsy in individuals who show typical blood or skin immune responses to beryllium and who have typical clinical and radiographic findings. It is important to note that pathologists cannot distinguish between sarcoidosis and CBD by light microscopy.

Diagnostic Evaluation

Historically, diagnostic criteria for CBD required the presence of four of six of the following criteria, including one of the first two: (1) a history of beryllium exposure, (2) elevated beryllium levels in tissue or urine, (3) characteristic chest radiographic abnormalities, (4) restrictive and/or obstructive physiology or a DL_{CO} defect, (5) pathology consistent with CBD, and (6) a clinical course consistent with a chronic respiratory disorder.[112] However, as indicated above, the clinical features, radiographic manifestations, physiologic abnormalities, and pathologic changes present in CBD are neither specific nor diagnostic. The measure of beryllium in tissue or urine does not establish disease and is fraught with technical and interpretive problems. Thus, these old diagnostic criteria probably underdiagnose CBD. By definition they miss those individuals with early stage disease. In addition, distinguishing CBD from other forms of granulomatous lung disease such as sarcoidosis or hypersensitivity pneumonitis is difficult using these criteria because of the lack of tests to lend specificity to the diagnosis.

In the 1980s, the introduction of transbronchial biopsy, BAL, and the blood and BAL BeLPT improved our ability to make a highly specific, accurate diagnosis of CBD. The diagnosis of CBD is now established by demonstrating a beryllium-specific immune response using the blood or BAL BeLPT or beryllium salt patch test plus pathologic changes consistent with CBD (see Table 18–2).[18,75,78] Thus, although a history of beryllium exposure is helpful if present, its documentation is no longer essential to establish a diagnosis of CBD because the BeLPT has been shown to be highly specific.[18,129] By using an immunologic criterion, even patients who have had seemingly small beryllium exposures can be diagnosed, as illustrated by a report of CBD in the spouse of a beryllium production worker.[130] A recent investigation detected CBD in office workers who were occupying a building that formerly housed beryllium-alloy machining operations. Such cases would not have been detected without the availability of immunologic testing for beryllium sensitization. Individuals may now be diagnosed with CBD at its early stages, sometimes prior to the appearance of clinical signs, symptoms, or radiographic or physiologic abnormalities. Early detection may improve disease prognosis. We observe that patients who are diagnosed only after they have developed conventional symptoms, radiographic changes, and lung function decrements are harder to treat and have a more complicated and severe course than those detected early and treated at the first evidence of clinical deterioration. The immunologic tests help distinguish CBD from other interstitial lung disorders, correct misdiagnoses, and direct appropriate therapeutic interventions. Table 18–3 compares CBD with hypersensitivity pneumonitis and sarcoidosis. Like all immunologic assays and most diagnostic tests, false negatives and false positive results occur. For example, the results of the BAL and the BAL BeLPT may be affected by smoking tobacco. Neither test is 100% sensitive.[20,129] The blood BeLPT detects approximately 70 to 94% of CBD cases. The BAL BeLPT, considered by some as the "gold standard," can, itself, give false negative results in patients who smoke, are immunosuppressed, or who have pulmonary infection. In cases in which the blood and BAL BeLPT are equivocal or thought to be falsely negative, beryllium patch testing can be used safely to confirm the diagnosis.[75,131,132] We recommend patch testing in those cases with a high suspicion of disease and a nondiagnostic blood or BAL BeLPT.[75]

Some individuals with CBD may have an abnormal blood BeLPT, BAL BeLPT, and BAL lymphocytosis but have nondiagnostic lung biopsies. Although transbronchial biopsy has improved our diagnostic capabilities, the small samples that are obtained render this procedure prone to sampling error. In such instances, a presumptive diagnosis of CBD can be made without tissue confirmation. Sometimes a repeat biopsy may be warranted if significant diagnostic uncertainty remains. If there is clinical and immunologic evidence of disease, pathology may not be necessary for diagnosis. Similarly, when an individual has an abnormal chest radiograph or an abnormal thin-section CT and has repeated abnormal blood BeLPTs but is unable to undergo bronchoscopy, the diagnosis should be based on the clinical findings and on the abnormal blood BeLPT. In such circumstances, the blood BeLPT is used to confirm the beryllium-specific immune response while the radiographic abnormalities confirm that there are underlying pathologic changes consistent with CBD.

NATURAL HISTORY OF CHRONIC BERYLLIUM DISEASE

The clinical course of CBD is variable. Some individuals remain clinically stable for many years; however, the majority experience a gradual worsening of symptoms and physiology. Another subset of patients suffers a rapidly progressive debilitating course, leading to respiratory failure within a few years of diagnosis. Mortality rates range from 5 to 38% and may be related to the type of exposure.[55,56,133] In general, CBD worsens if not treated. Rarely, patients may have a spontaneous improvement in their chest radiographic infiltrates or gas exchange after reduction or cessation of exposure.[134,135] In our experience, patients exposed principally to beryllium ceramics (beryllium oxide) tend to have a more severe clinical course than do patients exposed to metal dust. However this may be more a function of the dose of exposure rather than the form of the beryllium, because we have also observed very severe and even fatal disease in CBD patients exposed only to low percentage beryllium-copper alloy dust. Reduction of exposure or removal from exposure and medical treatment are recommended although the long-term impact of these interventions is unknown. The detection of CBD at an early stage improves our ability to intervene early and change the natural history and prognosis of CBD. A large longitudinal study that is currently in progress will address this issue.[56] Late recognition of this disease is associated with a worse clinical prognosis and higher mortality, especially if pulmonary hypertension and cor pulmonale are found.

TREATMENT AND FOLLOW-UP

Prevention is superior to treatment of CBD. Unfortunately for current cases, there is no cure for CBD, and, regrettably, the numbers of workers exposed to beryllium continue to increase, raising the size of the population that must be considered at risk. The goals of treatment are to reduce morbidity and mortality by inhibiting inflammation and slowing down the disease progression. Reduction of exposure or, in some cases, removal from exposure is advisable, although the medical evidence to support this prudent approach is limited. Corticosteroids are the first-line therapy for CBD although they have never been tested in a randomized fashion or against a control population. More than 25 published clinical case series and case reports of CBD over the span of 40 years have shown the efficacy of corticosteroids in reducing symptoms and improving lung function,[112,136–147] with relapse on drug withdrawal. It is not known to what extent corticosteroid treatment changes the course of surveillance-identified, early-stage CBD. Such patients are only placed on treatment if there is evidence of emerging symptoms, abnormal gas exchange, or interval decline in gas exchange or lung function.

Before starting corticosteroid therapy, we recommend a baseline evaluation consisting of chest radiography; thin-section CT; complete pulmonary function tests including lung volumes, spirometry, and DL_{CO}; exercise testing, ideally with arterial blood gas measurements; and baseline laboratory testing as described above. Clinical indications for treatment include: (1) severe symptoms, such as debilitating cough or dyspnea; (2) abnormal gas exchange, diminished exercise tolerance, or abnormal pulmonary physiology; (3) documented decline in these measures of impairment; or (4) evidence of pulmonary hypertension, cor pulmonale, or cardiac or extrathoracic involvement. Initial therapy should be similar to that used in sarcoidosis: oral prednisone (or an equivalent) at a dose of approximately 0.5 to 0.6 mg/kg body weight either daily or on alternate days. After 3 to 6 months, the response to therapy should be reassessed objectively before tapering the steroid dose gradually to the minimum dose required to maintain objective and symptomatic improvement. Therapy is usually continued lifelong because disease relapses occur after steroid withdrawal.[107–109] If corticosteroid therapy is not initiated (for example, in early stage or mild cases of CBD), follow-up examination and objective testing should be performed on a yearly basis to monitor for disease progression. Because of the need for lifelong treatment, patients should be informed of the long-term side effects of corticosteroids and be monitored and treated for steroid-related side effects.

In those patients who fail to respond to corticosteroids or who experience severe side effects, other immunosuppressive agents may prove efficacious. Our preliminary experience suggests that methotrexate (5 to 15 mg orally per week) has a significant steroid-sparing effect in CBD. In some cases, methotrexate alone has been used efficaciously.

Allogeneic single lung transplantation has been used successfully in some cases of severe end stage CBD.

Supplemental oxygen should be prescribed as needed to improve hypoxemia and treat pulmonary hypertension, cor pulmonale, and hypoxemia-related polycythemia. Diuretics may be necessary to treat right heart failure. Symptomatic obstructive physiology and cough may respond to inhaled bronchodilators and high-dose inhaled steroids. Regular immunization should be administered to prevent influenza and pneumococcal infections. Antibiotics may be needed to treat bouts of infection. Patients should be encouraged to maintain or improve physical conditioning and be enrolled in pulmonary rehabilitation programs as warranted by the severity of their condition.

Patients who are beryllium sensitized but do not yet have CBD should be followed up for evidence of CBD approximately every 2 years because of the risk of progression to disease. Repeat transbronchial biopsy and BAL can be used to detect progression. Typically, we first repeat the baseline tests described above and then determine whether repeat bronchoscopy is warranted to confirm disease progression.

LUNG CANCER

Animal studies have shown that beryllium induces cancer in many species.[70,72,73,148–150] Early studies showed that intravenous injection of beryllium induced osteogenic tumors in rabbits.[151] Rats develop lung cancer after inhalational administration of beryllium.[73,75,152,153] The histologic tumor types produced have varied from adenocarcinoma in some studies to predominantly bronchoalveolar cell carcinoma in others.[73]

Large epidemiologic studies have shown an increased risk of lung cancer among beryllium-exposed workers and among workers with acute beryllium disease, with standardized mortality ratios (SMR) of 1.37 to 1.97 for production workers and 3.14 for those with acute beryllium disease.[154–158] In a study of the US Beryllium Case Registry, an increased risk of lung cancer was found in those individuals with acute and chronic beryllium disease (overall SMR 2.00).[159] Those with acute disease had a higher risk (SMR 2.32) compared with those with CBD (SMR 1.57), suggesting a dose-response relationship.[159] An increased risk of lung cancer was observed in a separate study of beryllium-exposed workers, after adjusting for smoking.[160] In that study, the risk to the beryllium-exposed population was less than for those with beryllium lung disease (SMR 1.26).[160] The International Agency for Research on Cancer (IARC) has reclassified beryllium as a class 1 human carcinogen.[149,150]

SURVEILLANCE

Advances in immunology plus the beryllium epidemiologic studies of the past 2 decades have revolutionized the approach to the screening and surveillance of beryllium disease. As it may not be possible to eliminate all exposure, major beryllium users now conduct medical screening to identify individuals at early stages of disease and those who are sensitized and at increased risk of developing CBD. Historically, screening for CBD included nonspecific and insensitive tests, such as physical examination, spirometry, and chest radiography.[76,110] The blood BeLPT has made disease screening in the beryllium industry a much more specific and sensitive endeavor.[22,24,76,78] The blood BeLPT has a high positive predictive value and is more sensitive than clinical evaluation, spirometry, or chest radiography.[21,22,24,78] The blood test identifies approximately 70 to 94% of cases.[20–22,24,78,161] The chest radiograph catches a small number of additional cases that may be missed by the blood BeLPT.[21,22,78]

Beryllium-exposed workers should undergo periodic testing, approximately every 1 to 3 years, preferably scheduled on the basis of whether they work in high- or low-exposure areas. High-risk areas are identified by analyzing the frequency of disease or sensitization, by job task, title, building, and so on. For example, machinists may warrant yearly or alternate year testing whereas office workers might be tested every 3 years. In addition to discovering new cases of disease and sensitization, such periodic screening can help identify high-risk processes in manufacturing areas, leading to better engineering controls.

PREVENTION

The current Occupational Safety and Health Administration (OSHA) standard may be sufficient to prevent most cases of acute beryllium disease; however, adherence to this exposure standard does not prevent CBD. Early studies suggested that some neighborhood cases developed disease at ambient air levels as low as 0.01 µg/m^3.[7,8] Case series in Japan have documented cases of CBD that occurred below the 2 µg/m^3 threshold limit value,[162–164] consistent with recent cases that have occurred in nonoccupationally exposed individuals[23,72,115] and among occupationally exposed secretaries and security guards.[21,22] In recent epidemiologic studies, CBD cases have occurred at levels below the OSHA standard.[16,24,38] Using historic industrial hygiene data, Kreiss and colleagues showed that many workers in a modern beryllium ceramics plant developed sensitization and disease at median air concentrations below 2 µg/m^3, raising significant concern about the efficacy of the current standard.[24] Adherence to the 2 µg/m^3 limit is not sufficiently protective. The threshold limit below which no cases of CBD occur is not known.[38] However, given that genetic susceptibility markers and exposure might contribute independently to disease risk, it is likely that the number of CBD cases can be decreased by reducing exposure to as low as reasonably achievable. Clinicians should consider all beryllium exposure histories to be significant and rule out CBD in any case of sarcoidosis or interstitial lung disease in which prior beryllium exposure could have occurred.

REFERENCES

1. Weber H, Engelhardt WE. Anwendung bei der Untersuchungen von Stauben aus der Berylliumgewinnung. Zentralbl Gewerbehyg Unfallverhuet 1993;10:41.
2. Gelman I. Poisoning by vapors of beryllium oxyfluoride. J Ind Hyg Toxicol 1936;18:371–99.
3. Berkovits M, Izrael B. Changes in the lungs by beryllium oxyfluoride poisoning. Klin Med 1940;18:117–22.
4. Van Ordstrand HS, Hughes F, DeNardi JM, Carmody MG. Beryllium poisoning. JAMA 1945;129:1084–90.
5. Hardy HL, Tabershaw IR. Delayed chemical pneumonitis in workers exposed to beryllium compounds. J Ind Hyg Toxicol 1946;28:197–211.
6. Hardy HL, Rabe EW, Lorch S. U.S. Beryllium Case Registry (1952–1966): review of its methods and utility. J Occup Med 1967;9:271–6.
7. Eisenbud M, Wanta RC, Dustan C, et al. Non-occupational berylliosis. J Ind Hyg Toxicol 1949;31:281–94.
8. Sterner JH, Eisenbud M. Epidemiology of beryllium intoxication. Arch Ind Hyg Occup Med 1951;4:123–51.
9. Lieben J, Metzner F. Epidemiological findings associated with beryllium extraction. Am Ind Hyg Assoc J 1959;20:494–99.
10. Sussman VH, Lieben J, Cleland JG. An air pollution study of a community surrounding a beryllium plant. Am Ind Hyg Assoc J 1959;20:504–8.
11. Newman LS, Kreiss K. Non-occupational chronic beryllium disease masquerading as sarcoidosis: identification by blood lymphocyte proliferative response to beryllium. Am Rev Respir Dis 1992;145:1212–4.
12. Rom WN, Lockey JE, Bang KM. Reversible beryllium sensitization in a prospective study of beryllium workers. Arch Environ Health 1983;38:302–7.
13. Epstein PE, Dauber JH, Rossman MD, Daniele RP. Bronchoalveolar lavage in a patient with chronic berylliosis: evidence for hypersensitivity pneumonitis. Ann Intern Med 1982;97:213–6.
14. Bargon J, Kronenberger H, Bergmann L, et al. Lymphocyte transformation test in a group of foundry workers exposed to beryllium and non-exposed controls. Eur J Respir Dis 1986;69 Suppl 136:211–5.
15. Aronchick JM, Rossman MD, Miller WT. Chronic beryllium disease: diagnosis, radiographic findings, and correlation with pulmonary function tests. Radiology 1987;163:677–82.
16. Cullen MR, Kominsky JR, Rossman MD, et al. Chronic beryllium disease in a precious metal refinery: clinical, epidemiologic, and immunologic evidence for continuing risk from exposure to low level beryllium fume. Am Rev Respir Dis 1987;135:201–8.
17. Rossman MD, Kern JA, Elias JA, et al. Proliferative response of bronchoalveolar lymphocytes to beryllium: a test for chronic beryllium disease. Ann Intern Med 1988;108:687–93.
18. Newman LS, Kreiss K, King TE Jr, et al. Pathologic and immunologic alterations in early stages of beryllium disease. Am Rev Respir Dis 1989;139:1479–86.
19. Saltini C, Winestock K, Kirby M, et al. Maintenance of alveolitis in patients with chronic beryllium disease by beryllium-specific helper T cells. N Engl J Med 1989;320:1103–9.
20. Mroz MM, Kreiss K, Lezotte DC, et al. Reexamination of the blood lymphocyte transformation test in the diagnosis of chronic beryllium disease. J Allergy Clin Immunol 1991;88(1):54–60.
21. Kreiss K, Mroz MM, Zhen B, et al. Epidemiology of beryllium sensitization and disease in nuclear workers. Am Rev Respir Dis 1993;148:985–91.
22. Kreiss K, Wasserman S, Mroz MM, Newman LS. Beryllium disease screening in the ceramics industry. Blood lymphocyte test performance and exposure-disease relations. J Occup Med 1993;35(3):267–74.
23. Newman LS, Bobka C, Schumacher B, et al. Compartmentalized immune response reflects clinical severity of beryllium disease. Am J Respir Crit Care Med 1994;150:135–42.
24. Kreiss K, Mroz MM, Newman LS, et al. Machining risk of beryllium disease and sensitization with median exposures below 2 µg/m^3. Am J Industr Med 1996;30:16–25.
25. Yoshida T, Shima S, Nagaoka K, et al. A study on the beryllium lymphocyte transformation test and the beryllium levels in working environment. Ind Health 1997;35:374–9.
26. Kreiss K, Mroz MM, Zhen B, et al. Risks of beryllium disease related to work processes at a metal, alloy, and oxide production plant. Occup Environ Med 1997;54(8):605–12.
27. Balkissoon RC, Newman LS. Beryllium copper alloy (2%)

causes chronic beryllium disease. J Occup Environ Med 1999;41:304–8.

28. Schuler C, Deubner D, Henneberger P, Kreiss K. Population-based risk of beryllium disease at a beryllium copper alloy plant. Am J Respir Crit Care Med 2001;163(5):A242.

29. Newman LS, Mroz MM, Maier LA, et al. Efficacy of serial medical surveillance for chronic beryllium disease in a beryllium machining plant. J Occup Environ Med 2001; 43(3):231–7.

30. Henneberger PK, Cumro D, Deubner DD, et al. Beryllium sensitization and disease among long-term and short-term workers in a beryllium ceramics plant. Int Arch Occup Environ Health 2001;74(3):167–76.

31. Tarlo SM, Rhee K, Powell E, et al. Marked tachypnea in siblings with chronic beryllium disease due to copper-beryllium alloy. Chest 2001;119(2):647–50.

32. Stange AW, Hilmas DE, Furman FJ, Gatliffe TR. Beryllium sensitization and chronic beryllium disease at a former nuclear weapons facility. Appl Occup Environ Hyg 2001; 16(3):405–17.

33. (OSHA), US Department of Labor. O. S. a. H. A. (29 CFR 1910.1000). Air Contaminants; final rule. Federal Register 1989:54:2332–960.

34. American Conference of Governmental Industrial Hygienists: draft. Documentation of threshold limit values. Beryllium and compounds. Cincinnati (OH): ACGIH; 1998.

35. Izumi T, Kobara Y, Inuis S, et al. The first seven cases of chronic beryllium disease in ceramic factory workers in Japan. Ann N Y Acad Sci 1976;278:636–53.

36. Shima S, Watanabe K, Tachikawa S. Experimental study an oral administration of beryllium compounds. Rodo Kagaku 1983;59:463–73.

37. Wambach PF, Tuggle RM. Development of an eight-hour occupational exposure limit for beryllium. Appl Occup Environ Hyg 2000;15(7):581–7.

38. Kelleher PC, Martyny JW, Mroz MM, et al. Beryllium particulate exposure and disease relations in a beryllium machining plant. J Occup Environ Med 2001;43(3):238–49.

39. Jameson CW. Introduction to the conference on beryllium-related diseases. Environ Health Perspect 1996;104:935–6.

40. Eisenbud M, Lisson J. Epidemiological aspects of beryllium-induced non-malignant lung disease: a 30-year update. J Occup Med 1983;25:196–202.

41. Kriebel D, Brain JD, Sprince NL, Kazemi H. The pulmonary toxicity of beryllium. Am Rev Respir Dis 1988;137(2):464–73.

42. Grier R, Nash P, Freiman D. Skin lesions in persons exposed to beryllium compounds. J Ind Hyg Toxicol 1948;30:228.

43. NIOSH, Centers for Disease Control. N. I. f. O. S. a. H. Occupational exposure to beryllium: criteria for a recommended standard. US Department of Health, Education, and Welfare; Cincinnati, OH. 1972.

44. Epstein W. Cutaneous effects of beryllium. In: Rossman M, Preuss O, Powers M, editors. Beryllium biomedical and environmental aspects. Baltimore: Williams and Wilkins; 1991.

45. Martyny JW, Hoover MD, Mroz MM, et al. Aerosols generated during beryllium machining. J Occup Environ Med 2000;42(1):8–18.

46. Kent MS, Robins TG, Madl AK. Is total mass or mass of alveolar-deposited airborne particles of beryllium a better predictor of the prevalence of disease? A preliminary study of a beryllium processing facility. Appl Occup Environ Hyg 2001;16(5):539–58.

47. McCawley MA, Kent MS, Berakis MT. Ultrafine beryllium number concentration as a possible metric for chronic beryllium disease risk. Appl Occup Environ Hyg 2001; 16(5):631–8.

48. Reeves AL, Preuss OP. Immunotoxicity of beryllium. In: Dean JH, Luster MI, Munson AE, Amos H, editors. Immuno-toxicology and immunopharmacology. New York: Raven Press, 1985. p. 441–56.

49. Mroz M, Martyny J, Hoover M, et al. Exposure-response relationships for beryllium sensitization and disease. Am J Respir Crit Care Med 1997;155:A812.

50. Reeves A. Toxicokinetics. In: Rossman MD, Preuss OP, Powers MB, editors. Beryllium. Baltimore: Williams and Wilkins; 1991. p. 77–85.

51. Reeves AL. Toxicodynamics. In: Rossman MD, Preuss OP, Powers MB, editors. Beryllium: biomedical and environmental aspects. Baltimore; Williams and Wilkins; 1991. p. 87–93.

52. Richeldi L, Kreiss K, Mroz MM, et al. Interaction of genetic and exposure factors in the prevalence of berylliosis. Am J Ind Med 1997;32:337–40.

53. Shima S. Hygienic control of beryllium (translation from Japanese). Rodo Kagaku 1971;26:36–46.

54. Newman LS. Immunology, genetics, and epidemiology of beryllium disease. Chest 1996;109:40S–3S.

55. Newman LS. Significance of the blood beryllium lymphocyte proliferation test (BeLPT). Environ Health Perspect 1996; 104:953–6.

56. Newman LS, Lloyd J, Daniloff E. The natural history of beryllium sensitization and chronic beryllium disease. Environ Health Perspect 1996;104:937–43.

57. Freiman DG, Hardy HL. Beryllium disease: the relation of pulmonary pathology to clinical course and prognosis based on a study of 130 cases from the U.S. Beryllium Case Registry. Hum Pathol 1970;1:25–44.

58. Inoue Y, King TE Jr, Tinkle SS, et al. Human mast cell basic fibroblast growth factor in pulmonary fibrotic disorders. Am J Pathol 1996;149:2037–54.

59. Finkel AJ, Hamilton A, Hardy HL. Beryllium. In: Finkel AJ, editor. Hamilton and Hardy's industrial toxicology. 4th ed. Boston: John Wright; 1983. p. 26–36.

60. Newman LS, Kreiss K. Non-occupational beryllium disease identified by screening with blood lymphocyte transformation test. Am Rev Respir Dis Suppl 1992;145:1212–4.

61. Sprince NL, Kazemi H, Hardy HL. Current (1975) problems of differentiating between beryllium disease and sarcoidosis. Ann N Y Acad Sci 1976;278:654–64.

62. Sawyer RT, Maier LA, Kittle LA, Newman LS. Chronic beryllium disease: a model interaction between innate and acquired immunity. Int Immunopharmacol 2002;2:249–61.

63. Fontenot AP, Newman LS, Kotzin BL. Chronic beryllium disease: T cell recognition of a metal presented by HLA-DP. Clin Immunol 2001;100(1):4–14.

64. Barna BP, Deodhar SD, Chiang T, et al. Experimental beryllium-induced lung disease: I. differences in immunologic response to beryllium compounds in strains 2 and 13 guinea pigs. Int Arch Allergy Appl Immunol 1984;73:42–8.

65. Barna BP, Deodhar SD, Gautam S, et al. Experimental beryllium-induced lung disease: II. analyses of bronchial lavage cells in strains 2 and 13 guinea pigs. Int Arch Allergy Appl Immunol 1984;73:49–55.

66. Votto JJ, Barton RW, Gionfriddo MA, et al. A model of pulmonary granulomatosis induced by beryllium sulfate in the rat. Sarcoidosis 1987;4:71–6.

67. Haley PJ, Finch GL, Mewhinney JA, et al. A canine model of beryllium-induced granulomatous lung disease. Lab Invest 1989;61:219–27.

68. Haley PJ, Finch GL, Hoover MD, et al. Immunologic specificity of lymphocyte cell lines from dogs exposed to BO. In: Thomassen DG, Shyr LJ, Bechtold WE, Bradley PL, editors. Inhalation toxicology research institute annual report 1989–1990, LMF-129. Springfield: National Technical Information Service; 1990. p. 236–9.

69. Haley PJ. Mechanisms of granulomatous lung disease from inhaled beryllium: the role of antigenicity in granuloma formation. Toxicol Pathol 1991;19:514–25.

70. Reeves AL. Experimental pathology. In: Rossman MD, Preuss OP, Powers MB, editors. Beryllium: biomedical and environmental aspects. Baltimore: Williams and Wilkins; 1991. p. 59–76.

71. Huang H, Meyer KC, Kubai L, Aurbach R. An immune model of beryllium-induced pulmonary granulomata in mice: histopathology, immune reactivity, and flow cytometric analysis of bronchoalveolar lavage-derived cells. Lab Invest 1992;67:138–46.

72. Newman LS. Beryllium lung disease: the role of cell-mediated immunity in pathogenesis. In: Dean JH, Luster MI, Munson AE, Kimber I, editors. Immunotoxicology and immunopharmacology. 2nd ed. New York: Raven Press, Ltd.; 1994. p. 377–93.

73. Finch GL, Hoover MD, Hahn FF, et al. Animal models of beryllium-induced lung disease. Environ Health Perspect 1996;104:973–9.

74. Curtis GH. Cutaneous hypersensitivity due to beryllium: a study of thirteen cases. AMA Arch Dermatol Syph 1951; 64:470–82.

75. Bobka CA, Stewart LA, Engelken GJ, et al. Comparison of in vivo and in vitro measures of beryllium sensitization. J Occup Environ Med 1997;39:540–7.

76. Kreiss K, Newman LS, Mroz MM, Campbell PA. Screening blood test identifies subclinical beryllium disease. J Occup Med 1989;31:603–8.

77. Hanifin JM, Epstein WL, Cline MJ. In vitro studies of granulomatous hypersensitivity to beryllium. J Invest Dermatol 1970;55:284–8.

78. Kreiss K, Miller F, Newman LS, et al. Chronic beryllium disease: from the workplace to cellular immunology, molecular immunogenetics, and back. Clin Immunol Immunopathol 1994;71:123–9.

79. Williams WR, Jones Williams W. Comparison of lymphocyte transformation and macrophage migration inhibition tests in the detection of beryllium hypersensitivity. J Clin Pathol 1982;35:684–7.

80. Williams WR, Jones Williams WJ. Development of beryllium lymphocyte transformation tests in chronic beryllium disease. Int Arch Allergy Appl Immunol 1982;67:175–80.

81. Rossman MD. Chronic beryllium disease. In: Daniele RP, editor. Immunology and immunologic diseases of the lung. Boston (MA): Blackwell Scientific Publications; 1988. p. 351–9.

82. Newman LS. Significance of the blood beryllium lymphocyte proliferation test. Environ Health Perspect 1996;104:953–6.

83. Saltini C, Kirby M, Trapnell BC, et al. Biased accumulation of T lymphocytes with "memory"-type CD45 leukocyte common antigen gene expression on the epithelial surface of the human lung. J Exp Med 1990;171:1123–40.

84. Comment CE, Kotzin BL, Schumacher BA, Newman LS. Preferential use of T cell antigen receptors in beryllium disease. Am J Respir Crit Care Med 1994;149:A264.

85. Rossman MD, Yan H-C, Murray RK, et al. Chronic beryllium disease: an immune response by restricted subfamiles of T cells. Am Rev Respir Dis 1992;145:A415.

86. Fontenot AP, Newman LS, Kotzin BL. T cell clonal expansions and marked conservation of T cell receptor sequences in the lungs of patients with chronic beryllium disease (CBD). Am J Respir Crit Care Med 1997;155:A983.

87. Richeldi L, Sorrentino R, Saltini C. HLA-DPb1 glutamate 69: a genetic marker of beryllium disease. Science 1993; 262:242–4.

88. Newman LS. To Be2+ or not to Be2+: immunogenetics to occupational exposure. Science 1993;262:197–8.

89. Fontenot AP, Torres M, Marshall WH, et al. Beryllium presentation to CD4+ T cells underlies disease-susceptibility HLA-DP alleles in chronic beryllium disease. Proc Natl Acad Sci U S A 2000;97(23):12717–22.

90. Lombardi G, Germain C, Uren J, et al. HLA-DP allele-specific T cell responses to beryllium account for DP-associated susceptibility to chronic beryllium disease. J Immunol 2001;166(5):3549–55.

91. Bost TW, Riches DWH, Schumacher B, et al. Alveolar macrophages from patients with beryllium disease and sarcoidosis express mRNA for TNF-α and IL-6 but not IL-1β. Am J Respir Cell Mol Biol 1994;10:506–13.

92. Tinkle SS, Kittle LA, Schumacher BA, Newman LS. Beryllium induces IL-2 and IFN-gamma in berylliosis. J Immunol 1997;158(1):518–26.

93. Tinkle SS, Schwitters PW, Newman LS. Cytokine production by bronchoalveolar lavage cells in chronic beryllium disease. Environ Health Perspect 1996;104:969–71.

94. Fontenot AP, Kotzin BL, Comment CL, Newman LS. Expansions of T cell subsets expressing particular T cell receptor variable regions in chronic beryllium disease. Am J Respir Cell Mol Biol 1998;18(4):581–9.

95. Inoue Y, Barker E, Daniloff E, et al. Pulmonary epithelial cell injury and alveolar-capillary permeability in berylliosis. Am J Respir Crit Care Med 1997;156:109–15.

96. Inoue Y, Barker EA, Daniloff E, et al. Mast cell basic fibroblast growth factor in bronchiolitis obliterans organizing pneumonia and constrictive bronchiolitis. Am J Respir Crit Care Med 1997;155:A327.

97. Inoue Y, Newman LS. Regulation of basic fibroblast growth factor gene expression in human mast cell line. Am J Respir Crit Care Med 1997;155:A758.

98. Kittle LA, Sawyer RT, Fadok VA, et al. Beryllium induces apoptosis in human lung macrophages. Sarcoid Vasc Diffuse Lung Dis 2002;19(2):101–13.

99. McConnochie K, Williams WR, Kilpatrick GS, Jones Williams W. Chronic beryllium disease in identical twins. Br J Dis Chest 1988;82:431–5.

100. Wang Z, White P, Petrovic M, et al. Differential susceptibilities to chronic beryllium disease contributed by different Glu69 HLA-DPB1 and -DPA1 alleles. J Immunol 1999; 163:1647–53.

101. Wang Z, Farris GM, Newman LS, et al. Beryllium sensitivity is linked to HLA-DP genotype. Toxicology 2001;165(1): 27–38.

102. Maier LA, Lympany PA, McGrath DS, et al. Influence of MHC class II in susceptibility to beryllium sensitization and chronic beryllium disease. Am J Respir Crit Care Med 2001;163(5):A242.

103. Lympany PA, Southcott AM, Welsh K, du Bois RM. Lack of association between HLA-DPB phenotype and sarcoidosis. Am J Respir Crit Care Med 1994;149:A266.

104. Newman LS, Orton R, Kreiss K. Serum angiotensin converting enzyme activity in chronic beryllium disease. Am Rev Respir Dis 1992;146:39–42.

105. Maier LA, Barker EA, Raynolds MV, Newman LS. Angiotensin-1 converting enzyme polymorphisms in chronic beryllium disease. Am J Respir Crit Care Med 1999;159:1342–50.

106. Maier LA, Sawyer RT, Bauer RA, et al. High beryllium-stimulated TNF-alpha is associated with the -308 TNF-alpha promoter polymorphism and with clinical severity in chronic beryllium disease. Am J Respir Crit Care Med 2001;164(7):1192–9.

107. Finkel AJ, Hamilton A, Hardy HL. Hamilton and Hardy's industrial toxicology. In: Finkel AJ, editor. Hamilton and Hardy's industrial toxicology. 4th ed. Boston: John Wright; 1983. p. 1–428.

108. Hardy HL. Beryllium poisoning: lessons in control of man-made disease. N Engl J Med 1965;273:1188–99.

109. Tepper LB, Hardy HL, Chamberlin RI. Toxicity of beryllium compounds. In: Browning E, editor. Elsevier monographs on toxic agents. Amsterdam: Elsevier Publishing Company; 1961. p. 1–190.

110. Pappas GP, Newman LS. Early pulmonary physiologic abnor-

malities in beryllium disease. Am Rev Respir Dis 1993; 148:661–6.

111. Andrews JL, Kazemi H, Hardy H. Patterns of lung dysfunction in chronic beryllium disease. Am Rev Respir Dis 1969;100:791–800.

112. Stoeckle JD, Hardy HL, Weber AL. Chronic beryllium disease: Long-term follow-up of sixty cases and selective review of the literature. Am J Med 1969;46:545–61.

113. Robert AG. A consideration of the roentgen diagnosis of chronic pulmonary granulomatosis of beryllium workers. AJR Am J Rotentgenol 1950;63:467–87.

114. Weber AL, Stoeckle JD, Hardy HL. Roentgenologic patterns in long-standing beryllium disease: report of eight cases. AJR Am J Rotentgenol 1965;93:879–90.

115. Newman LS, Buschman DL, Newell JD Jr, Lynch DA. Beryllium disease: assessment with CT. Radiology 1994;190:835–40.

116. Wilson SA. Delayed chemical pneumonitis or diffuse granulomatosis of the lung due to beryllium. Radiology 1948;50: 770–9.

117. Daniloff EM, Lynch DA, Bucher Bartelson B, et al. Observer variation and relationship of computed tomography to severity of beryllium disease. Am J Respir Crit Care Med 1997;155:2047–56.

118. Harris KM, McConnochie K, Adams H. The computed tomographic appearances in chronic berylliosis. Clin Radiol 1993;47:26–31.

119. Newman LS. Beryllium disease and sarcoidosis: clinical and laboratory links. Sarcoidosis 1995;12:7–19.

120. Kelley WN, Goldfinger SE, Hardy HL. Hyperuricemia in chronic beryllium disease. Ann Intern Med 1969;70:977–83.

121. Deodhar SD, Barna B, Van Ordstrand HS. A study of the immunologic aspects of chronic berylliosis. Chest 1973; 63:309–13.

122. Sprince NL, Kazemi H, Fanburg BL. Serum angiotensin 1-converting enzyme in chronic beryllium disease. In: Jones Williams W, Davies BH, editors. Sarcoidosis and other granulomatous diseases. Cardiff, Wales: Alpha Omega Publishing, Ltd.; 1980. p. 287–300.

123. Harris J, Bucher Bartelson B, Barker E, et al. Serum neopterin in chronic beryllium disease. Am J Ind Med 1997;32:21–6.

124. Schepers GWH. The mineral content of the lung in chronic berylliosis. J Dis Chest 1962;42:600–7.

125. Jones-Williams W, Kelland D. New aid for diagnosing chronic beryllium disease (CBD): laser ion mass analysis (LIMA). J Clin Pathol 1986;39:900–1.

126. Jones-Williams W, Wallach ER. Laser microprobe mass spectrometry (LAMMS) analysis of beryllium, sarcoidosis, and other granulomatous diseases. Sarcoidosis 1989;6:111–7.

127. Dutra FR. The pneumonitis and granulomatosis peculiar to beryllium workers. Am J Pathol 1948;24:1137–65.

128. Jones-Williams W. United Kingdom Beryllium Registry: mortality and autopsy study. Environ Health Perspect 1996; 104:949–51.

129. Stokes RF, Rossman MD. Blood cell proliferation response to beryllium: analysis by receiver-operating characterisitics. J Occup Med 1991;33:23–8.

130. Newman LS, editor. Case reports in environmental medicine: beryllium toxicity. U.S. Public Health Service, Agency for Toxic Substances and Disease Registry; Atlanta, GA. 1992.

131. Haberman AL, Pratt M, Storrs FJ. Contact dermatitis from beryllium in dental alloys. Contact Dermatitis 1993;28:157–62.

132. Vilaplana J, Romaguera C, Grimalt F. Occupational and non-occupational allergic contact dermatitis from beryllium. Contact Dermatitis 1992;26:295–8.

133. Peyton MF, Worcester J. Exposure data and epidemiology of the beryllium case registry—1958. AMA Arch Ind Health 1959;19:94–9.

134. Nishikawa S, Hirata T, Kitaichi M, Izumi T. Three years prospective study of mantoux reactions in factory workers exposed to beryllium oxide. In: Jones Williams W, Davies BH, editors. Sarcoidosis and other granulomatous diseases. Cardiff, Wales: Alpha Omega Publishing, Ltd., 1980. p. 722–7.

135. Sprince NL, Kanarek DJ, Weber AL, et al. Reversible respiratory disease in beryllium workers. Am Rev Respir Dis 1978;117:1011–7.

136. DaHoli JA, Lieben J, Bisbing J. Chronic beryllium disease: a follow-up study. J Occup Med 1964;6:189–94.

137. DeNardi JM. Chronic pulmonary interstitial granulomatosis: preliminary report on two patients treated with ACTH. Arch Ind Hyg Occup Med 1951;3:543–6.

138. Gaensler EA, Verstraeten JM, Weil WB, et al. Respiratory pathophysiology in chronic beryllium disease: review of 30 cases with some observations after long term steroid therapy. AMA Arch Ind Health 1957;19:132–45.

139. Hall TC, Wood CH, Stoeckle JD, Tepper LB. Case data from the beryllium registry. AMA Arch Ind Health 1959;19:18–21.

140. Hardy HL. Epidemiology, clinical character, and treatment of beryllium poisoning. Arch Ind Health 1955;11:273.

141. Hardy HL, Wright G, Dubson RL, Aub, JC. General discussion on the treatment of chronic beryllium poisoning with ACTH and cortisone. Arch Ind Hyg Occup Med 1951; 3:629–30.

142. Kennedy BJ, Pare JAP, Pump KK, et al. Effect of adrenocorticotropic hormone (ACTH) on beryllium granulomatosis and silicosis. Am J Med 1951;10:134–55.

143. Kennedy BJ, Pare JAP, Pump KK, Standford RL. The effect of adrenocorticotropic hormone (ACTH) on beryllium granulomatosis. Can Med Assoc J 1950;62:426–8.

144. Kline EM, Moir TW. Long-term experience with beryllium disease. Arch Ind Health 1959;19:104–9.

145. Seeler AO. Treatment of chronic beryllium poisoning. AMA Arch Ind Health 1959;19:164–8.

146. Thorn GW, Forsham PH, Frawley TF, et al. The clinical usefulness of ACTH and cortisone. N Engl J Med 1950; 242:865–72.

147. Wright GW. Interpretation of results of ACTH and cortisone therapy in chronic beryllium poisoning. Arch Ind Hyg Occup Med 1951;3:617–21.

148. IARC, I. A. f. R. o. C. Monographs on the evaluation of the carcinogenic risk of chemicals to humans; beryllium, cadmium, mercury, and exposures in the glass manufacturing industry. Lyon, France: IARC Monographs, 1993.

149. 1980. International Agency for Research on Cancer (IARC). Monographs on the evaluation of the carcinogenic risk of chemicals to humans. Vol. 23. Some metals and metallic compounds. Lyon: IARC: 139–42; 205–323.

150. Meeting of the IARC working group on beryllium, cadmium, mercury, and exposures in the glass manufacturing industry. Scand J Work Environ Health 1993;19(5):360–3.

151. Gardner LU, Heslington HF. Osteosarcoma from intravenous beryllium compounds in rabbits. Fed Proc 1946;5:221.

152. Vorwald AJ, Reeves AL. Pathologic changes induced by beryllium compounds. Arch Industr Health 1959;19:190–9.

153. Vorwald AJ, Reeves AL, Urban EJ. Experimental beryllium toxicology. In: Stokinger HE, editor. Beryllium: its industrial hygiene aspects. New York: Academic Press; 1966. p. 201–34.

154. Infante PF, Wagoner JK, Sprince NL. Mortality patterns for lung cancer and non-neoplastic respiratory disease among white males in the Beryllium Case Registry. Environ Res 1980;21:35–43.

155. Mancuso TF. Occupational lung cancer among beryllium workers. In: Lemen R, Dement J, editors. Dust and diseases. Forest Park (IL): Pathotox Pub; 463–72.

156. Mancuso TF. Mortality study of beryllium industry workers' occupational lung cancer. Environ Res 1980;21:48–55.

157. Mancuso TF, El-Attar AA. Epidemiologic study of the beryllium industry. Cohort methodology and mortality studies. J Occup Med 1969;11:424–34.

158. Wagoner JK, Infante PF, Bayliss DL. Beryllium: an etiologic agent in the induction of lung cancer, non-neoplastic respiratory disease, and heart disease among industrially exposed workers. Environ Res 1980;21:15–34.

159. Steenland K, Ward E. Lung cancer incidence among patients with beryllium disease: a cohort mortality study. J Natl Cancer Inst 1991;83(19):1380–5.

160. Ward E, Okun A, Ruder A, et al. A mortality study of workers at seven beryllium processing plants. Am J Ind Med 1992;22:885–904.

161. Rossman MD. Differential diagnosis of chronic beryllium disease. In: Rossman MD, Preuss OP, Powers MB, editors. Beryllium: biomedical and environmental aspects. Baltimore: Williams & Wilkins; 1991. p. 167–75.

162. Izumi T, Nishikawa S. Chronic beryllium lung in Japan. Nikkyorin 1976;35:805–13.

163. Shima S. Proposal for the management and prevention of chronic beryllium lesions. Rodo Eisei 1974;8:12–24.

164. Shima S. Recommendations for the preventive maagement of chronic beryllium disorders. Rodo Eisei 1974;8:18–24.

19

HYPERSENSITIVITY PNEUMONITIS

MOISÉS SELMAN

Hypersensitivity pneumonitis (HP), also known as extrinsic allergic alveolitis, is a syndrome that results from repeated inhalation of finely dispersed antigens. These antigens encompass a wide variety of organic particles, such as mammalian and avian proteins, fungi, thermophilic bacteria, and certain small-molecular-weight volatile and nonvolatile chemical compounds. The disease is characterized by a diffuse and predominantly mononuclear cell inflammation of the small airways and pulmonary parenchyma.[1]

Hypersensitivity pneumonitis may occur in several clinical forms and may lead to irreversible pulmonary damage that depends on several factors including the amount and duration of exposure to the antigen, the nature of the inhaled dust, and the host response.

Although there is a wide spectrum of possible offending antigens, these disorders may potentially arise in any work or home environment where bacteria and fungi grow or where animals and pets are kept. Overall, however, the incidence of HP in the general population is low, suggesting that host susceptibility factors and other environmental conditions are necessary if the disease is to develop.

It is difficult to determine how many persons exposed to causative agents develop HP, given that the disease is often unrecognized or misdiagnosed. However, most experts agree that only 5 to 15% of persons exposed to high levels of etiologic agents associated with HP will develop the disease. The prevalence of HP among people exposed to relatively lower concentrations of antigens is unknown.

The sequence of immunopathologic events that contribute to HP remains poorly understood, and several mechanisms may operate simultaneously. Evidence supports a prominent role for T-cell hyperreactivity, although the deposit of immune complexes may participate in the acute form of the disease as well as in the early phases of the more chronic forms. Considering that only a small percentage of the total number of people exposed to potential disease-causing antigens develop the disease, a combination of factors must be considered as requisites.

HISTORICAL BACKGROUND

Given that man has a long history of cultivating grains and of living in the proximity of domesticated and wild animals, it is safe to assume that HP has probably existed since ancient times. One of the earliest recorded descriptions of the disease was made in 1713 by Ramazzini da Capri in *De Morbis Artificum Diatriba*, one of the most prominent treatises on early occupational medicine. In his seminal work, da Capri demonstrates the first link between inhaled small organic particles and human disease:

> I began to suspect that in that dust (grain) there must lurk minute worms imperceptible to our senses and that they are set in motion by the sifting and measuring of the grain and broadcast by the air ... Almost all who make a living by sifting or measuring grain are short of breath and cachectic and rarely reach old age.[2]

More than 200 years later, Campbell[3] presented the first detailed report of HP and the clinical features and occurrence of the disease among farmers exposed to the dusts of moldy hay. A few years later, Pickles[4] coined the term "farmer's lung" for this specific form of HP. Bagassosis was described soon thereafter in 1941 by Jamison and Hopkins,[5] and, in 1960, bird breeder's disease was first described by Pearsall and colleagues and Plessner.[6,7] In 1970, Banaszak and colleagues[8] described the occurrence of HP among office workers exposed to a thermophilic actinomycete contaminating a central air-conditioning system. This last report showed that HP should be suspected in cases of interstitial pneumonitis, even in the absence of clear-cut contact with organic dusts.

During the last 30 years, an extensive number of etiologic agents and sources of antigens capable of inducing HP have been described (Table 19–1). Unfortunately, however, its nomenclature was confusing as the names were assigned according to the sources of exposure. Thus, the literature is replete with a number of

TABLE 19–1   Etiologic Agents of Hypersensitivity Pneumonitis

Disease	Antigen	Source
Fungal and bacterial		
Farmer's lung	*Faeni rectivirgula*	Moldy hay, grain, silage
Ventilation pneumonitis; humidifier lung; air conditioner lung	*Thermoactinomyces vulgaris, Thermoactinomyces sacchari, Thermoactinomyces candidus Klebsiella oxytoca*	Contaminated forced-air systems; water reservoirs
Bagassosis	*T. vulgaris*	Moldy sugarcane (ie, bagasse)
Mushroom worker's lung	*T. sacchari*	Moldy mushroom compost
Suberosis	*Thermoactinomyces viridis Penicillium glabrum*	Moldy cork
Detergent lung; washing powder lung	*Bacillus subtilis* enzymes	Detergents (during processing or use)
Malt worker's lung	*Aspergillus fumigatus, Aspergillus clavatus*	Moldy barley
Sequoiosis	*Graphium, Pullularia,* and *Trichoderma* spp. *Aureobasidium pullulans*	Moldy wood dust
Maple bark stripper's lung	*Cryptostroma corticale*	Moldy maple bark
Cheese washer's lung	*Penicillium casei, A. clavatus*	Moldy cheese
Woodworker's lung	*Alternaria* spp., wood dust	Oak, cedar, and mahogany dust, pine and spruce pulp
Paprika slicer's lung	*Mucor stolonifer*	Moldy paprika pods
Sauna taker's lung	*Aureobasidium* spp., other sources	Contaminated sauna water
Familial HP	*B. subtilis*	Contaminated wood dust in walls
Wood trimmer's lung	*Rhizopus* spp., *Mucor* spp.	Contaminated wood trimmings
Composter's lung	*T. vulgaris, Aspergillus*	Compost
Basement shower HP	*Epicoccum nigrum*	Mold on unventilated shower
Hot tub lung	*Cladosporium* spp.	Hot tub mists; mold on ceiling
Wine maker's lung	*Botrytis cincrea*	Mold on grapes
Woodsman's disease	*Penicillium* spp.	Oak and maple trees
Thatched roof lung	*Sacchoromonospora viridis*	Dead grasses and leaves
Tobacco grower's lung	*Aspergillus* spp.	Tobacco plants
Potato riddler's lung	Thermophilic actinomycetes, *F. rectivirgula, T. vulgaris, Aspergillus* spp.	Moldy hay around potatoes
Summer-type pneumonitis	*Trichosporon cutaneum*	Contaminated old houses
Dry rot lung	*Merulius lacrymans*	Rotten wood
Stipatosis	*Aspergillus fumigatus; T. actinomycetes*	Esparto dust
Machine operator's lung	*Pseudomona fluorescens, mycobacterium* spp.??	Aerosolized metalworking fluid
Amebae		
Humidifier lung	*Naegleria gruberi, Acanthamoeba polyphaga, Acanthamoeba castellani*	Contaminated water
Animal proteins		
Pigeon breeder's or pigeon fancier's disease	Avian droppings, feathers, serum	Parakeets, budgerigars, pigeons, chickens, turkeys
Pituitary snuff taker's lung	Pituitary snuff	Bovine and porcine pituitary proteins
Fish meal worker's lung	Fish meal	Fish meal dust
Bat lung	Bat serum protein	Bat droppings
Furrier's lung	Animal fur dust	Animal pelts
Animal handler's lung; laboratory worker's lung	Rats, gerbils	Urine, serum, pelts, proteins
Insect proteins		
Miller's lung	*Sitophilus granarius* (ie, wheat weevil)	Dust-contaminated grain
Lycoperdonosis	Puffball spores	Lycoperdon puffballs

(continued)

TABLE 19–1 Etiologic Agents of Hypersensitivity Pneumonitis (*continued*)

Disease	Antigen	Source
Chemical		
Pauli's reagent alveolitis	Sodium diazobenzene sulfate	Laboratory reagent
Chemical worker's lung	Isocyanates; trimellitic anhydride	Polyurethane foams, spray paints, elastomers, special glues
Vineyard sprayer's lung	Copper sulfate	Bordeaux mixture
Pyrethrum HP	Pyrethrum	Pesticide
Epoxy resin lung	Phthalic anhydride	Heated epoxy resin
Unknown		
Bible printer's lung		Moldy typesetting water
Coptic lung (mummy handler's lung)		Cloth wrappings of mummies
Grain measurer's lung		Cereal grain
Coffee worker's lung		Coffee bean dust
Tap water lung		Contaminated tap water
Tea grower's lung		Tea plants
Mollusk shell HP		Sea snail shell
Swimming pool worker's lung		Aerosolized endotoxin from pool water sprays and fountains

HP = hypersensitivity pneumonitis.

HP-like disorders, with their own eponym. Often, the condition occurred in only a small number of individuals, occupationally or domestically exposed, and without clear confirmation. The two most adequately studied and best known forms of HP are farmers' lung and pigeon breeder's disease (PBD).

PATHOGENESIS

The pathogenesis of HP is intricate, and many of the immunopathologic processes—as well as the sequence of events involved in the development of alveolitis—are poorly understood.

Early investigations suggested that immune complexes provoked lung inflammation.[9] Evidence to support this theory included the presence of increased bronchoalveolar lavage (BAL) and systemic specific antibodies and immune complexes, positive Arthus-type skin reaction, and the acute form of the disease. Over time, however, a series of findings downplayed the role of this mechanism in causing tissue damage. For example, the presence of immune complexes in lungs of patients with HP is an unusual finding, and specific antibodies are present in some exposed asymptomatic subjects. Furthermore, HP has occurred in the presence of hypogammaglobulinemia.[10]

In the last 20 years, a strong body of evidence supporting a pivotal role of T-cell-mediated, delayed-type hypersensitivity in the pathogenesis of HP has surfaced.[11] Data to support this theory include histopathologic features; a significantly high number of T cells in BAL fluid; lymphokine production by antigen-stimulated lung T cells; and the reproduction of the disease in nonsensitized rabbits with the transfer of specifically sensitized T lymphocytes rather than with the passive transfer of immunoglobulins.[1,12–15] Murine models further support the etiologic role of an immune T cell response. In one study, HP was transferred by CD4+ cells whereas B cells and antibodies failed to provoke the disease in response to the sensitizing antigen.[16]

On the other hand, findings from acute HP clearly suggest a role for humoral mechanisms. Activated complement components and BAL neutrophilia are found in patients with the acute form of the disease and in those studied using antigen inhalation challenge.[17,18]

Thus, it is likely that both humoral and cellular mechanisms participate in the development of the lung lesion, but in different phases and clinical forms of the disease. In the early stages of alveolitis (hours after antigen challenge), or in the acute intermittent form, an immune-complex-mediated tissue injury seems to occur. In more advanced stages of the disease (acute progressive) and in the chronic form, a T-cell-mediated immune inflammatory response takes place.

In general, these studies—though limited—have helped us to understand the mechanisms associated with lung injury. Nevertheless, a number of important questions still remain to be resolved:[1]

1. Why do only a small number of exposed subjects develop the disease?
2. Why is the time of exposure, regardless of antigen levels, so variable and often so prolonged prior to the onset of clinical disease?
3. Why are the response rates associated with treatment and cessation of antigen exposure so variable?

In other words, why do some patients heal, whereas others evolve to fibrosis?

To answer these questions, a hypothetical sequence of events has been proposed.[1,19] A simplified scheme is summarized in Figure 19–1.

For inflammation to occur, the presence of an *inducing factor* (the inhaled antigen) and a *promoting factor(s)* are necessary. It is believed that alveolitis is triggered when both the inducing factor and promoting factor(s) converge. In the presence of *regression factors*, lung inflammation can be subsequently controlled and resolved. In contrast, inflammation autoperpetuates and evolves to fibrosis in the presence of *progression factors*. According to this hypothesis, the offending antigen is essential but not sufficient to initiate the disease process in the absence of a promoting factor.

Since the disease appears to be associated with a genetic predisposition linked to the major histocompatibility complex (MHC),[20–24] an uncontrolled immune response correlated to this system can be considered as a *host promoting factor*. Recently, the polymorphisms of MHC class II alleles and of tumor necrosis factor alpha (TNF-α) promoter were evaluated by polymerase chain reaction (PCR)-specific sequence oligonucleotide analysis and by amplification refractory mutation system PCR in patients with PBD.[24] Results showed the presence of several alleles and haplotypes that increase the susceptibility to develop the disease. Interestingly, patients exhibiting the TNF-2(-308) allele were younger and displayed more lymphocytes in their BAL fluids. These results strongly support that genetic factors located within the MHC region contribute to the development

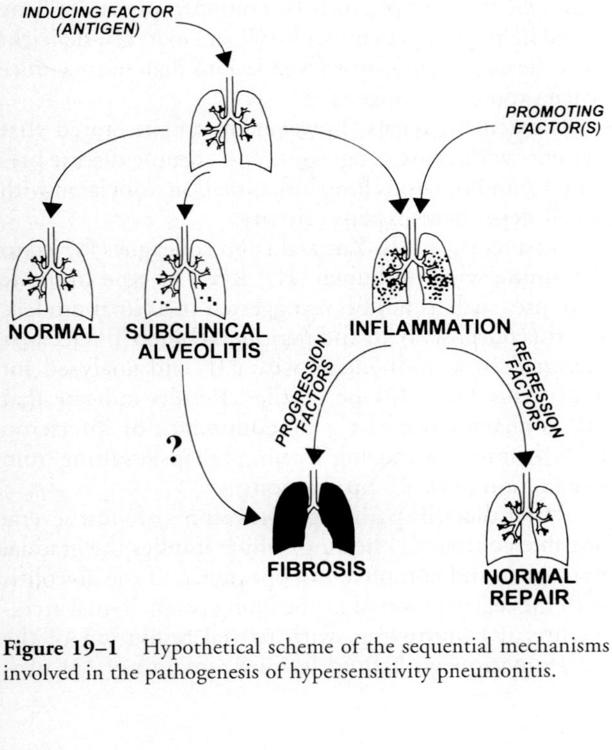

of HP. In another similar work, but performed in farmer's lung as well as in PBD, Schaaf and colleagues[25] genotyped the -308 TNF-α promoter polymorphism and the TNF-β intron 1 gene polymorphism. TNF bioactivity and the frequency for the TNFA2 allele, a genotype associated with increased TNF-α expression, was higher in farmer's lung patients than in controls or patients with PBD.

A disordered immunoregulation, represented primarily by an abrogation of T suppressor cell function, appears to be a leading component in the pathogenesis of HP.[26] A variety of studies conducted in humans and laboratory animals suggest that one of the most essential differences between exposed subjects who develop the disease and those who remain asymptomatic is the presence of a deficient or nonfunctional T-cell immunosuppression.[27,28]

It has been observed in a rabbit model, after a short-lived and modest lung inflammation, that alveolitis is rapidly abolished despite continued exposure to the antigen.[29] Throughout 30 weeks of study, the animals were unable to respond to either the specific initial antigen or a new, unrelated antigen. After this time, the rabbits became responsive to a second antigen but remained unresponsive to the initial antigen. These data suggest that animals maintain an antigen-specific suppression of pulmonary inflammation and present a possible model for understanding why many individuals remain asymptomatic despite exposure to an offending antigen. These data support evidence that asymptomatic dairy farmers may have persistent bronchoalveolar lymphocytosis without ever developing the disease, in spite of continued antigen exposure over several years.[30]

If this is truly the case, then there is at least one major paradox to solve, considering that patients with HP usually exhibit increased CD8+ immunosuppressive T cells in BAL fluid and lung tissues. Why do these patients have decreased suppressive activity? At first glance, increased CD8+ cells may be interpreted as an attempt to control the inflammation, although unsuccessfully. Nevertheless, there is now increasing evidence suggesting that CD8+ T lymphocytes may differentiate in at least two different phenotypes that exhibit a different cytokine pattern of secretion and cytolytic activity.[31] In the expanding universe of T-cell subsets, we do not yet know which subsets are present—and in what proportion—in the lung parenchyma of HP patients.

Interleukin(IL)-6, a cytokine commonly associated with an immune response, may be associated with lung protection. In patients with PBD, levels of IL-6 were significantly lower than asymptomatic controls.[32] Moreover, the use of a monoclonal antibody against IL-6 strongly potentiated the alveolitis and fibrotic response in an experimental model of HP.[33] Like many other cytokines, IL-6 is remarkable in its pleiotropy and redundancy and may exert so many different effects that it is difficult to pinpoint a definitive protective role.

Figure 19–1 Hypothetical scheme of the sequential mechanisms involved in the pathogenesis of hypersensitivity pneumonitis.

In general, it is believed that an inappropriate immunologic response, mainly related to antigen-specific suppressor cells, may constitute an important host-promoting factor in genetically susceptible individuals.

Some environmental factors could also be regarded as promoting factors. For example, Allen and colleagues[34] observed that seven members of two families developed PBD when they began to use a gamma isomer of hexachlorobenzene to eradicate parasites from birds. Similarly, unpublished individual observations suggest that some patients who remain asymptomatic despite long-time exposure to avian antigens manifest the disease only after they inhale a second agent such as an insecticide or a weed killer.

Superimposed viral infection may be another possible environmental promoting factor. Cormier and colleagues[35,36] reported two studies supporting the role of viruses in HP. The investigators, using a murine model of *Saccharopolyspora rectivirgula*–induced allergic alveolitis, compared a group of mice exposed to both parainfluenza 1 Sendai virus and the offending antigen to a group of mice exposed only to the offending antigen. In mice exposed to both the virus and the offending antigen, a markedly long-term enhancement of the lung inflammatory response measured by histopathologic changes, BAL cell subpopulations profile (increase of macrophages, lymphocytes, and neutrophils), and by cytokine production (increase of TNF-α and IL-1α) was reported. Viral infection increases both the early (neutrophilic) as well as the late (Th1-type granulomatous) inflammatory responses in experimental HP.[37]

In a recent study of human disease using PCR, an increase of influenza A virus was found in BAL macrophages. This documented, for the first time, the presence of viruses in the lower airways of patients with acute HP. This finding may imply a potential role for influenza A in the modulation of human HP during antigen exposure.[38] Several mechanisms may be implicated in the ability of a viral infection to enhance allergic alveolitis. One of them appears to be related to its capacity of upregulating the expression of B7 costimulatory molecules (CD80, CD86), which play a role in the antigen-presenting capacity by alveolar macrophages.[39]

Occasionally, the onset of the disease has been associated with the postpartum period.[40] This observation is similar to those described for some collagen vascular diseases and suggests that hormonal changes, which have a profound effect on the immune response, may be another promoting component.

In summary, it appears that a second independent host or environmental factor is necessary to provoke the onset of the disease in some patients. The convergence of the inducing factor plus the promoting factor(s) triggers a complex series of immunopathologic and nonspecific events, such as alternate complement pathway activation and an abnormal release of cytokines, enzymes, and oxygen free radicals, that result in lung damage.

In acute episodes, humoral mechanisms such as immune-complex formation and activated neutrophils releasing toxic oxygen metabolites and proteinases appear to play an important pathogenic role.[18,41] For example, hours after exposure to hay, the number of polymorphonuclear leukocytes liberated from the marginal pool is similar in both symptomatic farmers with farmer's lung and asymptomatic individuals. However, only neutrophils from patients with farmer's lung are primed for an enhanced respiratory burst.[41] These molecules may provoke serious lung damage by overwhelming the antiproteinase and antioxidant defense mechanisms.

In acute progressive and chronic disease, events involving cellular rather than humoral mechanisms (characterized by an exaggerated T-cell-mediated response) appear to play a pivotal role. Cellular adhesion between lymphocytes and antigen-presenting cells precedes antigen recognition and is an important step for the induction of the immune response by signal transmission and the induction of functional activity of the target cells. The intercellular adhesion molecule (ICAM)-1 has been shown to be up-regulated in macrophages from patients with HP, with an increased expression after antigen exposure, suggesting that up-regulation of ICAM-1 is the consequence of a specific immune response to an inhaled antigen.[42]

Alveolitis in acute progressive and chronic HP is provoked primarily by the expansion of different types of cytotoxic cells represented mainly by non-MHC-restricted cytotoxic lymphocytes and also by natural killer and lymphokine activated killer cells.[43] Overwhelming amounts of proinflammatory cytokines, oxidants, and proteases (produced mainly by activated macrophages) participate in the lung damage.

However, in the complicated concert of recruited cells and secreted cytokines, the pathogenic role of other cells is unclear. For example, increased numbers of mast cells are found in lungs of patients with HP, and mast cell-deficient mice develop significantly fewer lesions than normal mice when exposed to antigens.[44,45]

In general terms, however, it can be stated that patients with acute progressive and chronic disease present a granulomatous lung inflammation associated with T-cell-dependent hypersensitivity.

In a recent study, Yamasaki and colleagues[46] tried to determine whether human HP is a Th$_1$-type immune response, such as has been suggested in animal models. For this purpose, BAL and peripheral blood T cells were obtained from individuals with HP and analyzed for Th$_1$ versus Th$_2$ cytokine profiles. Results indicate that HP is characterized by a predominance of interferon (IFN)-gamma-producing T cells, perhaps resulting from a reduction in IL-10 production.

After that, the pathologic process may follow several possible courses: (1) healing, which implies the gradual resolution and complete disappearance of the alveolitis with the regeneration of normal lung parenchymal architecture; (2) improving, with partial resolution of the inflammation with lung lesions remaining; (3) progressing slowly toward pulmonary fibrosis; or (4) advancing rapidly toward pulmonary fibrosis.

Thus, it appears that the lung may respond in two ways following alveolitis (ie, improving or healing versus evolving to fibrosis). As a result, we propose the existance of *regression factors* and *progression factors* that might influence the healing or fibrotic sequelae.

Host regression factors should include T-cell-dependent immunoregulatory processes that lead to desensitization and regression of the alveolitis. Anti-inflammatory mechanisms, represented by the release of specific antioxidant enzymes and antiproteases, should also play a role. In addition, some situations related to medical assistance, such as avoidance of further antigen exposure and treatment with corticosteroids, may be considered as regression factors, because pulmonary manifestations may resolve with these interventions.

In contrast, additional or continued antigen inhalation and/or lack of effective therapy may be involved in the progression to fibrosis and could be considered as progression factors. It is important to note, however, that a subgroup of patients develop pulmonary fibrosis although they avoid further exposure and receive well-controlled therapy.

Host progression factors should include abnormalities in the behavior of lung cells, with the rising of aggressive subpopulations of mesenchymal cells followed by an abnormal collagen metabolism. It has been shown that alveolar macrophages and epithelial cells obtained from lungs of some patients with PBD produce platelet-derived growth factor, a potent mitogen for fibroblasts.[47] Similarly, in about 25% of patients with chronic HP, lung lymphocytes are able to stimulate an increased synthesis of collagens by fibroblasts.[48] In murine models of HP, a progressive increase of total lung transforming growth factor-β as well as lung fibroblast collagen synthesis, have also been found.[49] Transforming growth factor-β has powerful effects on extracellular matrix remodeling enhancing collagen synthesis, tissue inhibitor of metalloproteinase (TIMP)-1 production, and decreasing collagenase expression.

More recently, it was found that patients with chronic HP evolving to fibrosis exhibit an increased number of neutrophils in the lung tissue, many of them loaded with gelatinase B and collagenase-2.[50] This finding suggests that an exaggerated traffic of neutrophils with the secretion of some matrix metalloproteinases might participate in the fibrotic response.

Studies on lung collagen metabolism in patients with HP have shown that progression to fibrosis is accompanied by an increase in collagen synthesis and, more importantly, by a significant decrease in collagenolytic activity, which seems to be associated with an excessive production of collagenase inhibitors.[51,52]

Thus, an abnormal secretion of fibroblast growth factors, an increase in collagen synthesis, and a decrease in collagen degradation may be regarded as progression factors, rendering a potentially reversible disease into a progressive and irreversible disorder.

In summary, we propose that this sequence of events may at least partially explain the pathogenesis of the disease. The convergence of the inducing factor with one or more promoting factors provokes the propagation of an uncontrolled T-cell-dependent lung inflammation, and, thereafter, the balance between the action of progression factors or regression factors permits the development of fibrosis or healing.

The pathogenesis of the inflammatory and fibrotic response in HP is undoubtedly far more complex; the ultimate cellular and molecular mechanisms responsible for triggering these abnormalities are essentially unknown.

ANTIGENS

To produce allergic alveolitis in a susceptible host, it is essential to inhale particulate matter that is sufficiently small in aerodynamic diameter to reach the lung acinus. Particles smaller than 5 μm can penetrate the distal respiratory tract and are deposited by gravitational sedimentation. Extremely small particles (usually smaller than 0.5 μm) may be deposited by brownian diffusion as they are displaced by randomly moving gas molecules and ultimately collide with airway walls.

The antigens capable of provoking HP may be fungal, bacterial, protozoal, animal and insect proteins, and small molecular chemical compounds (see Table 19–1). In general, the most frequent forms of HP are provoked by thermophylic actinomycetes, fungi, and bird droppings.

Thermophilic Actinomycetes

Thermophilic actinomycetes (or spores of saprophytic fungi) are present in the atmosphere throughout the year. However, the disease is most often produced when individuals are exposed to a large number of particles associated with exuberant growth on decaying organic matter enhanced by appropriate conditions of temperature and humidity. These spores can heavily contaminate a wide variety of vegetables, wood, sawdust, and bark as well as water-reservoir humidifiers and air-conditioning systems.[53–72]

Thermophilic actinomycetes are bacteria with the morphology of fungi of less than 1 μm in size and are most commonly found in soil, grain, compost, fresh water, forced-air heating and cooling systems, humidifiers, and air-conditioning systems. The most common species implicated in HP include *Saccharopolyspora* or *Faeni rectivirgula* (formerly known as *Micropolyspora faeni*), *Thermoactinomyces vulgaris*, *Thermoactinomyces viridis*, *Thermoactinomyces saccharis*, and *Thermoactinomyces candidus*. They thrive best at 50 to 60°C, temperatures that are commonly reached during composting or in heating systems.

These organisms secrete multiple enzymes that cause the decay of vegetable matter. Moldy hay, a frequent trigger of HP, contains large amounts of thermophilic actinomycetes; if packed while damp or stored in humid environments, the mold on the hay thrives. Thus, when damp hay is stored in bins on a farm, the humidity and heat encourage these microorganisms to grow. When workers directly thresh and handle damp, moldy hay, disease-causing antigens are released from the packed vegetation into thresh clouds, and the workers can then inhale the particles.

Certain conditions contribute to the dispersion of high levels of thermophilic actinomycetes in the air. Thus, for example, the number of spores is higher in hay samples from large cylindrical bales compared with small prismatic bales and also when the stalls have poor ventilation. Likewise, some feeding practices, such as the manual handling of hay and the constant presence of hay in feeding corridors, enhance the spreading of spores.[73]

In these poorly ventilated areas, inadequately protected workers may inhale spores; farmers who work under such conditions may inhale and retain approximately 750,000 actinomycetes spores (0.5 to 1.3 μm in size) per minute.[74] The persistence of similar levels of incidence of farmer's lung throughout the years is clearly associated with inappropriate farmer practices, as recently reported in Ireland.[75]

Some nonthermophilic bacteria may produce the disease. For example, Bacillus subtilis has been identified as a causative antigen in some cases of HP.[76] Recently, the disease has been detected in workers in automobile parts manufacturing exposed to aerosolized metalworking fluid.[77] In the first report, patients demonstrated antibodies against several cultured microorganisms, but the most frequent positive precipitin response was found to be against Pseudomonas fluorescens.[77] Interestingly, the disease seems to be increasing in workers exposed to metal removal fluids, and several outbreaks have been recently described.[78,79] However, in these studies, antibody testing has failed to identify a specific single organism.[78,79] A recent study suggests the hypothesis that aerosolized mycobacteria colonizing the metal removal fluids likely cause the disease.[80] In general, these studies support the observation that HP in metalworking environments with water-based aerosols may be more common than usually recognized.

Bird Antigens

The most common form of avian-related HP develops among pigeon fanciers, but similar symptoms can occur after exposure to budgerigars, parakeets, chickens, ducks, turkeys, and other small caged birds such as finches and canaries.[81–86] Occasionally, native birds such as owls have been implicated in the development of HP.[87] Avian antigens represent a complex mixture of high- and low-molecular-weight proteins; patients usually become sensitized to a wide range of these antigens.[88] Thus, patients often have reactive serum precipitins to bird serum, feathers, egg white, and droppings. Precipitins often cross-react with antigens of different bird species.[89]

Avian albumin and gamma globulins were first suggested as antigens in avian materials. More recently, however, attention has focused predominantly on secretory immunoglobulin A (IgA) and its subfractions as the major antigenic components in pigeon secretory materials.[90,91] In this context, it has been suggested that bloom, a dust commonly found coating bird feathers that is composed of fine 1 mm particles of keratin covered with IgA, is a potent antigen.[92,93] Flying birds, particularly pigeons in peak racing condition, produce bloom in large amounts. This may explain why birds such as pigeons and parakeets seem to be more potent sensitizers than chickens and turkeys. In addition, pigeon intestinal mucin, a complex high-molecular-weight glycoprotein, has been described as a novel and key antigen in the development of pigeon breeder's lung.[94] Mucin and IgA are both found in secretions from birds' gastrointestinal and respiratory epithelia. Thus, if the mucin antigen is in feces, it may also be present on the feathers as a result of contamination. Actually, pigeon intestinal mucin is present in a variety of materials found in the environment of the pigeon loft, including droppings and bloom, in a form capable of reacting with antimucin antibodies in the sera of exposed individuals.[95]

Recent findings suggest that different IgG subclasses (ie, IgG1, -2, or -3) recognize different epitopes on mucin, and that epitopes recognized by major subclasses are present on O-linked oligosaccharides. Moreover, carbohydrate-specific antimucin antibodies produced by patients with HP may differ in their specificity from those found in individuals who have been exposed to antigens but remain asymptomatic.[96]

Interestingly enough, there is a recent report suggesting that exposure to wild pigeons may also provoke the disease.[97] In this study, the authors described a family in which the mother died of an unresolved lung disorder and whose five children were subsequently affected by HP that was putatively caused by wild city pigeons. This report brings to our attention the fact that nondomestic birds may cause the disease. A similar case was reported by Muramatsu and colleagues.[98]

In addition, HP could also be provoked by unusual sources of exposure such as wreathes of feathers or feather-down duvets and pillows.[99–101] Likewise, indirect exposure (eg, from clothing) to avian antigens through household contact between pigeon-exposed individuals and family members may also produce the disease.[102] Physicians should be aware of these possible sources of antigenic material.

Fungi and Other Antigens

Summer HP is the most prevalent distinctive type of HP in Japan. The disease is caused by Trichosporon cutaneum, and the causative antigens are present in a high-molecular-weight, polysaccharide-rich fraction of *T. cutaneum*.[103,104] More recently, it was demonstrated that *Cryptococcus albidus* may also be an important etiologic agent of the disease.[105] *C. albidus* strains were isolated in a high percent of patient's home environments, and furthermore, the amount of local IgA and IgM antibodies bound to *Cryptococcus neoformans* was significantly higher than that bound to *T. cutaneum* in a number of patients with summer-type HP.[105]

In general, fungi are important etiologic agents of HP in a variety of occupational conditions (see Table 19–1). Actually, in some HP strongly associated with thermophilic actinomycetes, such as farmer's lung, fungi are also implicated in a number of cases. Thus, for example, in a prospective case-control study performed in the east of France, corymbifera somatic antigen and to a lesser degree *Eurotium amstelodami* and *Wallemia sebi* were likely to be the main causes of farmer's lung.[106] Modifications in working conditions over time could explain the emergence of new contributing etiologies. Likewise, among Finnish farmers, the disease is associated with the fungus *Aspergillus umbrosus*.[107]

Fungi are also involved in nonoccupational outbreaks. Thus, for example, an outburst of allergic respiratory diseases, including HP, occurred in a new building that was characterized from initial residence by the presence of extensive visible mold (especially *Aspergillus versicolor*) on interior surfaces. After building restoration, the concentration of nonphylloplane fungi was reduced to the lowest feasible level, and no new or recrudescent cases occurred after building re-entry.[108]

Previously unrecognized work environments and new fungi are constantly being reported; for example, the disease has been described in workers of a peat moss packaging plant, where *Monocillium* spp. and *Penicillium citreonigrum* were identified.[109]

The disease is also associated with exposure to contaminated forced-air systems, such as home humidifiers and air conditioners as well as cool-mist vaporizers. Pools of stagnant water in these systems often provide ideal environments for the colonization of fungi, bacteria, and amebae. Moreover, the aerosol systems effectively disperse the offending antigens in droplets of the appropriate size.[8,110,111]

Protein antigens from bovine or porcine serum and pituitary powder may be inhaled by patients with diabetes insipidus and may result in HP. Other sources of antigens include certain drugs and highly reactive chemical compounds, such as toluene diisocyanate and trimellitic anhydride, widely used in the production of flexible and rigid foams, synthetic rubbers, adhesives, and paints.[112–121] Recently, it was found that 1,5-naphthalene-diisocyanate, an aromatic diisocyanate with a very low vapor pressure that is mainly used in the automotive industry, may also provoke HP.[122]

Other organic particles small enough to cause acinar disease may be derived from animal urine, dander, hair, or excreta.[123,124] In a few instances, HP has also been recorded following inhalation of organic and even inorganic vapors or fumes; for example, the disease has been diagnosed in individuals exposed to zirconium silicate.[125,126] The reaction presumably occurs as a result of hapten formation with lung proteins.

Although occupational exposure to recognized etiologic agents causes most cases of HP, the disease is also reported in individuals through avocational or environmental exposure.

Finally, exposure to antigens in such unexpected places as home saunas and enclosed hot tubs may also provoke the disease.[127,128] Interestingly, as mentioned for metalworking fluid-associated HP, nontuberculous mycobacteria may also be implicated in the hot tub disease. In a recent study, Khoor and colleagues described 10 immunocompetent healthy individuals with a history of hot tub exposure who developed HP.[129] All patients showed nonnecrotizing granulomatous inflammation in their lung biopsy, and, in all but 1 case, *Mycobacterium avium-intracellulare* complex was revealed by culture. Four patients were treated with antimycobacterial therapy, 4 patients received only oral corticosteroids, and 2 patients received both therapies. Independent of the type of treatment received, all patients experienced substantial improvement.

PREVALENCE

The prevalence of HP varies from country to country; even within a country the rate may vary due to the local climate, season, geographic conditions, local customs, and the presence of industrial manufacturing plants. The prevalence of HP is difficult to estimate accurately because allergic alveolitis represents a group of syndromes with different causative agents and epidemiologic studies lack uniform diagnostic criteria.

Grant and colleagues[130] estimated the prevalence of farmer's lung at approximately 9% in the humid zones of Scotland and 2.3% in the drier zones of East Lothian. Staines and Forman[131] estimated the prevalence of farmer's lung to be between 11.5 and 193 per 100,000 individuals in different zones of England. Other studies in different countries and in different regions within a country show prevalence rates between 4 and 170 per 1,000 farmers.[132,133] The incidence of farmer's lung is 2 to 4 per 10,000 farmers per year in Sweden and Finland.[134,135]

Farmer's lung shows both seasonal and geographic variations in incidence. The disease is most common in late winter when stored hay is used to feed cattle, and it is particularly common in years with excessive rainfall in late spring or summer when the hay is mowed and baled. Similarly, the disease occurs most frequently in regions with both heavy rainfall and harsh winter conditions.

The prevalence of clinical disease in pigeon fanciers may be between 10 and 20% in those regularly exposed to lofts with high antigen levels, but figures as low as 1.4 per 1,000 and 1 per 5,000 have been reported.[136,137]

In one study, the sensitization rate among pigeon fanciers was 32%.[138] The prevalence of pigeon breeder's lung among people with only a few birds at home is largely unknown; it appears that individuals exposed to chickens or turkeys rarely develop the disease.[139,140]

The geographic, seasonal, and climatic factors that contribute to the prevalence and periodicity of farmer's lung are absent in bird breeder's lung because birds are often kept in the home and are not subjected to drastic changes in these factors. On the other hand, subjects who have owned only one or two pet birds may develop the disease.

Summer-type HP is the most frequent allergic alveolitis in Japan.[141,142] A nationwide epidemiologic study that included 653 definite, 182 probable, and 99 possible cases of this disease demonstrated that approximately 75% had summer-type HP. Caused by seasonal mold contamination in home environments, summer-type HP is characterized by symptoms that appear during the hot and humid summer season that follows the rainy season.[143,144] The second most prevalent form of HP in Japan was farmer's lung, which was also the most prevalent form of occupational HP with 13.8% of reported cases.

An evaluation of workers in an office environment served by a contaminated forced-air system revealed an attack rate of 15%.[8] Some studies of HP outbreaks in office buildings and industrial settings describe attack rates as high as 70% of exposed individuals.[145]

The disease is infrequent in childhood, and, overall, pigeon breeder's lung is the most common form. Clinical behavior is similar to adult disease.[19]

SMOKING AND HYPERSENSITIVITY PNEUMONITIS

It has been known for a long time that farmer's lung and pigeon breeder's disease occur more frequently in nonsmokers than in smokers under the same risk of exposure.[132,146] Pigeon fanciers and farmers who smoke have lower levels of specific IgG antibodies than in nonsmokers.[147,148] Similar findings have also been reported in patients with HP provoked by the inhalation of aerosols of contaminated air conditioners. Baur and colleagues[149] showed that nonsmokers exposed to humidifier antigens have a significantly higher IgG response and more lung disease than smokers. Arima and colleagues[150] have reported that summer-type HP as well as the prevalence of anti–*T. cutaneum* antibodies are significantly lower in individuals who smoke. In another study that included 227 pigeon fanciers, smokers displayed a lower incidence of precipitating antibodies to pigeon antigens and lower titers of serum IgG and IgA antibodies to mucin and pigeon serum proteins compared with nonsmokers and ex-smokers.[151] In contrast, salivary IgA antibody titers to pigeon antigens were similar in smokers and non- or ex-smokers. Moreover, salivary IgA titers against pigeon mucin were significantly higher in asymptomatic individuals, suggesting a protective role for these antibodies.

Additional evidence regarding the clinical significance of smokers versus nonsmokers for the development of HP arises from an extensive study concerning the prevalence of farmer's lung conducted in 30 districts of the French Doubs province. The study was controlled for age, sex, smoking, and geographic (altitude) factors.[152] Dairy farms (n = 5,703) participated in the study by answering a medical questionnaire. The prevalence rates of chronic bronchitis and clinical farmer's lung were 9.3% and 1.4%, respectively. The risk of developing farmer's lung was significantly associated with nonsmokers ($p < .05$). Interestingly, a significant linear association between HP with altitude was also found.

In general, these findings strongly suggest that cigarette smoking has a suppressive effect that interferes with the immunopathologic processes that ultimately lead to HP. The reasons for this finding remain unclear. Cigarette smoking has several effects on the immunologic functions of the lung, which could account for this consistent observation. Smoking may, for example, interfere with energy-dependent processes involved in phagocytosis by alveolar macrophages as well as with the expression of surface Ia antigens by these cells.[153,154] In addition, smoking also decreases the capacity of human alveolar macrophages to produce IL-1 and TNF-α.[155,156] Cigarette smoking adversely affects cellular immunity by reducing the proliferative response of lung T cells to mitogens and altering the balance between helper/inducer and suppressor/cytotoxic T cells in BAL fluid.[157] Overall, cigarette smoking suppresses lymphocyte and macrophage activities and thus may prevent the exaggerated reaction necessary to develop HP.

On the other hand, smoking may affect the clinical behavior of the disease and may change the clinical course of HP to a more insidious and chronic form. Although farmer's lung occurs less frequently among farmers who smoke than in farmers who do not smoke, the prognosis is significantly worse in smokers than in nonsmokers. In farmers who smoke and develop HP, the 10-year survival rate is significantly lower than in farmers with HP who do not smoke.[158] In an experimental model, cigarette smoking decreased the initial inflammatory response but retarded the eventual recovery during continuous antigen exposure.[159]

Likewise, because alveolar macrophages in the lower respiratory tract of cigarette smokers can modify α_1-antitrypsin in the local milieu by oxidant mechanisms,[160] the sum of antigen exposure and tobacco smoke inhalation could provoke emphysematous changes as have been described in some chronic cases.[161]

CLINICAL FEATURES

The clinical features of the disease are usually similar, regardless of the type or nature of the inhaled dust. The interval between sensitization by antigen inhalation and the clinical onset of HP is unknown, but it appears to be extremely variable and may take many months or years after exposure.

Three clinically different presentations of HP have been described: acute, subacute, and chronic.[1,162–164] The differing manifestations are determined by the intensity and the frequency of antigen exposure, among other factors.

Acute Form

Episodes of the acute form result from intermittent and intense exposure of a known antigen in the domestic, occupational, or atmospheric environment. Symptoms of the acute disease occur 4 to 8 hours after exposure to the offending antigen and consist of the abrupt onset of a flu-like syndrome characterized by fever, chills, and malaise. Frontal headache, arthralgia, and myalgias are also common. Pulmonary symptoms include severe dyspnea, chest tightness, and a dry or mildly productive cough; hemoptysis is rare. These signs and symptoms gradually clear over the next 24 to 48 hours but often recur after the next inhalation of the causative antigen.

Subacute and Chronic Forms

The subacute and chronic forms result from continual low-level exposure to inhaled antigens, usually in the domestic environment. A classic example is the disease provoked by the exposure to domestic caged birds. In this case, prolonged inhalation of avian antigens from bird droppings and feathers results in pigeon breeder's lung. The onset of the disease may be insidious, with few—if any—symptoms during the early stages of the pathologic process. Thus, patients may delay getting medical care until several weeks or months after the onset of illness. The main symptoms are progressive dyspnea on exertion, fatigue, cough with mucoid sputum, anorexia, malaise, and weight loss. Occasionally, in the subacute form, patients may have fever at the onset of the illness.

Unrecognized and untreated subacute HP may progress to chronic HP. A number of patients with chronic disease develop irreversible lung changes due to interstitial fibrosis that progresses to right-sided heart failure. The insidious onset of symptoms and lack of acute episodes are often mistaken for other chronic interstitial lung diseases (ILDs) such as idiopathic pulmonary fibrosis (IPF). In a nationwide study performed in Japan,[165] two subgroups of chronic fibrotic HP were described, one of them was seen with chronic advanced disease whereas the other became chronic after repeated identifiable acute episodes.

Tachypnea and bibasilar crackles are the usual clinical findings in all forms of HP. Wheezing, provoked by small airway obstruction, is not a characteristic physical sign, but it occurs in some patients and may lead to an erroneous diagnostic approach. In chronic HP, overt manifestations of right-sided heart involvement and digital clubbing may be found. In a study by Sansores and colleagues,[166] digital clubbing was recorded in 51% of 82 patients with chronic PBD. Interestingly, 35% of patients with digital clubbing clinically deteriorated compared with only 13% of those without clubbing. Thus, it appears that digital clubbing occurs frequently, especially in the chronic form of HP, and may be predictive of clinical worsening.

Although the classification system described above is widely used, it can be misleading. Occasionally, for example, acute and chronic forms may coexist in a single patient. In addition, the complex spectrum of the clinical and functional presentation and variable clinical courses of the disease make this classification somewhat limited. Accordingly, a different system to define the clinical spectrum was proposed.[167] This classification takes into account the anatomic differences by which the disease manifests itself, the broad range of clinical and functional presentations, and the possible evolution of the disease. The following are some considerations of this new proposal.

Lung Structure Involvement: Hypersensitivity Pneumonitis versus "Hypersensitivity" Chronic Bronchitis

The disease may affect the lung parenchyma and cause the patient to present with typical HP, or it may affect the large airways and manifest as a chronic bronchitis or chronic airways obstruction.

In this context, it is important to emphasize that chronic bronchitis is a frequent problem in both the farm population and in pigeon breeders, and, interestingly, the risk of developing airways disease has been observed to be high in nonsmokers.[168,169] Moreover, organic dust and tobacco smoke are independent and additive causes of chronic bronchitis.[170] Of the pigeon fanciers surveyed, 8.5 to 12% had chronic bronchitis as their only manifestation of pigeon-related symptomatology[147,169]; the prevalence increased significantly in those who were sensitized. Bourke and colleagues[171] studied 287 pigeon fanciers and noted a 26% prevalence rate of chronic bronchitis in nonsmokers with an increasing prevalence as antibody levels rose. Moreover, chronic bronchitis was the only manifestation of the disease in 8.4% of the population surveyed. A recent clinical study involving 343 pigeon breeders found that while 8% met the criteria for HP, 15% suffered from chronic bronchitis.[172] In this study, increased levels of specific IgG were significantly associated with chronic airways disease.

Depierre and colleagues[132] reported a 50% prevalence rate of chronic bronchitis in patients with farmer's lung—regardless of their smoking history—compared with 8.6% in farmers without the disease. In addition to the presence of farmer's lung, a strong positive relationship has been found between chronic bronchitis and a previous history of acute respiratory syndromes during barn threshing.[173] Additionally, a risk of chronic bronchitis has been associated with male gender, age, and altitude.[152] Hasani and colleagues[174] have reported additional evidence of larger airways damage in PBD, consisting of impairment of lung mucociliary clearance in sensitized pigeon fanciers compared with precipitin-negative controls.

Clinical Behavior: Acute versus Chronic

Hypersensitivity pneumonitis, as a lung parenchymal disease, may be acute or chronic. The acute form can be *nonprogressive and intermittent*, with spontaneous improvement after antigen avoidance, or *acute progressive*, with coughing and dyspnea becoming persistent, requiring antigen avoidance and therapy with corticosteroids. When chronic, the disease may present as a *chronic nonprogressive* or as a *chronic progressive* disorder evolving until end-stage lung damage is present.

Acute and chronic refer to the type of reaction and the duration of HP. Acute HP is representative of a disease mediated by immune complexes and is characterized by influenza-like manifestations and pulmonary involvement several hours after each exposure. If the acute reaction disappears spontaneously but recurs several hours after the next exposure, an intermittent pattern is present. When T-cell immune mechanisms take place, the acute form may be progressive, requiring antigen avoidance and corticosteroids for resolution. Chronic HP presents as prolonged and persistent pneumonitis. Nonprogressive HP refers to whether the symptoms stabilize, improve, or disappear, either spontaneously or with treatment. Chronic progressive HP refers to symptoms evolving to diffuse fibrosis and end-stage lung disease.

This author suggests an alternate clinical classification of HP as follows: (a) acute nonprogressive and intermittent, (b) acute progressive (former subacute), (c) chronic nonprogressive, and (d) chronic progressive.

IMAGING APPROACHES

Chest Radiographs

The radiologic appearance and the type and distribution of shadowing vary with the different stages of the disease.[1] However, it is important to consider that a number of patients with acute and subacute (acute progressive) forms of HP may have normal chest radiographs.[175] It has been suggested that the sensitivity of chest radiographs for detecting HP has steadily declined over the last 30 years.[176] This is probably due to a higher index of suspi-

cion for the disease and to the increased sensitivity of other diagnostic techniques that lead to an earlier diagnosis, even when the chest roentgenogram may be normal. It is important to consider that HP is probably one of the most common ILDs displaying a normal chest radiograph, although the reason for this finding is unknown. In the classic paper by Epler and colleagues,[177] 38% of patients with allergic alveolitis showed a normal chest roentgenogram. The authors suggested that in a number of patients, the granulomas are too small and too few and the interstitial pneumonitis too inconspicuous to produce a visible increase in radiographic density.

In the acute form (*acute nonprogressive intermittent form*), a transient widespread diffuse ground-glass or air space consolidation is usually seen (Figure 19–2). In the subacute form (*acute progressive form*), the chest radiograph reveals a fine nodular or reticulonodular shadowing with some degree of ground-glass attenuation (Figure 19–3). The chronic stages are characterized by a predominantly reticular pattern, which, in the *progressive form*, evolves to a honeycomb pattern with cystic areas visible within the thickened interstitium (Figure 19–4).

The distribution of radiologic abnormalities is variable and may involve the upper two-thirds of the lungs with relative sparing of the basal segments. Alternately, it may show a middle- and lower-zone predominance.[178,179] Several factors may contribute to the topologic distribution of lung lesions and, consequently, to radiologic appearances; some of these factors are related to how the antigen deposits during inhalation and to the capacity of alveolar clearance in the local microenvironment. The distribution of inhaled particles is dependent on the following: breathing pattern; gravity; individual respiratory tract anatomy; antigenic load; average residence time of the antigen in the respiratory system; and characteristics of the organic dust including its size, density, electrical charge, and hygroscopic properties.[180,181] In addition, it has been suggested that the location of

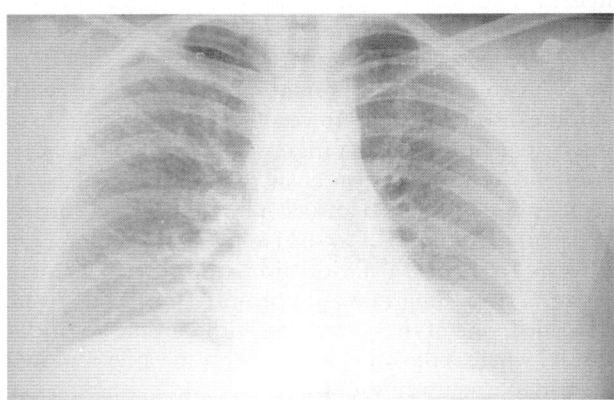

Figure 19–2   Chest radiograph from a patient with an acute form of hypersensitivity pneumonitis showing a moderate diffuse hazy opacity.

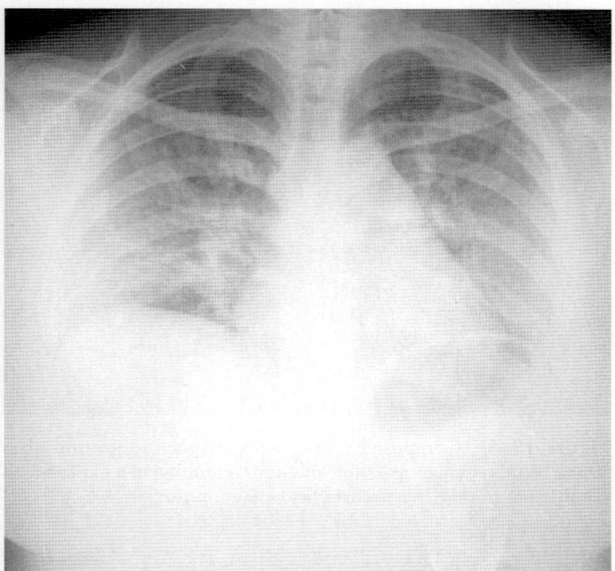

Figure 19–3 Chest radiograph exhibiting hazy opacities attenuation and diffuse, poorly marginated, small rounded opacities and reticular opacities in an acute progressive (subacute) patient with hypersensitivity pneumonitis.

radiologic abnormalities may differ as a function of disease, with a middle lung zone predominance in acute and acute progressive HP and an upper lung zone predominance in the chronic form.[179,182] The reason for this finding is unknown.

Radiologic changes are diffusely spread over both lungs and are usually without hilar adenopathy or pleural effusion. Occasionally, hilar and mediastinal lymphadenopathy has been described.[183] In this context, a study that used computed tomography in patients with ILD, including 17 patients with HP, demonstrated that enlarged mediastinal nodes can be found in about half of the patients with HP. In contrast to sarcoidosis,

only one or two nodes are usually enlarged, and their maximal short axis diameter is < 15 mm.[184]

Although pleural involvement is usually absent, McLoud and colleagues[185] found pleural effusion in 2 out of 27 patients studied.

Although it is not clear whether the extent and type of radiologic features correlate with the histopathologic severity or prognosis of the disease, the ground-glass appearance and nodular shadows are generally observed in acute and subacute forms, whereas the more coarse interstitial pattern is seen in the chronic form.

Computed Tomography

Computed tomography (CT) and high-resolution computed tomography (HRCT) display similar images as described for conventional chest radiographs, although HRCT provides a more precise and finer assessment of the pattern, extent, and distribution of the disease[186–188] and correlates better with clinical and functional parameters.

A population-based study in a group of swimming pool employees clearly demonstrated that the sensitivity of HRCT is greater than that of chest radiography.[189] As described in this report, HRCT facilitated the diagnosis of relatively mild disease, although it was also suggested that HP patients with pathologic evidence of interstitial lung disease may have normal HRCT findings.

In acute HP, HRCT features may include a diffuse and hazy increased parenchymal density (ground-glass attenuation) and patchy or widespread air space opacification (Figure 19–5). In subacute (acute progressive) HP, small rounded opacities (nodules) are usually seen in addition to the acute changes previously described (Figure 19–6). Patients with chronic disease have a nodular pattern with both fine and coarse reticular opacities that may eventually evolve to honeycombing (Figures 19–7 and 19–8).

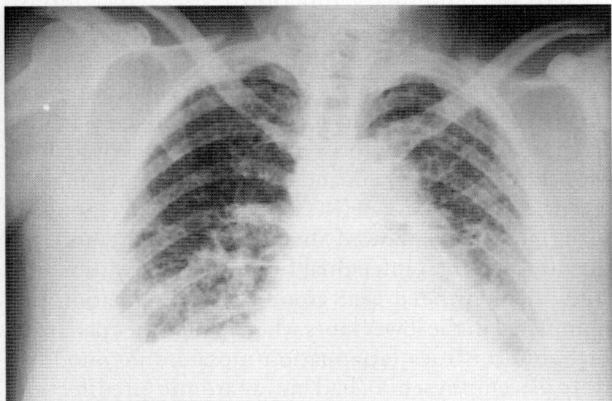

Figure 19–4 Chest radiograph showing fibrotic changes in a patient with chronic hypersensitivity pneumonitis. There is a lower-lobe coarse reticulonodular opacity with numerous irregular linear opacities, shortening of the lung fields, and pulmonary hypertension.

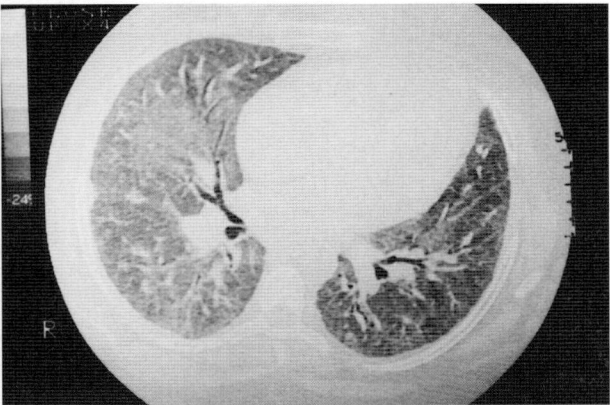

Figure 19–5 High-resolution computed tomography scan showing a diffuse increase of lung attenuation ground-glass opacities in acute hypersensitivity pneumonitis. Notice the marked contrast between the density of the lung parenchyma and air in the airways.

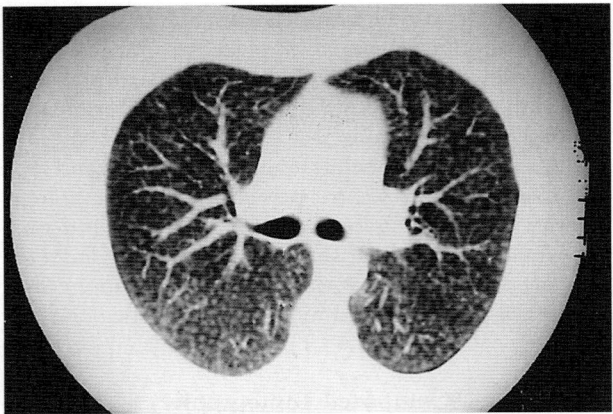

Figure 19–6   Computed tomography scan shows discrete ground-glass attenuation and, mostly, poorly defined micronodules diffusely distributed throughout both lungs in acute progressive (subacute) hypersensitivity pneumonitis.

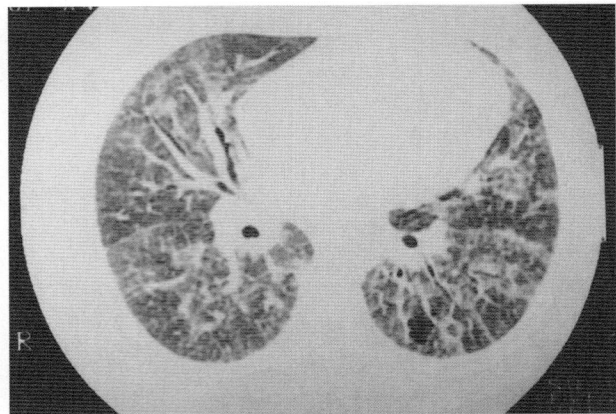

Figure 19–8   Computed tomography displaying ground-glass attenuation, reticular opacities, and honeycombing in a patient with chronic progressive hypersensitivity pneumonitis.

Ground-glass attenuation is generally bilateral and can be patchy or diffuse. The subtle increase in attenuation of the lung parenchyma, when virtually uniform in distribution throughout the lungs, is better appreciated by the abnormal prominence of bronchial walls and the marked contrast between the density of the lung parenchyma and air in the major airways.

The micronodular pattern is also bilateral and consists of poorly defined micronodules, usually less than 5 mm in diameter, that affect both the central and peripheral portions of the lung. Although the finding of centrilobular, peribronchiolar, indistinct nodules is not pathognomonic, it should suggest the diagnosis of chronic HP.[186] Actually, areas of ground-glass attenuation plus centrilobular nodules without air space consolidation are strongly suggestive of HP.[190] Nodules and ground-glass attenuation are also frequently present in the chronic form, both progressive and nonprogressive, suggesting acute changes superimposed on chronic disease.

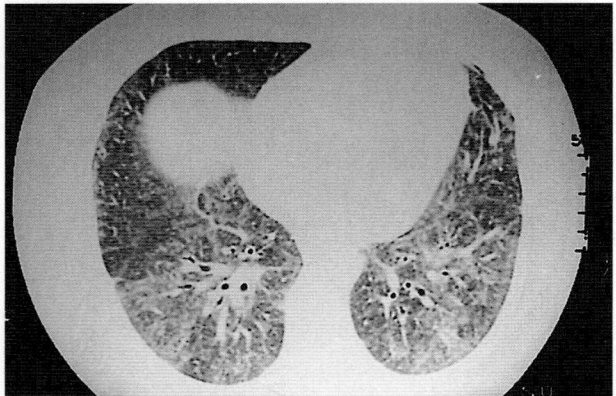

Figure 19–7   Computed tomography scan exhibiting a mixture of images including nodules, ground-glass opacities, and reticular images in chronic hypersensitivity pneumonitis.

In acute progressive disease, and in the chronic clinical forms, CT may exhibit focal air-trapping or emphysema as well as mild to severe fibrotic changes.[175]

In PBD, diffuse emphysematous changes have been described that are probably provoked by diffuse bronchiolar obstruction.[191] Moreover, in a study performed by Hansell and colleagues,[192] areas of *decreased attenuation* and mosaic perfusion were found to be a common CT pattern in both acute progressive (subacute) and chronic HP. A CT scan obtained at the end of expiration is useful to improve the visualization of the patchy air-trapping images. Decreased attenuation correlated with increased residual volume, suggesting that obstructive functional abnormalities caused by bronchiolitis might be responsible for this pattern. Images showing findings of infiltrative diffuse lung disease on inspiratory HRCT and air-trapping on expiratory HRCT are suggestive of a diagnosis of HP. In general, the extent of parenchymal abnormalities and air-trapping correlate with the presence of an obstructive/restrictive mixed pattern on pulmonary function tests.[193] In contrast, ground-glass opacification and reticulation correlated with restrictive lung function.

In summary, two kinds of CT images may be present: (a) those related to interstitial and intra-alveolar lung inflammation and fibrosis, and (b) those derived from bronchiolar involvement and emphysematous changes. A recent study evaluating HRCT findings at different phases of farmer's lung, showed that emphysema is more frequently seen than interstitial fibrosis.[194] In addition, this study demonstrated that ground-glass attenuation predominated in the lower lobes whereas the other parenchymal abnormalities (attenuation/mosaic, micronodules, fibrosis, emphysema) had no anatomic predilection. About one-third of patients exhibited mediastinal lymphadenopathy suggesting that this finding has no negative diagnostic value. Interestingly, some farmers persisted in working on dairy farms although the study supported the fact that contact avoidance allowed a better resolution of CT abnormalities than continued exposure.

In most patients with chronic HP and fibrosis, the irregular linear opacities involve either the middle lung zones or distribute evenly throughout the three lung zones; apices, costophrenic angles, and bases are relatively spared. This pattern may help in the differential diagnosis because it is distinct from the basal subpleural fibrosis commonly seen in idiopathic pulmonary fibrosis and from the middle to upper zone of peribronchovascular fibrosis seen in sarcoidosis.[195] Another study showed that peripheral- and lower-zone predominance is more suggestive of IPF than HP.[196] However, radiologic findings, including lung predominance, can be identical in both diseases.

Computed Tomography and Pathology

High-resolution computed tomography abnormalities may reflect the morphologic changes observed in lung biopsy specimens.[197] Thus, for example, ground-glass opacity, which represents a decrease in the air content of the lung parenchyma without totally obliterating the alveoli, appears to coincide with the presence of small granulomas within the alveolar septa and with the partial filling of air spaces with inflammatory cells. Nodular opacities with patchy air space opacification reflect the presence of interstitial pneumonitis, cellular bronchiolitis, and granulomas, whereas irregular linear opacities correspond to areas of fibrosis. In patients described by Buschman and colleagues[186] the characteristic small centrilobular nodules corresponded with polypoid intraluminal granulation tissue within the bronchioles and an active alveolitis filling alveoli around the central area of the lobules.

Follow-up CT scans have shown that the air space consolidation cleared first, followed by regression of increased lung density. Diffuse micronodules might remain even after clinical improvement.[198]

The comparison of CT findings with histologic abnormalities suggests that ground-glass attenuation might reflect reversible inflammatory changes. In fact, such opacities usually resolve following cessation of antigen exposure in both acute progressive and chronic forms of HP.[175] However, it is important to note that increased lung attenuation is occasionally related to diffuse interstitial fibrosis with minimal cellular infiltration, similar to that reported in progressive systemic sclerosis.[199] By contrast, honeycombing—areas of cystic spaces with thickened walls—represents an advanced stage of fibrosis in chronic progressive disease and is a poor predictor of therapeutic response.[200]

Magnetic Resonance Imaging

It is important to keep in mind that the use of repeated CT scans in the follow-up is limited by radiation risks.

The exact radiation dose depends on several factors, but a conventional CT exposure and HRCT yield radiation levels several times higher than that of standard chest films.[201] In this context, alternate imaging modalities have been assayed.

Although magnetic resonance imaging (MRI) is of lesser clinical value than CT in the anatomic assessment of lung parenchyma, it might be useful in detecting pulmonary infiltrates that decrease air spaces. The MRI scan makes sectional images of the body as does CT; its advantages are that ionizing radiation is not used, and it apparently has no known hazards or side effects. In addition, MRI can directly acquire sagittal and coronal imaging planes with spatial resolution equal to axial images and without reformatting.[202] However, the use of MRI in ILDs has been limited due to the low proton density of lung parenchyma, the loss of signal due to motion, and the difference in diamagnetic susceptibility between air and soft tissue.

In a report on 25 patients with different types of chronic ILDs, including 4 with HP, it was shown that areas of air space opacification observed on MRI corresponded to areas of active alveolitis or air space infiltration when studied by morphology (Figure 19–9).[203] In this study, CT was superior to MRI in the anatomic assessment of the lung parenchyma and in showing fibrosis. Areas of ground-glass opacities were, however, equally clear with either technique. This finding suggests that MRI may play a role in the study and follow-up of patients with air space opacification.

Primack and colleagues[204] compared MRI to pathologic findings on lung biopsy specimens in 22 patients with different ILDs, including 3 with HP. The predominant patterns of abnormality on MRI included parenchymal opacification (ground-glass intensity or consolidation), reticulation, nodularity, and interlobular septal thickening. Areas of parenchymal opacification were the main finding in the 3 patients with HP. In 12 out of 14 patients, the parenchymal opacification represented an active inflammatory process, including alve-

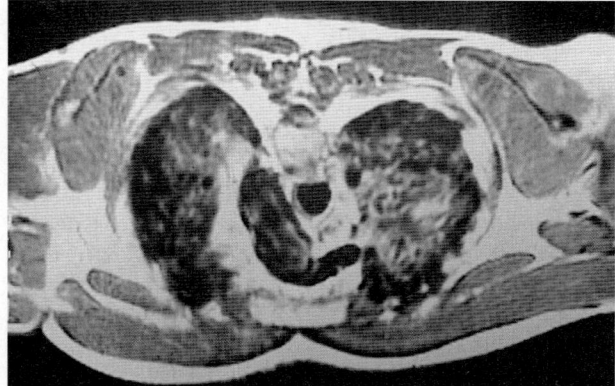

Figure 19–9 Magnetic resonance imaging showing areas of parenchymal opacification and nodular images. (Courtesy of Dr. N. L. Muller, Vancouver General Hospital.)

olitis and granulomas, and therefore a potentially treatable disease. Peripheral reticulation was identified on MRI in all 5 patients with IPF. In general, these results suggest that MRI findings correlate closely with those seen on lung biopsy. However, MRI has several limitations in the assessment of patients with ILDs, including its low spatial resolution compared with HRCT, and is therefore generally not recommended as a routine diagnostic tool in these patients.

Scintigraphic Studies

Gallium-67 lung scanning has been used to evaluate the extent and intensity of inflammatory changes in a number of interstitial pulmonary diseases.[205] In patients with allergic alveolitis, an abnormal lung gallium-67 accumulation that seemed to correlate with the clinical course has been reported. Specifically, patients who improved or remained stable showed the lowest gallium-67 index, whereas deteriorating patients usually showed a significantly higher gallium-67 uptake.[206]

Clearance from the lungs of micronic aerosols of technetium 99m-labeled diethylenetriamine pentaacetic acid (^{99m}Tc-DTPA) has been proposed to assess alveolar epithelial integrity by measuring permeability to small solutes. The tracer molecule, ^{99m}Tc-DTPA, has been used in several ILDs, including HP, and it has been postulated that an increased clearance rate of this aerosolized radionuclide through the alveolar epithelium may reflect, in a highly sensitive way, the extent of alveolar damage.[207] Bourke and colleagues[208] have found that both patients with PBD and asymptomatic pigeon breeders' with high specific antibody levels presented significantly increased rates of clearance of ^{99m}Tc-DTPA. Nonantigen-exposed individuals showed normal clearance, and asymptomatic (antigen exposed) subjects without sensitization had intermediate rates of clearance. This finding suggests that this test can identify an alteration in lung integrity more subtle than that found with conventional pulmonary function tests and may be useful in the earlier evolutionary stages of the disease. Moreover, the exquisite sensitivity of this measurement can detect lung alterations and alveolar disease in asymptomatic patients with a history of previous HP.[209] However, there have been reported overlaps in clearance rates of the radioisotope between patients with ILD and normal subjects, so it is difficult to determine the cutoff value for differentiating pathologic from normal permeability.[210] In addition, accelerated clearance of ^{99m}Tc-DTPA permeability has been observed in healthy persons breathing at increased lung volume, whether or not the increase in lung volume results from positive or negative (voluntary) pressure breathing.[211] Likewise, cigarette smoking increases the respiratory clearance of ^{99m}Tc-DTPA in healthy persons.[212] Therefore, it is difficult to ascertain the usefulness of ^{99m}Tc-DTPA clearance in routine clinical practice.

PULMONARY FUNCTION TESTS

Lung function abnormalities are neither specific nor diagnostic for HP because similar changes are found in many other ILDs. In general, the study of static respiratory mechanics exhibits a restrictive ventilatory defect with a loss of lung volume. This reduction is not uniform among all the compartments of lung volume, and the decrease is usually more significant in vital capacity than in total lung capacity, whereas the residual volume is relatively well preserved.

Patients display impaired gas exchange characterized by hypoxemia that usually worsens with exercise, normal or slightly decreased arterial carbon dioxide tension ($PaCO_2$), and an elevated alveolar-arterial oxygen gradient ($P_{(A-a)}O_2$).[213–215] Occasionally, in accordance with the extension and severity of lung lesions, or in early stages of the disease, patients may present normoxemia at rest; however, exercise always reveals hypoxemia. An early and sensitive functional abnormality is a reduction in the diffusing lung capacity for carbon monoxide (DL_{CO}), which appears to be a good predictor of arterial oxygen desaturation during exercise.

A classic restrictive pattern is usually seen in the acute intermittent form of the disease or following an antigen challenge. Occasionally, an immediate and short-lived obstructive airflow defect may precede the restrictive abnormality.

In acute progressive (subacute) and chronic HP, mechanical properties are characterized by a variable reduction in total and vital lung capacities. In addition, the static expiratory pressure-volume curve is shifted down and to the right of the normal curve, showing a decrease in lung compliance over the entire range of the reduced inspiratory capacity. If exposure to an offending antigen continues, deterioration can occur with an accelerated decline in serial lung function.[200]

Some degree of obstruction of the peripheral airways, as suggested by a decrease in the maximum to midflow rates and in the ratio of dynamic to static lung compliance, may be present due to bronchiolitis.[216] Additionally, a number of patients demonstrate hyperreactive airways.

The presence of bronchiolitis notwithstanding, airflow obstruction may not be detected by functional tests, perhaps because the damaged bronchioles and surrounding damaged parenchyma are excluded completely from pulmonary function tests, producing as a net result a predominantly restrictive pattern.[191] Furthermore, pulmonary function tests are unlikely to detect focal alteration in bronchioles, no matter how severe, nor are they sensitive to very mild diffuse disease.

However, the involvement of bronchioles is a frequent pathologic abnormality; in a number of chronic patients, functional defects reflecting bronchiolitis and emphysematous changes are dominant. In these cases, the pattern of lung function impairment may differ markedly from the typical restrictive figure, and decreased flow rates, increased lung compliance, and reduced elastic recoil are seen.

Therefore, after prolonged allergic alveolitis, the lungs may be repaired by fibrosis with a uniform increase in stiffness, or they may evolve to a different kind of tissue remodeling that results in cystic emphysematous space formation. Often, both pathologic processes are present in the lung parenchyma; the balance between them will determine the overall lung function.

The correlation between pulmonary functional abnormality and the severity or prognosis of HP is poor. Patients with a severe decrease in lung volume and DL_{CO} may recover fully, whereas others with relatively mild functional abnormalities at the onset of disease may develop progressive pulmonary fibrosis or airway obstruction and emphysematous changes.

In the patients who present a pressure-volume curve that is shifted down and to the right, it has been suggested that its exponential analysis could be useful in monitoring progression of the disease.[217] Theoretically, lung compliance can be decreased by inflammation, which produces patchy reductions in lung volume by replacing gas volume with cells and fluid, or by fibrosis, which destroys the alveolocapillary units, thus altering lung architecture. The exponential modeling of static lung compliance may help to differentiate both pathologic processes where a low constant k can indicate increased stiffness of the functioning alveoli by fibrosis rather than by a simple decrease of alveolar volume (Figure 19–10). In other words, the exponential modeling avoids the volume dependency of compliance. In this way, a low value of the constant k suggests a real change in the mechanical properties of the functional lung parenchyma, whereas a normal value accompanied by restriction suggests a loss of lung units without a change in the mechanical properties of the functioning units.[218]

PULMONARY CIRCULATION

Studies of hemodynamic characteristics of pulmonary circulation in HP are extremely limited. Some investigations have demonstrated an increase in the mean pulmonary arterial pressure, which is associated with high levels of pulmonary arteriolar resistance and total pulmonary vascular resistance, in otherwise cardiologically healthy patients with subacute and chronic PBD.[1,219] In these studies, pulmonary arterial hypertension has been associated with the levels of hypoxemia. As in other chronic ILDs, patients with chronic progressive HP develop clinical evidence of pulmonary hypertension, with right ventricular hypertrophy and right heart failure.

LABORATORY TESTS

Routine Laboratory Tests

There is no clinically useful diagnostic laboratory test at present, nor are there serologic markers to monitor disease activity or progression. In the acute intermittent or acute progressive forms, a slight or moderate neutrophilic leukocytosis with lymphopenia may occur. In chronic disease, leukocyte counts are usually normal. The erythrocyte sedimentation rate may be moderately elevated in some patients. Rheumatoid factor, C-reactive protein, immune complexes, and a mild increase in IgG and IgM have also been described as nonspecific findings.[1]

Recently, it has been suggested that the measurement of plasma lactate dehydrogenase (LDH) may be useful in assessing disease activity.[220] The LDH activity was higher in HP patients, and it decreased significantly with improving lung function.

Detection of Specific Antibodies

Serum-precipitating IgG antibodies against the offending antigen are usually detectable. However, the presence of these antibodies is considered to be of questionable clinical relevance for diagnosis, primarily because similar antibodies are present in sera from exposed but asymptomatic individuals. Thus, the presence of these antibodies merely represents exposure to the antigen, and approximately 10 to 50% (depending on the antigen investigated) of exposed but asymptomatic subjects have detectable antibodies in their serum.[221,222]

However, the presence of antibodies is still one of the diagnostic criteria for disease. Although false negatives might occur, HP can be ruled out in patients with ILD suspected of having the disease. By contrast, the presence of specific antibodies is another small piece of information favoring the diagnosis of HP. Enzyme-linked immunosorbent assay is a simple and very sensitive test for the detection of antibodies.[88]

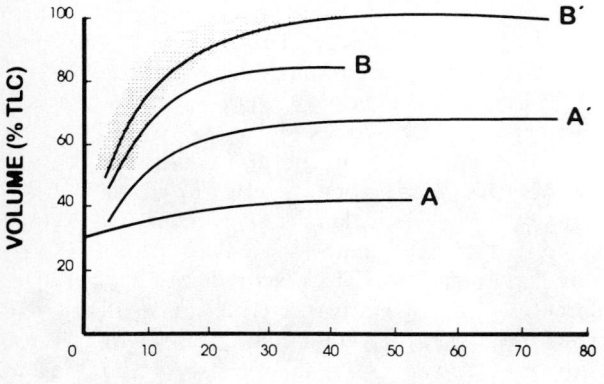

STATIC TRANSPULMONARY PRESSURE

Figure 19–10   Static expiratory pressure-volume curves for two patients with chronic hypersensitivity pneumonitis. Stippled area represents the normal range. After adjustment for the decrease in total lung capacity, the curve of patient B reaches the normal range (B'), whereas the curve of patient A is still shifted down and to the right (A').

The incidence of serum precipitins in asymptomatic bird breeders is higher than in farmers, perhaps because the exposure to pigeons tends to occur more continuously than the seasonal exposures experienced by farmers. Also, this could be one of the reasons why it is more common to find the chronic forms of the disease in the absence of acute attacks in patients with PBD. Specific precipitating antibodies have been detected in up to 40% of pigeon breeders regularly exposed to lofts where they inhale a high antigen load in contrast to approximately 9% in dairy farmers.[222,223]

In PBD, the number of epitopes that are recognized by antibodies present in serum and BAL fluid has demonstrated that patients react with an extensive variety of molecules bearing epitopes.[88]

In this sense, the presence of possible differences in the recognition of specific antigens in both symptomatic patients and exposed but asymptomatic individuals has been explored. Calvanico[224] has partially purified a 55 kD protein from pigeon droppings. This protein reacts with the sera of patients with PBD and not with the sera from asymptomatic pigeon breeders. De Beer and colleagues[225] have found that although sera from asymptomatic and symptomatic pigeon breeders react to antigens of high molecular weights (> 86 kD), only sera from patients with PBD recognize an antigen of an approximate molecular weight of 29 to 32 kD.

Another study demonstrated that IgG3 subclass reactivity specific to pigeon mucin is strongly associated with sera from patients with active lung disease, whereas it is found in less than 15% of healthy pigeon breeders.[226]

Further purification of these or other similar components of avian and other known antigens may lead to more sensitive laboratory tests that may be of diagnostic value for HP in the future.

Recently, it has been demonstrated that avian-antigen-specific IgG and IgA can be easily detectable in saliva samples.[227,228] Moreover, the levels of IgG antibody in saliva and in serum correlated significantly. Because collecting saliva is a noninvasive technique, these results suggest that saliva antibody measurement may be a suitable method for monitoring HP, especially in children, and can also facilitate sampling for epidemiologic studies of antibody prevalence.

Regarding the T-cell proliferative response, Mendoza and colleagues,[91] using avian-antigen-bearing nitrocellulosa particles derived from Western blots, found that a high-molecular-weight antigen (220 kD) was the only immunodominant antigen. By contrast, Hisauchi-Kojima and colleagues[229] identified a 21 kD protein that displayed a 57% identity to a *Saccharomyces cerevisiae* chromosome X reading frame. This protein, which was detected by immunoblotting, was the only one that recognized individuals exposed to pigeons. Only cells from patients with HP showed significant proliferation to this 21 kD protein and to the synthetic peptide on the basis of the N-terminal sequence of the native peptide.

Skin tests are not helpful for the diagnosis of HP. Moreover, suitable pure preparations for skin testing are scarce, and no reliable standardized antigens for skin tests that can be used routinely are available at present.

BRONCHOALVEOLAR LAVAGE

An extensive number of abnormalities both in cells and molecules are present in the fluid recovered from BAL of patients with HP. Unfortunately, many of them are also shared, to a lesser extent, by exposed but asymptomatic individuals.

Cell Profile

A significant increase in the total cell count is usually found, and a remarkable elevation in the percentage of lymphocytes, often over 50%, is seen (Figure 19–11); actually, a BAL lymphocyte count less than 30% should discard the diagnosis of HP. The majority of BAL lymphocytes are T cells.[43]

The analyses of T-cell surface phenotypes have revealed a strong predominance of the CD8+ T-lymphocyte subset, with an associated imbalance of the CD4 to CD8 ratio.[12,13,230] Although most authors agree with the concept that an increase of CD8 T cells with an inversion in the CD4/CD8 ratio is a feature of HP, we do not yet know whether this general assumption is universal or consistent. The CD4/CD8 ratio varied significantly with the type of disease in a nationwide study conducted in Japan.[231] This ratio was decreased in summer-type HP, almost normal in PBD and ventilation pneumonitis, and increased in patients with farmer's lung. Likewise, Cormier and colleagues[232] also found wide differences in T-cell subsets of patients with farmer's lung. The reason for these differences is

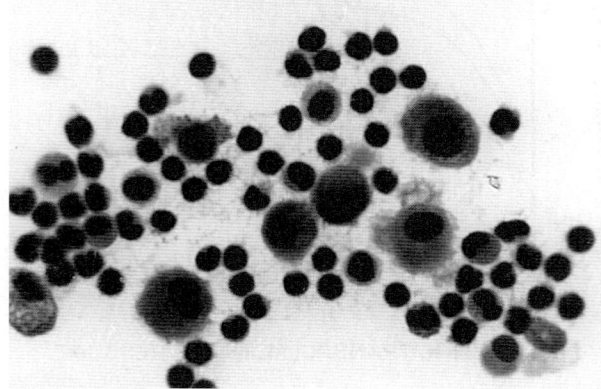

Figure 19–11 Light micrograph of a bronchoalveolar lavage cell population as usually observed in patients with acute progressive or chronic hypersensitivity pneumonitis. There is an increase in the percentage of lymphocytes (hematoxylin and eosin; ×250 original magnification).

unknown. The causative agent, the type of exposure (high concentration and intermittent versus low concentration and continuous), the genetic host response, the smoking habit, and the stage of the disease when the BAL is performed may account for such differences.

Interestingly, when CD3, CD4, and CD8 T-cell density have been investigated by flow cytometry, a significant increase in all these surface markers has been found in the T lymphocytes of patients with HP in comparison with patients with sarcoidosis, bronchiolitis obliterans with organizing pneumonia, and healthy controls. This suggests a high degree of T-cell activation.[233] Furthermore, an elevated number of BAL T lymphocytes express a variety of activation markers such as the p75 chain of IL-2 receptor, "very late activation antigen" (VLA-1), and human leukocyte antigen (HLA)-DR antigens.[234] Flow cytometry and PCR analyses of T-cell receptor β chain variable regions have demonstrated an overexpression of cells bearing Vβ2, Vβ3, Vβ5, Vβ6, and Vβ8 gene segments.[13] Additionally, studies using the Leu-15 surface marker have suggested that cytotoxic cell subpopulations (recognized as CD8+) are also increased.[230]

Increased natural killer cells, non-MHC-restricted cytotoxic lymphocytes, and lymphokine-activated killer cells are usually detected in BAL fluid from patients with HP.[14,235]

However, increased BAL lymphocytes and CD8+ T cells have also been found in some asymptomatic pigeon breeders and dairy farmers.[30,236,237] Moreover, bronchoalveolar lymphocytosis appears to be a persistent phenomenon in a large number of asymptomatic dairy farmers who do not develop the disease.[30] It is not known whether this finding represents an appropriate normal inflammatory response or whether the apparent "normal" individuals exposed to birds—or thermophilic actinomycetes—have a subclinical, low-intensity alveolitis.

In experimental HP induced by avian antigens as well as in human PBD, T-suppressor cells exhibited impaired function only in those subjects with disease.[27,28] However, it seems that a subgroup of asymptomatic pigeon breeders also show a low concanavalin A–induced suppression similar to that found in patients with signs of PBD.[238]

A few B lymphocytes that vary in maturation from small lymphocytes to mature plasma cells can be present in BAL fluid. Thus, small numbers of plasma cells are found in about half of patients, which may be a feature of recent antigen exposure and of active alveolitis.[239] Furthermore, patients with plasma cells in BAL fluid display signs of a more active inflammation, demonstrated by the increased number of lymphocytes, eosinophils, and mast cells, as well as by higher immunoglobulin levels, when compared with patients with HP whose BAL fluid contains no plasma cells.[240]

The percentage of BAL macrophages in HP is very low. (However, because there is a significant increase in the total number of cells recovered in BAL fluid, the absolute number of macrophages in patients with HP is comparable with those in controls.)

Several studies have shown that alveolar macrophages are in a high state of activation. Using flow cytometric methods, Haslam and associates[241] have demonstrated that alveolar macrophages from patients with HP exhibit a higher intensity expression of HLA-DQ and HLA-DP than those from patients with idiopathic fibrosing alveolitis or from healthy subjects, suggesting an enhanced antigen-presenting function of these cells in HP. Likewise, alveolar macrophages from patients with HP overexpress ICAM-1, an important cell surface glycoprotein that functions as an adhesion molecule.[242] In addition, an increase in the percentage of alveolar macrophages producing surfactant protein A (SP-A) has been found in patients with HP.[243]

With respect to polymorphonuclear leukocytes, a moderate but significant increase of the percentage of neutrophils has been found after inhalation challenge in HP patients (acute transient neutrophil alveolitis) and in half of the patients with chronic PBD (Figure 19–12).[17,244,245]

Increased numbers of mast cells, which resemble tissue mast cells, are also present in BAL fluid from patients with HP; these cells often appear degranulated. Coincidentally, BAL histamine levels are elevated as well.[244,246,247] Mast cells are also increased in lung tissues, and a significant correlation between BAL and tissue mast cells have been reported.[44] Nevertheless, an increase in the number of mast cells has been found in BAL fluid taken from farmers without clinical signs of farmer's lung.[248] Thus, the significance of these cells in the pathogenesis of this disorder or in disease activity is unclear.

The cell profile may be related to the time elapsed between the last antigen exposure and the obtaining of BAL fluid. Drent and colleagues[240] studied the BAL fluid

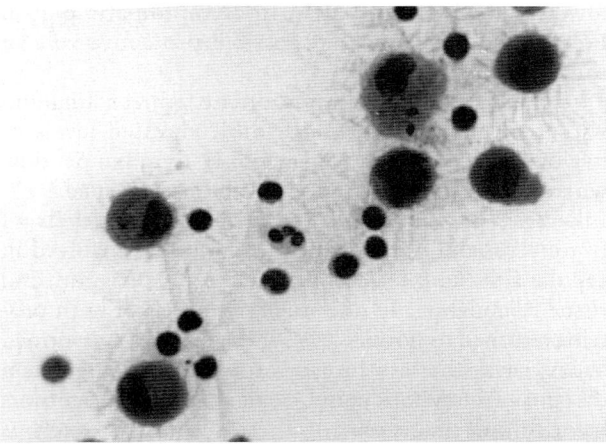

Figure 19–12   The presence of neutrophils within bronchoalveolar lavage lymphocytosis is detected in acute hypersensitivity pneumonitis and in a number of chronic HP patients (hematoxylin and eosin; ×250 original magnification).

from 59 nonsmoking patients with HP at various time points after termination of antigen exposure. Early after provocation (< 24 h), an increase in the relative numbers of lymphocytes, neutrophils, eosinophils, mast cells, and plasma cells was observed. After recent antigen exposure (2 to 7 days), a similar cell profile, with the exception of a drop in the percentage of polymorphonuclear cells, was detected. In BAL obtained from 1 week to several months after antigen exposure, cellular constituents showed a tendency to return to normal values. Lymphocyte levels, however, remained high. The timing of BAL sampling in relation to antigen exposure also affects the preponderance of the T-cell subsets. A persistent increase in CD8[+] cells with reversal of the CD4/CD8 ratio is seen in patients with regular exposure to specific antigens,[249] whereas a normalization of the T-lymphocyte subpopulations is observed in patients who avoid further exposure.

Because there is no unique finding for HP, BAL by itself does not play a pivotal role in the diagnosis, although it may eventually help to distinguish HP from other frequent ILDs. For example, Drent and colleagues,[250] were able to distinguish between patients with sarcoidosis, HP, and IPF using a discriminate analysis with selected variables such as yield of recovered BAL fluid, total cell count, and percentages of alveolar macrophages, lymphocytes, polymorphonuclear neutrophils, eosinophils, and plasma cells.

Molecular Constituents

Several acellular components of BAL fluids are also elevated in patients with HP. These molecules include IgG, IgM, IgA, immune complexes, leukotriene C4, and β_2-microglobulin.[221,251,252] In patients with PBD, it was found that levels of immunoglobulins and specific antibodies are significantly higher than in asymptomatic pigeon breeders.[253]

Interleukin-6 has been shown to be significantly lower in PBD patients than in asymptomatic pigeon breeders,[32] suggesting the possible protective role of this cytokine.

Patients with acute intermittent farmer's lung and with recent onset of PBD exhibit elevated levels of hyaluronic acid and procollagen 3 N-terminal peptide, whereas asymptomatic farmers' values are normal.[254,255] Likewise, patients with HP display high levels of fibronectin and vitronectin, two molecules involved in cellular adhesion, extracellular matrix organization, and tissue remodeling. In one study, the levels of both proteins returned to normal levels if the BAL was performed 5 days after the last antigen exposure; this suggests a dynamic accumulation and clearance.[256] Other authors have found that some of these molecules, such as hyaluronic acid, fibronectin, and fibroblast growth factor activity, remain abnormal in patients who have had farmer's lung yet remain asymptomatic despite daily contact with the farm environment.[257]

A mucin-like glycoprotein, KL-6, is increased in HP as well as in other ILDs. It is probably derived from damaged or regenerating type II alveolar epithelial cells.[258]

Additionally, the levels of SP-A in BAL fluid obtained from patients with acute farmer's lung are significantly higher than in asymptomatic dairy farmers, although this finding does not appear to correlate with either clinical abnormalities or the prognosis of the disease.[259,260]

DIFFERENTIAL DIAGNOSIS

Acute Hypersensitivity Pneumonitis

The diagnosis of acute *nonprogressive and intermittent* HP is often difficult to make and depends on the clinician's index of suspicion. Without a history of illness occurring within hours of exposure to an identifiable agent, the clinical syndrome is indistinguishable from an acute respiratory infection such as an episode of flu or from an atypical pneumonia caused by viral or mycoplasmal agents.[261] Furthermore, it has been described that patients with genuine HP may show a nonspecific rise of influenza viruses or *Mycoplasma pneumoniae* antibody titers.[262]

In farmers, the differential diagnosis must include the organic dust toxic syndrome (ODTS), which is usually associated with unloading silos.[263] In contrast to patients with acute HP, patients with ODTS generally have no precipitins to antigens of molds and usually present with normal clinical findings on respiratory examination and chest radiographs. The syndrome is characterized by fever or facial warmth without fever, chills, shivering, malaise, fatigue, muscle and joint aches, headache, with or without dry cough, nasal irritation, throat burning, mild dyspnea, chest tightness, and wheezing. Lung morphology exhibits acute neutrophilic inflammation in the terminal bronchioles and the alveolar septa without the typical features of HP.[264] Bacterial endotoxins and fungal toxins of moldy hay have been proposed as causative agents of ODTS.[263] It has been suggested that ODTS is associated with extreme exposure that occurs on a single day. By contrast, although the concentration of mold spores or actinomycetes are often found to be high, HP is associated with lower more prolonged exposure levels.[265] The toxic syndrome has a benign course without long-term effects.

Acute Progressive (Subacute) and Chronic Forms

The differential diagnosis of the acute progressive form of the disease includes some granulomatous lung infections such as tuberculosis and noninfectious granulomatous lung disorders, which is mainly sarcoidosis.[1,266,267] Some characteristics of a differential diagnosis are explained in Table 19–2.

TABLE 19–2   Differential Diagnosis between Hypersensitivity Pneumonitis, Tuberculosis, and Sarcoidosis

Findings	Hypersensitivity Pneumonitis	Tuberculosis	Sarcoidosis
Diffuse interstitial alveolitis	All cases	Uncommon	Uncommon
Granulomas	Poorly formed, around the airway walls	Caseating granulomas	Well defined, located along lymphatics
Fever	Rare	Common	Rare
PPD	Not relevant	Usually positive	Negative
BAL T cells	Increases of CD8+	Increases of CD4+	Increases of CD4+
CD4/CD8 ratio	Decreased	Increased	Increased
SACE	Usually negative	Occasionally positive	Usually positive
Hilar lymphadenopathy	Unfrequent	Occasionally (more often in primary TB)	Frequent (stages I and II)
Cavitation	Uncommon	Common	Uncommon

BAL = bronchoalveolar lavage; SACE = serum angiotensin converting enzyme; PPD = purified protein derivative; TB = tuberculosis.

On the other hand, subacute and chronic HP may be confused with virtually any ILD; lung biopsy is usually required for a precise diagnosis. The chronic progressive form may mimic IPF, one of the most common causes of ILD.

INHALATION CHALLENGE

When the diagnosis is uncertain, a provocation test may be performed using aerosolized materials of the suspected causative agent.[268–272] When indicated, the inhalation provocation study can either re-expose the patient to the suspected agent in the suspected causative natural environment, or it can be conducted in the hospital using controlled antigen inhalation.

Although provocation tests are widely used in asthma, their role for diagnosis in HP has not yet been fully established. Currently, no standardized, commercial source of purified antigens exists. As a result, aerosols prepared in medical laboratories may contain an imprecise mixture of the antigenic substances and may be contaminated with nonspecific irritants.

Patient response to the inhalation challenge may result in an immediate transient reaction. More commonly, however, a delayed response occurs several hours after exposure. The classic responses include fever, malaise, headache, gravity-dependent crackles, neutrophilia, and decreased forced vital capacity (FVC). In general, an accurate reproduction of acute HP symptoms, compounded by positive laboratory and functional test abnormalities, constitutes a positive test (Figure 19–13). With respect to neutrophilia, a considerable increase in blood leukocyte counts can be observed in farmer's lung patients as well as in asymptomatic farmers and normal individuals who are exposed to moldy hay inhalation. However, only patients with HP exhibit neutrophil activation measured through an enhanced respiratory burst.[273] Additionally, an early increase in

BAL total cells, lymphocytes, and neutrophils occurred in PBD postinhalation challenge.[274]

Chest radiographs may, occasionally, present an increase in haziness, density, or nodularity. Auscultatory and roentgenographic abnormalities as well as a reduction of diffusing capacity and hypoxemia may occur if the response is severe. Considering that a severe reaction may be harmful to patients, routine use of the inhalational challenge is not recommended. It should be used only when other assessments have failed and when a lung biopsy is not indicated. When it must be done, the test should always be conducted carefully to elicit a controlled, mild-to-moderate clinical and functional reaction. Results of the inhalational challenge must be interpreted cautiously, keeping in mind that not all patients with HP respond to the challenge.

Reynolds and colleagues[274] conducted a study on 12 patients with PBD who agreed to undergo the challenge, only 7 exhibited a positive response measured by body

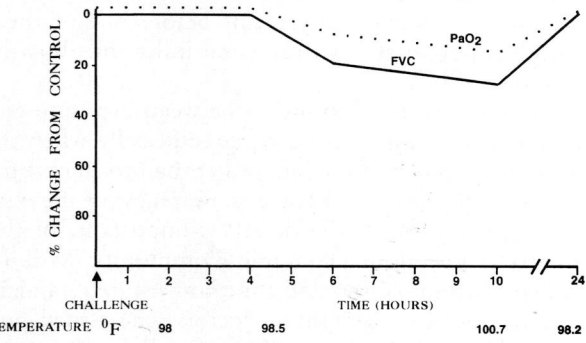

Figure 19–13 Typical findings in an inhalation provocation test. Impairment of lung mechanical function and gas exchange begin about 4 to 6 hours after antigen challenge, reach the maximum change at 8 to 12 hours, and resolve spontaneously 18 to 24 hours later. The lung response is paralleled by fever, a constant finding in a positive test.

temperature, spirometry, and white blood cell count. More recently, the diagnostic usefulness of a provocation test with avian antigens in patients with subacute/chronic PBD has also been determined.[275] The study included 17 patients with HP, 17 with other ILDs, and 5 healthy control subjects who were challenged with pigeon serum. After the inhalation challenge, an increase in body temperature and a significant decrease in FVC, PaO_2, and SO_2 were observed in all patients with PBD and in 3 with ILD. No reaction was noticed in healthy subjects. Receiver operating characteristic (ROC) curves showed that for FVC the best cut-point was a drop of 16% with sensitivity (S) of 76% and specificity (SP) of 81%. The positive predictive value (PPV) and negative predictive value (NPV) were over 80%. Similar results were obtained for a drop of 3 mm Hg in PaO_2 or 3% in SaO_2. The best indicator of a positive test was the body temperature. Thus, an increase in body temperature of > 0.5°C revealed the following: S, 100%; SP, 82%; PPV, 100%; NPV, 86%. A univariate regression analysis confirmed that changes in body temperature and FVC are predictive values for HP with a relative risk of 82.5 (CI, 10.43 to 651.76) and 1.21 (CI, 1.06 to 1.36), respectively. There were no challenge test complications. As mentioned, false negative results were obtained in approximately 20% of patients with other ILDs but not in healthy subjects, suggesting that provocation tests can properly identify patients with HP. In this study, complications of a challenge test were not encountered.

DIAGNOSTIC FORESIGHTS

A low index of suspicion for HP combined with overlapping clinical, radiologic, and functional features contribute to the difficulty of distinguishing this disease from other ILDs. Thus, the most important step is to include HP in the differential diagnosis of any diffuse ILD. An environmental antigen is essential for the development of HP and must be considered when reviewing a patients' clinical history. Some patients consult a number of physicians before one of them considers potential environmental links and thus the diagnosis of HP.

The temporal relationship between exposure and the onset of disease can be vague, especially when the exposure is related to hobbies rather than to an occupation. In addition, the physician's awareness of the etiologic agents associated with HP is important. In this context, a European Economic Community Working Party of epidemiologists and clinicians sent ten standard case histories to a sample of doctors who issued pulmonary-related death certificates in eight European countries.[276] The majority of the physicians certified farmer's lung as "interstitial lung disease." The proportion of physicians who stated farmer's lung as the diagnosis ranged from 0 to 70%; the overall rate of correct certification was only 26%.

In part, many of the diagnostic problems are due to the fact that there are no pathognomonic clinical, radiographic, or physiologic abnormalities for HP. Routine laboratory tests are not helpful, and specific serum precipitating antibodies can be present in a large number of exposed but asymptomatic subjects. Likewise, cellular analysis of BAL is characteristic but nonspecific. Finally, the interval between exposure and the onset of symptoms may be long, or the exposure history may be so subtle that the cause-and-effect relationship may not surface easily.

The diagnosis of HP relies on a cluster of findings that include a suggestive environmental history, symptoms, physical findings, radiographic abnormalities, pulmonary function and immunologic tests, and BAL results. Removing the patient from the suspected environment often results in spontaneous amelioration of symptoms; this finding is useful for orientation to the diagnosis. Likewise, an exacerbation of symptoms after the patient re-enters the suspected workplace or household environment provides strong evidence for establishing the diagnosis.

Inhalation challenge is investigational, but it can be performed in selected patients in whom the causal relationship between antigen and lung disease must be established definitively.

A lung biopsy specimen is required when the diagnosis is not apparent. In many countries, birds are commonly kept as pets. Therefore, a positive history of exposure to birds and the detection of specific antibodies in the sera may not be conclusive. In addition, because the exposure to avian antigens in the domestic environment is usually low grade and continuous, there may be a long latent period before the onset of symptoms, which makes it increasingly difficult to establish the relationship between antigen inhalation and disease. Despite exposure to birds, a patient with clinical, radiologic, and functional abnormalities of ILD may not necessarily have HP. In this context, the morphologic study can confirm the diagnosis. Similarly, unsuspected chronic HP was diagnosed only after biopsy sampling in a family with several cases of familial IPF.[277] Thus, our bias in the "to open or not to open" issue is "to open" and obtain a lung biopsy. In addition to providing a specific diagnosis by histologic features, lung biopsy also permits a better prognostic approach, particularly in chronic HP.

In general, evidence for the diagnosis of HP should include the following:

1. Antecedent of exposure and positive specific antibodies
2. BAL lymphocytes higher than 40%
3. Clinical behavior of an ILD
4. HRCT with ground-glass attenuation plus centrilobular nodules without air space consolidation
5. Positive inhalation challenge or compatible histopathologic findings

HISTOLOGY

The pathologic changes observed in HP are similar, regardless of the causative antigen, and depend largely on the stage of the disease. Because most patients have a biopsy taken in the acute progressive (subacute) and chronic stages, morphologically speaking, these are the best described. In contrast, relatively little is known about the pathology of acute HP, in which interstitial inflammation with deposition of immunoglobulins and complement and mild obstructive bronchiolitis have been described.

Typical pathologic features in acute progressive and chronic HP are represented by interstitial and luminal alveolitis, intra-alveolar exudate, non-necrotizing granulomas, and bronchiolitis; in the chronic form, interstitial fibrosis with collagenous thickening of alveolar septa is seen (Figures 19–14 to 19–17).[278] Additionally, intra-alveolar fibrinous and proteinaceous edema are usually observed in the early phases of HP.

The histologic hallmark of subacute and chronic HP is a granulomatous interstitial pneumonitis characterized by a prominent, often patchy, interstitial infiltrate that usually begins near the terminal bronchioles but may extend widely into the parenchyma. Alveolitis is composed predominantly of lymphocytes, plasma cells, monocytes, and macrophages. Foamy macrophages prevail in the air spaces, whereas lymphocytes are more abundant in the interstitium. In striking resemblance to BAL findings, the percentage of CD8[+] T-cell subsets is usually greater than that of CD4[+] helper cells in the pulmonary parenchyma, and a certain number of interstitial lymphocytes appear to coexpress both surface receptors.[279]

Striking aggregates of intra-alveolar and interstitial foam cells, which probably represent the foci of obstructive pneumonitis, are seen in a number of cases.[280]

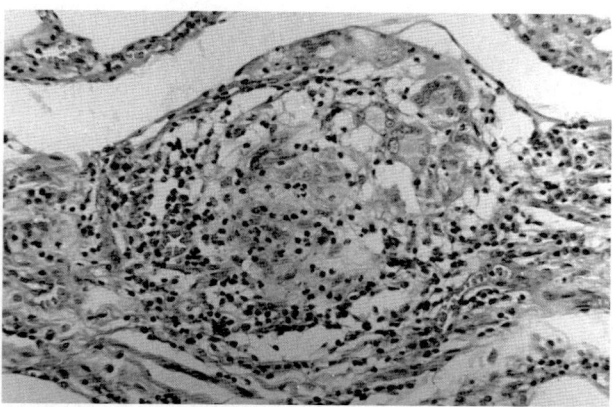

Figure 19–15 Micrograph of a noncaseating interstitial granuloma in a patient with acute progressive hypersensitivity pneumonitis (hematoxylin and eosin; ×100 original magnification).

Although the presence of granulomas is a classic histologic feature of HP, the granulomas differ from those of sarcoidosis. The granulomas seen in HP are usually small, poorly differentiated, loosely arranged, and contain a high concentration of lymphocytes. Their borders are usually blurred by surrounding lymphocytes and monocytes. In contrast, sarcoid granulomas are somewhat larger, rich in multinucleated giant cells, and have sharply defined perimeters; mononuclear inflammatory cells are less numerous and tend to be excluded from the granuloma. Rarely, a small area of necrosis may be present in the center of a granuloma, but caseation is virtually absent.

In the absence of granulomas, the histopathologic pattern in subacute/chronic HP can be very similar to that observed in nonspecific interstitial pneumonia.[281]

Bronchiolocentric lesions and the presence of some giant multinucleated cells may support the diagnosis of HP.

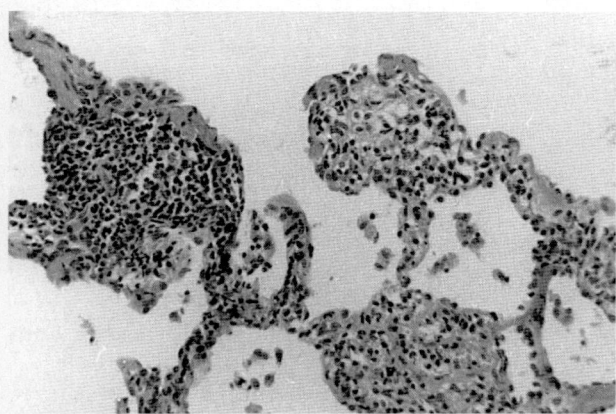

Figure 19–14 Lung sample micrograph from a patient with acute progressive (subacute) hypersensitivity pneumonitis showing diffuse mononuclear interstitial inflammation, two poorly formed noncaseating granulomas, and a lymphoid aggregate (hematoxylin and eosin; ×62.5 original magnification).

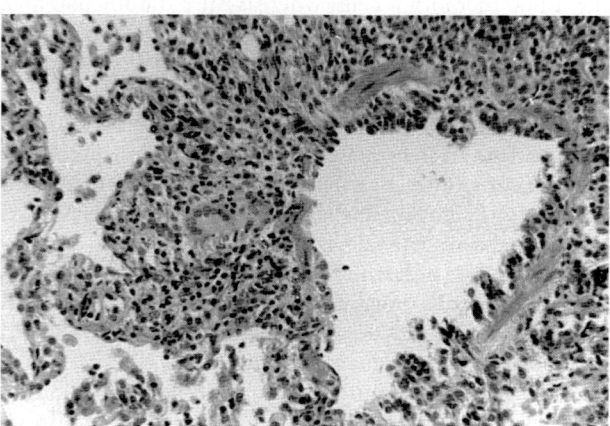

Figure 19–16 Micrograph of cellular bronchiolitis with some multinucleated cells (hematoxylin and eosin; ×62.5 original magnification).

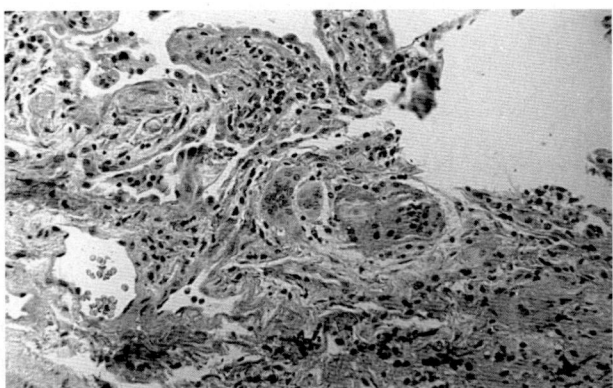

Figure 19–17   Micrograph of a lung sample of chronic hypersensitivity pneumonitis. In addition to the interstitial mononuclear infiltrate and a cluster of multinucleated giant cells, distortion of the lung architecture with increased matrix deposition is also noticed (hematoxylin and eosin; ×62.5 original magnification).

Small airways are usually involved in HP. However, bronchiolar abnormalities seem to vary and are dependent on the causative antigen. Thus, proliferative bronchiolitis obliterans, consisting of an intraluminal organizing exudate composed of fibroblasts, a mucopolysaccharide matrix, and mixed chronic inflammatory cells, has been described in farmer's lung.[282] In contrast, chronic PBD is associated with peribronchiolar inflammation and fibrosis. These changes, along with smooth muscle hypertrophy, produce a histopathologic picture suggestive of constrictive bronchiolitis.[167,191] Several factors could account for such differences, including the nature of the inhaled particles and the type of exposure. Additionally, peribronchiolar lymphoid aggregates and occasional hyperplasia of lymphoid follicles are also seen (see Figure 19–14). Recently, the presence of bronchus-associated lymphoid tissue was described in three out of five studied patients.[283] Analysis of the cellular composition revealed that the follicular area was composed of B lymphocytes, including memory B cells, whereas the parafollicular area was composed of T lymphocytes.

Vascular lesions similar to hypertensive pulmonary vascular disease, particularly medial hypertrophy in arteries and arterioles and, less frequently, cellular intimal proliferation in the smallest muscular arteries and arterioles, are sometimes seen in lung specimens obtained from patients with chronic HP (Figure 19–18).[284] Vasculitis is virtually absent, but it has been reported in a "hyperacute" fatal case of farmer's lung.[285]

A reversible, localized alveolar-septal amyloidosis was reported in a case of mollusk-shell allergic alveolitis,[286] but its significance is unknown.

As previously mentioned, variable degrees of fibrotic changes are histologic features of chronic HP; fibrosis can be a conspicuous histologic finding in the pulmonary parenchyma of advanced cases of HP, particularly in those with chronic progressive disease. When present, the association of mild or moderate infiltration with lymphocytes, some giant cells, and the occasional poorly formed granuloma indicates that the pulmonary fibrosis may be secondary to HP. Nevertheless, histologic changes in advanced chronic HP may not differ from those found in other fibrotic lung disorders. In this instance, the "nonspecific pulmonary fibrosis" reported by pathologists is often ambiguous because it may be a mere representation of an end histologic reaction of HP.

Emphysematous changes are usually related to the foci of fibrosis, which have also been described in chronic cases.[284]

In most cases, a specific etiologic diagnosis through histologic examination is not possible. Pathologic changes are strongly suggestive of HP, but the specific organic particle cannot be determined. Sporadically, it is possible to detect specific antibodies against avian antigens in the lung tissue of patients with PBD. It is also possible to find positive staining for *thermophilic actinomycetes* in biopsy specimens of farmer's lung or to find spores of *Cryptostroma corticale* within histiocytes or granulomas in maple bark stripper's disease.[287] However, the antigen responsible for the disease should be sought by a detailed clinical history and laboratory studies of circulating specific antibodies.

Ultrastructural studies have confirmed the features of mononuclear alveolitis and the presence of noncaseating granulomas and intra-alveolar buds. In addition, endothelial damage with swelling and bleb formation, thrombosis of capillaries, perivascular edema, loss of microvilli in the ciliated bronchiolar epithelium, and rarefaction and multilamellation of the basement membrane have been described.[288–290] In several areas, type I pneumocytes are separated from the alveolar wall, and there is hyperplasia of type II alveolar epithelial cells. Intra-alveolar clusters of loose connective tissue attached to alveolar walls by a stalk, containing small numbers of mononuclear phagocytes and mesenchymal cells, can be found. Eventually, the clusters incorporated into the alve-

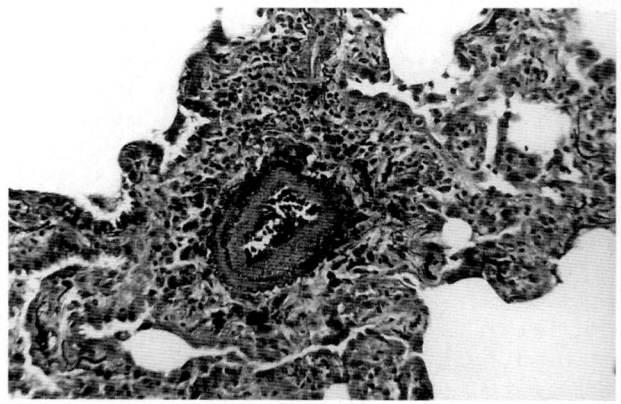

Figure 19–18   Micrograph of moderate vascular changes characterized by arteriolar proliferation of intimal cells in chronic hypersensitivity pneumonitis (Verhoeff-van Gieson; ×62.5 original magnification).

olar walls. Epithelial and endothelial damage are most often observed in inflammatory areas, whereas type II cell hyperplasia is mainly identified in fibrotic tissues.[291] Often, in lung tissue considered normal by light microscopy, the air-blood barrier is found to be damaged.

BRONCHIAL HYPERREACTIVITY, ASTHMA, AND HYPERSENSITIVITY PNEUMONITIS

It is not clear whether HP and asthma can coexist in the same patient. A number of patients with HP complain of wheezing, dry cough, or increased bronchial responsiveness to nonspecific stimuli. In our experience with PBD, this situation occurs in about 10% of nonasthmatic patients who develop HP. We have also found that during periods of exuberant lung inflammation or when the disease is healing, patients may develop bronchial symptoms including airway hyperreactivity (unpublished results).

Similarly, in farmer's lung, bronchial hyperresponsiveness has been demonstrated during the acute phase of the disease as well as in subjects with past histories of farmer's lung.[292,293] Occasionally, asthma has been diagnosed in patients with recurrent farmer's lung; in these cases, both diseases started at the same time.[294]

In a 5-year follow-up study of 101 patients with farmer's lung who did not have asthma at the time of the initial evaluation, it was found that 7 of the patients later developed asthma.[295] Thus, it seems possible that patients who have had an episode of HP may have an increased risk of developing subsequent asthma. Furthermore, challenge tests with crude extracts of antigens to which patients with HP are allergic may show an early or late asthmatic response instead of, or in addition to, the alveolar response.[167]

However, in another study involving dairy farmers,[296] it was found that bronchial hyperresponsiveness to methacholine may occur in patients with farmer's lung as well as in exposed but asymptomatic farmers with and without antibodies to *M. faeni* and/or *T. vulgaris*. This finding suggests that bronchial hyperreactivity among dairy farmers is not due to past episodes of farmer's lung or sensitization to mold antigens but may be due to the occupational environment of dairy farming.

On the other hand, it is known that exposure to some "classic" HP antigens can provoke an "asthmatic response" in some individuals, without provoking extrinsic alveolitis. For example, Pelikan and colleagues[297] found that 18 out of 160 (11.3%) patients with "allergic" asthma or "asthmatic bronchitis" without HP were regularly exposed to pigeons. Similarly, Hargreave and Pepys[271] reported that 18 asthmatics were reactive to bird antigens. When exposed to avian antigens, patients may exhibit either an early, late, or dual asthmatic reaction.

It is difficult to understand whether the same antigen is responsible for the asthma and HP, given that patients are often exposed to a mixture of antigens. Studies of individuals who inhale simple chemicals (eg, isocyanates and Pauli's reagent [sodium diazobenzenesulfonate]), strongly suggest that the same antigen can produce both conditions.[298–300] Similarly, a case of penicillin-induced occupational asthma coexisting with HP has been described.[301]

Considering the bronchiolitis usually observed in HP, it appears that there may be a link between this disease and bronchial hyperreactivity; the inflammatory response in the small airways can have a marked effect on airways' caliber and cause hyperresponsiveness and reversible obstruction of the airway. It has been suggested that chronic bronchiolitis is an important factor in determining airway obstruction in asthma.[302] In HP, on the other hand, increased numbers of mast cells and high levels of histamine and leukotriene C_4 have been reported; these substances may also play a role in narrowing the airways.[244,252,303,304]

TREATMENT

Early diagnosis and avoidance of antigen exposure are key elements and the mainstay of treatment regimens. In our experience with PBD, continued antigen inhalation is one of the identified causes of an adverse prognosis.

Recognition and prevention of occupation-related HP is relatively easy but those of domestic-related HP may be difficult due to the complexity of home environments.

The improvement of farm conditions has helped to decrease the incidence of farmer's lung. Likewise, when the colonizing of *T. cutaneum*—the causative agent of summer-type HP in Japan—was found in patients' homes, elimination of the yeast from the domestic environment proved to be efficacious.[305] However, in the case of PBD, high levels of bird antigen may persist for prolonged periods of time in the patient's home, despite removal of the offending birds and a complete environmental clean-up.[306] This finding may account for the persistence of the disease in some patients with HP.

On the other hand, it is important to point out that some patients report complete remission of the disease, despite subsequent exposure to the offending antigen. A 10-year follow-up of patients who had suffered the acute intermittent form of the disease showed a favorable prognosis in spite of continuing avian antigen exposure.[307] There are also data to support the notion that many farmers reluctant to change their occupation or location do not progress to disabling pulmonary fibrosis; this suggests that with appropriate care, most patients with farmer's lung can continue farming.[148] It has been demonstrated in a rabbit model of acute HP that acute alveolitis resulting from antigen challenge does not result in chronic alveolitis in animals repeatedly challenged with the offending antigen. These data suggest a rapid development of antigen-specific desensitization or immunologic tolerance.[308] This response constitutes an intriguing observation that must be investigated further. In spite of this, the primary focus in the treatment of HP is avoidance of further exposure to the organic particle. In this context, a change in patient's habits, occupation, or environment to avoid future contact with the offending antigen should be considered.

Dust masks with filters that can remove the antigenic particles, appropriate ventilation facilities in work areas, mechanization of the feeding process on farms, industrial hygiene, and alterations in forced-air ventilatory systems may be necessary to achieve adequate control. The use of dust masks, for example, has been shown to significantly reduce acute episodes of farmer's lung.[309] However, it is important to consider the practicality of using a mask (ie, comfort) during antigen exposure.

In farmer's lung, it has been shown that the decision to quit farming is usually based on cognitive and behavioral motives rather than direct physiologic limitations the disease may have caused.[310]

Corticosteroids are recommended in acute, severe, and progressive disease. Long-term efficacy of these agents has yet to be determined. In acute farmer's lung, pulmonary function improves after an 8-week course of prednisolone, when compared with placebo. However, this scheme did not influence the long-term clinical and functional behavior of the disease.[311]

Initial high doses of corticosteroids followed by gradual tapering once clinical improvement has begun, is the usual regimen. Although long-term efficacy of corticosteroid therapy in acute progressive and chronic HP remains to be definitively established, this treatment is often used. The empiric scheme is similar to those recommended for other chronic, noninfectious, non-neoplastic ILDs and consists of 1 mg per kg per day of prednisone for a month followed by a gradual reduction until a maintenance dose of 10 to 15 mg per day is reached. Prednisone is discontinued when the patient is considered to be healed or when there is no clinical and/or functional response. If pulmonary abnormalities recur or deteriorate during the prednisone taper, the maintenance regimen should be prolonged indefinitely.

Inhaled steroids could theoretically be used to reduce the severe side effects of prolonged systemic steroid therapy. However, there is very little experience with this approach.[312,313] A study of patients with subacute and chronic HP suggested that high doses of inhaled beclomethasone may achieve similar benefits as that of oral prednisone without systemic adverse effects.[312]

In a murine model of HP, it was found that liposome-encapsulated dexamethasone had a greater effect on several parameters, such as BAL abnormalities and lung index, than standard free dexamethasone. Liposomal dexamethasone did not inhibit adrenocorticotropic hormone (ACTH) secretions as compared with standard dexamethasone.[314]

In patients with documented hyperreactive airways, the use of inhaled bronchodilators is appropriate. Finally, some encouraging results are emerging regarding the use of cyclosporine and lipoxygenase inhibitors, at least in experimental HP as well as in other experimentally induced granulomatous lung disorders. To date however, no data in human subjects are available.

PROGNOSIS AND SURVIVAL

The long term outcome of HP varies greatly from patient to patient and depends on several factors: the type and duration of antigen exposure, the dose and chemical composition of the inhaled antigen, and the lung-host response to the immunopathologic damage.

Data on mortality rates associated with HP are limited and often contradictory. For example, there were no reported HP-related deaths in any of several long-term clinical studies.[148,315,316] In one retrospective study that examined a large pool of death certificates and incidence data, the mortality rate associated with HP was approximately 1%.[317] Other retrospective studies have reported HP-associated mortality in patients with chronic disease[284,318]; three fatal cases among Canadian farmers with progressive pulmonary fibrosis due to chronic farmer's lung provoked by *Penicillium brevicompactum* have been recently reported.[319]

Acute PBD appears to have a favorable prognosis. A long-term follow-up of 24 patients demonstrated that the majority of patients surveyed reported clinical improvements, in spite of continual exposure to antigens. The study, which provided a follow-up window of 10 years, did not report any acute PBD-related deaths.[307]

A different impression emerged from our studies in chronic PBD.[200] In a cohort of 78 patients with chronic PBD, approximately 25% of surveyed patients died within 5 years of the initial diagnosis of chronic PBD. In the absence of typical acute symptoms, patients with an insidious onset of the disease may evolve to progressive and irreversible pulmonary damage, and a fairly large percentage risk death as a consequence of diffuse lung fibrosis.

Other studies have shown that airflow obstruction with or without emphysema, is an important long-term sequela of farmer's lung, yet they have not provided definitive mortality data.[316,320,321]

In a recent study,[322] the long-term outcome of 88 patients with farmer's lung and 83 matched control farmers was evaluated using HRCT and functional tests. Most of the studied subjects were nonsmokers. Emphysema was found significantly more often (23%) in patients with farmer's lung than in control farmers (7%). The presence of emphysema was most frequent in smokers. Patients with recurrent attacks of farmer's lung tended to have emphysema more often than patients who had experienced only a single attack. No differences were observed in relation to fibrosis. In general, all these studies strongly suggest that whereas chronic PBD may evolve to fibrosis, farmer's lung disease seems to be associated with an increased risk of developing emphysema.

In the case of a fibrotic response, the best predictors of mortality are the severity of fibrosis revealed on open lung biopsy, the presence of honeycombing on chest radiograph, and digital clubbing.[166,200]

Although it has been suggested that the presence of BAL fibrosing factors such as hyaluronic acid, type III procollagen, fibronectin, and fibroblast growth factors may reflect early fibrosis, these parameters do not correlate with long-term outcome and do not appear to have any predictive value.[316] Likewise, antibody activities of IgG and IgA subclasses, as well as BAL lymphocytosis are considered to be useless in determining the progression or disappearance of HP.[232,323] Data concerning T-cell subsets are controversial. According to one study, continuous exposure is accompanied by a persistent high-intensity alveolitis, characterized by an increase in CD8[+] cells and a persistent low CD4[+]/CD8[+] ratio.[215] Other authors, however, have reported that an insidious onset with a relatively increased CD4[+] subset are seen in patients evolving to fibrosis, whereas an acute onset with increased CD8[+] occur in HP unaccompanied by lung fibrosis.[324]

REFERENCES

1. Selman M, Chapela R, Salas J, et al. Hypersensitivity pneumonitis: clinical approach and an integral concept about its pathogenesis. A Mexican point of view. In: Selman M, Barrios R, editors. Interstitial pulmonary diseases: selected topics. Boca Raton (FL): CRC Press; 1991. p. 171–98.
2. Ramazzini da Capri B. De Morbis Artificum Diatriba, 1713. Translation. Chicago (IL): University of Chicago Press; 1940.
3. Campbell JA. Acute symptoms following work with hay. BMJ 1932;2:1143–4.
4. Pickles WW. Farmer's lung. Public Health (Lond) 1944;58:2–4.
5. Jamison SG, Hopkins J. Bagassosis: a fungus disease of the lung. N Ore Med Surg 1941;93:580–2.
6. Pearsall HR, Morgan EH, Teslu H, et al. Parakeet dander pneumonitis: acute psittaco-kerato-pneumoconiosis. Bull Mason Clin 1960;14:127–37.
7. Plessner MM. Une maladie des trieurs de plumes: la fievre de canard. Arch Mal Praf 1960;21:67–71.
8. Banaszak EF, Thiede WH, Fink JN. Hypersensitivity pneumonitis due to contamination of an air conditioner. N Engl J Med 1970;283:271–6.
9. Daniele RP, Henson PM, Fantone JC, et al. Immune complex injury of the lung. Am Rev Respir Dis 1981;124:738–55.
10. Schkade PA, Routes JM. Hypersensitivity pneumonitis in a patient with hypogammaglobulinemia. J Allergy Clin Immunol 1996;98:710–2.
11. Salvaggio JE, Millhollon BW. Allergic alveolitis: new insights into old mysteries. Respir Med 1993;87:495–501.
12. Costabel U, Bross KJ, Marxen J, Matthys H. T-lymphocytosis in bronchoalveolar lavage fluid of hypersensitivity pneumonitis. Chest 1984;85:514–8.
13. Trentin L, Zambello R, Facco M, et al. Selection of T lymphocytes bearing limited TCR-Vβ regions in the lung of hypersensitivity pneumonitis and sarcoidosis. Am J Respir Crit Care Med 1997;155:587–96.
14. Semenzato G, Trentin L, Zambello R, et al. Different types of cytotoxic lymphocytes recovered from the lungs of patients with hypersensitivity pneumonitis. Am Rev Respir Dis 1988;137:70–4.
15. Bice D, Salvaggio JE, Hoffman E. Passive transfer of experimental hypersensitivity pneumonitis with lymphoid cells in the rabbit. J Allergy Clin Immunol 1976;58:250–62.
16. Schuyler M, Shopp G, Crooks L. CD31 and CD41 cells adoptively transfer experimental hypersensitivity pneumonitis. Am Rev Respir Dis 1992;146:1582–8.
17. Fournier E, Tonnel AB, Gosset PH, et al. Early neutrophil alveolitis after antigen inhalation in hypersensitivity pneumonitis. Chest 1985;88:563–6.
18. Yoshizawa Y, Nomura A, Ohdama S, et al. The significance of complement activation in the pathogenesis of hypersensitivity pneumonitis; sequential changes of complement components and chemotactic activities in bronchoalveolar lavage fluids. Int Arch Allergy Appl Immunol 1988;87:417–23.
19. Grech V, Vella C, Lenicker H. Pigeon breeder's lung in childhood: varied clinical picture at presentation. Pediatr Pulmonol 2000;30:145–8.
20. Flaherty DK, Braun SR, Marx JJ, et al. Serologically detectable HLA-A, B, C loci antigens in farmer's lung disease. Am Rev Respir Dis 1980;122:437–43.
21. Ritner G, Sennenkamp J, Mollenhauer E, et al. Pigeon breeder's lung association with HLA-DR3. Tissue Antigens 1983;21:374–8.
22. Selman M, Teran L, Mendoza A, et al. Increase of HLA-DR7 in pigeon breeder's lung in a Mexican population. Clin Immunol Immunopathol 1987;44:63–70.
23. Ando M, Hirayama K, Soda K, et al. HLA-DQw3 in Japanese summer-type hypersensitivity pneumonitis induced by *Trichosporon cutaneum*. Am Rev Respir Dis 1989;140:948–50.
24. Camarena A, Juarez A, Mejia M, et al. Major histocompatibility complex and tumor necrosis factor-alpha polymorphisms in pigeon breeder's disease. Am J Respir Crit Care Med 2001;163:1528–33.
25. Schaaf BM, Seitzer U, Pravica V, et al. Tumor necrosis factor-alpha -308 promoter gene polymorphism and increased tumor necrosis factor serum bioactivity in farmer's lung patients. Am J Respir Crit Care Med 2001;163:379–82.
26. Salvaggio JE. Current concepts in the pathogenesis of occupationally induced allergic pneumonitis. Int Arch Allergy Appl Immunol 1987;82:424–34.
27. Keller RH, Swartz S, Schlueter DP, et al. Immunoregulation in hypersensitivity pneumonitis. Phenotypic and functional studies of bronchoalveolar lavage lymphocytes. Am Rev Respir Dis 1984;130:766–71.
28. Keller RH, Calvanico NJ, Stevens O. Hypersensitivity pneumonitis in nonhuman primates. 1. Studies on the relationship of immunoregulation and disease activity. J Immunol 1982;128:116–22.
29. Calvanico NJ, Garancis JC. Specificity and duration of postinflammatory suppression in rabbit lungs challenged with aerosolized antigen. Clin Exp Immunol 1985;59:336–41.
30. Cormier Y, Belanger J, Laviolette M. Persistent bronchoalveolar lymphocytosis in asymptomatic farmers. Am Rev Respir Dis 1986;133:843–7.
31. Mossmann TR, Subash S. The expanding universe of T-cell subsets: Th1, Th2 and more. Immunol Today 1996;17:138–46.
32. Jones KP, Reynolds SP, Capper S, et al. Measurement of interleukin-6 in bronchoalveolar lavage fluid by radioimmunoassay: differences between patients with interstitial lung disease and control subjects. Clin Exp Immunol 1991;83:30–4.
33. Denis M. Interleukin-6 in mouse hypersensitivity pneumonitis: changes in lung free cells following depletion of endogenous IL-6 or direct administration of IL-6. J Leukoc Biol 1992;52:197–201.
34. Allen DH, Basten A, Williams GV, Woolcock AJ. Familial hypersensitivity pneumonitis. Am J Med 1975;59:505–14.
35. Cormier Y, Israel-Assayag E, Fournie M, Tremblay GM. Mod-

ulation of experimental hypersensitivity pneumonitis by Sendai virus. J Lab Clin Med 1993;121:683–8.

36. Cormier Y, Tremblay GM, Fournier M, Israel-Assayag E. Long-term viral enhancement of lung response to *Saccharopolyspora rectivirgula*. Am J Respir Crit Care Med 1994; 149:490–4.

37. Gudmundsson G, Monick MM, Hunninghake GW. Viral infection modulates expression of hypersensitivity pneumonitis. J Immunol 1999;162:7397–401.

38. Dakhama A, Hegele RG, Laflamme G, et al. Common respiratory viruses in lower airways of patients with acute hypersensitivity pneumonitis. Am J Respir Crit Care Med 1999;159:1316–22.

39. Israel-Assayag E, Dakhama A, Lavigne S, et al. Expression of costimulatory molecules on alveolar macrophages in hypersensitivity pneumonitis. Am J Respir Crit Care Med 1999;159:1830–4.

40. Chapela R, Selman M, Salas J, et al. Influencia del embarazo y puerperio en el desarrollo de la alveolitis alérgica extrínseca. Allergol Immunopathol (Madr) 1985;13:305–9.

41. Vogelmeier C, Krombach F, Munzig S, et al. Activation of blood neutrophils in acute episodes of farmer's lung. Am Rev Respir Dis 1993;148:396–400.

42. Pforte A, Schiessler A, Gais P, et al. Expression of the adhesion molecule ICAM-1 on alveolar macrophages and in serum in extrinsic allergic alveolitis. Respiration 1993;60:221–6.

43. Semenzato G. Immunology of interstitial lung diseases: cellular events taking place in the lung of sarcoidosis, hypersensitivity pneumonitis and HIV infection. Eur Respir J 1991;4:94–102.

44. Pesci A, Bertorelli G, Olivieri D. Mast cells in bronchoalveolar lavage fluid and in transbronchial biopsy specimens of patients with farmer's lung disease. Chest 1991;100: 1197–202.

45. Takizawa H, Ohta K, Koichi H. Mast cells are important in the development of hypersensitivity pneumonitis. A study with mast cell-deficient mice. J Immunol 1989;143:1982–8.

46. Yamasaki H, Ando M, Brazer W, et al. Polarized type 1 cytokine profile in bronchoalveolar lavage T cells of patients with hypersensitivity pneumonitis. J Immunol 1999;163:3516–23.

47. Antoniades H, Bravo M, Galanopoulos T, Selman M. Molecular basis for the role of platelet-derived growth factor in pulmonary fibrosis. In: Selman M, Barrios R, editors. Interstitial pulmonary diseases. Selected topics. Boca Raton (FL): CRC Press; 1991. p. 35–46.

48. Selman M, González G, López JS, et al. Effect of lung T-lymphocytes on fibroblasts in idiopathic pulmonary fibrosis and allergic extrinsic alveolitis. Thorax 1990;45:451–5.

49. Denis M, Ghadirian E. Transforming growth factor-β is generated in the course of hypersensitivity pneumonitis: contribution to collagen synthesis. Am J Respir Cell Mol Biol 1992;7:156–60.

50. Pardo A, Barrios R, Gaxiola M, et al. Increase of lung neutrophils in hypersensitivity pneumonitis is associated with lung fibrosis. Am J Respir Crit Care Med 2000;161: 1698–704.

51. Selman M, Montaño M, Ramos C, et al. Lung collagen metabolism and the clinical course of hypersensitivity pneumonitis. Chest 1988;94:347–53.

52. Montaño M, Ramos C, González G, et al. Lung collagenase inhibitors and spontaneous and latent collagenase activity in idiopathic pulmonary fibrosis and hypersensitivity pneumonitis. Chest 1989;96:1115–9.

53. Lacey J, Crook B. Fungal and actinomycete spores as pollutants of the workplace and occupational allergens. Ann Occup Hyg 1988;32:515–33.

54. Cohen HI, Merigan TC, Kosek JC, Eldridge F. Sequoisis. A granulomatous pneumonitis associated with redwood sawdust inhalation. Am J Med 1967;43:785–94.

55. Avilia R, Lacey J. The role of *Penicillium frequentans* in suberosis (respiratory disease in workers in the cork industry). Clin Allergy 1974;4:109–17.

56. Wenzel FJ, Emanuel DA. The epidemiology of maple bark disease. Arch Environ Health 1967;14:385–9.

57. Belin L. Sawmill alveolitis in Sweden. Int Arch Allergy Appl Immunol 1987;82:440–3.

58. Enarson DA, Chan-Yeung M. Characterization of health effects of wood dust exposures. Am J Ind Med 1990;17:33–8.

59. Gregory PM, Lacey ME. Mycological examination of the dust from mouldy hay associated with farmer's lung disease. J Gen Microbiol 1963;30:75–84.

60. Buechner H, Prevatt A, Thompson J, Blitz O. Bagassosis: review with further historical data, studies of pulmonary function, results of adrenal steroid therapy. Am J Med 1958;25:234–47.

61. Bringhurst L, Byrne R, Bershon-Cohen J. Respiratory disease of mushroom workers. JAMA 1959;171:15–8.

62. Riddle HF, Channel S, Blyth W. Allergic alveolitis in a malt-worker. Thorax 1968;23:271–80.

63. Schlueter D. Cheesewasher's disease: a new occupational hazard? Ann Intern Med 1973;78:606–13.

64. Sosman AJ, Schlueter DP, Fink JN, Barboriak JJ. Hypersensitivity to wood dust. N Engl J Med 1969;281:977–80.

65. Emanuel DA, Wenzel FJ, Lawton BR. Pneumonitis due to *Cryptostroma corticale* (maple bark disease). N Engl J Med 1966;274:1413–8.

66. Dykewicz MS, Laufer P, Patterson R, et al. Woodman's disease: hypersensitivity pneumonitis from cutting live trees. J Allergy Clin Immunol 1988;81:455–60.

67. Fink JN, Banaszak EF, Barboriak JJ, et al. Interstitial lung disease due to contamination of forced air systems. Ann Intern Med 1976;84:406–13.

68. Fergusson RJ, Milne LJR, Crompton GK. Penicillium allergic alveolitis: faulty installation of central heating. Thorax 1987;42:32–7.

69. Kohler P, Gross G, Salvaggio J, Hawkins J. Humidifier lung: hypersensitivity pneumonitis related to thermotolerant bacterial aerosols. Chest 1976;69 Suppl:294–305.

70. Malmberg P, Rask-Andersen A. Natural and adoptive immune reactions to inhaled microorganisms in the lung of farmers. Scand J Work Environ Health 1988;14 Suppl 1:68–71.

71. Ganier M, Lieberman P, Fink JN, Lockwood DG. Humidifier lung. An outbreak in office workers. Chest 1980;77:183–7.

72. Hinojosa M, Fraj J, De la Hoz B, et al. Hypersensitivity pneumonitis in workers exposed to esparto grass (*Stipa tenacissima*) fibers. J Allergy Clin Immunol 1996;98:985–91.

73. Ranalli G, Grazia L, Roggeri A. The influence of hay-packing techniques on the presence of *Saccharopolyspora rectivirgula*. J Appl Microbiol 1999;87:359–65.

74. Lacey J, Lacey ME. Spore concentrations in the air of farm buildings. Trans Br Mycol Soc 1964;47:547–52.

75. McGrath DS, Kiely J, Cryan B, Bredin CP. Farmer's lung in Ireland (1983–1996) remains at a constant level. Ir J Med Sci 1999;168:21–4.

76. Franz T, McMurrain K, Brooks S, Bernstein I. Clinical, immunologic, physiologic observations in factory workers exposed to *B. subtilis* enzyme dust. J Allergy 1971;47:170–8.

77. Bernstein DI, Lummus ZL, Santilli G, et al. Machine operator's lung. A hypersensitivity pneumonitis disorder associated with exposure to metalworking fluid aerosols. Chest 1995;108:636–41.

78. Hodgson MJ, Bracker A, Yang C, et al. Hypersensitivity pneumonitis in a metal-working environment. Am J Ind Med 2001;39:616–28.

79. Fox J, Anderson H, Moen T, et al. Metal working fluid-associated hypersensitivity pneumonitis: an outbreak investigation and case-control study. Am J Ind Med 1999;35:58–67.

80. Shelton BG, Flanders WD, Morris GK. *Mycobacterium* sp. as a possible cause of hypersensitivity pneumonitis in machine workers. Emerg Infect Dis 1999;5:270–3.

81. Reed CE, Sosman AJ, Barbee RA. Pigeon breeder's lung. JAMA 1965;193:261–5.

82. Fink JN, Sosman AJ, Barboriak JJ, et al. Pigeon breeder's disease: a clinical study of a hypersensitivity pneumonitis. Ann Intern Med 1968;68:1205–19.

83. Warren CPW. Hypersensitivity pneumonitis due to exposure to budgerigars. Chest 1972;62:170–4.

84. Korn DS, Florman AL, Gribitz I. Recurrent pneumonitis with hypersensitivity pneumonitis to hen litter. JAMA 1968;205:114–5.

85. Boyer RS, Klock LE, Schmidt CD, et al. Hypersensitivity lung disease in the turkey-raising industry. Am Rev Respir Dis 1974;109:630–5.

86. Cunningham AL, Fink JN, Schlueter DP. Hypersensitivity pneumonitis due to dove. Pediatrics 1976;58:436–40.

87. Kokkarinen J, Tukiainen H, Seppa A, Terho EO. Hypersensitivity pneumonitis due to native birds in a bird ringer. Chest 1994;106:1269–71.

88. Sandoval J, Bañales JL, Cortés J, et al. Detection of antibodies against avian antigens in bronchoalveolar lavage from patients with pigeon breeder's disease: usefulness of enzyme-linked immunosorbent assay and enzyme immunotransfer blotting. J Clin Lab Anal 1990;4:81–5.

89. Sennenkamp J, Lange G, Nerger K, et al. Human antibodies against antigens of the sparrow, blackbird, weaver finch, canary, budgerigar, pigeon, and hen using the indirect immunofluorescent technique. Clin Allergy 1981;11:375–84.

90. Fredericks WW. Antigens in pigeon dropping extracts. J Allergy Immunol 1978;61:221–3.

91. Mendoza F, Melendro E, Baltazares M, et al. Cellular immune response to fractionated avian antigens by peripheral blood mononuclear cells from patients with pigeon breeder's disease. J Lab Clin Med 1996;127:23–8.

92. Longbottom JL. Pigeon breeder's disease: quantitative immunoelectrophoretic studies of pigeon bloom antigen. Clin Exp Allergy 1989;19:619–24.

93. Banham SW, McKenzie H, McSharry C, et al. Antibody against a pigeon bloom extract: a further antigen in pigeon breeder's lung. Clin Allergy 1982;12:173–8.

94. Todd A, Coan RM, Allen A. Pigeon breeder's lung: pigeon intestinal mucin, an antigen distinct from pigeon IgA. Clin Exp Immunol 1991;85:453–8.

95. Baldwin CI, Stevens B, Connors S, et al. Pigeon fanciers' lung: the mucin antigen is present in pigeon droppings and pigeon bloom. Int Arch Allergy Immunol 1998;117:187–93.

96. Baldwin CI, Todd A, Bourke SJ, et al. Pigeon fanciers' lung: identification of disease-associated carbohydrate epitopes on pigeon intestinal mucin. Clin Exp Immunol 1999;117:230–6.

97. du Marchie Sarvaas GJ, Merkus JFM, Jongste JC. A family with extrinsic allergic alveolitis caused by wild city pigeons: a case report. Pediatrics 2000;105:E62.

98. Muramatsu T, Miyazaki E, Sawabe T, et al. A case of chronic hypersensitivity pneumonitis due to wild pigeons. Nihon Kokyuki Gakkai Zasshi 2001;39:220–5.

99. Meyer FJ, Bauer PC, Costabel U. Feather wreath lung: chasing a dead bird. Eur Respir J 1996;9:1323–4.

100. Haitjema TJ, van Velzen-Blad H, van den Bosch JMM. Extrinsic allergic alveolitis caused by goose feathers in a duvet. Thorax 1992;47:990–1.

101. Kim K, Dalton JW, Klaustermeyer WB. Subacute hypersensitivity pneumonitis presenting with weight loss and dyspnea. Ann Allergy 1993;71:19–23.

102. Burdon JGW, Stone C. Bird fancier's lung after an unusual exposure to avian protein. Am Rev Respir Dis 1986;134:1319–20.

103. Shimazu K, Ando M, Sakata T, et al. Hypersensitivity pneumonitis induced by *Trichosporon cutaneum*. Am Rev Respir Dis 1984;130:407–11.

104. Mizobe T, Yamasaki H, Doi K, et al. Analysis of serotype-specific antibodies to *Trichosporon cutaneum* types I and II in patients with summer-type hypersensitivity pneumonitis with monoclonal antibodies to serotype-related polysaccharide antigens. J Clin Microbiol 1993;31:1949–51.

105. Miyagawa T, Hamagami S, Tanigawa N. *Cryptococcus albidus*-induced summer-type hypersensitivity pneumonitis. Am J Respir Crit Care Med 2000;161:961–6.

106. Reboux G, Piarroux R, Mauny F, et al. Role of molds in farmer's lung disease in eastern France. Am J Respir Crit Care Med 2001;163:1534–9.

107. Kaukonen K, Savolainen J, Viander M, Terho EO. Avidity of *Aspergillus umbrosus* IgG antibodies in farmer's lung disease. Clin Exp Immunol 1994;95:162–5.

108. Jarvis JQ, Morey PR. Allergic respiratory disease and fungal remediation in a building in a subtropical climate. Appl Occup Environ Hyg 2001;16:380–8.

109. Cormier Y, Israel-Assayag E, Bedard G, Duchaine C. Hypersensitivity pneumonitis in peat moss processing plant workers. Am J Respir Crit Care Med 1998;158:412–7.

110. Pitcher WD. Southwestern internal medicine conference: hypersensitivity pneumonitis. Am J Med Sci 1990;300:251–66.

111. Edwards JH, Griffiths AJ, Mullins J. Protozoa as sources of antigen in humidifier fever. Nature 1976;264:438–9.

112. Yoshizawa Y, Ohtsuka M, Noguchi K, et al. Hypersensitivity pneumonitis induced by toluene diisocyanate. Sequelae of continuous exposure. Ann Intern Med 1989;110:31–4.

113. Vandenplas O, Malo JL, Dugas M, et al. Hypersensitivity pneumonitis-like reaction among workers exposed to diphenylmethane diisocyanate (MDI). Am Rev Respir Dis 1993;147:338–46.

114. Baur X. Hypersensitivity pneumonitis (extrinsic allergic alveolitis) induced by isocyanates. J Allergy Clin Immunol 1995;95:1004–10.

115. Zeiss CR, Wolkonsky P, Chacon R, et al. Syndromes in workers exposed to trimellitic anhydride. A longitudinal clinical and immunologic study. Ann Intern Med 1983;98:8–12.

116. Guillon JM, Joly P, Autran B, et al. Minocycline-induced cell-mediated hypersensitivity pneumonitis. Ann Intern Med 1992;117:476–81.

117. Martin WJ. Pharmacologic and other chemical causes of interstitial lung disease. Chest 1991;100:241–3.

118. Crestani B, Jaccard A, Israel-Biet D, et al. Chlorambucil-associated pneumonitis. Chest 1994;105:634–6.

119. Venet A, Canbarrere I, Bonan G. Five cases of immune mediated amiodarone pneumonitis. Lancet 1984;i:962–3.

120. Lewis LD. Procarbazine associated alveolitis. Thorax 1984;39:206–7.

121. Foucher P, Biour M, Blayac JP, et al. Drugs that may injure the respiratory system. Eur Respir J 1997;10:265–79.

122. Baur X, Chen Z, Marczynski B. Respiratory diseases caused by occupational exposure to 1,5-naphthalene-diisocyanate (NDI): results of workplace-related challenge tests and antibody analyses. Am J Ind Med 2001;39:369–72.

123. Carroll KB, Pepys J, Longbotton JL, et al. Extrinsic allergic alveolitis due to rat serum proteins. Clin Allergy 1975;5:443–56.

124. Pimental JC. Furrier's lung. Thorax 1970;25:387–98.

125. Kotter JM, Ziegler G. Sarkoidale Granulomatose nach mehrjahriger Zirkoniumexposition, eine "Zirkoniumlunge." Pathologe 1992;13:104–9.

126. Liippo KK, Anttila SL, Taikina-Aho O, et al. Hypersensitivity pneumonitis and exposure to zirconium silicate in a young ceramic tile worker. Am Rev Respir Dis 1993;148:1089–92.

127. Metzger WJ, Patterson R, Fink J, et al. Sauna-takers disease: hypersensitivity pneumonitis due to contaminated water in a home sauna. JAMA 1976;236:2209–11.

128. Jacobs RL, Thorner RE, Holcomb JR, et al. Hypersensitivity pneumonitis caused by *Cladosporium* in an enclosed hot-tub area. Ann Intern Med 1986;105:204–6.

129. Khoor A, Leslie KO, Tazelaar HD, et al. Diffuse pulmonary disease caused by nontuberculous mycobacteria in immunocompetent people (hot tub lung). Am J Clin Pathol 2001;115:755–62.

130. Grant IWB, Blyth W, Wardrop VE, et al. Prevalence of farmer's lung in Scotland; a pilot survey. BMJ 1972;1:530–4.

131. Staines FH, Forman JAS. A survey of farmer's lung. J Coll Gen Pract 1961;4:351–6.

132. Depierre A, Dalphin JC, Pernet D, et al. Epidemiological study of farmer's lung in five districts of the French Doubs province. Thorax 1988;43:429–35.

133. Gruchow HW, Hoffmann RG, Marx JJ, et al. Precipitating antibodies to farmer's lung antigens in a Wisconsin farming population. Am Rev Respir Dis 1981;124:411–5.

134. Malmberg P, Rask-Anderson A, Palmgren V, et al. Incidence of organic dust toxic syndrome and allergic alveolitis in Swedish farmers. Int Arch Allergy Appl Immunol 1988;87:47–54.

135. Terho ED, Heinonen OP, Lammi S. Incidence of clinically confirmed farmer's lung disease in Finland. Am J Ind Med 1986;10:330–3.

136. Christensen LT, Schmidt CD, Robbins L. Pigeon breeder's disease. A prevalence study and review. Clin Allergy 1975;5:417–22.

137. Turner-Warwick M. Extrinsic allergic bronchiolo-alveolitis. In: Current topics in immunlogy. Series No. 10. Immunology of the lung. London: Edward Arnold; 1978. p. 165–90.

138. Carrillo T, Rodríguez de Castro F, Cuevas M, et al. Effect of cigarette smoking on the humoral immune response in pigeon fanciers. Allergy 1991;46:241–6.

139. Elman AJ, Tebo T, Fink J, et al. Reactions of poultry farmers against chicken antigens. Arch Environ Health 1968;17:98–100.

140. Warren CPW, Tse KS. Extrinsic allergic alveolitis owing to hypersensitivity to chickens. Significance of sputum precipitins. Am Rev Respir Dis 1974;109:672–7.

141. Yoshida K, Suga M, Nishiura Y, et al. Occupational hypersensitivity pneumonitis in Japan: data on a nationwide epidemiological study. Occup Environ Med 1995;52:570–4.

142. Ando M, Arima K, Yoneda R, Tamura M. Japanese summer-type hypersensitivity pneumonitis. Am Rev Respir Dis 1991;144:765–9.

143. Shimazu K, Ando M, Sakata T, et al. Hypersensitivity pneumonitis induced by *Trichosporon cutaneum*. Am Rev Respir Dis 1984;130:407–11.

144. Ando M, Suga M, Nishiura Y, Miyajima M. Summer-type hypersensitivity pneumonitis. Intern Med 1995;34:707–12.

145. Kreiss K, Hodgson MJ. Building-associated epidemics. In: Walsh PJ, Dudney CS, Copenhaver ED, editors. Indoor air quality. Boca Raton (FL): CRC Press; 1984. p. 87–108.

146. Warren CPW. Extrinsic allergic alveolitis: a disease commoner in non-smokers. Thorax 1977;32:567–9.

147. Carrillo T, Rodríguez de Castro F, Cuevas M, et al. Effect of cigarette smoking on the humoral immune response in pigeon fanciers. Allergy 1991;46:241–6.

148. Cormier Y, Belanger J. Long-term physiologic outcome after acute farmer's lung. Chest 1985;87:796–800.

149. Baur X, Richter G, Pethran A, Czuppon AB. Increased prevalence of IgG-induced sensitization and hypersensitivity pneumonitis (humidifier lung) in nonsmokers exposed to aerosols of a contaminated air conditioner. Respiration 1992;59:211–4.

150. Arima K, Ando M, Ito K, et al. Effect of cigarette smoking on prevalence of summer-type hypersensitivity pneumonitis caused by *Trichosporon cutaneum*. Arch Environ Health 1992;47:274–8.

151. Baldwin CI, Todd A, Bourke S, et al. Pigeon fanciers' lung: effects of smoking on serum and salivary antibody responses to pigeon antigens. Clin Exp Immunol 1998;113:166–72.

152. Dalphin JC, Debieuvre D, Pernet D, et al. Prevalence and risk factors for chronic bronchitis and farmer's lung in French dairy farmers. Br J Ind Med 1993;50:941–4.

153. Hocking WG, Golde DW. The pulmonary alveolar macrophage. N Engl J Med 1979;301:580–7.

154. Lawrence EC, Fox TB, Hall BT, Martin RR. Deleterious effect of cigarette smoking on expression of Ia antigens by human pulmonary alveolar macrophages. Clin Res 1983;31:418A.

155. Brown GP, Iwamoto GK, Monick MM, Hunninghake GW. Cigarette smoking decreases interleukin 1 release by human alveolar macrophages. Am J Physiol 1989;256:C260–6.

156. Yamaguchi E, Itoh A, Furuya K, et al. Release of tumor necrosis factor-alpha from human alveolar macrophages is decreased in smokers. Chest 1993;103:479–83.

157. Costabel EA, Bross KJ, Reuter C, et al. Alterations in immunoregulatory T-cell subsets in cigarette smokers: a phenotypic analysis of bronchoalveolar and blood lymphocytes. Chest 1986;90:39–44.

158. Ohtsuka Y, Munakata M, Tanimura K, et al. Smoking promotes insidious and chronic farmer's lung disease, deteriorates the clinical outcome. Intern Med 1995;34:966–71.

159. Cormier Y, Gagnon L, Berube-Genest F, Fournier M. Sequential bronchoalveolar lavage in experimental extrinsic allergic alveolitis. Am Rev Respir Dis 1988;137:1104–9.

160. Hubbard RC, Ogushi F, Fells GA, et al. Oxidants spontaneously released by alveolar macrophages of cigarette smokers can inactivate the active site of α2-antitrypsin, rendering it ineffective as an inhibitor of neutrophil elastase. J Clin Invest 1987;80:1289–95.

161. Emanuel DA, Wenzel FJ, Bowerman CI, et al. Farmer's lung: clinical, pathologic and immunologic study of 24 patients. Am J Med 1964;37:392–401.

162. Selman M, Chapela R, Raghu G. Hypersensitivity pneumonitis: clinical manifestations, pathogenesis, diagnosis, therapeutic strategies. Semin Respir Med 1993;14:353–64.

163. Sharma OP, Fujimura N. Hypersensitivity pneumonitis: a noninfectious granulomatosis. Semin Respir Infect 1995;10:96–106.

164. Fink JN. Hypersensitivity pneumonitis. Clin Chest Med 1992;13:303–9.

165. Yoshizawa Y, Ohtani Y, Hayakawa H, et al. Chronic hypersensitivity pneumonitis in Japan: a nationwide epidemiologic survey. J Allergy Clin Immunol 1999;103:315–20.

166. Sansores R, Salas J, Chapela R, et al. Clubbing in hypersensitivity pneumonitis. Its prevalence and possible prognostic role. Arch Intern Med 1990;150:1849–51.

167. Selman M, Pérez-Padilla R. Airflow obstruction and airway lesions in hypersensitivity pneumonitis. Clin Chest Med 1993;14:699–714.

168. Dalphin JC, Bildstein F, Pernet D, et al. Prevalence of chronic bronchitis and respiratory function in a group of dairy farmers in the French Doubs province. Chest 1989;95:1244–7.

169. Bourke S, Anderson K, Lynch P, et al. Chronic simple bronchitis in pigeon fanciers: relationship of cough with expectoration to avian exposure and pigeon breeder's disease. Chest 1989;95:598–601.

170. Malmberg P. Health effects of organic dust exposure in dairy farmers. Am J Ind Med 1990;17:7–15.

171. Bourke SJ, Carter R, Anderson K, et al. Obstructive airway disease in non-smoking patients with pigeon fancier's lung. Clin Exp Allergy 1989;19:629–33.

172. Rodríguez de Castro F, Carrillo T, Castillo R, et al. Relationships between characteristics of exposure to pigeon antigens. Chest 1993;103:1059–63.

173. Dalphin JC, Pernet D, Dubiez A, et al. Etiologic factors of chronic bronchitis in dairy farmers. Case control study in the Doubs region of France. Chest 1993;103:417–21.

174. Hasani A, Johnson M, Pavia D, et al. Impairment of lung mucociliary clearance in pigeon fanciers. Chest 1992;102:887–91.

175. Remy-Jardin M, Remy J, Wallaert B, Muller NL. Subacute and chronic bird breeder hypersensitivity pneumonitis: sequen-

tial evaluation with CT and correlation with lung function tests and bronchoalveolar lavage. Radiology 1993;189: 111–8.

176. Hodgson MJ, Parkinson DK, Karpf M. Chest x-rays in hypersensitivity pneumonitis: a metaanalysis of secular trend. Am J Ind Med 1989;16:5–53.

177. Epler GR, McLoud TC, Gaensler EA, et al. Normal chest roentgenograms in chronic diffuse infiltrative lung disease. N Engl J Med 1978;298:934–9.

178. Emanuel DA, Kryda MJ. Farmer's lung disease. Clin Rev Allergy 1983;1:509–32.

179. Cook PG, Wells IP, McGavin CR. The distribution of pulmonary shadowing in farmer's lung. Clin Radiol 1988;39: 21–7.

180. Brain JD, Valberg PA. Deposition of aerosol in the respiratory tract. Am Rev Respir Dis 1979;120:1325–73.

181. Schreck RM. Respiratory airway deposition of aerosols. In: McGath JJ, Barnes CD, editors. Air pollution: physiological effects. New York: Academic Press; 1982. p. 183–221.

182. Hargreave F, Hinson KF, Reid L, et al. The radiological appearances of allergic alveolitis due to bird sensitivity (bird fancier's lung). Clin Radiol 1972;23:1–6.

183. Yonemaru M, Mizuguchi Y, Kasuga I, et al. Hilar and mediastinal lymphadenopathy with hypersensitivity pneumonitis induced by penicillin. Chest 1992;102:1907–9.

184. Niimi H, Kang EY, Kwong JS, et al. CT of chronic infiltrative lung disease: prevalence of mediastinal lymphadenopathy. J Comput Assist Tomogr 1996;20:305–8.

185. McLoud TC, Carrington CB, Gaensler EA. Diffuse infiltrative lung disease: a new scheme for description. Radiology 1983;149:353–63.

186. Buschman DL, Gamsu G, Waldron JA, et al. Chronic hypersensitivity pneumonitis: use of CT in diagnosis. Am J Roentgenol 1992;159:957–60.

187. Silver SF, Muller NL, Miller RR, Lefcoe MS. Hypersensitivity pneumonitis: evaluation with CT. Radiology 1989;173: 441–5.

188. Hansell DM, Moskovic E. High-resolution computed tomography in extrinsic allergic alveolitis. Clin Radiol 1991;43: 8–12.

189. Lynch DA, Rose CS, Way D, King TE. Hypersensitivity pneumonitis: sensitivity of high-resolution CT in a population-based study. AJR Am J Roentgenol 1992;159:469–72.

190. Tomiyama N, Muller NL, Johkoh T, et al. Acute parenchymal lung disease in immunocompetent patients: diagnostic accuracy of high-resolution CT. AJR Am J Roentgenol 2000;174:1745–50.

191. Pérez-Padilla R, Gaxiola MN, Salas J, et al. Bronchiolitis in chronic pigeon breeder's disease. Morphologic evidence of a spectrum of small airway lesions in hypersensitivity pneumonitis induced by avian antigens. Chest 1996;110:371–7.

192. Hansell DM, Wells AU, Padley SPG, Muller NL. Hypersensitivity pneumonitis: correlation of individual patterns with functional abnormalities. Radiology 1996;199:123–8.

193. Chung MH, Edinburgh KJ, Webb EM, et al. Mixed infiltrative and obstructive disease on high-resolution CT: differential diagnosis and functional correlates in a consecutive series. J Thorac Imaging 2001;16:69–75.

194. Cormier Y, Brown M, Worthy S, et al. High-resolution computed tomographic characteristics in acute farmer's lung and in its follow-up. Eur Respir J 2000;16:56–60.

195. Adler BD, Padley SPG, Muller NL, et al. Chronic hypersensitivity pneumonitis: high-resolution CT and radiographic features in 16 patients. Radiology 1992;185:91–5.

196. Lynch DA, Newell JD, Logan PM, et al. Can CT distinguish hypersensitivity pneumonitis from idiopathic pulmonary fibrosis? AJR Am J Roentgenol 1995;165:807–11.

197. Nakata H, Kimoto T, Nakayama T, et al. Diffuse peripheral lung disease: evaluation by high-resolution computed tomography. Radiology 1985;157:181–5.

198. Akira M, Kita N, Higashihara T, et al. Summer-type hypersensitivity pneumonitis: comparison of high-resolution CT and plain radiographic findings. AJR Am J Roentgenol 1992;158:1223–8.

199. Remy-Jardin M, Remy J, Wallaert B, et al. Pulmonary involvement in progressive systemic sclerosis: sequential evaluation with CT, pulmonary function tests, bronchoalveolar lavage. Radiology 1993;188:499–506.

200. Pérez-Padilla R, Salas J, Chapela R, et al. Mortality in Mexican patients with chronic pigeon breeders lung compared to those with usual interstitial pneumonia. Am Rev Respir Dis 1993;148:49–53.

201. DiMarco AF, Briones BI. Chest CT performed too often? Chest 1993;103:985–6.

202. Gamsu G, Sostman D. Magnetic resonance imaging of the thorax. Am Rev Respir Dis 1989;139:254–74.

203. Muller NL, Mayo JR, Zwirewich CV. Value of MR imaging in the evaluation of chronic infiltrative lung diseases: comparison with CT. AJR Am J Roentgenol 1992;158:1205–9.

204. Primack SL, Mayo JR, Hartman TE, et al. MRI of infiltrative lung disease: comparison with pathologic findings. J Comput Assist Tomogr 1994;18:233–8.

205. Selman M. Pulmonary fibrosis: human and experimental disease. In: Rojkind M, editor. Focus on connective tissue in health and disease. Vol. I. Boca Raton, Florida: CRC Press; 1989. p. 123–88.

206. Vanderstappen M, Mornex JF, Lahneche B, et al. Gallium-67 scanning in the staging of cryptogenic fibrosing alveolitis and hypersensitivity pneumonitis. Eur Respir J 1988;1: 517–22.

207. Rinderknecht J, Shapiro L, Krauthammer M, et al. Accelerated clearance of small solutes from the lungs in interstitial lung disease. Am Rev Respir Dis 1980;121:105–17.

208. Bourke SJ, Banham SW, McKillop JH, Boyd G. Clearance of 99mTc-DTPA in pigeon fancier's hypersensitivity pneumonitis. Am Rev Respir Dis 1990;142:1168–71.

209. Schmekel B, Wollmer P, Venge P, et al. Transfer of 99mTc-DTPA and bronchoalveolar lavage findings in patients with asymptomatic extrinsic allergic alveolitis. Thorax 1990;45: 525–9.

210. Uh S, Lee SM, Kim HT, et al. The clearance rate of alveolar epithelium using 99mTc-DTPA in patients with diffuse infiltrative lung diseases. Chest 1994;106:161–5.

211. Marks JD, Luce JM, Lazar NM, et al. Effect of increases in lung volume on clearance of aerosolized solute from human lungs. J Appl Physiol 1985;59:1242–8.

212. Dusser DJ, Minty BD, Collignon MAG, et al. Regional respiratory clearance of aerosolized 99mTc-DTPA: posture and smoking effects. J Appl Physiol 1986;60:2000–6.

213. Boyd G. Clinical and immunological studies in pulmonary extrinsic allergic alveolitis. Scott Med J 1978;23:267–76.

214. Warren CPW, Tse KS, Cherniak RM. Mechanical properties of the lung in extrinsic allergic alveolitis. Thorax 1978; 33:315–21.

215. Du Wayne Schmidt C, Jensen RL, Christensen LT, et al. Longitudinal pulmonary function changes in pigeon breeders. Chest 1988;93:359–63.

216. Pérez-Neria J, Selman M, Rubio H, et al. Relationship between lung inflammation or fibrosis and frequency dependence of compliance in interstitial pulmonary diseases. Respiration 1987;52:254–62.

217. Sansores R, Pérez-Padilla R, Pare P, Selman M. Exponential analysis of the lung pressure-volume curve in patients with chronic pigeon breeder's lung. Chest 1992;101:1352–6.

218. Sansores R, Ramírez A, Pérez-Padilla R, et al. Correlation between pulmonary fibrosis and the lung pressure-volume curve. Lung 1996;174:315–23.

219. Lupi E, Sandoval J, Bialostozky D, et al. Extrinsic allergic alveolitis caused by pigeon breeding at high altitude (2,240 meters). Hemodynamic behavior of pulmonary circulation. Am Rev Respir Dis 1981;124:602–7.

220. Matusiewiez SP, Williamson IJ, Sime PJ, et al. Plasma lactate dehydrogenase. A marker of disease activity in cryptogenic fibrosing alveolitis and extrinsic allergic alveolitis. Eur Respir J 1993;6:1282–6.

221. McSharry C, Banham SW, Lynch PP, Boyd G. Antibody measurement in extrinsic allergic alveolitis. Eur J Respir Dis 1984;65:259–65.

222. Cormier Y, Belanger J, Durand P. Factors influencing the development of serum precipitins to farmer's lung antigen in Quebec dairy farmers. Thorax 1985;40:138–42.

223. Fink JN, Schlueter DP, Sosman AJ, et al. Clinical survey of pigeon breeders. Chest 1972;62:277–81.

224. Calvanico NJ. A component of pigeon dropping extract that reacts specifically with sera of individuals with pigeon breeder's disease. Allergy Clin Immunol 1986;77:79–86.

225. De Beer PM, Bouic PJ, Joubert JR. Identification of a "disease-associated" antigen in pigeon breeder's disease by Western blotting. Int Arch Allergy Appl Immunol 1990;91:343–7.

226. Todd A, Coan R, Allen A. Pigeon breeder's lung; IgG subclasses to pigeon intestinal mucin and IgA antigens. Clin Exp Immunol 1993;92:494–9.

227. Mendoza F, Baltazares M, Ramírez A, et al. Detection of salivary and seric IgG and IgA antipooled pigeon sera activities in patients with pigeon breeder's disease. J Clin Lab Anal 1996;10:149–54.

228. McSharry C, MacLeod K, McGregor S, et al. Mucosal immunity in extrinsic allergic alveolitis: salivary immunoglobulins and antibody against inhaled avian antigens among pigeon breeders. Clin Exp Allergy 1999;29:957–64.

229. Hisauchi-Kojima K, Sumi Y, Miyashita Y, et al. Purification of the antigenic components of pigeon dropping extract, the responsible agent for cellular immunity in pigeon breeder's disease. J Allergy Clin Immunol 1999;103:1158–65.

230. Semenzato G, Agostini C, Zambello C, et al. Lung T cells in hypersensitivity pneumonitis: phenotypic and functional analyses. J Immunol 1986;137:1164–72.

231. Ando M, Konishi K, Yoneda R, Tamura M. Difference in the phenotypes of bronchoalveolar lavage lymphocytes in patients with summer-type hypersensitivity pneumonitis, farmer's lung, ventilation pneumonitis, bird fancier's lung: report of a nationwide epidemiologic study in Japan. J Allergy Clin Immunol 1991;87:1002–9.

232. Cormier Y, Belanger J, Laviolette M. Prognostic significance of bronchoalveolar lavage lymphocytosis in farmer's lung. Am Rev Respir Dis 1987;135:692–5.

233. Satake N, Nagai S, Kawatani A, et al. Density of phenotypic markers on BAL T-lymphocytes in hypersensitivity pneumonitis, pulmonary sarcoidosis and bronchiolitis obliterans with organizing pneumonia. Eur Respir J 1993;6:477–82.

234. Trentin L, Migone N, Zambello R, et al. Mechanisms accounting for lymphocytic alveolitis in hypersensitivity pneumonitis. J Immunol 1990;145:2147–54.

235. Semenzato G, Trentin L, Zambello R, et al. Cytotoxic lymphocytes in the lung of patients with hypersensitivity pneumonitis. Functional and molecular analysis. Ann N Y Acad Sci 1988;532:447–50.

236. Leatherman JW, Michael AF, Schwartz BA, Hoidal JR. Lung T cells in hypersensitivity pneumonitis. Ann Intern Med 1984;100:390–2.

237. Johnson MA, Nemeth A, Condez A, et al. Cell-mediated immunity in pigeon breeder's lung: the effect of removal from antigen exposure. Eur Respir J 1989;2:444–50.

238. Barquín N, Sansores R, Chapela R, et al. Immunoregulatory abnormalities in patients with pigeon breeder's disease. Lung 1990;168:103–10.

239. Drent M, van Velzen-Blad H, Diarnant M, et al. Differential diagnostic value of plasma cells in bronchoalveolar lavage fluid. Chest 1993;103:1720–4.

240. Drent M, Wagenaar SS, van Velzen-Blad H, et al. Relationship between plasma cell levels and profile of bronchoalveolar lavage fluid in patients with subacute extrinsic allergic alveolitis. Thorax 1993;48:835–9.

241. Haslam PL, Parker DJ, Townsend PJ. Increases in HLA-DQ, DP, DR, transferrin receptors on alveolar macrophages in sarcoidosis and allergic alveolitis compared with fibrosing alveolitis. Chest 1990;97:651–61.

242. Pforte A, Schiessler A, Gais P, et al. Expression of the adhesion molecule ICAM-1 on alveolar macrophages and in serum in extrinsic allergic alveolitis. Respiration 1993;60:221–6.

243. Guzman J, Wang YM, Kalaycioglu O, et al. Increased surfactant protein A content in human alveolar macrophages in hypersensitivity pneumonitis. Acta Cytol 1992;36:668–73.

244. Haslam PL, Dewar A, Butchers P, et al. Mast cells, atypical lymphocytes, neutrophils in bronchoalveolar lavage in extrinsic allergic alveolitis: comparison with other interstitial lung diseases. Am Rev Respir Dis 1987;135:35–47.

245. Drent M, van Velzen-Blad H, Diamant M, et al. Bronchoalveolar lavage in extrinsic allergic alveolitis: effect of time elapsed since antigen exposure. Eur Respir J 1993;6:1276–81.

246. Soler P, Nioche S, Valeyre D, et al. Role of mast cells in the pathogenesis of hypersensitivity pneumonitis. Thorax 1987;42:565–72.

247. Miadonna A, Pesci A, Tedeschi A, et al. Mast cell and histamine involvement in farmer's lung disease. Chest 1994;105:1184–9.

248. Laviolette M, Cormier Y, Loiseau A, et al. Bronchoalveolar mast cells in normal farmers and subjects with farmer's lung. Am Rev Respir Dis 1991;144:855–60.

249. Trentin L, Marcer G, Chilosi M, et al. Longitudinal study of alveolitis in hypersensitivity pneumonitis patients: an immunological evaluation. J Allergy Clin Immunol 1988;82:577–85.

250. Drent M, Mulder PGH, Wagenaar SS, et al. Differences in BAL fluid variables in interstitial lung diseases evaluated by discriminant analysis. Eur Respir J 1993;6:803–10.

251. Sansores R, Selman M, Martínez E, et al. Bronchoalveolar and serum elevated levels of beta-2-microglobulin in patients with hypersensitivity pneumonitis. Med Sci Res 1988;16:403–4.

252. Selman M, Barquín N, Sansores R, et al. Increased levels of leukotriene C4 in bronchoalveolar lavage from patients with pigeon breeder's disease. Arch Invest Med (Mex) 1988;19:127–33.

253. Reynolds SP, Edwards JH, Jones KP, Davies BH. Immunoglobulin and antibody levels in bronchoalveolar lavage fluid from symptomatic and asymptomatic pigeon breeders. Clin Exp Immunol 1991;86:278–85.

254. Larsson K, Eklund A, Malmberg P, et al. Hyaluronic acid (hyaluronan) in BAL fluid distinguishes farmers with allergic alveolitis from farmers with asymptomatic alveolitis. Chest 1992;101:109–14.

255. Teschler H, Thompson AB, Pohl WR, et al. Bronchoalveolar lavage procollagen-III-peptide in recent onset hypersensitivity pneumonitis: correlation with extracellular matrix components. Eur Respir J 1993;6:709–14.

256. Teschler H, Pohl WR, Thompson AB, et al. Elevated levels of bronchoalveolar lavage vitronectin in hypersensitivity pneumonitis. Am Rev Respir Dis 1993;147:332–7.

257. Cormier Y, Laviolette M, Cantin A, et al. Fibrogenic activities in bronchoalveolar lavage fluid of farmer's lung. Chest 104:1038–42.

258. Kohno N, Awaya Y, Oyama T, et al. KL-6 a mucin-like glycoprotein, in bronchoalveolar lavage fluid from patients with interstitial lung disease. Am Rev Respir Dis 1993;148:637–42.

259. Hamm H, Luhrs J, Guzman y Rotaeche J, et al. Elevated surfactant protein A in bronchoalveolar lavage fluids from sarcoidosis and hypersensitivity pneumonitis patients. Chest 1994;106:1766–70.

260. Cormier Y, Israel-Assayag E, Desmeules M, Lesur O. Effect of contact avoidance or treatment with oral prednisolone on bronchoalveolar lavage surfactant protein A levels in subjects with farmer's lung. Thorax 1996;51:1210–5.

261. Chryssanthopoulos C, Fink JN. Clinical-immunologic correlates: a differential diagnostic update. Hypersensitivity pneumonitis. J Asthma 1983;20:285–96.

262. Udwadia ZF, Wright MJ, McIntosh LG, Leitch AG. Confusing serological abnormalities in bird fancier's lung. BMJ 1990;300:1519–20.

263. Malmberg P. Health effects of organic dust exposure in dairy farmers. Am J Ind Med 1990;17:7–15.

264. Von Essen S, Robbins R, Thompson A, Rennard S. Organic dust toxic syndrome: an acute febrile reaction to organic dust exposure distinct from hypersensitivity pneumonitis. Clin Toxicol 1990;28:389–420.

265. Malmberg P, Rask-Andersen A, Rosenhall R. Exposure to microorganisms associated with allergic alveolitis and febrile reactions to mold dust in farmers. Chest 1993;103:1202–9.

266. Konig G, Baur X, Fruhman G. Sarcoidosis or extrinsic allergic alveolitis? Respiration 1981;42:150–4.

267. Forst LS, Abraham J. Hypersensitivity pneumonitis presenting as sarcoidosis. Br J Ind Med 1993;50:497–500.

268. Warren CPW, Tse KS. Extrinsic allergic alveolitis owing to hypersensitivity to chickens. Significance of sputum precipitins. Am Rev Respir Dis 1974;109:672–7.

269. Fink JN. The use of bronchoprovocation in the diagnosis of hypersensitivity pneumonitis. J Allergy Clin Immunol 1979;64 Part 2:590–1.

270. Hendrick DJ, Marshall R, Faux JA, Krall JM. Positive "alveolar" responses to antigen inhalation provocation tests: their validity and recognition. Thorax 1980;35:415–27.

271. Hargreave FE, Pepys J. Allergic respiratory reactions in bird fanciers provoked by allergen inhalation provocation tests. Relation to clinical features and allergic mechanisms. J Allergy Clin Immunol 1972;50:157–73.

272. Vogelmeier C, Baur X, Mauermayer R, Fruhmann G. Der Heustaubexpositionstest in der diagnostik der farmerlunge: Staubmessungen und testungen von kontrollpersonen. Prax Klin Pneumol 1988;42:749–52.

273. Vogelmeier C, Krombach F, Munzig S, et al. Activation of blood neutrophils in acute episodes of farmer's lung. Am Rev Respir Dis 1993;148:396–400.

274. Reynolds SP, Jones KP, Edwards JH, Davies BH. Inhalation challenge in pigeon breeder's disease: BAL fluid changes after 6 hours. Eur Respir J 1993;6:467–76.

275. Ramirez-Venegas A, Sansores RH, Perez-Padilla R, et al. Utility of a provocation test for diagnosis of chronic pigeon breeder's disease. Am J Respir Crit Care Med 1998;158:862–9.

276. Farebrother MJB, Kelson MC, Heller RF. Death certification of farmer's lung and chronic airway diseases in different countries of the EEC. Br J Dis Chest 1985;79:352–60.

277. van Valenberg PLJ, Lammers JWJ, van den Hout HA, et al. Chronic extrinsic allergic alveolitis in a family with idiopathic pulmonary fibrosis: the importance of histological diagnosis. Eur Respir J 1992;5:1154–7.

278. Coleman A, Colby TV. Histologic diagnosis of extrinsic allergic alveolitis. Am J Surg Pathol 1988;12:514–8.

279. Barrios R, Selman M, Franco R, et al. Subpopulations of T cells in lung biopsies from patients with pigeon breeder's disease. Lung 1987;165:181–7.

280. Hensley GT, Garancis JC, Cheravyl GD, et al. Lung biopsies of pigeon breeder's disease. Arch Pathol 1969;87:572–9.

281. Vourlekis JS, Brown KK, Cool CD, et al. Nonspecific interstitial pneumonitis (NSIP) can be the sole lesion of hypersensitivity pneumonitis (HP). Am J Respir Crit Care Med 2001;163:A982.

282. Reyes CN, Wenzel FJ, Lawton BR, et al. The pulmonary pathology of farmer's lung disease. Chest 1982;81:142–6.

283. Suda T, Chida K, Hayakawa H, et al. Development of bronchus-associated lymphoid tissue in chronic hypersensitivity pneumonitis. Chest 1999;115:357–63.

284. Seal RME, Hapke EJ, Thomas GO, et al. The pathology of the acute and chronic stages of farmer's lung. Thorax 1968;23:469–89.

285. Barrowcliff DF, Arblaster PG. Farmer's lung: a study of an early acute fatal case. Thorax 1968;23:490–500.

286. Orriols R, Aliaga JL, Rodrigo MJ, et al. Localised alveolar-septal amyloidosis with hypersensitivity pneumonitis. Lancet 1992;339:1261–2.

287. Katzenstein ALA, Askin FB. Immunologic lung disease. In: Katzenstein ALA, Askin FB, editors. Surgical pathology of non-neoplastic lung disease. Philadelphia: W.B. Saunders; 1990. p. 168–213.

288. Kawanami O, Basset F, Barrios R, et al. Hypersensitivity pneumonitis in man. Light and electron microscopy studies of 18 lung biopsies. Am J Pathol 1983;110:275–89.

289. Takemura T, Hiraga Y, Oomichi M, et al. Ultrastructural features of alveolitis in sarcoidosis. Am J Respir Crit Care Med 1995;152:360–6.

290. Reijula K, Sutinen S. Ultrastructure of extrinsic bronchiolo-alveolitis. Pathol Res Pract 1986;181:418–29.

291. Planes C, Valeyre D, Loiseau A, et al. Ultrastructural alterations of the air-blood barrier in sarcoidosis and hypersensitivity pneumonitis and their relation to lung histopathology. Am J Respir Crit Care Med 1994;150:1067–74.

292. Monkare S, Haahtela T, Ikonen M, Laitinen LA. Bronchial hyperreactivity to inhaled histamine in patients with farmer's lung. Lung 1981;159:145–51.

293. Freedman PM, Ault B. Bronchial hyperreactivity to methacholine in farmer's lung disease. J Allergy Clin Immunol 1981;67:59–63.

294. Karr RM, Kohler PF, Salvaggio JE. Hypersensitivity pneumonitis and extrinsic asthma. An unusual association. Chest 1978;74:98–102.

295. Kokkarinnen JI, Tukiainen HO, Terho EO. Recovery of pulmonary function in farmer's lung. A five-year follow-up study. Am Rev Respir Dis 1993;147:793–6.

296. Amishima M, Munakata M, Ohtsuka Y, et al. Dairy farmers have increased methacholine bronchial responsiveness independent of sensitization to mold antigens. Am J Respir Crit Care Med 1995;151:1794–8.

297. Pelikan Z, Schot JD, Koedijk FH. The late bronchusobstructive response to bronchial challenge with pigeon faeces and its correlation with precipitating antibodies (IgG) in the serum of patients having long-term contact with pigeons. Clin Allergy 1983;13:203–11.

298. Baur X, Dewair M, Rommelt H. Acute airway obstruction followed by hypersensitivity pneumonitis in an isocyanate worker. J Occup Med 1984;26:285–7.

299. Malo JL, Ouimet G, Cartier A, et al. Combined alveolitis and asthma due to hexamethylene diisocyanate (HDI), with demonstration of crossed respiratory and immunologic reactivities to diphenylmethane diisocyanate (MDI). J Allergy Clin Immunol 1983;72:413–9.

300. Evans WV, Seaton A. Hypersensitivity pneumonitis in a technician using Pauli's reagent. Thorax 1979;34:767–70.

301. De Hoyos A, Holness DL, Tarlo SM. Hypersensitivity pneumonitis and airways hyperreactivity induced by occupational exposure to penicillin. Chest 1993;103:303–4.

302. Hogg JC. Asthma as a bronchiolitis. Semin Respir Med 1992;13:114–8.

303. Soler P, Nioche S, Valeyre D, et al. Role of mast cells in the pathogenesis of hypersensitivity pneumonitis. Thorax 1987;42:565–72.

304. Miadonna A, Pesci A, Tedeschi A, et al. Mast cell and histamine involvement in farmer's lung disease. Chest 1994;105:1184–9.

305. Yoshida K, Ando M, Sakata T, Araki S. Prevention of summer-type hypersensitivity pneumonitis: effect of elimination of

Trichosporon cutaneum from the patient's homes. Arch Environ Health 1989;44:317–22.

306. Craig TJ, Hershey J, Engler RJM, et al. Bird antigen persistence in the home environment after removal of the bird. Ann Allergy 1992;69:510–2.

307. Bourke SJ, Banham SW, Carter R, et al. Longitudinal course of extrinsic allergic alveolitis in pigeon breeders. Thorax 1989;44:415–8.

308. Richerson HB, Richards DW, Swanson PA, et al. Antigen-specific desensitization in a rabbit model of acute hypersensitivity pneumonitis. J Allergy Clin Immunol 1981;68:226–34.

309. Kusaka H, Ogasawara H, Munakata M, et al. Two-year follow up on the protective value of dust masks against farmer's lung disease. Intern Med 1993;32:106–11.

310. Bouchard S, Morin F, Bedard G, et al. Farmer's lung and variables related to the decision to quit farming. Am J Respir Crit Care Med 1995;152:997–1002.

311. Kokkarinen JI, Tukiainen HO, Terho EO. Effect of corticosteroid treatment on the recovery of pulmonary function in farmer's lung. Am Rev Respir Dis 1992;145:3–5.

312. Ramírez A, Sansores R, Chapela R, et al. Inhaled beclomethasone versus oral prednisone. A clinical trial in patients with hypersensitivity pneumonitis. Am J Respir Crit Care Med 1995;151:A605.

313. Carlsen KH, Leegard J, Lund OD, Skjaervik H. Allergic alveolitis in a 12-year-old boy: treatment with budesonide nebulizing solution. Pediatr Pulmonol 1992;12:257–9.

314. Tremblay GM, Therien HM, Rocheleau H, Cormier Y. Liposomal dexamethasone effectiveness in the treatment of hypersensitivity pneumonitis in mice. Eur J Clin Invest 1993;23:656–61.

315. Kokkarinen JI, Tukiainen HO, Terho EO. Recovery of pulmonary function in farmer's lung. A five-year follow-up study. Am Rev Respir Dis 1993;147:793–6.

316. Lalancette M, Carrier G, Laviolette M, et al. Farmer's lung. Long-term outcome and lack of predictive value of bronchoalveolar lavage fibrosing factors. Am Rev Respir Dis 1993;148:216–21.

317. Kokkarinen J, Tukiainen H, Terho EO. Mortality due to farmer's lung in Finland. Chest 1994;106:509–12.

318. Barbee RA, Callies Q, Dickie HA, Rankin J. The long-term prognosis in farmer's lung. Am Rev Respir Dis 1968;97:223–31.

319. Nakagawa-Yoshida K, Ando M, Etches RI, Dosman JA. Fatal cases of farmer's lung in a Canadian family. Chest 1997;111:245–8.

320. Remy-Jardin M, Remy J, Wallaert B, Muller NL. Subacute and chronic bird breeder hypersensitivity pneumonitis: sequential evaluation with CT and correlation with lung function tests and bronchoalveolar lavage. Radiology 1993;189:111–8.

321. Hapke EJ, Seal RME, Thomas GO, et al. Farmer's lung. A clinical, radiographic, functional, serological correlation of acute and chronic stages. Thorax 1968;23:451–68.

322. Erkinjuntti-Pekkanen R, Rytkonen H, Kokkarinen JI, et al. Long-term risk of emphysema in patients with farmer's lung and matched control farmers. Am J Respir Crit Care Med 1998;158:662–5.

323. Yoshizawa Y, Miyashita Y, Inoue T, et al. Sequential evaluation of clinical and immunological findings in hypersensitivity pneumonitis: serial subclass distribution of antibodies. Clin Immunol Immunopathol 1994;73:330–7.

324. Murayama J, Yoshizawa Y, Ohtsuka M, Hasegawa S. Lung fibrosis in hypersensitivity pneumonitis. Association with CD4+ but not CD8+ cell dominant alveolitis and insidious onset. Chest 1993;104:38–43.

20

DRUG INDUCED INFILTRATIVE LUNG DISEASES

PHILIPPE CAMUS

In the past 50 years, drugs, radiation therapy, procedures, and transplantation have become a significant cause of lung disease.[1–79] The different types of involvement include diseases of the airways (laryngeal edema, cough, bronchospasm),[69,76] lung parenchyma (the interstitial lung diseases [ILD]),[75] pulmonary circulation (pulmonary hypertension, hyperpermeability, vasculitides),[80] pleura (effusions, thickening, the lupus syndrome),[32,70] lymph nodes (adenopathies, sarcoidosis, lymphoma),[81–83] and neuromuscular system (respiratory failure).[84,85] Among these, the ILDs are foremost in terms of diversity and frequency. Drugs are a common cause of ILD, the severity of which may range from an asymptomatic state, to transient pulmonary infiltrates, and, finally, to life-threatening acute respiratory distress syndrome (ARDS). The possible patterns for diffuse lung disease include

- *interstitial* changes, as occur in methotrexate pneumonitis or in eosinophilic pneumonia;
- *alveolar* changes, as occur in drug-induced pulmonary edema or hemorrhage, diffuse alveolar damage, amiodarone pneumonitis, or exogenous lipoid pneumonia; or
- *vascular* changes, as occur in drug-induced angiitides involving either large or small lung vessels.

Drug-induced ILDs are frequent and create significant problems for the practitioner. The diagnosis is made by excluding other causes. Drugs may induce lung diseases that closely resemble ILDs from other causes or idiopathic interstitial pneumonias. Being cognizant of drug-induced ILD enables the diagnosis to be suspected early and the causative drug withdrawn, which should translate into an improved prognosis. Although discontinuance of an offending drug often positively influences the clinical outcome of drug-induced lung disease, it may negatively impact on the underlying illness. Based on clinical status, corticosteroids may sometimes be avoided, and this will allow more accurate determination of the specific effects of drug withrawal. Several ILDs due to chemotherapeu-

tic agents or amiodarone may induce irreversible pulmonary fibrosis. This is usually not affected by drug withdrawal and moreover impacts the quality of life, and life expectancy. It is particularly tragic, when a child with a stabilized malignant brain tumor dies of nitrosourea-induced pulmonary fibrosis or when a patient with arrhythmia dies of pulmonary fibrosis from amiodarone toxicity. Although some risk factors have been identified, the development of drug-induced ILD is unpredictable.

Many drugs or agents cause ILD (Table 20–1).[65] Some drugs induce a distinctive pattern, making the recognition of lung disease possible in patients receiving the drug.

- Radiation pneumonitis often localizes preferentially to the irradiated area.[86]
- Nitrofurantoin occasions an acute form of ILD characterized by intense symptoms and minimal radiographic opacities or the distinctive histologic pattern of desquamative interstitial pneumonia.[87]
- Methotrexate may cause a characteristic granulomatous ILD, which mimicks diffuse infectious pneumonia.[74]
- Bleomycin causes basilar pulmonary infiltrates with volume loss or the pattern of multiple lung nodules.[88]
- Mitomycin is associated with the hemolytic uremic syndrome.[89]
- Amiodarone causes asymmetric pulmonary infiltrates and has characteristic histopathologic findings (foamy macrophages, organizing pneumonia).[90–92]
- Lipoid pneumonia has distinctive imaging characteristics[93–95] and demonstrates specific features in bronchoalveolar lavage (BAL) fluid[96] (see Chapter 31, "Miscellaneous Insterstitial Lung Diseases").
- Self-injection of elemental mercury opacifies the pulmonary arterial tree.[97]

Drug-induced lung disease often, but not always, shows a close temporal relationship between exposure and the onset of pulmonary disease. For instance, the administration of hydrochlorothiazide,[98] blood transfusion,[99] or

TABLE 20–1 Drugs Causing Interstitial Lung Disease and the Resulting Clinical, Radiographic, and Pathologic Patterns*

	Acute ILD	Subacute ILD	PIE	Granulomatous ILD	Organizing Pneumonia	DIP	Pulmonary Fibrosis	Shrinking Lung	Subclinical Involvement	Diffuse Calcifications	Lipoid Pneumonia	Lung Nodules	Transient Infiltrates	Pulmonary Edema	ARDS	HUS	DAH	SLE	PVOD	Pulmonary or Systemic Vasculitis	Fat Embolism	DIHSS	Opportunistic Infections
Abacavir		2			2												1	3				1	
Abciximab			1																				
Acebutolol			1																				
Acetaminophen														3									
Acetylsalicylic acid (aspirin)														2	1		1			1			
Acyclovir		1																		1		1	
Adrenalin (epinephrine)														1									
Albumin																							
Allopurinol																							
Aminoglutethimide			(1)																				
Amiodarone		4	1		3		3					2		1	2		1	2					
Amitriptyline																							
Amphotericin B		1			1									1	1								
Ampicillin		1	1											2	2								
Amrinone		1	2																				
Angiotensin convertase inhibitors		1					1																
Antazoline			2											2				2					
Antithymocyte globulin		2											1				1						
Atenolol		1	1																				
Aurothiopropanosulfonate (gold salt)	2	2	2	2	1		2										1			1			
Azapropazone		1																					
Azathioprine		2																					
Azithromycin																							
Barbiturates																							
BCG therapy (intravesical)	3	2	1	2/3	1										1								
Beclomethasone		2	1		1		1												1				
Bepridil																							
Betaxolol																							
Bicalutamide		1	1																				
Bleomycin		3	2		3		3					3		3	3				1				3
Blood transfusions			1			1	2								2								2
Bromocriptine																							
Bucillamine																							
Buprenorphine														2									
Busulfan		1					3												1				
Calcium salts										1													
Camprothecin			1											1									
Captopril		1	1												2								

TABLE 20–1 Continued

Drug	Acute ILD	Subacute ILD	PIE	Granulomatous ILD	Organizing Pneumonia	DIP	Pulmonary Fibrosis	Shrinking Lung	Subclinical Involvement	Diffuse Calcifications	Lipoid Pneumonia	Lung Nodules	Transient Infiltrates	Pulmonary Edema	ARDS	HUS	DAH	SLE	PVOD	Pulmonary or Systemic Vasculitis	Fat Embolism	DIHSS	Opportunistic Infections
Carbamazepine	2	2	2		1							1		1			1	1		1		2	
Carbimazole		2	1																				
Carmustine (BCNU)	1						3								3				1				
Cefotiam	1		1																				
Celiprolol			1																				
Cephalexin		1	1		1																		
Cephalosporins																							
Chlorambucil							2								1								
Chlorhexidine															1								
Chloroquine			1																			1	
Chlorozotocin (DCNU)																							
Chlorpromazine														1				1				1	
Chlorpropamide			1																				
Cladribine			1																				
Clindamycin			1																				
Clofazimine			1						1														
Clofibrate			1											2	1			1					
Clomiphene																		1					
Clonidine																		1					
Clopidogrel																	1						
Clozapine		1	1											1								1	
Colchicine	1														1								
Contraceptives (oral)		1	1											1				1	1			1	
Co-trimoxazole		1	1											1								1	
Cromoglycate		1																					
Cyclophosphamide		2	1		1		2				1			1	2								2
Cyclosporine		1												1									2
Cyproterone acetate		1																					
Cytosine arabinoside (ara-C)							1							2	2		1					1	
Danazol			1														1						
Dapsone															1							1	
Deferoxamine			1											1			1						
Desipramine														1						1			
Dextran			1											1			1						
Diclofenac		1	1																				
Diflunisal			1																				
Dihydroergocryptine					1																		
Dihydroergotamine					1																		

TABLE 20-1 Continued

	Acute ILD	Subacute ILD	PIE	Granulomatous ILD	Organizing Pneumonia	DIP	Pulmonary Fibrosis	Shrinking Lung	Subclinical Involvement	Diffuse Calcifications	Lipoid Pneumonia	Lung Nodules	Transient Infiltrates	Pulmonary Edema	ARDS	HUS	DAH	SLE	PVOD	Pulmonary or Systemic Vasculitis	Fat Embolism	DIHSS	Opportunistic Infections
Diltiazem	1	1											1	1			1						
Dimethyl sulfoxide (DMSO)		1												1	1		1						
Docetaxel																							
Dothiepin																							
Efavirenz		1												1								1	
Epoprostenol (see prostacyclin)			1											1									
Ergometrine																							
Ergotamine							1																
Erythromycin														1	1								
Estrogens																			1				
Etanercept																		1		1			1
Ethambutol		1	1																				
Ethchlorvynol														2									
Etoposide														1	1								
Etretinate																							
Febarbamate			1																				
Fenbufen			1																				
Fenfluramine/dexfenfluramine		1			1																		
Fenoprofen			1																				
Fibrinolytics (including RTPA)																	2						
fk-506	1	2												1			1						
Flecainide		1													1								
Floxuridine		1																					
Fludarabine																							
Fluorescein															1								
5-Fluorouracil		1																					
Fluoxetine		1					1																
Flutamide																							
Fluvastatin															1			1					
Fosinopril			1																			1	
Fotemustine							1								2								
Furazolidone																							
G/GM-CSF															2								
Gemcitabine		1	1										2		2								
Glafenine		1	1																				
Glibenclamide																							
Haloperidol		1	1												1							1	
Heparins															2		1						

TABLE 20–1   Continued

	Acute ILD	Subacute ILD	PIE	Granulomatous ILD	Organizing Pneumonia	DIP	Pulmonary Fibrosis	Shrinking Lung	Subclinical Involvement	Diffuse Calcifications	Lipoid Pneumonia	Lung Nodules	Transient Infiltrates	Pulmonary Edema	ARDS	HUS	DAH	SLE	PVOD	Pulmonary or Systemic Vasculitis	Fat Embolism	DIHSS	Opportunistic Infections
Heroin		1			(3)									3									
Hexamethonium (discontinued)		1	1		1										2		1	2					
Hydralazine/dihydralazine		1												3									
Hydrochlorothiazide		1					1																
Hydroxyquinoline		1	1											1	1								
Hydroxyurea			1											1	1								
Ibuprofen		1	1												1								
Ifosfamide																							
Imipramine														1									
Immunoglobulins (IVIG)																							
Indinavir																							
Indomethacin			1																				
Infliximab				1		1																	2
Insulin														1									
Interferon alpha		1	1																				
Interferon beta					1																		
Interleukin-2		1	1		1									3	2								
Irinotecan														2	2								
Isoniazid			1															2					
Isotretinoin																							
Ketamine																		2					
Labetalol														1				1					
L-Asparaginase		1												2									
L-Dopa							1								1								
Leukotriene antagonists		1	1																				
Leuprorelin			1																				
Levofloxacin																				2			
Lidocaine																							
IV lipids		1	1												1				1		1		
Lomustine CCNU		1	1				2								2								
Loxoprofen		1																					
Maprotiline					(2)																		
Mecamylamine							2								1								
Mefloquine		1	1																				
Melphalan		1																					
Mephenesin		1																					
6-Mercaptopurine			1																				
Mesalamine/mesalazine			2		2																		

TABLE 20–1 Continued

Drug	Acute ILD	Subacute ILD	PIE	Granulomatous ILD	Organizing Pneumonia	DIP	Pulmonary Fibrosis	Shrinking Lung	Subclinical Involvement	Diffuse Calcifications	Lipoid Pneumonia	Lung Nodules	Transient Infiltrates	Pulmonary Edema	ARDS	HUS	DAH	SLE	PVOD	Pulmonary or Systemic Vasculitis	Fat Embolism	DIHSS	Opportunistic Infections
Metapramine		1												1	2								
Metformin		1												2	2								
Methadone																							
Methotrexate	4	3	1	4			1								1		1						3
Methyldopa			1															2					
Methylphenidate																							
Methysergide							1†													1			
Metronidazole																							
Miconazole			1																				
Minocycline		1	3		1			1				1						2		1		2	
Mitomycin C		1					2							1	2	3	2						
Mitoxantrone														2									
Montelukast																	1			2			
Moxalactam			1				1								1								
Mycophenolate mofetil		1																					
Nadolol														1									
Naphazoline														1									
Nalbuphine																							
Nalfon			1																				
Nalidixic acid			1															1					
Naloxone														1									
Naproxen		1	2																				
Nevirapine			1																			1	
Niflumic acid			1											1									
Nilutamide			1		1									1									
Niridazole														1									
Nitric oxide (NO)	1	3													1								
Nitrofurantoin	4	3	1		1	1	2	1	1				2		1		1	1		2		1	
Nitroglycerin		2												1						1			
Nitrosoureas		1					3								2				1				
Nomifensine			1																				
NSAIDS			3												1							2	
Noramidopyrine (metamizole)																							
OKT3																							
Olsalazine																							
Opioids (morphine agonist/antagonist)														3									
Oral anticoagulants																	2						
Ornipressin														1				1					

TABLE 20–1 Continued

Drug	Acute ILD	Subacute ILD	PIE	Granulomatous ILD	Organizing Pneumonia	DIP	Pulmonary Fibrosis	Shrinking Lung	Subclinical Involvement	Diffuse Calcifications	Lipoid Pneumonia	Lung Nodules	Transient Infiltrates	Pulmonary Edema	ARDS	HUS	DAH	SLE	PVOD	Pulmonary or Systemic Vasculitis	Fat Embolism	DIHSS	Opportunistic Infections
Oxprenolol		1	1																				
Oxyphenbutazone		1	2																				
Paclitaxel		1																					
Para(4)-aminosalicylic acid (PAS)			1																				
Paraffin (mineral oil)											4										2		
Parenteral nutrition			2										1	1									
Penicillamine		2	1		1		1										2			1			
Penicillins	1		1												1								
Pentamidine																							
Perindopril																							
Phenylbutazone			2											1								1	
Phenylephrine														1									
Phenytoin	1	2	1	1	1		1					1		1			1	1		1		1	
Pindolol																		1					
Piroxicam			1																				
Pituitary snuff		1												2									
Plasma (fresh frozen)																							
Practolol (recalled)		(1)					(1)																
Pranlukast																							
Pranoprofen																							
Pravastatin																							
Procainamide		1	1															2					
Procarbazine		1					1																
Propofol					1								1								1		
Propoxyphene			1											1									
Propranolol		1	1											1									
Propylthiouracil																	1	2		1			
Prostacyclin												1		2	1								
Protamine																							
Pyrimethamine-dapsone			1																				
Pyrimethamine-sulfadoxine		1	1																				
Quinidine		2													2			1		2			
Radiation therapy	2	1			2		4	2	2						2				2				1
Radiographic contrast media			1						2					2									
Raltitrexed															2								
Retinoic acid (ATRA)														2	2		1						
Rifampin			1														1						
Ritodrine														3			2						

TABLE 20–1 Continued

Drug	Acute ILD	Subacute ILD	PIE	Granulomatous ILD	Organizing Pneumonia	DIP	Pulmonary Fibrosis	Shrinking Lung	Subclinical Involvement	Diffuse Calcifications	Lipoid Pneumonia	Lung Nodules	Transient Infiltrates	Pulmonary Edema	ARDS	HUS	DAH	SLE	PVOD	Pulmonary or Systemic Vasculitis	Fat Embolism	DIHSS	Opportunistic Infections
Rituximab			1			1														1			
Roxithromycin			1																				
Salbutamol (infected)			1											3									
Serrapeptase			1																				
Sertraline																							
Simvastatin		1			1										1			1					
Sirolimus (rapamycin)		1			1												1						
Sotalol																							
β₂-agonists (administered IV in ob/gyn)														3									
Steroids																							3
Streptokinase															1		2						
Streptomycin															1								
Sulfamides-sulfonamides		1	1											1				1		2		1	
Sulfasalazine		1	2		1	1	1							1				1		1			
Sulindac			2																				
Tacrolimus			1											1									
Tamoxifen			1		1		1											2					
Tenidap																							
Terbutaline														3									
Tetracycline			2																				
Tiaprofenic acid		1	1																				
Ticlopidine			1																				
Tiopronin																							
Tirofiban																	1						
TNF-alpha		1	1		1		1							2			1						
Tocainide			1																				
Tolazamide																							
Tolfenamic acid																							
Topotecan													2		2								
Tosufloxacin			1											1									
Trazodone			1											2									
Triazolam																							
Tricyclic antidepressants																							
Trimipramine			1																				
Troglitazone														1									
Troleandomycin																							
L-tryptophan			(4)		(1)															(4)			
Urokinase																	2						

TABLE 20–1 Continued

	Acute ILD	Subacute ILD	PIE	Granulomatous ILD	Organizing Pneumonia	DIP	Pulmonary Fibrosis	Shrinking Lung	Subclinical Involvement	Diffuse Calcifications	Lipoid Pneumonia	Lung Nodules	Transient Infiltrates	Pulmonary Edema	ARDS	HUS	DAH	SLE	PVOD	Pulmonary or Systemic Vasculitis	Fat Embolism	DIHSS	Opportunistic Infections
Valproate (valproic acid)		1															1						
Valsartan			1											1									
Vasopressin	1																						
Venlafaxine														1	1								
Vinblastine												1		1	1	1							
Vindesine																							
Vinorelbine																							
Vitamin D										1													
Zafirlukast			1																	1			

Drugs that cause pulmonary edema or ARDS may also cause transient pulmonary infiltrates.

Figures in boxes indicate the frequency of the adverse effect: from 1 (rare) to 4 (common).

Empty boxes: adverse effect not reported.

Brackets indicate that the drug was recalled (eg, hexamethonium, practolol).

When most drugs in a therapeutic group induce similar adverse effects in the lung (eg, angiotensin-converting enzyme inhibitors, β-blockers, β_2-agonists, leukotriene antagonists, NSAIDs) the family of drugs is mentioned, not all specific drugs.

ILD = interstitial lung disease; PIE = pulmonary infiltrates and eosinophilia; DIP = desquamative interstitial pneumonia; ARDS = adult respiratory distress syndrome; HUS = hemolytic uremic syndrome; DAH = diffuse alveolar hemorrhage; SLE = systemic lupus erythematosus; PVOD = pulmonary veno-occlusive disease; DIHSS = drug-induced hypersensitivity syndrome (a multiorgan reaction to drugs); NSAIDs = nonsteroidal anti-inflammatory drugs.

(*See text for definitions of the patterns of ILD).

*The pulmonary fibrosis of methysergide and of other ergots is closely associated with pleural fibrosis, the predominant adverse effect from these drugs.

intravenous (IV) β_2-agonists to retard labor,[100] is acutely followed by the development of pulmonary infiltrates.

In other instances, the association between drug exposure and lung disease is less clear. For example, if a drug has been administered with no adverse consequences for many years and then lung disease develops, drug withdrawal may help determine whether the drug is responsible.

Regardless of the pattern of drug-induced ILD, it is important to exclude opportunistic pneumonias, because methotrexate, corticosteroids, immunosuppressives, and infliximab have been associated with the development of bacterial, fungal, parasitic (eg, *Pneumocystis carinii*, strongyloidiasis), and viral infections.[101]

There is no classification of drug-induced ILD that is ideal. We choose to rely on a dual classification. One relates to clinical patterns of drug-induced ILD (§ 5) and the other to specific drugs or agents (§ 6).

DRUGS CAUSING INTERSTITIAL LUNG DISEASE

A regularly updated list of drugs causing lung disease is available on the Web (see Table 20–1).[65] Drugs responsible for ILD are antibiotics, anticancer agents (bleomycin, busulfan, chlorambucil, cyclophosphamide, methotrexate, mitomycin, nitrosoureas), amiodarone, chrysotherapy, the nitro-bearing drugs nitrofurantoin and nilutamide, mineral oil, and nonsteroidal anti-inflammatory drugs (NSAIDs). More recently, all-*trans*-retinoic acid (ATRA); colony stimulating factors (CSFs); interferons; the novel anticancer agents docetaxel, gemcitabine, irinotecan, and vinorelbine; cytokines; autologous or allogeneic blood, and proteins (eg, antithymocyte globulin) have also been shown to cause ILD.[65] In a few instances, the vehicle (eg, Cremophor, lipids, dimethyl sulfoxide) in which drugs are dissolved or suspended causes lung disease. In addition to approved drugs, herbs and plants (eg, *Sauropus* roots),[102] dietary food supplements (eg, L-tryptophan, in the recent past),[103] illicit or home synthesized drugs,[104] and pneumotoxic chemicals (paraquat, carbamates, rodenticides)[105,106] may also cause ILD. Accordingly, a careful history is required.

Almost any route of administration of a drug could increase the risk of developing ILD, including, by decreasing order of frequency, oral, IV–intramuscular (IM), inhaled, ophthalmic, intrathecal, intravesical, gynecologic, intranasal, peripheral intra-arterial, and transdermal. A few drugs intended for oral use cause lung damage if *aspirated* into the lung (eg, mineral oil,[93] shark oil,[94] Kayexalate,[107] psyllium[108]).

The incidence of drug-induced ILD for an individual drug is variable, from 0.0013% for nitrofurantoin,[109] to several percent in radiation- or amiodarone-treated patients,[110] and to 40 to 50% or more in women receiving agressive nitrosourea-based chemotherapy regimens for the treatment of high-risk breast carcinoma.[111] (See "one-star" and "four-star" drugs on the Pneumotox® Web site.[65])

Certain drugs tend to cause a stereotypical pattern of ILD in most or all affected patients. For instance, minocycline induces the syndrome of pulmonary infiltrates and eosinophilia (PIE),[50] and methotrexate can cause a form of acute hypersensitivity pneumonitis.[7,74] Others, such as amiodarone or bleomycin, may cause asymptomatic pulmonary infiltrates, symptomatic interstitial pneumonia, pulmonary infiltrates with eosinophilia, organizing pneumonia, multiple nodules, an ARDS picture, or irreversible pulmonary fibrosis.[65]

Drugs belonging to a therapeutic class may all induce similar adverse effects, suggesting a common cytopathic mechanism. Examples of this include the relationships of NSAIDs with eosinophilic pneumonia or asthma, angiotensin-converting enzyme inhibitor (ACEI) with eosinophilic pneumonia or cough, ergolines with pleural fibrosis, and alkylating agents with pneumocyte dysplasia and pulmonary fibrosis. In contrast, chemically-unrelated drugs can induce an identical pattern of nonspecific interstitial pneumonia, implying that the lung disease is unrelated to the specific pharmacologic action.

RISK FACTORS

A small number of risk factors have been identified, which are supported by animal studies. Nonspecific risk factors include prior lung disease, pneumonectomy, or abnormal baseline pulmonary physiology.[112] Renal failure increases the blood level and toxicity of bleomycin,[113,114] and atopy enhances the risk of eosinophilic pneumonia[50] or Churg-Strauss syndrome (CSS).[115]

For a few agents (amiodarone, bleomycin, the nitrosoureas, and radiation therapy), dose-related toxicity has been demonstrated. These include bleomycin (> 500 Units) and bischloroethyl nitrosourea (BCNU or carmustine) (> 1,000 to 1,200 mg/m^2).[116] Theoretically, this finding is important in regard to pathophysiology; however, several ILDs occur after lower doses of these agents.[117]

Concomitant or sequential pneumotoxic drugs, the combination of pneumotoxic drugs and CSFs, or the addition of radiation therapy to the chest may significantly enhance the likelihood of developing adverse pulmonary effects.[118] Administration of chemotherapeutic agents to patients who have received radiation therapy in the past may also "recall" a severe skin and/or lung reaction within the previously irradiated area.[119]

Oxygen therapy, administered for surgical procedures, may induce severe pulmonary infiltrates in patients who have previously received chemotherapeutic agents, radiation therapy, CSFs, or amiodarone.[120,121] The acetylator phenotype and certain human leukocyte antigen (HLA) haplotypes have been cited as risk factors, but evidence is questionable.

DIAGNOSTIC CRITERIA

The following five diagnostic criteria are gaining acceptance in the diagnosis of drug-induced lung disease.

There should be a History of Drug Exposure

A history should include approved and over-the-counter drugs, herbs, exotic compounds, and illicit substances, regardless of the route of administration. Of note, several case reports have mentioned that exposures to mineral oil, aspirin, hydrochlorothiazide, nitrofurantoin, or illicit drugs have been overlooked. Establishing drug use is often difficult in obtunded patients, in patients with psychiatric illness, and in illicit drug abusers.

Temporally, drug-induced ILD may develop within minutes, such as hydrochlorothiazide-induced pulmonary edema.[98] Time to onset of several years is seen in patients with amiodarone or chemotherapy lung.[122] Generally, drug-induced ILD develops after a few weeks to a few months. A few reports have described the onset of lung disease years *after* cessation of exposure to the drug. Examples include patients with lung fibrosis, who had received nitrosoureas for the treatment of childhood brain tumor.[123]

Clinical, Imaging, and Pathologic Pattern of Lung Involvement should Conform to Earlier Observations with the Drug

Drugs that have been shown to cause lung disease and their clinical and pathologic features are shown in Table 20–1 and are available on the Pneumotox Web site.[65]

Etiology of Lung Disease Other than Drugs should be Ruled Out

Causes for lung disease other than drugs generally fit into four main categories.

- Infection: The exclusion of infection is essential, especially in patients with acute febrile ILD and in those receiving immunosuppressive drugs.[124]
- Hemodynamic: Diuresis is usually performed to evaluate this hypothesis. However, diuretic therapy may attenuate the density of nonhemodynamic ILD. Therefore, opacities should clear completely for the diagnosis of pulmonary edema to be considered. Additional investigations include cardiac echography or invasive hemodynamic measurements.
- Pulmonary involvement caused by an underlying disease (eg, connective tissue disease,[125,126] inflammatory bowel disease,[127,128] cancer, lymphoma): This represents the most difficult distinction, and even tissue evaluation may not answer this question.

Improvement should Follow Discontinuation of Suspected Drug

Withdrawal of drugs such as amiodarone, the antineoplastic agent methotrexate, or bowel disease–modifying drugs should be done cautiously to avoid a flare of the underlying disease. Removal of a drug is generally followed by improvement of symptoms. Patients with mild-to-moderate inflammatory ILD will respond quickly, whereas this may not be the case with drugs that cause acute interstitial reactions (eg, methotrexate pneumonitis) or pulmonary fibrosis. In this situation, corticosteroids are often used in conjunction with drug discontinuation. Discontinuation is more complex in patients on multiple drugs. In this case, sequential discontinuation is sometimes performed beginning with the drug most likely to have caused the syndrome and then withdrawing the others until improvement occurs.

Symptoms should Recur on Rechallenge

Rechallenge of patients with drug-induced pulmonary fibrosis is generally considered unethical as the pulmonary changes are largely irreversible, and this increases the risk to the patient. Rechallenge is also problematic in patients with acute ILD as the relapse may be more severe. Indeed, fatalities have been recorded following rechallenge of patients with methotrexate.[74] Rechallenge was performed safely in several patients with eosinophilic pneumonia,[50] and this confirmed the diagnosis. There is currently no agreed protocol for rechallenge. Dosages to be used, tools to monitor relapse (symptoms, blood tests, imaging, or BAL), and criteria for a positive rechallenge have not been defined.

Nevertheless, rechallenge may be considered if four conditions are present: (1) there remains a doubt as regards the role of the drug, (2) the drug is essential to the management of the patient, (3) no other drug can be used as a substitute, and (4) no reported adverse effects following rechallenge with the drug are known. For the latter criterion to be satisfied, the literature, Drug Safety Agencies, and the drug manufacturer should be consulted.

Practically, start with a small dose, and then increase the dose under strict medical supervision. If no symptoms have developed after approximately 1 week, the patient is discharged with instructions to report any symptoms. The duration of rechallenge remains unestablished as some patients have relapsed after up to several weeks.[129]

For patients taking more than one drug at the time of onset of ILD, indirect rechallenge may be performed starting with the least likely drug responsible.

Potentially diagnostic tests include inhibition of macrophage migration,[130] lymphocyte proliferation, and basophil degranulation. These have no established role in the diagnosis of drug-related conditions. The presence of antinuclear antibodies (ANA), antineutrophil cytoplasmic antibodies (ANCA), anti-Jo-1 antibodies, and antiphospholipid antibodies may suggest drug-related autoimmune conditions, especially if there is a temporal association between exposure to the drug and changes in antibody levels.

CLINICAL, PATHOLOGIC, AND IMAGING PATTERNS

The diverse clinical, pathologic, and imaging patterns of drug-induced ILD often relate to specific families of drugs.

Cellular Pneumonitis

Cellular pneumonitis (also called alveolitis or hypersensitivity pneumonitis) is the most common drug-induced ILD. Gold, methotrexate, nilutamide, nitrofurantoin, and many others cause the reaction.[65] Amiodarone induces a distinctive form of ILD that is detailed below.

Time to onset of the pneumonitis varies from a few days to several years. Onset of the disease is unpredictable, except for nilutamide pneumonitis and gold lung, which develop electively within the first 6 months of treatment. Onset of the disease is often progressive over a few weeks, and symptoms include dyspnea, a dry cough, fever, and sometimes a skin rash or hypotension. Mild changes in liver chemistry may be present as an associated feature, especially with nilutamide and nitrofurantoin.[131,132] The spectrum of severity ranges from vague pulmonary infiltrates and mild symptoms to acute ILD and respiratory failure (eg, methotrexate).

Radiographic studies indicate bilateral, somewhat symmetric, interstitial, and alveolar opacities (Figure 20–1). A miliary pattern is unusual but has been reported with the use of chrysotherapy, methotrexate, and intravesical bacille Calmette-Guérin (BCG). Infiltrates may localize in the lung bases or middle lung zones or may be diffuse.[133] The radiographic density can be a discrete haze or may show ground-glass or dense bilateral alveolar consolidation with air bronchograms (see Figure 20–1). Pleural effusion and mediastinal lymphadenopathy are occasional findings. The computed tomography (CT) scan can show interstitial septal lines or a ground-glass, crazy-paving, or mosaic pattern and, in cases with extensive disease, diffuse, patchy, or dense alveolar shadows (Figure 20–2).

Restrictive pulmonary functions and hypoxemia are usually present, and these correlate with the extent of radiographic involvement.[134] Azathioprine is the exception, because restrictive physiology and hypoxemia coexist with mild radiographic changes.[135]

Fiberoptic bronchoscopy and BAL are often indicated to exclude an opportunistic infection. Appropriate stains, cultures, and molecular techniques should be negative in BAL and other fluids. In drug-induced lung disease, the BAL usually shows a lymphocyte predominance. The contribution of lymphocyte typing is unclear, because increases in CD4+, or CD8+ subsets have been observed.[112,136,137] Although an increase in lymphocytes is the most common pattern in BAL fluid, neutrophilic and mixed patterns have also been reported.[133,138]

A lung biopsy may also be required in some cases. The main histologic features include a cellular interstitial pneumonia or nonspecific interstitial pneumonia and mild-to-moderate interstitial edema (Figures 20–3 and 20–4).[48] Organizing pneumonia[139] or interstitial fibrosis may also be seen.[74] Granulomas are decribed with methotrexate, interferon, highly active antiretroviral therapy, and intravesical BCG (Figures 20–3 and 20–5).[74,140] A pattern of desquamative interstitial pneumonia (DIP) is rare and suggests exposure to nitrofurantoin.[141] A pattern of perivascular cellular infiltrates is also unusual.[142] Alveolar edema or hemorrhage may be evidenced in patients with severe drug reactions (eg, from gold,[143] methotrexate,[144] or nitrofurantoin[145]). Corticosteroids are often required in patients with gas exchange impairment and respiratory failure. Initial high-dose boluses of methylprednisolone have been advocated in patients with respiratory failure. The overall prognosis of cellular drug-induced pneumonitis is good; however, fatalities have been reported in patients with severe respiratory failure,[74,130] and in those who did not receive corticosteroids.[146] The development of lung fibrosis following recognition and treatment of this problem is unusual. Rechallenge with the drug will often lead to relapse,[147] and proper instructions should be given to avoid inadvertent re-exposure to the drug or its related compounds.

Pulmonary Infiltrates and Eosinophilia or Eosinophilic Pneumonia

In a manner similar to the liver or gut, the lung may be the target organ for drug-induced tissue eosinophilia. Drug-induced PIE was first described following the use of sulfonamides, and, currently, more than 100 drugs are recognized to cause this syndrome.[65] Drugs causing PIE belong to five therapeutic classes: anticonvulsants (eg, carbamazepine), antibiotics (eg, minocycline, sulfasalazine, sulfamethoxypyridazine, sulfamethoxazole), ACEIs, NSAIDs, and antidepressants (imipramine). A typical form of drug-induced PIE results from exposure of young individuals to minocycline for the treatment of acne vulgaris.[50] Amiodarone, bleomycin, chloroquine, methotrexate, nilutamide, nitrofurantoin, and several other drugs cause PIE less frequently (see Table 20–1).[65] In the late 1980s, an epidemic of systemic eosinophilic disease resulted from the use of L-tryptophan, a popular dietary supplement at the time.[148] More recently, there is the concern that asthmatics receiving leukotriene inhibitors may develop PIE or eosinophilic angiitis (the CSS; see below under "DI angiitides").[149,150]

Generally, patients are still receiving the offending drug when the symptoms of PIE develop. Onset more than a few days after termination of treatment is

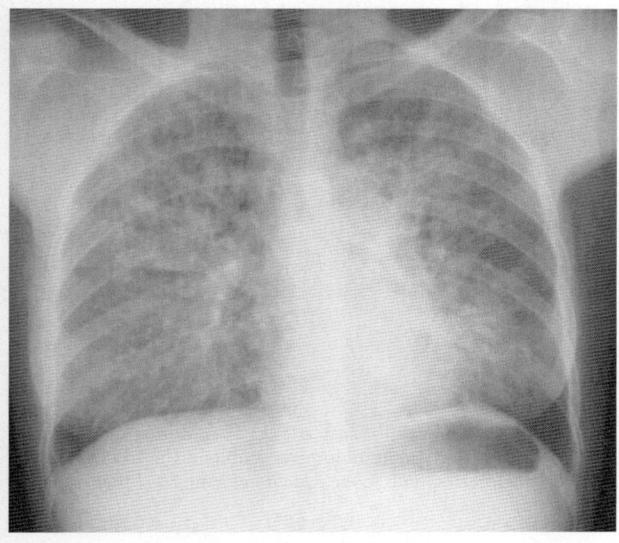

A

Figure 20–1   Chest radiographs of cellular drug-induced pneumonitis (methotrexate-induced). A young lady received weekly methotrexate for the treatment of molar pregnancy. *A*, She insidiously developed cough, fever, dyspnea, interstitial pulmonary infiltrates, and hypoxemia. *B, C,* The disease accelerated producing acute interstitial lung disease and respiratory failure. The open lung biopsy disclosed granulomatous interstitial pneumonitis (see Figures 20–3 and 20–5) and pulmonary edema. The patient improved following discontinuance of the drug and oxygen. Although not used in this particular case, corticosteroids are indicated in severe drug-induced pneumonitides, provided an infection has been ruled out.

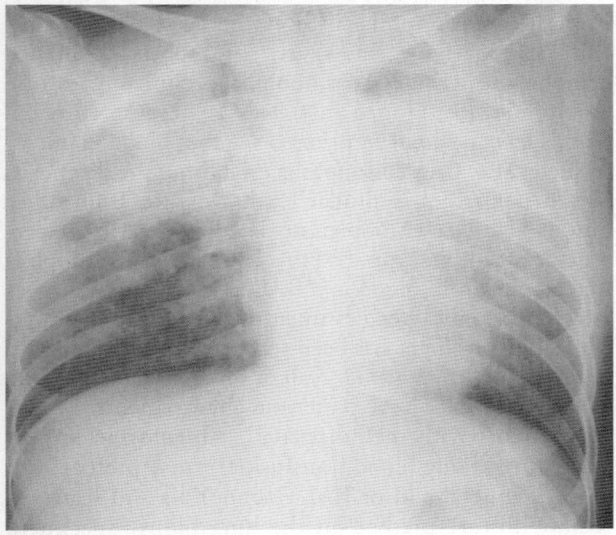

B

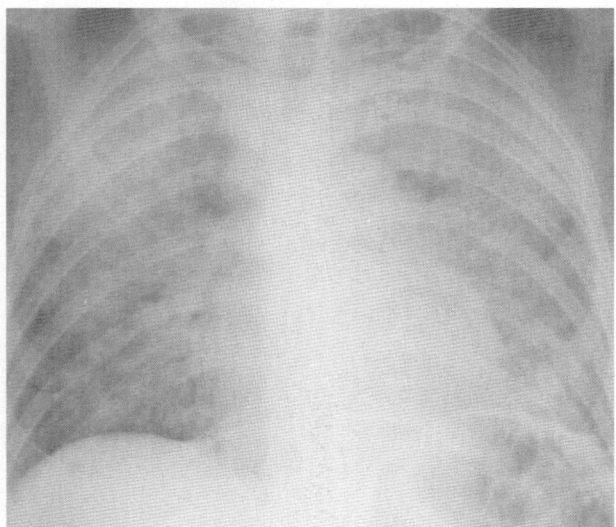

C

unusual. In the majority of cases, the drug was taken orally, but IV or topical minocycline or gynecologic applications of sulfonamides have been cited. Inhaled pentamidine or illicit drugs (eg, cocaine)[151,152] may also cause eosinophilic pneumonia.

Risk factors include prior atopy or asthma and repeated courses of treatment (eg, minocycline), which may sensitize the patient.[50] Rapid tapering or withdrawal of corticosteroids, especially in asthmatics, is also suspected as the origin of eosinophilic pneumonia.[153] Overall, the onset of eosinophilic pneumonia is difficult to predict, except with minocycline lung, which develops after 2 to 3 weeks.[50]

Typical respiratory symptoms include fever and dyspnea and sometimes chest pain or a skin rash. The intensity of respiratory symptoms depends on the extent of pulmonary shadowing and the presence of associated eosinophilic bronchitis, which may cause wheezing. Moderate pleural and/or pericardial effusion may occur, as well as skin, heart, liver, neurologic, kidney, or brain involvement. The constellation of pulmonary and extrapulmonary involvement, sometimes severe, have been referred to as the drug-induced hypersensitivity syndrome (DIHSS) or drug-rash and eosinophilia systemic syndrome (DRESS). This is a potentially life-threatening situation due to a systemic reaction with eosinophilia that has been reported with anticonvulsants, aspirin, or minocycline.[154–160] Other patterns of drug-induced eosinophilic disease include isolated blood eosinophilia, acute eosinophilic pneumonia,[161] and the CSS.[162]

Circulating eosinophils can be > 20,000/µL, and the percentage of eosinophils may reach 50% or more. This is often associated with raised IgE levels. Not uncommonly, blood eosinophil levels continue to increase *after* drug discontinuation, although respiratory symptoms and pulmonary infiltrates improve.[50]

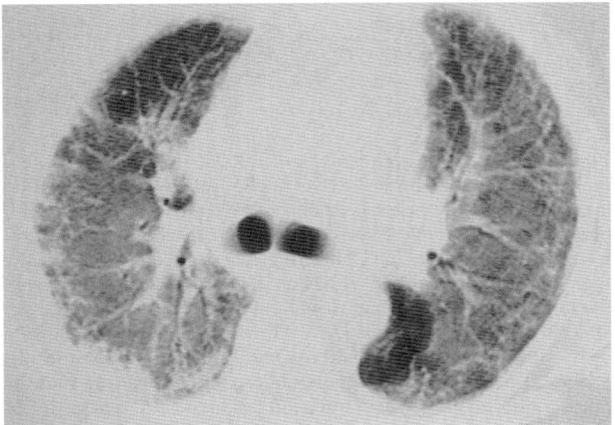

A

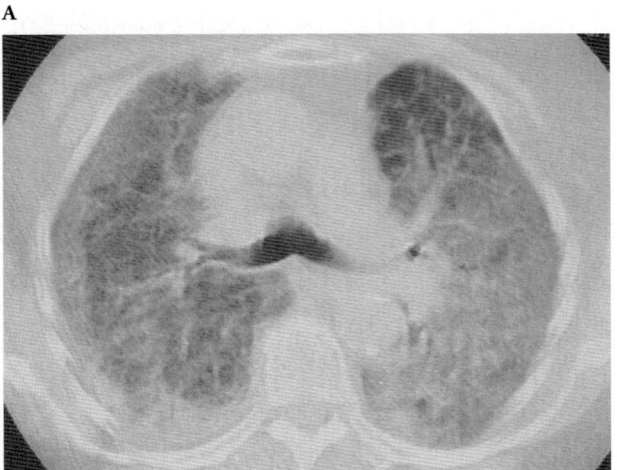

B

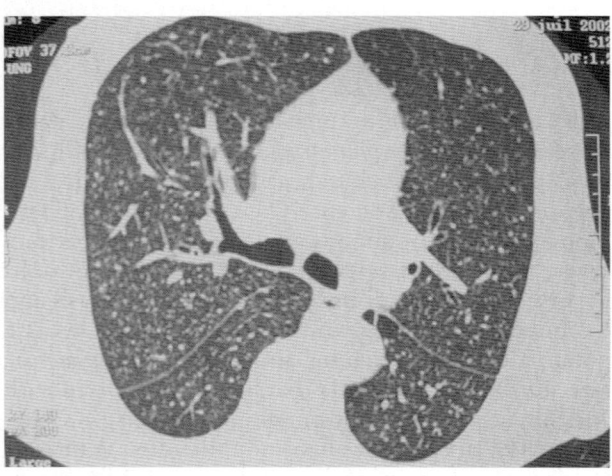

C

Figure 20–2   High-resolution computed tomography in cellular drug-induced interstitial pneumonitis reveals *A*, ground-glass densities (methotrexate), *B*, diffuse haze (nitrofurantoin), or, less commonly, *C*, a miliary pattern (bacille Calmette-Guérin therapy).

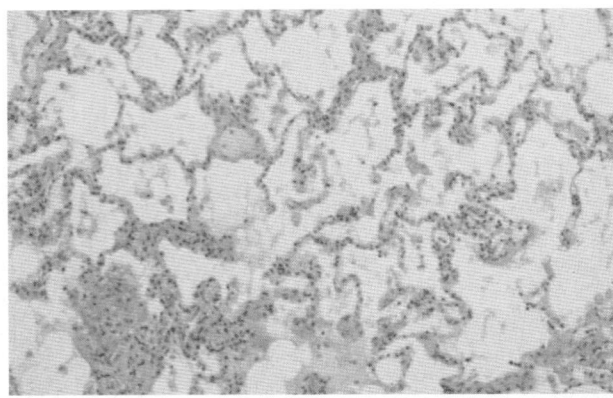

Figure 20–3   Mild cellular interstitial pneumonitis (methotrexate lung). A loosely-formed granuloma is visible in the left lower area. This specimen corresponds to the patient in Figure 20–1 (hematoxylin-eosin-safranin stain).

The diagnosis of PIE is established by the demonstration of eosinophilia in bone marrow, blood, BAL, and/or lung tissue. However, some patients do not demonstrate peripheral eosinophilia, presumably because eosinophils are trapped in tissues or because corticosteroids have been given prior to the first blood count.[163] In such cases, BAL eosinophilia establishes the diagnosis. The BAL pattern is similar to that of PIE from other causes[164] with a commonly associated increase in the percentage of lymphocytes.[50,164] In a few patients, eosinophils were absent from blood *and* BAL, and the diagnosis was established only after examination of lung tissue. Subclinical involvement has been suspected on the basis of a positive gallium 67 (^{67}Ga) scan or on the isolated finding of an eosinophilic BAL pattern in a few patients.

Patients with methotrexate[7] or bleomycin lung[165] or those receiving blood transfusion[166] may present with mild peripheral and/or BAL eosinophilia and scattered eosinophils are present on the lung biopsy specimen. These patients do not strictly meet the definition of PIE.

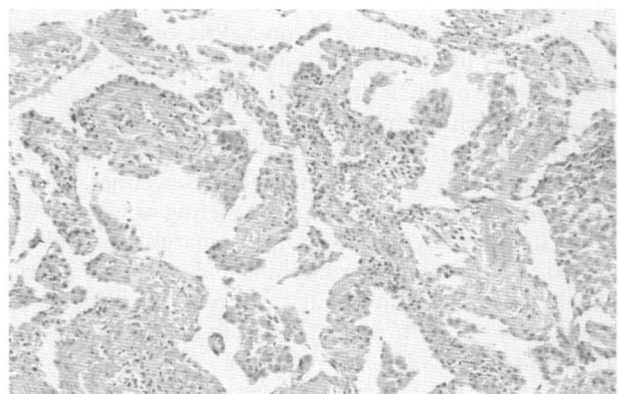

Figure 20–4   Moderate cellular interstitial pneumonitis induced by acebutolol. A florid mononuclear cell interstitial infiltrate in present (hematoxylin-eosin-safranin stain).

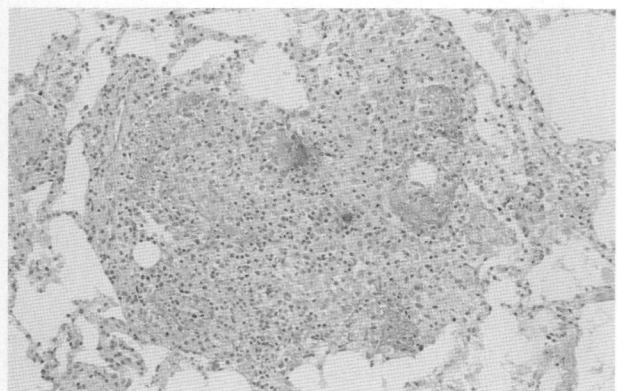

Figure 20–5 Well-formed granulomas are a feature of adverse pulmonary reactions to methotrexate (as in the present case), interferon, and bacille Calmette-Guérin therapy (hematoxylin-eosin-safranin stain).

There are also patients with pulmonary infiltrates and peripheral eosinophilia without eosinophils in the lung.

On imaging, the pulmonary infiltrates of drug-induced PIE are typically alveolar and symmetric. The peripheral pattern of "photographic negative of pulmonary edema" is distinctive; however, it is present in less than half of the cases. In fact, the opacities of PIE may localize to the bases and posteriorly,[50] have a "batwing" pattern, or be scattered, diffuse,[163] asymmetric[50] (Figure 20–6), or migratory.[167] Many appear as faint shadowing, discrete ground-glass, and limited or diffuse opacification. Intestitial Kerley's B lines have been reported in several instances.[168] On CT, opacities tend to be symmetric and dense, localize subpleurally, and range in density from a discrete haze to diffuse alveolar shad-

owing (Figure 20–7).[50,163] Shaggy nodules[169] or enlargement of hilar or mediastinal lymph nodes[82,170] are possible but unusual features.

The diagnosis of drug-induced PIE is facilitated in patients exposed to a single agent. The diagnosis is more complex in the context of a systemic disease or in patients receiving treatment with corticosteroids, immunosuppressive agents, sulfasalazine, or mesalazine. Opportunistic infections, pulmonary involvement from an underlying disease, and drug-induced reactions should be considered. A parasitic infestation is also a possibility.

A lung biopsy is rarely needed to establish PIE except when peripheral and BAL eosinophilia are lacking or if systemic symptoms point to the possibility of an eosinophilic angiitis. On histology, an interstitial infiltrate of mononuclear cells admixed with eosinophils is seen (Figure 20–8) and may localize around small pulmonary vessels. There may be occasional foci of organizing pneumonia.[48,50]

Drug withdrawal is generally followed by a marked improvement in clinical symptoms within a few days. Corticosteroids are given to patients with acute eosinophilic pneumonia and are very effective in reversing the clinical and radiographic abnormalities. Moderate peripheral eosinophilia may persist for several weeks.

Deliberate rechallenge, although usually unnecessary, has been safely performed in several patients. Recurrence of symptoms, eosinophilia, and sometimes pulmonary opacities or BAL cell derangements developed shortly after reintroduction of minocycline, para-aminosalicylic acid (PAS), sulfonamides, or chloroquine.[127,171–173] Despite the apparent safety in reported cases, the diagnostic contribution of rechallenge tests remains questionable. Patients with inflammatory bowel

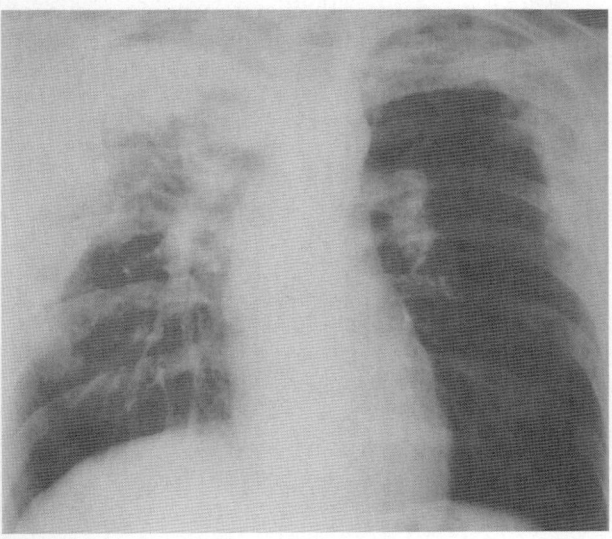

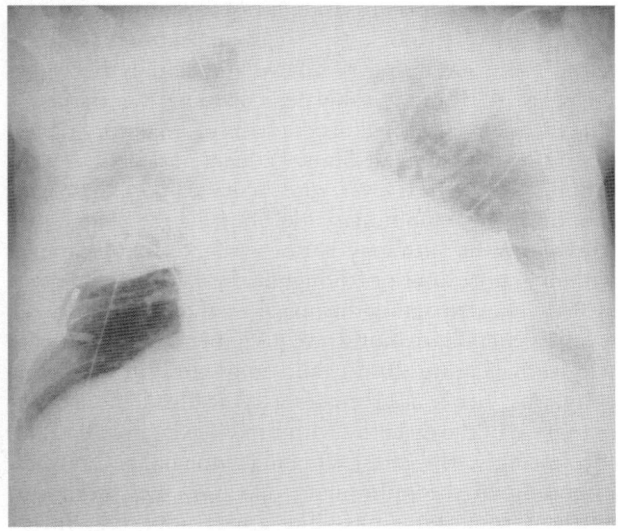

A

B

Figure 20–6 Chest radiographs of drug-induced eosinophilic pneumonia. *A,* The opacities of drug-induced eosinophilic pneumonia characteristically localize in the apices (minocycline). *B,* However, the opacities often localize elsewhere in the lung or are diffuse (angiotensin-converting enzyme inhibitor induced).

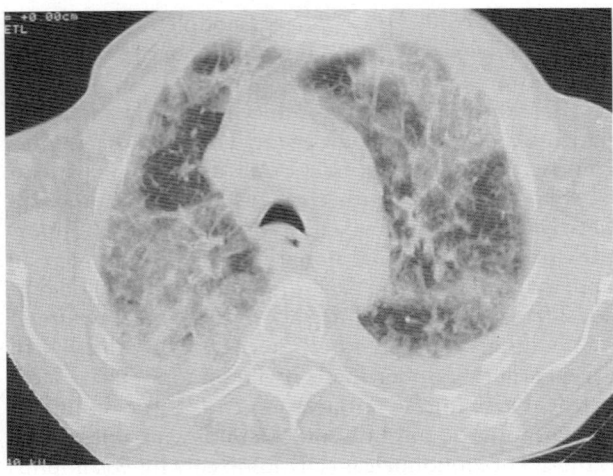

A

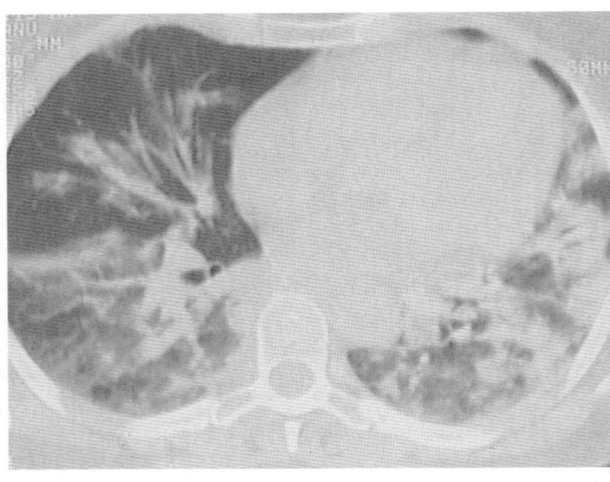

B

Figure 20–7   High-resolution computed tomography in eosinophilic pneumonia shows *A*, lobular ground-glass opacities and thickening of interlobular septa (angiotensin-converting enzyme inhibitor-induced; corresponds to Figure 20–6B) or *B*, dense masses or nodules that contain air bronchograms (nonsteroidal anti-inflammatory drug-induced).

disease and sulfasalazine-induced PIE are the exception, particularly if no alternate drug is effective. Rechallenge with a therapeutic intent has been successfully performed by giving incremental doses of the causative drug. This has resulted in desensitization and reinstatement of the drug.[127,128,174,175]

Organizing Pneumonia

Organizing pneumonia[176] was initially described in patients treated with hexamethonium for systemic hypertension who developed a fatal form of "fibrinous pneumonitis."[177] Today, organizing pneumonia is seen with unrelated drug classes such as amiodarone,[139,178,179] bleomycin,[180] β-blockers,[178] carbamazepine,[181] interferon,[182] nitrofurantoin,[183] following radiation therapy to the breast,[184,185] and possibly penicillamine[186] or statins.[187] The disease is suspected on the basis of migratory opacities on sequential chest films. Patients may present with dyspnea, moderate fever, and acute chest pain corresponding to the pulmonary foci abutting the pleural surface. However, histology is not available in all patients with migratory opacities thought to be caused by drugs.[188]

On chest imaging, the opacities of organizing pneumonia generally demonstrate a segmental or lobar distribution (Figure 20–9), and may contain air bronchograms. Sequential imaging typically demonstrates migration of the opacities with time (see Figure 20–9).[178] Interestingly, the chest film may normalize between migration of the pulmonary opacities. Less common patterns include a mass-like appearance (eg, interferon),[182] multiple peribronchovascular shadows (eg, nitrofurantoin) (Figure 20–10),[183] dense subpleural opacities (eg, mesalazine) (see Figure 20–9C and 20–10B), ill-defined infiltrates (eg, bleomycin, inter-

feron), multiple well-defined nodules (eg, carbamazepine,[181] bleomycin; see "Bleomycin Lung" to follow[180]), or diffuse infiltrates.[189]

There is no specific BAL pattern of drug-induced organizing pneumonia.[190] Histology reveals intra-alveolar connective tissue, interstitial inflammation (Figure 20–11),[178] and sometimes a mild eosinophilic infiltrate. Tissue eosinophilia of significant degree makes the differentiation of *organizing* from *eosinophilic* pneumonia difficult, and patients may present with overlapping features of the two conditions.[180,191] A histologic pattern of organizing pneumonia may appear as multiple nodules in patients receiving bleomycin, which raises the possibility of pulmonary metastases.[180]

Whether patients with migratory pulmonary opacities and a background of compatible drug exposure should undergo a lung biopsy or simply be observed

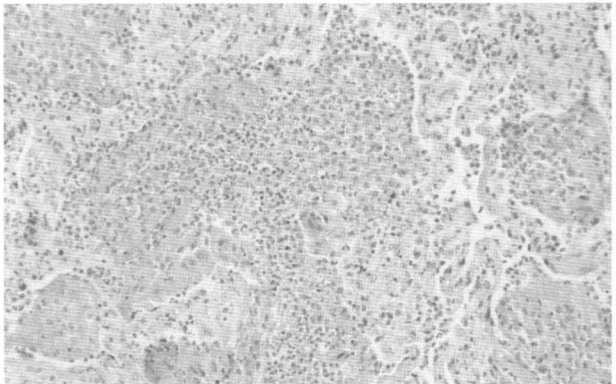

Figure 20–8   The infiltrate in drug-induced eosinophilic pneumonia (acebutolol in the present case) resembles that in eosinophilic pneumonia from other causes and consists of mononuclear cells and eosinophils. The latter are best seen on a May-Grünwald-Giemsa stain (hematoxylin-eosin-safranin stain).

after withdrawal of the agent is unknown.[188] Organizing pneumonia due to amiodarone differs from that of other drugs because of the persistence of amiodarone in the lung. This predisposes to relapses, which occur after drug withdrawal. In this case, extended use of or reinitiation of corticosteroid therapy is indicated.

There are cases that are thought to be cryptogenic organizing pneumonia, because the association with the drug was not made. Until the association was established and the drug withdrawn, multiple relapses occurred requiring repeated courses of corticosteroids.

Chemotherapy Lung

Chemotherapy lung refers to a noninfectious, nonneoplastic pulmonary complication that develops during or after the administration of single- (eg, BCNU or other nitrosoureas, bleomycin, busulfan, chlorambucil, cyclophosphamide, melphalan, mitomycin) or multiagent cytostatic chemotherapy with or without associated radiation therapy to the chest.[192–197] The increased complexity of multimodality treatments and high-dose protocols designed to augment antineoplastic efficacy have translated into an increased incidence of pulmonary complications and mortality.[198] Patients treated for leukemia, Hodgkin's disease, non-Hodgkin's lymphoma, and breast carcinoma and bone marrow transplant recipients are at risk.

Depending on the patient and the time of diagnosis, chemotherapy lung may have overlapping features with pulmonary edema, diffuse alveolar damage, pulmonary fibrosis, nonspecific interstitial pneumonia, or, less likely, eosinophilic pneumonia. The term chemotherapy

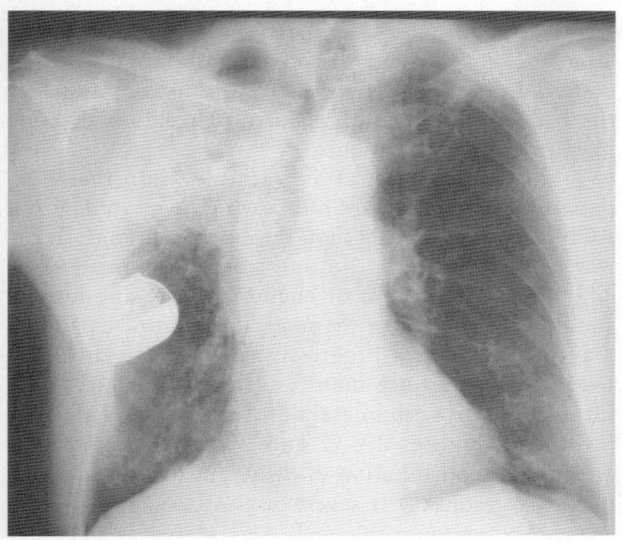

A

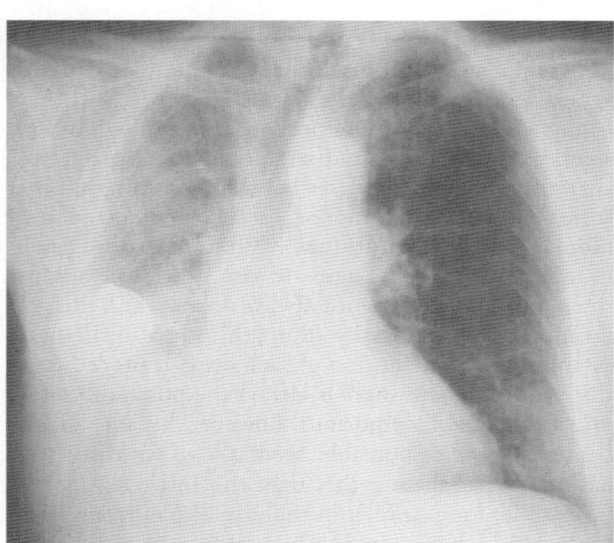

B

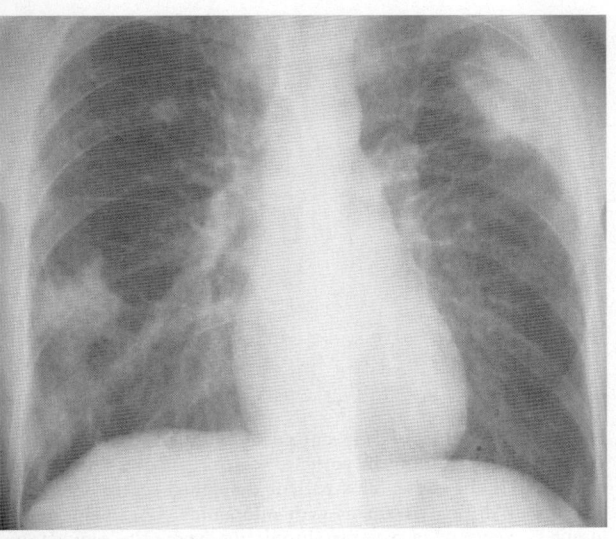

C

Figure 20–9   *A, B,* The opacities of drug-induced organizing pneumonia are typically alveolar and migrate on sequential chest radiographs (amiodarone induced; same patient taken a few weeks apart). *C,* Other patterns include nonmigratory subpleural masses (mesalazine induced) or diffuse involvement. Organizing pneumonia may occur as a complication of radiation therapy to the breast.

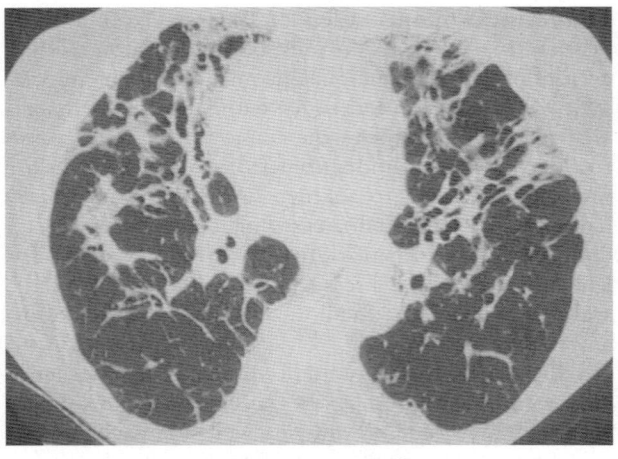

A

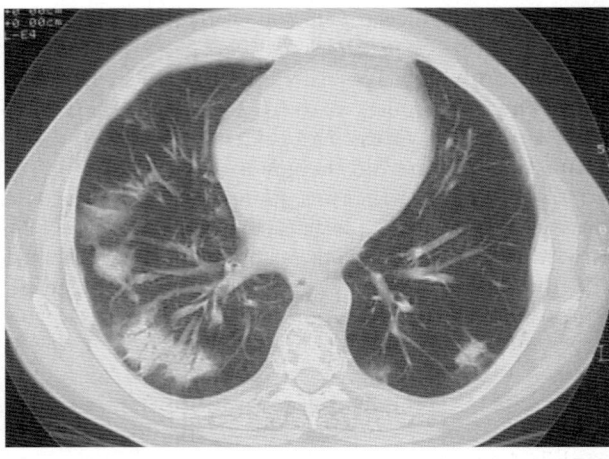

B

Figure 20–10   High-resolution computed tomography patterns in organizing pneumonia include *A*, multiple opacities around the bronchovascular bundles (nitrofurantoin induced), *B*, subpleural masses (interferon induced), or multiple areas of ground-glass opacities.

lung is not ideal, because other pneumotoxic drugs or agents such as colony stimulating factors (CSFs), oxygen, blood transfusions, proteins, immunoglobulins, stem cell infusion, and radiation therapy may trigger or aggravate the syndrome (see below). Accordingly, other terms have been proposed including delayed pulmonary toxicity syndrome[199,200] or idiopathic pneumonia syndrome.[201] These are also not ideal, because the manifestations are not always delayed and the syndrome is not necessarily idiopathic. It is difficult to establish the contribution of each drug or procedure to this syndrome and there is always the possibility of an infection. This is important, however, because identification of the responsible agent allows for discontinuation of that agent rather than the entire regimen. It is possible, for example, in the case of methotrexate or bleomycin, that a distinctive pattern of pulmonary involvement evolves, although other agents were administered. For instance, non-Hodgkin's lymphoma patients who received methotrexate, bleomycin, doxorubicin (Adriamycin), cyclophosphamide, vincristine (Oncovin), and dexamethasone (M-BACOD) or methotrexate, doxorubicin (Adriamycin), cyclophosphamide, vincristine (Oncovin), and dexamethasone (M-ACOD) regimens developed a picture similar to methotrexate lung, whereas no pulmonary infiltrates were observed in patients receiving a cyclophosphamide, doxorubicin, vincristine (Oncovin), and prednisone (CHOP) regimen.[202] Similarly, the difference in pulmonary events in two arms of a therapeutic regimen that differed by one drug (eg, with/without bleomycin, BCNU, CSF, or radiation therapy) or by the dosage of one drug (eg, low vs high BCNU)[203] points to the cause of the lung disease.

In addition to the intrinsic risk of cytoxic drugs,[65] other risk factors include advanced age, a history of smoking, drug dosage, the combination of drugs or radi-

ation therapy, oxygen, CSF, rapid withdrawal of corticosteroids, the type of bone marrow transplantation and the background of graft-versus-host reaction in bone marrow transplant patients.[119,204–209]

The time to onset is variable. For instance, patients with breast carcinoma who are treated with a BCNU-containing regimen develop pulmonary infiltrates after 3 weeks to 3 months of treatment.[194,200,210] The clinical evolution of chemoradiotherapy lung is variable. At one end of the spectrum, dyspneic patients may present with a progressive decrease in diffusing capacity as the only manifestation of toxicity.[118,199] Others present with bilateral, interstitial, and alveolar infiltrates (Figures 20–12 and 20–13A) that reverse after the discontinuation of drugs and/or the addition of corticosteroids.[200] In severe cases ARDS appears.[211,212]

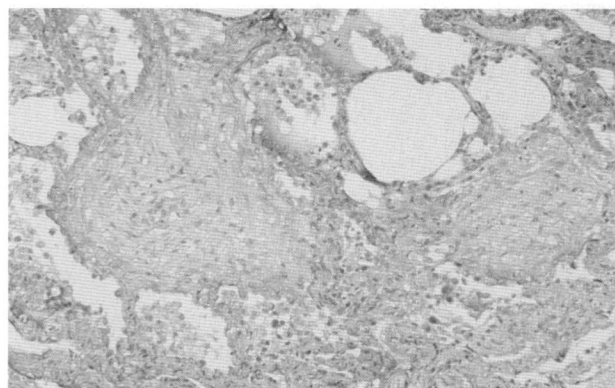

Figure 20–11   Buds of connective tissue within distal air spaces are a characteristic finding in patients with organizing pneumonia, regardless of the cause. This patient developed severe organizing pneumonia during treatment with nilutamide. Organizing pneumonia is common in patients chronically exposed to amiodarone (orcein stain).

High-resolution computed tomography (HRCT) shows scattered ground-glass opacities,[78] and increased thickness of the intralobular septa.[134] Sometimes a thoracic deformity develops in children following chemotherapy in addition to more typical changes of pleural and/or pulmonary fibrosis (Figure 20–13B).[213] Restrictive physiology and hypoxemia are typical. The diffusing capacity is decreased, and often the decrease will predate symptoms.[118] There is a decrease in the capillary volume (Vc) component of the diffusing capacity, possibly reflecting vascular injury during the early phase of the disease, whereas later on there is a preferential decrease in the membrane component (Dm) reflecting parenchymal fibrotic changes.[214] Bronchoalveolar lavage findings include increases in neutrophils, lymphocytes, or both cell types.[199] These cells are activated and have been shown to release interleukin (IL)-6 and -8.[199]

Evaluation for infection should include examination of the sputum, BAL, blood, and other fluids. If this is unrevealing, the diagnosis of chemotherapy lung is likely. The suspected drug is withdrawn, and corticosteroids should be administered.[200] A lung biopsy may be reserved for patients with an atypical presentation or those who do not improve on empiric treatment.[215] Histopathologic features of chemotherapy lung include (1) *interstitial* changes of edema, fibrosis, fibroblast proliferation, and (2) *alveolar* changes of atelectasis, exudation, filling by proteinaceous material (ie, alveolar edema), organized alveolar fibrin (organizing pneumonia), increased numbers of macrophages within the alveolar spaces, hyaline membranes, dysplasia/atypia of type II pneumocytes (Figure 20–14),[48] or a pattern of alveolar proteinosis.[216] There is usually little or no inflammation, except in patients with methotrexate lung in whom inflammation is the dominant feature (see Figures 20–3 and 20–5). Taken together, the above changes, although

nonspecific, suggest chemotherapy lung. Occasionally, vascular changes are present, especially in patients receiving bleomycin. In the setting of chemotherapy, the respective benefit of a minimally invasive approach with empiric treatment (antibiotic coverage and corticosteroids),[194] as opposed to the more invasive approach,[217] remains unclear.

Many patients will respond favorably to drug discontinuation and corticosteroid drugs, especially if the condition is recognized early.[218,219] In a series of 65 patients with hematologic malignancies who had received a carmustine-based conditioning regimen prior to bone marrow transplantation, 17 (26%) developed pulmonary infiltrates thought to be drug induced. Of the 17 patients, 15 responded to corticosteroids, and 1 died of interstitial pneumonitis.[207] In patients who respond favorably, corticosteroids should be tapered slowly to avoid recurrence.[204] The recurrence may not be sensitive to corticosteroids and evolve into fatal respiratory failure.[220] A few patients require chronic corticosteroid therapy because attempts at withdrawal are followed by relapse or deterioration. A fraction of patients are refractory to corticosteroids and deteriorate with rapidly evolving ARDS or later on, with progressive pulmonary fibrosis.[33,45] Patients who recover from chemotherapy lung may have a mild reduction of vital capacity and/or of diffusing capacity that persists.[221] Moreover, the likelihood of permanent physiologic impairment is greater in smokers.[222] Patients who receive alkylating agents for Hodgkin's or non-Hodgkin's lymphoma should be discouraged from smoking as this greatly increases the likelihood of late chemotherapy-related lung cancer.[223]

The high incidence, severity, and unpredictability of chemotherapy lung has led investigators to determine whether earlier detection of the disease is possible with pulmonary function tests or imaging techniques.

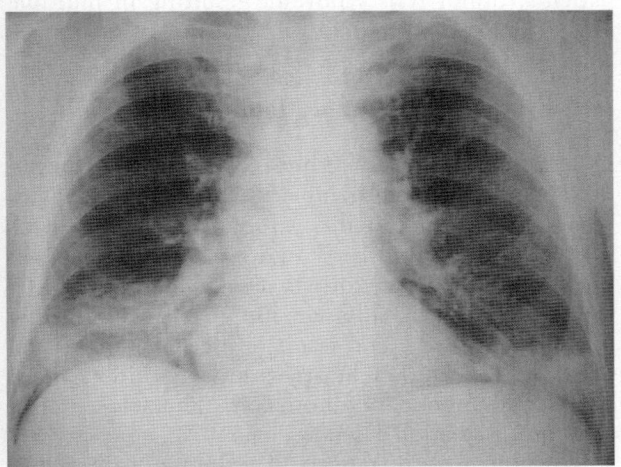

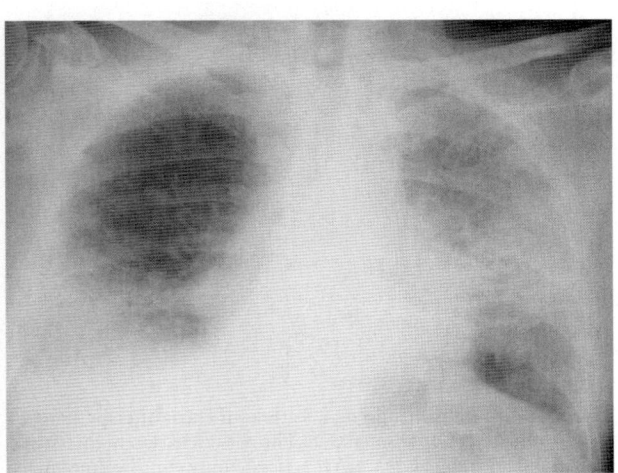

A   **B**

Figure 20–12   The opacities on chest radiographs of chemotherapy lung have a predilection to localize in *A*, the bases (busulfan induced) or *B*, are diffuse (mitomycin and chest irradiation in combination).

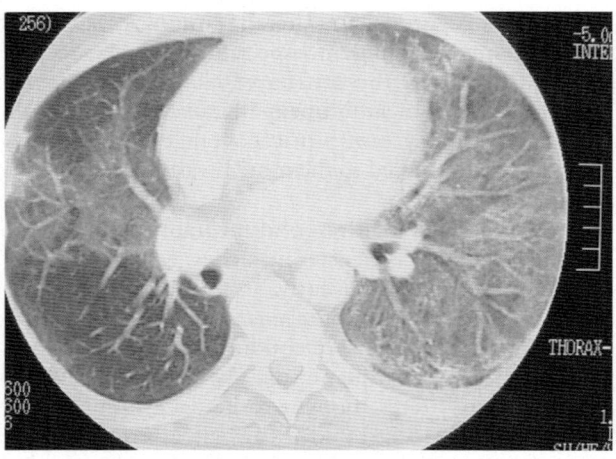
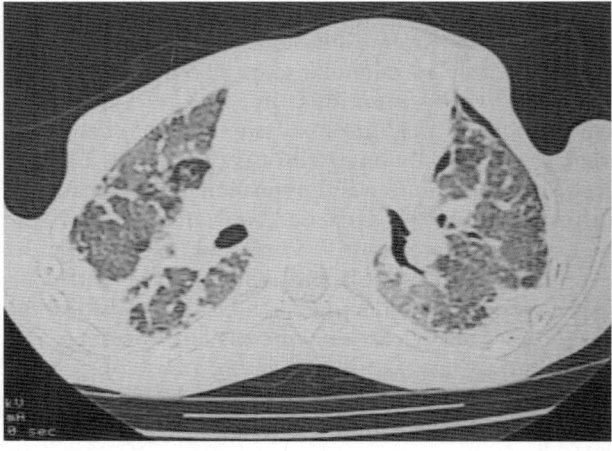

A   **B**

Figure 20–13   In chemotherapy lung, high-resolution computed tomography shows *A*, diffuse ground-glass or haze (corresponding to Figure 20–12B) or fibrosis. *B*, In patients who received chemotherapy in childhood, late changes may develop in the form of chest deformity in addition to ground-glass opacities, interstitial fibrosis, and pleural thickening (late changes following chemotherapy for non-Hodgkin's lymphoma in childhood).

- Some believe it is prudent to discontinue chemotherapy once the diffusing capacity has decreased to 50% of pretherapy values. Others do not rely on this measurement because it is their belief that the diffusing capacity does not necessarily equate to toxicity and, there is a risk involved in withdrawing chemotherapy.[224] A rapid decrease in the diffusing capacity, as a function of time, may indicate impending toxicity. When radiation therapy is planned after the administration of chemotherapeutic agents, it is advisable to wait for any chemotherapy-induced decrease in the diffusing capacity to stabilize or show a trend toward improvement.[118]

- It is difficult to rely on imaging to detect meaningful pulmonary toxicity from chemotherapeutic agents. Patients on chemotherapy may develop new opacities on CT although they never develop symptomatic disease.[225]
- Relying solely on clinical symptoms is also not satisfactory.

Currently, there is no agreement how patients on chemotherapy should be monitored to reliably and cost-effectively detect therapy-induced pulmonary complications.

A peculiar form of chemotherapy lung is known to develop after the first course of chemotherapy in patients with acute leukemia with high blast cell counts. Massive lysis of leukemic cells within pulmonary capillaries induces acute respiratory failure, ARDS, and, in some patients, tumor lysis syndrome resulting in multiple organ dysfunction.[226,227]

Pulmonary Fibrosis

Drug-induced pulmonary fibrosis complicates prolonged therapy with chemotherapeutic agents (bleomycin, busulfan, chlorambucil, cyclophosphamide, nitrosoureas),[21,49] amiodarone,[228] and nitrofurantoin[229] and, less frequently, noncytotoxic agents such as gold,[130] methotrexate,[74] or sulfasalazine.[127,128] Occasionally, fibrosis may be the end result of a cellular interstitial pneumonia. Radiation therapy induces a distinct pattern of localized pulmonary fibrosis (see "Thoracic Complications of Radiation Therapy" below).[86]

Although the diagnosis of pulmonary fibrosis is established by clinical, imaging, and functional criteria, the relationship to a specific drug is more difficult. Arguments that favor drug-induced fibrosis include the

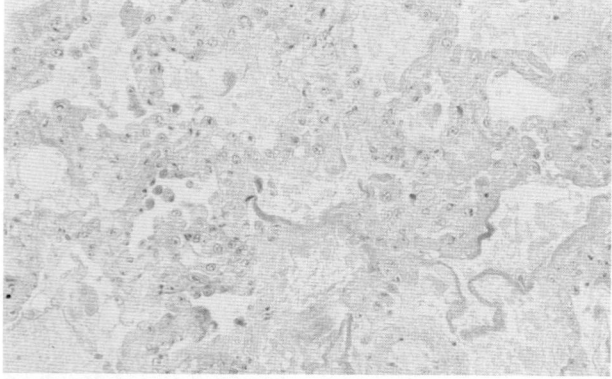

Figure 20–14   Histopathologic features of chemotherapy lung, in this case due to cyclophosphamide. The concatenation of interstitial edema and fibrosis, atypia of type II pneumocytes, hyaline membranes (diffuse alveolar damage), and intra-alveolar debris is suggestive. Patients may recover, develop an ARDS picture, or evolve toward pulmonary fibrosis (see Figure 20–16) (hematoxylin-eosin-safranin stain).

absence of symptoms, and a normal chest radiograph prior to institution of treatment.

The clinical onset is usually insidious but can be accelerated (Hamman-Rich-like)[230,231] and includes dyspnea, a dry cough, fever, and, with busulfan, hyperpigmentation of the skin.[33] Scattered coarse interstitial opacities are present on the chest radiograph (Figure 20–15A) and, on CT, coarse lines and areas of ground-glass density coexist with areas of unaffected lung (Figure 20–15B).[78,79] Honeycombing is unusual at this stage and may develop months or years later. Histology indicates fibrosis, sparse mononuclear interstitial infiltrates, interstitial edema, and reactive type II pneumocytes (Figure 20–16).[232]

Cessation of the drug is indicated but is rarely followed by measurable beneficial effects. Corticosteroids may be temporarily effective. The prognosis is similar to idiopathic pulmonary fibrosis, with inexorable progression but at a variable rate. Some patients have years of stabilization, and others will survive only for a few months following diagnosis. Transplantation has been carried out in patients in whom the primary diesease is considered cured.

Transient Pulmonary Infiltrates

A syndrome of transient pulmonary infiltrates that is usually self-limiting and benign and may occur following the administration of ATRA[233]; hydrochlorothiazide[98]; nitrofurantoin[234]; the newer antineoplastic agents docetaxel, gemcitabine, and Taxotere[235]; growth factors (CSFs[236]); autologous or allogeneic material (blood, bone marrow, stem cells, and immunoglobulins[237]); heterologous proteins (antithymocyte globulins[238]); interleukin-2; or tumor necrosis factor.[239] Transient pulmonary infil-

trates are generally well-tolerated, although they transiently alter gas exchange but are short-lived (Figure 20–17). A few patients underwent a lung biopsy, and there was evidence the transient infiltrates represented rapidly-evolving edema, diffuse alveolar damage, hyaline membranes, vasculitis, or interstitial pneumonia.[240–242] The pattern of transient pulmonary infiltrates may represent an attenuated form of drug-induced pulmonary edema or chemotherapy lung. Resumption of the causative agent is generally followed by recurrence.[98] Thus, caution is required if resumption of the drug is planned. In a few patients the pulmonary infiltrates did not recur following re-exposure.[235] Other patients received prophylactic corticosteroids, and the infiltrates did not recur.[243]

Pulmonary Edema

Drug-induced pulmonary edema[43] (PE) is characterized by increases in the alveolar-capillary permeability and lung water. Early reports described PE following heroin use in drug abusers.[244,245] Later, drug-induced PE was reported as a complication of the administration of a number of chemically unrelated drugs[43,51] and after bone marrow transplantation.[246] The general mechanisms by which drugs induce pulmonary edema include (1) excessive infusion of fluid (solutes, blood; "overload pulmonary edema"), (2) depression of myocardial function (Isoptin), (3) generalized vasoconstriction (epinephrine, vasopressin, ergometrine), (4) immunologic (anaphylaxis or transfusion of blood or its derivatives: platelets, immunoglobulins, fresh frozen plasma), (5) cell aggregation in the pulmonary circulation (ATRA, CSF), (6) hypersensitivity

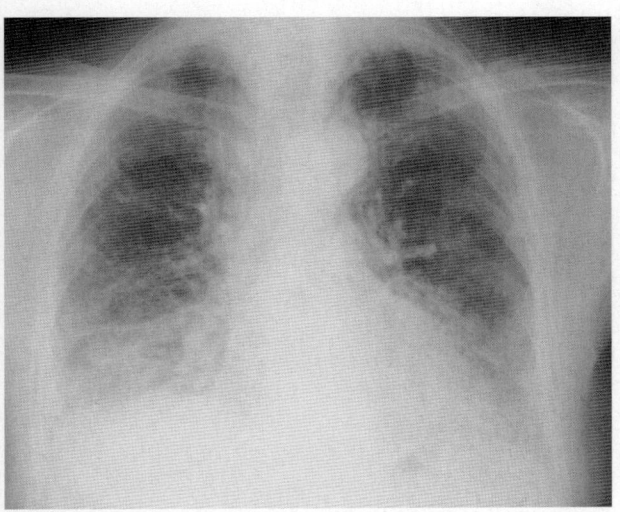

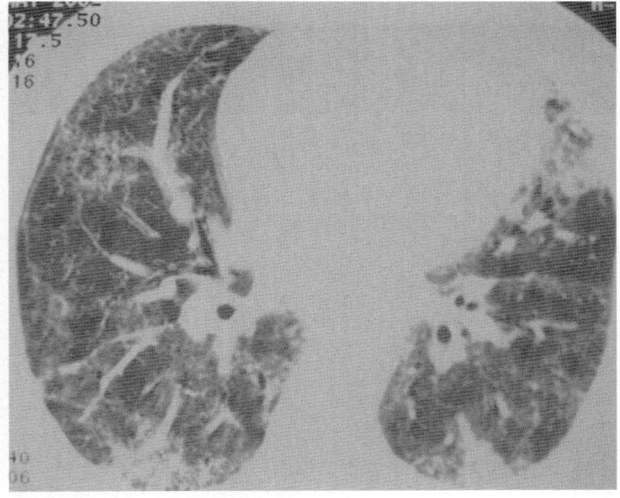

A   **B**

Figure 20–15 Drug-induced pulmonary fibrosis. A 75 year-old man developed dyspnea, crackles, pulmonary infiltrates and hypoxemia during treatment with amiodarone. The chest radiograph was normal prior to institution of treatment with amiodarone. *A*, At the time of diagnosis, there were coarse basilar opacities and evidence for volume loss. *B*, These changes are confirmed on a computed tomography scan. Honeycombing is generally absent at the time of diagnosis and may develop later on. Chemotherapeutic agents and nitrofurantoin also cause pulmonary fibrosis.

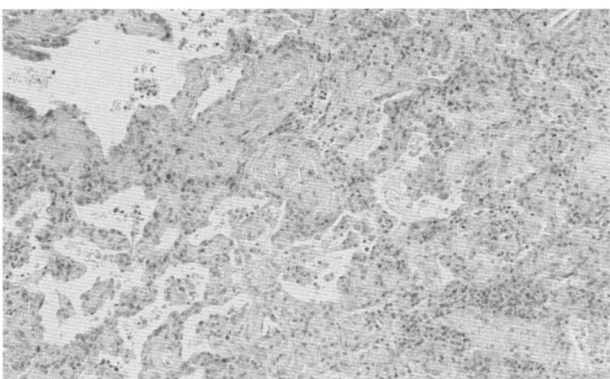

Figure 20–16 Drug-induced pulmonary fibrosis mitomycin. The patient developed progressive basilar changes following local instillations of mitomycin C for the treatment of bladder carcinoma. The clinical condition and pulmonary physiology stabilized after drug discontinuation (hematoxylin-eosin-safranin stain).

(hydrochlorothiazide, radiographic contrast material), (7) vascular leakage (interleukin-2, tumor necrosis factor [TNF]), (8) toxic (overdoses of carbamazepine, opiates, or tricyclics), (9) associated with severe drug-induced pneumonitis (gold, methotrexate, nitrofurantoin), and (10) unknown (cytarabine [ara-C], β_2-agonists, methotrexate, opiates, radiographic contrast media, vinorelbine). Drug-induced pulmonary edema is temporally related to the initiation of treatment as opposed to the interstitial pneumonias, which develop after longer periods of use. For instance, hydrochlorothiazide-induced edema developed after a mean of 44 minutes following injection.[98] In one patient, drug-induced pulmonary edema developed after the injection of radiographic contrast material. On the CT

scan, there was radiographic evidence of edema in 25 seconds and interstitial pulmonary edema in 15 min.[247] Acetylsalicylic acid (ASA) is one exception; pulmonary edema may develop with chronic exposure to the drug.[248] Clinical examination reveals crackles and wheezes and, in cases with severe edema, cyanosis, arterial hypoxemia, hypotension or shock, and cough productive of abundant frothy sputum appear. Radiographs show bilateral interstitial or alveolar shadows (Figure 20–18), thickened septa, and sometimes pleural effusion. Distension of septa, a ground-glass pattern or alveolar shadows are seen on the CT scan.[249] In one patient with drug-induced pulmonary edema, pulmonary angiography showed extravasation of the contrast material. In most cases of drug-induced pulmonary edema, the pulmonary capillary wedge pressure and cardiac echography are normal.

Histopathologic material, although rarely available, shows alveolar flooding by proteinaceous fluid and sometimes hyaline membranes, alveolar hemorrhage, and interstitial edema.[106,211,233,250,251] On discontinuation of the causative agent, corticosteroids, and mechanical ventilation (if needed), the pulmonary opacities clear within a few days. A fraction of patients develop ARDS. Because drug-induced pulmonary edema is of noncardiogenic origin, diuretic drugs are generally not recommended except in women with β_2-agonist edema.[100]

A few drugs or agents deserve special mention.

β2-Agonists

The β_2-agonists terbutaline, isoxsuprine, ritodrine, and salbutamol are used to retard labor. β_2-agonist-induced pulmonary edema appears unique to the pregnant state

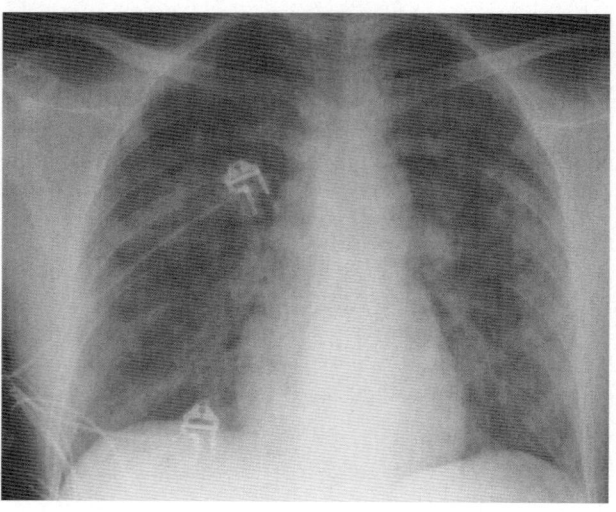

A

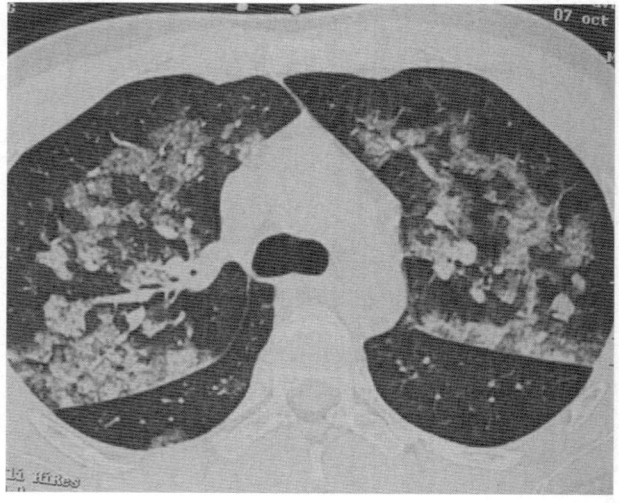

B

Figure 20–17 *A*, Radiograph of drug-induced transient pulmonary infiltrates that developed shortly after the IV administration of lidocaine and adrenaline during minor surgery in a young patient. *B*, High-resolution computed tomography scan reveals scattered lobular ground-glass opacities and moderate thickening of adjacent interlobular septa. The opacities cleared in a few days. The histopathologic features of transient pulmonary infiltrates are poorly known because a lung biopsy is rarely performed.

as it has not been reported when these drugs are used to treat other conditions. Risk factors include multiparity, twin pregnancy, and maternal infection. β_2-agonist edema generally develops acutely in patients who have received tocolytic agents intravenously with fluids for an average of 2 to 3 days (see Figure 20–18A). In one patient, β_2-agonist edema was precipitated by ergometrine. β_2-agonist edema responds promptly to drug discontinuation, oxygen, and diuretics. Mechanical ventilation is required in a minority of patients, and the prognosis in both the mother and child is good.[100]

Ovarian Stimulators

The ovarian hyperstimulation syndrome is observed in women undergoing induction of ovulation with clomiphene citrate, and gonadotropins. In a few patients, a syndrome of vascular leakage occurs. These patients usually present with exudative pleural effusion or ascites, and a fraction develop pulmonary edema or an ARDS picture.[252,253]

Acetylsalicylic Acid

Salicylate pulmonary edema is a complication of excessive intake of ASA, occurring more frequently in older patients. Clues to the diagnosis include confusion, lactic acidosis, and proteinuria. The latter may reflect an increase in capillary permeability. The diagnosis is supported by measurements of blood salicylate levels, which should be obtained as early as possible. Salicylate levels above 40 mg/dL are consistent with the diagnosis. The disease may recur on rechallenge with ASA.[248]

Hydrochlorothiazide

Hydrochlorothiazide may induce a picture of severe, allergic pulmonary edema, which often develops after the first exposure to the drug. The peculiarities of hydrochlorothiazide-induced edema are its immediate severity, tendency to recur on rechallenge, and the frequency at which the offending drug was not considered.[98]

Transfusion Products

Transfusion of whole blood, platelets, plasma components, or immunogobulins (IVIG) may induce pulmonary infiltrates believed to reflect pulmonary edema. The syndrome is referred to as TRALI, or transfusion-related acute lung injury (see Figure 20–18B).[166] Symptoms develop within a few hours of the transfusion. Transient hypoxemia following transfusion in patients on a respirator may correspond to attenuated forms of TRALI. The syndrome is thought to result from the passive transfer of complement-activating human leukocyte antigen (HLA) class I or II granulocyte-specific or lymphocytotoxic antibodies of donor origin. These antibodies presumably agglutinate and activate neutrophils, which damage the pulmonary microcirculation.

Retrospective investigation of TRALI demonstrated an antibody in the donor, generally a multiparous woman, in 85% of cases. Other mechanisms for TRALI include the accumulation of platelet activating factor-like substances in stored blood. Most patients recover within 96 hours. Recognition of TRALI is essential and should occasion the examination of the donor product for antibodies and subsequent elimination of the impli-

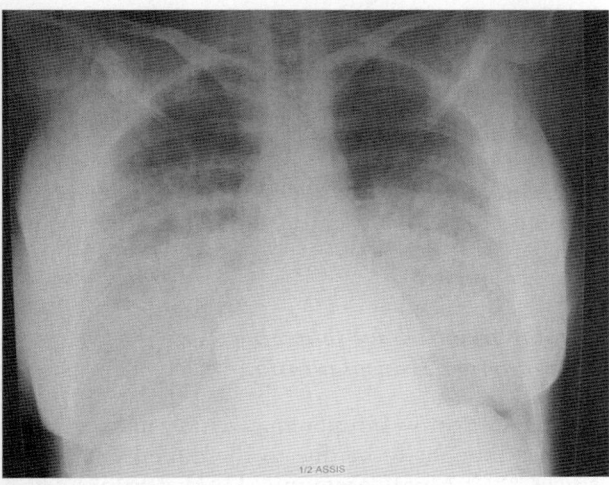
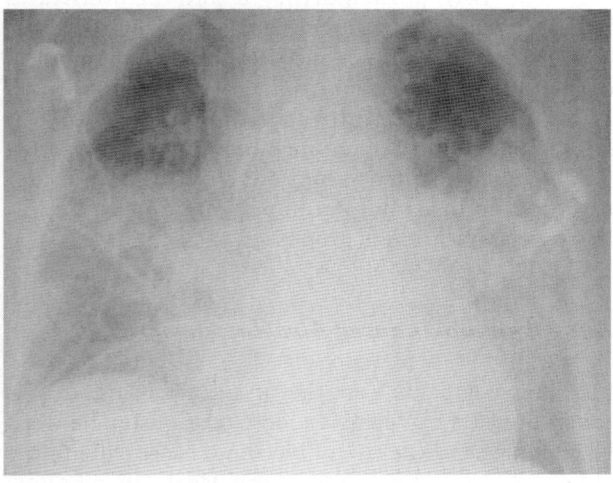

A   **B**

Figure 20–18   Radiographs of drug-induced pulmonary edema. *A*, Alveolar opacities developed in a young parturient who had received IV β_2-agonists and fluids to retard labor. Evidence of increased lung water was present in this case in the form of enlarged main and accessory fissures. The patient was mechanically ventilated for 2 days and responded promptly to discontinuation of the drug and administration of diuretics. *B*, Alveolar opacities thought to represent pulmonary edema developed shortly after blood transfusion (TRALI syndrome). The patient recovered in 2 days.

cated donor from the donor pool. A recent study indicates that TRALI is under-reported and that measures to withdraw the donor from the donor pool can be improved.[237]

Pulmonary Vasodilators

Recently, pulmonary edema has occurred in patients with pulmonary hypertension or veno-occlusive disease after administration of the pulmonary vasodilators nifedipine, prostacyclin, or nitric oxide.[254,255]

Alveolar Hemorrhage

Drug-induced alveolar hemorrhage is a diffuse and synchronous bleeding from the pulmonary capillary bed, which may be associated with histologically demonstrable capillaritis. The syndrome is unusual and requires expeditious management to avoid irreversible respiratory failure. The spectrum of severity of drug-induced diffuse alveolar hemorrhage (DAH) ranges from subclinical opacities on the chest radiograph or the incidental finding of iron-laden macrophages in the BAL fluid in patients on chronic oral anticoagulants to life-threatening ARDS. In some cases, the disease is heralded by unexplained anemia or transient episodes of hypoxemia. Full-blown disease causes dyspnea and interstitial infiltrates and in advanced cases alveolar infiltrates, which may assume a batwing distribution, and anemia are present (Figure 20–19). Hemoptysis is not a constant feature, even in patients with significant anemia. An increase in the diffusing capacity is not present in all patients with active bleeding. The BAL is hemorrhagic and demonstrates increased bleeding in sequential aliquots. Microscopic examination of the BAL fluid shows increased numbers of hemosiderin-laden macrophages in addition to red cells. A search for autoantibodies (ANA, ANCA, anti–glomerular basement membrane antibodies [anti-GBM]) is mandatory to look for a cause, or to recognize drug-induced autoimmune conditions. The following classification is proposed.

Anticoagulant-Induced Alveolar Hemorrhage

Oral anticoagulants were the first drugs recognized as causes of DAH.[256] There is a loose relationship between drug dosage and the risk of bleeding. Most patients are either taking too much drug, have inadequate monitoring of the therapeutic effects of the drug, or are taking drugs that enhance the anticoagulant effect. Clotting studies are well above therapeutic levels, and resolution occurs after cessation of exposure and replacement therapy with vitamin K in the case of coumadin.

Heparin,[257] tissue plasminogen activator,[258] intravenous or intra-arterial streptokinase, or urokinase,[259] also are associated with DAH. More recently, the platelet glycoprotein IIb/III inhibitor (abciximab),[260] and an inhibitor of platelet aggregation (clopidogrel)[257] have also been shown to induce alveolar hemorrhage.

The incidence of drug-induced DAH is low: 0.4% after thrombolysis and 0.19% after abciximab. Left ventricular failure or the presence of active lung disease may increase the risk of drug-induced bleeding. There is no current evidence that anticoagulant-induced DAH is due to capillaritis or is immune mediated.

Drug-Induced Alveolar Hemorrhage and Capillaritis

Drug-induced alveolar hemorrhage and capillaritis often occur in the setting of ANCA and associated systemic disease, including glomerulonephritis and the small vessel vasculitis pulmonary capillaritis, as the cause of the alveolar hemorrhage (See Chapter 23 "Diffuse Alveolar Hemorrhage"). Tretinoin (ATRA),[261] propylthiouracil,[262] allogeneic or autologous bone marrow transplantation,[263] and possibly phenytoin[264] and mitomycin[265] have been associated with this entity. A decrease in ANCA titers following withdrawal of the drug supports the drug etiology.

Alveolar Hemorrhage as a Manifestation of Severe Drug-Induced Pneumonitis

A subset of patients with severe drug-induced pneumonitis (eg, due to gold, methotrexate, or nitrofurantoin) develop DAH.[145] This may dominate the clinical scenario. In this case the underlying lesion is extensive diffuse alveolar damage (see Chapter 23 "Diffuse Alveolar Hemorrhage").

Drug-Induced Thrombocytopenia and Alveolar Hemorrhage

Severe thrombocytopenia and DAH have been reported after quinidine, valproate, and chemotherapeutic agents.[266,267]

Alveolar Hemorrhage following Bone Marrow Transplantation

Autologous marrow infusion may acutely induce DAH, which is thought to be due to the dimethylsulfoxide vehicle.[268–271] More commonly, DAH develops a few weeks after allogeneic or autologous bone marrow transplantation. The DAH occurs alone or in the context of infection[268] or diffuse microangiopathy with multiorgan involvement. The incidence is higher in recipients of allogeneic marrow (as opposed to autologous marrow) and in those patients in whom drugs (as opposed to T-cell depletion) were employed for graft-versus-host disease prophylaxis. This has also been described after infusion of stem cells or cord blood. The prognosis is poor.

Penicillamine-Induced Alveolar Hemorrhage

Penicillamine can induce a Goodpasture's-like syndrome.[272] Patients on high dosages of the drug (eg, for Wilson's disease) presented with anti-GBM–negative alveolar hemorrhage, glomerulonephritis, and renal failure. Corticosteroids, immunosuppression, and plasmapheresis reversed the condition. Since the drug is now less commonly used, there are no recent reports.

Mitomycin-Induced Hemolytic and Uremic Syndrome with Alveolar Hemorrhage

See "Mitomycin Lung" below.

Alveolar Hemorrhage Induced by Miscellaneous Drugs

Coagulation disturbances induced by moxalactam may induce alveolar hemorrhage.[273] Alveolar hemorrhage has been described after hysteroscopic examination using dextran 70. Extravasation of the compound induced a severe coagulopathic state complicated by pulmonary bleeding.[274] Treatments with tumor necrosis (TNF) or sirolimus may also cause DAH.[65,274]

Self-Induced Alveolar Hemorrhage

Patients who deliberately ingest rodenticides develop severe vitamin K depletion, with DAH as a complication.[275] Rodenticides are potent, longlasting vitamin K depleting agents. A history of intake may not be readily obtained because the patients are too ill.

Vascular Injury

In addition to the clinical patterns of pulmonary edema, alveolar hemorrhage, and capillaritis described above and acute nitrofurantoin lung described in "Nitrofurantoin Lung" below, drugs may have other effects on the vpulmonary vasculature.

Pulmonary Vasculitis and Related Diseases

Drugs have long been implicated in the development of systemic vasculitis. Several drugs including sulfonamides, allopurinol, phenytoin, thiourea, propylthiouracil, minocycline, immunizations, and vaccines have

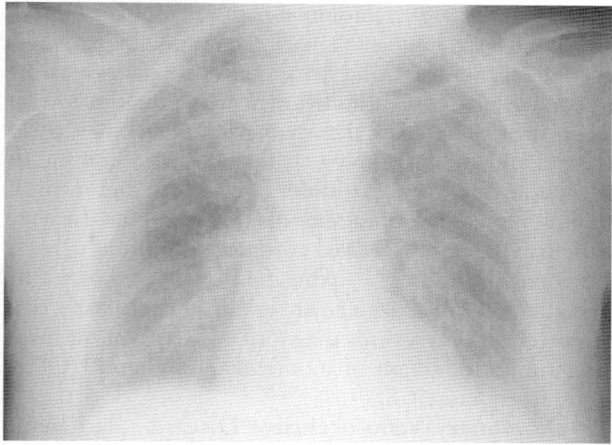

A

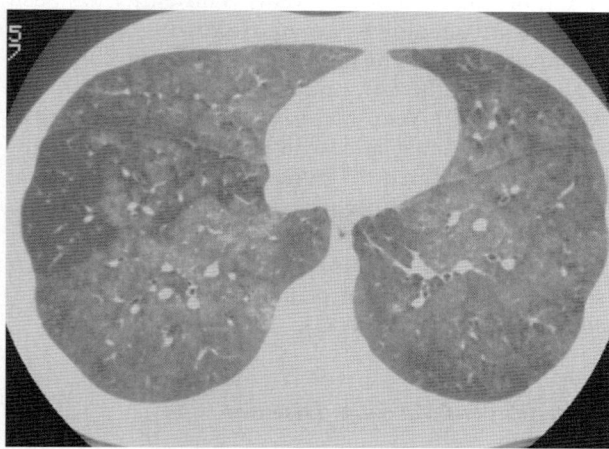

B

Figure 20–19 Coumadin-induced alveolar hemorrhage. *A*, The chest radiograph reveals diffuse ground-glass opacities. *B*, The high-resolution computed tomography scan discloses alveolar shadows with ill-defined margins. The diagnosis was confirmed by bronchoalveolar lavage. The patient recovered after drug discontinuation.

been implied in the development of systemic vasculitis-like disease with involvement of either large or small vessels, including the microcirculation[167,276–289]

Systemic Polyarteritis. The antithyroid drugs propylthiouracil and thiamazole,[287,290] can produce a small vessel vasculitis. Although the condition mimics Wegener's granulomatosis, the ANCA demonstrate perinuclear staining and antimyeloperoxidase specificity as opposed to the cytoplasmic distribution and antiproteinase 3 specificity seen in Wegener's granulomatosis.[291] The clinical and immunologic changes reverse on withdrawal of the drug.[291] Patients on propylthiouracil may have antimyeloperoxidase antibodies without clinical disease.[292]

The Churg-Strauss Syndrome. The use of leukotriene antagonists in the treatment of asthma have been associated with the development of the CSS.[150,153,162,293–295] Patients present with pulmonary infiltrates (Figure 20–20), cardiomyopathy, neurologic impairment, and eosinophilia, following the introduction of these agents. It is not clear whether this is a true increase in the incidence of CSS. In addition to the possible role of leukotriene antagonists, these patients have an atopic background and are undergoing corticosteroid withdrawal. It is possible that the higher doses of corticosteroid medication prevented the appearance of CSS. However, there are patients who never received corticosteroid drugs or were off corticosteroids,[162,295] who developed CSS after the introduction of leukotriene antagonists. There was a case reported with a previous diagnosis of CSS who relapsed after the introduction of montelukast sodium.[296] Other drugs rarely cause CSS.[115,152,286,297]

Pulmonary Veno-occlusive Disease.   Iatrogenic veno-occlusive disease is rare. It refers to fibrous obliteration of small pulmonary veins. This entity has been reported in oncology patients following the use of bleomycin, carmustine, gemcitabine, mitomycin, vinca alkaloids, radiotherapy, and after bone marrow transplantation.[298–300] Veno-occlusive disease also occurs in the liver,[299] and may appear in patients with malignancies prior to treatment.[301] Patients present with dyspnea, ill-defined interstitial markings, and Kerley's B lines. Postcapillary pulmonary hypertension and right heart failure eventually develop. The contribution of drugs, radiation therapy, or transplantation *versus* the underlying malignancy is not clear.

Miscellaneous Vascular Diseases

Patients sometimes develop thromboembolism after radiographic or surgical procedures. Biologic glue[302–304] or cement[305] can access the pulmonary vasculature and induce pulmonary infarction. The clinical findings include pleuritic chest pain and subpleural pulmonary infiltrates. Endogenous fat embolism is a rare complication of liposuction[306] and treatment with lipid-containing drugs (eg, propofol).[307]

Occasionally stem cell recipients present with fever and pulmonary nodules 2 to 3 months after transplantation. Histologic studies indicate sterile necrotic leukocyte aggregates and disrupted endothelium. The lesions are named pulmonary cytolytic thrombi.[308]

Other Drug-Induced Systemic Conditions

Lupus Erythematosus and Lupus-Like Syndromes. In the 1950s, a lupus-like syndrome was recognized with sulfonamides, hydrazides hydralazine and isoniazide, and procainamide. Other drugs causing the syndrome include amiodarone, angiotensin converting enzyme, ß-blockers (acebutolol, labetalol, pindolol, practolol [recalled in 1976], propranolol), carbamazepine, etanercept, gold, nitrofurantoin, olsalazine, phenytoin, quinidine, simvastatin, sulfonamides, and tetracyclines.[2,309,310] The pleuropulmonary manifestations of drug-induced systemic lupus erythematosus (SLE) are indistinguishable from those of spontaneous lupus.[2] The onset is insidious, and symptoms include moderate fever, weight loss, arthralgias, dyspnea, a hacking cough, chest pain, and, less frequently, myocarditis and pericardial tamponade or constriction. Radiographic studies indicate pleural thickening or effusion[311–313] (Figure 20–21), with or without pulmonary infiltrates, a shrinking lung,[314] or ARDS.[315] Pulmonary thromboembolism occurred in association with drug induced-SLE and anti-cardiolipin antibodies.[316] Antinuclear and antihistone antibodies are typically present in high titers, whereas antideoxyribonucleic acid [anti-DNA] antibodies are

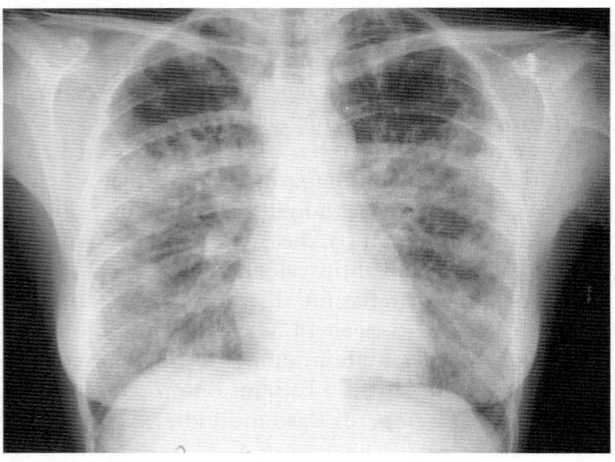

A

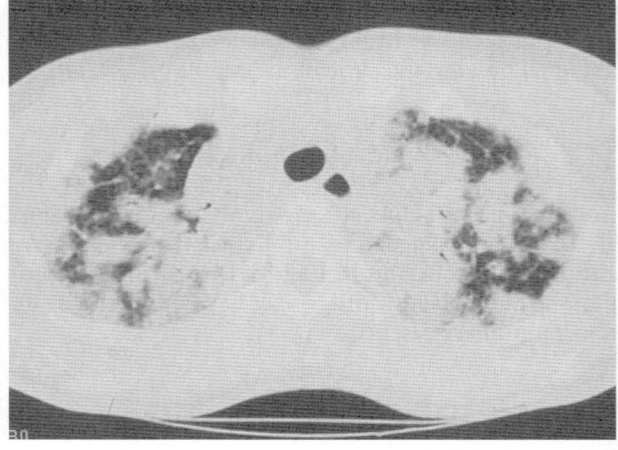

B

Figure 20–20   Drug-induced angiitis. *A*, Radiograph of diffuse pulmonary infiltrates, respiratory failure, and skin rash that developed during treatment with penicillin in a young lady. *B*, High-resolution computed tomography shows multiple dense lobular opacities. Eosinophilic angiitis (Churg-Strauss syndrome) was confirmed on histology of the lung.

rarely found.[2,309,310] Discontinuance of the SLE-inducing drug is associated with improvement and a resolution of the ANA with time.

Some patients with clinical findings of drug-induced SLE do not have ANA, and the disease is named lupus-like or LE-like syndrome.[315,317–319] In other patients with cellular pneumonitis induced by drugs (eg, gold, nitrofurantoin) ANA are present, but there is no extrapulmonary involvement.[130] Asymptomatic patients on drugs may develop ANA, but withdrawal is not indicated unless clinical symptoms develop.

L-Tryptophan and Eosinophilia-Myalgia Syndrome. Intake of excessive amounts of L-tryptophan was associated with an epidemic of systemic eosinophilic reactions called the "eosinophilia-myalgia syndrome.[148,320–322] Affected patients presented with an insidious or rapid onset of constitutional symptoms, myalgias, skin changes, neurologic, and cardiac involvement. Respiratory involvement included pulmonary infiltrates, pulmonary hypertension, pleural effusion, and acute respiratory failure. Histology of the lung showed eosinophilic infiltrates and angiitis. On discontinuance of the agent, symptoms improved, but residual disease persisted in many patients in the form of a scleroderma-like skin involvement, persistent neurologic symptoms, pulmonary hypertension, and peripheral eosinophilia. Some eventually died from the disease. A detailed epidemiologic and analytic investigation blamed ethylene-bis-tryptophan, a contaminant that was formed during the manufacturing process of L-tryptophan in one plant. No further cases were recorded following the recall of L-tryptophan.[103,323]

Other Systemic Diseases with Pulmonary Involvement. Statins and valsartan cause pulmonary involvement as well as polymyalgia, polymyositis, or the anti-synthetase syndrome.[324–326]

INTERSTITIAL LUNG DISEASE RELATED TO SPECIFIC DRUGS

Amiodarone Pneumonitis or Amiodarone Lung

More than 20 years after the original description of this condition,[327] amiodarone pneumonitis remains a frequent, distinctive, and potentially life-threatening illness. There is a high indicence of pulmonary toxicity, and pneumonitis is one of the leading causes for adverse effect–related discontinuation of the drug.[328] Both the structure and pharmacokinetics of amiodarone are distinctive and this impacts on the clinical, imaging, and pathologic features of pulmonary and other adverse effects from the drug.

Pharmacology

Amiodarone, and its principal metabolite, desethyl-amiodarone (DEAm), are cationic amphiphilic compounds that are toxic to lung cells.[329] They accumulate extensively in tissues during chronic treatment, with a lung tissue-to-plasma ratio of 100 to 500, respectively.[330,331]

Amiodarone and DEAm accumulate preferentially in the lung, liver, and skin, particularly the discolored skin of chronically-treated patients.[332] It is, therefore, conceivable that the adverse effects of amiodarone have a predilection to localize in tissues where amiodarone and/or DEAm are stored. Although plasma levels of amiodarone do not predict the occurrence of amiodarone pneumonitis, DEAm levels have been found to be higher in amiodarone pneumonitis as compared with unaffected patients.[333]

Amiodarone and DEAm localize in cell lysosomes and block the turnover of endogenous phospholipids. This

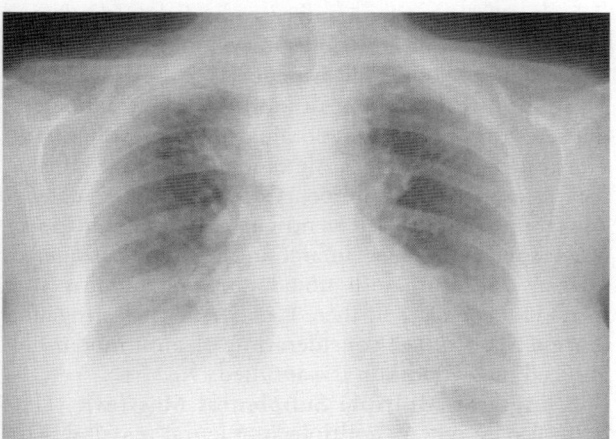

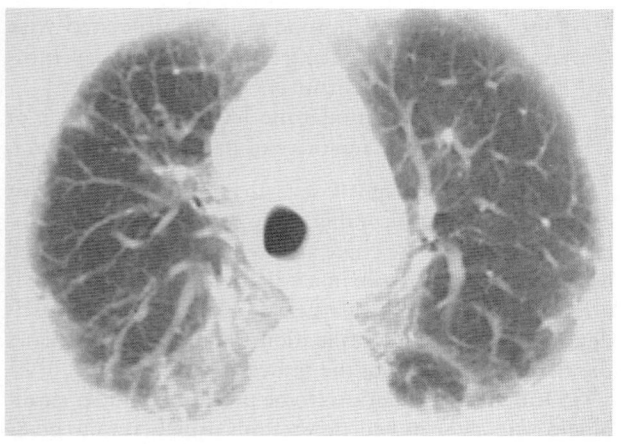

A   **B**

Figure 20–21 Pulmonary infiltrates, pleural thickening, and pleural effusion are seen in about half the patients with lupus erythematosus syndrome induced by drugs. Dyspnea, cough, and pulmonary infiltrates developed in a middle-aged woman treated with a ß-blocker agent. There was no pericardial effusion. Antinuclear and antihistone antibodies were strongly positive. All manifestations of the disease disappeared slowly after drug discontinuation.

explains the common finding of increased numbers of foamy or lipid-laden macrophages in the BAL fluid of any treated patients and it is considered a hallmark of both the pneumonitis and treated but unaffected patients.[334] In contrast, the accumulation of excessive numbers of foamy cells in lung tissue is a distinctive histologic feature of amiodarone pulmonary toxicity and is specifically found in amiodarone pneumonitis.[334] Interstitial inflammation and organizing pneumonia are also found.[334,335]

The clearance of amiodarone and DEAm from the lung is slow.[336] Autopsy studies have shown that significant amounts of both the drug and metabolite are still present in lung tissue up to 1 year after cessation of treatment. The clinical correlates of these pharmacokinetic features include the fact that discontinuation of amiodarone as the sole intervention is rarely followed by resolution of pulmonary infiltrates.[337,338] Moreover, if corticosteroids are withdrawn after 2 to 3 months in responsive patients, the disease may recur without reinstating treatment.[339]

Each molecule of amiodarone and DEAm contains two iodines, which explains the common finding of increased liver CT density and increased density of pulmonary infiltrates in patients with amiodarone pulmonary toxicity.[340]

Clinical Features

A strong cause-and-effect relationship between amiodarone and ILD exists.[341]

- There is a statistical association between exposure to the drug and the likelihood of developing ILD.
- The likelihood of developing pneumonitis increases with the degree of exposure to the drug (ie, dose and duration of treatment).
- The histopathologic features of amiodarone pneumonitis are often quite distinctive.[335]
- Discontinuation of amiodarone is associated with improvement or clearing of the pulmonary infiltrates in some patients.
- Reinitiation of amiodarone leads to recurrence of the disease in the majority of patients challenged.

The literature reports several hundred cases of this complication. In spite of this, there are difficulties in establishing the diagnosis. There are no diagnostic criteria, and because of increased risk in cardiac patients, lung tissue is often not available. Nevertheless, a definite diagnosis is desirable, because discontinuation of amiodarone increases the risk of recurrence of the underlying arrhythmia.[342]

Drug discontinuation (to be performed under cardiologic guidance) and corticosteroids usually lead to gradual,[343] but definite improvement of the radiographic and physiologic abnormalities.[344] However, in a small number of patients, irreversible sequellae will persist,[345] or the disease will progress.[232] Overall, the mortality rate of amiodarone pneumonitis is in the 20 to 30% range.[346]

Amiodarone pneumonitis is more frequent in males and is unusual below the age of 40 years. Rare reports have described its occurrence in children.[347] The incidence varies from 0.1% in patients receiving low doses of the drug to 50% in patients receiving high-dose regimens (eg, 1,200 mg daily). On the average, it will develop in 5 to 15% of patients on ≥ 500 mg amiodarone daily[344] versus 0.1 to 0.5% in those treated with ≤ 200 mg daily. Although low-dose regimens have decreased the incidence, the impression is that disease severity has not been altered.

Amiodarone pneumonitis may develop at any time ranging from a few days after an initial loading dose[348] to after a decade of treatment. Most cases develop at some point during the first year of treatment. In a few patients, amiodarone pneumonitis developed up to 3 months after cessation of treatment,[349] reflecting the storage and slow release from the lung.

Older patients are at greater risk for this complication. Exposure to high concentrations of oxygen in patients on amiodarone can lead to diffuse alveolar damage and ARDS. This has been described following cardiac and pulmonary surgery.[350] The common denominator appears to be exposure to high intraoperative concentrations of oxygen.[350] These observations are similar to that seen with bleomycin and radiation toxicity.

Clinical and Radiographic Patterns

Several clinical and radiographic patterns of amiodarone pneumonitis have been recognized.

Subacute Amiodarone Pneumonitis. Subacute amiodarone pneumonitis appears as a patchy or diffuse ILD involving both lung fields.[57,63,122,179] An alveolar, ground glass, or mottled pattern with high attenuation usually indicates a more acute presentation.[351] The opacities may be diffuse or localized to the lung bases (Figure 20–22).[352] Unexplicably, there is an impression that the right lung is more frequently involved than the left.[338] Alveolar shadowing and moderate volume loss of the right upper lobe developing in a patient taking the drug are suggestive of this condition. Although the chest radiograph indicates that one side predominates, HRCT often indicates bilateral disease.[179] An exudative pleural effusion may accompany the pulmonary disease.[353] When considering the diagnosis, left ventricular dysfunction, pneumonia, and pulmonary infarction should be considered. Diuresis will distinguish amiodarone pneumonitis from interstitial edema.[348] If there is only partial clearing after diuresis, continued consideration of an amiodarone-induced lung condition is warranted.

Single or Multiple Subpleural Mass(es). The pattern of single or multiple subpleural mass(es) with increased attenuation on HRCT can be seen (Figure 20–23).[354] They generally abut the pleura, which can be thickened. Clinically, pleuritic chest pain and a friction rub may be present. The masses can localize anywhere in the subpleural region of the lung and may

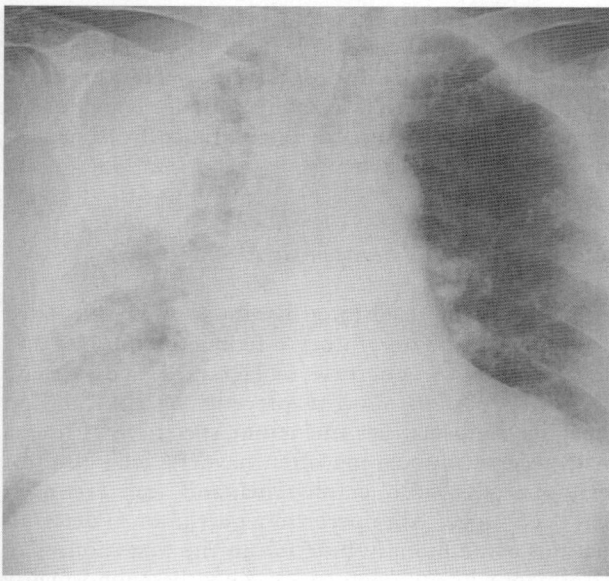 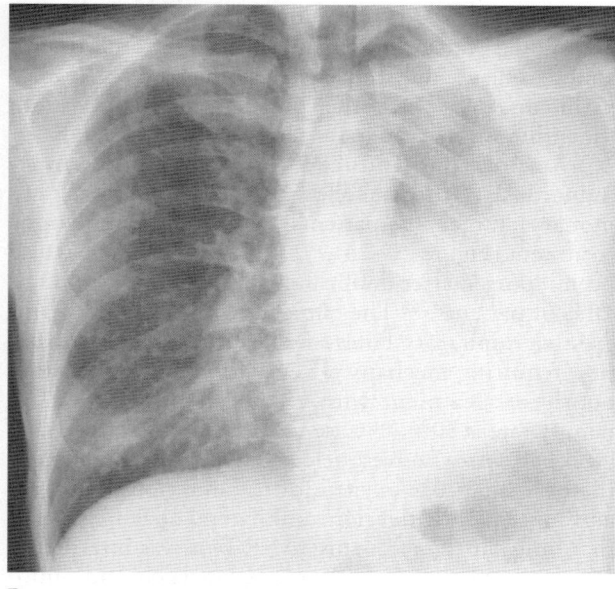

A   B

Figure 20–22   *A, B,* Radiographs of pulmonary infiltrates, which are often asymmetric in amiodarone pneumonitis. When symmetric, the pulmonary infiltrates localize in bases or apices of the lung.

simulate pulmonary infarction, pneumonia, carcinoma, or lymphoma.

Amiodarone-Induced Pulmonary Fibrosis. Amiodarone-induced pulmonary fibrosis is an uncommon pattern (see Figure 20–15) with an estimated frequency of 0.1%.[355] Amiodarone fibrosis may develop following an episode of amiodarone pneumonitis or as a de novo phenomenon. Criteria for the diagnosis include (1) the onset of the disease during or shortly after termination of treatment with amiodarone, (2) a more rapid progression of symptoms compared to idiopathic pulmonary fibrosis, (3) the absence of other

causes, and (4) a prior history of amiodarone pneumonitis with incomplete resolution. There are dense bibasilar reticular opacities in a dyspneic patient with coarse crackles, hypoxemia, and weight loss. On HRCT, there are coarse interstitial reticular and perilobular opacities that prevail at the lung bases. Honeycombing is unusual at the time of diagnosis. Amiodarone-induced fibrosis is irreversible, the response to corticosteroids is limited, and a poor outcome is to be expected.

Organizing Pneumonia.   Amiodarone may cause migratory or fixed alveolar opacities or nodules, which correspond to the histologic pattern of organizing

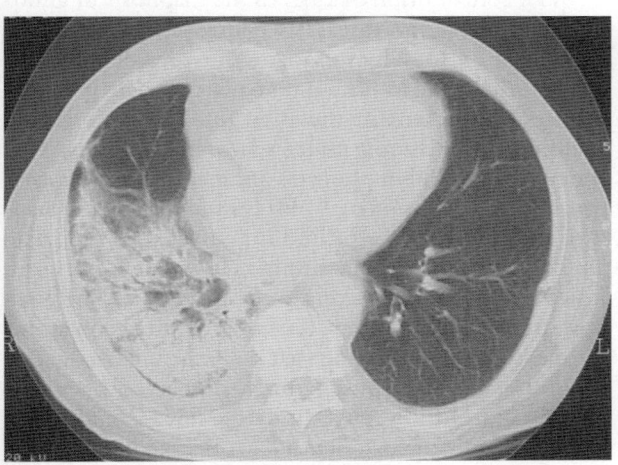 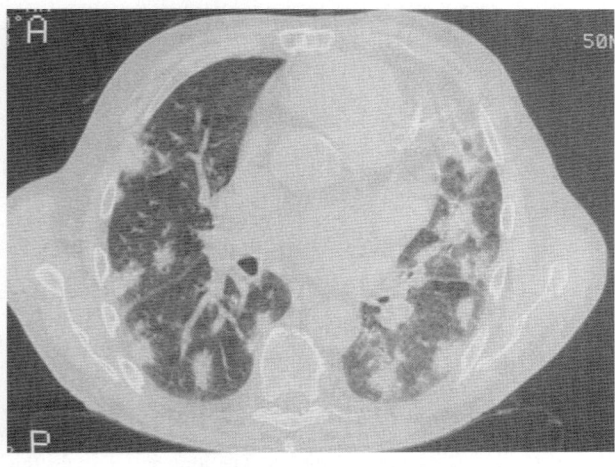

A   B

Figure 20–23   High-resolution computed tomography in amiodarone pneumonitis discloses focal areas of high attenuation with or without recognizable lobar distribution. *A,* Masses corresponding to amiodarone pneumonitis typically abut the pleura, which can be thickened. *B,* Multiple shaggy nodules as a manifestation of amiodarone pneumonitis are uncommon.

pneumonia.[139,178,356] The clinical, imaging, and histo-pathologic features of organizing penumonia due to amiodarone are indistiguishable from those of the idiopathic disease.[178] Over the course of this complication, the infiltrates may migrate (see Figure 20–9).[178]

Amiodarone-Induced ARDS. Amiodarone-induced ARDS occurs following thoracic (cardiac, pulmonary) surgery in patients on chronic amiodarone treatment (Figure 20–24).[357–359] The syndrome has also been reported after defibrillator implantation in up to 10% of patients.[360] The clinical picture is rapidly progressive respiratory failure with diffuse alveolar opacities, requiring mechanical ventilation and responding poorly to treatment with corticosteroid drugs. The fatality rate is 50%.[361] Case records have described surgical patients who were selectively intubated and ventilated with 100% oxygen for the duration of surgery and subsequently developed unilateral opacification of that lung shortly after surgery.[362] This was interpreted as a unilateral form of combined oxygen and amiodarone pulmonary toxicity. Similarly, patients who undergo a lung biopsy for establishing the diagnosis of amiodarone toxicity often deteriorate postprocedure.[338] This is an important consideration when contemplating a surgical biopsy to diagnose one of the amiodarone-associated lung conditions.

Subclinical Amiodarone Pneumonitis. Subclinical amiodarone pneumonitis occurs in patients on chronic amiodarone therapy in face of a normal chest radiograph. The HRCT indicates ground-glass densities, small alveolar opacities,[354] or septal lines.[363] These correspond histologically to aggregates of mural or alveolar foam cells or to alveolitis.[334,363] In addition, increased inflammatory cells in the BAL fluid, and positive gallium scans have been reported.[364] Subclinical amiodarone pulmonary toxicity is reversible on cessation of the drug. However, the significance of subclinical toxicity is unclear. It is not known if these patients will progress to overt disease.

Amiodarone-Induced Alveolar Hemorrhage. Amiodarone-induced alveolar hemorrhage is an unusual complication and must be differentiated from hemorrhagic pulmonary edema.[365]

Diagnostic and Therapeutic Management

Amiodarone-induced lung disease is often associated with an increased erythrocyte sedimentation rate and leukocytosis. An increase in lactate dehydrogenase (LDH) has been found to precede the clinical, and imaging abnormalities but is not specific.[366] Patients who receive amiodarone often have a background of exposure to tobacco, emphysema, and heart failure. It has been suggested to perform repeat (3 or 4) determinations of pulmonary function in the first months of treatment with amiodarone.[348] The earliest abnormality in amiodarone pulmonary toxicity is a consistent decrease in the diffusing capacity.[348] Chronic left heart failure does not significantly alter this test.[367] Using diffusion capacity as a surrogate marker of amiodarone pulmonary toxicity, Magro and colleagues have determined that the best sensitivity and specificity corresponded to a fall of ≥ 15 and 30%, respectively.[348] However, an isolated decrease of the diffusing capacity does not necessarily indicate clinically apparent disease, and overt disease will develop in only a third of these patients.[348] In practice, a reduction of the diffusing capacity should not prompt discontinuation of the drug unless there is clinical or imaging evidence of pneumonitis.[368] Conversely, a stable diffusing capacity is considered to indicate the lack of clinically meaningful amiodarone pulmonary toxicity.[369] Patients who develop amiodarone pulmonary toxicity demonstrate a precipitous decrease in this measurement.

The contribution of BAL to the diagnosis of amiodarone-related lung disease is controversial. Increased numbers of CD8+ lymphocytes are found; however, other studies have indicated that a wide range of abnormalities are present in the BAL fluid in amiodarone pneumonitis, including an increase in neutrophils, lymphocytes, in both lymphocytes and neutrophils, or even a normal distribution.[345,369,370] Eosinophilia as an isolated finding in the BAL fluid is a unusual feature. The time of onset of the pneumonitis tends to be shorter in patients with lymphocytosis in the BAL fluid. The presence of foam cells in the BAL fluid of patients on amiodarone is a routine finding that does not indicate amiodarone toxicity.[334] Hemosiderin-laden macrophages have been described in the BAL fluid in a few instances.[370]

The histopathologic appearance of amiodarone pneumonitis and subpleural masses includes septal thickening, interstitial edema, nonspecific inflammation, and fibrosis as well as the presence of lipids within interstitial and endothelial cells (Figure 20–25).[335,338,342,369] Foamy intra-

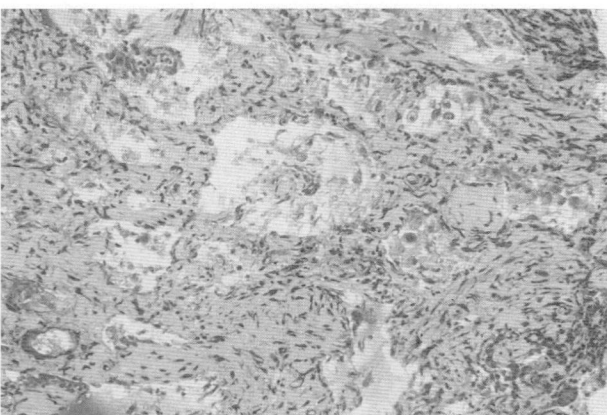

Figure 20–24 Drug-induced ARDS. The lung specimen in this patient exposed to long-term amiodarone, reveals interstitial fibrosis and dysplasia of type II pneumocytes. ARDS developed immediately after cardiac surgery, a known triggering factor for severe amiodarone pneumonitis (Masson trichrome stain).

alveolar macrophages are also seen (see Figure 20–25) and must be differentiated from desquamative interstitial pneumonia.[228] Other findings include organizing pneumonia,[139,178] type II cell hyperplasia (the latter correlates positively with the presence of interstitial fibrosis),[334] and free extracellular lipids. Active or resolving diffuse alveolar damage and hyaline membranes represent those cases with ARDS.[360] The histopathologic features of amiodarone-induced fibrosis are those of severe interstitial fibrosis with thickened alveolar septa, type II cell hyperplasia or dysplasia, and the accumulation of alveolar macrophages.[371] Foam cells may be seen depending on the time from discontinuation of the drug to biopsy.

Clinical improvement and clearing of pulmonary opacities often requires 2 to 3 months.[338] Discontinuation of amiodarone as the sole therapeutic measure may be sufficient if the disease is mild. However, discontinuation of amiodarone is rarely followed by convincing improvement in patients with advanced disease and corticosteroids are indicated.[330] Despite the lack of controlled studies, evidence has accumulated supporting the beneficial effects of corticosteroid treatment.

- Early mortality has been observed in patients in whom corticosteroids were not used[337,372] or used too late.[348]
- In some patients amiodarone withdrawal alone is not associated with improvement, and the patients deteriorated unless corticosteroids were given.[373]
- Early withdrawal of corticosteroids has been associated with recurrence, and, in some patients, a catastrophic course ensued.[339]

Improvement of imaging and pulmonary function generally lags behind clinical improvement.[344] A persistent decrease in diffusing capacity can occur, probably due to a combined effect of amiodarone pneumonitis

and previous smoking history. Prevention of arrhythmia recurrences relies on other antiarrhythmic agents or the insertion of an automatic defibrillator. In a few patients with arrhythmia and amiodarone pneumonitis, the drug dosage was decreased and corticosteroids were given with satisfactory control of both conditions.[374] Corticosteroids need to be administered for extended periods of time, otherwise, recurrences may develop during corticosteroid tapering up to 8 months after withdrawal. The pattern of recurrence may be more severe than the initial episode of amiodarone pneumonitis, and uncontrollable respiratory failure and death may develop.[375] Thus, although no controlled studies are available, corticosteroids are often given in the following way: (1) a sufficient initial dosage should be given (eg, 0.75 to 1 mg/kg prednisolone, or equivalent), (2) the initial dosage should be maintained until a definite clinical and radiographic response is obtained, (3) corticosteroid tapering should be gradual, (4) a reasonable estimate of the duration of treatment is 6 months, but more often it is 1 year, (5) patients should be carefully monitored after discontinuation of corticosteroids for possible recurrence of the disease. Patients who demonstrate recurrences or those with amiodarone-induced fibrosis may require long-term corticosteroids.

Mortality in amiodarone pneumonitis is substantial and ranges between 21 and 33%.[330,345,346,376] The prognosis is worse when amiodarone pneumonitis occurs on a background of chronic obstructive pulmonary disease.[368]

Resumption for amiodarone for the control of refractory arrhythmias is followed within a short period of time by the recurrence of clinical symptoms[377,378] and radiographic abnormalities in about two-thirds of patients. Monitoring of the diffusing capacity may enable the earlier detection of recurrence, and gallium scanning may be used as a confirmatory test.[377]

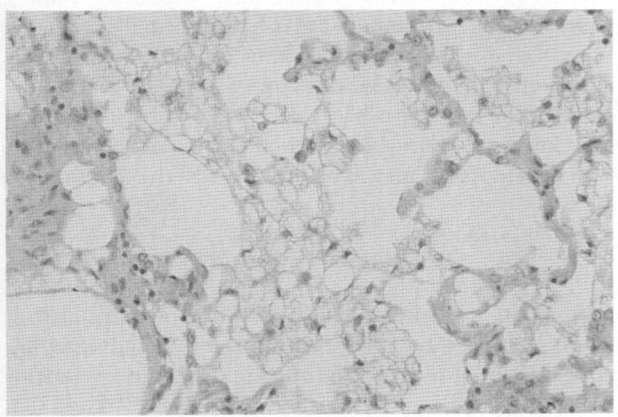

A

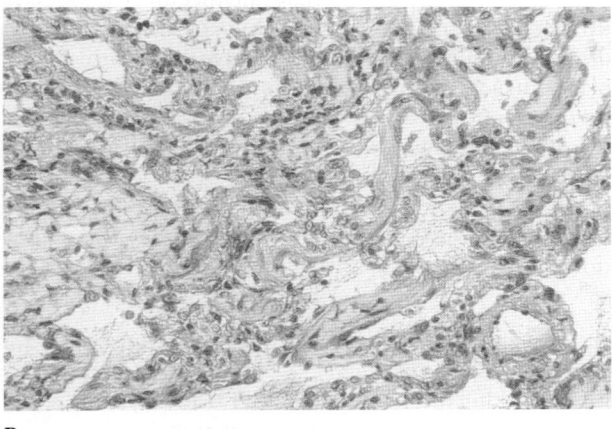

B

Figure 20–25   The accumulation of large foamy macrophages (also called vacuolated macrophages or foam cells) is a suggestive finding in patients with amiodarone pneumonitis. *A*, Foamy macrophages occur rarely as an isolated finding in amiodarone pneumonitis, and are often associated with *B*, interstitial inflammation or fibrosis and with dysplasia of type II pneumocytes. Lipid deposits may also be seen in resident cells of the lung (pneumocytes, endothelial cells) (hematoxylin-eosin-safranin stain).

All-*trans*-retinoic Acid

All-*trans*-retinoic acid (ATRA) accelerates the differentiation and maturation of promyelocytic cells in promyelocytic leukemia and reduced the hemorrhagic complications of the disease. The administration of ATRA is followed by an increase in the number of circulating myeloid cells, and this is temporally associated in some patients with the development of fever, pleural or pericardial effusion, lower extremity edema, dyspnea, pulmonary infiltrates, pulmonary edema or hemorrhage, or ARDS.[233,261] The syndrome is named ATRA or the retinoic acid syndrome. In a series of 35 patients receiving ATRA, 9 developed acute respiratory distress, which was preceded by an increase in peripheral neutrophils in 6. Radiographic studies indicate ill-defined infiltrates, ground-glass opacities, nodules, or diffuse alveolar shadows.[379] In one patient, blasts and promyelocytes with Auer rods were retrieved in the BAL fluid.[380] Patients improved on high-dose corticosteroids.[233] Postmortem examination of lung tissue showed maturing and mature myeloid cells within the interstitium.[233] One patient presented with diffuse alveolar hemorrhage, and capillaritis was seen in lung tissue.[261] Prophylactic administration of corticosteroids has decreased the incidence of the syndrome.[243]

Bacille Galmette-Guérin

Complications develop mainly in patients with bladder carcinoma who receive intravesical Bacille Galmette-Guérin (BCG). BCG causes granulomatous infiltrative lung disease[381] or miliary BCG infection.[140] The granulomatous form typically develops after the fifth or sixth instillation and manifests with dyspnea, fever, respiratory failure, or an ARDS picture.[382] Patients who have received BCG in the past are at risk. The chest radiograph and CT scan typically show a miliary pattern (see Figure 2C).[382] There is a predominance of lymphocytes in the BAL fluid,[383,384] and histologic features include diffuse granulomas,[384,385] and, in severe cases, diffuse alveolar damage.[386] No reliable clinical, radiographic, or histologic features can distinguish BCG granulomatosis from infection, except the identification of mycobacterial DNA sequences in lung tissue[387] or a positive culture of *Mycobacterium bovis* from a lung sample.[388] Patients are often treated with antituberculous chemotherapy in addition to corticosteroids until an infection is ruled out.

Bischoloroethyl Nitrosoura and Other Nitrosoureas

Bischloroethyl nitrosourea (BCNU) is an alkylating agent introduced in 1963 for the treatment of malignant central nervous system (CNS) tumors, because of its low molecular weight, and ability to reach the CNS.[45,389] Pulmonary complications from BCNU have been described in children and in adults. Currently, BCNU is used for the treatment of high-risk breast carcinoma[118] and as precondition therapy for bone marrow transplantation. BCNU has caused pulmonary toxicity more often than the other nitrosoureas (CCNU [lomustine], DCNU [chlorozotocin], methyl-CCNU, streptozocin, and fotemustine).[24,45]

Several cases of carmustine toxicity were reported in children with glioblastoma.[116] In most cases it is dose related[390] and ranges between 1 and 10% of treated patients.[391] BCNU pulmonary toxicity resembles the pneumonitis induced by bleomycin, busulfan, chlorambucil, cyclophosphamide, and mitomycin.[45] A total dose of 1,000 to 1,200 mg/m² is considered the threshold above which the incidence of pulmonary toxicity increases sharply.[116] The incidence increases nearly tenfold when cyclophosphamide or radiation therapy are employed.[392]

Clinically, patients present (1) early on with acute toxicity,[393] the form of BCNU lung that is more responsive to corticosteroid therapy,[194,220,394] thereby having an improved prognosis or (2) with late toxicity, which is characterized by pulmonary fibrosis and poor therapeutic response.[395–398] There are patients who develop late onset pulmonary complications of nitrosoureas, months to years following completion of treatment.[123,399] Most patients who develop late BCNU toxicity have progressive disease, evolving to respiratory failure.[400]

The histopathologic features of BCNU lung are those of chemotherapy lung. There is interstitial fibrosis, diffuse alveolar damage, and prominent dysplasia of type II pneumocytes.[401] Unusual features include pleural fibrosis, vascular thrombosis, veno-occlusive disease, or alveolar proteinosis. Electron microscopy shows a loss of myelinic figures in type II cells suggesting alteration in surfactant, which may aggravate alveolar instability.

A cohort of 8 adolescents and young adults who had been treated with nitrosourea and craniospinal irradiation for a childhood brain tumor developed chronic respiratory insufficiency up to 17 years following treatment.[123] Progressive upper-lobe fibrosis was a characteristic feature in 6, but 2 had a normal chest radiograph despite histologic evidence for pulmonary fibrosis. In all patients, BAL cell counts were normal. Since none of the 8 patients had a decrease in diffusing capacity, extrapulmonary factors such as alterations in chest wall development may explain the restrictive physiology.

Bleomycin Lung

Bleomycin was one of the first drugs recognized as a cause of lung disease.[402] The clinical and radiographic appearances of bleomycin lung are distinctive,[25] particularly bleomycin-induced lung nodules.[403,404]

Although early reports warned of the possibility of bleomycin pneumonitis after low cumulative doses of the drug,[405] for many years there was the belief that bleomycin caused pulmonary toxicity only if > 500 mg had been received. In fact, there is little correlation between dose and the likelihood of developing bleomycin lung. Slow infusions or intramuscular injections of the drug are associated with less toxicity opposed to rapid IV infusions. Previous use of bleomycin may increase the risk of pulmonary toxicity,[406] and this should be considered in those patients requiring retreatment. Concomitant irradiation,[407] treatment with cyclophosphamide,[408] and inhalation of oxygen-enriched gas mixtures may trigger the onset of acute bleomycin pneumonitis.[409] Anesthesiologists should be warned of the possible risk of oxygen therapy during the perioperative period.

The incidence of bleomycin pneumonitis is approximately 3%.[410] A 2.3 % fatality rate has been reported in patients exposed to bleomycin.[114] In patients with severe bleomycin pulmonary toxicity, the mortality rate was 60%.[410] The mortality rate is greater in older patients and in those with renal failure.[114]

Clinically, bleomycin presents acutely or subacutely,[25,411] with dyspnea and sometimes chest pain.[412] The finding of crackles on auscultation often precedes the radiographic changes of bleomycin lung toxicity. Imaging studies indicate greater involvement of the lung bases, costophrenic angles, and subpleural regions, as well as volume loss.[25] Retrospective review of chest radiographs may show the gradual development of these changes (Figure 20–26). A diffuse ill-defined ground-glass pattern is seen in some patients. Pleural thickening or effusion is unusual. Some patients develop acute alveolar opacities or the radiographic pattern of ARDS. HRCT in patients with moderate bleomycin toxicity showed alveolar infiltrates, discrete subpleural crescent-like opacities, peripheral masses abutting the pleura, or a diffuse haze (Figure 20–27).[413–415] These CT findings are common during treatment occuring in 15 of 18 patients.[416] However, none developed overt bleomycin toxicity. Bleomycin induces pleural-based or parenchymal pulmonary nodules in some patients, and this raises the possibility of pulmonary metastases (see Figure 20–27 and 20–28).[180] The nodules correspond to the histologic pattern of organizing pneumonia (see Figure 20–28), which progresses to nodular fibrosis.

Patients have a restrictive functional defect and hypoxemia. The question of whether serial pulmonary function testing is useful in identifying patients who will develop bleomycin pulmonary toxicity was assesed by Wolkowicz and colleagues.[225] Fifty-nine men with non-seminomatous testicular carcinoma, who received a three-course chemotherapy regimen consisting of vinblastine, bleomycin, and platinum, were evaluated. The average dose of bleomycin was 555.5 units, and pulmonary physiology was serially evaluated prior to each treatment course. They showed that the diffusing capacity fell significantly with bleomycin treatment, and this was regarded as the most sensitive indicator of pulmonary toxicity. However, the diffusing capacity failed to predict which patients would develop clinical toxicity. Reduction in the total lung capacity had a better correlation with clinical toxicity. Despite the inability of the diffusing capacity to detect patients who will develop clinical toxicity,[417] the test is still performed in this population.[418] It should be remembered that diffusing capacity decreases in 75% of patients on bleomycin, and in only a few will clinical toxicity develop.[418]

The BAL pattern is neutrophilic.[419] The histopathologic features are those seen with the other chemotherapeutic agents such as BCNU, busulfan, chlorambucil, and cyclophosphamide.

A sizable fraction of patients with bleomycin lung have reversible disease, despite evidence for histologic fibrosis.[420] Corticosteroids have been employed in nearly all patients and are beneficial.[410] It is thought that if a patient survives the initial episode of bleomycin pulmonary toxicity, they are likely to recover. Early withdrawal of corticosteroids leads to relapse.[410] As in many other drug-induced lung diseases, a slow taper is rec-

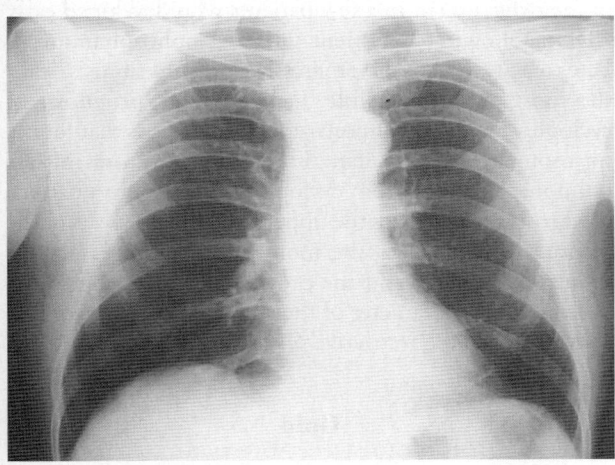
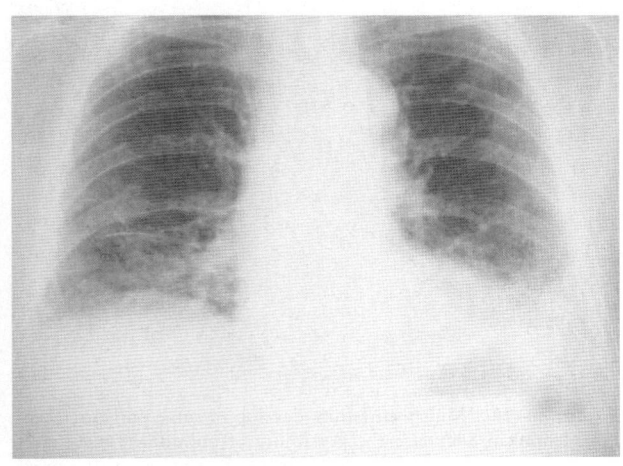

A **B**

Figure 20–26 Chest radiographs of a middle–aged man with laryngeal carcinoma *A*, before and *B*, after five courses of bleomycin. Bleomycin pulmonary toxicity has a predilection to involve the bases and costophrenic angles and is associated with volume loss.

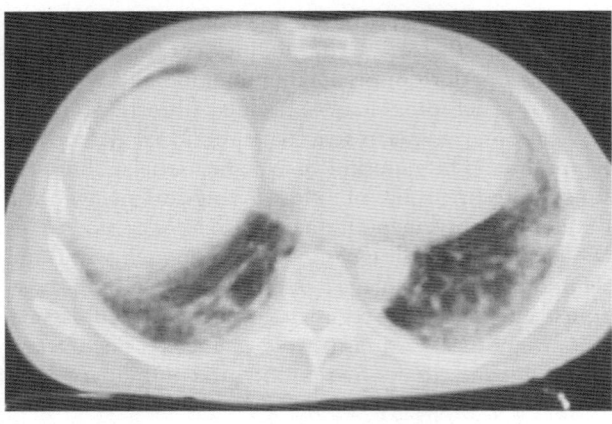

A

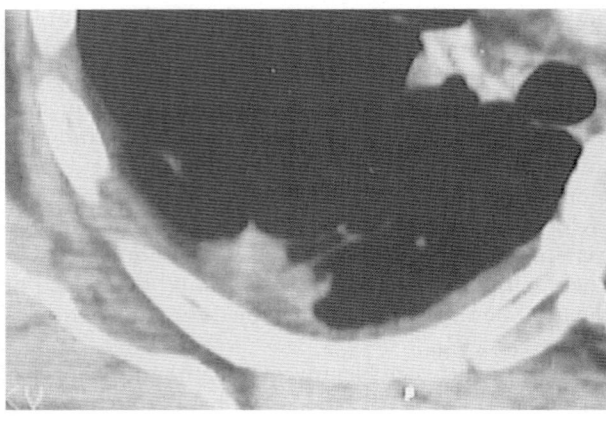

B

Figure 20–27 High-resolution computed tomography in bleomycin pulmonary toxicity often discloses *A*, subpleural opacities. Similar changes may occur in asymptomatic patients. *B*, Parenchymal or subpleural lung nodules can be observed in some patients, and this raises the possibility of pulmonary metastases.

ommended. There are patients, however, who develop irreversible pulmonary fibrosis and honeycomb lung and die from late bleomycin lung.[410]

Colony Stimulating Factors

Colony stimulating factors (CSF) are used to restore peripheral neutrophil counts in patients who are receiving myeloablative chemotherapy, and this increases the incidence of pulmonary infiltrates. In a series of 36 patients with non-Hodgkin's lymphoma receiving a bleomycin, Adriamycin (doxorubicin), cyclophosphamide, vincristine, and prednisone (BACOP) regimen, 12 received recombinant granulocyte (G)-CSF. Of these, 4 developed respiratory complications (3 died), as opposed to 1 of 24 patients not receiving CSF.[421] Other reports have confirmed the occurrence acute respiratory failure in patients receiving

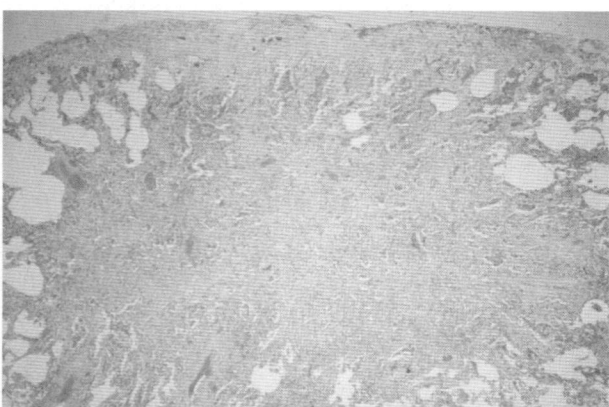

Figure 20–28 Multiple nodules develop in some patients receiving bleomycin and raise the possibility of pulmonary metastases. The nodules correspond to round-shaped foci of organizing pneumonia and pigmented macrophages. The nodules disappear or leave residual foci of apparently inert fibrosis. This particular nodule was adjacent to the pleural surface (*on top*) (Masson trichrome stain).

CSF for neoplastic and non-neoplastic conditions.[422] However, a randomized study in patients with germ cell tumors failed to demonstrate a difference in the incidence of bleomycin pulmonary toxicity in patients exposed versus not exposed to G-CSF. In several patients the pulmonary infiltrates developed concomitant with the CSF-induced increase in peripheral neutrophils.[212] There was an increase in lymphocytes in the BAL fluid.[423] The clinical severity ranged from transient subclinical hypoxemia to diffuse pulmonary infiltrates or an ARDS picture. The infiltrates clear over a few days or persist for several weeks. The mortality rate is about 20%, and the prognosis is improved on corticosteroids.[424]

Cyclophosphamide

Like busulfan and the nitrosoureas, cyclophosphamide is an alkylating agent that can induce early or late pulmonary toxicity.[213] Early toxicity is largely reversible after removal of the drug, except in a few patients who developed early ARDS following treatment with cyclophosphamide.[425] Late toxicity, because of progressive indolent fibrosis, is for the most part irreversible.[213] The overall prognosis of cyclophosphamide pulmonary toxicity exceeds that for the nitrosoureas and busulfan. The peculiar features of late pulmonary toxicity from cyclophosphamide are a pattern of fibrosis that involves the upper and lateral aspects of the pleura, in addition to the more typical changes of pulmonary fibrosis,[213] and the progressive narrowing of the anteroposterior diameter of the thorax in children, which contributes to the restrictive physiology later in life.[426]

Gold

Gold salts (thiomalate, thioglucose) and auranofin were also among the first drugs recognized as being responsible for lung disease. Gold lung has received increasing attention following the paper by Winterbauer and colleagues[427] and has been the subject of a recent review summarizing 140 cases of lung toxicity, which were compared with 208 cases of rheumatoid lung.[130]

Gold lung will become less frequent with the use of newer therapies for rheumatoid arthritis. Patients with gold lung (mostly women) tend to develop the disease within the first 6 months of treatment having received less than 1,300 mg (range 30 to 3,000 mg, average 677 mg of drug). Symptoms appear within the first 6 months of treatment and include the rapid onset of dyspnea, cough, fever, and a skin rash in 38%. A restrictive physiology, decreased diffusing capacity, and hypoxemia were common. Chest imaging shows bibasilar butterfly-shaped or diffuse opacities centered along the bronchovascular bundles. Peripheral eosinophilia appears in 39% of cases, but does not necessarily indicate eosinophilic pneumonia. BAL findings show an increased lymphocyte count in two-thirds of cases, with an inverted CD4+/CD8+ ratio in 78%.[130]

Pathology was available in 85 of the 140 cases reviewed by Tomioka and King.[130] The patterns of septal inflammation (which would probably now be called nonspecific interstitial pneumonia-cellular) and eosinophilic or organizing pneumonia have been reported.

In all patients therapy was discontinued, and corticosteroids induced complete remission in two-thirds of the cases. The mortality rate was 12% from progressive respiratory failure.[130] However, one confounding issue concerning the diagnosis and recognition of gold lung in patients with rheumatoid arthritis and methotrexate pneumonitis in patients with polymyositis is the concommitant use of NSAIDs. NSAIDS can cause eosinophilic pneumonia, which may be difficult to differentiate from gold lung.[428]

Interferon

Interferons are used to treat hematologic malignancies and to manage hepatitis C virus infection. The clinical, radiographic, and pathologic patterns of interferon-induced pulmonary complications include (1) diffuse ILD (cellular or, less often, fibrotic),[429] (2) organizing pneumonia (see Figure 20–10B),[182,430] or (3) a sarcoid-like reaction in mediastinal lymph nodes, or in the lung parenchyma.[431] Interferon-induced lung disease improves following a reduction in drug dosage and treatment with corticosteroids.

Methotrexate Pneumonitis or Methotrexate Lung

Methotrexate pneumonitis complicates the treatment of various neoplastic and non-neoplastic conditions in approximately 3% of patients.[432] Methotrexate lung is characterized by the insidious onset of cough, fever, and

dyspnea accompanied by diffuse pulmonary infiltrates and sometimes acute respiratory failure.[7] The combination of drug withdrawal and high-dose corticosteroids is associated with a favorable outcome, and sequellae are unusual. Rechallenge of patients should be avoided as it may lead to fatal respiratory disease.[147]

The first report of methotrexate pneumonitis was by Clarysse and colleagues in 1969.[433] They described an acute pulmonary event in 7 children while in clinical remission from the hematologic malignancy. The disease was life-threatening in 6, and the open lung biopsy showed granulomas and interstitial pneumonitis. Both cessation of the drug and corticosteroid therapy were effective; however, methotrexate was continued in some patients.

By the year 2000, 123 cases of methotrexate lung were recorded in the literature.[74] Methotrexate pneumonitis develops after treatment of leukemia, solid tumors, rheumatoid arthritis, psoriasis, primary biliary cirrhosis, asthma, and molar or ectopic pregnancy. The more recent cases appeared after long-term use of methotrexate for the treatment of rheumatoid arthritis.

The majority of patients are women (62%). Methotrexate pneumonitis developed after administration of doses ranging from 2.5 to 1,400 mg/week. The duration of treatment was diverse (from a single exposure to 5 years), although half developed the disease within the first 32 weeks of treatment.[434] The development of methotrexate pneumonitis is unpredictable; there is no correlation between the dose and time to onset or clinical severity. Indeed, fatal methotrexate pneumonitis can appear with low-dose methotrexate, as has occurred during the treatment of rheumatoid arthritis. All routes of administration expose patients to the risk of developing methotrexate pneumonitis, including oral, parenteral, and intrathecal. The vast majority of patients are still on the drug at the time of onset of the disease, although rare cases of delayed onset have been reported.[435] The incidence rate of methotrexate pneumonitis ranges between 0.3 and 11.6%. Risk factors may include male gender and prior pulmonary disease.[74]

Onset is insidious, occuring over days or weeks, and presenting with dyspnea, cough, sometimes mouth ulcers, or a skin rash. The disease can accelerate causing fever and the rapid development of acute ILD and respiratory failure. Severe hypoxia is consistently reported. It must be distinguished from opportunistic infections and from an acute immunologic pneumonia, which can complicate a collagen vascular disease. Patients who have received methotrexate intrathecally may develop ARDS, which has a poor outcome.[436] Unusual patterns of methotrexate lung include a subacute presentation, pulmonary infiltrates and eosinophilia, pulmonary fibrosis, pleuritic chest pain, and a lone cough.

Mild peripheral eosinophilia is present in about 40% of patients, but methotrexate pneumonitis is not an eosinophilic pneumonia.[7] Although eosinophils are present in lung tissue, they are not a predominant feature.[437]

Radiographic studies show a diffuse and symmetric interstitial opacification of both lung fields and, in severe cases, the pattern of dense bilateral alveolar opacities with air bronchograms (see Figure 20–1).[438] Pulmonary function tests are restrictive with a low diffusing capacity. Pulmonary function has been prospectively studied in patients receiving methotrexate, and, as opposed to alkylating agents, there is no consistent decrease in the diffusing capacity.[432] Both the percentage and number of lymphocytes are increased in the BAL. Lymphocytes are either a CD4+ or CD8+ phenotype.[136,137,439]

Histologic findings are available in 49 reports and include interstitial inflammation, interstitial fibrosis, granuloma formation, and increased number of tissue eosinophils in 71, 59, 35, and 18% of cases, respectively. The granulomas in methotrexate pneumonitis are typically small and ill-defined, and sterile necrosis of granulomas is unusual (see Figures 20–3 and 20–5). In patients with a predominantly granulomatous pattern, the disease is patchy and intervening areas of normal lung tissue remain.[437] Type II cell hyperplasia is a notable feature of methotrexate lung, as it is in pulmonary complications from other chemotherapeutic agents. Alveolar edema, diffuse alveolar damage, hyaline membranes, and DAH are unusual features and are seen in patients with severe disease. Rare histologic appearances include desquamative interstitial pneumonia, a sarcoidosis-like patterns, or acute interstitial pneumonia.[440]

The differential diagnosis of methotrexate lung is difficult, especially in oncology patients. The symptoms of methotrexate pneumonitis cannot be distinguished from those of opportunistic infections, which methotrexate can also predispose to. Thus, in considering the diagnosis of methotrexate pneumonitis, a workup for opportunistic infection is required. Moreover, other pneumotoxic drugs in addition to methotrexate may have been used. However, the clinical and pathologic pattern of a granulomatous pneumonitis with mild blood eosinophilia is distinctive, as opposed to that of other chemotherapeutic agents.[74] The background diseases, such as rheumatoid arthritis, cancers, or inflammatory bowel disease, also involve the lung.

The management of methotrexate pneumonitis includes drug discontinuation and corticosteroid therapy. Methotrexate pneumonitis responds to corticosteroids even with continuation of treatment.[74,441] Both the dose and duration of corticosteroid treatment has not been determined. Obviously, the clinical, physiologic, and radiographic responses dictate dosage and duration. Radiographic improvement is paralleled by functional improvement, which may require up to several months to be complete. Eighty-five percent of patients will recover fully. Fibrosis of the lung after methotrexate is unusual.[74] Overall, the mortality rate is 15% from progressive respiratory failure.[442]

Rechallenge with methotrexate may not cause recurrence in all patients. However, the disease will relapse in up to 66% of patients who are rechallenged, and this increases mortality.[147]

Mitomycin Lung

Mitomycin is used for the treatment of lung gastric carcinoma and, superficial bladder carcinoma.[443] The drug may induce two distinct patterns of pulmonary disease.

Mitomycin Pneumonitis

Mitomycin pneumonitis is similar to other chemotherapeutic agents and is primarily a fibrotic disease.[218,444] Mitomycin-induced pneumonitis and fibrosis develop in about 5% of patients, generally after at least 40 to 50 mg/m². The features include dyspnea, cough, fever, and diffuse pulmonary infiltrates. The histologic features include interstitial fibrosis and bizarre pneumocytes. Prospective studies with serial pulmonary function tests, including measurements of diffusing capacity, or serial CT scans do not predict the development of mitomycin lung. Corticosteroids have been effective in several patients.[218]

Mitomycin-Induced Hemolytic Uremic Syndrome

The hemolytic uremic syndrome (HUS)[445–448] is specific for mitomycin, as opposed to other chemotherapeutic agents.[449] The syndrome usually develops 4 to 8 weeks after completion of a mitomycin-based chemotherapy regimen, the average time of onset being 11.5 months from the beginning of chemotherapy. However, some patients developed the disease after a latent period of up to 9 months after termination of treatment.[447] The incidence ranges between 2 and 10%. After a total dose of mitomycin of ≥ 20 mg/m² (often in combination with vindesine), patients rapidly develop hemolytic anemia, red cell fragmentation, thrombocytopenia, reticulocytosis, systemic hyper- or hypotension, obtundation, seizures, neurologic deficits, renal failure, pulmonary edema (usually noncardiogenic), alveolar hemorrhage, and pulmonary hypertension.[447,448] All features may not be present. Interestingly, blood transfusions, even in small amounts, or the addition of vindesine to mitomycin may trigger the onset of HUS. Transfusions are contraindicated as they can aggravate or lead to relapse of the syndrome.[447] Patients with the HUS may develop ARDS from noncardiogenic pulmonary edema or hemorrhage, and in this case the mortality is 95%.[447] Histology of the lung shows intravascular fibrin thrombi and/or evidence of pulmonary embolism, along with alveolar edema or hemorrhage.[447] In addition to supportive care, treatment consists of removal of the drug, plasmapheresis, and high-dose corticosteroids. In patients receiving mitomycin, renal function and urinalysis should be monitored since subtle changes may indicate early mitomycin toxiciy and precede the onset of clinical disease.[447]

Nitrofurantoin Lung

As early as 1967, articles detailed the essentials of nitrofurantoin lung, and, grouped together, there are approximately 1,000 case reports.[234,450–453] Several features are characteristic of nitrofurantoin lung.

• The disease may present in an acute or chronic form, and one does not necessarily follow the other. The acute form is more prevalent (3:1) and has a better prognosis.
• Rechallenge of patients after an episode of acute nitrofurantoin lung almost invariably leads to relapse.
• The chronic form of nitrofurantoin lung develops incideously after months to years of therapy. It presents as interstitial pneumonitis or fibrosis[454] and, less often, desquamative interstitial pneumonia (DIP).[455]

Nitrofurantoin lung primarily occurs in women (75%). Interestingly, vitamin C added to nitrofurantoin to acidify the urine has decreased the incidence of nitrofurantoin lung.[241] Nitrofurantoin lung remains prevalent because of its use in chronic suppression of bladder infection in women.

Acute nitrofurantoin lung can occur within several days of initiation of therapy or even after a single dose in patients with prior, even uneventful, course(s) with the drug. Subacute and chronic nitrofurantoin lung develop after months to years.

Acute nitrofurantoin lung is characterized by the rapid or sudden development of fever, chills, dyspnea, cough, wheezing, myalgias, chest pain, and a cutaneous rash. The symptoms of acute nitrofurantoin lung may be alarming and mimick severe asthma, pulmonary edema, pulmonary embolism, or myocardial infarction. Symptoms are out of proportion to the radiographic changes, which are modest. Although an increase in blood eosinophils is commonly observed, these cells are not prominent in lung tissue, which differentiates acute nitrofurantoin lung from eosinophilic pneumonia.[456]

Chronic nitrofurantoin lung does not develop after the acute form of the disease. These patients gradually develop cough and dyspnea, and sometimes it is an incidental finding on the chest radiograph.[457] Some patients with subclinical nitrofurantoin lung were diagnosed on the basis of an abnormal BAL fluid.[458]

Radiographic abnormalities are present in about three-quarters of patients with acute nitrofurantoin lung, in the form of faint, discrete, bibasilar markings or Kerley's B lines.[87] These changes are more prominently seen on CT. Moderate pleural effusions are occasionally present. The chest radiograph may be normal in spite of the presence of clinical symptoms.[87] In contrast, patients with chronic nitrofurantoin lung present with reticular infiltrates, coarse central lines converging to the hili, subpleural lines, or thickened peribronchovascular areas and, sometimes, reduced lung volumes. Peribronchovascular involvement (see Figure 20–10A) may correspond to the histopathologic pattern of organizing pneumonia.[459] The rare patient with nitrofurantoin-induced DAH presents with alveolar shadows in a batwing distribution.[460]

Laboratory investigation demonstrated an increased erythrocyte sedimentation rate in nearly all patients with acute nitrofurantoin lung and mild peripheral eosinophilia in approximately two-thirds.[461] These findings are uncommon in the chronic form. An increased ANA titer is found in a minority of patients with chronic nitrofurantoin lung.[459,462]

Acute nitrofurantoin lung is a vasculitic process involving small pulmonary vessels.[283] In the few cases for which pathologic material was available, there was a perivascular influx of inflammatory cells, fibrin thrombi within pulmonary arterioles, and evidence for alveolar exudation. More severe or advanced cases demonstrated changes consistent with alveolar edema, hyaline membranes, and diffuse alveolar damage.[240,463,464] Despite peripheral eosinophilia, tissue eosinophils are inconspicuous. In contrast, the histopathologic features of chronic nitrofurantoin lung best correspond to nonspecific interstitial pneumonia, fibrosis, or organizing pneumonia. Uncommonly reported are eosinophilic pneumonia and desquamative interstitial pneumonia.[141,229,459,465]

In almost all published cases the drug was discontinued. This is of clear benefit in acute cases. Inadvertent rechallenge leads to recurrence of clinical symptoms, eosinophilia, and sometimes radiographic opacities in patients with acute nitrofurantoin lung.[466] The role of corticosteroids for the immediate management of acute nitrofurantoin lung remains unclear as the disease is short-lived and responds to discontinuation of the drug. In patients with respiratory failure, corticosteroids are recommended. Corticosteroids are a useful adjunct to drug withdrawal in patients with chronic nitrofurantoin lung. The indication for their use is similar to that for other chronic infiltrative lung diseases. Cessation of the drug is also required. Continuation and rechallenge has led to fatal consequences in some patients with acute or chronic nitrofurantoin lung.[467]

THORACIC COMPLICATIONS OF RADIATION THERAPY

Thoracic radiation has long been known to cause respiratory complications. In their classic 1940 paper, Warren and Spencer[468] established that (1) although there was a relation with dose, this was not absolute, (2) the disease was characterized by cough, which developed at the height of the skin reaction, and diminished thereafter, and (3) the pathologic changes, which included bizarre type II cells, hyaline membranes, edema, and eventually fibrosis, were typical. However, the radiomimetic and alkylating drugs were not in clinical use, and it was later realized that the pathologic changes induced by these drugs mimic those of radiation therapy. Early clinical observations also showed that corticosteroid drugs benefit patients with the early stages of radiation pneumonitis.

Most commonly, radiation lung injury develops in patients with lung or breast carcinoma, Hodgkin's or non-Hodgkin's lymphomas, or total body irradiation prior to bone marrow transplantation. Since lung radiation injury depends on the direction of the radiation beam, the distribution of radiation-induced changes depends on treatment delivery and port. For instance, radiation therapy for lung cancer tends to induce predominantly unilateral changes (Figure 20–29),[86] whereas mantle-field irradiation of Hodgkin's disease preferentially induces upper chest, and paramediastinal changes (Figures 20–30 and 20–31).[469] Radiation therapy may also induce changes in areas of the lung remote from the radiation beam, as shown by the fact that BAL lymphocytes are increased, or gallium is taken up in the nonirradiated as well as in the irradiated lung.[470] Similarly, organizing pneumonia following breast radiation therapy may develop in apparently nonirradiated areas of the lung.[184,185] Radiation therapy may also affect the pleura, heart, pericardium, large vessels, mediastinum, lymphatic vessels, and nerves. Accordingly, symptomatic pleural effusion, valvular stenosis/insufficiency, congestive heart failure, atrioventricular block, pericardial effusion (early or late), constrictive pericarditis, coronary artery disease, pulmonary artery stenosis, fibrosing mediastinitis, chylothorax, and diaphragmatic or left vocal cord palsy have been observed in association with the lung changes.[86,471–485]

In addition to individual susceptibility, the risk of radiation pneumonitis depends on the dose delivered to the lung (including previous radiation), the daily or fractionation of the dose, and the coadministration of chemotherapeutic agents, interferon-gamma, or oxygen. Other factors include advanced age, abrupt withdrawal of corticosteroids, and a low baseline arterial oxygen pressure (PaO_2). Recent pneumonectomy is a potential risk factor because more remaining lung is exposed to radiation as the postpneumonectomy hemithorax contracts. In contrast, smoking may have a protective effect.

Several clinical and imaging patterns of radiation pneumonitis are recognized.

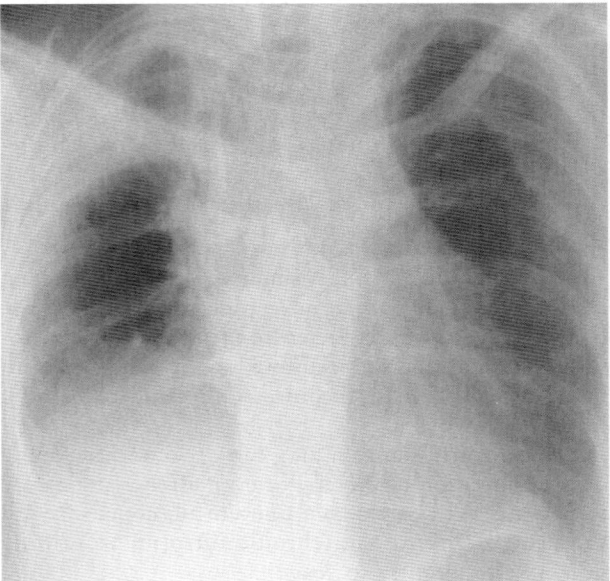

A

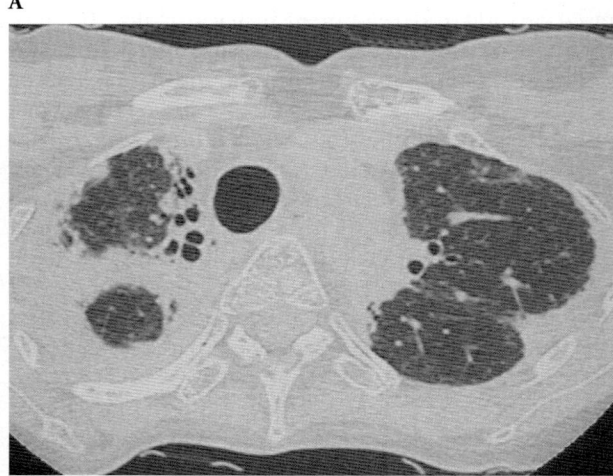

B

Figure 20–30 Thoracic changes induced by mantle irradiation have a predilection to localize in the mediastinum in the superior sulci and in the paramediastinal regions of the lung. This results in a distinctive Y-shaped pattern of pleuropulmonary and mediastinal fibrosis. (This 27-year-old woman had received radiation therapy for Hodgkin's disease in childhood and developed severe restrictive lung function).

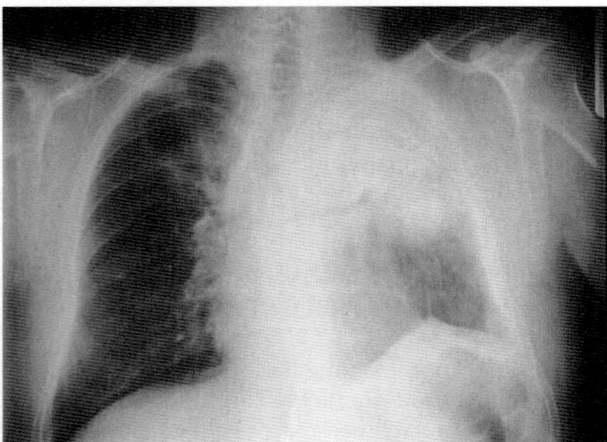

Figure 20–29 Pulmonary changes following chest irradiation often conform to the radiation portal, as seen in this radiograph of a patient who received radiation therapy for epidermoid carcinoma of the left upper lobe bronchus.

- Classic radiation pneumonitis[86] is the most common pattern of radiation-induced damage to the chest, and approximately 10% of patients develop this. The symptoms of radiation pneumonitis include a dry hacking cough, moderate fever, and dyspnea. On imaging, findings typically develop 1 to 2 months after the onset of treatment and include a discrete haze, ill-defined patchy nodules, or an area of condensation (see Figure 20–29). These changes usually predominate in the irradiated area, usually reverse within 6 months, or slowly progress toward a sharply-demarcated area of fibrosis, with volume loss and bronchiectasis. Mild-to-moderate restrictive lung function develops early in the course of radiation pneumonitis and normalizes within 18 to 24 months. A lung biopsy is rarely needed to establish the diagnosis. Histologic features include interstitial edema, hemorrhage, and a fibrinous exudate in the early stage of the disease and later, distortion, fibrosis, and pneumocyte dysplasia. Although patients usually respond well to the administration of corticosteroids, these drugs are not required in all cases, and treatment is guided by the severity of symptoms and gas exchange abnormalities. Late complications of chronic radiation pneumonitis are unusual and include pneumothorax or colonization by *Aspergillus*. Changes in the heart or pleura may be present in association with chronic radiation pneumonitis and may lead to chronic pleural effusions or to irreversible and progressive cardiorespiratory failure (see Figure 20–31).[472,486]
- In rare instances, the infiltrates of radiation pneumonitis extend outside the radiation field. This is associated with significant clinical symptoms, and in some patients respiratory failure or ARDS will develop.[487] Most patients, however, respond satisfactorily to the administration of corticosteroids. Acute radiation pneumonitis uncommonly develops in bone marrow transplant patients following the concomitant administration of total body irradiation and the conditioning chemotherapy regimen.
- Organizing pneumonia induced by radiation therapy to the breast is typically diagnosed on imaging studies. Migratory opacities develop a few weeks to a few months after treatment in the context of mild respiratory and constitutional symptoms (see under 'organizing pneumonia'). The disease is well controlled by corticosteroids.[488]
- Patients irradiated in the past for mediastinal lymphoma or Hodgkin's disease may develop paramediastinal fibrosis later in life.[489,490] The fibrosis localizes in the superior sulci of the lung, in the mediastinum, and in paramediastinal regions of the lung. This results in a distinctive Y-shaped pattern on the chest radiograph and severe restriction (see Figures 20–30 and 20–31). The loss of lung function is even greater when radiation therapy was delivered in childhood, possibly because, in addition to fibrosis, radiation therapy may impact on growth and development of the lung and chest wall.
- Other late radiation-induced changes include lung cancers or, less often, pleural mesothelioma. Smoking cessation should be encouraged in all patients irradiated in the past.[223]
- Endobronchial brachytherapy, given for the treatment of bronchial carcinoma, may dose-dependently induce endobronchial inflammation, stenosis, and/or necrosis of bronchial walls. There is a cutoff value of 12.5 Gy, above which the incidence of complications increases abruptly. Perforation of

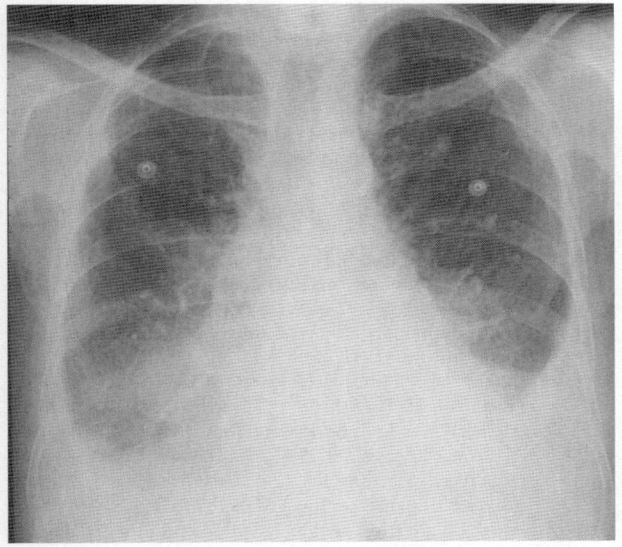

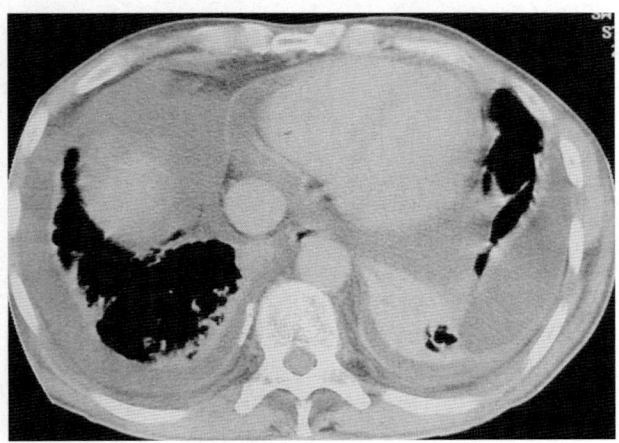

A   **B**

Figure 20–31   Radiation therapy to the chest can damage the heart (myocardial fibrosis, valvular stenosis or incompetence) or pleura (late effusions, chylothorax). These changes aggravate the lung dysfunction. This 60-year-old man developed exudative pleural effusions, myocardial dysfunction, pericardial effusion, and cardiorespiratory failure 35 years after radiation therapy for Hodgkin's disease (*B*, pleural calcification is present on right in this high-resolution computed tomography scan).

the bronchial wall and of nearby vessels may develop as a complication, with massive, usually fatal, hemoptysis as a result.[491]

- The administration of therapeutic doses of microspheres containing iodine 131 or yttrium 90 via the IV or intra-arterial route has been developed as a treatment for thyroid or hepatocellular carcinoma. Considerable irradiation of the lung may follow due to overspill and localization of the radioactive microspheres in the pulmonary circulation, where they persist. Transient or, more often, irreversible pulmonary changes develop in 5 to 10% of patients after one or more treatment courses. This is in the form of pulmonary infiltrates and progressive respiratory failure or an ARDS picture (Figure 20–32). On CT scan, distinctive changes of symmetric "parachute-like" opacities are seen at a distance of both the pleura and the hilum (see Figure 20–32).[492,493]

CONCLUSION

Drugs frequently cause diverse and distinctive patterns of ILD. Withdrawal of the drug is often followed by improvement, and corticosteroids prove beneficial in most patients who fail to improve after discontinuation of the agent. In a minority of patients sequellae will persist. Drug-induced lung disease requires a constant review of the literature as the field continues to expand. Drug-induced lung disease is well suited to Web technology, which enables access to updated information on novel drugs, agents, and clinical patterns.[65]

ACKNOWLEDGMENTS

The author acknowledges Kjetil Ask and Claudio Rabec for their help in the preparation of this manuscript and Pascal Foucher for the construction and maintenance of the Pneumotox Web site.

The author is very grateful to Marvin Schwarz, MD, Talmadge King Jr, MD, and Clio Camus, MD.

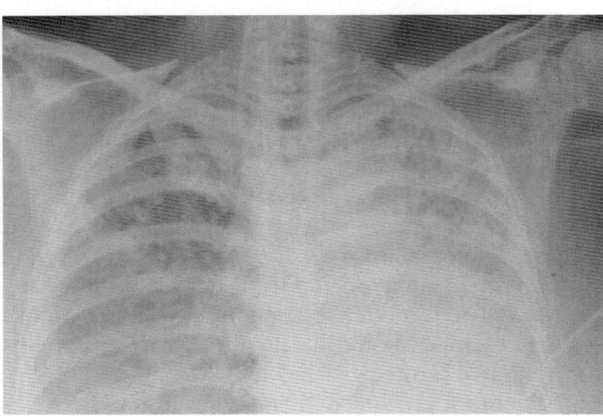

A

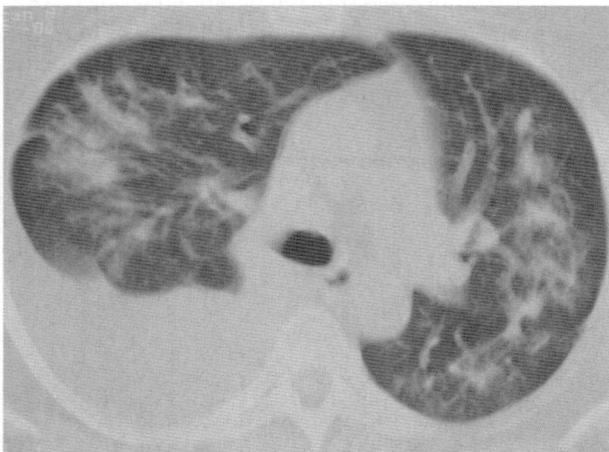

B

Figure 20–32 Instillation of therapeutic doses of microspheres containing radioactive iodine in patients with hepatocellular carcinoma can induce severe radiation pneumonitis, and an ARDS picture. The presumed mechanism consists of spillage of the radioactive material across the tumor, followed by localization of the radioactive microspheres in the pulmonary circulation. *B*, High-resolution computed tomography discloses symmetric "parachute-like" opacities at a distance of the pleura and hilum (57-year-old woman with liver cirrhosis, and hepatocellular carcinoma who had received 2 × 60 mCi [131]iodine).

REFERENCES

1. Siegel M, Lee SL, Peress NS. The epidemiology of drug-induced systemic lupus erythematosus. Arthritis Rheum 1967;10:407–15.
2. Alarcon-Segovia D. Drug-induced lupus syndromes. Mayo Clin Proc 1969;44:664–81.
3. Ansell G. Radiological manifestations of drug-induced disease. Clin Radiol 1969;20:133–48.
4. Rosenow ECI. The spectrum of drug-induced pulmonary disease. Ann Intern Med 1972;77:977–91.
5. Whitcomb ME. Drug-induced lung disease. Chest 1973; 63:418–22.
6. Kormano M. Drug-induced radiographic pulmonary changes. Duodecim 1974;90:1129–33.
7. Sostman HD, Matthay RA, Putman CE, Walker Smith GJ. Methotrexate-induced pneumonitis. Medicine (Baltimore) 1976;55:371–88.
8. Cole P. Drug-induced lung disease. Drugs 1977;13:422–44.
9. Green MR. Pulmonary toxicity of antineoplastic agents. West J Med 1977;127:292–8.
10. Gross NJ. Pulmonary effects of radiation therapy. Ann Intern Med 1977;86:81–92.
11. Lippmann ML. Pulmonary reactions to drugs. Med Clin North Am 1977;61:1353–67.
12. Roswit B, White DC. Severe radiation injuries of the lung. AJR Am J Roentgenol 1977;129:127–36.
13. Sostman HD, Matthay RA, Putman CE. Cytotoxic drug-induced lung disease. Am J Med 1977;62:608–15.
14. Rosenow ECI. Drugs that may induce pulmonary disease. Geriatrics 1978;33:64–73.
15. Whitcomb ME, Domby WR. Drug-induced lung disease. Prim Care 1978;5:411–23.
16. Willson JKV. Pulmonary toxicity of antineoplastic drugs. Cancer Treat Rep 1978;62:2003–8.
17. Demeter SL, Ahmad M, Tomashefski JF. Drug-induced pul-

monary disease. Part I. Patterns of response. Cleve Clin Q 1979;46:89–99.

18. Demeter SL, Ahmad M, Tomashefski JF. Drug-induced pulmonary disease. Part II. Categories of drugs. Cleve Clin Q 1979;46:100–12.

19. Demeter SL, Ahmad M, Tomashefski JF. Drug-induced pulmonary disease. Part III. Agents used to treat neoplasms or alter the immune system including a brief review of radiation therapy. Cleve Clin Q 1979;46:113–24.

20. Filipek WJ. Drug-induced pulmonary disease. Postgrad Med 1979;65:131–6, 139–40.

21. Rosenow EC. Chemotherapeutic drug-induced pulmonary disease. Semin Respir Med 1980;2:89–96.

22. Weiss RB, Muggia FM. Cytotoxic drug-induced pulmonary disease: update 1980. Am J Med 1980;68:259–66.

23. Sostman HD, Putman CE, Gamsu G. Diagnosis of chemotherapy lung. AJR Am J Roentgenol 1981;136:33–40.

24. Weiss RB, Poster DS, Penta JS. The nitrosoureas and pulmonary toxicity. Cancer Treat Rev 1981;8:111–25.

25. Balikian JP, Jochelson MS, Bauer KA, et al. Pulmonary complications of chemotherapy regimens containing bleomycin. AJR Am J Roentgenol 1982;139:455–61.

26. Muggia FM, Louie AC, Sikic Bl. Pulmonary toxicity of antitumour agents. Cancer Treat Rev 1983;10:221–43.

27. Bargon G. Drug-induced changes in the lungs. Rontgenblatter 1984;37:261–5.

28. White JP, Ward MJ. Drug-induced adverse pulmonary reactions. Adv Drug React Acute Pois Rev 1985;4:183–211.

29. Cooper JAD, White DA, Matthay RA. Drug-induced pulmonary disease. Part I: cytotoxic drugs. Am Rev Respir Dis 1986;133:321–40.

30. Cooper JAD, White DA, Matthay RA. Drug-induced pulmonary disease. Part II: noncytotoxic drugs. Am Rev Respir Dis 1986;133:488–505.

31. Cooper JAD, Matthay RA. Drug-induced pulmonary disease. Dis Mon 1987;33:61–120.

32. Rosenow ECI. Drug-induced bronchopulmonary pleural disease. J Allergy Clin Immunol 1987;80:780–7.

33. Massin F, Fur A, Reybet-Degat O, et al. La pneumopathie du busulfan. Rev Mal Respir 1987;4:3–10.

34. Martin WJ. Pulmonary toxicity induced by chemical agents. Eur Respir J 1990;3:375–6.

35. Prakash UBS. Pulmonary complications from ophthalmic preparations. Mayo Clin Proc 1990;65:521–9.

36. Walker-Smith GJ. The histopathology of pulmonary reactions to drugs. Clin Chest Med 1990;31:95–118.

37. Zitnik RJ, Cooper JAD. Pulmonary disease due to antirheumatic agents. Clin Chest Med 1990;11:139–50.

38. Bush WH, Swanson DP. Acute reactions to intravascular contrast media: types, risk factors, recognition, and specific treatment. AJR Am J Roentgenol 1991;157:1153–61.

39. Gregory SA, Gripp MA. The clinical diagnosis of drug-induced pulmonary disorders. J Thorac Imaging 1991;6:8–18.

40. Kuhlman JE. The role of chest computed tomography in the diagnosis of drug-related reactions. J Thorac Imaging 1991;6:52–61.

41. McCarroll KA, Roszler MH. Lung disorders due to drug abuse. J Thorac Imaging 1991;6:30–5.

42. Obermiller T, Lakshminarayan S. Drug-induced hypersensitivity reactions in the lung. Immunol Allergy Clin North Am 1991;11:575–94.

43. Reed CR, Glauser FL. Drug-induced non cardiogenic pulmonary edema. Chest 1991;100:1120–4.

44. Bryant DH. Drug-induced pulmonary disease. Med J Aust 1992;156:802–5.

45. Massin F, Coudert B, Foucher P, et al. La pneumopathie des nitrosourées. Rev Mal Respir 1992;9:575–82.

46. Rosenow ECI, Myers JL, Swensen SJ, Pisani RJ. Drug-induced pulmonary disease: an update. Chest 1992;102:239–50.

47. Russi E. Toxic and drug-induced lesions of the pulmonary parenchyma. Schweiz Rundsch Med Prax 1992;81:618–21.

48. Myers JL. Diagnosis of drug reactions in the lung. Monogr Pathol 1993;36:32–53.

49. Rosenow ECI. Drug-induced pulmonary disease. Dis Mon 1994;40:253–312.

50. Sitbon O, Bidel N, Dussopt C, et al. Minocycline pneumonitis and eosinophilia: a report on 8 patients. Arch Intern Med 1994;154:1633–40.

51. Albertson TE, Walby WF, Derlet RW. Stimulant-induced pulmonary toxicity. Chest 1995;108:1140–9.

52. Aronchick JM, Gefter WB. Drug-induced pulmonary disorders. Semin Roentgenol 1995;30:18–34.

53. Haim DY, Lippmann ML, Goldberg SK, Walkenstein MD. The pulmonary complications of crack cocaine. A comprehensive review. Chest 1995;107:233–40.

54. O'Donnell AE, Selig J, Aravamuthan M, Richardson MSA. Pulmonary complications associated with illicit drug use. An update. Chest 1995;108:460–3.

55. Zitnik RJ. Drug-induced lung disease: cancer chemotherapy agents. J Respir Dis 1995;16:855–65.

56. Zitnik RJ. Drug-induced lung disease: an overview of common causes. J Respir Dis 1995;16:552–62.

57. Zitnik RJ. Drug-induced lung disease: cardiovascular agents. J Respir Dis 1995;17:293–8.

58. Zitnik RJ. Drug-induced lung disease: antimicrobial agents. J Respir Dis 1995;17:592–601.

59. Zitnik RJ. Drug-induced lung disease: antiarrhythmic agents. J Respir Dis 1995;17:254–70.

60. Pfitzenmeyer P, Foucher P, Dennewald G, et al. Pleuropulmonary changes induced by ergoline drugs. Eur Respir J 1996;9:1013–9.

61. Albertson TE, Walby WF. Respiratory toxicities from stimulant use. Clin Rev Allergy Immunol 1997;15:221–41.

62. Camus P. Respiratory disease induced by drugs. Eur Respir J 1997;10:260–4.

63. Cooper JAJ. Drug-induced lung disease. Adv Intern Med 1997;42:231–68.

64. Foucher P, Biour M, Blayac JP, et al. Drugs that may injure the respiratory system. Eur Respir J 1997;10:265–79.

65. Foucher P, Camus P. Pneumotox®. 1997. Available at http://www.pneumotox.com (accessed September 2002).

66. Movsas B, Raffin TA, Epstein AH, Link CJ. Pulmonary radiation injury. Chest 1997;111:1061–76.

67. Roux F, Zitnik RJ. Drug-induced lung disease: antirheumatic agents. J Respir Dis 1997;18:431–46.

68. Jessurun GAJ, Boermsa WG, Crijns HJGM. Amiodarone-induced pulmonary toxicity. Predisposing factors, clinical symptoms and treatment. Drug Saf 1998;18:339–44.

69. Trottier M, Vaillancourt R. Drug-induced asthma. Can Pharm J 1998;131:30–7.

70. Morelock SY, Sahn SA. Drugs and the pleura. Chest 1999;116:212–21.

71. Babu KS, Salvi SS. Aspirin and asthma. Chest 2000;118:1470–6.

72. Ben-Noun LL. Drug-induced respiratory disorders. Incidence, prevention and management. Drug Saf 2000;23:145–64.

73. Ellis SJ, Cleverley JR, Müller NL. Drug-induced lung disease: high-resolution CT findings. AJR Am J Roentgenol 2000;175:1019–24.

74. Imokawa S, Colby TV, Leslie KO, Helmers RA. Methotrexate pneumonitis: review of the literature and histopathological findings in nine patients. Eur Respir J 2000;15:373–81.

75. Camus P, Foucher P, Bonniaud P, Ask K. Drug-induced infiltrative lung disease. Eur Respir J 2001;32:93S–100S.

76. Vaszar LT, Stevenson DD. Aspirin-induced asthma. Clin Rev Allergy Immunol 2001;21:71–87.

77. Schneider RK, Levenson JL, Schnoll SH. Update in addiction medicine. Ann Intern Med 2001;134:387–95.

78. Erasmus JJ, McAdams HP, Rossi SE. High-resolution CT of drug-induced lung disease. Radiol Clin North Am 2002;40:61–72.

79. Erasmus JJ, McAdams HP, Rossi SE. Drug-induced lung injury. Semin Roentgenol 2002;37:72–81.

80. Simonneau G, Fartoukh M, Sitbon O, et al. Primary pulmonary hypertension associated with the use of fenfluramine derivatives. Chest 1998;114:195S–9S.

81. Anonymous. Clinicopathologic conference. Lymphoma or drug reaction occurring during hydantoin therapy for epilepsy. Am J Med 1962;32:286–97.

82. Yonemaru M, Mizuguchi Y, Kasuga I, et al. Hilar and mediastinal lymphadenopathy with hypersensitivity pneumonitis induced by penicillin. Chest 1992;102:1907–9.

83. Krehmeier H. Sarcoidosis after interferon-alpha in hepatitis-C. Dtsch Med Wochenschr 2001;126:460.

84. Similowski T, Straus C, Attali V, et al. Neuromuscular blockade with acute respiratory failure in a patient receiving cibenzoline. Thorax 1997;52:582–4.

85. Oshima Y, Takahashi S, Nagayama H, et al. Fatal GVHD demonstrating an involvement of respiratory muscle following donor leukocyte transfusion (DLT). Bone Marrow Transplant 1997;19:737–40.

86. Abratt RP, Morgan GW. Lung toxicity following chest irradiation in patients with lung cancer. Lung Cancer 2002; 35:103–9.

87. Holmberg L, Boman G. Pulmonary reactions to nitrofurantoin. 447 cases reported to the Swedish Adverse Drug Reaction Committee 1966–1976. Eur J Respir Dis 1981;62:180–9.

88. Sleijfer S. Bleomycin pneumonitis. Chest 2001;120:617–24.

89. Verweij J, van der Burg MEL, Pinedo HM. Mitomycin C-induced hemolytic uremic syndrome. Six case reports and review of the literature on renal, pulmonary and cardiac side effects of the drug. Radiother Oncol 1987;8:33–41.

90. Martin WJI, Rosenow ECI. Amiodarone pulmonary toxicity. Recognition and pathogenesis (part 1). Chest 1988;93: 1067–75.

91. Martin WJI, Rosenow ECI. Amiodarone pulmonary toxicity. Recognition and pathogenesis (part 2). Chest 1988;93: 1242–8.

92. Siniakowicz RM, Narula D, Suster B, Steinberg JS. Diagnosis of amiodarone pulmonary toxicity with high-resolution computerized tomographic scan. J Cardiovasc Electrophysiol 2001;12:431–6.

93. Gondouin A, Manzoni P, Ranfaing E, et al. Exogenous lipid pneumonia: a retrospective multicentre study of 44 cases in France. Eur Respir J 1996;9:1463–9.

94. Lee JY, Lee KS, Kim TS, et al. Squalene-induced extrinsic lipoid pneumonia: serial radiologic findings in nine patients. J Comput Assist Tomogr 1999;23:730–5.

95. Gentina T, Tillié-Leblond I, Birolleau S, et al. Fire-eater's lung. Seventeen cases and a review of the literature. Medicine (Baltimore) 2001;80:291–7.

96. Midulla F, Strappini PM, Ascoli V, et al. Bronchoalveolar lavage cell analysis in a child with chronic lipid pneumonia. Eur Respir J 1998;11:239–42.

97. Gutiérrez F, Leon L. Elemental mercury embolism to the lung. N Engl J Med 2000;342:1791.

98. Biron P, Dessureault J, Napke E. Acute allergic interstitial pneumonitis induced by hydrochlorothiazide. Can Med Assoc J 1991;145:28–34.

99. Popovsky MA. Transfusion-related acute lung injury (TRALI). Vox Sang 2001;81:274–5.

100. Pisani RJ, Rosenow ECI. Pulmonary edema associated with tocolytic therapy. Ann Intern Med 1989;110:714–8.

101. Ullmer E, Mayr M, Binet I, et al. Granulomatous *Pneumocystis carinii* pneumonia in Wegener's granulomatosis. Eur Respir J 2000;15:213–6.

102. Higenbottam TW. Bronchiolitis obliterans following the ingestion of an Asian shrub leaf. Thorax 1997;52:S68–72.

103. Kilbourne EM, Philen RM, Kamb ML, Falk H. Tryptophan produced by Showa Denko and epidemic eosinophilia-myalgia syndrome. J Rheumatol 1996;23:81–8.

104. Gaine SP, Rubin LJ, Kmetzo JJ, et al. Recreational use of aminorex and pulmonary hypertension. Chest 2000;118: 1496–500.

105. Kao CH, Hsieh JF, Ho YJ, et al. Acute paraquat intoxication. Using nuclear pulmonary studies to predict patient outcome. Chest 1999;116:709–14.

106. Park CH, Kim KI, Park SK, Lee CH. Carbamate poisoning: high resolution CT and pathologic findings. J Comput Assist Tomogr 2000;24:52–4.

107. Fenton JJ, Johnson FB, Przygodzk RM, et al. Sodium polystyrene sulfonate (Kayexalate) aspiration. Histologic appearance and infrared microspectrophotometric analysis of two cases. Arch Pathol Lab Med 1996;120:967–9.

108. Janoski MM, Raymond GS, Puttagunta L, et al. Psyllium aspiration causing bronchiolitis: radiographic, high-resolution CT, and pathologic findings. AJR Am J Roentgenol 2000;174:799–801.

109. Schattner A, Von der Walde J, Kozak N, et al. Nitrofurantoin-induced immune-mediated lung and liver disease. Am J Med Sci 1999;317:336–40.

110. Vrobel TR, Miller PE, Mostow ND, Rakita L. A general overview of amiodarone toxicity: its prevention, detection and management. Progr Cardiovasc Dis 1989;31:393–426.

111. Cherniack RM, Abrams J, Kalica AR. Pulmonary disease associated with breast cancer therapy. Am J Resp Crit Care Med 1994;150:1169–73.

112. Salaffi F, Manganelli P, Carotti M, et al. Methotrexate-induced pneumonitis in patients with rheumatoid arthritis and psoriatic arthritis: report of five cases and review of the literature. Clin Rheumatol 1997;16:296–304.

113. Sleijfer S, van der Mark TW, Schraffordt Koops H, Mulder NH. Enhanced effects of bleomycin on pulmonary function disturbances in patients with decreased renal function due to cisplatin. Eur J Cancer 1996;32A:550–2.

114. Simpson AB, Paul J, Graham J, Kaye SB. Fatal bleomycin pulmonary toxicity in the west of Scotland 1991–95: a review of patients with germ cell tumours. Br J Cancer 1998;78: 1061–6.

115. Hübner C, Dietz A, Stremmel W, et al. Macrolide-induced Churg-Strauss syndrome in patient with atopy. Lancet 1997;ii:1552.

116. Aronin PA, Mahaley MSJ, Rudnick SA, et al. Prediction of BCNU pulmonary toxicity in patients with malignant gliomas: an assessment of risk factors. N Engl J Med 1980;303:183–8.

117. Real E, Roca MJ, Vinuales A, et al. Life threatening lung toxicity induced by low doses of bleomycin in a patient with Hodgkin's disease. Haematologica 1999;84:667–8.

118. Lind PA, Marks LB, Jamieson TA, et al. Predictors for pneumonitis during locoregional radiotherapy in high-risk patients with breast carcinoma treated with high-dose chemotherapy and stem-cell rescue. Cancer 2002;94: 2821–9.

119. Schweitzer VG, Juillard GJF, Bajada CL, Parker RG. Radiation recall dermatitis and pneumonitis in a patient treated with paclitaxel. Cancer 1995;76:1069–72.

120. Nalos PC, Kass RM, Gang ES, et al. Life-threatening postoperative pulmonary complications in patients with previous amiodarone pulmonary toxicity undergoing cardiothoracic operations. J Thorac Cardiovasc Surg 1987;93:904–12.

121. Ingrassia TSI, Ryu JH, Trastek VF, Rosenow ECI. Oxygen-exacerbated bleomycin pulmonary toxicity. Mayo Clin Proc 1991;66:173–8.

122. Kanji Z, Sunderji R, Gin K. Amiodarone-induced pulmonary toxicity. Pharmacotherapy 1999;19:1463–6.

123. O'Driscoll BR, Hasleton PS, Taylor PM, et al. Active lung fibrosis up to 17 years after chemotherapy with carmustine (BCNU) in childhood. N Engl J Med 1990;323:378–82.

124. Thomas E, Mazyad H, Olive P, Blotman F. Cytomegalovirus-induced pneumonia in a rheumatoid arthritis patient treated with low dose methotrexate. Clin Exp Rheumatol 1997;15:583–4.

125. Keane MP, Lynch JP. Pleuropulmonary manifestations of systemic lupus erythematosus. Thorax 2000;55:159–66.

126. Mayberry JP, Primack SL, Müller NL. Thoracic manifestations of systemic autoimmune diseases: radiographic and high-resolution CT findings. Radiographics 2000;20:1623–35.

127. Camus P, Piard F, Ashcroft T, et al. The lung in inflammatory bowel disease. Medicine (Baltimore) 1993;72:151–83.

128. Parry SD, Barbatzas C, Peel ET, Barton JR. Sulphasalazine and lung toxicity. Eur Respir J 2002;19:756–64.

129. Lombard JN, Bonnotte B, Maynadié M, et al. Celiprolol pneumonitis. Eur Respir J 1993;9:588–91.

130. Tomioka H, King TEJ. Gold-induced pulmonary disease: clinical features, outcome, and differentiation from rheumatoid lung disease. Am J Resp Crit Care Med 1997;155:1011–20.

131. Gomez JL, Dupont A, Cusan L, et al. Simultaneous liver and lung toxicity related to the nonsteroidal antiandrogen nilutamide (Anandron): a case report. Am J Med 1992;92:563–6.

132. Yalçin S, Sahin A, Yalçin B, Altinok G. Nitrofurantoin toxicity to both liver and lungs. Liver 1997;17:166–7.

133. Pfitzenmeyer P, Foucher P, Piard F, et al. Nilutamide pneumonitis: a report on eight patients. Thorax 1992;47:622–7.

134. Akira M, Ishikawa H, Yamamoto S. Drug-induced pneumonitis: thin-section CT findings in 60 patients. Radiology 2002;224:852–60.

135. Rubin G, Baume P, Vandenberg R. Azathioprine and acute restrictive lung disease. Aust N Z J Med 1973;3:272–4.

136. White DA, Rankin JA, Stover DE, et al. Methotrexate pneumonitis: bronchoalveolar lavage findings suggest an immunologic disorder. Am Rev Respir Dis 1989;139:18–21.

137. Fuhrman C, Parrot A, Wislez M, et al. Spectrum of CD4 to CD8 T-cell ratios in lymphocytic alveolitis associated with methotrexate-induced pneumonitis. Am J Respir Crit Care Med 2001;164:1186–91.

138. Leduc D, De Vuyst P, Lheureux P, et al. Pneumonitis complicating low-dose methotrexate therapy for rheumatoid arthritis. Chest 1993;104:1620–3.

139. Beasley MB, Franks TJ, Galvin JR, et al. Acute fibrinous and organizing pneumonia. Arch Pathol Lab Med 2002;126:1064–70.

140. Rabe J, Neff KW, Lehmann KJ, et al. Miliary tuberculosis after intravesical bacille Calmette-Guérin immunotherapy for carcinoma of the bladder. Am J Roentgenol 1999;172:748–50.

141. Bone RC, Wolfe J, Sobonya RE. Desquamative interstitial pneumonia following chronic nitrofurantoin therapy. Chest 1976;69:296–7.

142. Salerno SM, Ormseth EJ, Roth BJ, et al. Sulfasalazine pulmonary toxicity in ulcerative colitis mimicking clinical features of Wegener's granulomatosis. Chest 1996;110:556–9.

143. Noseworthy TW, Davey RS, Percy JS, King EG. Hypoxemic respiratory failure in rheumatoid arthritis: gold related? Crit Care Med 1983;11:761–2.

144. Lisbona A, Schwartz J, Lachance C, et al. Methotrexate-induced pulmonary disease. J Can Assoc Radiol 1973;24:215–20.

145. Bucknall CE, Adamson MR, Banham SW. Non fatal pulmonary haemorrhage associated with nitrofurantoin. Thorax 1987;42:475–6.

146. Smith RL, Alexander RF, Aranda CP. Pulmonary granulomata. A complication on intravesical administration of bacillus Calmette-Guérin for superficial bladder carcinoma. Cancer 1993;71:1846–7.

147. Kremer JM, Alarcon GS, Weinblatt ME, et al. Clinical, laboratory, radiographic, and histopathologic features of methotrexate-associated lung injury in patients with rheumatoid arthritis. Arthritis Rheum 1997;40:1829–37.

148. Hess EV. Eosinophilia-myalgia syndrome: opportunities realized and missed. J Rheumatol 1997;24:1239–40.

149. Weller PF, Plaut M, Taggart V, Trontell A. The relationship of asthma therapy and Churg-Strauss syndrome: NIH workshop summary report. J Allergy Clin Immunol 2001;108:175–83.

150. Lilly CM, Churg A, Lazarovich M, et al. Asthma therapies and Churg-Strauss syndrome. J Allergy Clin Immunol 2002;109:S1–S19.

151. Dupon M, Malou M, Rogues AM, Lacut JY. Acute eosinophilic pneumonia induced by inhaled pentamidine isethionate. BMJ 1993;306:109.

152. Orriols R, Munoz X, Ferrer J, et al. Cocaine-induced Churg-Strauss vasculitis. Eur Respir J 1995;9:175–7.

153. Wechsler ME, Pauwels R, Drazen JM. Leukotriene modifiers and Churg-Strauss syndrome. Adverse effect or response to corticosteroid withdrawal? Drug Safe 1999;21:241–51.

154. Kaufman D, Pichler W, Beer JH. Severe episode of high fever with rash, lymphadenopathy, neutropenia, and eosinophilia after minocycline therapy for acne. Arch Intern Med 1994;154:1983–4.

155. de Vriese ASP, Philippe J, Van Renterghem DM, et al. Carbamazepine hypersensitivity syndrome: report of 4 cases and review of the literature. Medicine (Baltimore) 1995;74:144–50.

156. Bourezane Y, Salard D, Hoen B, et al. DRESS (Drug Rash with Eosinophilia and Systemic Symptoms) syndrome associated with nevirapine therapy. Clin Infect Dis 1998;27:1321–2.

157. Eland IA, Dofferhoff ASM, Vink R, et al. Colitis may be part of the antiepileptic drug hypersensitivity syndrome. Epilepsia 1999;40:1780–3.

158. Choquet-Kastylevsky G, Intrator L, Chenal C, et al. Increased levels of interleukin 5 are associated with the generation of eosinophilia in drug-induced hypersensitivity syndrome. Br J Dermatol 1998;139:1026–32.

159. Kettaneh A, Fain O, Ziol M, et al. Minocycline-induced systemic adverse reaction with liver and bone marrow granulomas and Sezary-like cells. Am J Med 2000;108:353–4.

160. Tröger U, Brandt W, Rose W. Development of a pulmonary phenytoin-associated hypersensitivity reaction despite concomitant dexamethasone and prednisolone administration. Int J Clin Pharmacol Ther 2000;38:452–6.

161. Noh H, Lee YK, Kang SW, et al. Acute eosinophilic pneumonia associated with amitriptyline in a hemodialysis patient. Yonsei Med J 2001;42:357–9.

162. Green RL, Vayonis AG. Churg-Strauss syndrome after zafirlukast in two patients not receiving systemic steroid treatment. Lancet 1999;353:729–30.

163. Benzaquen-Forner H, Dournovo P, Tandjaoui-Lambiotte H, et al. Pneumopathie hypoxémiante sous traitement par IEC. Rev Mal Respir 1998;15:804–10.

164. Fujimura M, Yasui M, Shinagawa S, et al. Bronchoalveolar lavage cell findings in three types of eosinophilic pneumonia: acute, chronic and drug-induced eosinophilic pneumonia. Respir Med 1998;92:743–9.

165. Yousem SA, Lifson JD, Colby TV. Chemotherapy-induced eosinophilic pneumonia. Relation to bleomycin. Chest 1985;88:103–6.

166. Popovsky MA. Transfusion and lung injury. Transfus Clin Biol 2001;8:272–7.

167. Fiegenberg DS, Weiss H, Kirshman H. Migratory pneumonia with eosinophilia. Associated with sulfonamide administration. Arch Intern Med 1967;120:85–9.

168. Pfitzenmeyer P, Meier M, Zuck P, et al. Piroxicam-induced pulmonary infiltrates and eosinophilia. J Rheumatol 1994;21:1573–7.

169. Kameya T, Morita T, Tanaka I, et al. A case of minocycline-induced hypersensitivity pneumonitis with radiographic finding of multiple nodules. Nippon Naika Gakkai Zasshi 1994;83:1991–2.

170. Oishi Y, Sando Y, Tajima S, et al. Indomethacin induced bulky lymphadenopathy and eosinophilic pneumonia. Respirology 2001;6:57–60.

171. Begbie S, Burgess KR. Maloprim-induced pulmonary eosinophilia. Chest 1993;103:305–6.

172. Dykhuizen RS, Zaidi AM, Godden DJ, et al. Minocycline and pulmonary eosinophilia. BMJ 1995;i:1520–1.

173. Jedynak U, Ciezarek M, Kopinski P. Pulmonary infiltrates with masto- and lymphocytosis in BALF associated with Arechine. Pol J Pathol 1997;48:63–7.

174. Sullivan SN. Sulfasalazine lung. Desensitization to sulfasalazine and treatment with acrylic coated 5-ASA and azodisalicylate. J Clin Gastroenterol 1987;9:461–3.

175. Greenberger P. Desensitization and test-dosing for the drug-allergic patient. Ann Allergy Asthma Immunol 2000;85:250–1.

176. Hollingsworth HM. Drug-related bronchiolitis-obliterans organizing pneumonia. Diseases of the bronchioles. In: Epler GR, editor. Diseases of the bronchioles. New York: Raven Press, Ltd; 1994. p. 367–76.

177. Doniach I, Morrison B, Steiner RE. Lung changes during hexamethonium therapy for hypertension. Br Heart J 1954;16:101–8.

178. Camus P, Lombard JN, Perrichon M, et al. Bronchiolitis obliterans organising pneumonia in patients taking acebutolol or amiodarone. Thorax 1989;44:711–5.

179. Rossi SE, Erasmus JJ, McAdams P, et al. Pulmonary drug toxicity: radiologic and pathologic manifestations. Radiographics 2000;5:1245–59.

180. Santrach PJ, Askin FB, Wells RJ, et al. Nodular form of bleomycin-related pulmonary injury in patients with osteogenic sarcoma. Cancer 1989;64:806–11.

181. Milesi-Lecat A-M, Schmidt J, Aumaître O, et al. Lupus and pulmonary nodules consistent with bronchiolitis obliterans organizing pneumonia induced by carbamazepine. Mayo Clin Proc 1997;72:1145–7.

182. Ferriby D, Stojkovic T. Bronchiolitis obliterans with organizing pneumonia during interferon ß-1a treatment. Lancet 2001;357:751.

183. Fawcett IW, Ibrahim NBN. BOOP associated with nitrofurantoin. Thorax 2001;56:161.

184. Crestani B, Valeyre D, Roden S, et al. Bronchiolitis obliterans organizing pneumonia syndrome primed by radiation therapy to the breast. Am J Respir Crit Care Med 1998;158:1929–35.

185. Stover DE, Milite F, Zakowski M. A newly recognized syndrome—radiation related bronchiolitis obliterans and organizing pneumonia. Respiration 2001;68:540–4.

186. Lohr RH, Boland BJ, Douglas WW, et al. Organizing pneumonia. Features and prognosis of cryptogenic, secondary, and focal variants. Arch Intern Med 1997;157:1323–9.

187. Nizami IY, Kissner DG, Vissher DW, Dubaybo BA. Idiopathic bronchiolitis obliterans with organizing pneumonia. An acute and life-threatening syndrome. Chest 1995;108:271–7.

188. Portel L, Hilbert G, Gruson D, et al. Migratory pulmonary infiltrates in a patient treated with sotalol. Eur Respir J 1998;12:259–60.

189. Cohen AJ, King TE Jr, Downey GP. Rapidly progressive bronchiolitis obliterans with organizing pneumonia. Am J Respir Crit Care Med 1994;149:1670–5.

190. Majori M, Poletti V, Curti A, et al. Bronchoalveolar lavage in bronchiolitis obliterans organizing pneumonia primed by radiation therapy to the breast. J Allergy Clin Immunol 2000;105:239–44.

191. Faller M, Quoix E, Popin E, et al. Migratory pulmonary infiltrates in a patient treated with sotalol. Eur Respir J 1997;10:2159–62.

192. Weiner RS, Bortin MM, Gale RP, et al. Interstitial pneumonitis after bone marrow transplantation. Assessment of risk factors. Ann Intern Med 1986;10:168–75.

193. Seiden MV, Elias A, Ayash L, et al. Pulmonary toxicity associated with high-dose chemotherapy in the treatment of solid tumors with autologous marrow transplant: an analysis of four chemotherapy regimens. Bone Marrow Tranplant 1992;10:57–63.

194. Chap L, Shpiner R, Levine M, et al. Pulmonary toxicity of high-dose chemotherapy for breast cancer: a non-invasive approach to diagnosis and treatment. Bone Marrow Transplant 1997;20:1063–7.

195. Fanfulla F, Locatelli F, Zoia MC, et al. Pulmonary complications and respiratory function changes after bone marrow transplantation in children. Eur Respir J 1997;10:2301–6.

196. Rubio C, Hill ME, Milan S, et al. Idiopathic pneumonia syndrome after high dose chemotherapy for relapsed Hodgkin's disease. Br J Cancer 1997;75:1044–8.

197. Taghian AG, Assaad SI, Niemierko A, et al. Risk of pneumonitis in breast cancer patients treated with radiation therapy and combination chemotherapy with paclitaxel. J Natl Cancer Inst 2001;93:1806–11.

198. Gérard B, Aamdal S, Lee S-M, et al. Activity and unexpected lung toxicity of the sequential administration of two alkylating agents-dacarbazine and fotemustine-in patients with melanoma. Eur J Cancer 1993;29A:711–9.

199. Bhalla KS, Wilczynski SW, Abushamaa AM, et al. Pulmonary toxicity of induction chemotherapy prior to standard or high-dose chemotherapy with autologous hematopoietic support. Am J Respir Crit Care Med 2000;161:17–25.

200. Wilczynski SW, Erasmus JJ, Petros WP, et al. Delayed pulmonary toxicity syndrome following high-dose chemotherapy and bone marrow transplantation for breast cancer. Am J Respir Crit Care Med 1998;157:565–73.

201. Shankar G, Cohen DA. Idiopathic pneumonia syndrome after bone marrow transplantation: the role of pre-transplant radiation conditioning and local cytokine dysregulation in promoting lung inflammation and fibrosis. Int J Exp Pathol 2001;82:101–13.

202. Shapiro CL, Yeap DY, Godleski J, et al. Drug-related pulmonary toxicity in non-Hodgkin's lymphoma. Comparative results with three different treatment regimens. Cancer 1991;68:699–705.

203. Moormeier JA, Williams SF, Kaminer LS, et al. High-dose trialkylator chemotherapy with autologous stem cell rescue in patients with refractory malignancies. J Natl Cancer Inst 1990;82:29–34.

204. White DA, Orenstein M, Godwin TA, Stover DE. Chemotherapy-associated pulmonary toxic reactions during treatment for breast cancer. Arch Intern Med 1984;144:953–6.

205. Bentzen SM, Skoczylas JZ, Overgaard M, Overgaard J. Radiotherapy-related lung fibrosis enhanced by tamoxifen. J Natl Cancer Inst 1996;88:918–22.

206. Segawa Y, Takigawa N, Kataoka M, et al. Risk factors for development of radiation pneumonitis following radiation therapy with or without chemotherapy for lung cancer. Int J Radiation Oncol Biol Phys 1997;39:91–8.

207. Alessandrino EP, Bernasconi P, Colombo A, et al. Pulmonary toxicity following carmustine-based preparative regimens and autologous peripheral blood progenitor cell transplantation in hematological malignancies. Bone Marrow Transplant 2000;25:309–13.

208. Briasoulis E, Froudarakis M, Milionis H, et al. Chemotherapy-induced noncardiogenic pulmonary edema related to gemcitabine plus docetaxel combination with granulocyte colony-stimulating factor support. Respiration 2000;67:680–3.

209. Chen CI, Abraham R, Tsang R, et al. Radiation-associated pneumonitis following autologous stem cell transplantation: predictive factors, disease characteristics and treatment outcomes. Bone Marrow Transplant 2001;27:177–82.

210. Todd NW, Peters WP, Ost AH, et al. Pulmonary drug toxicity in patients with primary breast cancer treated with high-dose combination chemotherapy and autologous bone marrow transplantation. Am Rev Respir Dis 1993;147:1264–70.

211. Pavlakis N, Bell DR, Millward MJ, Levi JA. Fatal pulmonary toxicity resulting from treatment with gemcitabine. Cancer 1997;80:286–91.

212. Takatsuka H, Takemoto Y, Mori A, et al. Common features in the onset of ARDS after administration of granulocyte colony-stimulating factor. Chest 2002;121:1716–20.

213. Malik SW, Myers JL, DeRemee RA, Specks U. Lung toxicity associated with cyclophosphamide use. Two distinct patterns. Am J Respir Crit Care Med 1996;154:1851–6.

214. van Barneveld PWC, Mulder NH, Sleijfer DT, et al. A reduction in pulmonary capillary blood volume in patients with disseminated testicular carcinoma. Eur J Cancer Clin Oncol 1985;21:675–9.

215. Dai MS, Lee SC, Ho CL, et al. Impact of open lung biopsy for undiagnosed pulmonary infiltrates in patients with hematological malignancies. Am J Hematol 2001;68:87–90.

216. Aymard JP, Gyger M, Lavallee R, et al. A case of pulmonary alveolar proteinosis complicating chronic myelogenous leukemia. A peculiar pathologic aspect of busulfan lung? Cancer 1984;53:954–6.

217. White DA, Wong PW, Downey R. The utility of open lung biopsy in patients with hematologic malignancies. Am J Respir Crit Care Med 2000;161:723–9.

218. Chang AYC, Kuebler JP, Pandya KJ, et al. Pulmonary toxicity induced by mitomycin C is highly responsive to glucocorticoids. Cancer 1986;57:2285–90.

219. Wong MK, Bjarnason GA, Hrushesky WJ, et al. Steroid-responsive interstitial lung disease in patients receiving 2′-deoxy-5-fluorouridine-infusion chemotherapy. Cancer 1995;75:2558–64.

220. Richter JE, Hastedt R, Dalton JF, et al. Pulmonary toxicity of bischloronitrosourea. Report of a case with transient response to corticosteroid therapy. Cancer 1979;43:1607–12.

221. Bossi G, Cerveri I, Volpini E, et al. Long-term pulmonary sequelae after treatment of childhood Hodgkin's disease. Ann Oncol 1997;8:19–24.

222. Jensen BV, Carlsen NLT, Groth S, Nissen NI. Late effects on pulmonary function of mantle-field irradiation, chemotherapy or combined modality therapy for Hodgkin's disease. Eur J Haematol 1990;44:165–71.

223. van Leeuwen FE, Klokman WJ, Stovall M, et al. Roles of radiotherapy and smoking in lung cancer following Hodgkin's disease. J Natl Cancer Inst 1995;87:1530–7.

224. Bell MR, Meredith DJ, Gill PG. Role of carbon monoxide diffusing capacity in the early detection of major bleomycin-induced pulmonary toxicity. Aust N Z J Med 1985;15:235–40.

225. Wolkowicz J, Sturgeon J, Rawji M, Chan CK. Bleomycin-induced pulmonary function abnormalities. Chest 1992;101:97–101.

226. Tryka AF, Godleski JJ, Fanta CH. Leukemic cell lysis pneumopathy. A complication of treated myeloblastic leukemia. Cancer 1982;50:2763–70.

227. Lester WA, Hull DR, Fegan CD, Morris TCM. Respiratory failure during induction chemotherapy for acute myelomonocytic leukaemia (FAB M4Eo) with Ara-C and all-trans retinoic acid. Br J Haematol 2000;109:847–50.

228. Morera J, Vidal R, Morell F, et al. Pulmonary fibrosis and amiodarone. BMJ 1983;ii:895.

229. Willcox PA, Maze SS, Sandler M, Benatar SR. Pulmonary fibrosis following long-term nitrofurantoin therapy. S Afr Med J 1982;61:714–7.

230. Jacobs S. The Hamman-Rich syndrome following treatment of lymphoma with chlorambucil. J La State Med Soc 1975;127:311–5.

231. Wharton SP, Rogers TK. Hamman-Rich syndrome 'primed' by radiation therapy. Respir Med 1999;93:136–40.

232. Kharabsheh S, Abendroth CS, Kozak M. Fatal pulmonary toxicity occurring within two weeks of initiation of amiodarone. Am J Cardiol 2002;89:896–8.

233. Frankel SR, Eardley A, Lauwers G, et al. The "retinoic acid syndrome" in acute promyelocytic leukemia. Ann Intern Med 1992;117:292–6.

234. DeMasi CJ. Allergic pulmonary infiltrates probably due to nitrofurantoin. Arch Intern Med 1967;120:631–4.

235. Ramanathan RK, Belani CP. Transient pulmonary infiltrates: a hypersensitivity reaction to Paclitaxel. Ann Intern Med 1996;124:278.

236. Heyll A, Aul C, Gogolin F, et al. Granulocyte colony-stimulating factor (G-CSF) treatment in a neutropenic leukemia patient with diffuse interstitial pulmonary infiltrates. Ann Hematol 1991;63:328–32.

237. Kopko PM, Marshall CS, MacKenzie MR, et al. Transfusion-related acute lung injury—report of a clinical look-back investigation. JAMA 2002;287:1968–71.

238. Maillard N, Foucher P, Caillot D, et al. Transient pulmonary infiltrates during treatment with anti-thymocyte globulin. Respiration 1999;66:279–82.

239. Villani F, Galimberti M, Rizzi M, Manzi R. Pulmonary toxicity of recombinant interleukin-2 plus lymphokine-activated killer cell therapy. Eur Respir J 1993;6:828–33.

240. Geller M, Dickie HA, Kass DA, et al. The histopathology of acute nitrofurantoin-associated pneumonitis. Ann Allergy 1976;37:275–9.

241. Sovijärvi ARA, Lemola M, Stenius B, Idänpään-Heikkilä J. Nitrofurantoin-induced acute, subacute and chronic pulmonary reactions. A report of 66 cases. Scand J Respir Dis 1977;58:41–50.

242. Taskinen E, Tukainen P, Sovijärvi ARA. Nitrofurantoin-induced alterations in pulmonary tissue. Acta Pathol Microbiol Scand A 1977;85:713–20.

243. Wiley JS, Firkin FC. Reduction of pulmonary toxicity by prednisolone prophylaxis during all-*trans* retinoic acid treatment of acute promyelocytic leukemia. Leukemia 1995;9:774–8.

244. Silber R, Clerkin EP. Pulmonary edema in acute heroin poisoning. Report of four cases. Am J Med 1959;27:187–92.

245. Sporer KA, Dorn E. Heroin-related noncardiogenic pulmonary edema—a case series. Chest 2001;120:1628–32.

246. Khouri NF, Saral R, Armstrong EM, et al. Pulmonary interstitial changes following bone marrow transplantation. Radiology 1979;133:587–92.

247. Bristedt P, Tylén U. Pulmonary edema following intravenous injection of nonionic low-osmolar contrast medium—appearance on HRCT. A case report. Acta Radiol 1998;39:81–3.

248. Heffner JE, Sahn SA. Salicylate-induced pulmonary edema: clinical features and prognosis. Ann Intern Med 1981;95:405–9.

249. Bernal C, Patarca R. Hydrochlorothiazide-induced pulmonary edema and associated immunologic changes. Ann Pharmacother 1999;33:172–4.

250. Rao SX, Ramaswany G, Levin M, McCravey JW. Fatal acute respiratory failure after vinblastine-mitomycine therapy in lung carcinoma. Arch Intern Med 1985;145:1905–7.

251. Maruchella A, Fiorenzano G, Merizzi A, et al. Diffuse alveolar damage in a patient treated with gemcitabine. Eur Respir J 1998;11:504–6

252. Zosmer A, Katz Z, Lancet M, et al. Adult respiratory distress syndrome complicating ovarian hyperstimulation syndrome. Fertil Steril 1987;47:524–6.

253. Abramov Y, Elchalal U, Schenker JG. Pulmonary manifestations of severe ovarian hyperstimulation syndrome: a multicenter study. Fertil Steril 1999;71:645–51.

254. Palmer SM, Robinson LJ, Wang AD, et al. Massive pulmonary edema and death after prostacyclin infusion in a patient with pulmonary veno-occlusive disease. Chest 1998;113:237–40.

255. Humbert M, Sanchez O, Fartoukh M, et al. Short-term and long-term epoprostenol (prostacyclin) therapy in pulmonary hypertension secondary to connective tissue diseases: results of a pilot study. Eur Respir J 1999;13:1351–6.

256. Drent M, Wessels S, Jacobs JA, Thijssen H. Association of diffuse alveolar haemorrhage with acquired vitamin K deficiency. Respiration 2000;67:697.

257. Kilraru PK, Schweiger MJ, Hozman HA, Weil TR. Diffuse alveolar hemorrhage after clopidogrel use. J Invas Cardiol 2001;13:535–7.

258. Gopalakrishnan D, Tioran T, Emanuel C, Clark V L. Diffuse pulmonary hemorrhage complicating thrombolytic therapy for acute myocardial infarction. Clin Cardiol 1997;20:298–300.

259. Masip J, Vecilla F, Paez J. Diffuse pulmonary hemorrhage after fibrinolytic therapy for acute myocardial infarction. Int J Cardiol 1998;63:95–7.

260. Kalra S, Bell MR, Rihal CS. Alveolar hemorrhage as a complication of treatment with abciximab. Chest 2001;120:126–31.

261. Nicolls MR, Terada LS, Tuder RM, et al. Diffuse alveolar hemorrhage with underlying pulmonary capillaritis in the retinoic acid syndrome. Am J Respir Crit Care Med 1998;158:1302–5.

262. Dhillon SS, Singh D, Doe N, et al. Diffuse alveolar hemorrhage and pulmonary capillaritis due to propylthiouracil. Chest 1999;116:1485–8.

263. Srivastava A, Gottlieb D, Bradstock KF. Diffuse alveolar haemorrhage associated with microangiopathy after allogeneic bone marrow transplantation. Bone Marrow Transplant 1995;15:863–7.

264. Polman AJ, van der Werf TS, Tiebosch ATMC, Zijlstra JG. Early-onset phenytoin toxicity mimicking a renopulmonary syndrome. Eur Respir J 1998;11:501–3.

265. Chang-Poon WY-H, Hwang WS, Wong A, et al. Pulmonary angiomatoid vascular changes in mitomycin C-associated hemolytic-uremic syndrome. Arch Pathol Lab Med 1985;109:877–8.

266. Creech RH, Tritchler D, Ettinger DS, et al. Phase II study of PALA, amsacrine, teniposide, and zinostatin in small cell lung carcinoma (EST 2579). Cancer Treat Rep 1984;68:1183–4.

267. Sleiman C, Raffy O, Roué C, Mal H. Fatal pulmonary hemorrhage during high-dose valproate monotherapy. Chest 2000;117:613.

268. Agusti C, Ramirez J, Picado C, et al. Diffuse alveolar hemorrhage in allogeneic bone marrow transplantation. Am J Respir Crit Care Med 1995;151:1006–10.

269. Lewis ID, Defor T, Weisdorf DJ. Increasing incidence of diffuse alveolar hemorrhage following allogeneic bone marrow transplantation: cryptic etiology and uncertain therapy. Bone Marrow Transplant 2000;26:539–43.

270. Raanani P, Segal E, Levi I, et al. Diffuse alveolar hemorrhage in acute promyelocytic leukemia patients treated with ATRA—a manifestation of the basic disease or the treatment. Leukemia Lymphoma 2000;37:605–10.

271. Capizzi SA, Kumar S, Huneke NE, et al. Peri-engraftment respiratory distress syndrome during autologous hematopoietic stem cell transplantation. Bone Marrow Transplant 2001;27:1299–303.

272. Lauque D, Courtin JP, Fournie B, et al. Syndrome pneumo-rénal induit par la d-pénicillamine: syndrome de Goodpasture ou polyartérite microscopique? Rev Med Interne 1990;11:168–71.

273. Brandstetter RD, Tamarin FM, Rangraj MS, et al. Moxalactam disodium-induced pulmonary hemorrhage. Chest 1984;86:644–5.

274. Brandt RR, Dunn WF, Ory SJ. Dextran 70 embolization. Another cause of pulmonary hemorrhage, coagulopathy, and rhabdomyolysis. Chest 1993;104:631–3.

275. Palmer RB, Alakija P, de Baca JE, Nolte KB. Fatal brodifacoum rodenticide poisoning: autopsy and toxicologic findings. J Forensic Sci 1999;44:851–5.

276. Gibson PC, Quinlan JT. Periarteritis nodosa in thiourea therapy. Lancet 1945;ii:108–10.

277. Tompson RT, Zeek PM. Acute necrotizing angiitis due to hypersensitivity following sulfonamide therapy. Ohio State Med J 1945;41:824–5.

278. Kjellbo H, Stakeberg H. Possibly thiazide-induced renal necrotising vasculitis. Lancet 1965;i:1034–5.

279. Haas P. Über einen perakut verlaufenden Fall von Periarteritis nododa nach Diphentlhydantoin. Wien Klin Wochenschr 1967;79:56–8.

280. Jarzobski J, Ferry J, Wombolt D, et al. Vasculitis with allopurinol therapy. Am Heart J 1970;79:116–21.

281. Houston D, Crouch M, Brick J, DiBartolomeo A. Apparent vaculitis associated with PTU use. Arthritis Rheum 1979;22:925–8.

282. Michael JR, Rudin ML. Acute pulmonary disease caused by phenytoin. Ann Intern Med 1981;95:452–4.

283. Magee F, Wright JL, Chan N, et al. Two unusual pathological reactions to nitrofurantoin: case reports. Histopathology 1986;10:701–6.

284. Ohtsuka M, Yamashita Y, Doi M, Hasegawa S. Propylthiouracil-induced alveolar haemorrhage associated with antineutrophil cytoplasmic antibody. Eur Respir J 1997;10:1405–7.

285. Choi HK, Merkel PA, Niles JL. ANCA-positive vasculitis associated with allopurinol therapy. Clin Exp Rheumatol 1998;16:743–4.

286. Vanoli M, Gambini D, Scorza R. A case of Churg-Strauss vasculitis after hepatitis B vaccination. Ann Rheum Dis 1998;57:256–7.

287. Gunton JE, Stiel J, Caterson RJ, McElduff A. Anti-thyroid drugs and antineutrophil cytoplasmic antibody positive vasculitis. A case report and review of the literature. J Clin Endocrinol Metab 1999;84:13–6.

288. Yamada K, Sugimoto K, Matsumoto T, Narumi K, Oshimi K. All-*trans* retinoic acid-induced vasculitis and hemonecrosis of the ileum in a patient with acute promyelocytic leukemia. Leukemia 1999;13:647–8.

289. Schneider F, Meziani F, Chartier C, Jaeger A. Fatal allergic vasculitis associated with celecoxib. Lancet 2002;359:852–3.

290. Morita S, Ueda Y, Eguchi K. Anti-thyroid drug-induced ANCA-associated vasculitis: a case report and review of the literature. Endocrine J 2000;47:467–70.

291. Choi HK, Merkel PA, Cohen-Tervaert JW, et al. Alternating antineutrophil cytoplasmic antibody specificity. Drug-induced vasculitis in a patient with Wegener's granulomatosis. Arthritis Rheum 1999;42:384–8.

292. Noh JY, Asari T, Hamada N, et al. Frequency of appearance of myeloperoxidase-antineutrophil cytoplasmic antibody (MPO-ANCA) in Graves' disease patients treated with propylthiouracil and the relationship between MPO-ANCA and clinical manifestations. Clin Endocrinol 2001;54:651–4.

293. Wechsler ME, Garpestad E, Flier SR, et al. Pulmonary infiltrates, eosinophilia, and cardiomyopathy following corticosteroid withdrawal in patients with asthma receiving zafirlukast. JAMA 1998;279:455–7.

294. Pedvis S, Anastakis D, Inman R. Churg-Strauss syndrome associated with zafirlukast. J Rheumatol 1999;26:1630.

295. Stirling RG, Chung KF. Leukotriene antagonists and Churg-Strauss syndrome: the smoking gun. Thorax 1999;54:865–6.

296. Solans R, Bosch JA, Selva A, et al. Montelukast and Churg-Strauss syndrome. Thorax 2002;57:183–5.

297. Schmitz Schumann M, Palca A, Simon U, Blaser K. Aspirin-induced asthma and Churg-Strauss-syndrome. Eur J Clin Invest 1998;28 Suppl 1:A49.

298. Rose AG. Pulmonary veno-occlusive disease due to bleomycin therapy for lymphoma. S Afr Med J 1983;64:636–8.

299. Or R, Nagler A, Elad S, et al. Noncardiogenic pulmonary congestion following bone marrow transplantation. Respiration 1997;64:170–2.

300. Vansteenkiste JF, Bomans P, Verbeken EK, et al. Fatal pulmonary veno-occlusive disease possibly related to gemcitabine. Lung Cancer 2001;31:83–5.

301. Capewell SJ, Wright AJ, Ellis DA. Pulmonary veno-occlusive disease in association with Hodgkin's disease. Thorax 1984;39:554–6.

302. Pelz DM, Lownie SP, Fox AJ, Hutton LC. Symptomatic pulmonary complications from liquid acrylate embolization of brain arteriovenous malformations. Am J Neuroradiol 1995;16:19–26.

303. Lee DW, White RI, Egglin TK, et al. Embolotherapy of large pulmonary arteriovenous malformations: Long-term results. Ann Thorac Surg 1997;64:930–9.

304. Palejwala AA, Smart HL, Hughes M. Multiple pulmonary

glue emboli following gastric variceal obliteration. Endoscopy 2000;32:S1–2.

305. Padovani B, Kasriel O, Brunner P, Peretti-Viton P. Pulmonary embolism caused by acrylic cement: a rare complication of percutaneous vertebroplasty. Am J Neuroradiol 1999;20: 375–7.

306. Fourme T, Vieillard-Baron A, Loubières Y, et al. Early fat embolism after liposuction. Anesthesiology 1998;89:782–4.

307. Bairaktari A, Raitsiou B, Kokolaki M, et al. Respiratory failure after pneumonectomy in a patient with unknown hyperlipidemia. Respiratory failure after propofol infusion. Anesth Anal 2001;93:292–3.

308. Woodard JP, Gulbahce E, Shreve M, et al. Pulmonary cytolytic thrombi: a newly recognized complication of stem cell transplantation. Bone Marrow Transplant 2000;25:293–300.

309. Alarcon-Segovia D, Fishbein E, Reyes PA, et al. Antinuclear antibodies in patients on anticonvulsant therapy. Clin Exp Immunol 1972;12:39–47.

310. Skaer TL. Medication-induced systemic lupus erythematosus. Clin Ther 1992;14:496–506.

311. Takeda A, Ikegame K, Kimura Y, et al. Pleural effusion during interferon treatment for chronic hepatitis C. Hepatogastroenterology 2000;47:1431–5.

312. Verma SP, Yunis N, Lekos A, Crausman RS. Carbamazepine-induced systemic lupus erythematosus presenting as cardiac tamponade. Chest 2000;117:597–8.

313. Sheikhzadeh A, Schafer U, Schnabel A. Drug-induced lupus erythematosus by amiodarone. Arch Intern Med 2002;162: 834–6.

314. Christodoulou CS, Emmanuel P, Ray RA, et al. Respiratory distress due to minocycline-induced pulmonary lupus. Chest 1999;115:1471–3.

315. Sridhar MK, Abdulla A. Fatal lupus-like syndrome and ARDS induced by fluvastatin. Lancet 1998;352:114.

316. Roche-Bayard P, Rossi R, Mann JM, et al. Left pulmonary artery thrombosis in chlorpromazine-induced lupus. Chest 1990;98:1545.

317. Pelayo M, Vargas V, Gonzales A, et al. Drug-induced lupus-like reaction and captopril. Ann Pharmacother 1993;27:1541–2.

318. Knowles SR, Shapiro L, Shear NH. Serious adverse reactions induced by minocycline: report of 13 patients and review of the literature. Arch Dermatol 1996;132:934–9.

319. Herlin T, Birkebaek NH, Wolthers OD, et al. Anti-neutrophil cytoplasmic autoantibody (ANCA) profiles in propylthiouracil-induced lupus-like manifestations in monozygotic triplets with hyperthyroidism. Scand J Rheumatol 2002; 31:46–9.

320. Tazelaar HD, Myers JL, Strickler JG, et al. Tryptophan-induced lung disease: an immunophenotypic, immunofluorescent, and electron microscopic study. Mod Pathol 1993;6:56–60.

321. Hertzman PA, Clauw DJ, Kaufman LD, et al. The eosinophilia-myalgia syndrome: status of 205 patients and results of treatment 2 years after onset. Arch Intern Med 1995;122:851–5.

322. Pincus T. Eosinophilia-myalgia syndrome: patient status 2–4 years after onset. J Rheumatol 1996;23 Suppl 46:19–24.

323. Buss WC, Stepanek J, Bankhurst AD, et al. EBT, a tryptophan contaminant associated with eosinophilia myalgia syndrome, is incorporated into proteins during translation as an amino acid analog. Autoimmunity 1996;25:33–45.

324. Hill C, Zeitz C, Kirkham B. Dermatomyositis with lung involvement in a patient treated with simvastatin. Aust N Z J Med 1995;25:745–6.

325. Thickett DR, Millar AB. Drug-induced antisynthetase syndrome. Postgrad Med J 1997;73:165–6.

326. Liebhaber MI, Wright RS, Gelberg HJ, et al. Polymyalgia, hypersensitivity pneumonitis and other reactions in patients receiving HMG-CoA reductase inhibitors. Chest 1999;115:886–9.

327. Rotmensch HH, Liron M, Tupilsky M, Laniado S. Possible association of pneumonitis with amiodarone therapy. Am Heart J 1980;100:412–3.

328. Weinberg BA, Miles WM, Klein LS, et al. Five-year follow-up of 589 patients treated with amiodarone. Am Heart J 1993;125:109–20.

329. Martin WJ, Howard DM. Amiodarone-induced lung toxicity. In vitro evidence for the direct toxicity of the drug. Am J Pathol 1985;120:344–50.

330. Darmanata JI, Van Zandwijk N, Düren DR, et al. Amiodarone pneumonitis: three further cases with a review of published reports. Thorax 1984;39:57–64.

331. Camus P, Coudert B, d'Athis P, et al. Pharmacokinetics of amiodarone in the isolated rat lung. J Pharmacol Exp Ther 1990;254:336–43.

332. Adams PC, Holt DW, Storey GC, et al. Amiodarone and its desethyl metabolite: tissue distribution and morphologic changes during long-term therapy. Circulation 1985;72: 1064–75.

333. Pollak PT, Sharma AD, Carruthers SG. Relation of amiodarone hepatic and pulmonary toxicity to serum drug concentrations and superoxide dismutase activity. Am J Cardiol 1990;65:1185–91.

334. Bedrossian CW, Warren CJ, Ohar J, Bhan R. Amiodarone pulmonary toxicity: cytopathology, ultrastructure, and immunocytochemistry. Ann Diagn Pathol 1997;1:47–56.

335. Myers JL, Kennedy JI, Plumb VJ. Amiodarone lung: pathologic findings in clinically toxic patients. Hum Pathol 1987;18:349–54.

336. Esinger W, Schleiffer T, Leinberger H, et al. Steroidrefraktäre Lungenfibrose durch Amiodaron. Klinik und Morphologie nach einem amiodaronfreien Intervall von 3 Monaten. Dtsch Med Wochenschr 1988;113:1638–41.

337. Sobol SM, Rakita L. Pneumonitis and pulmonary fibrosis associated with amiodarone treatment: a possible complication of a new antiarrhythmic drug. Circulation 1982;65:819–24.

338. Marchlinski FE, Gansler TS, Waxman HL, Josephson ME. Amiodarone pulmonary toxicity. Ann Intern Med 1982;97:839–45.

339. Parra O, Ruiz J, Ojanguren I, et al. Amiodarone toxicity: recurrence of interstitial pneumonitis after withdrawal of the drug. Eur Respir J 1989;2:905–7.

340. Hopper KD, Potock PS. Hepatic and pulmonary accumulation of amiodarone. AJR Am J Roentgenol 1994;162:1149–450.

341. Vorperian VR, Havighurst TC, Miller S, January CT. Adverse effects of low dose amiodarone: a meta-analysis. J Am Coll Cardiol 1997;30:791–8.

342. Dean PJ, Groshart KD, Porterfield JG, et al. Amiodarone-associated pulmonary toxicity. A clinical and pathologic study of eleven cases. Am J Clin Pathol 1987;87:7–13.

343. Cazzadori A, Braggio P, Barbieri E, Ganassini A. Amiodarone-induced pulmonary toxicity. Respiration 1986;49:157–60.

344. Olson LK, Forrest JV, Friedman PJ, et al. Pneumonitis after amiodarone therapy. Radiology 1983;150:327–30.

345. Coudert B, Bailly F, André F, et al. Amiodarone pneumonitis: bronchoalveolar lavage findings in 15 patients and review of the literature. Chest 1992;102:1005–12.

346. Dunn M, Glassroth J. Pulmonary complications of amiodarone toxicity. Prog Cardiovasc Dis 1988;31:447–53.

347. Bowers PN, Fields J, Schwartz D, et al. Amiodarone induced pulmonary fibrosis in infancy. PACE 1998;21:1665–7.

348. Magro SA, Lawrence EC, Wheeler SH, et al. Amiodarone pulmonary toxicity: prospective evaluation of serial pulmonary function tests. J Am Coll Cardiol 1988;12:781–8.

349. Wilhelm JM, Thannberger P, Derragui A, et al. Pneumopathie interstitielle survenue 2 mois après arrêt d'un traitement par amiodarone. Presse Med 1999;28:2040.

350. Kay GN, Epstein AE, Kirklin JK, et al. Fatal postoperative amiodarone pulmonary toxicity. Am J Cardiol 1988;62:490–2.

351. Torres Romero J, Asin Guillén JM, Peral Martinez JI, et al. Fibrosis pulmonar inducida por amiodarona. Rev Esp Cardiol 1983;37:142–4.

352. Gefter WB, Epstein DM, Pietra GG, Miller WT. Lung disease caused by amiodarone, a new antiarrhythmic agent. Radiology 1983;147:339–44.

353. Clarke B, Ward DE, Honey M. Pneumonitis with pleural and pericardial effusion and neuropathy during amiodarone therapy. Int J Cardiol 1985;8:81–8.

354. Standertskjöld-Nordenstam CG, Wandtke JC, Hood WJ Jr, et al. Amiodarone pulmonary toxicity. Chest radiography and CT in asymptomatic patients. Chest 1985;88:143–5.

355. Morera J, Vidal R, Morell F, et al. Amiodarone and pulmonary fibrosis. Eur J Clin Pharmacol 1983;24:591–3.

356. Aranda EA, Basanez RA, Jimenez YL. Bronchiolitis obliterans organising pneumonia secondary to amiodarone treatment. Neth J Med 1998;53:109–12.

357. van Mieghem W, Coolen L, Malysse I, et al. Amiodarone and the development of ARDS after lung surgery. Chest 1994;105:1642–5.

358. Donaldson L, Grant IS, Naysmith MR, Thomas JS. Acute amiodarone-induced lung toxicity. Intensive Care Med 1998;24:626–30.

359. Ashrafian H, Davey P. Is amiodarone an underrecognized cause of acute respiratory failure in the ICU? Chest 2001; 120:275–82.

360. Liverani E, Armuzzi A, Mormile F, et al. Amiodarone-induced adult respiratory distress syndrome after nonthoracotomy subcutaneous defibrillator implantation. J Intern Med 2001;249:565–6.

361. Greenspon AJ, Kidwell GA, Hurley W, Mannion J. Amiodarone-related postoperative adult respiratory distress syndrome. Circulation 1991;84 Suppl III:407–15.

362. Herndon JC, Cook AO, Ramsay MAE, et al. Postoperative unilateral pulmonary edema: possible amiodarone pulmonary toxicity. Anesthesiology 1992;76:308–12.

363. Ren H, Kuhlman JE, Hruban RH, et al. CT-pathology correlation of amiodarone lung. J Comput Assist Tomogr 1990;14:760–5.

364. van Rooij WJ, van der Meer SC, van Royen EA, et al. Pulmonary gallium-67 uptake in amiodarone pneumonitis. J Nucl Med 1984;25:211–3.

365. Ravishankar R, Samuels LE, Kaufman MS, et al. Amiodarone-associated hemoptysis. Am J Med Sci 1998;316:390–2.

366. Drent M, Cobben NAM, Dieijen-Visser MP, et al. Serum lactate dehydrogenase activity: indicator of the development of pneumonitis induced by amiodarone. Eur Heart J 1998;19:969–70.

367. Mettauer B, Lampert E, Charloux A, et al. Lung membrane diffusing capacity, heart failure, and heart transplantation. Am J Cardiol 1999;83:62–7.

368. Ohar JA, Jackson F, Redd RM, et al. Usefulness of serial pulmonary function testing as an indicator of amiodarone toxicity. Am J Cardiol 1989;64:1322–6.

369. Adams PC, Gibson GJ, Morley AR, et al. Amiodarone pulmonary toxicity: clinical and subclinical features. QJM 1986;59:449–71.

370. Xaubet A, Roca J, Rodriguez-Roisin R, et al. Bronchoalveolar lavage cellular analysis and gallium lung scan in the assessment of patients with amiodarone-induced pneumonitis. Respiration 1987;52:272–80.

371. Lengyel C, Boros I, Varkonyi T, et al. Amiodarone-induced pulmonary fibrosis (see comments). Orv Hetil 1996;137: 1759–62.

372. Bates N, Dawson J. Suspected amiodarone-hypersensitivity pneumonitis. Can J Hosp Pharm 1998;51:117–21.

373. Butland RJA, Milliard FJC. Fibrosing alveolitis associated with amiodarone. Eur J Respir Dis 1984;65:616–9.

374. Zaher C, Hamer A, Peter T, Mandel W. Low-dose steroid therapy for prophylaxis of amiodarone-induced pulmonary infiltrates. N Engl J Med 1983;308:779.

375. Chendrasekhar A, Barke RA, Druck P. Recurrent amiodarone pulmonary toxicity. South Med J 1996;89:85–6.

376. Biour M, Hugues FC, Hamel JD, Cheymol G. Les effets indésirables pulmonaires de l'amiodarone. Analyse de 162 observations. Therapie 1984;40:343–8.

377. van Zandwijk N, Darmanata JI, Düren DR, et al. Amiodarone pneumonitis. Eur Respir J 1983;64:313–7.

378. Veltri EP, Reid PR. Amiodarone pulmonary toxicity: early changes in pulmonary function tests during amiodarone rechallenge. J Am Coll Cardiol 1985;6:802–5.

379. Davis BA, Cervi P, Amin Z, et al. Retinoic acid syndrome: pulmonary computed tomography (CT) findings. Leuk Lymphoma 1996;23:113–7.

380. Maloisel F, Petit T, Kessler R, Oberling F. Cytologic examination of broncho-alveolar fluid during the retinoic acid syndrome. Eur J Haematol 1996;56:319–20.

381. Lamm DL, van der Meijden APM, Morales A, et al. Incidence and treatment of complications of bacillus Calmette-Guérin intravesical therapy in superficial bladder cancer. J Urol 1992;147:596–600.

382. Kesten S, Title L, Mullen B, Grossman R. Pulmonary disease following intravesical BCG treatment. Thorax 1990;45: 709–10.

383. Israel-Biet D, Venet A, Sandron D, et al. Pulmonary complications of bacille Calmette-Guérin immunotherapy. Am Rev Respir Dis 1987;135:763–5.

384. de Diego A, Rogado MC, Prieto M, et al. Disseminated pulmonary granulomas after intravesical bacillus Calmette-Guérin immunotherapy. Respiration 1997;64:304–6.

385. Sicard D, Steg A, Leleu C, et al. "BCGite," une complication systémique de la thérapeutique par le BCG intravésical pour tumeur de vessie. Ann Med Interne 1987;138:555–6.

386. Tan L, Testa G, Yung T. Diffuse alveolar damage in BCGosis: a rare complication of intravesical bacillus Calmette-Guérin therapy for transitional cell carcinoma. Pathology 1999;31:55–6.

387. Kritjansson M, Green P, Manning HL, et al. Molecular confirmation of bacillus Calmette-Guérin as the cause of pulmonary infection following urinary tract instillation. Clin Infect Dis 1993;17:228–30.

388. McParland C, Cotton DJ, Gowda KS, et al. Miliary *Mycobacterium bovis* induced by intravesical bacille Calmette-Guérin immunotherapy. Am Rev Respir Dis 1992;146:1330–3.

389. Kaplan RL. Pulmonary effects of carmustine (bischloroethylnitrosourea, BCNU). Ann Intern Med 1979;91:131.

390. Selker RG, Jacobs SA, Moore PB, et al. 1,3-Bis(2-chloroethyl)-1-nitrosourea (BCNU)-induced pulmonary fibrosis. Neurosurgery 1980;7:560–5.

391. Phillips GL, Fay JW, Herzig GP, et al. Intensive 1,3-bis(2-chloroethyl)-1-nitrosourea (BCNU), NSC # 4366650 and cryopreserved autologous marrow transplantation for refractory cancer. Cancer 1983;52:1792–802.

392. Durant JR, Norgard MJ, Murad TM, et al. Pulmonary toxicity associated with bischloroethylnitrosourea (BCNU). Ann Intern Med 1979;90:191–4.

393. Litam JP, Dail DH, Spitzer G, et al. Early pulmonary toxicity after administration of high-dose BCNU. Cancer Treat Rep 1981;65:39–43.

394. Kalaycioglu M, Kavuru M, Tuason L, Bolwell B. Empiric prednisone therapy for pulmonary toxic reaction after high-dose chemotherapy containing carmustine. Chest 1995;107:482–7.

395. Crittenden D, Tranum BL, Haut A. Pulmonary fibrosis after prolonged therapy with 1,3-bis (2-chloroethyl)-1-nitrosourea. Chest 1977;72:372–3.

396. Ryan BR, Walters TR. Pulmonary fibrosis: a complication of 1 3-bis(2-chloroethyl)-1-nitrosourea (BCNU) therapy. Cancer 1981;48:909–11.

397. Mitsudo SM, Greenwald ES, Banerji B, Koss LG. BCNU (1 3-bis-(2-chloroethyl)-1-nitrosourea) lung. Cancer 1984; 54:751–5.

398. Schmitz N, Diehl V. Carmustine and the lungs. Lancet 1997;349:1712–3.

399. Tucci E, Verdiani P, Di Carlo S, Sforza V. Lomustine (CCNU)-induced pulmonary fibrosis. Tumori 1986;72:95–8.

400. Hundley RF, Lukens JN. Nitrosourea-associated pulmonary fibrosis. Cancer Treat Rep 1979;63:2128–30.

401. Bellot PA, Valdiserri RO. Multiple pulmonary lesions in a patient treated with BCNU (1,3-bis(2-chloroethyl)-1-nitrosourea) for glioblastoma multiforme. Cancer 1979;43:46–50.

402. Ishizuka M, Takayama H, Takeuchi T, Umezawa H. Activity and toxicity of bleomycin. J Antibiot (Tokyo) 1967; 20:15–24.

403. Zucker PK, Khouri NF, Rosenshein NB. Bleomycin-induced pulmonary nodules: a variant of bleomycin pulmonary toxicity. Gynecol Oncol 1987;28:284–91.

404. Trump DL, Bartel E, Pozniak M. Nodular pneumonitis after chemotherapy for germ cell tumors. Ann Intern Med 1988;109:431–2.

405. Iacovino JR, Leitner J, Abbas AK, et al. Fatal pulmonary reaction from low doses of bleomycin: an idiosyncratic tissue response. JAMA 1976;235:1253–5.

406. Crooke ST, Einhorn LH, Comis RL, et al. The effects of prior exposure to bleomycin on the incidence of pulmonary toxicities in a group of patients with disseminated testicular carcinomas. Med Pediatr Oncol 1978;5:93–8.

407. Einhorn L, Krause M, Hornbarck N, Furnas B. Enhanced pulmonary toxicity with bleomycin and radiotherapy in oat cell lung cancer. Cancer 1976;37:2414–6.

408. Krous HF, Hamlin WB. Pulmonary toxicity due to bleomycin. Report of a case. Arch Pathol 1973;95:407–10.

409. Toledo CH, Ross WE, Hood CI, Block ER. Potentiation of bleomycin toxicity by oxygen. Cancer Treat Rep 1982;66: 359–62.

410. White DA, Stover DE. Severe bleomycin-induced pneumonitis. Clinical features and response to corticosteroids. Chest 1984;86:723–8.

411. Ganick DJ, Peters ME, Hafez G-R. Acute bleomycin toxicity. Am J Pediatr Hematol Oncol 1980;2:249–52.

412. White DA, Schwartzberg LS, Kris MG, Bosl GJ. Acute chest pain syndrome during bleomycin infusions. Cancer 1987;59:1582–5.

413. Lien HH, Brodahl U, Telhaug R, et al. Pulmonary changes at computed tomography in patients with testicular carcinoma treated with cis-platinum, vinblastine and bleomycin. Acta Radiol Diagn 1985;26:507–10.

414. Bellamy EA, Nicholas D, Husband JE. Quantitative assessment of lung damage due to bleomycin using computed tomography. Br J Radiol 1987;60:1205–9.

415. Mills P, Husband J. Computed tomography of pulmonary bleomycin toxicity. Semin Ultrasound CT MR 1990;11: 417–22.

416. Rimmer MJ, Dixon AK, Flower CDR, Sikora K. Bleomycin lung: computed tomographic observations. Br J Radiol 1985;58:1041–5.

417. Lewis BM, Izbicki R. Routine pulmonary function tests during bleomycin therapy. Tests may be ineffective and potentially misleading. JAMA 1980;243:347–51.

418. Maher J, Daly PA. Severe bleomycin lung toxicity: reversal with high dose corticosteroids. Thorax 1993;48:92–4.

419. White DA, Kris MG, Stover DE. Bronchoalveolar lavage cell populations in bleomycin lung toxicity. Thorax 1987; 42:551–2.

420. O'Neill TJ, Kardinal CG, Tierney LM. Reversible interstitial pneumonitis associated with low-dose bleomycin. Chest 1975;68:265–7.

421. Lei KIK, Leung WT, Johnson PJ. Serious pulmonary complications in patients receiving recombinant granulocyte colony-stimulating factor during BACOP chemotherapy for agressive non-Hodgkin's lymphoma. Br J Cancer 1994;70:1009–13.

422. Gertz MA, Lacy MQ, Bjornsson J, Litzow MR. Fatal pulmonary toxicity related to the administration of granulocyte colony-stimulating factor in amyloidosis: a report and review of growth factor-induced pulmonary toxicity. J Hematother Stem Cell Res 2000;9:635–43.

423. Philippe B, Couderc LJ, Balloul-Delclaux E, et al. Pulmonary toxicity of chemotherapy and GM-CSF. Respir Med 1994;88:715.

424. Yokose N, Ogata K, Tamura H, et al. Pulmonary toxicity after granulocyte colony stimulating factor-combined chemotherapy for non-Hodgkin's lymphoma. Br J Cancer 1998;77:2286–90.

425. Woolley J, Collett J, Goldstein D. Diffuse alveolar damage following a single administration of a cyclophosphamide containing chemotherapy regimen. Aust N Z J Med 1997; 27:605–6.

426. Tucker AS, Newman AJ, Alvorado C. Pulmonary, pleural and thoracic changes complicating chemotherapy. Radiology 1977;125:805–9.

427. Winterbauer RH, Wilske KR, Wheelis RF. Diffuse pulmonary injury associated with gold treatment. N Engl J Med 1976;294:919–21.

428. McFadden RG, Fraher LJ, Thompson JM. Gold-naproxen pneumonitis. A toxic drug interaction? Chest 1989;96:216–8.

429. Kamisako T, Adachi Y, Chihara J, Yamamoto T. Interstitial pneumonitis and interferon-alfa. BMJ 1993;306:896.

430. Patel M, Ezzat W, Pauw KL, Lowsky R. Bronchiolitis obliterans organizing pneumonia in a patient with chronic myelogenous leukemia developing after initiation of interferon and cytosine arabinoside. Eur J Haematol 2001;67:318–21.

431. Hoffmann RM, Jung MC, Motz R, et al. Sarcoidosis associated with interferon-alpha therapy for chronic hepatitis C. J Hepatol 1998;28:1058–63.

432. Cottin V, Tébib J, Massonnet B, et al. Pulmonary function in patients receiving long-term low-dose methotrexate. Chest 1996;109:933–8.

433. Clarysse AM, Cathey WJ, Cartwright GE, Wintrobe MM. Pulmonary disease complicating intermittent therapy with methotrexate. JAMA 1969;209:1861–4.

434. Kremer JM, Joong KL. The safety and efficacy of the use of methotrexate in long term therapy for rheumatoid arthritis. Arthritis Rheum 1986;29:822–31.

435. Pourel J, Guillemin F, Fener P, et al. Delayed methotrexate pneumonitis in rheumatoid arthritis. J Rheumatol 1991; 18:303–4.

436. Dai MS, Ho CL, Chen YC, et al. Acute respiratory distress syndrome following intrathecal methotrexate administration: a case report and review of literature. Ann Hematol 2000;79:696–9.

437. Imokawa S, Sato A, Hayakawa H, et al. Possible involvement of an environmental agent in the development of acute eosinophilic pneumonia. Ann Allergy Asthma Immunol 1996;76:419–22.

438. Everts CS, Wescott JL, Bragg DG. Methotrexate therapy and pulmonary disease. Radiology 1973;107:539–43.

439. Akoun GM, Mayaud CM, Touboul JL, et al. Use of bronchoalveolar lavage in the evaluation of methotrexate lung disease. Thorax 1987;42:652–5.

440. Bedrossian CWM, Miller WC, Luna MA. Methotrexate-induced diffuse interstitial pulmonary fibrosis. South Med J 1979;72:313–8.

441. Massin F, Coudert B, Marot JP, et al. La pneumopathie du méthotrexate. Rev Mal Respir 1990;7:5–15.

442. Newman ED, Harrington TM. Fatal methotrexate pneumonitis in rheumatoid arthritis. Arthritis Rheum 1988;31:1585–6.

443. Cantrell JE, Phillips TM, Schein PS. Carcinoma-associated hemolytic-uremic syndrome: a complication of mitomycin C chemotherapy. J Clin Oncol 1985;3:723–34.

444. Linette DC, McGee KH, McFarland JA. Mitomycin-induced pulmonary toxicity: case report and review of the literature. Ann Pharmacother 1992;26:481–4.

445. Rabadi SJ, Khandekar JD, Miller HJ. Mitomycin-induced hemolytic uremic syndrome: case presentation and review of the literature. Cancer Treat Rep 1982;66:1244–7.

446. Lyman NW, Michaelson R, Viscuso RL, et al. Mitomycin-induced hemolytic-uremic syndrome. Successful treatment with corticosteroids and intense plasme exchange. Arch Intern Med 1983;143:1617–8.

447. Lesesne JB, Rotschild N, Erickson B, et al. Cancer-associated hemolytic-uremic syndrome: analysis of 85 cases from a National Registry. J Clin Oncol 1989;7:781–9.

448. Torra R, Poch E, Torras A, et al. Pulmonary hemorrhage as a clinical manifestation of hemolytic-uremic syndrome associated with mitomycin C therapy. Chemotherapy 1993;39:453–6.

449. van der Heijden M, Ackland SP, Deveridge S. Haemolytic uraemic syndrome associated with bleomycin, epirubicin and cisplatin chemotherapy — a case report and review of the literature. Acta Oncol 1998;37:107–9.

450. Deodhar SD, Bhagwat AG. Desquamative interstitial pneumonia-like syndrome in rabbits. Produced experimentally by Freund's adjuvant. Arch Pathol 1967;84:54–8.

451. Frankenfeld RH. Pulmonary edema caused by nitrofurantoin. Ann Intern Med 1967;66:1055.

452. Morris AJ. Pulmonary and eosinophilic reaction to nitrofurantoin. Del Med J 1967;39:299–301.

453. Strauss WG, Griffin LM. Nitrofurantoin pneumonia. JAMA 1967;199:175–6.

454. Sheehan RE, Wells AU, Milne DG, Hansell DM. Nitrofurantoin-induced lung disease: two cases demonstrating resolution of apparently irreversible CT abnormalities. J Comput Assist Tomogr 2000;24:259–61.

455. Bone RC, Wolfe J, Sobonya RE, et al. Desquamative interstitial pneumonia following long-term nitrofurantoin therapy. Am J Med 1976;60:697–701.

456. Cameron C, Bayliff CD, Patterson NAM. Nitrofurantoin-associated acute pulmonary toxicity. Can J Hosp Pharm 1999;52:83–6.

457. Hailey FJ, Glascock HWJ, Hewitt WF. Pleuropneumonic reactions to nitrofurantoin. N Engl J Med 1969;281:1087–90.

458. Akoun GM, Milleron B, El Gharbi N, Malka M. Le lavage bronchoalvéolaire dans la pneumopathie de la nitrofuran-toïne. Sem Hop Paris 1985;61:2443–6.

459. Cameron RJ, Kolbe J, Wilsher ML, Lambie N. Bronchiolitis obliterans organising pneumonia associated with the use of nitrofurantoin. Thorax 2000;55:249–351.

460. Averbuch SD, Yungbluth P. Fatal pulmonary hemorrhage due to nitrofurantoin. Arch Intern Med 1980;140:271–3.

461. Allen RW, Holt AH, Brown MG. Acute pulmonary sensitivity to nitrofurantoin. AJR Am J Roentgenol 1968;104:784–6.

462. Bayliff CD, Sobiera CJ, Paterson NAM. Nitrofurantoin induced acute pneumonitis. A review of three cases. Can J Hosp Pharm 1997;50:247.

463. Mulberg AE, Bell LM. Fatal cholestatic hepatitis and multi-system failure associated with nitrofurantoin. J Pediatr Gastroenterol Nutr 1993;17:307–9.

464. Meyer MM, Meyer RJ. Nitrofurantoin-induced pulmonary hemorrhage in a renal transplant recipient receiving immunosuppressive therapy: case report and review of the literature. J Urol 1994;152:938–40.

465. Formgren H, Lindgren S, Ahlstedt S, et al. Histopathological findings and immune response to nitrofurantoin in drug intolerance pneumonitis. Br J Dis Chest 1979;73:420.

466. Israel HL, Diamond P. Recurrent pulmonary infiltration and pleural effusion due to nitrofurantoin sensitivity. N Engl J Med 1962;266:1024–6.

467. Kursch ED, Mostyn EM, Persky L, et al. Nitrofurantoin pulmonary complications. J Urol 1975;113:392–5.

468. Warren S, Spencer J. Radiation reactions in the lung. AJR Am J Roentgenol 1940;43:682–701.

469. Jochelson MS, Tarbell NJ, Weinstein HJ. Unusual thoracic radiographic findings in children treated for Hodgkin's disease. J Clin Oncol 1986;4:874–82.

470. Gibson PG, Bryant DH, Morgan GW, et al. Radiation-induced pneumonitis: a hypersensitivity pneumonitis? Ann Intern Med 1988;109:288–91.

471. Whitcomb ME, Schwarz MI. Pleural effusion complicating intensive mediastinal radiation therapy. Am Rev Respir Dis 1971;103:100–7.

472. Greenwood RD, Rosenthal A, Cassady R, et al. Constrictive pericarditis in childhood due to mediastinal irradiation. Circulation 1974;50:1033–9.

473. Schneider JS, Edwards JE. Irradiation-induced pericarditis. Chest 1979;75:560–4.

474. Applefeld MM, Wiernik PH. Cardiac disease after radiation therapy for Hodgkin's disease: analysis of 48 patients. Am J Cardiol 1983;51:1679–81.

475. Rowinsky EK, Abeloff MD, Wharam MD. Spontaneous pneumothorax following thoracic radiation. Chest 1985;88:703–8.

476. Morgan GW, Freeman AP, McLean RG, et al. Late cardiac, thyroid, and pulmonary sequelae of mantle radiotherapy for Hodgkin's disease. Int J Radiation Oncol Biol Phys 1985;11:1925–31.

477. Rodriguez-Garcia JL, Fraile G, Moreno MA, et al. Recurrent massive pleural effusion as a late complication of radiotherapy in Hodgkin's disease. Chest 1991;100:1165–6.

478. Benoff LJ, Schweitzer P. Radiation therapy-induced cardiac injury. Am Heart J 1995;129:1193–6.

479. Knight CJ, Sutton GC. Complete heart block and severe tricuspid regurgitation after radiotherapy. Chest 1995;108:1748–51.

480. King V, Constine LS, Clark D, et al. Symptomatic coronary artery disease after mantle irradiation for Hodgkin's disease. Int J Radiat Oncol Biol Phys 1996;36:881–9.

481. Perrin C, Mouroux J, Tamisier R, et al. Un chylothorax d'origine particulière: la fibrose médiastino-pulmonaire post-radique. Presse Med 1996;25:259.

482. de Vito EL, Quadrelli SA, Montiel GC, Roncoroni AJ. Bilateral diaphragmatic paralysis after mediastinal radiotherapy. Respiration 1996;63:187–90.

483. Lund MB, Kongerud J, Boe J, et al. Cardiopulmonary sequelae after treatment for Hodgkin's disease: increased risk in females? Ann Oncol 1996;7:257–64.

484. Hurkmans CW, Borger JH, Bos LJ, et al. Cardiac and lung complication probabilities after breast cancer irradiation. Radiother Oncol 2000;55:145–51.

485. Johansson S, Lofroth PO, Denekamp J. Left sided vocal cord paralysis: a newly recognized late complication of mediastinal irradiation. Radiother Oncol 2001;58:287–94.

486. Donaldson SS, Kaplan HS. Complications of treatment of Hodgkin's disease in children. Cancer Treat Rep 1982;66:977–89.

487. Goldman AL, Enquist R. Hyperacute radiation pneumonitis. Chest 1975;67:613–5.

488. Crestani B, Kambouchner M, Soler P, et al. Migratory bronchiolitis obliterans organizing pneumonia after unilateral radiation therapy for breast carcinoma. Eur Respir J 1995;8:318–21.

489. Dechambre S, Dorzee J, Fastrez J, et al. Bronchial stenosis and sclerosing mediastinitis: an uncommon complication of external thoracic radiotherapy. Eur Respir J 1998;11:1188–90.

490. Loyer E, Fuller L, Libshitz HI, Palmer JL. Radiographic appearance of the chest following therapy for Hodgkin disease. Eur J Radiol 2000;35:136–48.

491. Speiser BL, Spratling L. Radiation bronchitis and stenosis secondary to high dose rate endobronchial irradiation. Int J Radiat Oncol Biol Phys 1993;25:586–97.

492. Rall JE, Alpers JB, Lewallen CG, et al. Radiation pneumonitis and fibrosis: a complication of radioiodine treatment of pulmonary metastases from cancer of the thyroid. J Clin Endocrinol Metab 1957;17:1263–76.

493. Lin M. Radiation pneumonitis caused by Yttrium-90 microspheres: radiologic findings. AJR Am J Roentgenol 1994;162:1300–02.

21 CONNECTIVE TISSUE DISEASES

MICHELLE M. FREEMER
TALMADGE E. KING JR

The connective tissue disorders are a heterogeneous group of immunologically mediated inflammatory diseases. These disorders are clearly multifactorial in origin, with genetic and environmental factors contributing to their development. The specific etiology and pathogenesis of each connective tissue disorder, as well as what determines the type and degree of pulmonary involvement, remains poorly understood.

It is not surprising that, by virtue of their abundant connective tissue and blood supply, the lungs are frequently involved in these disorders.[1–9] Consequently, the connective tissue diseases affect all areas of the lung (ie, the airways, alveoli, vascular system, and pleura), and do so in various degrees and combinations (Table 21–1). Chapters 8 to 11 describe the pathogenetic mechanisms that likely underlie the lung fibrosis found in patients with and without connective tissue diseases. The focus of this chapter is on diffuse interstitial lung disease in connective tissue disorders; other thoracic disease found in these disorders will be only briefly reviewed.

GENERAL CONSIDERATIONS

The association of connective tissue diseases and interstitial lung disease (ILD) is well established.[2,10] ILD complicating connective tissue diseases accounts for 414 deaths per year in the United States.[11] This number represents approximately 25% of all ILD mortality and 2% of all respiratory deaths.[12]

Until recently, most of the studies of lung involvement in the connective tissue diseases relied on clinical, physiologic, and radiologic data to define the presence of disease, determine the clinical course, and assess the prognosis of the lung involvement. In fact, very few patients had lung biopsies performed to better define the pattern of injury present. Consequently, our understanding of lung involvement in the connective tissue diseases remains incomplete.

First, the previous approach to assessing and describing the pulmonary manifestation in the connective tissue diseases was too simplistic. In particular, many reports included a heterogeneous group of patients, with multiple types of connective tissue diseases described. Additional studies are needed to better understand lung involvement in these diseases. Second, changes in the classification of idiopathic interstitial pneumonias (IIP), by definition, exclude patients with connective tissue disease contrary to the previous practice of including patients with and without connective tissue disease (see Chapter 25, "Idiopathic Interstitial Pneumonias").[13] Third, most studies that used radiographic features to diagnose or follow the course of the disease did not use high-resolution computed tomography (HRCT) scanning of the lung. Fourth, no pathologic findings are pathognomonic for the connective tissue diseases. Indeed, similar histopathologic patterns of lung repair can be seen in patients with and without autoimmune diseases. Although the presence of lymphoid follicles or aggregates on lung biopsy appears to be a characteristic feature associated with connective tissue disease, this finding is not specific and has no prognostic significance. Furthermore, of the few pathologic studies of patients with connective tissue diseases, most used the old terminology for describing the histopathologic patterns; for example, most cases that described an inflammatory-fibrotic pattern were called usual interstitial pneumonia. We now know that the usual interstitial pneumonia pattern is not commonly found. Nonspecific interstitial pneumonia is a more frequent pattern in many forms of connective tissue disease.[14–17]

In this chapter, where possible, we will use the current definitions for the histologic patterns when describing interstitial lung involvement in these diseases. Some authors have suggested a separate classification system for patients with rheumatologic disease, relying on statistical analysis to define patterns of disease.[18] However, the usefulness of this, or other classification systems, remains to be defined.

RHEUMATOID ARTHRITIS

Definition and General Features

Rheumatoid arthritis (RA) is characterized by a symmetric inflammatory arthropathy associated with a

TABLE 21–1   Clinical and Pathologic Pulmonary Manifestations in Connective Tissue Disease*

Manifestation	Rheumatoid Arthritis	Systemic Lupus Erythematosus	Progressive Systemic Sclerosis	Polymyositis Dermatomyositis	Sjögren's Syndrome	Mixed Connective Tissue Disease	Ankylosing Spondylitis
Pleural inflammation, fibrosis, effusions	X	X	X				
Airway disease, inflammation, obstrution, lymphoid hyperplasia (follicular bronchiolitis)	X	X	X		X		
Interstitial disease	X	X	X	X	X	X	
Diffuse alveolar damage		X		X		X	
Diffuse alveolar hemorrhage (bland)		X				X	
Diffuse alveolar hemorrhage and capillaritis	X	X	X	X		X	
Organizing pneumonia	X	X	X	X	X		
Chronic cellular and fibrosing (nonspecific interstitial pneumonia pattern)	X	X	X	X	X		
Honeycomb lung	X	X	X	X	X	X	X
Eosinophilic infiltrates	X						
Vascular disease							
Hypertension/vasculitis	X	X	X		X	X	
Parenchymal nodules	X						
Apical fibrobullous disease	X						X
Lymphoid proliferations					X		
Respiratory muscle dysfunction		X		X		X	
Aspiration pneumonitis			X	X		X	

*Modified from Colby TV, et al.[811]

female preponderance.[19] The clinical course is variable: 75% of patients experience a chronic and relatively indolent course and 15% a more progressive and disabling one. Despite the prominence of articular manifestations, extra-articular lesions may occur in up to three-fourths of patients with severe RA, especially in those with active erosive disease, high-titer rheumatoid factor (RF), and circulating immune complexes. The extra-articular lesions include subcutaneous nodules, ocular inflammation, pericarditis, lymphadenopathy, splenomegaly, Felty's syndrome, cutaneous ulceration, and a variety of pleuropulmonary lesions.[20–22] Not surprisingly, the 5-year mortality rate among patients with extra-articular involvement is twice that of individuals without extra-articular manifestations.[20] A wide variety of pulmonary lesions are seen in patients with RA (Table 21–2).[5,23–26]

Pleuropulmonary Manifestations in Rheumatoid Arthritis

Interstitial Lung Disease

Epidemiology.   Although RA was described by Landre-Beauvais in the year 1800 and perhaps identified by Sydenham in 1676,[27] it remained for Ellman and Ball in 1948 to delineate the association between ILD and RA.[28] This delay in recognition of an association suggests that the association is either uncommon or clinically silent. The incidence of ILD in RA depends on the methods of its detection (clinical, radiologic, physiologic, or pathologic) and the population selected for study (mild versus severe disease, inpatient versus outpatient, or autopsy series).[29–41]

In contrast to the predilection of RA for women, RA associated with pulmonary disease is more common in men (ratio of 3:1)[4] and occurs most often in those patients with late-onset RA. Although occasionally found in children, it appears more frequently in the fourth through eighth decades, with the majority of cases occurring between the ages of 50 to 60 years.[31,42–47]

Roentgenographic surveys for the presence of lung involvement in RA are insensitive and imprecise.[48] Nonetheless, in groups of rheumatoid patients, roentgenographic evidence of ILD is found in as many as 20%.[30–32,38,41,48–51] Patients with high-titer RF are even more likely to have an abnormal chest roentgenogram.

Physiologic screening suggests a higher incidence of ILD in RA.[37,39,40,50,52] Among patients with definite RA, a reduction in the vital capacity (VC) or the carbon monoxide diffusing capacity (DL_{CO}) is frequently present. Further, patients with physiologic abnormalities are more likely to have histologic evidence of interstitial pneumonitis and fibrosis. A history of cigarette

TABLE 21–2   Pleuropulmonary Manifestations of Rheumatoid Arthritis

Parenchymal pulmonary disease
  Usual interstitial pneumonia
  Nonspecific interstitial pneumonia
  Organizing pneumonia
  Lymphocytic interstitial pneumonia
  Chronic eosinophilic pneumonia
  Apical fibrobullous disease
  Rheumatoid (necrobiotic) nodules, pneumoconiotic nodules
    (Caplan's syndrome)
  Drug-induced lung disease
    Penicillamine
    Methotrexate
    Gold[158]
    Celecoxib[188]
  Respiratory tract infection, especially typical and atypical
    tuberculosis
  Amyloid
  Pulmonary vascular lesions and pulmonary hypertension
Airway disease
  Upper airway dysfunction secondary to cricoarytenoid arthritis
  Bronchiectasis
  Bronchiolitis obliterans
  Follicular bronchiolitis
  Diffuse panbronchiolitis
Pleural disease
  Pleuritis with or without effusion
  Sterile or septic empyema
  Necrobiotic rheumatoid nodules associated with bronchopleural
    fistula
  Pyopneumothorax
Thoracic cage immobility

smoking is a significant confounding factor in the identification of lung disease in patients with RA.[53] Smoking is positively correlated with seropositivity, higher RF nephelometric values, and pulmonary disease, particularly in male patients with RA.[54] In addition, RA disease severity, assessed by radiography (Larsen scores), is significantly associated with the duration of smoking (< 20 years versus > 20 years) after adjustment for age, disease duration, and RF level. British investigators have provided a potential pathogenetic explanation for the relationship between smoking and RA disease severity. Polymorphisms of the glutathione S-transferase (GST) M1 locus, an enzyme which detoxifies carcinogens in tobacco smoke, appear to determine the association between smoking and RA disease severity as well as RF level.[55] The RF level and RA disease severity were associated with smoking only in the RA patients with GST M1 null alleles.[55]

Gabbay and associates determined the prevalence of ILD associated with RA patients who had joint disease of less than 2 years' duration using a number of newer more sensitive techniques.[56] Patients who met American Rheumatism Association (ARA) criteria for the diagnosis of RA were recruited from community-based and hospital rheumatologists to participate in the study. The cases were assessed using the following measures: clinical, lung physiology, radiology (chest radiography,

HRCT), bronchoalveolar lavage (BAL), and technetium Tc 99m diethylenetriamine pentaacetic acid (99mTc-DTPA) nuclear scan.[56] Abnormalities consistent with ILD (defined as an abnormality in one or more of the study parameters) were found in 58% of the subjects: lung physiology in 22%, chest radiography in 6%, HRCT in 33%, BAL in 52%, and 99mTc-DTPA nuclear scan in 15%. Based on clinical and physiologic results, 14% of the subjects had clinically significant ILD; 44% had abnormalities compatible with ILD but no clinically significant ILD, and 42% had no abnormalities compatible with ILD. Thus, this study suggests that changes consistent with ILD are frequent in the early phases of RA. The significance of these changes remain unknown. Only male gender was associated with clinically significant ILD.[56]

Pathogenesis.   Current speculation suggests that RA represents a persistent immunologic response to an unidentified antigen in a genetically susceptible host. Potential antigenic sources include components of synovial tissue, cartilage, native or aggregated immunoglobulin (Ig)G, mycoplasma, viruses, and bacterial peptidoglycans.[57,58] The association of seropositive RA with human leukocyte antigen (HLA)-DRw4 and HLA-Dw4, the cellular sensitivity to types II and III collagen, and the evidence of an altered response to infection with Epstein-Barr virus have all been described, although the significance is unknown.[59–62]

Whatever its origin, the translation of the initial immunologic insult into articular and extra-articular injury would seem to involve both cellular hypersensitivity and the production of intra- and extravascular immune complexes.[63] As with other forms of extra-articular disease, the interstitial disease has been associated with RF positivity.[31,33,49,64] There is little evidence to suggest a primary pathogenic role for IgM RF; it may enhance the pathogenicity of other immune complexes by facilitating aggregation or by entrapment within the vasculature.[65,66] The administration of IgM RF (but not IgM) accentuates the inflammatory injury in a rabbit model of proliferative lung disease.[67] Further support for immune complex–mediated injury in RA ILD includes an association with circulating intermediate (9-15S) complexes, as well as elevated C1q binding. IgM and RF deposit in rheumatoid lung tissue studied by immunofluorescence, and soluble immune complexes are present in BAL fluids.[67,68]

The cellular and noncellular abnormalities found in BAL have unclear implications for the pathogenesis of ILD in patients with RA. Collectively, these findings support the hypothesis that alveolar macrophage dysfunction precedes the recruitment of inflammatory and immune effector cells, such as neutrophils and lymphocytes, to the lung. These findings of activated alveolar macrophages in subclinical and clinical pulmonary inflammation are not specific for rheumatoid arthritis but can be seen in other connective tissue diseases.[69] The T lymphocyte abnormality in RA patients may be a marker of disease activity and predict those patients that will experience clinical progression and evolution to ILD.[70]

The report of a familial association of RA and ILD, as well as the demonstration of an increase in the α_1-antitrypsin (α_1-AT) MZ phenotype in individuals with fibrosing alveolitis with and without RA suggest the possibility of a genetic predisposition.[71,72] The α_1-AT Pi type might conceivably determine whether subclinical injurious events could progress to overt alveolar damage. A unifying explanation would be that RA patients possess a heightened susceptibility to lung injury (possibly related to the presence of RF of the Pi type) with either an endogenous (immune complex) or exogenous (occupational agents, cigarette smoke) insult resulting in injury to the parenchyma.[73]

Clinical Manifestations. The clinical manifestations of ILD in RA resemble those of the IIP (see Chapter 25, "Idiopathic Interstitial Pneumonias").[45,49] Patients may be asymptomatic, even with extensive roentgenographic findings.[5,74] Conversely, symptoms may antedate roentgenographic abnormalities.[75] Most commonly, dyspnea at rest or with exertion and a nonproductive cough are noted. Exertional dyspnea may be masked by the immobility of the arthritic patient. Less frequently, pleuritic and nonpleuritic chest pain, fever, and hemoptysis may occur, although these may be related to coexistent nodular or pleural disease.[35,49,76]

Physical signs of respiratory involvement may be minimal or absent despite roentgenographic abnormalities.[31,77] Tachypnea and bibasilar rales are common. Associated pleural rubs may be heard, and, with more advanced disease, cyanosis, edema, and signs of pulmonary hypertension are present.[76-80] Clubbing occurs in as many as 75% of cases, but the full picture of hypertrophic osteoarthropathy is rarely seen.[49,77,81] In one series comparing patients with IPF with those with RA-associated usual interstitial pneumonia (UIP), clubbing was seen significantly more frequently in those with IPF.[82]

The temporal relationship of the pulmonary and articular disease is variable.[31,35,37,83-86] Although pulmonary symptoms most often follow the arthritis, simultaneous onset or exacerbations may occur, and in one-fifth of the cases the lung disease precedes the joint manifestations. As a rule, joint and lung symptoms tend to develop within 5 years of each other. The severity of the pulmonary disease does not necessarily correlate with the extent and severity of the underlying arthritis. Although high titers of RF favor the development of pulmonary fibrosis, the incidence of seropositivity is similar for those patients who do or do not develop interstitial disease.[30,33,87] Increased titers of antinuclear antibodies and cryoglobulins have been associated with more severe pulmonary lesions.[40,87]

Roentgenographic Features. Early findings on chest radiographs include bibasilar patchy alveolar or hazy opacities (see Chapter 1, Figures 1–23 and 1–32). With more advanced disease, a dense reticular or nodular pattern supervenes (Figure 21–1). With exacerbations, new, soft opacities can become superimposed on fibrotic areas.

The following computed tomography (CT) abnormalities were found with a significantly higher frequency among patients with respiratory symptoms: rounded areas of attenuation and areas of ground-glass attenuation (Figure 21–2).[88] Three major radiographic patterns of disease have been identified in symptomatic patients who developed lung disease prior to or following the diagnosis of RA.[86] These included reticulation with or without honeycombing (66% patients), centrilobular branching lines with or without bronchial dilatation (17%), and consolidation (17%). Although HRCT is superior to chest radiographs for the detection of interstitial disease,[48,89,90] chest radiographic findings are consistent with the HRCT findings in approximately 50% of patients with ILD.[89] Unfortunately, no radiographic features were able to distinguish between patients with IPF or those with RA and UIP.[82]

Goupille and coworkers failed to show an advantage for using J001X scintigraphy (a fully characterized acylated poly(1,3)galactoside isolated from *Klebsiella* membranes that is able to bind recruited macrophages after aerosol administration) in the imaging of pulmonary disease in RA when compared to HRCT, pulmonary function tests, and BAL.[91] Similarly, technetium lung clearance scans cannot distinguish between patients with idiopathic pulmonary fibrosis (IPF) or those with RA and UIP.[82]

Other radiographic features may include emphysematous bullae, evidence of air trapping, mosaic perfusion, and nodules.[48] Pleural disease accompanies interstitial lung disease in 20% of patients.[35] Cardiomegaly and pulmonary artery hypertension may ensue with the onset of cor pulmonale (see Figure 21–1).

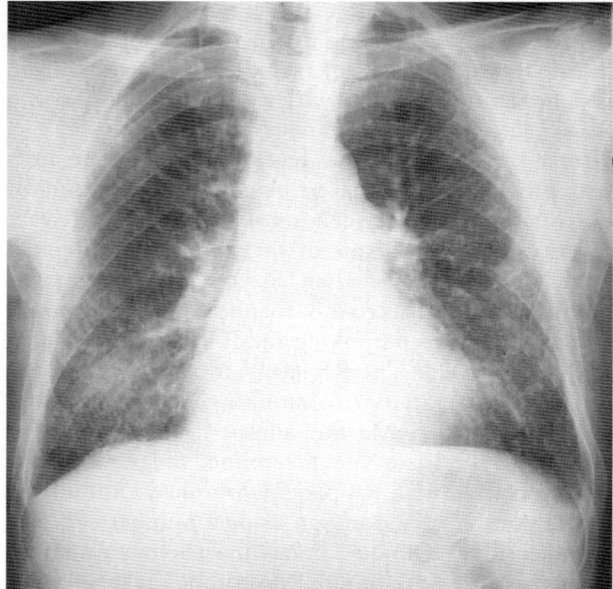

Figure 21–1 Rheumatoid arthritis. The chest radiograph shows severe diffuse reticular opacities, large pulmonary arteries, and cardiomegaly. The cor pulmonale resulted from longstanding interstitial lung disease.

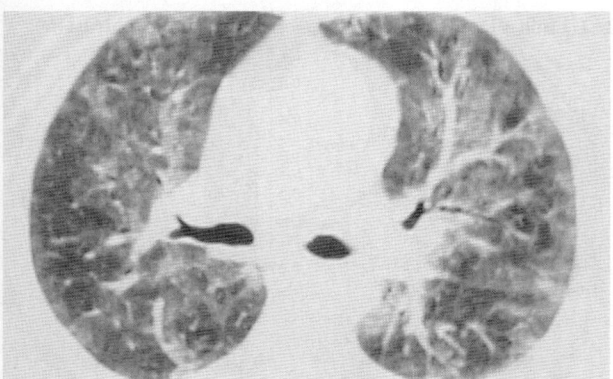

Figure 21–2   53-year-old woman with rheumatoid arthritis. This high-resolution computed tomography scan shows diffuse ground-glass attenuation. An open lung biopsy showed a pattern of nonspecific interstitial pneumonia with areas of organizing pneumonia. Prominent lymphoid follicles with germinal centers were also present. Her symptoms improved dramatically with corticosteroid therapy. However, there was only partial clearing of her radiographic abnormalities.

Physiologic Features.   The physiologic abnormalities of rheumatoid ILD are identical to the other fibrosing lung diseases.[30,80,87] There is a reduction in pulmonary compliance and lung volumes, abnormalities of gas transfer including a low DL_{CO}, a low or normal resting arterial CO_2 pressure ($PaCO_2$), and a normal or near normal arterial O_2 pressure (PaO_2), which falls with exercise. Abnormal pulmonary function may be found in individuals with normal chest roentgenograms.[50] Conversely, the pulmonary function tests may be normal despite the presence of ILD on biopsy.[40] Several studies have suggested a high prevalence of obstructive lung disease in patients with RA.[92,93]

Bronchoalveolar Lavage.   Bronchoalveolar lavage fluid and cellular abnormalities are common in patients with RA independent of the presence or absence of clinical lung disease (Table 21–3).[94,95] Patients with RA *and* clinical lung disease (either chest symptoms or physiologic abnormality) tend to have an alveolitis characterized by an increase in lavage macrophages and neutrophils.[70,96–102] A subset of patients with RA but *without* clinical lung disease have a BAL lymphocytosis.[69,70,95,97]

Garcia and colleagues[97] performed BAL in 24 patients with RA. Of these patients, 9 had evidence of clinical ILD (defined as an abnormality on chest roentgenogram consistent with an interstitial process and/or a restrictive pattern on functional testing) (group I, RA-ILD). Fifteen patients with RA had no evidence of interstitial lung involvement although five of these subjects had an abnormal BAL (group II). The remaining 10 patients with RA had no evidence of clinical ILD and had normal BAL findings as well (group III). The BAL findings of the three groups of subjects from this study are shown in Figure 21–3. Patients with RA-ILD (group I) had significantly increased numbers of neutrophils recovered in BAL fluid compared with those without ILD ($p < .05$). In contrast, a lavage lymphocytosis was found in a subset of patients with normal lung function and chest roentgenogram. Other abnormalities included an elevated level of IgM and a reduced helper/suppressor T-cell ratio (T-lymphocyte Leu 3/Leu 2A ratio).[97] Conversely, the patients with abnormal BAL findings without lung disease (group II) not only had a BAL lymphocytosis but also had an increase in BAL IgM and an elevated helper/suppressor T-cell ratio. Unlike the other groups, these group II patients had these BAL abnormalities reflected in their peripheral blood with an elevated Leu 3/Leu 2A ratio found. The significance of these findings are unclear.

Several biochemical markers of ongoing inflammation and injury have been identified in the BAL fluid of RA patients. The BAL fluid histamine level was significantly greater in patients with RA, especially those with active parenchymal lung disease, compared with normal subjects.[100] A marked increase in neutrophils and an active type I collagenase of neutrophil origin was found in BAL fluid recovered from patients with RA-associated ILD.[99] In contrast, this collagenase was not found in RA patients without lung disease. Gilligan and coworkers[101] demonstrated that patients with established ILD had a greater procollagen peptide concentration and collagenase activity in BAL fluid than either the control group or those with early disease. Alveolar macrophages from RA patients without detectable ILD released increased amounts of superoxide anion, fibronectin, and

TABLE 21–3   Bronchoalveolar Lavage Cytology in Connective Tissue Disease with and without Associated Interstitial Lung Disease*

Disease	With ILD	Without ILD
Progressive systemic sclerosis	Neutrophils, eosinophils	Neutrophils, eosinophils
Rheumatoid arthritis	Neutrophils, lymphocytes	Lymphocytes (CD4⁺, T519)
Primary Sjögren's syndrome	Neutrophils, lymphocytes (CD8⁺)	Lymphocytes (CD4⁺)
Systemic lupus erythematosus	Neutrophils, lymphocytes	Lymphocytes
Dermatopolymyositis	Neutrophils	Neutrophils
Mixed connective tissue disease	Neutrophils	Neutrophils
Secondary Sjögren's syndrome	Neutrophils, lymphocytes (CD8⁺)	Neutrophils, lymphocytes (CD8⁺)

Reproduced with permission from Wallaert B et al.[812]
ILD = interstitial lung disease.
*Presence of ILD is judged by clinical and radiologic findings.

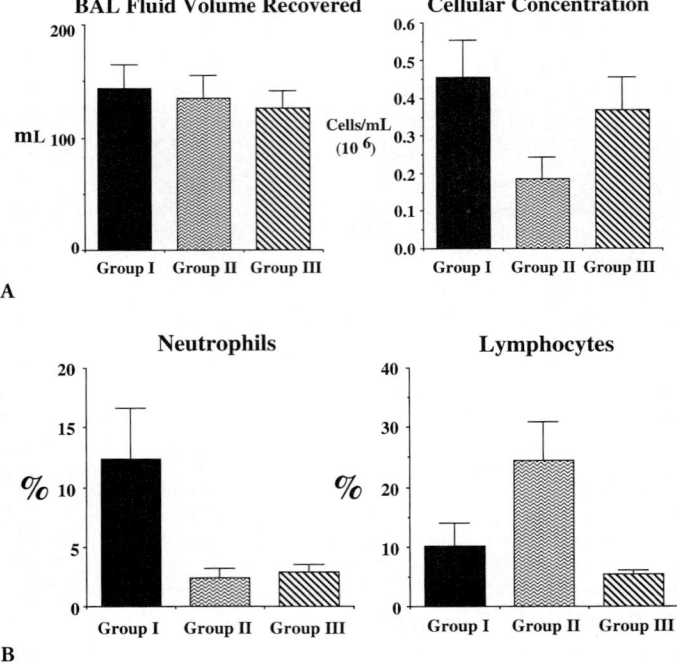

Figure 21–3 Rheumatoid arthritis (RA): bronchoalveolar lavage (BAL) cellular differentials. *A*, BAL fluid volume recovered (left panel) was not significantly different between the three groups of patients with RA. Patients with interstitial lung disease (ILD) (group I) had the highest concentration of cells (right panel) recovered but was not significantly different from the other groups. *B*, Patients with ILD had a significant increase in neutrophils compared with the other groups of RA patients (left panel). In contrast, all patients in group II, with normal functional and roentgenographic parameters, had elevated BAL lymphocytes compared with group I ($p > .05$) and group III ($p < .01$) (right panel). Definitions: group I, 5 RA patients with ILD; group II, 5 RA patients with abnormal BAL fluid but no evidence of clinical disease; group III, 5 RA patients with no clinical disease and normal BAL fluid. Reproduced with permission from Garcia JGN et al.[97]

neutrophil chemotactic factor.[70] The presence of increased amounts of superoxide anion in BAL fluid correlated with the percentage of neutrophils in BAL. Tumor necrosis factor alpha production by alveolar macrophages is increased in RA patients with and without ILD.[102] Interleukin-1 (IL-1) beta production was not different in these groups. Interestingly, RA patients with established ILD have a markedly increased ratio of local immune complex to albumin in BAL.

Histopathology Features. Few studies have examined lung specimens from surgical lung biopsies in patients with RA. Even fewer have done so using the recent criteria for defining the pattern of lung injury.[103]

Usual Interstitial Pneumonia. The classic features of UIP are not commonly found in patients with RA. In patients dying following rapid radiographic disease progression in the absence of cardiac failure or infection, diffuse alveolar damage may be superimposed on a UIP pattern.[48] Several features tend to differentiate the interstitial inflammation and fibrosis pattern found in patients with RA from those of classic UIP found in patients with idiopathic pulmonary fibrosis. A lymphocytic infiltrate consisting of small lymphocytes, plasma cells, and histiocytes is most marked around airways and adjacent alveolar walls. When extensive, this lesion correlates with the presence of ground-glass opacities on the HRCT scan.[104] Hyperplastic lymphoid follicles with reactive germinal centers are commonly found adjacent to small airways. This latter process may be prominent, and it is termed "follicular bronchitis or bronchiolitis" (see "Follicular Bronchiolitis" to follow).[5,30,45,75,104,105] As the UIP lesion advances, extensive fibrosis and distortion of the alveo-

lar septa occurs. The development of cystic spaces up to 2 cm in size, lined by flat, cuboidal, or columnar epithelium, signals end-stage or honeycombed lung.[106] A leiomyomatous change may occur as well as cuboidalization of the alveolar epithelium. An acute bronchiolitis may be noted, and frank bronchiolitis obliterans with endobronchial polyps occur. The small arteries demonstrate subintimal fibrosis and medial hyperplasia. Rheumatoid nodules, pleural fibrosis, and adhesions are also found in RA (see "Rheumatoid Nodules" to follow).

Lymphocytic Interstitial Pneumonia. Lymphocytic interstitial pneumonia (LIP) is part of a spectrum of pulmonary lymphoid proliferations, ranging from follicular bronchitis/bronchiolitis to low-grade malignant lymphoma. As noted above, LIP-like lesions are frequently found in patients with RA. LIP is characterized by a diffuse, prominent interstitial lymphoid infiltrate. The infiltrate diffusely invades alveolar septa and consists of lymphocytes and variable numbers of plasma cells. An autoimmune etiology for LIP is proposed given its association with many autoimmune processes (especially those with dysproteinemias) (see Chapter 27, "Lymphoplasmacytic Infiltrations of the Lung"). Sjögren's syndrome is associated with approximately one-fourth of reported cases of LIP (see "Sjögren's Syndrome" to follow).

Organizing Pneumonia. Organizing pneumonia (OP), characterized by abundant organizing granulation tissue within air spaces, may also be a component of the ILD of RA (see Chapter 2, Figure 2–11).[105,107–109] This was the histologic pattern of disease in symptomatic RA patients with consolidation as seen by HRCT.[48] Notably, one of these patients, with chronic eosinophilic pneumonia as well as OP, progressed to respiratory failure with pulmonary findings at autopsy included honey-combing.[48] OP has a much better overall prognosis than other forms of lung injury in this setting. However, rheumatoid patients with OP are prone to develop a rapidly progressive and fatal form of OP.[109–112] This entity is discussed in more detail elsewhere in this text (see Chapter 25, "Idiopathic Interstitial Pneumonias").

Granulomatous Inflammation. An apparent association of RA and sarcoidosis has been reported.[113,114]

Prognosis and Management. Any estimate of the prognosis, and hence the necessity of therapeutic intervention in RA ILD, is clouded by the clinical heterogeneity of this disorder. Although many have suggested that UIP in RA patients is indolent and less severe than IPF, recent data indicate that the prognosis of RA patients with UIP is no different than patients with IPF. (It should be noted that the power to detect a difference between groups in this study was limited by small sample sizes. In addition, histopathologic confirmation of diagnosis was not provided).[115] Progressive and rapid deterioration (Hamman-Rich syndrome) also has been reported.[28,106] In general, survival of patients with RA ILD is decreased by 3.5 to 4.9 years.[45,112]

Response to treatment is also difficult to determine because of small numbers of cases, uncontrolled studies, dissimilar modes of therapy, and different criteria for assessing therapeutic response. Subjective response to corticosteroids has been anecdotally reported, both with and without objective improvement. In 1962, Doctor and Snider suggested that the response to corticosteroids depended on the maturity of the fibrotic process rather than disease duration. They noted marked physiologic improvement when the lung tissue was highly cellular.[84] Reviewing the literature available in 1968, Walker and Wright noted that among 25 cases treated with corticosteroids, 44% had objective but often temporary evidence of improvement.[49] Turner-Warwick and Evans found no complete remissions among 23 patients after corticosteroid therapy. However, improved exercise tolerance occurred in 43% and objective roentgenographic improvement in 22%. Lung biopsy in two subjects showed a predominantly cellular pattern.[45] In a series of 15 patients with connective tissue disease and pulmonary fibrosis, two-thirds of whom had RA, corticosteroid therapy resulted in a reduction of the total cells, neutrophil percentage, and immune complexes in BAL fluid, though improvement in DL_{CO} was noted in only seven.[68]

The experience with other therapies is limited. Cyclophosphamide, effective in articular and vasculitic disease, would seem to be a likely supplemental or an alternative agent.[116] Azathioprine,[117] methotrexate,[118] hydroxychloroquine sulfate,[49] penicillamine,[119] and cyclosporine[120] have been found useful in case reports.

Given the relative uncertainty of therapy and its potential adverse effects, the decision to treat should be based on firm physiologic, and probably histologic, data, taking into consideration the overall clinical status of the patient. A reasonable approach would be to periodically screen patients with simple spirometry, DL_{CO}, and a chest roentgenogram. Should abnormalities be found or should symptoms be present, more extensive evaluation of lung function, to include lung volumes and exercise studies, should be obtained. Evidence of significant restriction, with abnormalities of gas transfer or serial studies showing progressive deterioration in a young patient with articular functional class I or II disease and hence the most to be gained from improved exercise tolerance, would suggest the advisability of therapy. Prior to treatment, a lung biopsy is desirable, not only to assess cellularity but also to define the primary histologic pattern, which may correspond poorly to roentgenographic changes.

Airway Disease In Rheumatoid Arthritis

Epidemiology. Airway disease is more frequent among patients with RA than in other rheumatologic disorders.[121] Obstructive pulmonary disease has been increasingly noted in patients with RA.[30,50,52,92,122,123] Geddes and coworkers studied 100 consecutive patients with RA who had normal chest roentgenograms.[93] They compared these patients with a control group matched for age, sex, and smoking habit and demonstrated that patients with RA had a remarkably high prevalence of airflow obstruction (one-third of RA patients). This suggested that airway obstruction may be the most common form of lung involvement in RA. Other studies have confirmed the increased prevalence of airway obstruction in RA.[124,125] For example, in a recent study of patients with newly diagnosed RA, 36% of patients had either airway hyperreactivity or obstructive physiology despite a lack of symptoms in the majority of patients.[126]

Pathogenesis. The mechanism of the airways obstruction in patients with RA remains unclear. Collins and colleagues suggested that the combination of tobacco smoking and rheumatoid disease was associated with a much higher occurrence of obstructive pulmonary disease than with either of these factors alone.[92] In support of a potential interaction between smoking and RA, investigators demonstrated that one in five newly diagnosed RA patients had coexisting lung disease at the time of diagnosis, with chronic obstructive pulmonary disease (COPD) accounting for the majority of pulmonary disease.[127] However, another recent study indicated that 24% of newly diagnosed RA patients had airway hyperreactivity without any association with the number of pack-years smoked.[126] Protease inhibition deficiency has been suggested.[92,93] Recurrent respiratory tract infection has also been postulated largely because of Walker's[124] suggestion that patients with RA are more prone to such illness.

Clinical Manifestations. *Cricoarytenoid Arthritis.* Upper airway obstruction may be a vexing and life-threatening complication in RA. It can result from synovitis of the cricoarytenoid joint,[128–130] rheumatoid nodules of the larynx,[131] or arteritis of the vasa nervorum of the recurrent laryngeal and vagus nerves.[24]

Although involvement of the cricoarytenoid joints may be seen in gout, systemic lupus erythematosus, and Reiter's syndrome, the most common association is with RA. One-fourth of patients with RA demonstrate signs and symptoms of cricoarytenoid disease.[129] However; it is more common in advanced RA. Although patients with cricoarytenoid arthritis may be asymptomatic, often it is manifested by varying combinations of a foreign body sensation or pain in the throat, hoarseness, dyspnea with exertion, ear pain, inspiratory stridor especially at night, dysphagia, odynophagia, or profound upper airway obstruction.[128,129] Cricoarytenoid arthritis may be slightly more common and more severe in women. Recognition is important since acute laryngeal obstruction may occur.[128]

Bronchiectasis.   Bronchiectasis can be a feature of RA and is often found in patients with severe, long-standing nodular disease.[132,133] The prevalence is unknown and in case series has varied between 0 to 10%.[133] In HRCT studies of patients with RA, up to 30% were noted to have bronchiectasis unassociated with ILD (see Chapter 4, Figures 4–37).[88,90,134,135] In most patients bronchiectasis does not appear to be clinically significant.

In a recent case series, productive cough, hemoptysis, and dyspnea were the most common respiratory symptoms and were present for an average of 4.3 years prior to the diagnosis of bronchiectasis.[132] The most common radiographic abnormalities were bibasilar diffusely increased interstitial markings and focal opacities, although nodules, bullae, cysts, and air-fluid levels were found. Obstructive or restrictive findings can be found in these patients.[132]

An increased proportion of RA patients with bronchiectasis have the protease inhibitor phenotype MM and are HLA-DR4–antigen positive.[134] Hillarby and associates examined HLA-DR, -DQA, and -DQB variants in controls and subjects with RA without extra-articular features and in subjects with rheumatoid pulmonary complications of interstitial fibrosis, peripheral airways disease, and in subjects with RA and bronchiectasis.[136] Subjects with RA alone showed the expected association with HLA-DR4 (79%) but those with RA and coexistent pulmonary fibrosis were less likely to be DR4 positive (61%). No other HLA-DR variants were significantly increased in the different disease groups. The HLA-DQB1*0501, serologic type DQw1, was higher in patients with RA with peripheral airways disease as compared with those with normal lung function, but these differences were not statistically significant. The DQB1*0601 was increased in subjects with bronchiectasis with or without RA (but only significantly so in RA and bronchiectasis subjects). The frequencies of DQB1*0301, DQB1*0201, and DQA1*0501 were also increased in subjects with RA and bronchiectasis as compared with those with RA alone.[136]

In RA patients with bronchiectasis, recurrent pulmonary infections and respiratory failure occur and may be fatal.[132]

Bronchiolitis Obliterans.   Bronchiolitis obliterans with airway obstruction is an increasingly recognized complication in RA. This association is described in Chapter 26, "Bronchiolitis."

Follicular Bronchiolitis.   Follicular bronchitis and bronchiolitis may occur in patients with RA, Sjögren's syndrome, juvenile RA, immunodeficiency syndromes, familial lung disorders, chronic infection, and a heterogeneous group of patients with a hypersensitivity-type reaction.[104,137,138]

Patients with RA usually present with dyspnea (100%); fever and cough occur occasionally. A positive RF is present, often at high levels (1:640 to 1:2,560). The chest radiograph is abnormal, showing bilateral reticular or nodular opacities. The most common CT scan findings are bilateral, diffuse centrilobular nodular opacities (usually less than 3 mm) and ground-glass opacity.[104] Mosaic perfusion or honeycombing is not present.[104]

Arterial blood gases demonstrate hypoxemia, hypocapnia, and a widened alveolar-arterial oxygen gradient. Both obstructive and restrictive patterns have been identified by spirometry, but the restrictive pattern appears to be more common. Immunofluorescence studies are negative.

The lesions of follicular bronchiolitis produce obstruction by external compression of the bronchioles, rather than by direct luminal occlusion, as is characteristic for proliferative bronchiolitis obliterans. In almost all cases, a concentric inflammatory infiltrate of lymphocytes and plasma cells surrounds the bronchiole. Abundant germinal centers in the peribronchiolar regions are present and are characterized by hyperplastic follicles located between bronchioles and pulmonary arteries. The bronchiolar lumen is often compressed into a slit-like or fish-mouth shape. Some have suggested that follicular bronchiolitis may be the precursor of interstitial lymphoid pneumonia or pseudolymphoma.

Treatment with corticosteroids has yielded variable results. Erythromycin may be useful for the management of this process.[139]

Diffuse Panbronchiolitis.   Diffuse panbronchiolitis (DPB) accompanying RA has been reported in Japanese patients (see Chapter 26, "Bronchiolitis").[140,141] In these patients, the predominant lesion shows lymphocytic, histiocytic, and plasma cell infiltration of the respiratory bronchiole resulting in thickening of the wall. Consequently, the proximal terminal bronchiole also become ectatic.

Both RA and DPB have been associated with the HLA-DR4 and B54 haplotype, and this potential association was supported by HLA antigen analysis in two RA patients with DPB.[140] Japanese investigators have observed the difficulty of distinguishing DPB from other bronchiolar disease (cellular bronchiolitis, follicular bronchiolitis, and obliterative bronchiolitis) in RA patients.[142] In their study, the RA patients with bronchiolar disease were significantly older, more dyspneic, more hypoxic, and more likely to be RF positive than the Japanese patients with DPB. Those with DPB, however, were more likely to have small nodules on chest radiography and respond to erythromycin treatment (as determined by a change in FEV_1) compared with bronchiolar disease patients with RA. Successful treatment of DPB in an RA patient has been described.[140]

Fibrobullous Disease

Apical fibrobullous changes (ie, a reticular pattern in the upper lung zones associated with emphysematous bullae) are most frequently reported in association with ankylosing spondylitis, but have also been found in seropositive RA, occasionally preceding signs of arthritis,[48,143] and occurring in the absence of HLA-B27.[144]

Rheumatoid Nodules

Rheumatoid (necrobiotic) nodules are the most common lesions found at open lung biopsy and are the only pleuropulmonary manifestation specific for RA.[105] They are either located in the interlobular septa or in a subpleural location. They may also occur in the lung parenchyma and may antedate the onset of arthritis.[145,146] Parenchymal necrobiotic nodules can be single or multiple, can cavitate, and must be differentiated from a pulmonary neoplasm (Figure 21–4).[83,87,147–149] Most patients are asymptomatic; however, hemoptysis (from cavitation of the nodule) and pneumothorax (from erosion into the pleural space) can be seen.[24] Recent HRCT studies show that pulmonary nodules (22%) and subpleural micronodules or pseudoplaques (17%) are more common than previously thought.[88,135] The finding of a solitary pulmonary density or nodule in a patient with RA provides no assurance that the lesion is benign,[149,150] especially given that the presence of nodules has been associated with a current or former smoker status as well as years of smoking.[54]

In 1953, Caplan described multiple rounded peripheral opacities from 0.5 to 5.0 cm in diameter in 25% of Welsh coal miners with RA.[151] These pneumoconiotic nodules appear rapidly and often cavitate. Subsequently, other occupational dust exposures have been associated with the syndrome. Interestingly, the syndrome appears uncommon in the United States.[152] Histologically, the Caplan's lesion resembles the nonpneumoconiotic nodule with the additional finding of dust particles.[153]

Pulmonary Infection

Respiratory tract infection is common in patients with RA. Indeed, respiratory infection has been demonstrated to cause 15 to 19% of deaths in these patients, exceed-

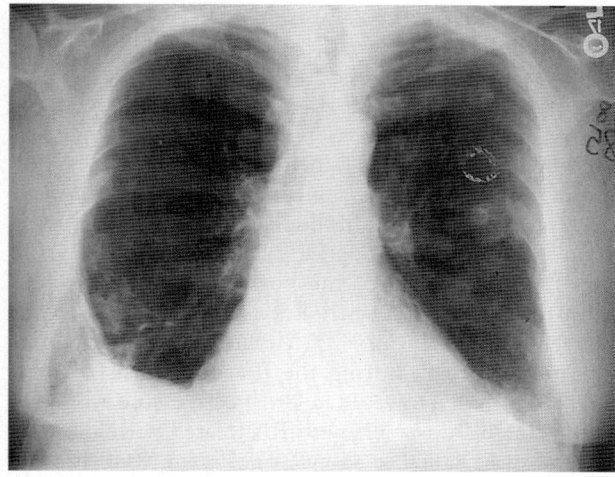

A

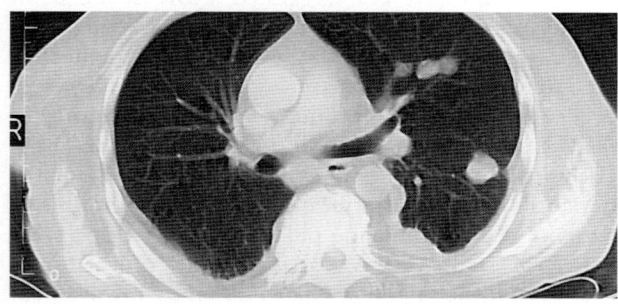

B

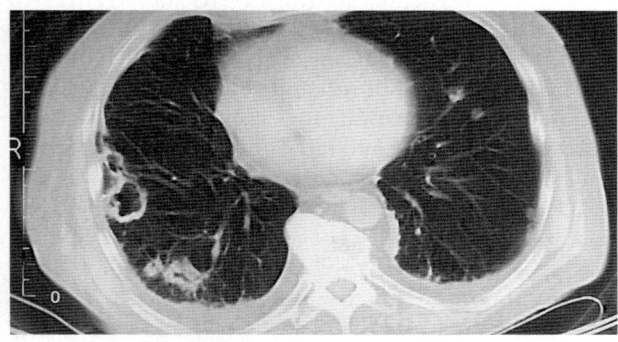

C

Figure 21–4   Rheumatoid arthritis: rheumatoid (necrobiotic) nodules. *A*, Posteroanterior chest roentgenogram reveals bilateral pulmonary nodules and bilateral pleural reaction. *B*, Computed tomography (CT) scan shows multiple well-circumscribed nodules in the left lung. *C*, CT scan shows thick-walled cavitary nodules in the right lung. Additional nodules are also seen in the left lung.

ing the expected rate for matched controls.[154–156] Tuberculosis should be excluded in these patients.

Amyloidosis

A case of diffuse interstitial pulmonary amyloidosis in a patient with long standing RA has been reported (see Chapter 31, "Miscellaneous Interstitial Lung Diseases").[157]

Drug-Induced Lung Disease in Rheumatoid Arthritis

The treatment of RA involves several drugs that can cause lung injury. This is particularly true of gold,[158] methotrexate,[159–173] and D-penicillamine.[174–181] The pulmonary manifestations resulting from these drugs are discussed elsewhere in this book (see Chapter 20, "Drug Induced Infiltrative Lung Diseases").

The prevalence of methotrexate-induced pneumonitis in patients with RA is estimated to range between 0.3 and 18%.[182–185] Methotrexate pneumonitis commonly occurs during the first 6 months of therapy.[167,182,183,186] However, a prospective study of lung involvement in patients with RA treated with low-dose methotrexate failed to show a significant association of this therapy with the development of chronic ILD.[185] Other studies have also suggested a low incidence of methotrexate-induced lung disease in this setting.[163,168] The most critical criteria for the diagnosis of methotrexate-induced pneumonitis are: an appropriate history of exposure, pulmonary opacities on chest radiography or HRCT, and exclusion of other pulmonary diseases, especially infections.[172,187] The strongest predictors for the development of methotrexate-induced pneumonitis in patients with RA include older age (odds ratio [OR], 5.1; 95% CI, 1.2 to 21.1), diabetes (OR, 35.6; CI, 1.3 to infinity), rheumatoid pleuropulmonary involvement (OR, 7.1; CI, 1.1 to 45.4), previous use of disease-modifying antirheumatic drugs (OR, 5.6; CI, 1.2 to 27.0), and hypoalbuminemia (OR, 19.5; CI, 3.5 to 109.7).[171] The typical clinical symptoms include progressive shortness of breath and cough, often associated with fever. Chest examination often reveals inspiratory crackles. Hypoxemia and tachypnea are commonly present. The peripheral blood eosinophil count was elevated in a minority of patients. Chest radiography reveals diffuse interstitial or mixed interstitial and alveolar opacities, with a predilection for the lower lung fields. Pulmonary function tests show a restrictive pattern with reduced diffusion capacity. Lung biopsy may reveal several patterns of lung injury: cellular interstitial infiltrates, granulomas, or a diffuse alveolar damage pattern accompanied by perivascular inflammation.[172]

Patients with RA receiving treatment with several newer agents have developed pulmonary complications, such as, fleeting pulmonary infiltrates associated with the cyclooxygenase-2 inhibitor celecoxib[188]; adult respiratory distress syndrome associated with infliximab therapy,[189] and pulmonary miliary tuberculosis in a patient treated with tumor necrosis factor-alpha blockade.[190]

Pulmonary Vascular Disease

Systemic rheumatoid vasculitis defined clinically by the presence of deep cutaneous ulcers, peripheral gangrene, acute peripheral neuropathy or mononeuritis, or digital or nailfold infarcts has been described.[116,118,191] Primary pulmonary vascular disease causing pulmonary hypertension in the absence of fibrotic parenchymal changes is uncommon in RA and is characterized by medial hypertrophy with intimal fibrosis.[192,193] Recent echocardiographic data in a cohort of RA patients showed that the prevalence of pulmonary hypertension was 31%. The majority of these patients (66%) had no evidence of cardiac dysfunction or pulmonary physiologic deficits as assessed by pulmonary function testing.[194] Aside from the presence of coexisting RA, these lesions may clinically and pathologically resemble primary pulmonary hypertension.[4] Veno-occlusive disease has also been reported in a patient with Felty's syndrome.[195] True pulmonary vasculitis with fibrinoid necrosis of vessel walls was not seen in a recent study of lung biopsies in RA.[105] Alveolar hemorrhage (often with capillaritis) can be found in RA (see Chapter 23, "Diffuse Alveolar Hemorrhage").[196]

Pleural Disease

Epidemiology.   Pleural disease is one of the most common pulmonary complications of RA (Table 21–4). Pleural involvement is found at autopsy in 38 to 73% of patients, although symptomatic pleurisy is less frequent.[49,197–199] Biopsy reveals nonspecific chronic inflammation and fibrosis, although typical rheumatoid nodules may be seen.[6] Approximately 20% of patients with RA will report a history of pleurisy. Pleural effusions are clinically evident in only 5% of patients and may occasionally antedate the onset of articular disease.[49,198–201] However, pleural effusions are more common in men with longstanding articular disease (frequently during a period of active articular disease) and in patients with subcutaneous nodules.[49,202–204] Hakala and coworkers showed that HLA-B8 antigen was strongly associated with the presence of pleural effusion in patients with RA.[205]

Clinical Manifestations.   The patient can present without symptoms with the effusion being discovered on routine chest radiograph. When symptomatic, the patient usually presents with symptoms mimicking bacterial pneumonia or with intermittent nonspecific chest discomfort.[203] Usually the pleural effusions are of small to moderate volume and unilateral. Presentations with massive effusions have been reported.[206,207] The effusion can be transient, chronic, or recurrent.[203] The pleural disease may be seen in the presence of interstitial lung disease or necrobiotic nodules in 30% of patients.[203]

Typically, the pleural effusion is an exudate; however, it may appear serous, turbid, yellow-green, or milky.[198,199] Cholesterol pleural effusions are uncommon.[203,208–210] The effusion demonstrates glucose levels less than 30 mg/dL in 70 to 80% of cases.[202] This low glucose level is secondary to impaired membrane transport of glucose.[208] Other biochemical findings include a total protein content usually exceeding 3.5 g/dL, a lactate dehydrogenase (LDH) greater that 1,000 U/L, and a pH of approximately 7.00.[198,199] Reduced levels of both complement and immune complexes are found in the pleural fluid when compared with levels in the serum.[211,212] The RF is increased in the pleural fluid usually greater than or equal to 1:320 and greater than that found in the serum.[198,199]

The triad of giant multinucleated macrophages, elongated macrophages, and a background of granular debris is characteristic of the pleural fluid cytologic examination in rheumatoid pleural effusions.[203,213] RA cells are seen but are not diagnostic since they can be found in tuberculous pleurisy.[203] Thoracoscopy is often useful in evaluating patients with suspected rheumatoid pleural disease.[214–216] The parietal pleura has a characteristic "gritty" or frozen appearance.[203] Microscopic examination shows loss of the mesothelial layer and replacement with a pseudostratified layer of epithelial cells.[203,213] The visceral pleural surface shows varying degrees of nonspecific inflammation.[203] Rheumatoid granulomata are rarely identified on pleural biopsy.

Both sterile and septic empyemas have been described in 16% of cases.[217,218] In some cases, necrosis and cavitation of a necrobiotic pleural nodule lead to a

TABLE 21–4   Pleural Lesions and Effusions in Connective Tissue Diseases*

Disease	Pleural Lesions/ Symptoms	Incidence	Probable Pathogenesis	Pleural Fluid Characteristics	Comments
Rheumatoid arthritis	Chest pain Pleural thickening Serous effusions Blood stained effusions	20% 38–70% (PM) 5% Rare	Local immune pleuritis Trapped lung	Exudative, PMN, or mononuclear predominant; glucose <30 mg/dL, pH 7.00; LDH >1000 IU/L; complement low; IC present; RF >1:320; pH and glucose low in 80%	Bloody effusion indicates vasculitis of pleura or infarction of lung; can be recurrent; some require decortication
	Empyema-like fluid	Several reports	Necrosis of nodule, massive exudation of white cells	Sterile empyemas; yellow to green; low pH; low glucose; very high LDH	Empyema-like fluid may resolve with corticosteroids
	Empyema (infected)	Several reports	Bronchopleural fistula	Culture/Gram stain positive	Antibiotic/tube drainage
	Cholesterol effusion	Several reports	Cholesterol from senile cells and granulomas	Milky, high cholesterol, occasionally cholesterol crystals seen	If persistent and symptomatic, requires decortication or pleurodesis
	Chylous effusions	3 case reports	Lymphatic obstruction from amyloidosis	Increased triglycerides	
Systemic lupus erythematosus	Chest pain Effusion Acute fibrinous pleuritis Fibrosis	75% 50% 40% (PM) 30% (PM)	Local immune pleuritis	Exudative, serous or bloody; PMN or mononuclear predominant; pH and glucose low in 20%; complement low; IC present; ANA >1:160; LE cells diagnostic	Responds to corticosteroids; alternatives for steroid-resistant cases include tetracycline or talc pleurodesis, IV, immunoglobulins, and pleurectomy
Wegener's granulomatosis	Chest pain Effusion	20–56% 5–55%	Vasculitis and infarction of subpleural parenchyma	Small unilateral effusion; PMN predominance in exudate	No clinical importance, resolves spontaneously or with cyclophosphamide/ corticosteroids
Mixed connective tissue disease	Chest pain Effusion	40% <6%	Unknown	Small, unilateral or bilateral effusions; serous; normal glucose and complement	No clinical importance

(continued)

TABLE 21–4   Pleural Lesions and Effusions in Connective Tissue Diseases* (*continued*)

Disease	Pleural Lesions/ Symptoms	Incidence	Probable Pathogenesis	Pleural Fluid Characteristics	Comments
Sjögren's syndrome	Effusion	<1%	Lymphocytic infiltration of pleura; local immune pleuritis	Analysis not reported	May require pleurodesis
Polymyositis/ dermatomyositis	Effusion Fibrosis	Rare (PM) Rare (PM)	Lymphocytic or plasma cell infiltration of pleura	Small volume noted postmortem	No clinical importance
Scleroderma	Pleural adhesions Pleural fibrosis Effusions	67% (PM) 86% (PM) Rare	Direct pleural involvement by systemic disease	Analysis not reported	No clinical importance
Ankylosing spondylitis	Effusion Fibrosis Pneumothorax	Rare Common 8%	Subpleural infection; noninfectious inflammation; *Aspergillus* colonization; rupture of subpleural bullae	Small to moderate Serous exudate Normal glucose	No clinical importance
Churg-Strauss syndrome	Effusion	29%	Inflammation of pleura or pulmonary infarction	Serous-bloody Eosinophilia	Responds to corticosteroids
Behçet's syndrome	Effusion Chylothorax	< 5% Several reports	SVC obstruction Thoracic duct rupture	Transudate Chylothorax	Resistant cases require chemical pleurodesis

Reproduced with permission from Sahn SA.[198]

ANA = antinuclear antibody; IC = immune complex; IV = intravenous; LDH = lactate dehydrogenase; PM = postmortem; PMN = polymorphonuclear leukocyte; RF = rheumatoid factor; SVC = superior vena cava; LE = lupus erythematosus.

bronchopleural fistula and pyopneumothorax. In other cases, empyema develops in the face of active articular disease, suggesting a direct role of the rheumatic process in its development.

Treatment and Prognosis.   Most rheumatoid pleural effusions are small and do not cause significant symptoms; therefore, no specific treatment is necessary. The rheumatoid pleural effusion usually resolves over several months (usually within an average of 14 months) and often with no serious complications developing after the pleurisy.[215] Rarely, the patient may develop a trapped lung.[203] Rheumatoid pleural effusions respond to corticosteroids and other immunosuppressive agents.[203] Repeated thoracentesis and intrapleural instillation of corticosteroids may be effective in the management of large or recurrent symptomatic effusions.[219,220]

Spontaneous pneumothorax is a complication of RA.[221,222] It is due to the rupture of a necrobiotic nodule and may lead to a bronchopleural fistula that is difficult to treat, requiring prolonged chest tube drainage or surgical intervention.[223] The triad of rheumatoid lung disease, pneumothorax, and peripheral eosinophilia has been described.[224,225] Secondary pneumothorax has also been reported following the initiation of treatment (methotrexate) for rheumatoid nodules.[226] Finally, spon-

taneous pneumomediastinum in a patient with RA has also been presented.[227]

Thoracic Cage Immobility

Although thoracic cage immobility is more characteristic of ankylosing spondylitis, the potential for abnormal thoracic mechanics exists in RA because of increased thoracic rigidity, pleurisy, and/or rheumatoid myopathy.[52,228]

SYSTEMIC LUPUS ERYTHEMATOSUS

General Features

Systemic lupus erythematosus (SLE) is an autoimmune disease with protean manifestations in each organ system (Table 21–5).[229–235] Although a wide array of laboratory abnormalities may be found in SLE, most characteristic is the demonstration of antibodies reactive to nuclear and extractable nuclear antigens including antibodies to single- and double-stranded deoxyribonucleic acid (DNA), nuclear ribonucleoprotein, Smith (Sm) antigen, Ro/SS-A, and La/SS-B/Ha.[236–243] Antibodies to phospholipids may also occur in patients with SLE, leading to thrombophilia.

The original description of SLE is credited to Kaposi in 1872.[244] Soon thereafter, Osler described a 24-year-old female with progressive pulmonary consolidation complicating an erythematous and purpuric skin eruption, she later succumbed to an acute nephritis. He wrote, "It is likely that the recurring skin lesions, the pleuro-pneumonia, the phlebitis, the general glandular enlargement, and the fatal nephritis were due to one and the same poison."[245] Since that time, it has become apparent that any portion of the respiratory tract as well as the pleura may be involved in patients with SLE (Table 21–6). The specific pathologic patterns of disease in SLE have not been described using current ILD terminology.[103] The patterns of interstitial lung disease listed in Table 21–6 include those for which well-documented histologic descriptions or pathologic specimens have been reported.

Pleuropulmonary Manifestations of Systemic Lupus Erythematosus

Interstitial Lung Disease

Epidemiology. Since Osler's original description of pulmonary consolidation in SLE, numerous reports of parenchymal abnormalities have appeared.[245] In the 1940s, these were variously described as "...long bouts of waxing and waning, migratory bronchopneumonia...,"[246] "....atelectising pneumonitis,"[247] and a "...focal allergic pneumonia."[248] Early roentgenographic series noted acute, recurrent, and migratory pneumonic opacities in 15 to 68% of cases.[249–255] Such reports demonstrate both the challenge that clinicians face when determining the etiology of radiographic opacities in a patient with SLE, and the confusion that persists with respect to the pathogenesis of parenchymal lung involvement in SLE.

Some form of pleuropulmonary disease is found in 38 to 89% of cases at some point in their disease course.[254,256–258] The exact form of pulmonary disease is difficult to determine in an individual patient with SLE, partially accounting for the discrepancy in the reported frequency of disease. Three pathologic patterns of ILD have been recognized in patients with SLE: acute lupus pneumonitis (acute interstitial pneumonia or diffuse alveolar damage), chronic interstitial pneumonia (nonspecific interstitial pneumonia), and LIP.

Pathogenesis. Systemic lupus erythematosus is characterized by B-cell hyperactivity, multiple autoantibodies directed against lymphocytes, and impaired T-lymphocyte functions. Although the etiology of SLE is unclear, the mechanism of tissue injury, especially in the kidney and blood vessels, most likely involves immune complexes.[259,260] Elevated levels of antinative DNA antibodies precede disease flares, while reduced anti-ds DNA levels and serum complement are associated with active renal disease, presumably because of deposition and/or consumption at the time of active disease.[261,262] In addition, the renal deposition of immunoglobulin and complement has been identified by immunofluorescence, and both DNA and antinative DNA antibodies have been eluted from the glomeruli of patients with SLE nephritis.[263,264] Elevated levels of circulating immune complexes may be related to an associated defect in Fc-receptor function, thereby prolonging the circulation of such complexes and potentially aggravating tissue damage.[265–268]

Investigations into the pathogenesis of extrarenal lesions are less extensive, in part because of the inaccessibility of tissue.[269] Nonetheless, several lines of evidence tend to implicate immune complexes in the pathogenesis of lupus-related lung disease.

First, experimental models of immune complex pulmonary injury have been developed that resemble the human disease. In the rat, an acute, hemorrhagic, neu-

---

TABLE 21–5 Systemic Lupus Erythematosus: Clinical Manifestations by Organ System

Organ System	Manifestation
Skin/mucosa	Butterfly rash, photosensitivity, Raynaud's phenomenon, discoid lesions, alopecia, erythematous maculopapular eruptions, urticaria, mucosal ulceration
Bone	Nonerosive arthropathy, arthralgias
Cardiovascular	Pericarditis, myocarditis, endocarditis, coronary artery disease, vasculitis
Renal	Glomerulonephritis, interstitial nephritis
Central nervous system	Stroke, seizure, psychosis or other psychiatric disease
Miscellaneous	Myositis, splenic disease, cytopenias

TABLE 21–6 Pleuropulmonary Manifestations of Systemic Lupus Erythematosus

Interstitial lung disease
  Acute lupus pneumonitis
  Nonspecific interstitial pneumonia
  Organizing pneumonia
  Lymphocytic interstitial pneumonia
  Diffuse alveolar hemorrhage

Airway disease
  Upper airway dysfunction
    (epiglottitis, laryngitis, cricoarytenoid arthritis)
  Bronchiectasis
  Bronchiolitis obliterans

Diaphragmatic disease
  Diaphragmatic dysfunction
  Shrinking lungs

Pleural disease
  Pleurisy with or without pleural effusion

Pulmonary vascular disease
  Thromboembolic disease
  Vasculitis
  Pulmonary hypertension

Mediastinal and axillary lymphadenopathy

Infection

trophil-rich injury is generated after the intrabronchial administration of heterologous antibody and intravenous administration of antigen. Both antigen and antibody are demonstrated in the alveoli and interstitium by immunofluorescence.[270] A more chronic and occasionally fibrotic interstitial pneumonitis is produced in rabbits after chronic intravenous administration of bovine serum albumin. Antigens, immunoglobulins, and smaller amounts of complement (C)3 deposit in the alveolar capillaries and interstitium.[271] Most interesting is the presence of coarse deposits of immunoglobulin (but not C3) in the perivascular, peribronchial, and interstitial areas in NZB (New Zealand black) or NZW (New Zealand white) mice, which, on light microscopy, demonstrate a lymphoplasmacytic interstitial infiltrate.[272]

Second, specific autoantibodies have been associated with some of the pulmonary manifestations of SLE. Interstitial pneumonitis, for example, has been associated with SS-A,[273,274] leading to speculation that immune complexes with anti–SS-A (Ro) antibodies might be selectively deposited within the lung and responsible for initiating the inflammatory response. In addition, specific autoantibodies may provide part of the explanation for a given SLE patient's pulmonary disease. Although SSA is frequently found in patients with pneumonitis, it is rarely found in patients with serositis/pleuritis.[275] Interestingly, plasmapheresis has been an effective therapy in case reports of patients with SLE with acute lupus pneumonitis or alveolar hemorrhage, further suggesting the importance of circulating immune complexes in mediating such lung disease.[276–278] However, other serologic markers suggestive of immune complex mediation of disease, such as complement levels,[279,280] have not consistently been associated with pulmonary disease activity.

Third, demonstration of pulmonary immune deposits in human SLE provides circumstantial evidence of their involvement in this process. Immunoglobulin with and without complement has been found within the alveolar walls and capillaries in patients with interstitial pneumonitis.[281–283] The antinuclear antibody concentration of immunoglobulin eluded from lung (and spleen) appears higher than in serum, suggesting an enrichment at these sites, perhaps related to the local presence of nuclear antigen.[283] This increased antinuclear antibody concentration in the lung would seem consistent with the demonstration of DNA, IgG, and C3 by immunofluorescence in lung tissue from acute lupus pneumonitis associated with the elution of antibody with anti-DNA activity from the tissue.[284] Similarly, immune complex deposition within alveolar septae as well as along the alveolar membrane, the capillary basement membranes and subendothelium, large blood vessels, and bronchioles has been demonstrated by both immunofluorescence and electron microscopy in individuals with SLE-associated pulmonary hemorrhage.[285–289] Immune complexes in pleural fluid have been described as well.[212] Furthermore, recent compar-

ison of patients with SLE renal disease and alveolar hemorrhage demonstrated immune complex deposition mediating microvascular damage and induction of apoptosis in both the lung and the kidney.[290] However, other studies have failed to find interstitial deposition of immunoglobulin both in SLE pneumonitis and in pulmonary hemorrhage.[281,291,292]

Acute Lupus Pneumonitis.   *Clinical Features.* Acute lupus pneumonitis is characterized by the acute or subacute onset of tachycardia, tachypnea, dyspnea, cyanosis, and cough.[253,284] Fever is common, but hemoptysis is infrequent, and clubbing is absent.[251,284,293] The mean age in one series was 38 years with a mean duration of known SLE of 16 months (range 0 to 48 months).[293] In 50% of these patients, pneumonitis was the presenting manifestation of their SLE. Chest examination may reveal fine or coarse rales, but signs of pleurisy are rare. In severe cases, evidence of right ventricular overload may appear.

Roentgenographic Features.   The chest radiograph plays a limited role in the differential diagnosis of pulmonary complications of SLE. The most common findings in patients with SLE are nonspecific areas of air space consolidation.[294] The consolidation may be unilateral or bilateral and focal or diffuse, but it tends to involve mainly the lower lung zones. The most common cause of consolidation is pneumonia.[294,295] However, acute lupus pneumonitis, pulmonary hemorrhage, and, occasionally, OP can result in similar radiologic findings.

Chest roentgenograms in the acute lupus syndrome demonstrate diffuse or patchy opacities that are predominantly basilar, although the middle and upper zones may be affected.[245,284,293] Usually bilateral, the opacities may be accompanied by pleural effusion and cardiomegaly. A recent case report described acute lupus pneumonitis in a patient with a normal chest radiograph and HRCT scan.[296] Subacute cases may demonstrate the migratory, recurrent, polymorphic densities discussed previously.

Physiologic Features.   Marked hypoxemia and hyperventilation are often described in acute pneumonitis.[297] Such deficits, in particular an elevation of the alveolar-arterial gradient, persist in the majority (of a small number) of patients despite the apparent resolution of their lung disease.[297]

Histopathologic Features.   The histopathologic pattern most common in acute lupus pneumonitis syndrome is that of diffuse alveolar damage characterized by interstitial edema and hyaline membrane formation.[153,293] A mononuclear cell infiltration of the interstitium may also be present, whereas vasculitis is uncommon.[284,293,298,299]

Other pathologic patterns may be seen in a patient with SLE presenting with an acute or subacute illness, including organizing pneumonia, lymphoplasmacytic infiltrate with lymphoid nodules and germinal centers, desquamative interstitial pneumonia, pulmonary infarction, and hemorrhage.[281,300]

Diagnosis.   Patients with SLE can develop acute respiratory failure from infection, congestive heart failure, uremia, drug reactions, and diffuse pulmonary hemorrhage. For this reason, lung biopsies can be very helpful to distinguish infection from underlying disease because the choice between antibiotic versus immunosuppressive therapy is critical.

The major differential diagnosis is that of an infectious pneumonia. An aggressive diagnostic approach should be undertaken using appropriate stains, cultures, and serologic tests to rule out this possibility. In milder cases it is often difficult to determine when to obtain these tests because spontaneous clearing of opacities[301] or a rapid response to corticosteroids has been noted.[302] BAL and transbronchial biopsy should be considered in the immunosuppressed lupus patient or in any patient that shows progression of the disease over 24 to 72 hours following presentation. Surgical (open or thoracoscopic) lung biopsy should be considered prior to the initiation of high-dose corticosteroid or immunosuppressive therapy (unless this therapy is indicated for management of other major organ system disease). Serial pulmonary function evaluation (before, during, after therapy) is invaluable in assessing the objective response.

Management and Prognosis.   Corticosteroids are reported to be effective in some cases of acute lupus pneumonitis, yet clinical deterioration while on corticosteroids also occurs.[293,301,303,304] Azathioprine, cyclophosphamide, or methotrexate may be a useful adjunctive agent in patients unresponsive to corticosteroids.[293,305–307] Therefore, employment of high-dose corticosteroids seems reasonable in severely ill patients with acute pneumonitis, adding azathioprine early for refractory cases. Beginning both agents simultaneously may be justified in severely impaired patients. Plasmapheresis, in conjunction with both high-dose parenteral steroids and cyclophosphamide, has been reported effective in a single case unresponsive to corticosteroids.[278]

Harvey and coworkers reported 3 of 38 deaths (7.9%) from lupus pneumonitis (2 were acute lupus pneumonitis),[251] more recent reviews either do not mention lupus pneumonitis as a cause of death or note lupus pneumonitis and/or acute pulmonary hemorrhage as causing death in only 2.5% of cases.[255,308] Matthay and colleagues recorded a 50% mortality rate from acute lupus pneumonitis, emphasizing the lethal potential of this syndrome.[293] Among the survivors, persistent ventilatory impairment was common. The progression of recurrent acute lupus pneumonitis to chronic ILD occurs, although the low incidence of chronic fibrotic disease would suggest that this progression is unusual. This lack of progression to chronic disease may relate to the shortened survival of patients with acute pneumonitis, the use of intensive corticosteroid therapy, or a propensity to recovery among survivors.

Chronic Interstitial Pneumonia.   *Clinical Features.*   Chronic ILD is an uncommon manifestation of SLE. Most investigators believe that there is an evolution from acute to chronic ILD because there are examples of persistent disease after an acute onset,

mixed acute and chronic roentgenographic patterns, histopathologic evidence of transition from an inflammatory cellular infiltrate to a fibrotic lesion, and the somewhat younger ages of the acute (mean age 38 years) as apposed to the chronic (mean age 46 years) cases.[248,253,293,309,310] Histologically, a cellular interstitial pneumonitis is far more prominent than is the fibrotic stage, even in autopsy studies.[299,311]

The mean age at presentation in one series was 46 years, with duration of SLE of 9.6 years (range 3 to 23 years). Dyspnea, cough, and pleuritic chest discomfort are common presentation manifestations. Examination demonstrates rapid, shallow breathing, decreased thoracic expansion, basilar dullness, and basilar or diffuse dry rales. Cyanosis is occasionally seen, as is clubbing, but the latter appears to be less common than in RA interstitial disease.[49,300,310,312] Cor pulmonale may also occur.

Roentgenographic Features.   Evidence of chronic interstitial opacities is found on the chest radiograph in approximately 3% of patients with SLE. However, several studies have demonstrated a considerably higher prevalence of chronic interstitial changes on HRCT, even in asymptomatic patients without known lung involvement (Table 21–7).[313–315] Multiple patterns have been reported.[282,310] The most common findings are intralobular interstitial thickening and irregular thickening of the interlobular septa that are predominantly or exclusively found in the lower lobes.[314,315] Other common findings seen on HRCT include traction bronchiectasis (architectural distortion and bronchial dilatation secondary to the fibrosis), small foci of air space consolidation, and areas of ground-glass attenuation.[313–315] Honeycomb changes may be present. Both pleural effusions and cardiomegaly may be noted.[246] Enlargement of the pulmonary arteries accompanies cor pulmonale.[282]

Quantitative gallium-67 lung scanning and technetium Tc-99m hexamethylpropyleneamine oxime uptake may have a limited role in identifying the severity of lung injury in SLE.[316,317]

Physiologic Features.   The detection of subclinical interstitial disease by physiologic testing is complicated by the potential presence of many pleuropulmonary, neuromuscular, and vascular lesions that may coexist in SLE. Nevertheless, several studies indicate that physiologic abnormalities (eg, DL_{CO}, lung volumes, or compliance) are more common than clinical or roentgenographic changes.[318–321]

The most common physiologic deficit in patients with SLE is the reduction in diffusing capacity with or without decreased total lung capacity.[279,320,322,323]

Among patients with normal chest roentgenograms, a reduction in VC was noted in 27% and in DL_{CO} in 67%.[324] In two series of unselected patients, a reduction in DL_{CO} occurred more frequently (72 to 80%) than did volume restriction (43 to 49%) or roentgenographic abnormalities (30 to 50%).[279,325] Thus, it appears that a subpopulation of patients with SLE manifests functional defects without clinically obvious pulmonary disease.

TABLE 21–7   Systemic Lupus Erythematosus: High-Resolution Computed Tomography Findings

	Bankier (1995)[313]	Fenlon (1996)[314]	Ooi (1997)[315]
Demographic information			
Number of subjects	48	34	10
Symptomatic patients (% of subjects)	0	23	100
Computed tomography features (% of subjects)			
Pleural thickening	13	15	80
Interlobular septal thickening	33	44	21
Bronchiectasis	18	21	13
Ground-glass opacities	13	6	94
Consolidation	7	6	7

Whether these individuals represent subclinical ILD is unclear. Pathologic confirmation or long-term follow-up will be necessary to clarify this point.

In a study that examined the CT appearance of early lung involvement in SLE of 45 patients with normal chest radiographs, 17 (38%) had abnormal CT findings.[313] The extent of disease was statistically significantly correlated with the duration of clinical history ($r = .93$) and a decreased single-breath diffusing capacity for carbon monoxide ($r = .8$) and ratio of forced expiratory volume in 1 second to forced vital capacity ($r = .77$).[313]

The few reports of exercise testing in patients with SLE demonstrate decreased aerobic capacity, regardless of patients' symptoms. Although this is not consistently attributable to respiratory limitations, multiple studies demonstrate that patients with SLE have a resting respiratory alkalosis and excessive ventilation for a given workload.[321,326]

Bronchoalveolar Lavage.   Few studies have assessed BAL findings in patients with SLE (see Table 21–3).[327–330] Table 21–8 presents the lavage findings in 26 patients with SLE without pulmonary dysfunction.[328] The cellular findings are not different from that commonly found in normal subjects. The CD4+/CD8+ ratio was significantly reduced in SLE compared with normal.[330] In patients with SLE with mild to severe pulmonary function abnormalities, the lymphocyte number and percentage was reduced compared with healthy controls.[331] Moreover, there was a significant correlation between diffusing capacity and BAL lymphocyte phenotype number and proportions. Wallaert and coworkers[328] demonstrated that the antibacterial activity of alveolar macrophages was abnormal in the presence of a normal respiratory burst (O_2 release) when compared with that from control subjects.

Histopathologic Features.   The pathology of the chronic interstitial disease remains poorly defined with several patterns being found: nonspecific interstitial pneumonia (NSIP), UIP, and LIP (Figure 21–5). More advanced disease results in fibrosis, parenchymal destruction, and cystic change (honeycomb lung).[310,312] A classic UIP pattern is very unusual in SLE. However, cases with a histologic pattern resembling NSIP have been

reported.[332,333] Several cases of OP have been described in SLE.[334,335] A variety of lymphoid lesions have been reported in patients with SLE, including LIP,[336] nodular lymphoid hyperplasia,[337] bronchus-associated lymphoid tissue (BALT) hyperplasia, and malignant lymphoma.[338]

Management and Prognosis.   Little is known about the therapeutic responsiveness of chronic interstitial disease. The response is thought to be poor.[304,312] We are aware of no documented cases of death due solely from chronic interstitial disease in SLE, although it may be contributory in some instances.[312]

Airway Disease in Systemic Lupus Erythematosus

Upper Airway Disease.   An acute epiglottiditis, laryngitis, cricoarytenoid arthritis, vocal cord edema, and necrotizing tracheitis have all been described.[234,339]

Bronchiectasis and Bronchiolitis.   Large airway obstruction is uncommon in SLE, although physiologic evidence of subclinical respiratory dysfunction, such as small airway disease, has been demonstrated.[322,340,341] Lung function abnormalities consistent with small airway disease were the only parameters that demonstrated a decline in patients with SLE followed over at least 2 years.[322] Chest HRCT in SLE has identified bronchiectasis in a greater number of subjects than previously suspected.[314] Steroid responsive bronchiolitis obliterans has also been reported.[342]

Pleural Disease

Chest pain is common in patients with SLE (~50% of patients) and most often results from musculoskeletal problems. Pleural disease (ie, adhesions, thickening, or effusions) may be found at autopsy in up to 93% of cases[234]; however, clinically apparent disease is less frequent.[203] Pleurisy with or without effusion occurs in up to half of patients with SLE during the course of their illness.[234,238,239,242–245,250,254,256,257,339,343–345] Pleuritic pain is common and usually present when there is an effusion.[198,199]

The pleural effusions found in SLE are usually bilateral and are an exudate (see Table 21–3). Higher glucose

TABLE 21–8   Systemic Lupus Erythematosus: Bronchoalveolar Lavage Cellular Data

	Wallaert (1987)[328]	Martinot (1989)[329]	Nagai (1989)[330]
Clinical parameters			
n	17	4	5
Age, yr	29	34	
Gender F/M	13/4	4/0	
Smoking history	17 nonsmoker	4 nonsmoker	5 nonsmoker
Bronchoalveolar lavage findings *			
Total cell count, x10^4/mL	16.1 ± 11.7	6.4 ± 1.8	35.9 ± 0.92
Macrophages, %	88.2 ± 8.8	80.8 ± 7.8	
Lymphocytes, %	10 ± 8.1	16.2 ± 8.3	49.3 ± 9.5
Neutrophils, %	1.2 ± 1.5	3 ± 2	1.6 ± 0.7
Eosinophils, %	0	0	0.8 ± 0.8
CD4$^+$/CD8$^+$			0.54 ± 0.14

*Data presented as mean ± SD.

(greater than 60 mg/dL) and lower lactate dehydrogenase (LDH less than 500 U/L) levels are found in SLE compared with that found in RA[198,199,212]; antinuclear antibodies and antinative DNA antibodies may be found in the fluid, as well as LE cells.[346–348] The latter are highly specific for lupus pleuritis. Although the levels of immune complexes in pleural fluid from SLE correspond to serum levels, complement may be relatively lower and the antinuclear antibody titer higher.[211,212,344] This difference between the serum and pleural fluid suggests a local intrapleural immunologic reaction. Spontaneous hemothorax with underlying subpleural hemorrhage and hemopneumothorax have also been described.[349,350] Lupus pleuritis/pleural effusion responds quite well to nonsteroidal anti-inflammatory drugs and corticosteroids. Spontaneous pneumothorax is very rare in SLE.[351]

Pulmonary Vascular Disease

Vasculitis.   Although features of cor pulmonale may complicate both acute and chronic pneumonitis in SLE, descriptions of a primary pulmonary vascular disease without parenchymal disease are infrequent.[282,293,352] However, pulmonary hypertension has been uncommonly reported in association with vascular lesions and is characterized by necrosis, intimal fibrosis, thickening, and muscular hypertrophy.[353,354] Thrombotic changes (intimal thickening, occlusion with recanalization, and new thrombi) associated with plexiform lesions have been described.[352] Raynaud's phenomenon is almost uniformly present in such cases.[353,355] Notably, small vessel vasculitis may occur in patients with antiphospholipid antibody syndrome (APS) alone, even in the absence of SLE.[356]

Pulmonary Hypertension.   Pulmonary hypertension may be seen in SLE patients, either associated with or without the APS. In those patients with SLE with APS, the prevalence of pulmonary hypertension is 1.8%, and the majority of cases (80%) are not attributable to thromboembolic disease.[357] Patients with SLE with antitopoisomerase I antibodies (in the absence of evidence of systemic sclerosis) are also at significantly increased risk for pulmonary hypertension.[358]

Control of the underlying disease activity appears key in the management of pulmonary hypertension in patients with SLE. Patients with SLE refractory to standard treatment for pulmonary hypertension, may respond to immunosuppressants (steroids and cyclophosphamide).[359]

Thromboembolism.   Thromboembolism occurs in up to 25% of patients with SLE and is a major cause of death. Pulmonary emboli may be associated with pulmonary vascular disease, and an association between the lupus anticoagulant and thromboembolism has been reported.[360,361] Pulmonary complications associated with presence of antiphospholipid antibodies (lupus anticoagulant and anticardiolipin) include pulmonary embolism and infarction, both thromboembolic and perhaps nonthromboembolic pulmonary hypertension, pulmonary arterial thrombosis, pulmonary microthrombosis, adult respiratory distress syndrome, intra-alveolar pulmonary hemorrhage, as well as a postpartum syndrome characterized by spiking fever, pleuritic chest pain, dyspnea, pleural effusion, and patchy opacities on the chest radiograph.[362] Optimal therapy is unknown; however, most patients are treated with long-term anticoagulant therapy.

Acute Reversible Hypoxemia Syndrome.   A syndrome of acute reversible hypoxemia in acutely ill, hospitalized patients has been recently reported.[280,363] No association with parenchymal lung disease was identified. The widened A-aO$_2$ gradient found in these patients was associated with diffusion abnormalities. It is postulated that complement-activated neutrophil aggregation in the pulmonary vasculature is the major mechanism leading to these abnormalities. Elevated

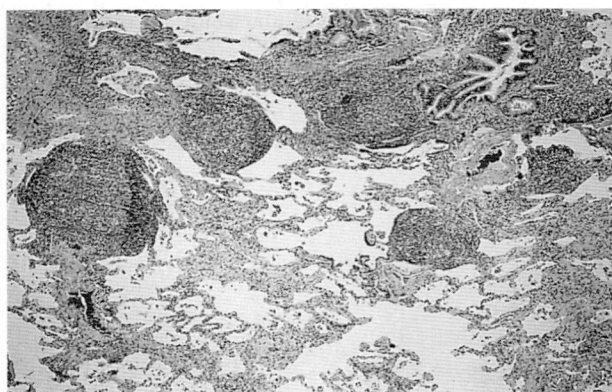

Figure 21–5   Systemic lupus erythematosus. Chronic cellular and fibrosing interstitial infiltrate in a woman with longstanding systemic lupus erythematosus. There are areas of lymphoid hyperplasia and an interstitial infiltrate of chronic inflammatory and immune effector cells with interstitial fibrosis (hematoxylin and eosin).

plasma levels of complement split products have been identified. In addition, up-regulation of endothelial cell adhesion molecules (E-selectin, vascular cell adhesion molecule 1 [VCAM-1], and intercellular adhesion molecule 1 [ICAM-1]) is most marked in patients with active disease characterized by significant elevations of the complement split product C3a desArg.[364] These investigators suggested that in certain patients with SLE, excessive complement activation in association with primed endothelial cells induces leukocyte-endothelial cell adhesion and leuko-occlusive vasculopathy.[364] A good response to high-dose corticosteroid therapy is usually found. Treatment with high-dose aspirin and moderate to low doses of corticosteroids may be sufficient to improve the pulmonary manifestations but may not be adequate to control the systemic activity of the disease.[363]

Pulmonary Hemorrhage

Epidemiology.   Pulmonary hemorrhage occurs infrequently (< 5% in general) in patients with SLE, although the reported frequency of disease varies with the population studied and the definition of disease.[250,251,277,285–288,291,365–373] In a study from the University of Colorado, there were 19 episodes of diffuse alveolar hemorrhage (DAH) over a 10-year period, which represented 3.7% of the admissions for complications of SLE.[374] The majority of patients were young women.

Clinical Manifestations.   (See Chapter 23, "Diffuse Alveolar Hemorrhage.") Pulmonary hemorrhage may be the primary or sole manifestation of SLE. In 11 to 20% of patients, pulmonary hemorrhage was the initial manifestation of SLE.[374] However, recent reports in a Korean cohort indicated that 83% of patients presenting with DAH had not been previously diagnosed with SLE.[277] It is certain, however, that patients may present at any time after their diagnosis of SLE.

The onset is often abrupt: < 3 days.[374] Temperature elevation (> 38°C) occurs infrequently (26%). Hemoptysis is present in 42 to 66% of patients at presentation.[374] It will develop in all patients during the clinical course. Thus, the absence of hemoptysis should not exclude this diagnosis, particularly in those patients who experience an acute pulmonary syndrome with new radiographic infiltrates accompanied by a falling hematocrit and the presence of a hemorrhagic BAL fluid.[374] A history lupus nephritis is seen in virtually all patients.[277,373,374]

Diagnosis.   Bronchoalveolar lavage may be useful in suggesting the diagnosis of pulmonary hemorrhage by finding frank blood or blood-tinged BAL fluid, free red blood cells, red blood cells inside alveolar macrophages, or hemosiderin-laden macrophages.[375,376] A hemosiderin scoring system has been developed that is useful in defining the intensity of the hemosiderin content, (score > 100) which correlates with the presence of significant pulmonary hemorrhage.[377–379] Hemosiderin-laden macrophages appear approximately 48 hours following the onset of pulmonary hemorrhage.[380]

Roentgenographic Features.   Chest radiographs and CT scans show extensive alveolar opacities (see Chapter 23, Figure 23–8).[381,382] In addition to the presence of intra-alveolar erythrocytes and hemosiderin-laden macrophages, the pattern of diffuse alveolar damage has been reported. Alveolar septal fibrosis may follow repeated episodes of pulmonary hemorrhage. Pulmonary capillaritis accompanies pulmonary hemorrhage in many patients and appears to be more frequent than previously reported.[374] Focal polymorphonuclear infiltration of arterioles and venules with associated alveolar wall destruction has been described, although most studies note an absence of vasculitis.

Management and Prognosis.   Although respiratory failure and death occur frequently, responses to corticosteroids and/or immunosuppressive agents have been reported. Treatment with plasmapheresis may benefit some patients but the use of plasmapheresis does not appear to improve survival in most patients.[374,383,384] Early treatment (within the first 48 h after the onset of the acute event) and high-dose methylprednisolone (> 4 g) treatment seem to improve outcome.[385]

Although complete resolution of pulmonary hemorrhage and a 75% survival rate was found in a recent study,[371] this is in marked contrast to previous reports where the overall survival rate was 38.2 to 50.0%.[277,374,385] Factors associated with an increased mortality include the need for mechanical ventilation, the presence of infection, and the need for cyclophosphamide therapy.

Diaphragmatic Dysfunction and "Shrinking Lung Syndrome"

Clinical Manifestations.   Diaphragmatic dysfunction characterized clinically by dyspnea, sometimes progressive in nature, and radiographically by poor motion and elevation of the diaphragm associated with the basilar atelectasis, is a well-recognized syndrome in SLE (so-called "shrinking" or "vanishing" lung syndrome).[257,386-388] Recent review of 49 documented cases of shrinking lung syndrome in the literature revealed that it was infrequently the presenting manifestation of SLE.[389] The most common symptoms included dyspnea and pleuritic chest pain.[389,390] In only a third of patients is there evidence of a myopathy.[389] A high rate of SS-A positivity has also been reported.[390,391]

Physiologic Features. The demonstration of restrictive impairment is usually present.[389,390] Studies of respiratory mechanics in SLE have demonstrated the frequent occurrence of inspiratory and expiratory muscle weakness, with a reduction in maximal transdiaphragmatic pressures.[325,392-395]

Roentgenographic Features. The hallmark of disease is elevation of the hemidiaphragms radiographically, usually in the absence of parenchymal lung disease.[390]

Management and Prognosis. Improvement has been reported with inhaled beta-agonist[396] and theophylline therapy.[397] In the follow-up of patients with SLE with shrinking lung syndrome, stabilization or improvement in disease has also been reported with the use of corticosteroids, methotrexate, cyclophosphamide, or azathioprine.[390]

Atelectasis

Atelectasis has long been noted at necropsy in SLE, and plate-like or linear basilar shadows are frequently described roentgenographically.[347,250,253,254,257,301,309,398,399] Atelectasis can be seen in the absence of diaphragmatic elevation. The mechanisms responsible are not known.

Pulmonary Infection

Pulmonary infections outnumber clinically significant SLE pneumonitis 34:1 and are an important cause of mortality.[251,324] The necessity of excluding infection as the cause of a pleuropulmonary abnormality in a patient with SLE cannot be overemphasized, especially in the face of corticosteroid therapy or renal insufficiency.[251,400-402] Recent investigations have assessed noninvasive techniques (serum procalcitonin levels or neutrophil CD64 expression) as a means of making the critical distinction between infectious and noninfectious inflammation in patients with SLE.[403,404]

PROGRESSIVE SYSTEMIC SCLEROSIS (SCLERODERMA)

Definition and General Features

Scleroderma (progressive systemic sclerosis [PSS]) is a systemic disease characterized by a progressive dermatologic abnormality. Scleroderma is not a common disorder, with an annual incidence rate of 1 to 2 cases per 100,000 population and a US prevalence rate of 26 cases per 100,000 population.[405] It is one-fourth as common as SLE, one-half as common as temporal arteritis, but more common than either polymyositis or polyarteritis.[406] Although more females are diagnosed with scleroderma than males (female to male ratio 6–8:1), males tend to have more extensive disease (female to male ratio 3:1 for diffuse disease).[407,408]

The hallmark of scleroderma is cutaneous involvement, which is commonly accompanied by Raynaud's phenomenon.[63,407,409-411] The extent of skin involvement determines the classification of patients' disease (Table 21–9).

Overall, patients with scleroderma have an increased mortality rate compared with population-matched controls.[408] Limited cutaneous scleroderma has a significantly better prognosis (than diffuse disease or diffuse and intermediate disease) with less internal organ involvement.[407,408,412,413] The 10-year mortality rates for patients with diffuse cutaneous sclerosis range between 38 to 79%.[408]

Although skin involvement serves as a marker for more severe disease, the cause of death in scleroderma patients is usually related to internal organ disease.[407,408,412,413] Systemic involvement in systemic sclerosis may include proliferative vascular and obliterative microvascular abnormalities as well as esophageal and other gastrointestinal involvement (hypomotility or malabsorption), pulmonary, cardiac (pericarditis, congestive heart failure, conduction abnormalities or arrhythmias), renal (renal crisis, renal failure or insufficiency), muscle (weakness associated with elevated serum creatinine kinase with or without electromyographic or histologic evidence of myopathy), and bone disease (arthralgia, stiffness, synovitis).[63,407,408,411-415]

Both the pattern and the rate of development of the organ involvement are determined in part by the subtype of scleroderma present. The diffuse cutaneous disorder is associated with the early appearance of visceral disease, most frequently renal and cardiac.[63,410,411,416,417] The so-called CREST syndrome, denoting *c*alcinosis, *R*aynaud's phenomenon, *e*sophageal dysmotility, *s*clerodactyly, and *t*elangiectasia, is characterized by more restricted skin involvement. Often considered a more indolent variant of scleroderma, the CREST syndrome is nonetheless associated with significant visceral disease, most typically pulmonary hypertension, occurring in the absence of interstitial disease in 8 to 12% of affected individuals.[416-420]

Pathogenesis

Genetics Factors. A wide variety of potential mechanisms have been considered in regard to the pathogenesis of scleroderma. Familial studies of three large US cohorts revealed familial relative risk in intragenerational siblings (lambda) of 15, with the highest familial risk seen in African Americans (lambda = 26).[405] Various HLA class II alleles have been associated with scleroderma in different ethnic groups: DR2 suballeles DRB1*1502 and DRB1*1602 were seen in Japanese and Chocotaw patients, while DRB1*1101-*1104 was seen more frequently in Whites.[421] Similarly the DRB1*11 group was more common in African Americans with scleroderma compared with controls (although not significantly),[421] and DRB1*1104 has also been robustly associated with scleroderma in Greek patients.[422] Angiotensin converting enzyme and endothelial nitric oxide synthase polymorphisms have also been associated with scleroderma.[423] In addition, ethnicity has been associated with lung involvement in scleroderma patients; Japanese and Black North Americans had significantly more lung involvement and a greater decline in pulmonary function than their White counterparts.[421] A positive family history of scleroderma is the strongest risk factor yet identified for scleroderma; however, the absolute risk for each family member remains quite low.[405]

Role of Collagen.   An increase in skin collagen has long been recognized[424]; the skin changes are due to an increase in skin thickness with a proportional increase in collagen.[410] Potential explanations for this phenomenon have included an increase in the synthesis of collagen by fibroblasts,[425,426] an increase in the synthesis of hyaluronic acid,[427] and a lack of inhibition of collagen production.[428] Serum levels of the cross-linked carboxyterminal telopeptide of collagen I (a collagen metabolite) have been shown to be elevated in patients with scleroderma and are inversely correlated with DL_{CO}.[429] The potential contribution of immunologic abnormalities is suggested by the association of scleroderma with other autoimmune disorders, as well as by the presence of antinuclear antibodies in almost all patients.[5,430] Further evidence includes the presence of a lymphocytic infiltrate in scleroderma skin and lung,[424,431,432] evidence of cellular hypersensitivity to collagen,[433] and to extracts of normal and sclerodermatous skin.[434] Moreover, antibodies to fibrillin-1 (an extracellular matrix protein) have been found more frequently in scleroderma patients than in controls (including polymyositis/dermatomyositis patients with or without

ILD).[435] Similarly, antibodies to fibroblasts are also present in the sera of scleroderma patients, particularly those with diffuse disease.[436] The demonstration of lymphokine-enhanced collagen accumulation by fibroblasts in vitro might produce a cyclic process whereby cell-mediated immunity to collagen or other skin components leads to lymphokine production, thus further stimulating collagen synthesis.[437] In addition, the occurrence of a scleroderma-like syndrome in the presumably T-cell mediated chronic graft-versus-host disease has been described.[438]

The presence of vascular and microvascular lesions in multiple organs, as well as the occurrence of sclerosis and parenchymal atrophy as consequences of vascular dysfunction, suggest that the vasculature is an important target organ. LeRoy has postulated that scleroderma may represent repeated episodes of endothelial injury, with the resulting platelet aggregation and mediator release promoting inward migration of smooth muscle cells from the media and intima (the myointimal cell) with subsequent connective tissue deposition.[411] An alternative possibility would relate to interstitial inflammation in the perivascular space, promoting both sclerosis of the interstitium as well as vascular proliferation.[439] The demonstration of a serum factor with selective cytotoxicity for endothelial cells in scleroderma provides a mechanism for microvascular injury, although other investigators have questioned its specificity for scleroderma and the vascular endothelium.[440–442] Another hypothesis invokes the failure of vasoregulation, which leads to hypertension followed by exudation, capillary dilatation, and arterial intimal fibrosis, thereby leading to vascular insufficiency and so causing changes in the connective tissue.[443] Pulmonary capillary endothelial dysfunction has also been associated with decreased endothelial-bound angiotensin converting enzyme activity in patients with scleroderma.[444]

Pleuropulmonary Manifestations of Scleroderma

Pulmonary involvement is common in scleroderma, with clinical and/or roentgenographic evidence of lung

---

TABLE 21–9   Clinical Classification of Progressive Systemic Sclerosis

Classification	Distribution of Skin Changes
Cutaneous subset model	
Limited cutaneous scleroderma	Finger sclerosis, with or without neck or face involvement
Intermediate cutaneous involvement	Sclerosis of the limbs, face, and neck, without truncal involvement
Diffuse cutaneous sclerosis	Distal and truncal sclerosis
Cutaneous subset model	
Limited cutaneous scleroderma	Sclerosis of the distal extremities below the elbows and knees, with or without sclerosis of the neck and face
Diffuse cutaneous scleroderma	Sclerosis of the distal and proximal extremities, with or without truncal involvement
Sine scleroderma (systemic sclerosis)	No cutaneous sclerosis in a patient with typical systemic sclerosis organ involvement, capillary changes, and serum autoantibodies

Reproduced with permission from Ferri C et al.[407]

disease appearing in the majority of patients (Table 21–10).[4,63,445–447] The lung ranks fourth behind the skin, peripheral vasculature, and esophagus in frequency of involvement. With a decline in mortality secondary to renal involvement, lung disease is becoming an important cause of mortality.[411] Multiple studies using a variety of measures of lung involvement, including insensitive tests such as plain chest radiography, show that pulmonary involvement is an important factor in predicting survival (Table 21–10).

Interstitial Lung Disease

Epidemiology. In contrast to other connective tissue diseases, diffuse ILD is the most common pulmonary manifestation of scleroderma, although other lesions can also occur (Table 21–11).[411] Estimates of the incidence of interstitial disease in scleroderma depend on the methods used for its detection. Although neither the absence of symptoms nor roentgenographic signs rule out ILD, both symptoms and roentgenographic changes occur frequently in scleroderma.[448] Traditionally, lung involvement in patients with scleroderma has been defined by physiologic or plain chest radiographic abnormalities.[407,408,413,415]

In spite of such insensitive measures, pulmonary involvement is seen in up to 80% of patients.[407] Roentgenogram surveys in scleroderma have noted interstitial changes in 14 to 67% of cases.[414,448–455] A reduction of the total lung capacity (TLC) has been noted in 32 to 67% with diminution in VC in 11 to 77% of scleroderma patients.[456–459] An increase in static recoil pressure and abnormalities of DL_{CO} have been reported to occur in over 90% of patients.[459–462] As many as 60% of scleroderma patients present with some lung involvement (radiographic disease, restrictive pulmonary function tests, or pulmonary hypertension), with 80% of patients demonstrating lung disease at some point in the course of their disease.[407] Although less extensively studied, decreases in O_2 saturation during exercise have been noted in 27 to 67% of subjects.[460,463] As might be expected, autopsy series reveal a higher incidence of interstitial disease (60 to 100% of cases) and are by their nature more specific than either clinicoradiologic or physiologic surveys.[448,464]

With the exception of involvement of the right side of the heart consistent with cor pulmonale, the degree of pulmonary involvement by PSS is not correlated with the extent of extrapulmonary involvement.[465] However, pulmonary function deficits (in lung volume and diffusion capacity) have a significantly greater rate of decline in patients with persistently positive antitopoisomerase antibodies, as opposed to those whose seropositivity becomes negative over time.[466] Antitopoisomerase antibody as well as antiribonucleic acid (anti-RNA) polymerase are both associated with right-sided heart failure.[415]

Pathogenesis of Pulmonary Fibrosis in Scleroderma. Inflammatory-immunologic factors have been implicated in the pathogenesis of ILD in patients with scleroderma. In a disease in which circulating immunocomplexes are not considered important, patients with

---

TABLE 21–10   Progressive Systemic Sclerosis: Predictors of Outcome

Study	Number of Subjects	Type of Study	Disease Duration before Enrollment	Independent Predictors of Survival
Bryan (1999)[413]	280	Prospective	17 months	DL_{CO} < 70% of predicted ESR Urine protein
Geirsson (2001)[412]	100	Retrospective	5 years	Low TLC Low VC Low static lung compliance Age Skin score
Jacobsen (2001)[415]	174	Retrospective	3.4 years	Restrictive lung disease Right ventricular failure
Ferri (2002)[407]	1,012	Retrospective	0	Pulmonary involvement (fibrosis by chest radiography, restriction on pulmonary function testing, or pulmonary hypertension) Age Renal involvement Cardiac involvement Skin classification
Scussel-Lonzetti (2002)[408]	309	Prospective	0	DL_{CO} < 70% of predicted Age Trunk involvement Anemia Elevated ESR

DL_{CO} = diffusing capacity of carbon monoxide; ESR = erythrocyte sedimentation rate; TLC = total lung capacity; VC = vital capacity.

scleroderma with such complexes have been shown to have an increased incidence of pulmonary disease.[467,468] In addition, a significant increase in anti-Scl-70 antibodies has been noted in scleroderma lung disease.[469] Lung disease in scleroderma has also been correlated with parity, suggesting that microchimerism resulting from the transfer of fetal or maternal cells during pregnancy affects the subsequent pulmonary involvement. The data regarding such an association are conflicting, however, with some investigators noting that patients with more severe lung disease have more children[470] and others finding greater lung disease in women who were never pregnant.[405]

Immune Complexes and Cytokines. Elevations of IgG and immune complexes have also been identified in BAL fluid of patients with scleroderma.[471–473] Collagenase activity is increased in the BAL fluid of patients with elevated BAL lymphocyte/neutrophil counts.[474] CD8+ T lymphocytes from the BAL fluid of patients with scleroderma produce equal amounts of type II cytokines (including interferon (IFN)-γ, Il-4, and IL-5) as compared with the unopposed production of IFN-γ in controls.[475] The production of IL-4 and IL-5 was associated with a subsequent decline in lung function.

The level of fibronectin released from cultured alveolar macrophages from patients with scleroderma is increased[69,476–478] and correlates with the percentage of polymorphonuclear leukocytes and the number of cells/mL: recovered in the lavage.[477,478] In addition, alveolar macrophages from patients with scleroderma have been shown to be activated as assessed by the detection of neutrophil chemotactic activity and the spontaneous release of increased amounts of superoxide anion.[69] Alveolar macrophages of patients with ILD and scleroderma spontaneously release more alveolar-macrophage–derived growth factor (AMDGF) than normal subjects[476] and show significant increases in the expression of specific extracellular matrix receptors, adhesion receptors, and receptors involved in signal transduction or inflamma-

TABLE 21–11   Pleuropulmonary Manifestations of Progressive Systemic Sclerosis

Parenchymal lung disease
  Nonspecific interstitial pneumonia
  Usual interstitial pneumonia
  Diffuse alveolar damage
  Aspiration pneumonia
Airway disease
  Obstructive lung disease
  Bronchiolitis
Vascular disease
  Pulmonary hypertension
  Pulmonary hemorrhage
Pleural disease
  Pleuritis
Miscellaneous
  Spontaneous pneumothorax
  Pulmonary scar carcinoma (bronchogenic carcinoma)

tion.[479] We have recently demonstrated increased expression of IL-8 mRNA and IL-8 protein by alveolar macrophages from patients with IPF and lung fibrosis associated with connective tissue disease, particularly scleroderma.[480] These findings suggest that IL-8 derived from alveolar macrophages is responsible for neutrophil recruitment and activation and further supports the neutrophil's role in the pathogenesis of lung injury.[481] Furthermore, the presence of alveolar-macrophage–derived fibronectin provides a mechanism for the chemoattraction and growth of fibroblasts in the lungs of these patients. In addition, more of the alveolar macrophages of scleroderma patients with fibrosing alveolitis secrete tumor necrosis factor (TNF)-α, and they do so at higher levels than controls or scleroderma patients without fibrosing alveolitis.[482] Macrophage inflammatory protein 1α (MIP-1α) and monocyte chemoattractant factor (MCF-1) are elevated in the serum of scleroderma patients, with significant association with the presence of pulmonary fibrosis.[483]

Collagen and Fibroblast Function. Investigation of the collagen composition in scleroderma interstitial disease notes a similar proportion of types I and III collagen as found in normal lungs.[484] This would seem interesting in view of an increase in type I collagen at the expense of type III seen in IPF,[484] suggesting a slight but basic difference in the fibrotic mechanisms. Also, serum type III procollagen an aminopropeptide of type III collagen, released during conversion into collagen by specific proteases, is increased in patients with scleroderma.[485]

Lung fibroblast function, specifically thrombin regulation of extracellular matrix protein tenascin-C production by protein kinase C, is altered in patients with scleroderma.[486] In addition, protein kinase C is bound to smooth muscle α actin in scleroderma patients, rather than requiring thrombin induction of binding as in normal lung fibroblasts.[487]

Serum Markers. Serum levels of surfactant proteins (SP) A and D are elevated in scleroderma patients with lung disease compared with healthy controls. Interestingly, the levels are highest in those with more severe radiographic disease (lung disease detectable by chest radiography as well as CT as opposed to CT alone), presumably corresponding to the release of SP-A and SP-D into the circulation during epithelial injury. SP-D levels were higher in scleroderma patients' serum than SP-A levels, with elevated SP-D levels having a 77% sensitivity and 83% specificity for CT-demonstrated ILD. The combination of chest radiography demonstrating ILD and SP-D being elevated lead to a sensitivity of 97% and a corresponding specificity of 83%.[488] Other studies comparing the operating characteristics of SP-D to KL-6, a mucin-like glycoprotein expressed on type II pneumocytes as well as bronchiolar epithelial cells, demonstrate equivalent sensitivity and specificity for diagnosing ILD in scleroderma.[489] Other investigators have also shown the utility of KL-6 as a marker of disease activity and pulmonary function in scleroderma patients.[490,491] von Willebrand factor propeptide, as a marker of endothelial activation, may serve as a useful marker of early lung disease in scleroderma patients.[492] This constellation of findings collectively support the hypothesis that inflammatory and immune effector cells modulate the injury and repair process occurring in scleroderma-associated pulmonary fibrosis.

Clinical Manifestations.   Interstitial lung disease in scleroderma is manifested by dyspnea, initially with exertion and later at rest.[449,452,493–495] Because of the marked limitation of physical activity, dyspnea may be denied.[410] Cough, either nonproductive or productive of mucoid or mucopurulent sputum, may be present.[1,5,414,496] Hemoptysis, pleurisy, and fever are uncommon.[7,497]

Physical examination may reveal basilar end-inspiratory rales, and, in those rare individuals with pleurisy, friction rubs may be appreciated. Clubbing, because of the cutaneous restriction and reduction of digital blood flow, is uncommon.[452,493] With advanced ILD, signs of cor pulmonale appear. Pulmonary hypertension may occur in the absence of pulmonary fibrosis and is often the cause of cor pulmonale.[498]

The percentage of patients with lung involvement is significantly greater in those patients with more extensive skin involvement, ranging from 10% of patients with systemic sclerosis without skin involvement to 52% of patients with diffuse cutaneous scleroderma at the time of presentation.[407,408] Although respiratory symptoms commonly follow cutaneous involvement, there are numerous instances of pulmonary symptoms antedating either Raynaud's phenomenon or cutaneous sclerosis.[493,496,499] Intervals as long as 14 years have been reported.[500]

Roentgenographic Features.   Early in ILD, the chest radiograph may be normal or show diffuse mottling with linear densities in the lower lung zones, subsequently giving way to diffuse symmetric reticular opacities (Figure 21–6).[495,499] A picture of recurring opacities with gradual progression has also been described.[450] Reticular or nodular densities may be noted in both CREST syndrome and diffuse scleroderma; a mixed reticular and nodular pattern is more predominant (Figure 21–7). The ILD tends to be basilar in location with sparing of the apices.[495] Areas of cyst formation (honeycombing) may be noted (see Chapter 1, Figure 1–22). On tomography, these cysts are multiple and range in size from a few millimeters up to 2.0 cm.[499] These may rupture, producing spontaneous pneumothorax.[450,495] Parenchymal pulmonary calcification has been described,[1,495] and, in the CREST syndrome, a strikingly high incidence of calcified granulomata has been noted (67%), compared with a 14% incidence in diffuse scleroderma.[455] Pleural effusions and/or pleural thickening are found in 10 to 25% of cases and prominence of the pulmonary arteries in 50%.[448,452,455] There is a poor correlation among the extent of cutaneous disease, symptoms, and the degree of roentgenographic involvement.[445,446,451] Rarely, patients with scleroderma will present with lung involvement prior to the development of classic sclerodermous cutaneous involvement.[501] Serial CT scans may be the best method to assess the disease course in PSS (see Chapter 4, Figure 4–1).[502] In one longitudinal CT series of 40 patients, initially a variety of radiologic features were found including ground-glass opacification (100%), irregular linear opacities (90%), small nodules (70%), honeycombing (33%), traction bronchiectasis (68%), bilateral pleural thickening (45%), and enlarged mediastinal lymph nodes (15%). After a mean follow-up of 40 months, regardless of the initial findings or presence of treatment, the extent of parenchymal disease, including ground-glass opacity and honeycombing, significantly increased with concomitant declines in forced expiratory volume in 1 second (FEV_1), and forced vital capacity (FVC) (without significant change in DL_{CO}).[503]

Physiologic Features.   The pulmonary physiologic abnormalities consist of a restrictive ventilatory defect with impairment of gas exchange.[5,458,460,463] Expiratory flow rates are preserved or reduced commensurate with the low lung volumes. The static compliance of the lung is reduced and is not due to skin tightening of the chest wall.[449,456,496,504] In addition, a reduction in muscle strength is common in scleroderma.[460,505] The major determinant of functional impairment in PSS is the extent of fibrosing alveolitis on CT.[506] Preservation of total lung capacity and depression of KCO are each associated with a history of cigarette smoking.[506]

Abnormalities of the DL_{CO} are sensitive indicators of underlying pathology even in the absence of volume restriction or roentgenographic changes.[63,414,455,459,460,507] The percent predicted DL_{CO} best reflects the extent of fibrosing alveolitis in PSS.[506] Interestingly, variations in the DL_{CO} measurement have been described with changes in the ambient temperature.[508] This is consistent with the reduction in perfusion noted on radionuclide scan after cold exposure, suggesting an intrapulmonary Raynaud's phenomenon.[509]

Arterial blood gases demonstrate normal or reduced O_2 and CO_2 tensions at rest, widening of the alveolar-arterial O_2 gradient, and arterial desaturation on exercise.[1,5,451,459,460,504] Exercise performance is impaired in scleroderma and is associated with an abnormally high ventilatory response to exercise.[458,463,504,506,510] Occult pulmonary impairment is best recognized during cardiopulmonary exercise testing.[510] Also, it is difficult to predict the presence or absence of exercise impairment from the resting blood gas or lung function data in patients with systemic sclerosis.[510] Evaluation of the pulmonary vasculature by right-heart catheterization has demonstrated an increase in pulmonary vascular resistance even in individuals without overt cor pulmonale.[460]

When the functional abnormalities of individuals with diffuse scleroderma and the CREST syndrome are compared, a similar frequency and severity of involvement is seen.[446,455] A tendency toward a lower mean DL_{CO} and a higher VC in the CREST group suggest primary pulmonary vascular disease.[455]

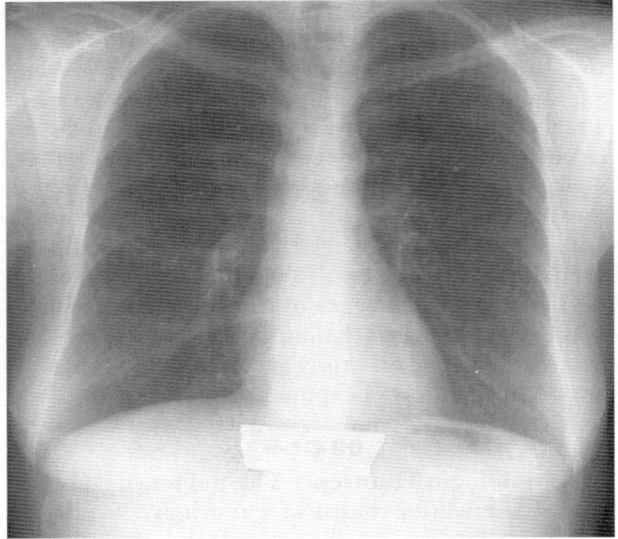

A

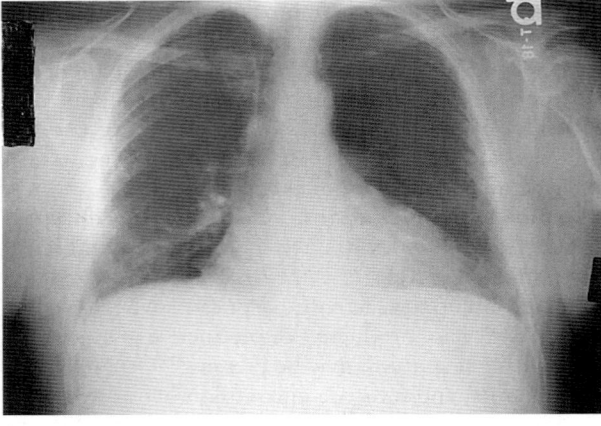

A

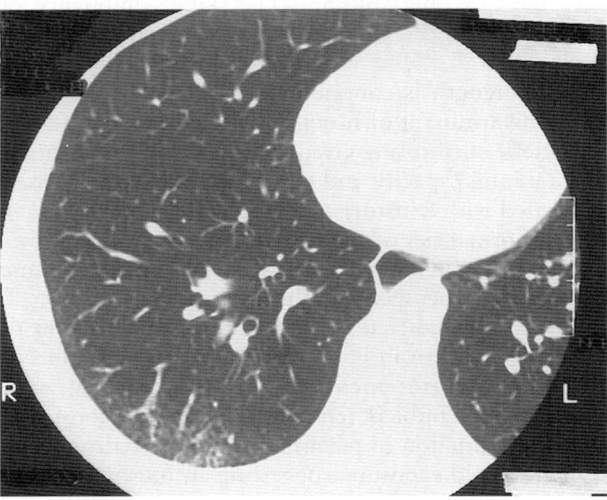

B

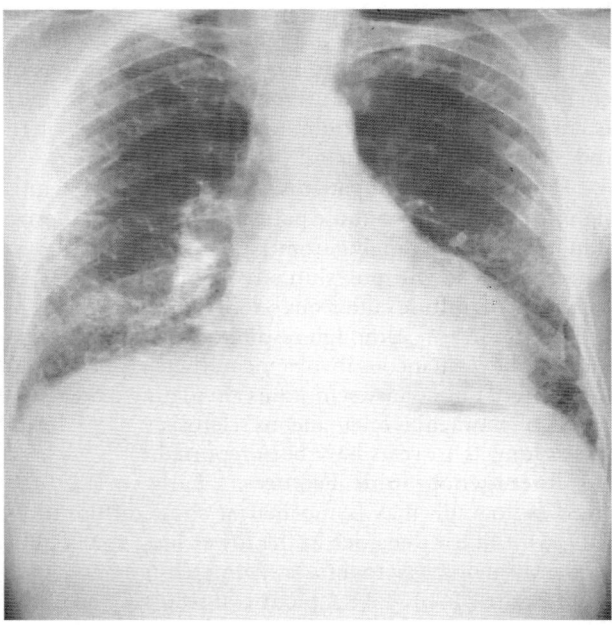

B

Figure 21–6 Progressive systemic sclerosis (scleroderma). *A,* Normal chest roentgenogram in a 34-year-old woman who denied dyspnea and had a normal physical examination. *B,* High-resolution computed tomography scan of the right lower lobe demonstrates fine subpleural reticulation. Bronchoalveolar lavage demonstrated a marked lymphocytosis. She has experienced progressive lung disease.

Figure 21–7 Progressive systemic sclerosis (scleroderma). *A,* Chest roentgenogram showing a mild reticulonodular and interstitial pattern at the bases and mild cardiomegaly. *B,* Chest roentgenogram 6 years later reveals progression of the interstitial opacities with honeycomb changes and pulmonary hypertension.

Bronchoalveolar Lavage.   Bronchoalveolar lavage studies in scleroderma have demonstrated active "alveolitis" (ie, hypercellularity with an increased recovery in the percentage or number of neutrophils, eosinophils, and/or lymphocytes compared with normal controls).[17,511,512] In a series of 103 symptomatic patients, 67% demonstrated elevated neutrophil or eosinophil levels.[512] Shown in Figure 21–8 are lavage differential counts from 115 subjects collected from the literature. Notably, while 11% of scleroderma patients with BAL fluid indicative of alveolitis have normal CT scans,[511] neutrophil percentages or absolute counts were strongly

correlated with the extent of radiographic disease in the lavaged lobe, while eosinophils were not related to the radiographic disease.[513] As can be seen, the PSS patients have a greater proportion of neutrophils and eosinophils recovered in their lavage fluid than normal subjects, especially those patients with evidence of pulmonary dysfunction. A subset of scleroderma patients have a BAL lymphocytosis.[474,514–517] Interestingly, this lymphocytic alveolitis appeared most often in patients prior to[514] or soon after the onset of pulmonary symptoms (< 1 y).[515] In addition,[20] scleroderma patients were shown to have radiographic disease, despite a normal BAL.[511] Thus, BAL findings and radiographic changes should be viewed as complementary in determining the pulmonary involvement in scleroderma patients.

Correlation of Bronchoalveolar Lavage Cellular Findings With Disease Activity.   Few studies have found clear correlations between BAL cellular findings and others measurements of disease activity or response to therapy. BAL abnormalities may precede radiographic and physiologic abnormalities.[518] Patients with abnormal chest radiographs are more likely to have lavage abnormalities than those without radiographic abnormalities.[511,518] However, there is evidence that BAL findings can predict patients' course. For example, the presence of BAL neutrophilia, in those patients with scleroderma for greater than 1 year, is associated with a decreased DL_{CO} and more advanced radiographic features of ILD.[471] In addition, BAL neutrophilia is associated with a lower DL_{CO} than BAL lymphocytosis in scleroderma patients.[511] Furthermore, in a 2-year follow-up of scleroderma patients, only 9% of patients with normal BAL cell counts had a decline in DL_{CO}, whereas those with a baseline BAL granulocytosis had a decline in DL_{CO} over the 2-year period.[511] Moreover, in untreated scleroderma patients followed over a minimum of 6 months, those with alveolitis (defined as neutrophils > 3% or eosinophils > 2%) underwent a significant decline in FVC and DL_{CO} compared with those without alveolitis.[512]

A significant correlation between BAL cellular recovery and the single-breath DL_{CO} has been demonstrated.[515] Wells and associates showed that BAL neutrophilia is generally associated with extensive fibrotic disease, whereas a BAL eosinophilia is often seen in less advanced disease, particularly when CT appearances suggest lung inflammation.[519] No relationship has been demonstrated between the presence of esophageal disease and abnormalities in the BAL cellular constituents.[514,515] Serial lavages in 23 patients receiving 6 months of cyclophosphamide for active alveolitis, demonstrated no differences in the cellularity or differential of BAL fluid.[520] In general, if alveolitis is present at presentation it usually is persistent despite treatment and if the BAL is normal at presentation the patient is not likely to experience rapid declines in lung function.[474,476,478,515,518,521] Despite these nonspecific findings, BAL analysis appears to be one of the best methods available for monitoring the pulmonary disease in these patients.[517]

Histopathologic Features.   *Nonspecific Interstitial Pneumonia.*   In the series of 80 scleroderma patients undergoing lung biopsy at the Brompton Hospital in London, 78% of patients had an NSIP pattern.[17] Of these patients with NSIP, a cellular pattern was seen in a minority of patients (24 versus 76% with a fibrotic pattern). The BAL fluid for patients with a cellular versus a fibrotic pattern demonstrated a significantly higher percentage of lymphocytes, although all patients with NSIP had more eosinophils at BAL than those with UIP or end-stage lung disease. Two retrospective studies of biopsy specimens in 9 Japanese scleroderma patients and 18 Korean patients revealed NSIP in 56% and 72% of

patients, respectively.[15,16] In the latter study there were no cases of purely cellular NSIP, and BAL did not distinguish between patients with NSIP versus UIP.

Usual Interstitial Pneumonitis.   A typical UIP pattern is uncommonly found in scleroderma patients undergoing lung biopsy.[15,17] Notably, in Japanese patients with PSS and histologic finding of UIP, there was radiographic evidence of honeycombing.[15] With progressive disease, extensive parenchymal distortion may supervene, with coalescence of alveolar spaces to form cysts of varying size surrounded by fibrous tissue.[153,414,476,522–525] These lesions, analogous to honeycombing, range in size from 0.2 to 2.0 cm. They may be lined with cuboidal, columnar, or ciliated epithelium or may be acellular. It has been suggested that these cysts communicate with bronchi; hence, they may arise because of bronchiolectasis, which itself may be due to traction or fibrosis of the airway wall.[448,496,524]

Other Histologic Patterns in Scleroderma.   In the Brompton Hospital series, an additional 8% of patients had end-stage lung disease of undetermined etiology; respiratory bronchiolitis associated interstitial lung disease (RB-ILD) was seen in four scleroderma patients who were smokers and granulomatous lesions were seen in a patient with known sarcoidosis.[17] OP was demonstrated in a patient receiving penicillamine.[17] A single patient from the Japanese series revealed diffuse alveolar damage, although the patient had a clinical diagnosis of bronchopneumonia while on the ventilator.[15]

Aspiration Pneumonia

Esophageal dysmotility predisposes to aspiration pneumonitis.[7] However, this is not thought to contribute greatly to the development of pulmonary fibrosis in these patients.[495] Recent data suggest that gastroesophageal reflux is common in PSS, and chest CT scans have demonstrated that the prevalence of asymptomatic esophageal dilatation is high.[526] However, there are conflicting data as to the relationship of gastroesophageal reflux to the development of lung disease. A correlation has been suggested between the severity of reflux and the severity of the lung disease.[527,528] Recently, Troshinsky and colleagues examined the relationship between esophageal dysfunction, gastroesophageal reflux, and lung involvement in patients with systemic sclerosis. Esophageal manometry, dual-probe (distal and proximal) esophageal 24-hour pH measurements, and pulmonary function studies (FVC, FEV_1, TLC, and single-breath DL_{CO}) were studied. They found that the measures of lung volume indicative of ILD (TLC, FVC) did not appear to be related to abnormal gastroesophageal acid reflux in patients with PSS.[529]

Airways Disease

An obstructive ventilatory defect with a reduction in maximum breathing capacity, an elevation in residual

Figure 21–8 Progressive systemic sclerosis: bronchoalveolar lavage cellular findings. There is no significant difference in the percentage of macrophages, lymphocytes, neutrophils, or eosinophils among progressive systemic sclerosis (PSS) patients with and without evidence of pulmonary dysfunction. The data is shown as the mean ± SEM. Data identification and data extraction: six major published reports that included 10 or more patients with PSS (with or without lung disease) were reviewed.[471,472,474,477,514,521] The data for normal subjects were obtained from the BAL Cooperative Group study.[813] These works were critically reviewed for information on the clinical, physiologic, radiologic, and lavage findings of PSS. Definition: normal subjects (n = 191) had no evidence of lung disease by absence of symptom, physiologic, or radiographic abnormalities. Patients with PSS were divided into two groups based on presence (lung disease, n = 80) or absence of lung disease (no lung disease, n = 35). Lung disease was present if the total lung capacity was reduced below 80% of predicted or if the diffusing capacity for carbon monoxide was reduced below 75% of predicted or if radiographic evidence of interstitial lung disease was present.

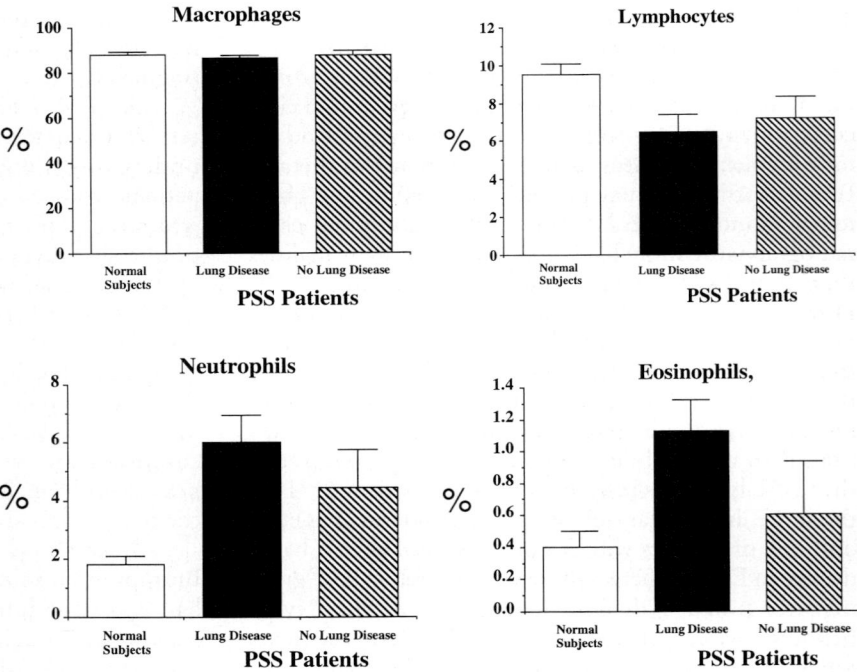

volume (RV) and the RV/TLC ratio, and a reduction in the FEV_1/FVC ratio occur in some individuals and are more often related to tobacco abuse and not to the underlying disease.[414,445,446,455,462,500,518,530–532] Focal lymphoid hyperplasia (follicular bronchiolitis) was identified in 23% of open lung biopsies from patients with scleroderma.[533] D-Penicillamine–associated bronchiolitis obliterans is a rare pulmonary complication in patients with RA or PSS treated with this drug (see Chapter 26, "Broncholitis").[534]

Pulmonary Vascular Disease

Pulmonary hypertension occurs in approximately 10% of patients with the CREST variant of scleroderma.[419,420,535] This rate of occurrence is more frequent than in diffuse scleroderma.[416,417] This is a primary form of pulmonary hypertension and occurs independent of roentgenographic or clinical evidence of pulmonary fibrosis (Figure 21–9).[7,536] Rarely, in < 0.45% of the 2,500 scleroderma patients receiving care at one university, pulmonary hypertension may be seen in a patient with renal crisis.[537] Patients with scleroderma-associated pulmonary hypertension showed a predominance of obliterative-concentric lesions on lung biopsy, with relatively few of the plexiform or combined lesions commonly seen in other forms of primary pulmonary hypertension.[538] In patients with parenchymal disease and pulmonary hypertension, the large pulmonary arteries may show dilatation, intimal plaques, and intimal and/or medial proliferation, whereas the small muscular

arteries and arterioles demonstrate fibromuscular hypertrophy of the media, concentric intimal proliferation, and fibrosis associated with a minor degree of adventitial thickening.[452,464,539,540] A necrotizing arteritis is not evident.[464,541] Cases of veno-occlusive disease as well as capillary hemangiomatosis have been reported in patients with scleroderma.[542] The subset of patients with PSS and antibodies to centromere and histone in serum samples appears to be the most likely to develop severe pulmonary or vascular disease.

Management and Prognosis.   In the absence of any prospectively evaluated and consistently effective treatment for scleroderma, a highly individualized approach to the evaluation and therapy of scleroderma interstitial disease is appropriate. Many therapeutic agents have been employed in scleroderma. In regard to the pulmonary disease, corticosteroids, cyclophosphamide, and D-penicillamine are worthy of mention. No data are available to document a favorable long-term effect of corticosteroid therapy as a single agent.

Cyclophosphamide has shown the most promise in changing the outcome of scleroderma patients with ILD.[543] Steen and coworkers showed that cyclophosphamide treatment resulted in significantly more improvement in lung function than did treatment with high-dose prednisone, D-penicillamine, or no drug in a retrospective observational study.[544] Patients with early disease had the greatest likelihood of responding to any drug. Similarly, Silver and coworkers showed that patients with PSS with ILD who were treated with oral cyclophosphamide (1–2 mg/kg/d) and low dose prednisone (< 10 mg/d) developed significant improvement in lung function after 6 months compared with entry values and the improvement was maintained at 12 months.[545] Additional retrospective analysis of the use of cyclophosphamide for active alveolitis in symptomatic patients with scleroderma, revealed that treatment significantly influenced patients' outcome in terms of pulmonary function and survival compared with patients with active alveolitis who were not treated.[512] Subsequently, in an additional uncontrolled study of cyclophosphamide for alveolitis in 23 patients, no significant change in lung function, radiographic disease, or alteration in the cellularity or differential of BAL was observed after 6 months of therapy.[520] However, issues in this study include the definitions of a significant response. For example, 21 of 23 patients had either a stable or improved FVC. The interpretation of this is limited by the lack of a control group. However, presumably based on prior data,[512] if patients were not treated they would have declined significantly. A third uncontrolled, open-label trial of cyclophosphamide and low- or high-dose prednisone for clinically diagnosed ILD in patients with scleroderma revealed physiologic, radiologic, and clinical improvement for the high-dose group only.[543] Notably, although statistical differences in radiographic scores were not seen between the low- and high-dose groups, 42% of patients in low dose, (nonresponding group) demonstrated honeycombing, which may be an indication of underlying UIP rather than NSIP.[503]

D-Penicillamine, a drug that inhibits intra- and intermolecular cross-linking of collagen and has anti-inflammatory and immunosuppressive properties, has also been tried.[446,546–548] The most impressive data are those of Steen and associates that retrospectively document a reduction in skin thickness, a diminished rate of new visceral disease, and improved 5-year survival in patients who had received D-penicillamine early in the course of their disease.[547] When serial pulmonary function was reviewed, the DL_{CO} was noted to improve in the treated individuals (76 to 87% of predicted) but was essentially unchanged in the untreated controls.[445] In those individuals with abnormal function initially, 79% and 32% of the treated group had a greater than or equal to 15% increase in DL_{CO} and FVC, respectively, as opposed to a 40% and 17% improvement in the untreated group. In addition, a significantly higher proportion of untreated patients demonstrated progression of dyspnea, rales, and roentgenographic findings suggestive of fibrosis. Although such data are clearly preliminary, they would suggest a preventive role for D-penicillamine in the management of scleroderma pulmonary disease. Side effects of therapy occurred in 47%. However, discontinuation of D-penicillamine was required in only 29%. The overall frequency of side effects did not differ from patients with RA treated with D-penicillamine, although pemphigus and myasthenia gravis seemed to occur more frequently in patients with scleroderma.[549] A more recent study of high- and low-dose penicillamine for scleroderma over 2 years revealed no change in DL_{CO} or FVC with therapy (no control group)[550]

Although pulmonary hypertension in patients with scleroderma may result from a variety of causes, individual patients (including those with secondary hypertension due to ILD) may have a significant pulmonary vasodilation with the use of epoprostenol.[551]

Single and double lung transplantation has been successfully performed in patients with PSS without disproportionate untoward complications relative to lung transplantation for other indications.[552,553] The use of autologous stem cell transplant for systemic sclerosis has not been shown to improve lung function, although pulmonary hypertension (in five patients) did not progress.[554]

The prognosis of scleroderma is determined by a variety of factors. Whereas overall survival ranges from 79 to 94% at 5 years,[408,412,413] males and patients with diffuse disease consistently have reduced survival relative to age- or population-matched controls as well as females and patients with limited scleroderma. The presence of renal, cardiac, or pulmonary disease also exerts a profound adverse effect; the 5-year survival rate after lung involvement ranges from 38 to 45%.[416,555–558] Pulmonary function abnormalities affect prognosis, with a 5-year survival rate greater than 90% in those with normal function, 58% in

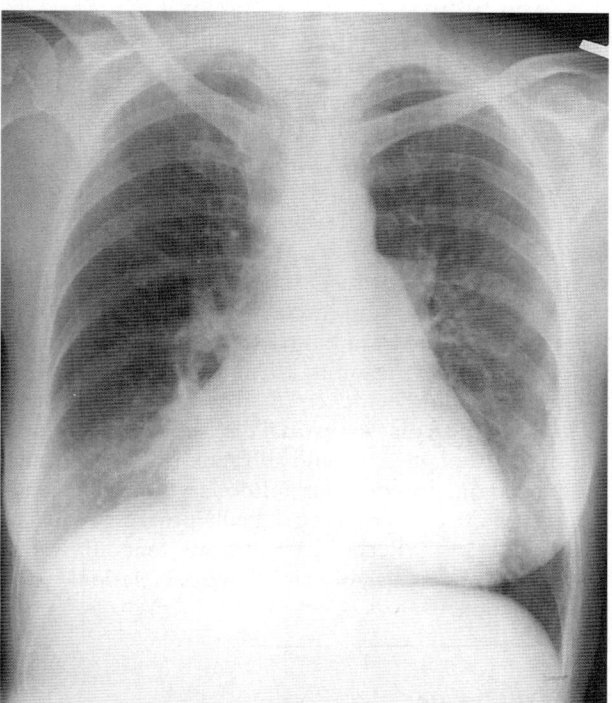

Figure 21–9   Progressive systemic sclerosis (scleroderma). Young woman with CREST syndrome and roentgenographic evidence of pulmonary hypertension without evidence of interstitial lung disease.

those with restrictive spirometry, and a dismal 9% survival rate of those with a DL_{CO} of less than 40% of predicted.[446,558] The presence of proteinuria, erythrocyte sedimentation rate (ESR) > 25, and DL_{CO} < 70% at presentation with scleroderma predicts a 5-year survival rate.[413]

It remains unclear whether fibrosing alveolitis associated with systemic sclerosis, histologically identical to UIP, has a different prognosis to that seen in patients with IPF. The only large study of biopsies in patients with scleroderma demonstrated that NSIP, rather than UIP, is the most common histologic pattern in scleroderma.[17] No comparison was made between scleroderma-associated NSIP and idiopathic NSIP in that series. Historic comparison with these authors' series of 28 patients with cellular and fibrotic idiopathic NSIP and that of the National Heart, Lung, and Blood Institute (NHLBI) series of 39 patients with NSIP (fibrotic and cellular groups), reveals that the 90% 5-year survival in NSIP associated with scleroderma[17] is comparable to Brompton's cellular NSIP patients (100% survival) and NHLBI cellular and fibrotic cases (90–100%).[559,560] The patients with idiopathic fibrotic NSIP from the Brompton series, however, had < 50% survival, making the survival of patients with scleroderma with fibrotic NSIP far better.[560] In patients with scleroderma, the prognosis with NSIP was no different from those with UIP; however, the study had insufficient power to detect all but large (> 50%) differences between these groups' survival.[17] In the Korean cohort of patients with scleroderma, those with NSIP had significantly better improvement (as assessed by the clinical-physiologic-radiologic score) after 12 months of cyclophosphamide therapy compared with their counterparts with UIP.[16]

Despite such prognostic considerations, it may be questioned as to whether pulmonary disease itself causes death or merely reflects widespread systemic disease. Published series report death due to pulmonary fibrosis in up to 17%.[414,448,555] A recent series composed equally of patients with diffuse scleroderma and CREST reported mortality from interstitial fibrosis in 5% (4 to 6 years after the onset of lung disease) and from primary pulmonary hypertension in 19%.[446] In the same series, roentgenographic evidence of fibrosis was present in 27%, suggesting that interstitial disease is often not progressive. Although acute and subacute progression may occur, examination of serial pulmonary functions tends to support the concept of a gradually progressive loss of function.[496,561–565] Recent data indicate that survival in scleroderma bears a significant (inverse) relationship to lung function.[412]

Pleural Disease

Pleural disease rarely presents as acute pleuritic pain or pleural effusions and is usually an incidental autopsy finding.[63,411,414,498,500] Only 7% of one 40-patient cohort demonstrated pleural effusions.[566] Spontaneous pneumothorax is a rarely reported complication.[452] Gross examination of the lungs often reveals thickening of the pleura as well as adhesions and effusion, with air-filled cystic structures projecting outward through the visceral pleura.[5]

Bronchogenic Carcinoma

There is a significant association of chronic pulmonary fibrosis and the development of bronchogenic carcinoma in scleroderma.[567] Carcinoma is thought to arise from the intense epithelial proliferation that accompanies the fibrotic process.[63] An extensive review has documented 44 such cases, the majority of which were either bronchoalveolar cell or adenocarcinomas.[568] Another recent review also demonstrated that the majority of lung cancers reported in patients with connective tissue disease are found in scleroderma patients. Furthermore, these scleroderma patients with lung cancer were predominantly nonsmokers. The frequency of bronchoalveolar carcinoma (BAC) in patients with scleroderma was significantly higher than the proportion of patients with BAC and RA, polymyositis/dermatomyositis (PM/DM), SLE, or Sjögrens syndrome.[569] Rosenthal and associates showed in an epidemiologic study from the six-county Uppsala health care region of Sweden for the period 1955 to 1984 that the standardized incidence ratio (SIR) for all cancers among patients with PSS was significantly increased.[570] The standardized incidence ratios for lung cancer (SIR = 7.8; 95% CI = 2.5 to 18.2) and non-Hodgkin's lymphoma (SIR = 9.6; 95% CI = 1.1 to 34.5) were also significantly increased.

POLYMYOSITIS AND DERMATOMYOSITIS

Definition and General Features

Polymyositis and dermatomyositis are inflammatory conditions involving muscle and dermis as a primary disease or in association with the other connective tissue diseases.[571] Both processes are characterized by skeletal muscle weakness, which results from a nonsuppurative, lymphocyte-predominant, inflammatory process. This inflammatory process in turn leads to muscle damage and loss of function. Patients with dermatomyositis also have a characteristic skin rash. The classification of various subgroups of these disorders has been controversial (Table 21–12).[572]

The incidence of polymyositis and dermatomyositis is unknown, but is probably between two and five cases per million population per year.[571] Because of the heterogeneity in presentation, diagnosis is often difficult. Polymyositis and dermatomyositis may occur at any age although the mean age in adults is 50 years. It is twice as common in females, and familial cases have been reported.[573,574] The insidious onset of muscle weakness, with or without myalgia, is present in nearly all patients and is the first manifestation of polymyositis and dermatomyositis in the majority of cases. Typically, the muscle weakness begins in either the lower or upper limbs, and the patient complains of difficulty running, climbing stairs, and getting out of a chair. Upper limb weakness (usually proximal) is also often reported and is associated with loss of strength of the shoulder girdle and weakness of the anterior neck muscles. Occasionally, there is involvement of the posterior pharyngeal muscle, leading to dysphagia and dysphonia. In about half the patients, there is pain and tenderness in the affected muscle groups. Difficulty in chewing and swallowing may be present in 20% of the patients, and weight loss often occurs. Most patients have symptoms for 3 to 6 months prior to seeking medical attention. Infrequently, the onset is more acute.

In dermatomyositis, the relative degree of skin and muscle involvement varies considerably. Occasionally, patients with extensive skin lesions have no evidence of muscle dysfunction, and in other cases the reverse is true. The skin and mucous membranes demonstrate a bright red hyperemic rash that occasionally leaves the skin shiny and atrophic. When the rash is florid, there may be accompanying edema and pain. Infrequently, desquamation occurs, and the rash is usually not pruritic. There is a predisposition for the eyelids, the cheeks, the bridge of the nose, the front and back of the chest, the extensor surfaces of the elbows and knees, the malleoli of the ankle, and the knuckles of the fingers. Gottron's sign is said to be pathognomonic and consists of erythema, scaling, dermal atrophy, and dusky red patches of linear streaks over the areas listed previously. Raynaud's phenomenon has been found in as high as 55% of reported cases.[572,575–578] However, recent evidence suggests that the incidence is closer to 10 to 20% in patients with the primary process.[577] Arthralgias and myalgias are seen in approximately 25% of patients.[575,578] Cardiac complications (tachyarrhythmias, conduction abnormalities, right- or left-sided failure) are common and may be a cause of death.

The ESR is elevated in approximately 50% of patients and may be high (ie, greater than 50 mm per hour) in one-fifth of the patients.[579] Although commonly elevated, the ESR does not correlate with the clinical course nor is it a useful test to follow response to treatment. Serum enzymes released from inflamed skeletal muscle are elevated in all patients at some point in their clinical course. It is thought that the level of elevation correlates with the acuteness and extent of the muscle damage. The serum creatine phosphokinase (CPK) level is the most reliable of the serum enzymes and correlates best with the clinical course and other parameters of disease activity.[580] The level is usually 10 times the normal range, although it may be as high as 80 times. The serum transaminases and aldolase are elevated but are not thought to be as sensitive a parameter of disease activity as the CPK. Although patients have been reported with this disease without elevation of these serum enzymes, it is thought to be unusual. Patients who have inactive disease or have widespread muscle atrophy and loss of muscle mass may demonstrate normal enzyme levels; in the latter case this represents a potentially poor prognostic sign.[580]

The serologic pattern in polymyositis and dermatomyositis often reflects an associated connective tissue disease. The antinuclear antibody is present in approximately 25% and the RF in up to 40% of polymyositis cases. However, in polymyositis and dermatomyositis not associated with another connective tissue disease, these antibodies are found in only 10% of the cases. The association of the anti-Jo-1 antibody in patients with IPF and PM/DM suggests that it may be a specific marker for ILD.

An open-muscle biopsy of adequate size is necessary to diagnose these patients. The site must be carefully selected and should be a moderately weak but unwasted muscle.

Pleuropulmonary Manifestations of Polymyositis and Dermatomyositis

Pulmonary complications are important determinants of the clinical course of polymyositis and dermatomyositis (Table 21–13).

Interstitial Lung Disease

Epidemiology. Mills and Mathews are credited with the first report of interstitial pneumonitis associated with polymyositis and dermatomyositis.[581] The existence of ILD in polymyositis and dermatomyositis is well established, although epidemiologic data to determine the incidence and natural history are not available since no prospective cohort analysis has been performed.[582–587] In two retrospective studies of large populations of patients with polymyositis and dermatomyositis using roentgenographic criteria only, lung disease was found in

TABLE 21–12   Classification of Polymositis and Dermatomyositis

Group 1	Primary idiopathic polymyositis
Group 2	Primary idiopathic dermatomyositis
Group 3	Dermatomyositis (or polymyositis) associated with neoplasia
Group 4	Childhood dermatomyositis (or polymyositis) associated with vasculitis
Group 5	Polymyositis or dermatomyositis associated with connective tissue disease (overlap group)

Adapted from Bohan A and Peter JB.[572]

5% and 9%.[588,589] If physiologic screening is used, the incidence of lung impairment (and presumably ILD) increases to 30%.[585] Another retrospective series combining physiologic and radiographic criteria for the diagnosis of lung disease, reported that 18% of patients with DM/PM had ILD.[590] In spite of this, many large series of polymyositis and dermatomyositis fail to even mention the presence of lung impairment or ILD.[575,578,591,592]

Pathogenesis.   The etiology of polymyositis and dermatomyositis is unknown. It is felt that a cell-mediated immunopathologic mechanism occurs.[593] T lymphocytes from patients with polymyositis and dermatomyositis are myotoxic to myoblasts and fibroblasts in tissue culture.[594] It is unclear whether the degree of cytotoxicity of these lymphocytes correlates with disease activity or response to therapy. In addition, it has been shown that lymphocyte transformation occurs in response to skeletal muscle antigens. Humoral immunity is altered in polymyositis and dermatomyositis; that is, serum immunoglobulins are occasionally increased, several nuclear and cytoplasmic antibodies are found in the sera (such as anti-Jo-1, anti-PL-7, anti-PL-12, anti-Mi-2 and anti-PM Sci), and immune complexes are deposited in skeletal muscle and blood vessel walls. Nonetheless, it is felt that these diseases result primarily from a cell-mediated process and are not related to antibody production.[572,595,596] Complement-fixing antitoxoplasma antibodies are found in one-fourth of adults with polymyositis.[572]

Clinical Features.   The presentation of ILD is variable, but respiratory signs and symptoms often dominate the clinical picture. Progressive dyspnea on exertion, a nonproductive cough, and bibasilar rales are common. Clubbing is very rare.[597] Some patients may present with a rapidly progressive illness and their muscle disease may be completely missed because of the severity of the lung impairment and limited exercise. More commonly, however, patients have slowly progressive dyspnea on exertion with a nonproductive cough. The lung disease may precede (months to years) the muscle complaints or may be superimposed on established muscle disease (Figure 21–10). In one series of 55 patients with DM/PM, 16% of patients developed ILD in a mean of 6 months after the rheumatologic disease. However, 20% of patients developed ILD prior to the rheumatologic disease diagnosis.[598] Occasionally, asymptomatic patients demonstrate significant physiologic and roentgenographic abnormalities consistent with ILD. There is no correlation between the severity or duration of the muscular disease and the ILD. Raynaud's phenomenon, arthralgia, and arthritis commonly occur in this group as well.

Laboratory Findings.   The serologic and laboratory findings described above for polymyositis and dermatomyositis are commonly present in patients with ILD as well. There has been no consistent relationship between the level of serum muscle enzymes and the presence of lung disease. The antinuclear antibody titer is usually negative in these patients in the absence of

another connective tissue disease. The precipitating antibody to an acidic nuclear protein antigen, the Jo-1 antigen, has been reported to be a marker for a subset of patients with polymyositis who have ILD.[584,599,600] Fifty to 64% of patients with ILD have the anti-Jo-1 antibody as compared with 13 to 18% of patients who are negative, but still have ILD. The relevance of this association is not clear. Several other myositis-specific autoantibodies have been associated with ILD: anti-PL-7, anti-PL-12, anti-isoleucyl-tRNA synthetase, antiglycyl-tRNA synthetase, and anti-KJ.[601]

Roentgenographic Findings.   The chest roentgenogram in polymyositis and dermatomyositis is similar to that seen in other ILDs (see Chapter 1, Figure 1–28). There are diffuse reticular or nodular opacities with a predilection for the lung bases. A pattern of mixed alveolar and interstitial opacities may occur, which is thought to represent the early stage of lung involvement.[582] Patients with advanced disease may progress to end-stage honeycomb lung (Figure 21–11). A recent review of 57 DM/PM patients' chest radiographs demonstrated bilateral lower-lobe irregular linear opacities in nearly all (95%) patients, whereas only a quarter of patients had consolidation, and a minority (4%) of patients had honeycombing or effusions.[14] HRCT scan findings of lung disease in patients with polymyositis and dermatomyositis include: irregular linear opacities with bilateral and lower-lung predominance (63 to 92% of subjects), consolidation (52 to 53% of subjects), ground-glass opacities (43 to 92% of subjects), micronodules (28% of subjects), and honeycombing (16% of subjects).[14,602] In Ikezoe and colleagues' examination of HRCT findings, air space consolidation was associated with diffuse alveolar damage or OP (see "Organizing Pneumonia" to follow).[602] The patients with honeycombing all had UIP noted on biopsy.[602]

TABLE 21–13   Pleuropulmonary Manifestations of Polymyositis and Dermatomyositis

Parenchymal lung disease
  Nonspecific interstitial pneumonia
  Diffuse alveolar damage
  Organizing pneumonia
  Pulmonary alveolar proteinosis
  Complications of polymyositis/dermatomyositis
    Aspiration pneumonitis secondary to pharyngeal and esophageal disorder
    Hypostatis pneumonia and respiratory failure secondary to respiratory muscle dysfunction and hypoventilation

Vascular disease
  Pulmonary hypertension

Complications of treatment
  Drug-induced pneumonitis (eg, methotrexate)
  Opportunistic infections

Malignancy (primary or metastastic)

Pleural disease
  Spontaneous pneumothorax
  Pleural disease

Physiologic Testing. These patients usually have evidence of a restrictive ventilatory pattern with reductions in VC and TLC. In addition, the DL_{CO} may also be reduced. The profound respiratory muscle weakness, which may often complicate these patient's courses, may be demonstrated by a decrease in maximal inspiratory pressure, maximal inspiratory flow rate, and maximal voluntary ventilation. Many patients have resting arterial hypoxemia, which is made worse with exercise.

Bronchoalveolar Lavage. Few studies reporting BAL findings in patients with PM/DM have been presented (see Table 21–3). Therefore, it is difficult to draw any conclusions regarding the role of BAL in the assessment of the lung disease in these patients.[69,327,329,330] In two small series (17 patients total), DM/PM patients with ILD had increases in the percentage of lymphocytes.[603,604] A third small series of PM/DM patients (n = 8) with no radiographic evidence of ILD demonstrated equal numbers of patients with neutrophilic or lymphocytic lavage findings.[598] Notably, following 10 months of treatment with prednisone, these abnormalities in BAL resolved along with improvements in pulmonary function and associated symptoms. However, all patients with radiographic disease and neutrophilic lavage findings deteriorated (clinically, physiologically, and radiographically). In flow cytometric studies, CD8+ T cells accounted for the majority of the lymphocytes in those with a lymphocytic alveolitis.[603] The CD4+/CD8+ ratio was significantly reduced (< 1, n=12) in DM/PM compared with normal.[330,605]

Histopathologic Findings. Multiple histologic patterns may be seen in PM/DM including NSIP, UIP, diffuse alveolar damage, and OP (See Chapter 2; Figures 2–9, 2–11, 2–12, 2–14 to 2–16). In a recent Mayo Clinic retrospective review of 22 biopsies from patients with DM/PM, 82% of the patients had NSIP. Of these, one-third were purely cellular NSIP. The remainder of the patients had other histologic patterns including diffuse alveolar damage, OP, or UIP.[14] Combining this data with a second series of 8 additional biopsies from

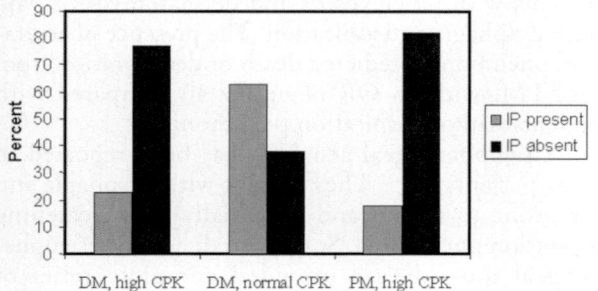

Figure 21–10 The frequency of interstitial pneumonia in polymyositis or dermatomyositis. The overall frequency in this series of 111 patients with polymyositis (PM) or dermatomyositis (DM) was 32.4%. The highest rate of interstitial pneumonia (IP) occurred in those with DM and normal serum creatine phosphokinase (CPK) levels at the onset of IP. Reproduced with permission from Nawata Y et al.[608]

patients with DM/PM, NSIP is clearly the most common pattern in these patients.

Pulmonary vascular inflammation is uncommon, with no evidence of vasculitis in a recent biopsy series.[598] However, medial or intimal thickening of small pulmonary arteries and arterioles consistent with secondary pulmonary hypertension is common. Pleural disease is distinctly uncommon. Interstitial ossification has been reported rarely.[582]

Prognosis and Management. Pulmonary involvement has repeatedly been shown to be a negative prognostic factor and significant cause of death in patients with PM/DM.[590,598] In a cohort of 9 patients with PM/DM and ILD, the mean survival was 5.5 years.[598] However, in the Mayo Clinic series of 58 patients with PM/DM and ILD, the 5-year survival was 60%.[14] This survival was similar to that of patients with idiopathic NSIP and significantly better than that of patients with UIP (Figure 21–12). It has been suggested that the presence of active inflammation on lung biopsy, especially OP, is predictive of a good therapeutic response. In addition, the patients are often younger among the responders compared with nonresponders. Fifty percent of patients who responded have decreased dyspnea, clearing of their chest roentgenogram, and improvement in their pulmonary function tests. Patients with diffuse alveolar damage have a uniformly poor prognosis.[606] Much of the morbidity and mortality of polymyositis and dermatomyositis is associated with the presence and severity of pulmonary disease, especially respiratory insufficiency and/or repeated aspiration and cardiac involvement.

The natural history of untreated ILD in polymyositis and dermatomyositis is unknown. Based on the lack of temporal correlation between myositis and pulmonary involvement, it is not surprising that active alveolitis (defined as hypercellularity and lymphocytosis on BAL) has been demonstrated in patients completing courses of immunosuppression with effective control of their muscular disease.[604] Although such information is problematic (unknown BAL prior to therapy), it seems likely that many patients with DM/PM will require therapy for parenchymal lung disease despite otherwise quiescent disease. Corticosteroids have caused remission with stabilization or improvement in the symptomatic, roentgenographic, and physiologic abnormalities in up to 40% of patients (Figure 21–13). Two groups have advocated the use of cyclosporine treatment to rescue the deteriorating patients with interstitial pneumonitis.[607,608] Others have observed the efficacy of tacrolimus in treating ILD in patients with myositis who are refractory to other immunosuppressive agents.[609]

Recently investigated serologic markers of disease activity have included KL-6, which, while (99%) specific for the presence of ILD in rheumatologic disorders, is not unique to PM/DM.[610,611] The KL-6 levels have no correlation with CPK levels in myositis patients.[610] Serum levels of cytokeratin 19 fragment, a cytoskeletal structure of epithelium, have also been found to paral-

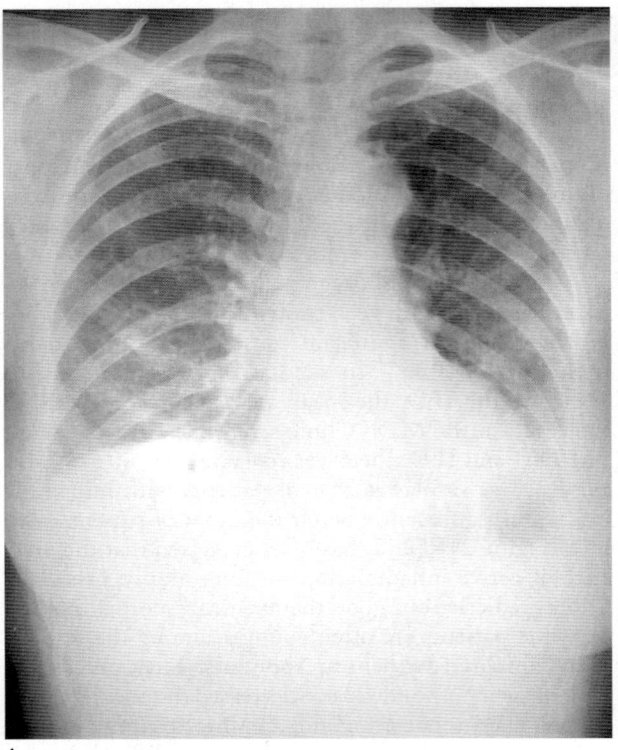
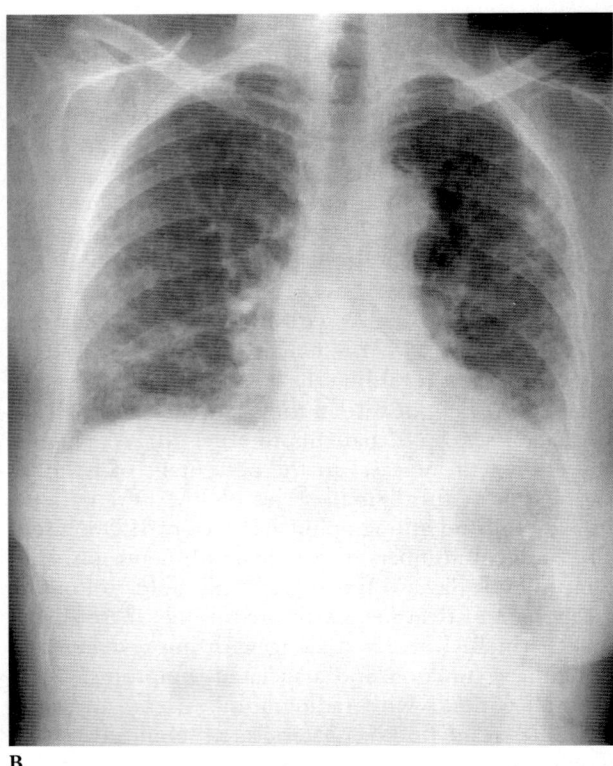

A   B

Figure 21–11   Polymyositis. *A*, Chest roentgenogram in a patient with polymyositis. Diffuse reticular opacities are present in association with a left pleural reaction. *B*, Chest roentgenogram of progression of the interstitial lung disease over a 2-year period with evidence of loss of volume and pulmonary hypertension now evident.

lel disease activity in DM/PM, during both clinical deterioration and response to therapy. Interestingly, immunohistologic staining in an autopsy case demonstrated cytokeratin 19 positivity in hyperplastic type II pneumocytes as well as hyaline membranes.[612]

At this time, clinical, physiologic, and radiographic follow up of patients is warranted for individual decision making until controlled trials of therapy are available for these rare diseases.

Organizing Pneumonia

Organizing pneumonia is a well-described histologic pattern identified in patients with PM/DM (see Chapter 2, Figures 2–11).[582,606,613,614] Patients with OP present with cough, fever, and dyspnea in addition to the proximal muscle weakness, malaise, and rash commonly found in this disease. Chest radiograph and HRCT scanning usually show air space consolidation or ground-glass opacities (Figure 21–14).[602] This lesion is responsive to corticosteroid and cyclophosphamide therapy.[614,615]

Aspiration Pneumonitis

Aspiration pneumonia is the most important pulmonary disease in polymyositis and dermatomyositis

due to its prevalence, associated morbidity and mortality, as well as preventability.[590,616–620] Respiratory muscle weakness, a poor cough reflex, and immunosuppression (as a result of corticosteroid or immunosuppressive therapy) are factors that contribute to the development of lung infections. Patients with polymyositis and dermatomyositis have an impaired cough reflex because of weakness of the striated muscle of the soft palate, pharynx, and upper esophagus. Thus, protection of the airways is important for patients with polymyositis and dermatomyositis who have dysphagia and aspiration. The presence of aspiration pneumonia predicted death or deterioration from DM/PM, with an OR of nearly 30 compared with patients without aspiration pneumonia.[590]

Cricopharyngeal achalasia has been reported in these patients.[621,622] They present with dysphagia and are prone to serious and potentially life-threatening aspiration pneumonia. Surgery to divide the cricopharyngeal musculature provided complete relief of symptoms in two patients with cricopharyngeal achalasia.[622] The exact incidence of dysphagia as a presenting manifestation of polymyositis and dermatomyositis is not clear but has been reported in up to 67% of patients in a large series. Manometric studies and radiographic studies are often useful in defining this problem since they often show an absence of

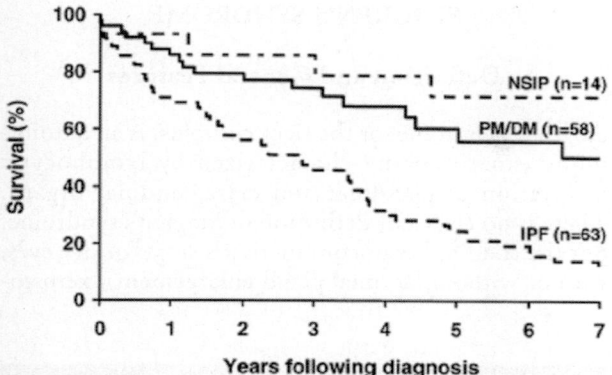

Figure 21–12   Dermatomyositis. Overall survival for 58 patients with polymyositis or dermatomyositis and associated interstitial lung disease (PM/DM/ILD), compared with 63 historic control patients with biopsy-proven idiopathic pulmonary fibrosis (IPF)/usual interstitial pneumonia and 14 patients with biopsy-proven idiopathic nonspecific interstitial pneumonia (NSIP). We included only those patients whose initial diagnosis of diffuse lung disease was made by chest radiography at the Mayo Clinic, Rochester within 1 month of the start of the study period. One-year survival for patients with PM/DM/ILD was 85.8%, 3-yr survival was 74.7%, and 5-yr survival was 60.4%. Survival is better ($p < .001$) for the PM/DM/ILD group when compared with the group with IPF and is not different from the group with idiopathic NSIP ($p = .247$). Reproduced with permission from Douglas W et al.[14]

swallowing responses in the pharynx, cricopharyngeal sphincter, and proximal esophagus or they radiographically show vallecular pooling, pharyngeal reflux, disorganized pharyngeal emptying, and occasional tracheal aspiration of barium.[572,585]

Pulmonary Hypertension

Pulmonary hypertension associated with polymyositis and dermatomyositis is rare.[623] It often occurs secondary to ILD or chronic ventilatory insufficiency.[624,625] A recent echocardiographic/Doppler study found that 7 of 11 patients with polymyositis had evidence of pulmonary hypertension.[626] Consequently, pulmonary vascular involvement may be more common than originally suspected because it is masked by the patient's peripheral muscle weakness that limits exercise.

Diffuse Alveolar Hemorrhage

Schwarz and coworkers recently described pulmonary capillaritis and DAH as the primary manifestation of polymyositis in two patients (see Chapter 2, Figure 2–10).[627] Concomitant with their muscle disease, they developed respiratory failure.

Drug-Induced Lung Disease

The immunosuppressive agents used in the treatment of polymyositis and dermatomyositis include methotrexate, azathioprine, and cyclophosphamide. These agents are associated with the development of ILD and thus carry the risk of this occurrence in patients with polymyositis and dermatomyositis treated with these agents (see "Drug-Induced Lung Disease in Rheumatoid Arthritis," above). Opportunistic infections also can result from the immunosuppression that is induced by these agents.[585]

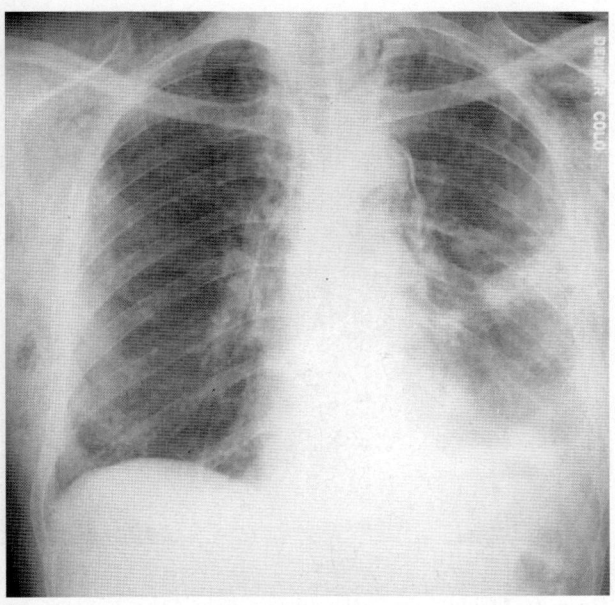

A

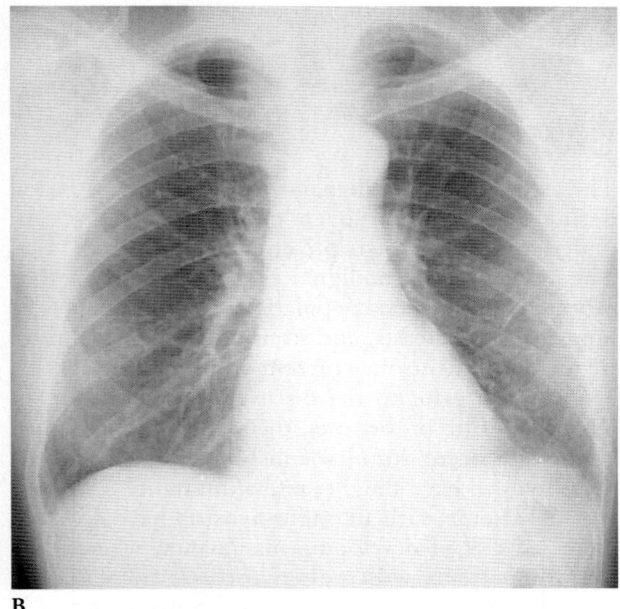

B

Figure 21–13   Dermatomyositis. *A,* Chest roentgenogram in a patient with dermatomyositis reveals diffuse reticular opacities, left pleural effusion, and subcutaneous emphysema secondary to pneumothorax. *B,* Follow-up chest roentgenogram after corticosteroid treatment demonstrates improvement with marked clearing of the interstitial opacities and left pleural process.

Adult Respiratory Distress Syndrome

The adult respiratory distress syndrome has been seen in polymyositis patients with a positive anti-Jo-1 antibody.[628]

Respiratory Muscle Dysfunction

Respiratory failure secondary to generalized respiratory muscle dysfunction occurs in less than 10% of cases. However, lesser degrees of respiratory impairment are common and often are only diagnosed after specific tests are performed to identify these patients.[585,592,617,629,630] Subclinical respiratory muscle weakness may not cause alveolar hypoventilation, but may be responsible for a reduction in the cough reflex. The ventilatory insufficiency of polymyositis and dermatomyositis is characterized by both inspiratory and expiratory dysfunction.[630,631] Patients often develop atelectasis because their muscle weakness makes it impossible for them to breath deeply (ie, sigh). The chest roentgenogram frequently reveals elevation of the diaphragm with a reduced lung volume and plate-like bibasilar atelectasis. As the disease advances, progressive hypoxemia occurs because of inspiratory dysfunction. With expiratory muscle dysfunction, hypoventilation occurs and respiratory failure results. Measurement of maximal inspiratory and expiratory pressures to estimate respiratory muscle power has been shown to be of benefit in monitoring the clinical course and the response to therapy in these patients.[632]

Pleural Disease

Spontaneous pneumothorax and pleural effusions are found infrequently.[633–635]

Malignancy

The association of malignancy with polymyositis and dermatomyositis has been controversial.[636–638] An underlying neoplasm is present in 5 to 8% of cases. The incidence of malignancy is higher than that expected in the general population. Malignancies of the lungs, ovaries, breasts, and stomach are reported most frequently. Patients may present with muscle weakness 1 to 2 years prior to the discovery of the tumor. In about one-third of the cases, the malignancy and muscle disease occur simultaneously. Patients with dermatomyositis have a higher rate of mortality from cancer.[638] Patients with dermatomyositis have a 3-fold increased risk of developing malignancy, whereas the risk for patients with polymyositis is increased by 30%.[639] Males over 40 years are most commonly affected. Patients with polymyositis and dermatomyositis and malignancy do not respond as well to corticosteroid treatment as those without malignancy.

SJÖGREN'S SYNDROME

Definition and General Features

Sjögren's syndrome, or the sicca complex, is an autoimmune exocrinopathy characterized by lymphocytic infiltration of glandular and extraglandular organs. There is no clear-cut definition of Sjögren's syndrome, but the triad of keratoconjunctivitis sicca (or dry eyes, with or without lacrimal gland enlargement), xerosto-

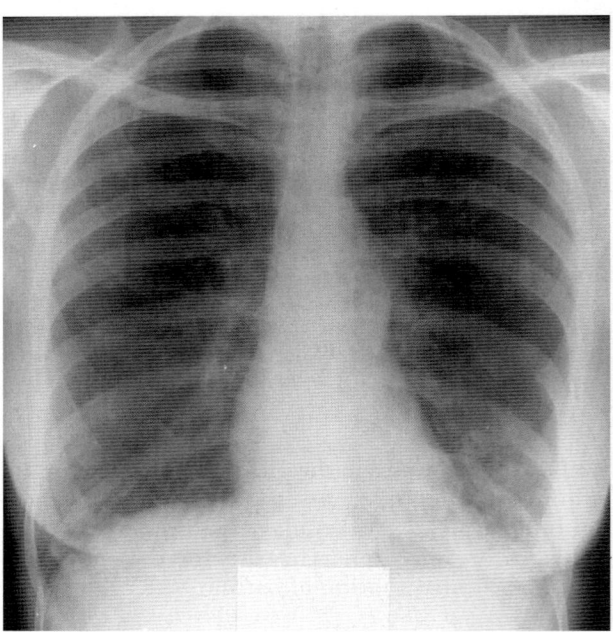

A

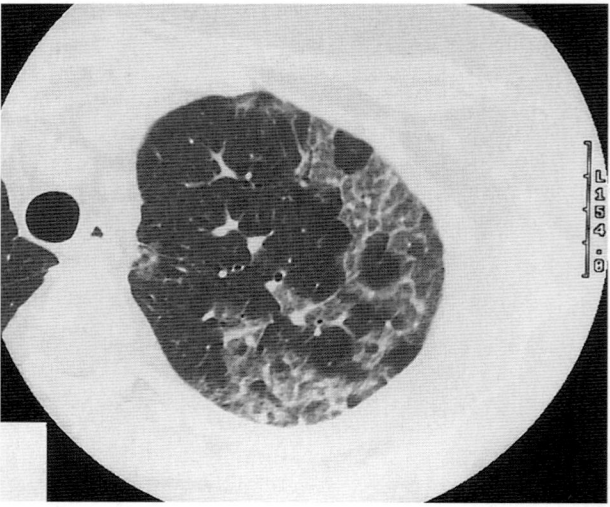

B

Figure 21–14   Polymyositis/dermatomyositis. *A*, Chest roentgenogram shows bilateral diffuse alveolar and interstitial opacities. *B*, High-resolution computed tomography scan shows predominent ground-glass opacities. A thoracoscopic lung biopsy showed an organizing pneumonia pattern.

mia (dry mouth, with or without salivary gland enlargement), and the presence of a connective tissue disease, usually RA, serves most clinical purposes. Sjögren's syndrome is classified as "primary" (a disease predominantly of postmenopausal women older than 40 years) or "secondary" (if it occurs with a connective tissue disease). In addition to RA, Sjögren's syndrome is found in SLE, PSS, polyarteritis nodosa, mixed connective tissue disease, or polymyositis.[640,641] Approximately 50 to 66% of Sjögren's syndrome is the secondary form.[641] Primary Sjögren's syndrome has an annual incidence rate of 4 cases per 100,000 in Olmstead county residents.[642]

Keratoconjunctivitis results in a diminished tear secretion and a punctuate or filamentary keratitis. In addition to the sicca complex, the exocrine glands of the skin, lung, gastrointestinal tract, and vagina have diminished secretions as well. Keratoconjunctivitis sicca is defined by the presence of at least two abnormal tests: (1) Schirmer's test: a crude test for tear secretion, which uses a standardized strip of blotting paper inserted into the lower conjunctival fornix. After 5 minutes, the strip is removed and the length of the wetted part measured from the fold. A normal individual should have wet 15 mm or more of the standard filter strip. (2) Break-up time: the interval between a complete blink and the appearance of the first dry spot on the cornea, and (3) van Bijsterveld score (quantitative rose bengal dye test: an estimate of the degree of staining of denuded areas of the cornea).[640]

The symptoms and signs of keratoconjunctivitis sicca include a foreign body sensation, burning, tiredness with or without difficulty in opening the eyes, dry feeling (with or without a poor response to physical or chemical irritants and emotions), redness, difficulty seeing, itchiness, aches, soreness or pain, and photosensitivity. Photophobia is the most common sign. Mild dysphagia is due to dryness of the pharynx and esophagus, which makes the passage of food difficult. In addition, postcricoid webs are sometimes seen. Abnormal esophageal motility has been reported in the sicca syndrome. Dryness of the skin, parotid gland enlargement, purpura, Raynaud's phenomenon, lymphadenopathy, splenomegaly, myositis, and renal involvement (manifested by hyposthenuria, renal tubular acidosis [usually type II], nephrogenic diabetes insipidus, or Franconi's syndrome) are present in Sjögren's syndrome and more commonly in the primary disease.[643]

A mild anemia is often seen and leukopenia occurs especially in the presence of an associated connective tissue disease. Eosinophilia and thrombocytopenia have also been reported. Hypergammaglobulinemia, polyclonal or monoclonal, is a common finding. Interestingly, the development of hypogammaglobulinemia may herald the development of a malignant lymphoma. Cryoglobulins, and most commonly RF, are found frequently in the sera.[644] A number of other autoantibodies have been observed in patients with Sjögren's syndrome, among them antinuclear antibodies, antisalivary

duct antibodies, as well as SS-A and SS-B, although none of these are specific to Sjögren's syndrome.

Primary Sjögren's syndrome appears to have a strong association with hereditary factors encoded by the MHC[645]; specifically, a higher frequency of HLA-DR2 and HLA-DR3 (50 to 80% of patients) and a decreased frequency of HLA-DR4 is seen in these patients. In contrast, the Sjögren's syndrome associated with connective tissue disease has a frequency of HLA-DR4, HLA-DR2, and HLA-DR3 levels similar to control populations. However, given that the production of the antibodies SS-A/Ro or SS-B/La is also thought to be under the control of HLA class II markers, recent authors have raised the possibility that the only significant association of Sjögren's syndrome with HLA markers is in those patients who are SS-A or SS-B positive.[646] It has also been suggested that there is a striking association between these antibodies, especially anti-SS-A/Ro antibodies, with extraglandular disease (vasculitis, purpura, and lymphadenopathy), hematologic abnormalities (anemia, leukopenia, and thrombocytopenia), and immune phenomenon (hyperglobulinemia, elevated antinuclear antibody and RF titers, cryoglobulinemia, and hypocomplementemia).[647,648] Interestingly, organ-specific autoantibodies, such as the antisalivary gland antibody are infrequent in primary Sjögren's syndrome, but have been reported in the majority of patients with secondary Sjögren's syndrome, suggesting an epiphenomenon. In addition to the increased frequency of eosinophilia, patients with Sjögren's syndrome seem to be more allergic to drugs especially penicillin and gold.[640]

Despite these findings, the pathogenesis remains unknown. The disease appears to result from an aggressive T- and B-lymphocyte infiltration of exocrine glands. Recent studies examining the lymphocyte subsets in affected tissues have demonstrated infiltrates of T cells with helper or inducer activity and a high frequency of activation antigens. It has also been demonstrated that natural killer cell activity is reduced in patients with Sjögren's syndrome. This defective natural killer cell function is secondary to an abnormal production of IL-2.[649] What role the low natural killer cell activity in primary Sjögren's syndrome plays in the development of lymphoma is unknown. The current view of pathogenesis of Sjögren's syndrome is that an inciting injury, possibly a viral infection (Epstein-Barr virus and cytomegalovirus are the leading candidates), causes a disruption of the host cell with the release of autoantigens that generate the accumulation of lymphocytes (both T cells and B cells) that induce local immunoglobulin synthesis. These immunoglobulins lead to the formation of immune complexes that further activate lymphocyte function and so lead to chronic stimulation of B cells, which are responsible for the hyperglobulinemia and increased autoantibodies that are found in these patients. The actual mechanism for the destruction of salivary and lacrimal glands is unknown. But it is likely due to the infiltrated cells causing a cell-to-cell interaction leading to cell-mediated destruction of the tissue.[649]

Pleuropulmonary Manifestations of Sjögren's Syndrome

Pulmonary manifestations occur frequently in Sjögren's syndrome.[650-656] However, because of the frequently associated connective tissue disease, it has been difficult to determine which of the pulmonary manifestations is the result of Sjögren's syndrome and not of the underlying associated connective tissue disease. The pleural and pulmonary manifestations of Sjögren's syndrome are outlined in Table 21–14.

Interstitial Lung Disease

Diffuse ILD is probably the most common functional abnormality identified in patients with primary Sjögren's syndrome and lung involvement.[651,657-662] The etiology of ILD associated with Sjögren's syndrome is unknown, and it appears that lymphocytic pneumonitis represents only one pole of the spectrum of diseases, which includes pseudolymphomas and malignant lymphomas. ILD occurs more often in patients with extraglandular manifestations than in those with glandular disease alone.

Clinical Manifestations. Lung involvement in Sjögren's syndrome is manifested by cough and dyspnea, although some patients may be asymptomatic and present with a normal chest roentgenogram. In a series of 61 consecutive patients diagnosed with primary Sjögren's syndrome, 41% noted a "sicca cough" whereas only 7% noted dyspnea with exertion.[663] Although bibasilar rales may frequently be present on physical examination, in the previously mentioned series, only 14% had bibasilar rales noted on examination.[663]

Although lung involvement is more common in patients with more severe and extraglandular disease with signs of immunologic derangement, no serologic marker of pulmonary manifestations has been isolated as yet. The course of primary Sjögren's syndrome with lung involvement, even considering the more specific anti SS-B (anti-La) and SS-A (anti-Ro) immunologic profile, is similar to that of patients without lung disease.[662]

The chest roentgenogram usually reveals a fine reticular or nodular pattern.[663] ILD and bronchiolar inflammatory changes are common abnormal findings seen on HRCT scans in primary Sjögren's syndrome.[653,664] For example, 20% of patients with primary Sjögren's syndrome undergoing HRCT had bronchial wall thickening with either ground-glass opacification or a small nodular pattern in the majority of these cases.[663]

In patients with interstitial opacities on their chest radiograph, a restrictive pattern with a low diffusion capacity is commonly found on lung function tests.[662] When compared with secondary Sjögren's syndrome, there was a higher incidence of such a pattern in primary Sjögren's syndrome, whereas an obstructive ventilatory defect was more common in secondary Sjögren's syndrome or RA alone. The significance of diffusion deficits

in patients with primary Sjögren's syndrome remains of uncertain significance; in a 10-year follow-up of pulmonary involvement in 30 patients, a significant decline in diffusion was seen at 4 years followed by a significant improvement at 10 years, in the absence of any intervention (there was a single death in a patient with ILD).[665]

Bronchoalveolar Lavage. Bronchoalveolar lavage fluid in patients with primary Sjögren's syndrome demonstrated an alveolitis characterized by an increase in the cells recovered and a predominance of lymphocytes in the cellular differential (see Table 21–3).[661] Those patients with the lymphocytic alveolitis had more frequent cough, dyspnea, roentgenologic evidence of ILD, and abnormal pulmonary function (lower TLC and diffusing capacity). Lymphocyte subtyping studies revealed a reduced T-helper/suppressor (CD4/CD8) ratio than those primary Sjögren's syndrome patients without alveolitis or normal nonsmoking healthy volunteers. In a more recent series of 18 patients with primary Sjögren's syndrome but no radiographic disease or respiratory symptoms, 88% patients had a pure lymphocytic alveolitis, whereas 22% had a mixed neutrophilic and lymphocytic alveolitis.[666] On repeat BAL after 2 years' observation, nearly half of the patients with lymphocytosis had a normal differential whereas the remainder of patients (with a lymphocytic alveolitis or mixed alveolitis) had no change in their differential. At the time of the second lavage, those patients with abnormal HRCT scans had greater BAL cellularity, a greater percentage of neutrophils and lymphocytes, but no difference in the CD4/CD8 ratio or percentage of activated (DR+) lymphocytes.[666] Notably, the patients with the lymphocytic alveolitis had a smaller loss of their DL_{CO} 2 years later compared with those patients with a mixed (neutrophilic and lymphocytic) alveolitis. Otherwise there were no differences in patients' extraglandular involvement or serologies based on BAL (cell differential) or radiographic (disease present or absent) differences. In a series of studies, Wallaert and colleagues have examined patients with primary and secondary Sjögren's syndrome with and without clinical pulmonary disease.[69,329,521,667] Half of the patients with primary Sjögren's syndrome without clinical, radiographic, or lung function evidence of pulmonary disease had an abnormal lavage cellular differential. Two patterns of BAL cellular yield were identified: a pure lymphocyte predominant (>18% lymphocytes in 69% of the abnormal lavages) and a mixed neutrophil and lymphocytic alveolitis (> 4% neutrophils in 25% of the abnormal lavages). The patients with abnormal BAL findings tended to have more severe Sjögren's disease with extensive extraglandular disease (myositis, lymphadenopathy, renal or hepatic involvement), higher serum gamma globulin and serum beta-2-microglobulin, and higher prevalence of RF and antinuclear antibodies.

Nonsmokers with secondary Sjögren's syndrome associated with biliary cirrhosis and secondary Sjögren's syndrome associated with a defined connective tissue dis-

TABLE 21–14 Pleuropulmonary Manifestations of Sjögren's Syndrome

Parenchymal lung disease
  Nonspecific interstitial pneumonia
  Organizing pneumonia
  Usual interstitial pneumonia
  Lymphocytic interstitial pneumonia (ie, pseudolymphoma, malignant lymphoma)
  Amyloidosis
  Recurrent bronchopneumonia
Airway disease: desiccation of the tracheobronchial tree
  Atrophic rhinitis
  Xerostomia (dry mouth)
  Xerotrachea (chronic dry cough)
  Chronic bronchitis with cough and production of tenacious sputum
  Atelectasis, middle-lobe collapse
Pulmonary vascular disease
  Pulmonary vasculitis
  Pulmonary hypertension
Pleural disease
  Pleurisy with or without effusion

ease in the absence of clinical or radiographic evidence of pulmonary disease had a significantly increased percentage of lymphocytes in BAL fluid.[98,667] In particular, patients with primary Sjögren's syndrome had an increase in T4+ helper/inducer and T8+ cytotoxic/suppressor cells in the lungs similar to findings reported from other mucous surfaces of these patients. A particularly interesting finding in this study was the demonstration that patients with a neutrophilic alveolitis tended to have a marked increase in the T8 suppressor/cytotoxic population in their BAL fluid. In addition, alveolar macrophages from patients with primary Sjögren's syndrome are activated as assessed by the detection of neutrophil chemotactic activity from alveolar macrophage in culture; fibronectin secretion; and spontaneous release of increased amounts of superoxide anion.[69] Unfortunately, it is not known if these abnormalities predict the development of clinically relevant lung disease.

The value of BAL alveolitis in Sjögren's syndrome is unknown. None of the patients with an abnormal BAL fluid at presentation was shown to develop clinical evidence of lung disease.[521] Even when ILD is present, a lavage lymphocytosis tends to predict a relatively good prognosis.[666] In contrast, patients with other defined connective tissue diseases had a neutrophil alveolitis often associated with a poorer clinical outcome and clinical deterioration in untreated patients. Thus the detection of these forms of pulmonary inflammation may be useful in the management of these disease processes.[521,666]

Histopathologic Features. The major changes are ILD and airway disease with involvement of the small airways. A spectrum of histopathologic lesions are found in Sjögren's syndrome including bronchiolitis obliterans either with granulation tissue plugs or with fibrotic obliteration or stenosis ("constrictive bronchiolitis"), LIP (see Figure 27–4), UIP, OP,[668] and a distinctive patchy lymphoid infiltrate associated with large numbers of histocytes aggregating into granulomas.[669,670]

Pseudolymphoma (ie, extensive diffuse or focal nodular opacities of mononuclear cells, predominantly lymphocytes) has been frequently reported.[651,659,671–674] Some patients have an associated lymphadenopathy and/or salivary gland swelling as well. Pseudolymphoma tends to develop in patients with sicca syndrome alone and can regress with corticosteroid or immunosuppressive treatment or may progress to frank lymphoma (quite rare), although the exact behavior of pseudolymphoma is unknown.[3,658,675] Sutinen and colleagues[676] have presented ultrastructural data suggesting the presence of virus-like particles in the bronchial epithelium of a patient with Sjögren's syndrome and LIP, thus lending some support to the theory that viral infection may be a stimulus for the immunologic abnormality observed in patients with this combination of findings.[676]

Treatment. Corticosteroid and immunosuppressive drugs are reserved for patients with extraglandular involvement. Deheinzelin and associates treated 11 patients with an azathioprine-based regimen and found a significant improvement in the FVC after at least 6 months when compared with nontreated patients.[662] Unfortunately, no control studies have been done; thus therapy has been empiric to this point. Our experience suggests that patients with LIP or OP respond well to corticosteroid or immunosuppressive therapy.

Desiccation of the Tracheobronchial Tree

Involvement of the nasal mucosa causes dryness and crusting, which leads to abnormalities in taste and smell. Obstruction of the eustachian tube often leads to conduction deafness secondary to otitis media.[677] Upper airway tract drying of the nasal passages occurs in approximately 50% of patients with primary Sjögren's syndrome. The dryness and crusting of the nose may cause epistaxis and septal perforation. Xerotrachea, manifested by a dry cough without other symptoms or chest roentgenogram changes, occurs in 25% of patients, and bronchoscopic examination usually reveals dry, inflamed bronchial mucosa.[678] Recent evaluation of a cohort of 61 patients with primary Sjögren's syndrome revealed that 41% had a dry cough.[663]

Newball and Brahim described chronic obstructive airway disease in Sjögren's syndrome.[679] Six of their 13 patients showed evidence of airflow obstruction in the absence of cigarette smoking or chest roentgenogram abnormalities. No associated chronic bronchitis or asthma occurred in these patients, and the history did not suggest bronchiectasis, bronchiolitis, or cystic fibrosis. Lung biopsy was performed in two of these patients and revealed a mononuclear cell infiltration centered around narrowed small airways.

Pulmonary hyperinflation associated with diminished peripheral spirometric flow values is frequently found in patients with primary Sjögren's syndrome.[654,655]Fairfax and coworkers[680] measured mucociliary clearance in patients with Sjögren's syndrome using technetium 99m–labeled polystyrene particles. Mucociliary clearance rate was found to be normal from central airways, and the whole lung clearance rate was significantly increased in patients with Sjögren's syndrome compared with normal controls.[680,681] It was felt that this increase was due to failure of penetration of the radioaerosol into the periphery of the lung consistent with obstruction of the small airways. Bariffi and colleagues studied 18 female nonsmokers with Sjögren's syndrome. They found that 13 of the 18 had an FEV_1:FVC ratio of less than 80% and 7 of 18 had an FEV_1 of less than 80%, whereas 9 of 14 had a maximum flow at 25% of VC (MEF_{25}) of less than 80%.[682] In addition, these investigators found abnormalities in diffusing capacity. Constantopoulos and colleagues, in a study of 36 patients with primary Sjögren's syndrome demonstrated that 75% of these patients had evidence of respiratory involvement and 30% had signs of airway disease involving both large and small airways.[683] Similarly, of 61 patients with primary Sjögren's syndrome, at least 50% of patients had a decline in either MEF_{25} or MEF_{50}, whereas only 10% had a low FEV_1.[663] In this same series, in those patients with radiographic disease, 10 of 11 patients undergoing transbronchial biopsies (with or with out endobronchial biopsy) showed submucosal mononuclear infiltrates in small and large bronchi. However, other investigators performed a longitudinal study of 18 asymptomatic, nonsmoking women with normal chest radiographs. In this group, baseline FEV_1/FVC, FVC, and TLC were normal in all patients. Only 17% had a diffusion deficit. None of these patients had any change in function when pulmonary function tests were repeated 2 years later (other than that expected for age).[666] Thus, whether these minor abnormalities in lung function are of clinical significance is not clear. There is a similar incidence of small airways disease in patients with RA without Sjögren's syndrome and in age- and sex-matched control subjects.[684]

Cavitary Lung Disease

Young and colleagues have described a patient with Sjögren's syndrome and Wegener's granulomatosis who presented with cavitary lung disease.[685]

Amyloidosis

Amyloidosis has been identified in a few of these patients with nodular opacities as well.[677,686–688]

Pulmonary Vascular Disease

Pulmonary vasculitis and pulmonary hypertension are extremely rare manifestations of this disease.[3,678,689]

Recurrent Bronchopneumonia

Patients frequently have recurrent bronchial pneumonia that are thought to be due to inspissated mucus secretions that plug the bronchial tree.

Pleural Disease

Pleurisy and/or pleural effusions, pleural thickening, and pleural adhesions have been reported often in association with recurrent pneumonias and atelectasis and in patients with an associated connective tissue disease.[659,677,683,684] Pleural effusion accompanying alveolitis has been described in a patient with primary Sjögren's syndrome.[665]

Shrinking Lung Syndrome

The shrinking lung syndrome has been most commonly reported in patients with SLE. The case of a woman with primary Sjögren's syndrome who developed shrinking lung (a normal lung parenchyma with right hemidiaphragm elevation and abnormal nerve conduction studies of the phrenic nerve) has been reported.[690,691]

MIXED CONNECTIVE TISSUE DISEASE

Definition and General Features

Sharp and his coworkers suggested in 1972 that patients with features of SLE, PSS, Sjögren's syndrome, and polymyositis constituted a distinctly different rheumatologic syndrome, which they labeled mixed connective tissue disease.[692] The unifying feature in these patients was the presence of a hemagglutinating antibody to an extractable nuclear antigen (ENA), which consisted mainly of protein and RNA, the latter being sensitive to ribonuclease.[692,693] Thus, the presence of antibodies to ribonucleoprotein (RNP) (often positive at high dilutions greater than 1:10,000) is generally considered a *sine qua non* of the diagnosis of mixed connective tissue disease. However, many patients with mixed connective tissue disease have the clinical syndrome yet lack anti-RNP antibodies. In addition, anti-RNP antibodies are not specific for mixed connective tissue disease; they can be found in the serum from patients with a wide variety of rheumatic diseases, especially classic scleroderma and SLE. A number of other serologic findings have been found with mixed connective tissue disease including hyperglobulinemia, lymphocytoxic antibodies, circulating immune complexes, positive direct Coomb's test, false-positive VDRL (test for syphilis), hypocomplementemia, positive RF, elevated ESR, and antibodies to ssDNA.[694,695]

The incidence of mixed connective tissue disease is unknown. It is thought to be slightly more frequent than scleroderma and polymyositis.[693] There is an 8:1 female to male ratio and no racial predilection.

It has been stated that the presenting features of this disease are vague, with arthralgia, myalgia, fatigability, and Raynaud's phenomenon being common. In addition, swollen hands, esophageal dysfunction, lymphadenopathy, myositis, renal disease, and central nervous system involvement are clinical features. The skin is almost always involved in mixed connective tissue disease, including Raynaud's phenomenon, alopecia, hand swelling, sclerodactyly, cutaneous lupus erythematosus, periungual telangiectasia, dyspigmentation, photosensitivity, or vasculitis.[694,696] Arthralgia and arthritis occur in most patients. In fact, the arthritis is more severe in mixed connective tissue disease than in SLE and produces a typical swan neck deformity, ulnar deviation, and boutonniere changes.[694,697] The most frequently involved joints are the proximal interphalangeal and distal interphalangeal joints of the hands, the feet, and the wrist joints.[697] An inflammatory myopathy involving the proximal muscle groups is present in 66% and is clinically and histologically identical to polymyositis.[694,696] Pericarditis is the most common clinically significant cardiac abnormality in mixed connective tissue disease. However, involvement of the myocardium may be more common than was initially appreciated after autopsy series revealed frequent evidence of cardiac fibrosis, infarction, and arteritis.[698,699] Diminished esophageal motility has been observed in as many as 80% of patients with high titer anti-RNP antibodies.[694,696,697] Twenty-five percent of patients have renal involvement, most commonly a membranous glomerular nephritis.[700,701] There is a high incidence of neuropsychiatric problems, commonly headaches. Trigeminal neuropathy is the most common neurologic problem.[694,697] Unexplained fever often occurs.

An anemia of chronic disease is present in a majority of patients with mixed connective tissue disease and 60% of patients have positive Coomb's tests. Leukopenia (white blood cell count less than 4,000 per mm³) is present at some time in the course of disease in these patients in approximately 75% and may correlate with disease activity. Although thrombocytopenia is rare, a false positive VDRL occurs in 10% of patients. Most patients have hypergammaglobulinemia. The ESR may be elevated and parallel disease activity. The CPK is elevated in about 50% of these patients and is often associated with inflammatory myopathy.

Pleuropulmonary Manifestations of Mixed Connective Tissue Disease

Pleuropulmonary disease commonly complicates the course of mixed connective tissue disease (Table 21–15).[700,702–704] Up to 82% of patients with mixed connective tissue disease have evidence of pulmonary dysfunction.[705] All symptomatic patients have an abnormal chest roentgenogram and abnormal pulmonary function tests.[705] Abnormal pulmonary functions and chest roentgenograms occur in two-thirds of patients without pulmonary symptoms.

Interstitial Lung Disease

Epidemiology.   The prevalence and incidence of lung involvement in mixed connective tissue disease remains ill-defined. It is generally felt that interstitial parenchymal disease is common in patients with mixed connective disease but is often subclinical and only identified by roentgenograph, abnormalities in pulmonary function testing, or physical examination in asymptomatic patients. This is supported by the radiographic findings described below; however, the size of the population from which patients were selected in unclear. There is a female predominance.[706]

Clinical Manifestations.   Dyspnea, pleuritic pain, bibasilar rales, increased P_2, and cough are the most frequent pulmonary manifestations. A third of the patients with evidence of lung involvement are asymptomatic. Clubbing is not seen in mixed connective tissue disease.

Roentgenographic Features.   One-third of patients with mixed connective tissue disease had initial chest roentgenograms that were abnormal, demonstrating small irregular opacities involving the lung bases (Figure 21–15).[707] HRCT findings of pulmonary involvement in mixed connective tissue disease have been characterized as the presence of ground-glass attenuation, nonseptal linear opacities, with a peripheral and lower-lobe predominance (Table 21–16).[708]

Physiologic Features.   Pulmonary function abnormalities include a reduction of the DL_{CO}, a decreased VC, TLC, and FEV_1 (Figure 21–16). Resting hypoxemia was present in 21% (Figure 21–17).[707] There is no correlation between the level of extractable nuclear antigen and pulmonary function abnormalities.[709]

Histopathologic Features.   There have been very limited reports of the histopathologic finding in the lungs of patients with mixed connective tissue disease. It is speculated that the major findings are similar to those of PSS (see "Progressive Systemic Sclerosis," above). Given the HRCT findings in these patients, we can speculate that the major lung injury patterns include NSIP and UIP.[708]

Management and Prognosis.   In an effort to prevent disease progression, evidence of early interstitial pulmonary disease should be sought and corticosteroid and/or immunosuppressive therapy instituted. However, no studies have definitely demonstrated that such therapy will prevent progression to irreversible pulmonary fibrosis.

Obstructive Lung Disease

Izumiyama and colleagues studied pulmonary function in 17 women with mixed connective tissue disease.[710] They showed that VC and DL_{CO} were reduced in 35% and 47% of the patients, respectively. The ratio of FEV_1 to VC was normal in all the patients, but pulmonary resistance and static compliance were abnormal in 35% and 59% of the patients, respectively. The reductions in DL_{CO} correlated with the disease duration. They concluded that small airway obstruction is an early and frequent indication of functional pulmonary impairment, and that impairment of alveolar gas exchange is progressive in patients with mixed connective tissue disease.[710] Radiographic evidence of airway involvement is infrequent.

Chronic Aspiration Pneumonitis

Esophageal dysmotility is present in approximately 80% of patients with mixed connective tissue disease, and aspiration pneumonitis often occurs.[707,711]

Pulmonary Hemorrhage

Germain and Davidman[701] described a patient with mixed connective tissue disease who developed pulmonary hemorrhage and acute renal failure. Schwarz and colleagues presented a case of diffuse alveolar pulmonary hemorrhage due to pulmonary capillaritis in a patient with mixed connective tissue disease.[712] The capillaritis was not part of a systemic vasculitis at the time of the diffuse alveolar pulmonary hemorrhage episode but rather represented an isolated small-vessel vasculitis of the lungs in this group of patients. Immune complex deposition may be involved in the pathogenesis.

Pulmonary Hypertension

Pulmonary artery hypertension occurs in mixed connective tissue disease and is a potentially fatal complication of this disease.[697,699,704,705,713–716] The onset is insidious.

The pulmonary hypertension can be the result of several processes: as a secondary event in patients with interstitial pulmonary fibrosis, as a primary vascular event caused by bland intimal proliferation of the lung arterioles, by a plexogenic angiopathy, or by chronic pulmonary emboli.[700,717,718] Fatal pulmonary hypertension in mixed connective tissue disease was identified in 11 cases in the literature. Interestingly, all were young women, ranging in age from 14 to 34 years. All had histopathologic findings consistent with marked intimal proliferation and medial hypertrophy of pulmonary arteries and arterioles with consequent narrowing of the vascular lumens in nine cases, pulmonary thromboembolic disease in one, and pulmonary vasculitis in the other case.[697,700,707,719–721] What the etiology of the pulmonary hypertension is in the nine cases with plexogenic pulmonary arteriopathy is not clear; however, it is suspected that it may be due to vasoconstriction evoked by the hyperactivity of the pulmonary vessels.[721] Interestingly, in many cases the severity of the proliferative vascular lesion paralleled the severity of the pulmonary hypertension found by right-heart catheterization.[707]

Treatment of this complication in mixed connective tissue disease is difficult. Rosenberg and colleagues

TABLE 21–15　Pleuropulmonary Manifestations of Mixed Connective Tissue Disease

Parenchymal lung disease
   Interstitial pneumonitis and fibrosis
   Chronic aspiration pneumonitis
Pulmonary vascular disease
   Hemorrhage
   Pulmonary hypertension
   Vasculitis (pulmonary capillaritis)
   Multiple pulmonary cysts
Airway disease
   Obstructive lung disease
Pleurisy with or without pleural effusion
Diaphragm dysfunction

reported a case of pulmonary hypertension caused by vasculitis in an 11-year-old girl who responded to a combination of prednisone and cyclophosphamide therapy.[717]

Pleurisy With or Without Pleural Effusion

Pleuritis was reported in 35% of patients and pleuritic chest pain in 40% evaluated by Sullivan and coworkers in a prospective study that emphasized pulmonary involvement.[707] Pleural thickening was identified in only one of 33 chest radiographs examined. Bilateral exudative pleuritis may be the initial manifestation of mixed connective tissue disease.[722] A case report describes a man with mixed connective tissue disease who presented with a left-sided pleural effusion.[723] However, by HRCT evaluation, pleural thickening is quite frequently seen (see Table 21–16).

ANKYLOSING SPONDYLITIS

Definition and General Features

The diagnosis of ankylosing spondylitis is dependent on a clinical suspicion, history, clinical evaluation, and radiologic confirmation demonstrating sacroiliitis.[724,725] The onset is insidious and occurs in persons under the age of 40 years. There is an equal gender distribution but women tend to have milder and more peripheral disease with fewer roentgenographic changes in the spine. The disease is rare in nonwhites.

Back pain and morning stiffness that improve with exercise are characteristic features useful in differentiating ankylosing spondylitis from mechanical spinal arthritis. These symptoms usually begin in the early twenties. During sleep or on awakening these patients complain of pain on inspiration. This pain is due to insertional tendonitis of the costochondral and costovertebral muscle insertions. The pain is poorly characterized, but the radiation may be diffuse. Physical examination may reveal paravertebral muscle spasm, loss of lumbar lordosis, and/or restriction of spinal mobility, which is often symmetrically decreased

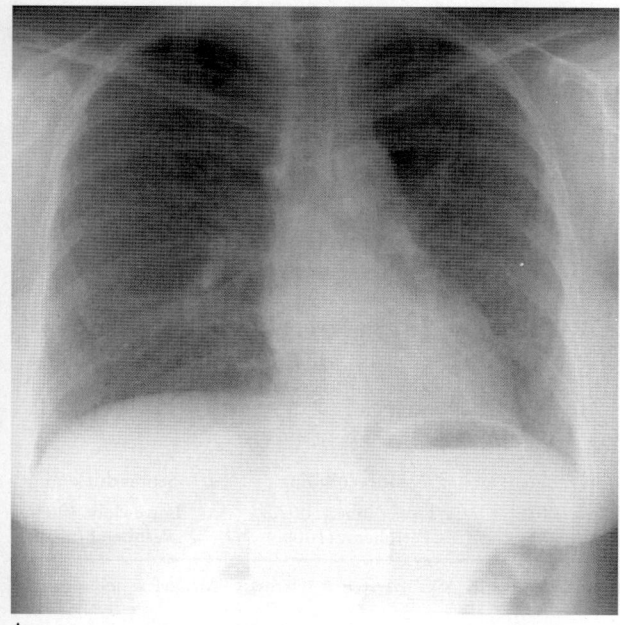

A

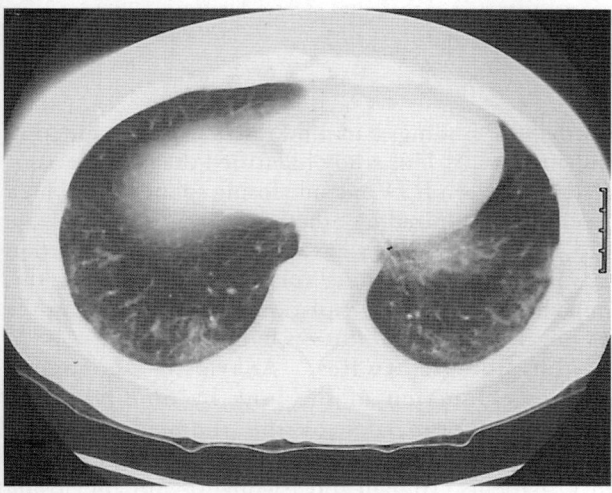

B

Figure 21–15   Mixed connective tissue disease. *A*, A 35-year-old African American woman with a 6-month history of exertional dyspnea. Chest roentgenogram shows bilateral diffuse reticular opacities in the mid-to-lower lung zones. *B*, Computed tomography scan shows predominant subpleural reticular opacities. Lung biopsy showed chronic fibrosing alveolitis characterized by a moderately cellular mural lymphoplasmacytic inflammatory infiltrate. There was a component of bronchiolitis obliterans with luminal distortion with mural fibrosis and smooth muscle hypertrophy involving terminal and respiratory bronchioles. There were foci of intraluminal granulation tissue in affected bronchioles.

and results in restriction of chest expansion. Extra-articular disease was thought to be uncommon in ankylosing spondylitis.[724] However, it is now recognized that constitutional features, such as fatigue, weight loss, and low-grade fever occur. In addition, 25% of patients have uveitis and conjunctivitis after an extended period of

active disease. Chronic prostatism has been identified in 80% of men with ankylosing spondylitis. The onset of prostatism does not seem to be related to the severity of the joint disease in ankylosing spondylitis. Cardiovascular involvement includes cardiac conduction defects, aortitis, and aortic insufficiency in 20% of patients. The cauda equina syndrome, spinal stenosis, and spinal fractures are other complications of this disease.

Laboratory abnormalities are relatively uncommon in ankylosing spondylitis, but include an increased alkaline phosphatase in 50% of patients, an increased serum CPK, and an elevated ESR. None of these abnormalities correlate with disease activity. Circulating immune complexes have also been identified in these patients. The clinical course of ankylosing spondylitis is generally benign with less than 20% of these patients becoming severely disabled, even after three decades of disease. Early involvement of the hip joint is thought to be associated with more extensive involvement of the spine and extremities and a worse long-term outcome.

The cause of ankylosing spondylitis remains unknown. Ankylosing spondylitis has a definite association with the histocompatibility antigen HLA-B27, with more than 90% of Whites with ankylosing spondylitis having HLA-B27 positivity. HLA-B27 is inherited as an autosomal codominant characteristic, and 50% of first-degree relatives of probands with HLA-B27 possess this antigen. Yet only about 20% of patients with HLA-B27 positivity develop ankylosing spondylitis.

Pleuropulmonary Manifestations of Ankylosing Spondylitis

The incidence of pleuropulmonary involvement in ankylosing spondylitis is unknown. It has been estimated to occur in up to 30% although a recent review by Rosenow and associates at the Mayo Clinic suggests that the frequency is less than 2%.[726,727] A number of different pleural and pulmonary manifestations have been seen and are outlined in Table 21–12.[727,728]

Interstitial Lung Disease

Epidemiology.   Apical fibrobullous disease is the most often described pulmonary complication of ankylosing spondylitis.[724,726,729–739] The true incidence of pleuropulmonary manifestations in ankylosing spondylitis is unknown; however, a comprehensive review of 2,080 patients identified an incidence of 1.3%.[727] It is predominantly seen in adult male subjects with a male to female ratio of 50:1.[740,741]

Clinical Manifestations.   Patients who present with apical fibrobullous disease usually have advanced ankylosing spondylitis. The disease is usually bilateral but may involve a single lung initially. Patients may complain of cough, sputum, and dyspnea, but they are often asymptomatic. Clubbing does not occur. Most

TABLE 21–16   Frequency of HRCT Findings in MCTD Compared with SSC and PM/DM*

HRCT Feature	MCTD Kozuka (2001)[708] (n = 41)	MCTD[†] Saito (2002)[706] (n = 35)	Scleroderma Saito (2002)[706] (n = 35)	PM/DM Saito (2002)[706] (n = 42)
Ground-glass opacities	100	11	44	33
Nodules	98	94	91	74
Consolidation	27	0	0	2
Interlobular septal thickening	32	100	97	100
Bronchial wall thickening*	32	3	6	0
Traction bronchiectasis	44			
Cyst	17			
Honeycombing	37	51	80	19
Emphysema	20	9	8	7
Pleural thickening		66	71	76
Predominant abnormality		Septal thickening	Honeycombing	Septal thickening
Predominant zonal distribution	Lower lobe (95%) Peripheral (98%)	Lower lobe (100%) Peripheral (97%)	Lower lobe (100%) Peripheral (100%)	Lower lobe (90%) Perpheral (97%)

HRCT = high-resolution computed tomography; MCTD = mixed connective tissue disease; SSC = systemic sclerosis; PM/DM = polymyositis/dermatomyositis; CTD = connective tissue disease.
*Inclusion of patients in these studies required the diagnosis of a CTD and an abnormal HRCT. Therefore, they are not representative of the group of CTD patients as a whole but intended to convey and compare the radiographic patterns seen in the setting of these diseases.
†Data includes 12 of 35 patients with Sjögren's syndrome associated with MCTD.

patients had the onset of their ankylosing spondylitis early in adult life.

Roentgenographic Features. The chest roentgenogram reveals diffuse reticular or nodular opacities in the upper lung zones. These opacities progress and eventually cause widespread fibrosis and cyst formation in the upper lobes because of the parenchymal destruction. The fibrous portion of the fibrobullous lesions appears as increased interstitial markings. With time, there is complete distortion and destruction of the involved lung and retraction of the hilum toward the apex. In advanced disease, the process can be complicated by a secondary infection, often by the invasion of aspergilli. The changes, in general, mimic those found in pulmonary tuberculosis.

HRCT scanning shows that the plain chest radiograph is insensitive as a measure of lung involvement (Figure 21–18). A study of 26 patients, 4 of whom had an abnormal plain chest radiograph, show frequent abnormalities (70% of the patients).[742] The abnormalities included interstitial lung disease (n = 4), bronchiectasis (n = 6), emphysema (n = 4), apical fibrosis (n = 2), mycetoma (n = 1), and nonspecific ILD (n = 12). Turetschek and coworkers examined thin-section CT in 21 patients; 15 (71%) had abnormalities.[743] The most frequent abnormalities were thickening of the interlobular septa in 33%, mild bronchial wall thickening in 29%, pleural thickening and pleuropulmonary irregularities (both 29%), and linear septal thickening (29%). In 6 patients there were no signs of pleuropulmonary involvement. Eight of 15 patients (53%) with abnormal and 4 of 6 patients (67%) with

normal CT findings had mild restrictive lung function impairment.[743] This study identified the possible association between ILD and ankylosing spondylitis, which has been recognized by others.[744]

Ventilation studies have demonstrated a reduction in ventilation to the lung apices and suggest that this impairment of apical ventilation may be a factor in the pathogenesis of apical fibrosis in this disease.[745]

Physiologic Studies. Ankylosing spondylitis alters the function of the lung by modifying the mechanical properties of the thoracic cage (see below).[746,747] Static pulmonary mechanics were studied in 17 patients (16 men and 1 woman) with ankylosing spondylitis and no obvious clinical or radiologic evidence of pulmonary involvement.[747] TLC was reduced in one and static lung compliance (Cst) in nine (52.9%) of the patients. Four (23.5%) patients had normal TLC, but Cst and shape constant (K) were reduced. Five (29.4%) patients had reduced TLS and Cst; four of them had a low K. The authors concluded that pulmonary involvement in patients with ankylosing spondylitis is probably diffuse and begins much earlier than generally presumed.[747]

Bronchoalveolar Lavage. Bronchoalveolar lavage was performed in 14 patients with spondyloarthropathies.[748] Only two were found to have abnormalities: one revealed lymphocytosis and increased neutrophils in a smoker and an isolated lymphocytosis in another patient with restrictive syndrome and radiographic apical fibrosis. Transbronchial biopsies showed interstitial fibrosis in these patients. Interestingly, unlike other connective tissue disease, subclinical alveolitis was

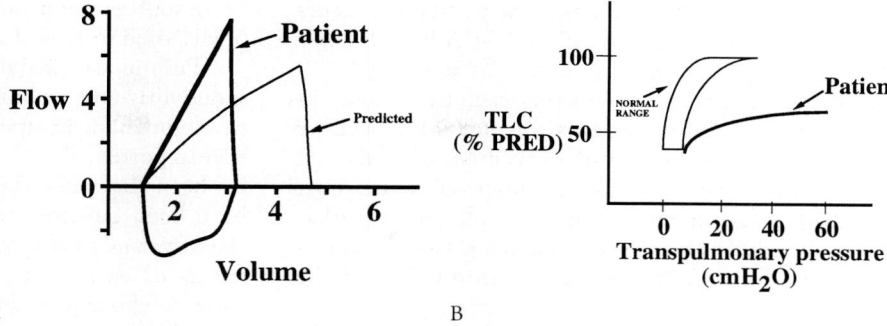

TLC 5 3.37 L (69% of predicted)
TGV 5 1.31 L (49% of predicted)

FVC 5 2.24 L (61% of predicted)
FEV₁ 5 1.96 L (61% of predicted)
FEV₁/FVC 5 87%

DL_CO 5 40% of predicted
DL_CO/VA 5 75% of predicted

Figure 21–16   Mixed connective tissue disease. Same patient as in Figure 21–15. *A*, Flow-volume relationship and lung volume determination revealed moderately severe restriction. The diffusing capacity for carbon monoxide was reduced. *B*, The relationship of the static deflation volume and transthoracic pressure in the same patient is compared with the normal range. This patient's curve is shifted down and to the right due to lung stiffness. The coefficient of elastic retraction (P_{ST} max/TLC) was 18.94 cm H_2O/L (upper limit of normal ~8 cm H_2O/L). TLC = total lung capacity; FVC = forced vital capacity; FEV_1 = forced expiratory volume in 1 second; DL_{CO} = diffusing capacity of carbon monoxide; TGV = thoracic gas volume; VA = alveolar volume; P_{ST} = maximal static transpulmonary pressure.

absent.[748] Wendling and coworkers in another study of bronchoalveolar lavage in 15 patients with ankylosing spondylitis also failed to show evidence of any subclinical alveolitis.[749]

Histopathologic Features.   Pathologically, the early changes are consistent with a patchy pneumonic process, with round cell and fibroblastic infiltration that progresses in time to extensive fibrosis. Usually, dense pleural and pulmonary fibrosis are associated. Bronchiectasis may also occur.

Abnormal Chest Wall and Respiratory Muscle Mobility

The most common thoracic complication is fixation of the thoracic cage because of costovertebral ankylosis. Because of the severity of the thoracic joint involvement in patients with ankylosing spondylitis, it has been thought that this would lead to significant impairment of lung function. Consequently, a number of studies have examined the gas exchange and lung mechanics in ankylosing spondylitis with conflicting results.[746,750,751] In general, it has been determined that there are decreases in VC and TLC and increases in RV and functional residual capacity (FRC). Most of these abnormalities have occurred in patients with advanced disease. On the other hand, flow measurements (ie, FEV, maximum ventilatory capacity, and maximum midexpiratory flow rates) have been consistently normal. The total respiratory resistance is normal and there is a small decrease in reactance at the lowest frequency (between 2–26 Hz as measured by the forced oscillation technique).[746] There is evidence that the changes in total respiratory resistance and reactance is mainly attributable to an increase in chest wall resistance and a decrease in chest wall compliance.[746]

Most studies of gas exchange in these patients have been normal. Renzetti and coworkers demonstrated

mild arterial O_2 desaturation at rest and after exercise in 50% of their patients.[728] An increase in the physiologic dead space was found in all the patients studied. The $PaCO_2$ and alveolar ventilation was normal. It was felt that the increase in the physiologic dead space was secondary to ventilation and perfusion abnormalities. Studies examining the partitioning of the contribution of the rib cage and abdomen to ventilation in ankylosing spondylitis have demonstrated that a greater than

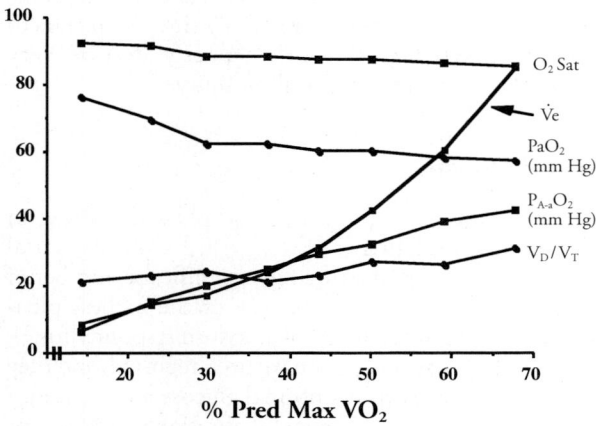

Figure 21–17   Mixed connective tissue disease: respiratory response to exercise. Same patient as in Figures 21–15 and 21–16. Her arterial blood gases at rest were normal ($PaO_2 = 83$; $PaCO_2 = 34$; pH = 7.44; O_2 Sat = 94%; $P_{(A-a)}O_2 < 5$), but a severe gas exchange abnormality developed with mild exercise. Shown is PaO_2, $P_{(A-a)}O_2$, V_D/V_T, $\dot{V}e$, and O_2 saturation obtained during maximal exercise on a bicycle ergometer, while breathing room air at 5,000 ft elevation. She achieved 105 watts (79% of predicted maximum), stopping because of breathlessness and moderate leg fatigue. The PaO_2 decreased, $P_{(A-a)}O_2$ increased, $\dot{V}e$ increased excessively, and V_D/V_T increased, with increasing exercise loads, as expressed by the percent of predicted maximum oxygen uptake ($\dot{V}O_2$ max). Importantly, the severity of her lung disease was much better appreciated after these data were obtained. Her gas exchange remained relatively stable after 4 years of treatment with prednisone, cyclophosphamide, and colchicine. V_D = deadspace volume; T_T = tidal volume; $\dot{V}e$ = minute ventilation.

normal increase of the diaphragmatic excursions occurs at rest and in exercise, especially in patients with abolished or markedly reduced chest wall mobility.[752–754] Seckin and coworkers showed that exercise capacity in ankylosing spondylitis patients was not influenced by the limitation of chest wall movements.[755] Also, it appears that peripheral muscle function is the most important determinant of exercise intolerance in ankylosing spondylitis patients, suggesting that deconditioning is the main factor in the production of the reduced aerobic capacity.[756]

In summary, ankylosing spondylitis causes a slight to moderate decrease in lung volumes (TLC and VC) with a maintenance of expiratory flow rates within the normal limits; FRC and RV are either normal or slightly increased, and gas exchange is usually normal. It is believed that this relative maintenance of the lung function in ankylosing spondylitis results from the fixation of the thorax at high lung volumes and the decrease in chest wall compliance, which contrasts with the abnormalities that occur in kyphoscoliosis, where there is a greater loss in lung volumes and thus does not allow the diaphragm to take over more function of the thoracic muscles. Consequently, hypoventilation, cor pulmonale, and respiratory failure result in those circumstances, but not in ankylosing spondylitis. Significant pulmonary insufficiency does not occur in uncomplicated ankylosing spondylitis despite the severe symmetric deformity and impaired mobility of the chest wall that occurs. Also, it has been recommended that patients undertake a modest amount of exercise regularly since it appears to maintain a satisfactory work capacity despite very restricted spinal and chest wall mobility.[757]

Pleural Disease

Pleural disease is an uncommon associated finding in ankylosing spondylitis.[726,727,729,730,738,758] Apical pleural thickening has been identified in a significant number of patients and is thought to be one of the earliest pleuropulmonary manifestations of ankylosing spondylitis.[727] Pleural effusions are rare, but have been reported, and they are usually exudates with a normal glucose and occasionally are empyemas.[727,759] Pleural calcifications, unrelated to previous occupational exposures, have also been identified. However, their significance is unclear.[735] Spontaneous pneumothorax occurs in about 8% of patients with ankylosing spondylitis and probably results from the rupture of cysts in patients with apical fibrobullous disease.[203]

Infectious Complications

Early reports suggested an association of ankylosing spondylitis with tuberculosis. However, a number of patients who were thought to have tuberculosis never had positive sputum cultures nor did they respond to antituberculous therapy. Nevertheless, it appears from a number of sources that patients with ankylosing spondylitis are predisposed to typical and atypical tuberculosis.[750,760,761]

Pulmonary cavitations (cysts) occur in ankylosing spondylitis and colonization of these cavities with the development of an aspergilloma as a late complication has been reported.[734,760,762,763] The most common organism has been *Aspergillus fumigatus*; however, other organisms have been cultured including *Aspergillus terreus* and *Metschnikowia pulcherrima*. Postoperative bronchopleural fistula or empyema complicates the management of patients who require thoracotomy for the management of aspergillomas; thus, it has been recommended that thoracotomy be avoided in patients with ankylosing spondylitis unless the hemoptysis from an aspergilloma is life threatening.[727,730,735,762,764,765]

Miscellaneous Pulmonary Complications

Cricoarytenoid Arthritis.   Cricoarytenoid arthritis has been described in ankylosing spondylitis and has been associated with acute respiratory failure and cor pulmonale.[766,767] Cricoarytenoid arthritis is a well-recognized complication of RA. This process is associated with upper airway obstruction and causes concern when fiberoptic laryngoscopy, bronchoscopy, or endotracheal intubation are indicated. Experienced personnel should intubate with the aid of a flexible fiberoptic bronchoscope.[768]

Bronchocentric Granulomatosis.   Rohatgi and Turrisi[769] presented a case report of the simultaneous occurrence of bronchocentric granulomatosis and ankylosing spondylitis in a 49-year-old white male who had a 25-year history of ankylosing spondylitis.[769] This patient had ankylosing spondylitis and apical fibrocystic disease and developed a progressive left upper lobe cavitating infiltrate with hemoptysis.

Organizing Pneumonia.   Turner and Enzenauer reported a case of ankylosing spondylitis with organizing pneumonia.[770]

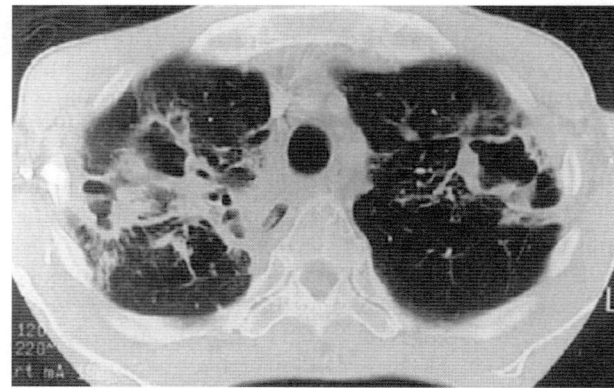

Figure 21–18   Fibrocavitary disease in ankylosing spondylitis. Contrast-enhanced chest computed tomography scan shows distortion of the lung architecture with bilateral upper-lobe cavitation and bronchial thickening. Reproduced with permission from Thai D et al.[741]

Obstructive Lung Disease. Bronchiectasis and emphysema were identified in 23% and 15% of patients, respectively, in an HRCT study of idiopathic ankylosing spondylitis.[742]

Malignancy. Because of the severe scarring process that occurs in some patients with ankylosing spondylitis, the development of a scar carcinoma is not unexpected; cases of both adenocarcinoma and squamous cell carcinoma of the lung thought be to be associated with a scar have been reported.[737,771]

Amyloidosis. Blavia and colleagues reported a case of primary pulmonary diffuse amyloidosis and ankylosing spondylitis.[772]

Drug-Induced Lung Disease. Treatment of patients with ankylosing spondylitis with infliximab has been complicated by the development of systemic tuberculosis and allergic granulomatosis of the lung.[773]

PSORIATIC ARTHRITIS

Definition and General Features

Psoriatic arthritis is an inflammatory arthritis occurring in 7% of patients with psoriasis. Although originally thought to represent RA, psoriatic arthritis is a distinct clinical entity characterized by involvement of the distal interphalangeal and all proximal interphalangeal joints of the hands and feet and by the absence of RF.[774] Kammer and colleagues[775] identified three groups based on the distribution of the arthritis that occurred during the course of the disease: asymmetric oligoarticular arthritis involving any joint especially the distal interphalangeal and the proximal interphalangeal joints of the hands and feet; symmetric arthritis affecting any pair of joints; spondyloarthritis consisting of sacroiliitis and/or ankylosing spondylitis with or without associated peripheral arthritis. An intermittent, oligoarticular, asymmetric synovitis is most frequent. In general, patients with psoriatic spondylitis had an increased association with HLA-B27. Patients with more severe skin disease and with pitting of the nails had a greater risk of developing joint disease. Many patients have hyperuricemia and/or hypercomplementemia; the hyperuricemia is not associated with gout.

Pleuropulmonary Manifestations of Psoriatic Arthritis

Few studies have examined lung function in patients with psoriatic arthritis. Scherak and coworkers examined BAL fluid in 13 asymptomatic patients with serologically negative arthritis (RF); (6 with peripheral psoriatic arthritis, 2 with axial psoriatic arthritis, 3 with ankylosing spondylitis, and 2 with sacroiliitis).[776] BAL revealed a significant decrease of neutrophil granulocytes and an increase of B lymphocytes in patients with seronegative arthritis in comparison with 64 patients with RA (RA; 24 seronegative, 39 seropositive) and 15 healthy controls. Patients with seronegative arthritis had a significant increase in lymphocytes, especially T, T helper, and activated cells. Transbronchial biopsy was performed on 9 patients with seronegative arthritis with abnormal histologic features of lung tissue observed in 4 patients (2 with fibrosis, 1 with follicular lymphoid hyperplasia, and 1 with desquamative interstitial pneumonitis). The significance of these findings is unknown. An advanced nongranulomatous upper lobe pulmonary fibrosis has been described in psoriatic spondylitis.[777] Because of the similarities between psoriatic spondylitis and ankylosing spondylitis, the pulmonary diseases are also likely to be similar. Hiki and associates reported a case of severe IgA nephropathy associated with psoriatic arthritis and idiopathic interstitial pneumonia.[778]

BEHÇET'S DISEASE

Definition and General Features

Behçet's disease is a multisystem disorder characterized by ulcers of the mouth and genitalia, relapsing iritis, joint manifestations, thrombophlebitis, migraines, erythema nodosum, and central nervous system abnormalities (meningoencephalitis).[779] In general, the diagnosis of Behçet's disease requires the presence of three of the following: (1) recurrent aphthous stomatitis, (2) genital aphthous ulcers, (3) uveitis, (4) synovitis, (5) cutaneous vasculitis, and (6) meningoencephalitis. Vascular involvement is common in Behçet's disease and is characterized by thrombosis of larger veins and arteries and arterial aneurysms. Obstruction of the inferior or superior vena cava occurs with relative frequency.[780–784]

Pleuropulmonary Manifestations of Behçet's Disease

Pulmonary involvement is uncommon in Behçet's disease.[784–792] Intrathoracic manifestations of Behçet's disease consist mainly of thromboembolism of the superior vena cava and/or other mediastinal veins; aneurysms of the aorta and pulmonary arteries; pulmonary infarct and hemorrhage; pleural effusion; and, rarely, myocardial or pericardial involvement, cor pulmonale, and mediastinal or hilar lymphadenopathy.[784]

Clinical Manifestations

Erkan and Cavdar reported the clinical findings of 12 patients with Behçet's disease and lung involvement.[793] The male to female ratio was 11 to 1, mean age was 35.3 ± 8.8 yr. All patients had at least four other organ manifestations of vasculitis, either in their history or during the period of lung involvement. The main complaint was hemoptysis of varying degree in 11 of the 12 patients. This was likely due to bronchial erosion secondary to the aneurysms. A leukocytoclastic vasculitis of the pulmonary arteries has been identified and is felt to be secondary to immune complex deposition.[783,794] The Hughes-Stovin syndrome is thought to be a manifestation of Behçet's disease, and venous thrombosis and pulmonary aneurysms are common to both processes.[795,796]

A report of 14 nonsmoking, asymptomatic patients with Behçet's disease and normal chest radiographs, demonstrated no difference in static lung volumes relative to healthy controls.[797] However, $P_{(A-a)}O_2$ gradient and VD/VT were higher than control values, whereas the PaO_2 was lower.

Roentgenographic Features

The chest radiographs in the study by Erkan and Cavdar showed unilateral hilar enlargements in six patients, diaphragm elevation in four, horizontally or obliquely oriented linear opacities in three, diffuse, ill-defined opacities in upper and lower zones in three, wedge-shaped peripheral opacities in one, and bilateral pleural effusion in one patient.[793] Computed tomography of the chest performed in nine patients revealed aneurysms, narrowings, and cutoffs of the main, lobar, segmental, or peripheral branches of the pulmonary artery and irregular configuration of other pulmonary vessels. Perfusion scans demonstrated defects of various sizes in all patients. Pulmonary angiography performed in only two patients showed amputation of branches of the pulmonary artery and aneurysmal dilatations.[793]

Because aneurysms may develop at the arterial puncture sites and veins may be quickly thrombosed after injection of contrast material, angiography and venography should be avoided whenever possible.[784] Although little data exist, CT and magnetic resonance angiography appear to be the imaging techniques of choice for evaluating vascular involvement.[784] Iodine 123-metaiodobenzylguanidine techniques to assess endothelial injury are being considered for use in Behçet's disease.[798]

Management

Treatment with corticosteroids, cyclophosphamide, and/or colchicine has been helpful in patients with active lung disease, as well as disease at other sites.[782,793,794,799] Cyclosporin treatment was used in a patient with rapidly progressive pulmonary thromboembolic Behçet's disease.[800] Koga and coworkers used FK506, a novel immunosuppressive agent, as a treatment in a 21–year-old woman who presented with repeated oral and genital ulcers, folliculitis, panuveitis, and localized pulmonary opacities on her chest radiograph.[801] These pulmonary opacities, skin lesions, and uveitis improved after the oral administration of FK506 for 8 weeks.[801]

RELAPSING POLYCHONDRITIS

Definition and General Features

Relapsing polychondritis is a chronic, episodic, systemic disorder characterized by recurrent widespread and potentially destructive inflammatory lesions that involve cartilaginous structures of the external ear, the joints, the nose, and the respiratory tract.[802,803] Approximately 25% of patients with relapsing polychondritis have a coexistent connective tissue disease such as adult and juvenile RA. Sjögren's syndrome, SLE, Reiter's syndrome, psoriatic arthritis, and ankylosing spondylitis.

The disease occurs predominantly in Whites and has an equal gender predilection with no apparent familial predisposition. Onset occurs between the ages of 40 and 60 years. Typically, pain and tenderness start suddenly in association with a violaceous erythematous swelling of one or both external ears. Two-thirds of the patients develop nasal chondritis, which often occurs suddenly and may result in cartilaginous destruction and deformity of the nose. Ocular inflammation including episcleritis, scleritis, conjunctivitis, and iritis occur in two-thirds of patients. The majority of patients develop an arthropathy characterized as an episodic, asymmetric, nonerosive, and nondeforming arthritis. Vasculitis with involvement of the medium and large vessels is common in many patients and is manifested by aneurysm formation as well as thrombosis. The vasculitis may be focal or diffuse, indolent or fulminate, and rapidly fatal. Cardiovascular and respiratory tract complications are the most common cause of death.[803,804] Cardiovascular complications occur in 25%, mainly men, and consist of an aortic insufficiency secondary to progressive dilatation of the aortic ring in the ascending aorta. Mitral and tricuspid insufficiency occurs but less frequently. In addition, aneurysms involving the ascending, thoracic, and abdominal aortas may rupture and cause sudden death. Pericarditis and myocarditis with conduction disturbances, endocarditis, and myocardial infarction may be seen less frequently.

Pleuropulmonary Manifestations of Relapsing Polychondritis

Clinical Manifestations

Pulmonary disease occurs in patients who have recurrent involvement of the laryngotracheal bronchial structures, causing obstruction of the upper airways and secondary pneumonia. Hoarseness and laryngeal tenderness over the thyroid cartilage and anterior trachea are common presenting symptoms. A nonproductive cough, dyspnea, aphonia, inspiratory stridor, or rarely hemoptysis should also alert the physician to the possibility of this life-threatening complication.

Roentgenographic Features

Tracheal tomography, cinebronchography, and computer tomography scans may be useful in identifying obstruction of the anatomic airways. The chest roentgenogram may sometimes reveal atelectasis, pneumonia, or widening of the aortic arch or of the ascending or descending aorta.

Physiologic Features

Studies of maximal expiratory and inspiratory flow volume curves and airway resistance are often useful in providing information on the site and nature of the obstructive process. They can differentiate between fixed and dynamic large airway obstruction as well as help in the localization of the obstruction to intrathoracic or extrathoracic airways.[805,806] Patients with expiratory obstruction do not have evidence of a loss of elastic forces.[807] Burlew and coworkers reported a case with pulmonary opacities and pulmonary function studies suggestive of small airways disease.[808]

Management and Prognosis

The management of patients with relapsing polychondritis is directed primarily at maintaining adequate ventilation. Tracheostomy is required if the larynx is significantly involved. Occasionally, surgical treatment of the collapsed airways may be successful. The use of multiple metallic stents to relieve severe airway obstruction has been described.[809] Corticosteroids and immunosuppressive agents have been used in the management of acute inflammatory episodes and are probably helpful especially in the extrapulmonary manifestations that occur. It is not clear whether corticosteroid treatment alters the natural course of this disease.[802,803,810]

A recent study of survival in relapsing polychondritis demonstrated that infection, systemic vasculitis, and malignancy were the most common causes of death. Respiratory tract involvement was only considered the cause of death in 10%.[810] Death due to respiratory tract involvement usually occurs because of recurrent attacks that lead to destruction of the cartilage of the tracheal and bronchial rings, causing collapse of these structures with inflammation, edema, and cicatrization. This cartilaginous destruction may lead to severe focal or diffuse airway collapse with inadequate ventilation that often is not corrected by tracheostomy and mechanical ventilation. Thus death can occur from asphyxiation.

REFERENCES

1. Divertie MB. Lung involvement in the connective tissue disorders. Med Clin North Am 1964;48:1015–30.
2. Turner-Warwick M. Immunologic aspects of systemic diseases of the lung. Proc R Soc Med 1974;67:541–7.
3. Matthay RA, Schwarz MI, Petty TL. Pleuro-pulmonary manifestations of connective tissue diseases. Clin Notes Respir Dis 1977;16:3–9.
4. Hunninghake GW, Fauci AS. Pulmonary involvement in the collagen vascular diseases. Am Rev Respir Dis 1979;119:471–503.
5. Eisenberg H. The interstitial lung diseases associated with the collagen-vascular disorders. Clin Chest Med 1982;3:565–78.
6. Stanford RE. Rheumatoid and other collagen lung diseases. Semin Respir Med 1982;4:107–13.
7. Doll NJ, Salvaggio JE. Pulmonary manifestations of the collagen vascular diseases. Semin Respir Dis 1984;5:273–81.
8. Lamblin C, Bergoin C, Saelens T, Wallaert B. Interstitial lung diseases in collagen vascular diseases. Eur Respir J Suppl 2001;32:69S–80S.
9. Wiedemann HP, Matthay RA. Pulmonary manifestations of the collagen vascular diseases. Clin Chest Med 1989;10:677–722.
10. Crystal RG, Fulmer JD, Roberts WC, et al. Idiopathic pulmonary fibrosis: clinical, histologic, radiographic, physiologic, scintigraphic, cytologic and biochemical aspects. Ann Intern Med 1976;85:769–88.
11. Centers for Disease Control. CDC surveillance for AIDS: defining opportunistic illnesses 1992–1997. MMWR Morb Mortal Wkly Rep 1999;48:1.
12. Black LF, Katz S. Respiratory disease: task force report on problems, research approaches, needs. National Heart and Lung Institute; 1977 DHEW Publication No.: NIH77–1248, Washington, DC.
13. American Thoracic Society. Idiopathic pulmonary fibrosis: diagnosis and treatment. International consensus statement. American Thoracic Society (ATS), and the European Respiratory Society (ERS). Am J Respir Crit Care Med 2000;161:646–64.
14. Douglas WW, Tazelaar HD, Hartman TE, et al. Polymyositis-dermatomyositis-associated interstitial lung disease. Am J Respir Crit Care Med 2001;164:1182–5.
15. Fujita J, Yoshinouchi T, Ohtsuki Y, et al. Non-specific interstitial pneumonia as pulmonary involvement of systemic sclerosis. Ann Rheum Dis 2001;60:281–3.
16. Kim DS, Yoo B, Lee JS, et al. The major histopathologic pattern of pulmonary fibrosis in scleroderma is nonspecific interstitial pneumonia. Sarcoid Vasc Diffuse Lung Dis 2002;19:121–7.
17. Bouros D, Wells AU, Nicholson AG, et al. Histopathologic subsets of fibrosing alveolitis in patients with systemic sclerosis and their relationship to outcome. Am J Respir Crit Care Med 2002;165:1581–6.
18. Salaffi F, Manganelli P, Carotti M, Baldelli S. The differing patterns of subclinical pulmonary involvement in connective tissue diseases as shown by application of factor analysis. Clin Rheumatol 2000;19:35–41.
19. Page SA, Gobosky A. Immunopathogenesis of rheumatoid arthritis. Am J Med 1979;67:961–70.
20. Gordon DA, Stein JL, Broder I. The extra-articular features of rheumatoid arthritis. Am J Med 1973;54:445–52.
21. Hurd ER. Extra-articular manifestations of rheumatoid arthritis. Semin Arthritis Rheum 1979;8:151–76.
22. Shannon TM, Gale ME. Noncardiac manifestations of rheumatoid arthritis in the thorax. J Thorac Imaging 1992;7:19–29.
23. Scott DGI, Bacon PA, Tribe CR. Systemic rheumatoid vasculitis: a clinical and laboratory study of 50 cases. Medicine 1981;60(4):288–97.
24. Gordon DA, Broder I, Hyland RH. Rheumatoid arthritis. In: Cannon GW, Zimmerman GA, editors. The lung in rheumatic diseases. New York: Marcel Dekker, Inc.; 1990. p. 229.
25. Anaya JM, Diethelm L, Ortiz LA, et al. Pulmonary involvement in rheumatoid arthritis. Semin Arthritis Rheum 1995;24:242–54.

26. Morrison SC, Mody GM, Benatar SR, Meyers OL. The lungs in rheumatoid arthritis—a clinical, radiographic and pulmonary function study. S Afr Med J 1996;86:829–33.

27. Short CL. The antiquity of rheumatoid arthritis. Arthritis Rheum 1974;17:193–205.

28. Ellman P, Ball RE. "Rheumatoid disease" with joint and pulmonary manifestations. BMJ 1948;2:816–20.

29. Harris EDJ. Rheumatoid arthritis: the clinical spectrum. In: Kelley WN, Harris ED Jr, Ruddy S, Sledge CB, editors. Textbook of rheumatology. Philadelphia: W.B. Saunders; 1985. p. 915.

30. Patterson CD, Harrille WE, Pierce JA. Rheumatoid lung disease. Ann Intern Med 1965;62:685–97.

31. Stack BHR, Grant JWB. Rheumatoid interstital lung disease. Br J Dis Chest 1965;59:202–11.

32. Bain LS, Robertson PD. Rheumatoid lung disease. Ann Phys Med 1967;9:110–6.

33. Tomasi TB, Fudenberg HH, Finby N. Possible relationship of rheumatoid factors and pulmonary disease. Am J Med 1962;33:243–348.

34. Waaler E. The visceral lesion in rheumatoid arthritis. Acta Rheumatol Scand 1967;13:20–41.

35. Brannen HM, Good CA, Divertie MB, Baggenstoss AH. Pulmonary disease associated with rheumatoid arthritis. JAMA 1964;189:914–8.

36. Talbott JA, Calkins E. Pulmonary involvement in rheumatoid arthritis. JAMA 1964;189:135–7.

37. Popper MS, Bogdonoff ML, Hughes RL. Interstitial rheumatoid lung disease. Chest 1972;62:243–50.

38. Salorinne Y, Laitinen O, Taskinen E, Tukiainen P. Lung involvement in rheumatoid arthritis. Scand J Rheumatol 1975;8 Suppl:65.

39. Whorwell PJ, Wojtulewski JA, Lacey BW. Respiratory function in rheumatoid arthritis. BMJ 1975;2:175.

40. Cervantes-Perez P, Toro-Perez AH, Rodriguez-Jurado P. Pulmonary involvement in rheumatoid arthritis. JAMA 1980;243:1715–9.

41. Jurik AG, Davidsen D, Graudal H. Prevalence of pulmonary involvement in rheumatoid patients and its relationship to some characteristics of the patients. Scand J Rheumatol 1982;11:217–24.

42. Brinkman GL, Chaikof L. Rheumatoid lung disease. Report of a case which developed in childhood. Am Rev Respir Dis 1959;80:732–7.

43. Jordon JD, Snyder CH. Rheumatoid disease of the lung and cor pulmonale. Am J Dis Child 1964;108:174–80.

44. Walker WC, Walker V. Diffuse interstitial pulmonary fibrosis and rheumatoid arthritis. Ann Rheum Dis 1969;28:252–8.

45. Turner-Warwick M, Evans RC. Pulmonary manifestations of rheumatoid disease. Clin Rheum Dis 1977;3:549–64.

46. MacFarlane JD, Dieppe PA, Rigden BG, Clark TJH. Pulmonary and pleural lesions in rheumatoid disease. Br J Dis Chest 1978;72:288–300.

47. Athreya BH, Doughty RA, Bookspan M, et al. Pulmonary manifestations of juvenile rheumatoid arthritis. A report of eight cases and review. Clin Chest Med 1980;1:361–74.

48. Dawson JK, Fewins HE, Desmond J, et al. Fibrosing alveolitis in patients with rheumatoid arthritis as assessed by high resolution computed tomography, chest radiography, and pulmonary function tests. Thorax 2001;56:622–7.

49. Walker WC, Wright V. Pulmonary lesions and rheumatoid arthritis. Medicine 1968;48:501–20.

50. Frank ST, Weg JG, Harkleroad LE, Fitch RF. Pulmonary dysfunction in rheumatoid disease. Chest 1973;63:27–34.

51. Dawson JK, Fewins HE, Desmond J, et al. Predictors of progression of HRCT diagnosed fibrosing alveolitis in patients with rheumatoid arthritis. Ann Rheum Dis 2002;61:517–21.

52. Schernthaner G, Scherak O, Kolarz G, Kummer F. Seropositive rheumatoid arthritis associated with decreased diffusion capacity of the lung. Ann Rheum Dis 1976;35:258–62.

53. Saag KG, Kolluri S, Koehnke RK, et al. Rheumatoid arthritis lung disease. Determinants of radiographic and physiologic abnormalities. Arthritis Rheum 1996;39:1711–9.

54. Wolfe F. The effect of smoking on clinical, laboratory, and radiographic status in rheumatoid arthritis. J Rheumatol 2000;27:630–7.

55. Mattey DL, Hutchinson D, Dawes PT, et al. Smoking and disease severity in rheumatoid arthritis: association with polymorphism at the glutathione S-transferase M1 locus. Arthritis Rheum 2002;46:640–6.

56. Gabbay E, Tarala R, Will R, et al. Interstitial lung disease in recent onset rheumatoid arthritis. Am J Respir Crit Care Med 1997;156:528–35.

57. Cudkowicz L, Madoff IM, Adelmann WH. Rheumatoid lung disease. Br J Dis Chest 1961;55:35–40.

58. Bennett JC. The infectious etiology of rheumatoid arthritis. Arthritis Rheum 1978;21:531–8.

59. Stastny P. Association of the B-cell alloantigen DRw4 with rheumatoid arthritis. N Engl J Med 1978;298:869–71.

60. Trentham DE, Dynesius RA, Rocklin RE, David JR. Cellular sensitivity to collagen in rheumatoid arthritis. N Engl J Med 1978;299:327–32.

61. Ferrell PB, Aiteson CT, Pearson GR, Tan EM. Seroepidemiological study of relationships between Epstein–Barr virus and rheumatoid arthritis. J Clin Invest 1981;67:681–7.

62. Alarcon GS, Koopman WJ, Acton RJ, Barger BO. Seronegative rheumatoid arthritis: a distinct immunogenetic disease? Arthritis Rheum 1982;35:502–7.

63. Rodnan GP, Schumacher HR, Zvaifler NJ. Primer on the rheumatic diseases. Atlanta: Arthritis Foundation; 1983.

64. Sievers K, Aho K, Hurri L, Perttla Y. Studies of rheumatoid pulmonary disease: a comparison of roentgenological findings among patients with rheumatoid factor titers and with completely negative reactions. Acta Tuberc Scand 1964; 35:21–34.

65. Baum J, Stastny P, Ziff M. Effects of the rheumatoid factor and antigen-antibody complexes on the vessels of the rat mesentery. J Immunol 1964;93:985–92.

66. Zubler RH, Nydegger U, Perrin LH, et al. Circulating and intra-articular immune complexes in patients with rheumatoid arthritis. J Clin Invest 1976;57:1308–19.

67. DeHoratius RJ, Williams RCJ. Rheumatoid factor accentuation of pulmonary lesions associated with experimental diffuse proliferative lung disease. Arthritis Rheum 1972;15:293–301.

68. Jansen JM, Schutte AJH, Elema ID, Giessen MVD. Local immune complexes and inflammatory response in patients with chronic interstitial pulmonary disorders associated with collagen vascular diseases. Clin Exp Immunol 1984;56:311–20.

69. Wallaert B, Bart F, Aerts C, et al. Activated alveolar macrophages in subclinical pulmonary involvement in collagen vascular diseases. Thorax 1988;43:24–30.

70. Perez T, Farre JM, Gosset P, et al. Subclinical alveolar inflammation in rheumatoid arthritis: superoxide anion, neutrophil chemotactic activity and fibronectin generation by alveolar macrophages. Eur Respir J 1989;2:7–13.

71. Hilton RC, Pitkeathly DA. Familial association of rheumatoid arthritis and fibrosing alveolitis. Ann Rheum Dis 1974;33:191–5.

72. Geddes DM, Brewerton DA, Webley M, et al. Alpha-1-antitrypsin phenotypes in fibrosing alveolitis and rheumatoid arthritis. Lancet 1977;ii:1049–51.

73. Hyland RH, Gordon DA, Broder I, et al. A systematic controlled study of pulmonary abnormalities in rheumatoid arthritis. J Rheumatol 1983;10:395–405.

74. Locke GB. Rheumatoid lung. Clin Radiol 1963;14:43–53.

75. Edge JR, Rickards AG. Rheumatoid arthritis with lung lesions. Thorax 1957;12:352–7.

76. Rubin EH. Pulmonary lesions in "rheumatoid disease" with remarks on diffuse interstitial pulmonary fibrosis. Am J Med 1955;19:569–82.

77. Lee FI, Brain AT. Chronic diffuse interstitial pulmonary fibrosis and rheumatoid arthritis. Lancet 1962;ii:693–5.

78. Cruickshank B. Interstitial pneumonia and its consequences in rheumatoid disease. Br J Dis Chest 1959;53:226–36.

79. Ognibene AJ. Systemic "rheumatoid disease" with interstitial pulmonary fibrosis. Arch Intern Med 1960;105:762–9.

80. Morgan WK, Wolfel DA. The lungs and pleura in rheumatoid arthritis. Am J Roentgenol Radiol Ther 1966;98:334–42.

81. Schechter SL, Bole GG. Hypertrophic osteothropathy and rheumatoid arthritis. Arthritis Rheum 1976;19:639–44.

82. Rajasekaran BA, Shovlin D, Lord P, Kelly CA. Interstitial lung disease in patients with rheumatoid arthritis: a comparison with cryptogenic fibrosing alveolitis. Rheumatology (Oxford) 2001;40:1022–5.

83. Flatley FJ. Rheumatoid pulmonary disease. N Engl J Med 1959;261:1105–8.

84. Doctor L, Snider GL. Diffuse interstitial pulmonary fibrosis associated with arthritis. Am Rev Respir Dis 1962;85:413–22.

85. Frayha R, Ayyash R, Gehshan A, Gemayel N. Rheumatoid disease without arthritis. Johns Hopkins Med J 1976;139:69–72.

86. Akira M, Sakatani M, Hara H. Thin-section CT findings in rheumatoid arthritis-associated lung disease: CT patterns and their courses. J Comput Assist Tomogr 1999;23:941–8.

87. Martel W, Abell MR, Mikkelsen WM, Whitehouse WM. Pulmonary and pleural lesions in rheumatoid disease. Radiology 1968;90:641–53.

88. Remy-Jardin M, Remy J, Cortet B, et al. Lung changes in rheumatoid arthritis: CT findings. Radiology 1994;193:375–82.

89. Fujii M, Adachi S, Shimizu T, et al. Interstitial lung disease in rheumatoid arthritis: assessment with high-resolution computed tomography. J Thorac Imaging 1993;8:54–62.

90. McDonagh J, Greaves M, Wright AR, et al. High resolution computed tomography of the lungs in patients with rheumatoid arthritis and interstitial lung disease. Br J Rheumatol 1994;33:118–22.

91. Goupille P, Diot P, Valat JP, et al. Imaging of pulmonary disease in rheumatoid arthritis using J001X scintigraphy: preliminary results. Eur J Nucl Med 1995;22:1411–5.

92. Collins RL, Turner RA, Johnson AM, et al. Obstructive pulmonary disease in rheumatoid arthritis. Arthritis Rheum 1976;19:623–8.

93. Geddes DM, Webley M, Emerson PA. Airways obstruction in rheumatoid arthritis. Ann Rheum Dis 1979;38:222–5.

94. Kolarz G, Scherak O, Popp W, et al. Bronchoalveolar lavage in rheumatoid arthritis. Br J Rheumatol 1993;32:556–61.

95. Scherak O, Popp W, Kolarz G, et al. Bronchoalveolar lavage and lung biopsy in rheumatoid arthritis. In vivo effects of disease modifying antirheumatic drugs. J Rheumatol 1993;20:944–9.

96. Tishler M, Grief J, Fireman E, et al. Bronchoalveolar lavage—a sensitive tool for early diagnosis of pulmonary involvement in rheumatoid arthritis. J Rheumatol 1986;13:547–50.

97. Garcia JG, Parhami N, Killam D, et al. Bronchoalveolar lavage fluid evaluation in rheumatoid arthritis. Am Rev Respir Dis 1986;133:450–4.

98. Wallaert B, Prin L, Hatron P, et al. Lymphocyte subpopulations in bronchoalveolar lavage in Sjögren's syndrome. Chest 1987;92:1025–31.

99. Weiland JE, Garcia JG, Davis WB, Gadek JE. Neutrophil collagenase in rheumatoid interstitial lung disease. J Appl Physiol 1987;62:628–33.

100. Casale TB, Little MM, Furst D, et al. Elevated BAL fluid histamine levels and parenchymal pulmonary disease in rheumatoid arthritis. Chest 1989;96:1016–21.

101. Gilligan DM, O'Connor CM, Ward K, et al. Bronchoalveolar lavage in patients with mild and severe rheumatoid lung disease. Thorax 1990;45:591–6.

102. Gosset P, Perez T, Lassalle P, et al. Increased TNF-alpha secretion by alveolar macrophages from patients with rheumatoid arthritis. Am Rev Respir Dis 1991;143:593–7.

103. American Thoracic Society/European Respiratory Society. International multidisciplinary consensus classification of the idiopathic interstitial pneumonias. Am J Respir Crit Care Med 2002;165:277–304.

104. Howling SJ, Hansell DM, Wells AU, et al. Follicular bronchiolitis: thin-section CT and histologic findings. Radiology 1999;212:637–42.

105. Yousem SA, Colby TV, Carrington CB. Lung biopsy in rheumatoid arthritis. Am Rev Respir Dis 1985;131:770–7.

106. Dixon AS, Dixon J, Ball J. Honeycomb lung and chronic rheumatoid arthritis. Ann Rheum Dis 1957;16:241–5.

107. Epler GR, Colby TV, McLoud TC, et al. Bronchiolitis obliterans organizing pneumonia. N Engl J Med 1985;312:152–8.

108. Ippolito JA, Palmer L, Spector S, et al. Bronchiolitis obliterans organizing pneumonia and rheumatoid arthritis. Semin Arthritis Rheum 1993;23:70–8.

109. Cohen AJ, King TE Jr, Downey GP. Rapidly progressive bronchiolitis obliterans with organizing pneumonia. Am J Respir Crit Care Med 1994;149:1670–5.

110. Hamman L, Rich AR. Fulminating diffuse interstitial fibrosis of the lungs. Trans Am Clin Climatol Assoc 1935;51:154–63.

111. Hamman L, Rich AR. Acute diffuse interstitial fibrosis of the lungs. Bull Johns Hopkins Hosp 1944;74:177–212.

112. Hakala M. Poor prognosis in patients with rheumatoid arthritis hospitalized for interstitial lung fibrosis. Chest 1988;93:114–8.

113. Kucera RF. A possible association of rheumatoid arthritis and sarcoidosis. Chest 1989;95:604–6.

114. Fellbaum C, Domej W, Popper H. Rheumatoid arthritis with extensive lung lesions. Thorax 1989;44:70–1.

115. Hubbard R, Venn A. The impact of coexisting connective tissue disease on survival in patients with fibrosing alveolitis. Rheumatology (Oxford) 2002;41:676–9.

116. Abel T, Andrews BS, Cunningham PH, et al. Rheumatoid vasculitis: effect of cyclophosphamide on the clinical course and levels of circulating immune complexes. Ann Intern Med 1980;93:407–13.

117. Cohen JM, Miller A, Spiera H. Interstitial pneumonitis complicating rheumatoid arthritis: sustained remission with azathioprine therapy. Chest 1977;72:521–4.

118. Scott DGI, Bacon PA. Response to methotrexate in fibrosing alveolitis associated with connective tissue disease. Thorax 1980;35:725–31.

119. Lorber A. Penicillamine therapy for rheumatoid lung disease: effects on protein sulfhydryl groups. Nature 1966;210:1235–7.

120. Puttick MP, Klinkhoff AV, Chalmers A, Ostrow DN. Treatment of progressive rheumatoid interstitial lung disease with cyclosporine. J Rheumatol 1995;22:2163–5.

121. Vergnenègre A, Pugnere N, Antonini MT, et al. Airway obstruction and rheumatoid arthritis. Europ Respir J 1997;10:1072–8.

122. Davidson C, Brook AGF, Bacon PA. Lung function in rheumatoid arthritis. Ann Rheumatic Dis 1974;33:293–7.

123. Begin R, Masse S, Cantin A, et al. Airway disease in a subset of nonsmoking rheumatoid patients. Characterization of the disease and evidence for an autoimmune pathogenesis. Am J Med 1982;72:743–50.

124. Walker WC. Pulmonary infection and rheumatoid arthritis. QJM 1967;36:239–51.

125. Vest JV, Smith TW, Gorman JC, et al. Airways abnormalities in non-smokers with rheumatoid arthritis. Am Rev Respir Dis 1980;121:202A.

126. Doyle JJ, Eliasson AH, Argyros GJ, et al. Prevalence of pulmonary disorders in patients with newly diagnosed rheumatoid arthritis. Clin Rheumatol 2000;19:217–21.

127. Kroot EJ, van Gestel AM, Swinkels HL, et al. Chronic comor-

bidity in patients with early rheumatoid arthritis: a descriptive study. J Rheumatol 2001;28:1511–7.

128. Polisar IA, Burbank B, Levitt L, et al. Bilateral midline fixation of cricoarytenoid joints as a serious medical emergency. JAMA 1960;75:901–6.

129. Lofgren RH, Montgomery WW. Incidence of laryngeal involvement in rheumatoid arthritis. N Engl J Med 1962;267:193–5.

130. Geterud A, Ejnell H, Mansson I, et al. Severe airway obstruction caused by laryngeal rheumatoid arthritis. J Rheumatol 1986;13:948–51.

131. Friedman BA, Rice DH. Rheumatoid nodules of the larynx. Arch Otolaryngol 1975;101:361–3.

132. Shadick NA, Fanta CH, Weinblatt ME, et al. Bronchiectasis. A late feature of severe rheumatoid arthritis. Medicine 1994;73:161–70.

133. Despaux J, Polio JC, Toussirot E, et al. Rheumatoid arthritis and bronchiectasis. A retrospective study of fourteen cases. Rev Rhum Engl Ed 1996;63:801–8.

134. Hassan WU, Keaney NP, Holland CD, Kelly CA. High resolution computed tomography of the lung in lifelong non-smoking patients with rheumatoid arthritis. Ann Rheum Dis 1995;54:308–10.

135. Cortet B, Flipo RM, Rémy-Jardin M, et al. Use of high resolution computed tomography of the lungs in patients with rheumatoid arthritis. Ann Rheum Dis 1995;54:815–9.

136. Hillarby MC, McMahon MJ, Grennan DM, et al. HLA associations in subjects with rheumatoid arthritis and bronchiectasis but not with other pulmonary complications of rheumatoid disease. Br J Rheumatol 1993;32:794–7.

137. Fortoul TI, Cano-Valle F, Oliva E, Barrios R. Follicular bronchiolitis in association with connective tissue diseases. Lung 1985;163:305–14.

138. Yousem SA, Colby TV, Carrington CB. Follicular bronchitis/bronchiolitis. Hum Pathol 1985;16:700–6.

139. Hayakawa H, Sato A, Imokawa S, et al. Bronchiolar disease in rheumatoid arthritis. Am J Respir Crit Care Med 1996; 154:1531–6.

140. Sugiyama Y, Ohno S, Kano S, et al. Diffuse panbronchiolitis and rheumatoid arthritis: a possible correlation with HLA-B54. Intern Med 1994;33:612–4.

141. Homma S, Kawabata M, Kishi K, et al. Diffuse panbronchiolitis in rheumatoid arthritis. Eur Respir J 1998;12:444–52.

142. Hayakawa H, Sato A, Imokawa S, et al. Diffuse panbronchiolitis and rheumatoid arthritis-associated bronchiolar disease: similarities and differences. Intern Med 1998;37:504–8.

143. Petrie GR, Bloomfield P, Grant IWB, Crompton GK. Upper lobe fibrosis and cavitation in rheumatoid disease. Br J Dis Chest 1980;74:263–7.

144. Strohl KP, Feldman NT, Ingram RH. Apical fibrobullous disease with rheumatoid disease. Chest 1979;75:739–41.

145. Scadding JG. The lungs in rheumatoid arthritis. Proc R Soc Med 1969;62:227–38.

146. Nüsslein HG, Rödl W, Giedel J, et al. Multiple peripheral pulmonary nodules preceding rheumatoid arthritis. Rheumatol Int 1987;7:89–91.

147. Ramirez J, Campbell GD. Rheumatoid disease of the lung with cavitation. Dis Chest 1966;50:544–7.

148. Blodgett RC, Cera PJ, Jones FL. Alveolar cell carcinoma associated with rheumatoid nodule. Chest 1972;62:625–7.

149. Jolles H, Moseley PL, Peterson MW. Nodular pulmonary opacities in patients with rheumatoid arthritis. A diagnostic dilemma. Chest 1989;96:1022–5.

150. Byrd RW, Byrd RP Jr, Roy TM. Rheumatoid arthritis and the pulmonary nodule. J Ky Med Assoc 1997;95:19–22.

151. Caplan A. Certain unusual radiographic appearances in the chest of coal-miners suffering from rheumatoid arthritis. Thorax 1953;8:19–37.

152. Aronoff A, Bywaters EGL, Fearnley GR. Lung lesions in rheumatoid arthritis. BMJ 1955;1:228–32.

153. Katzenstein AL, Askin FB. Surgical pathology of non-neoplastic lung disease. Miscellaneous I. Specific diseases of uncertain etiology. Philadelphia: W.B. Saunders; 1982. p. 347.

154. Mutru O, Koota K, Isomaki H. Causes of death in autopsied RA patients. Scand J Rheumatol 1976;5:239–40.

155. Koota K, Isomaki H, Mutru O. Death rate and causes of death in RA patients during a period of five years. Scand J Rheumtol 1977;6:241–4.

156. Shiel WC, Prete PE. Pleuropulmonary manifestations of rheumatoid arthritis. Semin Arthritis Rheum 1984;13:235–43.

157. Sumiya M, Ohya N, Shinoura H, et al. Diffuse interstitial pulmonary amyloidosis in rheumatoid arthritis. J Rheumatol 1996;23:933–6.

158. Tomioka H, King TE Jr. Gold-induced pulmonary disease: clinical features, outcome, and differentiation from rheumatoid lung disease. Am J Respir Crit Care Med 1997;155:1011–20.

159. Sostman HD, Matthay RA, Putman CE, Smith GJ. Methotrexate-induced pneumonitis. Medicine (Baltimore) 1976;55:371–88.

160. Searles G, McKendry RJR. Methotrexate pneumonitis in rheumatoid arthritis: potential risk factors. Four case reports and a review of the literature. J Rheumatol 1987;14:1164–71.

161. Pelucchi A, Lomater C, Gerloni V, et al. Lung function and diffusing capacity for carbon monoxide in patients with juvenile chronic arthritis: effect of disease activity and low dose methotrexate therapy. Clin Exp Rheumatol 1994;12:675–9.

162. Cottin V, Tébib J, Massonnet B, et al. Pulmonary function in patients receiving long-term low-dose methotrexate. Chest 1996;109:933–8.

163. Dayton CS, Schwartz DA, Sprince NL, et al. Low-dose methotrexate may cause air trapping in patients with rheumatoid arthritis. Am J Respir Crit Care Med 1995; 151:1189–93.

164. Leduc D, De Vuyst P, L'heureux P, et al. Pneumonitis complicating low-dose methotrexate therapy for rheumatoid arthritis. Discrepancies between lung biopsy and bronchoalveolar lavage findings. Chest 1993;104:1620–3.

165. Golden MR, Katz RS, Balk RA, Golden HE. The relationship of preexisting lung disease to the development of methotrexate pneumonitis in patients with rheumatoid arthritis. J Rheumatol 1995;22:1043–7.

166. Sharma A, Provenzale D, McKusick A, Kaplan MM. Interstitial pneumonitis after low-dose methotrexate therapy in primary biliary cirrhosis. Gastroenterology 1994;107:266–70.

167. Hilliquin P, Renoux M, Perrot S, et al. Occurrence of pulmonary complications during methotrexate therapy in rheumatoid arthritis. Br J Rheumatol 1996;35:441–5.

168. Beyeler C, Jordi B, Gerber NJ, Im Hof V. Pulmonary function in rheumatoid arthritis treated with low-dose methotrexate: a longitudinal study. Br J Rheumatol 1996;35:446–52.

169. Schnabel A, Dalhoff K, Bauerfeind S, et al. Sustained cough in methotrexate therapy for rheumatoid arthritis. Clin Rheumatol 1996;15:277–82.

170. Kremer JM, Alarcon GS, Weinblatt ME, et al. Clinical, laboratory, radiographic, and histopathologic features of methotrexate-associated lung injury in patients with rheumatoid arthritis: a multicenter study with literature review. Arthritis Rheum 1997;40:1829–37.

171. Alarcon GS, Kremer JM, Macaluso M, et al. Risk factors for methotrexate-induced lung injury in patients with rheumatoid arthritis. A multicenter, case-control study. Methotrexate-Lung Study Group. Ann Intern Med 1997;127:356–64.

172. Imokawa S, Colby TV, Leslie KO, Helmers RA. Methotrexate pneumonitis: review of the literature and histopathological findings in nine patients. Eur Respir J 2000;15:373–81.

173. Fuhrman C, Parrot A, Wislez M, et al. Spectrum of CD4 to CD8 T-cell ratios in lymphocytic alveolitis associated with methotrexate-induced pneumonitis. Am J Respir Crit Care Med 2001;164:1186–91.

174. Camus P, Degat R, Justrabe E, Jeannin L. D-penicillamine-induced severe pneumonitis. Chest 1982;81:376–8.

175. Chebat J, Seigneur F, Lechien J, et al. Obliterating bronchiolitis during D-penicillamine treatments [letter]. Nouv Presse Med 1980;9:2655.

176. Eastmond CJ. Diffuse alveolitis as complication of penicillamine treatment for rheumatoid arthritis. BMJ 1976;i:1506.

177. Hill HFH. Penicillamine in rheumatoid arthritis-adverse effects. Scand J Rheumatol 1979;28:94–8.

178. Lyle WH. D-penicillamine and fatal obliterative bronchiolitis. BMJ 1977;1:105.

179. Murphy KC, Atkins CJ, Offer RC, et al. Obliterative bronchiolitis in two rheumatoid arthritis patients treated with penicillamine. Arthritis Rheum 1981;24:557–60.

180. Yam LY, Wong R. Bronchiolitis obliterans and rheumatoid arthritis. Report of a case in a Chinese patient on D-penicillamine and review of the literature. Ann Acad Med Singapore 1993;22:365–8.

181. Haerden J, Coolen L, Dequeker J. The effect of D-penicillamine on lung function parameters (diffusion capacity) in rheumatoid arthritis. Clin Exp Rheumatol 1993;11:509–13.

182. Barrera P, Laan RF, van Riel PL, et al. Methotrexate-related pulmonary complications in rheumatoid arthritis. Ann Rheum Dis 1994;53:434–9.

183. Barrera P, Van Ede A, Laan RF, et al. Methotrexate-related pulmonary complications in patients with rheumatoid arthritis: cluster of five cases in a period of three months. Ann Rheum Dis 1994;53:479–80.

184. Salaffi F, Manganelli P, Carotti M, et al. Methotrexate-induced pneumonitis in patients with rheumatoid arthritis and psoriatic arthritis: report of five cases and review of the literature. Clin Rheumatol 1997;16:296–304.

185. Dawson JK, Graham DR, Desmond J, et al. Investigation of the chronic pulmonary effects of low-dose oral methotrexate in patients with rheumatoid arthritis: a prospective study incorporating HRCT scanning and pulmonary function tests. Rheumatology (Oxford) 2002;41:262–7.

186. van der Veen MJ, Dekker JJ, Dinant HJ, et al. Fatal pulmonary fibrosis complicating low dose methotrexate therapy for rheumatoid arthritis. J Rheumatol 1995;22:1766–8.

187. Cannon GW. Methotrexate pulmonary toxicity. Rheum Dis Clin North Am 1997;23:917–37.

188. Mehandru S, Smith RL, Sidhu GS, et al. Migratory pulmonary infiltrates in a patient with rheumatoid arthritis. Thorax 2002;57:465–7.

189. Riegert-Johnson DL, Godfrey JA, Myers JL, et al. Delayed hypersensitivity reaction and acute respiratory distress syndrome following infliximab infusion. Inflamm Bowel Dis 2002;8:186–91.

190. Mayordomo L, Marenco JL, Gomez-Mateos J, Rejon E. Pulmonary miliary tuberculosis in a patient with anti-TNF-alpha treatment. Scand J Rheumatol 2002;31:44–5.

191. Glass D, Soter NA, Schur PH. Rheumatoid vasculitis. Arthritis Rheum 1976;19(5):950–2.

192. Kay JM, Banik S. Unexplained pulmonary hypertension with pulmonary arteritis in rheumatoid disease. Br J Dis Chest 1977;71:53–9.

193. Balagopal VP, da Costa P, Greenstone MA. Fatal pulmonary hypertension and rheumatoid vasculitis. Eur Respir J 1995;8:331–3.

194. Dawson JK, Goodson NG, Graham DR, Lynch MP. Raised pulmonary artery pressures measured with Doppler echocardiography in rheumatoid arthritis patients. Rheumatology (Oxford) 2000;39:1320–5.

195. Devereux G, Evans MJ, Kerr KM, Legge JS. Pulmonary veno-occlusive disease complicating Felty's syndrome. Respir Med 1998;92:1089–91.

196. Torralbo A, Herrero JA, Portolés J, Barrientos A. Alveolar hemorrhage associated with antineutrophil cytoplasmic antibodies in rheumatoid arthritis. Chest 1994;105:1590–2.

197. Johnson PM, Faulk WP. Rheumatoid factor: its nature, specificity and production in rheumatoid arthritis. Clin Immunol Immunopathol 1976;6:414–30.

198. Sahn SA. Pathogenesis of pleural effusions and pleural lesions. In: Cannon GW, Zimmerman GA, editors. The lung in rheumatic disease. New York: Marcel Dekker; 1990. p. 27–45.

199. Sahn SA. The pathophysiology of pleural effusions. Annu Rev Med 1990;41:7–13.

200. Horler AR, Thompson M. The pleural and pulmonary complications of rheumatoid arthritis. Ann Intern Med 1959;51:1179–203.

201. Chou CW, Chang SC. Pleuritis as a presenting manifestation of rheumatoid arthritis: diagnostic clues in pleural fluid cytology. Am J Med Sci 2002;323:158–61.

202. Lillington GA, Carr DT, Mayne JG. Rheumatoid pleurisy with effusion. Arch Intern Med 1971;128:764–8.

203. Joseph J, Sahn SA. Connective tissue disease and the pleura. Chest 1993;104:262–70.

204. Stanek KA, Mills K. Pleural effusion with rheumatoid arthritis. S D J Med 1991;44:61–3.

205. Hakala M, Tiilikainen A, Hämeenkorpi R, et al. Rheumatoid arthritis with pleural effusion includes a subgroup with autoimmune features and HLA-B8, Dw3 association. Scand J Rheumatol 1986;15:290–6.

206. Brennan SR, Daly JJ. Large pleural effusions in rheumatoid arthritis. Br J Dis Chest 1979;73:133–40.

207. Pritikin JD, Jensen WA, Yenokida GG, et al. Respiratory failure due to a massive rheumatoid pleural effusion. J Rheumatol 1990;17:673–5.

208. Dodson WH, Hollingsworth JW. Pleural effusion in rheumatoid arthritis. N Engl J Med 1966;275:1337–42.

209. Ferguson GC. Cholesterol pleural effusion in rheumatoid lung disease. Thorax 1966;21:577–82.

210. Bower GC. Chyliform pleural effusion in rheumatoid arthritis. Am Rev Respir Dis 1968;97:455–9.

211. Hunder GG, McDuffie FC, Hepper NGG. Pleural fluid complement in systemic lupus erythematosus and rheumatoid arthritis. Ann Intern Med 1972;76:357–63.

212. Halla JT, Schrohenloher RE, Volanakis JE. Immune complexes and other laboratory features of pleural effusions: a comparison of rheumatoid arthritis, systemic lupus erythematosus, and other diseases. Ann Intern Med 1980;92:748–52.

213. Aru A, Engel U, Francis D. Characteristic and specific histological findings in rheumatoid pleurisy. Acta Pathol Microbiol Immunol Scand A Pathol 1986;94:57–62.

214. Faurschou P. Rheumatoid pleuritis and thoracoscopy. Scand J Respir Dis 1974;55:277–83.

215. Faurschou P, Francis D, Faarup P. Thoracoscopic, histological, and clinical findings in nine cases of rheumatoid pleural effusion. Thorax 1985;40:371–5.

216. Faurschou P. Thoracoscopy in rheumatoid pleural effusion. Pneumologie 1989;43:69–71.

217. Jones FL, Blodgett RC. Empyema in rheumatoid pleuropulmonary disease. Ann Intern Med 1971;74:665–71.

218. Dieppe PA. Empyema in rheumatoid arthritis. Ann Rheum Dis 1975;34:181–5.

219. Russell ML, Gladman DD, Mintz S. Rheumatoid pleural effusion: lack of response to intrapleural corticosteroid. J Rheumatol 1986;13:412–5.

220. Chapman PT, O'Donnell JL, Moller P. Rheumatoid pleural effusion: response to intrapleural corticosteroid. J Rheumatol 1992;19:478–80.

221. Ayzenberg O, Reiff DB, Levin L. Bilateral pneumothoraces and pleural effusions complicating rheumatoid lung disease. Thorax 1983;38:159–60.

222. Adelman HM, Dupont EL, Flannery MT, Wallach PM. Case report: recurrent pneumothorax in a patient with rheumatoid arthritis. Am J Med Sci 1994;308:171–2.

223. Sharma SS, Reynolds PM. Broncho-pleural fistula complicating rheumatoid lung disease. Postgrad Med J 1982;58:187–9.

224. Portner MM, Gracie WA Jr. Rheumatoid lung disease with cavitary nodules, pneumothorax and eosinophilia. New Engl J Med 1966;275:697–700.

225. Crisp AJ, Armstrong RD, Grahame R, Dussek JE. Rheumatoid lung disease, pneumothorax, and eosinophilia. Ann Rheum Dis 1982;41:137–40.

226. Gotsman I, Goral A, Nusair S. Secondary spontaneous pneumothorax in a patient with pulmonary rheumatoid nodules during treatment with methotrexate. Rheumatology (Oxford) 2001;40:350–1.

227. Patel A, Kesler B, Wise RA. Persistent pneumomediastinum in interstitial fibrosis associated with rheumatoid arthritis: treatment with high-concentration oxygen. Chest 2000; 117:1809–13.

228. Huang CT, Lyons HA. Comparison of pulmonary function in patients with systemic lupus erythematosus, scleroderma, and rheumatoid arthritis. Am Rev Respir Dis 1966; 93:865–75.

229. Dubois EL, Tufanelli DL. Clinical manifestations of systemic lupus erythematosus. JAMA 1964;190:104–11.

230. Tufanelli DL, Dubois EL. Cutaneous manifestations of systemic lupus erythematosus. Arch Dermatol 1964;90:337–86.

231. Labowitz R, Schumacher HRJ. Articular manifestations of systemic lupus erythematosus. Ann Intern Med 1971; 74:911–21.

232. Brentjens JR, Sepulveda M, Baliah T, et al. Interstitial immune complex nephritis in patients with systemic lupus erythematosus. Kidney Int 1975;7:342–50.

233. Feinglass EJ, Arnett FC, Dorsch CA, et al. Neuropsychiatric manifestations of systemic lupus erythematosus: clinic spectrum and relationship to other features of the disease. Medicine 1976;55:323–39.

234. Ropes MW. Systemic lupus erythematosus. Cambridge: Harvard University Press; 1976.

235. Pirani CL, Pollack VE. Systemic lupus erythematosus glomerulonephritis. In: McClusky RT, Andres GA, editors. Immunologically mediated renal diseases: criteria for diagnosis and treatment. New York: Marcel Dekker; 1978. p. 19.

236. Hargraves MD, Richmond H, Morton R. Presentation of two bone marrow elements: the "tart" cel and the "L.E." cell. Proc Staff Meet Mayo Clin 1948;23:25–8.

237. Holman HR, Kunkel HG. Affinity between the lupus erythematosus serum factor and cell nuclei and nucleoprotein. Science 1957;126:162–3.

238. Tan EM, Kunkel HG. Characteristics of a soluble nuclear antigen precipitating with sera of patients with systemic lupus erythematosus. J Immunol 1966;96:464–71.

239. Clark G, Reichlin M, Tomasi TBJ. Characterization of a soluble cytoplasmic antigen reactive with sera from patients with systemic lupus erythematosus. J Immunol 1969;102:117–22.

240. Koffler D, Carr RI, Agnello V, et al. Antibodies to polynucleotides; distribution in human serums. Science 1969; 166:1648–9.

241. Mattioli M, Reichlin M. Characterization of a soluble nuclear ribonucleoprotein antigen reactive with SLE sera. J Immunol 1971;107:1281–90.

242. Mattioli M, Reichlin M. Heterogeneity of RNA protein antigens reactive with sera of patients with systemic lupus erythematosus: description of a cytoplasmic nonribosomal antigen. Arthritis Rheum 1974;17:421–9.

243. Alspaugh MA, Tan EM. Antibodies to cellular antigens in Sjögren's syndrome. J Clin Invest 1975;55:1067–73.

244. Kaposi MK. Neue Beitrage zur Kenntniss des Lupus Erythematosus. Arch Dermatol Syph 1872;4:36–78.

245. Osler W. On the visceral manifestations of the erythema group of skin diseases. Am J Med Sci 1904;127:1–23.

246. Klemperer P, Pollack AD, Brehr G. Pathology of disseminated lupus erythematosus. Arch Pathol 1941;32:569–631.

247. Foldes J. Acute systemic lupus erythematosus. Am J Clin Pathol 1946;16:160–73.

248. Teilum G. Pathogenetic studies on lupus erythematosus disseminatus and related diseases. Acta Med Scand 1946; 74:126–42.

249. Israel HL. The pulmonary manifestations of disseminated lupus erythematosus. Am J Med Sci 1953;226:387–92.

250. Gould DM, Daves ML. Roentgenologic findings in systemic lupus erythematosus. J Chronic Dis 1955;2:136–45.

251. Harvey AM, Shulman LE, Tumulty PA, et al. Systemic lupus erythematosus: review of the literature and clinical analysis of 138 cases. Medicine (Baltimore) 1954;33:291–437.

252. Garland LH, Sisson MA. Roentgen findings in the "collagen" diseases. AJR Am J Roentgenol 1954;71:581–98.

253. Bulgrin JG, Dubois EL, Jacobson G. Chest roentgenographic changes in systemic lupus erythematosus. Radiology 1960; 74:42–9.

254. Alarcon-Segovia D, Alarcon DG. Pleuro-pulmonary manifestations of systemic lupus erythematosus. Dis Chest 1961; 39:7–17.

255. Estes D. The natural history of systemic lupus erythematosus by prospective analysis. Medicine (Baltimore) 1971;50: 85–95.

256. Jessar RA, Lamont-Havers RW, Ragan C. Natural history of lupus erythematosus disseminatus. Ann Intern Med 1953; 38:717–31.

257. Myhre JR. Pleuropulmonary manifestations in lupus erythematosus disseminatus. Acta Med Scand 1959;165:55–60.

258. Orens JB, Martinez FJ, Lynch JP 3rd. Pleuropulmonary manifestations of systemic lupus erythematosus. Rheum Dis Clin North Am 1994;20:159–93.

259. Decker JL, Steinberg AD, Reinertsen JL, et al. Systemic lupus erythematosus: evolving concepts. Ann Intern Med 1979;91:587–604.

260. Zvaifler NJ, Woods VLJ. Etiology and pathogenesis of systemic lupus erythematosus. In: Kelley WN, Harris EDJ, Ruddy S, Sledge CB, editors. Textbook of rheumatology. Philadelphia: W.B. Saunders; 1985. p. 1042.

261. Ho A, Magder LS, Barr SG, Petri M. Decreases in anti-double-stranded DNA levels are associated with concurrent flares in patients with systemic lupus erythematosus. Arthritis Rheum 2001;44:2342–9.

262. Ho A, Barr SG, Magder LS, Petri M. A decrease in complement is associated with increased renal and hematologic activity in patients with systemic lupus erythematosus. Arthritis Rheum 2001;44:2350–7.

263. Koffler D, Schur PH, Kunkel HG. Immunological studies concerning the nephritis of systemic lupus erythematosus. J Exp Med 1967;126:607–23.

264. Verroust PJ, Wilson CB, Cooper NR, et al. Glomerular complement components in human glomerulonephritis. J Clin Invest 1974;53:77–84.

265. Frank MM, Hamburger MI, Lawley TJ, et al. Defective reticuloendothelial system Fc-receptor function in systemic lupus erythematosus. N Engl J Med 1979;300:518–20.

266. Rascu A, Repp R, Westerdaal NA, et al. Clinical relevance of Fc gamma receptor polymorphisms. Ann N Y Acad Sci 1997;815:282–95.

267. Deo YM, Graziano RF, Repp R, van de Winkel JG. Clinical significance of IgG Fc receptors and Fc gamma R-directed immunotherapies. Immunol Today 1997;18:127–35.

268. Seligman VA, Suarez C, Lum R, et al. The Fc gamma receptor IIIA-158F allele is a major risk factor for the development of lupus nephritis among Caucasians but not non-Caucasians. Arthritis Rheum 2001;44:618–25.

269. Brentjens JR, Andres GA. The pathogenesis of extrarenal lesions in systemic lupus erythematosus. Arthritis Rheum 1982;25:880–6.

270. Johnson KJ, Ward PA. Acute immunologic pulmonary alveolitis. J Clin Invest 1974;54:349–57.

271. Brentjens JR, O'Connell DW, Pawlowski IB, et al. Experimental immune complex disease of the lung: the patho-

genesis of a laboratory model resembling certain human interstital lung diseases. J Exp Med 1974;140:105–25.

272. Eisenberg H, Simmons DH, Abe C, et al. Immune complex in the New Zealand black/white hybrid mouse lung. Chest 1976;69S:284–6.

273. Boulware DW, Hedgpeth MT. Lupus pneumonitis and anti-SSA(Ro) antibodies. J Rheumatol 1989;16:479–81.

274. Mochizuki T, Aotsuka S, Satoh T. Clinical and laboratory features of lupus patients with complicating pulmonary disease. Respir Med 1999;93:95–101.

275. Swaak AJ, Huysen V, Nossent JC, Smeenk RJ. Antinuclear antibody profiles in relation to specific disease manifestations of systemic lupus erythematosus. Clin Rheumatol 1990;9:82–94.

276. Schroeder JO, Euler HH, Loffler H. Synchronization of plasmapheresis and pulse cyclophosphamide in severe systemic lupus erythematosus. Ann Intern Med 1987;107:344–6.

277. Lee CK, Koh JH, Cha HS, et al. Pulmonary alveolar hemorrhage in patients with rheumatic diseases in Korea. Scand J Rheumatol 2000;29:288–94.

278. Isbister JP, Talston M, Hayes JM, Wright R. Fulminant lupus pneumonitis with acute renal failure and RBC aplasia: successful management with plasmapheresis and immunosuppression. Arch Intern Med 1981;141:1081–3.

279. Silberstein SL, Barland P, Grayzel AI, Koerner SK. Pulmonary dysfunction in systemic lupus erythematosus: prevalence, classification, and correlation with other organ involvement. J Rheumatol 1980;7:187–95.

280. Abramson SB, Dobro J, Eberle MA, et al. Acute reversible hypoxemia in systemic lupus erythematosus. Ann Intern Med 1991;114:941–7.

281. Pertschuk LP, Moccia LF, Rosen Y, et al. Acute pulmonary complications in systemic lupus erythematosus: immunofluorescence and light microscopic study. Am J Clin Pathol 1977;68:553–7.

282. Yeo PPB, Sinniah R. Lupus cor pulmonale with electron microscope and immunofluorescent antibody studies. Ann Rheum Dis 1975;34:457–60.

283. Brentjens J, Ossi E, Albini B, et al. Disseminated immune deposits in lupus erythematosus. Arthritis Rheum 1977;20:962–8.

284. Inoue T, Kanayama Y, Ohe A, et al. Immunopathologic studies of pneumonitis in systemic lupus erythematosus. Ann Intern Med 1979;91:30–4.

285. Elliot ML, Kuhn C. Idiopathic pulmonary hemosiderosis: ultrastructural abnormalities in the capillary walls. Am Rev Respir Dis 1970;102:895–904.

286. Rodriguez-Iturbe B, Garcia R, Rubio L, Serano H. Immunohistologic findings in the lung in systemic lupus erythematosus. Arch Pathol Lab Med 1977;101:342–4.

287. Eagen JW, Memoli VA, Roberts JL, et al. Pulmonary hemorrhage in systemic lupus erythematosus. Medicine (Baltimore) 1978;57:545–60.

288. Churg A, Franklin W, Chan KL, et al. Pulmonary hemorrhage and immune complex deposition in the lung. Arch Pathol Lab Med 1980;104:388–91.

289. Myers JL, Katzenstein AA. Microangiitis in lupus-induced pulmonary hemorrhage. Am J Clin Pathol 1986;85:552–6.

290. Hughson MD, He Z, Henegar J, McMurray R. Alveolar hemorrhage and renal microangiopathy in systemic lupus erythematosus. Arch Pathol Lab Med 2001;125:475–83.

291. Marino CT, Pertschuk LP. Pulmonary hemorrhage in systemic lupus erythematosus. Arch Intern Med 1981;57:545–60.

292. Desnoyers MR, Bernstein S, Cooper AG, Kopelman RI. Pulmonary hemorrhage in lupus erythematosus without evidence of an immunologic cause. Arch Intern Med 1984;144:1398–400.

293. Matthay RA, Schwarz MI, Petty TL, et al. Pulmonary manifestations of systemic lupus erythematosus: review of twelve cases of acute lupus pneumonitis. Medicine (Baltimore) 1975;54:397–409.

294. Primack SL, Muller NL. Radiologic manifestations of the systemic autoimmune diseases. Clin Chest Med 1998;19:573–86.

295. Wiedemann HP, Matthay RA. Pulmonary manifestations of systemic lupus erythematosus. J Thorac Imaging 1992;7:1–18.

296. Susanto I, Peters JI. Acute lupus pneumonitis with normal chest radiograph. Chest 1997;111:1781–3.

297. Matthay RA, Hudson LD, Petty TL. Acute lupus pneumonitis: response to azathioprine therapy. Chest 1973;69:117–20.

298. Gross M, Esterly JR, Earle RH. Pulmonary alterations in systemic lupus erythematosus. Am Rev Respir Dis 1972;105:572–7.

299. Haupt HM, Moore GM, Hutchins GM. The lung in systemic lupus erythematosus: analysis of the pathologic changes in 120 patients. Am J Med 1981;72:791–7.

300. Sperryn PN, Mace BEW. Systemic lupus erythematosus with fibrosing alveolitis. Proc R Soc Med 1971;64:58–9.

301. Levin DC. Proper interpretation of pulmonary roentgen changes in systemic lupus erythematosus. AJR Am J Roentgenol 1971;3:510–7.

302. Steinberg AD. Management of systemic lupus erythematosus. In: Kelley WN, Harris EDJ, Ruddy S, Sledge CB, editors. Textbook of rheumatology. Philadelphia: W.B. Saunders; 1985. p. 1098.

303. Newcomer AD, Miller RD, Hepper NGG, Carter ET. Pulmonary dysfunction in rheumatoid arthritis and systemic lupus erythematosus. Dis Chest 1964;46:562–70.

304. Holgate ST, Galss DN, Haslam P, et al. Respiratory involvement in systemic lupus erythematosus: a clinical and immunological study. Clin Exp Immunol 1976;24:385–95.

305. Ellman P. The pleural and pulmonary lesions of systemic lupus erythematosus. Proc R Soc Med 1958;51:654.

306. Fink SD, Kremer JM. Successful treatment of interstitial lung disease in systemic lupus erythematosus with methotrexate. J Rheumatol 1995;22:967–9.

307. Eiser AR, Shanies HM. Treatment of lupus interstitial lung disease with intravenous cyclophosphamide. Arthritis Rheum 1994;37:428–31.

308. Rosner S, Ginzler EM, Diamond HS, et al. A multicenter study of outcome in systemic lupus erythematosus: II. Causes of death. Arthritis Rheum 1982;25:612–7.

309. Taylor TL, Ostrum H. The roentgenologic evaluation of systemic lupus erythematosus. AJR Am J Roentgenol 1959;82:95–107.

310. Eisenberg H, Dubois EL, Sherwin RP, Balchum OJ. Diffuse interstitial lung disease in systemic lupus erythematosus. Ann Intern Med 1973;79:37–45.

311. Miller LR, Greenberg SD, McLarty JW. Lupus lung. Chest 1985;88:265–9.

312. Holden M. Massive pulmonary fibrosis due to systemic lupus erythematosus. N Y State J Med 1973;73:462–5.

313. Bankier AA, Kiener HP, Wiesmayr MN, et al. Discrete lung involvement in systemic lupus erythematosus: CT assessment. Radiology 1995;196:835–40.

314. Fenlon HM, Doran M, Sant SM, Breatnach E. High-resolution chest CT in systemic lupus erythematosus. AJR Am J Roentgenol 1996;166:301–7.

315. Ooi GC, Ngan H, Peh WC, et al. Systemic lupus erythematosus patients with respiratory symptoms: the value of HRCT. Clin Radiol 1997;52:775–81.

316. Kao CH, Lin HT, Yu YSL, et al. Lung inflammation in patients with systemic lupus erythematosus detected by quantitative 67Ga-citrate lung scanning. Nucl Med Commun 1994;15:928–31.

317. Shih CM, Shiau YC, Wang JJ, et al. Increased lung uptake of technetium-99m hexamethylpropylene amine oxime in systemic lupus erythematosus. Respiration 2002;69:143–7.

318. Huang CT, Hennigar GR, Lyons HA. Pulmonary dysfunction in systemic lupus erythematosus. N Engl J Med 1965;272:288–93.

319. Arnalich F, Ruiz de Andres S, Gil A, et al. Pulmonary function in systemic lupus erythematosus patients without respiratory symptoms. Bull Eur Physiopathol Respir 1979;15:649–57.

320. Chick TW, DeHoratius RJ, Skipper BE, Messner RP. Pulmonary dysfunction in systemic lupus erythematosus without pulmonary symptoms. J Rheumatol 1976;3:262–8.

321. Hellman DB, Kirsch CM, Whiting-O'Keefe Q, et al. Dyspnea in ambulatory patients with SLE: prevalence, severity, and correlation with incremental exercise testing. J Rheumatol 1995;22:455–61.

322. Eichacker PQ, Pinsker K, Epstein A, et al. Serial pulmonary function testing in patients with systemic lupus erythematosus. Chest 1988;94(1):129–32.

323. Groen H, ter Borg EJ, Postma DS, et al. Pulmonary function in systemic lupus erythematosus is related to distinct clinical, serologic, and nailfold capillary patterns. Am J Med 1992;93:619–27.

324. Dubois EL. Lupus erythematosus: a review of the current status of discoid and systemic lupus erythematosus and their variants. Los Angeles: University of Southern California Press; 1976.

325. Gibson GJ, Edmonds JP, Hughes ERV. Diaphragm function and lung involvement in systemic lupus erythematosus. Am J Med 1977;63:926–32.

326. Forte S, Carlone S, Vaccaro F, et al. Pulmonary gas exchange and exercise capacity in patients with systemic lupus erythematosus. J Rheumatol 1999;26:2591–4.

327. Greene NB, Solinger AM, Baughman RP. Patients with collagen vascular disease and dyspnea: the value of gallium scanning and bronchoalveolar lavage in predicting response to steroid therapy and clinical outcome. Chest 1987;91:698–703.

328. Wallaert B, Aerts C, Bart F, et al. Alveolar macrophage dysfunction in systemic lupus erythematosus. Am Rev Respir Dis 1987;136:293–7.

329. Martinot JB, Wallaert B, Hatron PY, et al. Clinical and subclinical alveolitis in collagen vascular diseases: contribution of alpha 2-macroglobulin levels in BAL fluid. Eur Respir J 1989;2:437–43.

330. Nagai N. The value of BALF cell findings for differentiation of idiopathic UIP, BOOP, and interstitial pneumonia associated with collagen vascular disease. In: Harasawa M, Fukuchi Y, Morinari H, editors. Interstitial pneumonia of unknown etiology. Vol. 27. Tokyo: University of Tokyo Press; 1989. p. 131–6.

331. Groen H, Aslander M, Bootsma H, et al. Bronchoalveolar lavage cell analysis and lung function impairment in patients with systemic lupus erythematosus (SLE). Clin Exp Immunol 1993;94:127–33.

332. Katzenstein AL, Fiorelli RF. Nonspecific interstitial pneumonia/fibrosis. Histologic features and clinical significance. Am J Surg Pathol 1994;18:136–47.

333. Murin S, Wiedemann HP, Matthay RA. Pulmonary manifestations of systemic lupus erythematosus. Clin Chest Med 1998;19:641–65.

334. Gammon RB, Bridges TA, al-Nezir H, et al. Bronchiolitis obliterans organizing pneumonia associated with systemic lupus erythematosus. Chest 1992;102:1171–4.

335. Mana F, Mets T, Vincken W, et al. The association of bronchiolitis obliterans organizing pneumonia, systemic lupus erythematosus, and Hunner's cystitis. Chest 1993;104:642–4.

336. Benisch B, Peison B. The association of lymphocytic interstitial pneumonitis and systemic lupus erythematosus. Mt Sinai J Med 1979;46:398–401.

337. Yum MN, Ziegler JR, Walker PD, et al. Pseudolymphoma of the lung in a patient with systemic lupus erythematosus. Am J Med 1979;66:172–6.

338. Milligan DW, Chang JG. Systemic lupus erythematosus and lymphoma. Acta Haematol 1980;64:109–10.

339. Toomey JM, Snyder GGI, Maenza RM, Rothfield NF. Acute epiglottitis due to systemic lupus erythematosus. Laryngoscope 1974;84:522–7.

340. Wohlgelernter D, Loke J, Matthay RA, Siegel NJ. Systemic and discoid lupus erythematosus: analysis of pulmonary function. Yale J Biol Med 1978;51:157–64.

341. Andonopoulos AP, Constantopoulos SH, Galanopoulou V, et al. Pulmonary function of nonsmoking patients with systemic lupus erythematosus. Chest 1988;94:312–5.

342. Kinney WW, Angelillo VA. Bronchiolitis in systemic lupus erythematosus. Chest 1982;82:646–9.

343. Carr DT, Lillington GA, Mayne JG. Pleural-fluid glucose in systemic lupus erythematosus. Mayo Clin Proc 1970; 45:409–12.

344. Good JT, King TE, Antony VB, Sahn SA. Lupus pleuritis. Clinical features and pleural fluid characteristics with special reference to pleural fluid antinuclear antibodies. Chest l983;84:714–8.

345. Rothfield N. Clinical features of systemic lupus erythematosus. In: Kelley WN, Harris EDJ, Ruddy S, Sledge CB, editors. Textbook of rheumatology. Phildelphia: W.B. Saunders; 1985. p. 1070.

346. Pandya MR, Agus B, Grady RF. In vivo LE phenomenon in pleural fluid. Arthritis Rheum 1976;19:962–3.

347. Riska H, Fyhrquist F, Selander RK, Hellstrom PE. Systemic lupus erythematosus and DNA antibodies in pleural effusions. Scand J Rheumatol 1978;7:159–60.

348. Leechawengwong M, Berger HW, Sukumaran M. Diagnostic significance of antinuclear antibodies in pleural effusion. Mt Sinai J Med 1979;46:137–9.

349. Mulkey D, Hudons L. Massive spontaneous unilateral hemothorax in systemic lupus erythematosus. Am J Med 1974;56:570–4.

350. Passero FC, Myers AR. Hemopneumothorax in systemic lupus erythematosus. J Rheumatol 1980;7:183–6.

351. Masuda A, Tsushima T, Shizume K, et al. Recurrent pneumothoraces and mediastinal emphysema in systemic lupus erythematosus. J Rheumatol 1990;17:544–8.

352. Yokoi T, Tomita Y, Fukaya M, et al. Pulmonary hypertension associated with systemic lupus erythematosus: predominantly thrombotic arteriopathy accompanied by plexiform lesions. Arch Pathol Lab Med 1998;122:467–70.

353. Aitchison JD, Williams AW. Pulmonary changes in disseminating lupus erythematosus. Ann Rheum Dis 1956;15:26–32.

354. Sivaramkrishnan SN, Askari AD, Popelka CG, Kleinerman JF. Pulmonary hypertension and systemic lupus erythematosus. Arch Intern Med 1980;140:109–11.

355. Perez HD, Kramer N. Pulmonary hypertension in systemic lupus erythematosus: report of four cases and review of the literature. Semin Arthritis Rheum 1981;11:177–81.

356. Crausman RS, Achenbach GA, Pluss WT, et al. Pulmonary capillaritis and alveolar hemorrhage associated with the antiphospholipid antibody syndrome. J Rheumatol 1995;22:554–6.

357. Alarcon-Segovia D, Deleze M, Oria CV, et al. Antiphospholipid antibodies and the antiphospholipid syndrome in systemic lupus erythematosus. A prospective analysis of 500 consecutive patients. Medicine (Baltimore) 1989;68: 353–65.

358. Gussin HA, Ignat GP, Varga J, Teodorescu M. Anti-topoisomerase I (anti-Scl-70) antibodies in patients with systemic lupus erythematosus. Arthritis Rheum 2001;44:376–83.

359. Tanaka E, Harigai M, Tanaka M, et al. Pulmonary hypertension in systemic lupus erythematosus: evaluation of clinical characteristics and response to immunosuppressive treatment. J Rheumatol 2002;29:282–7.

360. Gladman DD, Urowitz MB. Venous syndromes and pulmonary embolism in systemic lupus erythematosus. Ann Rheum Dis 1980;39:340–3.

361. Pines A, Kaplinsky N, Olchovsky D, et al. Pleuro-pulmonary manifestations of systemic lupus erythematosus: clinical features of its subgroups. Chest 1985;88:129–35.

362. Asherson RA, Cervera R. Review: antiphospholipid antibodies and the lung. J Rheumatol 1995;22:62–6.

363. Martinez-Taboada VM, Blanco R, Armona J, et al. Acute reversible hypoxemia in systemic lupus erythematosus: a new syndrome or an index of disease activity? Lupus 1995;4:259–62.

364. Belmont HM, Buyon J, Giorno R, Abramson S. Up-regulation of endothelial cell adhesion molecules characterizes disease activity in systemic lupus erythematosus. The Shwartzman phenomenon revisited. Arthritis Rheum 1994;37:376–83.

365. Byrd RB, Trunk G. Systemic lupus erythematosus presenting as pulmonary hemosiderosis. Chest 1973;64:128–9.

366. Lewis EJ, Schur PH, Busch GJ, et al. Immunopathologic features of a patient with glomerulonephritis and pulmonary hemorrhage. Am J Med 1973;54:507–13.

367. Mintz G, Galindo LF, Fernandez-Diez J, et al. Acute massive pulmonary hemorrhage in systemic lupus erythematosus. J Rheumatol 1978;5:39–50.

368. Green RJ, Ruoss SJ, Kraft SA, et al. Pulmonary capillaritis and alveolar hemorrhage. Update on diagnosis and management. Chest 1996;110:1305–16.

369. Blanche P, Krebs S, Renaud B, et al. Systemic lupus erythematosus presenting as iron deficiency anemia due to pulmonary alveolar hemorrhage. Clin Exp Rheumatol 1996;14:228.

370. Makino Y, Ogawa M, Ueda S, Ohto M. CT appearance of diffuse alveolar hemorrhage in a patient with systemic lupus erythematosus. Acta Radiol 1993;34:634–5.

371. Schwab EP, Schumacher HR Jr, Freundlich B, Callegari PE. Pulmonary alveolar hemorrhage in systemic lupus erythematosus. Semin Arthritis Rheum 1993;23:8–15.

372. Travis WD, Colby TV, Lombard C, Carpenter H. A clinicopathologic study of 34 cases of diffuse pulmonary hemorrhage with lung biopsy confirmation. Am J Surg Pathol 1990;14:1112–25.

373. Liu MF, Lee JH, Weng TH, Lee YY. Clinical experience of 13 cases with severe pulmonary hemorrhage in systemic lupus erythematosus with active nephritis. Scand J Rheumatol 1998;27:291–5.

374. Zamora MR, Warner ML, Tuder R, Schwarz MI. Diffuse alveolar hemorrhage and systemic lupus erythematosus. Clinical presentation, histology, survival, and outcome. Medicine 1997;76:192–202.

375. Elstad MR. Lung biopsy, bronchoalveolar lavage, and gallium scanning. In: Cannon GW, Zimmerman GA, editors. The lung in rheumatic diseases. Vol 45. New York: Marcel Dekker Inc.; 1990. p. 117–43.

376. Klech H, Hutter C. Clinical guidelines and indications for bronchoalveolar lavage (BAL): report of the European Society of Pneumology Task Force on BAL. Eur Respir J 1990;3:937–74.

377. Golde D, Drew L, Klein H, et al. Occult pulmonary hemorrhage in leukemia. BMJ 1975;2:166–8.

378. Drew L, Finley T, Golde D. Diagnostic lavage and occult pulmonary hemorrhage in thrombocytopenic immunocompromised patients. Am Rev Respir Dis 1977;116:215–21.

379. Kahn F, Jones J, England D. Diagnosis of pulmonary hemorrhage in the immunocompromised host. Am Rev Respir Dis 1987;136:155–60.

380. Sherman J, Winnie G, Thomassen MJ, et al. Time course of hemosiderin production and clearance by human pulmonary macrophages. Chest 1984;86:409–11.

381. Onomura K, Nakata H, Tanaka Y, Tsuda T. Pulmonary hemorrhage in patients with systemic lupus erythematosus. J Thorac Imaging 1991;6:57–61.

382. Hsu BY, Edwards DK 3d, Trambert MA. Pulmonary hemorrhage complicating systemic lupus erythematosus: role of MR imaging in diagnosis. Am J Roentgenol 1992; 158:519–20.

383. Erickson RW, Franklin WA, Emlen W. Treatment of hemorrhagic lupus pneumonitis with plasmapheresis. Semin Arthritis Rheum 1994;24:114–23.

384. Huang DF, Tsai ST, Wang SR. Recovery of both acute massive pulmonary hemorrhage and acute renal failure in a systemic lupus erythematosus patient with lupus anticoagulant by the combined therapy of plasmapheresis plus cyclophosphamide. Transfus Sci 1994;15:283–8.

385. Barile LA, Jara LJ, Medina-Rodriguez F, et al. Pulmonary hemorrhage in systemic lupus erythematosus. Lupus 1997;6:445–8.

386. Thompson PJ, Dhillon DP, Ledingham J, Turner-Warwick M. Shrinking lungs, diaphragmatic dysfunction, and systemic lupus erythematosus. Am Rev Respir Dis 1985;132: 926–8.

387. Walz-Leblanc BA, Urowitz MB, Gladman DD, Hanly PJ. The "shrinking lungs syndrome" in systemic lupus erythematosus—improvement with corticosteroid therapy. J Rheumatol 1992;19:1970–2.

388. Soubrier M, Dubost JJ, Piette JC, et al. Shrinking lung syndrome in systemic lupus erythematosus. A report of three cases. Rev Rhum Engl Ed 1995;62:395–8.

389. Warrington KJ, Moder KG, Brutinel WM. The shrinking lungs syndrome in systemic lupus erythematosus. Mayo Clin Proc 2000;75:467–72.

390. Karim MY, Miranda LC, Tench CM, et al. Presentation and prognosis of the shrinking lung syndrome in systemic lupus erythematosus. Semin Arthritis Rheum 2002;31:289–98.

391. Ishii M, Uda H, Yamagami T, Katada Y. Possible association of "shrinking lung" and anti-Ro/SSA antibody. Arthritis Rheum 2000;43:2612–3.

392. Hoffbrand BI, Beck ER. "Unexplained" dyspnoea and shrinking lungs in systemic lupus erythematosus. BJM 1965;1:1273–7.

393. Martens J, Demedts M, Vanmeenen MT, Dequeker J. Respiratory muscle dysfunction in systemic lupus erythematosus. Chest 1984;84:170–5.

394. Jacobelli S, Moreno R, Massardo L, et al. Inspiratory muscle dysfunction and unexplained dyspnea in systemic lupus erythematosus. Arthritis Rheum 1985;28(7):781–8.

395. Worth H, Grahn S, Lakomek HJ, et al. Lung function disturbances versus respiratory muscle fatigue in patients with systemic lupus erythematosus. Respiration 1988;53:81–90.

396. Muñoz-Rodríguez FJ, Font J, Badia JR, et al. Shrinking lungs syndrome in systemic lupus erythematosus: improvement with inhaled beta-agonist therapy. Lupus 1997;6:412–4.

397. Van Veen S, Peeters AJ, Sterk PJ, Breedveld FC. The "shrinking lung syndrome" in SLE, treatment with theophylline. Clin Rheumatol 1993;12:462–5.

398. Rakov HL, Taylor JS. Acute disseminated lupus erythematosus without cutaneous involvement and with heretofore undescribed pulmonary lesions. Arch Intern Med 1942;70:88–100.

399. Purnell DC, Baggenstoss AH, Olsen AM. Pulmonary lesions in disseminated lupus erythematosus. Ann Intern Med 1955;42:619–28.

400. Staples PJ, Gerding DN, Decker JL, Gordon RSJ. Incidence of infection in systemic lupus erythematosus. Arthritis Rheum 1974;17:1–10.

401. Ginzler E, Diamond H, Kaplan D, et al. Computer analysis of factors influencing frequency of infection in systemic lupus erythematosus. Arthritis Rheum 1978;21:37–44.

402. Segal AM, Calabrese LH, Ahmad M, et al. The pulmonary manifestations of systemic lupus erythematosus. Semin Arthritis Rheum 1985;14:202–24.

403. Allen E, Bakke AC, Purtzer MZ, Deodhar A. Neutrophil CD64 expression: distinguishing acute inflammatory autoimmune disease from systemic infections. Ann Rheum Dis 2002;61:522–5.

404. Eberhard OK, Haubitz M, Brunkhorst FM, et al. Usefulness of procalcitonin for differentiation between activity of systemic autoimmune disease (systemic lupus erythematosus/ systemic antineutrophil cytoplasmic antibody-associated vasculitis) and invasive bacterial infection. Arthritis Rheum 1997;40:1250–6.

405. Arnett FC, Cho M, Chatterjee S, et al. Familial occurrence frequencies and relative risks for systemic sclerosis (scleroderma) in three United States cohorts. Arthritis Rheum 2001;44:1359–62.

406. Kurland LT, Hauser WA, Ferguson RH, Holley KE. Epidemiologic features of diffuse connective tissue disorders in Rochester, Minn., 1951 through 1967, with special reference to systemic lupus erythematosus. Mayo Clin Proc 1969;44:649–63.

407. Ferri C, Valentini G, Cozzi F, et al. Systemic sclerosis: demographic, clinical, and serologic features and survival in 1,012 Italian patients. Medicine (Baltimore) 2002;81:139–53.

408. Scussel-Lonzetti L, Joyal F, Raynauld JP, et al. Predicting mortality in systemic sclerosis: analysis of a cohort of 309 French Canadian patients with emphasis on features at diagnosis as predictive factors for survival. Medicine (Baltimore) 2002;81:154–67.

409. Tuffanelli DL, Winklemann RK. Systemic scleroderma: a clinical study of 727 cases. Arch Dermatol 1961;84:359–71.

410. Rodnan GP. Progressive systemic sclerosis (scleroderma). In: McCarty DJ, editor. Arthritis and allied conditions. Philedelphia: Lea and Febiger; 1979. p. 762.

411. LeRoy EC. Scleroderma (systemic sclerosis). In: Kelley WN, Harris EDJ, Ruddy S, Sledge CB, editors. Textbook of rheumatology. Philadelphia: W.B. Saunders; 1985. p. 1183.

412. Geirsson AJ, Wollheim FA, Akesson A. Disease severity of 100 patients with systemic sclerosis over a period of 14 years: using a modified Medsger scale. Ann Rheum Dis 2001;60:1117–22.

413. Bryan C, Knight C, Black CM, Silman AJ. Prediction of five-year survival following presentation with scleroderma: development of a simple model using three disease factors at first visit. Arthritis Rheum 1999;42:2660–5.

414. Rodnan GP. The natural history of progressive systemic sclerosis (diffuse scleroderma). Bull Rheum Dis 1963;13:301–4.

415. Jacobsen S, Ullman S, Shen GQ, et al. Influence of clinical features, serum antinuclear antibodies, and lung function on survival of patients with systemic sclerosis. J Rheumatol 2001;28:2454–9.

416. Medsger TAJ. Progressive systemic sclerosis. Clin Rheum Dis 1983;8:655–70.

417. Steen VD, Medsger TAJ, Siegler G, Rodnan GP. Clinical comparison of two variants of progressive systemic sclerosis: diffuse scleroderma and CREST syndrome. Arthritis Rheum 1980;23S:752.

418. Winterbauer RH. Multiple telangiectasia. Raynaud's phenomenon, sclerodactyly, and subcutaneous calcinosis: a syndrome mimicking hereditary hemorrhagic telangiectasia. Bull Johns Hopkins Hosp 1964;114:361–83.

419. Rodnan GP, Medsger TAJ, Buckingham RB. Progressive systemic sclerosis-CREST syndrome: observations on natural history and late complications in 90 patients. Arthritis Rheum 1975;18S:423.

420. Salerni R, Rodnan GP, Leon DF, Shaver JA. Pulmonary hypertension in the CREST syndrome variant of progressive systemic sclerosis (scleroderma). Ann Intern Med 1977;86:394–9.

421. Kuwana M, Kaburaki J, Arnett FC, et al. Influence of ethnic background on clinical and serologic features in patients with systemic sclerosis and anti-DNA topoisomerase I antibody. Arthritis Rheum 1999;42:465–74.

422. Vlachoyiannopoulos PG, Dafni UG, Pakas I, et al. Systemic scleroderma in Greece: low mortality and strong linkage with HLA-DRB1*1104 allele. Ann Rheum Dis 2000;59:359–67.

423. Fatini C, Gensini F, Sticchi E, et al. High prevalence of polymorphisms of angiotensin-converting enzyme (I/D) and endothelial nitric oxide synthase (Glu298Asp) in patients with systemic sclerosis. Am J Med 2002;112:540–4.

424. Fisher ER, Rodnan GP. Pathologic observations concerning the cutaneous lesion of progressive systemic sclerosis: an electron microscope, histochemical, and immunohistochemical study. Arthritis Rheum 1960;3:536–45.

425. LeRoy EC. Increased collagen synthesis by scleroderma skin fibroblasts in vitro. J Clin Invest 1974;54:880–9.

426. Buckingham RB, Prince RK, Rodnan GP, Taylor F. Increased collagen accumulation in dermal fibroblast cultures from patients with progressive systemic sclerosis (scleroderma). J Lab Clin Med 1978;92:5–21.

427. Cabral A, Castor CW. Connective tissue activation: XXVII. The behavior of skin fibroblasts from patients with scleroderma. Arthritis Rheum 1983;26:1362–9.

428. Perlish JS, Timpl R, Fleischmajer R. Collagen synthesis regulation by the aminopeptide of procollagen I in normal and scleroderma fibroblasts. Arthritis Rheum 1985;28:647–51.

429. Scheja A, Wildt M, Wollheim FA, et al. Circulating collagen metabolites in systemic sclerosis. Differences between limited and diffuse form and relationship with pulmonary involvement. Rheumatology (Oxford) 2000;39:1110–3.

430. Bernstein RM, Steigerwald JC, Tan EM. Association of antinuclear and antinucleolar antibodies in progressive systemic sclerosis. Clin Exp Immunol 1982;48:43–51.

431. Fleischmajer R, Perlish JS, Reeves JRT. Cellular infiltrates in scleroderma skin. Arthritis Rheum 1977;20:975–84.

432. Fleischmajer R, Gay S, Meigel WN, Perlish JS. Collagen in the cellular and fibrotic states of scleroderma. Arthritis Rheum 1978;21:418–28.

433. Stuart JM, Postlethwaire AE, Kang AH. Evidence of cell-mediated immunity to collagen in progressive systemic sclerosis. J Lab Clin Med 1976;88:601–7.

434. Kondo H, Rabin BS, Rodnan GP. Cutaneous antigen-stimulating lymphokine production by lymphocytes of patients with progressive systemic sclerosis (scleroderma). J Clin Invest 1976;58:1388–94.

435. Tan FK, Arnett FC, Reveille JD, et al. Autoantibodies to fibrillin 1 in systemic sclerosis: ethnic differences in antigen recognition and lack of correlation with specific clinical features or HLA alleles. Arthritis Rheum 2000;43:2464–71.

436. Chizzolini C, Raschi E, Rezzonico R, et al. Autoantibodies to fibroblasts induce a proadhesive and proinflammatory fibroblast phenotype in patients with systemic sclerosis. Arthritis Rheum 2002;46:1602–13.

437. Johnson RL, Ziff M. Lymphokine stimulation of collagen accumulation. J Clin Invest 1976;58:240–52.

438. Lawley TJ, Peck GL, Moutsopoulos HM, et al. Scleroderma, Sjögren-like syndrome and chornic graft-versus-host disease. Ann Intern Med 1977;87:707–9.

439. Campbell PM, Leroy EC. Pathogenesis of systemic sclerosis: a vascular hypothesis. Semin Arthritis Rheum 1975;4:351–8.

440. Kahaleh MB, Sherer GK, LeRoy EC. Endothelial injury in scleroderma. J Exp Med 1979;14:1326–35.

441. Shanahan WRJ, Korn JH. Cytotoxic activity of sera from scleroderma and other connective tissue diseases: lack of cellular and disease specificity. Arthritis Rheum 1982;25:1391–5.

442. Cohen S, Johnson AR, Hurd E. Cytotoxicity of sera from patients with scleroderma: effects on human endothelial cells and fibroblasts in culture. Arthritis Rheum 1983;26:170–8.

443. Fries JF. The microvascular pathogenesis of scleroderma: an hypothesis. Ann Intern Med 1979;91:788–9.

444. Orfanos SE, Psevdi E, Stratigis N, et al. Pulmonary capillary endothelial dysfunction in early systemic sclerosis. Arthritis Rheum 2001;44:902–11.

445. Steen VD, Owens GR, Redmond C, et al. The effect of D-penicillamine on pulmonary findings in systemic sclerosis. Arthritis Rheum 1985;28:882–8.

446. Steen VD, Owens GR, Fino GJ, et al. Pulmonary involvement in systemic sclerosis (scleroderma). Arthritis Rheum 1985;28:759–67.

447. Jacobsen S, Halberg P, Ullman S, et al. A longitudinal study of pulmonary function in Danish patients with systemic sclerosis. Clin Rheumatol 1997;16:384–90.

448. Weaver AL, Divertie MB, Titus JL. Pulmonary scleroderma. Dis Chest 1968;54:490–8.

449. Shuford WH, Seaman WB, Goldman A. Pulmonary manifestations of scleroderma. Arch Intern Med 1953;92:85–97.

450. Boyd JA, Patrick SI, Reeves RJ. Roentgen changes observed in generalized scleroderma. Arch Intern Med 1954;94:248–58.

451. Miller RD, Fowler WS, Helmholz FHJ. Scleroderma of the lungs. Staff Meet Mayo Clin 1959;34:66–75.

452. Sackner MA. Scleroderma. New York: Grune and Stratton; 1966.

453. Farmer RG, Gifford RWJ, Hines EAJ. Prognostic significance of Raynaud's phenomenon and other clinical characteristics of systemic scleroderma. Circulation 1969;21:1088–95.

454. Taormina VJ, Miller WT, Gefter WB, Epstein DM. Progressive systemic sclerosis subgroups: variable pulmonary features. AJR Am J Roentgenol 1981;137:277–85.

455. Owens GR, Fino GJ, Herbert DL, et al. Pulmonary function in progressive systemic sclerosis. Comparison of CREST syndrome variant with diffuse scleroderma. Chest 1983;84:546–50.

456. Adhikari PK, Bianchi FA, Boushy SF, et al. Pulmonary function in scleroderma. Am Rev Respir Dis 1962;86:823–31.

457. Hughes DTD, Lee FI. Lung function in patients with systemic sclerosis. Thorax 1963;18:16–20.

458. Ritchie B. Pulmonary function in scleroderma. Thorax 1964;19:28–36.

459. Wilson RJ, Rodnan GP, Robin ED. An early pulmonary physiologic abnormality in progressive systemic sclerosis (diffuse scleroderma). Am J Med 1964;36:361–9.

460. Sackner MA, Akgun N, Kimbel P, Lewis DH. The pathophysiology of scleroderma involving the heart and respiratory system. Ann Intern Med 1964;60:611–30.

461. DeMuth GR, Furstenberg NA, Dabich L, Zarafonetis CJD. Pulmonary manifestations of progressive systemic sclerosis. Am J Med Sci 1968;255:94–104.

462. Bjerke RD, Tashkin DP, Clements DJ, et al. Small airways in progressive systemic sclerosis. Am J Med 1979;66:201–9.

463. Godfrey S, Bluestone R, Higgs BE. Lung function and the response to exercise in systemic sclerosis. Thorax 1969;24:427–34.

464. Young RH, Mark GJ. Pulmonary vascular changes in scleroderma. Am J Med 1978;64:998–1003.

465. Tashkin DP, Clements PJ, Wright RS, et al. Interrelationships between pulmonary and extrapulmonary involvement in systemic sclerosis. A longitudinal analysis. Chest 1994;105:489–95.

466. Kuwana M, Kaburaki J, Mimori T, et al. Longitudinal analysis of autoantibody response to topoisomerase I in systemic sclerosis. Arthritis Rheum 2000;43:1074–84.

467. Siminovitch K, Klein M, Pruzanski W, et al. Circulating immune complexes in patients with progressive systemic sclerosis. Arthritis Rheum 1982;25:1174–9.

468. Seibold JR, Medsger TAJ, Winkelstein A, et al. Immune complexes in progressive systemic sclerosis (scleroderma). Arthritis Rheum 1982;25:1167–73.

469. Catoggio LJ, Bernstein RM, Black CM, et al. Serological markers in progressive systemic sclerosis: clinical correlation. Ann Rheum Dis 1983;42:23–7.

470. Launay D, Hebbar M, Hatron PY, et al. Relationship between parity and clinical and biological features in patients with systemic sclerosis. J Rheumatol 2001;28:509–13.

471. Silver RM, Metcalf JF, Stanley JH, LeRoy EC. Interstitial lung disease in scleroderma. Analysis by bronchoalveolar lavage. Arthritis Rheum 1984;27:1254–62.

472. Silver RM, Metcalf JF, LeRoy EC. Interstitial lung disease in scleroderma. Immune complexes in sera and bronchoalveolar lavage fluid. Arthritis Rheum 1986;29:525–31.

473. Silver RM, Miller KS. Lung involvement in systemic sclerosis. Rheum Dis Clin North Am 1990;16:199–216.

474. Konig G, Luderschmidt C, Hammer C, et al. Lung involvement in scleroderma. Chest 1984;85:318–24.

475. Atamas SP, Yurovsky VV, Wise R, et al. Production of type 2 cytokines by CD8+ lung cells is associated with greater decline in pulmonary function in patients with systemic sclerosis. Arthritis Rheum 1999;42:1168–78.

476. Rossi GA, Bitterman PB, Rennard SI, et al. Evidence for chronic inflammation as a component of the interstitial lung disease associated with progressive systemic sclerosis. Am Rev Respir Dis 1985;131:612–7.

477. Kinsella MB, Smith EA, Miller KS, et al. Spontaneous production of fibronectin by alveolar macrophages in patients with scleroderma. Arthritis Rheum 1989;32:577–83.

478. Silver RM, Miller KS, Kinsella MB, et al. Evaluation and management of scleroderma lung disease using bronchoalveolar lavage. Am J Med 1990;88:470–6.

479. Taylor ML, Noble PW, White B, et al. Extensive surface phenotyping of alveolar macrophages in interstitial lung disease. Clin Immunol 2000;94:33–41.

480. Carre PC, Mortenson RL, King TE Jr, et al. Overexpression of interleukin 8 gene by alveolar macrophages in idiopathic pulmonary fibrosis: a potential mechanism for the recruitment and activation of neutrophils in lung fibrosis. J Clin Invest 1991;88:1802–10.

481. Crestani B, Seta N, Palazzo E, et al. Interleukin-8 and neutrophils in systemic sclerosis with lung involvement. Am J Respir Crit Care Med 1994;150:1363–7.

482. Pantelidis P, McGrath DS, Southcott AM, et al. Tumour necrosis factor-alpha production in fibrosing alveolitis is macrophage subset specific. Respir Res 2001;2:365–72.

483. Hasegawa M, Sato S, Takehara K. Augmented production of chemokines (monocyte chemotactic protein-1 (MCP-1), macrophage inflammatory protein-1alpha (MIP-1alpha) and MIP-1beta in patients with systemic sclerosis: MCP-1 and MIP-1alpha may be involved in the development of pulmonary fibrosis. Clin Exp Immunol 1999;117:159–65.

484. Seyer JM, Kang AH, Rodnan G. Investigation of type I and III collagens of the lung in progressive systemic sclerosis. Arthritis Rheum 1981;24:625–31.

485. Diot E, Diot P, Valat C, et al. Predictive value of serum III procollagen for diagnosis of pulmonary involvement in patients with scleroderma. Eur Respir J 1995;8:1559–65.

486. Tourkina E, Hoffman S, Fenton JW 2nd, et al. Depletion of protein kinase C epsilon in normal and scleroderma lung fibroblasts has opposite effects on tenascin expression. Arthritis Rheum 2001;44:1370–81.

487. Bogatkevich GS, Tourkina E, Silver RM, Ludwicka-Bradley A. Thrombin differentiates normal lung fibroblasts to a myofibroblast phenotype via the proteolytically activated receptor-1 and a protein kinase C-dependent pathway. J Biol Chem 2001;276:45184–92.

488. Takahashi H, Kuroki Y, Tanaka H, et al. Serum levels of surfactant proteins A and D are useful biomarkers for interstitial lung disease in patients with progressive systemic sclerosis. Am J Respir Crit Care Med 2000;162:258–63.

489. Asano Y, Ihn H, Yamane K, et al. Clinical significance of surfactant protein D as a serum marker for evaluating pulmonary fibrosis in patients with systemic sclerosis. Arthritis Rheum 2001;44:1363–9.

490. Yamane K, Ihn H, Kubo M, et al. Serum levels of KL-6 as a useful marker for evaluating pulmonary fibrosis in patients with systemic sclerosis. J Rheumatol 2000;27:930–4.

491. Sato S, Nagaoka T, Hasegawa M, et al. Elevated serum KL-6 levels in patients with systemic sclerosis: association with the severity of pulmonary fibrosis. Dermatology 2000;200:196–201.

492. Scheja A, Akesson A, Geborek P, et al. Von Willebrand factor propeptide as a marker of disease activity in systemic sclerosis (scleroderma). Arthritis Res 2001;3:178–82.

493. Wigley JEM, Edmunds V, Bradley R. Pulmonary fibrosis in scleroderma. Br J Dermatol Syphilis 1949;61:324–7.

494. Orabona ML, Albano O. Systemic progressive sclerosis (or visceral scleroderma): review of the literature and report of cases. Acta Med Scand 1958;160 Suppl 333:1–170.

495. Weaver AL, Divertie MB, Titus JL. The lung in scleroderma. Mayo Clin Proc 1967;42:754–66.

496. Spain DM, Thomas AG. The pulmonary manifestations of scleroderma: an anatomic-physiologic correlation. Ann Intern Med 1950;32:152–61.

497. Church RE, Ellis ARP. Cystic pulmonary fibrosis in generalized scleroderma. Lancet 1950;i:392–4.

498. Guttadauria M, Ellman H, Kaplan D. Progressive systemic sclerosis: pulmonary involvement. Clin Rheum Dis 1979; 5:151–66.

499. Hayman LD, Hunt RE. Pulmonary fibrosis in generalized scleroderma: report of a case and review of the literature. Dis Chest 1952;21:691–704.

500. Opie LH. The pulmonary manifestations of generalized scleroderma (progressive systemic sclerosis). Dis Chest 1955;28:665–80.

501. Lomeo RM, Cornella RJ, Schabel SI, Silver RM. Progressive systemic sclerosis sine scleroderma presenting as pulmonary interstitial fibrosis. Am J Med 1989;87:525–7.

502. Remy-Jardin M, Remy J, Wallaert B, et al. Pulmonary involvement in progressive systemic sclerosis: sequential evaluation with CT, pulmonary function tests, and bronchoalveolar lavage. Radiology 1993;188:499–506.

503. Kim EA, Johkoh T, Lee KS, et al. Interstitial pneumonia in progressive systemic sclerosis: serial high-resolution CT findings with functional correlation. J Comput Assist Tomogr 2001;25:757–63.

504. Blom-Bulow B, Jonson B, Bauer K. Factors limiting exercise performance in progressive systemic sclerosis. Semin Arthritis Rheum 1983;13:174–81.

505. Medsger TAJ, Rodnan GP, Moossy J, Vester JW. Skeletal muscle involvement in progressive systemic sclerosis (scleroderma). Arthritis Rheum 1968;11:554–68.

506. Wells AU, Hansell DM, Rubens MB, et al. Fibrosing alveolitis in systemic sclerosis: indices of lung function in relation to extent of disease on computed tomography. Arthritis Rheum 1997;40:1229–36.

507. Scheja A, Akesson A, Wollmer P, Wollheim FA. Early pulmonary disease in systemic sclerosis: a comparison between carbon monoxide transfer factor and static lung compliance. Ann Rheum Dis 1993;52:725–9.

508. Emmanuel G, Saroja D, Gopinathan K, et al. Environmental factors and the diffusing capacity of the lung in progressive systemic sclerosis. Chest 1976;69S:304–6.

509. Furst DE, Davis JA, Clements PJ, et al. Abnormalities of pulmonary vascular dynamics and inflammation in early progressive systemic sclerosis. Arthritis Rheum 1981;24:1403–8.

510. Schwaiblmair M, Behr J, Fruhmann G. Cardiorespiratory responses to incremental exercise in patients with systemic sclerosis. Chest 1996;110:1520–5.

511. Witt C, Borges AC, John M, et al. Pulmonary involvement in diffuse cutaneous systemic sclerosis: broncheoalveolar fluid granulocytosis predicts progression of fibrosing alveolitis. Ann Rheum Dis 1999;58:635–40.

512. White B, Moore WC, Wigley FM, et al. Cyclophosphamide is associated with pulmonary function and survival benefit in patients with scleroderma and alveolitis. Ann Intern Med 2000;132:947–54.

513. Wells AU, Hansell DM, Haslam PL, et al. Bronchoalveolar lavage cellularity: lone cryptogenic fibrosing alveolitis compared with the fibrosing alveolitis of systemic sclerosis. Am J Respir Crit Care Med 1998;157:1474–82.

514. Edelson JD, Hyland RH, Ramsden M, et al. Lung inflammation in scleroderma: clinical, radiographic, physiologic and cytopathological features. J Rheumatol 1985;12:957–63.

515. Owens GR, Paradis IL, Gryzan S, et al. Role of inflammation in the lung disease of systemic sclerosis: comparison with idiopathic pulmonary fibrosis. J Lab Clin Med 1986;107: 253–60.

516. Pesci A, Bertorelli G, Manganelli P, Ambanelli U. Bronchoalveolar lavage analysis of interstitial lung disease in CREST syndrome. Clin Exp Rheumatol 1986;4:121–4.

517. Behr J, Vogelmeier C, Beinert T, et al. Bronchoalveolar lavage for evaluation and management of scleroderma disease of the lung. Am J Respir Crit Care Med 1996;154:400–6.

518. Harrison NK, Glanville AR, Strickland B, et al. Pulmonary involvement in systemic sclerosis: the detection of early changes by thin section CT scan, bronchoalveolar lavage and 99mTc-DTPA clearance. Respir Med 1989;83:403–14.

519. Wells AU, Hansell DM, Rubens MB, et al. Fibrosing alveolitis in systemic sclerosis. Bronchoalveolar lavage findings in relation to computed tomographic appearance. Am J Respir Crit Care Med 1994;150:462–8.

520. Giacomelli R, Valentini G, Salsano F, et al. Cyclophosphamide pulse regimen in the treatment of alveolitis in systemic sclerosis. J Rheumatol 2002;29:731–6.

521. Wallaert B, Hatron PY, Grosbois JM, et al. Subclinical pulmonary involvement in collagen-vascular diseases assessed by bronchoalveolar lavage. Relationship between alveolitis and subsequent changes in lung function. Am Rev Respir Dis 1986;133:574–80.

522. Dostrovsky A. Progressive scleroderma of the skin with cystic scleroderal changes of the lungs. Arch Dermatol Syphilol 1947;55:1–11.

523. Piper WN, Helwig EB. Progressive systemic sclerosis: visceral manifestations in generalized scleroderma. Arch Dermatol 1955;72:535–46.

524. Caplan H. Honeycomb lungs and malignant pulmonary adenomatosis in scleroderma. Thorax 1959;14:89–96.

525. Kallenberg CGM, Jansen HM, Elema JD, The TH. Steroid-responsive interstitial pulmonary disease in systemic sclerosis: monitoring by bronchoalveolar lavage. Chest 1984;86:489–92.

526. Bhalla M, Silver RM, Shepard J-AO, McLoud TC. Chest CT in patients with scleroderma: prevalence of asymptomatic esophageal dilatation and mediastinal lymphadenopathy. AJR Am J Roentgenol 1993;161:269–72.

527. Denis P, Ducrotte P, Pasquis P, Lefrancois R. Esophageal motility and pulmonary function in progressive systemic sclerosis. Respiration 1981;42:21–4.

528. Johnson DA, Drane WE, Curran J, et al. Pulmonary disease in progressive systemic sclerosis. A complication of gastroesophageal reflux and occult aspiration? Arch Intern Med 1989;149:589–93.

529. Troshinsky MB, Kane GC, Varga J, et al. Pulmonary function and gastroesophageal reflux in systemic sclerosis. Ann Intern Med 1994;121:6–10.

530. Guttadauria M, Sarojo D, Gopintham P, et al. Small airway disease in scleroderma. Arthritis Rheum 1975;18S:283–4.

531. Guttadauria M, Ellman H, Emmanuel G, et al. Pulmonary function in scleroderma. Arthritis Rheum 1977;20:1071–9.

532. Greenwald GI, Tashkin DP, Gong H, et al. Longitudinal changes in lung function and respiratory symptoms in progressive systemic sclerosis. Prospective study. Am J Med 1987;83:83–92.

533. Harrison NK, Myers AR, Corrin B, et al. Structural features of interstitial lung disease in systemic sclerosis. Am Rev Respir Dis 1991;144:706–13.

534. Boehler A, Vogt P, Speich R, et al. Bronchiolitis obliterans in a patient with localized scleroderma treated with D-penicillamine. Eur Respir J 1996;9:1317–9.

535. Murata I, Takenaka K, Yoshinoya S, et al. Clinical evaluation of pulmonary hypertension in systemic sclerosis and related disorders. A Doppler echocardiographic study of 135 Japanese patients. Chest 1997;111:36–43.

536. Cailes JB, du Bois RM, Hansell DM. Density gradient of the lung parenchyma at computed tomographic scanning in

patients with pulmonary hypertension and systemic sclerosis. Acad Radiol 1996;3:724–30.

537. Gunduz OH, Fertig N, Lucas M, Medsger TA Jr. Systemic sclerosis with renal crisis and pulmonary hypertension: a report of eleven cases. Arthritis Rheum 2001;44:1663–6.

538. Cool CD, Kennedy D, Voelkel NF, Tuder RM. Pathogenesis and evolution of plexiform lesions in pulmonary hypertension associated with scleroderma and human immunodeficiency virus infection. Hum Pathol 1997;28:434–42.

539. Baldwin ED, Cournand A, Richards DW Jr. Pulmonary insufficiency: II. A study of thirty-one cases of pulmonary fibrosis. Medicine (Baltimore) 1949;28:1–25.

540. Trell E, Lindstron C. Pulmonary hypertension in systemic sclerosis. Ann Rheum Dis 1971;30:390–400.

541. Martin L, Pauls JD, Ryan JP, Fritzler MJ. Identification of a subset of patients with scleroderma with severe pulmonary and vascular disease by the presence of autoantibodies to centromere and histone [see comments]. Ann Rheum Dis 1993;52:780–4.

542. Gugnani MK, Pierson C, Vanderheide R, Girgis RE. Pulmonary edema complicating prostacyclin therapy in pulmonary hypertension associated with scleroderma: a case of pulmonary capillary hemangiomatosis. Arthritis Rheum 2000;43:699–703.

543. Pakas I, Ioannidis JP, Malagari K, et al. Cyclophosphamide with low or high dose prednisolone for systemic sclerosis lung disease. J Rheumatol 2002;29:298–304.

544. Steen VD, Lanz JK Jr, Conte C, et al. Therapy for severe interstitial lung disease in systemic sclerosis. A retrospective study [see comments]. Arthritis Rheum 1994;37:1290–6.

545. Silver RM, Warrick JH, Kinsella MB, et al. Cyclophosphamide and low-dose prednisone therapy in patients with systemic sclerosis (scleroderma) with interstitial lung disease. J Rheumatol 1993;20:838–44.

546. Kang B, Veres-Thorner C, Heredia R, et al. Successful treatment of far-advanced progressive systemic sclerosis by D-penicillamine. J Allergy Clin Immunol 1982;69:297–305.

547. Steen VD, Medsger TAJ, Rodnan GP. D-penicillamine therapy in progressive systemic sclerosis: a retrospective analysis. Ann Intern Med 1982;97:652–9.

548. Jimenez SA, Sigal SH. A 15-year prospective study of treatment of rapidly progressive systemic sclerosis with D-penicillamine. J Rheumatol 1991;18:1496–503.

549. Steen VD, Blair S, Medsger TAJ. The toxicity of D-penicillamine in systemic sclerosis. Ann Intern Med 1986;104:699–705.

550. Clements PJ, Furst DE, Wong WK, et al. High-dose versus low-dose D-penicillamine in early diffuse systemic sclerosis: analysis of a two-year, double-blind, randomized, controlled clinical trial. Arthritis Rheum 1999;42:1194–203.

551. Strange C, Bolster M, Mazur J, et al. Hemodynamic effects of epoprostenol in patients with systemic sclerosis and pulmonary hypertension. Chest 2000;118:1077–82.

552. Levine SM, Anzueto A, Peters JI, et al. Single lung transplantation in patients with systemic disease. Chest 1994;105:837–41.

553. Kubo M, Vensak J, Dauber J, et al. Lung transplantation in patients with scleroderma. J Heart Lung Transplant 2001;20:174–5.

554. Binks M, Passweg JR, Furst D, et al. Phase I/II trial of autologous stem cell transplantation in systemic sclerosis: procedure related mortality and impact on skin disease. Ann Rheum Dis 2001;60:577–84.

555. Bennett R, Bluestone R, Holt PJL, Bywaters EGL. Survival in scleroderma. Ann Rheum Dis 1971;30:581–8.

556. Medsger TAJ, Masi AT, Rodnan GP, et al. Survival with systemic sclerosis (scleroderma). Ann Intern Med 1971;75:369–76.

557. Eason RJ, Tan PL, Gow PJ. Progressive systemic sclerosis in Auckland: a ten year review with emphasis on prognostic features. Aust N Z J Med 1981;11:657–62.

558. Peters GM, Wise RA, Hochberg MC, et al. Carbon monoxide diffusing capacity as predictor of outcome in systemic sclerosis. Am J Med 1984;77:1027–34.

559. Travis WD, Matsui K, Moss J, Ferrans VJ. Idiopathic nonspecific interstitial pneumonia: prognostic significance of cellular and fibrosing patterns: survival comparison with usual interstitial pneumonia and desquamative interstitial pneumonia. Am J Surg Pathol 2000;24:19–33.

560. Nicholson AG, Colby TV, Dubois RM, et al. The prognostic significance of the histologic pattern of interstitial pneumonia in patients presenting with the clinical entity of cryptogenic fibrosing alveolitis. Am J Respir Crit Care Med 2000;162:2213–7.

561. Linenthal H, Talkov R. Pulmonary fibrosis in Raynaud's disease. N Engl J Med 1941;224:682–4.

562. Colp CR, Riker J, Williams MHJ. Serial changes in scleroderma and idiopathic interstitial lung disease. Arch Intern Med 1973;132:506–15.

563. Bettman MA, Kantrowitz F. Rapid onset of lung involvement in progressive sclerosis. Chest 1979;75:509–10.

564. Bag LR, Hughes DTD. Serial pulmonary function tests in progressive systemic sclerosis. Thorax 1979;34:224–8.

565. Schneider PD, Wise RA, Hochberg MC, Wigley FM. Serial pulmonary function in systemic sclerosis. Am J Med 1982;73:385–94.

566. Thompson AE, Pope JE. A study of the frequency of pericardial and pleural effusions in scleroderma. Br J Rheumatol 1998;37:1320–3.

567. Abu-Shakra M, Guillemin F, Lee P. Cancer in systemic sclerosis. Arthritis Rheum 1993;36:460–4.

568. Talbott JH, Barrocas M. Carcinoma of the lung in systemic sclerosis: a tabular review of the literature and a detailed report of the roentgenographic changes in two cases. Semin Arthritis Rheum 1980;9:191–217.

569. Yang Y, Fujita J, Tokuda M, et al. Lung cancer associated with several connective tissue diseases: with a review of literature. Rheumatol Int 2001;21:106–11.

570. Rosenthal AK, McLaughlin JK, Linet MS, Persson I. Scleroderma and malignancy: an epidemiological study. Ann Rheum Dis 1993;52:531–3.

571. Bradley JD, Pinals RS, Gupta RC. Chronic active hepatitis associated with polymyositis. Association with precipitating mitochondrial M-B antibody. J Rheumatol 1985;12:368–71.

572. Bohan A, Peter JB. Polymyositis and dermatomyositis. N Engl J Med 1975;292:344–7, 403–7.

573. Lambie JA, Duff IF. Familial occurrence of dermatomyositis. Case reports and a family survey. Ann Intern Med 1963;59:839–47.

574. Harati Y, Niakan E, Bergman EW. Childhood dermatomyositis in monozygotic twins. Neurology 1986;36:721–3.

575. Pearson CM. Polymyositis. Annu Rev Med 1966;65:63–82.

576. Logan RG, Bandera JM, Mikkelsen WM, Duff IF. Polymyositis: a clinical study. Ann Intern Med 1966;65:996–1007.

577. Pearson CM, Bohan A. The spectrum of polymyositis and dermatomyositis. Med Clin North Am 1977;61:439–57.

578. Bohan A, Peter JB, Bowman RL, Pearson CM. Computer-assisted analysis of 153 patients with polymyositis and dermatomyositis. Medicine (Baltimore) 1977;56:255–86.

579. Diessner GR, Howard FMJ, Winkelmann RK, et al. Laboratory tests in polymyositis. Arch Intern Med 1966;117:757–63.

580. Fudman EJ, Schnitzer TJ. Dermatomyositis without creatine kinase elevation. A poor prognostic sign. Am J Med 1986;80:329–32.

581. Mills ES, Mathews WH. Interstitial penumonitis in dermatomyositis. JAMA 1956;160:1467–70.

582. Schwarz MI, Matthay RA, Sahn SA, et al. Interstitial lung disease in polymyositis and dermatomyositis: analysis of six cases and review of the literature. Medicine 1976;55:89–104.

583. Kamin EJ, Southgate MT, Cook RW, et al. A case of dermatomyositis. JAMA 1975;233:66–74.

584. Yoshii A, Kitamura M, Komeji S, et al. Interstitial lung disease in polymyositis and dermatomyositis (PM-DM)-clinical and immunological studies [author's translation]. Nippon Naika Gakkai Zasshi 1981;70:1380–7.

585. Dickey BF, Myers AR. Pulmonary disease in polymyositis/dermatomyositis. Semin Arthritis Rheum 1984;14:60–76.

586. Lambie PB, Quismorio FP Jr. Interstitial lung disease and cryoglobulinemia in polymyositis. J Rheumatol 1991;18:468–9.

587. Forster BB, Blackie SP, Müller NL, et al. A 50-year-old woman with polymyositis and chronic bibasilar lung disease [clinical conference]. Can Assoc Radiol J 1990;41:45–8.

588. Frazier AR, Miller RD. Interstitial penumonitis in association with polymyositis and dermatomyositis. Chest 1974;65:403–7.

589. Salmeron G, Greenberg SD, Lidsky MD. Polymyositis and diffuse interstitial lung disease. A review of the pulmonary histopathologic findings. Arch Intern Med 1981;141:1005–10.

590. Marie I, Hachulla E, Hatron PY, et al. Polymyositis and dermatomyositis: short term and longterm outcome, and predictive factors of prognosis. J Rheumatol 2001;28:2230–7.

591. Christianson HB, Brunsting LA, Perry HO. Dermatomyositis: unusual features, complications, and treatment. Arch Dermatol 1956;74:581–4.

592. Rose AL, Walton JN. Polymyositis: a survey of 89 cases with particular reference to treatment and prognosis. Brain 1966;89:747–68.

593. Currie S, Saunders M, Knowles M, Brown AE. Immunological aspects of polymyositis. QJM 1971;40:63–84.

594. Dawkins RL, Mastaglia FL. Cell-mediated cytotoxicity to muscle in polymyositis: effect of immunosuppression. N Engl J Med 1973;288:434–8.

595. Caspary EA, Gubbay SS, Stern GM. Circulating antibodies in polymyositis and other muscle-wasting disorders. Lancet 1964;ii:941.

596. Whitaker JN, Engel WK. Mechanism of muscle injury in idiopathic inflammatory myopathy. N Engl J Med 1973;289:107–8.

597. Grathwohl KW, Thompson JW, Riordan KK, et al. Digital clubbing associated with polymyositis and interstitial lung disease. Chest 1995;108:1751–2.

598. Marie I, Hatron PY, Hachulla E, et al. Pulmonary involvement in polymyositis and in dermatomyositis. J Rheumatol 1998;25:1336–43.

599. Wasicek CA, Reichlin M, Montes M, Raahu G. Polymyositis and interstitial lung disease in a patient with anti-Jo-1 prototype. Am J Med 1984;76:538–44.

600. Saito E, Yoshimoto Y, Oshima H, et al. Fluorescent antibodies in polymyositis using cultured human skin fibroblasts: granular perinuclear cytoplasmic staining pattern by sera from patients with polymyositis and pulmonary fibrosis. J Rheumatol 1989;16:47–54.

601. Plotz PH, Dalakas M, Leff RL, et al. Current concepts in the idiopathic inflammatory myopathies: polymyositis, dermatomyositis, and related disorders. Ann Intern Med 1989;111:143–57.

602. Ikezoe J, Johkoh T, Kohno N, et al. High-resolution CT findings of lung disease in patients with polymyositis and dermatomyositis. J Thorac Imaging 1996;11:250–9.

603. Kourakata H, Takada T, Suzuki E, et al. Flow cytometric analysis of bronchoalveolar lavage fluid cells in polymyositis/dermatomyositis with interstitial pneumonia. Respirology 1999;4:223–8.

604. Komocsi A, Kumanovics G, Zibotics H, Czirjak L. Alveolitis may persist during treatment that sufficiently controls muscle inflammation in myositis. Rheumatol Int 2001;20:113–8.

605. Yamadori I, Fujita J, Kajitani H, et al. Lymphocyte subsets in lung tissues of interstitial pneumonia associated with untreated polymyositis/dermatomyositis. Rheumatol Int 2001;21:89–93.

606. Tazelaar HD, Viggiano RW, Pickersgill J, Colby TV. Interstitial lung disease in polymyositis and dermatomyositis. Clinical features and prognosis as correlated with histologic findings. Am Rev Respir Dis 1990;141:727–33.

607. Maeda K, Kimura R, Komuta K, Igarashi T. Cyclosporine treatment for polymyositis/dermatomyositis: is it possible to rescue the deteriorating cases with interstitial pneumonitis? Scand J Rheumatol 1997;26:24–9.

608. Nawata Y, Kurasawa K, Takabayashi K, et al. Corticosteroid resistant interstitial pneumonitis in dermatomyositis/polymyositis: prediction and treatment with cyclosporine. J Rheumatol 1999;26:1527–33.

609. Oddis CV, Sciurba FC, Elmagd KA, Starzl TE. Tacrolimus in refractory polymyositis with interstitial lung disease. Lancet 1999;353:1762–3.

610. Nakajima H, Harigai M, Hara M, et al. KL-6 as a novel serum marker for interstitial pneumonia associated with collagen diseases. J Rheumatol 2000;27:1164–70.

611. Kubo M, Ihn H, Yamane K, et al. Serum KL-6 in adult patients with polymyositis and dermatomyositis. Rheumatology (Oxford) 2000;39:632–6.

612. Fujita J, Yamadori I, Suemitsu I, et al. Clinical features of nonspecific interstitial pneumonia. Respir Med 1999;93:113–8.

613. Hsue YT, Paulus HE, Coulson WF. Bronchiolitis obliterans organizing pneumonia in polymyositis. A case report with longterm survival. J Rheumatol 1993;20:877–9.

614. Fata F, Rathore R, Schiff C, Herzlich BC. Bronchiolitis obliterans organizing pneumonia as the first manifestation of polymyositis. South Med J 1997;90:227–30.

615. Shinohara T, Hidaka T, Matsuki Y, et al. Rapidly progressive interstitial lung disease associated with dermatomyositis responding to intravenous cyclophosphamide pulse therapy [see comments]. Intern Med 1997;36:519–23.

616. Medsger TAJ, Robinson H, Masi AT. Factors affecting survivorship in polymyositis. A life-table study of 124 patients. Arthritis Rheum 1971;14:249–58.

617. O'Leary PA, Waisman M. Dermatomyositis: a study of forty cases. Arch Dermatol Syph 1940;41:1001–19.

618. Hepper NG, Ferguson RH, Howard FM. Three types of pulmonary involvement in polymyositis. Med Clin North Am 1964;48:1031–42.

619. Winkelmann GR, Muldetl DW, Lambert EH, et al. Course of dermatomyositis-polymyositis: comparison of untreated and cortisone-treated patients. Mayo Clin Proc 1968;43:545–56.

620. Benbassat J, Gelfel D, Larholt K, et al. Prognostic factors in polymyositis/dermatomyositis. A computer-assisted analysis of ninety-two cases. Arthritis Rheum 1985;28:249–55.

621. Porubsky ES, Murray JP, Pratt LL. Cricopharyngeal achalasia in dermatomyositis. Arch Otolaryngol 1973;98:428–9.

622. Kagen LJ, Hochman RB, Strong EN. Cricopharyngeal obsruction in inflammatory myopathy (polymyositis/dermatomyositis). Report of three cases and review of the literature. Arthritis Rheum 1985;28:630–6.

623. Grateau G, Roux ME, Franck N, et al. Pulmonary hypertension in a case of dermatomyositis [letter]. J Rheumatol 1993;20:1452–3.

624. Caldwell IW, Aitchison JD. Pulmonary hypertension in dermatomyositis. Br Heart J 1956;18:273–6.

625. Bunch TW. Prednisone and azathioprine for polymyositis. Longterm follow-up. Arthritis Rheum 1981;24:45–8.

626. Hebert CA, Byrnes TJ, Baethge BA, et al. Exercise limitation in patients with polymyositis. Chest 1990;98:352–7.

627. Schwarz MI, Sutarik JM, Nick JA, et al. Pulmonary capillaritis and diffuse alveolar hemorrhage. A primary manifestation of polymyositis. Am J Respir Crit Care Med 1995;151:2037–40.

628. Clawson K, Oddis CV. Adult respiratory distress syndrome in polymyositis patients with the anti-Jo-1 antibody. Arthritis Rheum 1995;38:1519–23.

629. DeVere R, Bradley WG. Polymyositis: its presentation, morbidity and mortality. Brain 1975;98:637–66.

630. Blumbergs PC, Byrne E, Kakulas BA. Polymyositis presenting with respiratory failure. J Neurol Sci 1984;65:221–9.

631. Braum NM, Aurora NS, Rochester DF. Respiratory muscle and pulmonary function in polymyositis and other proximal myopathies. Thorax 1983;38:616–23.

632. Black LF, Hyatt RE. Maximal statis respiratory pressures in generalized neuromuscular disease. Am Rev Respir Dis 1971;103:641–50.

633. Domzalski CA, Morgan VC. Dermatomyositis: diagnostic features and therapeutic pitfalls. Am J Med 1955;19:370–82.

634. Singsen BH, Tedford JC, Platzker AC, Hanson V. Spontaneous pneumothorax: a complication of juvenile dermatomyositis. Pediatrics 1978;92:771–4.

635. Roach DG, Salter WM. Polymyositis with pulmonary infiltrate and pleural effusion. Minn Med 1980;63:277–9, 281.

636. Williams RCJ. Dermatomyositis and malignancy: a review of the literature. Ann Intern Med 1959;50:1174–81.

637. Manchul LA, Jin A, Pritchard KI, et al. The frequency of malignant neoplasm in patients with polymyositis-dermatomyositis. Arch Intern Med 1985;145:1835–9.

638. Sigurgeirsson B, Lindelof B, Edhag O, Allander E. Risk of cancer in patients with dermatomyositis or polymyositis. N Engl J Med 1992;326:363–7.

639. Hill CL, Zhang Y, Sigurgeirsson B, et al. Frequency of specific cancer types in dermatomyositis and polymyositis: a population-based study. Lancet 2001;357:96–100.

640. Manthorpe R, Frost-Larsen K, Isager H, Prause JU. Sjögren's syndrome. A review with emphasis on immunological features. Allergy 1981;36:139–53.

641. Whaley K, Alspaugh MA. Sjögren's syndrome. In: Kelley WN, Harris EDJ, Ruddy S, Sledge CB, editors. Textbook of rheumatology. Philadelphia: W.B. Saunders; 1985. p. 956.

642. Pillemer SR, Matteson EL, Jacobsson LT, et al. Incidence of physician-diagnosed primary Sjögren syndrome in residents of Olmsted County, Minnesota. Mayo Clin Proc 2001;76:593–9.

643. Malinow KL, Molina R, Gordon B, et al. Neuropsychiatric dysfunction in primary Sjögren's syndrome. Ann Intern Med 1985;103:344–9.

644. Fischbach M, Char D, Christensen M, et al. Immune complexes in Sjögren's syndrome. Arthritis Rheum 1980;23:791–5.

645. Reveille JD, Wilson RW, Provost TT, et al. Primary Sjögren's syndrome and other autoimmune diseases in families. Prevalence and immunogenetic studies of six kindreds. Ann Intern Med 1984;101:748–56.

646. Bolstad AI, Wassmuth R, Haga HJ, Jonsson R. HLA markers and clinical characteristics in Caucasians with primary Sjögren's syndrome. J Rheumatol 2001;28:1554–62.

647. Alexander EL, Arnett FC, Provost TT, Stevens MB. Sjögren's syndrome: association of anti-Ro (SS-A) antibodies with vasculitis, hematologic abnormalities, and serologic hyperreactivity. Ann Intern Med 1983;98:155–9.

648. Thomsen BS, Oxholm P, Manthorpe R, Nielsen H. Complement C3b receptors on erythrocytes, circulating immune complexes and complement C3 split products in patients with primary Sjögren's syndrome. Arthritis Rheum 1986;29:857–62.

649. Pedersen BK, Oxholm P, Manthorpe R, Andersen V. Interleukin 2 augmentation of the defective natural killer cell activity in patients with primary Sjögren's syndrome. Clin Exp Immunol 1986;63:1–7.

650. Wigely SC, Egan JB. Pulmonary infection in Sjögren's disease (peratoconjunctivitis sicca): a report of a fatal case. Med J Aust 1955;2:371–4.

651. Snider GL, Weiss MA. Pulmonary infiltrates in a woman with Sjögren's syndrome. Case records of the Massachusetts General hospital. Case 28-1975. N Engl J Med 1975;293:136–44.

652. Mialon P, Barthélémy L, Sébert P, et al. A longitudinal study of lung impairment in patients with primary Sjögren's syndrome. Clin Exp Rheumatol 1997;15:349–54.

653. Franquet T, Giménez A, Monill JM, et al. Primary Sjögren's syndrome and associated lung disease: CT findings in 50 patients. AJR Am J Roentgenol 1997;169:655–8.

654. Lahdensuo A, Korpela M. Pulmonary findings in patients with primary Sjögren's syndrome. Chest 1995;108:316–9.

655. Martínez-Cordero E, Andrade-Ortega L, Martínez-Miranda E. Pulmonary function abnormalities in patients with primary Sjögren's syndrome. J Invest Allergol Clin Immunol 1993;3:205–9.

656. Gardiner P, Ward C, Allison A, et al. Pleuropulmonary abnormalities in primary Sjögren's syndrome. J Rheumatol 1993;20:831–7.

657. Karlish AJ. Lung changes in Sjögren's syndrome. Proc R Soc Med 1969;62:1042–3.

658. Liebow AA, Carrington CB. Diffuse pulmonary lymphoreticular infiltrations associated with dysproteinemia. Med Clin North Am 1973;57:809–43.

659. Strimlan CV, Rosenow EC, Divertie MB, Harrison EG. Pulmonary manifestations of Sjögren's syndrome. Chest 1976;70:354–61.

660. Oxholm P, Bundgaard A, Birk-Madsen E, et al. Pulmonary function in patients with primary Sjögren's syndrome. Rheumatol Int 1982;2:179–81.

661. Dalavanga YA, Constantopoulos SH, Galanopoulou V, et al. Alveolitis correlates with clinical pulmonary involvement in primary Sjögren's syndrome. Chest 1991;99:1394–7.

662. Deheinzelin D, Capelozzi VL, Kairalla RA, et al. Interstitial lung disease in primary Sjögren's syndrome. Clinicopathological evaluation and response to treatment. Am J Respir Crit Care Med 1996;154:794–9.

663. Papiris SA, Maniati M, Constantopoulos SH, et al. Lung involvement in primary Sjögren's syndrome is mainly related to the small airway disease. Ann Rheum Dis 1999;58:61–4.

664. Meyer CA, Pina JS, Taillon D, Godwin JD. Inspiratory and expiratory high-resolution CT findings in a patient with Sjögren's syndrome and cystic lung disease. AJR Am J Roentgenol 1997;168:101–3.

665. Davidson BK, Kelly CA, Griffiths ID. Ten year follow up of pulmonary function in patients with primary Sjögren's syndrome. Ann Rheum Dis 2000;59:709–12.

666. Salaffi F, Manganelli P, Carotti M, et al. A longitudinal study of pulmonary involvement in primary Sjögren's syndrome: relationship between alveolitis and subsequent lung changes on high-resolution computed tomography. Br J Rheumatol 1998;37:263–9.

667. Hatron PY, Wallaert B, Gosset D, et al. Subclinical lung inflammation in primary Sjögren's syndrome. Relationship between bronchoalveolar lavage cellular analysis findings and characteristics of the disease. Arthritis Rheum 1987;30:1226–31.

668. Matteson EL, Ike RW. Bronchiolitis obliterans organizing pneumonia and Sjögren's syndrome. J Rheumatol 1990;17:676–9.

669. Colby TV, Koss MN, Travis WD. Lymphoreticular disorders. In: Colby TV, Koss MN, Travis WD, editors. Atlas of tumor pathology. Tumors of the lower respiratory tract. Washington (DC): Armed Forces Institute of Pathology; 1994. p. 419–64.

670. Kadota J, Kusano S, Kawakami K, et al. Usual interstitial pneumonia associated with primary Sjögren's syndrome. Chest 1995;108:1756–8.

671. Ellman P, Weber FP, Goudier TEW. A contribution to the pathology of Sjögren's disease. QJM 1951;20:33–42.

672. Talal N, Sokoloff L, Barth WF. Extrasalivary lymphoid abnormalities in Sjögren's syndrome (reticulum cell sarcoma, "pseudolymphoma," macroglobulinemia). Am J Med 1967;43:50–65.

673. Anderson LG, Talal N. The spectrum of benign to malignant lymphoproliferation in Sjögren's syndrome. Clin Exp Immunol 1972;10:199–221.

674. Tsuzaka K, Akama H, Yamada H, et al. Pulmonary pseudolymphoma presented with a mass lesion in a patient

with primary Sjögren's syndrome: beneficial effect of intermittent intravenous cyclophosphamide. Scand J Rheumatol 1993;22:90–3.

675. Kassam S, Thomas T, Moutsopolous H, et al. Increased risk of lymphoma in sicca syndrome. Ann Intern Med 1978; 89:888–92.

676. Sutinen S, Sutinen S, Huhti E. Ultrastructure of lymphoid interstitial pneumonia: virus-like particles in bronchiolar epithelium of a patient with Sjögren's syndrome. Am J Clin Pathol 1977;67:328–33.

677. Block KJ, Buchanan WW, Wohl MJ, Bunim JJ. Sjögren's syndrome: a clinical, pathological, and serological study of sixty-two cases. Medicine 1965;44:187–231.

678. Constantopoulos SH, Drosos AA, Maddison PJ, Moutsopoulos HM. Xerotrachea and interstitial lung disease in primary Sjögren's syndrome. Respiration 1984;46:310–4.

679. Newball HH, Brahim SA. Chronic obstructive airway disease in patients with Sjögren's syndrome. Am Rev Respir Dis 1977;115:295–304.

680. Fairfax AJ, Haslam LP, Pavia D, et al. Pulmonary disorders associated with Sjögren's syndrome. QJM 1981;50:279–95.

681. Mathieu A, Cauli A, Pala R, et al. Tracheo-bronchial mucociliary clearance in patients with primary and secondary Sjögren's syndrome. Scand J Rheumatol 1995;24:300–4.

682. Bariffi F, Pesci A, Vertorelli G, et al. Pulmonary involvement in Sjögren's syndrome. Respiration 1984;46:82–7.

683. Constantopoulos SH, Papdimitrious CS, Moutsopoulos HM. Respiratory manifestations in primary Sjögren's syndrome. Chest 1985;88:226–9.

684. Papathanasiou MP, Constantopoulos SH, Tsampoulas C, et al. Reappraisal of respiratory abnormalities in primary and secondary Sjögren's syndrome. Chest 1986;90:370–4.

685. Young C, Hunt S, Watkinson A, Beynon H. Sjögren's syndrome, cavitating lung disease and high sustained levels of antibodies to serine proteinase 3. Scand J Rheumatol 2000;29:267–9.

686. Bonner H Jr, Ennis RS, Geelhoed GW, Tarpley TM Jr. Lymphoid infiltration and amyloidosis of lung in Sjögren's syndrome. Arch Pathol 1973;95:42–4.

687. Milburn JM, Kay D, Ridpath C. Pulmonary nodular amyloidosis in a patient with Sjögren's syndrome diagnosed by transthoracic biopsy. J Louisiana State Med Soc 1994; 146:395–8.

688. Wong BC, Wong KL, Ip IMS, et al. Sjögren's syndrome with amyloid A presenting as multiple pulmonary nodules. J Rheumatol 1994;21:165–7.

689. Fox RI, Howell FV, Bone RC, Michelson P. Primary Sjögren's syndrome: clinical and immunopathological features. Semin Arthritis Rheum 1984;14:77–105.

690. Tavoni A, Vitali C, Cirigliano G, et al. Shrinking lung in primary Sjögren's syndrome. Arthritis Rheum 1999;42: 2249–50.

691. Ahmed S, Herrick A, O'Driscoll BR. Shrinking lung syndrome in patients without systemic lupus erythematosus: comment on the concise communication by Tavoni et al. Arthritis Rheum 2001;44:243–5.

692. Sharp GC, Irvin WS, Tan EM, et al. Mixed connective tissue disease—an apparently distinct rheumatic disease syndrome associated with a specific antibody to an extractable nuclear antigen (ENA). Am J Med 1972;52:148–59.

693. Mattioli M, Reichlin M. Physical association of two nuclear antigens and the mutual occurrence of their antibodies: the relationship of the Sm and RNA protein (Mo) systems in SLE sera. J Immunol 1977;110:1318–24.

694. Bennett RM. Mixed connective tissue disease and other overlap syndromes. In: Kelley WN, Harris ED Jr, Ruddy S, Sledge CB, editors. Textbook of rheumatology. Philadelphia: W.B. Saunders; 1985. p. 1115.

695. Reichlin M. Mixed connective tissue disease. In: Hughes GRV, editor. Modern topics in rheumatology. London: Heinemann; 1976. p. 157.

696. Sharp GC. Mixed connective tissue disease. Bull Rheum Dis 1975;25:828–31.

697. Bennett RM, O'Connell DJ. Mixed connective tissue disease: a clinicopathologic study of 20 cases. Semin Arthritis Rheum 1980;10:25–51.

698. Singsen BH, Bernstein BH, Kornreich HK, et al. Mixed connective tissue disease in childhood. A clinical and serological survey. J Pediatr 1977;90:893–900.

699. Oetgen WJ, Mutter ML, Lawless OJ, Davia JE. Cardiac abnormalties in mixed connective tissue disease. Chest 1983; 83:185–8.

700. Jones MB, Osterholm RK, Wilson RB, et al. Fatal pulmonary hypertension and resolving immune-complex glomerulonephritis in mixed connective tissue disease. A case report and review of the literature. Am J Med 1978;65:855–63.

701. Germain MJ, Davidman M. Pulmonary hemorrhage and acute renal failure in a patient with mixed connective tissue disease. Am J Kidney Dis 1984;3:420–4.

702. Udoff EJ, Gerant HK, Kozin F, Ginsberg M. MCTD: the spectrum of radiologic manifestations. Radiology 1977; 124:613–8.

703. Prakash UB. Lungs in mixed connective tissue disease. J Thorac Imaging 1992;7:55–61.

704. Yazdy AM, Park MC, Supinski G. Restrictive ventilatory defect associated with pulmonary hypertension in mixed connective tissue disease [letter; comment]. J Rheumatol 1990;17:121–3.

705. Harmon C, Wolfe F, Lillard S, et al. Pulmonary involvement in mixed connective tissue disease (MCTD). Arthritis Rheum 1976;19:801(A).

706. Saito Y, Terada M, Takada T, et al. Pulmonary involvement in mixed connective tissue disease: comparison with other collagen vascular diseases using high resolution CT. J Comput Assist Tomogr 2002;26:349–57.

707. Sullivan WD, Hurst DJ, Harmon CE, et al. A prospective evaluation emphasizing pulmonary involvement in patients with mixed connective tissue disease. Medicine 1984;63:92–107.

708. Kozuka T, Johkoh T, Honda O, et al. Pulmonary involvement in mixed connective tissue disease: high-resolution CT findings in 41 patients. J Thorac Imaging 2001;16:94–8.

709. Derderian SS, Tellis CJ, Abbrecht PH, et al. Pulmonary involvement in mixed connective tissue disease. Chest 1985;88:45–8.

710. Izumiyama T, Hida W, Ichinose M, et al. Small airway involvement in mixed connective tissue disease. Tohoku J Exp Med 1993;170:273–83.

711. Cryer PE, Kissane JM. Clinicopathologic conference: mixed connective tissue disease. Am J Med 1978;65:833–42.

712. Schwarz MI, Zamora MR, Hodges TN, et al. Isolated pulmonary capillaritis and diffuse alveolar hemorrhage in rheumatoid arthritis and mixed connective tissue disease. Chest 1998;113:1609–15.

713. Sharp GC, Irvin WS, May CM, et al. Association of antibodies to ribonucleoprotein and Sm antigens with mixed connective tissue disease, systemic lupus erythematosus, and other rheumatic diseases. N Engl J Med 1976;295:1149–54.

714. Hosoda Y, Yoshida S, Mimori T, et al. Polymyositis associated with interstitial pulmonary fibrosis and glomerulonephritis. A report of two autopsy cases. Ryumachi 1981;21(S):183–8.

715. Yoshida S, Katayama M. [Pulmonary hypertension in patients with connective tissue diseases.] Nippon Rinsho 2001; 59:1164–7.

716. Andersen GN, Vasko J. Scleroderma renal crisis and concurrent isolated pulmonary hypertension in mixed connective tissue disease and overlap syndrome: report of two cases. Clin Rheumatol 2002;21:164–9.

717. Rosenberg AM, Petty RE, Cumming GR, Koehler BE. Pulmonary hypertension in a child with mixed connective tissue disease. J Rheumatol 1979;6:700–4.

718. Addison HM Jr, Levitin PM. Fatal pulmonary hypertension in

a patient with mixed connective tissue disease. N C Med J 1983;44:719–20.

719. Manthorpe R, Elling H, van der Meulen JR, Sorensen S. Two fatal cases of mixed connective tissue disease. Scand J Rheum 1980;9:7–10.

720. Weiner-Kronish JP, Solinder AM, Warnock ML, et al. Severe pulmonary involvement in mixed connective tissue disease. Am Rev Respir Dis 1981;124:499–503.

721. Ueda N, Mimura K, Maeda H, et al. Mixed connective tissue disease with fatal pulmonary hypertension and a review of literature. Virchows Arch (Pathol Anat) 1984;404:335–40.

722. Hoogsten HC, van Dongen JJ, van der Kwast TH, et al. Bilateral exudative pleuritis, an unusual pulmonary onset of mixed connective disease. Respiration 1985;48:164–7.

723. Ilan Y, Ben-Yehuda A, Okon E, Breuer R. Mixed connective tissue disease presenting as a left sided pleural effusion. Ann Rheum Dis 1992;51:1157–8.

724. Luthra HS. Extra-articular manifestations of ankylosing spondylitis [editorial]. Mayo Clin Proc 1977;52:655–6.

725. Calin A. Ankylosing spondylitis. In: Kelley WN, Harris ED Jr, Ruddy S, Sledge CB, editors. Textbook of rheumatology. Philadelphia: W.B. Saunders; 1985. p. 993.

726. Hamilton KA. Pulmonary disease manifestations of ankylosing spondylarthritis. Ann Intern Med 1949;31:216–27.

727. Rosenow E, Strimlan CV, Muhm JR, Ferguson RH. Pleuropulmonary manifestations of ankylosing spondylitis. Mayo Clin Proc 1977;52:641–9.

728. Renzetti DAJ, Nicholas W, Du Hon REJ, Jiroff L. Some effects of ankylosing spondylitis on pulmonary gas exchange. N Engl J Med 1960;262:215–8.

729. Travis DM, Cook CD, Julian DG, et al. The lungs in rheumatoid spondylitis. Gas exchange and lung mechanics in a form of restrictive pulmonary disease. Am J Med 1960;29:623–32.

730. Campbell AH, MacDonald CB. Upper lobe fibrosis associated with ankylosing spondylitis. Br J Dis Chest 1965;59:90–101.

731. Krohn J, Halvorsen JH. Aspergilloma of the lung in ankylosing spondylitis. Scand J Respir Dis 1968;S63:131–3.

732. Davies D. Ankylosing spondylitis and lung fibrosis. QJM 1972;41:395–417.

733. Davies D. Lung fibrosis in ankylosing spondylitis. Thorax 1972;27:262.

734. Krohn J, Johannessen H. Pulmonary aspergillosis and ankylosing spondylitis [abstract]. Br Thorac Tuberc Assoc Rev (Edinb) 1973;3:33.

735. Crompton GK, Cameron SJ, Langlands AD. Pulmonary fibrosis, pulmonary tuberculosis and ankylosing spondylitis. Br J Dis Chest 1974;68:51–6.

736. Parkin A, Robinson PJ, Hickling P. Regional lung ventilation in ankylosing spondylitis. Br J Radiol 1982;55:833–6.

737. Shankar PS. Ankylosing spondylitis with fibrosis and carcinoma of the lung. CA Cancer J Clin 1982;32:177–9.

738. Hrslev-Petersen K, Helen P. HLA-B27: a risk factor for lung disease? [letter]. Lancet 1984;i:104.

739. Hakala M, Kontkanen E, Koivisto O. Simultaneous presentation of upper lobe fibrobullous disease and spinal pseudarthrosis in a patient with ankylosing spondylitis. Ann Rheum Dis 1990;49:728–9.

740. Boulware DW, Weissman DN, Doll NJ. Pulmonary manifestations of the rheumatic diseases. Clin Rev Allergy 1985;3:249–67.

741. Thai D, Ratani RS, Salama S, Steiner RM. Upper lobe fibrocavitary disease in a patient with back pain and stiffness. Chest 2000;118:1814–6.

742. Casserly IP, Fenlon HM, Breatnach E, Sant SM. Lung findings on high-resolution computed tomography in idiopathic ankylosing spondylitis—correlation with clinical findings, pulmonary function testing and plain radiography. Br J Rheumatol 1997;36:677–82.

743. Turetschek K, Ebner W, Fleischmann D, et al. Early pulmonary involvement in ankylosing spondylitis: assessment with thin-section CT. Clin Radiol 2000;55:632–6.

744. Ferdoutsis M, Bouros D, Meletis G, et al. Diffuse interstitial lung disease as an early manifestation of ankylosing spondylitis. Respiration 1995;62:286–9.

745. Stewart RM, Ridyard JB, Pearson JD. Regional lung function in ankylosing spondylitis. Thorax 1976;31:433–7.

746. van Noord JA, Cauberghs M, Van de Woestijne KP, Demedts M. Total respiratory resistance and reactance in ankylosing spondylitis and kyphoscoliosis. Eur Respir J 1991;4:945–51.

747. Aggarwal AN, Gupta D, Wanchu A, Jindal SK. Use of static lung mechanics to identify early pulmonary involvement in patients with ankylosing spondylitis. J Postgrad Med 2001;47:89–94.

748. Kchir MM, Mtimet S, Kochbati S, et al. Bronchoalveolar lavage and transbronchial biopsy in spondyloarthropathies. J Rheumatol 1992;19:913–6.

749. Wendling D, Dalphin JC, Toson B, et al. Bronchoalveolar lavage in ankylosing spondylitis. Ann Rheum Dis 1990;49:325–6.

750. Hart FD, Bogdanovitch A, Nichol WD. The thorax in ankylosing spondylitis. Ann Rheum Dis 1950;9:116–31.

751. Wilkinson M, Bywaters EGL. Clinical features and course of ankylosing spondylitis, as seen in a follow-up of 222 hospital referred cases. Ann Rheum Dis 1958;17:209–28.

752. Josenhans WT, Wang CS, Josenhans G, Woodbury JF. Diaphragmatic contribution to ventilation in patients with ankylosing spondylitis. Respiration 1971;28:331–46.

753. Hauge BN. Diaphragmatic movement and spirometric volume in patients with ankylosing spondylitis. Scand J Respir Dis 1973;54:38–44.

754. Grimby G, Fugl-Meyer AR, Blomstrand A. Partitioning of the contributions of rib cage and abdomen to ventilation in ankylosing spondylitis. Thorax 1974;29:179–84.

755. Seckin U, Bolukbasi N, Gursel G, et al. Relationship between pulmonary function and exercise tolerance in patients with ankylosing spondylitis. Clin Exp Rheumatol 2000;18:503–6.

756. Carter R, Riantawan P, Banham SW, Sturrock RD. An investigation of factors limiting aerobic capacity in patients with ankylosing spondylitis. Respir Med 1999;93:700–8.

757. Fisher LR, Cawley MI, Holgate ST. Relation between chest expansion, pulmonary function, and exercise tolerance in patients with ankylosing spondylitis. Ann Rheum Dis 1990;49:921–5.

758. Zorab PA. The lungs in ankylosing spondylitis. QJM 1962;31:267–81.

759. Kinnear WJ, Shneerson JM. Acute pleural effusions in inactive ankylosing spondylitis. Thorax 1985;40:150–1.

760. Gacad G, Massaro D. Pulmonary fibrosis and group IV mycobacteria infection of the lungs in ankylosing spondylitis. Am Rev Respir Dis 1974;109:274–8.

761. Hillerdal G. Ankylosing spondylitis lung disease—an under-diagnosed entity? Eur J Respir Dis 1983;64:437–41.

762. Wolson AH, Rohwedder JJ. Upper lobe fibrosis in ankylosing spondylitis. Am J Roentgenol Radium Ther Nucl Med 1975;124:466–71.

763. Srensen K, Schnheyder H. Ankylosing spondylitis associated with pulmonary aspergillosis. Ugeskr Laeger 1983;145:1308–9.

764. Jessamine AG. Upper lobe fibrosis in ankylosing spondylitis. Can Med Assoc J 1968;98:25–9.

765. Appelrouth D, Gottlieb NL. Pulmonary manifestations of ankylosing spondylitis. J Rheumatol 1975;2:446–53.

766. Beinenstock H, Lanyi VF. Cricoarytenoid arthritis in a patient with ankylosing spondylitis. Arch Otolaryngol 1977;103:738–9.

767. Libby DM, Schley WS, Smith JP. Cricoarytenoid arthritis in ankylosing spondylitis. A cause of acute respiratory failure and cor pulmonale. Chest 1981;80:641–2.

768. Sinclair JR, Mason RA. Ankylosing spondylitis. The case for awake intubation. Anaesthesia 1984;39:3–11.

769. Rohatgi PK, Turrisi BC. Bronchocentric granulomatosis and ankylosing spondylitis. Thorax 1984;39:317–8.

770. Turner JF, Enzenauer RJ. Bronchiolitis obliterans and organizing pneumonia associated with ankylosing spondylitis. Arthritis Rheum 1994;37:1557–9.

771. Ahern MJ, Maddison P, Mann S, Scott CA. Ankylosing spondylitis and adenocarcinoma of the lung. Ann Rheum Dis 1982;41:292–4.

772. Blavia R, Toda MR, Vidal F, et al. Pulmonary diffuse amyloidosis and ankylosing spondylitis. A rare association. Chest 1992;102:1608–10.

773. Braun J, Brandt J, Listing J, et al. Treatment of active ankylosing spondylitis with infliximab: a randomised controlled multicentre trial. Lancet 2002;359:1187–93.

774. Wright V. Psoriatic arthritis. In: Kelley WN, Harris EDJ, Ruddy S, Sledge CB, editors. Textbook of rheumatology. Philadelphia: W.B. Saunders; 1985. p. 1021.

775. Kammer GM, Soter NA, Gibson DJ, Schur PH. Psoriatic arthritis: a clinical immunologic and HLA study of 100 patients. Semin Arthritis Rheum 1979;9:75–97.

776. Scherak O, Kolarz G, Popp W, et al. Lung involvement in rheumatoid factor-negative arthritis. Scand J Rheumatol 1993;22:225–8.

777. Guzman LR, Gall EP, Pitt M, Lull G. Psoriatic spondylitis. Association with advanced nongranulomatous upper lobe pulmonary fibrosis. JAMA 1978;239:1416–7.

778. Hiki Y, Kokubo T, Horii A, et al. A case of severe IgA nephropathy associated with psoriatic arthritis and idiopathic interstitial pneumonia. Acta Pathol Jap 1993;43:522–8.

779. Koç Y, Güllü I, Akpek G, et al. Vascular involvement in Behçet's disease [see comments]. J Rheumatol 1992;19:402–10.

780. Kansu E, Ozer FL, Akalin E, et al. Behçet's syndrome with obstruction of the venae cavae. A report of seven cases. QJM 1972;41:151–68.

781. Davies JD. Behçet's syndrome with haemoptysis and pulmonary lesions. J Pathol 1973;109:351–6.

782. Cadman EC, Lundberg WB, Mitchell MS. Pulmonary manifestations in Behçet's syndrome: case report and review of the literature. Arch Intern Med 1976;136:944–7.

783. Gamble CN, Wiesner KB, Shapiro RF, Boyer WJ. The immune complex pathogenesis of glomerulonephritis and pulmonary vasculitis in Behçet's disease. Am J Med 1979;6:1031–9.

784. Tunaci A, Berkmen YM, Gökmen E. Thoracic involvement in Behçet's disease: pathologic, clinical, and imaging features. AJR Am J Roentgenol 1995;164:51–6.

785. Corren J. Acute interstitial pneumonia in a patient with Behçet's syndrome and common variable immunodeficiency [clinical conference]. Ann Allergy 1990;64:15–20.

786. el-Ramahi KM, Fawzy ME, Sieck JO, Vanhaleweyk G. Cardiac and pulmonary involvement in Behçet's disease. Scand J Rheumatol 1991;20:373–6.

787. Abadoglu O, Osma E, Uçan ES, et al. Behçet's disease with pulmonary involvement, superior vena cava syndrome, chyloptysis and chylous ascites. Respir Med 1996;90:429–31.

788. Hamzaoui A, Hamzaoui K, Chabbou A, Ayed K. Endothelin-1 expression in serum and bronchoalveolar lavage from patients with active Behçet's disease. Br J Rheumatol 1996;35:357–8.

789. Witt C, John M, Martin H, et al. Behçet's syndrome with pulmonary involvement-combined therapy for endobronchial stenosis using neodym-YAG laser, balloon dilation and immunosuppression. Respiration 1996;63:195–8.

790. Tüzün H, Yaman M, Gemicioglu B, et al. Behçet's disease presenting with a pulmonary mass lesion. Chest 1993;104:1635–6.

791. Almog Y, Polliack G, Dranitzki Elhalel M, et al. Bilateral pulmonary artery aneurysms in Behçet's disease [see comments]. Eur Respir J 1993;6:1067–9.

792. O'Duffy JD. Pulmonary involvement in Behçet's disease [editorial; comment]. Eur Respir J 1993;6:936–7.

793. Erkan F, Cavdar T. Pulmonary vasculitis in Behçet's disease. Am Rev Respir Dis 1992;146:232–9.

794. Efthimiou J, Johnston C, Spiro SG, Turner-Warwick M. Pulmonary disease in Behçet's syndrome. QJM 1986;58: 259–80.

795. Hughes JP, Stovin PGI. Segmental pulmonary artery aneurysms with peripheral venous thrombosis. Br J Dis Chest 1959;53:19–27.

796. Duriex P, Bletry O, Huchon G, et al. Multiple pulmonary artery aneurysms in Behçet's disease and Hughes-Stovin syndrome. Am J Med 1981;71:736–41.

797. Tatsis G, Vaiopoulos G, Tassiopoulos T, et al. Lung function in Adamantiades-Behçet disease. Rheumatology (Oxford) 1999;38:1018–9.

798. Unlu M, Akincioglu C, Yamac K, Onder M. Pulmonary involvement in Behçet's disease: evaluation of 123 I-MIBG retention. Nucl Med Commun 2001;22:1083–8.

799. Reza MJ, Demanes DJ. Behçet's disease: a case with hemoptysis, pseudotumor cerebi and arteritis. J Rheumatol 1978;5:320–6.

800. Vansteenkiste JF, Peene P, Verschakelen JA, van de Woestijne KP. Cyclosporin treatment in rapidly progressive pulmonary thromboembolic Behçet's disease. Thorax 1990;45:295–6.

801. Koga T, Yano T, Ichikawa Y, et al. Pulmonary infiltrates recovered by FK506 in a patient with Behçet's disease. Chest 1993;104:309–11.

802. Gibson GJ, Davis P. Respiratory complications of relapsing polychondritis. Thorax 1974;29:726–31.

803. Herman JH. Polychondritis. In: Kelley WN, Harris EDJ, Ruddy S, Sledge CB, editors. Textbook of rheumatology. Philadelphia: W.B. Saunders; 1985. p. 1458.

804. Higenbottom T, Dixon J. Chondritis associated with fatal intramural bronchial fibrosis. Thorax 1979;34:563–4.

805. Vaudour X, Payot J, Diebnold J, LeMelletier J. Les manifestations respiratoires de la polychondrite chronique atrophiante. J Fr Med Chir Thorae 1967;21:383–6.

806. Grilliat JP, Vautrin DA. Manifestations respiratoires de la polychondrite atrophiante chronique. Presse Med 1969;77: 1455–6.

807. Krell WS, Staats BA, Hyatt RE. Pulmonary function in relapsing polychondritis. Am Rev Respir Dis 1986;133: 1120–3.

808. Burlew BP, Lippton H, Klinestiver D, Haponik EJ. Relapsing polychondritis: new pulmonary manifestations. J Louisiana State Med Soc 1992;144:58–62.

809. Faul JL, Kee ST, Rizk NW. Endobronchial stenting for severe airway obstruction in relapsing polychondritis. Chest 1999;116:825–7.

810. Michet CJJ, McKenna CH, Luthra HS, O'Fallon WM. Relapsing polychondritis. Ann Intern Med 1986;104:74–8.

811. Colby TV, Lombard C, Yousem SA, Kitaichi M. Atlas of pulmonary surgical pathology. Philadelphia: W.B. Saunders, Co.; 1991. p. 380.

812. Wallaert B, Rossi GA, Sibille Y. Clinical guidelines and indications for bronchoalveolar lavage (BAL): collagen-vascular diseases. Eur Respir J 1990;3:942–3.

813. BAL Cooperative Group. Bronchoalveolar lavage constituents in healthy individuals, idiopathic pulmonary fibrosis, and selected comparison groups. Am Rev Respir Dis 1990; 141:S169–S202.

22 PULMONARY VASCULITIS

ULRICH SPECKS

This chapter focuses primarily on the respiratory manifestations of the various forms of vasculitis. Most of the diseases causing inflammation of pulmonary vessels are systemic illnesses, and the lung is usually only one of many organs involved in the disease process. The different syndromes that may cause pulmonary vasculitis will be discussed in the order of their likelihood of being encountered by the pulmonologist.

Because the etiology of all of these syndromes remains unknown to date, their nomenclature and classification have been subject to both change and dispute over time. This fact complicates the interpretation of the existing literature.

With emphasis on the recent developments in the field, this chapter will provide an overview of the information required for a differential diagnostic approach to the individual patient, discuss the current understanding of the pathogenesis of pulmonary vasculitis, and describe the various treatment options. Because the vasculitides associated with anti-neutrophil cytoplasmic antibodies (ANCA) are by far the most common forms of vasculitis (ie, Wegener's granulomatosis, microscopic polyangiitis, and Churg-Strauss syndrome) to be considered in the differential diagnostic reasoning of the practicing pulmonologist, the largest portion of this chapter is devoted to their discussion. A detailed description of the clinical utility of ANCA testing and the current understanding of the pathogenetic potential of ANCA is also provided in this context.

NOMENCLATURE, DISEASE CLASSIFICATIONS, AND DEFINITIONS

Vasculitis can be separated into primary and secondary vasculitis. Secondary vasculitis is due to or associated with another well-defined underlying illness that usually precedes the diagnosis of the complicating vasculitis. Secondary vasculitis may represent a predominant clinical management problem, such as the pulmonary capillaritis with alveolar hemorrhage that occurs in the context of systemic lupus erythematosus (SLE), or it may be a rather incidental finding, such as the vasculitis detected histopathologically in necrotizing sarcoid granulomatosis. The primary systemic vasculitides represent a heterogeneous group of syndromes with a wide spectrum of clinical manifestations. The complexity of the clinical and histopathologic features, as well as their potential overlap, may complicate the establishment of a certain specific diagnosis, particularly early in the course of the disease. At this time, the only common denominators of the primary systemic vasculitides are their unknown etiology and the fact that they are immune mediated and responsive to immunosuppressive therapy.

The purpose of creating classification schemes and defining the various forms of vasculitis is to improve and standardize the communication between physicians and investigators. Ideally, classification and definition of the vasculitides should reflect differences in their clinical presentation, histopathologic features, prognosis, therapeutic requirements, and underlying pathogenic mechanisms. Over time, as more and more clinical facets of different forms of vasculitis have been described and the understanding of the pathogenesis has improved, the classification of the vasculitides has changed.

Attempts to classify these syndromes were made as early as 1952 when Zeek published the first classification of necrotizing angiitis, grouping the vasculitides in five categories: periarteritis nodosa (PAN), hypersensitivity angiitis, rheumatic arteritis, temporal arteritis, and allergic granulomatosis arteritis.[1] Wegener's granulomatosis (WG) was absent from this classification because it was not described in the English literature until 1954.[2] A subsequent classification by Fauci and colleagues was practical and found widespread acceptance among clinicians, particularly in the United States.[3] However, the grouping of classic polyarteritis nodosa (PAN), Churg-Strauss syndrome, and overlap angiitis as the polyarteritis nodosa group has not withstood the test of time. Furthermore, the addition of lymphomatoid granulomatosis as a separate category of vasculitis is no longer tenable, because it has been clearly identified as a lymphoproliferative process.

In 1990, the American College of Rheumatology (ACR) developed diagnostic criteria for the classification of the vasculitides.[4] Although adhering largely to the classification by Fauci and colleagues, the ACR study was designed to identify clinical features that allow the separation of one form of vasculitis from another. The major drawbacks for the clinical application of the 1990 ACR criteria are that (1) the underlying data were collected before testing for ANCA became available, (2) these criteria are difficult to apply in some patients with WG who have predominant necrotizing granulomatous features without prominent vasculitis, and (3) they do not acknowledge the concept of microscopic polyangiitis, which has been widely accepted in Europe.[5–7] In the American literature, microscopic polyangiitis cases were either referred to as hypersensitivity vasculitis or were lumped with PAN.

These discrepancies between European and American classification schemes and definitions have been eliminated as a result of an international consensus conference on the nomenclature of systemic vasculitides held in 1992 in Chapel Hill, NC.[8] The Chapel Hill nomenclature (Table 22–1) is mainly based on histopathologic criteria, particularly the size of the vessels involved. It takes the presence or absence of ANCA into account and acknowledges the occasional need to change the diagnosis in certain patients as their clinical presentation changes over time. For instance, a patient who is originally diagnosed with microscopic polyangiitis may have to be diagnosed with WG when characteristic necrotizing granulomas develop, or a patient with cutaneous leukocytoclastic angiitis may later have to be diagnosed with microscopic polyangiitis or WG.[9,10] The term "hypersensitivity vasculitis" is no longer used, according to the Chapel Hill nomenclature. The specific definitions of each form of vasculitis will be discussed in more detail, together with the description of the clinical manifestations of each form of vasculitis and their differential diagnosis. The Chapel Hill nomenclature was initially criticized for its distinction of classic PAN from microscopic polyangiitis based solely on the absence of small vessel involvement in the former,

whereas the latter may show involvement of medium-sized vessels.[8,11,12] However, this distinction has found wide acceptance because it seems to reflect the differences in pathogenesis and therapeutic implications. To date, the Chapel Hill nomenclature remains the most clinically useful attempt to categorize the primary systemic vasculitides available. Its categories fit well with the clinical and histopathologic pulmonary features, are in accordance with the ANCA data, and facilitate the therapeutic approach to individual patients.

EPIDEMIOLOGY

The systemic vasculitides are rare syndromes (Table 22–2). Large case series are reported from tertiary referral centers or are the result of multicenter studies. These reports do not provide any information about the denominator population. The steadily increasing number of reports about these syndromes might suggest an increasing incidence. Alternatively, they may simply reflect earlier and more frequent recognition of patients with these illnesses by primary physicians, which in turn results in increased referral of these patients to specialized centers with experience in the management of these syndromes.

The few epidemiologic studies available that allow an estimation of the incidence of these diseases are not based on ethnically diverse populations and do not clarify the issue of whether more frequent recognition or true increased incidence are responsible for the rising numbers of recorded cases. In addition, their interpretation is complicated by the changing definitions of the syndromes.[13] For instance, if the ACR 1990 criteria for PAN are applied, the incidence of PAN would be 2.4 per million annually.[13] In contrast, if the Chapel Hill Consensus Conference definitions are applied, the incidence of microscopic polyangiitis would be 3.6 per million annually, and no patient meeting the definition of classic PAN would have been identified.[13] The apparent incidence of WG and microscopic polyangiitis may further be affected by the advent of ANCA testing.[14] The annual incidence of WG was estimated to be 0.5 to 0.7 per million during the 1970s and early 1980s.[14,15] It rose to 2.8 per million in the late 1980s following the introduction of ANCA testing.[14] For the adult population of 414,000 of the Norwich Health Authority, Watts and coworkers reported an annual incidence of WG of 8.7 per million for the years 1988 to 1992 and of 10.3 per million for the years 1993 to 1997.[16] A similar increase in annual incidence from 5.2 per million from 1984 through 1988 to 12.0 during the period 1994 through 1998 was observed in northern Norway.[17] Similar increases in annual incidence were observed for microscopic polyangiitis and Churg-Strauss syndrome.[14,16]

Giant cell arteritis remains the most frequent form of systemic vasculitis, with an annual incidence of 13 per million adults (40 per million over the age of 60) in

TABLE 22–1   Systemic Vasculitides*

Name	Vasculitic Lung Involvement	ANCA Findings
Large vessel vasculitis		
Giant cell (temporal) arteritis	Rare	No
Takayasu arteritis	Frequent	No
Medium-sized vessel vasculitis		
Polyarteritis nodosa	Rare	No
Kawasaki disease	No	No
Small vessel vasculitis		
WG	Frequent	PR3-ANCA
CSS	Frequent	MPO-ANCA or PR3-ANCA
MPA	Frequent	MPO-ANCA or PR3-ANCA
Henoch-Schönlein purpura	No	IgA-possible
Essential cryoglobulinemic vasculitis	No	No

*Systemic vasculitides as defined by the 1992 Chapel Hill international consensus conference on the nomenclature of systemic vasculitis.[8] ANCA = antineutrophil cytoplasmic antibodies; CSS = Churg-Strauss syndrome; MPA = microscopic polyangiitis; MPO = myeloperoxidase; PR3 = proteinase 3; WG = Wegener's granulomatosis.

TABLE 22–2 Estimated Annual Incidence of Systemic Vasculitides

Giant cell arteritis	13
Rheumatoid arthritis associated-vasculitis	12.5
WG	8.5–10.3
MPA	6.8–8.9
CSS	1.5–3.7

Incidence per million adult population.[13,16,21]

the United Kingdom.[18] In Olmsted County, Minnesota, the incidence of giant cell arteritis was found to be highly cyclical and increasing over time.[19] However, respiratory manifestations rarely represent significant management problems in these patients.[20] The annual incidence of systemic rheumatoid vasculitis and of SLE-associated vasculitis are reportedly 12.5 and 3.6 per million, respectively.[21]

Finally, there is an ethnic predilection for certain types of vasculitis. WG affects predominantly Whites, and northern Europeans appear more prone to develop WG; individuals of southern European and Mediterranean descent appear to be relatively more likely to develop microscopic polyangiitis.[22–24]

WEGENER'S GRANULOMATOSIS

Historic Background

In 1931 Klinger described the first case of this multisystem disorder as a "borderline form of polyarteritis nodosa."[25] Two additional separate single case reports of a similar syndrome appeared prior to Wegener's detailed analysis of three autopsy cases, an analysis which led him to believe that he had discovered a new and distinct syndrome.[26] Based on his autopsy findings and the historic clinical data available to him, Wegener came to understand the disease as a generalized process affecting the arteries and kidneys that originates as a granulomatous process in the upper respiratory tract.[27–29] In 1954 Godman and Churg reported a detailed account of 22 autopsy cases from the literature, together with 7 of their own.[2] From this first series in the English literature they derived what hence was to be known as the "classic Wegener's diagnostic triad," consisting of necrotizing granulomatous inflammation of the upper and lower respiratory tract, generalized necrotizing vasculitis involving the small arteries and veins, and necrotizing glomerulonephritis.[2] For many years it was thought that the diagnosis of WG could not be established without fulfilling the complete Wegener's triad, despite the fact that only 14 of the 29 cases reported in the series of Godman and Churg fulfilled the complete triad.[2] The concept of limited WG was introduced by Carrington and Liebow, who reported on patients with WG limited to the lung.[30] These patients were initially thought to respond more favorably to prednisone monotherapy but later were found to have a high rate of relapse. In 1975 DeRemee and coworkers proposed the ELK (ear, nose, and throat; lung; and kidney) classification of involvement based on a 10-year experience with 50 patients.[31] The identification of three major sites of involvement implies that any one site or a combination of sites can be involved. These observations unified the concepts of isolated midline granuloma, limited WG, and classic WG, which at the time were thought to be distinct entities, and led to our current understanding of the disease as a continuum. This concept has subsequently been validated by the discovery of ANCA, followed by the recognition of the high-specificity of the cytoplasmic (cANCA) variant reacting with proteinase 3 (PR3) for the clinical spectrum of WG.

In 1990 the ACR developed criteria for the classification of WG (Table 22–3).[32] These should not be used to establish the diagnosis of WG in any given patient, but are only meant to allow the differentiation of WG from other forms of vasculitis in patients with documented vasculitis.[33]

The Chapel Hill Consensus Conference (see Table 22–1) put forth the following definition of WG: "…granulomatous inflammation involving the respiratory tract, and necrotizing vasculitis affecting small to medium-sized vessels (ie, capillaries, venules, arterioles, and arteries)."[8] Of note is that the histopathologic documentation of granulomatous involvement of the respi-

TABLE 22–3 The ACR 1990 Criteria for the Classification of Wegener's Granulomatosis

Criterion	Definition
1. Nasal or oral inflammation	Development of painful oral ulcers or purulent or bloody nasal discharge
2. Abnormal chest radiograph	Nodules; fixed infiltrates or cavities
3. Urinary sediment	Microhematuria (>5 RBCs per high-power field) or red cell casts
4. Granulomatous inflammation	Histologic changes showing granulomatous on biopsy; inflammation within the wall of an artery or in the perivascular or extravascular area

A patient with vasculitis is said to have WG if two or more of the four criteria are present.[32] ACR = American College of Rheumatology; RBCs = red blood cells.

ratory tract is not explicitly required. Radiographic evidence or clinical examination findings highly predictive of such granulomatous pathology may be sufficient. Consequently, today more than ever, the diagnosis of WG depends on a correlation of clinical, pathologic, and serologic features.

Clinical Manifestations

WG usually affects the respiratory tract first. Symptoms caused by predominantly necrotizing granulomatous inflammation of the upper airways and/or the lung may predominate and persist for variable amounts of time (limited phase of the disease) before progressing to the generalized phase of the disease, during which the organ injury caused by small vessel vasculitis determines the clinical picture and outcome. The limited phase of the disease may be associated with minimal morbidity. Usually it is associated with few constitutional symptoms, and nonspecific markers of inflammatory activity such as the erythrocyte sedimentation rate (ESR) and the C-reactive protein are only minimally elevated. The generalized vasculitic phase of the disease is usually associated with prominent constitutional symptoms such as malaise, fevers, night sweats, and weight loss. The presence of migratory arthralgias affecting the large joints is also a sign of generalized disease. The ESR and the C-reactive protein level are markedly elevated, as are other markers of acute phase reaction. Although most patients, if untreated, will progress from limited disease to generalized disease with kidney involvement, this progression does not occur in every patient. The presence of cANCA appears to be a prognostic indicator in this context.[34] Because WG can affect any organ, and because the initial disease presentation may be quite heterogeneous, physicians from all specialties should be familiar with the multiple facets of this syndrome.

The clinical manifestations affecting the various organs are listed in Table 22–4, together with relevant references providing more detailed information on each of these aspects of the disease. At first, when all of these symptoms may occur in isolation, a positive test for PR3-ANCA may be the only indicator of an impending systemic disease.

TABLE 22–4 Organ Manifestations of Wegener's Granulomatosis

Organ	Symptoms or Findings	References
Eye	Conjunctivitis, episcleritis-scleritis, corneoscleral ulceration, uveitis, retinal vasculitis, ophthalmoplegia, optic neuropathy, central artery occlusion, orbital pseudotumor, dacryocystitis, dacryoadenitis, lacrimal duct stenosis	35, 37, 39–42, 97, 380, 381
Ear	Serous otitis, sensorineural hearing loss, chronic/subacute otitis or mastoiditis	44, 246, 382
Nose	Epistaxis, necrotizing inflammation with crusting, chondritis, septum perforation, saddle nose deformity	43, 112, 383, 384
Sinuses	Mucosal thickening, pansinusitis, bony destruction	43, 385
Oral cavity	Jaw pain, hyperplastic gingivitis ulcerations	46, 47, 68, 70
Salivary glands	Salivary gland swelling	49, 50, 386
Trachea, bronchi	Subglottic stenosis, mucosal ulceration, inflammatory pseudotumor, bronchomalacia	51–53, 89, 180, 387, 388
Lung	Solitary or multiple nodules, thick- or thin-walled cavities, localized or diffuse infiltrates, atelectasis, lobar collapse, alveolar hemorrhage	58, 59, 65, 87, 88, 95, 389–391
Pleura	Effusion, inflammatory pseudotumor	36, 60, 61, 88
Heart	Coronaritis, myocardial infarct, granulomatous valvulitis of aortic or mitral valves, pericarditis, pancarditis	36, 392–394
Kidney	Focal, segmental necrotizing glomerulonephritis, rapidly progressive glomerulonephritis (with crescent formation), periglomerular granulomatosis, renal insufficiency	81–86, 395–398
Genital tract	Orchitis, epididymitis, prostatitis	2, 50, 131, 399
Spleen	Splenomegaly, splenic infarcts	2, 27
Gastrointestinal tract	Erosive esophagitis, bowel perforation	399, 400
Joints	Arthralgias, symmetric polyarthritis of small and large joints, oligo- or monoarthritis, rarely erosive	36, 38, 399, 401–403
Skin	Urticaria, papules, vesicles, erythema, petechiae, ulcerations, pyoderma gangrenosum, palpable purpura	66–71
CNS	Multiple mononeuropathy, cranial nerve palsies, symmetric peripheral neuropathies, cerebral infarcts, seizures, transverse myelitis, meningeal involvement	72, 77–80, 98, 404, 405
Pituitary gland	Diabetes insipidus	73–76, 406–408

CNS = central-nervous system.

Eye involvement (Figure 22–1) occurs in about 40 to 70% of patients over the course of their disease.[35–40] The frequency and type of eye involvement do not appear to differ substantially between patients with limited and those with generalized disease.[37,40] Occasionally, the "red eye" may be the initial manifestation of the disease. Conjunctivitis, scleritis, episcleritis, corneal ulcerations, and uveitis may all persist as the only organ manifestation of the disease for protracted periods of time. Inflammatory pseudotumor of the orbit, associated with proptosis, lid swelling, chemosis, and limitations of ocular movement, can affect one or both eyes and needs to be differentiated from metastatic malignancies, lymphoma, and sarcoidosis of the orbit.[41] Retinal vasculitis and optic neuropathy are more frequently encountered in patients with generalized disease. Although some of the milder ophthalmologic manifestations of WG may be controlled with local steroid application, systemic immunosuppression is usually required to control the symptoms and prevent irreversible organ damage. In some patients, the eyes may represent treatment-refractory compartments, and there are no data in the literature that would suggest the advantage of one immunosuppressive regimen over another. Involvement of the nasolacrimal system can be the cause of epiphora, dacryocystitis, and draining fistulae.[35,42] It appears that early diagnosis of WG and its ocular manifestations has improved the visual prognosis by virtue of early intervention.[39]

Ninety-nine percent of patients with WG have ear, nose, and throat manifestations of the disease.[38] Most frequently, chronic rhinitis with or without epistaxis and nasal crusting, chronic sinusitis, and recurrent or chronic serous otitis are the first symptoms of the disease.[31,43–45] Destruction of the nasal cartilage may be the cause of the typical nasal septal perforation or saddle nose deformity

(Figure 22–2A).[43] Ulcerations of the oropharynx may also occur (Figure 22–2B).[46] Gingival hyperplasia with clefting and petechiae resulting from vasculitis of the interdental papillae, the so-called "strawberry" gingival hyperplasia, is a rare but almost pathognomonic manifestation of WG.[46,47] Salivary gland involvement is also not frequent, but if present may be a convenient site for a diagnostic tissue biopsy.[48–50]

Tracheobronchial involvement can cause symptoms that may initially be mistaken for asthma.[51–53] The inspiratory and expiratory flow-volume loop allows a preliminary determination of the location of the airway obstruction. The acute inflammation of the airways may present as tracheobronchial ulceration (Figure 22–3), intraluminal inflammatory pseudotumor (Figure 22–4), or, if the cartilage is involved, as bronchomalacia (Figure 22–5). The most frequent location of tracheobronchial involvement is the immediate subglottic area (Figure 22–6). For unknown reasons, subglottic stenosis preferentially affects younger patients.[52] The healing of tracheobronchial lesions may result in significant scarring, which in turn may be the cause of persistent morbidity such as airway obstruction, bronchomalacia, and recurrent postobstructive pneumonia.[51–53] The airway lesions observed in WG may be identical to those observed occasionally in microscopic polyangiitis and are difficult to differentiate from those associated with relapsing polychondritis.

Necrotizing granulomatous lesions of the lung may present as solitary pulmonary nodules or masses. More frequently these lesions are multiple, and, characteristically, they cavitate (Figure 22–7). As the lesions heal, the cavities may become more thin-walled before disappearing without remainder. Alternatively, the nodules may shrink, only rarely leaving residual areas of fibrotic scars. These granulomatous lesions of the lung can be the

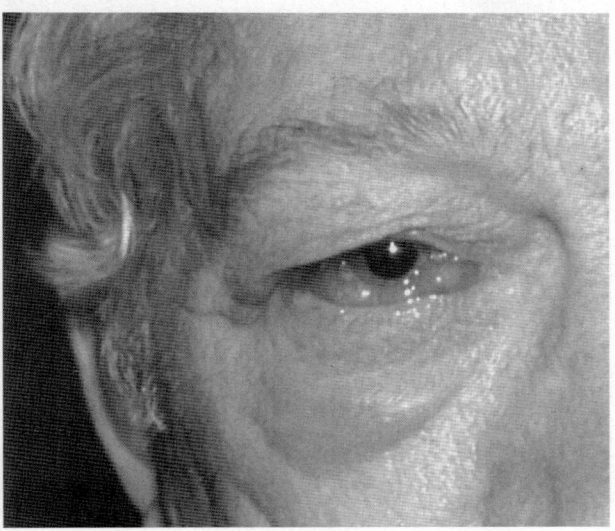

A

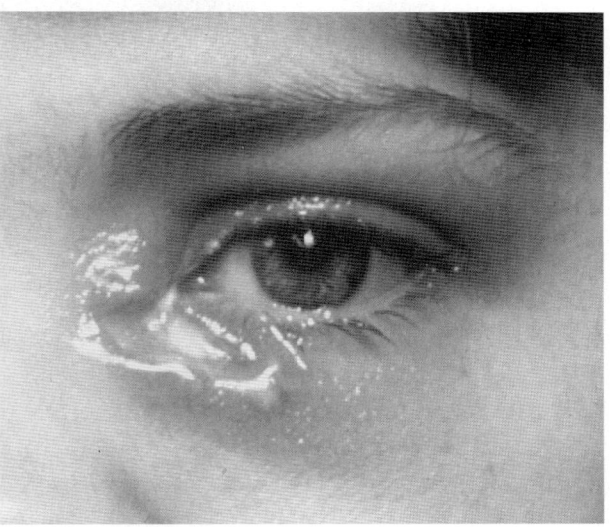

B

Figure 22–1 Ophthalmologic manifestations of Wegener's granulomatosis (WG). *A*, scleritis and orbital inflammation; *B*, destruction of the nasolacrimal duct.

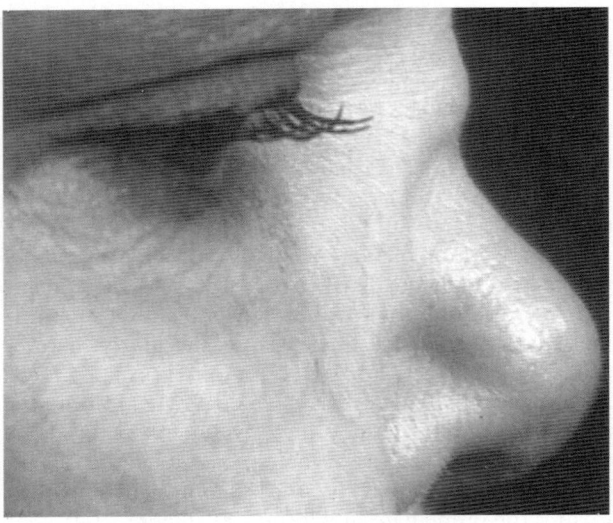

A

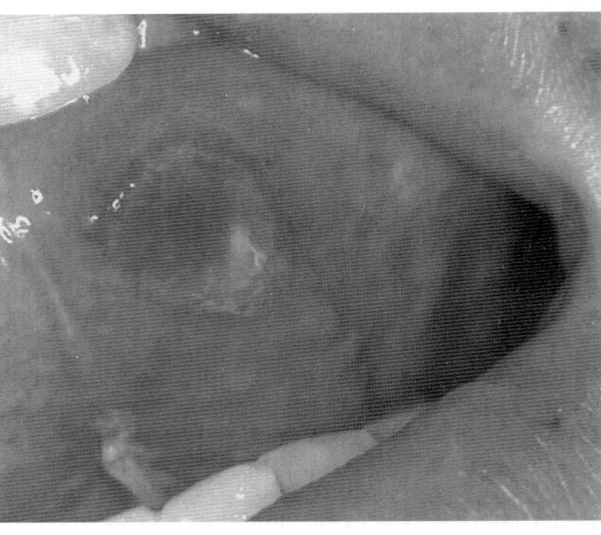

B

Figure 22–2   Characteristic saddle nose deformity of WG (*A*) and a sublingual mucosal ulcer (*B*).

cause of mild hemoptysis, but usually they are rather asymptomatic. The differential diagnosis of the lung nodules or masses of WG include primary or metastatic malignancies of the lung, including lymphomatoid granulomatosis, infectious processes such as fungal or *Nocardia* infections, and other idiopathic pulmonary processes such as necrotizing sarcoid granulomatosis.[54,55]

Alveolar hemorrhage as the result of capillaritis is a less frequent pulmonary manifestation of WG (Figure

22–8). It is a reflection of the generalized vasculitic phase of the disease, which may rapidly lead to respiratory failure, and is associated with a mortality of approximately 50%.[56–59] Although alveolar hemorrhage may occur as an isolated disease manifestation, it is usually associated with renal involvement. In the absence of other granulomatous features of WG, such a presentation is clinically indistinguishable from microscopic polyangiitis or Goodpasture's syndrome, and only the serologic detec-

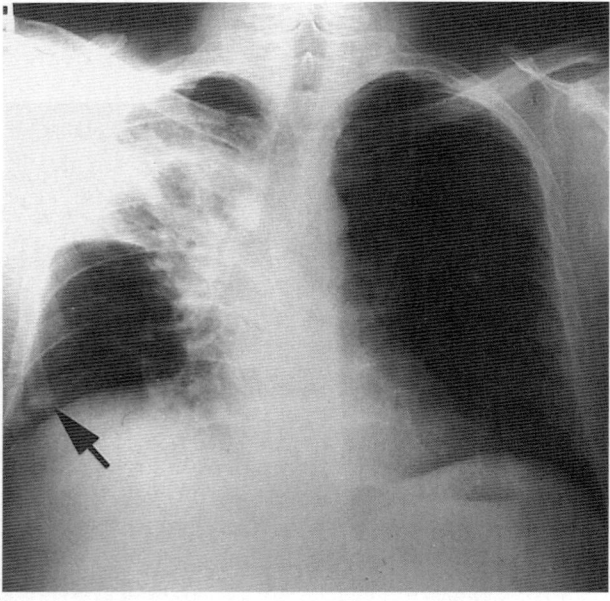

A

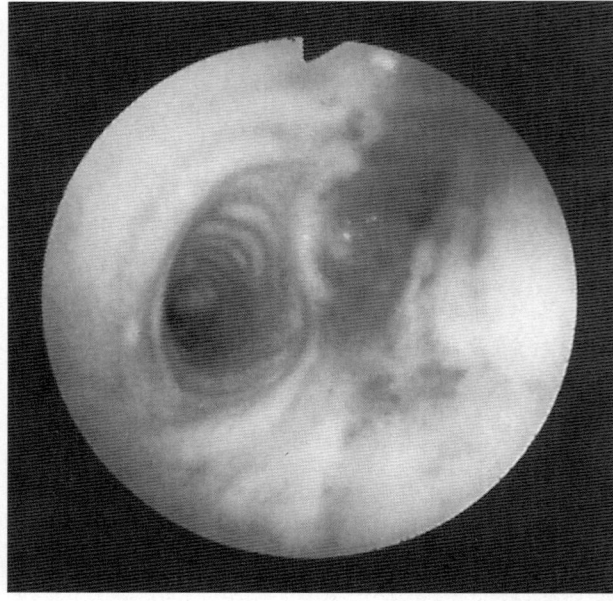

B

Figure 22–3   Post-obstructive pneumonia as a complication of WG. *A*, Chest radiograph showing right upper lobe infiltrates with volume loss. A nodular lesion in the right base is indicated by the arrow. *B*, Bronchoscopic view of ulcerating inflammatory lesion at the takeoff of the right upper lobe bronchus, resulting in significant stenosis of the lumen.

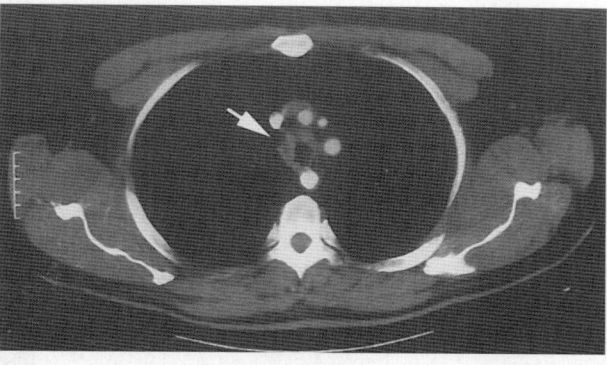

A

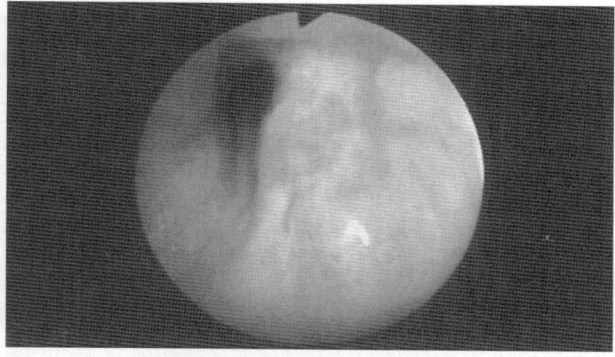

B

Figure 22–4   Inflammatory pseudotumor of the upper trachea. *A*, Computed tomogram section showing thickening of the tracheal wall with narrowing of the lumen (arrow). *B*, Bronchoscopic appearance of the same lesion. The bronchoscopic biopsy was diagnostic of WG.

tion of PR3-ANCA may allow a nosologic distinction from these other syndromes. (For a detailed discussion of the diffuse alveolar hemorrhage syndromes and their differential diagnosis and management, see Chapter 23, "Diffuse Alveolar Hemorrhage."

Other thoracic manifestations of WG include pleural effusions, pleural inflammatory pseudotumors, and hilar adenopathy. Pleural effusions occur in approximately 10% of patients and are usually small and clinically insignificant. They are exudates and are associated with other pulmonary manifestations.[60] Pleural inflammatory pseudotumors have been reported as single case reports and can be mistaken for mesotheliomas.[61] Mediastinal adenopathy is usually not apparent on standard chest radiography, but computed tomography (CT) reveals that the mediastinal lymph nodes may be enlarged in less than 10% of cases. With very few exceptions, this enlargement is small and clinically insignificant.[62–65]

The full clinical spectrum of skin manifestations associated with WG has been described in detail in several large series (Figure 22–9).[66–71] Up to 50% of WG patients may develop skin involvement over the course of their disease.[36,38] In approximately 10% of patients, it is part of the initial presentation.[36,38] Leukocytoclastic vasculitis presenting as palpable purpura with or without petechial lesions is the most common manifestation and is usually an indicator of the generalized phase of the disease.[69] The presence of PR3 and ANCA in patients with isolated leukocytoclastic vasculitis can predict the later development of other characteristic lesions of WG.[69] Necrotizing granulomatous lesions of the skin or pyoderma gangrenosum-like lesions are rarely encountered.[69]

Nervous system involvement is rarely an initial presentation of WG, but during the course of the disease it may affect up to 40% of patients.[36,38,72] Peripheral neuropathy, frequently in the form of multiple mononeuropathy, is the most frequent abnormality, followed by cranial neuropathies.[72] The neuropathy of WG is thought to be caused by vasculitis of the vasa nervorum and thus to be an indicator of generalized disease. Con-

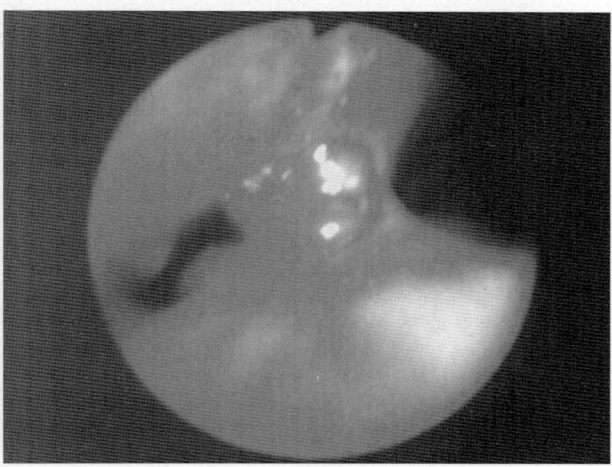

A

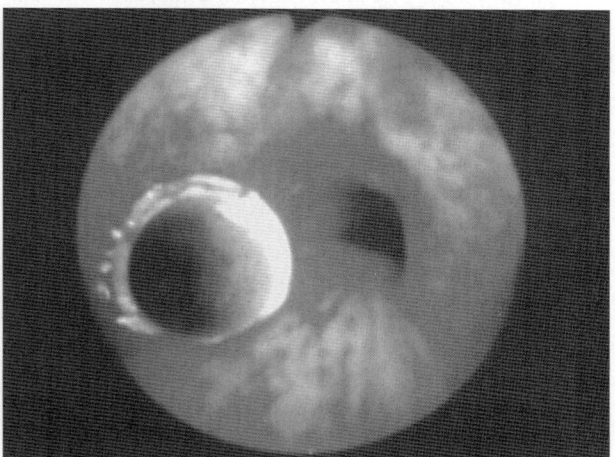

B

Figure 22–5   Inflammation of the mucosa and bronchomalacia of the left main-stem bronchus, resulting in partial collapse of the lumen before (*A*) and after (*B*) Silastic stent placement.

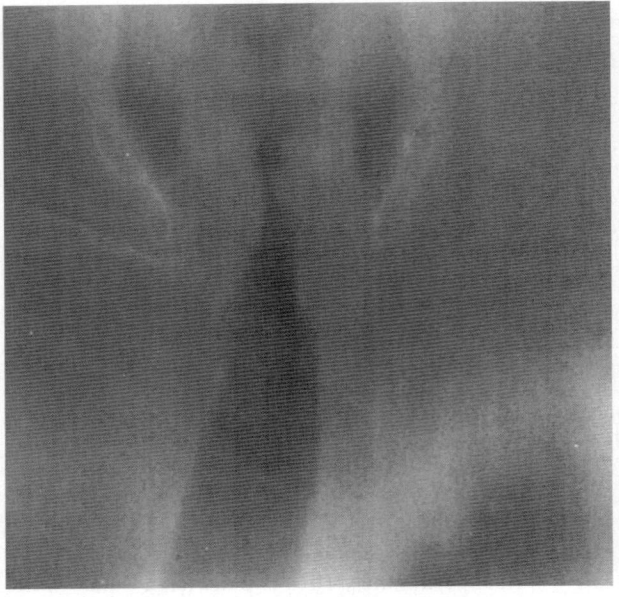
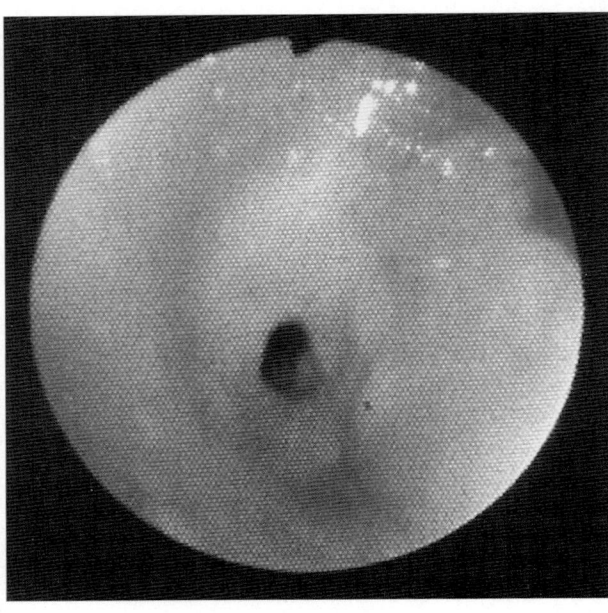

A   **B**

Figure 22–6   Subglottic stenosis of WG. *A*, Tracheal tomogram showing segmental narrowing in the immediate subglottic region. *B*, Bronchoscopic appearance of a healed subglottic lesion that resulted in cicatricial scarring with significant stenosis.

tiguous spread of the granulomatous inflammation from the respiratory tract can also lead to neurologic symptoms, particularly cranial nerve palsies.[72] Granulomatous infiltration of the pituitary gland can cause diabetes insipidus.[73–76] Cerebrovascular events, seizures, and meningeal involvement are other rare manifestations of nervous system involvement in WG.[72,77–80] The pachymeninges may be the site of compartmentalized disease activity, causing severe headaches.[80]

Renal involvement occurs in up to 80% of patients with WG.[36,38] It is the result of capillaritis and indicates that the patient has generalized disease requiring immunosuppressive therapy to prevent irreversible loss of renal function. The characteristic renal lesion is focal,

segmental necrotizing glomerulonephritis (Figure 22–10), with or without crescent formation. This lesion is not specific for WG and is also found in microscopic polyangiitis, Goodpasture's syndrome, or SLE.[81,82] Immunofluorescence microscopy shows no or only scant immune deposits in WG and microscopic polyangiitis (pauci-immune glomerulonephritis) in contrast to the linear distribution of immune deposits along the basement membranes in Goodpasture's syndrome or the granular immune-complex deposits in SLE and other forms of glomerulonephritis. Granulomatous lesions that would allow a distinction between WG and microscopic polyangiitis are rarely detected in renal biopsy specimens.[83] Reports of WG with renal

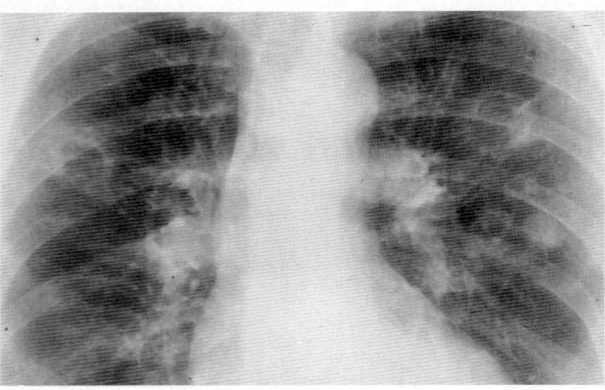
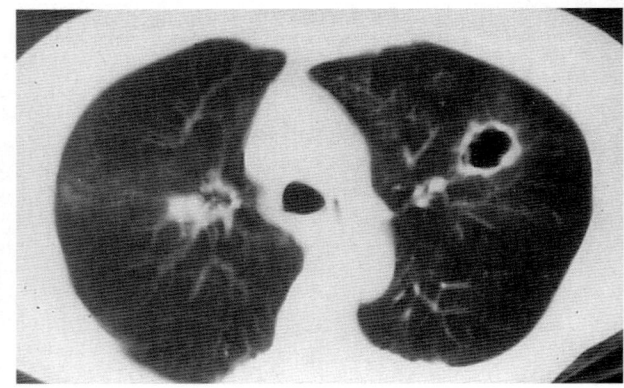

A   **B**

Figure 22–7   Necrotizing granulomatous lung lesions characteristic of WG. *A*, Appearance on standard chest roentgenogram; *B*, corresponding appearance on CT of the chest.

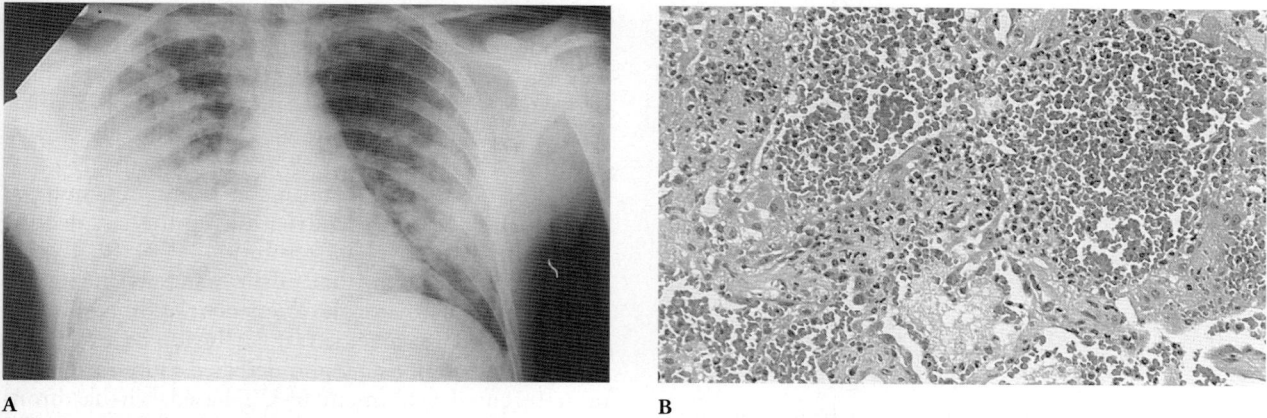

Figure 22–8 Alveolar hemorrhage resulting from capillaritis of the lung. *A*, Chest radiograph showing diffuse bilateral alveolar infiltrates. *B*, Open lung biopsy specimen showing filling of the alveolar spaces with red blood cells and thickening of the interstitium caused by infiltration with inflammatory cells, which are predominantly neutrophils. Although the clinical presentation and histopathologic appearance are not specific for any particular type of pulmonary vasculitis, they are the most frequent pulmonary presentation of microscopic polyangiitis.

artery involvement and aneurysm formation, such as is characteristically found in classic PAN, are anecdotal.[84] On rare occasions, renal involvement precedes other specific organ manifestations of WG.[85,86] The presence

of PR3-ANCA in patients with isolated pauci-immune glomerulonephritis should alert to that possibility.

Other organ manifestations of WG are rare. Any organ can be involved with the necrotizing granulomatous

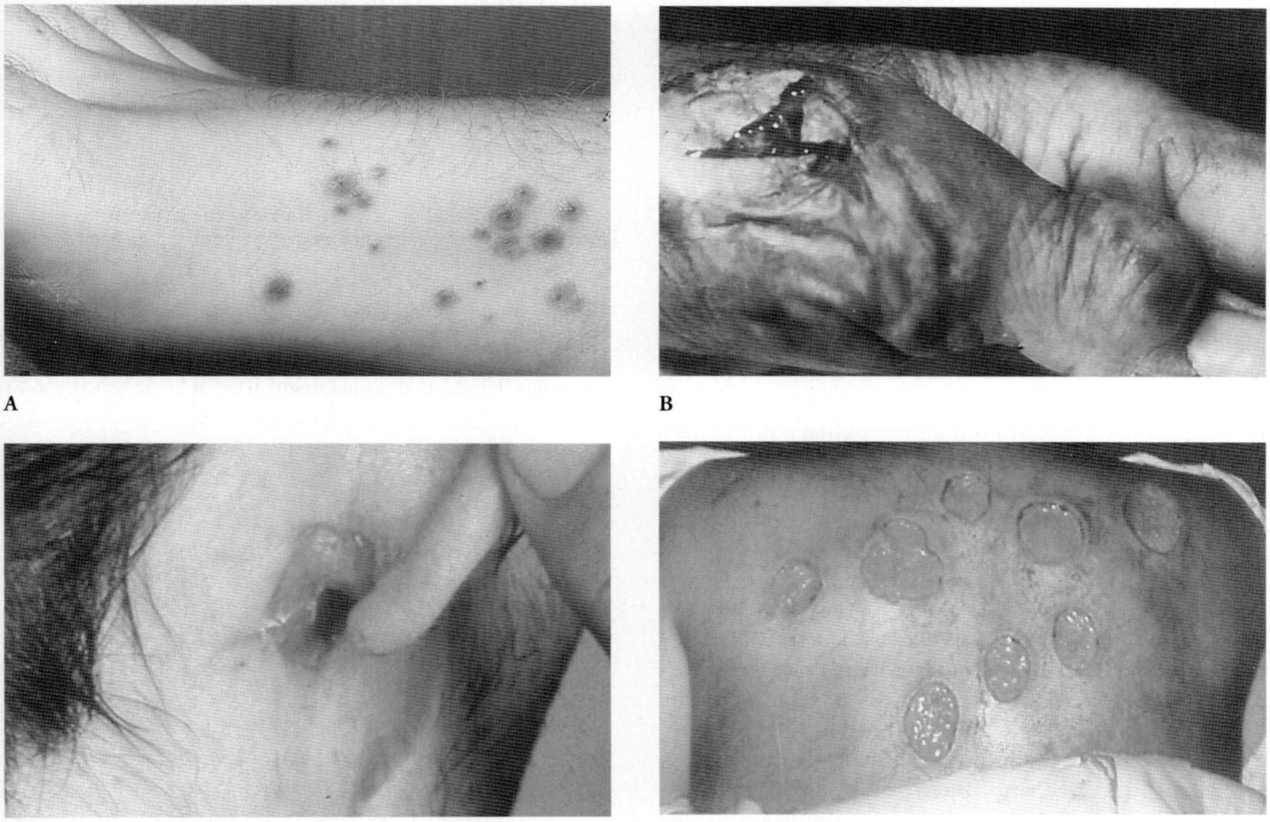

Figure 22–9 Skin manifestations of WG. *A*, Leukocytoclastic vasculitis causing palpable purpura, the most frequent skin manifestation of WG, and a sign of the generalized vasculitic phase of the disease. This lesion also be encountered in microscopic polyangiitis and other forms of vasculitis. *B*, Necrotizing granuloma of the skin. *C* and *D*, Pyoderma gangrenosum-like lesions in patients with WG.

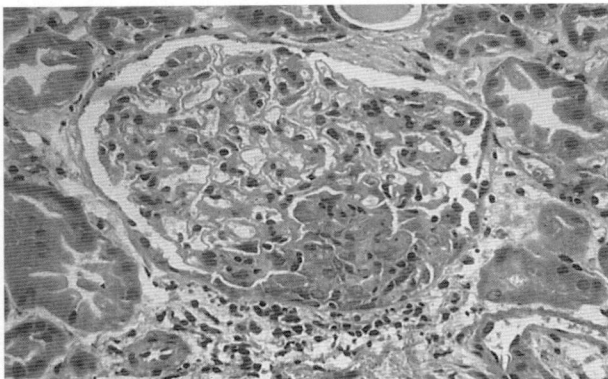

Figure 22–10 Focal segmental necrotizing glomerulonephritis. This renal lesion is typical but not specific for WG and microscopic polyangiitis.

inflammation, causing differential diagnostic consideration of malignant or infectious processes (see Table 22–4).

Diagnosis

Imaging Studies

The chest radiographic features caused directly by WG (Table 22–5) are either the result of the necrotizing granulomatous inflammation or a consequence of capillaritis. In addition, chest radiographic abnormalities caused by secondary complications of the illness or its therapy need to be considered.

Nodules or masses with or without cavitation are the most characteristic abnormality caused by the granulomatous inflammation of the lung parenchyma (see Figure 22–7). These changes are also the most frequent abnormality encountered.[87] The severity of the radiographic appearance of these granulomatous lesions is frequently out of proportion to the paucity of respiratory symptoms or lung function test abnormalities. Solitary pulmonary nodules or mass lesions and pleural or mediastinal pseudotumors are rare.[61,87] Small and clinically insignificant pleural effusions are incidental findings on chest radiograph in about 10% of cases.[88,89] When the inflammatory process leads to obstruction of a major bronchus, atelectasis or a postobstructive pneumonia may be the result (see Figure 22–3A).[53,88–90] Apical cavities, when isolated, can mimic tuberculous lesions.[88] If all other potential causes of cardiomegaly have been excluded, peri- or pancarditis as rare manifestation of WG should be considered.[36,38]

Diffuse alveolar infiltrates are usually a result of alveolar hemorrhage as a consequence of capillaritis (see Figure 22–8). They are associated with dyspnea and low hemoglobin levels and represent a life-threatening situation that should prompt initiation of high-dose intravenous corticosteroid therapy. If diffuse infiltrates occur in patients who already are on immunosuppressive therapy, the exclu-

sion of an infectious process is imperative. Cyclophosphamide toxicity is a rare pulmonary complication that may be the cause of diffuse reticulonodular interstitial infiltrates.[91] The occurrence of diffuse pulmonary infiltrates in patients on methotrexate (MTX) should raise suspicion about infections as well as drug toxicity.[92–94]

The role of CT scanning in the mangement of patients with WG has evolved during the last decade. The sensitivity of the high-resolution CT (HRCT) scan in WG is higher than that of the standard chest radiograph, particularly for the assessment of bronchial and peribronchial involvement.[65,95] Residuals of healed inflammatory lesions are also detected more easily. The most recent development of CT-based "virtual bronchoscopy" may facilitate the management of patients with tracheobronchial involvement.[96] Sometimes the CT scan detects an unsuspected involvement of vital mediastinal structures that is not clearly apparent on standard chest radiograph (Figure 22–11).

For the evaluation of neurologic symptoms in patients with WG, magnetic resonance imaging (MRI) has become an indispensable tool.[77–80,97–99]

Bronchoscopic Manifestations

Flexible fiberoptic bronchoscopy is useful in establishing the diagnosis and assessing disease activity.[53,89] Ulcerating tracheobronchitis is the most frequent finding in patients with WG (see Figure 22–3B). "Cobblestoning"

TABLE 22–5 Chest Radiographic Findings

Localization	Findings	Estimated Frequency		
		WG	MPA	CSS
Trachea/ bronchi	Subglottic stenosis	>15%	<10%	–
	Tracheal pseudotumor	SC	–	–
	Bronchial stenosis with lobar collapse	SC	–	–
Lung parenchyma	Multiple nodules	>30%	–	<10%
	Solitary nodules	>15	–	–
	Cavitation	>30%	–	–
	Localized infiltrates	>30%	>15%	–
	Lobar infiltrates	<10%	–	–
	Diffuse alveolar infiltrates	>15%	>50%	SC
	Transient/patchy infiltrates	SC	>15%	>30%
Mediastinum	Hilar/paratracheal mass	SC	–	SC
Pleura	Pleural effusion	<10%	–	>15%
	Pleural thickening	SC	–	–
	Pleural mass	SC	–	–
Heart	Cardiomegaly	SC	–	>15%

Frequency of chest radiographic findings in WG, MPA, and CSS. SC = single cases reported; – = not reported.

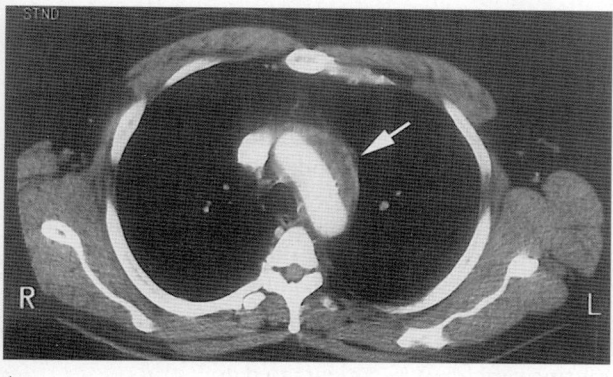
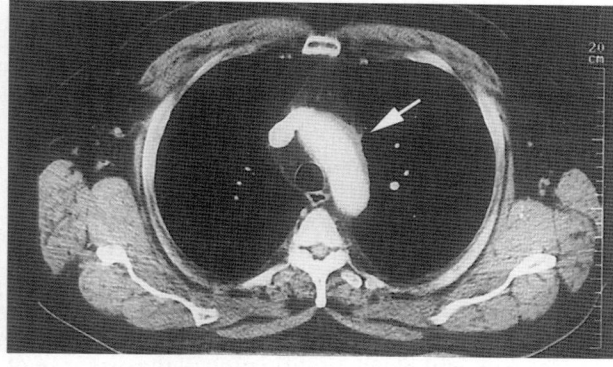

A

B

Figure 22–11   Inflammatory pseudotumor involving the wall of the aortic arch (arrow) in a patient with WG before (*A*) and after (*B*) 4 months of therapy with prednisone and cyclophosphamide. The lesion subsequently disappeared completely.

of the mucosa and/or inflammatory pseudotumors can also be encountered (see Figure 22–4B). These lesions may acutely cause stenoses of the airways or bronchomalacia (see Figure 22–5A). Healing of such lesions frequently results in permanent cicatricial stenoses (see Figure 22–6B). Endobronchial lesions of WG were found in all patients with symptoms, suggesting the possibility of an airway abnormality such as hemoptysis, dyspnea on exertion, stridor, or wheezing.[53] However, such lesions were also found in one-third of patients lacking such symptoms who underwent bronchoscopy for further evaluation of a radiographic abnormality.[53]

Only 20% of the biopsy specimens obtained by bronchoscopy may be diagnostic of WG. However, in conjunction with other clinical or serologic findings supportive of WG, the diagnosis can be established in up to half of the patients, thus sparing the patient an open lung biopsy.[53]

Bronchoscopy, in conjunction with bronchoalveolar lavage as part of the evaluation of diffuse pulmonary infiltrates in patients with WG, is indicated either to document alveolar hemorrhage or to allow the identification of pathogenic organisms.

Histopathologic Spectrum

The histopathologic features of WG (Figure 22–12) have been reviewed in detail elsewhere.[100] The characteristic histopathologic features of WG are (1) vasculitis, (2) necrosis, and (3) an inflammatory background. The vasculitis typically involves medium-sized and small vessels, including arteries, arterioles, capillaries, venules, and veins (Figure 22–12A). The large vessels are rarely affected. There may be simply a mural cellular infiltrate or fibrinoid necrosis. More frequently, an intramural eccentric necrotizing granulomatous lesion is found. The capillaritis may be neutrophilic or, rarely, granulomatous. The necrosis is granulomatous in nature. Small microabscesses appear to be the initial lesion (see Figure 22–12B). They enlarge and coalesce until the typical geographic and basophilic appearance of the necrosis has developed (Figure 22–12C). The necrotic center is surrounded by palisading histiocytes and scattered giant cells. Occasionally, the necrosis may be bronchocentric. The inflammatory background of the granulomatous necrosis and vasculitis can cause extensive parenchymal consolidation, mimicking organizing pneumonia. The

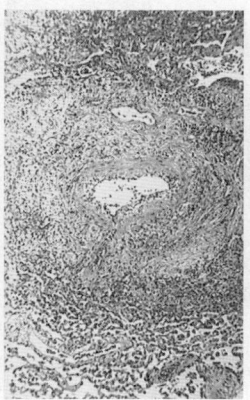
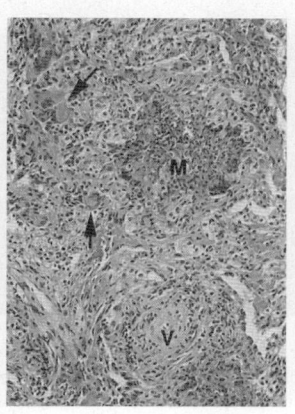

A

B

C

Figure 22–12   Histopathologic features of WG. *A*, Open lung biopsy specimen showing a small artery with transmural infiltration by inflammatory cells, which are predominantly neutrophils. *B*, Transbronchial lung biopsy specimen showing diagnostic features of WG microabscess formation (M) and multinucleated giant cells (arrows) in association with vasculitis (V). *C*, Open lung biopsy specimen showing the characteristic so-called geographic necrosis.

cellular infiltrates are mixed, consisting of lymphocytes, plasma cells, scattered giant cells, and eosinophils. Sarcoid-like nonnecrotizing granulomas are lacking. Other atypical patterns including capillaritis and hemorrhage without necrosis or classic vasculitis; neutrophilic air space infiltrates; pleural, septal, or bronchocentric predominance; isolated focal intimal vasculitis only; fibrinoid necrotizing vasculitis; extensive organizing pneumonia including a bronchiolitis obliterans organizing pneumonia (BOOP)-like variant; localized or infiltrative extravascular tumefactions; as well as marked eosinophilic infiltration have also been described.[101–108]

The histopathologic confirmation of the diagnosis of WG is still considered the gold standard. The original description of the histopathologic picture of WG was based on autopsy findings obtained from patients who had died of the disease without treatment. However, when interpreting histopathologic specimens from patients with suspected WG, limitations of its sensitivity need to be considered. It is affected by the biopsy site and the size of the specimen.[100] Furthermore, the findings may have been affected by immunosuppressive therapy.[109]

Biopsies from the lung and upper respiratory tract have the highest sensitivity and specificity.[48,103,110–113] Because the histopathologic features of kidney biopsies are nonspecific, a renal biopsy is not helpful for the distinction of WG from other small vessel vasculitides such as microscopic polyangiitis or Churg-Strauss syndrome. However, immunofluorescence microscopy performed on a renal biopsy specimen may be crucial to the separation of WG or microscopic polyangiitis from antiglomerular basement membrane (GBM)- or immune complex-mediated disease.

Laboratory Testing

Laboratory tests that should be obtained on all patients with suspected WG, microscopic polyangiitis, or Churg-Strauss syndrome include an ESR, a complete blood count, a serum chemistry group, urinalysis, and microscopy. In addition to the ESR, the determination of the C-reactive protein can serve as another nonspecific marker of inflammation. If renal involvement becomes apparent on urine testing or if impaired renal function is suspected based on serum chemistry abnormalities, the renal function should be assessed quantitatively, for instance, by determining a short iothalamate clearance. In patients with limited-phase WG, most of these parameters are within normal limits, with the exception of a mildly elevated ESR or C-reactive protein. Patients with active small vessel vasculitis (ie, generalized-phase WG or microscopic polyangiitis) usually display a high ESR (~100 mm/hour) as well as mild anemia, elevated white blood cell and platelet counts, an abnormal urinary sediment including red cells of glomerular origin and red cell casts, as well as various degrees of impairment of renal function.

The greatest advance in laboratory testing for WG and microscopic polyangiitis has come about with the discovery of ANCA (Figure 22–13).[114–116] Because ANCA testing has become such a critical component of the evaluation of patients with suspected WG and microscopic polyangiitis and because ANCA have been implicated in the pathogenesis of these syndromes, a separate extended paragraph is devoted to this topic.

Markers of vascular endothelial activation and injury such as thrombomodulin, soluble endothelial adhesion molecules, and others have been proposed as additional markers of disease activity but have not become part of routine care for WG patients to date.[117–120]

Differential Diagnosis

The differential diagnosis of WG is determined by the initial symptoms of each individual patient at presentation. If the symptomatology is caused primarily by necrotizing granulomatous inflammation confined to the upper and/or lower respiratory tract, the differentiation from granulomatous infections, particularly fungal or mycobacterial infections, becomes crucial. In most instances, histopathologic examination of the granulomatous lesion allows the differentiation of a granulomatous infection from WG.[100] Special stains and cultures of tissue specimens should be obtained whenever possible, especially if treatment with immunosuppressive agents is considered. Certain ophthalmologic features and ear, nose, and throat symptoms, particularly salivary gland swelling, require differentiation from sarcoidosis.[121]

Isolated necrotizing inflammation affecting the nose and resulting in nasal septal perforations may be difficult to differentiate from cocaine-induced midline destructive lesions (CIMDLs).[122] In contrast to WG, CIMDLs are characterized by the stark discrepancy between the

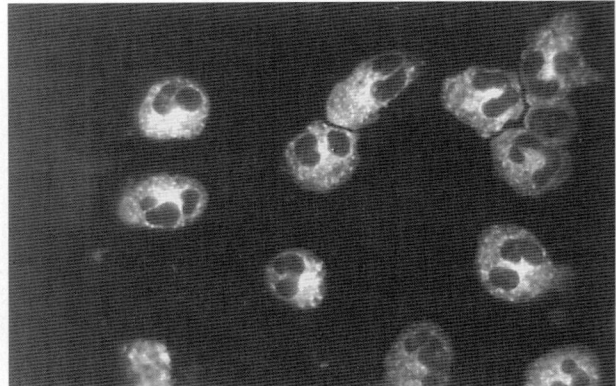

Figure 22–13   Indirect immunofluorescence microscopy image of ethanol-fixed neutrophil cytospin preparations displaying the characteristic granular centrally accentuated fluorescence pattern caused by cANCA.

severity of the localized destruction and the absence of any systemic involvement.[122] Only the presence of extravascular necrotizing granulomas and giant cells in WG can be used to distinguish the two lesions histopathologically.[122] Inflammatory changes of vessels can be encountered in both. Atypical ANCA are also frequent in CIMDLs and may not always be distinguishable from those of WG by routine methods.[122]

Relapsing polychondritis is a consideration in patients with saddle nose deformity and tracheobronchial disease. The characteristic ear cartilage involvement seen in relapsing polychondritis is not a feature of WG. Because ANCA have also been described in relapsing polychondritis and because patients with active limited WG have a 30% chance of being ANCA-negative, this laboratory test does not always allow the distinction between WG and relapsing polychondritis. Based on these observations, the possibility of overlap between relapsing polychondritis and WG has been discussed in the literature.[123–127]

WG of the upper and/or lower respiratory tract also needs to be differentiated from other pulmonary angiitis and granulomatosis syndromes. Although WG can resemble lymphomatoid granulomatosis clinically, the histopathologic differentiation from this lymphoproliferative process rarely presents a problem. The finding of bronchocentric granulomatosis may represent more of a challenge. Bronchocentric granulomatosis is more a reaction pattern than a separate disease entity. It may be encountered in the setting of WG, granulomatous infections, and as a result of allergic bronchopulmonary aspergillosis.[100,106]

If the primary clinical presentation is that of a diffuse alveolar hemorrhage syndrome with or without associated glomerulonephritis, other forms of autoimmune-mediated diffuse alveolar hemorrhage, such as anti-GBM disease, SLE, microscopic polyangiitis, and idiopathic pulmonary hemosiderosis, need to be excluded.[128]

Therapy

General Concepts and Historic Background

Over the course of the last decade, the general concept of therapy for WG has evolved. It is now understood that the treatment needs to be individualized according to the patient's disease acuity and extent at the time of presentation. Furthermore, remission-induction therapy is separated from remission-maintenance therapy. Finally, special attention needs to be given to the prevention of side effects from therapy because the morbidity and mortality resulting from complications of therapy rival and sometimes outweigh those of the underlying disease.[38,129,130]

WG was originally described as a universally fatal disease.[2,27,131] The introduction of immunosuppressive therapy regimens based on the combination of prednisone and cyclophosphamide has improved the prog-

nosis substantially, and the median survival after diagnosis is now 22 years.[36,38,132]

Remission Induction

To facilitate therapeutic decisions, patients are categorized as those with limited disease and those with severe or generalized disease. The use of the term limited disease and its implications have evolved over the last two decades. The term has frequently been used for patients lacking renal involvement. It must be stressed that even in the absence of renal involvement, patients with limited WG may have life-threatening disease manifestations (eg, capillaritis causing alveolar hemorrhage) that require aggressive immunosuppressive treatment. Consequently, today, limited WG implies that (1) there is predominantly necrotizing granulomatous pathology and no substantial vasculitic component and (2) that there is no disease manifestation that puts the affected organ at risk for irreversible damage. If the symptomatology is caused primarily by inflammation of the small vessels and capillaries (ie, alveolar hemorrhage, focal segmental necrotizing glomerulonephritis, scleritis, sensorineural hearing loss, mononeuritis multiplex, central nervous system involvement, and leukocytoclastic vasculitis of the skin), patients should be considered to have severe or generalized disease because the patient's life or the function of a significant organ are acutely threatened. Rarely, even localized necrotizing granulomatous lesions may be in life-threatening locations, prompting the more aggressive treatment approach used for severe disease.

The prevailing standard regimen for severe or generalized disease consists of the combined use of oral cyclophosphamide (2 mg/kg/day) and prednisone (1 mg/kg/day).[36,132] Once the patient responds to this regimen, prednisone is tapered over the following 2 to 3 months. If remission persists, the prednisone is discontinued, and cyclophosphamide is continued for another 3 months and then replaced by remission-maintenance therapy. In case of relapse, the standard protocol is re-initiated. A complete remission can be induced with this regimen in 75 to 93% of patients.[36,38,132,133] Unfortunately, the prolonged prednisone and cyclophosphamide use in WG is associated with substantial morbidity and mortality.[36,38,133] Up to 46% of patients treated with this regimen suffered serious infectious complications, up to 50% experienced hemorrhagic cystitis, up to 11% bladder cancer, and up to 8% myelodysplasia.[36,38,134,135] Osteoporosis as a consequence of prolonged corticosteroid therapy is also a major problem in WG patients.[136] Cyclophosphamide-induced infertility is another issue to be addressed with both young men and women.

Concern over the toxicity of prolonged oral cyclophosphamide use has prompted the search for equally effective but better-tolerated immunosuppressive regimens. In an attempt to reduce the cumulative cyclophosphamide dose, intermittent high-dose (pulse) intravenous cyclophosphamide in conjunction with oral prednisone has been used by several investigators.[137–143] These studies do not have enough power to allow firm conclusions, and the reported results are inconsistent. A recent meta-analysis of these data concludes that intravenous pulse cyclophosphamide may be somewhat more effective in inducing remission, and the overall side-effect rate may be lower.[144] However, the mortality associated with either treatment modality and the frequency of end-stage renal disease are the same, whereas the relapse rate is substantially higher after intravenous pulse therapy. Furthermore, the likelihood of response to pulse cyclophosphamide seems to be inversely proportional to the severity of the disease.[138] Consequently, the use of pulse cyclophosphamide seems advantageous only in select subsets of patients, such as young women in whom the overall cumulative cyclophosphamide dose is the crucial factor determining the likelihood of future fertility.[145,146]

For limited disease, MTX has replaced cyclophosphamide in remission-induction regimens. First reported to be effective for WG in the 1970s, an open-label study conducted at the National Institutes of Health showed that remission could be induced in 71% of patients.[147,148] Half of the patients had side effects that prompted MTX dosage reduction or discontinuation. Most significant was the occurrence of *Pneumocystis carinii* pneumonia in four (10%) patients, which resulted in two deaths. Because *P. carinii* is a complication of low-dose MTX therapy as well as of prednisone therapy and is not to be underestimated, prophylaxis with trimethoprim-sulfamethoxazole (T/S) or other agents is now considered mandatory.[92,149] Supplementation with folic acid at a dose of 1 mg/day can prevent MTX toxicity while preserving its efficacy.[150] Subsequent studies have confirmed the efficacy of this approach and indicated a lower rate of side effects.[151,152]

Remission Maintenance

Concern about the toxicity of longterm cyclophosphamide use has prompted the evaluation of alternative remission-maintenance regimens. An NIH study has shown that MTX can be used for remission maintenance with an efficacy similar to that observed in historic controls maintained on oral cyclophosphamide.[153] However, other studies have indicated a high relapse rate during or shortly after MTX remission-maintenance therapy (36.6 to 57%).[152,154] A randomized trial performed by the European Vasculitis Study Group has shown that azathioprine was equally effective in maintaining remission throughout the study period of 18 months.[133] In view of the high rate of renal relapse observed under remission-maintenance therapy with MTX, azathioprine may be the preferred remission-maintenance drug, not only for patients with impaired renal function.[154] The safety of azathioprine can be substantially increased by testing patients for thiopurine methyl-transferase deficiency prior to starting azathioprine.[155–157] For patients intolerant of azathioprine

or who suffered a relapse on azathioprine, mycophenolate mofetil and leflunomide may emerge as alternative agents for remission maintenance.[158,159]

Salvage Therapy and Novel Immune Response Modifying Agents

Patients with generalized disease who do not respond to immunosuppressive therapy represent a significant management problem. Several uncontrolled small studies, as well as a few randomized controlled trials, suggest a benefit from the addition of plasma exchange, particularly in patients with renal disease requiring dialysis.[160] The theoretical rationale of this treatment modality is based on the removal of inflammatory and immune mediators, particularly ANCA.

Based on the rationale that pooled gamma globulin preparations contain anti-ANCA idiotypic antibodies, intravenous immunoglobulin has been tried in several patients who did not respond to standard immunosuppression.[161–166] In some patients this therapy resulted in complete remission, whereas in others only an improvement in single disease manifestations or no improvement could be achieved, and the duration of benefit of a single course does not appear to exceed 3 months.[166] The observed differences in effectiveness seem to be related to batch-to-batch variability, as well as to variability between the preparations from different manufacturers.[167]

Novel immune response-modifying agents have become available in recent years. The humanized monoclonal antibody infliximab and the recombinant fusion protein etanercept are antagonists of tumor necrosis factor (TNF)-α, because TNF-α represents an attractive target for therapy in WG. TNF-α plays a significant role in granuloma formation because elevated TNF-α levels have been documented in active WG, and because TNF-α is thought to play a significant role in the priming of neutrophils and monocytes, a mechanism that is thought to be instrumental in allowing ANCA to exert their pro-inflammatory effects.[168–172] Anecdotal reports of the successful addition of infliximab treatment in patients failing standard therapy have emerged.[159] Etanercept seems to be safe when added to other immunosuppressive agents in WG and holds promise as an adjuvant to standard therapy.[173] Its efficacy as an adjuvant for remission induction and remission maintenance is the subject of the first multicenter randomized placebo-controlled trial of its use in vasculitis.[174] Another promising agent for remission induction in treatment-refractory cases that is currently undergoing further investigation is the humanized anti-CD20 monoclonal antibody rituximab, which effectively eliminates B lymphocytes.[175] Because of the unknown long-term side effect profile and substantial cost of these and other new immune response-modifying agents, it is crucial that they are carefully studied in formal trials before they are widely used for the treatment of the small vessel vasculitides.

Management of Disease Sequelae

Many patients suffer substantial permanent damage as a result of scarring that occurs during the healing of the active inflammatory lesions. The saddle nose deformity, large airway obstruction including subglottic stenosis, and end-stage renal disease all fall into this category and deserve special therapeutic attention. When patients are in stable remission, the reconstruction of nasal deformities is safe and effective.[176] Similarly, restoration of naso-lacrimal duct patency is an option for patients with epiphora.[177–179] Subglottic stenosis frequently occurs after disease activity has been controlled elsewhere, and by the time dyspnea and stridor call for medical attention, the area of stenosis lacks signs of mucosal inflammation (see Figure 22–6B). Tracheostomy has frequently been required to secure the airways. This may be avoided if intratracheal dilation, combined with local injection of long-acting glucocorticoids, is performed in a timely fashion.[180] If tracheostomy can not be avoided, tracheal reconstruction surgery can be performed when the disease is in remission.[181,182] Stenotic lesions may also occur at lower levels of the tracheobronchial tree where they may cause postobstructive pneumonia (see Figure 22–3). Patency of the trachea or mainstem bronchi may be restored by placement of Silastic airway stents (see Figure 22–5B).[53] Careful balloon dilation procedures may also restore airway patency at the segmental level. These procedures should only be performed by ear, nose, and throat surgeons and interventional bronchoscopists who are members of experienced interdisciplinary care teams for WG.

Because renal transplantation improves the quality of life and prognosis of patients more than does continued dialysis, renal transplantation should be considered for all patients with end-stage renal disease resulting from ANCA-associated vasculitis once a stable remission has been reached. A pooled analysis of all case series of renal transplantation in ANCA-associated vasculitis comprising 217 patients documents a cumulative disease relapse rate of 17.3% and a renal relapse rate of 9.5%.[183] The persistent presence of ANCA prior to transplantation does not seem to affect the postoperative relapse rate.[183] The overall relapse rate is lower than the 30 to 45% reported for patients not undergoing transplantation.[183,184] This may be the result of continued post-transplant immunosuppression, which may be sufficient to prevent a relapse in most patients.[185] In those patients who do suffer a relapse after transplantation, the addition of cyclophosphamide or azathioprine to the regimen has resulted in the induction of remission again.[185–187]

The Role of Trimethoprim-Sulfamethoxazole in the Therapy of WG

In 1985 DeRemee and colleagues first reported on the efficacy of T/S in the treatment of WG.[188] Subsequent anecdotal reports and small series have confirmed these original observations.[189–193] The use of T/S as the only agent may be effective against or at least temporize the disease in patients with limited disease of the upper and/or lower respiratory tract. T/S induced complete remission in 24 of 27 such patients.[194] A prospective study confirmed that T/S is effective as the sole agent in some patients with limited disease (11 of 19 patients had sustained complete remission).[195] However, T/S does not seem to be effective in patients with generalized vasculitis and kidney involvement, and it may not reliably prevent relapse in such patients.[195] In a follow-up report, the authors compared T/S treatment ($n = 24$) to low-dose weekly intravenous MTX ($n = 22$) in their respective abilities to maintain complete remission in patients with generalized disease.[196] Complete remission was maintained in only 58% of patients on T/S compared to 86% of patients on MTX. Drug side effects occurred in 12.5% of patients receiving T/S and in 27.2% receiving MTX. A large prospective, randomized, double-blind, placebo-controlled study indicated that the relapse rate of WG can be reduced by 50% if T/S is used continuously.[197] These data suggest that T/S is a safe adjunct that should be part of the regimen for all patients with WG unless they are allergic to the drug.

Approximately 10% of patients develop a skin reaction that requires discontinuation of T/S. Desensitization using oral pediatric T/S solution in gradual increments, from a single drop on day 1 to 21 drops on day 21 (the equivalent of a single strength tablet) is usually successful and allows the reinstitution of T/S in such patients. If MTX is part of the regimen, the T/S dose used should not exceed *P. carinii* pneumonia prophylaxis doses, and folic acid supplementation is imperative.

To date, the mechanisms by which T/S affects the course of WG are unclear. It may exert its effect as an antimicrobial agent on an infectious process that triggers the autoimmune cascade of WG, or it may have immunomodulatory effects on neutrophils, macrophages, and lymphocytes.[198–203]

MICROSCOPIC POLYANGIITIS

Clinical Presentation and Differential Diagnosis

The diagnostic term "microscopic polyarteritis" and its distinction from classic PAN goes back to the first description by Davson and coworkers of a microscopic variant of PAN.[5] These authors suggested that the necrotizing glomerulonephritis that occurs in patients with this form of disease is the result of capillaritis and that this feature distinguishes it from the PAN described by Kussmaul and Maier.[204] The category of microscopic polyarteritis was subsequently accepted in Great Britain and used for patients presenting with clinical and histopathologic features of necrotizing small vessel vasculitis associated with focal segmental necrotizing glomerulonephritis.[6] It has been separated from WG

TABLE 22–6   Frequency of Organ Involvement

Organ(s)	WG	MPA	CSS
Ear, nose, and throat	92–99%	61%	
Eye	50–60%	1%	–
Lung	66–85%	25%	38%
Kidney	70–80%	80%	26%
Gastrointestinal	very rare	31%	33%
Skin	33–46%	62%	57%
Nervous system	20–50%	60%	76%

Frequency of organ involvement in WG, MPA, and CSS.[36,38,220,242]

essentially by the lack of granulomatous respiratory tract involvement, and the pathologic distinction between these two syndromes may not always be clear-cut.[6] Many patients classified as having polyarteritis nodosa in the American literature (particularly those reported to have lung involvement) and others designated as having unclassified necrotizing small vessel vasculitis or hypersensitivity vasculitis probably represented cases of microscopic polyangiitis.

Microscopic polyangiitis has been defined by the Chapel Hill Consensus Conference as follows: "…necrotizing vasculitis with few or no immune deposits, affecting small vessels (ie, capillaries, venules, or arterioles). Necrotizing arteritis involving small and medium-sized arteries may be present. Necrotizing glomerulonephritis is very common; pulmonary capillaritis resulting in alveolar hemorrhage occurs frequently."[8] Microscopic polyangiitis is ANCA associated.[7,205,206] Patients may have perinuclear ANCA (pANCA) with specificity for myeloperoxidase (MPO) or, less frequently, cANCA with specificity for PR3. Some patients may initially present with microscopic polyangiitis and develop characteristic granulomatous lesions, allowing the diagnosis of WG at a later stage.[8] This is much more likely to occur in microscopic polyangiitis patients with cANCA than in those with pANCA.[207]

The differentiation of microscopic polyangiitis from classic PAN is felt to be essential for therapeutic and prognostic reasons.[12] Histologically, the necrotizing vasculitis in classic PAN affects the small and medium-sized muscular arteries and sometimes the arterioles, whereas in microscopic polyangiitis, it is predominantly the small vessels (capillaries) that are affected, although the small and medium-sized arteries may also be involved.[208,209] Classic PAN usually affects the renal vessels, causing renovascular hypertension, microaneurysms, and renal infarcts. These features are absent in microscopic polyangiitis. The rapidly progressive glomerulonephritis that is a characteristic manifestation of the capillaritis in microscopic polyangiitis is not seen in classic PAN. Similarly, pulmonary capillaritis leading to alveolar hemorrhage (see Figure 22–8) is common in microscopic polyangiitis but is not a feature of classic PAN. If classic PAN affects the lung, it is in the form of vasculitis of the bronchial or bronchiolar arteries.[210,211] Only one case of PAN affecting the medium-sized muscular pulmonary arteries has been described.[212]

Relapses are frequent in microscopic polyangiitis but rare in classic PAN.[213] Therefore, it has been suggested that immunosuppressive therapy in classic PAN be limited to 1 year in duration.[12] Classic PAN associated with viral infections, particularly hepatitis B or C virus, may respond to antiviral therapy aimed at reducing the viral replication when combined with plasmapheresis aimed at the elimination of circulating immune complexes.[12]

The presence of ANCA has also been proposed as a feature helpful in distinguishing between microscopic polyangiitis and classic PAN.[192] Although ANCA are detected in most patients with microscopic polyangiitis (> 85%), their presence is rare (10 to 20%) in classic PAN.[208,209,213–215] The controversy regarding whether patients with classic PAN (as defined by the Chapel Hill classification) who also have ANCA actually have microscopic polyangiitis or whether they represent an overlap syndrome will probably remain unresolved until specific etiologic agents are identified. With more widespread use of the definitions of the Chapel Hill classification and ANCA testing, it has become apparent that, in contrast to microscopic polyangiitis, classic PAN is exceedingly rare.[216–219]

A recent analysis of 85 patients indicates that renal involvement is the most frequent organ manifestation, occurring in 79% of patients, followed by skin (62.4%), peripheral nerve (57.6%), and gastrointestinal involvement (30.6%) (Table 22–6).[221] Lung involvement occurred only in 25% of patients, and less than half of these had alveolar hemorrhage.[220] Other clinical manifestations that can be part of the clinical presentation of microscopic polyangiitis are central nervous system vasculitis, sensorineural hearing loss, and, occasionally, subglottic stenosis (see Figure 22–6). These symptoms are indistinguishable from those observed in WG, because the underlying small vessel vasculitis and capillaritis is indistinguishable histopathologically.

Occasionally, microscopic polyangiitis may be associated with pulmonary fibrosis, either in the form of acute interstitial pneumonitis or resembling idiopathic pulmonary fibrosis.[222–224] Microscopic polyangiitis in association with severe obstructive airways disease or bronchiectases has also been reported.[225,226]

Prognosis and Therapy

The reported overall 5-year survival for microscopic polyangiitis is 74%.[220] In a prospective study of 107 patients with ANCA-associated microscopic polyangiitis and glomerulonephritis, Hogan and coworkers identified the following prognostic markers[227]: (1) the presence of pulmonary hemorrhage at presentation was the most significant negative prognostic factor, increasing

TABLE 22–7 Terminology and Target Antigens of ANCAs

Acronym	Staining*	Target Antigens	References
cANCA (formerly ACPA)	Cytoplasmic	PR3	272–274, 278
		MPO (rarely)	409
pANCA	Perinuclear	MPO	7, 205
		Elastase	122, 410–412
		Cathepsin G	413, 414
		Azurocidin	415, 416
		Lactoferrin	417, 418
		Lysozyme	414
		Enolase	419
		BPI	415, 420–422
		PR3 (rarely)	122, 278, 423
	Atypical cytoplasmic	BPI, others	415, 420, 422

*Immunofluorescence staining on ethanol-fixed neutrophils. BPI = bacteriocidal/permeability increasing protein; cANCA = cytoplasmic staining ANCA; pANCA = perinuclear staining ANCA.

the relative risk of death 8.6-fold compared to the absence of alveolar hemorrhage and (2) patients with a cANCA pattern had a 3.8-fold higher risk of death than patients with a pANCA pattern. Treatment with cyclophosphamide in addition to prednisone improves patient survival, the initial remission rate, and the relative risk for relapse.[220,227,228] Remission can be induced with combined corticosteroid and cyclophosphamide therapy in up to 93% of patients.[133] Twenty-five to thirty percent experience a relapse 18 to 24 months after the completion of initial therapy.[220,228,229] Most respond well to retreatment. Alveolar hemorrhage occurring in the context of microscopic polyangiitis is the most dramatic initial presentation of the disease and is associated with a high mortality. The overall mortality was 31% in a cohort of 29 patients recently reported from France.[129] The 5-year survival rate of

68% was similar to that of microscopic polyangiitis in general.[118] The general consensus is to treat microscopic polyangiitis according to the same principles used for generalized WG as described above.

CHURG-STRAUSS SYNDROME

Evolution of Disease Definitions and Diagnostic Criteria

In 1951 Jacob Churg and Lotte Strauss described the clinical and autopsy findings of 13 patients with a syndrome of allergic granulomatosis and angiitis, which quickly came to bear their name.[230] The authors thought this syndrome was related to, yet clearly distinct from, classic polyarteritis nodosa.[230] The syndrome was originally defined by severe asthma, fever, and hypereosinophilia in association with a systemic vasculitis.[230] The histopathologic features are necrosis in association with an eosinophilic exudate, severe "fibrinoid" collagen alteration, and granuloma formation with accumulation of epithelioid and giant cells, which the authors termed allergic granuloma (Figure 22–14). These granulomatous changes could be found in the connective tissue of any organ, as well as in vessel walls. The histopathologic features of the 30 cases reviewed at the Mayo Clinic consisted of prominent eosinophilia of vessels and perivascular tissues, with accompanying lymphocytes, plasma cells, and some histiocytes in all patients. Necrotizing vasculitis of the small arteries and veins was found in all patients, necrotizing extravascular granulomatosis in 22 patients, and fibrinoid necrosis of vessel walls in 12 patients.[231]

For several reasons it is impossible to establish the diagnosis of Churg-Strauss syndrome based on histopathologic findings alone. The allergic Churg-Strauss granuloma may occur as a nonspecific cutaneous reaction in association with a wide range of systemic diseases.[232] At times Churg-Strauss syndrome may be associated with eosinophilic pulmonary infiltrates indistinguishable from those of Löffler's eosinophilic

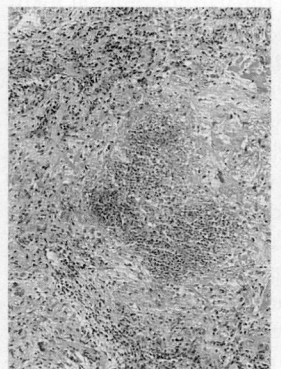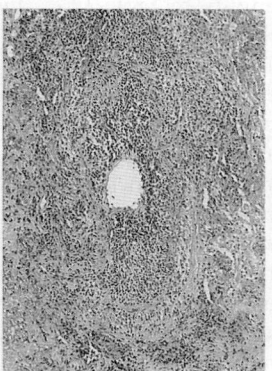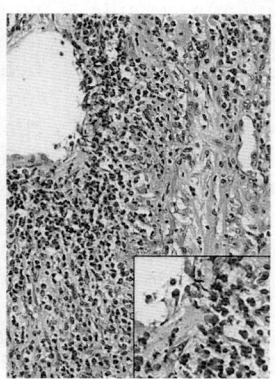

Figure 22–14 Histopathologic features of Churg-Strauss syndrome. Open lung biopsy specimen showing necrotizing granuloma formation (*A*) and vasculitis (*B*). Higher magnification reveals that the inflammatory cells are predominantly eosinophils (*C*).

A

B

C

pneumonia or chronic eosinophilic pneumonia.[230] Lie described several cases with eosinophilic vasculitis and/or extravascular granuloma in isolated organs or tissues, particularly the gastrointestinal tract, without evidence of systemic disease and proposed the use of the term "limited forms of Churg-Strauss syndrome" for such cases.[233] Furthermore, the necrotizing vasculitis of Churg-Strauss syndrome may be indistinguishable from that of microscopic polyangiitis or WG, and prominent tissue eosinophilia has been described in some cases of WG.[8,104] Finally, the classic histopathologic manifestations of Churg-Strauss syndrome are frequently altered by therapy or may be missed because of the small size of biopsy specimens obtained.[234] The use of corticosteroids for asthma may delay the manifestations of tissue eosinophilia and vasculitis until they are tapered. Such "formes frustes" of Churg-Strauss syndrome are recognized with increasing frequency.[235,236]

Based on a series of 16 patients and a review of another 138 reported in the literature, Lanham and coworkers gave a detailed description of the clinical features and course of the disease.[220] They confirmed that the classic histopathologic picture consisting of necrotizing vasculitis, eosinophilic tissue infiltration, and extravascular granulomas is not found in all cases and is not pathognomonic of the condition. Consequently, they proposed a clinical definition of the syndrome requiring the presence of asthma, peripheral eosinophilia in excess of 1.5×10^9/L, and systemic vasculitis involving two or more extrapulmonary organs as the basis of the diagnosis. They concluded that the clinical pattern of the disease is distinctive enough to justify the recognition of Churg-Strauss syndrome on clinical grounds. Furthermore, Lanham and associates identified three phases of the disease.[237] The first is a prodromal phase, which may persist for years, and consists of allergic disease (ie, allergic rhinitis, nasal polyposis), frequently followed by asthma. The second phase of the disease is characterized by the onset of peripheral blood and tissue eosinophilia, frequently causing a picture resembling Löffler's syndrome, chronic eosinophilic pneumonia, or eosinophilic gastroenteritis. The eosinophilic infiltrative disease may remit and recur over years before the third phase, which consists of a life-threatening systemic vasculitis, is reached. However, these three phases do not necessarily have to follow one another in this order; in 6 of 30 cases reported by Chumbley et al, asthma, eosinophilia, and vasculitis erupted simultaneously.[231] Guillevin and colleagues reported a wide variability between the onset of asthma and that of vasculitis, ranging from 0 to 61 years; in four patients, asthma developed after the onset of the vasculitic phase of Churg-Strauss syndrome.

The ACR study showed that the criteria proposed by Lanham and coworkers were more than 95% sensitive and specific for Churg-Strauss syndrome in patients with vasculitis.[238] The six ACR diagnostic criteria, of which a patient must meet at least four to be classified as having Churg-Strauss syndrome rather than another form of vasculitis, are (1) asthma, (2) eosinophilia (>10% on differential white blood count), (3) mono- or polyneuropathy attributable to a systemic vasculitis, (4) migratory or transient pulmonary infiltrates, (5) paranasal sinus abnormalities, and (6) extravascular eosinophils on biopsy, including an artery, arteriole, or venule tissue.

At the Chapel Hill Consensus Conference, Churg-Strauss syndrome was defined as "an eosinophil-rich and granulomatous inflammation involving the respiratory tract, and necrotizing vasculitis affecting small to medium-sized vessels, and associated with asthma and eosinophilia."[8] For patients to fulfill the Chapel Hill Consensus Conference definition of Churg-Strauss syndrome, surrogate markers for granulomatous inflammation of airways (ie, sinusitis or pulmonary infiltrates) and for vasculitis (ie, neurologic, cardiac, or renal disease consistent with a vasculitic cause) usually need to be accepted.[8,218,239]

Epidemiology of Churg-Strauss Syndrome

Even though Churg-Strauss syndrome appears to be diagnosed more frequently, it remains distinctly rare, and reliable epidemiologic data are scarce. Only 20 of the 807 patients with vasculitic syndromes submitted to the ACR classification study had Churg-Strauss syndrome.[238] Between 1950 and 1992, 77 patients have been diagnosed with Churg-Strauss syndrome at the Mayo Clinic, compared to 99 cases between 1990 and 2000.[231,239,240] A population-based study from England reports a 2.5-fold increase in the annual incidence over the course of the 10-year time span (1988 to 1997) to about 4 cases per million.[16] A recent study estimates the incidence of Churg-Strauss syndrome among asthmatics between zero (90%, CI 0–23) and 67 (90%, CI 22.5–160.6), depending on the disease definition used.[241]

Clinical Manifestations and Differential Diagnosis

The chest radiographic findings of Churg-Strauss syndrome are compared to those of WG and microscopic polyangiitis in Table 22–5, and the various clinical manifestations of Churg-Strauss syndrome and their reported frequencies are listed in Table 22–7.[231,237,242–244] The differentiation from WG or microscopic polyangiitis on clinical grounds is usually not difficult. An allergic background is no more frequent in these disorders than in the general population. Peripheral blood eosinophilia is only an occasional and minimal finding in Wegener's granulomatosis or microscopic polyangiitis, and whereas in Churg-Strauss syndrome the upper respiratory tract frequently manifests allergic rhinitis, necrotizing lesions as characteristically seen in WG are rare. In contrast to WG, the typical chest radiographic manifestation of Churg-Strauss syndrome consists of transient, usually alveolar-type, infiltrates.[242,245] Nodular lesions are less frequent, and alveolar hemorrhage is very rare.[242] Renal involvement in Churg-Strauss syndrome also appears to be less prominent than in WG or microscopic polyangiitis and rarely leads to renal failure.[231,237,242–244] Whereas renal involvement and lung involvement appear to be major negative prognostic factors in WG, most deaths from Churg-Strauss syndrome occur as a result of cardiac involvement.[231,237,242] Neurologic involvement is very common in Churg-Strauss syndrome, occurring in between 60 and 80% of patients.[237,240,242–244] Peripheral neuropathy is the most common finding, usually in the form of multiple mononeuropathy. Cerebral infarction is a rare feature of Churg-Strauss syndrome (<10%). In contrast to WG but similar to microscopic polyangiitis, gastrointestinal symptoms resulting from mesenteric vasculitis occur in one-third of patients.[231,237,239,242] Ocular, orbital, and otologic disease manifestations are well described, but in contrast to the other ANCA-associated vasculitides, they seem to be much less frequent.[246–249]

Churg-Strauss syndrome also needs to be differentiated from other eosinophilic pulmonary disorders. Particularly in the prevasculitic phases of the disease, the differentiation from chronic eosinophilic pneumonia, allergic bronchopulmonary aspergillosis, or hypereosinophilic syndrome may be challenging.

Pathogenesis

Very little is known about the pathogenesis of Churg-Strauss syndrome. The elevated IgE levels found in most patients may simply reflect the allergic background of these patients. The eosinophil seems to play a significant role in the pathogenesis. Serum markers of eosinophil activation, such as eosinophil cationic protein, parallel disease activity and may even predict relapse.[250,251] Elevated urinary excretion of eosinophil-derived neurotoxin is another marker of ongoing eosinophil activation that is found in patients with active Churg-Strauss syndrome.[252,253] Recent histopathologic studies suggest a direct link between degranulation of activated eosinophils and tissue injury.[254,255] However, activated neutrophils may also contribute.[255] There is growing evidence that Churg-Strauss syndrome is a Th2-mediated disease in which activated Th2-type lymphocytes predominate and may be responsible for the observed eosinophil activation with secondary tissue injury. Markers of T-cell activation such as soluble interleukin (IL)-2 receptor are elevated in active disease and also correlate with markers of endothelial cell damage (soluble thrombomodulin).[250] Furthermore, in Churg-Strauss syndrome, activated T lymphocytes preferentially express Th2-type cytokines (IL-4 and IL-13), and IL-4 production correlates with eosinophil counts.[256] Furthermore, aberrant CD95 function has been identified as a possible important pathogenic mechanism in Churg-Strauss syndrome.[257] Alternative splicing of the CD95 results in increased levels of the soluble isoform of CD95, which neutralizes CD95 ligand and thus functions as an inhibitor of CD95-mediated lymphocyte and eosinophil apoptosis. This mechanism may allow for clonal expansion of autoaggressive T-cell clones and enhance survival of eosinophils in Churg-Strauss syndrome. In the same study, clonally expanded T cells from Churg-Strauss syndrome patients were shown to have preferential V-gene usage for a gene from the Vβ21family and similar T-cell receptor specificities.[257] This suggests a limited number of common antigens in the patients studied and supports a previous clinical observation suggesting inhaled antigen(s) as a trigger of Churg-Strauss syndrome.[258]

ANCA and Churg-Strauss Syndrome

ANCA are detectable in 50 to 80% of patients with Churg-Strauss syndrome.[239,242–244,259] Most of these are pANCA reacting with MPO. cANCA reacting with PR3 are rare exceptions, and the differentiation of such cases from WG may be more difficult.[215,239,242–244,259] In our own analysis, the clinical presentation or treatment response did not differ between ANCA-positive and ANCA-negative Churg-Strauss syndrome patients.[239] In patients, MPO-ANCA (ANCA directed against MPO) levels appear to correlate with disease activity.[7,239,259]

Leukotriene Receptor Antagonists and Churg-Strauss Syndrome

In recent years, leukotriene receptor antagonists have become part of standard therapy for asthma. Several case reports of their use being associated with the onset of Churg-Strauss syndrome have emerged.[236,260–266] However, the onset of Churg-Strauss syndrome has also been reported in association with other drugs that allowed a corticosteroid taper.[235,267] Data presented at a recent National Institutes of Health workshop indicated that 88% of patients developed Churg-Strauss syndrome during the period of decreasing corticosteroid usage, and no single compound or class of antiasthmatic agents was associated with Churg-Strauss syndrome.[268] It is therefore more likely that the steroid taper allowed by leukotriene receptor antagonists may promote the unmasking of "formes frustes" of the Churg-Strauss syndrome.[235] This conclusion is also supported by the most recent analysis of all leukotriene antagonist-associated cases reported as of October 2000.[269]

Treatment and Prognosis of Churg-Strauss Syndrome

The systemic vasculitis of Churg-Strauss syndrome generally responds well to glucocorticoids. The role of cytotoxic agents such as cyclophosphamide is not as clearly defined as in WG.[231,237,240,242] Guillevin and colleagues did not detect a significant outcomes benefit from the addition of cyclophosphamide to corticosteroids.[242] However, in patients with cardiac and neurologic involvement, this drug should be considered early on to help induce remission according to the standard recommendations outlined above for the treatment of WG and microscopic polyangiitis. A small subset of patients may remain refractory to this aggressive treatment approach.[242] Interferon-γ is a promising alternative for such patients.[270,271] In an analogy to hypereosinophilic syndrome, hydroxyurea has also been used in cases with prominent hypereosinophilia.

ANCA

The discovery of ANCA and their association with WG in the early 1980s had a major impact on the diagnostic evaluation of patients with suspected small vessel vasculitis.[114–116] It has also stimulated research efforts into the pathogenesis of these disorders. Because WG, microscopic polyangiitis, and Churg-Strauss syndrome are the most frequent forms of vasculitis affecting the lung, it is appropriate to review the clinical utility of testing for ANCA and the pathogenic potential of ANCA in some detail here.

Terminology, Target Antigens, and Methodology

ANCA were first described as a cause of diffuse granular cytoplasmic immunofluorescent staining (cANCA; originally also referred to as ACPA) on ethanol-fixed neutrophils in association with glomerulonephritis, vasculitis, and WG. PR3 was subsequently identified as the principal target antigen for these ANCA.[272–274] At the same time, ANCA reacting with MPO, causing a perinuclear immunofluorescence staining pattern on ethanol-fixed neutrophils (pANCA), were found in patients with microscopic polyangiitis, its renal-limited variant, pauci-immune glomerulonephritis, and, less frequently, in WG (see Table 22–7).[123,205,275] Multiple other neutrophil granule constituents have since been identified as potential targets for ANCA in a variety of disorders (see Table 22–7). However, ANCA directed against target antigens other than PR3 or MPO have not been found to be associated with defined clinical entities with any degree of clinically useful sensitivity or specificity.[276] Over the last 5 years, a multitude of test systems allowing target antigen-specific ANCA detection have become available. Most are solid-phase assay systems in which the purified target antigen is coated to the ELISA plate directly or via an antigen-specific monoclonal capturing antibody (capture ELISA). The analytical sensitivity and specificity of these assay systems may vary widely, and frequently this information is not disclosed by the manufacturers.[277–280] This has prompted consensus statements calling for dual analysis of all serum samples from patients suspected of having WG, microscopic polyangiitis, or Churg-Strauss syndrome by both indirect immunofluorescence and target antigen-specific solid-phase assay in order to optimize the positive and negative predictive value of ANCA test results.[281–283] More recent studies have indicated that screening by immunofluorescence followed by confirmation of positive results with PR3- and MPO-ANCA-specific solid-phase assay, or vice versa, may be sufficient.[280,284] However, because the quality of ANCA testing, and hence its clinical utility, remain highly dependent on methodology, the test algorithms used need to be validated by the laboratories offering the service, and the data need to be available to the clinician interpreting the test results.

Clinical Utility of ANCA Testing

Most patients with active WG or microscopic polyangiitis have either cANCA/PR3-ANCA or pANCA/MPO-ANCA. cANCA/PR3-ANCA occur in approximately 75 to 90% of patients with active WG and in 10 to 50 % of patients with microscopic polyangiitis.[36,38,126,281,285] In contrast, pANCA reacting with MPO are found in up to 20% of patients with WG and in up to 80% of patients with microscopic polyangiitis.[7,171,205,220,281] Up to 80% of patients with active Churg-Strauss syndrome have ANCA, mostly of the pANCA/MPO-ANCA type.[239] The sensitivity of ANCA testing is affected by methodology (outlined above) and by the disease activity and extent at the time of sampling.[126,239]

Provided that rigorous test methods are used, false positive cANCA/PR3-ANCA or pANCA/MPO-ANCA combinations are rare.[280,281,284,286–288] Positive pANCA/MPO-ANCA test results can be found in patients with unclassified forms of small vessel vasculitis, drug-induced vasculitis, and, rarely, in patients with collagen vascular diseases.[284,287,288] Occasionally, cANCA/PR3-ANCA are also found in patients with subacute bacterial endocarditis.[289] Other reports of cANCA/PR3-ANCA in patients with invasive amebiasis and hepatitis C have not been confirmed by experienced ANCA laboratories.[290,291] However, patients with cocaine-induced destructive midline lesions may have cANCA/PR3-ANCA indistinguishable by routine methods from the ANCA found in WG.[115]

In addition, the diagnostic accuracy of ANCA testing depends on the pretest probability of a positive test result in any given patient population. The more indiscriminately ANCA testing is applied, the higher the chance of a false positive test result.[292] A positive ANCA test result should not be viewed as a surrogate for histopathologic confirmation of the diagnosis. Yet, as an indispensable piece of the diagnostic puzzle, it carries a weight similar to that of clinical symptoms and radiographic and histopathologic findings; therefore, it has become a widely accepted diagnostic tool.

Early studies found a correlation between ANCA levels and disease activity in patients.[116,126,285] One small prospective study even suggested that treatment based on the recurrence of ANCA could prevent relapses.[293] Unfortunately, the correlation between disease activity and ANCA levels is not apparent in all patients.[294,295] Nevertheless, the persistence or recurrence of ANCA, as well as a significant ANCA titer rise, indicate that a patient is at risk for a clinical relapse, even though the exact timing of it cannot be predicted in any given patient.[197,295] Consequently, for as long as therapy consists of immunosuppression with an associated high risk of toxicity, treatment decisions should not be made based on ANCA levels alone.

Because ANCA testing is frequently used in the differential diagnostic evaluation of patients with pulmonary–renal syndromes, the occurrence of ANCA in anti-GBM disease (Goodpasture's syndrome) and SLE needs to be addressed briefly. Several studies have confirmed that up to 38% of sera positive for anti-GBM disease may also contain ANCA.[296–300] Most of these ANCA are of the pANCA variety. The simultaneous occurrence of anti-GBM disease and cANCA is rare. If it does occur, such patients have classic clinical features of WG at some point or other during the course of their disease.[297,298] Similarly, patients with high levels of MPO-ANCA and anti-GBM disease usually have clinical features of systemic small vessel vasculitis.[301] However, the majority of patients with anti-GBM disease with ANCA have pANCA directed against antigens other than MPO or low levels of MPO-ANCA. These patients usually do not have any clinical symptoms suggesting the coexistence of vasculitis, but rather manifest the symptoms of classic anti-GBM disease.[297] Occasionally patients may develop ANCA-associated pauci-immune glomerulonephritis and true anti-GBM disease sequentially.[302]

Several studies have analyzed ANCA in SLE using reliable and validated ANCA test methods. Schnabel and coworkers studied 120 patients with SLE and found ANCA in 25%.[286] None of these ANCA were directed against PR3 or MPO. The detected ANCA also failed to identify a certain clinical subset of lupus patients with lupus vasculitis or glomerulonephritis. Similarly, Merkel and associates found only one patient (1.4%) with MPO-ANCA among 22 (31.4%) of 70 SLE patients who had pANCA.[287] No cANCA or PR3-ANCA were detected in these SLE patients.

Potential Role of ANCA in the Pathogenesis of Vasculitis

Many clinical observations and experimental data support a pathogenic role for ANCA in the development of vasculitis. In WG, the presence of PR3-ANCA appears most closely related to the development of vasculitic complications. Patients with biopsy-proven WG limited to the respiratory tract who remain PR3-ANCA negative have a good prognosis, do not develop vasculitic complications without seroconversion, and generally do not require aggressive immunosuppressive therapy[34] In contrast, most patients with similar initial clinical manifestations and PR3-ANCA eventually required immunosuppressive therapy for the control of symptoms and prevention of progression to severe systemic vasculitis.[34] Furthermore, systemic vasculitic relapses without recurrence of ANCA are extremely rare.[295] Yet, remission may be maintained for extended periods of time in up to half of patients despite the presence of ANCA. Taken together, the clinical observations suggest that the mere presence of ANCA alone is not sufficient to cause disease activity, but ANCA seem to be required for the development of the vasculitic complications of WG and systemic relapses.

Many in vitro studies have demonstrated the proinflammatory effects of PR3-ANCA and MPO-ANCA on neutrophils, monocytes, and endothelial cells, effects which enhance and perpetuate endothelial cell and tissue damage.[288] ANCA may increase the adhesion of neutrophils to endothelial cells by enhancing the expression of cell adhesion molecules on endothelial cells. ANCA seem to contribute to tissue damage by activating primed neutrophils, resulting in the release of oxygen radicals and proteolytic enzymes. The latter may in turn induce endothelial cell apoptosis. ANCA-mediated neutrophil activation involves both Fcγ-receptor engagement and recognition of expressed target antigen on the surface of primed neutrophils. ANCA may also cause endothelial cell damage by direct cytotoxicity or by localized immune complex formation, with target antigens bound to the endothelial cell surface. The latter may initiate localized complement activation. Finally, ANCA are thought to contribute to the recruitment of more inflammatory cells to the area of tissue injury by stimulating the release of chemotactic chemokines and agents from neutrophils, monocytes, and endothelial cells. For a detailed description of pathways and mechanisms by which ANCA may directly and indirectly contribute to damage of the vascular endothelium, the reader is referred to recent reviews.[303–305]

Most ANCA-mediated effects on neutrophils and monocytes require priming of the cells. This cytokine-dependent process is not unique to vasculitis. Cytokine stimulation of neutrophils and monocytes, typically by TNF, with resulting increased surface expression of ANCA target antigens occurs normally in the context of infections. Patients with active vasculitis have indeed been shown to have both increased expression of ANCA target antigens on the surface of their neutrophils and elevated levels of TNF.[169,306–308] In combination, these observations allow the hypothesis that the neutrophil priming that occurs in response to cytokine stimulation during infection enables ANCA to interact with their target antigen on the neutrophil surface. This in turn sets the documented pro-inflammatory effects of ANCA in motion, which aggravate and perpetuate the inflammatory reaction at the endothelial cell interphase. This concept may explain why some patients relate the onset or recurrence of disease activity to preceding infectious episodes.[309]

The pathogenic role of ANCA in the development of vasculitis is also supported by animal models of MPO-ANCA-associated vasculitis.[310,311] They clearly indicate that ANCA contribute directly to the development of vasculitis and glomerulonephritis and that the interaction of ANCA with their target antigen is required for the development of lesions. Furthermore, the localization of lesions is determined by the site of this interaction. At the same time, animal models support the significance of genetic determinants for the development of autoimmunity, vasculitis, and a specific phenotype with characteristic organ involvement and histopathologic features. Finally, animal model studies indicate that infection may be a significant disease modifier.[312,313]

To date, the causes of the production and persistence of ANCA remain poorly understood. ANCA directed against a broad variety of target antigens have been documented in association with viral, fungal, bacterial, and protozoal infections.[276,289] In the rare instances in which cANCA/PR3-ANCA are observed in infections, the ANCA disappear with appropriate antimicrobial therapy.[289,290] These observations may suggest that ANCA can occur transiently in the setting of infection and that the persistent ANCA response in patients with vasculitis may be the result of molecular mimicry in susceptible hosts.[314] Subsequent diversification of T- and B-cell responses (epitope spreading) may lead to responses against different epitopes on the same target molecule (intramolecular spreading) or extend to other molecules (intermolecular spreading).[315,316]

It is also hypothesized that bacterial superantigens play a significant role in the pathogenesis of ANCA-associated vasculitis. WG patients colonized with superantigen-producing *Staphylococcus aureus* are at a higher risk for relapse than those with superantigen-negative *S. aureus*.[198,317] In addition, the expansion of T cells expressing Vβ segments specific for *S. aureus* superantigens occurred more frequently in patients than in controls.[318] This evidence supports the theory that *S. aureus* contributes to the pathogenesis of vasculitis. By inducing potent T- and B-cell activity, superantigens produced during a *S. aureus* infection could initiate and maintain both ANCA production and cytokine release, thought to be required for the cascade that results in necrotizing granulomatous inflammation and vasculitis.

In summary, the clinical observations and experimental data accumulated over the last two decades support the theory that infections may give rise to ANCA via molecular mimicry and contribute to their persistence via T- and B-cell stimulation by microbial superantigens. A predisposition of the patient to develop autoimmune disease may also be required. Infections or other inflammatory stimuli may cause cytokine-mediated neutrophil and monocyte activation, which are, in turn, required for certain types of ANCA (PR3-ANCA and MPO-ANCA in particular) to interact with their target antigens expressed on the surface of these cells. This interaction of PR3-ANCA and MPO-ANCA with primed mononuclear cells is thought to prompt multiple pro-inflammatory effects that together result in small vessel vasculitis.

GIANT CELL ARTERITIS

Giant cell arteritis, which is a generalized inflammatory disorder involving large and medium-sized arteries, is the most common form of vasculitis in the White population and appears to predominantly affect elderly patients. Although an epidemiologic study would suggest the presence of respiratory symptoms in as many as 25% of patients, practicing pulmonologists see few patients with giant cell arteritis for the management of respiratory complications of this illness.[319] The respiratory symptoms may consist of cough, hoarseness, or throat pain, which generally resolve promptly with prednisone therapy. Chest radiographs are usually normal, and pulmonary function tests do not differ significantly from matched control populations. Because respiratory symptoms may be the initial manifestations of giant cell arteritis, this possibility should be considered in any elderly patient with new onset of cough, hoarseness, or throat pain without other identifiable cause.[20,320] Pleural effusion as a respiratory manifestation of giant cell arteritis has also been reported.[321]

A patient with multinodular pulmonary lesions has also been reported.[322] Such an observation should raise the question about an overlap syndrome or a mistaken diagnosis of WG.[323,324]

TAKAYASU'S ARTERITIS

Takayasu's arteritis is a form of vasculitis that predominantly affects the aorta and its major branches in young patients. Females of Asian descent are more frequently affected.[325] Pulmonary complications are the result of a unique arteriopathy characterized by progressive defects in the outer media of the arteries and ingrowth of granulation tissuelike capillaries associated with thickened intima with subendothelial smooth muscle proliferation.[326] The large and medium-sized pulmonary vessels are most commonly affected.[327] Clinically, the involvement of pulmonary arteries is usually occult, but angiographic, perfusion scan, and magnetic resonance (MR) angiography studies have documented pulmonary artery stenoses and occlusion in up to half of all patients.[328–332] CT may show areas of low attenuation thought to represent regional hypoperfusion, subpleural reticulolinear changes, and pleural thickening.[333] Mild to moderate pulmonary hypertension is not uncommon.[334] Fistula formation between pulmonary artery branches and bronchial arteries, as well as nonspecific inflammatory interstitial lung disease, have also been reported. Therapy consists primarily of immunosuppression with glucocorticoids.[325] MTX may have to be added in refractory or relapsing cases.[335] Vascular bypass procedures may be beneficial in severe disease.[336] ANCA are not found in Takayasu's arteritis, but overlap cases with WG have been reported.[337–341]

BEHÇET'S DISEASE

Behçet's disease is a rare chronic relapsing disorder characterized by recurrent aphthous oral ulcers and at least two or more of the following: aphthous genital ulcers, uveitis, cutaneous nodules or pustules, or meningoencephalitis.[342] Pulmonary complications of Behçet's disease manifest themselves as cough, hemoptysis, fever, chest pains, and dyspnea.[343,344] The hemoptysis may be massive and has been reported to be fatal in up to 39% of instances.[343]

The vasculitis of Behçet's disease is felt to be immune complex mediated because immune deposits such as IgG, C3, and C4 have been detected in the walls of affected vessels.[344,345] Histopathologic evaluation revealed that vasculitis can affect vessels of all sizes. Vasculitic involvement of the veins frequently leads to secondary thrombosis with major venous occlusion. This type of thrombosis may not be preventable by anticoagulation.[342] Destruction of the elastic lamina of pulmonary arteries can lead to the characteristic aneurysm formation, secondary erosion of bronchi, and arterial–bronchial fistulae, which cause massive hemoptysis. Recurrent pneumonia and bronchial obstruction as a consequence of mucosal inflammation have also been described.[346,347]

Pulmonary angiography for the diagnosis of pulmonary artery aneurysms has largely been replaced by CT and MR angiography.[348,349] Immunosuppressive therapy is indicated in all patients with active Behçet's syndrome. Prednisone alone may not be sufficient to control the vasculitis, and the addition of other drugs, such as colchicine, chlorambucil, MTX, cyclosporin or azathioprine, has been recommended.[342] Particularly, the addition of azathioprine or cyclophosphamide to glucocorticoids has resulted in the resolution of pulmonary aneurysms.[350–352] Although anticoagulation should be avoided once pulmonary arteritis has been documented, aspirin at a dose of 80 mg/day may be considered for prevention of the secondary thromboses.[342] The prognosis with pulmonary involvement is poor. Of patients with pulmonary involvement reported by Raz, 16 of 49 died, most from fatal pulmonary hemorrhage, within 2 years of developing pulmonary involvement.[344] Embolization therapy may prevent and treat hemorrhage from pulmonary artery aneurysms.[353–355]

PULMONARY VASCULITIS ASSOCIATED WITH CONNECTIVE TISSUE DISORDERS

Vasculitis is most commonly associated with rheumatoid arthritis and SLE. In contrast to the vasculitis in WG, microscopic polyangiitis, or Churg-Strauss syndrome, the small vessel vasculitis of rheumatoid arthritis and SLE is immune complex mediated. Rheumatoid pulmonary arteritis can be the cause of pulmonary hypertension in some patients with normal chest radiographs.[356] Rheumatoid nodules frequently show necrotizing granulomatous features and vasculitis.[357] If pulmonary vasculitis is documented in patients with active rheumatoid arthritis, it is usually a subordinate phenomenon, and the mode of therapy should be decided according to the overall disease activity. However, pulmonary capillaritis and alveolar hemorrhage may be an isolated feature of rheumatoid arthritis, part of a systemic vasculitic complication of rheumatoid arthritis, or even an early manifestation of the disease.[358–360]

Immune complex-mediated capillaritis in lupus erythematosus may be the rare cause of diffuse alveolar hemorrhage. In most instances, pulmonary capillaritis associated with a neutrophil-mediated disruption of alveolar and capillary basement membranes is the characteristic histopathologic finding.[361] However, bland alveolar wall changes without immune complex deposition can also be found.[362] Other signs of the disease usually precede the hemorrhage. In the past, the outcome has been fatal despite high-dose steroid therapy.[356,363,364] In the more recent series reported from Denver University Hospital, the mortality still exceeded 50%.[361] Alveolar hemorrhage accounted for 22% of all pulmonary complications and 3.7% of all lupus-related hospital admissions.[361] It was the initial manifestation of SLE in 11% of cases.[361] Intravenous pulse cyclophosphamide and the prompt initiation of plasmapheresis have been reported as more effective treatment modalities.[365] The efficacy of the synchronized combination of plasmapheresis and pulse cyclophosphamide therapy in severe lupus erythematosus is currently being evaluated in a multicenter trial.[366] The rationale behind this approach is the assumption that plasmapheresis induces a compensatory rebound proliferation of pathogenic antibody-producing clones. These would be attacked by the pulse cyclophosphamide given immediately following the plasmapheresis, when these clones are the most vulnerable. Treatment-free remissions lasting up to 7 years have been reported with this approach.[366,367] However, this regimen has not been successful in preventing renal failure in patients with lupus nephritis.[368]

Pulmonary capillaritis and alveolar hemorrhage can also be associated with the antiphospholipid syndrome, mixed connective tissue disorder, scleroderma, and polymyositis.[359,369–375] These associations and the wide spectrum of other respiratory manifestations of collagen vascular disease are reviewed in detail elswhere in this book.

NECROTIZING SARCOID GRANULOMATOSIS

Vasculitis is a prominent histopathologic feature of necrotizing sarcoid granulomatosis. The disease, which is usually limited to the lungs, was first described as a separate entity in 1973 by Liebow.[376] The characteristic pulmonary nodules are usually bilateral and may be an incidental finding in asymptomatic patients. Alternatively, patients may complain of cough, dyspnea, or phlegm production. Generalized constitutional symptoms occur rarely.

Histopathologically, there are characteristic necrotizing epithelioid granulomas that may form aggregates. In contrast to WG, these granulomas are well circumscribed. Vasculitis is a central feature of necrotizing sarcoid granulomatosis. Three types of vasculitis have been described: an epithelioid-granulomatous form; a form reminiscent of giant cell arteritis with prominent histiocytes and multinucleated giant cells in the inflammatory infiltrate of the vessel wall; and a lymphocytic form lacking granuloma formation and giant cells.[376]

The differential diagnosis primarily includes infectious processes. Special sputum and tissue stains and cultures should always be obtained to exclude mycobacterial or fungal disease. The separation from sarcoidosis is somewhat controversial. However, the following features are thought to distinguish necrotizing sarcoid granulomatosis from sarcoidosis. First, the extensive vasculitis and necrosis would be unusual for sarcoidosis, even though vascular involvement is frequently seen in sarcoidosis. Furthermore, the chest radiographic appearance of pulmonary nodules or masses and the presence of pleural involvement are unusual for sarcoidosis.[377] Finally, extrapulmonary involvement has only rarely been documented in necrotizing sarcoid granulomatosis.[378,379]

It is debatable whether necrotizing sarcoid granulomatosis should be included with the primary systemic vasculitides. Most authors would argue against this inclusion because of its limitation to the lungs and good prognosis (spontaneous remission may occur). Therapeutically, necrotizing sarcoid granulomatosis can be approached as cases with chronic pulmonary sarcoidosis. Decisions about the use of oral steroid therapy should be individualized based on symptoms, pulmonary function data, and their evolution over time.

REFERENCES

1. Zeek PM. Periarteritis nodosa—a critical review. Am J Clin Pathol 1952;22:777–90.
2. Godman GC, Churg J. Wegener's granulomatosis. Pathology and review of the literature. AMA Arch Pathol 1954;58: 533–53.
3. Fauci AS, Haynes BF, Katz P. The spectrum of vasculitis: clinical, pathologic, immunologic, and therapeutic considerations. Ann Intern Med 1978;89:660–76.
4. Hunder GG, Arend WP, Bloch DA, et al. The American College of Rheumatology 1990 criteria for the classification of vasculitis: introduction. Arthritis Rheum 1990;33:1101–7.
5. Davson J, Ball J, Platt R. The kidney in periarteritis nodosa. Q J Med 1948;17:175–202.
6. Savage COS, Winearls CG, Evans DJ, et al. Microscopic polyarteritis: presentation, pathology and prognosis. Q J Med 1985;56:467–83.
7. Cohen Tervaert JW, Goldschmeding R, Elema JD, et al. Association of autoantibodies to myeloperoxidase with different forms of vasculitis. Arthritis Rheum 1990;33:1264–72.
8. Jennette JC, Falk RJ, Andrassy K, et al. Nomenclature of systemic vasculitides: the proposal of an international consensus conference. Arthritis Rheum 1994;37:187–92.
9. Bosch X. Microscopic polyangiitis (microscopic polyarteritis) with late emergence of generalised Wegener's granulomatosis. Ann Rheum Dis 1999;58:644–7.
10. Daoud MS, Gibson LE, Specks U. Cutaneous leukocytoclastic vasculitis with positive anti-neutrophil cytoplasmic antibodies. Acta Derm Venereol 1999;79:328–9.
11. Lie JT. Nomenclature and classification of vasculitis: plus ça change, plus c'est la meme chose. Arthritis Rheum 1994; 37:181–6.
12. Guillevin L, Lhote F. Distinguishing polyarteritis nodosa from microscopic polyangiitis and implications for treatment. Curr Opin Rheumatol 1995;7:20–4.
13. Watts RA, Jolliffe VA, Carruthers DM, et al. Effect of classification on the incidence of polyarteritis nodosa and microscopic polyangiitis. Arthritis Rheum 1996;39:1208–12.
14. Andrews M, Edmunds M, Campbell A. Systemic vasculitis in the 1980's—is there an increasing incidence of Wegener's granulomatosis and microscopic polyarteritis? J R C Physicians 1990;24:284–8.
15. Scott DG, Bacon PA, Elliott PJ, et al. Systemic vasculitis in a district general hospital 1972–1980: clinical and laboratory features, classification and prognosis of 80 cases. Q J Med 1982;51:292–311.
16. Watts RA, Lane SE, Bentham G, Scott DG. Epidemiology of systemic vasculitis: a ten-year study in the United Kingdom. Arthritis Rheum 2000;43:414–9.
17. Koldingsnes W, Nossent H. Epidemiology of Wegener's granulomatosis in northern Norway. Arthritis Rheum 2000;43:2481–7.
18. Jonasson F, Cullen JF, Elton RA. Temporal arteritis: a 14-year epidemiological, clinical and prognostic study. Scott Med J 1979;24:292–311.
19. Salvarani C, Gabriel SE, O'Fallon WM, Hunder GG. The incidence of giant cell arteritis in Olmsted County, Minnesota: apparent fluctuations in a cyclical pattern. Ann Intern Med 1995;123:192–4.
20. Larson TS, Hall S, Hepper NGG, Hunder GG. Respiratory tract symptoms as a clue to giant cell arteritis. Ann Intern Med 1984;101:594–7.
21. Watts RA, Carruthers DM, Scott DGI. Epidemiology of systemic vasculitis: changing incidence or definition? Sem Arthritis Rheum 1995;25:28–34.
22. Carruthers DM, Watts RA, Symmons DPM, Scott DGI. Wegener's granulomatosis—increased incidence or increased recognition? Br J Rheumatol 1996;35:142–5.
23. Cotch MF, Hoffman GS, Yerg DE, et al. The epidemiology of Wegener's granulomatosis. Estimates of the five-year-period prevalence, annual mortality, and geographic disease distribution from population-based data sources. Arthritis Rheum 1996;39:87–92.
24. Watts RA, Gonzalez-Gay MA, Lane SE, et al. Geoepidemiology of systemic vasculitis: comparison of the incidence in two regions of Europe. Ann Rheum Dis 2001;60:170–2.
25. Klinger H. Grenzformen der periarteriitis nodosa. Franfurter Zeitschrift für Pathologie 1931;42:455–80.
26. Wegener F. Über generalisierte septische Gefässerkrankungen. Verhandl Dtsch Gesell Pathol 1936;29:202–9.
27. Wegener F. Über eine eigenartige rhinogene Granulomatose mit besonderer Beteiligung des Arteriensystems und der Nieren. Beitr Pathol Anat 1939;109:36–68.
28. Wegener F. On generalised septic vessel diseases. Thorax 1987; 42:918–9.
29. Wegener F. Wegener's granulomatosis. Thoughts and observations of a pathologist. Eur Arch Otorhinolarygol 1990; 247:133–42.
30. Carrington CB, Liebow AA. Limited forms of angiitis and granulomatosis of Wegener's type. Am J Med 1966;41:497–527.
31. DeRemee RA, McDonald TJ, Harrison EG, Coles DT.

Wegener's granulomatosis. Anatomic correlates, a proposed classification. Mayo Clin Proc 1975;51:777–81.

32. Leavitt RY, Fauci AS, Bloch DA, et al. The American College of Rheumatology 1990 criteria for the classification of Wegener's granulomatosis. Arthritis Rheum 1990;33: 1101–7.

33. Hunder GG. The use and misuse of classification and diagnostic criteria for complex diseases. Ann Intern Med 1998;129:417–8.

34. Chiba M, Specks U. Prognosis of Wegener's granulomatosis limited to the respiratory tract: significance of c-ANCA [abstract]. Chest 1996;11:25S.

35. Bullen CL, Liesegang TJ, McDonald TJ, DeRemee RA. Ocular complications of Wegener's granulomatosis. Ophthalmology 1983;90:279–90.

36. Hoffman GS, Kerr GS, Leavitt RY, et al. Wegener granulomatosis: an analysis of 158 patients. Ann Intern Med 1992;116:488–98.

37. Stavrou P, Deutsch J, Rene C, et al. Ocular manifestations of classical and limited Wegener's granulomatosis. Q J Med 1993;86:719–25.

38. Reinhold-Keller E, Beuge N, Latza U, et al. An interdisciplinary approach to the care of patients with Wegener's granulomatosis: long-term outcome in 155 patients. Arthritis Rheum 2000;43:1021–32.

39. Sadiq SA, Jennings CR, Jones NS, Downes RN. Wegener's granulomatosis: the ocular manifestations revisited. Orbit 2000;19:253–61.

40. Harper SL, Letko E, Samson CM, et al. Wegener's granulomatosis: the relationship between ocular and systemic disease. J Rheumatol 2001;28:1025–32.

41. Kalina PH, Garrity JA, Herman DC, et al. The role of testing for anticytoplasmic autoantibodies in the differential diagnosis of scleritis and orbital pseudotumor. Mayo Clin Proc 1990;65:1110–7.

42. Boukes RJ, de Vries-Knoppert WA. Lacrimal gland enlargement as one of the ocular manifestations of Wegener's granulomatosis. Doc Ophthalmol 1985;59:21–6.

43. McDonald TJ, DeRemee RA, Kern EB, Harrison EGJ. Nasal manifestations of Wegener's granulomatosis. Laryngoscope 1974;84:2101–11.

44. McCaffrey TV, McDonald TJ, Facer GW, DeRemee RA. Otologic manifestations of Wegener's granulomatosis. Otolaryngol Head Neck Surg 1980;88:586–93.

45. Hoffman GS, Leavitt RY, Kerr GS, Fauci AS. The treatment of Wegener's granulomatosis with glucocorticoids, and MTX. Arthritis Rheum 1992;35:1322–9.

46. Handlers JP, Waterman J, Abrams AM, Melrose RJ. Oral features of Wegener's granulomatosis. Arch Otolaryngol 1985;111:267–70.

47. Knight JM, Hayduk MJ, Summerlin DJ, Mirowski GW. "Strawberry" gingival hyperplasia: a pathognomonic mucocutaneous finding in Wegener granulomatosis. Arch Dermatol 2000;136:171–3.

48. Devaney KO, Travis WD, Hoffman G, et al. Interpretation of head and neck biopsies in Wegener's granulomatosis. Am J Surg Pathol 1990;14:555–64.

49. Murty GE, Mains BT, Bennett MK. Salivary gland involvement in Wegener's granulomatosis. J Laryngol Otol 1990;104:259–61.

50. Specks U, Colby TV, Olsen KD, DeRemee RA. Submandibular gland involvement in Wegener's granulomatosis. Arch Otolaryngol Head Neck Surg 1991;117:218–23.

51. McDonald TJ, Neel HBI, DeRemee RA. Wegener's granulomatosis of the subglottis and the upper portion of the trachea. Ann Otol Rhinol Laryngol 1982;91:588–92.

52. Lebovics RS, Hoffman GS, Leavitt RY, et al. The management of subglottic stenosis in patients with Wegener's granulomatosis. Laryngoscope 1992;102:1341–5.

53. Daum DE, Specks U, Colby TV, et al. Tracheobronchial

involvement in Wegener's granulomatosis. Am J Respir Crit Care Med 1995;151:522–6.

54. Ulbright TM, Katzenstein A-LA. Solitary necrotizing granulomas of the lung. Differentiating features and etiology. Am J Surg Pathol 1980;4:13–28.

55. Katzenstein A-LA. Necrotizing granulomas of the lung. Hum Pathol 1980;11:596–7.

56. Leatherman JW, Sibley RK, Scott FD. Diffuse intrapulmonary hemorrhage and glomerulonephritis unrelated to anti-glomerular basement membrane antibody. Am J Med 1982;72:401–10.

57. Haworth SJ, Savage COS, Carr D, et al. Pulmonary haemorrhage complicating Wegener's granulomatosis and microscopic polyarteritis. Br J Med 1985;290:1775–8.

58. Travis WD, Carpeter HA, Lie JT. Diffuse pulmonary hemorrhage. An uncommon manifestation of Wegener's granulomatosis. Am J Surg Pathol 1987;11:702–8.

59. Myers JL, Katzenstein A-LA. Wegener's granulomatosis presenting with massive pulmonary hemorrhage and capillaritis. Am J Surg Pathol 1987;11:895–8.

60. Lhote F, Cohen P, Chemlal K, et al. Les manifestations pleurales au cours de la périartérite noueuse de la maladie de Wegener et du pupus érythémateux systémique. Ann Med Interne 1992;143:228–32.

61. England DM, Unger JM. Pleural-based mass in an elderly man with arthralgias. Chest 1987;91:603–4.

62. Aberle DR, Gamsu G, Lynch D. Thoracic manifestations of Wegener granulomatosis: diagnosis and course. Radiology 1990;174:703–9.

63. Papiris SA, Manoussakis MN, Drosos AA. Imaging of thoracic Wegener's granulomatosis: the computed tomographic appearance. Am J Med 1992;93:529–36.

64. Weir IH, Müller NI, Chiles C, et al. Wegener's granulomatosis: findings from computed tomography of the chest in 10 patients. Can Assoc Radiol J 1992;43:31–4.

65. Maskell GF, Lockwood CM, Flower CDR. CT of the lung in Wegener's granulomatosis. Clin Radiol 1993;48:377–80.

66. Reed WB, Jensen AK, Konwaler BE, Hunter D. The cutaneous manifestations in Wegener's granulomatosis. Acta Dermato-Venereologica 1963;43:250–64.

67. Hu C-H, O'Loughlin S, Winkelmann RK. Cutaneous manifestations of Wegener granulomatosis. Arch Dermatol 1977;113:175–82.

68. Patten SF, Tomecki KJ. Wegener's granulomatosis: cutaneous and oral mucosal disease. J Am Acad Dermatol 1993; 28:710–8.

69. Daoud MS, Gibson LE, DeRemee RA, et al. Cutaneous Wegener's granulomatosis: clinical, histopathologic, and immunopathologic features of thirty patients. J Am Acad Dermatol 1994;31:605–12.

70. Francès C, Du LHT, Piette J-H, et al. Wegener's granulomatosis. Dermatologic manifestations in 75 cases with clinicopathologic correlation. Arch Dermatol 1994;130: 861–7.

71. Barksdale SK, Hallahan CW, Keer GS, et al. Cutaneous pathology in Wegener's granulomatosis. A clinicopathologic study of 75 biopsies in 46 patients. Am J Surg Pathol 1995;19:161–72.

72. Nishino H, Rubino FA, DeRemee RA, et al. Neurologic involvement in Wegener's granulomatosis: an analysis of 324 consecutive patients at the Mayo Clinic. Ann Neurol 1993;33:4–9.

73. Rosete A, Cabral R, Kraus A, Alarcón-Segovia D. Diabetes insipidus secondary to Wegener's granulomatosis: report and review of the literature. J Rheumatol 1991;18:761–5.

74. Roberts GA, Eren E, Sinclair H, et al. Two cases of Wegener's granulomatosis involving the pituitary. Clin Endocrinol 1995;42:323–8.

75. Czarnecki EJ, Spickler EM. MR demonstration of Wegener granulomatosis of the infundibulum, a cause of diabetes insipidus. AJNR Am J Neuroradiol 1995;16:968–70.

76. Garovic VD, Clarke BL, Chilson TS, Specks U. Diabetes insipidus and anterior pituitary insufficiency as presenting features of Wegener's granulomatosis [abstract]. Am J Kidney Dis 2001;37:E5.

77. Miller KS, Miller JM. Wegener's granulomatosis presenting as a primary seizure disorder with brain lesions demonstrated by magnetic resonance imaging. Chest 1993;103:316–8.

78. Vaile JH, Owen ET, Rhodes HC, et al. A granulomatous meningeal mass as the initial presentation of Wegener's granulomatosis. Aust N Z J Med 1995;25:369–70.

79. Jinnah HA, Dixon A, Brat DJ, Hellmann DB. Chronic meningitis with cranial neuropathies in Wegener's granulomatosis. Arthritis Rheum 1997;40:573–7.

80. Specks U, Moder KG, McDonald TJ. Meningeal involvement in Wegener granulomatosis. Mayo Clin Proc 2000;75:856–9.

81. Weiss MA, Crissman JD. Segmental necrotizing glomerulonephritis: diagnostic, prognostic, and therapeutic significance. Am J Kidney Dis 1985;4:199–211.

82. Furlong TJ, Ibels LS, Eckstein RP. The clinical spectrum of necrotizing glomerulonephritis. Medicine 1987;66:192–201.

83. Oliet A, Praga M, Vidaur F, et al. Periglomerular granulomatosis. A limited form of Wegener's granulomatosis with exclusive renal involvement? Arch Intern Med 1988;148:1377–9.

84. Baker SB, Robinson DR. Unusual renal manifestations of Wegener's granulomatosis. Report of two cases. Am J Med 1978;64:883–9.

85. van der Woude FJ, Hoorntje SJ, Weening JJ, et al. Renal involvement in Wegener's granulomatosis. Report of three unusual cases. Nephron 1982;32:185–7.

86. Woodworth TG, Abuelo JG, Austin HA, Esparza A. Severe glomerulonephritis with late emergence of classic Wegener's granulomatosis. Report of 4 cases and review of the literature. Medicine 1987;66:181–91.

87. Landman S, Burgener F. Pulmonary manifestations in Wegener's granulomatosis. Am J Roentgenol 1974;172:750–7.

88. Maguire R, Fauci AS, Doppman JL, Wolff SM. Unusual radiographic features of Wegener's granulomatosis. AJR Am J Roentgenol 1978;130:233–8.

89. Cordier J-F, Valeyre D, Guillevin L, et al. Pulmonary Wegener's granulomatosis. A clinical and imaging study of 77 cases. Chest 1990;97:906–12.

90. Amin R. Endobronchial involvement in Wegener's granulomatosis. Postgrad Med J 1983;59:452–4.

91. Malik SW, Myers JL, DeRemee RA, Specks U. Lung toxicity associated with cyclophosphamide use: two distinct patterns. Am J Respir Crit Care Med 1996;154:1851–6.

92. Yale SH, Limper AH. *Pneumocystis carinii* pneumonia in patients without acquired immunodeficiency syndrome: associated illnesses and prior corticosteroid therapy. Mayo Clin Proc 1996;71:5–13.

93. Kremer JM, Alarcon GS, Weinblatt ME, et al. Clinical, laboratory, radiographic, and histopathologic features of methotrexate-associated lung injury in patients with rheumatoid arthritis: a multicenter study with literature review [see comments]. Arthritis Rheum 1997;40:1829–37.

94. Alarcon GS, Kremer JM, Macaluso M, et al. Risk factors for methotrexate-induced lung injury in patients with rheumatoid arthritis. A multicenter, case-control study. Methotrexate-Lung Study Group. Ann Intern Med 1997;127:356–64.

95. von Schubert F, Muhle C, Schnabel A, et al. High-resolution CT (HRCT) der Lunge bei Wegenerscher Granulomatose. Fortschr Röntgenstr 1994;161:19–24.

96. Summers RM, Aggarwal NR, Sneller MC, et al. CT virtual bronchoscopy of the central airways in patients with Wegener's granulomatosis. Chest 2002;121:242–50.

97. Belden CJ, Hamed LM, Mancuso AA. Bilateral isolated retrobulbar optic neuropathy in limited Wegener's granulomatosis. J Clin Neuroophthalmol 1993;13:119–23.

98. Newman NJ, Slamovits TL, Friedland S, Wilson WB. Neuroophthalmic manifestations of meningocerebral inflammation from the limited form of Wegener's granulomatosis. Am J Ophthalmol 1995;120:613–21.

99. Calabrese LH. Diagnostic strategies in vasculitis affecting the central nervous system. Cleve Clin J Med 2002;69: SII105–108.

100. Colby TV, Specks U. Wegener's granulomatosis in the 1990s—a pulmonary pathologist's perspective. Monogr Pathol 1993;36:195–218.

101. Fienberg R. The protracted superficial phenomenon in pathergic (Wegener's) granulomatosis. Hum Pathol 1980;12: 458–67.

102. Yoshikawa Y, Watanabe T. Pulmonary lesions in Wegener's granulomatosis: a clinicopathologic study of 22 autopsy cases. Hum Pathol 1986;17:401–10.

103. Mark EJ, Matsubara O, Tan-Liu NS, Fienberg R. The pulmonary biopsy in the early diagnosis of Wegener's (pathergic) granulomatosis: a study based on 35 open lung biopsies. Hum Pathol 1988;19:1065–71.

104. Yousem SA, Lombard CM. The eosinophilic variant of Wegener's granulomatosis. Hum Pathol 1988;19:682–8.

105. Travis WD, Colby TV, Lombard C, Carpenter HA. A clinicopathologic study of 34 cases of diffuse pulmonary hemorrhage with lung biopsy confirmation. Am J Surg Pathol 1990;14:1112–25.

106. Yousem SA. Bronchocentric injury in Wegener's granulomatosis: a report of five cases. Hum Pathol 1991;22:535–40.

107. Goulart RA, Mark EJ, Rosen S. Tumefactions as an extravascular manifestation of Wegener's granulomatosis. Am J Surg Pathol 1995;19:145–53.

108. Uner AH, Rozum-Slota B, Katzenstein A-L. Bronchiolitis obliterans-organizing pneumonia (BOOP)-like variant of Wegener's granulomatosis. A clinicopathologic study of 16 cases. Am J Surg Pathol 1996;20:794–801.

109. Mark EJ, Flieder DB, Matsubara O. Treated Wegener's granulomatosis: distinctive pathological findings in the lungs of 20 patients and what they tell us about the natural history of the disease. Hum Pathol 1997;28:450–8.

110. Del Buono EA, Flint A. Diagnostic usefulness of nasal biopsy in Wegener's granulomatosis. Hum Pathol 1991;22:107–10.

111. Travis WD, Hoffman GS, Leavitt RY, et al. Surgical pathology of the lung in Wegener's granulomatosis. Am J Surg Pathol 1991;15:315–33.

112. Colby TV, Tazelaar H, Specks U, DeRemee RA. Nasal biopsy in Wegener's granulomatosis. Hum Pathol 1991;22:101–4.

113. Katzenstein ALA, Locke WK. Solitary lung lesions in Wegener's granulomatosis—pathologic findings and clinical significance in 25 cases. Am J Surg Pathol 1995;19:545–52.

114. Davies DJ, Moran JE, Niall JF, Ryan GB. Segmental necrotising glomerulonephritis with antineutrophil antibody: possible arbovirus aetiology. Br Med J 1982;285:606.

115. Hall JB, Wadham BM, Wood CJ, et al. Vasculitis and glomerulonephritis: a subgroup with an antineutrophil cytoplasmic antibody. Aust N Z J Med 1984;14:277–8.

116. van der Woude FJ, Rasmussen N, Lobatto S, et al. Autoantibodies against neutrophils and monocytes: tool for diagnosis and marker of disease activity in Wegener's granulomatosis. Lancet 1985;i:425–9.

117. Ohdama S, Matsubara O, Aoki N. Plasma thrombomodulin in Wegener's granulomatosis as an indicator of vascular injuries. Chest 1994;106:666–71.

118. Boehme MW, Schmitt WH, Youinou P, et al. Clinical relevance of elevated serum thrombomodulin and soluble E-selectin in patients with Wegener's granulomatosis and other systemic vasculitides. Am J Med 1996;101:387–94.

119. Mrowka C, Sieberth HG. Circulating adhesion molecules ICAM-1, VCAM-1 and E-selectin in systemic vasculitis: marked differences between Wegener's granulomatosis and SLE. Clin Invest 1994;72:762–8.

120. Westphal JR, Boerbooms AMT, Schalkwijk CJM, et al. Anti-endothelial cell antibodies in sera of patients with autoim-

mune diseases: comparison between ELISA and FACS analysis. Clin Exp Immunol 1994;96:444–9.

121. DeRemee RA. Sarcoidosis and Wegener's granulomatosis: a comparative analysis. Sarcoidosis 1994;11:7–18.

122. Trimarchi M, Gregorini G, Facchetti F, et al. Cocaine-induced midline destructive lesions: clinical, radiographic, histopathologic, and serologic features and their differentiation from Wegener's granulomatosis. Medicine (Baltimore) 2001;80:391–404.

123. Specks U, Wheatley CL, McDonald TJ, et al. Anticytoplasmic autoantibodies in the diagnosis and follow-up of Wegener's granulomatosis. Mayo Clin Proc 1989;64:28–36.

124. Papo T, Piette JC, Du LTH, et al. Antineutrophil cytoplasmic antibodies in polychondritis. Ann Rheum Dis 1993;52:384–5.

125. Piette JC, Papo T, Du LTH, Meyer O. Relapsing polychondritis as a secondary phenomenon of primary systemic vasculitis. Ann Rheum Dis 1993;52:896–7.

126. Nölle B, Specks U, Lüdemann J, et al. Anticytoplasmic autoantibodies: their immunodiagnostic value. Ann Intern Med 1989;111:28–40.

127. Handrock K, Gross WL. Relapsing polychondritis as a secondary phenomenon of primary systemic vasculitis. Ann Rheum Dis 1993;52:895–6.

128. Specks U. Diffuse alveolar hemorrhage syndromes. Curr Opin Rheumatol 2001;13:12–7.

129. Lauque D, Cadranel J, Lazor R, et al. Microscopic polyangiitis with alveolar hemorrhage. A study of 29 cases and review of the literature. Medicine (Baltimore) 2000;79:222–33.

130. Gallagher H, Kwan JT, Jayne DR. Pulmonary renal syndrome: a 4-year, single-center experience. Am J Kidney Dis 2002;39:42–7.

131. Walton EW. Giant-cell granuloma of the respiratory tract (Wegener's granulomatosis). Br Med J 1958;2:265–70.

132. Fauci AS, Haynes BF, Katz P, Wolff SM. Wegener's granulomatosis: prospective clinical and therapeutic experience with 85 patients for 21 years. Ann Intern Med 1983;98:76–85.

133. Jayne D. Update on the European vasculitis study group trials. Curr Opin Rheumatol 2001;13:48–55.

134. Talar-Williams C, Hijazi YM, Walther MM, et al. Cyclophosphamide-induced cystitis and bladder cancer in patients with Wegener granulomatosis. Ann Intern Med 1996;124:477–84.

135. Stillwell TJ, Benson RC Jr, DeRemee RA, et al. Cyclophosphamide-induced bladder toxicity in Wegener's granulomatosis. Arthritis Rheum 1988;31:465–70.

136. Boomsma MM, Stegeman CA, Kramer AB, et al. Prevalence of reduced bone mineral density in patients with antineutrophil cytoplasmic antibody associated vasculitis and the role of immunosuppressive therapy: a cross-sectional study. Osteoporos Int 2002;13:74–82.

137. Hoffman GS, Leavitt RY, Fleisher TA, et al. Treatment of Wegener's granulomatosis with intermittent high-dose intravenous cyclophosphamide. Am J Med 1990;89:403–10.

138. Reinhold-Keller E, Kekow J, Schnabel A, et al. Influence of disease manifestation and antineutrophil cytoplasmic antibody titer on the response to pulse cyclophosphamide therapy in patients with Wegener's granulomatosis. Arthritis Rheum 1994;37:919–24.

139. Généreau T, Lortholary O, Leclerq P, et al. Treatment of systemic vasculitis with cyclophosphamide and steroids: daily oral low-dose cyclophosphamide administration after failure of a pulse intravenous high-dose regimen in four patients. Br J Rheumatol 1994;33:959–62.

140. Guillevin L, Cordier JF, Lhote F, et al. A prospective, multicenter, randomized trial comparing steroids and pulse cyclophosphamide versus steroids and oral cyclophosphamide in the treatment of generalized Wegener's granulomatosis. Arthritis Rheum 1997;40:2187–98.

141. Gayraud M, Guillevin L, Cohen P, et al. Treatment of good-prognosis polyarteritis nodosa and Churg-Strauss syndrome: comparison of steroids and oral or pulse cyclophosphamide in 25 patients. French Cooperative Study Group for Vasculitides. Br J Rheumatol 1997;36:1290–1297.

142. Adu D, Pall A, Luqmani RA, et al. Controlled trial of pulse versus continuous prednisolone and cyclophosphamide in the treatment of systemic vasculitis. Q J Med 1997;90:401–9.

143. Haubitz M, Schellong S, Göbel Y, et al. Intravenous pulse administration of cyclophosphamide versus daily oral treatment in patients with antineutrophil cytoplasmic antibody-associated vasculitis and renal involvement. Arthritis Rheum 1998;41:1835–44.

144. de Groot K, Adu D, Savage CO. The value of pulse cyclophosphamide in ANCA-associated vasculitis: meta-analysis and critical review. Nephrol Dial Transplant 2001;16:2018–27.

145. Langevitz P, Klein L, Pras M, Many A. The effect of cyclophosphamide pulses on fertility in patients with lupus nephritis. Am J Reprod Immunol 1992;28:157–8.

146. Boumpas DT, Austin HA III, Vaughan EM, et al. Risk for sustained amenorrhea in patients with systemic lupus erythematosus receiving intermittent pulse cyclophosphamide therapy. Ann Intern Med 1993;119:366–9.

147. Capizzi RL, Bertino JR. Methotrexate therapy of Wegener's granulomatosis. Ann Intern Med 1971;74:74–9.

148. Sneller MC, Hoffman GW, Talar-Williams C, et al. An analysis of forty-two Wegener's granulomatosis patients treated with methotrexate and prednisone. Arthritis Rheum 1995;38:608–13.

149. Godeau B, Coutant-Perrone V, Le Thi Huong D, et al. *Pneumocystis carinii* pneumonia in the course of connective tissue disease: report of 34 cases. J Rheumatol 1994;21:246–51.

150. Morgan SL, Baggott JE, Vaughn WH, et al. Supplementation with folic acid during methotrexate therapy for rheumatoid arthritis. Ann Intern Med 1994;121:833–41.

151. de Groot K, Muhler M, Reinhold-Keller E, et al. Induction of remission in Wegener's granulomatosis with low dose methotrexate. J Rheumatol 1998;25:492–5.

152. Stone JH, Tun W, Hellman DB. Treatment of non-life threatening Wegener's granulomatosis with methotrexate and daily prednisone as the initial therapy of choice. J Rheumatol 1999;26:1134–9.

153. Langford CA, Talar-Williams C, Barron KS, Sneller MC. A staged approach to the treatment of Wegener's granulomatosis: induction of remission with glucocorticoids and daily cyclophosphamide switching to methotrexate for remission maintenance. Arthritis Rheum 1999;42:2666–73.

154. Reinhold-Keller E, Fink CO, Herlyn K, et al. High rate of renal relapse in 71 patients with Wegener's granulomatosis under maintenance of remission with low-dose methotrexate. Arthritis Rheum 2002;47:326–32.

155. Lennard L, Van Loon JA, Weinshilboum RM. Pharmacogenetics of acute azathioprine toxicity: relationship to thiopurine methyltransferase genetic polymorphism. Clin Pharmacol Ther 1989;46:149–54.

156. Stolk JN, Boerbooms AMT, De Abreu RA, et al. Reduced thiopurine methyltransferase activity and development of side effects of azathioprine treatment in patients with rheumatoid arthritis. Arthritis Rheum 1998;41:1858–66.

157. Yates CR, Krynetski EY, Loennechen T, et al. Molecular diagnosis of thiopurine S-methyltransferase deficiency: genetic basis for azathioprine and mercaptopurine intolerance. Ann Intern Med 1997;126:608–14.

158. Nowack R, Göbel U, Klooker P, et al. Mycophenolate mofetil for maintenance therapy of Wegener's granulomatosis and microscopic polyangiitis: a pilot study in 11 patients with renal involvement. J Am Soc Nephrol 1999;10:1965–71.

159. Gross WL. New concepts in treatment protocols for severe systemic vasculitis. Curr Opin Rheumatol 1999;11:41–6.

160. Gaskin G, Pusey CD. Plasmapheresis in antineutrophil cytoplasmic antibody-associated systemic vasculitis. Ther Apher 2001;5:176–81.

161. Jayne DR, Black CM, Davies M, Lockwood CM. Treatment of systemic vasculitis with pooled intravenous immunoglobulin. Lancet 1991;337:1137–9.

162. Tuso P, Moudgil A, Hay J, et al. Treatment of antineutrophil cytoplasmic autoantibody-positive systemic vasculitis and glomerulonephritis with pooled intravenous gammaglobulin. Am J Kidney Dis 1992;20:504–8.

163. Jayne DR, Esnault V, Lockwood CM. ANCA anti-idiotype antibodies and the treatment of systemic vasculitis with intravenous immunoglobulin. J Autoimmun 1993;6:207–19.

164. Richter C, Schnabel A, Csernok E, et al. Treatment of Wegener's granulomatosis with intravenous immunoglobulin. Adv Exp Med Biol 1993;336:487–9.

165. Jayne DR, Lockwood CM. Intravenous immunoglobulin as sole therapy for systemic vasculitis. Br J Rheumatol 1996;35:1150–3.

166. Jayne DR, Chapel H, Adu D, et al. Intravenous immunoglobulin for ANCA-associated systemic vasculitis with persistent disease activity. Q J Med 2000;93:433–9.

167. Pall AA, Varagunam M, Adu D, et al. Anti-idiotypic activity against anti-myeloperoxidase antibodies in pooled human immunoglobulin. Clin Exp Immunol 1994;95:257–62.

168. Kindler V, Sappino AP, Grau GE, et al. The inducing role of tumor necrosis factor in the development of bactericidal granulomas during BCG infection. Cell 1989;56:731–40.

169. Nassonov EL, Samsonov MY, Tilz GP, et al. Serum concentrations of neopterin, soluble interleukin 2 receptor, and soluble tumor necrosis factor receptor in Wegener's granulomatosis. J Rheumatol 1997;24:666–70.

170. Jonasdottir O, Petersen J, Bendtzen K. Tumour necrosis factor-alpha (TNF), lymphotoxin and TNF receptor levels in serum from patients with Wegener's granulomatosis. Apmis 2001;109:781–6.

171. Falk RJ, Hogan S, Carey TS, et al. Clinical course of antineutrophil cytoplasmic autoantibody-associated glomerulonephritis and systemic vasculitis. Ann Intern Med 1990;113:656–63.

172. Reumaux D, Vossebeld PJM, Roos D, Verhoeven AJ. Effect of tumor necrosis factor-induced integrin activation on Fcg receptor II-mediated signal transduction: relevance for activation of neutrophils by anti-proteinase 3 or anti-myeloperoxidase antibodies. Blood 1995;86:3189–95.

173. Stone JH, Uhlfelder ML, Hellmann DB, et al. Etanercept combined with conventional treatment in Wegener's granulomatosis: a six-month open-label trial to evaluate safety. Arthritis Rheum 2001;44:1149–54.

174. The WGET Research Group. Design of the Wegener's granulomatosis etanercept trial (WGET). Control Clin Trials 2002;23:450–68.

175. Specks U, Fervenza FC, McDonald TJ, Hogan MC. Response of Wegener's granulomatosis to anti-CD20 chimeric monoclonal antibody therapy. Arthritis Rheum 2001;44:2836–40.

176. Congdon D, Sherris DA, Specks U, McDonald T. Long-term follow-up of repair of external nasal deformities in patients with Wegener's granulomatosis. Laryngoscope 2002;112:731–7.

177. Hardwig PW, Bartley GB, Garrity JA. Surgical management of nasolacrimal duct obstruction in patients with Wegener's granulomatosis. Ophthalmology 1992;99:133–9.

178. Wong RJ, Gliklich RE, Rubin PA, Goodman M. Bilateral nasolacrimal duct obstruction managed with endoscopic techniques. Arch Otolaryngol Head Neck Surg 1998;124:703–6.

179. Kwan AS, Rose GE. Lacrimal drainage surgery in Wegener's granulomatosis. Br J Ophthalmol 2000;84:329–31.

180. Langford CA, Sneller MC, Hallahan CW, et al. Clinical features and therapeutic management of subglottic stenosis in patients with Wegener's granulomatosis. Arthritis Rheum 1996;39:1754–60.

181. McCaffrey TV. Management of subglottic stenosis in the adult. Ann Otol Rhinol Laryngol 1991;100:90–4.

182. Herridge MS, Pearson FG, Downey GP. Subglottic stenosis complicating Wegener's granulomatosis: surgical repair as a viable treatment option. J Thorac Cardiovasc Surg 1996;111:961–6.

183. Nachman PH, Sejelmark M, Westman K, et al. Recurrent ANCA-associated small vessel vasculitis after transplantation: a pooled analysis. Kidney Int 1999;56:1544–50.

184. Westman KW, Bygren PG, Olsson H, et al. Relapse rate, renal survival, and cancer morbidity in patients with Wegener's granulomatosis or microscopic polyangiitis with renal involvement. J Am Soc Nephrol 1998;9:842–52.

185. Schmitt WH, Haubitz M, Mistry N, et al. Renal transplantation in Wegener's granulomatosis. Lancet 1993;342:860.

186. Clarke AE, Bitton A, Eappen R, et al. Treatment of Wegener's granulomatosis after renal transplantation. Is cyclosporine the preferred treatment? Transplantation 1990;50:1047–51.

187. Boubenider SA, Akhtar M, Alfurayh O, et al. Late recurrence of Wegener's granulomatosis presenting as tracheal stenosis in a renal transplant patient. Clin Transplantation 1994;8:5–9.

188. DeRemee RA, McDonald TJ, Weiland LH. Wegener's granulomatosis: observations on treatment with antimicrobial agents. Mayo Clin Proc 1985;60:27–32.

189. Israel HL. Sulfamethoxazole-trimethoprim therapy for Wegener's granulomatosis. Arch Intern Med 1988;148:2293–5.

190. Fukuda K, Yuasa K, Uchizono A, et al. Three cases of Wegener's granulomatosis treated with an antimicrobial agent. Arch Otolaryngol Head Neck Surg 1989;115:515–8.

191. Georgi J, Ulmer JG, Gross WL. Co-trimoxazol bei Wegenerscher Granulomatose—eine prospektive Studie. Immun Inekt 1991;19:97–8.

192. McRae D, Buchanan G. Long-term sulfamethoxazole-trimethoprim in Wegener's granulomatosis. Arch Otolaryngol Head Neck Surg 1993;119:103–5.

193. Valeriano-Marcet J, Spiera H. Treatment of Wegener's granulomatosis with sulfamethoxazole-trimethoprim. Arch Intern Med 1991;151:1649–52.

194. DeRemee RA. Wegener's granulomatosis. Ann Intern Med 1992;117:619–20.

195. Reinhold-Keller E, De Groot K, Rudert H, et al. Response to trimethoprim/sulfamethoxazole in Wegener's granulomatosis depends on the phase of disease. Q J Med 1996;89:15–23.

196. de Groot K, Reinhold-Keller E, Tatsis E, et al. Therapy for the maintenance of remission in sixty-five patients with generalized Wegener's granulomatosis. Methotrexate versus trimethoprim/sulfamethoxazole. Arthritis Rheum 1996;39:2052–61.

197. Stegeman CA, Tervaert JWC, Kallenberg CGM. Co-trimoxazole in Wegener's granulomatosis—reply. N Engl J Med 1996;335:1770.

198. Stegeman CA, Cohen Tervaert JW, Sluiter WJ, et al. Association of chronic nasal carriage of *Staphylococcus aureus* and higher relapse rates in Wegener granulomatosis. Ann Intern Med 1994;120:12–7.

199. Welch WD, Davis D, Thrupp LD. Effect of antimicrobial agents on human polymorphonuclear leukocyte microbicidal function. Antimicrob Agents Chemother 1981;20:15–20.

200. Siegel JP, Remington JS. Effect of antimicrobial agents on chemiluminescence of human polymorphonuclear leukocytes in response to phagocytosis. J Antimicrob Chemother 1982;10:505–15.

201. Voisin C, Carré P, Piva F, Wallaert B. Macrophages alvéolaires et antibiotiques. Pathol Biol 1987;35:1412–7.

202. Carré P, Forgue MF, Pipy B, et al. Effets du cotrimoxazole sur certaines fonctions de macrophages: microbicidie, tumoricidie, production de radicaux libres oxygénés, de prostaglandines et de leucotriènes. Pathol Biol 1990;38:289–93.

203. Gaylarde PM, Sarkany I. Suppression of thymidine uptake of human lymphocytes by co-trimoxazole. Br Med J 1972;3:144–6.

204. Kussmaul A, Maier R. Über eine bisher nicht beschriebene eigenthümliche Arterienerkrankung (Periarteritis nodosa), die mit Morbus Brightii und rapid fortschreitender allge-

meiner Muskellähmung einhergeht. Dtsch Arch Klin Med 1866;1:484–514.

205. Falk RJ, Jennette JC. Anti-neutrophil cytoplasmic autoantibodies with specificity for myeloperoxidase in patients with systemic vasculitis and idiopathic necrotizing and crescentic glomerulonephritis. N Engl J Med 1988;25:1651–7.

206. Savage COS, Winearls CG, Jones S, et al. Prospective study of radioimmunoassay for antibodies against neutrophil cytoplasm in diagnosis of systemic vasculitis. Lancet 1987;i:1389–93.

207. Kallenberg CGM, Brouwer E, Weening JJ, Cohen Tervaert JW. Anti-neutrophil cytoplasmic antibodies: current diagnostic and pathophysiological potential. Kidney Int 1994;46:1–5.

208. Jennette JC, Falk RJ. Clinical and pathological classification of ANCA-associated vasculitis: what are the controversies? Clin Exp Immunol 1995;101 Suppl 1:18–22.

209. Kirkland GS, Savige J, Wilson D, et al. Classical polyarteritis nodosa and microscopic polyarteritis with medium vessel involvement—a comparison of the clinical and laboratory features. Clin Nephrol 1997;47:176–80.

210. Matsumoto T, Homma S, Okada M, et al. The lung in polyarteritis nodosa: a pathologic study of 10 cases. Hum Pathol 1993;24:717–24.

211. Fisher RG, Graham DY, Granmayeh M, Trabanino JG. Polyarteritis nodosa and hepatitis-B surface antigen: role of angiography in diagnosis. AJR Am J Roentgenol 1977;129:77–81.

212. Nick J, Tuder R, May R, Fisher J. Polyarteritis nodosa with pulmonary vasculitis. Am J Respir Crit Care Med 1996;153:450–3.

213. Gayraud M, Guillevin L, le Toumelin P, et al. Long-term followup of polyarteritis nodosa, microscopic polyangiitis, and Churg-Strauss syndrome: analysis of four prospective trials including 278 patients. Arthritis Rheum 2001;44:666–75.

214. Guillevin L, Visser H, Noel LH, et al. Antineutrophil cytoplasm antibodies in systemic polyarteritis nodosa with and without hepatitis B virus infection and Churg-Strauss syndrome —62 patients. J Rheumatol 1993;20:1345–9.

215. Hauschild S, Csernok E, Schmitt WH, Gross WL. Antineutrophil cytoplasmic antibodies in systemic polyarteritis nodosa with and without hepatitis B virus infection and Churg-Strauss syndrome—62 patients. J Rheumatol 1994;21:1173–4.

216. Baranger TAR, Audrain MAP, Testa A, et al. Anti-neutrophil cytoplasm antibodies in patients with ACR criteria for polyarteritis nodosa: help for systemic vasculitis classification? Autoimmunity 1995;20:33–7.

217. Bruce IN, Bell AL. A comparison of two nomenclature systems for primary systemic vasculitis. Br J Rheumatol 1997;36:453–8.

218. Sorensen SF, Slot O, Tvede N, Petersen J. A prospective study of vasculitis patients collected in a five-year period: evaluation of the Chapel Hill nomenclature. Ann Rheum Dis 2000;59:478–82.

219. Lane SE, Scott DG, Heaton A, Watts RA. Primary renal vasculitis in Norfolk—increasing incidence or increasing recognition? Nephrol Dial Transplant 2000;15:23–7.

220. Guillevin L, Durand-Gasselin B, Cevallos R, et al. Microscopic polyangiitis: clinical and laboratory findings in eighty-five patients. Arthritis Rheum 1999;42:421–30.

221. Akikusa B, Kondo Y, Irabu N, et al. Six cases of microscopic polyarteritis exhibiting acute interstitial pneumonia. Pathol Int 1995;45:580–8.

222. Nada AK, Torres VE, Ryu JH, et al. Pulmonary fibrosis as an unusual clinical manifestation of a pulmonary–renal vasculitis in elderly patients. Mayo Clin Proc 1990;65:847–56.

223. Hiromura K, Nojima Y, Kitahara T, et al. Four cases of antimyeloperoxidase antibody-related rapidly progressive glomerulonephritis during the course of idiopathic pulmonary fibrosis. Clin Nephrol 2000;53:384–9.

224. Souid M, Terki NH, Nochy D, Hillion D. Myeloperoxidase anti-neutrophil cytoplasmic autoantibodies (MPO-ANCA)- related rapidly progressive glomerulonephritis (RPGN) and pulmonary fibrosis (PF) with dissociated evolution. Clin Nephrol 2001;55:337–8.

225. Brugiere O, Raffy O, Sleiman C, et al. Progressive obstructive lung disease associated with microscopic polyangiitis. Am J Respir Crit Care Med 1997;155:739–42.

226. McKane WS, Velasco N, Farrington K. ANCA-positive crescentic glomerulonephritis in chronic bronchiectasis. Nephrol Dial Transplant 1995;10:1447–50.

227. Hogan SL, Nachman PH, Wilkman AS, et al. Prognostic markers in patients with antineutrophil cytoplasmic autoantibody-associated microscopic polyangiitis and glomerulonephritis. J Am Soc Nephrol 1996;7:23–32.

228. Nachman PH, Hogan SL, Jennette JC, Falk RJ. Treatment response and relapse in antineutrophil cytoplasmic autoantibody-associated microscopic polyangiitis and glomerulonephritis. J Am Soc Nephrol 1996;7:33–9.

229. Gordon M, Luqmani RA, Adu D, et al. Relapses in patients with a systemic vasculitis. Q J Med 1993;86:779–89.

230. Churg JC, Strauss L. Allergic granulomatosis, allergic angiitis and periarteritis nodosa. Am J Pathol 1951;27:277–301.

231. Chumbley LC, Harrison EG, DeRemee RA. Allergic granulomatosis and angiitis (Churg-Strauss syndrome). Mayo Clin Proc 1977;52:477–84.

232. Finan MC, Winkelmann RK. The cutaneous extravascular necrotizing granuloma (Churg-Strauss granuloma) and systemic disease: a review of 27 cases. Medicine 1983;62:142–58.

233. Lie JT. Limited forms of Churg-Strauss syndrome. Pathology Annual 1993;28:199–220.

234. Churg A. Recent advances in the diagnosis of Churg-Strauss syndrome. Mod Pathol 2001;14:1284–93.

235. Churg A, Brallas M, Cronin SR, Churg J. Formes frustes of Churg-Strauss syndrome. Chest 1995;108:320–3.

236. Wechsler ME, Garpestad E, Flier SR, et al. Pulmonary infiltrates, eosinophilia, and cardiomyopathy following corticosteroid withdrawal in patients with asthma receiving zafirlukast. JAMA 1998;279:455–7.

237. Lanham JG, Elkon KB, Pusey CD, Hughes GR. Systemic vasculitis with asthma and eosinophilia: a clinical approach to the Churg-Strauss syndrome. Medicine 1984;63:65–81.

238. Masi AT, Hunder GG, Lie JT, et al. The American College of Rheumatology 1990 criteria for the classification of Churg-Strauss syndrome (allergic granulomatosis and angiitis). Arthritis Rheum 1990;33:1094–100.

239. Keogh K, Specks U. Churg-Strauss syndrome in the 1990's: the pathogenic role of ANCA and leukotriene receptor antagonists remain unclear. Am J Med 2002;Submitted.

240. Sehgal M, Swanson JW, DeRemee RA, Colby TV. Neurologic manifestations of Churg-Strauss syndrome. Mayo Clin Proc 1995;70:337–41.

241. Loughlin JE, Cole JA, Rothman KJ, Johnson ES. Prevalence of serious eosinophilia and incidence of Churg-Strauss syndrome in a cohort of asthma patients. Ann Allergy Asthma Immunol 2002;88:319–25.

242. Guillevin L, Cohen P, Gayraud M, et al. Churg-Strauss syndrome. Clinical study and long-term follow-up of 96 patients. Medicine 1999;78:26–37.

243. Reid AJC, Harrison BDW, Watts RA, et al. Churg-Strauss syndrome in a district hospital. Q J Med 1998;91:219–29.

244. Solans R, Bosch JA, Perez-Bocanegra C, et al. Churg-Strauss syndrome: outcome and long-term follow-up of 32 patients. Rheumatology (Oxford) 2001;40:763–71.

245. Choi YH, Im JG, Han BK, et al. Thoracic manifestation of Churg-Strauss syndrome: radiologic and clinical findings. Chest 2000;117:117–24.

246. Ishiyama A, Canalis RF. Otological manifestations of Churg-Strauss syndrome. Laryngoscope 2001;111:1619–24.

247. Robin JB, Schanzlin DJ, Meisler DM, et al. Ocular involve-

ment in the respiratory vasculitides. Surv Ophthalmol 1985;30:127–40.

248. Takanashi T, Uchida S, Arita M, et al. Orbital inflammatory pseudotumor and ischemic vasculitis in Churg-Strauss syndrome: report of two cases and review of the literature. Ophthalmology 2001;108:1129–33.

249. Vitali C, Genovesi-Ebert F, Romani A, et al. Ophthalmological and neuro-ophthalmological involvement in Churg–Strauss syndrome: a case report. Graefe's Arch Clin Exp Ophthalmol 1996;234:404–8.

250. Schmitt WH, Csernok E, Kobayashi S, et al. Churg-Strauss syndrome. Serum markers of lymphocyte activation and endothelial damage. Arthritis Rheum 1998;41:445–52.

251. Hurst S, Chizzolini C, Dayer JM, et al. Usefulness of serum eosinophil cationic protein (ECP) in predicting relapse of Churg and Strauss vasculitis. Clin Exp Rheumatol 2000; 18:784–5.

252. Cottin V, Tardy F, Gindre D, et al. Urinary eosinophil-derived neurotoxin in Churg-Strauss syndrome. J Allergy Clin Immunol 1995;96:261–4.

253. Kurosawa M, Nakagami R, Morioka J, et al. Interleukins in Churg-Strauss syndrome. Allergy 2000;55:785–7.

254. Peen E, Hahn P, Lauwers G, et al. Churg-Strauss syndrome: localization of eosinophil major basic protein in damaged tissues. Arthritis Rheum 2000;43:1897–900.

255. Drage LA, Davis MD, De Castro F, et al. Evidence for pathogenic involvement of eosinophils and neutrophils in Churg-Strauss syndrome. J Am Acad Dermatol 2002;47: 209–16.

256. Kiene M, Csernok E, Muller A, et al. Elevated interleukin-4 and interleukin-13 production by T cell lines from patients with Churg-Strauss syndrome. Arthritis Rheum 2001;44: 469–73.

257. Muschen M, Warskulat U, Perniok A, et al. Involvement of soluble CD95 in Churg-Strauss syndrome. Am J Pathol 1999;155:915–25.

258. Guillevin L, Amouroux J, Arbeille B, Boura R. Churg-Strauss angiitis. Arguments favoring the responsibility of inhaled antigens. Chest 1991;100:1472–3.

259. Cohen Tervaert JW, Kallenberg CGM. Anti-myeloperoxidase antibodies in Churg-Strauss syndrome. J Neurol 1993; 240:449–52.

260. Potter MB, Fincher RK, Finger DR. Eosinophilia in Wegener's granulomatosis. Chest 1999;116:1480–3.

261. Franco J, Artes MJ. Pulmonary eosinophilia associated with montelukast. Thorax 1999;54:558–60.

262. Green RL, Vayonis AG. Churg-Strauss syndrome after zafirlukast in two patients not receiving systemic steroid treatment. Lancet 1999;353:725–6.

263. Kinoshita M, Shiraishi T, Koga T, et al. Churg-Strauss syndrome after corticosteroid withdrawal in an asthmatic patient treated with pranlukast. J Allergy Clin Immunol 1999;103:534–5.

264. Knoell DL, Lucas J, Allen JN. Churg-Strauss syndrome associated with Zafirlukast. Chest 1998;114:332–4.

265. Tuggey JM, Hosker HS. Churg-Strauss syndrome associated with montelukast therapy. Thorax 2000;55:805–6.

266. Wechsler ME, Finn D, Gunawardena D, et al. Churg-Strauss syndrome in patients receiving montelukast as treatment for asthma. Chest 2000;117:708–13.

267. Le Gall C, Pham S, Vignes S, et al. Inhaled corticosteroids and Churg-Strauss syndrome: a report of five cases. Eur Respir J 2000;15:978–81.

268. Weller PF, Plaut M, Taggart V, Trontell A. The relationship of asthma therapy and Churg-Strauss syndrome: NIH workshop summary report. J Allergy Clin Immunol 2001;108: 175–83.

269. Jamaleddine G, Diab K, Tabbarah Z, et al. Leukotriene antagonists and the Churg-Strauss syndrome. Semin Arthritis Rheum 2002;31:218–27.

270. Tatsis E, Schnabel A, Gross WL. Interferon-α treatment of four patients with the Churg-Strauss syndrome. Ann Intern Med 1998;129:370–4.

271. Termeer CC, Simon JC, Schopf E. Low-dose interferon-α–2b for the treatment of Churg-Strauss syndrome with prominent skin involvement. Arch Dermatol 2001;137:136–8.

272. Jenne DE, Tschopp J, Lüdemann J, et al. Wegener's autoantigen decoded. Nature 1990;346:520.

273. Lüdemann J, Utecht B, Gross WL. Anti-neutrophil cytoplasm antibodies in Wegener's granulomatosis recognize an elastinolytic enzyme. J Exp Med 1990;171:357–62.

274. Niles JL, Ahmad MR, McCluskey RT, Arnaout MA. Specificity of anti-neutrophil cytoplasmic autoantibodies for proteinase 3. Blood 1990;75:2264.

275. Wiik A, van der Woude FJ. The new ACPA/ANCA nomenclature. Neth J Med 1990;35:107–8.

276. Hoffman GS, Specks U. Anti-neutrophil cytoplasmic antibodies. Arthritis Rheum 1998;41:1521–37.

277. Wang G, Csernok E, de Groot K, Gross WL. Comparison of eight commercial kits for quantitation of antineutrophil cytoplasmic antibodies (ANCA). J Immunol Methods 1997;208:203–11.

278. Specks U, Wiegert EM, Homburger HA. Human mast cells expressing recombinant proteinase 3 (PR3) as substrate for clinical testing for anti-neutrophil cytoplasmic antibodies (ANCA). Clin Exp Immunol 1997;109:286–95.

279. Lim LC, Taylor JG III, Schmitz JL, et al. Diagnostic usefulness of antineutrophil cytoplasmic autoantibody serology. Comparative evaluation of commercial indirect fluorescent antibody kits and enzyme immunoassay kits. Am J Clin Pathol 1999;111:363–9.

280. Stone JH, Talor M, Stebbing J, et al. Test characteristics of immunofluorescence and ELISA tests in 856 consecutive patients with possible ANCA-associated conditions. Arthritis Care Res 2000;13:424–34.

281. Hagen EC, Daha MR, Hermans J, et al. Diagnostic value of standardized assays for anti-neutrophil cytoplasmic antibodies in idiopathic systemic vasculitis. EC/BCR project for ANCA assay standardization. Kidney Int 1998;53:743–53.

282. Savige J, Gillis D, Benson E, et al. International consensus statement on testing and reporting of antineutrophil cytoplasmic antibodies (ANCA). Am J Clin Pathol 1999;111:507–13.

283. Savige J, Davies D, Falk RJ, et al. Antineutrophil cytoplasmic antibodies and associated diseases: a review of the clinical and laboratory features. Kidney Int 2000;57:846–62.

284. Russell KA, Wiegert E, Schroeder DR, et al. Detection of antineutrophil cytoplasmic antibodies under actual clinical testing conditions. Clin Immunol 2002;103:196–203.

285. Cohen Tervaert JW, van der Woude FJ, Fauci AS, et al. Association between active Wegener's granulomatosis and anticytoplasmic antibodies. Arch Intern Med 1989;149:2461–5.

286. Schnabel A, Csernok E, Isenberg DA, et al. Antineutrophil cytoplasmic antibodies in systemic lupus erythematosus. Arthritis Rheum 1995;38:633–7.

287. Merkel PA, Polisson RP, Chang Y, et al. Prevalence of antineutrophil cytoplasmic antibodies in a large inception cohort of patients with connective tissue disease. Ann Intern Med 1997;126:866–73.

288. Choi HK, Merkel PA, Walker AM, Niles JL. Drug-associated antineutrophil cytoplasmic antibody-positive vasculitis: prevalence among patients with high titers of antimyeloperoxidase antibodies. Arthritis Rheum 2000;43:405–13.

289. Choi HK, Lamprecht P, Niles JL, et al. Subacute bacterial endocarditis with positive cytoplasmic antineutrophil cytoplasmic antibodies and anti-proteinase 3 antibodies. Arthritis Rheum 2000;43:226–31.

290. Pudifin DJ, Duursma J, Gathiram V, Jackson TFHG. Invasive amoebiasis is associated with the development of anti–neutrophil cytoplasmic antibody. Clin Ex Immunol 1994; 97:48–51.

291. Wu YY, Hsu TC, Chen TY, et al. Proteinase 3 and dihydrolipoamide dehydrogenase (E3) are major autoantigens in hepatitis C virus (HCV) infection. Clin Exp Immunol 2002;128:347–52.

292. Langford CA. The diagnostic utility of c-ANCA in Wegener's granulomatosis. Cleve Clin J Med 1998;65:135–40.

293. Cohen Tervaert JW, Huitema MG, Hené RJ, et al. Prevention of relapses in Wegener's granulomatosis by treatment based on antineutrophil cytoplasmic antibody titre. Lancet 1990;336:709–11.

294. Kerr GS, Fleisher TA, Hallahan CW, et al. Limited prognostic value of changes in antineutrophil cytoplasmic antibody titer in patients with Wegener's granulomatosis. Arthritis Rheum 1993;36:365–71.

295. Boomsma MM, Stegeman CA, van der Leij MJ, et al. Prediction of relapses in Wegener's granulomatosis by measurement of antineutrophil cytoplasmic antibody levels. A prospective study. Arthritis Rheum 2000;43:2025–33.

296. Jayne DRW, Marshall PD, Jones SJ, Lockwood CM. Autoantibodies to GBM and neutrophil cytoplasm in rapidly progressive glomerulonephritis. Kidney Int 1990;37:956–70.

297. Weber MFA, Andrassy K, Pullig O, et al. Antineutrophil-cytoplasmic antibodies and antiglomerular basement membrane antibodies in Goodpasture's syndrome and in Wegener's granulomatosis. J Am Soc Nephrol 1992;2:1227–34.

298. Bygren P, Rasmussen N, Isaksson B, Wieslander J. Antineutrophil cytoplasm antibodies, anti-GBM antibodies and anti-dsDNA antibodies in glomerulonephritis. Eur J Clin Invest 1992;22:783–92.

299. Short AK, Esnault VLM, Lockwood CM. Anti-neutrophil cytoplasm antibodies and anti–glomerular basement membrane antibodies: two coexisting distinct autoreactivities detectable in patients with rapidly progressive glomerulonephritis. Am J Kidney Dis 1995;26:439–45.

300. Hellmark T, Niles JL, Collins AB, et al. Comparison of anti-GBM antibodies in sera with or without ANCA. J Am Soc Nephrol 1997;8:376–85.

301. Bosch X, Mirapeix E, Font J, et al. Prognostic implication of anti-neutrophil cytoplasmic autoantibodies with myeloperoxidase specificity in anti-glomerular basement membrane disease. Clin Neph 1991;36:107–13.

302. Verburgh CA, Bruijn JA, Daha MR, van Es LA. Sequential development of anti-GBM nephritis and ANCA-associated pauci-immune glomerulonephritis. Am J Kidney Dis 1999;34:344–8.

303. Russell KA, Specks U. Are antineutrophil cytoplasmic antibodies pathogenic? Experimental approaches to understand the antineutrophil cytoplasmic antibody phenomenon. Rheum Dis Clin North Am 2001;27:815–32, vii.

304. Hewins P, Tervaert JW, Savage CO, Kallenberg CG. Is Wegener's granulomatosis an autoimmune disease? Curr Opin Rheumatol 2000;12:3–10.

305. Savage CO, Harper L, Holland M. New findings in pathogenesis of antineutrophil cytoplasm antibody-associated vasculitis. Curr Opin Rheumatol 2002;14:15–22.

306. Noronha IL, Krüger C, Andrassy K, et al. In situ production of TNF-α, IL-1β and IL-2R in ANCA-positive glomerulonephritis. Kidney Int 1993;43:682–92.

307. Csernok E, Ernst M, Schmitt W, et al. Activated neutrophils express proteinase 3 on their plasma membrane in vitro and in vivo. Clin Exp Immunol 1994;95:244–50.

308. Witko-Sarsat V, Lesavre P, Lopez S, et al. A large subset of neutrophils expressing membrane proteinase 3 is a risk factor for vasculitis and rheumatoid arthritis. J Am Soc Nephrol 1999;10:1224–33.

309. Pinching AJ, Rees AJ, Pussell BA, et al. Relapses in Wegener's granulomatosis: the role of infection. Br Med J 1980;281:836–8.

310. Heeringa P, Brouwer E, Cohen Tervaert JW, et al. Animal models of anti-neutrophil cytoplasmic antibody associated vasculitis. Kidney Int 1998;53:253–63.

311. Specks U. Are animal models of vasculitis suitable tools? Curr Opin Rheumatol 2000;12:11–9.

312. Harper JM, Thiru S, Lockwood CM, Cooke A. Myeloperoxidase autoantibodies distinguish vasculitis mediated by anti-neutrophil cytoplasm antibodies from immune complex disease in MRL/Mp-*Ipr/Ipr* mice: a spontaneous model for human microscopic angiitis. Eur J Immunol 1998;28:2217–26.

313. Mathieson PW, Thiru S, Oliveira DB. Mercuric chloride-treated brown Norway rats develop widespread tissue injury including necrotizing vasculitis. Lab Invest 1992;67:121–9.

314. Albert LJ, Inman RD. Molecular mimicry and autoimmunity. N Engl J Med 1999;341:2068–74.

315. Craft J, Fatenejad S. Self antigens and epitope spreading in systemic autoimmunity. Arthritis Rheum 1997;40:1374–82.

316. Vanderlugt CJ, Miller SD. Epitope spreading. Curr Opin Immunol 1996;8:831–6.

317. Cohen Tervaert JW, Stegeman CA, Bakker H, et al. *Staphylococcus aureus* superantigens: a risk factor for disease reactivation in Wegener's granulomatosis [abstract]. FASEB J 1998;12:A488.

318. Popa ER, Stegeman CA, Bos NA, et al. T-cell activation and TCR Vb skewing in Wegener's granulomatosis: indicators for superantigen activation? Clin Exp Immunol 1998;112 Suppl 1:16.

319. Machado EB, Michet CJ, Ballard DJ, et al. Trends in incidence and clinical presentation of temporal arteritis in Olmsted County, Minnesota, 1950–1985. Arthritis Rheum 1988;31:745–9.

320. Olopade CO, Sekosan M, Schraufnagel DE. Giant cell arteritis manifesting as chronic cough and fever of unknown origin. Mayo Clin Proc 1997;72:1048–50.

321. Gur H, Ehrenfeld M, Izsak E. Pleural effusion as a presenting manifestation of giant cell arteritis. Clin Rheumatol 1996;15:200–3.

322. Kramer MR, Melzer E, Nesher G, Sonnenblick M. Pulmonary manifestations of temporal arteritis. Eur J Respir Dis 1987;71:430–3.

323. Palaic M, Yeadon C, Moore S, Cashman N. Wegener's granulomatosis mimicking temporal arteritis. Neurology 1991;41:1694–5.

324. Nishino H, DeRemee RA, Rubino FA, Parisi JE. Wegener's granulomatosis associated with vasculitis of the temporal artery: report of five cases. Mayo Clin Proc 1993;68:115–21.

325. Kerr GS, Hallahan CW, Giordano J, et al. Takayasu arteritis. Ann Intern Med 1994;120:919–29.

326. Rose AG, Halper J, Factor SM. Primary arteriopathy in Takayasu's disease. Arch Pathol Lab Med 1984;108:644–8.

327. Lie JT. Isolated pulmonary Takayasu arteritis: clinicopathologic characteristics. Mod Pathol 1996;9:469–74.

328. Lupi E, Sanchez G, Horwitz S, Gutierrez E. Pulmonary artery involvement in Takayasu's arteritis. Chest 1975;67:69–74.

329. Ogawa Y, Hayashi K, Sakamoto I, Matsunaga N. Pulmonary arterial lesions in Takayasu arteritis: relationship of inflammatory activity to scintigraphic findings and sequential changes. Ann Nucl Med 1996;10:219–23.

330. Elsasser S, Soler M, Bolliger C, et al. Takayasu disease with predominant pulmonary involvement. Respiration 2000;67:213–5.

331. Yamada I, Nakagawa T, Himeno Y, et al. Takayasu arteritis: diagnosis with breath-hold contrast-enhanced three-dimensional MR angiography. J Magn Reson Imaging 2000;11:481–7.

332. Castellani M, Vanoli M, Cali G, et al. Ventilation-perfusion lung scan for the detection of pulmonary involvement in Takayasu's arteritis. Eur J Nucl Med 2001;28:1801–5.

333. Takahashi K, Honda M, Furuse M, et al. CT findings of pul-

monary parenchyma in Takayasu arteritis. J Comput Assist Tomogr 1996;20:742–8.

334. Hall S, Barr W, Lie JT. Takayasu's arteritis. A study of 32 North American patients. Medicine 1985;64:89–99.

335. Hoffman GS, Leavitt RY, Kerr GS, et al. Treatment of glucocorticoid-resistant or relapsing Takayasu arteritis with methotrexate. Arthritis Rheum 1994;37:578–82.

336. Miyata T, Ohara N, Shigematsu H, et al. Endovascular stent graft repair of aortopulmonary fistula. J Vasc Surg 1999;29:557–60.

337. Schwarz-Eywill M, Breitbart A, Csernok E, et al. Treatment modalities and ANCA in Takayasu's arteritis. Adv Exp Med Biol 1993;336:497–501.

338. Garcia-Torres R, Noel LH, Reyes PA, et al. Absence of ANCA in Mexican patients with Takayasu's arteritis. Scand J Rheumatol 1997;26:55–7.

339. Dabague J, Arevola RM, Garciatorres R, Reyes PA. Takayasu's arteritis and Wegener's granulomatosis—a coincidental case. Clin Exp Rheumatol 1995;13:413–4.

340. Mejia-Hernandez C, Alvarez-Mendoza A, DeLeon-Bojorge B. Takayasu's arteritis coexisting with Wegener's granulomatosis in a teenager with renal insufficiency: case report. Pediatr Dev Pathol 1999;2:385–8.

341. Yamasaki S, Eguchi K, Kawabe Y, et al. Wegener's granulomatosis overlapped with Takayasu arteritis. Clin Rheumatol 1996;15:303–6.

342. O'Duffy JD. Vasculitis in Behçet's disease. Rheum Dis Clin North Am 1990;16:423–31.

343. Efthimiou J, Johnston C, Spiro SG, Turner-Warwick M. Pulmonary disease in Behçet's syndrome. Q J Med 1986; 58:259–80.

344. Raz I, Okon E, Chajek-Shaul T. Pulmonary manifestations in Behçet's syndrome. Chest 1989;95:585–9.

345. Slavin RF, de Groot WJ. Pathology of the lung in Behçet's disease: case report and review of the literature. Am J Surg Pathol 1981;5:779–88.

346. Petty TL, Scoggin CH, Good JT. Recurrent pneumonia in Behçet's syndrome: roentgenographic documentation during 13 years. JAMA 1977;238:2529–30.

347. Davies JD. Behçet's syndrome with haemoptysis and pulmonary lesions. J Pathol 1973;109:351–6.

348. Winer-Muram HT, Gavant ML. Pulmonary CT findings in Behçet's disease. J Comput Assist Tomogr 1989;13:346–7.

349. Berkmen T. MR angiography of aneurysms in Behçet disease: a report of four cases. J Comput Assist Tomogr 1998;22:202–6.

350. Tunaci M, Ozkorkmaz B, Tunaci A, et al. CT findings of pulmonary artery aneurysms during treatment for Behçet's disease. AJR Am J Roentgenol 1999;172:729–33.

351. Acican T, Gurkan OU. Azathiopine-steroid combination therapy for pulmonary arterial aneurysms in Behçet's disease. Rheumatol Int 2001;20:171–4.

352. Aktogu S, Erer OF, Urpek G, et al. Multiple pulmonary arterial aneurysms in Behçet's disease: clinical and radiologic remission after cyclophosphamide and corticosteroid therapy. Respiration 2002;69:178–81.

353. Lacombe P, Qanadli SD, Jondeau G, et al. Treatment of hemoptysis in Behçet syndrome with pulmonary and bronchial embolization. J Vasc Interv Radiol 1997;8:1043–7.

354. Bozkurt AK. Embolisation in Behçet's disease. Thorax 2002; 57:469–70.

355. Cantasdemir M, Kantarci F, Mihmanli I, et al. Emergency endovascular management of pulmonary artery aneurysms in Behçet's disease: report of two cases and a review of the literature. Cardiovasc Intervent Radiol 2002;25:4.

356. Hunninghake GW, Fauci AS. Pulmonary involvement in the collagen vascular diseases. Am Rev Respir Dis 1979; 119:471–503.

357. Churg A. Pulmonary angiitis and granulomatosis revisited. Hum Pathol 1983;14:868–83.

358. Lemley DE, Katz P. Rheumatoid-like arthritis presenting as idiopathic pulmonary hemosiderosis: a report and review of the literature. J Rheumatol 1986;13:954–7.

359. Schwarz MI, Zamora MR, Hodges TN, et al. Isolated pulmonary capillaritis and diffuse alveolar hemorrhage in rheumatoid arthritis and mixed connective tissue disease. Chest 1998;113:1609–15.

360. Naschitz JE, Yeshurun D, Scharf Y, et al. Recurrent massive alveolar hemorrhage, crescentic glomerulonephritis, and necrotizing vasculitis in a patient with rheumatoid arthritis. Arch Intern Med 1989;149:406–8.

361. Zamora MR, Warner ML, Tuder R, Schwarz MI. Diffuse alveolar hemorrhage and systemic lupus erythematosus. Clinical presentation, histology, survival, and outcome. Medicine (Baltimore) 1997;76:192–202.

362. Hughson MD, He Z, Henegar J, McMurray R. Alveolar hemorrhage and renal microangiopathy in systemic lupus erythematosus. Arch Pathol Lab Med 2001;125:475–83.

363. Gould DB, Soriano RZ. Acute alveolar hemorrhage in lupus erythematosus. Ann Intern Med 1975;83:836–7.

364. Marino CT, Pertschuk LP. Pulmonary hemorrhage in SLE. Arch Intern Med 1981;141:201–3.

365. Erickson RW, Franklin WA, Emlen W. Treatment of hemorrhagic lupus pneumonitis with plasmapheresis. Sem Arthritis Rheum 1994;24:114–23.

366. Euler HH, Guillevin L. Plasmapheresis and subsequent pulse cyclophosphamide in severe systemic lupus erythematosus. Ann Med Interne 1994;145:296–302.

367. Euler HH, Schroeder JO, Harten P, et al. Treatment-free remission in severe systemic lupus erythematosus following synchronization of plasmapheresis with subsequent pulse cyclophosphamide. Arthritis Rheum 1994;37:1784–94.

368. Wallace DJ, Goldfinger D, Pepkowitz SH, et al. Randomized controlled trial of pulse/synchronization cyclophosphamide/apheresis for proliferative lupus nephritis. J Clin Apheresis 1998;13:163–6.

369. Crausman RS, Achenbach GA, Pluss WT, et al. Pulmonary capillaritis and alveolar hemorrhage associated with the antiphospholipid antibody syndrome. J Rheumatol 1995; 22:554–6.

370. Asherson RA, Cervera R, Piette JC, et al. Catastrophic antiphospholipid syndrome. Clinical and laboratory features of 50 patients. Medicine (Baltimore) 1998;77:195–207.

371. Gertner E. Diffuse alveolar hemorrhage in the antiphospolipid syndrome: spectrum of disease and treatment. J Rheumatol 1999;26:805–7.

372. Horiki T, Fuyuno G, Ishii M, et al. Fatal alveolar hemorrhage in a patient with mixed connective tissue disease presenting polymyositis features. Intern Med 1998;37:554–60.

373. Griffin MT, Robb JD, Martin JR. Diffuse alveolar haemorrhage associated with progressive systemic sclerosis. Thorax 1990;45:903–4.

374. Vazquez-Del Mercado M, Mendoza-Topete A, Best-Aguilera CR, Garcia-De La Torre I. Diffuse alveolar hemorrhage in limited cutaneous systemic sclerosis with positive perinuclear antineutrophil cytoplasmic antibodies. J Rheumatol 1996;23:1821–3.

375. Schwarz MI, Sutarik JM, Nick JA, et al. Pulmonary capillaritis and diffuse alveolar hemorrhage. A primary manifestation of polymyositis. Am J Respir Crit Care Med 1995; 151:2037–40.

376. Liebow AA. The J. Burns Amberson lecture —pulmonary angiitis and granulomatosis. Am Rev Respir Dis 1973; 108:178–82.

377. Chittock DR, Joseph MG, Paterson NA, McFadden RG. Necrotizing sarcoid granulomatosis with pleural involvement. Clinical and radiographic features. Chest 1994;106:672–6.

378. Dykhuizen RS, Smith CC, Kennedy MM, et al. Necrotizing sarcoid granulomatosis with extrapulmonary involvement. Eur Respir J 1997;10:245–7.

379. Strickland-Marmol LB, Fessler RG, Rojiani AM. Necrotizing

sarcoid granulomatosis mimicking an intracranial neoplasm: clinicopathologic features and review of the literature. Mod Pathol 2000;13:909–13.

380. Foster WP, Greene JS, Millman B. Wegener's granulomatosis presenting as ophthalmoplegia and optic neuropathy. Otolaryngol Head Neck Surg 1995;112:758–62.

381. Sneller MC. Ocular manifestations of Wegener's granulomatosis—reply source. JAMA 1995;274:1200.

382. Dagum P, Roberson JB Jr. Otologic Wegener's granulomatosis with facial nerve palsy. Ann Otol Rhinol Laryngol 1998;107:555–9.

383. Devaney KO, Ferlito A, Hunter BC, et al. Wegener's granulomatosis of the head and neck. Ann Otol Rhinol Laryngol 1998;107:439–45.

384. Rasmussen N. Management of the ear, nose, and throat manifestations of Wegener granulomatosis: an otorhinolaryngologist's perspective. Curr Opin Rheumatol 2001;13:3–11.

385. Halstead LA, Karmody CS, Wolff SM. Presentation of Wegener's granulomatosis in young patients. Otolaryngol Head Neck Surg 1986;94:368–71.

386. Lustmann J, Segal N, Markitziu A. Salivary gland involvement in Wegener's granulomatosis. A case report and review of the literature. Oral Surg Oral Med Oral Pathol 1994;77:254–9.

387. Arauz JC, Fonseca R. Wegener's granulomatosis appearing initially in the trachea. Ann Otol Rhinol Laryngol 1982;91: 593–4.

388. Bohlman ME, Ensor RE, Goldman SM. Primary Wegener's granulomatosis of the trachea: radiologic manifestations. South Med J 1984;77:1318–9.

389. McGregor MBB, Sandler G. Wegener's granulomatosis. A clinical and radiological survey. Br J Radiol 1964;37:430–9.

390. Israel HL, Patchefsky AS. Wegener's granulomatosis of lung: diagnosis and treatment. Experience with 12 cases. Ann Intern Med 1971;74:881–91.

391. Gohel VK, Dalinka MK, Israel HL. The radiological manifestations of Wegener's granulomatosis. Br J Radiol 1973;16: 427–32.

392. Gatenby PA, Lytton DG, Bulteau VG, et al. Myocardial infarction in Wegener's granulomatosis. Aust N Z J Med 1976; 6:336–40.

393. Davenport A, Goodfellow J, Goel S, et al. Aortic valve disease in patients with Wegener's granulomatosis. Am J Kidney Dis 1994;24:205–8.

394. Fox AD, Robbins SE. Aortic valvulitis complicating Wegener's granulomatosis. Thorax 1994;49:1176–7.

395. Horn RG, Fauci AS, Rosenthal AS, Wolff SM. Renal biopsy pathology in Wegener's granulomatosis. Am J Pathol 1974; 74:423–40.

396. Pinching AJ, Lockwood CM, Pussell BA, et al. Wegener's granulomatosis: observations on 18 patients with severe renal disease. Q J Med 1983;208:435–60.

397. ten Berge IJM, Wilmink JM, Meyer CJLM, et al. Clinical and immunological follow-up of patients with severe renal disease in Wegener's granulomatosis. Am J Nephrol 1985;5:21–9.

398. Falk RJ, Moore DT, Hogan SL, Jennette JC. A renal biopsy is essential for the management of ANCA-positive patients with glomerulonephritis. Sarcoidosis Vasc Diffuse Lung Dis 1996;13:230–1.

399. DeRemee RA. Extrapulmonary manifestations of Wegener's granulomatosis. Semin Respir Med 1988;9:403–8.

400. Spiera RF, Filippa DA, Bains MS, Paget SA. Esophageal involvement in Wegener's granulomatosis. Arthritis Rheum 1994;37:1404–7.

401. Pritchard MH, Gow PJ. Wegener's granulomatosis presenting as rheumatoid arthritis (two cases). Proc R Soc Med 1976; 69:501–4.

402. Jacobs RP, Moore M, Brower A. Wegener's granulomatosis presenting with erosive arthritis. Arthritis Rheum 1987;30: 943–6.

403. ter Borg EJ, Disch FJM, Kallenberg CGM. Erosive polyarthritis as presenting manifestation of Wegener's granulomatosis. Clin Rheumatol 1995;14:551–3.

404. Drachman DD. Neurological complications of Wegener's granulomatosis. Arch Neurol 1963;8:145–55.

405. Nishino H, Rubino FA, Parisi JE. The spectrum of neurologic involvement in Wegener's granulomatosis. Neurology 1993;43:1334–7.

406. Haynes BF, Fauci AS. Diabetes insipidus associated with Wegener's granulomatosis successfully treated with cyclophosphamide. N Engl J Med 1978;299:764.

407. Hurst NP, Dunn NA, Chalmers TM. Wegener's granulomatosis complicated by diabetes insipidus. Ann Rheum Dis 1983;42:600–1.

408. Lohr KL, Ryan LM, Toohill RJ, Anderson T. Anterior pituitary involvement in Wegener's granulomatosis. J Rheumatol 1988;15:855–61.

409. Segelmark M, Baslund B, Weislander J. Some patients with anti-myeloperoxidase autoantibodies have a c-ANCA pattern. Clin Exp Immunol 1994;96:458–65.

410. Cohen Tervaert JW, Mulder L, Stegeman C, et al. Occurrence of autoantibodies to human leucocyte elastase in Wegener's granulomatosis and other inflammatory disorders. Ann Rheum Dis 1993;52:115–20.

411. Nässberger L, Jonsson H, Sjöholm AG, Sturfelt G. Circulating anti-elastase in systemic lupus erythematosus. Lancet 1989;i:509.

412. Apenberg S, Andrassy K, Wörner I, et al. Antibodies to neutrophil elastase: a study in patients with vasculitis. Am J Kidney Dis 1996;28:178–85.

413. Halbwachs-Mecarelli L, Nusbaum P, Noël LH, et al. Anti-neutrophil cytoplasmic antibodies (ANCA) directed against cathepsin G in ulcerative colitis, Crohn's disease and primary sclerosing cholangitis. Clin Exp Immunol 1992;90:79–84.

414. Gross WL, Schmitt WH, Csernok E. ANCA and associated diseases: immunodiagnostic and pathogenetic aspects. Clin Exp Immunol 1993;91:1–12.

415. Yang JJ, Tuttle R, Falk RJ, Jennette JC. Frequency of anti-bactericidal/permeability–increasing protein (BPI) and anti-azurocidin in patients with renal disease. Clin Exp Immunol 1996;105:125–31.

416. Zhao MH, Lockwood CM. Azurocidin is a novel antigen for anti-neutrophil cytoplasmic autoantibodies (ANCA) in systemic vasculitis. Clin Exp Immunol 1996;103:397–402.

417. Mulder AHL, Broekroelofs J, Horst G, et al. Anti-neutrophil cytoplasmic antibodies (ANCA) in inflammatory bowel disease: characterization and clinical correlates. Clin Exp Immunol 1994;95:490–97.

418. Broekroelofs J, Mulder AHL, Nelis GF, et al. Anti-neutrophil cytoplasmic antibodies (ANCA) in sera from patients with inflammatory bowel disease (IBD). Relation to disease pattern and disease activity. Dig Dis Sci 1994;39:545–9.

419. Moodie FDL, Leaker B, Cambridge G, et al. α-Enolase: a novel cytosolic autoantigen in ANCA positive vasculitis. Kidney Int 1993;43:675–81.

420. Zhao MH, Jones SJ, Lockwood CM. Bacteriocidal/permeability-increasing protein (BPI) is an important antigen for anti-neutrophil cytoplasm autoantibodies (ANCA) in vasculitis. Clin Exp Immunol 1996;99:49–56.

421. Zhao MH, Jayne DR, Ardiles LG, et al. Autoantibodies against bactericidal/permeability-increasing protein in patients with cystic fibrosis. Q J Med 1996;89:259–65.

422. Stoffel MP, Csernok E, Herzberg C, et al. Anti-neutrophil cytoplasmic antibodies (ANCA) directed against bactericidal/permeability increasing protein (BPI): a new seromarker for inflammatory bowel disease and associated disorders. Clin Exp Immunol 1996;104:54–9.

423. Jennings JG, Chang L, Savige JA. Anti-proteinase 3 antibodies, their characterization and disease associations. Clin Exp Immunol 1994;95:251–6.

23

DIFFUSE ALVEOLAR HEMORRHAGE

ANDREW P. FONTENOT
MARVIN I. SCHWARZ

Diffuse alveolar hemorrhage (DAH) refers to a clinicopathologic syndrome defined by diffuse intra-alveolar bleeding. The intra-alveolar red blood cells originate from the alveolar capillaries and less frequently from the precapillary arterioles and postcapillary venules. The clinical syndrome is characterized by hemoptysis, anemia, diffuse radiographic pulmonary infiltrates, and hypoxemic respiratory failure often necessitating ventilatory support. The presence of a hemorrhagic bronchoalveolar lavage (BAL) in serial BAL samples is characteristic. Moreover, several of the etiologies of DAH can cause recurrent episodes. Diffuse alveolar hemorrhage has many clinical etiologies as well as a variety of underlying histologic patterns (Table 23–1).[1–6] Diffuse alveolar hemorrhage is recognized by the presence of red blood cells and fibrin within the alveolar spaces followed by the accumulation of intra-alveolar hemosiderin-containing macrophages (Figure 23–1). Free hemosiderin also appears within the lung parenchyma, particularly if the DAH is chronic and recurrent (Figure 23–2). Organizing pneumonia (organizing diffuse alveolar hemorrhage), representing an attempt at repair, is commonly present. With repeated episodes, interstitial fibrosis may develop (Figure 23–3).

HISTOLOGY

Pulmonary capillaritis, first described by Spencer in 1957,[7] is the most frequent underlying histologic pattern associated with the clinical syndrome of DAH. Pulmonary capillaritis is recognized by the disruption of the interstitium including the alveolar capillaries. Red blood cells and fibrin subsequently leak into the alveolar spaces through the damaged alveolar-capillary basement membranes resulting in DAH (Figure 23–4).[8–10] The alveolar interstitium is broadened by the presence of edema, fibrinoid necrosis, infiltrating inflammatory cells, and free interstitial red blood cells. In severe cases, there is total destruction of the alveolar walls with replacement by necrotic tissue. The other characteristic feature of pulmonary capillaritis is a striking neutrophilic interstitial infiltration; many of these cells appear fragmented (leukocytoclasis) and pyknotic (Figure 23–5). This programmed cell death (apoptosis) causes nuclear debris (dust) to accumulate in the necrotic edematous interstitium as well as within the alveolar spaces. Fragmented neutrophils accompany the fibrin and red blood cells into the alveolar spaces as a result of disruption of the alveolar wall. Other histologic features of pulmonary capillaritis and DAH include capillary and sometimes arteriolar thrombosis, organizing pneumonia, and type II epithelial cell hyperplasia.

It is likely that the cytokine priming and neutrophil activation that leads to their eventual destruction is also responsible for the alveolar wall damage and subsequent DAH. Neutrophils react by undergoing both a respiratory burst with the release of reactive oxygen species and cytoplasmic degranulation with the release of tissue injuring proteolytic enzymes into the surrounding tissue. These events lead to lung matrix injury, endothelial injury, and increased vascular permeability. The triggers for this event remain unknown. In florid cases of necrotizing pulmonary capillaritis, neutrophils can be seen "lining up" within the alveolar walls in relatively spared areas of the lung. These structures otherwise appear normal, suggesting that the neutrophils are present prior to alveolar wall necrosis (Figure 23–6). Most cases of pulmonary capillaritis are associated with either a systemic vasculitis, a collagen vascular disease, or another autoimmune disease process (see Table 23–1). Antineutrophil cytoplasmic antibodies (ANCA) are believed to play a role in the pathogenesis of some cases of necrotizing pulmonary capillaritis, particularly those caused by a systemic vasculitis such as Wegener's granulomatosis or microscopic polyangiitis. This is due in part to the ability of this antibody to activate circulating neutrophils as well as the antibodies' tendency to bind to endothelial cell surfaces and facilitate the production of immune complexes in vitro.[11–13] There are, however, diseases associated with pulmonary capillaritis in which serum ANCA are not present. These include cases of isolated

TABLE 23–1   Causes and Underlying Histologies Associated With Diffuse Alveolar Hemorrhage

Pulmonary capillaritis
  Wegener's granulomatosis
  Microscopic polyangiitis
  Isolated pulmonary capillaritis (ANCA positive)
  Isolated pulmonary capillaritis (ANCA negative)
  *Systemic lupus erythematosus
  Rheumatoid arthritis
  Mixed connective tissue disease
  Scleroderma
  Polymyositis
  Primary antiphospholipid antibody syndrome
  Henoch-Schönlein purpura
  Behçet's syndrome
  IgA nephropathy
  *Goodpasture's syndrome
  Idiopathic glomerulonephritis (pauci-immune or immune-
    complex related)
  Acute lung transplant rejection
  Idiopathic pulmonary fibrosis
  Diphenylhydantoin
  Retinoic acid toxicity
  Autologous bone marrow transplantation
  Myasthenia gravis
  Cryoglobulinemia
  Ulcerative colitis
  Propylthiouracil

Bland pulmonary hemorrhage
  Idiopathic pulmonary hemosiderosis
  *Goodpasture's syndrome
  *Systemic lupus erythematosus
  Coagulation disorders
  Trimellitic anhydride
  Isocyanate exposure
  Penicillamine
  Amiodarone
  Nitrofurantoin
  Mitral stenosis
  Subacute bacterial endocarditis
  Polyglandular autoimmune syndrome
  Multiple myeloma

Diffuse alveolar damage
  Bone marrow transplantation (idiopathic pneumonia
    syndrome)
  Crack cocaine inhalation
  Cytotoxic drug therapy
  *Systemic lupus erythematosus
  Radiation therapy
  Acute respiratory distress syndrome

Miscellaneous histologies
  Lymphangioleiomyomatosis
  Pulmonary veno-occlusive disease
  Pulmonary capillary hemangiomatosis
  Obstructive sleep apnea
  Fibrillary glomerulonephritis
  Metastatic renal cell carcinoma
  Epithelioid hemangioepithelioma
  Angiosarcoma
  Choriocarcinoma syndrome

*Entities with several underlying histologies possible.

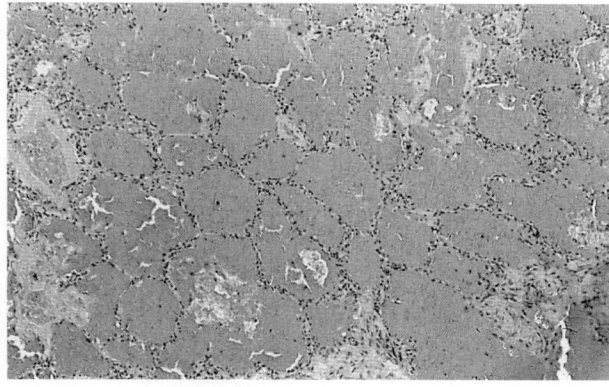

Figure 23–1   DAH due to bland alveolar hemorrhage in a patient with Goodpasture's syndrome. The alveolar spaces are packed with red blood cells, but the alveolar walls (interstitium) appear normal except for type II epithelial cell hyperplasia (hematoxylin and eosin; ×20 original magnification).

pauci-immune pulmonary capillaritis[14] and pulmonary capillaritis that complicates the collagen vascular diseases. There is a single report of a case of rheumatoid arthritis–associated DAH with underlying bland hemorrhage in which ANCA are directed against neutrophil cytoplasmic myeloperoxidase (p-ANCA).[15] Although 25% of patients with systemic lupus erythematosus (SLE) have p-ANCA positivity, these antibodies are not directed against myeloperoxidase, and no correlation between the clinical appearance of lupus vasculitis and the presence of these antibodies has been established.[16] There is also no correlation between the development of DAH in SLE and the presence of ANCA.[17]

It is possible that pulmonary capillaritis results from the deposition of immune complexes in the capillary endothelium. Immune complexes activate complement and influence the migration of neutrophils to the lung.[18,19] In some diseases associated with pulmonary capillaritis, including SLE,[20–24] Henoch-Schönlein purpura,[25,26] immunoglobulin A (IgA) nephropathy,[27]

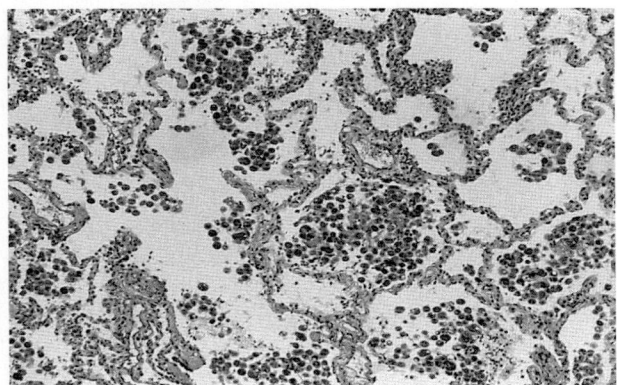

Figure 23–2   DAH resolving phase. The alveolar spaces are filled with hemosiderin-laden macrophages (hematoxylin and eosin, ×40 original magnification).

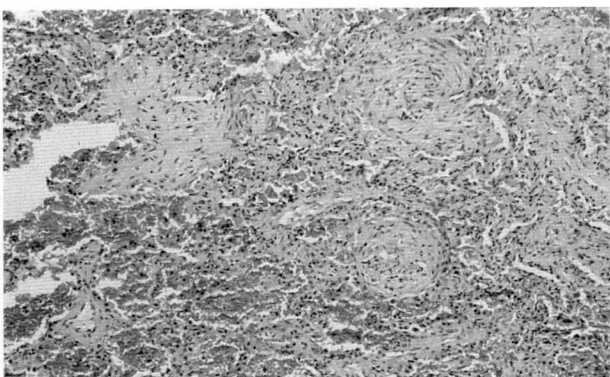

Figure 23–3   Organizing DAH in a patient with pulmonary capillaritis secondary to Wegener's granulomatosis. Note the residual alveolar hemorrhage and the proliferating fibroblasts as well as loose, new connective tissue within the distal air spaces (hematoxylin and eosin; ×40 original magnification).

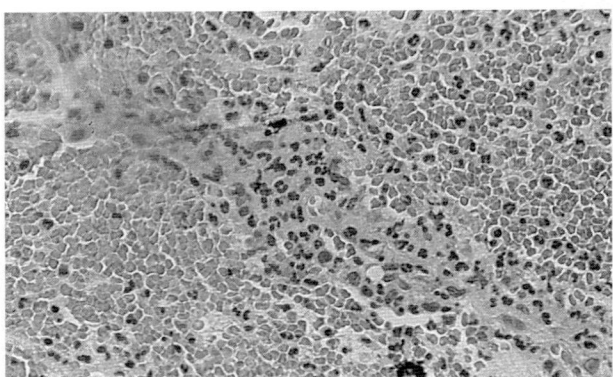

Figure 23–5   DAH due to pulmonary capillaritis. Fragmented neutrophils are expanding the alveolar wall. Note the dense pyknotic appearance of some of these cells as well as the appearance of the fragmented neutrophils and red blood cells in the alveolar spaces (hematoxylin and eosin; ×40 original magnification).

Goodpasture's syndrome,[28–30] and Behçet's syndrome,[31] immune complexes are detected in the alveolar interstitium by both light and electron microscopy. Due to the absence of immune complex deposition, other entities associated with pulmonary capillaritis and DAH such as Wegener's granulomatosis, microscopic polyangiitis, isolated pulmonary capillaritis, and some forms of idiopathic glomerulonephritis are considered to be pauci-immune but conceivably could have been immune-complex induced.[32]

In addition to the development of interstitial fibrosis following recurrent episodes of DAH, another consequence is the development of a progressive obstructive lung disease.[33,34] Three cases of pulmonary capillaritis with recurrent DAH due to microscopic polyangiitis developed severe, irreversible airflow limitation and hyperinflation ten years following the initial episode of DAH. Physiologic testing and high-resolution com-

puted tomographic scans showed the development of emphysema. It is possible that the repeated neutrophilic infiltration of the alveolar walls and their subsequent death with the release of oxygen radicals and proteolytic enzymes led to the development of emphysema.[33,34] Significant airflow limitation has also been seen many years after the episode(s) of recurrent DAH, which accompanies idiopathic pulmonary hemosiderosis. In this case, the underlying histology is bland pulmonary hemorrhage.[35] These patients were hyperinflated and had low diffusing capacities for carbon monoxide, which also suggested emphysema. In some of these cases, the diagnosis of idiopathic pulmonary hemosiderosis was established solely on clinical grounds, and therefore the possibility of an underlying isolated pulmonary capillaritis exists.[36] Further, the lesion of pulmonary capillaritis has only recently been widely recognized by pathologists. Thus, some adult cases of idiopathic pulmonary hemo-

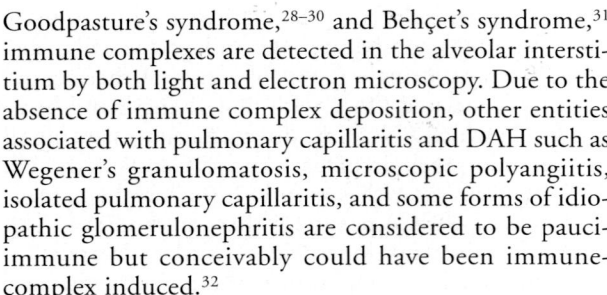

Figure 23–4   DAH due to pulmonary capillaritis secondary to microscopic polyangiitis. Note the broadening and disruption of the alveolar walls as well as neutrophilic infiltration. The interstitium is necrotic in some areas (hematoxylin and eosin; ×40 original magnification).

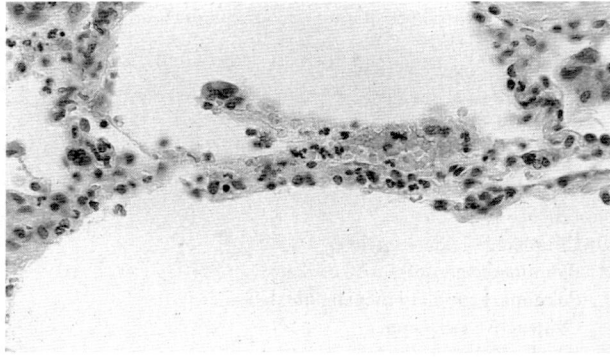

Figure 23–6   Early pulmonary capillaritis. Neutrophils are lining up within the alveolar interstitium. DAH may be beginning in one area, but the remainder of the alveolar spaces appear normal. In other portions of this biopsy in this patient with isolated pulmonary capillaritis, florid DAH and capillaritis were seen (hematoxylin and eosin; ×100 original magnification).

siderosis previously thought to have underlying bland hemorrhage, are now being reclassified as pulmonary capillaritis.[9]

The histologic appearance of bland pulmonary hemorrhage is identical to that of DAH (see Figures 23–1 and 23–2). In this case, the alveolar interstitium is not inflamed, edematous, or necrotic. There is only type II epithelial cell hyperplasia, and interstitial fibrosis develops after repeated episodes.[37] The common etiologies of bland pulmonary hemorrhage include Goodpasture's syndrome, idiopathic pulmonary hemosiderosis, and SLE. Goodpasture's syndrome and SLE are also associated with pulmonary capillaritis.[17,37] For bland pulmonary hemorrhage (no interstitial inflammation), the pathogenesis of DAH is even more elusive. In idiopathic pulmonary hemosiderosis, electron microscopic studies have demonstrated abnormalities in the continuity and integrity of the alveolar-capillary membrane[38–41]; immune complexes are present in both Goodpasture's syndrome[28–30] and SLE.[20–24]

Diffuse alveolar damage (DAD) complicating bone marrow transplantation, cytotoxic drug therapy, crack cocaine inhalation, and acute interstitial pneumonia accompanying collagen vascular diseases can produce the syndrome of DAH. Diffuse alveolar damage is diagnosed based on the presence of alveolar-septal and intra-alveolar edema, capillary congestion and microthrombi, and the characteristic intra-alveolar hyaline membrane formation in addition to the features of DAH (Figure 23–7).[42]

The miscellaneous histologies will be discussed under the specific disease entities (see Table 23–1).

CLINICAL PRESENTATION OF DIFFUSE ALVEOLAR HEMORRHAGE

Patients presenting with DAH often have a previously recognized predisposing condition such as a systemic vasculitis, collagen vascular disease, or mitral stenosis. In addition, many of the entities listed in Table 23–1 cause recurrent intra-alveolar bleeding. Diffuse alveolar hemorrhage, on the other hand, may be the initial manifestation of an underlying systemic disease, or at presentation it may be the only obvious manifestation of that disorder. Hemoptysis, the cardinal symptom of DAH, can be present intermittently for weeks prior to presentation, or, as often is the case, it appears in a more dramatic fashion over days or even hours. For example, crack cocaine inhalation with underlying diffuse alveolar damage has a very acute presentation.[43,44]

Patients can be of any age, but most of those with DAH due to pulmonary capillaritis are under 40 years of age. In one-third of cases of DAH from any cause, cough and dyspnea are present, but hemoptysis is absent in spite of extensive intra-alveolar bleeding.[17] In this situation, DAH is discovered following BAL, which reveals a sequential hemorrhagic return in the presence of a low

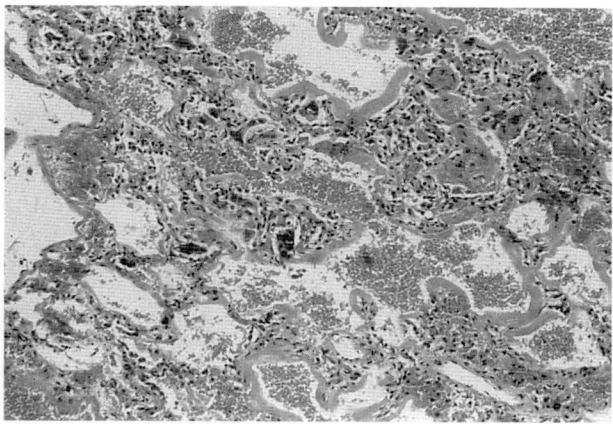

Figure 23–7 DAH secondary to diffuse alveolar damage in an autologous bone marrow transplant patient. There is alveolar hemorrhage and hyaline membrane formation (hematoxylin and eosin; ×40 original magnification).

and falling hemoglobin and a chest radiograph that demonstrates diffuse pulmonary infiltrates. Fever and nonspecific chest pain may accompany the cough, dyspnea, and hemoptysis. Other symptoms are usually related to the presence of the underlying systemic disease and include cutaneous leukocytoclastic vasculitis, sinusitis, inflammatory ocular disease, arthritis, myositis, and glomerulonephritis.

The immediate past history is important in the evaluation of a patient with DAH. Is there a history of a systemic or cardiac disease? Does the patient take any drugs such as phenytoin, penicillamine, propylthiouracil, cytotoxic drugs (carmustine, cyclophosphamide, busulfan, bleomycin, retinoic acid), or crack cocaine, that are associated with DAH? Does the patient have a coagulation disorder or an occupational exposure (trimellitic anhydride or isocyanates) that predisposes to DAH? In addition, cigarette smoking adversely affects the lung in Goodpasture's syndrome. For example, 100% of patients with antibasement membrane antibodies (ABMA) who smoke develop DAH compared with 20% of nonsmokers.[45] Physical examination is nonspecific, but may reveal fever, diffuse crackles, and possibly signs of consolidation. Other physical findings, such as palpable purpura (which indicates a cutaneous leukocytoclastic vasculitis), conjunctivitis, iridocyclitis, myositis, and synovitis, point to an underlying systemic disease.

The chest roentgenogram is nonspecific and shows alveolar infiltrates that range from a patchy focal process to diffuse alveolar filling (Figure 23–8). Unilateral and lobar infiltrates can be seen initially with a rapid progression to diffuse alveolar filling. The computed tomographic scan confirms the presence of air space filling but offers no advantage over the standard chest radiograph other than a more dramatic demonstration of the extent of involvement. With recurrent and chronic DAH, interstitial infiltrates may appear and persist on the chest radiograph as fibrosis develops. Dense scarring can occur with time.[46] The discovery of radiographic Kerley's B lines in the setting of DAH suggests either mitral stenosis or pulmonary veno-occlusive disease. If either of these are suspected, particularly in a patient with DAH without extrapulmonary disease, echocardiography and eventually a right-heart catheterization are indicated. Kerley's B lines may occasionally accompany DAH due to systemic vasculitis or the collagen vascular diseases. The most likely explanation is the presence of associated myocarditis with left ventricular dysfunction. As previously mentioned, obstructive lung disease appearing as radiographic hyperinflation can also evolve following years of repeated bouts of DAH.[33,34]

Diffuse alveolar hemorrhage is characterized by a low or decreasing hemoglobin and hematocrit. If the bleeding is recurrent, iron deficiency, as measured by a reduced serum iron concentration and an increased serum iron binding capacity, will develop. Nonspecific elevations of the white blood cell and platelet counts are the rule, although thrombocytopenia may be present when the DAH is caused by idiopathic thrombocytopenic purpura, thrombotic thrombocytopenic purpura, disseminated intravascular coagulation, leukemia, or anticoagulation and thrombolytic therapy.[47–54] All of these conditions have been associated with DAH and bland pulmonary hemorrhage. If thrombocytopenia accompanies the DAH, the possibility of SLE or primary antiphospholipid syndrome should be entertained.[55,56] An elevation of the erythrocyte sedimentation rate in the absence of infection (> 60 mm) suggests a systemic vasculitis. An abnormal urinalysis showing proteinuria, microscopic hematuria, and red blood cell casts suggests an underlying glomerulonephritis. This is usually due to focal segmental necrotizing glomerulonephritis, the common renal lesion of the systemic vasculitides, Goodpasture's syndrome, SLE, and idiopathic pauci-immune or immune-complex-related glomerulonephritis. This

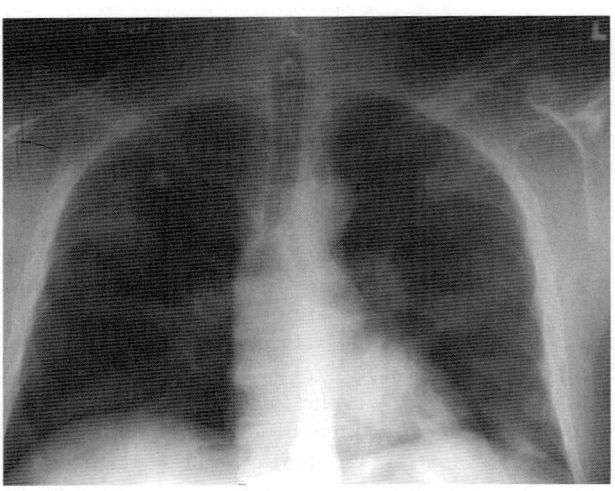

A

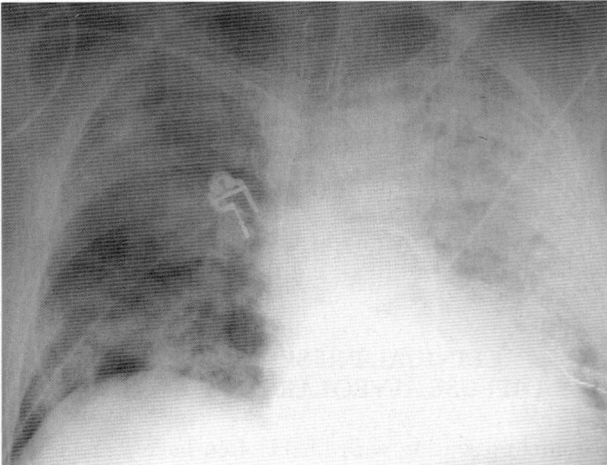

C

Figure 23–8   Chest radiographs of a patient with SLE with DAH. *A,* On admission (February 28), there are bilateral patchy alveolar infiltrates. *B,* By March 2, these infiltrates are more dense with areas of consolidation. *C,* The next day, there are diffuse alveolar infiltrates, more dense on the left, and the patient is intubated.

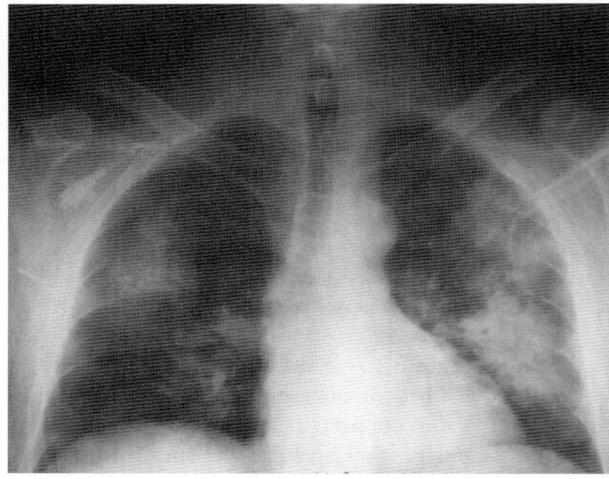

B

rapidly progressive glomerulonephritis can quickly result in chronic renal insufficiency and end-stage renal failure. The presence of renal insufficiency in a patient with DAH dictates immediate and aggressive treatment.

Hypoxemia can be severe and often requires mechanical ventilation. In less dramatic cases, hemoptysis as well as other symptoms can be minimal and intermittent, producing a subacute course. In such cases, there may be little interference with gas exchange. Symptoms can, however, accelerate at any time. The sequential increase in the diffusing capacity for carbon monoxide on serial measurement is a sensitive test for intra-alveolar bleeding.[57] Measurement of the diffusing capacity can be used to detect more subtle presentations of DAH or early exacerbations in established cases. This unexpected finding is explained by the increased availability of intra-alveolar hemoglobin for combination with carbon monoxide. As mentioned above, after recurrent episodes of DAH, serial pulmonary function testing may demonstrate the development of either an obstructive or a restrictive lung process. The development of interstitial fibrosis causing restrictive lung disease after repeated episodes of DAH poses a number of intriguing questions. Since excessive amounts of intraparenchymal iron are present in the lung, is this the putative factor? This is unlikely, because in primary hemochromatosis there is excessive deposition of iron into all tissues, but pulmonary fibrosis has not been described. Could the fibrogenicity be related to the presence of free tissue hemoglobin or some other component of the red blood cell? Hemoglobin has great affinity for nitric oxide, which has significant antimitotic and antiproliferative effects.[58-60] Free hemoglobin could effectively remove nitric oxide, which would favor unopposed cellular proliferation and fibrosis. The red blood cell is also a rich source of endothelin, a potent vasoconstrictor substance, and vanadate, which catalyses many oxidant reactions and affects the activity of protein kinase.[61,62] On the other hand, the red blood cell is also a source of the antioxidants superoxide dismutase and catalase.

DIAGNOSIS

The discovery of a hemorrhagic BAL in a patient without hemoptysis could be the first indication of DAH. A BAL should always be considered in patients who present with nonspecific symptoms and signs as well as radiographic findings that point to an atypical pneumonia. A low and falling hematocrit supports the diagnosis of DAH. Goodpasture's syndrome is confirmed by the presence of ABMA in the serum or by the linear deposition of immunoglobulin and complement within alveolar and glomerular basement membranes (Figure 23–9).[1,63] In 5 to 10% of patients with Goodpasture's syndrome, DAH occurs without clinical renal disease.[64-70] In this case, diagnosis can be made only by demonstrating ABMA in the tissue, because the antibody may not be present in the serum. Lung tissue

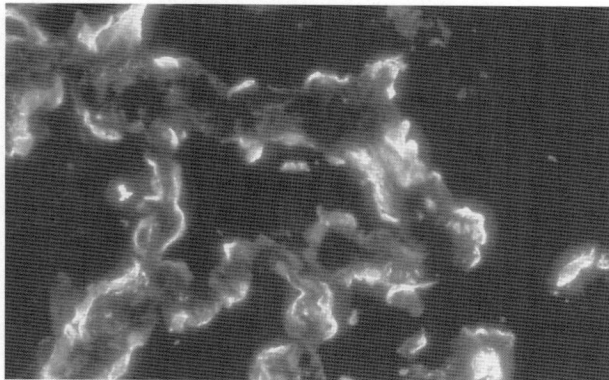

Figure 23–9   Goodpasture's syndrome; immunofluorescence of lung. There is antibody directed against IgG deposited along the alveolar-capillary basement membrane in a linear fashion (hematoxylin and eosin; ×100 original magnification).

demonstrates the antibody and renal tissue, even without clinical evidence of an active glomerulonephritis, also stains positively.

Diffuse alveolar hemorrhage that complicates SLE occurs in an established case in most instances. In up to 20% of cases, DAH is the presenting and the first clinical manifestation of this disease.[17,22,71-73] In this instance, a low serum complement, a positive serum antinuclear factor, and the presence of double-stranded antideoxyribonucleic acid (anti-DNA) antibodies in the serum point to the diagnosis. Granular deposition of IgG and complement representing immune complexes in pulmonary or renal tissue also support the diagnosis of SLE (Figure 23–10).[20,22-24,71] Granular deposition of IgA in the lungs and kidneys is found in both Henoch-Schönlein purpura and IgA nephropathy.[25,26,74-77] IgA immune complexes are also present in the serum of patients with these disorders. Isolated pulmonary capillaritis, Wegener's granulomatosis, microscopic polyangiitis, and most types of idiopathic glomerulonephritis are

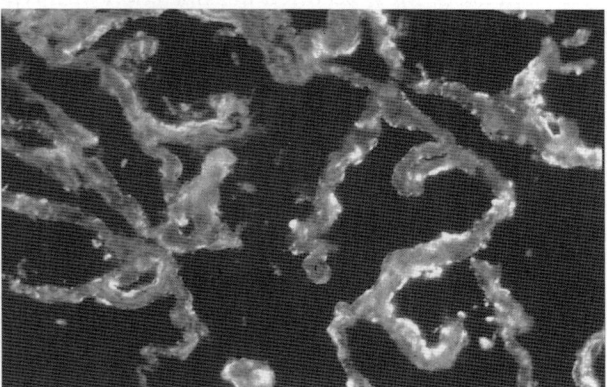

Figure 23–10   SLE; lung immunofluorescence. There is deposition of antibody to IgG at the alveolar-capillary interface in a granular fashion (hematoxylin and eosin; ×100 original magnification).

pauci-immune. In patients with recurrent thrombophlebitis and thrombocytopenia, primary antiphospholipid syndrome should be suspected, and serum anticardiolipin antibodies should be measured.[55,56]

Serum ANCA positivity limits the diagnostic possibilities. For a complete discussion of ANCA see Chapter 22. Serum c-ANCA positivity (antiproteinase 3 antibody) supports the diagnosis of Wegener's granulomatosis, and p-ANCA (antimyeloperoxidase antibody) positivity suggests either microscopic polyangiitis or pauci-immune idiopathic glomerulonephritis.[78–86] In one type of isolated pulmonary capillaritis, p-ANCA levels are also elevated.[87,88] Although the presence of c-ANCA is highly specific for Wegener's granulomatosis, the sensitivity of this test is only 63%.[89,90] Of note, these results refer to a general vasculitic population rather than to patients who presented with DAH.

The presence of subclinical alveolar bleeding is a common finding in ANCA-associated vasculitides. Schnabel and colleagues[91] reported that 95% of patients with ANCA-associated vasculitis have greater than 5% hemosiderin-laden alveolar macrophages as compared to less than 5% of individuals with lung disease due to collagen vascular diseases. Other serum markers of endothelial cell injury such as thrombomodulin elevation and the appearance of antiendothelial cell antibodies are found in patients with systemic vasculitis.[92–94] These assays are not clinically available and do not point to a specific etiology.

WEGENER'S GRANULOMATOSIS

Diffuse alveolar hemorrhage resulting from pulmonary capillaritis in Wegener's granulomatosis can be the presenting manifestation of the disease.[95–107] In addition, DAH can occur in the setting of a more typical clinical presentation with associated necrotizing granulomatous vasculitis, or it may occur for the first time during an exacerbation in an established case.[106–108] Cordier and colleagues[101] identified pulmonary capillaritis in 31% of the open lung biopsies in patients with Wegener's granulomatosis. Most occurred in association with typical granulomatous vasculitic lesions involving small- and medium-sized vessels. However, in three cases, pulmonary capillaritis was an isolated finding. There was inadequate clinical information to determine whether these patients presented with DAH. In another series, pulmonary capillaritis was found in 17% of 35 patients but was never an isolated finding.[109] In a postmortem study of 22 patients, examination of the lungs showed pulmonary capillaritis in seven patients, and capillaritis was the sole finding and the immediate cause of death in three patients. This shows that DAH can first appear during an exacerbation in a well-established case, and its presence increases the acute mortality. The DAH may sometimes dominate the clinical picture in patients with Wegener's granulomatosis who present with the more typical clinical and histologic findings. Moreover, the

development of the more recognizable features of Wegener's granulomatosis can be delayed for months or years in patients who present with DAH.[1,110]

There are over 40 patients reported with Wegener's granulomatosis in whom DAH was present and pulmonary capillaritis was the only histologic finding in the lung.[95–107,111] Other systemic vasculitic involvement, particularly evidence for a focal segmental necrotizing glomerulonephritis, is almost always present. However, this presentation is difficult to differentiate from microscopic polyangiitis. The presence of serum c-ANCA helps to distinguish between these two entities, but there are cases of pulmonary capillaritis in Wegener's granulomatosis with p-ANCA positivity.[78–85,112,113] Only with the development of the more typical clinical-radiographic-histologic picture can the diagnosis of Wegener's granulomatosis be confirmed.

An association between lymphoid malignancies and DAH due to c-ANCA–mediated vasculitis has recently been reported,[114] and the occurrence of vasculitis was thought to represent a paraneoplastic syndrome. Other malignancies, including renal cell carcinoma[115] and Hodgkin's disease[116] have also occurred in association with ANCA vasculitis.

The presence of DAH increases early mortality to 37%. When compared with more classic presentations of Wegener's granulomatosis, this is considerably higher.[1,4,79,96–100] The immediate cause of death is either renal or respiratory failure, although superimposed infections contribute to this mortality. The treatment of DAH complicating Wegener's granulomatosis is similar to that of standard Wegener's granulomatosis and consists of corticosteroids and cyclophosphamide. Azathioprine can be substituted for cyclophosphamide. Plasmapheresis, intravenous IgG, and trimethoprim/sulfamethoxazole are not recommended for DAH in Wegener's granulomatosis. Erythrocyte sedimentation rates, ANCA levels, diffusing capacity, and urinalysis should be monitored because recurrences commonly occur.

MICROSCOPIC POLYANGIITIS

Microscopic polyangiitis (MPA), previously referred to as microscopic polyarteritis, is considered by some to be a variant of classic polyarteritis nodosa. It can be differentiated from the classic form by the lack of involvement of medium-sized blood vessels and the absence of asthma and systemic hypertension. Moreover, the prominent gastrointestinal tract involvement and the absence of upper respiratory tract involvement help to distinguish MPA from Wegener's granulomatosis. In addition, the classic form of polyarteritis nodosa rarely involves the lungs, but DAH and underlying pulmonary capillaritis occur in up to one-third of patients with microscopic polyangiitis.[1,8,9,88,112,113,117–129]

All patients with MPA have a focal segmental necrotizing glomerulonephritis, the renal lesion common to all systemic vasculitides. Other manifestations include arthritis, myositis, gastrointestinal bleeding secondary to an intestinal mucosal vasculitis, and peripheral neuropathy.[121,127] As with Wegener's granulomatosis, the erythrocyte sedimentation rate is high, and nonspecific increases in both serum antinuclear antibodies and rheumatoid factors may be present. Circulating immune complexes have been reported to occur in 45% of patients, but tissue localization is rarely seen. Therefore, MPA is considered to be a pauci-immune vasculitis. Antibodies to hepatitis B and particularly hepatitis C antigens are present in up to 33% of patients.[122,130,131]

Antineutrophil cytoplasmic antibodies are frequently present in patients with microscopic polyangiitis. Guillevin and colleagues[128] reported that ANCA were present in 75% of patients with MPA, of which 85% were p-ANCA. Thus, the presence of c-ANCA cannot be used to differentiate Wegener's granulomatosis from MPA. In addition, a small number of patients with Wegener's granulomatosis will be p-ANCA positive. In this instance, the later development of a necrotizing granulomatous vasculitis helps in the differentiation. There is also a form of idiopathic glomerulonephritis with serum p-ANCA positivity in which DAH can develop.[122,132–134] Moreover, there are isolated cases of pulmonary capillaritis and DAH with serum p-ANCA positivity without extrapulmonary disease.[85,88]

Treatment of MPA is similar to that for Wegener's granulomatosis. Some authors recommend the addition of plasmapheresis, but its efficacy has not been definitively established.[102,120] The presence of DAH in patients with MPA contributes to an early mortality (25%).[1,3,10,102,118–121,135,136] However, the 5-year survival for all patients approaches 65%. As with other causes of pulmonary capillaritis, recurrences are expected, particularly during reduction or discontinuation of therapy. Both obstructive lung disease and pulmonary fibrosis have been reported to occur in MPA patients with recurrent bouts of DAH.[10,14,137]

ISOLATED PULMONARY CAPILLARITIS

Isolated pulmonary capillaritis with DAH occurs with or without serum ANCA.[14,87,88,138] Isolated pulmonary capillaritis refers to a small vessel vasculitis that is confined to the lungs. A series described 29 patients with DAH and biopsy-proven pulmonary capillaritis from all causes and 8 (28%) had isolated pulmonary capillaritis.[14] In this series, it was the most common cause of pulmonary capillaritis, followed by Wegener's granulomatosis and MPA. Unlike the systemic vasculitides, there were no clinical, serologic, or histologic features of an associated disease. Direct immunofluorescent studies of lung tissue were negative for immune complexes, making this a pauci-immune type of small vessel vasculitis. Six of the cases presented with respiratory failure and four required mechanical ventilation. There was one death during the

initial hospitalization, but seven survived. During a mean follow-up period of 43 months, no patient developed serologic or clinical evidence of an associated systemic disease. Two patients experienced recurrent DAH without the emergence of a systemic disease. The prognosis for this group of patients also appears to be favorable.

There is also a form of isolated pulmonary capillaritis in which serum p-ANCA positivity is present.[87,88] Follow-up data are inadequate to determine whether a systemic disease developed in these patients. In lieu of the p-ANCA positivity, it is possible that these cases represent a lung-limited form of MPA, which would be similar to the idiopathic form of glomerulonephritis associated with p-ANCA positivity. Both types of isolated pulmonary capillaritis respond favorably to standard vasculitis therapy with corticosteroids and cytotoxic drugs.

SYSTEMIC LUPUS ERYTHEMATOSUS

The noninfectious pleural-pulmonary complications of SLE occur in 50 to 70% of patients.[139,140] These include pleuritis and pleural effusions; interstitial lung disease including acute lupus pneumonitis and nonspecific intersitial pneumonitis; pulmonary embolism usually associated with antiphospholipid antibodies; pulmonary vascular disease including small- and medium-vessel vasculitis; and a primary form of pulmonary hypertension, diaphragmatic weakness, bronchiolitis, and DAH.[141–147] Diffuse alveolar hemorrhage occurs in approximately 4% of patients and is the most catastrophic pulmonary complication of SLE with a mortality rate approaching 50%.[17] In prior reports, the underlying histology of DAH in SLE was reported to be either bland pulmonary hemorrhage or DAH secondary to diffuse alveolar damage.[20,23,24,143,148–157] Several recent series have documented the presence of pulmonary capillaritis and microangiitis causing the DAH of SLE. The most current studies found that 80% of SLE patients with DAH had underlying pulmonary capillaritis.[17] Immune complexes are frequently present in the lung and were found in 10 of 13 cases in which they were sought.[20,23,24,42]

As expected, most patients with DAH and SLE are women, the mean age being 27 years.[17] The diagnosis of SLE is usually established prior to the onset of the DAH. Most patients who present with DAH also have lupus nephritis.[17,158,159] The majority of patients report hemoptysis at the time of presentation.

Diffuse alveolar hemorrhage in SLE must be distinguished from acute lupus pneumonitis. Although the clinical and radiographic appearances are similar, hemoptysis is seen in < 20% of cases of acute lupus pneumonitis.[150] In 50% of cases, acute lupus pneumonitis is the presenting manifestation of SLE, and the underlying histology shows either diffuse alveolar damage, organizing pneumonia, or a cellular nonspecific interstitial pneumonitis. Acute lupus pneumonitis is associated with a 50% mortality with some survivors progressing to pulmonary fibrosis.[150]

Mortality rates associated with DAH in SLE are extremely high, ranging from 52 to 92%.[17,149,151,158] However, a recent series reported a 100% survival.[159] The variable mortality rates in the DAH of SLE are influenced by the following: (1) the need for mechanical ventilation (62%) versus nonventilated patients (0%); (2) infection (78%) versus no infection (20%); and (3) the use of cyclophosphamide therapy for the acute DAH episode (70%) versus no cyclophosphamide therapy (20%). More recent reports show a higher incidence of co-infection than previously reported.[17] A possible explanation is the increased use of outpatient cyclophosphamide therapy for the treatment of lupus nephritis. Plasmapheresis has been used for DAH complicating SLE, but survival remains unchanged.[17] There is a similar lack of therapeutic efficacy of plasmapheresis for the treatment of lupus nephritis.[160]

OTHER COLLAGEN VASCULAR DISEASES

The development of DAH complicating other collagen vascular diseases is an uncommon but well-documented occurrence. A recent report describes the development of an acute pulmonary syndrome which coincided with the onset of muscle weakness in two patients with polymyositis.[161] Hemoptysis was absent in both patients. However, lung biopsy revealed pulmonary capillaritis with histologic evidence of DAH. Both patients were responsive to corticosteroid and immunosuppressive therapy. Therefore, acute lung disease in polymyositis can be due either to pulmonary capillaritis, bronchiolitis obliterans organizing pneumonia, diffuse alveolar damage, or a cellular nonspecific interstitial pneumonitis.[161,162] In a few cases, pulmonary capillaritis has been reported to complicate the course of scleroderma and mixed connective tissue disease.[163–168] Although alveolar hemorrhage has been described in patients with rheumatoid arthritis, either histology was not available, or was interpreted as showing bland pulmonary hemorrhage.[15,169–171] In a recent report, three patients with well-documented rheumatoid arthritis who developed DAH due to pulmonary capillaritis were described.[172] All patients responded to standard vasculitic treatment. There is even one case of DAH in rheumatoid arthritis in which p-ANCA was present in the serum.[15] However, lung biopsy demonstrated bland pulmonary hemorrhage.

Patients with primary antiphospholipid syndrome may develop DAH, with the episode of hemorrhage sometimes being the initial manifestation of the condition.[55,56,173–175] Symptoms at presentation range from cough, dyspnea, and fever (with or without hemoptysis) to acute respiratory failure. Thrombocytopenia is usually present at the time of the DAH episode. The histopathology shows evidence of pulmonary capillaritis with microvascular thrombosis.[55,56] Treatment with corticosteroids usually results in rapid improvement.

HENOCH-SCHÖNLEIN PURPURA AND IMMUNOGLOBULIN A NEPHROPATHY

Henoch-Schönlein purpura occurs in children and less commonly in adults.[176–179] As in the pediatric cases, adults present with the typical palpable purpuric rash and a focal segmental necrotizing glomerulonephritis. Synovitis and gastrointestinal tract manifestations are also common. There are several well-documented cases of pulmonary capillaritis with DAH in these patients.[25,26,77,180,181] In these cases, IgA immune complexes are present in the serum, lung, and kidney.[74–76] Corticosteroids are the recommended therapy. Immunoglobulin A nephropathy has some features in common with Henoch-Schönlein purpura. This is a very common form of glomerulonephritis characterized by the presence of IgA immune complexes in the serum and kidney, but DAH is rare.[182–184] However, several cases of pulmonary capillaritis have been described. Immunoglobulin A immune complexes were present in lung tissue in one case.[27,185] Both linear and granular IgA deposition have been described.[183,184] One patient with DAH secondary to pulmonary capillaritis without clinical evidence for glomerulonephritis has been reported. In this patient, a renal biopsy revealed glomerular IgA deposition.[185] Both Henoch-Schönlein purpura and IgA nephropathy lack IgA-specific ANCA in the serum.[186]

BEHÇET'S DISEASE

Behçet's disease is a chronic, relapsing illness characterized by oral and genital ulceration, iridocyclitis, thrombophlebitis, and a multisystem disease featuring cutaneous vasculitis, arthritis, meningoencephalitis, and a focal segmental necrotizing glomerulonephritis.[187–189] Immune complexes have been identified in the serum, kidneys, and lungs of these patients.[32,187,188]

Lung involvement occurs in 10% of cases and is characterized by a small vessel vasculitis manifested as pulmonary capillaritis, venulitis, and arteriolitis resulting in DAH.[190–195] Pulmonary hemorrhage can also occur secondary to involvement of larger vessels. Aneurysms of the pulmonary arteries can erode into bronchi causing massive hemorrhage and death. Pulmonary arterial occlusion with pulmonary infarction may also cause hemoptysis in Behçet's disease. It appears that pulmonary involvement occurs more frequently in men than in women with this syndrome. Pulmonary hemorrhage was the cause of death in 39% of 28 cases in one series.[193] Death usually occurred within 6 years of the first episode of hemoptysis. Other authors have confirmed the serious nature of hemoptysis. Treatment consists of corticosteroids and immunosuppressive therapy.[196]

CRYOGLOBULINEMIA

Mixed cryoglobulinemia is a systemic vasculitis of small- to medium-sized vessels due to the vascular deposition of immune complexes and complement.[197] The clinical features include purpura, synovitis, hepatitis, and glomerulonephritis. In the majority of cases, a causal link between infection with hepatitis B or C virus and the development of mixed cryoglobulinemia has been established.[198,199] Interstitial lung disease, characterized by cellular inflammation and fibrosis, has been reported and appears to be the most common lung manifestation.[200] The occurrence of DAH complicating mixed cryoglobulinemia is a rare event.[201–203] Its occurrence is thought to be secondary to immune complex deposition in alveolar capillary endothelium. There have been two documented cases of DAH from pulmonary capillaritis.[203,204] The renal involvement is a focal segmental necrotizing glomerulonephritis.

IDIOPATHIC GLOMERULONEPHRITIS

Idiopathic glomerulonephritis is a rapidly progressive, crescent forming, focal segmental necrotizing glomerulonephritis. There are three types: one is pauci-immune,[1,3,122,134,205] another is associated with granular immune complexes,[77,206,207] and the third is associated with the linear deposition of immune complexes in glomerular capillaries (Goodpasture's syndrome).[208] DAH can occur in all cases; therefore, differentiation is essential due to the differences in treatment and outcome. Pauci-immune idiopathic glomerulonephritis is associated with p-ANCA positivity and is considered to be a localized renal vasculitis analogous to isolated pulmonary capillaritis. Diffuse alveolar hemorrhage with underlying pulmonary capillaritis has been reported in up to 50% of patients with pauci-immune idiopathic glomerulonephritis.[1,134] Other manifestations of systemic vasculitis may appear; when they do, it is difficult to differentiate between MPA or another systemic vasculitis. Furthermore, 30 to 40% of patients with Goodpasture's syndrome have a positive serum p-ANCA.[208–211] Thus, it is imperative to seek a specific diagnosis by finding ABMA in the serum or in renal tissue. Treatment of idiopathic pauci-immune glomerulonephritis with or without DAH is similar to that of other vasculitides. An unusual form of idiopathic glomerulonephritis has granular immune complex deposits and is occasionally associated with DAH and pulmonary capillaritis. In patients with this entity, immune deposits are found in the kidney but not in lung tissue.[204,207]

ACUTE LUNG ALLOGRAFT REJECTION

Acute rejection following lung transplantation is a common problem and is usually recognized by perivascular mononuclear cell infiltrates. In five reported cases of patients with acute lung allograft rejection who were transplanted for a variety of underlying diseases, the open lung biopsy demonstrated pulmonary capillaritis.[212] Of these, DAH was histologically confirmed in four patients, of whom only two had hemoptysis. This complication occurred from several weeks to months following organ transplantation. All five were treated with intensification of immunosuppressive therapy, and two died. Plasmapheresis was carried out in two and coincided with temporary improvement, but its efficacy remains to be established. Two initially responded to treatment but had a subsequent recurrence of pulmonary capillaritis and DAH.

MISCELLANEOUS CAUSES OF PULMONARY CAPILLARITIS

There are numerous reports of pulmonary complications of ulcerative colitis, including bronchiolitis, bronchiolitis obliterans, panbronchiolitis, bronchiolitis obliterans organizing pneumonia, and an inflammatory interstitial lung disease as well as pulmonary fibrosis. There have been two cases of DAH and pulmonary capillaritis complicating ulcerative colitis.[213,214] Both had established colitis, and their lung disease responded to corticosteroids and cytotoxic therapy. Diffuse alveolar hemorrhage secondary to pulmonary capillaritis has also complicated a case of mild ocular myasthenia gravis.[215] Other unusual causes of pulmonary hemorrhage and capillaritis include toxicities due to diphenylhydantoin,[216,217] retinoic acid,[218–220] and propylthiouracil.[221–224] To date, there are five case reports of propylthiouracil-associated ANCA-positive syndrome with DAH.[217,223–226] Most of these patients had a preceding viral-like prodrome, and all improved with the discontinuation of propylthiouracil. Several of the patients also had focal crescentic glomerulonephritis.

GOODPASTURE'S SYNDROME (ANTIBASEMENT MEMBRANE ANTIBODY DISEASE)

In 1919, Goodpasture described an 18-year-old man who developed DAH following an influenza infection.[227] An autopsy revealed the presence of a systemic vasculitis. Thus, it is unlikely that the case originally described by Goodpasture represents Goodpasture's syndrome as we know it today. Rather, the original case may have been some form of systemic vasculitis, such as microscopic polyangiitis. In 1965, an antibody common to both glomerular and alveolar basement membranes was identified in the kidneys and lungs of some patients with DAH and glomerulonephritis.[228,229] Goodpasture's syndrome is part of a spectrum of diseases known as ABMA diseases. A diagnosis of Goodpasture's syndrome is reserved for those cases of DAH and glomerulonephritis in which this antibody is present in the serum.[230,231] The ABMA is identified in the kidney and the lung as a very distinct pattern of wavy, uninterrupted linear immunofluorescence to IgG along the basement membranes of glomerular tufts and alveolar walls (see Figure 23–9).[1,232] The level of ABMA in the serum correlates positively with the severity of the renal disease but not that of the lung disease.

Autoantibodies mediate the tissue injury in Goodpasture's syndrome. It has been shown in several animal models that basement membranes from different species can induce a glomerulonephritis characterized by epithelial crescent formation.[228,233,234] Moreover, passive transfer of ABMA from humans to other animals can induce a glomerulonephritis.[235] This autoantibody is directed against the noncollagenous domain (NC1) of type IV collagen, the major component of basement membranes.[236] More specifically, it is directed against the α-3 chain of type IV collagen.[237] Using epitope mapping, multiple studies have narrowed the antigenic epitope to the 230 amino acid COOH-terminal domain of the α-3 chain of type IV collagen.[238–241] In addition, the gene for the α-3 chain has been mapped to the long arm of chromosome 2.[242] Patients with Goodpasture's syndrome may also have antibodies directed against other components of basement membrane, but these are not considered pathogenic.[243] Although the clinical expression of Goodpasture's syndrome is confined to the kidneys and lung, distribution of type IV collagen is widespread throughout the body including the skin, eye, choroid plexus, small intestine, and placenta.[244,245] Not all patients who are diagnosed with Goodpasture's syndrome develop pulmonary hemorrhage. It is possible that an additional injury is necessary to increase alveolar capillary permeability and to permit the passage of the autoantibody.[246–248] For example, the clinical onset of DAH and sometimes its exacerbation have been associated with influenza A2 infection,[230] other respiratory tract infections,[28] volatile hydrocarbon exposure,[249,250] and cigarette smoking.[46,251]

Linear IgG deposition in renal basement membranes is not necessarily specific for Goodpasture's syndrome. It has been reported in lupus nephritis and diabetes mellitus.[252,253] Also, in one patient with IgA nephropathy, linear deposition of IgA was noted along the glomerular capillaries.[183] There is also a report of a patient with polyglandular autoimmune syndrome who developed DAH and whose lung biopsy demonstrated linear staining of IgG.[254]

In addition to environmental exposures, genetic susceptibility is an important variable in the immunopathogenesis of Goodpasture's syndrome, and susceptibility to Goodpasture's syndrome has been associated with particular human leukocyte antigen (HLA)-DR alleles.[241] The presence of HLA-DRB1*1501 is strongly associated with the development of disease, being present in approximately 90% of affected individuals.[255–257]

Convincing clinical data suggest that patients with Goodpasture's syndrome who possess this histocompatibility antigen experience severe renal disease and have a poor prognosis.[258]

In 60 to 80% of cases, the lung and renal disease occur simultaneously, and in 10 to 30%, glomerulonephritis is the sole manifestation.[1,28,246,259] In 5 to 10% of patients, DAH occurs alone, and clinical renal disease never becomes manifest.[64–70,260] In this case, a lung biopsy demonstrating the typical immunofluorescence pattern is diagnostic. Although renal disease may not be clinically apparent, renal biopsy will reveal the presence of the tissue antibody.[260] Men are two to three times more likely to develop this disease than women.[151,261,262] Most cases occur in the second and third decades. In older patients, the sex distribution equalizes, and the clinical expression is likely to be limited to the kidneys.[263] Patients who develop DAH are either smokers, have experienced a recent viral illness, or were exposed to volatile hydrocarbons.[28,46,249–251] Exacerbations of DAH are often associated with these events. In one study, 100% of smokers with Goodpasture's syndrome developed both DAH and glomerulonephritis; among nonsmokers, only 20% developed DAH.[46]

This disease has always been deemed monophasic. If patients survive the initial event, recurrences rarely occur, and if they do, they appear early on. There are, however, several documented cases of clinical and serologic recurrences of both the renal and the lung disease months to years after the initial episode.[264–267]

The clinical presentation of Goodpasture's syndrome is similar to other etiologies of DAH and glomerulonephritis. There are varying degrees of hemoptysis, cough, and dyspnea.[28,228,263] Fatigue due to both iron-deficiency anemia and renal failure may be the presenting symptom, particularly in those cases without DAH. Evidence of microscopic hematuria, proteinuria, and red blood cell casts as well as increases in the serum creatinine are common, but gross hematuria and systemic hypertension are unusual.[228,261,262] The radiograph shows patchy or diffuse alveolar infiltrates when lung involvement is present. Since the mortality rate is higher with deaths occurring earlier in Goodpasture's syndrome than in other causes of DAH and because recurrences are less frequent, evolution to radiographic interstitial infiltrates representing interstitial fibrosis is rarely, if ever, seen. The diffusing capacity is increased during periods of active bleeding. An increase of 30% above the baseline is highly suggestive of intra-alveolar bleeding. This bleeding could precede the development of hemoptysis or chest radiographic abnormalities and may be the first sign of an exacerbation.[268,269] Demonstration of serum or tissue ABMA establishes the diagnosis in a patient with either DAH, glomerulonephritis, or both.[262] The preferred method for the detection of ABMA is either radioimmunoassay or enzyme-linked immunosorbent assay (ELISA).[270] In a patient with Goodpasture's syndrome with renal dysfunction, a falling antibody titer following treatment is associated with improving renal function.[262] Up to 40% of patients with Goodpasture's syndrome have increased serum ANCA levels.[208–210] Some of these patients may have signs of a systemic vasculitis and represent a crossover between Goodpasture's syndrome and Wegener's granulomatosis or microscopic polyangiitis. For other causes of DAH, the presence of serum ANCA points to underlying pulmonary capillaritis. It is unclear whether this is also the case for Goodpasture's syndrome.

The DAH in Goodpasture's syndrome results from either bland pulmonary hemorrhage or pulmonary capillaritis. In those with pulmonary capillaritis, alveolar wall necrosis, which is commonly present in systemic vasculitis, is not seen.[39] As found in the systemic vasculitides and SLE, the renal histology is a focal segmental necrotizing glomerulonephritis with crescent formation. Clinically, this is a rapidly progressing glomerulonephritis. Immunofluorescent staining differentiates this form of rapidly progressive glomerulonephritis by demonstrating an uninterrupted linear deposition of immunoglobulin and sometimes complement along glomerular basement membranes.[66] Identical findings are present on the alveolar basement membrane.[29] Electron microscopic studies reveal basement membrane fragmentation and electron-dense deposits in the kidneys and lungs of these patients.[31,271]

Prior to the introduction of plasmapheresis for the treatment of Goodpasture's syndrome, the mortality or renal transplant rate was between 75 to 90%.[228,261,272] In patients with DAH alone, corticosteroids are very effective.[273,274] However, if glomerulonephritis with or without DAH is present, monotherapy is usually unsuccessful.[66,68,228,275] Cytotoxic agents, more specifically cyclophosphamide or azathioprine, may occasionally reverse the renal failure, but their main function is to control DAH.[261,276] However, the combination of plasmapheresis, corticosteroids, and a cytotoxic drug such as cyclophosphamide is quite effective, particularly for patients without oliguria who do not require dialysis.[277–284] Plasmapheresis (3 to 6 L/day) is generally continued for two weeks, in addition to various combinations of cyclophosphamide, azathioprine, and corticosteroids. A reduction in ABMA levels correlates with an improvement in renal function.[32] Some oliguric dialysis-dependent patients show a sufficient response to this combination therapy, such that dialysis can be discontinued.[278,279,282] Anuric patients, on the other hand, do not experience improvement in renal function, and continued dialysis is required; renal transplantation may be considered.[263,285] Up to 88% of nonoliguric patients who use this combination therapy can be expected to respond. In one study, only 31% of these required maintenance dialysis.[279,286] The 2-year survival for all patients is approximately 50%. The majority succumb during the first year due to DAH, often precipitated by a concomitant infection.[28,287,288] Severe renal failure that causes oliguria reduces the survival rate to 50% at 6 months.[289] Renal biopsy is not only diagnostic but also has prognostic value. In those

subjects in whom less than 30% of the glomeruli have undergone crescent formation in conjunction with fairly well-preserved renal function, significant response to therapy and prolonged survival can be expected.[278,284] However, when greater than 70% of the glomeruli are involved with crescent formation and there is clinical evidence of renal insufficiency, the renal disease is often progressive, requiring dialysis and possibly transplantation. Of all the causes of DAH, Goodpasture's syndrome remains the most difficult to treat and has the poorest prognosis and survival.

IDIOPATHIC PULMONARY HEMOSIDEROSIS

The diagnosis of idiopathic pulmonary hemosiderosis (IPH) is reserved for patients with DAH in whom all other causes have been excluded.[290] Clinically, this entity is characterized by recurrent episodes of DAH but without renal or other systemic involvement. Histologic examination of the lungs reveals bland pulmonary hemorrhage. Pulmonary fibrosis evolves with recurring episodes.[41,291] The etiology of this disease is poorly understood. Histologic examination reveals type II epithelial cell hyperplasia with capillary dilatation and tortuosity.[40,271,292] Hemosiderin-laden macrophages are seen within alveolar spaces as well as within the lung interstitium. Immune complexes are absent in this disease, and electron microscopy has revealed a degeneration of type I epithelial cells with exposure of the basement membrane. In addition, breaks in the continuity of the capillary basement membrane, thickening or duplication of the membrane, separation of the basement membrane with fibrillar material found in the separated areas, and focal ruptures of the basement membrane with excessive collagen deposition are found.[38–41,271,291–295] These findings show a form of diffuse lung injury. It is possible that IPH represents an autoimmune disorder since serum IgA levels are increased in 50% of children with this disease.[296] In a number of pediatric and adult patients, it is associated with celiac disease or jejunal villous atrophy.[36] Moreover, some patients demonstrate clinical responses to anti-inflammatory and cytotoxic therapy and even to plasmapheresis.[297]

The diagnosis of IPH in adults is a difficult one. Many cases of IPH were diagnosed before the ability to measure serum autoantibodies such as ABMA and ANCA. In some adult cases originally diagnosed with IPH, a systemic disease such as SLE or microscopic polyangiitis developed years later.[73,123,148] Histologic reclassification of cases of IPH have demonstrated the presence of pulmonary capillaritis, which could account for the fact that some cases respond to immunosuppressive treatment. It is likely that some of these cases represented isolated pulmonary capillaritis.[14,87,88,138] In one series of pulmonary capillaritis, the isolated form was the most common cause of DAH.[14] Previously, these cases would have been classified as IPH.

Idiopathic pulmonary hemosiderosis is predominately a disease of children, but 20% of cases occur in adults. Most adult cases appear between 20 and 40 years of age. Men are affected twice as frequently as women, and there are several reports of familial cases.[298–300] The clinical picture resembles other causes of DAH and ranges from minimal symptoms to severe respiratory failure requiring mechanical ventilation. Low-grade fever and cough often accompany hemoptysis. Other symptoms are related to iron-deficiency anemia. As in the other etiologies of DAH, hemoptysis may be absent at the time of admission, and only dyspnea, an abnormal chest radiograph, and anemia are present. In this case, a hemorrhagic BAL and the presence of hemosiderin-laden alveolar macrophages suggest the diagnosis of DAH. With repeated episodes of DAH, pulmonary fibrosis, chronic dyspnea, and finger clubbing appear,[290] as does a restrictive lung disease with a reduced diffusing capacity.[301] Some patients who experience recurrent episodes of DAH develop a severe obstructive lung disease resembling emphysema,[35,36] a finding that also has been reported in patients with microscopic polyangiitis and recurrent DAH.[33,34] Examination of the urine is negative. All serum antibody tests should be negative before this diagnosis can be entertained. An echocardiogram is indicated in some patients to exclude mitral valve disease.

It is recommended that patients suspected of having IPH undergo an open or thoracoscopic lung biopsy. Idiopathic pulmonary hemosiderosis must be differentiated from isolated pulmonary capillaritis and lung-limited Goodpasture's syndrome. Treatment, in addition to supportive therapy, includes anti-inflammatory and cytotoxic drugs.[290,297,298,302] One case was successfully treated with plasmapheresis.[303] It appears that adults with this diagnosis have a better prognosis than children.[304,305] Approximately 25% will be free of disease following the initial episode; another 25% will be free of active disease but will have persistent dyspnea and anemia; and another 25% will have persistent active disease that leads to fibrosis and restrictive lung disease. The remaining 25% have unresponsive disease with repeated, massive hemorrhage and an early respiratory death.[290,298,306]

PENICILLAMINE AND NONCYTOTOXIC DRUGS

Penicillamine is an unusual cause of DAH associated with underlying bland pulmonary hemorrhage. Diffuse alveolar hemorrhage has been reported in eight patients who received penicillamine for either rheumatoid arthritis, Wilson's disease, or primary biliary cirrhosis.[155,307–310] Diffuse alveolar hemorrhage usually occurs after twelve months of penicillamine therapy (1 g daily), but in one case it appeared after 20 years of treatment. All patients presented with DAH, and in one case this was the sole manifestation. In the rest, however, glomerulonephritis was also present. Systemic involvement other than the

kidney and the lung has not been found, leading some authors to call this entity penicillamine-induced Goodpasture's syndrome.[307,308,310,311] The pattern of deposition of tissue immunoglobulin clearly differentiates this entity from Goodpasture's syndrome. There is a granular as opposed to a linear deposition of IgG and complement.[312,313] Lung biopsy shows bland pulmonary hemorrhage. Although both renal and circulating immune complexes are described, pulmonary capillaritis has not been found. Three of the reported patients recovered following treatment with immunosuppressive therapy and plasmapheresis.[308,310]

Amiodarone-induced DAH can occur abruptly following 400 mg daily for at least 2 months.[314] Histology reveals bland pulmonary hemorrhage as well as nonspecific cellular interstitial pneumonitis, organizing pneumonia, and foamy macrophages with lamellar inclusions. Recently, the use of intravenous amiodarone also has been associated with DAH.[315] Rare cases of nitrofurantoin-induced DAH have been reported.[316,317] This results in bland pulmonary hemorrhage with a slow resolution following discontinuation of the drug.

TRIMELLITIC ANHYDRIDE AND PYROMELLITIC DIANHYDRIDE

The acid anhydrides, a family of reactive organic chemicals of low molecular weight, are necessary for the manufacture of alkyd and epoxy resins used in paint, varnishes, and plastics. Diffuse alveolar hemorrhage has been reported after the inhalation of fumes or dry powders of trimellitic anhydride.[318–320] Antibodies (IgG, IgE) to this compound can be found in the serum of affected workers, but DAH develops only following a latent period of 1 to 3 months. This is an isolated form of DAH, without renal or other systemic disease. Removal from exposure is the treatment, and persistent physiologic impairment should not occur. A report describes a patient who developed DAH after exposure to pyromellitic dianhydride, with antibodies (IgG) to pyromellitic dianhydride detected in the serum.[321] Lung tissue in acid anhydride injury has not been available for study, but the underlying histology is believed to be either bland alveolar hemorrhage or diffuse alveolar damage.

Diffuse alveolar hemorrhage has been described in a patient exposed to isocyanate.[322] The patient, a spray painter, developed serum antibodies directed against diisocyanates. The authors proposed that this entity was analogous to the DAH induced by trimellitic anhydride exposure.

MITRAL STENOSIS

Mitral stenosis must be considered in patients who present with DAH alone and without a history of exposure to drugs or toxins. Mitral stenosis can be relatively silent.

With the development of pulmonary venous hypertension, however, intermittent hemoptysis can occur.[323–325] When severe, this can result in significant blood gas abnormalities and radiographic infiltration due to DAH. With repeated episodes, pulmonary fibrosis can develop as it does in other causes of recurrent DAH. It is unclear whether the bleeding originates from the pulmonary microcirculation or from submucosal bronchial veins that are exposed to high pressures through anastomosis with the pulmonary veins.[326]

Hemoptysis and pulmonary hypertension with mitral regurgitation have also been reported.[327] Most patients with a mean pulmonary artery pressure that exceeds 35 mm Hg have reduced atrial compliance, exposing the microcirculation to this pressure elevation. In acute mitral regurgitation due to papillary muscle dysfunction or bacterial endocarditis, the sudden increase in pressure is transmitted to the pulmonary microcirculation and can lead to capillary rupture. Pulmonary interstitial edema and DAH have been reported in these cases.

COAGULATION DISORDERS

Coagulation disorders are another cause of DAH with underlying bland pulmonary hemorrhage.[47–54] Thrombocytopenia, either drug induced or secondary to idiopathic thrombocytopenic purpura or thrombotic thrombocytopenic purpura, are well-recognized causes of DAH.[50,51,54] Anticoagulation may be a subtle cause of alveolar hemorrhage. In anticoagulated patients, a syndrome characterized by dyspnea, unexplained anemia, and pulmonary infiltrates may evolve. Hemoptysis is often absent in these patients.[328] In this case as in other causes of DAH, BAL fluid demonstrating a hemorrhagic return as well as hemosiderin-laden macrophages help to make the diagnosis. Diffuse alveolar hemorrhage secondary to acquired vitamin K deficiency has been reported.[329,330] Treatment with vitamin K replacement results in resolution of the hemorrhage.

Diffuse alveolar hemorrhage is also seen complicating disseminated intravascular coagulation.[47] Individuals with acute leukemia who have undergone induction chemotherapy with resulting thrombocytopenia commonly develop DAH.[50,51,53] Although the thrombocytopenia in these patients can be quite profound, it is more likely that the hemorrhage is secondary to cytotoxic drug toxicity and underlying diffuse alveolar damage. In a patient with multiple myeloma due to an IgA paraprotein who initially presented with DAH,[331] examination of the lung biopsy did not show capillaritis nor did it reveal evidence of either protein deposition or alveolar-septal amyloid infiltration. Immunofluorescent studies also failed to show deposition of immunoglobulin or complement.

Diffuse alveolar hemorrhage is an infrequent complication of fibrinolytic therapy. Recently, tirofiban and abciximab, platelet membrane glycoprotein IIb/IIIa receptor blockers that are used in the treatment of acute coronary syndromes and complications of percutaneous coronary interventions, have been associated with DAH.[332,333]

DIFFUSE ALVEOLAR DAMAGE AND DIFFUSE ALVEOLAR HEMORRHAGE

Diffuse alveolar damage refers to a response of the lung to an acute injury from a variety of sources.[43,44,272,334–342] Histologically, this lesion is characterized by alveolar-septal and intra-alveolar edema, alveolar capillary congestion, microvascular thrombi, intra-alveolar hyaline membrane formation, and varying degrees of acute and chronic alveolar-septal inflammation.[335,336,339] Diffuse alveolar hemorrhage often accompanies DAD as a result of the widespread injury to the epithelial lining and alveolar-capillary basement membranes (see Figure 23–7). With extensive injury, red blood cells accompany serum into the alveolar spaces, which may result in hemoptysis or blood-tinged sputum. Often, however, a hemorrhagic BAL fluid is the only finding of the accompanying DAD.

Multiple causes of DAD include drugs (cytotoxic agents, crack cocaine, paraquat, acetylsalicylic acid, heroin, hydrochlorothiazide, ethylchlorvynol), acute respiratory distress syndrome (shock, trauma, aspiration, smoke inhalation, high altitude pulmonary edema, etc.), infectious pneumonias (mycoplasma, virus, legionella species, and pneumocystis), radiation, collagen vascular diseases (SLE, polymyositis, and mixed connective tissue disease), and acute (idiopathic) interstitial pneumonia also known as the Hamman-Rich syndrome. The most common causes of DAD, which also result in DAH, are cytotoxic chemotherapy for the treatment of acute leukemia and solid tumors,[312,313,340] as well as the preconditioning cytotoxic therapy given prior to bone marrow transplantation.[343–349] Crack cocaine toxicity is one of the completely reversible forms of drug-induced DAH secondary to DAD.[43,44,334,342]

Although DAH in patients undergoing autologous bone marrow transplantation is thought to be due to preconditioning chemotherapy, other etiologic factors include infection and previous radiation therapy.[345,346,348] The presence of DAH in an autologous bone marrow transplant recipient occurs in 10 to 20% of cases and is a poor prognostic indicator; mortality is reported to be as high as 50 to 100%.[344,350,351] High-dose corticosteroid therapy has met with variable success.[350] The DAH in this case is usually secondary to DAD but infection may be superimposed. Diagnosis is established after an acute pulmonary syndrome occurs, diffuse radiographic infiltrates appear, and BAL fluid reveals a sequential hemorrhagic return.[345]

Crack cocaine or free base smoking causes hemoptysis, diffuse pulmonary infiltrates, and DAH within hours of the event. Other pulmonary complications include acute noncardiogenic pulmonary edema, interstitial pneumonitis (including bronchiolitis obliterans organizing pneumonia), and pulmonary interstitial fibrosis.[342,352,353] A reduction in the diffusion capacity and increased alveolar epithelial permeability in long-term users point to the risk of chronic lung damage.[354,355]

LYMPHANGIOLEIOMYOMATOSIS AND TUBEROUS SCLEROSIS

Lymphangioleiomyomatosis (LAM) (see Chapter 29) describes a proliferation of normal-appearing smooth muscle within all elements of the lung that interferes with pulmonary function.[356–361] Proliferation of smooth muscle in the pulmonary lymphatics causes chylous pleural effusions. In the walls of the bronchioles, it leads to a progressive obstructive lung disease with parenchymal cyst formation and spontaneous pneumothorax. When the smooth muscle infiltrates the interstitium, an interstitial lung disease results.

Intermittent hemoptysis occur in 40% of patients due to the myoproliferative process in the walls of venules and small pulmonary veins, resulting in obstruction and eventually rupture. Lung biopsies in LAM demonstrate proliferating smooth muscle bundles and focal areas of alveolar hemorrhage and hemosiderin deposition. Recurrent episodes of self-limited hemoptysis in a premenopausal woman with obstructive physiology with or without a history of chylous pleural effusions should raise the suspicion of LAM.

Tuberous sclerosis (TS) (see Chapter 29) that affects the lungs is histologically identical to LAM, and intermittent hemoptysis is also possible. Although multiple extrapulmonary manifestations occur (mental retardation, epilepsy, dermal angiofibroma, renal angiomyolipomas, cardiac rhabdomyomas, and periungual fibromas), pulmonary involvement is usually evident only in women with TS.[362–367]

PULMONARY VENO-OCCLUSIVE DISEASE

Pulmonary veno-occlusive disease (PVOD) is characterized by fibrous obliteration of postcapillary venules as well as larger pulmonary veins.[368–377] It is an unusual cause of pulmonary hypertension and is seen in both children and adults and has an equal gender distribution. Although most cases are idiopathic, it has been described as a complication of chemotherapy for malignant disease and after preconditioning chemotherapy for bone marrow transplantation.[378–381] The chemotherapeutic agents most commonly implicated are bleomycin and carmustine. Pulmonary veno-occlusive disease has also been reported in patients with rheumatoid arthritis and SLE.[382,383] It has also been reported with Raynaud's phenomenon, arthritis, and elevated serum autoantibodies. In one case, pulmonary intraparenchymal electron-dense deposits were found.[384] Other associations include tho-

racic radiation and human immunodeficiency virus (HIV) positivity.[385,386]

As with other causes of primary pulmonary hypertension, patients with PVOD complain primarily of dyspnea and syncope and have pulmonary hypertension and, later, cor pulmonale. Hemoptysis is not unusual, but the full-blown syndrome of DAH occurs infrequently. The chest radiograph shows signs of pulmonary hypertension and in some cases interstitial lymphatic edema with Kerley's B lines. Rupture of pulmonary venules results in hemoptysis and sometimes the clinical and radiographic picture of DAH. Pulmonary function testing in these patients reveals progressive loss of the diffusing capacity for carbon monoxide, but lung volumes are usually preserved. Occasionally, a high probability ventilation-perfusion lung scan can be obtained in patients with PVOD.[387] A pulmonary artery catheter, if properly wedged, indicates a normal or decreased pulmonary capillary wedge pressure as well as pulmonary hypertension.[388,389] This occurs because the wedged catheter is adjacent to a static column of blood that extends from the central pulmonary veins into the left atrium, which is hemodynamically normal in PVOD.

The diagnosis of PVOD should be suspected in individuals with severe pulmonary arterial hypertension, radiographic evidence of pulmonary venous hypertension, and a normal pulmonary capillary wedge pressure.[377,389] However, a definitive diagnosis can be established only following a lung biopsy, which reveals diffuse fibrous obliteration of the venules and small veins with occasional acute or recanalized thrombi in their lumens (Figure 23–11). Evidence for bland, acute, or chronic (hemosiderin-laden macrophages) DAH is usually present.[370,374,377]

The prognosis of PVOD is dismal, with most patients dying within 2 years of the diagnosis.[377] Due to the rarity of the disorder, no randomized therapeutic trials have been performed. Treatment options include immunosuppressive agents such as corticos-

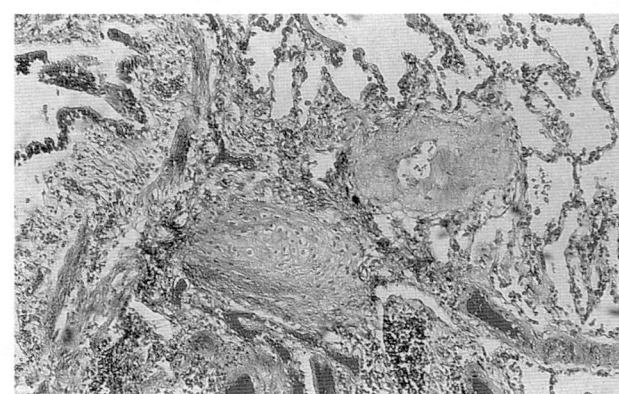

Figure 23–11   Pulmonary veno-occlusive disease. There is fibrous obliteration of two small intralobular septal pulmonary veins (hematoxylin and eosin; ×100 original magnification).

teroids[380] and azathioprine.[390] Other treatment modalities include anticoagulation, vasodilator therapy, and lung transplantation.[375,377,391]

PULMONARY CAPILLARY HEMANGIOMATOSIS

Pulmonary capillary hemangiomatosis is an unusual cause of pulmonary hypertension that is also associated with recurrent episodes of DAH.[392–398] This condition is characterized by a proliferation of capillaries within the interstitium of the lung that infringes on the alveolar spaces (Figure 23–12). There is also a proliferation of capillaries within the walls of small pulmonary veins; this eventually occludes these vessels, producing a postcapillary type of pulmonary hypertension. Familial cases of this disease have been reported.[393] These patients have symptoms of pulmonary hypertension (dyspnea, fatigue, and syncope) as well as recurrent hemoptysis. Occasionally, the syndrome of DAH occurs, due to extensive rupture of the capillaries in the interstitium of the lung. The clinical presentation mimics pulmonary veno-occlusive disease.[399] The chest radiograph demonstrates pulmonary hypertension, and, with episodes of DAH, diffuse alveolar filling is superimposed. In some cases, the interstitial capillary proliferation produces a diffuse interstitial infiltrate on the chest radiograph.[400] Survival following diagnosis is usually less than 5 years, although most cases are diagnosed only at autopsy. In one case treated with interferon alpha-2a, however, there was marked improvement in the clinical, radiologic, and physiologic picture.[401]

OBSTRUCTIVE SLEEP APNEA

The occurrence of pulmonary hemosiderosis and alveolar hemorrhage in individuals with sleep apnea/obesity hypoventilation syndrome has been reported.[402] These individuals had evidence of pulmonary hypertension with medial hypertrophy of the muscular pulmonary arteries and biventricular failure. Pathology showed capillary proliferation resembling pulmonary capillary hemangiomatosis. The distinction between capillary proliferation in these patients and capillary hemangiomatosis is the lack of angioinvasion and veno-occlusion in the sleep apnea/obesity hypoventilation syndrome, suggesting that capillary proliferation occurs as a direct response to hypoxia/anoxia.[402] Whether these findings are clinically relevant is yet to be determined, because patients with sleep apnea/obesity hypoventilation syndrome rarely present with DAH.

FIBRILLARY GLOMERULONEPHRITIS

Fibrillary glomerulonephritis is a unique renal disease characterized by infiltration of the mesangium and glomerular basement membrane by fibrillary deposits that consist of polyclonal immunoglobulins,[403] a material distinct from amyloid. Most cases have no extrarenal involvement, but there are reports of patients with fibrillary glomerulonephritis who present with a pulmonary-renal syndrome.[403,404] In one case, the fibrillary material also infiltrated the pulmonary capillaries. Because this pulmonary-renal syndrome is associated with recurrent DAH, it can be confused with Goodpasture's syndrome. Histology, in addition to the fibrillary material within the interstitium of the lung, shows acute and chronic pulmonary hemorrhage.

MALIGNANCY AND DIFFUSE ALVEOLAR HEMORRHAGE

Malignancies of the lung, including metastatic renal cell carcinoma and the choriocarcinoma syndrome (a germ cell tumor of the testes with metastatic tumor to the lung), are associated with DAH.[405,406] The DAH usually occurs prior to the discovery of the tumor, and the cause of the alveolar hemorrhage is recognized only at open lung biopsy. Epithelial hemangioepithelioma and angiosarcoma, which are primary tumors of the lung, can also result in DAH.[407] Epithelial hemangioepithelioma was previously known as the intravascular sclerosing bronchiolar alveolar tumor. Angiosarcoma of the lung results from prior radiation, particularly in women who were treated for breast cancer,[408] and these patients often present with DAH.

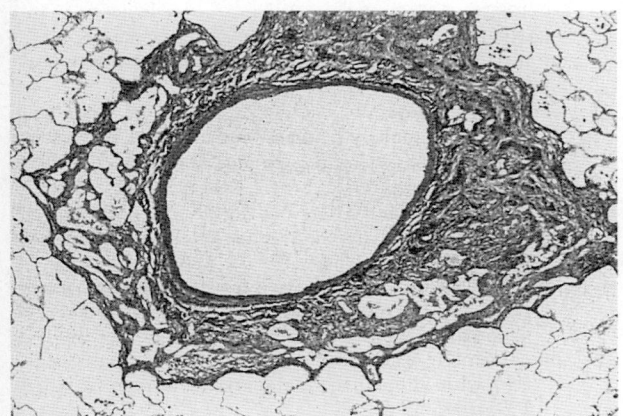

Figure 23–12 Capillary hemangiomatosis. There is capillary proliferation in the wall of a pulmonary vein without impingement of the lumen (hematoxylin and eosin; ×100 original magnification).

REFERENCES

1. Leatherman JW, Davies SF, Hoidal JR. Alveolar hemorrhage syndromes: diffuse microvascular lung hemorrhage in immune and idiopathic disorders. Medicine (Baltimore) 1984;63:343–61.

2. Leatherman JW. The lung in systemic vasculitis. Semin Respir Infect 1988;3:274–88.

3. Leatherman JW. Immune alveolar hemorrhage. Chest 1987; 91:891–7.

4. Schwarz MI, Cherniack R, King TEJ. Diffuse alveolar hemorrhage and other rare infiltrative dosorders. In: Murray JF, Nadel JA, Mason RJ, Boushey HA, editors. Textbook of respiratory medicine. Vol. 2. Philadelphia: WB Saunders; 2000. p. 1733–55.

5. Green RJ, Ruoss SJ, Kraft SA, et al. Pulmonary capillaritis and alveolar hemorrhage. Update on diagnosis and management. Chest 1996;110:1305–16.

6. Schwarz MI. Pulmonary capillaritis. Pulm Perspect 1994;11:4–6.

7. Spencer H. Pulmonary lesions in polyarteritis nodosa. Br J Tuberc Dis Chest 1957;51:123–30.

8. Mark EJ, Ramirez JF. Pulmonary capillaritis and hemorrhage in patients with systemic vasculitis. Arch Pathol Lab Med 1985;109:413–8.

9. Travis WD, Colby TV, Lombard C, Carpenter HA. A clinicopathologic study of 34 cases of diffuse pulmonary hemorrhage with lung biopsy confirmation. Am J Surg Pathol 1990;14:1112–25.

10. Katzenstein AL, Askin FB. Miscellaneous pulmonary angiitides. In: Katzenstein ALA, Askin FB, editors. Surgical pathology of non-neoplastic lung disease. Philadelphia: W.B. Saunders; 1990. p. 282–5.

11. Falk RJ, Terrell RS, Charles LA, Jennette JC. Anti-neutrophil cytoplasmic autoantibodies induce neutrophils to degranulate and produce oxygen radicals in vitro. Proc Natl Acad Sci U S A 1990;87:4115–9.

12. Jennette JC. Pathologic potential of anti-neutrophil cytoplasmic autoantibodies. Lab Invest 1994;70:135–7.

13. Gross WL, Schmitt WH, Csernok E. ANCA and associated diseases: immunodiagnostic and pathogenetic aspects. Clin Exp Immunol 1993;91:1–12.

14. Jennings CA, King TE Jr, Tuder R, et al. Diffuse alveolar hemorrhage with underlying isolated, pauciimmune pulmonary capillaritis. Am J Respir Crit Care Med 1997;155:1101–9.

15. Torralbo A, Herrero JA, Portoles J, Barrientos A. Alveolar hemorrhage associated with antineutrophil cytoplasmic antibodies in rheumatoid arthritis. Chest 1994;105:1590–2.

16. Schnabel A, Csernok E, Isenberg DA, et al. Antineutrophil cytoplasmic antibodies in systemic lupus erythematosus. Prevalence, specificities, and clinical significance. Arthritis Rheum 1995;38:633–7.

17. Zamora MR, Warner ML, Tuder R, Schwarz MI. Diffuse alveolar hemorrhage and systemic lupus erythematosus. Clinical presentation, histology, survival, and outcome. Medicine (Baltimore) 1997;76:192–202.

18. Fauci AS, Haynes B, Katz P. The spectrum of vasculitis: clinical, pathologic, immunologic and therapeutic considerations. Ann Intern Med 1978;89:660–76.

19. Leavitt RY, Fauci AS. Pulmonary vasculitis. Am Rev Respir Dis 1986;134:149–66.

20. Churg A, Franklin W, Chan KL, et al. Pulmonary hemorrhage and immune-complex deposition in the lung. Complications in a patient with systemic lupus erythematosus. Arch Pathol Lab Med 1980;104:388–91.

21. Eagen JW, Memoli VA, Roberts JL, et al. Pulmonary hemorrhage in systemic lupus erythematosus. Medicine (Baltimore) 1978;57:545–60.

22. Myers JL, Katzenstein AA. Microangiitis in lupus-induced pulmonary hemorrhage. Am J Clin Pathol 1986;85:552–6.

23. Gould DB, Soriano RZ. Acute alveolar hemorrhage in lupus erythematosus. Ann Intern Med 1975;83:836–7.

24. Rodriguez-Iturbe B, Garcia R, Rubio L, Serrano H. Immunohistologic findings in the lung in systemic lupus erythematosus. Arch Pathol Lab Med 1977;101:342–4.

25. Kathuria S, Cheifec G. Fatal pulmonary Henoch-Schönlein syndrome. Chest 1982;82:654–6.

26. Markus HS, Clark JV. Pulmonary haemorrhage in Henoch-Schönlein purpura. Thorax 1989;44:525–6.

27. Lai FM, Li EK, Suen MW, et al. Pulmonary hemorrhage. A fatal manifestation in IgA nephropathy. Arch Pathol Lab Med 1994;118:542–6.

28. Beirne GJ, Octaviano GN, Kopp WL, Burns RO. Immunohistology of the lung in Goodpasture's syndrome. Ann Intern Med 1968;69:1207–12.

29. Sisson S, Dysart NK Jr, Fish AJ, Vernier RL. Localization of the Goodpasture antigen by immunoelectron microscopy. Clin Immunol Immunopathol 1982;23:414–29.

30. Rees AJ. Pulmonary injury caused by anti-basement membrane antibodies. Semin Respir Dis 1984;5:264–72.

31. Gamble CN, Wiesner KB, Shapiro RF, Boyer WJ. The immune complex pathogenesis of glomerulonephritis and pulmonary vasculitis in Behçet's disease. Am J Med 1979;66:1031–9.

32. Shasby DM, Schwarz MI, Forstot JZ, et al. Pulmonary immune complex deposition in Wegener's granulomatosis. Chest 1982;81:338–40.

33. Schwarz MI, Mortenson RL, Colby TV, et al. Pulmonary capillaritis. The association with progressive irreversible airflow limitation and hyperinflation. Am Rev Respir Dis 1993;148:507–11.

34. Brugiere O, Raffy O, Sleiman C, et al. Progressive obstructive lung disease associated with microscopic polyangiitis. Am J Respir Crit Care Med 1997;155:739–42.

35. Wright PH, Buxton-Thomas M, Keeling PW, Kreel L. Adult idiopathic pulmonary haemosiderosis: a comparison of lung function changes and the distribution of pulmonary disease in patients with and without coeliac disease. Br J Dis Chest 1983;77:282–92.

36. Wright PH, Menzies IS, Pounder RE, Keeling PW. Adult idiopathic pulmonary haemosiderosis and coeliac disease. QJM 1981;50:95–102.

37. Lombard CM, Colby TV, Elliott CG. Surgical pathology of the lung in anti-basement membrane antibody-associated Goodpasture's syndrome. Hum Pathol 1989;20:445–51.

38. Hyatt RW, Adelstein ER, Halazun JF, Lukens JN. Ultrastructure of the lung in idiopathic pulmonary hemosiderosis. Am J Med 1972;52:822–9.

39. Gonzalez-Crussi F, Hull MT, Grosfeld JL. Idiopathic pulmonary hemosiderosis: evidence of capillary basement membrane abnormality. Am Rev Respir Dis 1976;114:689–98.

40. Yeager H Jr, Powell D, Weinberg RM, et al. Idiopathic pulmonary hemosiderosis: ultrastructural studies and responses to azathioprine. Arch Intern Med 1976;136:1145–9.

41. Katzenstein ALA. Idiopathic pulmonary hemosiderosis. In: Katzenstein ALA, Askin FB, editors. Surgical pathology of non-neoplastic lung disorders. Philadelphia: W.B. Saunders; 1982. p. 133.

42. Haselton PS. Adult respiratory distress syndrome. In: Haselton PS, editor. Spencers pathology of the lung: New York: McGraw-Hill; 1996. p. 375–400.

43. Forrester JM, Steele AW, Waldron JA, Parsons PE. Crack lung: an acute pulmonary syndrome with a spectrum of clinical and histopathologic findings. Am Rev Respir Dis 1990; 142:462–7.

44. Haim DY, Lippmann ML, Goldberg SK, Walkenstein MD. The pulmonary complications of crack cocaine. A comprehensive review. Chest 1995;107:233–40.

45. Donaghy M, Rees AJ. Cigarette smoking and lung haemorrhage in glomerulonephritis caused by autoantibodies to glomerular basement membrane. Lancet 1983;ii:1390–3.

46. Buschman DL, Ballard R. Progressive massive fibrosis associated with idiopathic pulmonary hemosiderosis. Chest 1993;104:293–5.

47. Robboy SJ, Minna JD, Colman RW, et al. Pulmonary hemorrhage syndrome as a manifestation of disseminated intravascular coagulation: analysis of ten cases. Chest 1973;63:718–21.

48. Buchanan GR, Moore GC. Pulmonary hemosiderosis and immune thrombocytopenia. Initial manifestations of collagen-vascular disease. JAMA 1981;246:861–4.

49. Martinez AJ, Maltby JD, Hurst DJ. Thrombotic thrombocytopenic purpura seen as pulmonary hemorrhage. Arch Intern Med 1983;143:1818–20.

50. Golde DW, Drew WL, Klein HZ, et al. Occult pulmonary haemorrhage in leukaemia. BMJ 1975;2:166–8.

51. Smith LJ, Katzenstein AL. Pathogenesis of massive pulmonary hemorrhage in acute leukemia. Arch Intern Med 1982; 142:2149–52.

52. Fireman Z, Yust I, Abramov AL. Lethal occult pulmonary hemorrhage in drug-induced thrombocytopenia. Chest 1981;79:358–9.

53. Papagiannis A, Smith AP, Hebden MW. Acute dyspnea, chest tightness, and anemia in a 33-year-old man. Chest 1995; 107:863–5.

54. Awadh N, Ronco JJ, Bernstein V, et al. Spontaneous pulmonary hemorrhage after thrombolytic therapy for acute myocardial infarction. Chest 1994;106:1622–4.

55. Gertner E, Lie JT. Pulmonary capillaritis, alveolar hemorrhage, and recurrent microvascular thrombosis in primary antiphospholipid syndrome. J Rheumatol 1993;20:1224–8.

56. Crausman RS, Achenbach GA, Pluss WT, et al. Pulmonary capillaritis and alveolar hemorrhage associated with the antiphospholipid antibody syndrome. J Rheumatol 1995; 22:554–6.

57. Greening AP, Hughes JM. Serial estimations of carbon monoxide diffusing capacity in intrapulmonary haemorrhage. Clin Sci (Colch) 1981;60:507–12.

58. Zapol WM, Rimar S, Gillis N, et al. Nitric oxide and the lung. Am J Respir Crit Care Med 1994;149:1375–80.

59. Adnot S, Raffestin B, Eddahibi S. NO in the lung. Respir Physiol 1995;101:109–20.

60. Mizutani T, Layon AJ. Clinical applications of nitric oxide. Chest 1996;110:506–24.

61. Voelkel NF, Czartolomna J. Vanadate potentiates hypoxic pulmonary vasoconstriction. J Pharmacol Exp Ther 1991;259: 666–72.

62. Hyslop S, DeNucci G. Vasoactive mediators released by endothelons. Pharmacol Res 1992;26:223–42.

63. Beechler CR, Enquist RW, Hunt KK, et al. Immunofluorescence of transbronchial biopsies in Goodpasture's syndrome. Am Rev Respir Dis 1980;121:869–72.

64. Mathew TH, Hobbs JB, Kalowski S, et al. Goodpasture's syndrome: normal renal diagnostic findings. Ann Intern Med 1975;82:215–8.

65. Abboud RT, Chase WH, Ballon HS, et al. Goodpasture's syndrome: diagnosis by transbronchial lung biopsy. Ann Intern Med 1978;89:635–8.

66. Zimmerman SW, Varanasi UR, Hoff B. Goodpasture's syndrome with normal renal function. Am J Med 1979;66:163–71.

67. Carre P, Lloveras JJ, Didier A, et al. Goodpasture's syndrome with normal renal function. Eur Respir J 1989;2:911–5.

68. Hamm H, Niedermeyer J, Krause J, Fabel H. [Anti-basement membrane antibody disease of the lungs without clinical kidney involvement.] Dtsch Med Wochenschr 1992;117: 858–62.

69. Tobler A, Schurch E, Altermatt HJ, Im Hof V. Anti-basement membrane antibody disease with severe pulmonary haemorrhage and normal renal function. Thorax 1991;46:68–70.

70. Ekholdt PF, Gulsvik A, Digranes S, et al. Recurrent diffuse pulmonary hemorrhage with minor kidney lesions. Eur J Respir Dis 1985;66:353–9.

71. Elliott ML, Kuhn C. Idiopathic pulmonary hemosiderosis. Ultrastructural abnormalities in the capillary walls. Am Rev Respir Dis 1970;102:895–904.

72. Abud-Mendoza C, Diaz-Jouanen E, Alarcon-Segovia D. Fatal pulmonary hemorrhage in systemic lupus erythematosus. Occurrence without hemoptysis. J Rheumatol 1985;12: 558–61.

73. Byrd RB, Trunk G. Systemic lupus erythematosus presenting as pulmonary hemosiderosis. Chest 1973;64:128–9.

74. Kauffmann RH, Herrmann WA, Meyer CJ, et al. Circulating IgA-immune complexes in Henoch-Schönlein purpura. A longitudinal study of their relationship to disease activity and vascular deposition of IgA. Am J Med 1980;69:859–66.

75. Faille-Kuyber EH, Kater L, Kooiker CJ, Dorhout Mees EJ. IgA-deposits in cutaneous blood-vessel walls and mesangium in Henoch-Schönlein syndrome. Lancet 1973;i:892–3.

76. Levinsky RJ, Barratt TM. IgA immune complexes in Henoch-Schönlein purpura. Lancet 1979;ii:1100–3.

77. Shichiri M, Tsutsumi K, Yamamoto I, et al. Diffuse intrapulmonary hemorrhage and renal failure in adult Henoch-Schönlein purpura. Am J Nephrol 1987;7:140–2.

78. Savige JA, Gallicchio M, Chang L, Parkin JD. Autoantibodies in systemic vasculitis. Aust N Z J Med 1991;21:433–7.

79. Hoffman GS, Kerr GS, Leavitt RY, et al. Wegener granulomatosis: an analysis of 158 patients. Ann Intern Med 1992; 116:488–98.

80. Bindi P, Mougenot B, Mentre F, et al. Necrotizing crescentic glomerulonephritis without significant immune deposits: a clinical and serological study. QJM 1993;86:55–68.

81. Gross WL, Ludemann G, Kiefer G, Lehmann H. Anticytoplasmic antibodies in Wegener's granulomatosis. Lancet 1986;i:806.

82. Andrassy K, Koderisch J, Waldherr R, Rufer M. Diagnostic significance of anticytoplasmatic antibodies (ACPA/ANCA) in detection of Wegener's granulomatosis and other forms of vasculitis. Nephron 1988;49:257–8.

83. Falk RJ, Jennette JC. Anti-neutrophil cytoplasmic autoantibodies with specificity for myeloperoxidase in patients with systemic vasculitis and idiopathic necrotizing and crescentic glomerulonephritis. N Engl J Med 1988;318:1651–7.

84. Goeken JA. Antineutrophil cytoplasmic antibody—a useful serological marker for vasculitis. J Clin Immunol 1991;11: 161–74.

85. Walters MD, Savage CO, Dillon MJ, et al. Antineutrophil cytoplasm antibody in crescentic glomerulonephritis. Arch Dis Child 1988;63:814–7.

86. Harper L, Savage CO. Pathogenesis of ANCA-associated systemic vasculitis. J Pathol 2000;190:349–59.

87. Bosch X, Font J, Mirapeix E, et al. Antimyeloperoxidase autoantibody-associated necrotizing alveolar capillaritis. Am Rev Respir Dis 1992;146:1326–9.

88. Bosch X, Lopez-Soto A, Mirapeix E, et al. Antineutrophil cytoplasmic autoantibody-associated alveolar capillaritis in patients presenting with pulmonary hemorrhage. Arch Pathol Lab Med 1994;118:517–22.

89. Rao JK, Weinberger M, Oddone EZ, et al. The role of antineutrophil cytoplasmic antibody (c-ANCA) testing in the diagnosis of Wegener granulomatosis. A literature review and meta-analysis. Ann Intern Med 1995;123:925–32.

90. Rao JK, Allen NB, Feussner JR, Weinberger M. A prospective study of antineutrophil cytoplasmic antibody (c-ANCA) and clinical criteria in diagnosing Wegener's granulomatosis. Lancet 1995;346:926–31.

91. Schnabel A, Reuter M, Csernok E, et al. Subclinical alveolar bleeding in pulmonary vasculitides: correlation with indices of disease activity. Eur Respir J 1999;14:118–24.

92. Salojin KV, Le Tonqueze M, Nassonov EL, et al. Anti-endothelial cell antibodies in patients with various forms of vasculitis. Clin Exp Rheumatol 1996;14:163–9.

93. Boehme MW, Schmitt WH, Youinou P, et al. Clinical relevance of elevated serum thrombomodulin and soluble E-selectin in patients with Wegener's granulomatosis and other systemic vasculitides. Am J Med 1996;101:387–94.

94. Ohdama S, Matsubara O, Aoki N. Plasma thrombomodulin in Wegener's granulomatosis as an indicator of vascular injuries. Chest 1994;106:666–71.

95. Kjellstrand CM, Simmons RL, Uranga VM, et al. Acute fulminant Wegener granulomatosis. Therapy with immunosuppression, hemodialysis, and renal transplantation. Arch Intern Med 1974;134:40–3.

96. Stokes TC, McCann BG, Rees RT, et al. Acute fulminating intrapulmonary haemorrhage in Wegener's granulomatosis. Thorax 1982;37:315–6.

97. Travis WD, Carpenter HA, Lie JT. Diffuse pulmonary hemorrhage. An uncommon manifestation of Wegener's granulomatosis. Am J Surg Pathol 1987;11:702–8.

98. Lenclud C, De Vuyst P, Dupont E, et al. Wegener's granulomatosis presenting as acute respiratory failure with anti-neutrophil-cytoplasm antibodies. Chest 1989;96:345–7.

99. Travis WD, Hoffman GS, Leavitt RY, et al. Surgical pathology of the lung in Wegener's granulomatosis. Review of 87 open lung biopsies from 67 patients. Am J Surg Pathol 1991;15:315–33.

100. Case records of the Massachusetts General Hospital. Weekly clinicopathological exercises. Case 12-1986. A 15-year-old boy with hemoptysis and occult blood in the urine. N Engl J Med 1986;314:834–44.

101. Cordier JF, Valeyre D, Guillevin L, et al. Pulmonary Wegener's granulomatosis. A clinical and imaging study of 77 cases. Chest 1990;97:906–12.

102. Haworth SJ, Savage CO, Carr D, et al. Pulmonary haemorrhage complicating Wegener's granulomatosis and microscopic polyarteritis. BMJ (Clin Res Ed) 1985;290:1775–8.

103. Brandwein S, Esdaile J, Danoff D, Tannenbaum H. Wegener's granulomatosis. Clinical features and outcome in 13 patients. Arch Intern Med 1983;143:476–9.

104. Sanchez-Masiques J, Ettensohn DB. Alveolar hemorrhage in Wegener's granulomatosis. Am J Med Sci 1989;297:390–3.

105. Case records of the Massachusetts General Hospital. Weekly clinicopathological exercises. Case 25-1989. A 56-year-old man with hemoptysis and microscopic hematuria. N Engl J Med 1989;320:1677–86.

106. Yoshimura N, Matsubara O, Tamura A, et al. Wegener's granulomatosis. Associated with diffuse pulmonary hemorrhage. Acta Pathol Jpn 1992;42:657–61.

107. Case records of the Massachusetts General Hospital. Weekly clinicopathological exercises. Case 52-1993. A 17-year-old girl with massive hemoptysis and acute oliguric renal failure. N Engl J Med 1993;329:2019–26.

108. Odeh M, Best LA, Kerner H, et al. Localized Wegener's granulomatosis relapsing as diffuse massive intra-alveolar hemorrhage. Chest 1993;104:955–6.

109. Mark EJ, Matsubara O, Tan-Liu NS, Fienberg R. The pulmonary biopsy in the early diagnosis of Wegener's (pathergic) granulomatosis: a study based on 35 open lung biopsies. Hum Pathol 1988;19:1065–71.

110. Bosch X. Microscopic polyangiitis (microscopic polyarteritis) with late emergence of generalised Wegener's granulomatosis. Ann Rheum Dis 1999;58:644–7.

111. Kikawada M, Ichinose Y, Minemura K, et al. Diffuse alveolar hemorrhage associated with proteinase 3-specific anti-neutrophil cytoplasmic antibodies. Intern Med 1997;36:430–4.

112. Gaudin PB, Askin FB, Falk RJ, Jennette JC. The pathologic spectrum of pulmonary lesions in patients with anti-neutrophil cytoplasmic autoantibodies specific for anti-proteinase 3 and anti-myeloperoxidase. Am J Clin Pathol 1995;104:7–16.

113. Niles JL, Bottinger EP, Saurina GR, et al. The syndrome of lung hemorrhage and nephritis is usually an ANCA-associated condition. Arch Intern Med 1996;156:440–5.

114. Hamidou MA, El Kouri D, Audrain M, Grolleau JY. Systemic antineutrophil cytoplasmic antibody vasculitis associated with lymphoid neoplasia. Ann Rheum Dis 2001;60:293–5.

115. Tatsis E, Reinhold-Keller E, Steindorf K, et al. Wegener's granulomatosis associated with renal cell carcinoma. Arthritis Rheum 1999;42:751–6.

116. Gratadour P, Fouque D, Laville M, et al. Wegener's granulomatosis with antiproteinase-3 antibodies occurring after Hodgkin's disease. Nephron 1993;64:456–61.

117. Imoto EM, Lombard CM, Sachs DP. Pulmonary capillaritis and hemorrhage. A clue to the diagnosis of systemic necrotizing vasculitis. Chest 1989;96:927–8.

118. Zashin S, Fattor R, Fortin D. Microscopic polyarteritis: a forgotten aetiology of haemoptysis and rapidly progressive glomerulonephritis. Ann Rheum Dis 1990;49:53–6.

119. Doebbeling BN, Bonsib SM, Walker WP. Pulmonary-renal syndrome with "triad" involvement due to small vessel vasculitis. J Rheumatol 1990;17:1087–90.

120. Savage CO, Winearls CG, Evans DJ, et al. Microscopic polyarteritis: presentation, pathology and prognosis. QJM 1985;56:467–83.

121. Bocanegra TS, Espinoza LR, Vasey FB, Germain BF. Pulmonary hemorrhage in systemic necrotizing vasculitis associated with hepatitis B. Chest 1981;80:102–3.

122. Sanchez M, Bosch X, Martinez C, et al. Idiopathic pulmonary-renal syndrome with antiproteinase 3 antibodies. Respiration 1994;61:295–9.

123. Leaker B, Cambridge G, du Bois RM, Neild GH. Idiopathic pulmonary haemosiderosis: a form of microscopic polyarteritis? Thorax 1992;47:988–90.

124. Li PK, Lui SF, Lai FM, et al. Microscopic polyarteritis has a poor prognosis in Chinese. J Rheumatol 1995;22:1295–9.

125. ter Maaten JC, Franssen CF, Gans RO, et al. Respiratory failure in ANCA-associated vasculitis. Chest 1996;110:357–62.

126. Akikusa B, Sato T, Ogawa M, et al. Necrotizing alveolar capillaritis in autopsy cases of microscopic polyangiitis. Incidence, histopathogenesis, and relationship with systemic vasculitis. Arch Pathol Lab Med 1997;121:144–9.

127. Lhote F, Guillevin L. Polyarteritis nodosa, microscopic polyangiitis, and Churg-Strauss syndrome. Semin Respir Crit Care Med 1998;19:27–45.

128. Guillevin L, Durand-Gasselin B, Cevallos R, et al. Microscopic polyangiitis: clinical and laboratory findings in eighty-five patients. Arthritis Rheum 1999;42:421–30.

129. Lauque D, Cadranel J, Lazor R, et al. Microscopic polyangiitis with alveolar hemorrhage. A study of 29 cases and review of the literature. Groupe d'Etudes et de Recherche sur les Maladies "Orphelines" Pulmonaires (GERM"O"P). Medicine (Baltimore) 2000;79:222–33.

130. Guillevin L, Lhote F, Cohen P, et al. Polyarteritis nodosa related to hepatitis B virus. A prospective study with long-term observation of 41 patients. Medicine (Baltimore) 1995;74:238–53.

131. Guillevin L, Lhote F, Gayraud M, et al. Prognostic factors in polyarteritis nodosa and Churg-Strauss syndrome. A prospective study in 342 patients. Medicine (Baltimore) 1996;75:17–28.

132. Proliferative glomerulonephritis and pulmonary hemorrhage. Am J Med 1973;55:199–210.

133. Lewis EJ, Schur PH, Busch GJ, et al. Immunopathologic features of a patient with glomerulonephritis and pulmonary hemorrhage. Am J Med 1973;54:507–13.

134. Leatherman JW, Sibley RK, Davies SF. Diffuse intrapulmonary hemorrhage and glomerulonephritis unrelated to anti-glomerular basement membrane antibody. Am J Med 1982;72:401–10.

135. Hall JB, Wadham BM, Wood CJ, et al. Vasculitis and glomerulonephritis: a subgroup with an antineutrophil cytoplasmic antibody. Aust N Z J Med 1984;14:277–8.

136. Thomashow BM, Felton CP, Navarro C. Diffuse intrapulmonary hemorrhage, renal failure and a systemic vasculitis. A case report and review of the literature. Am J Med 1980;68:299–304.

137. Nada AK, Torres VE, Ryu JH, et al. Pulmonary fibrosis as an unusual clinical manifestation of a pulmonary-renal vasculitis in elderly patients. Mayo Clin Proc 1990;65:847–56.

138. Nierman DM, Kalb TH, Ornstein MH, Gil J. A patient with antineutrophil cytoplasmic antibody-negative pulmonary capillaritis and circulating primed neutrophils. Arthritis Rheum 1995;38:1855–8.

139. Hunninghake GW, Fauci AS. Pulmonary involvement in the collagen vascular diseases. Am Rev Respir Dis 1979;119: 471–503.

140. Emlen W. Systemic lupus erythematosus and mixed connective tissue disease. Immunol Allergy Clin N Am 1993;13: 291–311.

141. Gross M, Esterly JR, Earle RH. Pulmonary alterations in systemic lupus erythematosus. Am Rev Respir Dis 1972;105: 572–7.

142. Eisenberg H, Dubois EL, Sherwin RP, Balchum OJ. Diffuse interstitial lung disease in systemic lupus erythematosus. Ann Intern Med 1973;79:37–45.

143. Menchaca JA, Boris G, Iacuone JJ, Bartholomew B. Glomerulonephritis and pulmonary hemorrhage. J Pediatr 1979;94: 507–8.

144. Kinney WW, Angelillo VA. Bronchiolitis in systemic lupus erythematosus. Chest 1982;82:646–9.

145. Asherson RA, Oakley CM. Pulmonary hypertension and systemic lupus erythematosus. J Rheumatol 1986;13:1–5.

146. Alarcon-Segovia D, Deleze M, Oria CV, et al. Antiphospholipid antibodies and the antiphospholipid syndrome in systemic lupus erythematosus. A prospective analysis of 500 consecutive patients. Medicine (Baltimore) 1989;68:353–65.

147. King TE Jr. Connective tissue disease. In: Schwarz MI, King TE Jr, editors. Interstitial lung disease. Hamilton: B.C. Decker; 1998. p. 451–505.

148. Kuhn C. Systemic lupus erythematosus in a patient with ultrastructural lesions of the pulmonary capillaries previously reported in the review as due to idiopathic pulmonary hemosiderosis. Am Rev Respir Dis 1972;106:931–2.

149. Marino CT, Pertschuk LP. Pulmonary hemorrhage in systemic lupus erythematosus. Arch Intern Med 1981;141: 201–3.

150. Matthay RA, Schwarz MI, Petty TL, et al. Pulmonary manifestations of systemic lupus erythematosus: review of twelve cases of acute lupus pneumonitis. Medicine (Baltimore) 1975;54:397–409.

151. Mintz G, Galindo LF, Fernandez-Diez J, et al. Acute massive pulmonary hemorrhage in systemic lupus erythematosus. J Rheumatol 1978;5:39–50.

152. Onomura K, Nakata H, Tanaka Y, Tsuda T. Pulmonary hemorrhage in patients with systemic lupus erythematosus. J Thorac Imaging 1991;6:57–61.

153. Schwab EP, Schumacher HR Jr, Freundlich B, Callegari PE. Pulmonary alveolar hemorrhage in systemic lupus erythematosus. Semin Arthritis Rheum 1993;23:8–15.

154. Carette S, Macher AM, Nussbaum A, Plotz PH. Severe, acute pulmonary disease in patients with systemic lupus erythematosus: ten years of experience at the National Institutes of Health. Semin Arthritis Rheum 1984;14:52–9.

155. Hill HF. Penicillamine in rheumatoid arthritis: adverse effects. Scand J Rheumatol Suppl 1979;28:94–9.

156. Millman RP, Cohen TB, Levinson AI, et al. Systemic lupus erythematosus complicated by acute pulmonary hemorrhage: recovery following plasmapheresis and cytotoxic therapy. J Rheumatol 1981;8:1021–3.

157. Hughson MD, He Z, Henegar J, McMurray R. Alveolar hemorrhage and renal microangiopathy in systemic lupus erythematosus. Arch Pathol Lab Med 2001;125:475–83.

158. Liu MF, Lee JH, Weng TH, Lee YY. Clinical experience of 13 cases with severe pulmonary hemorrhage in systemic lupus erythematosus with active nephritis. Scand J Rheumatol 1998;27:291–5.

159. Santos-Ocampo AS, Mandell BF, Fessler BJ. Alveolar hemorrhage in systemic lupus erythematosus: presentation and management. Chest 2000;118:1083–90.

160. Lewis EJ, Hunsicker LG, Lan SP, et al. A controlled trial of plasmapheresis therapy in severe lupus nephritis. The Lupus Nephritis Collaborative Study Group. N Engl J Med 1992;326:1373–9.

161. Schwarz MI, Sutarik JM, Nick JA, et al. Pulmonary capillaritis and diffuse alveolar hemorrhage. A primary manifestation of polymyositis. Am J Respir Crit Care Med 1995; 151:2037–40.

162. Tazelaar HD, Viggiano RW, Pickersgill J, Colby TV. Interstitial lung disease in polymyositis and dermatomyositis. Clinical features and prognosis as correlated with histologic findings. Am Rev Respir Dis 1990;141:727–33.

163. Kallenbach J, Prinsloo I, Zwi S. Progressive systemic sclerosis complicated by diffuse pulmonary haemorrhage. Thorax 1977;32:767–70.

164. Griffin MT, Robb JD, Martin JR. Diffuse alveolar haemorrhage associated with progressive systemic sclerosis. Thorax 1990;45:903–4.

165. Nishi K, Myou S, Ooka T, et al. Diffuse cutaneous systemic sclerosis associated with pan-serositis, disseminated intravascular coagulation, and diffuse alveolar haemorrhage. Respir Med 1994;88:471–3.

166. Bar J, Ehrenfeld M, Rozenman J, et al. Pulmonary-renal syndrome in systemic sclerosis. Semin Arthritis Rheum 2001; 30:403–10.

167. Germain MJ, Davidman M. Pulmonary hemorrhage and acute renal failure in a patient with mixed connective tissue disease. Am J Kidney Dis 1984;3:420–4.

168. Horiki T, Fuyuno G, Ishii M, et al. Fatal alveolar hemorrhage in a patient with mixed connective tissue disease presenting polymyositis features. Intern Med 1998;37:554–60.

169. Ognibene AJ, Dito WR. Rheumatoid disease with unusual pulmonary manifestations. Pulmonary hemosiderosis, fibrosis, and concretions. Arch Intern Med 1965;116:567–72.

170. Smith BS. Idiopathic pulmonary haemosiderosis and rheumatoid arthritis. BMJ 1966;5500:1403–4.

171. Naschitz JE, Yeshurun D, Scharf Y, et al. Recurrent massive alveolar hemorrhage, crescentic glomerulonephritis, and necrotizing vasculitis in a patient with rheumatoid arthritis. Arch Intern Med 1989;149:406–8.

172. Schwarz MI, Zamora MR, Hodges TN, et al. Isolated pulmonary capillaritis and diffuse alveolar hemorrhage in rheumatoid arthritis and mixed connective tissue disease. Chest 1998;113:1609–15.

173. Asherson RA, Cervera R, Piette JC, et al. Catastrophic antiphospholipid syndrome. Clinical and laboratory features of 50 patients. Medicine (Baltimore) 1998;77:195–207.

174. Gertner E. Diffuse alveolar hemorrhage in the antiphospholipid syndrome: spectrum of disease and treatment. J Rheumatol 1999;26:805–7.

175. Wiedermann FJ, Mayr A, Schobersberger W, et al. Acute respiratory failure associated with catastrophic antiphospholipid syndrome. J Intern Med 2000;247:723–30.

176. Cream JJ, Gumpel JM, Peachey RD. Schönlein-Henoch purpura in the adult. A study of 77 adults with anaphylactoid or Schönlein-Henoch purpura. QJM 1970;39:461–84.

177. Bar-On H, Rosenmann E. Schoenlein-Henoch syndrome in adults. A clinical and histological study of renal involvement. Isr J Med Sci 1972;8:1702–15.

178. Roth DA, Wilz DR, Theil GB. Schönlein-Henoch syndrome in adults. QJM 1985;55:145–52.

179. Counahan R, Cameron JS. Henoch-Schönlein nephritis. Contrib Nephrol 1977;7:143–65.

180. Weiss VF, Naidu S. Fatal pulmonary hemorrhage in Henoch-Schönlein purpura. Cutis 1979;23:687–8.

181. Yokose T, Aida J, Ito Y, et al. A case of pulmonary hemorrhage in Henoch-Schönlein purpura accompanied by polyarteritis nodosa in an elderly man. Respiration 1993;60:307–10.

182. Endo Y, Kanbayashi H. Etiology of IgA nephropathy syndrome. Pathol Int 1994;44:1–13.

183. Border WA, Baehler RW, Bhathena D, Glassock RJ. IgA antibasement membrane nephritis with pulmonary hemorrhage. Ann Intern Med 1979;91:21–5.

184. Harland RW, Becker CG, Brandes JC, et al. Immunoglobulin A (IgA) immune complex pneumonitis in a patient with IgA nephropathy. Ann Intern Med 1992;116:220–2.

185. Yum MN, Lampton LM, Bloom PM, Edwards JL. Asymptomatic IgA nephropathy associated with pulmonary hemosiderosis. Am J Med 1978;64:1056–60.

186. Sinico RA, Tadros M, Radice A, et al. Lack of IgA antineutrophil cytoplasmic antibodies in Henoch-Schönlein purpura and IgA nephropathy. Clin Immunol Immunopathol 1994;73:19–26.

187. O'Duffy JD, Carney JA, Deodhar S. Behçet's disease. Report of 10 cases, 3 with new manifestations. Ann Intern Med 1971;75:561–70.

188. Chajek T, Fainaru M. Behçet's disease. Report of 41 cases and a review of the literature. Medicine (Baltimore) 1975;54:179–96.

189. Yazici H, Yurdakul S, Hamuryudan V. Behçet disease. Curr Opin Rheumatol 2001;13:18–22.

190. Cadman EC, Lundberg WB, Mitchell MS. Pulmonary manifestations in Behçet syndrome. Case report and review of the literature. Arch Intern Med 1976;136:944–7.

191. Slavin RE, de Groot WJ. Pathology of the lung in Behçet's disease. Case report and review of the literature. Am J Surg Pathol 1981;5:779–88.

192. Raz I, Okon E, Chajek-Shaul T. Pulmonary manifestations in Behçet's syndrome. Chest 1989;95:585–9.

193. Efthimiou J, Johnston C, Spiro SG, Turner-Warwick M. Pulmonary disease in Behçet's syndrome. QJM 1986;58:259–80.

194. Stricker H, Malinverni R. Multiple, large aneurysms of pulmonary arteries in Behçet's disease. Clinical remission and radiologic resolution after corticosteroid therapy. Arch Intern Med 1989;149:925–7.

195. Erkan F. Pulmonary involvement in Behçet disease. Curr Opin Pulm Med 1999;5:314–8.

196. Yazici H, Pazarli H, Barnes CG, et al. A controlled trial of azathioprine in Behçet's syndrome. N Engl J Med 1990;322:281–5.

197. Ferri C, Zignego AL. Relation between infection and autoimmunity in mixed cryoglobulinemia. Curr Opin Rheumatol 2000;12:53–60.

198. Cacoub P, Maisonobe T, Thibault V, et al. Systemic vasculitis in patients with hepatitis C. J Rheumatol 2001;28:109–18.

199. Della Rossa A, Tavoni A, Baldini C, Bombardieri S. Mixed cryoglobulinemia and hepatitis C virus association: ten years later. Isr Med Assoc J 2001;3:430–4.

200. Bombardieri S, Paoletti P, Ferri C, et al. Lung involvement in essential mixed cryoglobulinemia. Am J Med 1979;66:748–56.

201. Madrenas J, Valles M, Ruiz Marcellan MC, et al. [Pulmonary hemorrhage and glomerulonephritis associated with essential mixed cryoglobulinemia.] Med Clin (Barc) 1989;93:262–4.

202. Frankel AH, Singer DR, Winearls CG, et al. Type II essential mixed cryoglobulinaemia: presentation, treatment and outcome in 13 patients. QJM 1992;82:101–24.

203. Gomez-Tello V, Onoro-Canaveral JJ, de la Casa Monje RM, et al. Diffuse recidivant alveolar hemorrhage in a patient with hepatitis C virus-related mixed cryoglobulinemia. Intensive Care Med 1999;25:319–22.

204. Clinical conference: mixed cryoimmunoglobulinemia. Am J Med 1976;61:95–102.

205. Couser WG. Idiopathic crescentic glomerulonephritis. In: Massry SG, Glassock RJ, editors. Textbook of nephrology. Baltimore: Williams & Wilkins; 1983. p. 6–52.

206. Loughlin GM, Taussig LM, Murphy SA, et al. Immune-complex-mediated glomerulonephritis and pulmonary hemorrhage simulating Goodpasture syndrome. J Pediatr 1978;93:181–4.

207. Beirne GJ, Kopp WL, Zimmerman SW. Goodpasture syndrome. Dissociation from antibodies to glomerular basement membrane. Arch Intern Med 1973;132:261–3.

208. Jayne DR, Marshall PD, Jones SJ, Lockwood CM. Autoantibodies to GBM and neutrophil cytoplasm in rapidly progressive glomerulonephritis. Kidney Int 1990;37:965–70.

209. O'Donoghue DJ, Short CD, Brenchley PE, et al. Sequential development of systemic vasculitis with anti-neutrophil cytoplasmic antibodies complicating anti-glomerular basement membrane disease. Clin Nephrol 1989;32:251–5.

210. Bosch X, Mirapeix E, Font J, et al. Prognostic implication of anti-neutrophil cytoplasmic autoantibodies with myeloperoxidase specificity in anti-glomerular basement membrane disease. Clin Nephrol 1991;36:107–13.

211. Heeringa P, Brouwer E, Klok PA, et al. Autoantibodies to myeloperoxidase aggravate mild anti-glomerular-basement-membrane-mediated glomerular injury in the rat. Am J Pathol 1996;149:1695–706.

212. Badesch DB, Zamora M, Fullerton D, et al. Pulmonary capillaritis: a possible histologic form of acute pulmonary allograft rejection. J Heart Lung Transplant 1998;17:415–22.

213. Isenberg JI, Goldstein H, Korn AR, et al. Pulmonary vasculitis—an uncommon complication of ulcerative colitis. Report of a case. N Engl J Med 1968;279:1376–7.

214. Sargent D, Sessions JT, Fairman RP. Pulmonary vasculitis complicating ulcerative colitis. South Med J 1985;78:624–5.

215. Kradin RL, Kiprov D, Dickersin GR, et al. Immune complex disease with fatal pulmonary hemorrhage: its occurrence in a patient with myasthenia gravis. Arch Pathol Lab Med 1981;105:582–5.

216. Yermakov VM, Hitti IF, Sutton AL. Necrotizing vasculitis associated with diphenylhydantoin: two fatal cases. Hum Pathol 1983;14:182–4.

217. Harper L, Cockwell P, Savage CO. Case of propylthiouracil-induced ANCA associated small vessel vasculitis. Nephrol Dial Transplant 1998;13:455–8.

218. Frankel SR, Eardley A, Lauwers G, et al. The "retinoic acid syndrome" in acute promyelocytic leukemia. Ann Intern Med 1992;117:292–6.

219. Nicolls MR, Terada LS, Tuder RM, et al. Diffuse alveolar hemorrhage with underlying pulmonary capillaritis in the retinoic acid syndrome. Am J Respir Crit Care Med 1998;158:1302–5.

220. Raanani P, Segal E, Levi II, et al. Diffuse alveolar hemorrhage in acute promyelocytic leukemia patients treated with atra—a manifestation of the basic disease or the treatment. Leuk Lymphoma 2000;37:605–10.

221. Stankus SJ, Johnson NT. Propylthiouracil-induced hypersensitivity vasculitis presenting as respiratory failure. Chest 1992;102:1595–6.

222. Dolman KM, Gans RO, Vervaat TJ, et al. Vasculitis and antineutrophil cytoplasmic autoantibodies associated with propylthiouracil therapy. Lancet 1993;342:651–2.

223. Ohtsuka M, Yamashita Y, Doi M, Hasegawa S. Propylthiouracil-induced alveolar haemorrhage associated with antineutrophil cytoplasmic antibody. Eur Respir J 1997;10:1405–7.

224. Dhillon SS, Singh D, Doe N, et al. Diffuse alveolar hemorrhage and pulmonary capillaritis due to propylthiouracil. Chest 1999;116:1485–8.

225. D'Cruz D, Chesser AM, Lightowler C, et al. Antineutrophil cytoplasmic antibody-positive crescentic glomerulonephritis associated with anti-thyroid drug treatment. Br J Rheumatol 1995;34:1090–1.

226. Romas E, Henderson DR, Kirkham BW. Propylthiouracil therapy: an unusual cause of antineutrophil cytoplasmic antibody associated alveolar hemorrhage. J Rheumatol 1995;22:803.

227. Goodpasture EW. The signficance of certain pulmonary lesions in relation to the etiology of influenza. Am J Med Sci 1919;158:863–70.

228. Duncan DA, Drummond KN, Michael AF, Vernier RL. Pulmonary hemorrhage and glomerulonephritis: report of six cases and study of the renal lesion by the fluorescent antibody technique and electron microscopy. Ann Intern Med 1965;62:920–38.

229. Sturgill BC, Westervelt FB. Immunofluorescence studies in a case of Goodpasture's syndrome. JAMA 1965;194:914–6.

230. Wilson CB, Smith RC. Goodpasture's syndrome associated with influenza A2 virus infection. Ann Intern Med 1972;76:91–4.

231. Simpson IJ, Doak PB, Williams LC, et al. Plasma exchange in Goodpasture's syndrome. Am J Nephrol 1982;2:301–11.

232. Martinez JS, Kohler PF. Variant "Goodpasture's syndrome"? The need for immunologic criteria in rapidly progressive glomerulonephritis and hemorrhagic pneumonitis. Ann Intern Med 1971;75:67–76.

233. Krakower CA, Greenspon SA. Localization of the nephrotoxic antigen with the isolated renal glomerulus. Arch Pathol Lab Med 1951;51:629–51.

234. Sleblay RW. Glomerulonephritis induced in sheep by injections of heterologous glomerular basement membrane and Freunds complete adjuvant. J Exp Med 1962;116:253–71.

235. Lerner RA, Glassock RJ, Dixon FJ. The role of anti-glomerular basement membrane antibody in the pathogenesis of human glomerulonephritis. J Exp Med 1967;126:989–1004.

236. Wieslander J, Barr JF, Butkowski RJ, et al. Goodpasture antigen of the glomerular basement membrane: localization to noncollagenous regions of type IV collagen. Proc Natl Acad Sci U S A 1984;81:3838–42.

237. Kalluri R, Gunwar S, Reeders ST, et al. Goodpasture syndrome. Localization of the epitope for the autoantibodies to the carboxyl-terminal region of the alpha 3(IV) chain of basement membrane collagen. J Biol Chem 1991;266:24018–24.

238. Hellmark T, Burkhardt H, Wieslander J. Goodpasture disease. Characterization of a single conformational epitope as the target of pathogenic autoantibodies. J Biol Chem 1999;274:25862–68.

239. Gunnarsson A, Hellmark T, Wieslander J. Molecular properties of the Goodpasture epitope. J Biol Chem 2000;275:30844–8.

240. Borza DB, Netzer KO, Leinonen A, et al. The Goodpasture autoantigen. Identification of multiple cryptic epitopes on the NC1 domain of the alpha3(IV) collagen chain. J Biol Chem 2000;275:6030–7.

241. Phelps RG, Rees AJ. The HLA complex in Goodpasture's disease: a model for analyzing susceptibility to autoimmunity. Kidney Int 1999;56:1638–53.

242. Turner N, Mason PJ, Brown R, et al. Molecular cloning of the human Goodpasture antigen demonstrates it to be the alpha 3 chain of type IV collagen. J Clin Invest 1992;89:592–601.

243. Hudson BG, Wieslander J, Wisdom BJ Jr, Noelken ME. Goodpasture syndrome: molecular architecture and function of basement membrane antigen. Lab Invest 1989;61:256–69.

244. McIntosh RM, Copack P, Chernack WB, et al. The human choroid plexus and autoimmune nephritis. Arch Pathol 1975;99:48–50.

245. Weber M, Pullig O. Different immunologic properties of the globular NC1 domain of collagen type IV isolated from various human basement membranes. Eur J Clin Invest 1992;22:138–46.

246. McPhaul JJ Jr, Mullins JD. Glomerulonephritis mediated by antibody to glomerular basement membrane. Immunological, clinical, and histopathological characteristics. J Clin Invest 1976;57:351–61.

247. Jennings L, Roholt OA, Pressman D, et al. Experimental antialveolar basement membrane antibody-mediated pneumonitis. I. The role of increased permeability of the alveolar capillary wall induced by oxygen. J Immunol 1981;127:129–34.

248. Salant DJ. Immunopathogenesis of crescentic glomerulonephritis and lung purpura. Kidney Int 1987;32:408–25.

249. Beirne GJ, Brennan JT. Glomerulonephritis associated with hydrocarbon solvents: mediated by antiglomerular basement membrane antibody. Arch Environ Health 1972;25:365–9.

250. Keogh AM, Ibels LS, Allen DH, et al. Exacerbation of Goodpasture's syndrome after inadvertent exposure to hydrocarbon fumes. BMJ (Clin Res Ed) 1984;288:188.

251. Jones JG, Minty BD, Lawler P, et al. Increased alveolar epithelial permeability in cigarette smokers. Lancet 1980;i:66–8.

252. Koffler D, Agnello V, Carr RI, Kunkel HG. Variable patterns of immunoglobulin and complement deposition in the kidneys of patients with systemic lupus erythematosus. Am J Pathol 1969;56:305–16.

253. Westberg NG, Michael AF. Immunohistopathology of diabetic glomerulosclerosis. Diabetes 1972;21:163–74.

254. Moss M, Neff TA, Colby TV, et al. Diffuse alveolar hemorrhage due to antibasement membrane antibody disease appearing with a polyglandular autoimmune syndrome. Chest 1994;105:296–8.

255. Rees AJ, Peters DK, Amos N, et al. The influence of HLA-linked genes on the severity of anti-GBM antibody-mediated nephritis. Kidney Int 1984;26:445–50.

256. Perl SI, Pussell BA, Charlesworth JA, et al. Goodpasture's (anti-GBM) disease and HLA-DRw2. N Engl J Med 1981;305:463–4.

257. Rees AJ, Peters DK, Compston DA, Batchelor JR. Strong association between HLA-DRW2 and antibody-mediated Goodpasture's syndrome. Lancet 1978;i:966–8.

258. Peters DK, Rees AJ, Lockwood CM, Pusey CD. Treatment and prognosis in antibasement membrane antibody-mediated nephritis. Transplant Proc 1982;14:513–21.

259. Holdsworth S, Boyce N, Thomson NM, Atkins RC. The clinical spectrum of acute glomerulonephritis and lung haemorrhage (Goodpasture's syndrome). QJM 1985;55:75–86.

260. Bell DD, Moffatt SL, Singer M, Munt PW. Antibasement membrane antibody disease without clinical evidence of renal disease. Am Rev Respir Dis 1990;142:234–7.

261. Proskey AJ, Weatherbee L, Easterling RE, et al. Goodpasture's syndrome. A report of five cases and review of the literature. Am J Med 1970;48:162–73.

262. Kelly PT, Haponik EF. Goodpasture syndrome: molecular and clinical advances. Medicine (Baltimore) 1994;73:171–85.

263. Teague CA, Doak PB, Simpson IJ, et al. Goodpasture's syndrome: an analysis of 29 cases. Kidney Int 1978;13:492–504.

264. Mehler PS, Brunvand MW, Hutt MP, Anderson RJ. Chronic recurrent Goodpasture's syndrome. Am J Med 1987;82:833–5.

265. Klasa RJ, Abboud RT, Ballon HS, Grossman L. Goodpasture's syndrome: recurrence after a five-year remission. Case report and review of the literature. Am J Med 1988;84:751–5.

266. Keller F, Nekarda H. Fatal relapse in Goodpasture's syndrome 3 years after plasma exchange. Respiration 1985;48:62–6.

267. Levy JB, Lachmann RH, Pusey CD. Recurrent Goodpasture's disease. Am J Kidney Dis 1996;27:573–8.

268. Ewan PW, Jones HA, Rhodes CG, Hughes JM. Detection of intrapulmonary hemorrhage with carbon monoxide uptake. Application in Goodpasture's syndrome. N Engl J Med 1976;295:1391–6.

269. Addleman M, Logan AS, Grossman RF. Monitoring intrapulmonary hemorrhage in Goodpasture's syndrome. Chest 1985;87:119–20.

270. Fish AJ, Kleppel M, Jeraj K, Michael AF. Enzyme immunoassay of anti-glomerular basement membrane antibodies. J Lab Clin Med 1985;105:700–5.

271. Donald KJ, Edwards RL, McEvoy JD. Alveolar capillary basement membrane lesions in Goodpasture's syndrome and idiopathic pulmonary hemosiderosis. Am J Med 1975;59:642–9.

272. Bils RF. Ultrastructural alterations of alveolar tissue of mice. 3. Ozone. Arch Environ Health 1970;20:468–80.

273. McCormick JR, Kass J, Skewes M. Goodpasture's syndrome. Compr Ther 1987;13:25–32.

274. Balow JE. Plasmapheresis: development and application in treatment of renal disorders. Artif Organs 1986;10:324–30.

275. Stanton MC, Tange JD. Goodpasture's syndrome. Aust Ann Med 1958;7:132–44.

276. Wilson CB, Dixon FJ. Anti-glomerular basement membrane antibody-induced glomerulonephritis. Kidney Int 1973;3:74–89.

277. Lockwood CM, Rees AJ, Pearson TA, et al. Immunosuppression and plasma-exchange in the treatment of Goodpasture's syndrome. Lancet 1976;i:711–5.

278. Keller F, Offermann G, Schultze G, et al. Membrane plasma exchange in Goodpasture's syndrome. Am J Med Sci 1984;287:32–6.

279. Rosenblatt SG, Knight W, Bannayan GA, et al. Treatment of Goodpasture's syndrome with plasmapheresis. A case report and review of the literature. Am J Med 1979;66:689–96.

280. Erickson SB, Kurtz SB, Donadio JV Jr, et al. Use of combined plasmapheresis and immunosuppression in the treatment of Goodpasture's syndrome. Mayo Clin Proc 1979;54:714–20.

281. Shumak KH, Rock GA. Therapeutic plasma exchange. N Engl J Med 1984;310:762–71.

282. Fort J, Espinel E, Rogriquez JA, et al. Partial recovery of renal function in an oligoanuric patient affected with Goodpasture's syndrome after treatment with steroids, immunosuppressives and plasmapheresis. Clin Nephrol 1984;22:211–2.

283. Bygren P, Freiburghaus C, Lindholm T, et al. Goodpasture's syndrome treated with staphylococcal protein A immunoadsorption. Lancet 1985;ii:1295–6.

284. Johnson JP, Moore J Jr, Austin HA 3rd, et al. Therapy of anti-glomerular basement membrane antibody disease: analysis of prognostic significance of clinical, pathologic and treatment factors. Medicine (Baltimore) 1985;64:219–27.

285. Walker RG, Scheinkestel C, Becker GJ, et al. Clinical and morphological aspects of the management of crescentic anti-glomerular basement membrane antibody (anti-GBM) nephritis/Goodpasture's syndrome. QJM 1985;54:75–89.

286. Hind CR, Paraskevakou H, Lockwood CM, et al. Prognosis after immunosuppression of patients with crescentic nephritis requiring dialysis. Lancet 1983;i:263–5.

287. Beirne GJ, Wagnild JP, Zimmerman SW, et al. Idiopathic crescentic glomerulonephritis. Medicine (Baltimore) 1977;56:349–81.

288. Rees AJ, Lockwood CM, Peters DK. Enhanced allergic tissue injury in Goodpasture's syndrome by intercurrent bacterial infection. BMJ 1977;2:723–6.

289. Mahieu P, Lambert PH, Miescher PA. Detection of anti-glomerular basement membrane antibodies by radioimmunological technique. Clinical application in human nephropathies. J Clin Invest 1974;54:128–37.

290. Cohen S. Idiopathic pulmonary hemosiderosis. Am J Med Sci 1999;317:67–74.

291. Case records of the Massachusetts General Hospital. Weekly clinicopathological exercises. Case 30-1979. N Engl J Med 1979;301:201–8.

292. Soergel KH, Sommers SC. The alveolar epithelial lesion of idiopathic pulmonary hemosiderosis. Am Rev Respir Dis 1962;85:540–52.

293. Irwin RS, Cottrell TS, Hsu KC, et al. Idiopathic pulmonary hemosiderosis: an electron microscopic and immunofluorescent study. Chest 1974;65:41–5.

294. Dolan CJ Jr, Srodes CH, Duffy FD. Idiopathic pulmonary hemosiderosis. Electron microscopic, immunofluorescent, and iron kinetic studies. Chest 1975;68:577–80.

295. Seiden MV, O'Donnell WJ, Weinblatt M, Licht J. Vasculitis with recurrent pulmonary hemorrhage in a long-term survivor after autologous bone marrow transplantation. Bone Marrow Transplant 1990;6:345–7.

296. Valassi-Adam H, Rouska A, Karpouzas J, Matsaniotis N. Raised IgA in idiopathic pulmonary haemosiderosis. Arch Dis Child 1975;50:320–2.

297. Byrd RB, Gracey DR. Immunosuppressive treatment of idiopathic pulmonary hemosiderosis. JAMA 1973;226:458–9.

298. Chryssanthopoulos C, Cassimos C, Panagiotidou C. Prognostic criteria in idiopathic pulmonary hemosiderosis in children. Eur J Pediatr 1983;140:123–5.

299. Beckerman RC, Taussig LM, Pinnas JL. Familial idiopathic pulmonary hemosiderosis. Am J Dis Child 1979;133:609–11.

300. Thaell JF, Greipp PR, Stubbs SE, Siegal GP. Idiopathic pulmonary hemosiderosis: two cases in a family. Mayo Clin Proc 1978;53:113–8.

301. Bowley NB, Hughes JM, Steiner RE. The chest x-ray in pulmonary capillary haemorrhage: correlation with carbon monoxide uptake. Clin Radiol 1979;30:413–7.

302. Kjellman B, Elinder G, Garwicz S, Svan H. Idiopathic pulmonary haemosiderosis in Swedish children. Acta Paediatr Scand 1984;73:584–8.

303. Pozo-Rodriguez F, Freire-Campo JM, Gutierrez-Millet V, et al. Idiopathic pulmonary haemosiderosis treated by plasmapheresis. Thorax 1980;35:399–400.

304. Saeed MM, Woo MS, MacLaughlin EF, et al. Prognosis in pediatric idiopathic pulmonary hemosiderosis. Chest 1999;116:721–5.

305. Le Clainche L, Le Bourgeois M, Fauroux B, et al. Long-term outcome of idiopathic pulmonary hemosiderosis in children. Medicine (Baltimore) 2000;79:318–26.

306. Albelda SM, Gefter WB, Epstein DM, Miller WT. Diffuse pulmonary hemorrhage: a review and classification. Radiology 1985;154:289–97.

307. Gavaghan TE, McNaught PJ, Ralston M, Hayes JM. Penicillamine-induced "Goodpasture's syndrome": successful treatment of a fulminant case. Aust N Z J Med 1981;11:261–5.

308. Sternlieb I, Bennett B, Scheinberg IH. D-penicillamine induced Goodpasture's syndrome in Wilson's disease. Ann Intern Med 1975;82:673–6.

309. Louie S, Gamble CN, Cross CE. Penicillamine associated pulmonary hemorrhage. J Rheumatol 1986;13:963–6.

310. Matloff DS, Kaplan MM. D-Penicillamine-induced Goodpasture's-like syndrome in primary biliary cirrhosis—successful treatment with plasmapheresis and immunosuppressives. Gastroenterology 1980;78:1046–9.

311. Gibson T, Burry HC, Ogg C. Goodpasture syndrome and D-penicillamine [letter]. Ann Intern Med 1976;84:100.

312. Israel-Biet D, Labrune S, Huchon GJ. Drug-induced lung disease: 1990 review. Eur Respir J 1991;4:465–78.

313. Pietra GG. Pathologic mechanisms of drug-induced lung disorders. J Thorac Imaging 1991;6:1–7.

314. Vizioli LD, Cho S. Amiodarone-associated hemoptysis. Chest 1994;105:305–6.

315. Iskander S, Raible DG, Brozena SC, et al. Acute alveolar hemorrhage and orthodeoxia induced by intravenous amiodarone. Cathet Cardiovasc Interv 1999;47:61–3.

316. Averbuch SD, Yungbluth P. Fatal pulmonary hemorrhage due to nitrofurantoin. Arch Intern Med 1980;140:271–3.

317. Bucknall CE, Adamson MR, Banham SW. Nonfatal pulmonary haemorrhage associated with nitrofurantoin. Thorax 1987;42:475–6.

318. Herbert FA, Orford R. Pulmonary hemorrhage and edema due to inhalation of resins containing tri-mellitic anhydride. Chest 1979;76:546–51.

319. Ahmad D, Morgan WK, Patterson R, et al. Pulmonary haemorrhage and haemolytic anaemia due to trimellitic anhydride. Lancet 1979;ii:328–30.

320. Zeiss CR, Wolkonsky P, Chacon R, et al. Syndromes in workers exposed to trimellitic anhydride. A longitudinal clinical and immunologic study. Ann Intern Med 1983;98:8–12.

321. Kaplan V, Baur X, Czuppon A, et al. Pulmonary hemorrhage due to inhalation of vapor containing pyromellitic dianhydride. Chest 1993;104:644–5.

322. Patterson R, Nugent KM, Harris KE, Eberle ME. Immunologic hemorrhagic pneumonia caused by isocyanates. Am Rev Respir Dis 1990;141:226–30.

323. Cortese DA. Pulmonary function in mitral stenosis. Mayo Clin Proc 1978;53:321–6.

324. Ramsey HW, De la Torre A, Bartley TD, Linhart JW. Intractable hemoptysis in mitral stenosis treated by emergency mitral commissurotomy. Ann Intern Med 1967;67:588–93.

325. Case records of the Massachusetts General Hospital. Weekly clinicopathological exercises. Case 17-1995. An 81-year-old woman with mitral regurgitation and a left-upper-lobe pulmonary infiltrate. N Engl J Med 1995;332:1566–72.

326. Gilroy JC, Marchand P, Wilson VH. The role of the bronchial veins in mitral stenosis. Lancet 1952;ii:957–9.

327. Spence TH, Connors JC. Diffuse alveolar hemorrhage syndrome due to 'silent' mitral valve regurgitation. South Med J 2000;93:65–7.

328. Finley TN, Aronow A, Cosentino AM, Golde DW. Occult pulmonary hemorrhage in anticoagulated patients. Am Rev Respir Dis 1975;112:23–9.

329. Barnett VT, Bergmann F, Humphrey H, Chediak J. Diffuse alveolar hemorrhage secondary to superwarfarin ingestion. Chest 1992;102:1301–2.

330. Drent M, Wessels S, Jacobs JA, Thijssen H. Association of diffuse alveolar haemorrhage with acquired vitamin K deficiency. Respiration 2000;67:697.

331. Russi E, Odermatt B, Joller-Jemelka HI, Spycher MA. Alveolar haemorrhage as a presenting feature of myeloma. Eur Respir J 1993;6:267–70.

332. Ali A, Patil S, Grady KJ, Schreiber TL. Diffuse alveolar hemorrhage following administration of tirofiban or abciximab: a nemesis of platelet glycoprotein IIb/IIIa inhibitors. Catheter Cardiovasc Interv 2000;49:181–4.

333. Kalra S, Bell MR, Rihal CS. Alveolar hemorrhage as a complication of treatment with abciximab. Chest 2001;120:126–31.

334. Murray RJ, Albin RJ, Mergner W, Criner GJ. Diffuse alveolar hemorrhage temporally related to cocaine smoking. Chest 1988;93:427–9.

335. Gross NJ. Pulmonary effects of radiation therapy. Ann Intern Med 1977;86:81–92.

336. Rosiello RA, Merrill WW, Rockwell S, et al. Radiation pneumonitis. Bronchoalveolar lavage assessment and modulation by a recombinant cytokine. Am Rev Respir Dis 1993; 148:1671–6.

337. Rebello G, Mason JK. Pulmonary histological appearances in fatal paraquat poisoning. Histopathology 1978;2:53–66.

338. Pratt PC. Pathology of pulmonary oxygen toxicity. Am Rev Respir Dis 1974;110:51–7.

339. Katzenstein AL, Bloor CM, Leibow AA. Diffuse alveolar damage—the role of oxygen, shock, and related factors. A review. Am J Pathol 1976;85:209–28.

340. Cooper JA Jr, White DA, Matthay RA. Drug-induced pulmonary disease. Part 1: cytotoxic drugs. Am Rev Respir Dis 1986;133:321–40.

341. Gross NJ. The pathogenesis of radiation-induced lung damage. Lung 1981;159:115–25.

342. Thadani PV. NIDA conference report on cardiopulmonary complications of "crack" cocaine use. Clinical manifestations and pathophysiology. Chest 1996;110:1072–6.

343. Sisson JH, Thompson AB, Anderson JR, et al. Airway inflammation predicts diffuse alveolar hemorrhage during bone marrow transplantation in patients with Hodgkin disease. Am Rev Respir Dis 1992;146:439–43.

344. Jules-Elysee K, Stover DE, Yahalom J, et al. Pulmonary complications in lymphoma patients treated with high-dose therapy autologous bone marrow transplantation. Am Rev Respir Dis 1992;146:485–91.

345. Robbins RA, Linder J, Stahl MG, et al. Diffuse alveolar hemorrhage in autologous bone marrow transplant recipients. Am J Med 1989;87:511–8.

346. Kahn FW, Jones JM, England DM. Diagnosis of pulmonary hemorrhage in the immunocompromised host. Am Rev Respir Dis 1987;136:155–60.

347. Koziel H, Haley K, Nasser I, Filderman AE. Pulmonary hemorrhage. An uncommon cause of pulmonary infiltrates in patients with AIDS. Chest 1994;106:1891–4.

348. Agusti C, Ramirez J, Picado C, et al. Diffuse alveolar hemorrhage in allogeneic bone marrow transplantation. A postmortem study. Am J Respir Crit Care Med 1995;151:1006–10.

349. De Lassence A, Fleury-Feith J, Escudier E, et al. Alveolar hemorrhage. Diagnostic criteria and results in 194 immunocompromised hosts. Am J Respir Crit Care Med 1995;151: 157–63.

350. Chao NJ, Duncan SR, Long GD, et al. Corticosteroid therapy for diffuse alveolar hemorrhage in autologous bone marrow transplant recipients. Ann Intern Med 1991;114:145–6.

351. Mulder PO, Meinesz AF, de Vries EG, Mulder NH. Diffuse alveolar hemorrhage in autologous bone marrow transplant recipients. Am J Med 1991;90:278–81.

352. Bailey ME, Fraire AE, Greenberg SD, et al. Pulmonary histopathology in cocaine abusers. Hum Pathol 1994;25: 203–7.

353. Laposata EA, Mayo GL. A review of pulmonary pathology and mechanisms associated with inhalation of freebase cocaine ("crack"). Am J Forensic Med Pathol 1993;14:1–9.

354. Susskind H, Weber DA, Volkow ND, Hitzemann R. Increased lung permeability following long-term use of free-base cocaine (crack). Chest 1991;100:903–9.

355. Tashkin DP, Khalsa ME, Gorelick D, et al. Pulmonary status of habitual cocaine smokers. Am Rev Respir Dis 1992;145: 92–100.

356. Carrington CB, Cugell DW, Gaensler EA, et al. Lymphangioleiomyomatosis. Physiologic-pathologic-radiologic correlations. Am Rev Respir Dis 1977;116:977–95.

357. El Allaf D, Borlee G, Hadjoudj H, et al. Pulmonary lymphangiomyomatosis. Eur J Respir Dis 1984;65:147–52.

358. Taylor JR, Ryu J, Colby TV, Raffin TA. Lymphangioleiomyomatosis. Clinical course in 32 patients. N Engl J Med 1990;323:1254–60.

359. Corrin B, Liebow AA, Friedman PJ. Pulmonary lymphangiomyomatosis. A review. Am J Pathol 1975;79:348–82.

360. NHLBI Workshop Summary. Report of workshop on lymphangioleiomyomatosis. National Heart, Lung, and Blood Institute. Am J Respir Crit Care Med 1999;159:679–83.

361. Kelly J, Moss J. Lymphangioleiomyomatosis. Am J Med Sci 2001;321:17–25.

362. Marshall D, Saul GB, Sach E. Tuberous sclerosis: a report of 16 cases in two family trees revealing genetic dominance. N Engl J Med 1959;261:1102–3.

363. Dwyer JM, Hickie JB, Garvan J. Pulmonary tuberous sclerosis. Report of three patients and a review of the literature. QJM 1971;40:115–25.

364. Medley BE, McLeod RA, Houser OW. Tuberous sclerosis. Semin Roentgenol 1976;11:35–54.

365. Capron F, Ameille J, Leclerc P, et al. Pulmonary lymphangioleiomyomatosis and Bourneville's tuberous sclerosis with pulmonary involvement: the same disease? Cancer 1983; 52:851–5.

366. Liberman BA, Chamberlain DW, Goldstein RS. Tuberous sclerosis with pulmonary involvement. Can Med Assoc J 1984;130:287–9.

367. Mestres CA, Catalan M, Letang E, et al. Tuberous sclerosis and associated pleuropulmonary lesions. Thorac Cardiovasc Surg 1983;31:243–6.

368. Rosenthal A, Vawter G, Wagenvoort CA. Intrapulmonary veno-occlusive disease. Am J Cardiol 1973;31:78–83.

369. Thadani U, Burrow C, Whitaker W, Heath D. Pulmonary veno-occlusive disease. QJM 1975;44:133–59.

370. Wagenvoort CA, Wagenvoort N, Takahashi T. Pulmonary veno-occlusive disease: involvement of pulmonary arteries and review of the literature. Hum Pathol 1985;16:1033–41.

371. Case records of the Massachusetts General Hospital. Weekly clinicopathological exercises. Case 21-1986. Recent development of pulmonary hypertension seven years after an aortic valve replacement. N Engl J Med 1986;314:1435–45.

372. Glassroth J, Woodford DW, Carrington CB, Gaensler EA. Pulmonary veno-occlusive disease in the middle-aged. Respiration 1985;47:309–21.

373. Bjornsson J, Edwards WD. Primary pulmonary hypertension: a histopathologic study of 80 cases. Mayo Clin Proc 1985; 60:16–25.

374. Pietra GG, Edwards WD, Kay JM, et al. Histopathology of primary pulmonary hypertension. A qualitative and quantitative study of pulmonary blood vessels from 58 patients in the National Heart, Lung, and Blood Institute, Primary Pulmonary Hypertension Registry. Circulation 1989;80:1198–206.

375. Palevsky HI, Pietra GG, Fishman AP. Pulmonary veno-occlusive disease and its response to vasodilator agents. Am Rev Respir Dis 1990;142:426–9.

376. Holcomb BW Jr, Loyd JE, Ely EW, et al. Pulmonary veno-occlusive disease: a case series and new observations. Chest 2000;118:1671–9.

377. Mandel J, Mark EJ, Hales CA. Pulmonary veno-occlusive disease. Am J Respir Crit Care Med 2000;162:1964–73.

378. Lombard CM, Churg A, Winokur S. Pulmonary veno-occlusive disease following therapy for malignant neoplasms. Chest 1987;92:871–6.

379. Troussard X, Bernaudin JF, Cordonnier C, et al. Pulmonary veno-occlusive disease after bone marrow transplantation. Thorax 1984;39:956–7.

380. Hackman RC, Madtes DK, Petersen FB, Clark JG. Pulmonary venoocclusive disease following bone marrow transplantation. Transplantation 1989;47:989–92.

381. Williams LM, Fussell S, Veith RW, et al. Pulmonary veno-occlusive disease in an adult following bone marrow transplantation. Case report and review of the literature. Chest 1996;109:1388–91.

382. Case records of the Massachusetts General Hospital. Weekly clinicopathological exercises. Case 37-1992. A 68-year-old woman with rheumatoid arthritis and pulmonary hypertension. N Engl J Med 1992;327:873–80.

383. Kishida Y, Kanai Y, Kuramochi S, Hosoda Y. Pulmonary venoocclusive disease in a patient with systemic lupus erythematosus. J Rheumatol 1993;20:2161–2.

384. Corrin B, Spencer H, Turner-Warwick M, et al. Pulmonary veno-occlusive. An immune complex disease? Virchows Arch 1974;364:81–6.

385. Kramer MR, Estenne M, Berkman N, et al. Radiation-induced pulmonary veno-occlusive disease. Chest 1993;104:1282–4.

386. Escamilla R, Hermant C, Berjaud J, et al. Pulmonary veno-occlusive disease in a HIV-infected intravenous drug abuser. Eur Respir J 1995;8:1982–4.

387. Bailey CL, Channick RN, Auger WR, et al. "High probability" perfusion lung scans in pulmonary venoocclusive disease. Am J Respir Crit Care Med 2000;162:1974–8.

388. Weed HG. Pulmonary "capillary" wedge pressure not the pressure in the pulmonary capillaries. Chest 1991;100:1138–40.

389. Rambihar VS, Fallen EL, Cairns JA. Pulmonary veno-occlusive disease: antemortem diagnosis from roentgenographic and hemodynamic findings. Can Med Assoc J 1979;120: 1519–22.

390. Sanderson JE, Spiro SG, Hendry AT, Turner-Warwick M. A case of pulmonary veno-occlusive disease responding to treatment with azathioprine. Thorax 1977;32:140–8.

391. Salzman GA, Rosa UW. Prolonged survival in pulmonary veno-occlusive disease treated with nifedipine. Chest 1989;95:1154–6.

392. Faber CN, Yousem SA, Dauber JH, et al. Pulmonary capillary hemangiomatosis. A report of three cases and a review of the literature. Am Rev Respir Dis 1989;140:808–13.

393. Langleben D, Heneghan JM, Batten AP, et al. Familial pulmonary capillary hemangiomatosis resulting in primary pulmonary hypertension. Ann Intern Med 1988;109:106–9.

394. Vevaina JR, Mark EJ. Thoracic hemangiomatosis masquerading as interstitial lung disease. Chest 1988;93:657–9.

395. Magee F, Wright JL, Kay JM, et al. Pulmonary capillary hemangiomatosis. Am Rev Respir Dis 1985;132:922–5.

396. Ishii H, Iwabuchi K, Kameya T, Koshino H. Pulmonary capillary haemangiomatosis. Histopathology 1996;29:275–8.

397. Domingo C, Encabo B, Roig J, et al. Pulmonary capillary hemangiomatosis: report of a case and review of the literature. Respiration 1992;59:178–80.

398. Case records of the Massachusetts General Hospital. Weekly clinicopathological exercises. Case 38-2000. A 45-year-old woman with exertional dyspnea, hemoptysis, and pulmonary nodulas. N Engl J Med 2000;343:1788–96.

399. Tron V, Magee F, Wright JL, et al. Pulmonary capillary hemangiomatosis. Hum Pathol 1986;17:1144–50.

400. Lippert JL, White CS, Cameron EW, et al. Pulmonary capillary hemangiomatosis: radiographic appearance. J Thorac Imaging 1998;13:49–51.

401. White CW, Sondheimer HM, Crouch EC, et al. Treatment of pulmonary hemangiomatosis with recombinant interferon alfa-2a. N Engl J Med 1989;320:1197–200.

402. Ahmed Q, Chung-Park M, Tomashefski JF Jr. Cardiopulmonary pathology in patients with sleep apnea/obesity hypoventilation syndrome. Hum Pathol 1997;28:264–9.

403. Masson RG, Rennke HG, Gottlieb MN. Pulmonary hemorrhage in a patient with fibrillary glomerulonephritis. N Engl J Med 1992;326:36–9.

404. Rovin BH, Bou-Khalil P, Sedmak D. Pulmonary-renal syndrome in a patient with fibrillary glomerulonephritis. Am J Kidney Dis 1993;22:713–6.

405. Benditt JO, Farber HW, Wright J, Karnad AB. Pulmonary hemorrhage with diffuse alveolar infiltrates in men with high-volume choriocarcinoma. Ann Intern Med 1988;109:674–5.

406. Durieu I, Berger N, Loire R, et al. Contralateral haemorrhagic pulmonary metastases ("choriocarcinoma syndrome") after pneumonectomy for primary pulmonary choriocarcinoma. Thorax 1994;49:523–4.

407. Carter EJ, Bradburne RM, Jhung JW, Ettensohn DB. Alveolar hemorrhage with epithelioid hemangioendothelioma. A previously unreported manifestation of a rare tumor. Am Rev Respir Dis 1990;142:700–1.

408. Segal SL, Lenchner GS, Cichelli AV, et al. Angiosarcoma presenting as diffuse alveolar hemorrhage. Chest 1988;94: 214–6.

24 EOSINOPHILIC PNEUMONIAS

JEAN-FRANÇOIS CORDIER

The eosinophilic pneumonias represent, in the vast group of interstitial lung diseases, a category of disorders defined by the prominent presence of one cell type, the eosinophil. Even when called chronic, the eosinophilic pneumonias usually last for only a few weeks before patients seek medical advice. Although when acute and severe they may be life-threatening, the eosinophilic pneumonias almost always respond dramatically to corticosteroids. Furthermore, despite an impressive initial impairment of lung function in some cases, they usually heal without any sequelae. The eosinophilic pneumonias therefore represent a very distinct and original type of interstitial lung disease.

THE EOSINOPHIL

Our knowledge of eosinophil biopathology has continuously increased over the last years, and its review, which is beyond the scope of this chapter, may be found in comprehensive papers.[1–13] The eosinophil, so termed by Paul Ehrlich in 1879[14] because of the avidity of its granules for eosin, is a bone-marrow derived polymorphonuclear leukocyte 12 to 15 µm in diameter that possesses two types of granules. The larger granules, which number about 200 per cell, have an electron-dense crystalloid matrix and contain the characteristic cationic proteins. The smaller granules are of an amorphous nature, and they contain arylsulfatase and acid phosphatase. After a maturation of about 5 days in the bone marrow under the promotion of cytokines and especially of interleukin (IL)-5 and granulocyte-macrophage colony–stimulating factor (GM-CSF), the eosinophil circulates in the blood for an average time of 1 day before migrating into the tissues, following complex mechanisms of adhesion and attraction, diapedesis, and chemotaxis. The eosinophil is capable of producing and releasing a wide range of inflammation mediators, including especially the specific nonenzymatic proteins consisting of major basic protein (MBP), eosinophil cationic protein (ECP), eosinophil-derived neurotoxin (EDN) otherwise called eosinophil-protein X (EPX), and the enzymatic protein eosinophil peroxidase (EPO). Once activated, the eosinophil degranulates with mor-

phologic evidence of the loss of granules and the release of the eosinophil specific proteins that may be found within biologic fluids. The morphologic evidence of degranulation is provided by the finding of vacuoles in the cytoplasm of the cells, and ultrastructural evidence of loss of electron density from the central core of the granules (inversion or disappearance of the core density) (Figure 24–1).[15–17] Although many biologic properties of the eosinophil are orchestrated by T helper lymphocytes, interactions with other cells including mast cells and basophils, endothelial cells, macrophages, platelets, and fibroblasts play a role in the diverse interventions of the eosinophil in the inflammatory processes.

The function of the eosinophil still remains unclear. Even its main and early supposed beneficial role in parasitic infestation is now debated. Nevertheless, there is no doubt that the eosinophil plays a role (either beneficial and/or detrimental) in a variety of inflammatory processes of determined or undetermined origin. Because it is easy to recognize when present in tissues or the biologic fluids, the eosinophil may be a clue to the identity of specific conditions or syndromes of clinical importance to the practitioner.

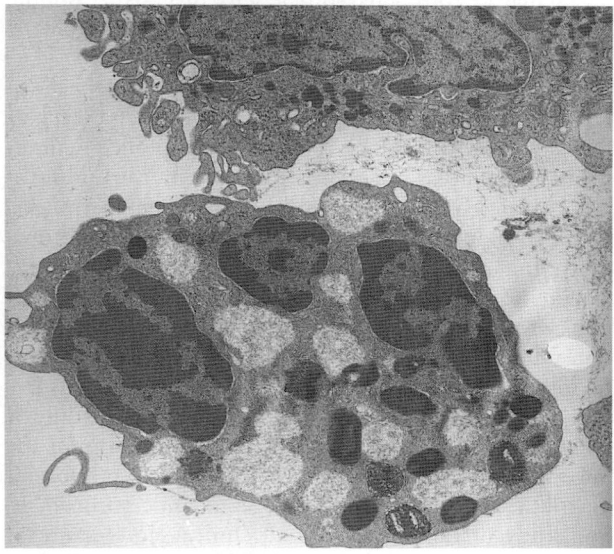

Figure 24–1 Idiopathic chronic eosinophilic pneumonia. Electron microscopy (×6610) of a degranulated eosinophil in bronchoalveolar lavage fluid. (Courtesy of D. Gindre, Department of Pathology, Louis Pradel Hospital, Lyon, France.)

This work was supported by grant HCL-PRNC 93.97-005 from Ministère de la Santé et de l'Action Humanitaire, France.

One striking mystery of eosinophil function is its dramatic disappearance from the bloodstream within a few hours after administration of corticosteroids.[9] The mechanism of this exclusion of eosinophils from the circulation is probably multifactorial, but likely implicates their sequestration in tissues and their further apoptotic or nonapoptotic (lytic) cell death. This rapid disappearance of blood eosinophilia within 24 hours may blur the clinical recognition of eosinophilic pulmonary disorders when corticosteroids unfortunately have been given before a differential blood cell count was done.

DEFINITION AND DIAGNOSTIC CRITERIA OF EOSINOPHILIC PNEUMONIA

Eosinophilic pneumonia is a pneumonia where the pulmonary parenchyma is infiltrated by inflammatory cells comprising conspicuous eosinophils. Although eosinophils are often the most prominent and immediately remarkable cells at histopathologic examination, they are generally associated with other inflammatory cells, especially lymphocytes and neutrophils. Pathologic examination of the lung is the only currently unquestionable means to define eosinophilic pneumonia. However, lung biopsy is seldom indicated in clinical practice by clinicians who have a good experience with such disorders, but in especially complex cases it remains the gold standard for both the diagnosis of eosinophilic pneumonia and its etiologic classification (for example by finding prominent necrotizing vasculitis or previously unsuspected intrapulmonary parasites). Open lung biopsy has been replaced by video-assisted thoracoscopic lung biopsy, which is a safe and less aggressive procedure.[18–21] Transbronchial lung biopsy may show characteristic features of eosinophilic pneumonia, which may be considered sufficient for diagnosis,[22] but the small size of the specimen often makes the pathologist reluctant to provide a definite diagnosis.

Because pulmonary biopsy to obtain a large piece of lung tissue has been a rather aggressive and rarely performed procedure, the diagnosis of eosinophilic pneumonia has been and is still commonly made on the finding of both radiographic pulmonary opacities and peripheral blood eosinophilia.[23,24] The most characteristic syndrome illustrating this diagnostic approach is Löffler's syndrome, as seen in ascariasis, which is defined by rather mild symptoms with a cough and wheezes, transient pulmonary infiltrates, and blood eosinophilia.[25–27] However, the finding of peripheral blood eosinophilia obviously does not prove that the observed pulmonary opacities correspond only or even mainly to eosinophilic pneumonia. Furthermore, the lower limit of peripheral eosinophilia for the purpose of diagnosing eosinophilic pneumonia is undetermined. In one study of the incidence and clinical significance of unsuspected eosinophilia discovered by automated white blood cell differential cell counting, eosinophilia was defined by absolute eosinophil counts exceeding 0.7×10^9/L.[28] In this study of ambulatory outpatients,

0.16% had eosinophilia that was not anticipated in 72% of them, and a specific medical condition as the causal factor could not be defined in 53% of these. In the group of patients with unanticipated eosinophilia, the eosinophil differential cell count ranged from 9 to 38%, with a mean percentage of 17.2%, and the absolute eosinophil count ranged from 1.08 to 3.8×10^9/L with a mean value of 1.58×10^9/L. This exemplifies that eosinophilia greater than 0.7×10^9/L is an uncommon but unspecific finding that may be encountered in individuals with no identifiable disease. Therefore, diagnosing eosinophilic pneumonia with confidence only on the finding of blood eosinophilia and pulmonary opacities requires a markedly elevated eosinophilia together with typical clinicoradiologic features. Even with these features, diagnosis must still remain presumptive, and any atypical evolution should prompt more secure diagnostic investigations.

Bronchoalveolar lavage (BAL) is currently widely used in the diagnosis of pulmonary infiltrative diseases, and it has become a key for the noninvasive diagnosis of eosinophilic pneumonia. In normal controls, BAL eosinophilia is lower than 1% of cells at differential count, with values slightly higher in exsmokers and smokers.[29] A study of sequential BAL to separate bronchial and alveolar samples did not mention the presence of eosinophils in both fractions.[30] BAL eosinophilia of or greater than 3% was found in 13.3% of a series of 1,084 BAL fluids.[31] Values between 3 and 9% had little diagnostic value and were found in various conditions mainly including idiopathic pulmonary fibrosis, connective tissue disorders associated pulmonary fibrosis, hypersensitivity pneumonitis, sarcoidosis, radiation pneumonitis, asthma, pneumoconioses, and infection. Values between 10 and 40% also were occasionally observed in the latter conditions, but these values were less common than an eosinophilia lower than 10%. BAL eosinophilia of greater than 40% was found mainly in patients with chronic eosinophilic pneumonia. In another series of 1,059 BAL fluids, 5% or more eosinophils were found in only 5% of cases, and this was associated with interstitial lung disease, acquired immunodeficiency syndrome (AIDS)-associated *Pneumocystis carinii* pneumonia, idiopathic eosinophilic pneumonia, and drug-induced lung disease.[32] Although no study definitely correlated the increased percentage of BAL eosinophils with pathologic evidence of eosinophilic pneumonia, BAL eosinophilia is currently considered as a valuable clue to the diagnosis of eosinophilic pneumonia in patients with infiltrates on pulmonary imaging.

CLASSIFICATION OF THE EOSINOPHILIC PNEUMONIAS

In 1952, Reeder and Goodrich[23] published a series of cases of pulmonary "infiltration with eosinophilia," a term with "descriptive appeal and when accompanied by primary, subsidiary, or modifying diagnosis, affords a clear word image." They mentioned that a differential diagnosis should include eosinophilic leukemia, pulmonary tuberculosis, and other diseases, including periarteritis nodosa that they noted as an "accompanying diagnosis." They reported eight cases, of which four were presented in detail. Two of these seem compatible with idiopathic chronic eosinophilic pneumonia, although there was no relapse after a rather short corticosteroid treatment. The other two patients probably had Churg-Strauss syndrome.

Crofton and colleagues[24] published in the same year a series of 16 cases of "pulmonary eosinophilia" with a review of 450 cases reported in the literature. Pulmonary eosinophilia was defined as a condition where pulmonary infiltration on the radiograph is accompanied by blood eosinophilia, but in which four conditions are excluded: the resolving stage of pneumonia, hydatid disease of the lung, Hodgkin's disease, and sarcoidosis. They suggested a classification as follows: (1) simple pulmonary eosinophilia (Löffler's syndrome), defined mainly by the paucity of symptoms and transient infiltrates; the cause was mainly parasitic, but the authors also mentioned sulfonamides as a possible cause; (2) prolonged pulmonary eosinophilia characterized by radiographic shadows persisting for over a month; involvement of other organs was mentioned; parasitic infestation and allergy were possible causes, but some cases were idiopathic; (3) tropical eosinophilia, which had been well studied previously; (4) pulmonary eosinophilia with asthma, a rather heterogeneous category, with some patients having "appearances intermediate between those of simple pulmonary eosinophilia and those of pure polyarteritis nodosa"; all of the patients who died had lesions in organs other than the lungs; and (5) polyarteritis nodosa. This meticulous study emphasized the diversity of the identified causes and the history of allergy in many patients. The authors also mentioned that "both clinically and pathologically there is a continuum from the simple and transient abnormalities of Löffler's syndrome to the severe and often fatal manifestations of polyarteritis nodosa."

In the following years, several syndromes were progressively individualized within the group of eosinophilic lung disorders.

McCarthy and Pepys[33] reported 27 cases of "cryptogenic pulmonary eosinophilias" that they compared to cases of allergic bronchopulmonary aspergillosis. Two patients with cryptogenic pulmonary eosinophilia in this series developed typical features of systemic vasculitis.

There is currently no definitely accepted classification of the eosinophilic pneumonias (ie, the pulmonary disorders characterized by a predominant eosinophilic infiltration of the pulmonary interstitial structures [alveoli, bronchioles, vessels]). For this chapter, the simple classification this author uses in clinical practice will be adopted (Table 24–1). It principally separates these disorders into two main categories: those where no etiologic agent is identified (undetermined origin) and those where a definite cause is found (determined origin). Looking carefully for a definite cause is essential in all patients presenting with eosinophilic pneumonia, because finding the cause almost always has immediate practical consequences (for example stopping a drug responsible for iatrogenic eosinophilic pneumonia). When no cause is found, the eosinophilic pneumonias may be included within the syndromes, which have been well characterized and individualized. Some other pulmonary disorders may comprise mild or moderate eosinophilia at blood cell count or at BAL, and because they may represent occasional differential diagnostic problems, they must be kept in mind. Furthermore, irrespective of their determined or undetermined origin, the eosinophilic pneumonias may manifest by different clinicoradiologic syndromes, namely Löffler's syndrome, chronic eosinophilic pneumonia, or acute eosinophilic pneumonia. Löffler's syndrome is defined by transient pulmonary infiltrates, often migratory, accompanied by blood eosinophilia and only mild symptoms. The most common cause of Löffler's syndrome is parasitic, but because of its poorly specific definition, Löffler's syndrome may result from many causes (for example, a reaction to a drug taken for a short time). Some cases of Löffler's syndrome remain idiopathic, but it is worthwhile commenting that usually only limited investigations are done in such cases because the clinical manifestations are minimal.

PATHOLOGY

Pathologic studies of eosinophilic pneumonia mainly have been done in patients with chronic pneumonia where no evident cause was found.[34–40] Therefore, most studies concern idiopathic chronic eosinophilic pneumonia, the diagnosis of which was initially obtained on pathologic analy-

---

TABLE 24–1   Classification of Eosinophilic Pneumonias in Clinical Practice

Eosinophilic pneumonias of undetermined origin
  Solitary idiopathic eosinophilic pneumonias*
    Chronic eosinophilic pneumonia
    Acute eosinophilic pneumonia
  Eosinophilic pneumonia in systemic syndromes
    Churg-Strauss syndrome
    Idiopathic hypereosinophilic syndrome
Eosinophilic pneumonias of determined origin
  Eosinophilic pneumonias of parasitic origin
  Eosinophilic pneumonias of other infectious causes
  Drug-induced eosinophilic pneumonias
  Allergic bronchopulmonary aspergillosis and related syndromes
    (including bronchocentric granulomatosis)
Other pulmonary syndromes with possible eosinophilia
  Bronchiolitis obliterans organizing pneumonia, asthma,
    idiopathic pulmonary fibrosis, Langerhans cell
    histiocytosis, malignancies, etc

---

*Löffler's syndrome may be idiopathic.

sis of a specimen obtained by open lung biopsy. On occasions when they are available, pathologic studies in eosinophilic pneumonias of determined origin have not shown strikingly specific features, except for a possible peculiar distribution of lesions (for example, bronchocentric) or the presence of causal agents such as parasites or fungal hyphae. The pathologic features of idiopathic eosinophilic pneumonia may be considered, with the exception of slight differences, as the common denominator of all categories of eosinophilic pneumonias, whatever their origin. Detailed pathologic descriptions of eosinophilic pneumonia may be found in pathology textbooks,[41–44] and these will only be summarized hereafter.

The most prominent and characteristic feature of chronic eosinophilic pneumonia is the filling of the alveolar spaces by eosinophils (when eosinophils are not numerous, the Giemsa stain may help in their identification) (Figures 24–2 and 24–3). Macrophages are also present, with varying proportions of eosinophils and macrophages. Some multinucleated giant cells are scattered in the infiltrate, and they may contain eosinophilic granules or Charcot-Leyden crystals, which also may be present in the cytoplasm of macrophages.[34] A proteinaceous and fibrinous exudate is usually present in the alveolar spaces adjacent to the cellular eosinophilic infiltrate. Some foci of necrotic intra-alveolar eosinophils may be surrounded by macrophages, which sometimes have the appearance of epithelioid cells with a palisading arrangement, forming a figure-denominated eosinophilic microabscess. Morphologic as well as immunohistochemical studies of major basic protein in chronic eosinophilic pneumonia (CEP) have shown that eosinophils degranulate.[45,46] Electron microscopic studies confirmed that eosinophils exhibit features of degranulation, and macrophages contain engulfed eosinophilic granules and fragments of eosinophils.[36]

An interstitial inflammatory cellular infiltrate is constant. It consists of eosinophils, lymphocytes, plasma cells, and histiocytes. Interstitial fibrosis is conspicuously absent, and the global architecture of the lung remains intact.

A mild vasculitis involving both small arteries and venules is common. It mainly consists of perivascular cuffing, with relatively few cells infiltrating the arterial media. In simple eosinophilic pneumonia, this vasculitis is non-necrotizing. Eosinophils accounting for approximately 90% of the cells within veins and capillaries has been reported in a patient with interstitial eosinophilic pneumonitis with a peripheral eosinophil count of only $0.8 \times 10^9/L$.[47] The mechanisms of chemotaxis and sequestration of the eosinophils within the lung structures are still poorly understood.

Organization of the alveolar inflammatory exudate is a rather common finding. It has been demonstrated in the early reported cases of CEP.[34,35] In the original paper of Carrington and colleagues,[34] a figure clearly showed organization with deposition of collagen in an alveolar duct. Bronchiolitis obliterans of the proliferative type may be an associated finding. These pathologic findings suggest a pathologic overlap between CEP and bronchiolitis obliterans organizing pneumonia (BOOP) in some cases. However, intraluminal organization of the distal air spaces is only sparse in CEP, and it does not represent the major pathologic feature in this condition. The comparison of eosinophil numbers and degranulation by immunofluorescent staining for eosinophil-derived major basic protein has shown that, although histologic overlap exists in about 10% of cases, CEP and idiopathic BOOP are quite distinct conditions.[45] Mucus plugs may cause obstruction of the small airways in CEP.[34]

Although the distribution of eosinophilic pneumonia is generally diffuse at histopathologic examination, it may be more focal in some cases. Furthermore, the lesions may have an angiocentric or bronchiolocentric pattern in some etiologic groups of eosinophilic pneumonia.

The hilar lymph nodes associated with CEP contain many eosinophils, and lymphoid hyperplasia is present.[34]

In idiopathic acute eosinophilic pneumonia, pathologic studies are scarce and have limited information when performed on specimens obtained by transbronchial lung biopsy.[48–50] No specific findings have been identified. The

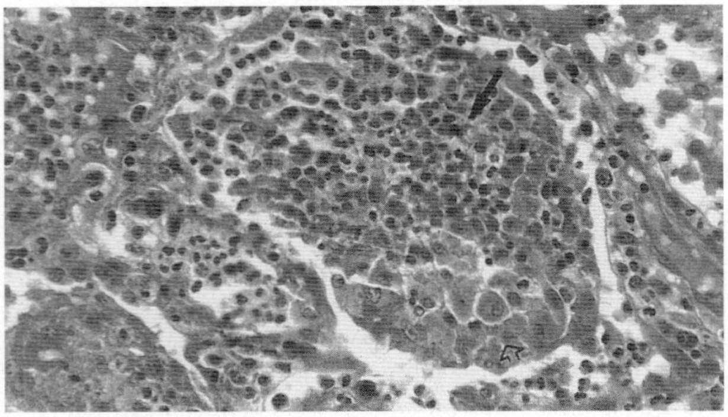

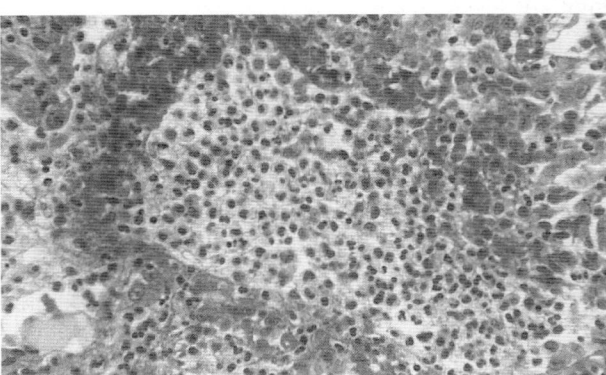

Figure 24–2 Idiopathic chronic eosinophilic pneumonia. The alveolar lumen is filled by eosinophils (*arrow*) and macrophages (*arrow head*) (hematoxylin, eosin, saffron; ×400 original magnification). (Courtesy of R. Loire, Department of Pathology, Louis Pradel Hospital, Lyon, France.)

Figure 24–3 Idiopathic chronic eosinophilic pneumonia. Filling of the alveolar lumen by eosinophils. The alveolar wall is thickened by inflammatory cells including histiocytes. (Courtesy of R. Loire, Department of Pathology, Louis Pradel Hospital, Lyon, France.)

reported features include intra-alveolar and interstitial eosinophilic infiltrates, diffuse alveolar edema, intra-alveolar fibrinous exudates, organizing pneumonia, and non-necrotizing vasculitis.[48-50] These features show that the acute inflammatory process probably comprises a permeability defect with extravasation of plasma proteins as occurs in the infectious pneumonias.

EOSINOPHILIC PNEUMONIAS OF UNDETERMINED ORIGIN

Eosinophilic pneumonias with no definite cause are quite characteristic of a "pure" eosinophilic disorder, therefore, they will be discussed first. The eosinophilic pneumonias of undetermined origin may occur as solitary pulmonary disorders: these are the idiopathic eosinophilic pneumonias, either chronic or acute. They also may be part of a systemic syndrome such as the Churg-Strauss syndrome or the hypereosinophilic syndrome.

Idiopathic Eosinophilic Pneumonias

Idiopathic eosinophilic pneumonias may present as either chronic or acute pneumonia. Chronic eosinophilic pneumonia is characterized by a progressive onset of symptoms leading within a few weeks to an infiltrative pulmonary disease with cough, increasing dyspnea, malaise, and weight loss. Acute eosinophilic pneumonia presents as an acute pneumonia with respiratory failure, often necessitating mechanical ventilation.

Chronic Eosinophilic Pneumonia

In 1952, Reeder and Goodrich[23] reported two cases of pulmonary infiltration on chest radiograph with associated blood eosinophilia, which improved with nebulized cortisone and adrenocorticotropic hormone (ACTH), respectively. Christoforidis and Molnar[35] reported, in 1960, two cases of long duration pulmonary infiltration associated with fever, malaise, and blood eosinophilia contrasting with Löffler's syndrome where the duration of pulmonary infiltration is short and the symptoms are mild or absent. Both patients were women. One recovered spontaneously, and the other received corticosteroids with a dramatic improvement of the radiologic and clinical findings and a rapid return of the eosinophil count to normal levels. The lung biopsy showed the characteristic features of eosinophilic pneumonia in both patients, with organization in the one where the disease lasted for more than three months.

Chronic eosinophilic pneumonia was subsequently individualized as an entity by Carrington and colleagues[34] who studied a series of 9 patients with clinical, radiologic, physiologic, and pathologic data. This study clearly defined a syndrome that was further confirmed and detailed by several series and numerous case reports.[38,51-55]

CEP occurs predominantly in women who are affected about twice as often as males.[38,55] Although CEP may occur in young people, only 6% of patients are less than 20 years old.[38] The peak incidence of CEP is among 30 to 39 year olds,[38] with a mean age at diagnosis of 45 years.[55] Except for a single report[56] in identical twins (who did not live together and had not visited each other or their parental home for several weeks before the onset of disease), there are currently no data to suggest a possible genetic factor in the pathogenesis of CEP.

A prior history of atopy is found in about half of the patients. Prior asthma was present in half of the patients of a large series,[38,55] with allergic rhinitis in 12[38] to 24%,[55] drug allergy in about 10%,[38,55] nasal polyps in 5[38] to 13%,[55] urticaria in 10%,[55] and eczema in 5%.[55] Prior asthma has also been reported in other series: 11 of 16 patients,[37] 4 of 12,[53] and 5 of 14,[54] but was absent from the 8 patients of another series.[52] Asthma also may occur concomitant with the diagnosis of CEP (in 15% of patients in our series), or develop after CEP (in 10% of patients in our series).[57] CEP may occur while asthmatic patients are on a desensitization program,[34,51,55,58] but there is no proof that this may contribute to the development of CEP. CEP was reported in a patient receiving montelukast, a leukotriene-receptor antagonist suspected of inducing Churg-Strauss syndrome; however, because corticosteroids were given while montelukast was withdrawn, the responsibility of the latter in CEP remains unproved.[59]

A majority of patients are nonsmokers,[38,53] with only 4 of 62 (6.5%) smokers in our series.[55] The rather high proportion of patients with a prior history of asthma, who are thus usually encouraged not to smoke, may explain in part the low prevalence of smokers in patients with CEP. However, because a low proportion of smokers has also been reported in other pulmonary disorders, such as hypersensitivity pneumonitis,[60] it is not excluded that smoking may prevent the development of CEP by unknown mechanisms.

The onset of CEP is progressive, with the diagnosis usually made several weeks or months after the first symptoms. The mean interval between the onset of symptoms and diagnosis varies from 7.7 months[38] to 4 months in a more recent series,[55] the reduction in diagnosis delay probably resulting from the increased awareness of physicians for the disease. The most common respiratory symptoms are cough in about 90% of patients, dyspnea in 57[38] to 92%[55] with sputum production in 33[38] to 42%,[55] and chest pain in 9[38] to 16%[55] of patients. Dyspnea usually is not severe, although the necessity for mechanical ventilation occasionally has been reported after several months of progression of the disease with increasing dyspnea.[61] Hemoptysis is less common and occurs in about 10% of cases.[38,55] Wheezes at physical examination are found in one-third of the patients,[38] and crackles in 38%.[55] Pleural effusion is uncommon and when present is usually small, although it may occasionally be massive and recurrent.[62] Upper respiratory tract symptoms of chronic rhinitis or sinusitis are present in about 20% of patients.[55]

Systemic symptoms are often prominent, with fever in about two-thirds of patients.[38,55] Weight loss is present in 57[38] to 75%[55] of patients, with loss of 10 kg or more in 13%.[55] Asthenia, malaise, fatigue, anorexia, weakness, and night sweats are common.[38,53–55]

The imaging features of CEP are rather characteristic (Figures 24–4 to 24–7). Peripheral infiltrates on the chest radiograph are present in almost all cases,[34,38,55,63–67] and these are migratory in a quarter of cases.[55] They usually consist of opacities with ill-defined margins, the density of which varies from ground glass to consolidation. The classic pattern of "photographic negative or reversal of the shadows usually seen in pulmonary edema"[65] is quite evocative of CEP,[51,65] but is seen in only a fourth of patients[38] and is not specific for CEP.

High-resolution computed tomography (HRCT) has further allowed the definition of some imaging features of CEP (see Figures 24–5B and 24–6B), and these were characteristic enough to allow the correct diagnosis in 78% of cases of CEP in a study of 111 patients with eosinophilic lung diseases.[67] The opacities are bilateral in at least 50% of cases on the chest radiograph,[38,53] but the proportion of bilateral opacities may increase from 80% on the chest radiograph to 97.5% with HRCT.[55] Opacities predominate in the upper parts of the lung,[38,55,63] are characteristically peripheral, with generally coexisting ground-glass and consolidation opacities on HRCT.[55,64,68] Ground-glass and dense opacities are each present in about three-quarters of cases.[55] Inhomogeneous consolidation and ground-glass opacities are located in the outer third of the lung parenchyma, with dense confluent consolidation in the lung periphery

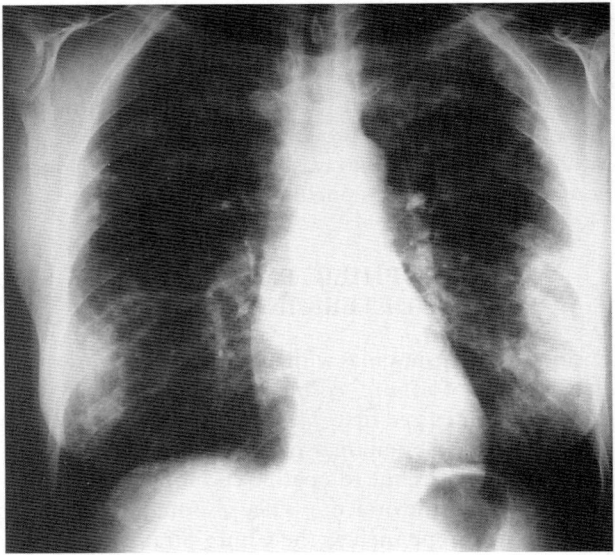

A

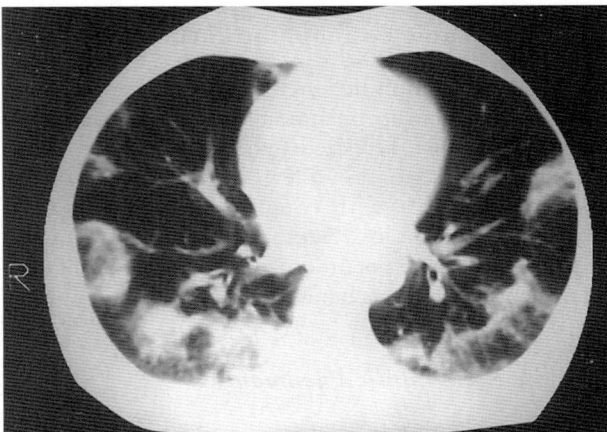

B

Figure 24–5   Idiopathic chronic eosinophilic pneumonia in a 55-year-old woman. *A*, Chest radiograph showing bilateral infiltrative opacities predominating in the lower parts of the lungs. *B*, CT scan in the same patient shows peripheral patchy alveolar opacities in the lower lobes.

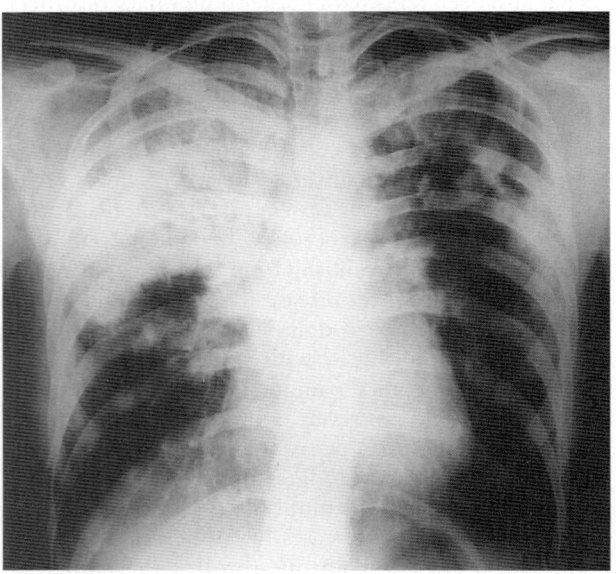

Figure 24–4   Chest radiograph of idiopathic chronic eosinophilic pneumonia in a 28-year-old woman. The alveolar opacities are bilateral but predominate in the right upper lobe.

adjacent to the pleura.[64] Consolidation with segmental or lobar atelectasis may be seen[64] and septal line thickening is common.[68] Streaky or band-like opacities parallel to the chest wall also may be present.[64] On corticosteroid treatment, consolidation and/or ground-glass opacities show a decrease in size and extent, with possible visualization or change from consolidation to ground-glass opacities, or inhomogeneous opacities and later streaky or band-like opacities.[64,69] Ground-glass opacities on HRCT are commonly missed on the chest radiograph.[55,64] CEP without radiographic pulmonary infiltrates has been reported,[70] but HRCT was not performed in this case. Cavitary lesions are extremely rare,[38,55,64] and these may correspond to the visualization

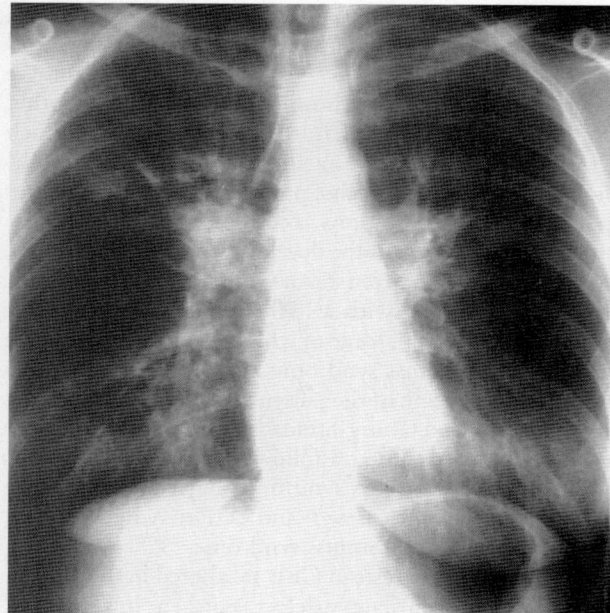

A

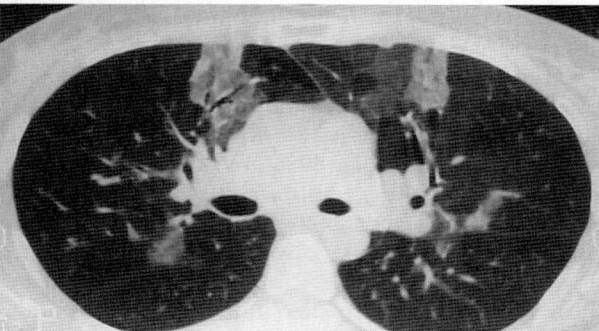

B

Figure 24–6 Idiopathic chronic eosinophilic pneumonia in a 45-year-old woman. *A*, The chest radiograph shows an unusual aspect of irregular hilar enlargement with interstitial opacities. *B*, On CT scan, anterior ground-glass and alveolar opacities are found, thus explaining the unusual radiologic features.

of previous bullae or pneumatocele as to real cavitation from pneumonia, which has not been convincingly pathologically documented in CEP. Small pleural effusions are present in up to 10% of cases on HRCT,[55] and mediastinal lymph node enlargement in 17%[55] to 50%.[63]

Gallium-67 pulmonary uptake has been reported in one case, and it was no longer present one month after corticosteroid treatment and radiographic normalization.[71] Technetium 99m glucoheptonate may show intense parenchymal uptake, which returns to normal after several weeks of corticosteroid treatment.[72]

Peripheral blood eosinophilia over 6% was present in 88% of 111 cases in the literature,[38] with an increased

white blood cell count in 63% of cases and a mean percentage of blood eosinophils on the differential count of 26%. Because peripheral blood eosinophilia is often a diagnostic criterion of CEP, the proportion of patients with CEP and a normal peripheral blood count is unknown. In our series where CEP was defined by blood eosinophilia $> 1.0 \times 10^9$/L and/or eosinophil percentage $> 40\%$ at bronchoalveolar differential count, the mean blood eosinophilia was 5.5×10^9/L, with eosinophils representing a mean of 32% of the total blood leukocyte count.[55] Thrombocytosis occasionally has been observed in CEP.[73]

Erythrocyte sedimentation rate is almost always increased,[38,53,55] with a mean value of about 60 mm at the first hour.[38,55] C-reactive protein is increased in 83% of cases.[55] Total blood immunoglobulin (Ig)E level is increased in 55% of cases and is greater than 2400 µg/L in 15%.[55] Increased IgE level returns to normal under corticosteroid treatment.[74,75] Circulating immune complexes have been reported in CEP in about one-third of patients,[55,76,77] and their significance in CEP is unknown. They might correlate with disease activity and flare-ups.[76] Antinuclear antibodies may occasionally be present.[55] Antineutrophil cytoplasmic antibodies (perinuclear pattern) were found in only 1 out of 32 patients tested.[55] Markedly increased urinary EDN levels are found in patients with CEP.[78,79]

Sputum eosinophilia has been mentioned in CEP[24,35,55] but has been found in less than one-half of the studied patients.[38] However, it was present in 63% of cases in one series.[54]

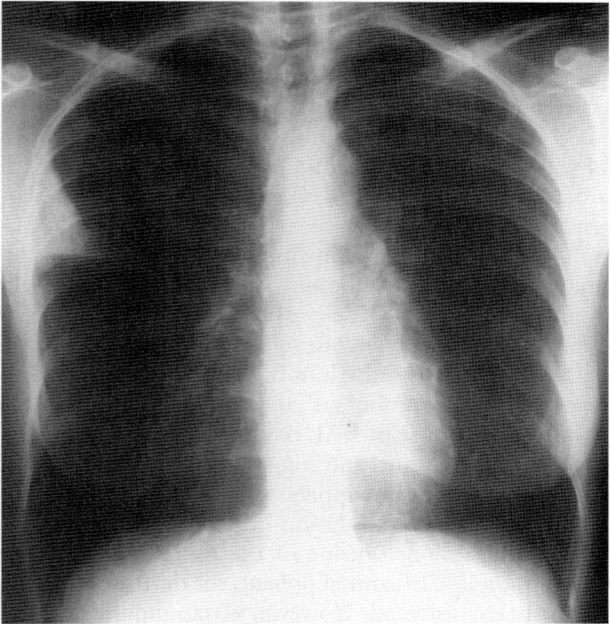

Figure 24–7 Chest radiograph of idiopathic chronic eosinophilic pneumonia in a 31-year-old woman. There is only a limited opacity in the right upper lobe.

BAL has progressively become a major diagnostic procedure in CEP, making lung biopsy unnecessary in most cases. Alveolar eosinophilia is a characteristic feature in CEP,[51,55,70,80-83] and CEP is the most common cause of alveolar eosinophilia, accounting for greater than 40% of cases.[31] BAL eosinophilia is present in all cases of CEP, with a mean of 58% on the differential cell count.[55] Alveolar eosinophilia may be associated with an increased percentage of neutrophils, mast cells, and lymphocytes.[55] Although the mean alveolar percentage of lymphocytes is normal, the absolute number of alveolar lymphocytes is increased.[84] The BAL eosinophil cell count drops under corticosteroid treatment.[85-87]

BAL eosinophils of patients with CEP show signs of activation with the release of eosinophil proteins and the evidence of uptake of MBP and ECP by macrophages.[88] ECP,[89-91] EDN,[90] and immunoglobulins[89] are increased in the BAL fluid of patients with CEP, with a correlation between ECP and eosinophil count[91] and between IgA and ECP levels.[89] Increased content of prostaglandins E_2 and F_2 alpha has been found in BAL fluid, with prostaglandin E_2 reverting to normal on corticosteroid treatment.[92] Expression of human leukocyte antigen (HLA)-DR in a patient with CEP was present in 86% of alveolar eosinophils in contrast to 7% of blood eosinophils, suggesting compartmentalization of eosinophilic activation within the lung.[93] Alveolar eosinophils in one patient with CEP produced high amounts of oxygen free radicals and exhibited an increased level of cyclic adenosine monophosphate (cAMP) phosphodiesterase activity compared with blood eosinophils from control or allergic subjects.[94] BAL lymphocytes are characterized by an accumulation of CD4+ cells[84,95] showing a phenotypic repertoire usually expressed by memory T cells.[84] The ratios of IL-2–receptor positive T cells and HLA-DR positive T cells in BAL fluid were decreased by corticosteroid therapy in two patients.[87] Overexpression of CD44 on alveolar eosinophils with high concentrations of soluble CD44 in BAL fluid has been reported, with a correlation between BAL IL-5 and soluble CD44 suggesting upregulation of the expression of CD44 by IL-5.[96] RANTES, a chemokine implicated in the migration and activation of eosinophils, is increased in BAL fluid and correlated with the proportion of eosinophils.[97] Eotaxin, a chemokine with selective chemotactic activity for eosinophils, is high in BAL, and its level is correlated with the number of eosinophils.[98] Study of the apoptotic response of BAL eosinophils has shown that they are Fas-resistant, and suggests that the apoptosis of eosinophils might be suppressed by cytokines like IL-5, leading to their accumulation in the lung.[99]

Manifestations outside of the respiratory tract are uncommon in CEP, and, if present, the diagnosis must be seriously reconsidered. However, extrapulmonary manifestations have been reported occasionally, including arthralgias, repolarization alterations of the electrocardiogram, pericarditis, altered liver biologic tests, eosinophilic lesions at liver biopsy, mononeuritis multiplex, diarrhea, skin nodule, immune complex vasculitis in the skin, and eosinophilic enteritis.[34,51,55,69,77,100-103] It is likely that these patients indeed have a disorder overlapping with other conditions such as the Churg-Strauss syndrome (such cases may also represent an initial stage of these conditions). Furthermore, because patients with CEP and extrapulmonary manifestations receive corticosteroid treatment, this may prevent the development of overt systemic manifestations characteristic of Churg-Strauss syndrome. In a series of CEP with a high frequency of extrapulmonary signs (30%), some of which being quite evocative of the Churg-Strauss syndrome (and especially the neurologic signs), none of the patients treated with corticosteroids developed Churg-Strauss syndrome or the hypereosinophilic syndrome on follow-up.[100] The frontiers of CEP and Churg-Strauss syndrome may thus be difficult to delineate in some cases,[104] and CEP may be a presenting feature of Churg-Strauss syndrome.[105-107]

Lung function tests in CEP are altered in most cases. An obstructive ventilatory defect is present in about half the patients,[38,55] a finding not restricted to patients with prior asthma. A restrictive ventilatory defect present in half of the cases.[55] The frequency of hypoxemia was 96% in one series,[38] and hypoxemia defined by a PaO_2 of 75 mm Hg or less was present in 64% of patients in another series.[55] A reduced transfer factor was found in 90% of cases in one series,[38] but a reduced transfer factor (defined as less than 80% predicted) was found in 52% in another series with a reduced transfer coefficient (defined as less than 80% predicted) in only 27%.[55] An increased alveoloarterial oxygen gradient has been reported in 90% of cases.[38] Improvement and further normalization of the impaired lung function tests under treatment is the rule in most patients.[38] However, a ventilatory obstructive defect may develop in some patients and especially in those with a markedly increased BAL eosinophilia at initial evaluation.[108]

The course of untreated CEP is not well known, and spontaneous resolution may occur.[36,38,52,55] Death resulting from CEP is extremely rare. A review of the literature recorded only seven deaths occurring during the follow-up of patients, with only one related to CEP.[38] Most deaths in patients with CEP cannot be related to CEP.[55,65] One untreated patient described by Liebow and Carrington had a syncopal episode and died with ventricular fibrillation; however, the cause of death was unclear because no significant heart lesions were found at autopsy. The autopsy also disclosed eosinophilic pneumonia with vasculitis and emphysema, and vasculitis was also found in an intercostal muscle, raising the possibility of systemic vasculitis.[37]

The dramatic response of CEP to corticosteroid treatment was observed shortly after these drugs became available.[38] Symptoms improve within 1 or 2 weeks,[38,52,53] and even within 48 hours[34,55] in about 80%[55] of cases. ACTH and cortisone[23] were the first drugs to be used, followed by prednisone and prednisolone, which are currently used. There is no study defining the optimal dose of corticosteroids, but the usual doses are between 20 to 60 mg/day.[53] The mean initial dose used in our series was about 1 mg/kg/day,[55] but this is probably too high and our current recommendation is to start with 0.75 mg/kg/day. Smaller doses are probably as efficient in most cases, but, because the condition of a large proportion of patients is often severely impaired, a rapid improvement is appreciable. The clearing of pulmonary opacities on imaging is rapid. They disappeared within 1 week in 69% of patients in our series of patients treated with a mean initial dose of 1 mg/kg/day.[55] However, the time required for the chest radiograph to clear may vary both with the dose of corticosteroids used and the frequency at which the radiographs are performed. Total clearing of opacities took less than 2 weeks in 55% of patients, but a slower clearing occurred in 45% in a series.[38] Most patients require prolonged treatment (ie, more than 6 months). In one series, recurrence occurred in 58% after corticosteroids were discontinued, and 21% relapsed while corticosteroids were being tapered.[38] In our series, relapses occurred in half of the patients after corticosteroids were weaned (the mean time between weaning and relapse was 72 weeks) or tapered (the mean dose of corticosteroids at the time of relapse was 11 mg).[55] Relapses, which again respond dramatically to corticosteroids, may occur in the same areas of the lungs or in different areas.[51,55]

The series where follow-up is available clearly show that most patients need prolonged corticosteroid treatment. In a series with a mean 10.2 years of follow-up, 10 of 12 patients were still receiving maintenance steroid therapy.[53] In our series with a mean 6.2 years of follow-up, only 31% were weaned at last control, and 9 of 14 of these required inhaled corticosteroids because of asthma; the causes for continuation of corticosteroids in the other patients were relapses of CEP, asthma, or both.[55] A relapse of CEP occurred in a pregnant woman, leading to an increase in the treatment dose of corticosteroids with no adverse consequences to the patient or her baby.[109]

Inhaled corticosteroids with high doses of beclomethasone dipropionate (1,500 µg/day) were effective in the long-term treatment of one patient; this allowed a reduction in oral corticosteroids and controlled relapses, either alone or with the addition of small doses (5 mg) of corticosteroids.[110] Inhaled corticosteroids have been reported to help in reducing the maintenance oral corticosteroid dose in CEP.[53] Relapses of CEP are less frequent in patients with a previous history of asthma, possibly because they receive inhaled corticosteroids after stopping oral corticosteroids.[57]

There are few radiologic sequelae from CEP, with almost all patients having a normal chest radiograph at their last follow-up.[55] Progression of a possible CEP to pulmonary fibrosis (desquamative interstitial pneumonia-like condition) with superimposed CEP has been reported in one case.[111]

Acute Eosinophilic Pneumonia

Idiopathic acute eosinophilic pneumonia (IAEP) has been recently individualized from the other eosinophilic pneumonias.[48,49,54,112–122] It differs from CEP mainly by its acute onset, the severity of hypoxemia, the usual lack of increased blood eosinophils at the onset of disease in contrast with a frank eosinophilic alveolitis in BAL fluid, and no relapse after recovery.

Pope-Harman and colleagues[114] proposed the following criteria for the diagnosis of IAEP: (1) acute onset (onset of any symptoms within 7 days before presentation); (2) fever; (3) bilateral infiltrates on chest film; (4) severe hypoxemia (PaO_2 on room air ≤ 60 mm Hg, oxygen saturation on room air $< 90\%$, or A-a gradient > 40 mm Hg); (5) lung eosinophilia (BAL differential count with $\geq 25\%$ eosinophils or predominance of eosinophils in open lung biopsy); and (6) no history of hypersensitivity to drugs, no historic or laboratory evidence of infection, and no other known cause of acute eosinophilic lung disease.[114] These criteria may be too restrictive, and we consider that, in some patients, IAEP may develop over 1 month.

The average age at presentation is about 30 years in the largest series[114,122]; several reported patients were 20 years old or less,[49,116–118] but IAEP also occurs in older patients, up to 86 years old in our series.[122] In contrast with CEP, there is a male predominance. No prior asthma history is found, although some patients may have a history of atopy.[54,119] Interestingly, some patients had peculiar outdoor activities within the days before the onset of disease, such as cave exploration, plant repotting, wood pile moving, smoke-house cleaning,[114] or a bicycle motorcross race in dusty conditions.[48] Four patients from our series[122] had been exposed to dusts from indoor renovation work (2 patients), gasoline tank cleaning, or explosion of a tear gas bomb.[122] The causative role of cigarette smoke has been discussed, as IAEP has developed soon after the initiation of smoking (especially when starting with large quantities) in some patients.[122–126] Interestingly, a challenge with cigarette smoking was positive in some patients,[122–126] but tolerance developed in some of them who resumed smoking.[124–126] IAEP after exposure to smoke from fireworks has also been reported.[127] Whether in such cases the smoke is really the specific cause of IAEP is unknown. Given the incidence of smoking and the rarity of IAEP, it is unlikely. However, inhalation of smoke or of any nonspecific injurious agent may initiate or contribute to the development of IAEP of some other unknown cause. Furthermore, some individuals may be intrinsically prone to develop eosinophilic reactions to nonspecific causative agents.

IAEP occurs acutely in previously healthy individuals. Symptoms at presentation consist of cough, dyspnea, fever, and chest pain. Abdominal complaints have been mentioned,[114,117] and this was the main symptom leading to hospitalization in one patient who developed respiratory failure in the following hours.[117] Myalgias may also be noted.[114] On physical examination, tachypnea and tachycardia are present, with crackles or less often wheezes on auscultation.

The chest radiograph shows bilateral infiltrates, with mixed alveolar or interstitial opacities or both (Figure 24–8A).[114,115,121] Bilateral pleural effusion and Kerley's B lines are common.[114] Radiographic signs consistent with pulmonary edema (including areas of opacity in the air spaces and interlobular thickening) and pleural effusion are characteristic.[128] The progression of findings is first, increased interstitial opacities, followed by alveolar infiltrates, and then interstitial opacities when the alveolar opacities rapidly clear.[114] Within 3 weeks the chest radiograph returns to normal,[114,115] with pleural effusions being the last abnormality to disappear.[114]

On CT imaging, ground-glass opacities and air space consolidation are the most common patterns of parenchymal lesions; poorly defined nodules and interlobular septal thickening are seen in a majority of patients; and pleural effusion is present in at least two-thirds of patients and is usually bilateral (Figure 24–8B).[67,114,115,122]

White blood cell count at presentation usually shows increased leukocytosis with a predominance of neutrophils, with eosinophils being rarely higher than 0.3×10^9/L.[114,129] However, the eosinophil count may rise to high values in the course of disease.[54,117–119,130]

BAL is the key to diagnosis of IAEP, by showing frank eosinophilic alveolitis with an average percentage of 37[114] to 54%.[122] Eosinophilia was found in the sputum of 6 of 9 patients.[54] After recovery, no eosinophilia was found in the BAL fluid,[114,116] even though it may have persisted for several weeks.[130]

The pleural fluid differential cell count shows eosinophilia, ranging from about 10 to 50%.[114,119,124] The IgE level is raised in some patients.[119] Increased levels of IL-5 (a cytokine active in the regulation of the eosinophil) in the blood and BAL fluid have been reported in IAEP.[130–135] IL-5, eotaxin, and GM-CSF levels are higher than those in CEP, and anti-IL-5 neutralizing antibody inhibits eosinophil chemotaxis.[135]

Hypoxemia may be severe and refractory to breathing 100% oxygen in some patients,[49,113] with mechanical ventilation, either noninvasive or with intubation, being necessary in a majority of patients.[114,122] Although most patients present with symptoms of acute lung injury or adult respiratory distress syndrome, shock is exceptional[136] and extrapulmonary organ failure is absent. The fraction of inspired oxygen (FiO_2) may be decreased within a few hours of steroid treatment in many patients initially requiring oxygen.[114] When performed, lung function tests have shown a mild restrictive ventilatory defect with a normal forced expiratory volume in 1 second/forced vital capacity (FEV_1/FVC) ratio (but with small airways dysfunction) and reduced transfer factor.[119] The alveolar-arterial oxygen gradient is increased.[114] Lung function tests done after recovery are normal in most patients, with possible restriction in some of them.[49,114,116]

When performed, lung biopsy shows acute and organizing diffuse alveolar damage together with inter-

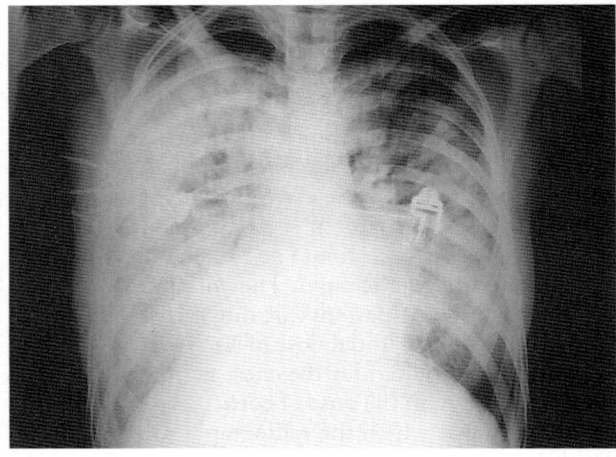

A

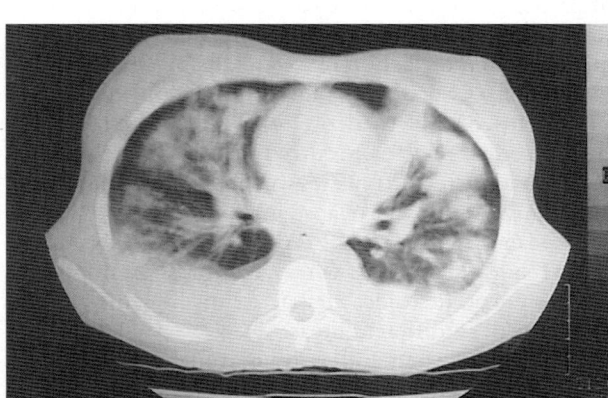

B

Figure 24–8 Idiopathic acute eosinophilic pneumonia in a 16-year-old girl. *A*, Chest radiograph show bilateral diffuse alveolar opacities. *B*, Bilateral alveolar opacities with associated pleural effusion are seen on CT scan.

stitial alveolar and bronchiolar infiltration by eosinophils, intra-alveolar eosinophils, and interstitial edema.[48,49,114,119,137] Eosinophil infiltration is also present in the bronchial wall.[119]

Recovery without corticosteroid treatment has been reported,[54,116,119] and occurred in up to 6 of 22 patients in our retrospective series.[122] Improvement concomitant with corticosteroid treatment cannot therefore be considered a diagnostic criterion of IAEP as it has been proposed.[137] However, in most cases once the diagnosis of IAEP is obtained, corticosteroid treatment is usually applied, initially intravenously (methyl prednisolone) then changed to oral therapy.[114] Steroids can be tapered over 2 to 4 weeks.[114] The response to corticosteroids occurs within 48 hours, allowing rapid weaning from the ventilator. Recovery is rapid with no significant clinical or imaging sequelae. In contrast with CEP, no relapse occurs after stopping corticosteroid treatment.

Thus, although IAEP presents clinically like acute lung injury or adult respiratory distress syndrome, its prognosis is much better. The key to diagnosis is eosinophilia in the BAL fluid since blood eosinophilia is usually initially absent. In typical cases, this author considers that lung biopsy is unnecessary. However, a careful search for a cause of AEP is mandatory, and especially infectious agents must be sought for in BAL fluid by cultures and appropriate staining. Drug-induced AEP must also be carefully excluded.[138,139]

Churg-Strauss Syndrome

In 1951, Churg and Strauss described, mainly from autopsied cases, the syndrome to which their name was given.[140] However, the subgroup of patients with periarteritis (polyarteritis) nodosa and associated asthma and eosinophilia had been previously characterized. Maybe the case presented by W. Osler in 1900 at a meeting of the Johns Hopkins Hospital Medical Society under the heading "Case of asthma with cyanosis, extensive purpura, painful muscles, and eosinophilia" was a case of Churg-Strauss syndrome.[141] In 1914, Lamb published a detailed study of two cases of periarteritis nodosa, one of which was clearly a case of Churg-Strauss syndrome with characteristic systemic involvement at autopsy, including pulmonary vascular involvement.[142] He further commented on the eosinophilia, already mentioned in two previous cases. Rackemann and Greene[143] reported eight patients with periarteritis nodosa and asthma, with eosinophilia in all eight cases, and they considered that "the development of the actual lesions in the arteries is the end stage of a process which in its beginning is common to many cases of asthma." Harkavy[144] reported eight cases of asthma with recurrent pulmonary infiltration and eosinophilic polyseritis. The pulmonary lesions were described as insidious in onset and migratory, with a miliary and interstitial appearance on chest radiograph. Wilson and Alexander[145] further detailed features of this peculiar type of periarteritis nodosa, and they stated that in almost every instance, asthma antedated periarteritis nodosa in the great majority of cases by a few years and sometimes by only a month or two. They also stated that only about 10% of cases occurred before the age of 21 years, and that only 6% of cases of periarteritis nodosa without asthma had eosinophilia, in distinction to 94% of the cases with associated asthma.

In their study, Churg and Strauss[140] reported cases of severe asthma that presented the clinical syndrome previously described by Rackemann and Greene[143] and by Harkavy,[144] and, which, on pathologic examination, exhibited granulomatous extravascular lesions as well as necrotizing, inflammatory, and granulomatous vascular changes. The lesions were characterized by an inflammatory exudate rich in eosinophils. Recurrent episodes of pneumonia were present in nearly every case, with some cases exhibiting the typical clinical and roentgenologic findings of Löffler's syndrome pulmonary infiltration. The most frequent site of inflammation was

the heart. Involvement of branches of the pulmonary artery was observed in six of nine cases. In approximately half of the cases a pneumonic process was found, with an eosinophil-rich exudate mixed with giant cells in the acute stage.

In the Chapel Hill Consensus Conference on the Nomenclature of Systemic Vasculitis, Churg-Strauss syndrome was included in the group of small vessel vasculitis, and defined as eosinophil-rich and granulomatous inflammation involving the respiratory tract, necrotizing vasculitis affecting small- to medium-sized vessels, and associated with asthma and eosinophilia.[146]

The pathologic lesions of Churg-Strauss syndrome associate both vasculitis (Figure 24–9) and granulomatous eosinophilic tissue infiltration.[44,150,147–150] Necrotizing giant cell eosinophilic vasculitis involves mainly the large- and medium-sized pulmonary arteries. The eosinophilic component is of varying intensity. The extravascular granuloma consists of palisading histiocytes and giant cells. However, all of these features are seldom found on a single biopsy. The pulmonary eosinophilic pneumonia in Churg-Strauss syndrome is similar to that of chronic eosinophilic pneumonia. Eosinophilic bronchial infiltration is common.

Isolated case reports and a few series delineated the clinical features of the Churg-Strauss syndrome.[147,151–154]

Churg-Strauss syndrome is a very rare vasculitis that occurs in adults,[147] although it has been occasionally reported in children and adolescents.[155–159] There is no gender predominance. The mean age of onset of vasculitis is 38[147] to 47,[154] 48,[159] or 49 years.[160]

Asthma is generally severe and becomes rapidly corticosteroid dependent. It may occasionally be absent.[161] Asthma occurs at a mean age of about 35 years[147,152] and precedes the onset of vasculitis by a mean of 3 to 8.9 years.[147,151–153,159] The interval between asthma and the onset of vasculitis may be much longer,[152,153] or contemporary.[151,153] The shortness of the interval might be an unfavorable prognostic factor.[153] Usually, the severity of

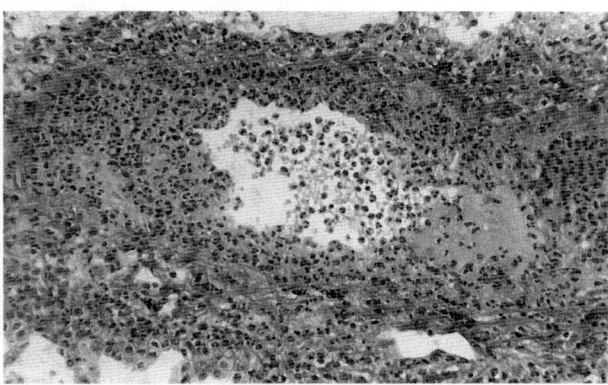

Figure 24–9 Churg-Strauss syndrome. The wall of a small arteriole is infiltrated by large numbers of eosinophils (hematoxylin, eosin, saffron; ×250 original magnification). (Courtesy of R. Loire, Department of Pathology, Louis Pradel Hospital, Lyon, France.)

asthma increases progressively until vasculitis develops, but it may paradoxically attenuate once vasculitis occurs only to further reappear when vasculitis abates.[147,151–153] Asthma may be severe and lead to death.[147,151,152,159]

Pulmonary infiltrates are the most typical abnormalities on the chest radiograph. They have been reported with varying frequency in 37%,[159] 51%,[160] or 72%[147] in large series. In the series by Guillevin and colleagues,[159] pulmonary infiltrates were noted in patients at presentation but did not develop in other patients during follow-up. The chest radiograph may be normal throughout the course of the disease. This was the case in other series for 4 of 10 patients,[151] 5 of 16 patients,[152] and 22 of 30 cases.[153] The pulmonary infiltrates usually consist of ill-defined opacities, sometimes migratory, transient, and of varying density.[144,147,151–153,158,162–167] Cavitation rarely has been observed,[163] in contrast to the pulmonary lesions in Wegener's granulomatosis where cavitary lesions are common (Figure 24–10).[168] Other abnormalities seen on the chest radiograph include mild pleural effusion[147,152,169,170] and phrenic nerve palsy.[152,170] Churg-Strauss syndrome presenting with bilateral massive pleural involvement (biopsy proven) has been reported.[171] The most common lesions on thin-section CT consist of areas of ground-glass attenuation or air space consolidation, with peripheral predominance or random distribution; less common findings are centrilobular nodules, bronchial wall thickening or dilatation, interlobular septal thickening, hilar or mediastinal adenopathy, pleural effusion, or pericardial effusion.[67,167,172] However, these abnormalities are not specific, and a correct diagnosis of Churg-Strauss syndrome was made in only 44% of cases in a series of 111 patients with eosinophilic lung diseases.[67]

Associated rhinitis is present in about three-quarters of the cases.[147,173] It is generally of the allergic type, often accompanied by relapsing sinusitis and/or polyps. Crusty rhinitis may be present. Although the rhinitis observed in the Churg-Strauss syndrome is usually much less severe than that seen in Wegener's granulomatosis, septal nasal perforation may occur.[173] Paranasal sinusitis has been reported in 61% of patients.[159]

Blood eosinophilia is a major feature of Churg-Strauss syndrome. It usually parallels the vasculitis activity but rapidly regresses with corticosteroids. Blood eosinophils are generally between 5 and 20×10^9/L, but they may reach or exceed 30×10^9/L or greater than 80% of the differential cell count.[147,151–153,159]

BAL fluid usually shows eosinophilia, sometimes greater than 60% on the differential cell count.[151,169,174] There is no strict correlation between blood and alveolar eosinophilia, the latter possibly persisting after blood eosinophilia has normalized.[174] Eosinophils represent generally more than 60% of the cells in pleural effusions.[144,169,175]

Antineutrophil cytoplasmic antibodies (ANCA) have been reported in Churg-Strauss syndrome, which is one of the pulmonary ANCA-associated vasculitides (together with Wegener's syndrome and microscopic polyangiitis), and these are mainly p-ANCA with

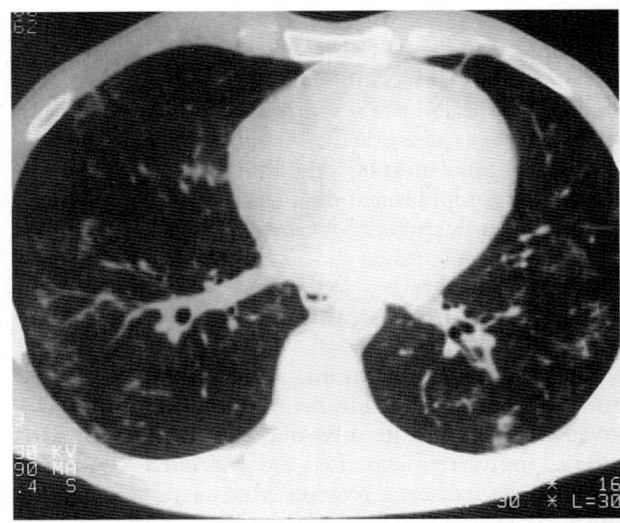

Figure 24–10   Churg-Strauss syndrome in a 33-year-old man with severe asthma, blood eosinophilia of 12×10^9 eosinophils/L, alveolar eosinophilia of 50% in the differential cell count. The CT scan shows bilateral reticulonodular opacities. Systemic involvement consisted of cardiac ischemia (further resulting in cardiomyopathy), sinusitis, mononeuritis multiplex, and cutaneous lesions. Vasculitis was controlled with corticosteroids only.

myeloperoxidase specificity (much less often c-ANCA with proteinase 3 specificity).[159,160,176–180] ANCA were present in 36% of patients in the series from the Mayo Clinic,[160] and 48% of patients in the series of Guillevin and colleagues.[159] IgE level is usually markedly increased.[157,151–153] The erythrocyte sedimentation rate is increased and anemia is common. High levels of urinary EDN have been reported, and these might represent an activity index of disease.[181,182]

The extrapulmonary manifestations of vasculitis developing in asthmatic patients are generally associated with asthenia, weight loss, fever, arthralgias, and myalgias, all of which are unusual in simple asthma.

Peripheral neurologic involvement typically consists of mononeuritis multiplex, present in 77% of patients,[159] or asymmetric polyneuropathy.[183] Cranial nerve palsies and central nervous system involvement are less common.[140,147,159] Heart involvement may be severe and lead to death.[147,153,159,160,184] Myocardial involvement is a consequence of eosinophilic myocarditis and/or coronary arteritis and is often insidious and asymptomatic, with the diagnosis made only at the stage of left ventricular failure and dilated cardiomyopathy.[144,147,185–187] This author considers that every patient with a possible diagnosis of Churg-Strauss syndrome should have a systematic cardiac evaluation in search of cardiac involvement. Cardiac involvement may result in heart failure requiring heart transplantation[188] with possible recurrence in the transplanted heart.[189] However, myocardial impairment as well as coronary arteritis may markedly improve with corticosteroid treatment.[190–196] Pericarditis is common, usually with limited effusion; however, pericardial effusion may be more important and occasionally give rise to tamponade.[197,198] Endomyocardial involvement is distinctly rare but has been responsible for restrictive myocardiopathy, with fibrosis at endomyocardial biopsy.[199] Mitral regurgitation, when present, suggests the presence of myocardial fibrosis.[200] Isolated electrocardiographic abnormalities are common. Digestive tract involvement is present in 31% of cases[159] and usually manifests as isolated abdominal pain, but intestinal or biliary tract vasculitis may be present. Diarrhea, ulcerative colitis, gastroduodenal ulcerations, perforations (esophageal, gastric, bowel), digestive hemorrhage (hematemesis, melena), and cholecystitis have also been reported.[147,153,166,201–203] Cutaneous lesions, present in 49% of patients,[159] mainly consist of palpable purpura of the extremities, nodules, erythematous rashes, and urticaria; and subcutaneous nodules of the scalp or of the extremities are evocative. A biopsy of the cutaneous lesions should be performed and is the most common and simple procedure to obtain pathologic evidence of vasculitis.[147,153,159,204–207] In contrast with periarteritis nodosa, renal involvement, present in 26% of cases, is usually mild, with only 5% of patients developing mild renal insufficiency.[159] Renal involvement may occasionally be severe, but the long-term renal outcome is usually very good under treatment.[208]

Although the cause of the Churg-Strauss syndrome is unknown, some triggering or adjuvant factors (as vaccines or desensitization) have been suspected.[152,159,185,209–211] The possible role of allergy is debated, because atopic familial antecedents are common and allergic-type rhinitis is present in many patients with Churg-Strauss syndrome. Some reported cases suggest the possible triggering role of *Aspergillus*,[212] allergic bronchopulmonary candidiasis,[213] *Ascaris*,[214] bird exposure,[215] or cocaine.[216] Interestingly, whereas the association between periarteritis nodosa and hepatitis B virus is well established, only a few cases of Churg-Strauss syndrome are associated with this virus.[210] Two patients with hepatitis C infection developed Churg-Strauss syndrome.[217] One patient with Churg-Strauss syndrome and antibodies to human immunodeficiency virus (HIV) and hepatitis B virus has been reported.[218] Much debate has centered on the possible responsibility of leukotriene-receptor antagonists (montelukast, zafirlukast, pranlukast) in the development of Churg-Strauss syndrome.[219–240] At the time of this writing, no direct responsibility of this family of drugs has been clearly established. Whether the association is coincidental, whether smoldering Churg-Strauss syndrome flares just because of reducing oral or inhaled corticosteroids[241,242] while coincidentally introducing leukotriene receptor antagonists, or whether the latter really exert a role on the pathogenesis of vasculitis is not known. This author considers that while awaiting further evidence, leukotriene receptor antagonists should be avoided in asthma patients with eosinophilia and/or extrapulmonary manifestations compatible with smoldering Churg-Strauss syndrome. Drug-induced eosinophilic vasculitis with pulmonary involvement has been reported in the past with sulfonamides used together with antiserum,[243] and later with diflunisal,[244] macrolides,[245,246] and diphenylhydantoin.[247] Churg-Strauss syndrome during pregnancy after steroid withdrawal[248] and severe pregnancy-related Churg-Strauss syndrome[248–250] have been reported.

The diagnosis of Churg-Strauss syndrome is difficult, because the clinician is currently more often confronted with patients with early and mild signs of vasculitis than with cases like those described by Churg and Strauss, where florid and overt disseminated vasculitis was much more evident. The evolution of Churg-Strauss syndrome generally follows three stages: initial allergic disease with asthma and rhinitis; pulmonary disease resembling chronic eosinophilic pneumonia; and extrapulmonary vasculitis. Diagnostic difficulties thus largely depend on the stage of disease when the patient is seen.

Lanham and colleagues[147] have proposed three diagnostic criteria: asthma; eosinophilia exceeding 1.5×10^9/L; and systemic vasculitis of two or more extrapulmonary organs. According to the classification (but not the diagnostic!) criteria of the American College of Rheumatology,[251] a sensitivity of 85% and a specificity of 99.7% are obtained if four or more of the six following criteria are present: asthma; eosinophilia greater than 10% in the differential blood cell count; mononeuritis (including multiplex) or polyneuropathy; fluctuating infiltrates on the chest radiograph; bilateral maxillary sinusal abnormalities; and the presence of extravascular eosinophils in a biopsy comprising a vessel. However, these diagnostic and classification criteria were proposed before ANCA were available. The presence of ANCA may probably be considered a major diagnostic criterion when present. The skin, nerve, and muscle are the most common sites where a pathologic diagnosis of vasculitis may be obtained.[159] A Lung biopsy is seldom done. Transbronchial biopsies usually do not show vasculitis or granulomata (merely sparse interstitial inflammation with eosinophils),[252] although one case of transbronchial biopsy providing granulomas and angiitis with focal necrosis and eosinophilic infiltration has been reported.[158]

The frontiers of the Churg-Strauss syndrome with both the other vasculitides and the other idiopathic eosinophilic syndromes are often difficult to delineate, and clearly occasional cases of overlap syndromes exist.

Distinguishing between Wegener granulomatosis and Churg-Strauss syndrome may be occasionally tricky,[253–256] and an eosinophilic variant of Wegener's granulomatosis has been individualized.[255] It has even been argued that Churg-Strauss syndrome could simply be Wegener's syndrome or periarteritis nodosa occurring in an asthmatic patient with eosinophilia.[257,258] Concurrent Churg-Strauss syndrome and pulmonary infiltrates and temporal arteritis (either with or without giant cells, either eosinophilic or not) has been described.[248,259–263] Alveolar hemorrhage, probably due to capillaritis, has been observed occasionally in Churg-Strauss syndrome.[147,264]

Distinguishing between Churg-Strauss syndrome and idiopathic chronic eosinophilic pneumonia with minor extrathoracic symptoms also may be difficult as mentioned above, but most often this has little if any importance because corticosteroid treatment is the common issue. Some mild vasculitis is common on pathologic examination of the lung in patients with CEP.[34] Furthermore, CEP may progress to Churg-Strauss syndrome.[105–107,265–267] Extrapulmonary manifestations may be present in patients with CEP. Some cases with "limited" Churg-Strauss syndrome have been reported[268] including those in the lung[169,268–271] and the heart.[149,272,273] Published formes frustes of Churg-Strauss syndrome consist of cases where the disease has been suppressed to a greater or lesser extent by corticosteroids given for asthma, and where the diagnosis of Churg-Strauss has been made only retrospectively or when the patients were at a terminal stage.[274]

Depending on the definition of both entities, some cases are difficult to classify as either Churg-Strauss syndrome or idiopathic hypereosinophilic syndrome. Careful clinical analysis, the presence of ANCA, and vasculitis and granulomatosis on biopsy help in determining the appropriate diagnosis.

The treatment of the Churg-Strauss syndrome is not well established. However, corticosteroids are clearly the mainstay of therapy and suffice in a large number of cases.[147,154,275] An initial methylprednisolone bolus is useful in the most severe cases, then oral treatment starts, usually with 1 mg/kg/day of prednisone. Treament is prolonged for several months with progressively reduced doses. Relapses are common, and asthma often persists (or reappears if it had disappeared during high-dose corticosteroid treatment). Distinguishing simple relapse or persistence of asthma from relapse or persistance of vasculitis requires very precise evaluation. The necessity of adding cytostatic drugs to corticosteroids is controversial. A study enrolling 342 patients with either polyarteritis nodosa (260 cases) or Churg-Strauss syndrome (82 cases),[154] identified parameters with significant pronostic value and higher mortality: proteinuria greater than 1 g/day; renal insufficiency with serum creatinine greater than 158 mg/L; and gastrointestinal tract involvement. Cardiomyopathy and central nervous system involvement were associated with a relative risk of mortality of 2.2 and 1.8, respectively (not statistically significant). Corticosteroids improve disease control, despite the associated infectious complications that could be decreased by using bolus cyclophosphamide administration.[276,277] Mortality is associated with disease severity, and treatment with cytotoxic agents does not prevent relapses.[278] Treatment must take the severity of disease into account, and treatment with corticosteroids alone should be reserved for patients without manifestations that could result in mortality or severe morbidity.[279] We are currently conducting a prospective study [Guillevin L, Cordier JF, coordinators] in polyarteritis nodosa and Churg-Strauss syndrome where patients with the criteria of a poor prognosis receive pulse cyclophosphamide and

corticosteroids, whereas patients with criteria of a good prognosis receive corticosteroids with immunosuppressants added only if the daily dose of corticosteroids necessary to control the vasculitis is above 20 mg.

Subcutaneous interferon alpha was successfully used mainly in patients with severe disease (including cardiac involvement), with a dose-dependent decrease in the blood eosinophil count.[280,281] High dose intravenous immunoglobulins[282,283] and cyclosporin[284] have been useful in occasional patients.

The prognosis of Churg-Strauss syndrome has considerably improved, with 79% of patients alive at 5 years.[154] Mortality is mainly due to delayed diagnosis and insufficient disease control.[151,152]

Idiopathic Hypereosinophilic Syndrome

The definition of the hypereosinophilic syndrome proposed by Chusid and colleagues[285] in 1975 was (1) a persistent eosinophilia of greater than 1.5×10^9 eosinophils/L for longer than 6 months, or death before 6 months associated with the signs and symptoms of hypereosinophilic disease; (2) a lack of evidence for parasitic, allergic, or other known causes of eosinophilia; and (3) presumptive signs and symptoms of organ involvement, including hepatosplenomegaly, organic heart murmur, congestive heart failure, diffuse or focal central nervous system abnormalities, pulmonary fibrosis, fever, weight loss, or anemia. Chusid and colleagues[285] reported 14 personal cases including 2 patients with "prolonged benign hypereosinophilia" (both with cutaneous lesions and abnormal electrocardiograms), 3 patients with eosinophilic leukemia, and 1 with possible Churg-Strauss syndrome. In subsequent studies,[286,287] some patients had allergic features or features of myeloproliferation. The published cases corresponding to the definition of the idiopathic hypereosinophilic syndrome are therefore heterogeneous. However, patients with typical chronic disease share common complications, especially cardiac involvement.

Advances in the comprehension of idiopathic hypereosinophilic syndrome came from the concept of clonality as a major pathogenetic mechanism. Whereas hypereosinophilia is, in a number of cases, a reactive nonclonal process (as in parasitic disorders), it may also result from a clonal proliferation of either the eosinophils themselves or of clonal lymphocytes producing chemokines active on the accumulation of eosinophils. Hematologic disorders with clonal eosinophilia are represented by the rare chronic or acute eosinophilic leukemia and other myeloproliferative conditions.[288–293]

The production of chemokines active on the accumulation of eosinophils (especially IL-5) by clonal Th_2 lymphocytes (as demonstrated by clonal rearrangement of the T-cell receptor) bearing an aberrant phenotype ($CD3^-$, $CD4^+$) has been demonstrated in patients with the idiopathic hypereosinophilic syndrome (usually associated with high levels of IgE).[294–296] The majority of these patients were recruited from dermatology clinics and had papules or urticarial plaques infiltrated by lymphocytes and eosinophils (and in some of them a cutaneous T-cell lymphoma or Sézary syndrome was ultimately present). In such cases, hypereosinophilic syndrome may be considered as a premalignant T-cell disorder.[294–296]

The pulmonary involvement in patients with eosinophilia of clonal origin has not been studied extensively. However, lung or pleural involvement has been mentioned in some cases,[294–297] and chronic eosinophilic pneumonia has been reported[298–300] in patients with clonal lymphoid proliferations. In patients with aggressive clonal hematologic disorders, eosinophilic pneumonia must be distinguished from malignant cell infiltration of the lung.[301] A case of eosinophilia with polyclonal aberrant T cells and elevated serum levels of IL-2 and IL-15, presenting with wheezing dyspnea and papules throughout the airways (consisting of eosinophils, lymphocytes, and macrophages on biopsy) has been reported.[302]

Ongoing cytogenetic and molecular biology studies will undoubtedly help in the classification of subgroups in the so-called idiopathic hypereosinophilic syndrome.

The following data derived from older studies may therefore need reconsideration in the future.

It is difficult to determine the frequency of pulmonary involvement, and especially that of the eosinophilic pneumonias, in idiopathic hypereosinophilic syndrome. Well-documented reports of eosinophilic pneumonia are surprisingly few, in contrast with the estimated frequency of pulmonary involvement in 49% of cases in the literature.[303]

The hypereosinophilic syndrome is more common in men than in women (9:1), and occurs at ages between 20 and 50 years.[303] Several cases have been reported in children.[304] The onset is generally insidious, with eosinophilia discovered incidentally in 12% of the patients.[17] The mean eosinophil count at presentation was 20.1×10^9/L, with an average highest value of 44.4×10^9/L in one series.[286] The majority of patients present with white blood cell counts between 10 and 30×10^9/L, and percentages of eosinophils between 30 and 70%.[285] Extremely high values of eosinophilia, in excess of 100×10^9/L are found in some patients.[285] The main presenting symptoms are weakness and fatigue (26%), cough (24%), and dyspnea (16%).[17] Cardiovascular involvement, present in 58% of the patients,[303] is characteristic and is a major cause of morbidity and mortality. Fibrotic thickening of the endocardium by collagen-rich connective tissue (endomyocardial fibrosis), initially reported as fibroplastic parietal endocarditis (endocarditis parietalis fibroplastica) by Löffler,[305] is the hallmark of cardiac disease in the idiopathic hypereosinophilic syndrome.[17,306] This late irreversible stage of cardiac fibrosis is preceded by an initial acute necrotic stage followed by a thrombotic stage.[303] Cardiac manifestations consist of dyspnea, con-

gestive heart failure, mitral regurgitation, and cardiomegaly.[17,287] Echocardiography demonstrates classic features of the idiopathic hypereosinophilic syndrome, consisting of mural thrombus, ventricular apical obliteration, and involvement of the posterior mitral leaflet.[307] The neurologic manifestations, present in 54% of the patients,[303] are thromboemboli, central nervous system dysfunction, and peripheral neuropathies. Cutaneous manifestations, present in 56% of the cases,[303] are generally of two types: erythematous pruritic papules and nodules, and urticaria and angioedema.[303,308]

The frequency of pulmonary involvement is about 40%,[17,285] including pleural effusion, pulmonary emboli, cough, and interstitial infiltrates. Pulmonary pathologic studies were reported in two cases from the series of Chusid and colleagues,[285] one with pulmonary emboli and otherwise normal lungs, and the other one with pulmonary fibrosis with scanty eosinophilic infiltrates. Severe coughing attacks were present in 40% of the cases in one series[286] with no other mention of bronchopulmonary disease. In another series,[287] cough was also the predominent feature, with bronchospasm and pulmonary infiltrates in 11 of 40 patients each. However, in the largest reported series[17,285–287] there was no precise analysis of the pulmonary manifestations allowing a definite diagnosis of eosinophilic pneumonia. CT findings in 5 patients consisted of small nodules with or without a halo of ground-glass attenuation and focal areas of ground-glass attenuation mainly in the lung periphery.[309] However, CT findings are poorly specific and a correct diagnosis was obtained in only one-third of patients with the hypereosinophilic syndrome in a series of 111 patients with eosinophilic diseases.[67]

Given the frequency of cardiac failure in patients with hypereosinophilic syndrome, many of the observed pulmonary radiologic changes may result from the consequences of pulmonary edema. In one patient with interstitial and alveolar edema on the chest radiograph, pulmonary edema was found at autopsy but eosinophilic pulmonary infiltration was not mentioned.[310] One patient with patchy pulmonary opacity was found to have necrotizing bronchitis with eosinophilic infiltrates at bronchoscopic biopsy and purulent bronchitis at open-lung biopsy.[310] However, pulmonary eosinophilic involvement in hypereosinophilic syndrome rarely has been reported. One patient with pulmonary crackles at auscultation and bibasal alveolar infiltrates had 73% eosinophils in the BAL fluid, and pulmonary manifestations improved with corticosteroid therapy.[311] Adult respiratory distress syndrome developed in a patient with hypereosinophilic syndrome, with more than 75% eosinophils in the BAL fluid, which improved with corticosteroids.[312] Another patient presenting with eosinophilic pneumonia healed with corticosteroids and remained well without corticosteroids for 3 years. He then presented again with pneumonia and neurologic signs. Control of eosinophilia was not obtained by corticosteroids but was achieved with hydroxyurea. CT findings of pulmonary involvement in a series of five patients included several small nodules with a halo of ground-glass attenuation.[309] Interestingly, whereas alveolar and blood eosinophilia are usually correlated, only mild eosinophilia in the BAL fluid contrasting with high blood eosinophilia has been reported in patients with the hypereosinophilic syndrome.[313,314] This suggests that, in some patients, eosinophilia may be compartmentalized in hypereosinophilic syndrome, with eosinophils predominating in the vascular compartment in contrast with only sparse parenchymal pulmonary eosinophilic infiltration. Therefore, BAL might be a useful tool to distinguish patients with eosinophilic pulmonary infiltrates in hypereosinophilic syndrome.[311]

Although occasional vasculitis may be present in patients with hypereosinophilic syndrome, it generally differentiates the latter from Churg-Strauss syndrome, but when no biopsy of involved organs is avalaible, the distinction between the two entities may be difficult.

The treatment of the idiopathic eosinophilic syndrome offers further proof of the heterogeneity of this condition. Less than half of the patients respond well to corticosteroids, which remain the first-line therapy[287,315] but others do not and especially those with criteria of myeloproliferative syndrome.[287] Other therapies are therefore necessary in patients with little or only transient response to corticosteroids. These include chemotherapeutic agents (hydroxyurea, vincristine, etoposide), cyclosporin,[286,303,315–318] and especially alpha-interferon, which is an effective treatment at the present time, either as monotherapy[319–322] or in association with hydroxyurea in the myeloproliferative subset of patients.[323,324]

Whereas cases of idiopathic hypereosinophilic syndromes reported before 1975 had an average survival of 9 months with a 3-year survival of only 12%,[285] the prognosis has improved markedly with about a 70% survival at 10 years in Fauci and colleague's series.[17] In the series of Lefebvre and colleagues,[287] there was an 80% survival at 5 years and 42% at 10 and 15 years, including patients with myeloproliferative features who represent a subset of patients with a poorer prognosis. Whether prognosis will be improved or not with the use of alpha-interferon is not known.

The theoretical possibility that alpha-interferon might promote the expansion of a T clone by protecting CD3⁻ CD4⁺ cells from spontaneous apoptosis has been evoked.[325,326]

EOSINOPHILIC PNEUMONIAS OF DETERMINED ORIGIN

Eosinophilic Pneumonias of Parasitic Origin

The eosinophilic pneumonias related to parasite infestation probably represent the most common cause of eosinophilic pneumonia in the world, but these are certainly underestimated for at least two reasons: most are common and benign thus discouraging medical investigations, and most occur in countries with only poor access to medical care. Parasitic eosinophilic pneumonia occurs mainly in humans following infection by helminths, which are large multicellular worms, and especially after infection by nematodes (roundworms). The parasites responsible for eosinophilic pneumonia may or may not be found on pathologic examination of the lung.[327–331]

Tropical Eosinophilia

Tropical eosinophilia was individualized by Weingarten as a syndrome characterized by severe spasmodic bronchitis, leukocytosis, and high blood eosinophilia, occurring in India and affecting people living near to the sea.[332] Affected individuals had fever, loss of appetite and weight, and developed a dry, hacking cough exacerbating at night and often associated with expiratory dyspnea and wheezing. Respiratory symptoms were regularly present every night, and especially between 1 and 5 am. Eosinophils, and sometimes Charcot-Leyden crystals, were found in the sputum. Massive blood eosinophilia, "higher than that of any other disease except eosinophilic leukemia," was present. On the chest radiograph, disseminated mottling of both lungs was observed. No etiology could be determined.

Subsequent studies established that tropical eosinophilia is caused by the filarial parasites *Wuchereria bancrofti* and *Brugia malayi*.[333–335] Filarial parasites are nematodes that infect more than 150 million persons in the world. The adult worms of *W. bancrofti* and *B. malayi* reside in the lymphatic vessels, resulting in lymphatic obstruction with subsequent elephantiasis. Humans are infected by infective larvae deposited in the skin by the mosquitoes *Culex, Anopheles, Aedes,* and *Mansonia.* Within 6 to 12 months, the parasites develop into mature male or female worms, which may remain viable for several years. First-stage larvae or microfilariae are released from the fecund female's uterus and circulate in the bloodstream where from they are ingested by the mosquitoes. Microfilariae have a periodicity with nyctohemeral variation of the density of microfiliarae in the blood (the maximal density being between 10 pm and 4 am).

Human filariasis caused by *W. bancrofti* and *B. malayi* is endemic in the tropical and subtropical areas of coastal regions of Asia, southern and western Pacific, and Africa. Isolated foci are found in South and Central America. Other worm (especially hookworm) infestations may be associated with tropical pulmonary eosinophilia.[336]

Patients with tropical pulmonary eosinophilia rarely have clinical features of lymphatic filariasis. Microfilariae are usually not found in the blood and only very occasionally in the lung at pathologic analysis.[337] It is currently admitted that circulating microfilariae are trapped in the lung vasculature where they degenerate and release their antigenic constituents that trigger the inflammatory pulmonary reaction. The lung is the main organ affeted by tropical eosinophilia.[338,339] The clinical features of tropical pulmonary eosinophilia are mainly considered to be the result of an immune response to infection.[333,338–341] This is in contrast with the minimal clinical and immunologic response seen in the majority of infected persons living in endemic areas. Furthermore, the immunologic response in patients with tropical pulmonary eosinophilia is not restricted to parasites, but results in polyclonal activation of B cells and hypergammaglobulinemia.

Pathologic studies in patients with tropical pulmonary eosinophilia have provided interesting findings, and especially the fact that although blood eosinophilia is very high at the early stage (less than 2 weeks) of pulmonary disease, no prominent eosinophilia is found in the lung.[342,343] At this early stage, there is dense infiltration with histiocytes. Later on (1 to 3 months), a pattern of eosinophilic pneumonia is found, with the formation of eosinophilic abscesses and granulomatous lesions characterized by the presence of foreign-body giant cells, fibroblasts, and epithelioid cells radiating from the necrotic center of the granuloma; heavy eosinophilic infiltration is present at the periphery of the granuloma.[337,342,344,345] Microfilariae or portions of microfilariae have been found in the center of granulomatous eosinophilic nodules.[337,344] In later stages (6 months to 5 years), a mixed cell or histiocytic pattern with fibrosis is found. Cases untreated for 5 years or more show pulmonary fibrosis with histiocytic infiltration.[342,343] Although possible, the demonstration of microfilariae in the lung is unusual.[337,343]

The clinical manifestations of tropical pulmonary eosinophilia occur mainly in the second and third decades of life, with a male predominance (about 4:1). Tropical pulmonary eosinophilia has been reported mostly in Indians, and in a study in Singapore, although the population was predominantly Chinese (78%), the disease occurred in Indians in 80% of cases, whereas Chinese and Europeans were rarely affected.[346] Although tropical pulmonary eosinophilia is observed in *W. bancrofti*–endemic areas of East Africa,[347] it seems to be rare.[348] Tropical eosinophilia has been reported in a patient living in Italy for 2 years.[349]

Malaise, low-grade fever, and weight loss are followed within a few days by a cough, which becomes characteristically nocturnal, paroxysmal, and is accompanied by dyspnea and wheezes. Some patients may be misdiagnosed as having asthma, as occured in a recent Asian immigrant to Upstate New York.[350] Although the chest radiograph may be normal in some patients, it usually shows infiltrative opacities predominating in the middle and lower fields. The most common pattern has been described as an increase in lung markings, with other findings consisting of mottlings, homogeneous opacities, and possible extensive changes combining all of these.[346,351] Whereas mottlings and areas of pneumonitis clear within a month after treatment, increased lung markings take longer to return to normal.[346] Per-

sisting irregular basilar opacities are present in about two-thirds of patients after one year.[352] A "reticulonodular pattern" on CT has been reported in a majority of patients, with other features consisting of bronchiectasis, air trapping, and adenopathy.[353] Extrapulmonary manifestations are rare[338,354] and occur mainly in children, with generalized lymphadenopathy, hepatomegaly, and splenomegaly.[354]

Blood eosinophilia is prominent, with more than 2×10^9 eosinophils/L in all cases, more than 4×10^9 in 90% of cases and up to 60×10^9 in some cases.[354]

IgE levels are increased, especially in patients with relapsing disease.[355] Antifilarial IgG antibodies are increased, as in all patients with filariasis. Increased total IgE levels are found in the lower respiratory tract epithelial lining fluid, along with high levels of filarial-specific IgG, IgM, and IgE; within 2 weeks after treatment, there is a marked reduction in parasite-specific IgG and IgE.[356]

BAL in patients with tropical pulmonary eosinophilia shows an intense alveolitis with a mean percentage of 54% of eosinophils. The concentration of eosinophils is 3- to 20-fold greater in epithelial lining fluid than in the blood, suggesting a selective process of accumulation in the lung. Eosinophils recovered in BAL fluid show marked degranulation with loss of the cores and the peripheral portions of the granules and loss of granules.[357] In patients treated with diethylcarbamazine, there is a drop of BAL eosinophils within 2 weeks; blood eosinophils also decrease rapidly.[357–360] At one month, the percentage of eosinophils in the differential cell count decreased from 44.6 to 5.5% in one study.[359] When evaluated one year later, patients still have a moderate eosinophilic alveolitis with a mean percentage of 6% eosinophils in the BAL differential count.[352] The presence of microfilariae of *W. bancrofti* has been reported in bronchial brushing cytology of pulmonary lesions in two cases.[361]

Lung function tests in patients with tropical pulmonary eosinophilia show a restrictive ventilatory defect, with a superimposed reversible obstructive ventilatory defect and hypoxemia in about a quarter of the patients.[343,362] The CO transfer factor is decreased,[359,362,363] due to a reduction in membrane diffusing capacity.[363] Although the CO transfer factor improves with treatment, it does not return to normal values,[352,362,363] possibly because of residual interstitial fibrosis.[362] No specific pattern of ventilation and perfusion has been observed at scintiscanning.[355]

Because microfilariae are not detectable in the blood of patients with tropical pulmonary eosinophilia, diagnosis is made in patients with residence for several months in an endemic area on the combination of the clinical, epidemiologic, and laboratory features including blood eosinophilia persisting for weeks with an absolute eosinophil count in the blood greater than 3×10^9/L, IgE levels exceeding 10,000 ng/mL, and markedly increased antifilarial IgG. Diagnosis is further supported by clinical improvement in the weeks following treatment.[334,354,364]

Diethylcarbamazine, which kills microfilariae and adult-stage worms, is the only effective drug for tropical pulmonary eosinophilia. The recommended dose is 6 mg/kg per day for 21 days.[333,334] Improvement is rapid, within a few days. However, unsatisfactory responses may occur, suggesting reinfection and relapses requiring repeated treatments. The persistence of mild alveolitis, fibrosis, and altered diffusing capacity may provide evidence that infection has triggered an immunologic process continuing after the live parasites have been eliminated. This suggests a possible benefit from corticosteroids in addition to diethylcarbamazine.[334] Indeed, treatment of tropical pulmonary eosinophilia with prednisolone for 1 week has resulted in a decrease of eosinophilia within 24 hours after the start of the drug, with the return to pretreatment levels after the drug was discontinued.[344]

The diagnostic criteria of tropical pulmonary eosinophilia have recently been re-examined leading to the proposal of the following criteria: cough worse at night; residence in a filarial endemic area; eosinophil count greater than 3,300 cells/mm³; clinical and hematologic response to diethylcarbamazine.[365]

Ascaris Pneumonia

Pulmonary infiltrates with eosinophilia may develop during the migration of the larvae of the parasite through the lung.

Ascaris lumbricoides, a nematode or roundworm, is the most common helminthic infection in humans with an estimated prevalence of 1 billion.[366] It is a cosmopolitan parasitosis, which is most common in the tropical and subtropical areas. It affects mainly children, but eosinophilic pneumonia due to infection by this parasite has been reported in an 80-year-old woman.[367]

Mature females in the human intestine release large numbers of eggs, which are expulsed with stools. These are able to survive for several months or years, even in an unfavorable environment. The transmission of disease is through a fecal-oral route via eggs present in food or water contaminated by human feces. After ingestion, the infective larvae formed within eggs develop in the small intestine and within 5 to 10 days penetrate through the intestinal wall and migrate through the venous circulation to the lungs where they break out into the alveoli. They then migrate through the bronchi and trachea, are swallowed, and mature into adult worms in the small intestine. The time to produce a mature female is about 2 months.[366,368,369]

Pulmonary manifestations at the time of larval migration to the lungs is of varying severity, depending on the initial amount of ingested eggs.

Usually, pulmonary symptoms are mild, with cough and wheezing, transient pulmonary infiltrates, and eosinophilia. This is the typical presentation of Löffler's syndrome. Löffler[25] estimated that 23 out of 100 of his cases were caused by ascariasis. The majority of patients are febrile, with possible pruritic eruption within the first 4 or 5 days of respiratory symptoms.[370] Blood eosinophilia may reach values as high as 22×10^9/L.[370] Diagnosis may be obtained by the finding of larvae in the sputum or gastric aspirates (within 8 to 16 days after the ingestion of eggs)[366,370,371] but is more commonly obtained by the delayed finding of the worm or ova in the stool within 3 months of the pulmonary manifestations.[366,372] The enormous amount of eggs released by the female worm makes diagnosis easy on direct smears of fecal material. Larvae have been found in the occasional lung biopsy.[366] Pulmonary biopsy during the early convalescence of patients showed only minimal changes with interstitial edema and scattered perivascular accumulation of eosinophils.[370] Pulmonary ascariasis with eosinophilic pneumonia may occasionally result in death.[373]

Intestinal ascariasis is treated with mebendazole for 3 days.[366,369] In severe cases, associated corticosteroids produce a dramatic diminution in symptoms, a decrease in temperature, and a drop in the eosinophilia.[370] Other agents active on ascariasis are pyrantel pamoate and albendazole.[368]

Ascaris suum, a parasite of the pig, has been reported to produce severe pulmonary infiltrates with eosinophilia. This occurred during a winter carnival in Canada when four students ingested a "festive meal maliciously seasoned with large quantities of embryonated *Ascaris suum* ova."[374] Three of the students presented, respectively, 3 days, 10 days, and 2 weeks later with acute respiratory failure and massive pulmonary alveolar opacities on their chest radiograph. Their initial PaO$_2$ was respectively 37, 34, and 48 mm Hg. Two of them had no blood eosinophilia and the other had an eosinophilia of 2.9×10^9/L. However, all three had eosinophil counts greater than 2×10^9/L during the recovery phase of the illness. Dramatic improvement of all three patients followed corticosteroid treatment. Worm larvae were found in the sputum and/or gastric washings of three of the four contaminated patients. The two patients with the most widespread pulmonary infiltrates also had elevated IgE levels, IgM precipitating antibodies to *A. suum* antigen, and the higher eosinophilia.

Eosinophilic Pneumonia in Larva Migrans Syndrome

Humans are not permissive for the normal progression of the canine nematode *Toxocara canis* through each of its developmental stages.[375,376] Visceral larva migrans, a terminology proposed by Beaver and colleagues,[377] is a zoonotic infection caused in humans by *T. canis,* which infects dogs and other canines. Toxocariasis occurs in all temperate and tropical areas of the world. A large proportion of dogs is infected, and the soil of public playgrounds in urban areas is often contaminated with eggs of *Toxocara*. Children playing in contaminated areas are the primary victims of visceral larva migrans syndrome, especially when they practice geophagia.[375,378] Eggs released by female worms pass in feces of infected dogs.

Eggs ingested by humans hatch in the intestine, migrate through the portal circulation, and invade the liver, lung, and other organs. However, the development of the parasite is blocked at the larval stage.[375]

Visceral larva migrans occurs predominantly in children. The majority of infected children remain asymptomatic. The symptomatic patients present with fever, pulmonary manifestations, seizures, and fatigue. Pulmonary manifestations occur in approximately 80% of cases, generally consisting of mild cough, wheezes, and dyspnea, with pulmonary infiltrates on the chest radiograph, which are present in approximately half of the patients with pulmonary symptoms.[376,377] However, severe pulmonary involvement occurs in about 17% of cases and may benefit from corticosteroids.[379]

Toxocariasis is uncommon in adults, but is nevertheless a possible cause of pulmonary disease with eosinophilia. Some cases correspond to mild disease,[358] whereas in other patients, pulmonary involvement may be severe[380–384] and necessitate mechanical ventilation.[381] Patients present with fever, dyspnea, and pulmonary infiltrates on the chest radiograph. However, the initial chest radiograph may be normal.[383] Wheezes or crackles are present at pulmonary auscultation. Blood eosinophilia may be present initially,[380,382,383] or may develop only in the following days.[381] BAL fluid shows a marked eosinophilia, ranging from 55 to 75%.[380–382]

The diagnosis of toxocariasis is obtained by serologic methods and especially by enzyme-linked immunosorbent assay (ELISA), with a sensitivity and specificity of 91% and 86%, respectively.[385] As the worm does not develop in humans, eggs are not found in the stools of patients. *Toxocara* was found in a small brown itchy nodule of the ankle in a patient with larva migrans who had multiple lung nodules on the CT scan and extensive eosinophilic infiltration on transbronchial biopsy.[386]

Visceral larva migrans is usually a self-limiting disease requiring only symptomatic treatment. The use of anthelmintics is controversial.[387] Corticosteroids seem beneficial in cases with severe pulmonary involvement.[379,381–383]

Strongyloides stercoralis *Infection*

The intestinal nematode *Strongyloides stercoralis* may cause severe autoinfection in immunocompromised patients. Strongyloidiasis is widely distributed in the tropics and subtropics, with a prevalence estimated at 50 to 100 million.[366] The most common route of human infection is through the skin by contact with the soil of beaches or mud. The larvae pass through the circulation to the lungs where they break into the alveoli, ascend the trachea, are swallowed, and reside in the small intestine where they mature. Females deposit eggs that hatch into larvae and pass with feces. Infected patients usually have eosinophilia, but it is frequently absent in disseminated disease.[388] Because of its capacity to replicate within the host, *S. stercoralis* may persist for years in infected people and give rise to the hyperinfection syndrome (severe

disseminated strongyloidiasis which may affect all organs) when immunosupppression occurs.[389] Immunocompromised individuals at risk of disseminated disease in endemic areas comprise children with malnutrition, patients treated with corticosteroids or cytotoxic drugs, transplant recipients, and patients with AIDS.

About 20% of hospitalized patients with strongyloidiasis have coexisting chronic lung disease.[390] Many patients with chronic obstructive pulmonary disease receive corticosteroids, therefore, they are at risk of hyperinfection syndrome.[390–393] Opportunistic pulmonary strongyloidiasis may also complicate asthma treated with corticosteroids.[394] Pulmonary strongyloidiasis may be confused with asthma, and if corticosteroids are given the hyperinfection syndrome may develop.[390]

Pulmonary manifestations of Löffler's syndrome occur when larvae migrate through the lungs after acute infection.[366,395,396] The finding of peripheral blood eosinophilia, in association with pneumonia, bronchospasm, or bronchitis and abdominal pain or diarrhea, should suggest strongyloidiasis in patients living, or having traveled, in endemic areas.[389,395,397] Chronic infections are usually asymptomatic.

Massive larval infection of the lungs (hyperinfection syndrome) is seen in patients with immunosuppression,[389,398–400] who present with fever, abdominal pain, ileus or small bowel obstruction, jaundice, or meningitis. Bacterial infection by enteric bacteria may supervene, due to gut flora leaking from the bowel damaged by the invasive larvae. Eosinophilia may or may not be present. Cough, wheezing, and dyspnea are associated with bilateral patchy infiltrates. Rhabdoid larvae have been recovered in the BAL fluid or bronchial washing (Figure 24–11)[389,393,401] or in the sputum,[402–404] but despite of the presence of larvae in the lungs, blood, and BAL fluid, eosinophilia may be absent, possibly because of previous corticosteroid treatment in some cases.[393] Eosinophil counts greater than 8% are associated with a better prognosis.[388]

Diagnosis of strongyloidiasis depends on the demonstration of larvae in the feces or in any secretion or tissue specimen, including sputum and BAL fluid.[399,404–406] Immunodiagnostic assays by ELISA methods may be useful for diagnosis (and screening), but cross-reactivity with other parasitic infections exists.[390,407]

Because of the risk of hyperinfection syndrome, all diagnosed infected patients should be treated. The classic effective agent is thiabendazole given for 2 days, but continued for 2 to 3 weeks in patients with the hyperinfection syndrome.[407,408]

Eosinophilic Pneumonias in Other Parasitic Infections

The dog hookworm *Ancylostoma braziliense* is the cause of cutaneous helminthiasis (creeping eruption) characterized by serpiginous elevated reddish tunnels or burrows on the exposed surfaces of the skin and produced within a few hours or days after the larvae present in the soil have penetrated the skin. It may produce, in 50% of the cases, a typical Löffler's syndrome with transitory migratory pulmonary infiltration and peripheral eosinophilia, with almost complete absence of clinical signs or symptoms of systemic disease.[409,410] Pulmonary manifestations develop after the seventh day of cutaneous eruption.[409] Sputum eosinophil count is high in 90% of cases.[409] The degree of eosinophilia approximates the extent of the pulmonary consolidation and tends to persist (as well as sputum eosinophilia) for 4 to 6 weeks after the consolidation has subsided.[409] Humans are dead-end hosts, and the pathogenesis of pulmonary manifestations is unclear. The human hookworms *Ancylostoma duodenale* and *Necator americanus* are possible causes of Löffler's syndrome, but pulmonary manifestations are much less common than in other migrating nematode infections.[366]

Schistosomiasis affects about 200 million people worldwide, especially throughout Africa, South and Central America, and parts of the Middle East. Pulmonary disease occurs with three of the five major species of *Schistosoma* that infect humans: mainly *S. mansoni, S. haematobium*, and *S. japonicum*.[372,411] In early acute schistosomiasis, patients may develop multiple transient small pulmonary nodules on the chest radiograph and eosinophilia[372,411,412]; a greater number of nodules may be detected on the CT scan.[412] In chronic schistosomiasis, embolization of ova in small arteries in the lungs results in granuloma formation, occlusion of pulmonary arteries, and further pulmonary hypertension, which is the most conspicuous type of pulmonary disease in schistosomiasis. The characteristic granuloma comprises lymphocytes, eosinophils, and giant cells. In addition to these pulmonary manifestations, a post-treatment eosinophilic pneumonitis (variously described under the names of lung shift, verminous pneumonia, reactionary Löffler-like pneumonitis) may develop.[413] The pathogenesis of this syndrome is unclear. It could result from parasitic antigen release following treatment. In a reported case after oxam-

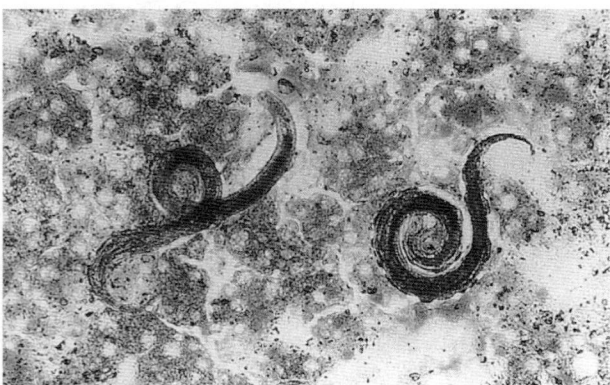

Figure 24–11   *Strongyloides stercoralis* in bronchoalveolar lavage fluid (Methenamine silver; ×250 original magnification). (Courtesy of M.A. Piens, Department of Parasitology, Claude Bernard University, Lyon, France.)

inquine treatment, diffuse reticulonodular infiltrates were present on chest radiograph, and eosinophilic pneumonia was proved by BAL and transbronchial biopsy.[413]

The filarial parasite of the dog *Dirofilaria immitis* (the pulmonary fluke), common in the southern United States, may occasionally develop into adult worms in the lungs after inoculation of infective larvae by mosquitoes. It manifests mainly as solitary pulmonary nodules or masses with or without eosinophilia,[414–417] but eosinophilic pulmonary infiltrates have been reported.[383,418]

Paragonimus westermani, an oval trematode, is present in East Asia, Japan, India, West Africa, and South America. The majority of infected patients have mild or no symptoms, but others develop pulmonary infection with cough, hemoptysis, and pulmonary opacities on imaging. Multiple thin-walled cavities are the most characteristic pulmonary feature, but patchy densities may be present. Eosinophilia is variable.[128,339,419–421]

Eosinophilic pneumonia has been convincingly reported with the presence of both eosinophilia and parasites in the lung in *Trichomonas tenax* pulmonary infection[422] and in *Angiostrongylus*-like nematode pulmonary infection.[423]

Pulmonary infiltrates with blood eosinophilia have been reported in *Loa loa* infection.[424] Löffler's syndrome has been reported in trichiniasis.[425] Capillariasis, due to the helminth *Capillaria aerophila* infecting carnivores and ingested with contaminated soil, has occasionally been reported as a cause of eosinophilic pneumonia.[426,427] Eosinophilia and pulmonary infiltrates were reported in China in patients with infection by the parasite *Clonorchis sinensis* (*Opisthorchis sinensis*).[428]

Eosinophilic Pneumonias of Other Infectious Causes

Infection with the fungus *Coccidioides immitis* is a well-established cause of eosinophilia,[429–433] especially in patients with disseminated disease.[433] Pulmonary eosinophilia has been demonstrated on lung biopsy.[434] Biopsy of skin lesions in patients with eosinophilia and pulmonary infiltrates may provide a clue to the diagnosis.[435] *Coccidioides* grew on culture of BAL fluid in a patient with eosinophilic pneumonia.[436] Disseminated infection with blood eosinophilia and pulmonary consolidation due to the fungi *Bipolaris australiensis* and *Bipolaris spicifera* has been reported in a young immunocompetent man and in an asthmatic patient, respectively.[437,438]

BAL eosinophilia (with possibly greater than 40% eosinophils in differential cell count values) has been reported in *Pneumocystis carinii* pneumonitis in patients with AIDS.[32,439,440] However, pulmonary eosinophilia is not usually conspicuous on lung biopsies of patients with AIDS and *P. carinii* pneumonia.[441] Cellular infiltrates consisting of histiocytes and eosinophils were found at autopsy in a child with sex-linked agammaglobulinemia and fatal *P. carinii* pneumonia.[442]

Bacterial pulmonary infection may occasionally be a cause of eosinophilic pneumonia (Figure 24–12). This has been reported in *Corynebacterium pseudotuberculosis* infection in a veterinary medical student (this bacteria is a common pathogen of livestock, occasionally reported as a cause of infection in humans).[443] Eosinophilic pneumonia was demonstrated in a lung biopsy in a patient with *Mycobacterium simiae* infection.[444] Pulmonary eosinophilia has also been reported in tuberculosis,[445] and pneumonia with blood eosinophilia has been reported in chronic brucellosis.[446]

Allergic Bronchopulmonary Aspergillosis and Related Syndromes

Allergic Bronchopulmonary Aspergillosis

Allergic bronchopulmonary aspergillosis (ABPA) accounts for most of the currently diagnosed allergic bronchopulmonary mycoses. ABPA is distinct from the other pulmonary manifestations due to *Aspergillus,* such as invasive pulmonary aspergillosis (where blood and tissue eosinophilia is conspicuously absent) occurring especially in immunocompromised patients or aspergilloma developing in pre-existent pulmonary cavities.[447–451] ABPA is characterized by asthma, eosinophilia, and bronchopulmonary lesions with bronchiectasis secondary to a complex type of allergic and immune response to the presence of *Aspergillus* in the airways. ABPA is also distinct from fungal asthma.[452] ABPA occurs mainly in adults, but it has been reported in childhood.[453] It is also a well-recognized complication in up to about 10% of patients with cystic fibrosis[454,455]; in a large American database, the prevalence of ABPA was 2% in 14,210 eligible patients, suggesting that ABPA is underdiagnosed in the cystic fibrosis population.[456] The prevalence of ABPA in cystic fibrosis patients may differ largely according to the diagnostic criteria used to diagnose it. ABPA may be associated with allergic *Aspergillus* sinusitis,[457,458] a condition that has been considered as the nasal correlate of ABPA, a proposition that is still debated.[459–464] ABPA may have an occupational dimension as suggested by a study of workers in the bagasse-containing sites in sugar cane mills.[465] *Aspergillus fumigatus* was the preponderant organism found at aeromycologic study, and was frequently isolated from the sputum cultures of the mill workers. During a survey of 238 workers having chronic respiratory problems, a diagnosis of ABPA was made on positive clinical and laboratory findings in 7% of them.

ABPA is considered to be the result of an immunologic inflammatory reaction in the bronchi and the surrounding parenchyma in response to antigens from *Aspergillus* growing in mucus plugs in the airways of asthmatics. The immunologic response of the host includes a type I hypersensitivity (anaphylactic type) mediated by IgE antibodies, and type III hypersensitivity (immune complex-mediated) with the participation of IgG and IgA antibodies. The associated inflammatory reaction results in damage to the bronchial epithelium, submucosa, and adjacent pulmonary parenchyma.[452,466]

The criteria for the diagnosis of ABPA have been different in the United Kingdom and the United States. The British criteria for diagnosis were the presence of asthma, pulmonary eosinophilia (fleeting shadow on the chest radiograph in association with a peripheral blood or airway eosinophilia), and a positive immediate skin prick test to *A. fumigatus.*[454,467] The American primary criteria include asthma, a history of pulmonary infiltrates, proximal bronchiectasis, elevated serum IgE, and an immunologic hypersensitivity to *A. fumigatus,* such as an immediate reaction to prick test for *Aspergillus* antigen, precipitating antibodies against *A. fumigatus,* or elevated specific IgE against *A. fumigatus.*[468,469] Other common findings in patients with ABPA include the expectoration of plugs, the presence of *Aspergillus* in sputum, and late skin reactivity to *Aspergillus* antigen.[468] Five stages of disease have been individualized: acute, remission, recurrent exacerbations, corticosteroid-dependent asthma, and fibrotic end stage.[470,471] Allergic bronchopulmonary fungal (and especially ABPA) disease has been reported occasionally in patients without clinical asthma.[472,473]

It is clear that damage by exaggerated inflammation to the large bronchi is the major feature of the disease, with mucus plugs containing *Aspergillus* obstructing the airways with subsequent atelectasis and bronchial wall damage resulting in central bronchiectasis predominating in the upper lobes, which are well visualized on the CT scan.[320,454,474–484] In asthmatic patients, bronchiectasis affecting three or more lobes, centrilobular nodules, and mucoid impaction on the CT scan are highly suggestive of ABPA[485]; the correct diagnosis of ABPA

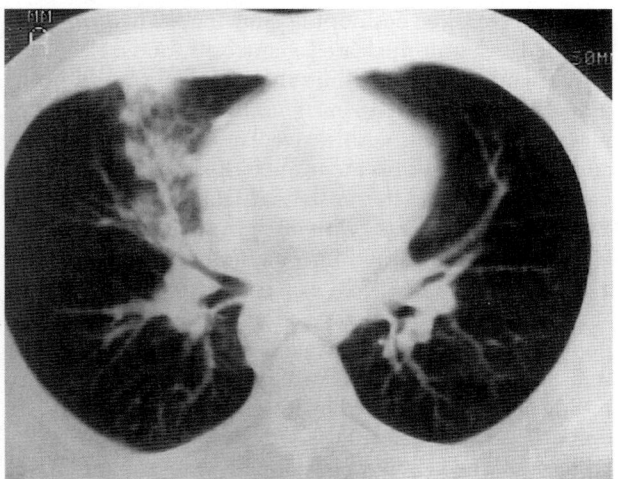

Figure 24–12 CT scan of a middle lobe pulmonary infiltrate in a 28-year-old man. The blood eosinophil count was 1.44 × 10⁹/L, and the alveolar differential eosinophil count was 37%. *Mycobacterium chelonae* was cultured from bronchoalveolar lavage fluid and was considered to be the cause of the pulmonary eosinophilia.

was made on the CT scan in 84% of cases of ABPA in a series of patients with eosinophilic lung diseases.[67] It has been suggested that testing positive to the *A. fumigatus* skin prick could be a screening test for ABPA in asthma patients, as it was found to be positive in about 20% of patients of whom 25 to 40% had features of ABPA on the CT scan.[486]

Although eosinophilic pneumonia is not a major finding in patients with ABPA,[487] it may have been underestimated, especially at the early stage of disease (ie, before the development of overt bronchiectasis). Eosinophilic pneumonia may be found in resection specimens from patients with asthma and ABPA with pulmonary consolidation.[488] Pathologic analysis of pulmonary surgical specimens of ABPA obtained for a diagnosis of recurrent or persistent chest infiltrates found, in addition to bronchial and bronchiolar lesions, areas diagnosable as eosinophilic pneumonia in the distal lung parenchyma in 8 of 15 patients.[474] Eosinophils were always present within the inflammatory infiltrates of the bronchi and bronchioles and in the infiltrate surrounding bronchocentric granulomas with the focal filling of alveolar spaces by eosinophils.[474] In patients with mucoid impaction of the bronchi, which occurs mainly in asthmatics, eosinophils are present in the bronchial walls in more than 50% of cases, with bronchiectasis and chronic pneumonitis with alveoli filled with eosinophils in one-third of the cases.[489] The peribronchial inflammation in ABPA may be prominent in the peripheral parts of the bronchial tree, giving an appearance of "allergic bronchopneumonia."[479] The same bronchocentric pattern was found in a patient with ABPA complicating cystic fibrosis, together with the demonstration of septate hyphae in the granulomatous inflammation.[490] Eosinophilic pneumonia prominent on lung biopsy in one patient with ABPA[491] was characterized by necrotizing granulomatous bronchiolitis, parenchymal granulomas with clustered eosinophils showing necrosis and surrounded by multinucleated giant cells, and epithelioid cells resembling eosinophilic abscesses. The center of the granulomas contained *Aspergillus*. Organizing pneumonia and eosinophils within alveolar spaces were present, and vasculitis was also mentioned. Eosinophil infiltrates have been reported in transbronchial biopsy in ABPA.[492] Bronchiolitis obliterans with organizing pneumonia overlapping chronic eosinophilic pneumonia, consistent with a clinical diagnosis of ABPA, has been reported.[493]

The variety of lung reactions to *Aspergillus* is still poorly understood, as demonstrated by a report of two immunocompetent brothers who were both exposed to moldy hay and developed hypersensitivity lung disease in one, and invasive aspergillosis with bronchoalveolar lavage eosinophilia and *Aspergillus* suppurative-type granulomata with prominent tissue eosinophilia in the other.[494] Another case of acute eosinophilic pneumonia was reported in an 11-year-old boy who had played in a compost pile.[495] He developed diffuse pulmonary infiltrates with 27% eosinophils in the BAL fluid. After a transient improvement with corticosteroids, he deteriorated again and lung biopsy demonstrated numerous palisading granulomas with necrotic centers containing eosinophils, neutrophils, and *Aspergillus* hyphae. The patient died soon thereafter, and, at autopsy, nearly confluent granulomas containing fungal hyphae and parenchymal destruction with vascular invasion were found. The reason(s) why some patients respond to *Aspergillus* with an allergic and immune reaction whereas others develop severe aspergillosis is unclear. The use of corticosteroids in patients with *Aspergillus* reactions to the lung must therefore remain cautious in acute situations, in order to avoid the progression of infectious fungal disease when it occurs.

In ABPA, the acute stage of disease is characterized on imaging by either fleeting infiltrates due to eosinophilic pneumonia, or mucus plugging with segmental, lobar, or even whole lung atelectasis. Fever is present. Blood eosinophilia is generally over $1 \times 10^9/L$. Sputum and expectorated plugs of laminated exudate contain eosinophils and Charcot-Leyden crystals.[454,468,475,478,481,496–502] Mucoid impaction is typically characterized by atelectasis and a V-shaped lesion with the vertex pointing toward the hilum.[468,489,502–504] In later stages of ABPA, imaging findings are mainly those of bronchiectasis (Figure 24–13), and lung opacities susceptible of corresponding to eosinophilic pneumonia (Figure 24–14) are less common than in the early stage.

Treatment of ABPA mainly relies on corticosteroids during attacks, with long-term corticosteroids only in patients with frequent symptomatic attacks and in patients with evidence of progressive lung damage.[454,505] Management of episodes of pulmonary consolidation may prevent the progression of ABPA to the fibrotic end stage.[506] Inhaled corticosteroids may limit the need for oral corticosteroids.[507,508] Oral itraconazole has been considered as a possible useful adjunct to corticosteroids, especially allowing reduction of the doses of corticosteroids.[509–512] The remission of relapses of ABPA with itraconazole without corticosteroids has been reported.[513] A double-blind, randomized, placebo-controlled study indicated that patients with corticosteroid-dependent ABPA generally benefit from concurrent itraconazole treatment; improvements included the immunologic and physiologic criteria and the corticosteroid dose, but there was no significant effect on pulmonary infiltrates.[514]

Other Allergic Bronchopulmonary Syndromes Associated with Fungi or Yeasts

Yeasts and fungi other than *Aspergillus* have also been reported to produce a similar pattern of allergic bronchopulmonary disease.[515] These include *Pseudallescheria boydii*,[516] *Cladosporium herbarum*,[517] *Candida albicans*,[518–521] *Stemphylium* species,[522] *Torulopsis* species,[470] *Curvularia lunata*,[523] *Bipolaris* species,[472,523–525] *Rhizopus* species,[526] *Trichosporon terrestre*,[527] *Fusarium vasinfectum*,[528,529] and *Helminthosporium* species.[530–532] Mixed allergic bronchopulmonary fungal disease may associate with different species of fungi.[533] In some yeast or fungal allergic bronchopulmonary diseases, signs suggestive of eosinophilic pneumonia were present.[472,516,517,527]

A case of eosinophilic pneumonia attributed to *Candida albicans* has been reported.[534]

Bronchocentric Granulomatosis

Bronchocentric granulomatosis, first described by Liebow,[535] is an inflammatory process beginning within the bronchiole walls, and in which, although the destruction may extend into the surrounding parenchyma, the peribronchiolar distribution of the lesions remains constant.[44] At the early stage, the bronchiolar mucosa is replaced by epithelioid histiocytes often palisading around the lumen. Then a granulomatous inflammatory process destroys both the mucosa and walls of the bronchiole. The necrotic zones resulting from the destroyed bronchioles are often surrounded by palisading histiocytes.[44,536] In patients (generally asthmatics) with eosinophils comprising the major component of the cellular infiltrate, Giemsa stain shows clumps of conglutinated cellular debris consisting of granules and fragmented eosinophils. Transfer of granules from eosinophils to the cytoplasm of large mononuclear cells may be observed. Scattered fungal hyphae may be demonstrated by the Grocott silver stain in some patients. A dense inflammatory infiltrate is, in most cases, present in the immediate peribronchial tissue but may occasionally extend into distal parenchyma. In asthmatic patients with bronchocentric granulomatosis, eosinophils comprise the major proportion of the infiltrate and may give rise to the characteristic lesions of eosinophilic pneumonia. Other possible changes include vascular inflammation and mucoid impaction.[44,537]

About half the patients with bronchocentric granulomatosis on lung pathologic examination are asthmat-

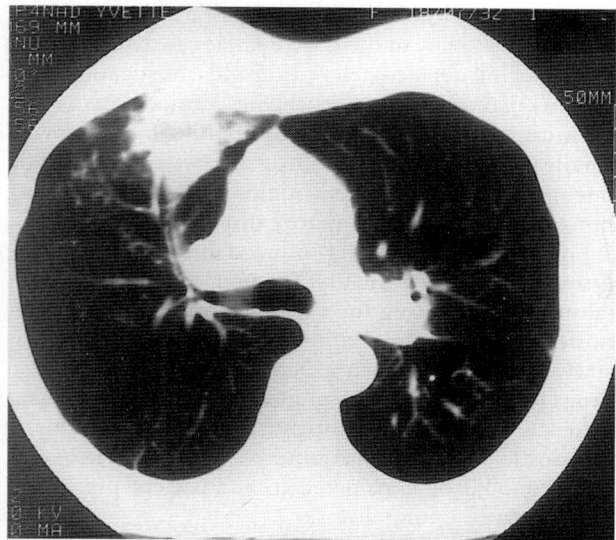

Figure 24–14   CT scan of pulmonary consolidation in a patient with allergic bronchopulmonary aspergillosis.

ics who present with fever and cough in addition to symptoms of asthma. A peripheral blood eosinophilia is common, generally exceeding 1×10^9 eosinophils/L.[44,537] The radiographic features consist of mass lesions, alveolar infiltrates or pneumonic consolidation, or reticulonodular opacities, which predominate in the upper lobes and are unilateral in a majority of patients.[538,539] Bilateral multiple cavitating nodules have been reported.[536] Most of these patients fulfill the criteria for ABPA, and corticosteroids are the treatment of choice, with an excellent prognosis although recurrences are common.[44]

Bronchocentric granulomatosis may also occur in nonasthmatic patients.[44,537,540–542] Eosinophilia is usually not conspicuous. Clinical manifestations are heterogeneous, and an infectious cause may be found in some cases.[543]

The pathogenesis of bronchocentric granulomatosis in asthmatic patients may be considered as the tissue manifestation of ABPA, where bronchocentric granulomatosis may be a major finding.[44] The pathologic diagnosis of bronchocentric granulomatosis must be very strict, because serious pittfalls are possible (granulomatous vasculitis, infections).[44]

Drug-Induced Eosinophilic Pneumonias

A continuously increasing number of drugs are reported to have adverse effects on the lung. Several distinct syndromes of pulmonary iatrogenic reactions have been identified, with interstitial lung disease being one of the most common.[544] Iatrogenic eosinophilic pulmonary infiltrates were reported as early as the 1940s, when the first antibiotics became available. Up to now, over 80 drugs have been incriminated as a cause of eosinophilic

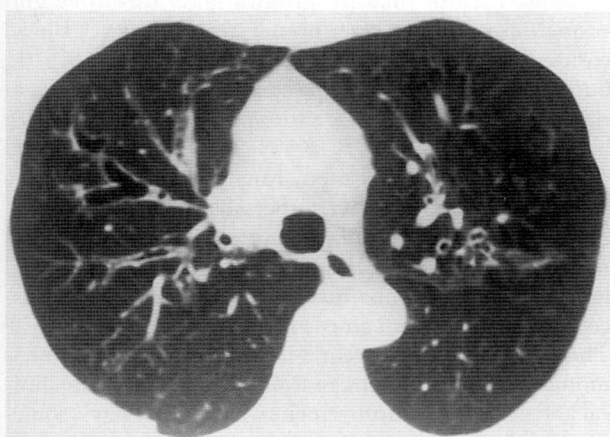

Figure 24–13   CT scan of bronchiectasis in a patient with allergic bronchopulmonary aspergillosis.

pulmonary infiltrates[138,139,244,545–653] (Table 24–2). However, because many of them were single case reports sometimes lacking detailed description and investigations, the number of drugs that can reliably be considered as a common cause of drug-induced eosinophilic pneumonia is smaller, about 20 to 30. Drug-induced eosinophilic pneumonias are mainly encountered in patients taking nonsteroidal anti-inflammatory drugs or antibiotics.

The diagnosis of drug-induced interstitial lung diseases is of varying difficulty. When it occurs in a patient taking only one drug for a benign condition, the diagnosis is often easy by eliminating the drug. On the contrary, when it occurs in a patient treated with several drugs for a systemic disease, itself capable of being associated with pulmonary interstitial involvement, many diagnostic pitfalls are encountered. However, iatrogenic causes should be considered in any patient presenting with interstitial lung disease.

The diagnosis of drug-induced interstitial lung disease may be discovered in three main clinical settings.[654] Many patients, after being on a drug for several months or years for a chronic condition, develop progressively increasing dyspnea with cough and mild fever. In other patients, the interstitial lung disease is discovered by systematic chest radiograph although no or minor pulmonary symptoms are present. Acute and severe interstitial lung disease, sometimes requiring mechanical ventilation, is the third clinical setting of interstitial drug-induced lung disease. In all of these settings, associated extrapulmonary iatrogenic manifestations may be present and especially cutaneous rashes.

Relating an interstitial lung disease to drug intake may be puzzling for many reasons. As mentioned above, the differential diagnosis includes the many causes of interstitial lung disease, such as pulmonary involvement in the connective tissue disorders, neoplasias, or infectious processes (for example, *P. carinii* in patients receiving immunosuppressors for systemic immune disorders). All the drugs taken in the weeks preceding the clinical syndrome must be carefully recorded, including illicit drugs (cocaine, heroin) (Figure 24–15) the intake of which may be denied by the patient. A further difficulty is the fact that a same drug may give rise to different pulmonary syndromes.

Transient interstitial infiltrates with eosinophilia, chronic eosinophilic pneumonia, and acute eosinophilic pneumonia have all been reported as drug-induced lung disease. Interestingly, even systemic eosinophilic vasculitis involving the lung (and thus closely resembling the Churg-Strauss syndrome) has been reported.[243,247]

The best clue to the diagnosis of drug-induced eosinophilic pneumonia is its regression after stopping the drug. However, this may take some time for drugs that are taken on a long-term basis. Therefore, in many reports, corticosteroids have been given concomitantly with drug withdrawal, and thus the responsibility of the drug cannot be reliably demonstrated. There is currently no confident biologic test to relate eosinophilic pneu-

monia to drugs. The only absolute proof of the drug responsibility is provided by its reintroduction resulting in a relapse of the pneumonia. This may be involuntary and accidental, especially when the initial eosinophilic pneumonia has not been properly attributed to the intake of a drug, the latter being reintroduced by either the physician or the patient. Otherwise, reintroducing a drug that has given rise to a serious pulmonary reaction may be dangerous and unethical if done only for scientific purposes. Careful reintroduction of the drug may be indicated only in patients requiring this specific drug when no alternative treatment is available.

The presentation of patients with eosinophilic drug-induced pneumonia has generally no specificity. When only isolated case reports have been published for a drug, it is not possible to determine the possible characteristic findings specific to this drug. However, greater numbers of well-studied cases may give a more comprehensive view of a peculiar drug-induced pulmonary eosinophilia. Furthermore, it is instructive since the cause of disease is known and the chronology of events after exposure to the drug may be determined exactly. This is the case for minocycline-induced eosinophilic pneumonia.[556,558,560–567] This semisynthetic tetracycline derivative is used mainly for the treatment of acne vulgaris or the treatment of urinary tract and respiratory infections. The duration of treatment before the onset of pulmonary symptoms varies from a few days to 6 weeks. Some patients had pulmonary symptoms during previous treatments with the drug, but the relationship of these symptoms to minocycline had been overlooked.[558–560] Atopy was present in some patients.[558,563] The onset of symptoms is subacute or acute, with dyspnea, cough, chest pain, fever, chills, and weight loss. The other symptoms include mainly fatigue, myalgias, and skin rashes.[558] Fine crackles and/or wheezes are present on lung auscultation. On chest imaging, most patients present with diffuse interstitial and/or ground-glass opacities, sometimes with Kerley's B lines,[557,563,564,566] although apical subpleural opacities more evocative of eosinophilic pneumonia may be present.[558,560] CT scan findings include mainly ground-glass opacities and bronchial wall and interlobular thickening.[563] Blood eosinophilia is usually increased between 1 and 2×10^9/L, but it may be absent[563] or peak 1 to 3 weeks after cessation of treatment.[558] BAL eosinophilia is constant, with mean percentages of 21[563] to 30% on the differential cell count.[558] When performed, lung function tests have shown a ventilatory defect, either obstructive, restrictive, or mixed.[558,563] Hypoxemia is constant, with some patients necessitating mechanical ventilation.[567] Transbronchial lung biopsy shows inflammatory interstitial and perivascular infiltration with an eosinophil predominance.[558,563] The outcome of minocycline-induced eosinophilic pneumonia is favorable after cessation of the drug, with clinical and radiologic improvement within a few days, sometimes with the addition of corticosteroids, especially in the most severely affected patients.[556,558,560,563,564,566] No clinical or imaging sequelae have been reported. A reduced

Table 24–2   Drugs that May Cause Eosinophilic Pneumonia

Drugs with typical pulmonary eosinophilia
  Acetylsalicylic[545,546]
  Captopril[547]
  Diclofenac[548]
  Ethambutol[549]
  Fenbufen[550]
  Granulocyte-macrophage colony–stimulating factor[551,552]
  Ibuprofen[553]
  L-Tryptophan[554,555]
  Minocycline[556–568]
  Naproxen[569]
  Para (4)-aminosalicylic acid[570,571]
  Penicillins[572,573]
  Phenylbutazone[574]
  Piroxicam[575]
  Pyrimethamine[652]
  Sulindac[577,578]
  Sulphamides-sulfonamides[579–582]
  Tolfenamic acid[583]
  Trimethoprim-sulfamethoxazole[584]
Drugs with occasional pulmonary eosinophilia
  Bleomycin[585]
  Carbamazepine[586]
  Chlorpromazine[587]
  Cocaine[588–591]
  Desipramine[545]
  Dapsone[592,643]
  Febarbamate[593]
  Gold salts[594,595]
  Heroin[596]
  Imipramine[597]
  Isoniazid[598]
  Loxoprofen[599,600]
  Mephenesin[601]
  Methotrexate[602]
  Methylphedinate[603]
  Nitrofurantoin[604]
  Nomifensine[605]
  Pentamidine[606]
  Perindopril[607]
  Phenytoin[608–610]
  Propranolol[594]

  Sulfasalazine[570,611–614]
  Trimipramine[615]
Drugs with exceptional eosinophilia
  Amiodarone[616]
  Aminoglutethimide[645]
  Ampicillin[617]
  Beclomethasone[618]
  Bicalutamide[644]
  Bucillamine[619]
  Cephalosporins[620]
  Chloroquine[653]
  Chlorpropamide[621]
  Clofibrate[622]
  Cromoglycate[623]
  Diflunisal[244]
  Erythromycin[624]
  Furazolidone[625]
  Glafenine[626]
  Indomethacin[646]
  Iodinated contrast medium[627]
  Levofloxacin[649]
  Maloprim[576]
  Maprotiline[647]
  Mesalazine (5-aminosalicylic acid)[650,651]
  Metronidazole[628]
  Nalidixic acid[629]
  Nilutamide[594,630]
  Paracetamol[631]
  Penicillamine[594,632–634]
  Procarbazine[635]
  Propylthiouracil[636]
  Ranitidine[138]
  Scotchguard[637]
  Streptomycin[545]
  Tenidap[638]
  Tetracycline[640]
  Tolazamide[639]
  Tosufloxacin tosilate[648]
  Trazodone[641]
  Troleandomycin[642]
  Venlafaxine[139]

transfer factor 2 months after discontinuation of the drug has been reported in one patient.[560]

Most reported cases of other drug-induced eosinophilic pneumonias fit well with the above description of minocycline eosinophilic pneumonia, with some slight differences or particularities. Acute respiratory failure has been reported with phenytoin,[655] as well as pulmonary vasculitis.[247] A clinical presentation with a predominance of asthma, with only an apical shadow, has been reported with carbamazepine,[656] whereas the same drug gave rise to a typical interstitial lung disease with crackles and hypoxemia together with erythroderma in another patient.[657] A patient developed eosinophilic pneumonia during *Mycoplasma pneumoniae* infection while on carbamazepine, raising the possibility that infection might enhance the development of the drug reaction.[586] Bulky intrathoracic lymphadenopathy and eosinophilic pneumonia attributed to indomethacin has been reported.[646]

Local extrapulmonary use of drugs may result in pulmonary infiltrates with eosinophilia as occurred in patients using a vaginal cream containing sulfanilamide, aminacrine, and allantoin with lactose in a water miscible base.[579,582]

In 1989, an outbreak of eosinophilia with myalgia and systemic symptoms (including respiratory manifestations in most patients) occured in the United States. The condition was subsequently denominated the eosinophilia-myalgia syndrome, and was subsequently proved to be related to the intake of contaminated preparations of L-tryptophan originating from a single manufacturer.[658–665] Evidence of eosinophil degranulation with markedly increased levels of serum and urine MBP and EDN suggest that eosinophil activation and degranulation play a role in the pathogenesis of this syndrome, together with fibroblasts.[662,663,666] In a large series of 205 patients, respiratory symptoms were present in 67%, with findings of interstitial lung

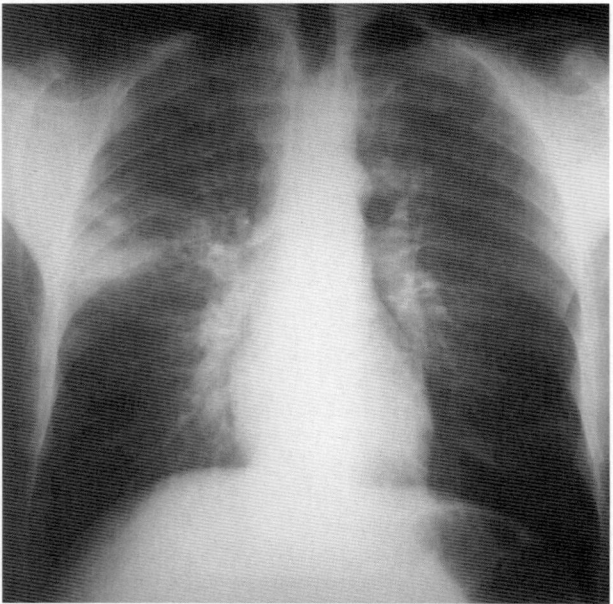

A

B

Figure 24–15   *A*, Chest radiograph of heroin-induced chronic eosinophilic pneumonia in a 36-year-old man who presented with patchy alveolar opacities predominating in the right upper lobe. The blood eosinophil count was 1.2×10^9/L. *B*, Many eosinophils and many Charcot-Leyden crystals (Papanicolau stain; ×1000 original magnification) were found in bronchial aspirates. The alveolar infiltrates cleared while the patient stopped inhaling heroin but relapsed as the patient started again to inhale the drug (BAL fluid at relapse found 30% eosinophils in the differential cell count).

disease or infiltrate in 13%, and pulmonary hypertension in 4%.[667] The mean eosinophil count in this series was 4.7×10^9/L, and the other symptoms observed in at least 60% of patients were myalgia (94%), fatigue (79%), rash (77%), paresthesia (62%), swelling (61%), and muscle weakness (60%). There are relatively few detailed studies of pulmonary manifestations in patients with the eosinophilia-myalgia syndrome.[554,668–672] Dyspnea and a nonproductive cough are the most common symptoms of pulmonary involvement, with rales on pulmonary auscultation. Diffuse interstitial infiltrates

are present on the chest radiograph. When performed, pulmonary function tests have shown a mild or moderate restriction.[668] Interestingly, whereas patients have a markedly increased blood eosinophilia, the findings in lung biopsy specimens are in contrast not typically those of eosinophilic pneumonia. The most conspicuous lesions are a small- to medium-vessel vasculitis with a mixed inflammatory cell infiltrate (primarily lymphocytes and eosinophils) involving both arteries and veins and a chronic interstitial pneumonia consisting of lymphocytes and eosinophils.[668,671] However, tissue eosinophilia is not a constantly prominent finding.[668] The evolution of respiratory symptoms is favorable in 74% of patients.[667] Improvement has been reported in 79% of patients with eosinophilia-myalgia syndrome receiving corticosteroids.[667]

The toxic oil syndrome, which manifested as an epidemic disease in Spain in 1981, was attributed to the ingestion of denatured cooking oil.[673] This sclerodermalike disorder affected about 20,000 persons. It was characterized by an interstitial-alveolar pattern on the chest radiograph and eosinophilia during the first 4 months. Pulmonary hypertension, scleroderma, hepatic disease, sicca syndrome, polyneuropathy, joint contractures, and chronic pulmonary sequelae characterized the chronic stage of the disease.[673–676] In the acute phase, death was mainly due to respiratory failure. The pathology of the pulmonary lesions was marked by vasculitis and vascular fibrosis, edema, interstitial infiltrates of mononuclear cells, and eosinophils in variable proportions. However, the pathologic findings consisted more of vascular disease with increased capillary permeability than of eosinophilic pneumonia.[676,677]

OTHER PULMONARY DISORDERS WITH EOSINOPHILIA

Eosinophilia in the peripheral blood and/or in BAL fluid may be encountered in several pulmonary disorders where eosinophilic pneumonia is not a major and usual feature. Nevertheless, these will be mentioned briefly mainly because they may occasionally present problems for the differential diagnosis.

Bronchiolitis Obliterans Organizing Pneumonia

BOOP is a pathologic syndrome defined by the presence of buds composed of inflammatory cells, fibroblasts, and connective tissue in variable proportions within the lumen of distal air spaces. It may be secondary to various causes (such as an infection or drug induced reactions) or idiopathic (and then the denomination of cryptogenic organizing pneumonia is preferred). The clinical and imaging features of BOOP are rather characteristic, especially in the most typical presentation of patchy alveolar infiltrates, which may closely mimic CEP.[678,679] There is some possible patho-logic overlap of BOOP and CEP, with foci of orga-nizing pneumonia in CEP and eosinophils in BOOP.[34,35,585,680,681] It has been suggested that, in some cases, BOOP may represent the evolution of an untreated CEP[678,680]; as mentioned above, foci of orga-nizing pneumonia may be present in idiopathic chronic eosinophilic pneumonia. Eosinophilia in BAL fluid may be present in BOOP but is usually less than 20% in the differential cell count.[679,682–684]

Asthma and Other Airways Eosinophilia

Infiltration of the airways by eosinophils is common in the eosinophilic pneumonias, but it may occur as an iso-lated phenomenon. The eosinophil has emerged as a key cell in the pathogenesis of asthma.[685] Eosinophilic inflam-mation of the airways is present in the submucosa and epithelium of patients with asthma,[686] and it is correlated with severity.[687] Furthermore, BAL fluid has shown mildly increased levels of eosinophils on the differential cell count in asthmatic patients (generally less than 5%, but occasionally higher).[688–693] Although alveolar sam-ples contain increased percentages of eosinophils, these are lower than those found in bronchial samples.[694] Bron-choprovocation with an allergen increases alveolar eosinophilia.[691,695] Severe bronchial eosinophilia was found at necropsy in 60% of patients dying during sta-tus asthmaticus.[696] Although asthma or symptoms of asthma are common in eosinophilic pneumonias, pul-monary opacities in patients with asthma and eosinophilia are in no way synonymous of eosinophilic pneumonia (for example these may result from simple mucus plugging or coincidental associated pulmonary disease). However, complex cases may be observed such as one of a patient with AIDS, asthma acute and chronic, mucus plugging, bronchiolitis obliterans, and chronic eosinophilic pneumonia.[697]

Eosinophilic bronchitis with a chronic cortico-steroid-responsive cough without asthma, but with a high percentage of eosinophils (about 40%) in the sputum, is a well-recognized cause of chronic cough.[698–702] The observed values of sputum eosinophils are much higher in eosinophilic bronchi-tis than in asthma.[702,703] The development of an irre-versible airflow obstruction in a patient with eosinophilic bronchitis without asthma has been reported.[704] Eosinophilic bronchitis induced by latex gloves has been reported in a nurse, which resulted in 80% eosinophils in the induced sputum. After corti-costeroid treatment and the disappearance of eosinophils in the induced sputum, a challenge test was done. This resulted in 90% eosinophils in the induced sputum 24 hours later.[705]

A case of eosinophilic bronchiolitis presenting with dyspnea has been reported[706]; airflow obstruction and blood and BAL eosinophilia were present; on the CT scan, poorly defined centrilobular nodules and thicken-ing of the bronchi and bronchioles were observed throughout the bilateral lung fields; on the lung biopsy, the alveolar interstitium was normal, but diffuse infil-trates of eosinophils, plasma cells, and lymphocytes with lymphoid follicles to the bronchiolar walls were present, with degenerated eosinophils and Charcot-Leyden crys-tals within the alveolar lumen.

Idiopathic Interstitial Pneumonias

Although eosinophils may be present in usual interstitial pneumonia, these are usually not numerous and eosinophilic pneumonia is not present.[44,707] Neverthe-less, mildly increased levels of eosinophils may be found in the BAL differential cell count.[31,32,708–716] Increases of BAL eosinophils relate to a poor clinical response to corticosteroids.[711,717,718] Focal eosinophilic pneumonia (without eosinophilia in the BAL fluid) has been reported in six cases of usual interstitial pneumonia, in the absence of any identified cause.[719]

Focal eosinophils are a minor feature of nonspecific interstitial pneumonia.[720]

Langerhans Cell Histiocytosis

Pulmonary Langerhans cell histiocytosis is a proliferative disease of Langerhans' cells, which has also been given the alternate names of pulmonary eosinophilic granu-loma and pulmonary histiocytosis X. The pulmonary pathologic lesions consist of nodules often assuming a stellate shape, which are composed of a mixture of Langerhans' cells and variable numbers of eosinophils, plasma cells, and lymphocytes. Eosinophils are usually present in the initial active stage, where they are the most characteristic histologic finding after the Langer-hans' cells (eosinophilic granuloma). They vary in num-ber, being numerous in about 25% of cases, and are usu-ally situated at the periphery of the lesions where they infiltrate the adjacent tissue. In more chronic disease, the eosinophils are scanty.[721–726] However, not only are eosinophils not necessary for the diagnosis, but they may even be absent.[44]

Malignancies

Malignant cells may produce cytokines that are active in the production of eosinophils, thus resulting in eosinophilia with possible eosinophilic pneumonia. Pulmonary opacities with blood eosinophilia may be lung cancers with associated widespread paraneoplas-tic eosinophilia due to the production of colony-stimulating factor.[727–729] Eosinophilic pneumonia was reported in a patient with gastric cancer producing GM-CSF and IL-5.[730]

Eosinophilic pneumonia may occur in patients with lymphomas.[299] It also may occur in patients with mycosis fungoides (cutaneous T-cell lymphoma) (Figure 24–16).[298] Clonal proliferation of type 2 helper T cells in a man with hypereosinophilic syndrome produced high levels of IL-4 and IL-5.[296] However, interstitial pulmonary opacities in a child with idiopathic hypereosinophilic syndrome terminating as disseminated T-cell lymphoma proved to be mononuclear cell inflammation without significant eosinophilia; whereas at the same time, the blood eosinophil cell count was 5.8×10^9/L. Eosinophilic pneumonia developed in a patient with Hodgkin's disease following autologous bone marrow transplantation.[731] A case of lymphomatoid papulosis associated with both severe hypereosinophilic syndrome (with pulmonary involvement) and large T-cell lymphoma 6 years later, has been reported.[732]

Pulmonary infiltration by leukemic cells may be observed in patients with eosinophilic leukemia.[301]

Miscellaneous Disorders

Sarcoidosis developed in a patient with eosinophilia and a previous history of asthma and eosinophilic pneumonia.[733] A case of overlapping idiopathic chronic eosinophilic pneumonia with features of sarcoidosis and Behçet syndrome has been reported.[734] Blood eosinophilia and tissue eosinophilia may be present in sarcoidosis, but it is usually mild.[735]

Eosinophilic pneumonia after professional exposure to sulfites has been reported.[736] Eosinophilia in the BAL fluid (62% in the differential cell count) was reported in a patient with professional heavy exposure to aluminium oxide.[737]

Pulmonary infiltrates with eosinophilia have rarely been reported in patients with inflammatory bowel disease who may or may not be taking drugs susceptible of causing eosinophilia.[570,738]

Chronic eosinophilic pneumonia developed in a 31-year-old patient with ataxia telangiectasia.[739]

Pulmonary infiltration with blood eosinophilia after a scorpion sting has been reported.[740] A case of acute eosinophilic pneumonia with hypersensitivity to "red spider" allergens with 61% eosinophils in the BAL fluid has been reported.[741]

CONCLUSION

There is currently no established clinical approach to the patient with suspected eosinophilic pneumonia because of the variety of causes and syndromes underlying eosinophilic pneumonia. However, some milestones on the way to diagnosis may be useful in clinical practice.

The first thing to remember is that eosinophilic pneumonia may manifest clinically by a pulmonary disease of varying severity, ranging from transient infiltrates with mild symptoms of Löffler's syndrome to acute severe eosinophilic pneumonia resembling acute respiratory distress syndrome. Although the peripheral alveolar infiltrates of CEP on imaging are quite evocative for the experienced clinician, much less typical pulmonary opacities may be encountered in eosinophilic pneumonias.

The second point is that blood eosinophilia may be reliably taken into account for diagnosis only for values of greater than 1×10^9 eosinophils/L, and preferably greater than 1.5×10^9/L. However, blood eosinophilia may be absent, especially in the early phase of IAEP. In

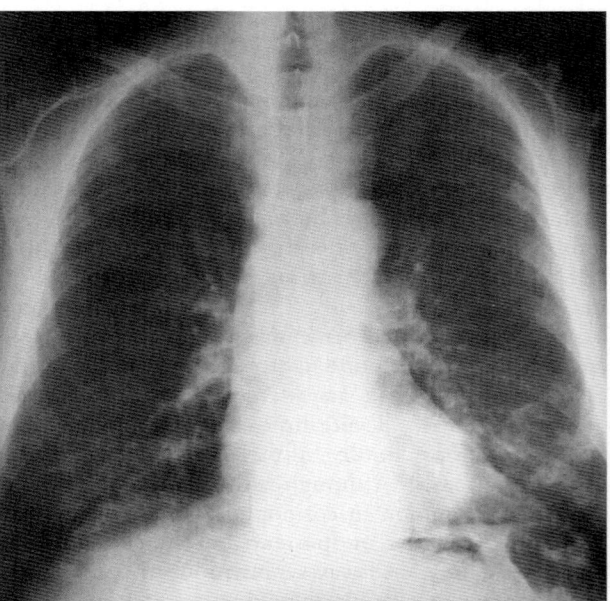

A

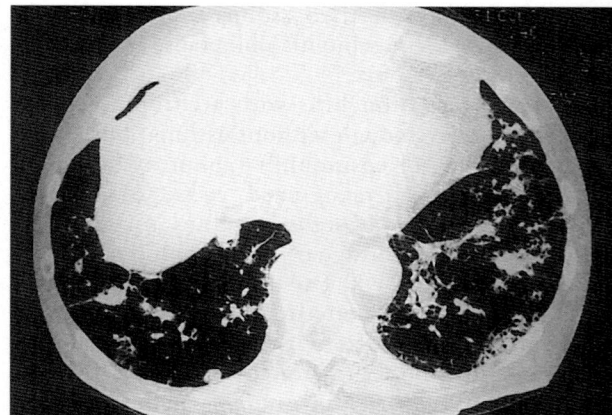

B

Figure 24–16   Chronic eosinophilic pneumonia in a 70-year-old man with cutaneous mycosis fungoides. *A*, Infiltrative opacities on chest radiograph predominating in lung lower fields. *B*, On high-resolution computed tomography, note the patchy peribronchovascular opacities, which, on pulmonary specimen obtained by video-assisted thoracoscopic biopsy, were composed of eosinophilic pneumonia only (without lymphoid infiltrates).

BAL fluid, mild eosinophilia (up to 10%) is of little diagnostic help and should not be considered as evidence of eosinophilic pneumonia. Moderate eosinophilia (10 to 25%) is compatible with eosinophilic pneumonia but not specific. High eosinophilia (greater than 25% and preferably over 40%) may be considered diagnostic of eosinophilic pneumonia in a compatible setting. A pulmonary biopsy may be avoided in almost all cases, but, if strictly necessary, it must be done without delay and before treatment to avoid major histopathologic changes due to corticosteroid treatment.

Once a diagnosis of eosinophilic pneumonia is made, the immediate question is that of its cause. Inquiry as to drug intake must be meticulous and any suspected drug withdrawn. Travel history or residence in areas at high risk of parasitic infestation must be recorded, even when several years earlier. Laboratory investigations for parasitic causes must be conducted with the help of specialists who know perfectly well the epidemiology of parasites throughout the world and the appropriate laboratory tests (stool examination is helpful in some parasitic infections, but it does not provide any clue to the diagnosis in other infections such as *Toxocara* larva migrans). The other known causes of eosinophilic pneumonia must also be systematically checked. If no cause is found, the eosinophilic pneumonia is considered idiopathic. It may be either solitary or part of a systemic syndrome. Extrathoracic manifestations must be carefully searched for because they may orient the diagnosis toward Churg-Strauss syndrome or idiopathic hypereosinophilic syndrome (and point to sites of possible biopsy for diagnosis in Churg-Strauss syndrome, for example).

Once the diagnosis of eosinophilic pneumonia has been made, and further classified into an etiologic category (determined origin or undetermined origin either solitary or part of a systemic disorder), treatment may be started. If a determined cause has been found, its treatment should provide improvement (eg, drug withdrawal in drug-induced disease, specific treatment for a parasitic infection). Corticosteroids remain the cornerstone of symptomatic treatment for eosinophilic disorders, and they may help in a large majority of patients with severe pulmonary impairment (provided that the treatment of the cause of eosinophilic pneumonia, when known, has been started). Corticosteroids are necessary in attacks of ABPA, idiopathic eosinophilic pneumonias, Churg-Strauss syndrome, and hypereosinophilic syndrome (with possible necessity for other drugs, especially immunosuppressants, in the latter two conditions). If corticosteroid treatment does not work, the diagnosis must be reconsidered seriously, especially because of the risk of an undiagnosed infection, which may be enhanced by corticosteroid treatment. If the response to corticosteroids is dramatic in the idiopathic chronic eosinophilic pneumonias and Churg-Strauss syndrome, relapses often occur when tapering the doses or stopping treatment.

The diagnosis and management of the eosinophilic pneumonias is usually devoid of major difficulties if the clinician makes a strict and simple synthesis of data obtained from the history and physical examination, imaging, and laboratory data.

REFERENCES

1. Anderson GP. Eosinophilia in genetically altered mice. Eur Respir Rev 1995;5:231–7.
2. Gleich GJ, Adolphson CR, Leiferman KM. The biology of the eosinophilic leukocyte. Annu Rev Med 1993;44:85–101.
3. Gleich GJ, Adolphson CR. The eosinophilic leukocyte: structure and function. Adv Immunol 1986;39:177–253.
4. Horie S, Gleich GJ, Kita H. Cytokines directly induce degranulation and superoxide production from human eosinophils. J Allergy Clin Immunol 1996;98:371–81.
5. Kroegel C, Virchow JC Jr, Luttmann W, et al. Pulmonary immune cells in health and disease: the eosinophil leucocyte (part I). Eur Respir J 1994;7:519–43.
6. Kroegel C, Warner JA, Virchow JC. Pulmonary immune cells in health and disease: the eosinophil leucocyte (Part 2). Eur Respir J 1994;7:743–60.
7. Popken-Harris P, Thomas L, Owvig C, et al. Biochemical properties, activities, and presence in biologic fluids of eosinophil granule major basic protein. J Allergy Clin Immunol 1994;94:1282–9.
8. Schatz M, Wasserman S, Patterson R. The eosinophil and the lung. Arch Intern Med 1982;142:1515–9.
9. Schleimer RP, Bochner BS. The effects of glucocorticoids on human eosinophils. J Allergy Clin Immunol 1994;94:1202–13.
10. Walker C, Braun RK, Boer C, et al. Cytokine control of eosinophils in pulmonary diseases. J Allergy Clin Immunol 1994;94:1262–71.
11. Weller PF. The immunobiology of eosinophils. N Engl J Med 1991;324:1110–8.
12. Resnik MB, Weller PF. Mechanisms of eosinophil recruitment. Am J Respir Cell Mol Biol 1993;8:349–55.
13. Allen JN, Davis WB. Eosinophils. In: Crystal RG, West JB, Weibel ER, Barnes PJ, editors. The lung: scientific foundations. 2nd ed. Philadelphia: Lippincott-Raven; 1997. p. 905–15.
14. Ehrlich P. Beiträge zur Kenntniss der granulirten Bindegewebszellen und der eosinophilen Leukocythen. Arch Anat Physiol 1879;3:166–82.
15. Tai PC, Spry CJF. The mechanisms which produce vacuolated and degranulated eosinophils. Br J Haematol 1981;49:219–26.
16. Torpier G, Colombel JF, Mathieu-Chandelier C, et al. Eosinophilic gastroenteritis: ultrastructural evidence for a selective release of eosinophil major basic protein. Clin Exp Immunol 1988;74:404–8.
17. Fauci AS, Harley JB, Roberts WC, et al. The idiopathic hypereosinophilic syndrome: clinical, pathophysiologic and therapeutic considerations. Ann Intern Med 1982;97:78–92.
18. Coltharp WH, Arnold JH, Alford WC, et al. Videothoracoscopy: improved technique and expanded indications. Ann Thorac Surg 1992;53:776–9.
19. Krasna MJ, White CS, Aisner SC, et al. The role of thoracoscopy in the diagnosis of interstitial lung disease. Ann Thorac Surg 1995;59:348–51.
20. Allen MS, Deschamps C, Jones DM, et al. Video-assisted thoracic surgical procedures: the Mayo experience. Mayo Clin Proc 1996;71:351–9.
21. Kadokura M, Colby TV, Myers JL, et al. Pathologic comparison of video-assisted thoracic surgical lung biopsy with traditional open lung biopsy. J Thorac Cardiovasc Surg 1995;109:494–8.
22. Umeki S. Reevaluation of eosinophilic pneumonia and its diagnostic criteria. Arch Intern Med 1992;152:1913–9.

23. Reeder WH, Goodrich BE. Pulmonary infiltration with eosinophilia (PIE syndrome). Ann Intern Med 1952;36:1217–40.

24. Crofton JW, Livingstone JL, Oswald NC, et al. Pulmonary eosinophilia. Thorax 1952;7:1–35.

25. Loeffler W. Infiltrations pulmonaires fugaces avec éosinophilie du sang (syndrome de Loeffler). Presse Med 1945;53:516–7.

26. Löffler W. Die flüchtigen Lungeninfiltrate mit Eosinophilie. Schweiz Med Wochenschr 1936;66:1069–78.

27. Löffler W. Zur differential-Diagnose der Lungeninfiltrierungen. Il Über flüchtige succedan-Infiltrate (mit Eosinophilie). Beitr Klinik Tuberk 1932;79:368–82.

28. Brigden ML, Horak MG. Incidence and clinical significance of unsuspected eosinophilia discovered by automated WBC differential counting. Lab Med 1993;24:173–6.

29. The BAL Cooperative Group Steering Committee. Bronchoalveolar lavage constituents in healthy individuals, idiopathic pulmonary fibrosis, and selected comparison groups. Am Rev Respir Dis 1990;141:S169–202.

30. Rennard SI, Ghafouri MO, Thompson AB, et al. Fractional processing of sequential bronchoalveolar lavage to separate bronchial and alveolar samples. Am Rev Respir Dis 1990;141:208–17.

31. Velay B, Pages J, Cordier JF, et al. Hyperéosinophilie du lavage broncho-alvéolaire. Valeur diagnostique et corrélations avec l'éosinophilie sanguine. Rev Mal Respir 1987;4:257–60.

32. Allen JN, Davis WB, Pacht ER. Diagnostic significance of increased bronchoalveolar lavage fluid eosinophils. Am Rev Respir Dis 1990;142:642–7.

33. McCarthy DS, Pepys J. Cryptogenic pulmonary eosinophilias. Clin Allergy 1973;3:339–51.

34. Carrington C, Addington W, Goff A, et al. Chronic eosinophilic pneumonia. N Engl J Med 1969;280:787–98.

35. Christoforidis AJ, Molnar W. Eosinophilic pneumonia: report of two cases with pulmonary biopsy. JAMA 1960;173:157–61.

36. Fox B, Seed W. Chronic eosinophilic pneumonia. Thorax 1980;35:570–80.

37. Liebow AA, Carrington CB. The eosinophilic pneumonias. Medicine 1969;48:251–85.

38. Jederlinic PJ, Sicilian L, Gaensler EA. Chronic eosinophilic pneumonia. A report of 19 cases and a review of the literature. Medicine 1988;67:154–62.

39. Case Records of the Massachusetts General Hospital. Case 29-1977. N Engl J Med 1977;297:155–61.

40. Bayley EC, Lindberg DON, Baggenstoss AH. Loeffler's syndrome. Report of a case with pathologic examination of the lungs. Arch Pathol 1945;40:376–81.

41. Griffiths MH, Hasleton PS. Eosinophilic pneumonia. In: Hasleton PS, editor. Spencer's pathology of the lung. New-York: McGraw-Hill; 1996. p. 449–59.

42. Dail DH. Eosinophilic infiltrates. In: Dail DH, Hammar SP, editors. Pulmonary pathology. New-York: Springer-Verlag; 1994. p. 537–66.

43. Flint AF, Colby TV. The pulmonary eosinophilias, hypersensitivity pneumonitis, and drug-induced lung diseases. In: Flint A, Colby TV, editors. Surgical pathology of diffuse infiltrative lung disease. Orlando, (FL): Grune & Stratton, Inc; 1987. p. 63–90.

44. Katzenstein AL, Askin FB. Katzenstein and Askin's surgical pathology of non-neoplastic lung disease. Philadelphia: W.B. Saunders; 1997.

45. Olopade CO, Crotty TB, Douglas WW, et al. Chronic eosinophilic pneumonia and idiopathic bronchiolitis obliterans organizing pneumonia: comparison of eosinophil number and degranulation by immunofluorescence staining for eosinophil-derived major basic protein. Mayo Clin Proc 1995;70:137–42.

46. Grantham J, Meadows J, Gleich G. Chronic eosinophilic pneumonia. Evidence for eosinophil degranulation and release of major basic protein. Am J Med 1986;80:89–94.

47. Case Records of the Massachusetts General Hospital. Case 1-1993. N Engl J Med 1993;328:48–55.

48. Badesch DB, King TE Jr, Schwarz MI. Acute eosinophilic pneumonia: a hypersensitivity phenomenon? Am Rev Respir Dis 1989;139:249–52.

49. Buchheit J, Eid N, Rodgers G, et al. Acute eosinophilic pneumonia with respiratory failure: a new syndrome? Am Rev Respir Dis 1992;145:716–8.

50. Lombard CM. Eosinophilic pneumonia. In: Saldana MJ, editor. Pathology of pulmonary disease. Philadelphia: J.B. Lippincott Company; 1994. p. 745–53.

51. Bancal C, Sadoun D, Valeyre D, et al. Pneumopathie chronique idiopathique à éosinophiles: maladie de Carrington. Presse Med 1989;18:1695–8.

52. Pearson DJ, Rosenow EC. Chronic eosinophilic pneumonia (Carrington's). A follow-up study. Mayo Clin Proc 1978;53:73–8.

53. Naughton M, Fahy J, FitzGerald MX. Chronic eosinophilic pneumonia. A long-term follow-up of 12 patients. Chest 1993;103:162–5.

54. Hayakawa H, Sato A, Toyoshima M, et al. A clinical study of idiopathic eosinophilic pneumonia. Chest 1994;105:1462–6.

55. Marchand E, Reynaud-Gaubert M, Lauque D, et al. Idiopathic chronic eosinophilic pneumonia. A clinical and follow-up study of 62 cases. Medicine (Baltimore) 1998;77:299–312.

56. Barnes N, Gray BJ, Heaton R, et al. Pulmonary eosinophilia in identical twins. Thorax 1983;38:318–9.

57. Marchand E, Etienne-Mastroianni B, Chanez P, et al. Asthma and chronic idiopathic eosinophilic pneumonia (CIEP). A study of 52 patients. Eur Respir J 2001;18:5S.

58. Rogers RM, Christiansen JR, Coalson JJ, et al. Eosinophilic pneumonia: physiologic response to steroid therapy and observations on light and electron microscopic findings. Chest 1975;68:665–71.

59. Franco J, Artes MJ. Pulmonary eosinophilia associated with montelukast. Thorax 1999;54:558–60.

60. Warren CP. Extrinsic allergic alveolitis: a disease commoner in non-smokers. Thorax 1977;32:567–9.

61. Libby DM, Murphy TF, Edwards A, et al. Chronic eosinophilic pneumonia: an unusual cause of acute respiratory failure. Am Rev Respir Dis 1980;122:497–500.

62. Samman YS, Wali SO, Abdelaal MA, et al. Chronic eosinophilic pneumonia presenting with recurrent massive bilateral pleural effusion. Chest 2001;119:968–70.

63. Mayo J, Müller N, Road J, et al. Chronic eosinophilic pneumonia. CT findings in six cases. AJR Am J Roentgenol 1989;153:727–30.

64. Ebara H, Ikezoe J, Johkoh T, et al. Chronic eosinophilic pneumonia: evolution of chest radiograms and CT features. J Comput Assist Tomogr 1994;18:737–44.

65. Gaensler EA, Carrington CB. Peripheral opacities in chronic eosinophilic pneumonia: the photographic negative of pulmonary edema. AJR Am J Roentgenol 1977;128:1–13.

66. Robertson CL, Shackelford GD, Armstrong JD. Chronic eosinophilic pneumonia. Radiology 1971;101:57–61.

67. Johkoh T, Muller NL, Akira M, et al. Eosinophilic lung diseases: diagnostic accuracy of thin-section CT in 111 patients. Radiology 2000;216:773–80.

68. Arakawa H, Kurihara Y, Niimi H, et al. Bronchiolitis obliterans with organizing pneumonia versus chronic eosinophilic pneumonia: high-resolution CT findings in 81 patients. AJR Am J Roentgenol 2001;176:1053–8.

69. Azar R, Brillet L, Poret E, et al. Pneumonie chronique à éosinophiles. Semin Hop Paris 1990;66:2491–4.

70. Dejaegher P, Dervaux L, Dubois P, et al. Eosinophilic pneumonia without radiographic pulmonary infiltrates. Chest 1983;84:637–8.

71. Morais J, Carrier L, Gariépy G, et al. Gallium-67 pulmonary uptake in eosinophilic pneumonia. Clin Nucl Med 1988;13:41–3.

72. Lieske TR, Sunderrajan EV, Passamonte PM. Bronchoalveolar lavage and technetium-99m glucoheptonate imaging in chronic eosinophilic pneumonia. Chest 1984;85:282–4.

73. Brezis M, Lafair J. Thrombocytosis in chronic eosinophilic pneumonia. Chest 1979;76:231–2.

74. Gonzalez EB, Hayes D, Weedn VW. Chronic eosinophilic pneumonia (Carrington's) with increased serum IgE levels. A distinct subset? Arch Intern Med 1988;148:2622–4.

75. McEvoy JDS, Donald KJ, Edward RL. Immunoglobulin levels and electron microscopy in eosinophilic pneumonia. Am J Med 1978;64:529–36.

76. Demedts M, De Man F. Circulating immune complexes in chronic eosinophilic pneumonia. Acta Clin Belg 1991;46:75–81.

77. Chan NH, Boyko WJ, Schellenberg RR, et al. A case of eosinophilic pneumonia. Unusual immune complex vasculitis in the skin. Chest 1982;82:113–5.

78. Cottin V, Deviller P, Tardy F, et al. Urinary eosinophil-derived neurotoxin/protein X: a simple method for assessing eosinophil degranulation in vivo. J Allergy Clin Immunol 1998;101:116–23.

79. Deviller P, Gruart V, Prin L, et al. Detection of an eosinophil derived neurotoxin in the urine of a patient with idiopathic chronic eosinophilic pneumonia. Clin Chim Acta 1991;201:105–12.

80. Olivieri D, Pesci A, Bertorelli G. Eosinophilic alveolitis in immunologic interstitial lung disorders. Lung 1990;168 Suppl:964–73.

81. Pesci A, Bertorelli G, Manganelli P, et al. Bronchoalveolar lavage in chronic eosinophilic pneumonia. Analysis of six cases in comparison with other interstitial lung diseases. Respiration 1988;54 Suppl 1:16–22.

82. Speich R, Hess T, Krestin GP, et al. The value of bronchoalveolar lavage for the diagnosis of eosinophilic pneumonias. Schweiz Med Wochenschr 1992;122:1005–10.

83. Greif J, Kivity S, Struhar D, et al. Bronchoalveolar lavage: a useful tool in the diagnosis of eosinophilic pneumonia. Isr J Med Sci 1986;22:479–80.

84. Albera C, Ghio P, Solidoro P, et al. Activated and memory alveolar T-lymphocytes in idiopathic eosinophilic pneumonia. Eur Respir J 1995;8:1281–5.

85. Dejaegher P, Demedts M. Bronchoalveolar lavage in eosinophilic pneumonia before and during corticosteroid therapy. Am Rev Respir Dis 1984;129:631–2.

86. Costabel U, Teschler H, Guzman J. Bronchiolitis obliterans organizing pneumonia (BOOP): the cytological and immunocytological profile of bronchoalveolar lavage. Eur Respir J 1992;5:791–7.

87. Takahashi H, Arakawa Y, Oki K, et al. Analysis of bronchoalveolar lavage cells in chronic eosinophilic pneumonia before and during corticosteroid therapy. Int Arch Allergy Immunol 1995;108 Suppl 1:2–5.

88. Janin A, Torpier G, Courtin P, et al. Segregation of eosinophil proteins in alveolar macrophage compartments in chronic eosinophilic pneumonia. Thorax 1993;48:57–62.

89. Boomars KA, van Velzen-Blad H, Mulder PG, et al. Eosinophil cationic protein and immunoglobulin levels in bronchoalveolar lavage fluid obtained from patients with chronic eosinophilic pneumonia. Eur Respir J 1996;9:2488–93.

90. Jorens PG, Van Overveld FJ, Van Meerbeeck JP, et al. Evidence for marked eosinophil degranulation in a case of eosinophilic pneumonia. Respir Med 1996;90:505–9.

91. Shijubo N, Shigehara K, Hirasawa M, et al. Eosinophilic cationic protein in chronic eosinophilic pneumonia and eosinophilic granuloma. Chest 1994;106:1481–6.

92. Ogushi F, Ozaki T, Kawano T. PGE2 and PGF2alpha content in bronchoalveolar lavage fluid obtained from patients with eosinophilic pneumonia. Chest 1987;91:204–6.

93. Beninati W, Derdak S, Dixon PF, et al. Pulmonary eosinophils express HLA-DR in chronic eosinophilic pneumonia. J Allergy Clin Immunol 1993;92:442–9.

94. Aloui R, Gormand F, Prigent AF, et al. Increased respiratory burst and phosphodiesterase activity in alveolar eosinophils in chronic eosinophilic pneumonia. Eur Respir J 1996;9:377–9.

95. Mukae H, Kadota JI, Kohno S, et al. Increase of activated T-cells in BAL fluid of Japanese patients with bronchiolitis obliterans organizing pneumonia and chronic eosinophilic pneumonia. Chest 1995;108:123–8.

96. Katoh S, Taniguchi H, Matsubara Y, et al. Overexpression of CD44 on alveolar eosinophils with high concentrations of soluble CD44 in bronchoalveolar lavage fluid in patients with eosinophilic pneumonia. Allergy 1999;54:1286–92.

97. Kurashima K, Mukaida N, Fujimura M, et al. A specific elevation of RANTES in bronchoalveolar lavage fluids of patients with chronic eosinophilic pneumonia. Lab Invest 1997;76:67–75.

98. Katoh S, Matsumoto N, Fukushima K, et al. Elevated chemokine levels in bronchoalveolar lavage fluid of patients with eosinophilic pneumonia. J Allergy Clin Immunol 2000;106:730–6.

99. Saita N, Yamanaka T, Kohrogi H, et al. Apoptotic response of eosinophils in chronic eosinophilic pneumonia. Eur Respir J 2001;17:190–4.

100. Weynants P, Riou R, Vergnon JM, et al. Pneumopathies chroniques idiopathiques à éosinophiles. Etude de 16 cas. Rev Mal Respir 1985;2:63–8.

101. Marnocha KE, Maglinte DDT, Kelvin FM, et al. Eosinophilic enteritis associated with chronic eosinophilic pneumonia. Am J Gastroenterol 1986;81:1205–8.

102. Vergnon JM, Vernet G, Court-Fortune I, et al. Pneumopathie chronique idiopathique à éosinophiles (PCIE) avec atteinte hépatique spécifique. Rev Mal Respir 1988;5:R59–60.

103. Miyazono T, Kawabata M, Higashimoto I, et al. Eosinophilic pneumonia with eosinophilic gastroenteritis. Intern Med 1999;38:450–3.

104. Case Records of the Massachusetts General Hospital. Case 46-1980. N Engl J Med 1980;303:1218–25.

105. Steinfeld S, Golstein M, De Vuyst P. Chronic eosinophilic pneumonia (CEP) as a presenting feature of Churg-Strauss syndrome (CSS). Eur Respir J 1994;7:2098.

106. Hueto-Perez-de-Heredia JJ, Dominguez-del-Valle FJ, Garcia E, et al. Chronic eosinophilic pneumonia as a presenting feature of Churg-Strauss syndrome. Eur Respir J 1994;7:1006–8.

107. Chaouat D, Gompel H, Vignaud O, et al. Pneumonie infiltrante chronique à éosinophiles suivie d'une angéite de type Churg et Strauss. Ann Med Interne (Paris) 1988;139:228–30.

108. Durieu J, Wallaert B, Tonnel AB. Long term follow-up of pulmonary function in chronic eosinophilic pneumonia. Groupe d'Etude en Pathologie Interstitielle de la Société de Pathologie Thoracique du Nord. Eur Respir J 1997;10:286–91.

109. Tosoni C, Faden D, Cattaneo R, et al. Idiopathic eosinophilic pneumonia and pregnancy: report of a case. Int Arch Allergy Immunol 1995;106:173–4.

110. Lavandier M, Carre P. Effectiveness of inhaled high-dose corticosteroid therapy in chronic eosinophilic pneumonia. Chest 1994;105:1913–4.

111. Yoshida K, Shijubo N, Koba H, et al. Chronic eosinophilic pneumonia progressing to lung fibrosis. Eur Respir J 1994;7:1541–4.

112. Davis WB, Wilson HE, Wall RL. Eosinophilic alveolitis in acute respiratory failure. A clinical marker for a non-infectious etiology. Chest 1986;90:7–10.

113. Allen JN, Pacht ER, Gadek JE, et al. Acute eosinophilic pneumonia as a reversible cause of non infectious respiratory failure. N Engl J Med 1989;321:569–74.

114. Pope-Harman AL, Davis WB, Allen ED, et al. Acute eosinophilic pneumonia. A summary of 15 cases and a review of the literature. Medicine 1996;75:334–42.

115. Cheon JE, Lee KS, Jung GS, et al. Acute eosinophilic pneumonia: radiographic and CT findings in six patients. AJR Am J Roentgenol 1996;167:1195–9.

116. Chiappini J, Arbib F, Heyraud JD, et al. Pneumopathie éosinophilique subaiguë idiopathique d'évolution favorable sans corticothérapie. Rev Mal Respir 1995;12:25–8.

117. Elcadi T, Morcos E, Lancrenon C, et al. Syndrome douloureux abdominal révélant une pneumonie aigue à éosinophiles. Presse Med 1997;26:416.

118. Balbi B, Fabiano F. A young man with fever, dyspnoea and nonproductive cough. Eur Respir J 1996;9:619–21.

119. Ogawa H, Fujimura M, Matsuda T, et al. Transient wheeze. Eosinophilic bronchobronchiolitis in acute eosinophilic pneumonia. Chest 1993;104:493–6.

120. Greenburg M, Schiffman RL, Geha DG. Acute eosinophilic pneumonia. N Engl J Med 1990;322:635.

121. King MA, Pope-Harman AL, Allen JN, et al. Acute eosinophilic pneumonia: radiologic and clinical features. Radiology 1997;203:715–9.

122. Philit F, Langevin B, Etienne B, et al. Acute eosinophilic pneumonia. A study of 22 patients. Am J Respir Crit Care Med 2001;163:A980.

123. Nakajima M, Manabe T, Niki Y, et al. Cigarette smoke-induced acute eosinophilic pneumonia. Radiology 1998;207:829–31.

124. Shintani H, Fujimura M, Yasui M, et al. Acute eosinophilic pneumonia caused by cigarette smoking. Intern Med 2000;39:66–8.

125. Shintani H, Fujimura M, Ishiura Y, et al. A case of cigarette smoking-induced acute eosinophilic pneumonia showing tolerance. Chest 2000;117:277–9.

126. Nakajima M, Manabe T, Niki Y, et al. A case of cigarette smoking-induced acute eosinophilic pneumonia showing tolerance. Chest 2000;118:1517–8.

127. Hirai K, Yamazaki Y, Okada K, et al. Acute eosinophilic pneumonia associated with smoke from fireworks. Intern Med 2000;39:401–3.

128. King CH. Pulmonary flukes. In: Mahmoud AAF, editor. Parasitic lung diseases. New-York: Marcel Dekker; 1997. p. 157–69.

129. Slabbynck H, Coeck C, Galdermans D, et al. Dyspnea, fever, and eosinophilia. Chest 1993;104:585–6.

130. Taniguchi H, Kadota J, Fujii T, et al. Activation of lymphocytes and increased interleukin-5 levels in bronchoalveolar lavage fluid in acute eosinophilic pneumonia. Eur Respir J 1999;13:217–20.

131. Godding V, Bodart E, Delos M, et al. Mechanisms of acute eosinophilic inflammation in a case of acute eosinophilic pneumonia in a 14-year-old girl. Clin Exp Allergy 1998; 28:504–9.

132. Okubo Y, Horie S, Hachiya T, et al. Predominant implication of IL-5 in acute eosinophilic pneumonia: comparison with chronic eosinophilic pneumonia. Int Arch Allergy Immunol 1998;116:76–80.

133. Okubo Y, Hossain M, Kai R, et al. Adhesion molecules on eosinophils in acute eosinophilic pneumonia. Am J Respir Crit Care Med 1995;151:1259–62.

134. Allen JN, Liao Z, Wewers MD, et al. Detection of IL-5 and IL-1 receptor antagonist in bronchoalveolar lavage fluid in acute eosinophilic pneumonia. J Allergy Clin Immunol 1996;97:1366–74.

135. Nakahara Y, Hayashi S, Fukuno Y, et al. Increased interleukin-5 levels in bronchoalveolar lavage fluid is a major factor for eosinophil accumulation in acute eosinophilic pneumonia. Respiration 2001;68:389–95.

136. Buddharaju VL, Saraceno JL, Rosen JM, et al. Acute eosinophilic pneumonia associated with shock. Crit Care Med 1999;27:2014–6.

137. Tazelaar HD, Linz LJ, Colby TV, et al. Acute eosinophilic pneumonia: histopathologic findings in nine patients. Am J Respir Crit Care Med 1997;155:296–302.

138. Andreu V, Bataller R, Caballeria J, et al. Acute eosinophilic pneumonia associated with ranitidine. J Clin Gastroenterol 1996;23:160–2.

139. Fleisch MC, Blauer F, Gubler JG, et al. Eosinophilic pneumonia and respiratory failure associated with venlafaxine treatment. Eur Respir J 2001;15:205–8.

140. Churg J, Strauss L. Allergic granulomatosis, allergic angiitis, and periarteritis nodosa. Am J Pathol 1951;27:277–301.

141. Warren P. Osler's unusual case—was it Churg-Strauss syndrome? Can Med Assoc J 1999;161:846–7.

142. Lamb AR. Periarteritis nodosa—a clinical and pathological review of the disease. With a report of two cases. Arch Intern Med 1914;14:481–516.

143. Rackemann FM, Greene JE. Periarteritis nodosa and asthma. Trans Assoc Am Phys 1939;54:112–8.

144. Harkavy J. Vascular allergy. Pathogenesis of bronchial asthma with recurrent pulmonary infiltrations and eosinophilic polyserositis. Arch Intern Med 1941;67:709–34.

145. Wilson KS, Alexander HL. The relation of periarteritis nodosa to bronchial asthma and other forms of human hypersensitiveness. J Lab Clin Med 1945;30:195–203.

146. Jennette JC, Falk RJ, Andrassy K, et al. Nomenclature of systemic vasculitides. Proposal of an international consensus conference. Arthritis Rheum 1994;37:187–92.

147. Lanham JG, Elkon K, Pusey C, et al. Systemic vasculitis with asthma and eosinophilia: a clinical approach to the Churg-Strauss syndrome. Medicine 1984;63:65–81.

148. Lie JT. The classification of vasculitis and a reappraisal of allergic granulomatosis and angiitis (Churg-Strauss syndrome). Mount Sinai J Med 1986;53:429–39.

149. Lie JT, Bayardo RJ. Isolated eosinophilic coronary arteritis and eosinophilic myocarditis. A limited form of Churg-Strauss syndrome. Arch Pathol Lab Med 1989;113:199–201.

150. Scolyer RA. Test and teach. Number ninety-four: part 1. Churg-Strauss syndrome. Pathology 1999;31:217–8.

151. Newinger G, Fournier E, Hatron PY, et al. Manifestations systémiques d'angéite avec asthme et hyperéosinophilie. Etude de 10 observations. Rev Med Interne 1984;5:165–71.

152. Haas C, Geneau C, Odinot JM, et al. L'angéite allergique avec granulomatose: syndrome de Churg et Strauss. Etude rétrospective de 16 observations. Ann Med Interne (Paris) 1991; 142:335–42.

153. Chumbley LC, Harrison EG, De Remee RA. Allergic granulomatosis and angiitis (Churg-Strauss syndrome). Report and analysis of 30 cases. Mayo Clin Proc 1977;52:477–84.

154. Guillevin L, Lhote F, Gayraud M, et al. Prognostic factors in polyarteritis nodosa and Churg-Strauss syndrome. A prospective study in 342 patients. Medicine 1996;75:17–28.

155. Rabusin M, Lepore L, Costantinides F, et al. A child with severe asthma. Lancet 1998;351:32.

156. Louthrenoo W, Norasetthada A, Khunamornpong S, et al. Childhood Churg-Strauss syndrome. J Rheumatol 1999; 26:1387–93.

157. Frayha RA. Churg-Strauss syndrome in a child. J Rheumatol 1982;9:807–9.

158. Treitman P, Herskowitz JL, Bass HN. Churg-Strauss syndrome in a 14 year-old boy diagnosed by transbronchial lung biopsy. Clin Pediatr 1991;30:502–5.

159. Guillevin L, Cohen P, Gayraud M, et al. Churg-Strauss syndrome. Clinical study and long-term follow-up of 96 patients. Medicine 1999;78:26–37.

160. Keogh KA, Specks U. Churg-Strauss syndrome in the 1990's: the pathogenic role of ANCA and leukotriene inhibitors remain unclear. Am J Respir Crit Care Med 2001;163:A557.

161. Chen KR, Ohata Y, Sakurai M, et al. Churg-Strauss syndrome: report of a case without preexisting asthma. J Dermatol 1992;19:40–7.

162. Li GW, Dickey BF, Green LK, et al. Recurrent asthma, sinusitis, and rash in a 63-year-old man. Chest 1995;108:1551–3.

163. Degesys GE, Mintzer RA, Vria RF. Allergic granulomatosis:

Churg-Strauss syndrome. AJR Am J Roentgenol 1980;135: 1281–2.

164. Murray NB, Barber FA, Murray KM. Asthma, eosinophilia and palpable purpura. Chest 1989;96:416–8.

165. Rose GA, Spencer H. Polyarteritis nodosa. QJM 1957;26:43–86.

166. Neef B, Horing E, von Gaisberg U, et al. Ulzeröse Kolitis als primäre Manifestation eines Churg-Strauss-Syndroms. Dtsch Med Wochenschr 1995;120:396–402.

167. Choi YH, Im JG, Han BK, et al. Thoracic manifestation of Churg-Strauss syndrome: radiologic and clinical findings. Chest 2000;117:117–24.

168. Cordier JF, Valeyre D, Guillevin L, et al. Pulmonary Wegener's granulomatosis. A clinical and imaging study of 77 cases. Chest 1990;97:906–12.

169. Erzurum SC, Underwood GA, Hamilos DL, et al. Pleural effusion in Churg-Strauss syndrome. Chest 1989;95:1357–9.

170. Herreman G, Ferme, I, Puech H, et al. Angéite granulomateuse allergique de Churg et Strauss avec paralysie phrénique. Deux observations. Nouv Presse Med 1980;9:3631.

171. Hirasaki S, Kamei T, Iwasaki Y, et al. Churg-Strauss syndrome with pleural involvement. Intern Med 2000;39:976–8.

172. Worthy SA, Muller NL, Hansell DM, et al. Churg-Strauss syndrome: the spectrum of pulmonary CT findings in 17 patients. AJR Am J Roentgenol 1998;170:297–300.

173. Olsen KD, Neel HB III, De Remee RA, et al. Nasal manifestations of allergic granulomatosis and angiitis (Churg Strauss syndrome). Otolaryngol Head Neck Surg 1995;88:85–9.

174. Wallaert B, Gosset P, Prin L, et al. Bronchoalveolar lavage in allergic granulomatosis and angiitis. Eur Respir J 1993;6:413–7.

175. Dujardin P, Cassuto JP, Audoly P, et al. Angéite granulomateuse allergique. A propos de 4 observations. Ann Med Interne (Paris) 1978;129:165–73.

176. Cohen Tervaert JW, Elema JD, Kallenberg CG. Clinical and histopathological association of 29kD-ANCA and MPO-ANCA. APMIS 1990;19 Suppl:35.

177. Cohen Tervaert JW, Limburg PC, Elema JD, et al. Detection of autoantibodies against myeloid lysosomal enzymes: a useful adjunct to classification of patients with biopsy-proven necrotizing arteritis. Am J Med 1991;91:59–66.

178. Harrison DJ, Simpson R, Kharbanda R, et al. Antibodies to neutrophil cytoplasmic antigens in Wegener's granulomatosis and other conditions. Thorax 1989;44:373–7.

179. Lee SS, Adu D, Thompson RA. Anti-myeloperoxidase antibodies in systemic vasculitis. Clin Exp Immunol 1990;79:41–6.

180. Hauschild S, Csernok E, Schmitt WH, et al. Antineutrophil cytoplasmic antibodies in systemic polyarteritis nodosa with and without hepatitis B virus infection and Churg-Strauss syndrome—62 patients. J Rheumatol 1994;21:1173–4.

181. Kurosawa M, Nakagami R, Morioka J, et al. Interleukins in Churg-Strauss syndrome. Allergy 2000;55:785–7.

182. Cottin V, Tardy F, Gindre D, et al. Urinary eosinophil-derived neurotoxin in Churg-Strauss syndrome. J Allergy Clin Immunol 1995;96:261–4.

183. Hattori N, Ichimura M, Nagamatsu M, et al. Clinicopathological features of Churg-Strauss syndrome-associated neuropathy. Brain 1999;122:427–39.

184. Reid AJC, Harrison BDW, Watts RA, et al. Churg-Strauss syndrome in a district hospital. QJM 1998;91:219–29.

185. Diebold J, Anteri L, Kalifat RS, et al. Angéite allergique granulomateuse avec manifestations pulmonaires et cardiaques prédominantes. Presse Med 1969;7:1211–2.

186. Kozak M, Gill EA, Green LS. The Churg-Strauss syndrome. A case report with angiographically documented coronary involvement and a review of the literature. Chest 1995; 107:578–80.

187. Terasaki F, Hayashi T, Hirota Y, et al. Evolution to dilated cardiomyopathy from acute eosinophilic pancarditis in Churg-Strauss syndrome. Heart Vessels 1997;12:43–8.

188. Thomson D, Chamsi-Pasha H, Hasleton P. Heart transplantation for Churg-Strauss syndrome. Br Heart J 1989;62: 409–10.

189. Henderson RA, Hasleton P, Hamid BNA. Recurrence of Churg Strauss vasculitis in a transplanted heart. Br Heart J 1993;70:553.

190. Azzopardi C, Montefort S, Mallia C. Cardiac involvement and left ventricular failure in a patient with the Churg-Strauss syndrome. Adv Exp Med Biol 1999;455:547–9.

191. Renaldini E, Spandrio S, Cerudelli B, et al. Cardiac involvement in Churg-Strauss syndrome: a follow-up of three cases. Eur Heart J 1993;14:1712–6.

192. Hellemans S, Dens J, Knockaert D. Coronary involvement in the Churg-Strauss syndrome. Heart 1997;77:576–8.

193. Isaka N, Araki S, Shibata M, et al. Reversal of coronary artery occlusions in allergic granulomatosis and angiitis (Churg-Strauss syndrome). Am Heart J 1994;128:609–13.

194. Balestrieri GP, Valentini U, Cerudelli B, et al. Reversible myocardial impairment in the Churg-Strauss syndrome: report of a case. Clin Exp Rheumatol 1992;10:75–7.

195. Takahashi N, Horita M, Tatsukawa M, et al. Allergic granulomatosis and angiitis with severe cardiac disease: a case in which cardiac function was extremely improved by long-term steroid therapy. Intern Med 1992;31:534–9.

196. Frustaci A, Gentiloni N, Chimenti C, et al. Necrotizing myocardial vasculitis in Churg-Strauss syndrome. Clinicohistologic evaluation of steroids and immunosuppressive therapy. Chest 1998;114:1484–9.

197. Hasley PB, Follansbee WP, Coulehan JL. Cardiac manifestations of Churg-Strauss syndrome: report of a case and review of the literature. Am Heart J 1990;120:996–9.

198. Peen E, Hahn P, Lauwers G, et al. Churg-Strauss syndrome: localization of eosinophil major basic protein in damaged tissues. Arthritis Rheum 2000;43:1897–900.

199. Leung W, Wong K, Lau C, et al. Myocardial involvement in Churg-Strauss syndrome: the role of endomyocardial biopsy. J Rheumatol 1989;16:828–31.

200. Morgan JM, Raposo L, Gibson DG. Cardiac involvement in Churg-Strauss syndrome shown by echocardiography. Br Heart J 1989;62:462–6.

201. Sharma MC, Safaya R, Sidhu BS. Perforation of small intestine caused by Churg-Strauss syndrome. J Clin Gastroenterol 1996;23:232–5.

202. Boggi U, Mosca M, Giulianotti PC, et al. Surviving catastrophic gastrointestinal involvement due to Churg-Strauss syndrome: report of a case. Hepatogastroenterology 1997; 44:1169–71.

203. Guillevin L, Lhote F, Gallais V, et al. Gastrointestinal tract involvement in polyarteritis nodosa and Churg-Strauss syndrome. Ann Med Interne (Paris) 1995;146:260–7.

204. Schwartz RA, Churg J. Churg-Strauss syndrome. Br J Dermatol 1992;127:199–204.

205. Finan MC, Winkelmann RK. The cutaneous extravascular necrotizing granuloma (Churg-Strauss granuloma) and systemic disease: a review of 27 cases. Medicine 1983;62: 142–58.

206. Piette WW. Primary systemic vasculitis. In: Sontheimer RD, Provost TT, editors. Cutaneous manifestations of rheumatic diseases. Baltimore: Williams & Wilkins; 1996. p. 177–232.

207. Crotty CP, DeRemee RA, Winkelmann RK. Cutaneous clinicopathologic correlation of allergic granulomatosis. J Am Acad Dermatol 1981;5:571–81.

208. Gaskin G, Clutterbuck EJ, Pusey CD. Renal disease in the Churg-Strauss syndrome. Diagnosis, management and outcome. Contrib Nephrol 1991;94:58–65.

209. Mouthon L, Khaled M, Cohen P, et al. Antigen inhalation as a triggering factor in systemic small-sized-vessel vasculitis. Four cases. Ann Med Interne (Paris) 2001;152:152–6.

210. Guillevin L, Guittard T, Bletry O, et al. Systemic necrotizing angiitis with asthma: causes and precipitating factors in 43 cases. Lung 1987;165:165–72.

211. Huong Du LT, Wechsler B, Ronco P, et al. Forme familiale

d'angéite nécrosante. Une observation chez deux frères. Semin Hop Paris 1988;64:179–82.

212. Stephens M, Reynolds S, Gibbs AR, et al. Allergic bronchopulmonary aspergillosis progressing to allergic granulomatosis and angiitis (Churg-Strauss syndrome). Am Rev Respir Dis 1988;137:1226–8.

213. Matsumoto H, Niimi A, Suzuki K, et al. Allergic granulomatous angiitis (Churg-Strauss syndrome) associated with allergic bronchopulmonary candidiasis. Respiration 2000;67:577–9.

214. Chauman A, Scott DGI, Neuberger J, et al. Churg-Strauss vasculitis and ascaris infection. Ann Rheum Dis 1990;49:320–2.

215. Guillevin L, Amouroux J, Arbeille B, et al. Churg-Strauss angiitis. Arguments favoring the responsibility of inhaled antigens. Chest 1991;100:1472–3.

216. Orriols R, Munoz X, Ferrer J, et al. Cocaine-induced Churg-Strauss vasculitis. Eur Respir J 1996;9:175–7.

217. Mercie P, Viallard JF, Faure I, et al. Hepatitis C virus infection with and without cryoglobulinemia as a case of Churg-Strauss syndrome. J Rheumatol 2000;27:814–7.

218. Cooper LM, Patterson JAK. Allergic granulomatosis and angiitis of Churg-Strauss. Case report in a patient with antibodies to human immunodeficiency virus and hepatitis B virus. Int J Dermatol 1989;28:597–9.

219. Case Records of the Massachusetts General Hospital. Case 30-2000. N Engl J Med 2000;343:953–61.

220. Wechsler ME, Drazen JM. Zafirlukast and Churg-Strauss syndrome. Chest 1999;116:266–7.

221. Stoloff S, Stempel DA. Churg-Strauss syndrome: is there an association with leukotriene modifiers? Chest 2000;118:1515–6.

222. Mukhopadhyay A, Stanley NN. Churg-Strauss syndrome associated with montelukast. Postgrad Med J 2001;77:390–1.

223. Goransson LG, Omdal R. A severe systemic inflammatory reaction following therapy with montelukast (Singulair). Nephrol Dial Transplant 2000;15:1054–5.

224. Weschler M. Churg-Strauss syndrome with montelukast. Thorax 2001;56:417.

225. Stirling RG, Chung KF. Leukotriene antagonists and Churg-Strauss syndrome: the smoking gun. Thorax 1999;54:865–6.

226. Churg A, Churg J. Steroids and Churg-Strauss syndrome. Lancet 1998;352:32–3.

227. Donohue JF. Montelukast and Churg-Strauss syndrome. Chest 2001;119:668.

228. Gruer P, Bold T, Vilardo L. Case 30-2000: Churg-Strauss syndrome. N Engl J Med 2001;344:858–9.

229. Wechsler M, Drazen JM. Churg-Strauss syndrome. Lancet 1999;353:1970–1.

230. Frosi A, Foresi A, Bozzoni M, et al. Churg-Strauss syndrome and antiasthma therapy. Lancet 1999;353:1102.

231. Tuggey JM, Hosker HS. Churg-Strauss syndrome associated with montelukast therapy. Thorax 2000;55:805–6.

232. Villena V, Hidalgo R, Sotelo MT, et al. Montelukast and Churg-Strauss syndrome. Eur Respir J 2000;15:626.

233. Lipworth BJ, Wilson AM. Montelukast and Churg-Strauss syndrome. Thorax 2001;56:244.

234. Wechsler ME, Garpestad E, Flier SR, et al. Pulmonary infiltrates, eosinophilia, and cardiomyopathy following corticosteroid withdrawal in patients with asthma receiving zarfirlukast. JAMA 1998;279:455–7.

235. Kinoshita M, Shiraishi T, Koga T, et al. Churg-Strauss syndrome after corticosteroid withdrawal in an asthmatic patient treated with pranlukast. J Allergy Clin Immunol 1999;103:534–5.

236. Wechsler ME, Finn D, Gunawardena D, et al. Churg-Strauss syndrome in patients receiving montelukast as treatment for asthma. Chest 2000;117:708–13.

237. Knoell DL, Lucas J, Allen JN. Churg-Strauss syndrome associated with zafirlukast. Chest 1998;114:332–4.

238. Green R, Vayonis AG. Churg-Strauss syndrome after zafirlukast in two patients not receiving systemic steroid treatment. Lancet 1999;353:725–6.

239. Hashimoto M, Fujishima T, Tanaka H, et al. Churg-Strauss syndrome after reduction of inhaled corticosteroid in a patient treated with pranlukast for asthma. Intern Med 2001;40:432–4.

240. Weller PF, Plaut M, Taggart V, et al. The relationship of asthma therapy and Churg-Strauss syndrome: NIH workshop summary report. J Allergy Clin Immunol 2001;108:175–83.

241. Le Gall C, Pham S, Vignes S, et al. Inhaled corticosteroids and Churg-Strauss syndrome: a report of five cases. Eur Respir J 2000;15:978–81.

242. Bili A, Condemi JJ, Bottone SM, et al. Seven cases of complete and incomplete forms of Churg-Strauss syndrome not related to leukotriene receptor antagonists. J Allergy Clin Immunol 1999;104:1060–5.

243. Rich AR. The role of hypersensitivity in periarteritis nodosa as indicated by seven cases developing during serum sickness and sulfonamide therapy. Bull Johns Hopkins Hosp 1942;71:123–41.

244. Rich MW, Thomas RA. A case of eosinophilic pneumonia and vasculitis induced by diflunisal. Chest 1997;111:1767–9.

245. Hubner C, Dietz A, Stremmel W, et al. Macrolide-induced Churg-Strauss syndrome in a patient with atopy. Lancet 1997;350:563.

246. Dietz A, Hubner C, Andrassy K. Makrolid-Antibiotika induzierte Vaskulitis (Churg-Strauss syndrom). Laryngorhinootologie 1998;77:111–4.

247. Yermakov VM, Hitti IF, Sutton AL. Necrotizing vasculitis associated with diphenylhydantoin: two fatal cases. Hum Pathol 1983;13:182–4.

248. Priori R, Tomassini M, Magrini L, et al. Churg-Strauss syndrome during pregnancy after steroid withdrawal. Lancet 1998;352:1599–600.

249. Connolly JO, Lanham JG, Partridge MR. Fulminant pregnancy-related Churg-Strauss syndrome. Br J Rheumatol 1994;33:776–7.

250. Barry C, Davis S, Garrard P, et al. Churg-Strauss disease: deterioration in a twin pregnancy. Successful outcome following treatment with corticosteroids and cyclophosphamide. Br J Obstet Gynaecol 1997;104:746–7.

251. Masi AT, Hunder GG, Lie JT, et al. The American College of Rheumatology 1990 criteria for the classification of Churg-Strauss syndrome (allergic granulomatosis and angiitis). Arthritis Rheum 1990;33:1094–100.

252. Schnabel A, Holl-Ulrich K, Dalhoff K, et al. Efficacy of transbronchial biopsy in pulmonary vasculitides. Eur Respir J 1997;10:2738–43.

253. Krupsky M, Landau Z, Lifschitz-Mercer B, et al. Wegener's granulomatosis with peripheral eosinophilia. Atypical variant of a classic disease. Chest 1993;104:1290–2.

254. Yousem SA. Overlap syndromes: Wegener's granulomatosis and Churg Strauss syndrome. Semin Respir Med 1989;10:162–6.

255. Yousem SA, Lombard CM. The eosinophilic variant of Wegener's granulomatosis. Hum Pathol 1988;19:682–8.

256. Potter MB, Fincher RK, Finger DR. Eosinophilia in Wegener's granulomatosis. Chest 1999;116:1480–3.

257. Case Records of the Massachusetts General Hospital. Case 18-1987. N Engl J Med 1987;316:1139–47.

258. Fienberg R, Mark EJ, Goodman M, et al. Correlation of antineutrophil cytoplasmic antibodies with the extrarenal histopathology of Wegener's (pathergic) granulomatosis and related forms of vasculitis. Hum Pathol 1993;24:160–8.

259. Lie JT, Nagpal S. Churg-Strauss syndrome with nongiant cell eosinophilic temporal arteritis. J Rheumatol 1994;21:366–7.

260. Vidal E, Liozon F, Rogues AM, et al. Concurrent temporal arteritis and Churg-Strauss syndrome. J Rheumatol 1992; 19:1312–4.

261. Amato MB, Barbas CS, Delmonte VC, et al. Concurrent Churg-Strauss syndrome and temporal arteritis in a young patient with pulmonary nodules. Am Rev Respir Dis 1989; 139:1539–42.

262. Endo T, Katsuta Y, Kimura Y, et al. A variant form of Churg-Strauss syndrome: initial temporal non-giant cell arteritis followed by asthma—is this a distinct clinicopathologic entity? Hum Pathol 2000;31:1169–71.

263. Grishman E, Wolfe D, Spiera H. Eosinophilic temporal and systemic arteritis. Hum Pathol 1995;26:241–4.

264. Clutterbuck EJ, Evans DJ, Pusey CD. Renal involvement in Churg-Strauss syndrome. Nephrol Dial Transplant 1990; 5:161–7.

265. Cogen FC, Mayock RL, Zweiman B. Chronic eosinophilic pneumonia followed by polyarteritis nodosa complicating the course of bronchial asthma. Report of a case. J Allergy Clin Immunol 1977;60:377–82.

266. De Toffol B, Gaymard B, Adam G, et al. Pneumonie infiltrante chronique à éosinophiles suivie d'une angéite de type Churg et Strauss. Ann Med Interne (Paris) 1989;140:334–5.

267. Kinsella DL, Simpson HN. Löffler's pneumonia terminating in fatal periarteritis nodosa. JAMA 1967;202:101–3.

268. Lie JT. Limited forms of Churg-Strauss syndrome. Pathol Annu 1993;28:199–220.

269. MacFadyen R, Tron, V, Keshmiri M, et al. Allergic angiitis of Churg and Strauss syndrome. Response to pulse methylprednisolone. Chest 1987;91:629–31.

270. Buschman DL, Waldron JA Jr, King TE Jr. Churg-Strauss pulmonary vasculitis. High-resolution computed tomography scanning and pathologic findings. Am Rev Respir Dis 1990;142:458–61.

271. Clausen KP, Bronstein H. Granulomatous pulmonary arteritis. A hypereosinophilic syndrome. Am J Clin Pathol 1974; 62:82–7.

272. Galiuto L, Enriquez-Sarano M, Reeder GS, et al. Eosinophilic myocarditis manifesting as myocardial infarction: early diagnosis and successful treatment. Mayo Clin Proc 1997; 72:603–10.

273. Hunsaker JC II, O'Connor WN, Lie JT. Spontaneous coronary arterial dissection and isolated eosinophilic coronary arteritis: sudden cardiac death in a patient with a limited variant of Churg-Strauss syndrome. Mayo Clin Proc 1992; 67:761–6.

274. Churg A, Brallas M, Cronin SR, et al. Formes frustes of Churg-Strauss syndrome. Chest 1995;108:320–3.

275. Abu-Shakra M, Smythe H, Lewtas J, et al. Outcome of polyarteritis nodosa and Churg-Strauss syndrome. Arthritis Rheum 1994;37:1798–803.

276. Chow CC, Mac-Moune Lai F. Allergic granulomatosis and angiitis (Churg-Strauss syndrome): response to "pulse" intravenous cyclophosphamide. Ann Rheum Dis 1989;48: 605–8.

277. Guillevin L, Lhote F, Jarrousse B, et al. Treatment of polyarteritis nodosa and Churg-Strauss syndrome. A meta-analysis of 3 prospective controlled trials including 182 patients over 12 years. Ann Med Interne (Paris) 1992;143:405–16.

278. Gayraud M, Guillevin L, le Toumelin P, et al. Long-term followup of polyarteritis nodosa, microscopic polyangiitis, and Churg-Strauss syndrome: analysis of four prospective trials including 278 patients. Arthritis Rheum 2001;44:666–75.

279. Langford CA. Treatment of polyarteritis nodosa, microscopic polyangiitis, and Churg-Strauss syndrome: where do we stand? Arthritis Rheum 2001;44:508–12.

280. Tatsis E, Schnabel A, Gross WL. Interferon-alpha treatment of four patients with the Churg-Strauss syndrome. Ann Intern Med 1998;129:370–4.

281. Seelbach H, Ehmann R, Simon HU, et al. Interferon-α in steroid-resistant aspirin-induced-asthma and Churg-Strauss syndrome. Am J Respir Crit Care Med 2000;161:A608.

282. Hamilos DL, Christensen J. Treatment of Churg-Strauss syndrome with high-dose intravenous immunoglobulin. J Allergy Clin Immunol 1991;88:823–4.

283. Levy Y, George J, Fabbrizzi F, et al. Marked improvement of Churg-Strauss vasculitis with intravenous gammaglobulins. South Med J 1999;92:412–4.

284. McDermott EM, Powell RJ. Cyclosporin in the treatment of Churg-Strauss syndrome. Ann Rheum Dis 1998;57:258–9.

285. Chusid MJ, Dale DC, West BC, et al. The hypereosinophilic syndrome: analysis of fourteen cases with review of the literature. Medicine 1975;54:1–27.

286. Spry CJF, Davies J, Tai PC, et al. Clinical features of fifteen patients with the hypereosinophilic syndrome. QJM 1983; 205:1–22.

287. Lefebvre C, Bletry O, Degoulet P, et al. Facteurs pronostiques du syndrome hyperéosinophilique. Etude de 40 observations. Ann Med Interne (Paris) 1989;140:253–7.

288. Bain BJ. Eosinophilic leukaemias and the idiopathic hypereosinophilic syndrome. Br J Haematol 1996;95:2–9.

289. Brito-Babapulle F. Clonal eosinophilic disorders and the hypereosinophilic syndrome. Blood Rev 1997;11:129–45.

290. Oliver JW, Deol I, Morgan DL, et al. Chronic eosinophilic leukemia and hypereosinophilic syndromes. Proposal for classification, literature review, and report of a case with a unique chromosomal abnormality. Cancer Genet Cytogenet 1998;107:111–7.

291. Schoffski P, Ganser A, Pascheberg U, et al. Complete haematological and cytogenetic response to interferon alpha-2a of a myeloproliferative disorder with eosinophilia associated with a unique t(4;7) aberration. Ann Hematol 2000;79:95–8.

292. Chang HW, Leong KH, Koh DR, et al. Clonality of isolated eosinophils in the hypereosinophilic syndrome. Blood 1999;93:1651–7.

293. Bigoni R, Cuneo A, Roberti MG, et al. Cytogenetic and molecular cytogenetic characterization of 6 new cases of idiopathic hypereosinophilic syndrome. Haematologica 2000; 85:486–91.

294. Simon HU, Plotz SG, Dummer R, et al. Abnormal clones of T cells producing interleukin-5 in idiopathic eosinophilia. N Engl J Med 1999;341:1112–20.

295. Roufosse F, Schandene L, Sibille C, et al. Clonal Th2 lymphocytes in patients with the idiopathic hypereosinophilic syndrome. Br J Haematol 2000;109:540–8.

296. Cogan E, Schandené L, Crusiaux A, et al. Clonal proliferation of type 2 helper T cells in a man with the hypereosinophilic syndrome. N Engl J Med 1994;330:535–8.

297. Herzig G, Glazer H, Orland M, et al. Pleural effusions and eosinophilia in a 63-year-old woman. Am J Med 1989;87: 316–24.

298. Mouly F, Rybojad M, Morel P. Syndrome hyperéosinophilique pulmonaire et hépatique au cours d'un mycosis fungoide. Ann Dermatol 1996;123:S36.

299. Kawasaki A, Mizushima Y, Matsui S, et al. A case of T-cell lymphoma accompanying marked eosinophilia, chronic eosinophilic pneumonia and eosinophilic pleural effusion. A case report. Tumori 1991;77:527–30.

300. Hirshberg B, Kramer MR, Lotem M, et al. Chronic eosinophilic pneumonia associated with cutaneous T-cell lymphoma. Am J Hematol 1999;60:143–7.

301. Bentley HP, Reardon AE, Knoedler JP, et al. Eosinophilic leukemia report of a case, with review and classification. Am J Med 1961;30:310–22.

302. Means-Markwell M, Burgess T, deKeratry D, et al. Eosinophilia with aberrant T cells and elevated serum levels of interleukin-2 and interleukin-15. N Engl J Med 2000;342:1568–71.

303. Weller PF, Bubley GJ. The idiopathic hypereosinophilic syndrome. Blood 1994;83:2759–79.

304. Alfaham MA, Ferguson SD, Sihra B, et al. The idiopathic hypereosinophilic syndrome. Arch Dis Child 1987;62:601–13.

305. Löffler W. Endocarditis parietalis fibroplastica mit Bluteosinophilie. Schweiz Med Wochenschr 1936;66:817–20.

306. Roberts WC, Ferrans VJ. Pathologic anatomy of the cardiomyopathies. Idiopathic dilated and hypertrophic types, infiltrative types, and endomyocardial disease with and without eosinophilia. Hum Pathol 1975;6:287–342.

307. Ommen SR, Seward JB, Tajik AJ. Clinical and echocardiographic features of hypereosinophilic syndromes. Am J Cardiol 2001;86:110–3.

308. Kazmierowski JA, Chusid MJ, Parrillo JE, et al. Dermatologic manifestations of the hypereosinophilic syndrome. Arch Dermatol 1978;114:531–5.

309. Kang EY, Shim JJ, Kim JS, et al. Pulmonary involvement of idiopathic hypereosinophilic syndrome: CT findings in five patients. J Comput Assist Tomogr 1997;21:612–5.

310. Epstein DM, Taormina V, Gefter WB, et al. The hypereosinophilic syndrome. Radiology 1981;140:59–62.

311. Slabbynck H, Impens N, Naegels S, et al. Idiopathic hypereosinophilic syndrome-related pulmonary involvement diagnosed by bronchoalveolar lavage. Chest 1992;101:1178–80.

312. Winn RE, Kollef MH, Meyer JI. Pulmonary involvement in the hypereosinophilic syndrome. Chest 1994;105:656–60.

313. Cordier JF, Faure M, Hermier C, et al. Pleural effusions in an overlap syndrome of idiopathic hypereosinophilic syndrome and erythema elevatum diutinum. Eur Respir J 1990;3:115–8.

314. Dussopt C, Schandené L, Perrin-Fayolle M, et al. Augmentation du taux d'interleukine 5 sérique au cours d'un syndrome hyperéosinophilique. Presse Med 1997;26:166.

315. Parrillo JE, Borer JS, Henry WL, et al. The cardiovascular manifestations of the hypereosinophilic syndrome. Prospective study of 26 patients, with review of the literature. Am J Med 1979;67:572–82.

316. Papo T, Piette JC, Hermine O. Treatment of the hypereosinophilic syndrome with interferon-α. Ann Intern Med 1995;123:155–6.

317. Bourrat E, Lebbe C, Calvo F. Etoposide for treating the hypereosinophilic syndrome. Ann Intern Med 1994;121:899–900.

318. Smit AJ, Van Essen LH, de Vries EGE. Successful long-term control of idiopathic hypereosinophilic syndrome with etoposide. Cancer 1991;67:2826–7.

319. Butterfield JH, Gleich GJ. Interferon-α treatment of six patients with the idiopathic hypereosinophilic syndrome. Ann Intern Med 1994;121:648–53.

320. Butterfield JH, Gleich GJ. Response of six patients with idiopathic hypereosinophilic syndrome to interferon alfa. J Allergy Clin Immunol 1994;94:1318–26.

321. Ceretelli S, Capochiani E, Petrini M. Interferon-alpha in the idiopathic hypereosinophilic syndrome: consideration of five cases. Ann Hematol 1998;77:161–4.

322. Yoon TY, Ahn GB, Chang SH. Complete remission of hypereosinophilic syndrome after interferon-alpha therapy: report of a case and literature review. J Dermatol 2000;27:110–5.

323. Coutant G, Bletry O, Prin L, et al. Traitement des syndromes hyperéosinophiliques à expression myéloproliférative par l'association hydroxyurée-interféron alpha. A propos de 7 observations. Ann Med Interne (Paris) 1993;144:243–50.

324. Malbrain ML, Zachee P. Combination of interferon-alpha and hydroxyurea in the treatment of idiopathic hypereosinophilic syndrome. Br J Haematol 1997;97:928–30.

325. Roufosse F, de Lavareille A, Schandené L, et al. Clones T chez des patients atteints du syndrome hyperéosinophilique idiopathique: implications pronostiques et thérapeutiques. Rev Fr Allergol Immunol Clin 2001;41:301–5.

326. Schandené L, Roufosse F, de Lavareille A, et al. Interferon alpha prevents spontaneous apoptosis of clonal Th2 cells associated with chronic hypereosinophilia. Blood 2000;96:4285–92.

327. Baird JK, Neafie RC, Marty AM. Parasitic infections. In: Dail DH, Hammar SP, editors. Pulmonary pathology. 2nd ed. New-York: Springer-Verlag; 1994. p. 491–536.

328. Corrin B. Parasitic diseases. In: Corrin B, editor: The lungs. London: Churchill Livingstone; 1990. p. 147–59.

329. Fraser RS. Protozoal and helminthic pulmonary infection. In: Thurlbeck WM, Churg AM, editors. Pathology of the lung. 2nd ed. New-York: Thieme Medical; 1995. p. 333–48.

330. Lucas SB, Schwartz DA, Hasleton PS. Parasitic lung disease. In: Hasleton PS, editor. Spencer's pathology of the lung. New-York: McGraw-Hill; 1996. p. 305–56.

331. Marty AM, Neafie RC. Protozoal and helminthic diseases. In: Saldana MJ, editor. Pathology of pulmonary disease. Philadelphia: J.B. Lippincott Company; 1994. p. 489–502.

332. Weingarten RJ. Tropical eosinophilia. Lancet 1943;i:103–5.

333. Ottesen EA, Neva FA, Paranjape RS, et al. Specific allergic sensitisation to filarial antigens in tropical eosinophilia syndrome. Lancet 1979;ii:1158–61.

334. Kazura JW. The filariases. In: Mahmoud AAF, editor. Parasitic lung diseases. New-York: Marcel Dekker; 1997. p. 109–24.

335. Ottesen EA. Filarial infections. Infect Dis Clin North Am 1993;7:619–33.

336. Ray D, Abel R. Pulmonary eosinophilia in children: report of a school survey in rural tamil nadu in India. J Trop Pediatr 1994;40:49–51.

337. Webb JKG, Job CK, Gault EW. Tropical eosinophilia. Demonstration of microfilariae in lung, liver, and lymph-nodes. Lancet 1960;1:835–42.

338. Dreyer G, Dreyer P, Piessens WF. Extralymphatic disease due to bancroftian filariasis. Braz J Med Biol Res 1999;32:1467–72.

339. Chitkara RK, Sarinas PS. Dirofilaria, visceral larva migrans, and tropical pulmonary eosinophilia. Semin Respir Infect 1997;12:138–48.

340. Marshall BG, Wilkinson RJ, Davidson RN. Pathogenesis of tropical pulmonary eosinophilia: parasitic alveolitis and parallels with asthma. Respir Med 1998;92:1–3.

341. Ong RK, Doyle RL. Tropical pulmonary eosinophilia. Chest 1998;113:1673–9.

342. Udwadia FE, Joshi VV. A study of tropical eosinophilia. Thorax 1964;19:548–54.

343. Udwadia FE. Tropical eosinophilia—a correlation of clinical, histopathologic, and lung function studies. Dis Chest 1967;52:531–8.

344. Danaraj TJ, Pacheco G, Shanmugaratnam K, et al. The etiology and pathology of eosinophilic lung (tropical eosinophilia). Am J Trop Med Hyg 1966;15:183–9.

345. Joshi VV, Udwadia FE, Gadgil RK. Etiology of tropical eosinophilia. A study of lung biopsies and review of published reports. Am J Trop Med Hyg 1969;18:231–40.

346. Khoo FY, Danaraj TJ. The roentgenographic appearance of eosinophilic lung (tropical eosinophilia). AJR Am J Roentgenol 1960;83:251–9.

347. Wilson HTH. Tropical eosinophilia in east Africa. BMJ 1947;7:801–4.

348. Magnussen P, Makunde W, Simonsen PE, et al. Chronic pulmonary disorders, including tropical pulmonary eosinophilia, in villages with endemic lymphatic filariasis in Tanga region and in Tanga town, Tanzania. Trans R Soc Trop Med Hyg 1995;89:406–9.

349. Bartoloni A, Dini F, Farese A, et al. Tropical pulmonary eosinophilia. Report of a case. Ann Med Interne (Paris) 1997;148:321–2.

350. Jiva TM, Israel RH, Poe RH. Tropical pulmonary eosinophilia masquerading as acute bronchial asthma. Respiration 1996;63:55–8.

351. Islam N, Huque KS. Radiological features of tropical eosinophilia. Am J Trop Med Hyg 1965;68:177–80.

352. Rom WN, Vijayan VK, Cornelius MJ, et al. Persistent lower respiratory tract inflammation associated with interstitial lung disease in patients with tropical pulmonary eosinophilia following conventional treatment with diethylcarbamazine. Am Rev Respir Dis 1990;142:1088–92.

353. Sandhu M, Mukhopadhyay S, Sharma SK. Tropical pulmonary eosinophilia: a comparative evaluation of plain chest radiography and computed tomography. Australas Radiol 1996;40:32–7.

354. Rohatgi PK, Smirniotopoulos TT. Tropical eosinophilia. Semin Respir Med 1991;12:98–106.

355. Ray D, Saha K. Serum immunoglobulin and complement levels in tropical pulmonary eosinophilia, and their correlation with primary and relapsing stages of the illness. Am J Trop Med Hyg 1978;27:503–7.

356. Nutman TB, Vijayan VK, Pinkston P, et al. Tropical pulmonary eosinophilia: analysis of antifilarial antibody localized to the lung. J Infect Dis 1989;160:1042–50.

357. Pinkston P, Vijayan VK, Nutman TB, et al. Acute tropical pulmonary eosinophilia. Characterization of the lower respiratory tract inflammation and its response to therapy. J Clin Invest 1987;80:216–25.

358. Vijayan VK, Kuppu Rao KV, Sankaran K, et al. Tropical eosinophilia: clinical and physiological response to diethylcarbamazine. Respir Med 1991;85:17–20.

359. Vijayan VK, Sankaran K, Venkatesan P, et al. Effect of diethylcarbamazine on the alveolitis of tropical eosinophilia. Respiration 1991;58:255–9.

360. Dreyer G, Noroes J, Rocha A, et al. Detection of living adult *Wuchereria bancrofti* in a patient with tropical pulmonary eosinophilia. Braz J Med Biol Res 1996;29:1005–8.

361. Anupindi L, Sahoo R, Rao RV, et al. Microfilariae in bronchial brushing cytology of symptomatic pulmonary lesions. A report of two cases. Acta Cytol 1991;37:397–9.

362. Poh SC. The course of lung function in treated tropical pulmonary eosinophilia. Thorax 1974;29:710–2.

363. Vijayan VK, Kuppuraou KV, Venkatesan P, et al. Pulmonary membrane diffusing capacity and capillary blood volume in tropical eosinophilia. Chest 1990;97:1386–9.

364. Neva FA, Ottesen EA. Tropical (filarial) eosinophilia. N Engl J Med 1978;298:1129–31.

365. Cooray JH, Ismail MM. Re-examination of the diagnostic criteria of tropical pulmonary eosinophilia. Respir Med 1999;93:655–9.

366. Salata RA. Intestinal nematodes. In: Mahmoud AAF, editor. Parasitic lung diseases. New-York: Marcel Dekker; 1997. p. 89–108.

367. Rexroth G, Keller C. Chronischer Verlauf einer eosinophilen Pneumonie bei Infektion mit *Ascaris lumbricoides*. Pneumologie 1995;49:77–83.

368. Khuroo MS. Ascariasis. Gastroenterol Clin North Am 1996; 25:553–77.

369. Sarinas PS, Chitkara RK. Ascariasis and hookworm. Semin Respir Infect 1997;12:130–7.

370. Gelpi AP, Mustafa A. Ascaris pneumonia. Am J Med 1968; 44:377–89.

371. Proffitt RD, Walton BC. Ascaris pneumonia in a two-year-old girl. N Engl J Med 1962;266:931–4.

372. Barrett-Connor E. Parasitic pulmonary disease. Am Rev Respir Dis 1982;126:558–63.

373. Piggott J, Hansbarger EA, Neafie RC. Human ascariasis. Am J Clin Pathol 1970;53:223–34.

374. Phills JA, Harold AJ, Whiteman GV, et al. Pulmonary infiltrates asthma and eosinophilia due to *Ascaris suum* infestation in man. N Engl J Med 1972;286:965–70.

375. Kazura JW. Visceral larva migrans and other tissue nematodes. In: Mahmoud AAF, editor. Parasitic lung diseases. New-York: Marcel Dekker; 1997. p. 125–33.

376. Schantz PM, Glickman LT. Current concepts in parasitology. Toxocaral visceral larva migrans. N Engl J Med 1978;298: 436–9.

377. Beaver PC, Snyder CH, Carrera GM, et al. Chronic eosinophilia due to visceral larva migrans. Report of three cases. Pediatrics 1952;9:7–19.

378. Huntley CC, Costas MC, Lyerly A. Visceral larva migrans syndrome: clinical characteristics and immunologic studies in 51 patients. Pediatrics 1965;36:523–36.

379. Beshear JR, Hendley JO. Severe pulmonary involvement in visceral larva migrans. Am J Dis Child 1973;125:599–600.

380. Roig J, Romeu J, Riera C, et al. Acute eosinophilic pneumonia due to toxocariasis with bronchoalveolar lavage findings. Chest 1992;102:294–6.

381. Schinkewitch P, Kessler R, Candolfi E, et al. Insuffisance respiratoire aiguë au cours d'une pneumopathie à éosinophiles parasitaire. Rev Mal Respir 1997;14:61–3.

382. Bouchard O, Arbib F, Paramelle B, et al. Pneumopathie éosinophilique aigue et syndrome de *larva migrans*. A propos d'un cas chez un adulte. Rev Mal Respir 1994;11:593–5.

383. Feldman GJ, Worth Parker H. Visceral larva migrans associated with the hypereosinophilic syndrome and the onset of severe asthma. Ann Intern Med 1992;116:838–42.

384. Bartelink AK, Kortbeek LM, Huidekoper HJ, et al. Acute respiratory failure due to toxocara infection. Lancet 1993; 342:1234.

385. Jacquier P, Gottstein B, Stingelin Y, et al. Immunodiagnosis of toxocarosis in humans: evaluation of a new enzyme-linked immunosorbent assay kit. J Clin Microbiol 1991;29: 1831–5.

386. Aragane K, Akao N, Matsuyama T, et al. Fever, cough, and nodules on ankles. Lancet 1999;354:1872.

387. Iwai K, Mori T, Yamada N, et al. Idiopathic pulmonary fibrosis. Epidemiologic approaches to occupational exposure. Am J Respir Crit Care Med 1994;150:670–5.

388. Igra-Siegman Y, Kapila R, Sen P, et al. Syndrome of hyperinfection with *Strongyloides stercoralis*. Rev Infect Dis 1981; 3:397–407.

389. Liu LX, Weller PF. Strongyloidiasis and other intestinal nematode infections. Infect Dis Clin North Am 1993;7:655–82.

390. Davidson RA. Infection due to *Strongyloides stercoralis* in patients with pulmonary disease. South Med J 1992;85:28–31.

391. Berk SL, Verghese A, Alvarez S, et al. Clinical and epidermiologic features of strongyloidiasis. A prospective study in rural Tennessee. Arch Intern Med 1987;147:1257–61.

392. Chu E, Whitlock W, Dietrich R. Pulmonary hyperinfection syndrome with *Strongyloides stercoralis*. Chest 1990;97:1475–7.

393. Williams J, Nunley D, Dralle W, et al. Diagnosis of pulmonary strongyloïdiasis by bronchoalveolar lavage. Chest 1988; 94:643–4.

394. Higenbottam TW, Heard BE. Opportunistic pulmonary strongyloidiasis complicating asthma treated with steroids. Thorax 1976;31:226–33.

395. Woodring JH, Halfhill H, Reed JC. Pulmonary strongyloidiasis: clinical and imaging features. AJR Am J Roentgenol 1994;162:537–42.

396. Miguérès J, Cantegril A, Séguéla JP, et al. Syndrome de Löffler dû à strongyloïde stercoralis (anguillulose). Rev Med Toulouse 1972;8:245–53.

397. Milder JE, Walzer PD, Kilgore G, et al. Clinical features of *Strongyloides stercoralis* infection in an endemic area of the United States. Gastroenterology 1981;80:1481–8.

398. Scowden EB, Schaffner W, Stone WJ. Overwhelming strongyloidiasis. An unappreciated opportunistic infection. Medicine 1978;57:527–44.

399. Makris AN, Sher S, Bertoli C, et al. Pulmonary strongyloidiasis: an unusual opportunistic pneumonia in a patient with AIDS. AJR Am J Roentgenol 1993;161:545–7.

400. Morgan JS, Schaffner W, Stone WJ. Opportunistic strongyloidiasis in renal transplant recipients. Transplantation 1986;42:518–24.

401. Jamil SA, Hilton E. The strongyloides hyperinfection syndrome. N Y State J Med 1992;92:67–8.

402. Harris RA, Musher DM, Fainstein V, et al. Disseminated strongyloidiasis. Diagnosis made by sputum examination. JAMA 1980;244:65–6.

403. Gage JG. A case of strongyloides intestinalis with larvae in the sputum. Arch Intern Med 1911;6:561–79.

404. Smith B, Verghese A, Guiterrez C, et al. Pulmonary strongyloidiasis. Diagnosis by sputum gram stain. Am J Med 1985;79:663–6.

405. Schainberg L, Scheinberg MA. Recovery of *Strongyloides stercoralis* by bronchoalveolar lavage in a patient with acquired immunodeficiency syndrome. Am J Med 1989;87:486.

406. Rassiga AL, Lowry JL, Forman WB. Diffuse pulmonary infection due to *Strongyloides stercoralis*. JAMA 1974;230:426–7.

407. Salata RA. Approach to diagnosis and management. In: Mahmoud AAF, editor. Parasitic lung diseases. New-York: Marcel Dekker; 1997. p. 191–210.

408. Wehner JH, Kirsch CM. Pulmonary manifestations of strongyloidiasis. Semin Respir Infect 1997;12:122–9.

409. Wright DO, Gold EM. Löffler's syndrome associated with creeping eruption (cutaneous helminthiasis): report of twenty-six cases. Arch Intern Med 1946;78:303–12.

410. Ambrus JL, Klein E. Löffler syndrome and *Ancylostomiasis brasiliensis*. N Y State J Med 1988;88:498–9.

411. King CL. Schistosomiasis. In: Mahmoud AAF, editor. Parasitic lung diseases. New-York: Marcel Dekker; 1997. p. 135–55.

412. Schwartz E, Rozenman J, Perelman M. Pulmonary manifestations of early schistosome infection among nonimmune travelers. Am J Med 2000;109:718–22.

413. Davidson BL, El-Kassimi F, Uz-Zaman A, et al. The "lung shift" in treated schistosomiasis. Bronchoalveolar lavage evidence of eosinophilic pneumonia. Chest 1986;89:455–7.

414. Robinson NB, Chavez CM, Conn JH. Pulmonary dirofilariasis in man. A case report and review of the literature. J Thorac Cardiovasc Surg 1977;74:403–8.

415. Asimacopoulos PJ, Katras A, Christie B. Pulmonary dirofilariasis.The largest single-hospital experience. Chest 1992;102:851–5.

416. Ciferri F. Human pulmonary dirofilariasis in the United States: a critical review. Am J Trop Med Hyg 1982;31:302–8.

417. Kido A, Ishida T, Oka T, et al. Pulmonary dirofilariasis causing a solitary lung mass and pleural effusion. Thorax 1991;46:608–9.

418. Gershwin LJ, Gershwin ME, Kritzman J. Human pulmonary dirofilariasis. Chest 1974;66:92–6.

419. Im JG, Whang HY, Kim WS, et al. Pleuropulmonary paragonimiasis: radiologic findings in 71 patients. AJR Am J Roentgenol 1992;159:39–43.

420. Johnson JR, Falk A, Iber C, et al. Paragonimiasis in the United States. A report of nine cases in hmong immigrants. Chest 1982;82:168–71.

421. Johnson RJ, Johnson JR. Paragonimiasis in Indochinese refugees. Roentgenographic findings with clinical correlations. Am Rev Respir Dis 1983;128:534–8.

422. El Kamel A, Rouetbi N, Chakroun M, et al. Pulmonary eosinophilia due to *Trichomonas tenax*. Thorax 1996;51:554–5.

423. Pirisi M, Gutierrez Y, Minini C, et al. Fatal human pulmonary infection caused by an *Angiostrongylus*-like nematode. Clin Infect Dis 1995;20:59–65.

424. Morel L, Delaude A, Girard M, et al. Infiltrats pulmonaires éosinophiliques au cours de filarioses de type Loa-Loa. Poumon Coeur 1967;23:685–94.

425. Slowey JF. A case of transient successive pulmonary infiltrations (Loeffler's syndrome) associated with trichiniasis. Ann Intern Med 1944;21:130–5.

426. Aftandelians R, Raafat F, Taffazoli M, et al. Pulmonary capillariasis in a child in Iran. Am J Trop Med Hyg 1977;26:64–71.

427. Coudert J, Despeignes J, Battesti MR. A propos d'un cas de capillariose pulmonaire. Bull Soc Pathol Exot Filiales 1972;65:841–8.

428. Li LY, Xue CS, Luo WC. Clinical analysis of 90 cases of eosinophilia and pulmonary infiltrates with peripheral eosinophilia. Zhonghua Nei Ke Za Zhi 1990;29:659–62.

429. Bayer AS. Fungal pneumonias; pulmonary coccidioidal syndromes (part 1). Primary and progressive primary coccidioidal pneumonias—diagnostic, therapeutic, and prognostic considerations. Chest 1981;79:575–83.

430. Bayer AS. Fungal pneumonias: pulmonary coccidioidal syndromes (part 2). Miliary, nodular, and cavitary coccidioidomycocis; chemotherapeutic and surgical considerations. Chest 1981;79:686–91.

431. Drutz DJ, Catanzaro A. Coccidioidomycosis (part I). Am Rev Respir Dis 1978;117:559–85.

432. Drutz DJ, Catanzaro A. Coccidioidomycosis (part II). Am Rev Respir Dis 1978;117:727–71.

433. Echols RM, Palmer DL, Long GW. Tissue eosinophilia in human coccidioidomycosis. Rev Infect Dis 1982;4:656–64.

434. Lombard CM, Tazelaar HD, Krasne DL. Pulmonary eosinophilia in coccidioidal infections. Chest 1987;91:734–6.

435. Jacobs SE, Whitlock WL, Dietrich RA. Pulmonary infiltrates, eosinophilia, and facial skin nodule. Chest 1990;97:476–8.

436. Whitlock WL, Dietrich RA, Tenholder MF. Acute eosinophilic pneumonia. N Engl J Med 1990;322:635.

437. Flanagan KL, Bryceson ADM. Disseminated infection due to *Bipolaris australiensis* in a young immunocompetent man: case report and review. Clin Infect Dis 1997;25:311–3.

438. Karim M, Sheikh H, Alam R, et al. Disseminated *Bipolaris* infection in an asthmatic patient: case report. Clin Infect Dis 1993;17:248–53.

439. Fleury-Feith J, Van Nhieu J, Picard C, et al. Bronchoalveolar lavage eosinophilia associated with *Pneumocystis carinii* pneumonitis in AIDS patients. Chest 1989;95:1198–201.

440. Llibre JM, Tor J, Milla F. Acute eosinophilic pneumonia. N Engl J Med 1990;322:634–6.

441. Travis WD, Pittaluga S, Lipschik GY, et al. Atypical pathologic manifestations of *Pneumocystis carinii* pneumonia in the acquired immune deficiency syndrome. Review of 123 lungs biopsies from 76 patients with emphasis on cysts, vascular invasion, vasculitis, and granulomas. Am J Surg Pathol 1990;14:615–25.

442. Jose DG, Gatti RA, Good RA. Eosinophilia with *Pneumocystis carinii* pneumonia and immune deficiency syndromes. J Pediatr 1971;79:748–54.

443. Keslin MH, McCoy EL, McCusker JJ, et al. *Corynebacterium pseudotuberculosis*. A new cause of infectious and eosinophilic pneumonia. Am J Med 1979;67:228–31.

444. Wright JL, Pare PD, Hammond M, et al. Eosinophilic pneumonia and atypical mycobacterial infection. Am Rev Respir Dis 1983;127:497–9.

445. Vijayan VK, Reetha AM, Jawahar MS, et al. Pulmonary eosinophilia in pulmonary tuberculosis. Chest 1992;101:1708–9.

446. Elsom KA, Ingelfinger FJ. Eosinophilia and pneumonitis in chronic brucellosis; a report of two cases. Ann Intern Med 1942;16:995–1002.

447. Addis B. Pulmonary mycotic disease. In: Hasleton PS, editor: Spencer's pathology of the lung. New-York: McGraw-Hill; 1996. p. 257–304.

448. Chandler FW, Watts JC. Fungal infections. In: Dail DH, Hammar SP, editors. Pulmonary pathology. New-York: Springer-Verlag; 1994. p. 351–427.

449. Corrin B. Fungal diseases. In: Corrin B, editor. The lungs. London: Churchill Livingstone; 1990. p. 125–45.

450. Marty AM, Neafie RC. Fungal diseases. In: Saldana MJ, editor. Pathology of pulmonary disease. Philadelphia: J.B. Lippincott Company; 1994. p. 477–87.

451. Sobonya RE. Fungal diseases, including allergic bronchopulmonary aspergillosis. In: Thurlbeck WM, Churg AM, editors. Pathology of the lung. 1995; New-York: Thieme Medical; 1995. p. 303–31.

452. Kauffman HF, Tomee JF, van der Werf TS, et al. Review of fungus-induced asthmatic reactions. Am J Respir Crit Care Med 1995;151:2109–16.

453. Caballero T, Ferrer A, Diaz-Pena JM, et al. Childhood allergic bronchopulmonary aspergillosis. J Allergy Clin Immunol 1995;95:1044–7.

454. Wardlaw A, Geddes DM. Allergic bronchopulmonary aspergillosis: a review. J R Soc Med 1992;85:747–51.

455. Mroueh S, Spock A. Allergic bronchopulmonary aspergillosis in patients with cystic fibrosis. Chest 1994;105:32–6.

456. Geller DE, Kaplowitz H, Light MJ, et al. Allergic bron-

chopulmonary aspergillosis in cystic fibrosis: reported prevalence, regional distribution, and patient characteristics. Scientific Advisory Group, Investigators, and Coordinators of the Epidemiologic Study of Cystic Fibrosis. Chest 1999;116:639–46.

457. Shah A, Khan ZU, Chaturvedi S, et al. Concomitant allergic *Aspergillus* sinusitis and allergic bronchopulmonary aspergillosis associated with familial occurrence of allergic bronchopulmonary aspergillosis. Ann Allergy 1990;64: 507–12.

458. Shah A, Bhagat R, Panchal N, et al. Allergic bronchopulmonary aspergillosis with middle lobe syndrome and allergic *Aspergillus* sinusitis. Eur Respir J 1993;6:917–8.

459. Marple BF. Allergic fungal rhinosinusitis: current theories and management strategies. Laryngoscope 2001;111:1006–19.

460. Ponikau JU, Sherris DA, Kern EB, et al. The diagnosis and incidence of allergic fungal sinusitis. Mayo Clin Proc 1999;74:877–84.

461. Torres C, Ro JY, el-Naggar AK, et al. Allergic fungal sinusitis: a clinicopathologic study of 16 cases. Hum Pathol 1996;27:793–9.

462. Khan DA, Cody DT, George TJ, et al. Allergic fungal sinusitis: an immunohistologic analysis. J Allergy Clin Immunol 2000;106:1096–101.

463. Schubert MS, Goetz DW. Evaluation and treatment of allergic fungal sinusitis. I. Demographics and diagnosis. J Allergy Clin Immunol 1998;102:387–94.

464. Schubert MS, Goetz DW. Evaluation and treatment of allergic fungal sinusitis. II. Treatment and follow-up. J Allergy Clin Immunol 1998;102:395–402.

465. Mehta SK, Sandhu RS. Immunological significance of *Aspergillus fumigatus* in cane-sugar mills. Arch Environ Health 1983;38:41–6.

466. Patterson R, Grammer LC. Immunopathogenesis of allergic bronchopulmonary aspergillosis. In: Patterson R, Greenberger PA, Roberts ML, editors. Allergic bronchopulmonary aspergillosis. Providence (RI): OceanSide Publications Inc; 1995. p. 35–8.

467. Malo JL, Hawkins R, Pepys J. Studies in chronic allergic bronchopulmonary aspergillosis. 1. Clinical and physiological findings. Thorax 1977;32:254–61.

468. Rosenberg M, Patterson R, Mintzer R, et al. Clinical and immunologic criteria for the diagnosis of allergic bronchopulmonary aspergillosis. Ann Intern Med 1977;86: 405–14.

469. Patterson R, Greenberger PA, Roberts M. The diagnosis of allergic bronchopulmonary aspergillosis. In: Patterson R, Greenberger PA, Roberts ML, editors. Allergic bronchopulmonary aspergillosis. Providence (RI): OceanSide Publications Inc; 1995. p. 1–3.

470. Patterson R, Greenberger PA, Radin RC, et al. Allergic bronchopulmonary aspergillosis: staging as an aid to management. Ann Intern Med 1982;96:286–91.

471. Patterson R, Roberts M. Classification and staging of allergic bronchopulmonary aspergillosis. In: Patterson R, Greenberger PA, Roberts ML, editors. Allergic bronchopulmonary aspergillosis. Providence (RI): OceanSide Publications Inc; 1995. p. 5–10.

472. Glancy JJ, Elder JL, McAleer R. Allergic bronchopulmonary fungal disease without clinical asthma. Thorax 1981; 36:345–9.

473. Hoshino H, Tagaki S, Kon H, et al. Allergic bronchopulmonary aspergillosis due to *Aspergillus niger* without bronchial asthma. Respiration 1999;66:369–72.

474. Bosken C, Myers J, Greenberger P, et al. Pathologic features of allergic bronchopulmonary aspergillosis. Am J Surg Pathol 1988;12:216–22.

475. Malo JL, Pepys J, Simon G. Studies in chronic allergic bronchopulmonary aspergillosis. 2. Radiological findings. Thorax 1977;32:262–8.

476. Malo JL, Longbottom J, Mitchell J, et al. Studies in chronic allergic bronchopulmonary aspergillosis. 3. Immunological findings. Thorax 1977;32:269–74.

477. Malo JL, Inouye T, Hawkins R, et al. Studies in chronic allergic bronchopulmonary aspergillosis. 4. Comparison with a group of asthmatics. Thorax 1977;32:275–80.

478. McCarthy DS. Bronchiectasis in allergic bronchopulmonary aspergillosis. Proc R Soc Med 1968;61:503–6.

479. Chan-Yeung M, Chase WH, Trapp W, et al. Allergic bronchopulmonary aspergillosis. Clinical and pathologic study of three cases. Chest 1971;59:33–9.

480. Neeld DA, Goodman LR, Gurney JW, et al. Computerized tomography in the evaluation of allergic bronchopulmonary aspergillosis. Am Rev Respir Dis 1990;142:1200–5.

481. Panchal N, Bhagat R, Pant C, et al. Allergic bronchopulmonary aspergillosis: the spectrum of computed tomography appearances. Respir Med 1997;91:213–9.

482. Angus RM, Davies ML, Cowan MD, et al. Computed tomographic scanning of the lung in patients with allergic bronchopulmonary aspergillosis and in asthmatic patients with a positive skin test to *Aspergillus fumigatus*. Thorax 1994;49:586–9.

483. Bain GA, Flower CDR. Pulmonary eosinophilia. Eur J Radiol 1996;23:3–8.

484. Kumar R, Gaur SN. Prevalence of allergic bronchopulmonary aspergillosis in patients with bronchial asthma. Asian Pac J Allergy Immunol 2000;18:181–5.

485. Ward S, Heyneman L, Lee MJ, et al. Accuracy of CT in the diagnosis of allergic bronchopulmonary aspergillosis in asthmatic patients. AJR Am J Roentgenol 1999;173:937–42.

486. Eaton T, Garrett J, Milne D, et al. Allergic bronchopulmonary aspergillosis in the asthma clinic. A prospective evaluation of CT in the diagnostic algorithm. Chest 2000;118:66–72.

487. Myers JL. Pathology of allergic bronchopulmonary aspergillosis. In: Patterson R, Greenberger PA, Roberts ML. Allergic bronchopulmonary aspergillosis. Providence (RI): OceanSide Publications Inc; 1995. p. 39–46.

488. McCarthy DS, Simon G, Hargreave FE. The radiological appearances in allergic bronchopulmonary aspergillosis. Clin Radiol 1970;21:366–75.

489. Urschel HC, Paulson DL, Chaw RR. Mucoid impaction of the bronchi. Ann Thorac Surg 1966;2:1–16.

490. Slavin RG, Bedrossian CW, Hutcheson BA, et al. A pathologic study of allergic bronchopulmonary aspergillosis. J Allergy Clin Immunol 1988;81:718–25.

491. Warnock ML, Fennessy J, Rippon J. Chronic eosinophilic pneumonia, a manifestation of allergic aspergillosis. Am J Clin Pathol 1974;62:73–81.

492. Kauffman HF, Koeter GH, van der Heide S, et al. Cellular and humoral observations in a patient with allergic bronchopulmonary aspergillosis during a nonasthmatic exacerbation. J Allergy Clin Immunol 1989;83:829–38.

493. Case Records of the Massachusetts General Hospital. Case 24-2001. N Engl J Med 2001;345:443–9.

494. Meeker DP, Gephardt GN, Cordasco EM Jr, et al. Hypersensitivity pneumonitis versus invasive pulmonary aspergillosis: two cases with unusual pathologic findings and review of the literature. Am Rev Respir Dis 1991;143:431–6.

495. Ricker DH, Taylor SR, Gartner JC, et al. Fatal pulmonary aspergillosis presenting as acute eosinophilic pneumonia in previously healthy child. Chest 1991;100:875–7.

496. Mendelson EB, Fisher MR, Mintzer RA, et al. Roentgenographic and clinical staging of allergic bronchopulmonary aspergillosis. Chest 1985;87:334–9.

497. Hinson KFW, Moon AJ, Plummer NS. Bronchopulmonary aspergillosis. A review and report of eight new cases. Thorax 1952;7:317–33.

498. Gefter WB, Epstein DM, Miller WT. Allergic bronchopulmonary aspergillosis: less common patterns. Radiology 1981;140:307–12.

499. Chapman BJ, Capewell S, Gibson R, et al. Pulmonary eosinophilia with and without allergic bronchopulmonary aspergillosis. Thorax 1989;44:919–24.

500. Sider L. Radiology of ABPA. In: Patterson R, Greenberger PA, Roberts ML, editors. Allergic bronchopulmonary aspergillosis. Providence (RI): OceanSide Publications Inc; 1995. p. 17–24.

501. Torrington KG, McEvoy PL. A middle-aged woman with chronic productive cough diagnosed using sputum wet mount examination. Chest 1998;113:1411–4.

502. Mintzer RA, Rogers LF, Kruglik GD, et al. The spectrum of radiologic findings in ABPA. Radiology 1978;127:301–7.

503. Sulavik S. Bronchocentric granulomatosis and allergic bronchopulmonary aspergillosis. Clin Chest Med 1988;9:609–21.

504. Cote CG, Cicchelli R, Hassoun PM. Hemoptysis and a lung mass in a 51-year-old patient with asthma. Chest 1998;114:1465–8.

505. Greenberger PA. Allergic fungal sinusitis. In: Patterson R, Greenberger PA, Roberts ML, editors. Allergic bronchopulmonary aspergillosis. Providence (RI): OceanSide Publications Inc; 1995. p. 53–9.

506. Patterson R, Greenberger PA, Lee TM, et al. Prolonged evaluation of patients with corticosteroid-dependent asthma stage of allergic bronchopulmonary aspergillosis. J Allergy Clin Immunol 1987;80:663–8.

507. Seaton A, Seaton RA, Wightman AJA. Management of allergic bronchopulmonary aspergillosis without maintenance oral corticosteroids: a fifteen-year follow-up. QJM 1994;87:529–37.

508. Balter MS, Rebuck AS. Treatment of allergic bronchopulmonary aspergillosis with inhaled corticosteroids. Respir Med 1992;86:441–2.

509. Denning DW, Van Wye JE, Lewiston NJ, et al. Adjunctive therapy of allergic bronchopulmonary aspergillosis with itraconazole. Chest 1991;100:813–9.

510. Mannes GPM, van der Heide S, Van Aalderen WMC, et al. Itraconazole and allergic bronchopulmonary aspergillosis in twin brothers with cystic fibrosis. Lancet 1993;341:492.

511. Wark PA, Gibson PG. Allergic bronchopulmonary aspergillosis: new concepts of pathogenesis and treatment. Respirology 2001;6:1–7.

512. Salez F, Brichet A, Desurmont S, et al. Effects of itraconazole therapy in allergic bronchopulmonary aspergillosis. Chest 1999;116:1665–8.

513. Nikaido Y, Nagata N, Yamamoto T, et al. A case of allergic bronchopulmonary aspergillosis successfully treated with itraconazole. Respir Med 1998;92:118–9.

514. Stevens DA, Schwartz HJ, Lee JY, et al. A randomized trial of itraconazole in allergic bronchopulmonary aspergillosis. N Engl J Med 2000;342:756–62.

515. Beth Hogan M. Other allergic bronchopulmonary mycoses. In: Patterson R, Greenberger PA, Roberts ML, editors. Allergic bronchopulmonary aspergillosis. Providence (RI): OceanSide Publications Inc; 1995. p. 57–9.

516. Miller MA, Greenberger PA, Amerian R, et al. Allergic bronchopulmonary mycosis caused by *Pseudallescheria boydii*. Am Rev Respir Dis 1993;148:810–2.

517. Moreno-Ancillo A, Diaz-Pena JM, Ferrer A, et al. Allergic bronchopulmonary cladosporiosis in a child. J Allergy Clin Immunol 1996;97:714–5.

518. Pinson P, Van der Straeten M. Fibrotic stage of allergic bronchopulmonary candidiasis. Chest 1991;100:565–7.

519. Akiyama K, Mathison DA, Riker JB, et al. Allergic bronchopulmonary candidiasis. Chest 1984;85:699–701.

520. Pepys J, Faux JA, Longbottom JL, et al. *Candida albicans* precipitins in respiratory disease in man. J Allergy 1968; 41:305–18.

521. Lee TM, Greenberger PA, Oh S, et al. Allergic bronchopulmonary candidiasis: case report and suggested diagnostic criteria. J Allergy Clin Immunol 1987;80:816–20.

522. Benatar SR, Allan B, Hewitson RP, et al. Allergic bronchopulmonary stemphyliosis. Thorax 1980;35:515–8.

523. McAleer R, Kroenert DB, Elder JL, et al. Allergic bronchopulmonary disease caused by *Curvularia lunata* and *Drechslera hawaiiensis*. Thorax 1981;36:338–44.

524. Saenz RE, Brown WD, Sanders CV. Allergic bronchopulmonary disease caused by *Bipolaris hawaiiensis* presenting as a necrotizing pneumonia: case report and review of literature. Am J Med Sci 2001;321:209–12.

525. Hendrick DJ, Ellithrope DB, Lyon F, et al. Allergic bronchopulmonary helminthosporiosis. Am Rev Respir Dis 1982;126:935–8.

526. Lirsac B, Godard P, Baconnier P, et al. Allergic bronchopulmonary rhizoposis. J Allergy Clin Immunol 1986;77:167.

527. Miyazaki E, Sugisaki K, Shigenaga T, et al. A case of acute eosinophilic pneumonia caused by inhalation of *Trichosporon terrestre*. Am J Respir Crit Care Med 1995;151:541–3.

528. Saini SK, Boas SR, Jerath A, et al. Allergic bronchopulmonary mycosis to *Fusarium vasinfectum* in a child. Ann Allergy Asthma Immunol 1998;80:377–80.

529. Backman KS, Roberts M, Patterson R. Allergic bronchopulmonary mycosis caused by *Fusarium vasinfectum*. Am J Respir Crit Care Med 1995;152:1379–81.

530. Halloran TJ. Allergic bronchopulmonary helminthosporiosis. Am Rev Respir Dis 1983;128:578.

531. Matthiesson AM. Allergic bronchopulmonary disease caused by fungi other than aspergillus. Thorax 1981;36:719–20.

532. Dolan CT, Weed LA, Dines DE. Bronchopulmonary helminthosporiosis. Am J Clin Pathol 1970;53:235–42.

533. Lake FR, Tribe AE, McAleer R, et al. Mixed allergic bronchopulmonary fungal disease due to *Pseudallescheria boydii* and *Aspergillus*. Thorax 1990;45:489–91.

534. Pacheco A, Cuevas M, Carbelo B, et al. Eosinophilic lung disease associated with *Candida albicans* allergy. Eur Respir J 1998;12:502–4.

535. Liebow AA. Pulmonary angiitis and granulomatosis. Am Rev Respir Dis 1973;108:1–18.

536. Meghjee S, Campbell A, Greenstone MA. Multiple cavitating nodules in a patient with hemoptysis. Chest 1999;115:1184–7.

537. Katzenstein AL, Liebow AA, Friedmann PJ. Bronchocentric granulomatosis, mucoid impaction and hypersensitivity reaction to fungi. Am Rev Respir Dis 1975;111:497–537.

538. Robinson RG, Wehnut WD, Tsou E, et al. Bronchocentric granulomatosis. Roentgenographic manifestations. Am Rev Respir Dis 1982;125:751–6.

539. Ward S, Heyneman LE, Flint JD, et al. Bronchocentric granulomatosis: computed tomographic findings in five patients. Clin Radiol 2000;55:296–300.

540. Myers JL. Bronchocentric granulomatosis. Disease or diagnosis? Chest 1989;96:3–4.

541. Tazelaar HD, Baird AM, Mill M, et al. Bronchocentric mycosis occurring in transplant recipients. Chest 1989;96:92–5.

542. Lee JH, Joihovsky T, Yan K. Bronchocentric granulomatosis: review of 14 patients. Thorax 1982;37:779.

543. Myers JL, Katzenstein AL. Granulomatous infection mimicking bronchocentric granulomatosis. Am J Surg Pathol 1986;10:317–22.

544. Foucher P, Biour M, Blayac JP, et al. Drugs that may injure the respiratory system. Eur Respir J 1997;10:265–79.

545. Mayock RL, Iozzo RV. The eosinophilic pneumonias. In: Fishman AP, editor. Pulmonary diseases and disorders. New York: McGraw Hill; 1988. p. 683–8.

546. Schatz M, Wasserman S, Patterson R. Eosinophils and immunologic lung disease. Med Clin North Am 1981;65:1055–71.

547. Schatz PH, Mesologites D, Hyun J, et al. Captopril-induced hypersensitivity lung disease. Chest 1989;95:685–7.

548. Khalil H, Molinary E, Stoller JK. Diclofenac (Voltaren)-induced eosinophilic pneumonitis. Arch Intern Med 1993;153:1649–52.

549. Wong PC, Yew WW, Wong CF, et al. Ethambutol-induced pulmonary infiltrates with eosinophilia and skin involvement. Eur Respir J 1995;8:866–8.

550. Burton GH. Rash and pulmonary eosinophilia associated with fenbufen. BMJ 1990;300:82–3.

551. Donhuijsen K, Haedicke C, Hattenberger S, et al. Granulocyte-macrophage colony–stimulating factor-related eosinophilia and Loeffler's endocarditis. Blood 1992;79:2798.

552. Seebach J, Speich R, Fehr J, et al. GM-CSF-induced acute eosinophilic pneumonia. Br J Haematol 1995;90:963–5.

553. Goodwin SD, Glenny RW. Nonsteroidal anti-inflammatory drug-associated pulmonary infiltrates with eosinophilia. Arch Intern Med 1992;152:1521–4.

554. Banner AS, Borochovitz D. Acute respiratory failure caused by pulmonary vasculitis after L-tryptophan ingestion. Am Rev Respir Dis 1991;143:661–4.

555. Campagna AC, Blanc PD, Criswell LA, et al. Pulmonary manifestations of the eosinophilia-myalgia syndrome associated with tryptophan ingestion. Chest 1992;101:1274–81.

556. Dussopt C, Mornex JF, Cordier JF, et al. Poumon éosinophile aigu après prise de minocycline. Rev Fr Mal Respir 1994; 11:67–70.

557. Otero M, Goodpasture H. Pulmonary infiltrates and eosinophilia from minocycline. JAMA 1983;250:2602.

558. Sitbon O, Bidel N, Dussopt C, et al. Minocycline pneumonitis and eosinophilia. A report on eight patients. Arch Intern Med 1994;154:1633–40.

559. Dykhuizen RS, Zaidi AM, Godden DJ, et al. Minocycline and pulmonary eosinophilia. BMJ 1995;310:1520–1.

560. Dykhuizen RS, Legge JS. Minocycline induced pulmonary eosinophilia. Respir Med 1995;89:61–2.

561. Yamaguchi S, Okubo Y, Hossain M, et al. IL–5 predominant in bronchoalveolar lavage fluid and peripheral blood in a patient with acute eosinophilic pneumonia. Intern Med 1995;34:65–8.

562. Kaufmann D, Pichler W, Beer JH. Severe episode of high fever with rash, lymphadenopathy, neutropenia, and eosinophilia after minocycline therapy for acne. Arch Intern Med 1994;154:1983–4.

563. Toyoshima M, Sato A, Hayakawa H, et al. A clinical study of minocycline-induced pneumonitis. Intern Med 1996; 35:176–9.

564. Cellerin L, Canfrere I, Ordronneau J, et al. Pneumopathie aiguë à éosinophiles induite par la minocycline. Rev Pneumol Clin 1994;50:325–8.

565. Dupont C, Rouveix E, Chinet T, et al. Syndrome de Löffler chez une patiente traitée par la minocycline. Ann Med Interne (Paris) 1993;144:76.

566. Marlier S, Carsuzaa F, Vauterin G. Poumon éosinophilique aigu au cours d'un traitement par minocycline. Presse Med 1996;25:1801.

567. Liegeon MN, de Blay F, Jaeger A, et al. Une cause de détresse respiratoire: la pneumopathie à éosinophiles de la minocycline. Rev Mal Respir 1996;13:517–9.

568. Bando T, Fujimura M, Noda Y, et al. Minocycline-induced pneumonitis with bilateral hilar lymphadenopathy and pleural effusion. Intern Med 1994;33:177–9.

569. Buscaglia AJ, Cowden FE, Brill H. Pulmonary infiltrates associated with naproxen. JAMA 1984;251:65–6.

570. Camus P, Piard F, Ashcroft T, et al. The lung in inflammatory bowel disease. Medicine 1993;72:151–83.

571. Simpson D, Walker J. Hypersensitivity to para-aminosalicylic acid. Am J Med 1960;29:297–306.

572. Reichlin S, Loveless M, Kane E. Loeffler's syndrome following penicillin therapy. Ann Intern Med 1953;38:113–20.

573. Falk MS, Newcomer VD. Loeffler's syndrome. Occurence in two patients with penicillin in oil and wax. JAMA 1949; 141:21–2.

574. Thuston JGB, Marks P, Trapnell D. Lung changes associated with phenylbutazone treatment. BMJ 1976;2:1422–3.

575. Pfitzenmeyer P, Meier M, Zuck P, et al. Piroxicam induced pulmonary infiltrates and eosinophilia. J Rheumatol 1994;21: 1573–7.

576. Begbie S, Burgess K. Maloprim-induced pulmonary eosinophilia. Chest 1993;103:305–6.

577. Fein M. Sulindac and pneumonitis. Ann Intern Med 1981; 95:245.

578. Sprung DJ. Sulindac causing a hypersensitivity reaction with peripheral and mediastinal lymphadenopathy. Ann Intern Med 1982;97:564–5.

579. Donlan CJ, Scutero JV. Transient eosinophilic pneumonia secondary to use of a vaginal cream. Chest 1975;67:232–3.

580. Fiegenberg DS, Weiss H, Kirshman H. Migratory pneumonia with eosinophilia associated with sulfamide administration. Arch Intern Med 1967;120:85–9.

581. Gascard E, Boutin C, Cargnino P, et al. Infiltrat labile provoqué par un sulfamide retard. Marseille Med 1969;106:891–3.

582. Klinghoffer JF. Löffler's syndrome following use of a vaginal cream. Ann Intern Med 1954;40:343–50.

583. Stromberg C, Palva E, Alhavae E. Pulmonary infiltrations induced by tolfenamic acid. Lancet 1987;ii:685.

584. Guerin JC, Chevalier JP, Kofmann J, et al. Pneumopathie interstitielle médicamenteuse après traitement par le cotrimoxazole. Deux observations. Nouv Presse Med 1980;9:2347.

585. Yousem SA, Lifson JD, Colby TV. Chemotherapy-induced eosinophilic pneumonia: relation to bleomycin. Chest 1985;88:103–6.

586. Stephan WC, Parks RD, Tempest B. Acute hypersensitivity pneumonitis associated with carbamazepine therapy. Chest 1978;74:463–4.

587. Shear MK. Chlorpromazine-induced PIE syndrome. Am J Psychiatry 1978;135:492–3.

588. Nadeem S, Nasir N, Israel RH. Loffler's syndrome secondary to crack cocaine. Chest 1994;105:1599–600.

589. Oh PI, Balter MS. Cocaine induced eosinophilic lung disease. Thorax 1992;47:478–9.

590. Anonymous. Respiratory failure and eosinophils in a young man. Am J Med 1993;94:533–42.

591. Kissner DG, Lawrence WD, Selis JE, et al. Crack lung: pulmonary disease caused by cocaine abuse. Am Rev Respir Dis 1987;136:1250–2.

592. Anier M, Guillevin L, Badillet G. Pulmonary eosinophilia associated with dapsone. Lancet 1994;343:860–1.

593. Gali JM, Vilanova JL, Mayo S, et al. Febarbamate induced-pulmonary eosinophilia: a case report. Respiration 1986; 49:231–4.

594. Akoun GM, Cadranel JL, Milleron BJ, et al. Bronchoalveolar lavage cell data in 19 patients with drug-associated pneumonitis (except amiodarone). Chest 1991;99:98–104.

595. Garrell M. Löffler's syndrome. Arch Intern Med 1960;106: 874–7.

596. Brander PE, Tukiainen P. Acute eosinophilic pneumonia in a heroin smoker. Eur Respir J 1993;6:750–2.

597. Wilson IC, Gambill JM, Sandifer MG. Loeffler's syndrome occurring during imipramine therapy. Am J Psychiatry 1963;119:892–3.

598. Perreau P, Fresneau M, Boumard B, et al. L'infiltrat pulmonaire avec éosinophilie au cours du traitement par l'isoniazide. Press Med 1955;63:1454–6.

599. Li T, Doutsu Y, Ashitani Jea. A case of loxoprofen-induced pulmonary eosinophilia. Nihon Kyobu Shikkan Gakkai Zasshi 1992;30:926–9.

600. Watanabe T, Sakata M, Shimabukuro Rea. Loxoprofen: another NSAID associated with acute asthmatic death. Clin Toxicol 1993;31:333–40.

601. Rodman T, Fraimow W, Myerson R. Löffler syndrome: report of a case associated with administration of mephenesin carbamate (tolseram). Ann Intern Med 1958;48:668.

602. White DA, Rankin JA, Stover DE, et al. Methotrexate pneumonitis: BAL findings suggest an immunologic disorder. Am Rev Respir Dis 1989;139:18–21.

603. Wolf J, Fein A, Fehrenbacher L. Eosinophilic syndrome with methylphenidate abuse. Ann Intern Med 1978;89:224–5.

604. Holmberg L, Boman G. Pulmonary reactions to nitrofurantoin. 447 cases reported to the Swedish adverse drug reaction committee 1966–1976. Eur J Respir Dis 1981;62:180–9.

605. Hamm H, Aumiller J, Bohmer R, et al. Alveolitis associated with nomifensine. Lancet 1985;i:1328–9.

606. Dupon M, Malou M, Rogues AM, et al. Acute eosinophilic pneumonia induced by inhaled pentamidine isethionate. BMJ 1993;306:109.

607. Melloni B, Vergnenegre A, Bonnaud F, et al. Pneumopathie induite par le perindopril. A propos d'un cas. Rev Fr Mal Respir 1994;11:308–11.

608. Bayer AS, Targan SR, Pitchon HE, et al. Dilantin toxicity: miliary pulmonary infiltrates and hypoxemia. Ann Intern Med 1976;85:475–6.

609. Michael J, Rudin M. Acute pulmonary disease caused by phenytoin. Ann Intern Med 1981;95:452–4.

610. Munn NJ, Baughman RP, Ploysongsang Y, et al. Bronchoalveolar lavage in acute drug-hypersensitivity pneumonitis probably caused by phenytoin. South Med J 1984;77:1594–5.

611. Williams T, Eidus L, Thomas P. Fibrosing alveolitis, bronchiolitis obliterans and sulfasalasine therapy. Chest 1982; 81:766–8.

612. Wang KK, Bowyer BA, Fleming CR, et al. Pulmonary infiltrates and eosinophilia associated with sulfasalazine. Mayo Clin Proc 1984;59:343–6.

613. Yamakado S, Yoshida Y, Yamada T, et al. Pulmonary infiltration and eosinophilia associated with sulfasalazine therapy for ulcerative colitis: a case report and review of literature. Intern Med 1992;31:108–13.

614. Peters FPJ, Engels LGJB, Moers AMJ. Pneumonitis induced by sulphasalazine. Postgrad Med J 1997;73:99–100.

615. Hatzinger M, Stohler R, Hoslboer-Trachsler E. Eosinophile Pleuritis und Hepatopathie unter Trimipramin-Therapie. Schweiz Med Wochenschr 1991;121:910–2.

616. Darmanata JI, Van Zandwijk N, Duren DR, et al. Amiodarone pneumonitis: three further cases with a review of published reports. Thorax 1984;39:57–64.

617. Poe RH, Condemi JJ, Weinstein SS, et al. Adult respiratory distress syndrome related to ampicillin sensitivity. Chest 1980;77:449–50.

618. Friedman H, Tworag F, Voss H, et al. Eosinophilic pneumonia in association with the use of beclomethasone dipropionate aerosol. J Allergy Clin Immunol 1978;61:150.

619. Ogawa H, Fujimura M, Heki U, et al. Eosinophilic bronchitis presenting with only severe dry cough due to bucillamine. Respir Med 1995;89:219–21.

620. Felman RH, Sutherland DB, Conklin JL, et al. Eosinophilic cholecystitis, appendiceal inflammation, pericarditis, and cephalosporin-associated eosinophilia. Dig Dis Sci 1994; 39:418–22.

621. Bell RJ. Pulmonary infiltration with eosinophils caused by chlorpropamide. Lancet 1964;i:1249–50.

622. Hendrickson R, Simpson F, Beach O. Clofibrate and eosinophilic pneumonia. JAMA 1982;247:3082.

623. Burgher LW, Kass I, Schenken JR. Pulmonary allergic granulomatosis: a possible drug reaction in a patient receiving cromolyn sodium. Chest 1974;66:84–6.

624. Abramov LA, Yust IC, Fierstater ED, et al. Acute respiratory distress caused by erythromycin hypersensitivity. Arch Intern Med 1978;138:1156–8.

625. Cortez LM, Pankey GA. Acute pulmonary hypersensitivity to furazolidone. Am Rev Respir Dis 1972;105:823–6.

626. Gheysens B, Van Mieghem W. Pulmonary infiltrates with eosinophilia due to glafenine. Eur J Respir Dis 1984;65: 456–9.

627. Jennings CA, Deveikis J, Azumi N, et al. Eosinophilic pneumonia associated with reaction to radiographic contrast medium. South Med J 1991;84:92–5.

628. Kristenson M, Fryden A. Pneumonitis caused by metronidazole. JAMA 1988;260:184.

629. Dan M, Aderka D, Topilsky M, et al. Hypersensitivity pneumonitis induced by nalidixic acid. Arch Intern Med 1986;146:1423–4.

630. Pfitzenmeyer P, Foucher P, Piard F, et al. Nilutamide pneumonitis: a report on eight patients. Thorax 1992;47:622–7.

631. Berrissoul F, Ang-Chin S, Mongin-Charpin D, et al. Pneumopathie à éosinophiles due au paracétamol. Rev Mal Respir 1986;3:282.

632. Akoun GM, Mayaud CM, Milleron BJ, et al. Pathologie pulmonaire d'origine médicamenteuse. 6019 ed. Paris: Encycl Med Chir; 1985.

633. Cooper JAD, White D, Matthay R. Drug-induced pulmonary disease. Part 2: noncytotoxic drugs. Am Rev Respir Dis 1986;133:488–505.

634. Davies D, Lloyd-Jones J. Pulmonary eosinophilia caused by penicillamine. Thorax 1980;35:957–8.

635. Ecker MD, Jay B, Keohane MF. Procarbazine lung. AJR Am J Roentgenol 1978;131:527–8.

636. Middleton K, Santella R, Couser JIJ. Eosinophilic pleuritis due to propylthiouracil. Chest 1993;103:955–6.

637. Kelly KJ, Ruffing R. Acute eosinophilic pneumonia following intentional inhalation of Scotchguard. Ann Allergy 1993; 71:358–61.

638. Martinez BM, Domingo P. Acute eosinophilic pneumonia associated with tenidap. BMJ 1997;314:349.

639. Bondi E, Slater S. Tolazamide-induced chronic eosinophilic pneumonia. Chest 1981;80:652.

640. Ho D, Tashkin D, Bein M, et al. Pulmonary infiltrates with eosinophilia associated with tetracycline. Chest 1979;76: 33–5.

641. Salerno SM, Strong JS, Roth BJ, et al. Eosinophilic pneumonia and respiratory failure associated with a trazodone overdose. Am J Respir Crit Care Med 1995;152:2170–2.

642. Ducolone A, Vandevenne A, Ringwald P, et al. Poumon éosinophile d'origine médicamenteuse. Semin Hop Paris 1986;62:1107–10.

643. Jaffuel D, Lebel B, Hillaire-Buys D, et al. Eosinophilic pneumonia induced by dapsone. BMJ 1998;317:181.

644. Wong P, Macris N, Difabrizio L, et al. Eosinophilic lung disease induced by bicalutamide. A case report and review of the medical literature. Chest 1998;113:548–50.

645. Bell SC, Anderson EG. Pulmonary eosinophilia associated with aminoglutethimide. Aust N Z J Med 1998;28:670–1.

646. Oishi Y, Sando Y, Tajima S, et al. Indomethacin induced bulky lymphadenopathy and eosinophilic pneumonia. Respirology 2001;6:57–60.

647. Gaudenz R, Hartmann K, Reinhart WH, et al. Extensive eosinophilic pulmonary infiltrates in a depressive patient treated with maprotiline. Schweiz Rundsch Med Prax 1999;88:1047–51.

648. Kimura N, Miyazaki E, Matsuno O, et al. Drug-induced pneumonitis with eosinophilic infiltration due to tosufloxacin tosilate. Nihon Kokyuki Gakkai Zasshi 1998; 36:618–22.

649. Fujimori K, Shimatsu Y, Suzuki E, et al. Levofloxacin-induced eosinophilic pneumonia complicated by bronchial asthma. Nihon Kokyuki Gakkai Zasshi 2000;38:385–90.

650. Saltzman K, Rossoff LJ, Gouda H, et al. Mesalazine-induced unilateral eosinophilic pneumonia. AJR Am J Roentgenol 2001;177:257.

651. Tanigawa K, Sugiyama K, Matsuyama H, et al. Mesalazine-induced eosinophilic pneumonia. Respiration 1999;66: 69–72.

652. Daniel PT, Holzschuh J, Berg PA. Sulfadoxine specific lymphocyte transformation in a patient with eosinophilic pneumonia induced by sulfadoxine-pyrimethamine (Fansidar). Thorax 1989;44:307–9.

653. Coetmeur D, Guivarch G, Briens E, et al. Acute eosinophilic

pneumonia. Possible role of chloroquine. Rev Mal Respir 1998;15:657–60.

654. Akoun GM, White JP, Dukes MNG, editors. Treatment-induced respiratory disorders. Amsterdam: Elsevier; 1989. p. 366.

655. Mahatma M, Haponik EF, Nelson S, et al. Phenytoin-induced acute respiratory failure with pulmonary eosinophilia. Am J Med 1989;87:93–4.

656. Lee T, Cochrane GM, Amlot P. Pulmonary eosinophilia and asthma associated with carbamazepine. BMJ 1981;282:440.

657. Cox NH, Johnston SRD, Marks J, et al. Extensive carbamazepine eruption with eosinophilia and pulmonary infiltrate. Postgrad Med J 1988;64:249–51.

658. Swygert LA, Maes EF, Sewell LE, et al. Eosinophilia-myalgia syndrome: results of national surveillance. JAMA 1990; 264:1698–703.

659. Kamb ML, Murphy JJ, Jones JL, et al. Eosinophilia myalgia syndrome in L-tryptophan-exposed patients. JAMA 1992;267:77–82.

660. Clauw DJ, Nashel DJ, Umhau A, et al. Tryptophan-associated eosinophilic connective-tissue disease. A new clinical entity? JAMA 1990;263:1502–6.

661. Philen RM, Hill RH, Flanders WD, et al. Tryptophan contaminants associated with eosinophilia-myalgia syndrome. Am J Epidemiol 1993;138:154–9.

662. Varga J, Peltonen J, Uitto J, et al. Development of diffuse fasciitis with eosinophilia during L-tryptophan treatment: demonstration of elevated type I collagen gene expression in affected tissues. A clinicopathologic study of four patients. Ann Intern Med 1990;112:344–51.

663. Belongia EA, Hedberg CW, Gleich GJ, et al. An investigation of the cause of the eosinophilia-myalgia syndrome associated with tryptophan use. N Engl J Med 1990;323:357–65.

664. Hertzman PA, Blevins WL, Mayer J, et al. Association of the eosinophilia-myalgia syndrome with the ingestion of tryptophan. N Engl J Med 1990;322:869–73.

665. Silver RM, Heyes MP, Maize JC, et al. Scleroderma, fasciitis, and eosinophilia associated with the ingestion of tryptophan. N Engl J Med 1990;322:874–81.

666. Martin RW, Duffy J, Engel AG, et al. The clinical spectrum of the eosinophilia-myalgia syndrome associated with L-tryptophan ingestion. Clinical features in 20 patients and aspects of pathophysiology. Ann Intern Med 1990;113:124–34.

667. Hertzman PA, Clauw DJ, Kaufman LD, et al. The eosinophilia-myalgia syndrome: status of 205 patients and results of treatment 2 years after onset. Ann Intern Med 1995;122:851–5.

668. Tazelaar HD, Myers JL, Drage CW, et al. Pulmonary disease associated with L-tryptophan-induced eosinophilic myalgia syndrome. Clinical and pathologic features. Chest 1990;97:1032–6.

669. Lakhanpal S, Duffy J, Engel AG. Eosinophilia associated with perimyositis and pneumonitis. Mayo Clin Proc 1988;63:37–41.

670. Bogaerts Y, Van Renterghem D, Vanvuchelen J, et al. Interstitial pneumonitis and pulmonary vasculitis in a patient taking an L-tryptophan preparation. Eur Respir J 1991;4:1033–6.

671. Strumpf IJ, Drucker RD, Anders KH, et al. Acute eosinophilic pulmonary disease associated with the ingestion of L-tryptophan containing products. Chest 1991;99:8–13.

672. Travis WD, Kalafer ME, Robin HS, et al. Hypersensitivity pneumonitis and pulmonary vasculitis with eosinophilia in a patient taking an L-tryptophan preparation. Ann Intern Med 1990;112:301–3.

673. Alonso-Ruiz A, Calabozo M, Perez-Ruiz F, et al. Toxic oil syndrome. A long-term follow-up of a cohort of 332 patients. Medicine 1993;72:285–95.

674. Martin-Escribano P, Diaz de Atauri MJ, Gomez-Sanchez MA. Persistence of respiratory abnormalities four years after the onset of toxic oil syndrome. Chest 1991;100:336–9.

675. Gomez-Sanchez MA, Saenz de la Calzada C, Gomez-Pajuelo C, et al. Clinical and pathologic manifestations of pulmonary vascular disease in the toxic oil syndrome. J Am Coll Cardiol 1991;18:1539–45.

676. Gomez-Sanchez MA, Mestre de Juan MJ, Gomez-Pajuelo C, et al. Pulmonary hypertension due to toxic oil syndrome. A clinicopathologic study. Chest 1989;95:325–31.

677. Martinez-Tello FJ, Navas-Palacios JJ, Ricoy JR, et al. Pathology of a new toxic syndrome caused by ingestion of adulterated oil in Spain. Virchows Arch A Pathol Anat Histopathol 1982;397:261–85.

678. Cordier JF. Cryptogenic organizing pneumonitis. Bronchiolitis obliterans organizing pneumonia. Clin Chest Med 1993;14:677–92.

679. Cordier JF, Loire R, Brune J. Idiopathic bronchiolitis obliterans organizing pneumonia. Definition of characteristic clinical profiles in a series of 16 patients. Chest 1989;96:999–1004.

680. Bartter T, Irwin RS, Nash G, et al. Idiopathic bronchiolitis obliterans organizing pneumonia with peripheral infiltrates on chest roentgenogram. Arch Intern Med 1989;149:273–9.

681. Cooney TP. Interrelationship of chronic eosinophilic pneumonia, bronchiolitis obliterans, and rheumatoid disease: a hypothesis. J Clin Pathol 1981;34:129–37.

682. Cohen AJ, King TE Jr, Downey GP. Rapidly progressive bronchiolitis obliterans with organizing pneumonia. Am J Respir Crit Care Med 1994;149:1670–5.

683. Izumi T, Kitaichi M, Nishimura K, et al. Bronchiolitis obliterans organizing pneumonia. Clinical features and differential diagnosis. Chest 1992;102:715–9.

684. Poletti V, Castrilli G, Romagna M, et al. Bronchoalveolar lavage, histological and immunohistochemical features in cryptogenic organizing pneumonia. Monaldi Arch Chest Dis 1996;51:289–95.

685. Bousquet J, Chanez P, Vignola AM, et al. Eosinophil inflammation in asthma. Am J Respir Crit Care Med 1994;150:S33–8.

686. Djukanovic R, Wilson JW, Britten KM, et al. Quantitation of mast cells and eosinophils in the bronchial mucosa of symptomatic atopic asthmatics and healthy control subjects using immunohistochemistry. Am Rev Respir Dis 1990;142:863–71.

687. Bousquet J, Chanez P, Lacoste JY, et al. Eosinophilic inflammation in asthma. N Engl J Med 1990;323:1033–9.

688. Adelroth E, Rosenhall L, Johansson SA, et al. Inflammatory cells and eosinophilic activity in asthmatics investigated by bronchoalveolar lavage. The effects of antiasthmatic treatment with budesonide or terbutaline. Am Rev Respir Dis 1990;142:91–9.

689. Foresi A, Pesci A, Pelucchi A, et al. Bronchial inflammation in mite-sensitive asthmatic subjects after 5 years of specific immunotherapy. Ann Allergy 1992;69:303–8.

690. Kirby JG, Hargreave FE, Gleich GJ, et al. Bronchoalveolar cell profiles of asthmatic and nonasthmatic subjects. Am Rev Respir Dis 1987;136:379–83.

691. Metzger WJ, Richerson HB, Worden K, et al. Bronchoalveolar lavage of allergic asthmatic patients following allergen bronchoprovocation. Chest 1986;89:477–83.

692. Smith DL, deShazo RD. Bronchoalveolar lavage in asthma. An update and perspective. Am Rev Respir Dis 1993;148:523–32.

693. Wardlaw AJ, Dunnette S, Gleisch JG, et al. Eosinophils and mast cells in bronchoalveolar lavage in subjects with mild asthma. Relationship to bronchial hyperreactivity. Am Rev Respir Dis 1988;137:62–9.

694. Van Vyve T, Chanez P, Lacoste JY, et al. Comparison between bronchial and alveolar samples of bronchoalveolar lavage fluid in asthma. Chest 1992;102:356–61.

695. Aalbers R, Kauffman HF, Vrugt B, et al. Bronchial lavage and bronchoalveolar lavage in allergen-induced single early and dual asthmatic responders. Am Rev Respir Dis 1993;147:76–81.

696. Messer JW, Peters GA, Bennett WA. Causes of death and pathologic findings in 304 cases of bronchial asthma. Dis Chest 1960;38:616–24.

697. Case Records of the Massachusetts General Hospital. Case 4-1997. N Engl J Med 1997;336:357–64.

698. Gibson PG, Hargreave FE, Girgis-Gabardo A, et al. Chronic cough with eosinophilic bronchitis: examination for variable airflow obstruction and response to corticosteroid. Clin Exp Allergy 1995;25:127–32.

699. Gibson PG, Dolovich J, Denburg J, et al. Chronic cough: eosinophilic bronchitis without asthma. Lancet 1989;i:1346–8.

700. Wong AG, Pavord ID, Sears MR, et al. A case for serial examination of sputum inflammatory cells. Eur Respir J 1996;9:2174–5.

701. Brightling CE, Pavord ID. Eosinophilic bronchitis: an important cause of prolonged cough. Ann Med 2000;32:446–51.

702. Niimi A, Amitani R, Suzuki K, et al. Eosinophilic inflammation in cough variant asthma. Eur Respir J 1998;11:1064–9.

703. Pizzichini E, Pizzichini MM, Efthimiadis A, et al. Measuring airway inflammation in asthma: eosinophils and eosinophilic cationic protein in induced sputum compared with peripheral blood. J Allergy Clin Immunol 1997;99:539–44.

704. Brightling CE, Woltmann G, Wardlaw AJ, et al. Development of irreversible airflow obstruction in a patient with eosinophilic bronchitis without asthma. Eur Respir J 1999;14:1228–30.

705. Quirce S, Fernandez-Nieto M, de Miguel J, et al. Chronic cough due to latex-induced eosinophilic bronchitis. J Allergy Clin Immunol 2001;108:143.

706. Takayanagi N, Kanazawa M, Kawabata Y, et al. Chronic bronchiolitis with associated eosinophilic lung disease (eosinophilic bronchiolitis). Respiration 2001;68:319–22.

707. Turner-Warwick M, Burrows B, Johnson A. Cryptogenic fibrosing alveolitis: clinical features and their influence on survival. Thorax 1980;35:171–80.

708. Boomars KA, Wagenaar SS, Mulder PGH, et al. Relationship between cells obtained by bronchoalveolar lavage and survival in idiopathic pulmonary fibrosis. Thorax 1995;50:1087–92.

709. Davis GS. Bronchoalveolar lavage in interstitial lung disease. Semin Respir Crit Care Med 1994;15:37–60.

710. Fujimoto K, Kubo K, Yamaguchi S, et al. Eosinophil activation in patients with pulmonary fibrosis. Chest 1995;108:48–54.

711. Haslam PL, Turton CWG, Lukoszek A, et al. Bronchoalveolar lavage fluid cell counts in cryptogenic fibrosing alveolitis and their relation to therapy. Thorax 1980;35:328–39.

712. Lapointe M, Laviolette M. Evaluation de l'éosinophilie pulmonaire dans les pathologies interstitielles. Rev Mal Respir 1988;5:R15–6.

713. Martin WJ, Williams DE, Dines DE, et al. Interstitial lung disease. Assessment by bronchoalveolar lavage. Mayo Clin Proc 1983;58:751–7.

714. Peterson MW, Monick M, Hunninghake GW. Prognostic role of eosinophils in pulmonary fibrosis. Chest 1987;92:51–6.

715. Watters LC, Schwarz MI, Cherniack RM, et al. Idiopathic pulmonary fibrosis: pretreatment bronchoalveolar lavage cellular constituents and their relationships with histopathology and clinical response to therapy. Am Rev Respir Dis 1987;135:696–704.

716. Hallgren R, Bjermer L, Lundgren R, et al. The eosinophil component of the alveolitis in idiopathic pulmonary fibrosis. Signs of eosinophil activation in the lung are related to impaired lung function. Am Rev Respir Dis 1989;139:373–7.

717. Turner-Warwick M, Haslam PL. The value of serial bronchoalveolar lavages in assessing the clinical progress of patients with cryptogenic fibrosing alveolitis. Am Rev Respir Dis 1987;135:26–34.

718. Rudd RM, Haslam PL, Turner-Warwick M. Cryptogenic fibrosing alveolitis: relationships of pulmonary physiology and bronchoalveolar lavage to response to treatment and prognosis. Am Rev Respir Dis 1981;124:1–8.

719. Yousem SA. Eosinophilic pneumonia-like areas in idiopathic usual interstitial pneumonia. Mod Pathol 2000;13:1280–4.

720. Travis WD, Matsui K, Moss J, et al. Idiopathic nonspecific interstitial pneumonia: prognostic significance of cellular and fibrosing patterns. Survival comparison with usual interstitial pneumonia and desquamative interstitial pneumonia. Am J Surg Pathol 2000;24:19–33.

721. Basset F, Corrin B, Spencer H, et al. Pulmonary histiocystosis X. Am Rev Respir Dis 1978;118:811–20.

722. Powers MA, Askin FB, Cresson DH. Pulmonary eosinophilic granuloma. 25-year follow-up. Am Rev Respir Dis 1984;129:503–7.

723. Fukuda Y, Basset F, Soler P, et al. Intraluminal fibrosis and elastic fiber degradation lead to lung remodeling in pulmonary Langerhans cell granulomatosis (histiocytosis X). Am J Pathol 1990;137:415–24.

724. Lieberman PH, Jones CR, Steinman RM, et al. Langerhans cell (eosinophilic) granulomatosis. A clinicopathologic study encompassing 50 years. Am J Surg Pathol 1996;20:519–52.

725. Friedman PJ, Liebow AA, Sokoloff J. Eosinophilic granuloma of the lung. Clinical aspects of primary pulmonary histiocytosis in the adult. Medicine 1981;60:385–96.

726. Travis WD, Borok Z, Roum JH, et al. Pulmonary Langerhans cell granulomatosis (histiocytosis X). A clinicopathologic study of 48 cases. Am J Surg Pathol 1993;17:971–86.

727. Kodama T, Takada K, Kameya T, et al. Large cell carcinoma of the lung associated with marked eosinophilia. A case report. Cancer 1984;54:2313–7.

728. Sawyers CL, Golde DW, Quan S, et al. Production of granulocyte-macrophage colony–stimulating factor in two patients with lung cancer, leukocytosis, and eosinophilia. Cancer 1992;69:1342–6.

729. Slungaard A, Ascensao J, Zanjani E, et al. Pulmonary carcinoma with eosinophilia. Demonstration of a tumor-derived eosinophilopoietic factor. N Engl J Med 1983;309:778–81.

730. Horie S, Okubo Y, Suzuki J, et al. An emaciated man with eosinophilic pneumonia. Lancet 1996;348:166.

731. Gross TG, Hoge FJ, Jackson JD, et al. Fatal eosinophilic disease following autologous bone marrow transplantation. Bone Marrow Transplant 1994;14:333–7.

732. Granel B, Serratrice J, Swiader L, et al. Lymphomatoid papulosis associated with both severe hypereosinophilic syndrome and CD30 positive large T-cell lymphoma. Cancer 2000;89:2138–43.

733. Anonymous. Asthma and eosinophilia in a 66-year-old woman. Am J Med 1989;87:439–44.

734. Shijubo N, Fujishima T, Morita S, et al. Idiopathic chronic eosinophilic pneumonia associated with noncaseating epithelioid granulomas. Eur Respir J 1995;8:327–30.

735. Renston JP, Goldman ES, Hsu RM, et al. Peripheral blood eosinophilia in association with sarcoidosis. Mayo Clin Proc 2000;75:586–90.

736. Marguerie C, Drouet M. Poumon eosinophile d'origine professionnelle chez un viticulteur: role des sulfites. Allerg Immunol 1995;27:163–7.

737. Schwarz YA, Kivity S, Fischbein A, et al. Eosinophilic lung reaction to aluminium and hard metal. Chest 1994;105:1261–3.

738. Ellis RV, Mckinlay CA. Allergic pneumonia. J Lab Clin Med 1941;26:1427–32.

739. Zagami AS, Colebatch HJH, Wakefield D. Chronic eosinophilic pneumonia in a patient with ataxia telangiectasia. Aust N Z J Med 1987;17:592–5.

740. Shah PK, Lakhotia M, Chittora M, et al. Pulmonary infiltration with blood eosinophilia after scorpion sting. Chest 1989;95:691–2.

741. Godeau B, Brochard L, Theodorou I, et al. A case of acute eosinophilic pneumonia with hypersensitivity to "red spider" allergens. J Allergy Clin Immunol 1995;95:1056–8.

25 IDIOPATHIC INTERSTITIAL PNEUMONIAS

TALMADGE E. KING JR

The diagnosis and management of the idiopathic interstitial pneumonias has been a challenge to physicians for over a century. When faced with a patient suspected of having idiopathic interstitial pneumonia, clinicians must have a rigorous and organized approach to its diagnosis (see Chapter 1, "Approach to the Evaluation and Diagnosis of Interstitial Lung Disease"). This fact remains unappreciated by many physicians, and, as a result, patients are often incompletely evaluated and empirically treated.

Our understanding of the idiopathic interstitial pneumonias has undergone dramatic change in the last decade.[1,2] The most important change has been greater appreciation of the clinical relevance of the different histopathologic subgroups that make up the idiopathic interstitial pneumonias. The level of evidence for the recommendations made in this chapter is largely that of expert opinion. There have been few randomized controlled clinical trials; consequently, the best evidence in the literature is from well-conducted cohort studies. In this chapter, we will review the epidemiology, clinical presentation, pathogenesis, diagnosis, and treatment of the idiopathic interstitial pneumonias. The chapter is divided into three sections: (1) a historical perspective of the idiopathic interstitial pneumonias, (2) a discussion of general issues that are common to all of these entities, and (3) a discussion of each specific entity.

IDIOPATHIC INTERSTITIAL PNEUMONIAS: A HISTORICAL PERSPECTIVE

In 1892, Osler described chronic interstitial pneumonia, also called cirrhosis of the lung, as "…a fibrinoid change, which may have its starting point in the tissue about the bronchi and blood-vessels, the interlobular septa, the alveolar walls or in the pleura. So diverse are the different forms and so varied the conditions under which this change occurs that a proper classification is extremely difficult."[3] In 1944, Hamman and Rich described four cases of acute diffuse interstitial fibrosis in which "…the lungs were the seats of a widespread connective tissue

hyperplasia throughout the interstitial structures. The alveolar walls were tremendously thickened; in the early stages of the process crowded with fibroblasts."[4] Although all four of their cases were acute in onset and rapidly progressive, the term "Hamman-Rich syndrome" was subsequently used to describe both acute and chronic diffuse idiopathic fibrotic lung diseases.[5,6] By the mid-1960s, significant progress in the subcategorization of interstitial lung disease (ILD) had been made, with drugs, occupational and environmental exposures, inherited conditions, and connective tissue diseases being recognized as potential etiologies or important associations.[7] Those conditions that remained idiopathic were collectively called by various names including idiopathic pulmonary fibrosis (IPF), cryptogenic fibrosing alveolitis, diffuse fibrosing alveolitis, chronic idiopathic interstitial fibrosis, diffuse interstitial fibrosis, Hamman-Rich syndrome, diffuse pulmonary alveolar fibrosis, and idiopathic interstitial pneumonia.

REDEFINING THE PATHOLOGIC CLASSIFICATION OF THE IDIOPATHIC INTERSTITIAL PNEUMONIAS

Liebow and Carrington Classification

In 1969, Liebow and Carrington described five histopathologic subgroups of chronic idiopathic interstitial pneumonia: undifferentiated or "usual" interstitial pneumonia (UIP), diffuse lesions similar to UIP with superimposed bronchiolitis obliterans (termed bronchiolitis interstitial pneumonia), desquamative interstitial pneumonia (DIP), lymphoid interstitial pneumonia (LIP), and giant cell interstitial pneumonia (Table 25–1).[8] Hamman-Rich disease was considered an acute form of UIP. Liebow emphasized "…that these (were) types of tissue response, and that no implication (was) intended that any is pathognomonic for a specific etiological factor. Nevertheless, histological characteristics may provide clues both to etiology and to pathogenesis and certainly to natural history and prognosis."[9]

Katzenstein and Meyers Classification

Over the last two decades, the subgroups described by Liebow and Carrington have evolved based on several findings. In many patients with interstitial pneumonia, the etiology was identified or at least presumed (viral pneumonias, drug reactions, and occupational exposures, eg, asbestosis). When no identifiable etiology was found, the term "idiopathic" was added to identify this subset of interstitial pneumonias. Subsequent studies showed that LIP represented a group of lymphoproliferative disorders and that most cases of giant cell interstitial pneumonia were associated with hard metal (cobalt) pneumoconiosis. Consequently, these entities were excluded from the group of idiopathic interstitial pneumonias. Also, the acute form of interstitial pneumonia (Hamman-Rich disease, diffuse alveolar damage) was originally lumped with UIP. It is now recognized that, in many instances, these cases corresponded to the acute respiratory distress syndrome (ARDS), in which there were no known predisposing factors (idiopathic ARDS).[10] Furthermore, the entity of UIP with bronchiolitis obliterans became known as bronchiolitis obliterans organizing pneumonia (BOOP), and many experts recommended excluding these cases from the interstitial pneumonias because they were predominantly an intraluminal, not an interstitial, process. Finally, other histologic subtypes were better characterized (eg, nonspecific interstitial pneumonia [NSIP] and respiratory bronchiolitis-associated ILD [RB-ILD]).

Consequently, Katzenstein and Myers proposed a change in the classification schema to include five histopathologically distinct subgroups: UIP, DIP and a closely related pattern termed RB-ILD, acute interstitial pneumonia (AIP; diffuse alveolar damage), and NSIP (see Table 25–1).[11] They noted that the previous inclusion of the different entities under a single designation (IPF) largely explained "…the perplexing variation in presentation, response to steroid therapy, and clinical course that has been noted in patients with IPF."[11] Importantly, Katzenstein and Myers emphasized that the pathologic criteria for the diagnosis of the interstitial pneumonias should not be confined to only the presence of fibrosis and inflammation in varying proportions, a finding shared by all of the idiopathic interstitial pneumonias. They emphasized that recognition of the qualitative differences in the nature of the fibrosis (collagen vs fibroblastic foci) and an appreciation of the temporal characteristics of these changes (uniform vs variegated) allowed their distinction from one another (Table 25–2). Most importantly, they recommended that the term "idiopathic pulmonary fibrosis" be reserved for cases with the lesion of UIP identified in tissue obtained by surgical lung biopsy.[11]

American Thoracic Society/European Respiratory Society Classification

The American Thoracic Society/European Respiratory Society (ATS/ERS) recently revised the classification schema of Katzenstein and Myers to emphasize the importance of an integrated clinical and pathologic approach to the diagnosis of idiopathic interstitial pneumonia (see Table 25–1).[2] The ATS/ERS classification combines the histopathologic pattern seen on lung biopsy with clinical and radiologic information to arrive at a final clinico-pathologic diagnosis. This approach allows for the preservation of existing histopathologic and clinical terms while precisely defining the relationship between them. When

TABLE 25–1   Classifications of Idiopathic Interstitial Pneumonias

| Liebow and Carrington (1969)* | Katzenstein (1997)† | ATS/ERS Classification‡ | |
		Histologic Pattern	CRP Diagnosis
UIP	UIP	UIP	IPF/Cryptogenic fibrosing alveolitis
	NSIP	NSIP	NSIP (provisional)
DIP	DIP/RB-ILD	DIP	DIP
		RB	RB-ILD
Bronchiolitis obliterans: interstitial pneumonia and diffuse alveolar damage			
		Organizing pneumonia	COP
	AIP	Diffuse alveolar damage	AIP
LIP		LIP	LIP
Giant cell interstitial pneumonia			

Classification was divided into acute and chronic forms. The chronic conditions are shown. AIP = acute interstitial pneumonia; ATS/ERS = American Thoracic Society/European Respiratory Society; COP = cryptogenic organizing pneumonia; CRP = clinical-radiologic-pathologic; DIP = desquamative interstitial pneumonia; ILD = interstitial lung disease; IPF = idiopathic pulmonary fibrosis; LIP = lymphoid interstitial pneumonia; NSIP = nonspecific interstitial pneumonia; RB = respiratory bronchiolitis; UIP = usual interstitial pneumonia.
See References *8; †636; and ‡2.

the terms are the same for the histopathologic pattern and for the clinical diagnosis (eg, DIP), it was recommended that the pathologist use the addendum "pattern" when referring to the appearance on lung biopsy (eg, DIP pattern), reserving the initial term for the final clinicopathologic diagnosis. It remains unsettled whether or not it is appropriate to include cryptogenic organizing pneumonia (COP) (because most of the connective tissue proliferation characteristic of this process is within air spaces rather than the interstitium) or LIP (because many of these cases are lymphoproliferative disorders) among the idiopathic interstitial pneumonias. Lymphoid interstitial pneumonia is discussed in Chapter 27, "Lymphoplasmocytic Infiltrations of the Lung."

GENERAL CONSIDERATIONS

Epidemiology

Population-based studies of the incidence and prevalence of the idiopathic interstitial pneumonias are few,

TABLE 25–2 Contrasting Pathologic Features of IIPs

Features	UIP	NSIP*	COP	DIP/RBILD	AIP†	LIP
Temporal appearance	Variegated	Uniform	Uniform	Uniform	Uniform	Uniform
Interstitial inflammation	Scant	Usually prominent	Usually prominent	Scant	Scant	Usually prominent Infiltrates comprise mostly T lymphocytes, plasma cells, and macrophages
Collagen fibrosis	Yes, patchy	Variable, diffuse	Not prominent	Variable, Diffuse (DIP) Focal, mild (RBILD)	No	No
Fibroblast foci	Prominent; typically scattered at edges of dense scars	Occasional, diffuse, or rare fibroblast foci	No	No	No	No
Organizing Pneumonia	No	Occasional, focal	Prominent intralumenal organizing fibrosis in distal airspaces (bronchioles, alveolar ducts, and alveoli)	No	Airspace organization (may be focal or diffuse)	No
Microscopic honeycomb change	Yes	Rare	No	No	No	No
Intra-alveolar macrophage accumulation	Occasional, focal	Occasional, patchy	No	Diffuse (DIP) Peribronchiolar (RBILD)	No	No
Hyaline membranes	No	No	No	No	Occasional, may be focal or diffuse	No
Other useful findings	Patchy lung involvement Frequent subpleural and paraseptal distribution	Lung architecture relatively preserved (elastic stains)	Patchy lung involvement Lung architecture relatively preserved (elastic stains)	Macrophages have dusty brown cytoplasm (may be positive for iron stains)	Diffuse distribution Alveolar septal thickening due to organizing fibrosis, usually diffuse	Predominantly alveolar septal distribution Lymphoid hyperplasia (mucosa associated lymphoid tissue hyperplasia)— frequent

Adapted from Katzenstein ALA and Myers JL[11] and Travis WD et al.[2]
*There is a spectrum from cellular to fibrosing patterns, with some cases showing a combination of cellular and fibrosing features.
†The histologic features are a spectrum of acute and/or organizing phases of diffuse alveolar damage. IIP = idiopathic interstitial pneumonia.

and the accuracy of the data is limited. Consequently, the prevalence of idiopathic interstitial pneumonias remains largely unknown. Earlier estimates have ranged from 3 to 6 cases per 100,000 persons in the population.[12,13] Coultas and colleagues, in a population-based study, established in 1988 in Bernalillo County, New Mexico, showed that the prevalence of ILD was higher in men (80.9 per 100,000) than in women (67.2 per 100,000).[14] For men and women, the overall prevalence rates for pulmonary fibrosis (including IPF) were 30.3 per 100,000 and 27.5 per 100,000, respectively.[14] Similarly, the overall incidence of ILD was slightly more common in men (31.5 per 100,000 per year) than in women (26.1 per 100,000 per year).

Vital statistics on pulmonary fibrosis are scant and known to be of limited value. In 1988, there were an estimated 30,000 hospitalizations (compared to 665,000 hospitalizations for chronic obstructive pulmonary disease and asthma) and 4,851 deaths in the United States attributed to pulmonary fibrosis.[14] Mannino and coworkers analyzed death certificate reports compiled by the National Center for Health Statistics from 1979 through 1991 for pulmonary fibrosis mortality.[15] They showed that the age-adjusted rate of pulmonary fibrosis among decedents in the United States increased from 48.6 per 1,000,000 in 1979 to 50.9 per 1,000,000 in 1991 among men and 21.4 per 1,000,00 to 27.2 per 1,000,000 in women. Also, the frequency with which pulmonary fibrosis was listed as the underlying cause of death increased from 40% in 1979 to 56% in 1991. Importantly, the age-adjusted mortality rates varied by state, with the lowest rates in the Midwest and Northeast and the highest rates in the West and Southwest.[15] Deaths from pulmonary fibrosis increase with increasing age (Figure 25–1). In Japan, the mortality rate for idiopathic interstitial pneumonias was estimated to be 3.3 per 100,000 in men and 2.5 per 100,000 in women, with an overall rate of 3.0 in both sexes.[16]

Diagnosis

The differential diagnosis of the idiopathic interstitial pneumonias is very extensive (see Chapter 1, "Approach to the Evaluation and Diagnosis of Interstitial Lung Disease") (Table 25–3). The term "idiopathic" (or cryptogenic) suggests that the etiologic agent is unknown. This should not detract from the fact that progress has been made in defining the characteristic clinical, radiologic, physiological (CRP), and pathologic manifestations that allow identification and separation of these entities. As emphasized by the ATS/ERS consensus statement, "The process of achieving a diagnosis…is dynamic, requiring close communication between the clinician, radiologist, and pathologist…the diagnosis may need to be revised, as more details of history are obtained, when new associations are discovered, or when results of bronchoalveolar lavage (BAL), transbronchial biopsy (where appropriate), and surgical lung biopsy become available."[2]

Table 25–4 shows the key clinical and radiologic features of the major idiopathic interstitial pneumonias. When a clinician is faced with a patient who is thought to have ILD, the most important initial step in the evaluation of such a patient is a carefully taken clinical history. Particular emphasis should be placed on possible occupational and environmental exposures. A strict chronologic listing of the patient's employment, including specific duties and known exposures to dust, gases, and chemicals, is important. Review of the home environment, especially as it relates to pets (especially birds), air conditioners, and humidifiers, is valuable. The specific diagnosis cannot rest on the exposure history alone but requires compatible symptoms, physical findings, and radiographic and pulmonary function abnormalities. Connective tissue diseases may be difficult to exclude because the pulmonary manifestations may precede the more typical systemic manifestations by months or years. Additionally, many primary ILDs (eg, sarcoidosis, eosinophilic granuloma,

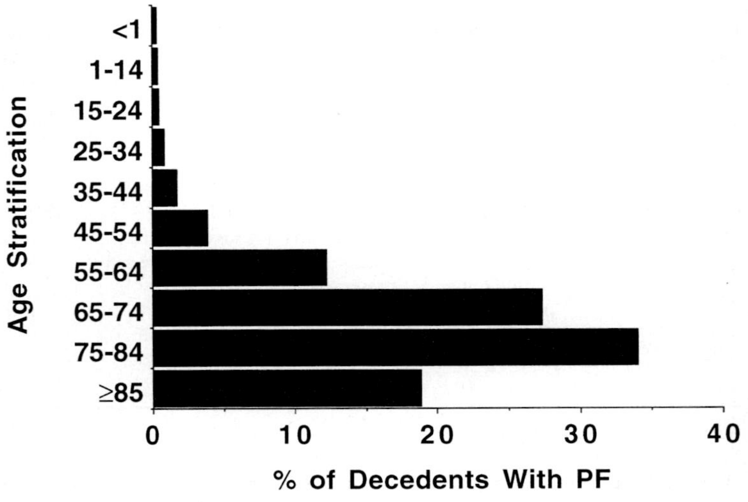

Figure 25–1 Age stratification of people who died with pulmonary fibrosis (PF). Results are from Internal Classification of Diseases codes 515 or 516.3 as a percentage of the deaths from PF. PF accounted for 40% of total deaths. Data were compiled from the multiple-cause mortality files, National Center for Health Statistics. Data from Mannino and coworkers.[15]

TABLE 25–3   Distinguishing Features of Common Diffuse Lung Diseases Confused with Idiopathic Interstitial Pneumonias

Disorders	Distinguishing Features	
	History/Physical	*Imaging*
Connective tissue disease		
Rheumatoid arthritis, scleroderma, polymyositis-dermatomyositis, lupus erythematosus, Sjögren's syndrome, Behçet's syndrome, mixed connective tissue disease, ankylosing spondylitis	Extrapulmonary manifestation; skin, joints; autoantibodies	Similar to IIP
Drug-induced disease		
Antineoplastic agents (bleomycin, busulphan, cyclophosphamide, methotrexate) Antibiotics (isoniazid, nitrofurantoin, sulphonamides) Miscellaneous	History of drug use; manifestations of primary disease	Similar to IIP
Pneumoconiosis (inorganic dust)		
Asbestosis	History of exposure; crackles and clubbing common	Pleural involvement
Hypersensitivity pneumonitis (organic dust)		
Farmer's lung	History of exposure; systemic symptoms; clubbing rare, crackles common	Fine nodularity; lack of subpleural predominance on HRCT
Primary lung disease		
Sarcoidosis	Extrapulmonary manifestation; little dyspnea in proportion to that expected from radiographs; clubbing rare, crackles uncommon	Hilar lymphadenopathy
Langerhans' pulmonary histiocytosis	Smokers Spontaneous pneumothorax	Cysts and nodules in upper and middle lung zones
Lymphangioleiomyomatosis	Spontaneous pneumothorax; women of reproductive age	Thin wall cystic spaces, diffuse throughout both lungs; increased lung volumes
Tuberous sclerosis	Disease affects brain and kidney; spontaneous pneumothorax	Same as lymphangioleiomyomatosis
Lymphangitis carcinomatosis	Symptoms of primary disease	Kerley B lines
Eosinophilic pneumonia	Peripheral-blood eosinophilia	Bilateral peripheral areas of consolidation

Adapted from: Chan-Yeung M, Müller N. Cryptogenic fibrosing alveolitis. Lancet 1997;350:651–656.[301]

lymphangitic carcinomatosis) can only be differentiated by their histologic appearance; therefore, a lung biopsy is often required.

Pathogenesis

The inciting factors in the development of idiopathic interstitial pneumonias are unknown. A widely held hypothesis is that these disorders occur in susceptible individuals following some unknown stimulus. Occupational or environmental exposures, viral infection, genetic factors, and immune-mediated processes are thought to play important roles in the development of the idiopathic interstitial pneumonias. The inciting agent(s) initiates a cascade of events that involves factors controlling inflammatory, immune, and fibrotic processes in the lung (see Chapters 8 "Inflammation in the Pathogenesis of Interstitial Lung Disease," Chapter 9 "Role of the Alveolar Epithelium in the Pathogenesis of Pulmonary Fibrosis," Chapter 10 "Cytokine Biology and the Pathogenesis of Interstitial Lung Disease," and Chapter 11 "Extracellular Matrix in the Pathogenesis of Lung Injury and Repair").

The main problem in the interpretation of data related to genetic risk, environmental exposure, and familial disease as possible etiologies for IPF is the high reliance in most reports on a clinical diagnosis of IPF, without confirmation by lung biopsy or high-resolution computed tomography (HRCT). In the absence of a definite diagnosis of IPF, the interpretation of most of these studies is difficult.

TABLE 25–4   Distinguishing Clinical Features of IIPs

	IPF/UIP	*NSIP*	*COP*	*DIP/RB-ILD*	*AIP*	*LIP*
Prodrome	Chronic (> 12 months)	Subacute to chronic (months to years)	Subacute (< 3 months)	Subacute (weeks to months); current or former smoker	Abrupt (1–2 weeks)	Chronic (> 12 months); Women
Chest radiograph	Bilateral reticular opacities in lower zones; volume loss; ± honeycombing	Bilateral hazy and reticular opacity	Patchy bilateral consolidation	Ground glass opacities in the lower zones	Diffuse, bilateral, ground glass opacities/ progression to consolidation	Reticular opacities, nodules
HRCT	Peripheral, subpleural, basal predominance Reticular opacities, Honeycombing Traction bronchiectasis/ bronchiolectasis; Architectural distortion Focal ground glass	Peripheral, subpleural, basal, symmetric Ground glass attenuation Consolidation Lower lobe volume loss	Subpleural/ peribronchial Patchy consolidation and/or nodules	DIP: Diffuse ground glass opacity in the middle and lower lung zones RB-ILD: bronchial wall thickening; centrilobular nodules; Patchy ground glass opacity	Diffuse, bilateral ground glass opacities often with lobular sparing	Diffuse Centrilobular nodules, Ground glass attenuation, Septal and bronchovascular thickening, Thin-walled cysts
Treatment	Poor response to corticosteroid or cytotoxic agents	Corticosteroid responsiveness	Corticosteroid responsiveness	Smoking cessation Corticosteroid responsiveness	Mechanical ventilation; Corticosteroid responsiveness unknown	Corticosteroid responsiveness
Prognosis	50–70% mortality in 5 years	Unclear; <10% mortality in 5 years	Rare deaths	5% mortality in 5 years	60% mortality in < 6 months	Not well defined.

IPF = idiopathic pulmonary fibrosis; UIP = usual interstitial pneumonia; NSIP = nonspecific interstitial pneumonia; DIP = desquamative interstitial pneumonia; RB-ILD = respiratory bronchiolitis-associated interstitial lung disease; AIP = acute interstitial pneumonia; HRCT = high-resolution computed tomography.

Environmental and Occupational Exposures

Cigarette Smoking.   Cigarette smoking is associated with a subtle form of pulmonary fibrosis (respiratory bronchiolitis) even in young asymptomatic individuals.[17] Several studies have reported a high percentage of current or former smokers ("ever smokers") among cases of idiopathic interstitial pneumonias, mostly cases of DIP, RB-ILD, and IPF. A small case-control study of 40 subjects with idiopathic interstitial pneumonias and 106 controls in England and Wales did not find a significant association between idiopathic interstitial pneumonias and cigarette smoking.[13] However, in a larger study conducted in the Trent region of the United Kingdom, this group found a higher risk for smokers.[18] In this study, there were 218 cases of idiopathic interstitial pneumonias (most were likely cases of IPF) and 569 controls (matched to age, sex, and location), and 77% of cases had a history of ever smoking compared to 71% of the controls. The odds ratio (OR) for ever smoking was 1.57 (95% CI, 1.01 to 2.43), and the risk increased with pack-years of smoking but was not significant (1.05; 95% CI, 0.99 to 1.12 for each additional pack-year of smoking).[18] Baum-

gartner and colleagues performed a multicenter case-control study of clinically and histologically diagnosed patients with idiopathic interstitial pneumonias.[19] There were 248 cases of idiopathic interstitial pneumonia (most were very likely cases of IPF) and 491 controls identified through random-digit dialing and matched to cases in age, sex, and geographic region. More cases (72%) than controls (63%) had a history of ever smoking. The OR for ever smokers was 1.6 (95% CI, 1.1 to 2.4). The risk was significantly elevated for former smokers (1.9; 95% CI, 1.3 to 2.9) and for smokers with histories of 21 to 40 pack-years (2.3; 95% CI, 1.3 to 3.8). There was no clear exposure-response pattern with cumulative consumption of cigarettes. These data suggest a role for cigarette smoking in causing or exacerbating the idiopathic interstitial pneumonias, in particular, DIP, RB-ILD, and IPF (Figure 25–2). Finally, whatever its role in the pathogenesis of the idiopathic interstitial pneumonias, smoking has a profound effect on the radiographic, physiological, and pathologic findings, as well as the natural history of these processes, especially IPF.[20–29]

Dusty Environments.   The role of occult environmental agents in the development of idiopathic interstitial pneumonias remains poorly defined (Table 25–5). Exposure to dusty environments, in particular, work with livestock (OR 2.2) and wood dust (OR 1.8) have been shown to be independent risk factors for idiopathic interstitial pneumonias.[30] The metal dust OR per work-year of exposure was 1.11 (95% CI, 1.06 to 1.16; $p < .001$) and for wood dust, the OR per work-year of exposure was 1.12 (95% CI, 1.02 to 1.24; $p < .02$).[18] The dust exposure started more than 5 years before diagnosis, and the median exposure history was 47.5 years for metal dust-exposed IPF patients and 45.5 years for wood dust-exposed patients. These data suggest that metal dust exposure may cause 10 to 13% and wood dust exposure 5 to 10% of the cases in the United Kingdom. Steel, brass, and lead were the most common metal dusts. Other studies have shown that metal dust exposures (usually prolonged and heavy exposure in a work environment) are associated with the development of pulmonary fibrosis. These include cobalt, aluminum (welders, polishers), zinc, cadmium, and mercury. Most of these associations have not been confirmed by adequately conducted studies.

Viral Factors

A few patients with idiopathic interstitial pneumonias, especially those with NSIP, COP, and AIP, date the onset of their symptoms to a flulike illness associated with chest symptoms.[31] Interestingly, respiratory viral infections were temporally related to onset of disease in at least three members of a family with familial pulmonary fibrosis.[32] To date, little culture, serologic, or morphologic evidence exists to support persistent or previous viral exposure as a causative factor in these processes.[33–39] However, pulmonary fibrosis has been documented to occur as a response to severe lung infections caused by a number of different viruses.[40] The role that adenovirus, cytomegalovirus or influenza, hepatitis C, or Epstein-Barr (EBV) viruses might may play in the etiology of idiopathic interstitial pneumonias is particularly intriguing.[41–43]

An association between idiopathic interstitial pneumonias and EBV has been suggested because increased serum antibodies to EBV and detectable immunoglob-

ulin (Ig)A against viral-capsid antigen are present in idiopathic interstitial pneumonias.[44] EBV viral-capsid antigen has been found in type II epithelial cells of lung tissue from patients with interstitial pneumonias when the tissue was analyzed with immunofluorescent staining.[45] Importantly, ultrastructural studies have largely failed to identify viral particles in the lung or pulmonary secretions.[35,37,38,46–51]

Serum antibodies to hepatitis C virus were increased in a group of Japanese patients with idiopathic interstitial pneumonias; however, a subsequent study in the United Kingdom using similar but improved techniques refuted this finding.[43,52] Meliconi and coworkers also found no evidence to support a causative relationship among Italian patients with idiopathic interstitial pneumonias.[53] They showed that the baseline prevalence of hepatitis C virus infection in the population studied strongly influenced the results. In the United States and western Europe, the prevalence of hepatitis C virus positivity is approximately 1%; in northern Italy it is 3.4, and in some parts of Japan it is as high as 30%.[40]

With nested polymerase chain reaction (PCR), Kuwano and colleagues showed, in studies performed on lung tissues obtained by transbronchial lung biopsy, adenovirus E1A DNA in pulmonary fibrosis.[54] However, they concluded that adenovirus E1A is unlikely to be etiologically involved in the pathogenesis of idiopathic interstitial pneumonias. Interestingly, their data suggested that a latent adenovirus infection may be reactivated or may newly infect the host following corticosteroid administration, because E1A adenovirus DNA was more prevalent in patients treated with corticosteroids (67%) than in those that were not (10%).

Genetic Factors

A genetic basis for idiopathic interstitial pneumonias is supported by several findings (see Chapter 7 "Genetic Basis of Interstitial Lung Disease").[55–59] Certain animal strains are susceptible to fibrotic agents, which suggests an inheritable predisposition. In humans, there is marked variation in the observed response to profibrotic agents such as asbestos despite similar levels of exposure.[59,60] Familial pulmonary fibrosis, including its description in

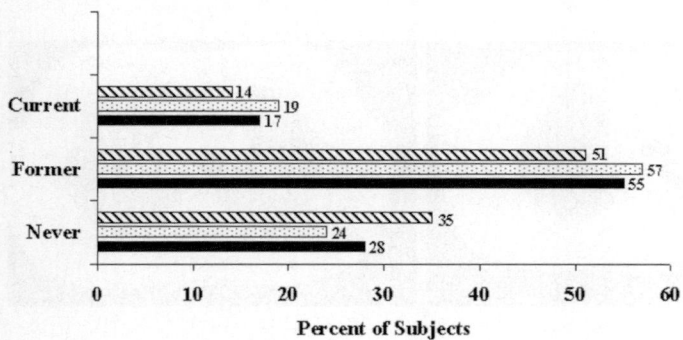

Figure 25–2 Smoking history in patients with idiopathic interstitial pneumonia (IIP). Three large studies show that ever-smoking (patients who have smoked at any time in their lives) is very common in patients with IIP, predominantly in cases of idiopathic pulmonary fibrosis (IPF). The data suggest a role for cigarette smoking in the cause or exacerbation of IIP, especially IPF. Hatched bars indicate data taken from King TE Jr et al[28]; stippled bars, data from Johnston et al[231]; solid bars, data from Baumgartner et al.[19]

TABLE 25–5   Risk Factors for Pulmonary Fibrosis

Exposure	Odds Ratios			
	Baumgartner[19]	Scott[13]	Hubbard[18]	Iwai[16]
Cigarette smoking	1.60	1.11	1.57	2.94
Wood fires	0.83	12.55		
Metal dust	10.82	0.97	1.68	1.34
Stone/sand	3.90	1.59	1.76	
Textile dust	1.89	0.90	1.80	
Wood dust		2.94	1.71	
Livestock	2.65	10.89		
Farming	1.50			3.01

Adapted from Verleden GM et al.[59]

identical twins (some of whom have been separated geographically for many years) has been reported (Figure 25–3).[5,6,32,60–95] Alveolar inflammation was identified in clinically unaffected family members of patients with familial pulmonary fibrosis.[90] These family members had increased numbers of neutrophils and activated macrophages that released one or more neutrophil chemoattractants and growth factors for lung fibroblasts, and they also had positive gallium 67 lung scans. The significance of these findings remains unknown, but researchers speculated that these unaffected family members might be at risk for the development of familial pulmonary fibrosis. The role of genetics in the pathogenesis of idiopathic interstitial pneumonias is further strengthened by the appearance of pulmonary fibrosis in association with inherited disorders such as neurofibromatosis, Hermansky-Pudlak syndrome, tuberous sclerosis, Gaucher's disease, lymphangiomyomatosis, and the hypocalciuric hypercalcemia syndrome.[96–111]

To date, over 68 kindreds presumed to have IPF have been reported.[32] Marshall and coworkers estimate that familial cases account for 0.5 to 2.2% of all patients with idiopathic interstitial pneumonias, with a prevalence of 1.34 cases per 10^6 population in the United Kingdom.[60] In Finland, it was estimated that the prevalence for familial IPF was 5.9 per million.[112] The familial form explained 3.3 to 3.7% of all Finnish cases of IPF diagnosed according to the revised ATS/ERS international guidelines. Geographic clustering has been noted, suggesting a recent founder effect in patients with familial IPF.[60,112]

The CRP, and morphologic manifestations of familial pulmonary fibrosis are similar to the nonfamilial forms of lung fibrosis. Patients with familial pulmonary fibrosis usually present at a younger age and appear to have more aggressive disease.[56,60,88] However, the longest survivals have been seen in those presenting between the ages of 10 and 20 years. This may have resulted from lead-time bias (eg, overestimation of survival duration resulting from earlier detection). There may be a slight male predominance, and women tend to have a more favorable prognosis.[32,60,88]

Figure 25–3 Familial pulmonary fibrosis in identical twins. Chest radiographs show a reticular pattern involving all lung zones (A). Computed tomography scans shows extensive parenchymal involvement, with irregular fibrotic changes (B).

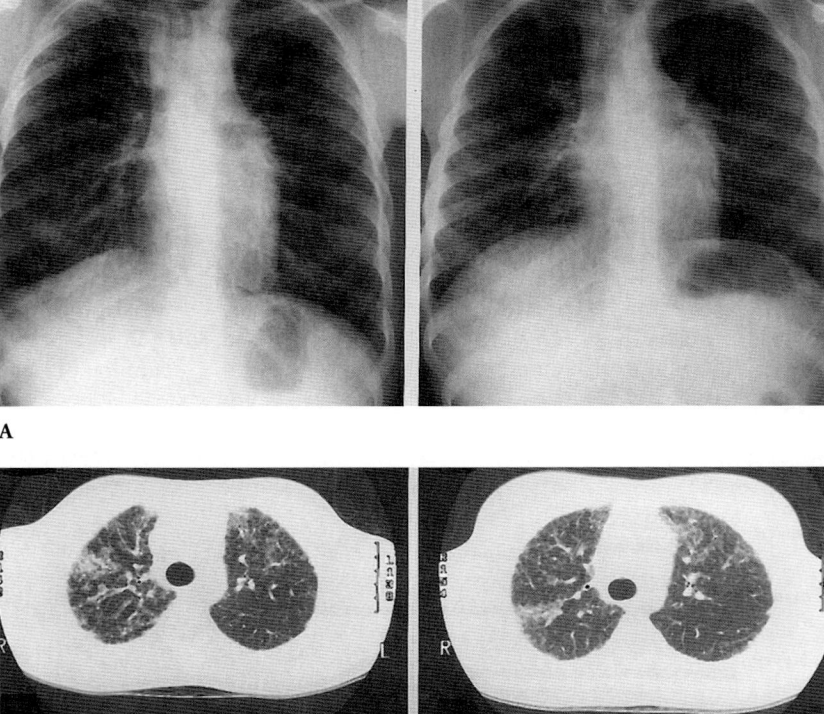

Familial pulmonary fibrosis has been associated with multiple pathologic subsets of the idiopathic interstitial pneumonias: DIP, LIP, and UIP.[32,113,114] Thomas and colleagues showed that mutations in the surfactant protein (SP)-C gene (*SFTpC*) are associated with familial desquamative and nonspecific interstitial pneumonitis and may cause type II cellular injury.[32] The mutation was not seen in control chromosomes and thus is not likely to be a polymorphism.[32] Electron microscopy of affected lung revealed alveolar type II cell atypia, with numerous abnormal lamellar bodies. The authors hypothesized that the presence of two different pathologic diagnoses in affected relatives sharing this mutation indicates that, in this kindred, these diseases may represent pleiotropic manifestations of the same central pathogenesis.[32] Multiple heterozygous mutations in the *SFTpC* gene have been reported in association with children suffering from ILD (DIP or NSIP), including familial and sporadic occurrences.[115,116] In addition, a deficiency of SP-C has been described in a small kindred suffering from a poorly defined form of interstitial pneumonitis, despite no sequence variation in the *SFTpC* gene.[117] Whitsett hypothesized that the nature and biology of the SP-C mutation, amount of production of the active SP-C peptide, the inheritance of other genetic modifiers, or exposure to environmental factors may influence the variability in histopathologic pattern among affected individuals.[118] Taken together, these findings support a model in which misfolded proSP-C or SP-C protein can cause type II alveolar cell injury that results in ILD.[118]

An autosomal dominant pattern of inheritance with reduced penetrance has been suggested for many examples of familial pulmonary fibrosis.[62–65,69,74,82,83,87,94,119] Linkage studies have suggested a link between the risk for familial pulmonary fibrosis and Ig-γ (Gm) allotypes.[89] The finding of a significant increase in non-MM protease inhibitor phenotypes, particularly MZ, in patients with idiopathic interstitial pneumonias is additional evidence for a role for chromosome 14 in the increased susceptibility of persons to the development of pulmonary fibrosis.[120,121] There is evidence of a genetic influence in sporadic cases, including conflicting evidence of an increased presence of human leukocyte antigen (HLA)-B8, HLA-B12, and HLA-B15; HLA-Dw6 and HLA-DR2 antigens; and a decrease incidence of HLA-Dw3 among patients with pulmonary fibrosis.[77,80,85,120] The strongest correlation described is that between HLA DR3/DRw52a and the susceptibility of patients with systemic sclerosis to develop lung fibrosis.[122] Despite these findings, it remains to be determined if a definite association between an HLA locus and idiopathic interstitial pneumonias exists.

Role Of Inflammatory, Fibrotic, and Immune Processes

An important advance in our understanding of ILDs has been the recognition of the central role of chronic inflammation (alveolitis) in the injury and fibrosis that occurs in the distal air spaces of these patients.[123,124] The mechanism by which these inflammatory and immune effector cells injure lung parenchymal cells and induce connective tissue proliferation is conjectural.[125–129] This inflammatory process often involves respiratory bronchioles and smaller airways as well as the alveolar walls and air spaces.[12,130] Studies aimed at understanding the inflammatory component of this disease have considerably increased our knowledge of the mechanisms of injury present in idiopathic interstitial pneumonias and other ILDs. Unfortunately, several major issues remain unresolved. Clearly, a shift in the types and quantity of inflammatory cells present in the lower respiratory tract occurs in patients with idiopathic interstitial pneumonias. However, considerable heterogeneity does occur, with most studies revealing a predominance of neutrophils and macrophages, whereas others suggest that the inflammation is actually the result of other cell types, for example, lymphocytes or mast cells.[12,31,130–136] Correlative studies of lung parenchymal inflammatory cells and the ultimate course of the disease have suggested that inflammation is a key factor in the prediction of therapeutic responsiveness in many of the idiopathic interstitial pneumonias; the exception is IPF/UIP.[12,55,130,137–141]

Much of our understanding of the mechanisms of pulmonary fibrosis comes from studies of bleomycin-induced lung fibrosis in animal models, especially in mice. The findings from these studies suggest that an initial alveolar injury triggers an inflammatory response and, subsequently, leads to fibrosis. Unfortunately, this model is not representative of the processes that appear to operate in the UIP pattern of lung injury.[142,143] The bleomycin-induced lung fibrosis actually resembles an NSIP pattern, because it has both mural incorporation-type and bud-type intra-alveolar fibroses and shows a tendency to recover.[143,144]

Patterns of injury similar to those of idiopathic interstitial pneumonia occur in several immune-mediated diseases, such as the connective tissue diseases, chronic active hepatitis, primary biliary cirrhosis, autoimmune hemolytic anemia, Hashimoto's disease, idiopathic thrombocytopenic purpura, mixed cryoglobulinemia, inflammatory bowel disease, myasthenia gravis, and renal tubular acidosis.[145–155] Furthermore, patients with idiopathic interstitial pneumonia uncommonly have systemic symptoms including fever, arthralgias, Raynaud's phenomenon, and digital vasculitis (the majority of these patients appear to have or will likely develop an associated connective tissue disease), as well as abnormal laboratory data (elevated erythrocyte sedimentation rate, hypergammaglobulinemia) and increased titers of antinuclear antibodies (7 to 25%), rheumatoid factors (14%), cryoimmunoglobulins (41%), positive lupus erythematosus cell preparations (3%), and depressed complement levels (6%).[156,157] In addition, immune complexes have been demonstrated in BAL fluid, in the circulation, and deposited in alveolar walls and capillaries in patients with idiopathic interstitial pneumonia. Most likely these are cases with NSIP.[131,132,138,139,158–164]

Clinical Findings

The typical patient presents with breathlessness or cough (Figure 25–4). Bibasilar end-inspiratory dry rales and clubbing are commonly found on physical examination (Figure 25–5). An elevated erythrocyte sedimentation rate, hypergammaglobulinemia, positive antinuclear antibodies (21% of patients with "lone" idiopathic interstitial pneumonias), rheumatoid factors, and circulating immune complexes have been identified in these patients.[138,165–171] Circulating cryoimmunoglobulins were found in 41% of patients with idiopathic interstitial pneumonias.[31] Only circulating immune complexes have been correlated with disease stage or prognosis.[138]

BAL

Bronchoalveolar lavage via the fiber-optic bronchoscope has gained widespread acceptance as a research and clinical tool since its introduction in the 1970s (see Chapter 5, "Bronchoalveolar Lavage"). It is easily performed, with good patient acceptance and extremely low morbidity. It has been suggested that the BAL fluid cellular constituents reflect the state of the pulmonary inflammatory response (staging). Early studies comparing BAL fluid cellular constituents to cells obtained from open lung biopsy suggested that cell types and their state of activation were similar.[134,172,173] Furthermore, cellular analysis of BAL fluid in different ILDs suggested that the patterns of inflammatory and immune effector cell changes are dissimilar; lymphocytes are increased in patients with hypersensitivity pneumonitis and sarcoidosis, whereas neutrophils and/or eosinophils are increased in IPF, asbestosis, and histiocytosis X (Figure 25–6).[134,173,174] Furthermore, it has been shown that in the active phases of the idiopathic interstitial pneumonias, there is a severalfold increase in the total number of inflammatory cells recovered from the respiratory tract. Thus, the inflammatory response in idiopathic interstitial pneumonias consists of increased numbers of several different effector cell types (Table 25–6). Unfortunately, many recent studies have failed to demonstrate a clear distinction between diseases based on the predominant cell type present in the lavage fluid.

Physiological Testing

The typical findings of pulmonary function tests are consistent with restrictive impairment (reduced vital capacity [VC]) and total lung capacity [TLC]). Unless a complicating airway disease occurs, isovolume flow rates are well maintained. The diffusing capacity of the lung for carbon monoxide (DL_{CO}) is reduced and may precede abnormalities in lung volume. The maximal breathing capacity is usually normal. The resting arterial blood gases may be normal or reveal hypoxemia (secondary to ventilation and perfusion mismatch) and respiratory alkalosis, and these abnormalities may be elicited or accentuated by exercise (see Chapter 3, "Physiology of Interstitial Lung Disease").

Chest Imaging Studies

Chest Radiograph

Often it is the radiographic changes that alert the physician to the presence of one of the idiopathic interstitial pneumonias. The chest radiograph is abnormal at presentation in most patients with idiopathic interstitial pneumonia (Figure 25–7). However, the conventional chest radiograph is of limited value in the imaging of diffuse lung diseases such as idiopathic interstitial pneumonias because

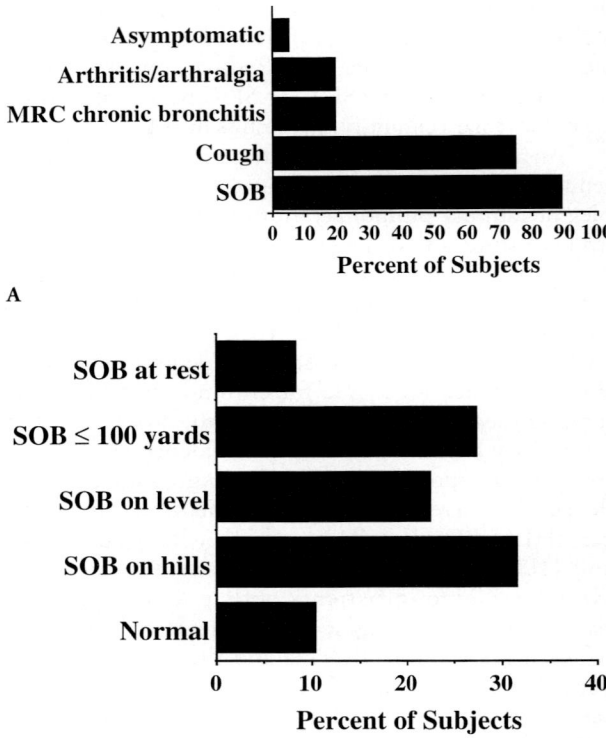

Figure 25–4 Presenting clinical manifestations in patients with IIP. Shortness of breath (SOB) and cough were the most common presenting symptoms (*n* = 588). Interestingly, 5% of patients were asymptomatic (no cough or SOB) at presentation (*A*). Ten percent of patients denied any degree of breathlessness. However, 36% were severely disabled by SOB, at rest or with minimal exertion (< 100 yards). Exercise tolerance was significantly worse in women. Median duration of SOB was 9 months before presentation (*B*). Data are from Johnston IDA et al.[231]

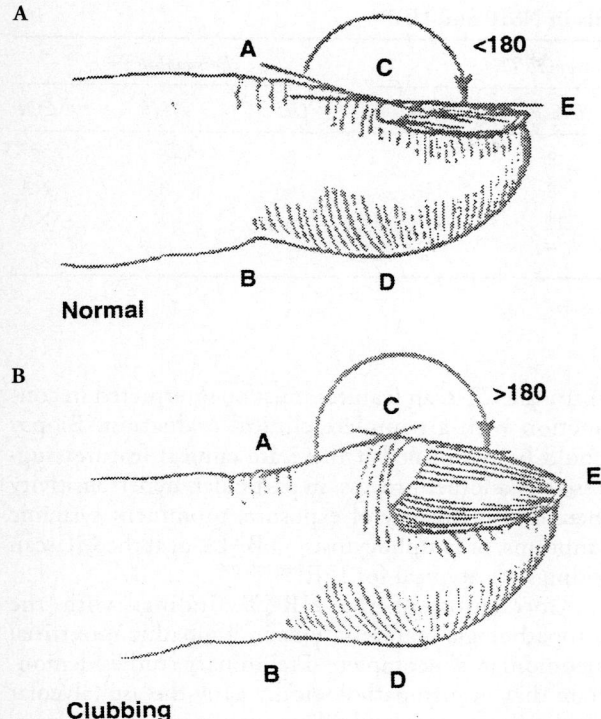

A

Normal

B

Clubbing

Figure 25–5 Clubbing of the fingers. In a normal finger (*top*), the length of the a perpendicular, which drops from point A to point B, should be greater than a similar line from C to D. In clubbing (*bottom*), the relationships are reversed (ie, distance from C to D is greater than the distance from A to B). The other important change is the angle described by A—C—E: in a normal finger, usually < 180°; in clubbing, > 180°. Reproduced with permission from: DeRemee RA.[654]

1. the terminology used to describe the radiographic features has been "inconsistent," "misleading," and "equivocal;"[175]
2. the distinction between interstitial and air space disease is relatively inaccurate, and there is a superimposition of anatomic structures[176];
3. there is no quantitative method for describing the extent and type of the parenchymal abnormalities;
4. the initial or serial chest radiographs do not correlate with the physiological abnormalities[31,177];
5. the chest radiograph does not correlate well with the histologic distribution and involvement; only honeycombing correlates with lung histopathology[141,176,178,179]; and
6. the chest radiograph lacks diagnostic specificity, with a correct diagnosis made in less than 50% of cases and only a 70% interobserver agreement as to the predominant findings or the degree of profusion.[175,180]

Sensitivity is better, but up to 10% of patients with histologically confirmed infiltrative lung disease will have normal chest radiographs.[33,175,180–182] In my experience, a normal chest radiograph is rare in idiopathic interstitial pneumonias and is more often present in

patients with hypersensitivity pneumonitis. Other ILDs with normal chest radiographs include scleroderma, von Recklinghausen's disease, and asbestosis.[165,182–187]

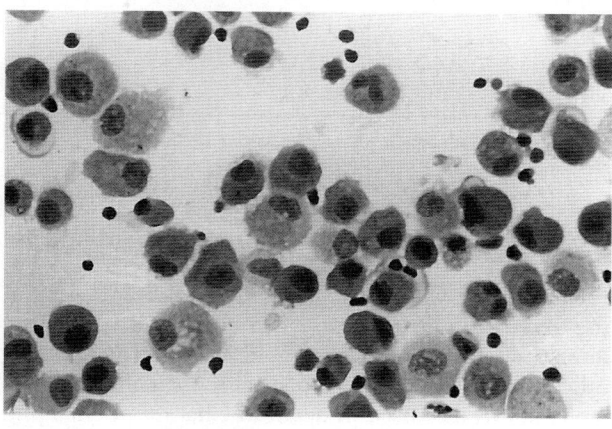

A

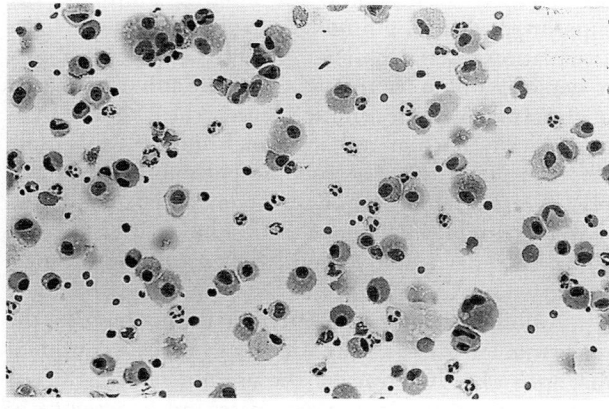

B

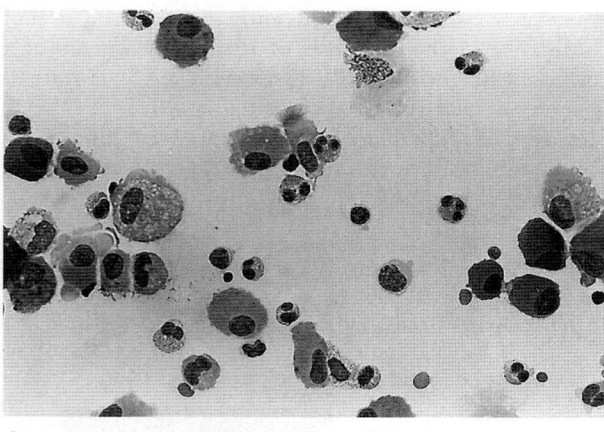

C

Figure 25–6 *A,* Bronchoalveolar lavage (BAL) fluid shows cells recovered from a normal subject (Diff-Quik stain; ×40 original magnification). *B,* Lavage fluid specimen from a patient with active untreated IPF shows increased numbers of total cells, predominantly neutrophils (Diff Quik stain; ×20 original magnification). *C,* Lavage fluid specimen from patient with progressive IPF shows an eosinophilia (Diff Quik stain; ×40 original magnification).

TABLE 25–6   BAL Fluid Cells in NSIP and UIP*

Study	Lymphocytes (%)			Neutrophils (%)			Eosinophils (%)		
	UIP	NSIP	COP	UIP	NSIP	COP	UIP	NSIP	COP
Nagai[411]	7	37	44	6	8	6	3	6	2
Daniil[413]	8	9	NA	10	8	NA	6	3	NA
Park[506]	3	25	NA	5	12	NA	3	2	NA
Suga[638]	7	21	38	3	7	7	2	3	4

*Data are mean values, given as percent of total cells
NA = not available

HRCT

HRCT shares with lung biopsy an important place in the evaluation of patients with suspected idiopathic interstitial pneumonia (see Table 25–4). HRCT is significantly more sensitive and specific than chest radiography and is discussed in detail in Chapter 4, "Imaging of Diffuse Parenchymal Lung Diseases" CT provides a direct visual window into the lung; it eliminates the superimposition of pulmonary structures and enhances attenuation discrimination.[176,188] HRCT has the ability to depict, without summation, the type and distribution of abnormal opacities and to identify the extent of radiographically normal and abnormal lung. HRCT more closely reflects the macroscopic pathologic anatomy; HRCT has a resolution of approximately 0.5 mm, and newer technology will make the resolution even smaller. Thus, it is particularly useful for examining the pulmonary parenchyma.[175,189–206]

Among the idiopathic interstitial pneumonias, the main role for HRCT is to attempt to make a confident diagnosis of IPF. However, the usefulness of HRCT is highly dependent on the expertise and experience of those who interpret the images. Compared to chest radiography, CT scanning significantly increases the level of confidence in the diagnosis of IPF. The accuracy of a confident diagnosis of IPF made with CT by a trained observer appears to be approximately 90%.[175,198,207,208] However, less experienced observers are substantially less accurate than more experienced observers. Most impor-

tantly, the CT scan features must be interpreted in conjunction with a complete clinical evaluation. Biopsy should be performed if there are clinical features suggestive of another process, in particular, hypersensitivity pneumonitis (history of exposure, prominent systemic symptoms, or lymphocytosis on BAL), or if the CT scan findings are atypical for IPF.[198,205,206]

Correlation of the HRCT findings with the histopathologic manifestations in idiopathic interstitial pneumonias is incomplete. Preliminary studies demonstrate that in histopathologically early disease (alveolar septal inflammation and filling of air spaces by mononuclear cells), a patchy, predominantly peripheral air space opacification (ie, opacified air spaces distinct from reticular densities of >1 cm in diameter and located away from the fissures) or a "hazy" increase in lung density or ground-glass opacities (ie, an increase in CT scan lung density which does not obscure the underlying lung parenchyma), thickened interlobular septa, and prominence of centrilobular core structures predominate[189,197,209,210] In some patients, ground-glass opacity on HRCT scans is associated with diffuse fine fibrosis on biopsy.[198] Patients who have ground-glass opacity resulting from lung fibrosis can often be identified by the presence of reticular lines and dilated bronchi or bronchioles (traction bronchiectasis or bronchiolectasis) within the area of increased density.[198] In more histopathologically advanced disease (ie, with a prominent fibrotic reaction), a lower lung zone predominant reticular pattern, consisting largely of thickened interlobular septa and intralobular lines, is commonly present. Honeycombing, traction bronchiectasis and subpleural fibrosis may also be present.

Gallium 67 Lung Scan

Gallium 67 lung scanning has been recommended as a noninvasive test for staging the alveolitis found in idiopathic interstitial pneumonias and other ILDs, particularly sarcoidosis (Figure 25–8). This cyclotron-produced nuclide localizes in inflammatory foci in the lung, whereas little gallium 67 accumulates in normal lungs.[211–214] Diffuse pulmonary uptake of gallium 67 has been reported in several interstitial lung disorders,

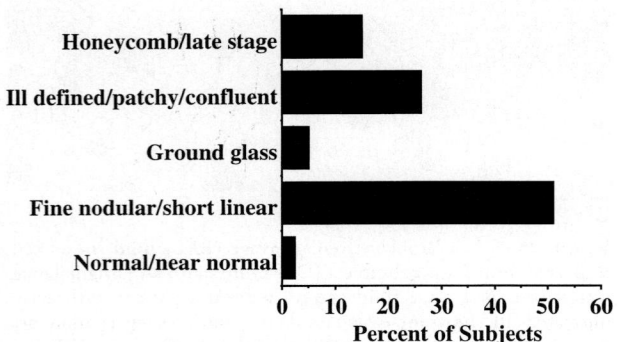

Figure 25–7   Chest radiograph findings on entry. Data are from Johnston IDA et al.[231]

including IPF (up to 70% of patients have a positive scan), sarcoidosis, pneumoconiosis, hypersensitivity pneumonitis, and in individuals exposed to asbestos and various drug-related lung disease.[31,130,212–223]

Early studies comparing the relationship between a visual index of gallium 67 uptake in the lung and the number of inflammatory cells recovered by BAL in patients with idiopathic interstitial pneumonias and sarcoidosis have suggested that a direct relationship exists; therefore, the uptake of gallium 67 may be useful in determining the degree of alveolar inflammation in such patients.[216,217,221–223] In theory, the uptake of gallium 67 into the lung would serve to differentiate active cellular diseases from fibrotic disease and so would be an important method for staging disease activity. Unfortunately, it has not been adequately demonstrated how or if the level of gallium 67 accumulation in the lung correlates with the inflammatory stage of idiopathic interstitial pneumonias, especially IPF.[216]

Role of Surgical Lung Biopsy in the Diagnosis of the Idiopathic Interstitial Pneumonias

After the initial evaluation, the next step is to diagnose and stage the disease so that prognostic and therapeutic decisions can be made. Surgical lung biopsy is necessary for a confident clinicopathologic diagnosis, except in certain cases with a typical picture of IPF/UIP.[2,206,207] Lung biopsy is indicated because (1) it provides an accurate diagnosis, (2) it excludes neoplastic and infectious processes that occasionally mimic chronic, progressive interstitial disease, (3) it occasionally identifies a more treatable process than originally suspected (eg, extrinsic allergic alveolitis), and (4) it provides a better assessment of disease activity.

Open lung biopsy is relatively safe, with little morbidity and less than 1% mortality.[224] A limited thoracotomy is usually performed under general anesthesia; following the procedure, a thoracostomy tube is required for 24 to 48 hours. Recovery is relatively quick, and patients frequently leave the hospital 4 to 7 days after surgery. Most clinicians do not perform open lung biopsy in the very elderly (> 75 years of age) or in patients with serious cardiovascular disease, radiographic evidence of diffuse honeycombing, severe pulmonary dysfunction, or other major operative risks. In these patients, a fiberoptic bronchoscopy with transbronchial biopsy is occasionally performed.

Open or video-assisted thoracoscopic (VATS) lung biopsy is preferred because of the larger quantity of tissue obtained and the ability to take biopsy specimens from more than one site. VATS lung biopsy is currently the preferred surgical approach to obtaining lung tissue. If properly performed, it allows complete inspection of the lung and can yield an adequate quantity of tissue from several lobes of the lung. This procedure provides an equivalent amount of tissue and similar diagnostic accuracy, and reduces the duration of chest tube drainage and length of hospital stay compared with thoracotomy.[225] Patients undergoing VATS lung biopsy must have sufficient pulmonary reserve to undergo unilateral ventilation for the duration of the procedure. It is important that the surgeon obtain an adequate sample. Specifically, the surgeon should avoid obtaining only subpleural tissue (especially if pleuritis is present) and avoid the dependent segments of the right middle lobe and lingula.[226–228] It is also important that samples be taken from two or more lobes; that is, an area of obvious but mild abnormality and one that appears normal. Areas with obvious severe fibrotic reaction should not be used because the pattern found will not help in the differential diagnosis. This approach decreases the sampling error that often occurs when a single small piece is obtained by open lung biopsy or the usually small crushed pieces obtained with transbronchial lung biopsy via the fiberoptic bronchoscope. More importantly, it allows the pathologist to better define the extent and severity of the inflammation and fibrosis, factors key to determining prognosis.[229] In most cases, the biopsy provides definitive classification of patients into the recognized histologic patterns. A small subset of patients with interstitial pneumonia remain unclassifiable after extensive clinical, radiologic, and/or pathologic examination. This situation often exists when some critical piece of data is unavailable or when there is a major discrepancy

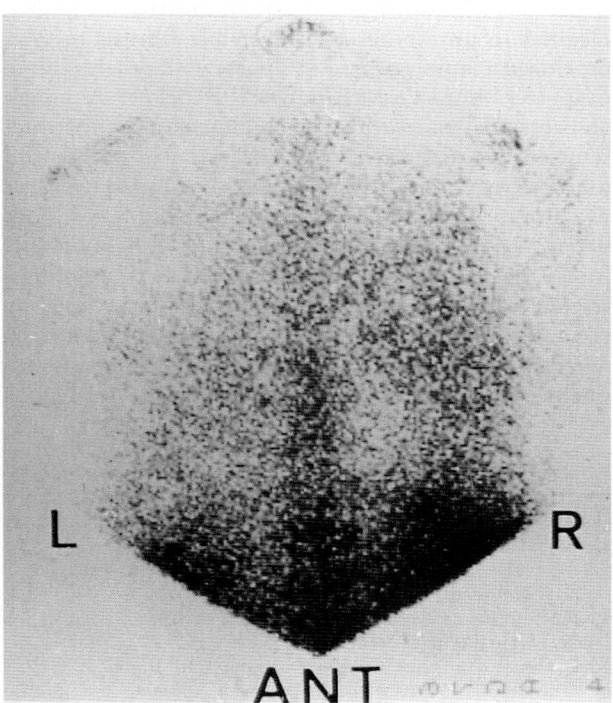

Figure 25–8 Gallium 67 (^{67}Ga) lung scintigraphy in a patient with IPF. ^{67}Ga uptake is increased in the lung, the right greater than the left. Normal lungs usually contain no more activity than do the shoulders.

between the clinical, radiologic, and/or pathologic information (Table 25–7).[2,230]

SELECTING PATIENTS WITH IDIOPATHIC INTERSTITIAL PNEUMONIA FOR TREATMENT

Before instituting any of the current treatments for the idiopathic interstitial pneumonias, it is important to inform the patient (and family) about the potential risks and side effects of the treatments, especially corticosteroids and cytotoxic therapy. Because the clinical course of the idiopathic interstitial pneumonias varies considerably, generalizations about the treatment program to be used in an individual patient is often difficult. Neither the patient nor the physician should be lulled into a sense of security by the insidious progression of the disease. This is especially true for patients with few or no symptoms or with slightly abnormal pulmonary function tests who were not treated early in their disease. Not only is disease progression often insidious, it may be difficult to detect progression based solely on the commonly employed parameters, such as symptomatology, chest radiographic findings, or spirometry. Both chest radiography and spirometry are insensitive parameters of change. Also, patients in this age group (the majority of patients are > 50 years old) often have difficulty discerning whether their functional limitations are the result of disease progression, deconditioning, or simply the aging process. The author has encountered numerous examples of patients with slowly progressive untreated disease that resulted in unresponsive, irreversible fibrosis or who developed a rapidly progressive phase with progression to death (see "Acute Exacerbation of IPF" below). Although an occasional patient may not require treatment at presentation, a carefully defined and executed program of follow-up at 3- to 6-month intervals is required to ensure the prompt institution of treatment at the first sign of deterioration. The view that patients with idiopathic interstitial pneumonias, in particular IPF, should be treated early in the clinical course is not widely held by clinicians (Figure 25–9). In fact, despite the high mortality associated with these diseases, treatment is frequently withheld, predominantly on the erroneous

grounds that either few or stable symptoms are present. Also, elderly patients are less likely to be treated at the time of presentation.[231] Figure 25–10 shows the common reasons that British physicians begin treatment in their patients with idiopathic interstitial pneumonia.

Equally difficult is the management of elderly patients in whom lung biopsy reveals predominantly fibrotic tissue and severe pulmonary function abnormalities. In general, these patients receive a brief treatment trial to determine if reversibility is feasible. Unfortunately, few if any of these patients are likely to have a significant objective response, and the risk of medication side effects is increased. I usually discontinue treatment if objective improvement is not clearly demonstrated at 12 to 16 weeks, especially in patients over age 70 years in whom the complications of the treatment may outweigh the potential benefits.

Common Treatment Modalities for the Idiopathic Interstitial Pneumonias

Corticosteroids (prednisone or equivalent) are the mainstay for the treatment of the idiopathic interstitial pneumonias.[137,141,232–238] The rationale for the use of corticosteroids in this disease is to stabilize or prevent disease progression by suppressing the chronic alveolitis. Alternative therapy to corticosteroids is frequently required because of the progression of the disease or patient intolerance of corticosteroid therapy. Cyclophosphamide or azathioprine is the usual second agent in the treatment regimen. In most instances, low-dose corticosteroid therapy (usually < 20 mg/day) is continued while adding one of these alternative therapies. A number of other drugs have been tried, and newer agents are being studied. Methotrexate, colchicine, penicillamine, and cyclosporine have been used only when the above-mentioned approaches have failed or are not tolerated by the patient. If these therapeutic approaches are ineffective or not tolerated, I recommend discontinuing the drugs. General recommendations regarding the use of the more common agents will be outlined here. Specific comments regarding the recommended treatment and discussion of new approaches for each of the specific idiopathic interstitial pneumonias will be discussed with each disease.

Corticosteroids

Corticosteroids (prednisone or equivalent) are highly effective for the treatment of some of the idiopathic interstitial pneumonias (eg, NSIP, COP, DIP/RB-ILD, and LIP) and ineffective in others (IPF and AIP; see Table 25–4).[239,240]

Mechanism of Action.   The mechanism by which corticosteroids affect the inflammatory immune effector cells is unknown. Data suggest that glucocorticoids work

---

TABLE 25–7   Unclassifiable Lung Fibrosis*

1. Inadequate clinical information
2. Inadequate radiologic data
3. An inadequate or nondiagnostic biopsy (eg, due to small size, poor sampling)
4. Previous therapy resulting in alterations in the radiologic or histologic findings
5. Existence of a major discrepancy among CRP findings
6. A discrepancy between histologic findings in different lobes that is not resolved after correlation with clinical and radiologic data

Adapted from Travis WD et al.[2]
*Table shows common reasons for a diagnosis of "unclassifiable" lung fibrosis.

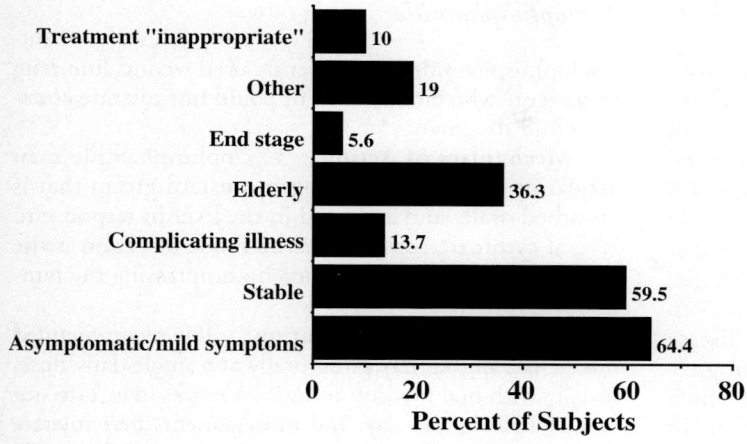

Figure 25–9   Reasons given by physicians for not beginning treatment in patients with IIP in the British Thoracic Society study. Data are from Johnston IDA et al.[231]

by suppressing neutrophil and lymphocyte migration to the lung, decreasing the level of immune complexes, altering alveolar macrophage function (eg, by inhibiting the secretion of proteolytic enzymes or decreasing the amount of chemotactic factors released), and altering the neutrophil adhesion to endothelial surfaces, probably mediated by a direct effect on the surface membrane configuration. Glucocorticoids exert their effects on target cells by interacting with specific intracellular receptors.[241] These receptors are members of a large family of nuclear proteins capable of binding to DNA and regulating expression of specific target genes. It is unclear why some patients respond to corticosteroids and others do not. It has been suggested that this may be related to the presence of glucocorticoid surface receptors on the parenchymal cells.[242,243] This hypothesis is potentially important because the effects of glucocorticoids on target cells are mediated by specific glucocorticoid receptors in the cells.

Dosage and Administration.   Initial therapy with prednisone is usually a relatively high dose, 0.5 to 1.0 mg/kg/day, and rarely is it necessary to exceed a total dose of 60 mg per day. This is given as a single oral dose in the morning. Alternate day therapy is not recommended as initial treatment because no data are available to suggest that it is effective. The patient should

return during the first 2 weeks to make sure he or she is tolerating the medication without any significant side effects. After approximately 2 to 3 months of daily prednisone therapy, reevaluation of chest radiographs and pulmonary physiological studies is performed. If the patient is responsive (ie, improved or stabilized), prednisone is tapered (by 1 to 2 mg per week) until a maintenance dose of 0.25 mg/kg/day is reached. This dose is continued for an additional 3 to 6 months, with the realization that with clinical and physiological deterioration, the prednisone dose may have to be raised to previous levels.

In general, it is unlikely that corticosteroid therapy can be discontinued, and patients are usually maintained on 0.25 mg/kg/day. In fact, no clear-cut guidelines exist for the length of therapy in idiopathic interstitial pneumonias. The author advocates 1 year of therapy, with or without another immunosuppressive agent, and then a gradual tapering with regular follow-up (3 to 6 months). Unfortunately, even after this prolonged therapy, one may find that the disease will flare up after several months or even years of stability. At this juncture, the author generally initiates repeat therapy with the same agent(s). Many clinicians feel that lifelong treatment is required in the management of idiopathic interstitial

Figure 25–10   Reasons given by physicians for initiating treatment in patients with IIP in the British Thoracic Society study. Data are from Johnston IDA et al.[231]

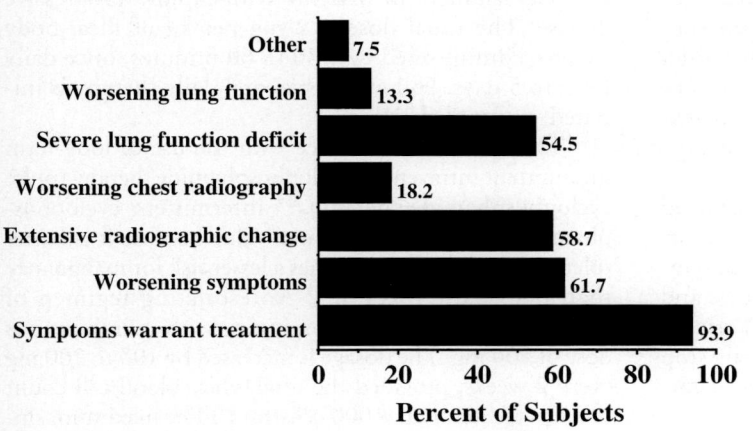

pneumonia, especially those that show response to treatment (a stable or improved course).

Intermittent, high-dose parenteral corticosteroid treatment (pulse corticosteroid therapy) has been used in patients with aggressive severe disease. Treatment with intravenous methylprednisolone, 2 g/week, plus oral prednisone, 0.25 mg/kg/day suppresses the neutrophil component of the alveolitis but has not been clearly shown to improve the lung disease. Initial treatment with intravenous high-dose corticosteroid therapy (ie, methylprednisolone, 250 mg every 6 hours for 3 to 5 days) has been used in an effort to control the disease as soon as possible in a patient who has rapidly progressive disease. No control trial exists to determine which of these methods of treatment is best. Nevertheless, in general, the higher doses appear to be somewhat more effective than the lower doses, although the incidence of complications may be higher.

Adverse Effects.   Significant complications can result from corticosteroid therapy.[244] The author's experience is that minor side effects are usual, and significant ones are uncommon in carefully managed patients. A study of 41 patients with IPF initially treated with at least 60 mg of prednisone daily found that 100% suffered at least one adverse reaction to the drug, most commonly insomnia, weight gain, skin changes, or irritability.[245] Weight gain and salt and water retention with exacerbation of cardiovascular disease (especially in elderly patients) can result in alterations of physiological measurements, making recognition of improvement difficult. Other significant side effects include (l) hyperglycemia and/or overt diabetes mellitus; (2) depression, hyperexcitability, or frank psychosis, especially in elderly women; (3) osteoporosis and joint destruction; (4) peptic ulcer disease; (5) immunosuppression leading to opportunistic infections; and (6) other side effects, such as hypokalemia, hypertension, renal lithiasis, poor wound healing, cataract, ecchymosis, phlebitis, and hirsutism.

A tuberculin skin test should be considered in patients starting on corticosteroids. Preventive therapy is recommended for persons with a positive tuberculin skin test or those at risk for tuberculosis (eg, individuals living in endemic areas) and, in particular, those patients taking > 15 mg of prednisone (or equivalent) daily for more than 3 weeks.[230] The routine use of trimethoprim/sulfamethoxazole (one single-strength tablet 3×/week) as prophylaxis against *Pneumocystis carinii* or isoniazid as prophylaxis against *Mycobacterium tuberculosis* in patients receiving immunosuppressive therapy may be considered.

It is important to remember that corticosteroid withdrawal may result in serious symptoms and morbidity (ie, fatigue, weakness, arthralgias, anorexia, nausea, desquamation of the skin, orthostatic dizziness and hypotension, fainting, and hypoglycemia). Patients should be appropriately cautioned not to suddenly stop therapy. Careful evaluation of patients during both corticosteroid therapy and withdrawal is important.

Cyclophosphamide

Cyclophosphamide is a frequently used second-line drug in patients who either failed or could not tolerate corticosteroid treatment.[246–249]

Mechanism of Action.   Cyclophosphamide is an alkylating agent of the nitrogen mustard group that is absorbed orally and activated in the liver in response to several cytotoxic compounds. Its mode of action is the depletion of lymphocytes, thereby suppressing the lymphocyte function.[246,248,250,251]

Dosage and Administration.   The recommended dosage is 2 mg/kg/day given orally as a single daily dose, usually with oral prednisone at 0.25 mg/kg/day. I do not exceed 150 mg per day, and most patients best tolerate dosages in the 75 to 100 mg per day range. We usually begin with 25 to 50 mg per day and increase gradually, by 25 mg increments, in order to maintain the white blood cell count at greater than 4,000 cells/mm³ (usually measured biweekly for the first 6 to 12 weeks and then at least monthly thereafter). Occasionally, the white blood cell count remains greater than 7,000 cells/mm³ despite increases in the cyclophosphamide dosage. In these instances, we do not raise the dosage above 100 mg per day. It is our clinical impression that cyclophosphamide responsiveness and reduced side effects occur at doses not exceeding 100 mg per day. Consequently, we do not exceed this dose, even if the white cell count remains above 7,000 cells/mm³. Forced diuresis, the drinking of eight or more glasses (8 oz each) of water daily, and monthly monitoring of the urine for red blood cells or other abnormalities is recommended in an attempt to prevent clinically significant hemorrhagic cystitis.

Few data are available on the appropriate length of therapy. In general, we do not expect to achieve a favorable response to cyclophosphamide therapy for at least 3 months after initiating treatment with this drug, with or without low-dose corticosteroids. Therapy should be given for not less than 3 months and probably for as long as 12 months in patients who appear to have stabilization or clinical improvement documented by follow-up studies.

Intravenous cyclophosphamide therapy has been used occasionally in patients with rapidly progressive disease. The usual dose is 2 mg per kg of ideal body weight, administered over 30 to 60 minutes, once daily for 3 to 5 days. Following this, oral daily therapy is initiated, as detailed above.

There is little experience with the use of long-term intermittent intravenous cyclophosphamide therapy (pulse cyclophosphamide therapy).[252] Intermittent cyclophosphamide therapy is of potential value because it is better tolerated, less toxic, and carries a lesser risk for malignancy than does daily therapy.[252] An escalating regimen of cyclophosphamide is used, beginning with an intravenous dose of 500 mg. The dosage is increased by 100 to 200 mg every 2 weeks, provided the total white blood cell count remains greater than 3,000 cells/mm³. The maximum single administered dose is 1,000 to 1,800 mg of cyclophosphamide, depending on body size. The patient is monitored for adverse side effects as noted below.

Adverse Effects.   The side effects of cyclophosphamide therapy include leukopenia, but careful monitoring of the blood counts allows adjustment of the dosage to an acceptable level. We generally aim to maintain a total white count of greater than 4,000 cells/mm^3 or a neutrophil count greater than 1,500/mm^3. If the white blood cell count decreases to less than 4,000/mm^3 and the platelet counts fall below 100,000/mm^3, then the cyclophosphamide should be stopped or the dosage lowered immediately by 50% until the hematologic abnormalities recover. Recovery of the white blood cell and platelet counts should be assessed weekly. If the counts do not recover, the medication should be completely discontinued until they improve. Zisman and colleagues[253] reported this toxicity in 68% of patients treated with cyclophosphamide. Gastrointestinal symptoms that required discontinuation of the drug (including nausea, vomiting, anorexia/weight loss, or diarrhea) were seen in 54% of those with toxicity. Thrombocytopenia, hematuria secondary to hemorrhagic cystitis (forced fluids and frequent bladder emptying are recommended to prevent this problem), bone marrow suppression, azoospermia and amenorrhea, infection, and the development of a hematological malignant disease are other possible complications.

Rarely, cyclophosphamide has been reported to cause interstitial pneumonitis and fibrosis.[254–257] These have been divided into two categories: early-onset pneumonitis, which is reversible and may respond to corticosteroid therapy, or late-onset pneumonitis, frequently associated with pleural thickening and which appears to be clinically distinct from IPF but with a chronically progressive course. It appears to be unresponsive to corticosteroid therapy.[256]

Azathioprine

Azathioprine is less toxic than cyclophosphamide and has been reported to be effective in the treatment of idiopathic interstitial pneumonias.

Mechanism of Action.   Azathioprine is a purine analogue that is slowly converted to mercaptopurine in body tissues; it appears to act by the substitution of purines in DNA synthesis and by inhibiting adenine deaminase, which results in an effect on lymphocytes, making them ineffective because they are so highly susceptible to adenine deaminase deficiency.[233,247,250,258] In addition to cytotoxic effects, azathioprine has been reported to suppress natural killer cell activity, antibody production, and antibody-dependent cellular cytotoxicity. Azathioprine also suppresses the production of autoantibodies in animal models of autoimmune disease, although the clinical relevance of these findings remains unknown.

Dosage and Administration.   The recommended dosage for azathioprine is approximately 2 mg per kg of body weight, although the optimal dosage for treatment is as yet undetermined. Generally, the dosage does not exceed 100 mg per day. As with cyclophosphamide, the maximal dose need not be adjusted to the lowering of the white blood cell count. If the white blood cell count decreases to less than 4,000 cells/mm^3 and the platelet counts fall below 100,000/mm^3, then the dose of azathioprine should be stopped or immediately lowered by 50% until these hematologic abnormalities recover. Recovery of the white blood cell and platelet counts should be assessed weekly. If the counts do not recover, the medication should be completely discontinued until they improve. A trial of at least 3 months duration is recommended to ensure an adequate opportunity for clinical response.

Adverse Effects.   Significant adverse drug reactions that result in discontinuance of azathioprine are reported in 20 to 30% of patients with rheumatoid arthritis. There is less data available regarding the tolerance of azathioprine in patients with idiopathic interstitial pneumonias. Hematologic adverse effects include leukopenia, anemia, thrombocytopenia, pure red cell aplasia, and pancytopenia. Gastrointestinal complaints are the most frequent side effects, including nausea and vomiting and, less commonly, peptic ulcer disease and diarrhea. Mild elevation of hepatic enzymes has been described in approximately 5% of patients treated with azathioprine, although reports of severe hepatitis, progressive hepatic cirrhosis, and cholestasis are rare.

Pulmonary complications of interstitial pneumonitis and diffuse alveolar damage have been reported in some renal transplant patients treated with azathioprine, however this has not been described in patients treated with azathioprine for IPF or connective tissue disorders. Although normal births have been reported in patients having received azathioprine during pregnancy, there are also reports of significant neonatal complications and chromosomal damage in the offspring of patients treated with azathioprine during pregnancy. The risk of malignancy is increased in renal transplant patients treated with azathioprine and corticosteroids. Although there is conflicting data regarding the carcinogenic potential of azathioprine in other disease processes, it appears to be similar to that seen in patients treated with cyclophosphamide.

Colchicine

Long used in the treatment of gout, colchicine has been tried as a treatment for fibrotic disorders, especially IPF. Several in vitro and animal model studies suggest that colchicine may be helpful in slowing the fibrotic process.[259–261]

Mechanism of Action.   Colchicine has multiple effects including the arrest of cell division, inhibition of granulocyte migration, and inhibition of the release of several proteins from cells, which blocks the release of some fibroblast growth and chemotactic factors.[261,262] It also may interfere with the secretion of collagen from fibroblasts and may increase collagen degradation by enhancing the action of collagenase.

Dosage and Administration.   I recommend an oral dose of 0.6 mg once or twice daily as tolerated.

Adverse Effects.   Colchicine is generally quite well tolerated. Side effects that may be encountered include nausea, vomiting, abdominal pain, and diarrhea.

Methotrexate

Methotrexate is used clinically for both its antineoplastic and immunosuppressive effects. Clinical experience with methotrexate in the treatment of ILD is limited. There have been several descriptions of its use in sarcoidosis, but very little has been written regarding its effectiveness in the idiopathic interstitial pneumonias. Scott and Bacon described three patients with the clinical diagnosis of fibrosing alveolitis associated with connective tissue disease who appeared to respond favorably to methotrexate.[263–267]

Mechanism of Action.   Methotrexate is a folic acid analog that inhibits the enzyme dihydrofolate reductase. Its immunosuppressive properties can likely be attributed to inhibition of the replication and function of T lymphocytes and possibly B lymphocytes. It may also interfere with neutrophil chemotaxis.

Dosage and Administration.   Methotrexate may be administered orally or intramuscularly. The recommended beginning dose is 7.5 mg per week. The dose is then gradually increased (eg, increments of 2.5 mg every 2 weeks) until a dose of 15 mg per week is achieved. A trial of methotrexate therapy should last at least 4 to 6 months to assess effectiveness.

Adverse Effects.   Liver function tests and white blood cell counts should be monitored monthly to assess toxicity. Because hepatic toxicity occurs in up to 10% of cases when the dose exceeds 5 g and may initially be clinically occult, some have advocated liver biopsy when the total dose exceeds 1 g or after 18 to 24 months of therapy, even in the absence of signs of hepatic injury. Other toxicities include bone marrow suppression, nausea, alopecia, and skin rash. Methotrexate is known to be teratogenic and may transiently suppress gonadal function. The oncogenic potential of methotrexate remains controversial.

Penicillamine

Several animal studies suggest a possible role for penicillamine in the treatment of fibrotic lung disorders.[268–271]

Mechanism of Action.   The postulated mechanisms through which penicillamine may affect the progression of idiopathic interstitial pneumonias include the inhibition of collagen synthesis by interference with the aldehyde groups involved in the intermolecular and intramolecular cross-linkages of mature collagen; it may also contribute to decrease abnormal collagen accumulation by inhibiting collagen biosynthesis and suppression of T cell function.[263]

Dosage and Administration.   The dosage I recommend is that used for the management of rheumatoid arthritis. The initial dose is 125 of 250 mg given as a daily oral dose. After 4 to 8 weeks, the dose is increased weekly to a final dose of 500 mg daily. Doses as high as 1,000 mg daily may be used if tolerated. A determination of effectiveness cannot be made before 3 to 6 months.

Adverse Effects.   Reported side effects include nausea, vomiting, diarrhea, dyspepsia, anorexia, transient loss of taste for sweet and salt, cutaneous lesions, hematologic toxicity (leukopenia, aplastic anemia, agranulocytopenia), renal toxicity (reversible proteinuria and hematuria, nephrotic syndrome), and myasthenia gravis. In the past, preparations of penicillamine contained trace amounts of penicillin. Although this is no longer the case, some of the reactions that occur may be explained by cross-reactivity with penicillin. Most side effects are experienced during the first 18 months of therapy. Concomitant drug therapy should be closely monitored because adverse reactions may occur.

Cyclosporine

The primary clinical indication for the use of cyclosporine is the prevention of allograft rejection. In addition, it may be effective in other T cell-mediated disorders such as uveitis, psoriasis, rheumatoid arthritis, and primary biliary cirrhosis. Because of the potential role of the T helper (Th)2 immune response in the pathogenesis of lung fibrosis, there is renewed interest in cyclosporine as a treatment for ILDs; however, the experience with this drug is limited.

Mechanism of Action.   Cyclosporine exerts an inhibitory effect on T cells. It is known to suppress antibody response to T cell-dependent antigens, delayed type hypersensitivity, and allograft rejection. There is apparently no myelotoxicity associated with the therapeutic use of cyclosporine. Cyclosporine A is a potent antagonist of transforming growth factor (TGF)-β activity in vitro.[272]

Dosage and Administration.   The optimal dose of cyclosporine is unknown. It is usually given in a once daily dose of 5 to 10 mg/kg/day for the first 3 to 9 months of treatment. The dose may be adjusted to maintain a blood level of 100 to 200 ng/mL. Maintenance therapy should be maintained at the lowest dose associated with stabilization of the disease activity, usually 3 to 5 mg/kg/day.

Adverse Effects.   The major adverse reactions are renal dysfunction, tremor, hirsutism, hypertension, and gum hyperplasia.

Assessing the Response to Treatment

Determining whether a treatment modality has produced the desired effect can be difficult. Subjective without objective improvement occurs frequently (up to 70% of treated patients). Objective improvement in physiological or radiographic abnormalities occurs in 20 to 30% of treated patients. Improvement is often found in only a subset of the tests used to evaluate response. For example, the chest radiograph or lung function test results are often divergent. The DL_{CO} may improve considerably, whereas lung volumes may not; the opposite may also occur.

In general, the responsive patient reports a decrease in symptoms (especially dyspnea or cough) and demonstrates radiographic clearing or physiological improvement (as assessed by measurement of forced vital capacity [FVC], TLC, DL_{CO}, and resting and exercise gas exchange). An absence of further decline in lung function or other parameters of disease activity for prolonged periods of time (3 to 6 months) is also considered a favorable response to treatment. Physiological improvement is commonly defined as a greater than 10% increase in TLC or VC, a 15% increase in single breath D_{CO}, and a reduction or normalization of oxygen desaturation during exercise. Even with these guidelines, determination of the therapeutic response is often difficult. Table 25–8 shows the key features associated with worsening of the disease in patients with one of the idiopathic interstitial pneumonias.

Watters and coworkers developed a composite CRP score that allows a quantification of the clinical course and the impact of therapy in individual patients.[179] It has been demonstrated that this composite CRP score correlates better than any single component with the histopathologic features present on lung biopsy, and that it is useful in estimation of the severity of the underlying pathologic derangement. Furthermore, it appears very useful for the longitudinal quantitative assessment of clinical impairment in patients with IPF. Although it has not been validated in a prospective study, others have shown it to be useful in the assessment of the disease course for patients with the idiopathic interstitial pneumonias.[273,274] The methods for calculating the CRP score are described by Watters and colleagues.[179] In general, CRP scores of 0 to 14 points are seen in relatively healthy individuals, scores of 15 to 29 are usually seen in patients able to carry on a fairly normal existence with full-time employment, and scores of 30 to 59 are associated with moderate impairment; scores of 60 to 79 are usually associated with severe impairment, often precluding continued employment; and scores greater than 80 are seen in patients confined to home and often to bed. In follow-up, improvement is defined as a greater than 10-point reduction in the CRP score and deterioration as a greater than 10-point increase in the CRP score. The patient is considered stable if the CRP score changes less than 10 points in either direction. This scoring system has not been validated by a longitudinal, prospective study but has been shown to be useful because it provides quantification of patient progress, and this simplifies the assessment of the patient's clinical course. This "original" CRP score has recently been shown to correlate with survival in patients with IPF.[28]

Lung Transplantation

Lung transplantation is the only therapeutic modality that has the potential to restore considerable physiological function in patients with end-stage idiopathic interstitial pneumonia. Improvements in donor and recipient selection, lung preservation, surgical techniques, postoperative management, and immunosuppression have made lung transplantation an effective treatment.[275–277] Transplantation should be considered for those patients who experience progressive physiological deterioration despite optimal medical management and who meet the criteria outlined in Table 25–9. Single lung transplantation is currently the preferred surgical procedure.[276–278]

ILDs, especially the idiopathic interstitial pneumonias, are the second most common indication for lung transplantation.[279] IPF accounts for 15% of all lung transplants. If lung transplantation is being considered, the patient should be referred as early as is feasible for further evaluation and counseling at a nearby center. The waiting time for procuring a suitable donor lung may exceed 2 years. Most patients with IPF (28 to 47%) die while waiting for lung transplant because of the progressive nature of this disease.[279]

After successful transplantation, arterial oxygen tension is frequently sufficiently improved to alleviate the

---

TABLE 25–8   Findings Suggestive of Disease Progression in Patients with Idiopathic Interstitial Pneumonia

Symptoms
  Increased breathlessness and/or cough
  Decreased exercise capacity

Physical findings
  Progression of crackles over all lung fields
  Worsening right ventricular failure
    Peripheral edema
    Increased pulmonic second sound
    Pulmonic insufficiency
  Digital clubbing
  Cyanosis

Pulmonary function
  Worsening hypoxemia and increased supplemental oxygen
    requirement
  Progressive restrictive disease and decreased D_{CO}
  Increased alveolar–arterial oxygen gradient at rest or with
    exercise
  Hypercapnia

Radiographic findings
  Progression of interstitial infiltrates with volume loss
  Development of honeycombing
  Enlarging heart
  Pulmonary hypertension

need for supplemental oxygen, lung volumes and DL_{CO} are increased, and pulmonary hypertension and right ventricular dysfunction are reversed.[280,281] The 1-year actuarial survival rate after single lung transplantation for pulmonary fibrosis varies from 57 to 73% among different centers.[281] Two-year survival is between 53 and 73%. Graft failure, infection, and heart failure are the most common causes of early mortality, whereas bronchiolitis obliterans, infection, and malignancy are responsible for most late mortality.[281] Disease recurrence in the lung allografts has been reported for a number of ILDs: sarcoidosis, lymphangioleiomyomatosis, pulmonary Langerhan cell histiocytosis, giant cell interstitial pneumonia, and DIP.[281,282–298] Interestingly, improvement in the primary disease in the native lung after single lung transplantation has been documented for UIP and AIP.[299,300]

IDEOPATHIC PULMONARY FIBROSIS

IPF is one of the more commonly occurring ILDs of unknown etiology.[146,301] The histologic lesion of UIP is required to confirm the diagnosis of IPF/UIP (see Table 25–2). The terms cryptogenic fibrosing alveolitis and IPF describe the same syndrome, and both are used.[230]

EPIDEMIOLOGY

Epidemiologic data related to IPF are scant and variable. The data suggest that it is among the most common idiopathic interstitial pneumonias (Table 25–10).[14,302] The incidence has been estimated at 10.7 cases per 100,000 per year for males and 7.4 cases per 100,000 per year for females.[14,302] The prevalence of IPF has been estimated at 20 cases per 100,000 for males and 13 cases per 100,000 for females.[14,302] The prevalence and incidence of IPF increases markedly with age; for example, among men and women 75 years of age or older, the prevalence of IPF is 250 per 100,000 and the incidence is 160 per 100,000/year. The nationwide prevalence of IPF in Finland as defined by the new ATS/ERS criteria was recently estimated to be 16 to 18 per 100,000.[112]

IPF has no distinct geographic distribution.[230] IPF does not appear to have a racial predilection; however, the majority of the patients reported are white.[16,19,28,303] Patients with IPF are often middle aged, usually between 50 and 70 years old (Figure 25–11). Approximately two-thirds of patients with IPF are over the age of 60 years at the time of presentation. There is a male predominance (1.5–1.7:1).[19,28,231] The majority of patients with IPF are former smokers (defined as not having smoked cigarettes in the past year) or current smokers (defined as those smoking cigarettes regularly within the year prior to diagnosis). Current smokers are younger at presentation than are former smokers or those who have never smoked (never smokers; Figure 25–12).

In the United States, IPF has been underreported as a cause of death, because it is not usually noted on death certificates, even in patients with a recognized primary respiratory death and a known diagnosis of IPF. IPF is estimated to have a 50 to 70% mortality 5 years after the diagnosis. Not only is the mortality associated with IPF likely to be grossly underreported, but also the consid-

TABLE 25–9 Lung Transplantation: Guidelines for Recipient Selection

General guidelines
  Severe end-stage lung disease with progression and life
    expectancy < 12–18 months, but longer than waiting time on
    transplant list (varies from 1 to 3 years).
  How disabled is the patient?
    Does the patient recognize the severity of the illness and
      the poor prognosis?
    What does the patient (and family) want?
  Medical therapy ineffective; no available alternative medical
    or surgical therapy
  Age < 65 years (single lung transplant)
  No other serious systemic disease, end-organ failure, or
    infection
  Normal body habitus (morbid obesity is a contraindication)
  Prednisone tapered to < 10–20 mg/day
  Adequate cardiac function
  Good general fitness and nutritional status
  Strong psychosocial and family support systems
  No recent alcohol, drug, or tobacco abuse
  Understanding of the transplantation procedure and ability to
    comply with medical and rehabilitation programs
  Substantial limitation in activities of daily living

Contraindications to transplantation:
  Absolute
    Presence of systemic disease that may complicate post-
      operative management
    Presence of significant psychosocial dysfunction
    Presence of significant secondary organ dysfunction
    Previous major cardiothoracic surgery
    Active malignancy within the past 2 years
    HIV infection
    Hepatitis B antigen positivity
    Hepatitis C with liver disease proven on liver biopsy
  Relative
    Presence of high-dose corticosteroid therapy (prednisone dose
      > 15 mg/day)
    Substance addiction: candidate should be free of tobacco,
      alchohol, and illicit drugs for at least 6 months

Objective parameters that correlate with end-stage disease:
  New York Heart Association functional class III or IV
    Class III: marked limitation of physical activity with ordinary
      activity resulting in fatigue, palpitation, dyspnea, or
      anginal pain
    Class IV: inability to carry on any physical activity without
      discomfort, often with discomfort even at rest
  Honeycombing and/or pulmonary hypertension on chest
    radiograph or CT scan
  Severe physiologic derangement
    TLC < 60% of predicted; FVC < 60% of predicted
    $DLCO_2/V_A$ < 50 % of predicted
    Resting hypoxemia (PaO_2 < 55 mm Hg); P(A-a)O_2 at rest >30
    Exercise desaturation score > 30*

*See Table 25–8. $DLCO_2/V_A$ = Diffusing capacity for carbon monoxide corrected for alveolar volume. FVC = forced vital capacity; P(A-a)O_2 = alveolar–arterial pressure difference for O_2; TLC = total lung capacity.

erable morbidity from this chronic disease is not defined by epidemiologic data.[304]

Etiology and Pathogenesis

The inciting factors in the development of IPF are unknown. General concepts regarding the pathogenesis of the idiopathic interstitial pneumonias are described in Chapter 25, "Idiopathic Interstitial Pneumonias," and additional discussion of the basic mechanism of lung fibrosis can be found in Part 2 (*"Basic Mechanisms"*) of the book.

It has been postulated that although chronic active inflammation may play a role in the pathogenesis of IPF/UIP, it is the fibrotic and destructive changes that distort the normal lung architecture and result in the high morbidity and mortality. In addition, it has been proposed that the fibroblastic foci are the primary sites of ongoing injury and repair in UIP (Figure 25–13).[126] These small aggregates of actively proliferating myofibroblasts and fibroblasts are located within the interstitial space directly beneath the alveolar epithelium. They are often at the interface between dense-collagenized and normal-appearing lung. These foci constitute many microscopic sites of ongoing alveolar epithelial injury and activation associated with evolving fibrosis.[126] Thus, emerging evidence suggests that UIP may be the result of disordered epithelial-fibroblast regulation.

Selman and colleagues hypothesize that UIP represents a model of abnormal wound healing in the lung, characterized by the absence of adequate reepithelialization and abnormalities in myofibroblast behavior.[126] Under this paradigm, the pathologic process of fibrosis is the result of persistent remodeling of the lung interstitium. Multiple microinjuries damage and activate alveolar epithelial cells, which in turn induce an antifibrinolytic environment in the alveolar spaces, enhancing wound clot formation. Alveolar epithelial cells secrete growth factors and induce migration and proliferation of fibroblasts and differentiation into myofibroblasts. Subepithelial myofibroblasts and alveolar epithelial cells produce gelatinases that may increase basement membrane disruption and allow fibroblast–myofibroblast migration. Angiogenic factors induce neovascularization. Both intra-alveolar and interstitial myofibroblasts secrete extracellular matrix proteins, mainly collagens. An imbalance between interstitial collagenases and tissue inhibitors of metalloproteinases provokes the progressive deposition of extracellular matrix. Signals responsible for myofibroblast apoptosis seem to be absent or delayed in UIP, increasing cell survival. Myofibroblasts produce angiotensinogen, which, as angiotensin II, provokes alveolar epithelial cell death, further impairing reepithelialization.[126] Barbas-Filho and

TABLE 25–10   Histopathologic Diagnosis in Case Series of IIP

Series	Design	Number of Patients	UIP	NSIP	DIP/ RB-ILD	AIP	Other*
Bjoraker and colleagues[398]	All patients previously diagnosed with IIP who had undergone open lung biopsy Study period: 1976 to 1985	104	62%	14%	10%	2%	12%
Nagai and colleagues[410]	All patients from a larger IIP cohort with a histopathologic diagnosis of UIP, NSIP, or BOOP Study period: not stated	111	58%	28%	0%	0%	14%
Travis and colleagues[411]	All patients from a larger IIP cohort with a histologic diagnosis of UIP, NSIP or DIP Study period: 1970 to 1992 Cases referred to Pulmonary Branch, NHLBI; Cases with BOOP, DAD, hypersensitivity pneumonitis were excluded.	101	55%	29%	16%	0%	0%
Nicholson and colleagues[413]	All patients previously diagnosed with IIP who had undergone open lung biopsy Study period: 1978 to 1989 A subset was previously reported as IPF[638]	78	47%	36%	17%	0%	0%
Park and colleagues[505]	All patients previously diagnosed with IIP who had undergone open lung biopsy Study period: 1984 to 1995	51	51%	16%	NR	NR	NR
Flaherty and colleagues[274]	All patients previously diagnosed with IIP who had undergone surgical lung biopsy Study period: 1989 to 2000 A subset was previously reported as IPF[245,273]	168	63%	20%	13%	0%	4%

Adapted from Nicholson AG et al[413] and Collard HR and King TE Jr.[409]

*Other includes hypersensitivity pneumonitis, bronchiolitis obliterans organizing pneumonia (BOOP), and unclassifiable ILDs. UIP = usual interstitial pneumonia; NSIP = nonspecific interstitial pneumonia; DIP/RBILD = desquamative interstitial pneumonia/respiratory bronchiolitis-associated interstitial lung disease; AIP = acute interstitial pneumonia; BOOP = bronchiolitis obliterans pneumonia; IIP = idiopathic interstitial pneumonia. NR = not reported.

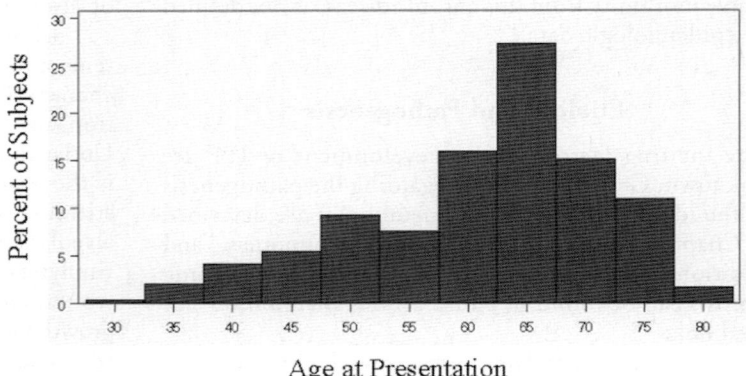

Figure 25–11   Age at presentation. Shown are prospectively enrolled patients with IPF/usual interstitial pneumonia (UIP) in Denver specialized center of research (SCOR) in interstitial lung disease (ILD) (*n* = 238, median age = 64 years). Data are from King TE Jr et al.[28]

coworkers showed that numerous type II pneumocytes from the normal alveoli of most patients with IPF/UIP actively undergo programmed cell death (apoptosis) and that this precedes the fibrotic response in the absence of an inflammatory reaction.[305] It is useful to compare the fibroproliferative process in organizing pneumonia (OP), a condition which is usually self-limited or reversible, to the intra-alveolar fibroblastic foci observed in UIP, which is progressive and irreversible.[126,144,306] It appears that OP represents the normal wound healing model in the lung, with appropriate extracellular matrix remodeling, fibroblast/myofibroblast apoptosis, and alveolar reepithelialization (Table 25–11).[144,306]

Although the molecular mechanisms that lead to end-stage pulmonary fibrosis in the idiopathic interstitial pneumonias are poorly understood, additional recent data suggest support for this "abnormal wound healing" hypothesis in UIP.[125,127] Zuo and colleagues analyzed gene expression patterns in lung samples from patients with histologically proven UIP using oligonucleotide microarrays.[307] Gene expression patterns clearly distinguished normal from fibrotic lungs. Many of the genes that were significantly increased in fibrotic lungs encoded proteins associated with extracellular matrix formation and degradation and proteins expressed in smooth muscle.[307] These investigators showed that matrilysin, a matrix metalloprotease not previously associated with pulmonary fibrosis, was the most informative

increased gene in their data set. Immunohistochemistry showed an increased expression of matrilysin protein in fibrotic lungs. Furthermore, matrilysin knockout mice were dramatically protected from pulmonary fibrosis resulting from intratracheal bleomycin. Their results identify matrilysin as a mediator of pulmonary fibrosis and a potential therapeutic target.

Clinical Findings

Patients with IPF commonly have an insidious onset of breathlessness with exertion and a nonproductive cough. Although patients may present with only a nonproductive cough, virtually all patients develop dyspnea with exertion as the disease progresses. A few patients with IPF present with constitutional symptoms: weight loss, fever, fatigue, myalgias, and arthralgias. Also, very rarely the onset is heralded by a flulike illness. Importantly, these features should suggest the presence of another disease, especially pulmonary fibrosis associated with connective tissue diseases, chronic COP, or viral or mycoplasmal infection.[308,309] The median duration of illness prior to diagnosis is 24 months.[28] A duration of symptoms less than 6 months before diagnosis is uncommon.

The physical examination is rarely normal, and a history of cigarette smoking alters the frequency of some findings. Most patients have a chest examination that

Figure 25–12   Smoking status at presentation. Current smokers presented at a younger age than former or never smokers. Data are from King TE Jr et al.[28]

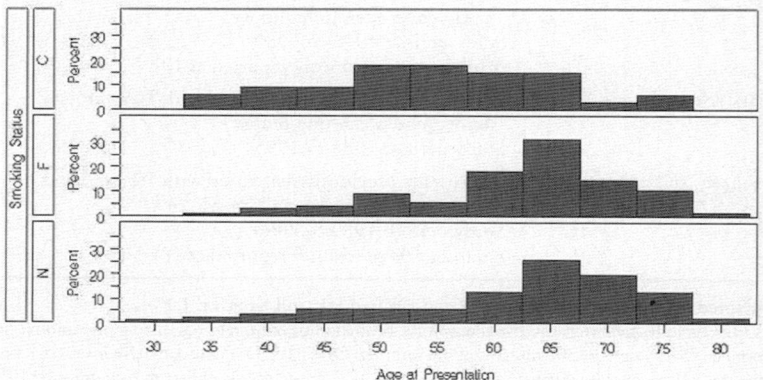

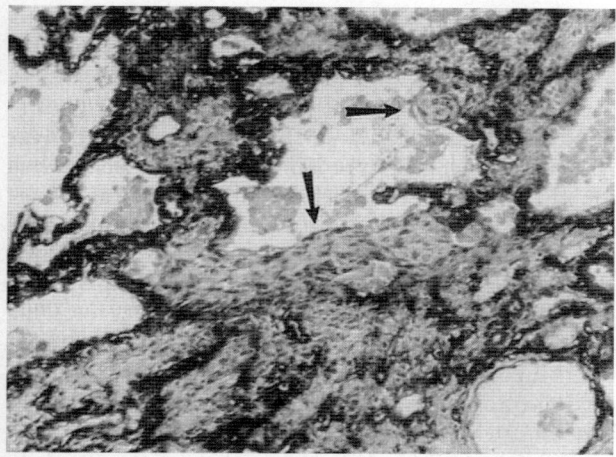

Figure 25–13   Fibroblastic foci in UIP. Two foci of active collagen synthesis (arrows) are illustrated at the edge of a badly distorted area of lung. Smudgy, discontinuous remnants of basal lamina are present beneath the fibroblasts, but none cover their surfaces, indicating that they are located in the lumen of an air space (Immunoperoxidase for procollagen type I and glucose oxidase for type IV collagen; ×230 original magnification). Reproduced with permission from Kuhn C.[621]

reveals late inspiratory fine crackles ("Velcro rales") at the lung bases. A higher proportion of current smokers have none or few crackles heard on chest examination compared to never and former smokers.[28] Clubbing of the fingers is relatively common (40 to 75%; see Figure 25–5).[28,165,234,237,309] Never smokers have significantly less frequent finger clubbing compared to former or current smokers.[28] In my experience, clubbing is a finding late in the course of the disease, and the full-blown picture

of hypertrophic pulmonary osteoarthropathy does not develop in most patients.[183] Cardiac examination is usually normal except in mid or late stages of the disease when findings of pulmonary hypertension (ie, augmented P2, right-sided lift, and S3 gallop) and cor pulmonale may become evident. Similarly, cyanosis is a late manifestation indicative of advanced disease. Spontaneous pneumothorax occurs, but is much less common in IPF than in other ILDs, such as eosinophilic granuloma and lymphangiomyomatosis.[137,177,311,312]

Laboratory Findings

Hypoxemia is a common manifestation of IPF; however, erythrocytosis is not. Total plasma lactate dehydrogenase (LDH) activity may be elevated in IPF, and LDH activity increases in IPF patients with deteriorating lung function.[313]

Bronchoalveolar Lavage

Cellular Analysis

It has been shown that there is no correlation between the percentage of various cell types found in the lavage fluid of patients with IPF and various clinical parameters, serum tests, or pulmonary function studies (see Table 25–6).[130] The relationship between cellular abnormalities in BAL fluid and clinical response to therapy has not been defined conclusively.[31,130,132,134,135,174,228,314] A strong correlation has been suggested between the per-

TABLE 25–11   Morphological Differences Between Fibroblast Foci and Organizing Pneumonia

Process	Fibroblast Foci (UIP-pattern)	Organizing Pneumonia (OP-pattern)	References
Inflammation	Minimal or absent inflammation	Mixed inflammatory cell population in the central region CD8-positive T-cell lymphocyte-dominant interstitial pneumonia	144,639,640
Fibroblasts cytoskeleton	Myofibroblasts do not express desmin	Fibroblasts undergo specific changes, (ie, express desmin)	640
Myofibroblasts	Prolonged survival Predominant localization of tissue inhibitor of metalloproteinases-2	Early apoptosis and disappearance Predominant localization of matrix metalloproteinases	306,641,642
Extracellular matrix	Imbalance between MMP and TIMP Progressive deposition of dense collagen	Loose mode of organization thus susceptible to degradation Myofibroblasts phagocytose collagen fibrils Bud-type intra-alveolar fibrosis shrunk and become collagen globules	144,307,639, 642,643
Reepithelialization	It is delayed or absent (by apoptosis and disruption of basement membrane) Type II pneumocytes in normal appearing alveoli undergo apoptosis	Occurs rapidly and basement membrane is not severely impaired Regenerated type I alveolar epithelial cells surround the residual collagen globule	305,306, 644–646
Neovascularization	New vessels are usually not found	Newly formed vessels with well-developed basement membranes	144,306,647

MMP = matrix metalloproteinases; TIMP = tissue inhibitors of metalloprteinases.

centage of neutrophils in lavage fluid and the prognosis of IPF (see Figure 25–6). It was further suggested that modification of therapy could be guided by the neutrophil percentage found in lavage fluid; but other investigators have found no difference in the lavage neutrophil percentage of patients who responded to corticosteroid therapy versus those who did not.[130,134,135,315] Lavage fluid eosinophilia in IPF has been reported to be associated with a poor response to corticosteroids.[134,135,316] The role and value of serial BAL in assessment of the clinical progress of patients with IPF has not been adequately studied.

Fluid Analysis

Alveolar type II cells are the dominant secretory cells (producing pulmonary surface-active material) in the distal air space (see Chapter 9, "Role of the Alveolar Epithelium in the Pathogenesis of Pulmonary Fibrosis"). Phospholipids (PLs) (dipalmitoylphosphatidylcholine [DPPC], phosphatidylglycerol [PGly], and phosphatidylinositol [PI]) are key components of cellular membranes, and certain phospholipids possess the ability to lower surface tension at air-water interfaces. Also, the protein secretory products of the alveolar type II cell, SP-A, -B, -C, and -D are important contributors to the function and metabolism of pulmonary surface-active material.[317–322] SP-A and SP-D also play major roles in host defenses. Therefore, because type II cell abnormalities are thought to play a major role in the pathogenesis of IPF, measurement of the lipids and proteins produced by these cells might provide insights into disease activity.[126]

The quantity and composition of pulmonary surfactant PLs recovered by BAL are abnormal in IPF as well as in other ILDs and animal models of fibrotic lung disease (see Chapter 9, "Role of the Alveolar Epithelium in the Pathogenesis of Pulmonary Fibrosis").[323–334] There is a reduced total recovery of surfactant PL, a reduction in the percentage of PGly and a slight increase in PI. There is no change in the percentage of saturated phosphatidylcholine. Because PGly and PI share a common precursor, CDP-diacylglycerol, their synthesis is related, and the ratio of these two PL species can be used as a marker of surfactant alterations in disease.[325,335] In IPF, changes in the PG:PI ratio are predictive of the cellularity and degree of fibrosis on histopathologic examination of open lung biopsies.[325] In addition, patients with higher levels of total PLs in lavage fluid improve with corticosteroid therapy, whereas those with more severe decreases in total PL do not.[325]

McCormack and colleagues have demonstrated that SP-A is reduced in IPF and that a decrease in its concentration, referenced to total PL (a marker of surfactant to normalize to the surface sampled by lavage and recovery), predicts an adverse clinical outcome.[329] The decrease in SP-A is not disease specific and is found in other ILDs.[329] In a subsequent study, it was shown that SP-A levels predicted survival in IPF.[330] SP-A and total PL were

measured in BAL fluid. The mean SP-A:PL ratio was lower in patients with IPF than in healthy volunteers (31.8 ± 2.8 vs 63.9 ± 6.4 μg/μmol, $p = .006$) and in patients who died within 2 years than in those who survived (23.4 ± 2.6 vs 37.5 ± 4.2 μg/μmol, $p = .015$) (Figure 25–14). Using Cox's proportional hazard model, they found that SP-A/PL modeled continuously was associated with survival time ($p = .002$). The 5-year survival of patients with SP-A/PL ratios above the median level for all patients with IPF (29.7 μg/μmol) was more than twice that of patients below the median (68 vs 30%, $p = .007$) (see Chapter 9, Figure 9–5). Notably, SP-A/PL improved upon prediction of survival modeled by most routine physiological variables, with the exception of % predicted TLC or the multifarious CRP score.[329]

SP-A and SP-D can be detected at very low levels in the serum of healthy individuals and are elevated in patients with certain inflammatory lung diseases, including IPF.[336–339] Although the exact mechanism for the increase in SP-A and SP-D in the circulation is not known, it is probably a combination of a loss of epithelial integrity due to injury, altered alveolar polarity for secretion, or an increased mass of type II cells due to hyperplasia.[337] Takahashi and coworkers showed that the levels of SP-A and SP-D in the sera of patients with IPF correlated with the extent of alveolitis (as assessed by the presence of ground-glass opacities on HRCT), whereas they did not correlate with the progression or extent of fibrosis (as assessed by the presence of honeycombing on HRCT). The serum SP-D concentration, unlike that of serum SP-A, was also related to rate of deterioration in pulmonary function; higher levels of SP-D at presentation, even in asymptomatic subjects, predicted declines in lung function. The concentrations of serum SP-A and SP-D in patients who died within 3 years were significantly higher than those in patients who were still alive after 3 years of follow-up.[340] Based on their criteria for diagnosis, it is possible that many of the cases with diffuse ground-glass opacities on HRCT have NSIP as the histologic pattern rather than UIP. Greene and coworkers also showed that serum SP-A and SP-D levels are elevated in patients with IPF and progressive systemic sclerosis and are not elevated in the other pulmonary diseases with less diffuse parenchymal involvement (Figure 25–15). In addition, these authors reported that serum SP-A and SP-D levels are highly predictive of survival in patients with IPF.[337]

Physiological Findings

Pulmonary function tests usually demonstrate a restrictive process with a reduced DL_{CO} and abnormal gas exchange.

Airways Mechanics

Patients with IPF are tachypneic, with rapid shallow breaths; therefore, the work of breathing is increased.[341,342]

This rapid respiratory rate is felt to be secondary to altered mechanical reflexes, because of the increased elastic load and/or vagal mechanisms because no defined chemical basis for the hyperventilation has been identified.[343-350] Expiratory flow rates, forced expiratory volume in 1 second (FEV_1) and FVC are often decreased because of the reduction in lung volume, but the FEV_1 to FVC ratio is maintained in IPF (Figure 25–16). However, because of the increased static elastic recoil found in these patients, flow rates, when compared to lung volumes, are often increased (Figure 25–17). Also, functional and pathologic alterations consistent with small airways disease have been described in patients with various interstitial pulmonary diseases, including IPF, but only rarely has chronic large airway airflow obstruction been reported in IPF.[341,342,351-355] Smoking status at presentation has a profound effect on lung function (Figure 25–18).[28] Never smokers have a significantly higher FEV_1 to FVC ratio than former smokers. Among current smokers, the FEV_1 to FVC ratio is significantly lower compared to that in never and former smokers.[28]

Lung Volumes

The lung volumes (TLC, functional residual capacity [FRC], and residual volume) are reduced at some point in the course of most patients with IPF. Early on, or more commonly in patients with superimposed chronic obstructive pulmonary disease, the lung volumes may be normal. Lung volumes are higher in current smokers at presentation compared to never smokers with IPF (Figure 25–19).[22,28]

Pressure-volume studies often yield a curve that is shifted downward and to the right, consistent with a stiff noncompliant lung (see Figure 25–17). In general,

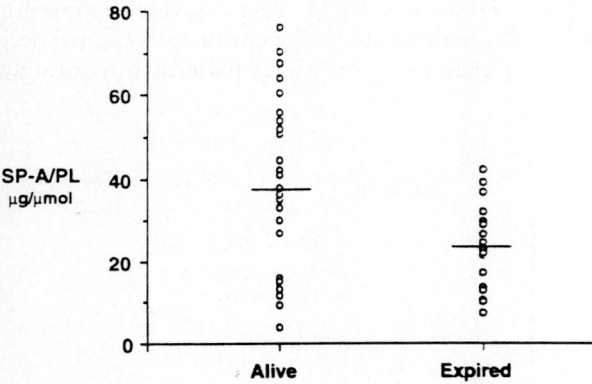

Figure 25–14   Relationship between surfactant protein (SP)-A and phospholipids (PLs) in bronchoalveolar lavage (BAL) fluid and survival in patients with IPF. SP-A content of the index lavage fluid was determined by ELISA and normalized to recovered lipid phosphorus as a marker of alveolar surface area sampled. Patients who died within 2 years (right) had a lower SP-A:PL ratio (23.4 ± 2.6 [SE], mg/mmol) than did those who survived (37.5 ± 4.2 [SE], mg/mmol). Reproduced with permission from McCormack FX et al.[330]

as the disease progresses, lung compliance decreases and lung volumes fall.[351,352,356-360] Smokers have a shift of the pressure-volume curve upwards and to the left, and the transpulmonary pressure at any given lung volume is significantly lower than that in nonsmokers with IPF.[22] As a result, the coefficient of elastic retraction of the lungs is lower in smokers than in nonsmokers with IPF (Figure 25–20).[22,28]

Gas Exchange at Rest and During Exercise

During exercise, the DL_{CO} is reduced and may actually precede the reduction of lung volume.[356,361] The reduction in the DL_{CO} is probably caused by both a contraction of the pulmonary capillary volume and by ventilation and perfusion abnormalities. The resting arterial blood gases may be normal initially or may reveal mild hypoxemia and respiratory alkalosis. The major cause of resting hypoxemia is ventilation and perfusion mismatching and does not result from either impaired oxygen diffusion as was originally suspected or anatomic shunts.[362,363] With exercise, the alveolar–arterial oxygen gradient, $P(A-a)O_2$, widens, and the arterial oxygen pressure (PaO_2) and arterial oxygen saturation (SaO_2) fall. During exercise, 20 to 30% of the exercise-induced widening of the $P(A-a)O_2$ may be caused by some impairment of oxygen diffusion.[364-366] Importantly, the abnormalities identified at rest do not accurately predict the magnitude of the abnormalities that may be seen with exercise.[367,368] Although these abnormalities can be assessed by oximetry saturation, it has been demonstrated that this method may not yield as dramatic or significant a change as that obtained by arterial blood gases. Thus, exercise testing is more sensitive than resting physiological testing in the detection of abnormalities in oxygen transfer, and exercise gas exchange has been demonstrated to be a sensitive parameter for following the clinical course (see Chapter 3, "Physiology of Interstitial Lung Disease" Figure 3–3).[360,369]

During exercise, patients with IPF increase their minute ventilation, primarily by increasing their respiratory frequency. This method of increase differs from normal subjects in whom increased ventilation during mild exercise occurs via an increase in the tidal volume (V_T) rather than the respiratory rate (see Chapter 3, Figure 3–3).[370] Thus, patients with IPF have elevated minute ventilation during exercise that is in part related to the increase in dead space (V_D) ventilation. The ratio of V_D to V_T ($V_D:V_T$) is increased at rest and is maintained or decreases with exercise (see Chapter 3, "Physiology of Interstitial Lung Disease" Figure 3–3). Occasionally, the $V_D:V_T$ ratio may increase in interstitial lung disorders that have a prominent pulmonary vascular component, such as scleroderma. In patients with IPF, an increase in the $V_D:V_T$ ratio should raise concern about pulmonary vascular disease, especially chronic pulmonary emboli or associated emphysema.

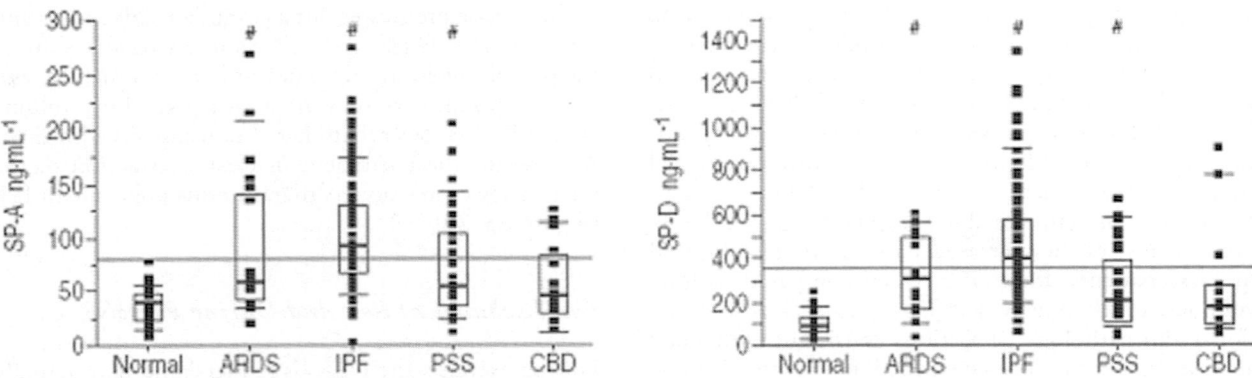

Figure 25–15   Serum concentrations of SP-A and SP-D in patients with ILD. SP-A (left) concentrations in serum from normal volunteers (n = 46), patients with acute respiratory distress syndrome (ARDS; n=21), IPF (n = 142), progressive systemic sclerosis (PSS; n = 37), and chronic beryllium disease (CBD; n = 19). SP-D (right) concentrations in serum from normal volunteers (n = 46), patients with ARDS (n = 21), IPF (n = 142), PSS (n = 37), and CBD (n = 19). Box plots show the 10th, 25th, 75th, and 90th percentiles and median. The solid horizontal line represents the 50th percentile. #p < .0001 vs normal subjects. Reproduced with permission from Greene et al.[338]

Pulmonary Hemodynamics

Pulmonary hypertension rarely occurs at rest in patients with early IPF, and cor pulmonale is a late sequela of the disease process.[5,177] Nevertheless, pulmonary hypertension during exercise is common even during the early stages of IPF.[371,372] When the VC is less than 50% of predicted or the D_{CO} falls below 45% of predicted, pulmonary hypertension at rest can be expected.[157] In 70% of patients with advanced pulmonary fibrosis, auscultatory findings consistent with pulmonary hypertension are present.[31,232] The mean pulmonary arterial pressure at rest ranges between 23 and 28 mm Hg and rarely exceeds 40 mm Hg.[371–374] A resting pulmonary arterial pressure greater than 30 mm Hg is associated with a poor prognosis.

The cause of pulmonary hypertension in IPF is unknown. Current data suggest that the etiology of pulmonary hypertension in ILD is multifactorial: (1) primary lesions of pulmonary vessels (eg, vasculitis); (2) compression and the destruction of pulmonary vessels by the interstitial process; (3) vasoconstriction of vessels mediated by hypoxia, acidosis, and autacoids; and (4) other factors that may be involved, such as pulmonary blood volume, pulmonary arterial compliance, lung water temperature, and left ventricular function.[372,375,376] It has been demonstrated that oxygen therapy at rest and during exercise improves pulmonary hemodynamics and likely improves exercise capacity and prognosis.[376–379] However, little data exist on the value of vasodilator therapy in the treatment of pulmonary hypertension in the ILDs.[374,376,377]

Sleep Disturbance

Patients with IPF, especially those with a daytime SaO_2 of less than 90% and/or a history of snoring during sleep, have been shown to develop sleep disturbances. These patients were found to have reduced rapid eye movement (REM) sleep, lighter and more fragmented sleep, and hypoxemia during REM sleep. Severe hypoxemia occurred even in the absence of obstructive or actual sleep apnea or changes in breathing pattern. Interestingly,

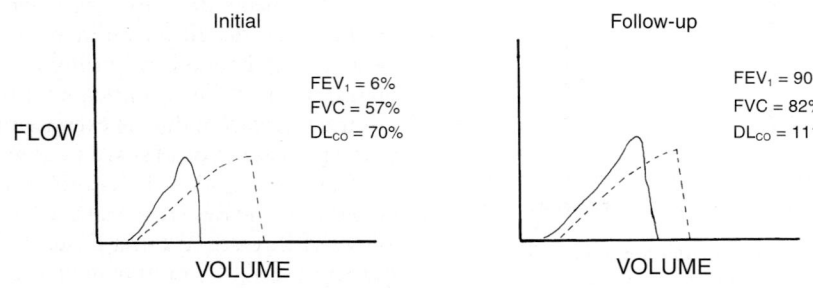

Figure 25–16   Maximal expiratory flow volume (MEFV) curve in IPF. MEFV curves at presentation (initial) and after 8 months of corticosteroid therapy (follow-up) in a 42-year-old male nonsmoker with IPF with a normal chest radiograph. A lung biopsy revealed moderate usual interstitial pneumonitis. The forced expiratory volume in 1 second (FEV_1) and forced vital capacity (FVC) values are low relative to the predicted values, but the FEV_1:FVC ratio is increased (ie, 83%). However, at any given lung volume, the flow rates are increased. These changes are even more evident after treatment. Broken lines = predicted MEFV curve. Solid lines = MEFV curve observed in this patient.

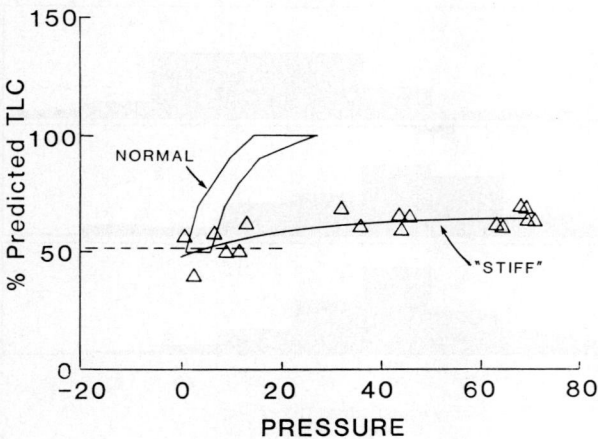

Figure 25–17   Relationship of the static deflation volume and pressure in a patient with IPF. The % predicted total lung capacity (TLC) is plotted against the static transpulmonary pressure (cmH$_2$O) for a patient with moderate to severe fibrosis and honeycombing. In general, the compliance, maximum cmH$_2$O, and the coefficient of retraction (maximum cmH$_2$O/TLC) tend to correlate with the extent of fibrosis observed on open lung biopsy.

patients with tachypnea while awake maintained their tachypnea during sleep. This maintenance of rapid breathing during sleep suggested that the reflexes causing the rapid shallow breathing were active during the sleep phase as well. Thus, identification and correction of the sleep disturbance may improve patient survival and so reduce morbidity, especially the pulmonary hypertension and cor pulmonale that develop in patients with IPF.[380,381]

Lung Imaging Studies

Chest Radiography

The most common radiographic abnormalities are reticular (netlike appearance of linear or curvilinear densities). These usually appear as diffuse opacities with a predilection for the lower lung zones (Figure 25–21). A

coarse reticular pattern and/or multiple cystic or honeycombed areas (ie, coarse reticular pattern with translucencies measuring 0.5 to 1.0 cm in diameter) is a late radiographic finding and portends a poor prognosis (Figure 25–22). Chest radiographic evidence of reduced lung volumes is usually present unless an associated obstructive airway disease occurs (Figure 25–23).

The correlation between the plain chest radiographic pattern and the stage of disease (clinical or histopathologic) is generally poor. Most commonly, early IPF is manifested radiographically by lesser extent and severity of reticular abnormalities. As the disease progresses, linear densities and reticulation become more extensive and eventually result in a honeycombed appearance. Pleural involvement is very uncommon in IPF; therefore, its presence suggests another diagnosis, such as collagen vascular disease (especially rheumatoid arthritis or systemic lupus erythematosus), mitral valve disease, congestive heart failure, asbestosis, infection, drug-induced lung disease, or lymphangitic carcinosis.

HRCT

The primary role of HRCT in a patient with suspected idiopathic interstitial pneumonia is to separate patients with typical findings of IPF/UIP from those with the less specific findings associated with other idiopathic interstitial pneumonias (Figure 25–24).[2,230] A confident diagnosis of IPF/UIP made with HRCT is based on the presence of a bilateral, predominantly basal, predominantly subpleural, reticular pattern associated with subpleural cysts (honeycombing) and/or traction bronchiectasis (see Chapter 4, "Imaging of Diffuse Parenchymal Lung Disease," Figures 4–9 and 4–20).[2,205,206,230] Consolidation and nodules are absent. When all of these radiologic features are present, the diagnosis of UIP is correct in more than 90% of cases; however, this radiologic pattern occurs in less than 50% of the cases proven to be IPF/UIP.[205,206] However, when the CT scan findings are not consistent with these features (eg, upper lobe or peribronchovascu-

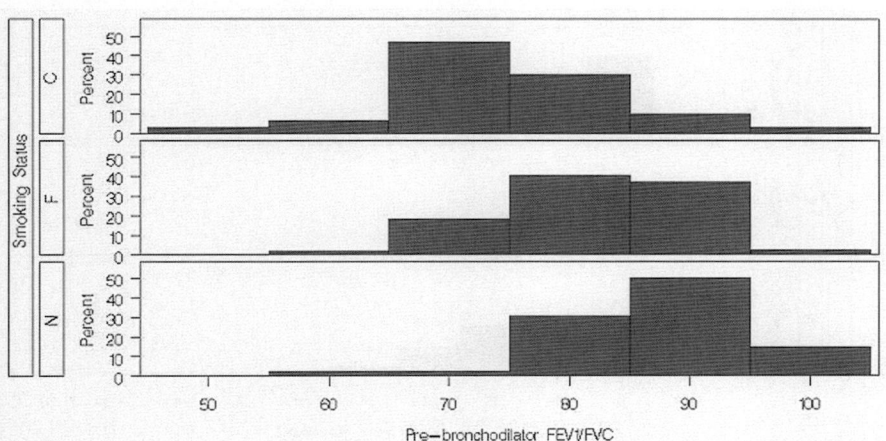

Figure 25–18   FEV$_1$:FVC ratio at presentation in patients with IPF/UIP divided according to smoking status. Never-smokers had a significantly higher FEV$_1$:FVC ratio ($n = 82$; median 87%; $p < .05$) than in former smokers ($n = 161$; median 82.5%; $p < .05$). Among current smokers, the FEV$_1$:FVC ratio ($n = 30$; median 73%; $p < .05$) was significantly lower compared with never- and former smokers. Data are from King TE Jr et al.[28]

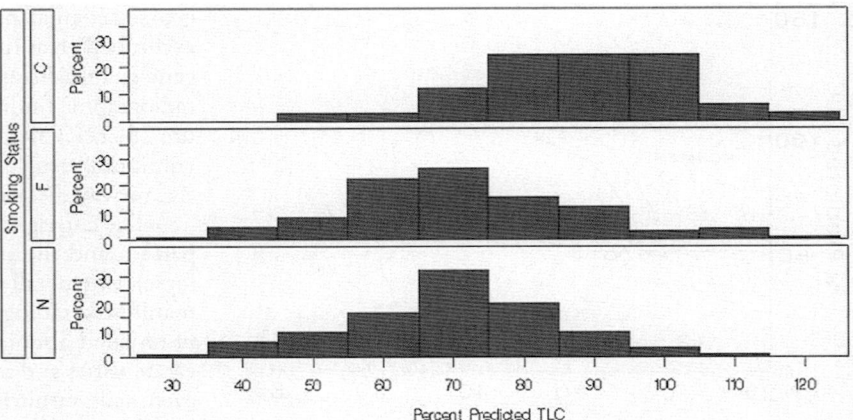

Figure 25–19 TLC at presentation in patients with IPF/UIP divided according to smoking status. TLC was significantly lower among never (*n* = 84; median 69%) and former (*n* = 120; median 69.5%) smokers compared with current (*n* = 33; median 89; *p* < .05) smokers. Data are from King TE Jr et al.[28]

lar predominance, predominant ground-glass abnormality or micronodules, presence of emphysema or cysts) or when there is one or more atypical clinical features (eg, young age, inconclusive exposure history, lack of dyspnea, absence of restrictive lung function defect, or presence of marked lymphocytosis on BAL), then biopsy is indicated (see Chapter 4, "Imaging of Diffuse Parenchymal Lung Diseases" Figures 4–4 to 4–40).[2,230]

The pattern found on HRCT scanning may correlate with histopathology and have prognostic significance.[274] Ground-glass opacity detected with CT is usually associated with interstitial inflammation, air space filling by macrophages, patchy fibrosis, or a combination of these features. One might expect that the presence of this finding in patients with IPF/UIP would be consistent with potentially reversible lung disease. However, frequently in IPF/UIP, this area of ground-glass opacity is associated with reticular lines, traction bronchiectasis, or bronchiolectasis. As a result, these changes are usually progressive and become reticular opacities or honeycombing on follow-up evaluation (Figure 25–25).[382] Some studies do show that ground-glass opacity predicts physiologic improvement following steroid treatment.[195] Reticular abnormality seen on HRCT scans

tends to correlate with fibrosis on histopathologic examination. Honeycombing visible on CT scans correlates with honeycombing on biopsy.[2] The majority of honeycomb cysts seen with HRCT in end-stage disease represent dilated bronchioles that communicate with the proximal airways and change in size with respiration.[383] Patients with predominant reticular opacity or honeycombing usually progress despite treatment.[195,384–386] Honeycomb cysts usually enlarge slowly over time.[2] The value of serial HRCT scans in the longitudinal assessment of IPF remains to be defined.

Several recent studies show that HRCT is very useful in achieving a confident diagnosis of IPF among a subset of cases of idiopathic interstitial pneumonia.[205,206] In general, the sensitivity for a confident diagnosis is low (~48%), but the specificity is high (~95%) (Table 25–12). Also, use of a semiquantitative HRCT scoring system may be very helpful in predicting the likely pathology present (UIP vs other idiopathic interstitial pneumonias) and in making the prognosis.[273] Flaherty and colleagues showed that scoring all lobes for the presence of ground-glass opacity on a scale of 0 to 5 and determining the total score for the entire lung was a very useful method to derive both prognostic and diagnostic information about

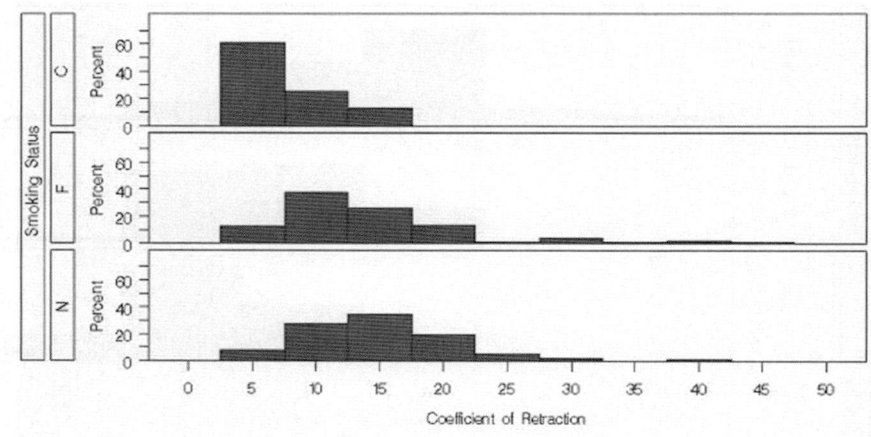

Figure 25–20 Coefficient of retraction at presentation in patients with IPF/UIP divided according to smoking status. The median coefficient of elastic retraction was significantly higher in never (*n* = 72; median 14.4) and former (*n* = 102; median 12.2) smokers than in current smokers (*n* = 31; median 6.6). The median for the latter was in the normal range (ie, 3–8 cmH$_2$O/lL). Data are from King TE Jr et al.[28]

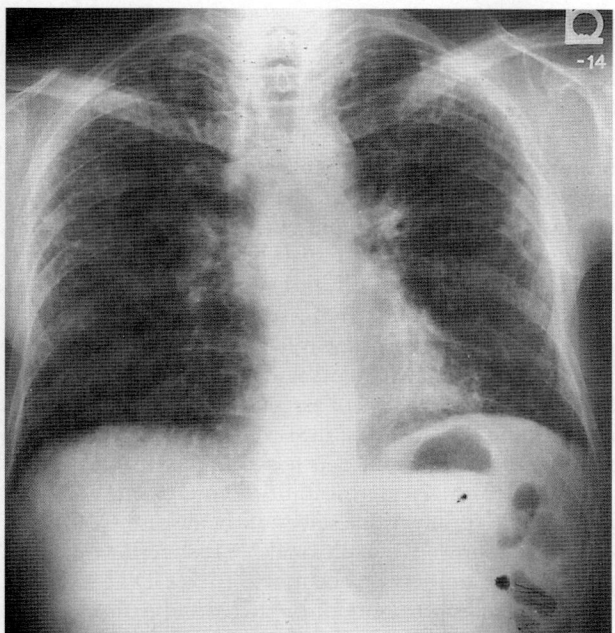

Figure 25–21   IPF. Patient with diffuse coarse reticular opacities, typical of the radiographic appearance of the mid-to late stage of pulmonary fibrosis.

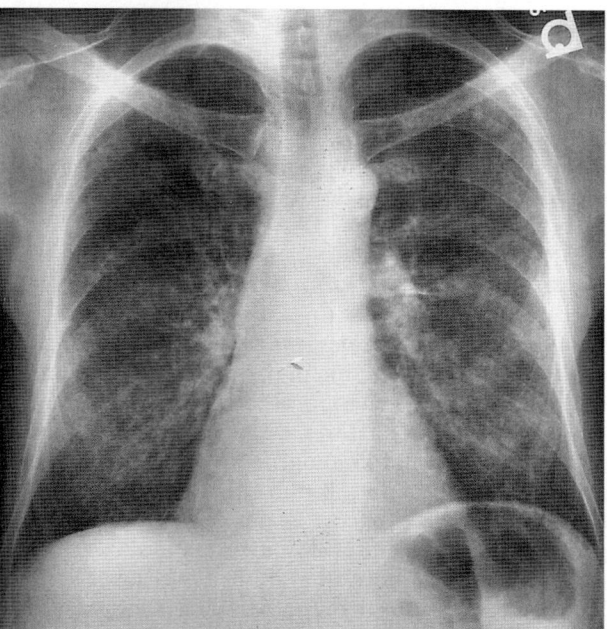

Figure 25–23   IPF. Patient with chronic obstructive lung disease and associated interstitial fibrosis. The lungs are hyperexpanded, which is atypical for IPF.

patients with idiopathic interstitial pneumonia.[274] An interstitial opacity score greater than 2 reliably identified patients with UIP. From their data, Flaherty and colleagues calculated that a surgical lung biopsy was warranted for patients without honeycombing on HRCT

because the absence of radiographic honeycombing does not exclude the pathologic diagnosis of UIP. In addition, they suggested that the usual diagnostic approach, combined with the use of a semiquantitative HRCT scoring system, would have resulted in a recommendation for surgical lung biopsy in 43% (54 of 126) of their patients; in

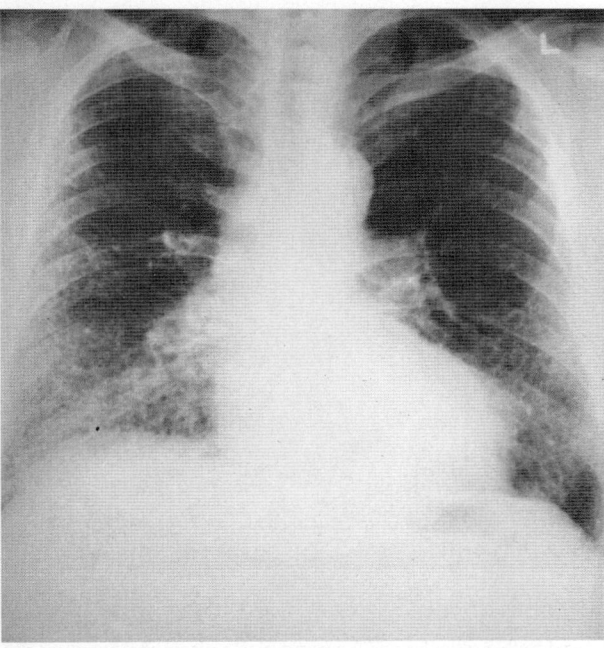

Figure 25–22   IPF. Patient with longstanding IPF and severe radiographic honeycombing.

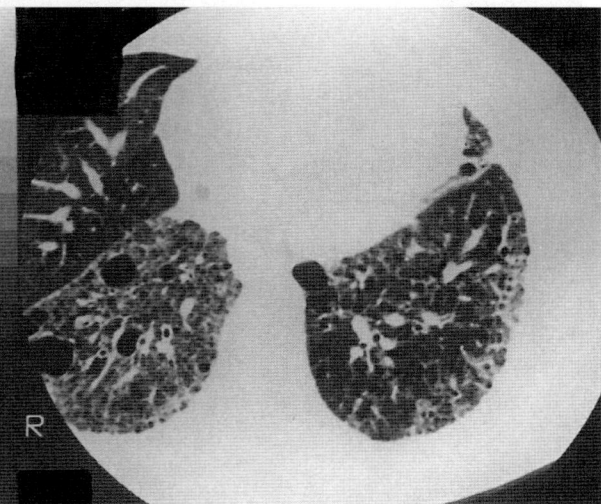

Figure 25–24   High-resolution (HR), thin-section computed tomography (CT) scan in late stage IPF. The chest radiograph showed a reticular pattern that involved the lung bases. CT scan reveals extensive parenchymal involvement with irregular fibrotic changes containing small honeycomb-like air spaces in the lower lung zones.

those patients in whom a biopsy would not be recommended, only 8% (6 of 72) would have been misclassified as having UIP.[274] Importantly, semiquantitative HRCT scoring is independent of a radiologist's interpretation of the pattern seen and exhibit good interobserver agreement among expert radiologists.[274] Additional prospective studies are required to confirm these findings.

Ventilation and Perfusion Scintiphotography

Ventilation and perfusion scanning provides information about pulmonary function in patients with IPF, but it is not recommended as a routine part of the evaluation. In most parenchymal diseases, ventilation and perfusion scanning reveals an inhomogeneous reduction of blood flow and/or ventilation. But in IPF, two types of perfusion abnormalities occur: (1) nonsegmental inhomogeneities, which are probably due to a localized loss of the capillary bed, most often in the lower lobes and (2) increased perfusion of the upper lung zones resulting from pulmonary hypertension, which induces an upward shift in the gradient of capillary perfusion. Ventilation scans generally reveal patchy nonsegmental areas of decreased ventilation, reflecting regions of airway obstruction or alveolar destruction. In general, patchy areas of high and low ventilation and perfusion matching usually occur, with a few areas of well-maintained ventilation and perfusion matching. These findings of mismatching of ventilation and blood flow explain the hypoxemia that occurs in these patients and suggest an anatomic reason for the high V_D to V_T ratio found in many of these patients at rest.[364,365]

Radioaerosol Studies

An accelerated clearance of soluble aerosolized hydrophilic radionuclides from the lungs of patients with IPF, sarcoidosis, pneumoconiosis, and scleroderma has been reported.[387,388] In patients with pulmonary alveolar proteinosis or chronic obstructive pulmonary disease, increased clearance is not present. The initial clearance of these small solutes occurs in part by diffusion through the epithelium of the alveoli and respiratory bronchioles. Although these results indicate an increased epithelial permeability in ILD, what role these findings may play in the evaluation of patients with IPF is not clear. These studies provide a means of assessing the activity of acute and chronic ILD, because the severity and rapidity of the movement of these solutes is related in part to the degree to which epithelial permeability is increased, and this increase differs at various stages of the disease. Wells and coworkers showed that normal [99m]Technetium-labeled diethylenetriaminepentaacetic acid (^{99m}Tc-DTPA) clearance at initial measurement predicted stable disease and that rapid clearance identified patients at risk for deterioration. Mogulkoc and colleagues showed that ^{99m}Tc-DTPA clearance measurements may predict survival in patients with IPF/UIP.[389,390]

Histopathologic Findings

The gross appearance of the lungs in IPF reveals a distinctive nodular pleural surface, sometimes with a marked "cirrhotic" appearance.[391–393] Histologically, patients with idiopathic interstitial pneumonia have a

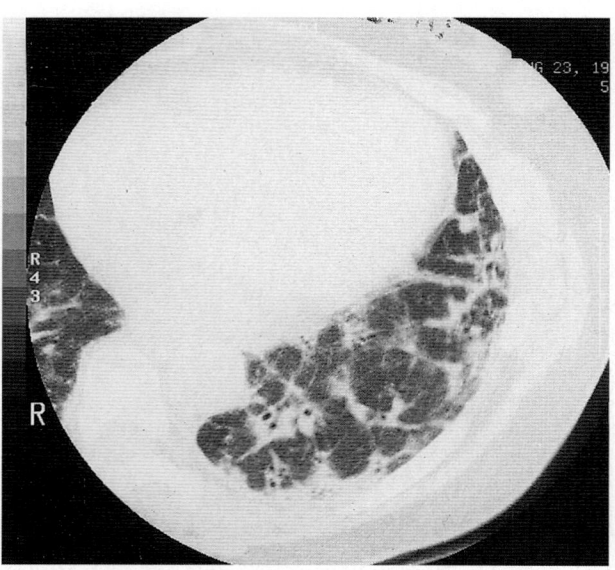

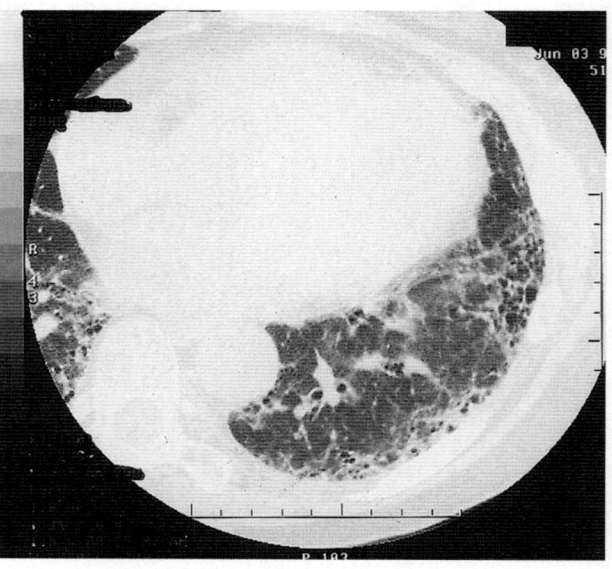

A

B

Figure 25–25   IPF: serial HRCT scans. *A,* The initial chest radiograph showed both a reticular and a ground-glass pattern that involved the lung bases. The corresponding CT scan shown here reveals ground-glass opacity in the lower lung zone. *B,* A follow-up CT scan 3 years later shows that the areas of ground-glass opacity have progressed to reticular opacity and honeycombing

Table 25–12   Accuracy of CT Diagnosis of IPF/UIP

Article	Total Patients (No. with IPF/UIP)	Study Design	Results*

Hunninghake and colleagues[206]	n = 91 (54)	Observers were provided no clinical information	Likely diagnosis of IPF:
			  sensitivity = 76%
			  specificity = 72%
			Certain diagnosis of IPF:
			  sensitivity = 48%
			  specificity = 97%

Raghu and colleagues[205]	n = 59 (29)	Observers knew only that the patients were referred for possible ILD	Diagnosis of UIP:
			  sensitivity = 78.5%
			  specificity = 90%

Johkoh and colleagues[648]	n = 129 (35)	Observers knew that the diagnosis was one of the 5 IIPs	Likely diagnosis of UIP:
			  sensitivity = 71%
			  specificity = 88%
			Certain diagnosis of UIP:
			  sensitivity = 43%
			  specificity = 95%

UIP = usual interstitial pneumonia; IPF = idiopathic pulmonary fibrosis; CT = computed tomography scan.

spectrum of findings (see Table 25–2). It has been shown that in IPF there is a broad range of extent and severity for most of the specific histopathologic abnormalities that make up the UIP-pattern. All patients have evidence of alveolar septal fibrosis. The smoking history alters the extent and the severity of the histopathologic changes. Occasionally, in patients who have undergone biopsies of multiple lobes of the lung, one lobe may show a pattern of ill-defined fibrosis simulating UIP and another lobe may show a specific lesion, such as a granulomatous reaction or asbestos bodies. In such a case, the diagnosis is the one most consistent with the specific histologic finding; that is, infection or sarcoidosis or hypersensitivity pneumonitis or asbestosis.[2]

Quantitative Method for the Assessment of Histopathologic Changes in IPF

Cherniack and colleagues have described a quantitative method for the assessment of the histopathologic changes found in IPF.[394] A principal component factor analysis of the means of the ratings of four pathologists for each of 14 specific histopathologic features resulted in the derivation of 4 factor scores:

1. the fibrosis factor (maximum score = 25), which takes into account the degree of interstitial fibrosis and the presence of honeycomb cysts, alveolar wall metaplastic cells lining the air spaces, metaplastic smooth muscle in the stroma, and myointimal mural thickening in the vessel walls;
2. the cellularity factor (maximum score = 10), taking into account the severity and extent of cellular infiltration of the alveolar walls;
3. the desquamation factor (maximum score = 10), which looks at the severity and extent of cellularity within the alveolar space; and

4. the granulation/connective tissue factor (maximum score = 9), which looks at interstitial "young connective tissue" and granulation tissue in the lumens of small airways and alveoli.

Each factor score was derived from the sum of the scores assigned to its components, and the total pathology score was derived from the sum of the four factor scores. The maximum total pathology score was 54. This quantitative method of assessment of the lung histology has proven very useful in determining the relationship between histopathology and physiology and survival.

Relationship between Histopathology and Physiology

It has been shown that there is a correlation between the quantitative analysis of structural changes in the lung and physiological abnormalities in patients with IPF.[395] In the study group as a whole, there was no significant relationship between the amount of fibrosis or the connective/granulation tissue factor and any of the physiological parameters. The DL_{CO} correlated with the desquamation and the total pathology scores (Figure 25–26), whereas the TLC and FVC correlated with the cellularity factor score (Figure 25–27). In current smokers, the coefficient of elastic retraction, DL_{CO}/V_A, and the FEV_1 to FVC ratio were significantly lower than in nonsmokers and ex-smokers, and TLC and FVC were higher than in nonsmokers. Also, the mean cellularity and granulation/connective tissue factor scores were significantly lower, and the desquamation factor score was significantly higher than in nonsmokers and ex-smokers. Both age and smoking status were significant for the cellularity factor score; for the connective/granulation tissue factor score, age was not significant but smoking status was. For the desquamation factor score, age was significant but

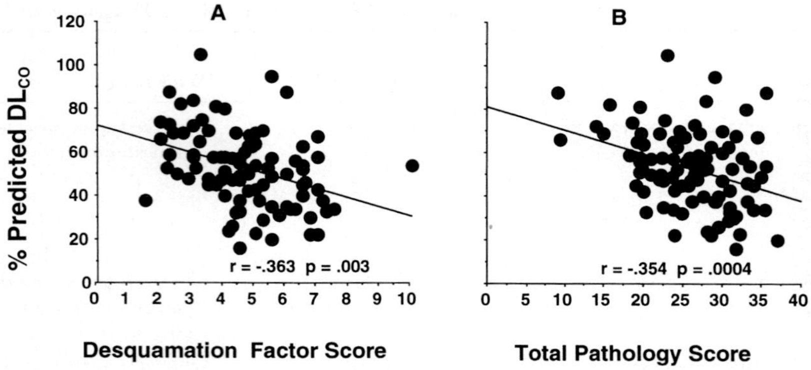

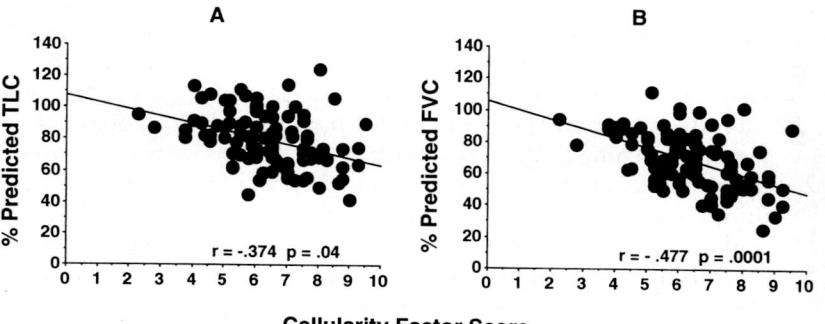

Figure 25–26   The relationship between the diffusing capacity of the lung for carbon monoxide (DL$_{CO}$) and the desquamation factor (*A*) and total pathology scores (*B*) in IPF. Reproduced with permission from Cherniack et al.[395]

smoking status was not. There were significant differences between never smokers and ever smokers in the slope of the relationship between the pathology factors (fibrosis and desquamation scores) and measurements of respiratory function (Figures 25–28 and 25–29). These differences may explain some of the widely recognized difficulties in assessing structure–function correlation in patients with IPF. In the nonsmokers, the correlations between structure and function were likely the direct result of IPF, per se. In the current smokers, bronchiolar and/or emphysematous changes associated with cigarette smoking may complicate the pathologic alterations of IPF and influence the functional derangements.

Relationship between Histopathology and Survival

Studies examining the relationship between outcome and histopathology have suggested that prognosis and response to therapy in IPF is determined by the extent of inflammation (cellularity) and interstitial fibrosis seen on biopsy. However, the widely held views that, in patients with UIP, it is the inflammatory response that drives the fibrogenic process and that successful suppression of the inflammation would prevent the progression to end-stage fibrosis appears to have limited support.[126,127,396] It has been proposed that the earliest and most characteristic manifestation of ongoing lung injury in UIP is the development of multiple fibroblastic foci.[11] Also, it is now recognized that many of this ear-

lier data were derived from the study of a heterogeneous population of patients with several histopathologic subtypes other than UIP (eg, DIP, RB-ILD, NSIP, and OP). Increasingly, it is being recognized that these are distinct clinical, radiographic, and histopathologic entities with different responses to therapy and different survival rates. Furthermore, the term "cellularity" was used indiscriminately for interstitial inflammation (common to OP and NSIP but often essentially absent in UIP), intra-alveolar macrophage accumulation (a smoking-related reaction commonly seen in DIP or RB-ILD), or a combination of both.[29] Finally, the term "fibrosis" has evolved such that a distinction is being made between fibrotic areas of the lesion characterized by old, relatively acellular collagen bundles and small aggregates of fibroblasts in myxoid connective tissue, so-called fibroblastic foci.[11,29,126,395,397–399]

Until recently, no specific histologic feature, other than end-stage fibrosis and honeycombing, has been shown to correlate with treatment response or prognosis in UIP.[29,125] King and coworkers, using the semi-quantitative grading of histopathologic abnormalities found in surgical lung biopsy specimens, determined the relationship between histopathology and survival.[29] A wide range of pathology factor scores were observed in patients with IPF/UIP. The median scores for each factor score for the entire group were cellularity, 6.3 (25th, 75th percentile; 5.5 to 7.1); alveolar space cellularity, 4.5 (3.5 to 5.5); fibrosis, 12.9 (9.8 to 16.5); granulation/connective tissue, 1.8 (1.0 to 2.7); and total pathology

Figure 25–27   The relationship between DL$_{CO}$ and the cellularity factor and TLC (*A*) and FVC scores (*B*) in IPF. Reproduced with permission from Cherniack et al.[395]

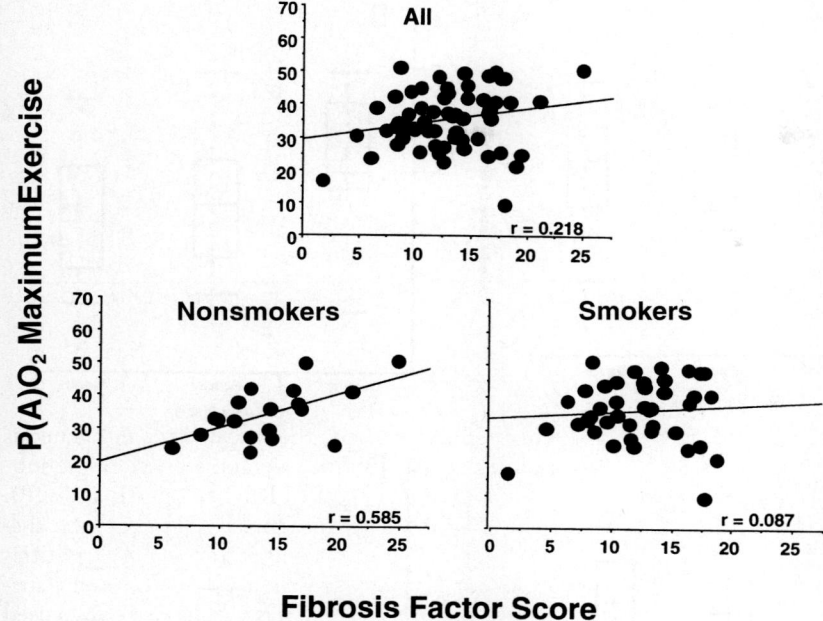

Figure 25–28   The relationship between the fibrosis factor score and the alveolar–arterial pressure difference for O_2 ($P(A$-$a)O_2$) score during maximal exercise in all patients with IPF, those who had never smoked, and those who had smoked chronically. Reproduced with permission from Cherniack et al.[395]

score, 26.0 (22.3 to 30.8).[29] Importantly, the smoking history at the time of presentation was related to the histopathologic abnormalities found at lung biopsy and to the ultimate survival in these patients. Current smokers had significantly lower degrees of cellularity and granulation/connective tissue and higher alveolar space cellularity than did former and never smokers (Figure 25–30).[29] The amount of fibrosis was not tied to smoking status.

They further examined the relative roles of the stage of fibrosis (mature collagen vs fibroblast foci) in determining survival. In this study, a distinction was made between interstitial fibrosis with extensive collagen deposition (including honeycomb change) and fibroblastic foci recognized as young connective tissue or connective tissue with granulation tissue type appearance. In survival analyses adjusted for age, sex, and smoking history, only the granulation/connective tissue score was a significant predictor of survival in patients with IPF.[29] A 1-unit increase in the granulation/connective tissue factor was associated with a 1.74-fold greater risk of death. Of the specific components that comprise the granulation/connective tissue factor scores, the degree of alveolar

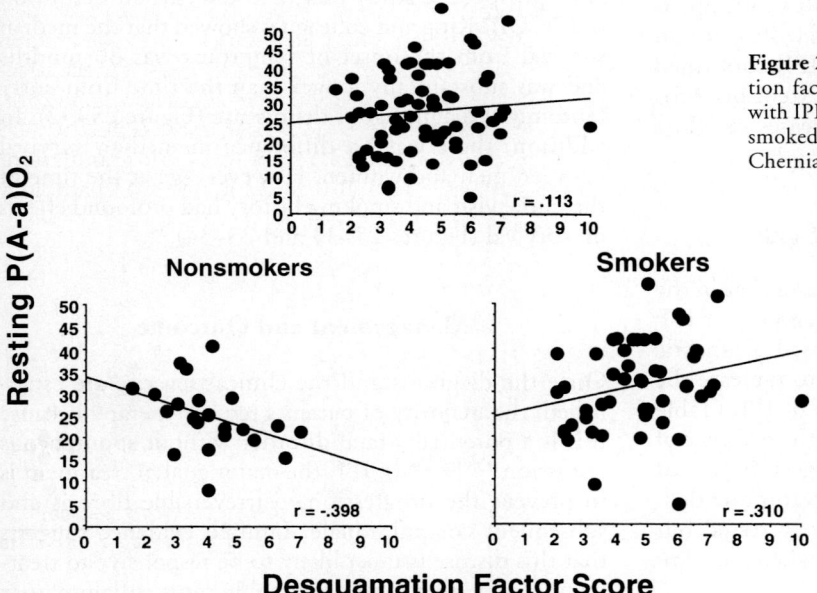

Figure 25–29   The relationship between the desquamation factor score and the resting $P(A$-$a)O_2$ in all patients with IPF, those who had never smoked, and those who had smoked chronically. Reproduced with permission from Cherniack et al.[395]

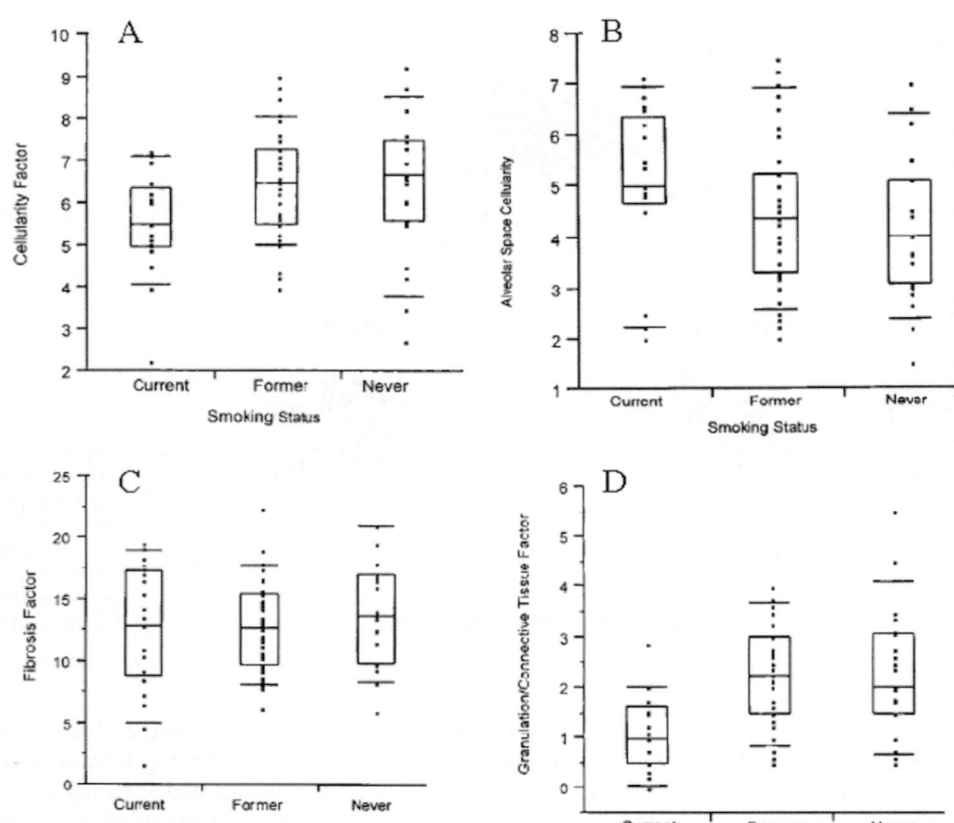

Figure 25–30 Influence of cigarette smoking on the histopathologic findings in patients with IPF. NS = not significant. *A*, Current smokers have lesser degrees of cellularity (*p* < .05) and *B*, slightly higher degrees of alveolar space cellularity *p* = NS). *C*, The degree of fibrosis is similar in all groups (*p* = NS). *D*, Current smokers have fewer granulation/young connective tissue abnormalities (*p* < .05). Reproduced with permission from King TE Jr et al.[29]

space granulation tissue and the fibrotic/reparative changes in young connective tissue were each significantly associated with survival. On the other hand, the airway lumenal granulation tissue extent of involvement was not associated with an increased risk of death. The Kaplan-Meier survival analysis for each factor score, dichotomized at the median for the entire group, is shown in Figure 25–31.[29] Nicholson and colleagues, in a retrospective study of 53 patients with IPF, confirmed a strong correlation between increasing extent of fibroblastic foci and both mortality and decreases in DL_{CO} and FVC at 6 and 12 months after biopsy.[400]

Confirming the Diagnosis of IPF

The ATS/ERS consensus panel on IPF states that in the absence of a surgical lung biopsy, the diagnosis of IPF remains uncertain. However, they proposed diagnostic criteria that could be used by clinicians to increase the likelihood of a correct clinical diagnosis of IPF (Table 25–13). In the immunocompetent adult, the presence of all of the major diagnostic criteria, along with at least three of the four minor criteria, was recommended. These criteria have not been prospectively tested but appear quite useful in those situations where surgical lung biopsy is not possible.

Natural History

The natural history of IPF has not been appropriately defined.[137,232,234,237,401–403] Data obtained from several reports indicate that the median survival after diagnosis, with or without treatment, is less than 5 years.[404] In a large prospective study that used the current definition of IPF/UIP, King and colleagues showed that the median survival from the onset of symptoms was 80 months and was substantially longer than the time from entry (and initial diagnosis) of the disease (Figure 25–32). In addition, there was no difference in median survival between men and women. However, age at the time of the initial visit and smoking history had profound effects on survival (Figures 25–33 and 25–34).[28]

Management and Outcome

Once the diagnosis and the clinical severity are established, the majority of patients require therapy because this is a potentially fatal disorder without spontaneous remission.[130,137,258] In IPF, the major goal of treatment is to prevent the progression to irreversible fibrosis and subsequent cor pulmonale. Limited evidence suggests that this disease is most likely to be responsive to treatment at an earlier (and presumably more inflammatory

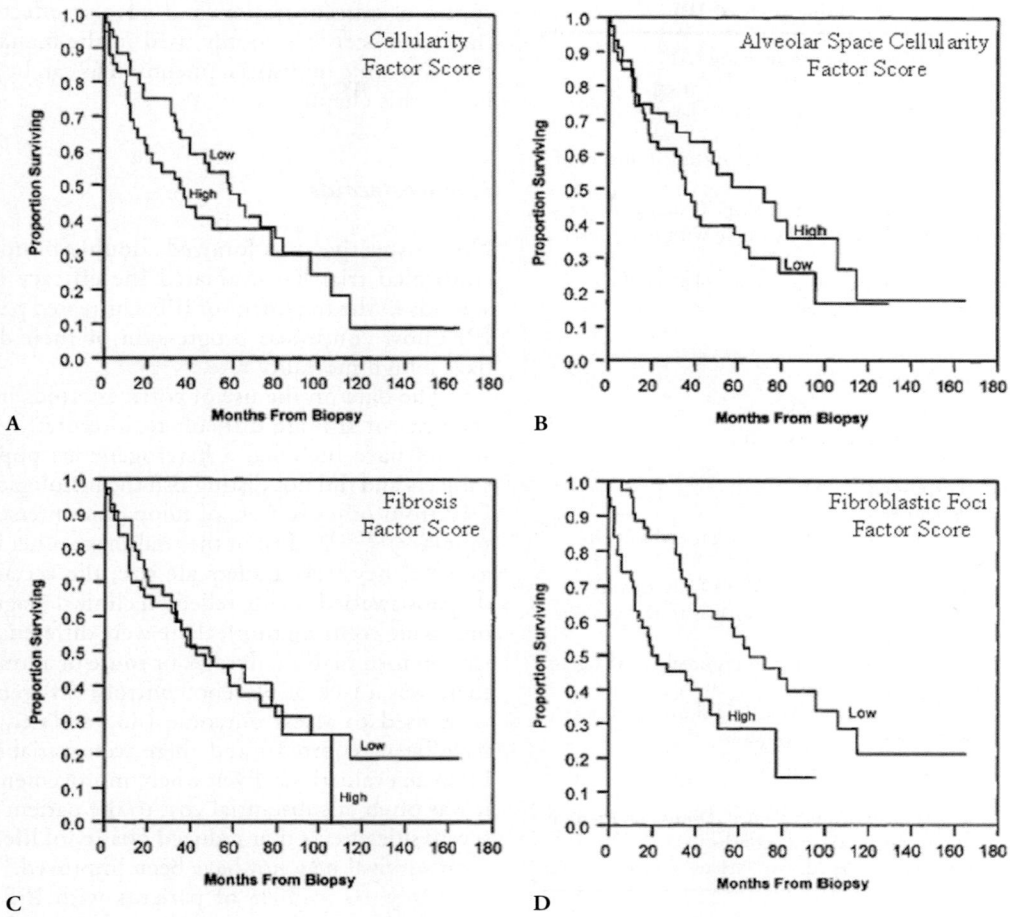

Figure 25–31 Kaplan-Meier survival analysis grouped by dichotomized factor score at the median for entire group. *A,* Cellularity. Survival tended to be longer in subjects with less cellularity. (Low: score range 2.25 to 6.25; median survival 59.2 months. High: score range 6.4 to 9.25; median survival 36.2 months; *p* = .46). *B,* Alveolar space cellularity. Survival tended to be better in subjects with greater degrees of alveolar space cellularity. (Low: score range 1.5 to 4.5; median survival 36.2 months. High: score range 4.6 to 7.5; median survival 73.4 months; *p* = .19). *C,* Fibrosis: Survival was not different in the two groups (Low: range of score, 1.6 to 12.9; median survival, 49.6 months; High: range of score, 13.0 to 24.8; median survival 43.4 months; *p* = .98). *D,* Fibroblastic foci (granulation/connective tissue). Survival was better in subjects with lesser degrees of granulation/connective tissue. (Low: score range 0 to 1.8; median survival 65.8 months. High: score range 2.0 to 5.5; median survival 22.8 months; *p* = .002). Reproduced with permission from King TE Jr et al.[29]

stage) rather than later in its course when the predominant histologic finding is that of fibrosis.[137,165,234,310,315] Thus, early diagnosis of IPF is important in order to initiate treatment before irreversible fibrosis develops. The current therapy for IPF, regardless of the agent used, requires 3 to 6 months of use before its effectiveness can be assessed. Importantly, randomized controlled clinical treatment trials of sufficient numbers of patients with IPF have not been performed. Consequently, conclusions drawn from the studies available need to be confirmed by more properly performed studies.

There is limited clinical evidence that any of the current treatments improve survival or the quality of life for patients with IPF.[230,405,406] However, because of the very poor prognosis for patients with IPF, any potential for a positive outcome has encouraged clinicians to treat these patients. The ATS/ERS consensus panel on IPF recommended that treatment not be given to all patients because the potential benefits of any current treatment protocol for an individual patient with IPF may be outweighed by the risk of treatment-related complications (eg, age >75 years, extreme obesity, concomitant major illness such as cardiac disease, diabetes mellitus, or osteoporosis, severe impairment in pulmonary function, end-stage honeycomb lung on radiographic evaluation).[230] The treatment recommendations from the ATS/ERS consensus panel on IPF are presented below in "ATS/ERS Treatment Recommendations for IPF." Most importantly, novel new approaches to the treatment of IPF are critical if we are to improve survival in patients with IPF.[230,405,406,] Descriptions of the mechanism of action, dosages, and

TABLE 25–13   Diagnosis of IPF

Definite diagnosis (with surgical biopsy showing UIP)
  Exclusion of other known causes of ILD
    drug toxicities, environmental exposures, collagen vascular diseases
  Abnormal pulmonary function studies that include evidence of restriction
    reduced VC (often with increased FEV_1:FVC ratio) and/or impaired gas exchange (increased $P(A-a)O_2$ with rest or exercise or decreased DL_{CO})
  Abnormalities on conventional chest radiographs or HRCT scans consistent with UIP pattern

Probable diagnosis (without surgical biopsy in an immunocompetent adult)

1. Major criteria (ALL must be present)
  A. Exclusion of other known causes of ILD
    drug toxicities
    environmenal exposures
    connective tissue diseases
  B. Abnormal pulmonary function studies that include evidence of restriction
    reduced VC (often with increased FEV_1:FVC ratio) and/or impaired gas exchange (increased $P(A-a)O_2$ with rest or exercise or decreased DL_{CO})
  C. Bibasilar reticular abnormalities with minimal-ground glass opacities on HRCT scan
  D. Transbronchial lung biopsy or BAL fluid showing no features to support an alternative diagnosis

2. Minor Criteria (3 of 4 must be present)
  A. Age 50 years
  B. Insidious onset of otherwise unexplained dyspnea on exertion
  C. Duration of illness longer than 3 months
  D. Bibasilar, inspiratory crackles (dry or "Velcro"-type in quality)

Adapted from: King TE Jr et al.[230]
FEV_1 = forced expiratory volume in 1 second; FVC = forced vital capacity.

routes of administration and adverse effects of drugs that have been commonly used in the management of the idiopathic interstitial pneumonias can be found earlier in this chapter.

Corticosteroids

No prospective, randomized, double-blind, placebo-controlled trial has evaluated the efficacy of corticosteroids in the treatment of IPF. Untreated patients with IPF show continued progression of their disease and have a high mortality rate.[137,310,407]

The data on the use of corticosteroids in the management of IPF are difficult to interpret. Most of the studies have included a heterogeneous population of subjects and did not distinguish the histologic pattern of UIP from other subsets of idiopathic interstitial pneumonias.[245,273,315] Most of the trials have other limitations as well: they lacked adequate size; the certainty of the diagnosis varied (many relied on clinical diagnosis without tissue confirmation); there were differences in medication formulation, dosage, or route of administration; there was a lack of placebo controls; different methods were used to assess outcome (no validated endpoints have been reported); and there were variable intervals between evaluations. Even when improvement occurred, it was often at substantial cost to the patient because of severe side effects that reduced quality of life, and long-term survival may not have been improved.[239,240,408,410]

Only 10 to 30% of patients with IPF appear to improve or at least survive longer when treated with corticosteroids (or in combination with immunosuppressive agents). Most investigators now concede that those stud-

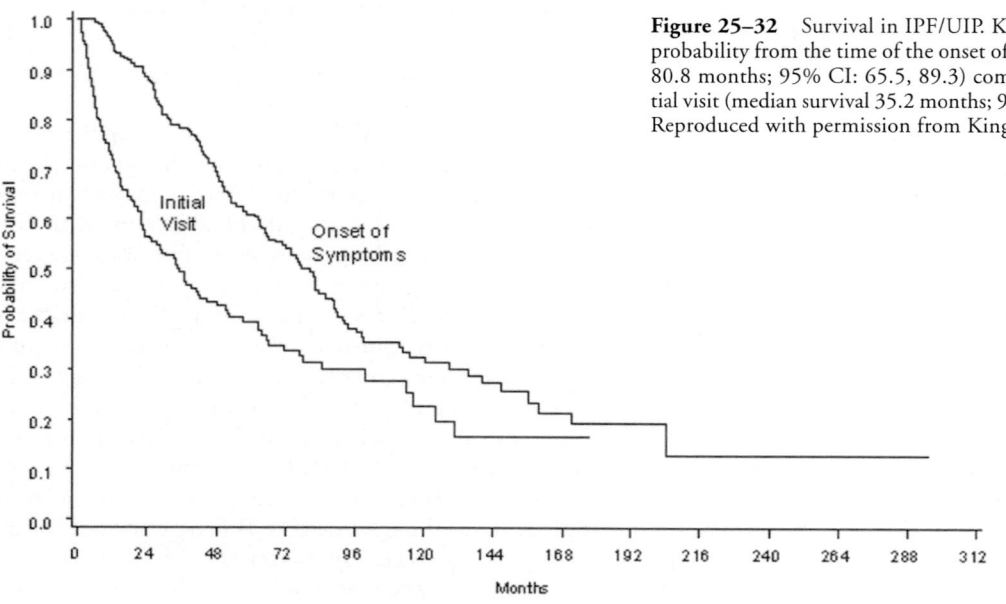

Figure 25–32   Survival in IPF/UIP. Kaplan-Meier plot of survival probability from the time of the onset of symptoms (median survival 80.8 months; 95% CI: 65.5, 89.3) compared to the time from initial visit (median survival 35.2 months; 95% CI: 23.2, 48.5; *n* = 238). Reproduced with permission from King TE Jr et al.[28]

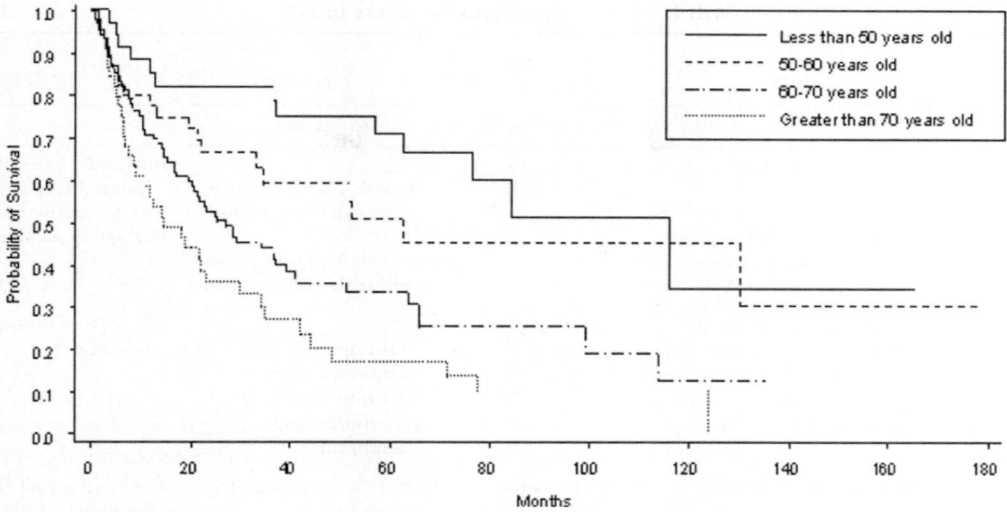

Figure 25–33 Kaplan-Meier plot of survival probability from the time of the initial visit, stratified by age group: < 50 years (*n* = 36); 50–60 years (*n* = 48); 60–70 years (*n* = 108); > 70 years (*n* = 46). The median survival time was 116.4, 62.8, 27.2, and 14.6 months, respectively. Reproduced with permission from King TE Jr et al.[28]

ies showing corticosteroid-responsive cases very likely included patients with NSIP, DIP/RB-ILD, chronic hypersensitivity pneumonitis, or COP.[141,245,273,315] In fact, in a minority of patients who underwent lung biopsy in many previous studies, the initial histopathologic descriptions have often been retrospectively reclassified (eg, UIP to NSIP) as the histopathologic criteria have evolved over time.[274,398,409–413] This reclassification on the basis of histologic pattern has clearly shown that the UIP-pattern as it is currently defined is associated with much worse clinical responsiveness (0 to 16%) and poorer survival (20 to

43% at 5 years) than any of the other patterns (NSIP, COP, DIP/RB-ILD, LIP).[240,274,398,409–413] Table 25–14 shows the clinical outcome of treatment trials that focused primarily on IPF cases defined by diagnostic criteria consistent with the ATS/ERS recommendations.[2,230]

For patients with acute exacerbation of IPF (see following text), 3 to 5 days of an intravenous pulse corticosteroid regimen, such as methylprednisolone at an intravenous dose of 250 mg every 6 hours can reverse this process. Therapy, as outlined above, for chronic disease is instituted once the course is stabilized.

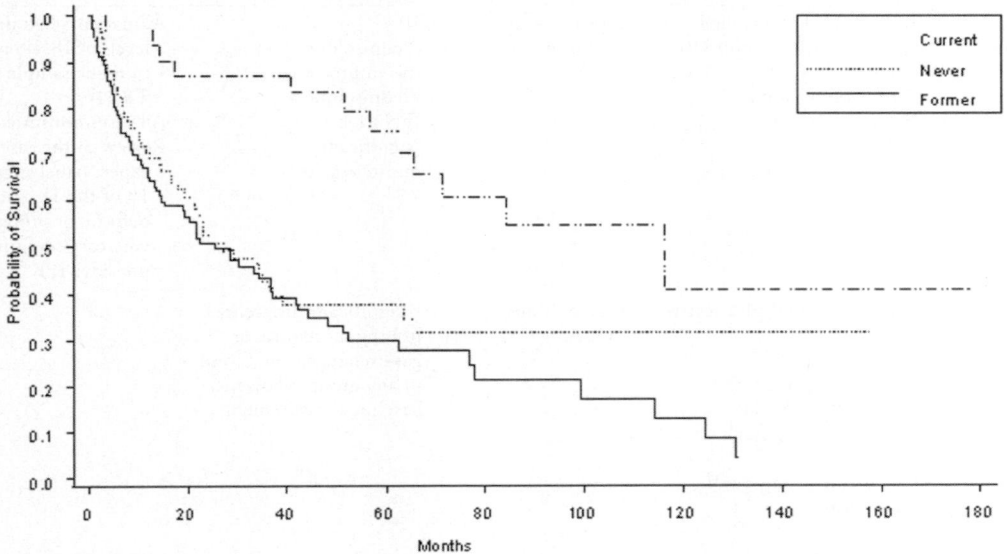

Figure 25–34 Kaplan-Meier plot of survival probability from the time of the initial visit, stratified by smoking group (current, *n* = 33; former, *n* = 121; never, *n* = 84). There was a significant difference (*p* < .0003) between the three smoking groups. The median survival time in current smokers was 116.4 months, 25.3 months in former smokers, and 27.2 months in never smokers. Reproduced with permission from King TE Jr et al.[28]

TABLE 25–14 Treatment Outcome in IPF

Author, Year	Study Design	Diagnostic Approach	Outcome	Comments
Corticosteroids with or without Cytotoxic Agents				
Carrington and colleagues, 1978[137]	Prospective case series: UIP, n = 53 DIP, n = 40 Prednisone, 30–60 mg/day tapered and maintained for 1 year	Type of biopsy: OLB, n = 86 Autopsy n = 7	UIP treated: 11.5% response untreated: 0% response DIP treated: 61.5% response untreated: 21.9% response	Included 2 cases of drug-induced ILD and 16 cases of connective tissue disease UIP group included cases of NSIP
Raghu and colleagues, 1991[417]	Prospective case series of (mostly) patients with UIP Prednisone; n = 13 Prednisone and azathioprine; n = 14	Type of biopsy: OLB, n = 23 TBB, n = 4	UIP 32% improved with prednisone alone 50% improved with prednisone and azathioprine	The type of fibrosis was not described.
Nicholson and colleagues, 2000[413]	Retrospective case series: UIP, n =37 NSIP, n = 28 DIP/RB-ILD, n = 13 Prednisone (60 mg tapered) or Prednisone (20 mg/day) plus cyclophosphamide (100–120 mg/day)	Type of biopsy: OLB, n = 78	UIP: 11% improved at 6 months+ NSIP: 29% improved at 6 months DIP/RBILD: 80% response at 6 months; none deteriorated	Used current ATS/ERS criteria for histologic diagnosis
Zisman and colleagues, 2000[253]	Prospective case series of patients with UIP who had failed prednisone, n = 19 Cyclophosphamide (2 mg/kg/day)	Type of biopsy: OLB, n = 19	UIP: 5% improved, 58% deteriorated	
Daniil and colleagues, 1999[412]	Retrospective case series: UIP, n = 15 NSIP, n = 15 Prednisone +/- azathioprine or cyclophosphamide (variable regimens)	Type of biopsy: OLB, n = 30	UIP: 8% improved, 77% deteriorated NSIP: 23% improved, 42% deteriorated	
Antifibrotic Agents with or without Corticosteroids				
Ziesche and colleagues, 1999[422]	Randomized, controlled trial of patients with UIP, n = 18 Prednisolone alone Prednisolone and IFN-γ1b (200 μg 3x/week)	Type of biopsy: OLB, n = 18	UIP Prednisolone: "no improvement" Prednisolone + IFN γ1-b: "significant improvement"	All patients had unmeasurable levels of IFN-γ mRNA in tissue sample from TBB All cases nonsmokers Review of the cases by an expert panel suggested that 15 of the 18 cases had definite or probable IPF, whereas 3 definitely did not have IPF
Selman and colleagues, 1998[262]	Nonrandomized prospective study, n = 56 Prednisone alone (1.0mg/kg/day for 1 month; biweekly taper to 15mg/day); n = 15 Colchicine (1 mg/day)/ prednisone; n = 14 D-penicillamine (600 mg/day)/ prednisone; n = 11 Colchicine/ D-penicillamine/ prednisone; n = 11	Type of biopsy: OLB, n = 51	No significant differences in lung mechanics or gas exchange were found in any group relative to baseline measurement	

TABLE 25–14 Continued

Author, Year	Study Design	Diagnostic Approach	Outcome	Comments
Douglas and colleagues, 1998[420]	Randomized trial of patients with UIP, n = 26 Prednisone alone (60 mg/day tapered over 1 year, n = 12); Colchicine (0.6–1.2 mg/day, n = 14)	Type of biopsy: OLB, n = 1 Rigorous clinical and radiologic criteria used HRCT scan in 96% of subjects	UIP Prednisone: 83% failure at 1 year Colchicine: 64% failure at 1 year	Failure = decreased FVC, drug intolerance, removal from study Colchicine had fewer side effects
Douglas and colleagues, 2000[421]	Retrospective review of patients with UIP, n = 487 Colchicine alone, n = 167 Prednisone (variable regimens, n = 54) Colchicine and prednisone, n = 71 Other treatments (including cyclophosphamide or azathioprine, n = 38) No treatment, n = 157	Type of biopsy: OLB, 23% Rigorous clinical and radiologic criteria used HRCT scan in 96% of subjects	No difference in survival among treated and untreated groups.	Some patients (51.3%) had received treatment prior to first study visit. Group likely included cases of NSIP Oxygen therapy did not improve survival

IFN = interferon; UIP = usual interstitial pneumonia; NSIP = nonspecific interstitial pneumonia; DIP/ RBILD = desquamative interstitial pneumonia/respiratory bronchiolitis-associated interstitial lung disease; OLB = open lung biopsy; TBB = transbronchial lung biopsy

Cyclophosphamide

Several reports suggest that cyclophosphamide (usually given with low-dose corticosteroids) may be beneficial in the treatment of IPF.[249,252,414,415] A randomized controlled trial comparing prednisolone alone with cyclophosphamide and low-dose prednisolone in combination showed a possible survival advantage for the group treated with both cyclophosphamide and low-dose prednisolone (Figure 25–35).[249] Cyclophosphamide showed limited efficacy and frequent adverse effects in patients with IPF who failed to respond or who experience adverse effects from corticosteroid treatment.[253,403] Intermittent intravenous cyclophosphamide pulse therapy may be a favorable regimen for certain patients with progressive IPF.[252,416]

Azathioprine

Azathioprine has been reported to be effective in the treatment of IPF.[141,233,236,247,258] Clinical experience suggests that azathioprine may not be as effective as cyclophosphamide, but its side effects may be more manageable. Recent studies on the use of azathioprine in a patient with IPF have shown encouraging results (Figure 25–36).[141,258,417]

Colchicine

Substantive data supporting the efficacy of colchicine as therapy for IPF are lacking. Its effectiveness appears to be similar to that of corticosteroids but with fewer and less severe side effects attributed to colchicine.[261,262,418–421] Interpretation of these data is very difficult because these studies were retrospective and largely without random-

ization. In addition, many patients were not diagnosed with the use of biopsy, and the use of other medications and the limited follow-up are problematic. A recent randomized prospective study failed to show a benefit to using colchicine rather than prednisone (Figure 25–37). Additional controlled trials are needed to determine the appropriate role for colchicine in the treatment of IPF.

Interferon-γ

A pilot study of interferon-γ1b by Ziesche and coworkers showed significantly better lung function at twelve months in patients treated with both interferon-γ1b and

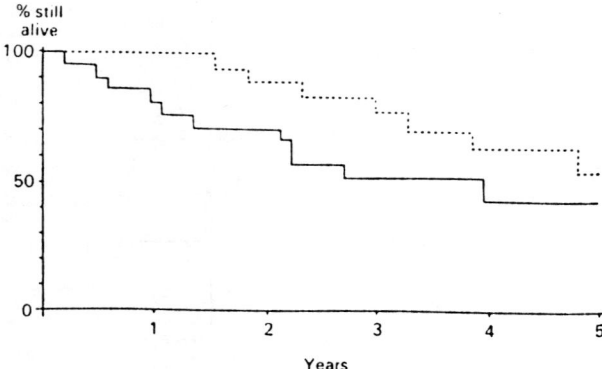

Figure 25–35 Cyclophosphamide treatment in IPF. Survival from allocation to treatment regimen until death in 22 patients receiving prednisolone only (——) and 21 receiving cyclophosphamide plus prednisolone (- - - -). There was a suggestion of improved survival in the patients treated with cyclophosphamide plus prednisolone, but this trend was not significant (*p* > .1). Reproduced with permission from Johnson MA et al.[249]

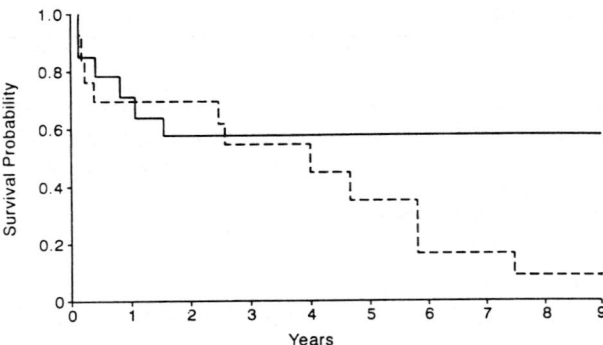

Figure 25–36 Reproduced with permission from Raghu et al.[417] Azathioprine treatment in IPF. Kaplan-Meier survival plots of patients who were randomized to therapy with azathioprine plus low-dose prednisone or prednisone alone. Age-adjusted analysis shows a significant survival advantage in the patients treated with combined azathioprine plus low-dose prednisone ($p = .02$)

prednisolone when compared to prednisolone alone.[423] Unfortunately, these findings must be viewed with caution, because there were a number of problems with the study design. First, not all of the patients studied had IPF. The histopathologic and HRCT criteria used to define IPF were incomplete. An expert panel reviewed each patient's surgical lung biopsy slides and photographs of the HRCT chest scans to reconfirm the diagnosis of IPF. Based on very strict diagnostic criteria for UIP on lung biopsy, correlated with confirmatory radiographic findings on HRCT chest scans, the panelists determined that 15 of the original 18 patients had either definite or probable IPF, whereas the remaining three patients definitely did not have IPF.[423] Second, this was a highly selective study population. Specifically, all 18 patients entered in the study were nonsmokers and all had undetectable levels of interferon-γ mRNA in tissue samples from transbronchial biopsies.[423] Third, the length of survival was atypical. These patients had not responded to more than 6 months of standard treat-

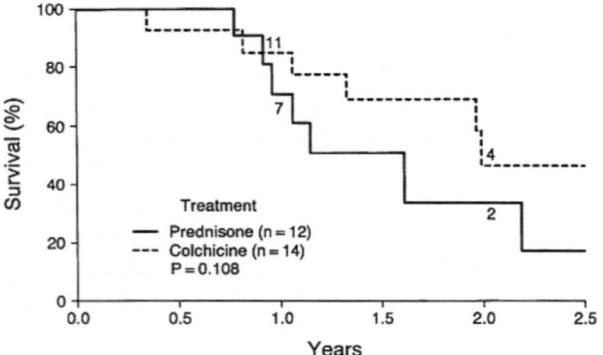

Figure 25–37 Survival after initiation of treatment of idiopathic usual interstitial pneumonitis, using either colchicine alone (broken lines) or prednisone alone (solid line). There was a trend for more prolonged survival in the colchicine-treated group, which was not statistically significant ($p = .108$). Reproduced with permission from Douglas WW et al.[420]

ment, and five required oxygen therapy. Given the enrollment criteria, it appears that patients were followed for from 3 to 7 years. In other studies of similar patients with IPF/UIP, there is invariably a subset of patients that progress to lung transplantation or death. Fourth, the treatment outcome was likely not clinically significant. The use of a change greater than 10% of that predicted (or an absolute change of 200 mL in the TLC) to define clinically significant improvement or decline in patients with IPF; there was no change in either the control group (prednisolone alone; 4% decline in TLC for the group) or treatment (interferon-γ1b and prednisolone; 9% increase in TLC for the group). The gas exchange data were also problematic. It is difficult to compare maximal exercise tests in a serial fashion because control for the level of work performed was not reported. The expert panel reviewed the data and used the published ATS/ERS/American College of Chest Physicians criteria to reassess the response to interferon-γ1b treatment (Table 25–15).[230] They used the following definitions for clinical change. For FVC and TLC, improvement was defined as an increase of more than 10% of the predicted value (or an increase of > 200 mL); a stable response was defined as a change in TLC or FVC no greater than ± 9% (or a change < 200 mL); and worsening was defined as a decrease in TLC or FVC of more than 10% (or a decrease > 200 mL). In the case of the $P(A-a)O_2$ gradient, improvement was defined as a decrease of more than 5 mm Hg from baseline, a stable response was defined as a change of less than ± 5 mm Hg, and worsening was defined as an increase of more than 5 mm Hg from baseline. Using these criteria and eliminating the patients who definitely did not have IPF, the panel reanalyzed the change at 12 months. They found that for FVC, five patients in the prednisolone-only group stabilized and three showed deterioration in lung function, while three patients in the interferon-γ1b plus prednisolone group improved and four stabilized; none of the patients treated with prednisolone alone improved, and none treated with interferon-γ1b deteriorated. Analysis of the change in $P(A-a)O_2$ gradient at 12 months showed that five patients in the prednisolone-only group stabilized, three deteriorated, and none improved, while all seven patients treated with interferon-γ1b and prednisolone improved. When the change in TLC was reanalyzed at 12 months, they found that none of the patients in the prednisolone-only group improved, six stabilized, and one deteriorated. In contrast, four patients in the interferon-γ1b plus prednisolone group improved, three stabilized, and none deteriorated. When the criteria included both FVC and $P(A-a)O_2$ gradient at 12 months, their analysis revealed that three patients in the interferon-γ1b and prednisolone group improved and six stabilized, with none worsening, while none in the prednisolone-only group improved, eight stabilized, and one deteriorated. The independent expert panel concluded that in this phase II clinical trial of patients with confirmed IPF, the

Table 25–15 Re-analysis of Data for Patients with Definite or Probable IPF

Response by Criterion Measured	Prednisolone Only	IFN-γ1b and Prednisolone
FVC at 12 months*		
Improved	0	3
Stable	5	4
Worse	3	0
TLC at 12 months*		
Improved	0	4
Stable	7	3
Worse	1	0
P(A-a)O₂ at 12 months*		
Improved	0	7
Stable	5	0
Worse	3	0
FVC + P(A-a)O₂ at 12 months*		
Improved	0	3
Stable	7	4
Worse	1	0
FVC on 2 consecutive measurements 3 months apart*		
Improved	0	3
Stable	6	4
Worse	2	0
AaPO₂ on 2 consecutive measurements 3 months apart*		
Improved	0	7
Stable	6	0
Worse	2	0

Reproduced with permission from Raghu G et al.[423]

$p < .05$ for patients treated with IFN-γ + prednisolone vs prednisolone only.

improvement of lung function was attributable to the combination of interferon-γ1b and prednisolone. Longer follow-up (average dureation 5 years) of the patients from this study was reported at the CHEST 2002 meeting in San Diego (November 6, 2002). Two of 9 (22%) IFN-γ1b and 7 of 9 (78%) control patients died during the follow-up period. Sixteen (9 of 9 IFN-γ1b and 7 of 9 control patients) of the original 18 study patients received one or more doses of IFN-γ1b following study completion and the duration of IFN-γ1b administration was similar across treatment groups. The Kaplan-Meier estimate of survival at 5 years was 77.8% in the IFN-γ1b group and 16.7% in the control group (log-rank test $p = .009$). The authors conclude that these results should be interpreted cautiously given the small sample size, open-label and single center study design, and baseline imbalances in time since IPF diagnosis, duration of immunosuppressive therapy, and lung function test that were observed at patient entry in the treatment groups.

Two additional pilot studies of interferon-γ1b treatment have been reported. Kalra and coworkers performed a retrospective review of 17 patients (15 males; mean age 67 years, range 52 to 80 years) treated between January 2000 and March 2002.[424] The diagnosis was based on clinical and HRCT scan criteria, and eight patients had VATS lung biopsy. All patients had severe impairment and had deteriorated while on previous treatment. No patient reported symptomatic improvement, and four stopped treatment because of continuing deterioration. Six (35%) died after an average of 5.7 months on treatment. Raghu and colleagues treated 33 terminally ill patients between March 2000 and May 2001 who had failed therapy (prednisone and azathioprine) and were ineligible for the phase III interferon-γ1b trial.[425] All patients required continuous supplemental oxygen. None of the patients improved; there were six deaths and three received lung transplants. These data suggest that interferon-γ1b is not effective in patients with advanced IPF. Preliminary data from a randomized, double-blind, placebo-controlled, phase 3 study of the safety and efficacy of subcutaneous recombinant interferon gamma-1b (IFN-γ1b) in 330 patients with IPF were reported at the 2002 European Respiratory Society meeting in Stockholm. Patients received either placebo or 200 µm of IFN-γ-1b injected subcutaneously three times per week. The primary endpoint was progression free survival defined as the first occurrence of one of the following: (A) a decrease in FVC of >10 percent, (B) an increase in P(A-a)O₂ gradient >5 mm Hg, or (C) death. the primary efficacy endpoint was not achieved. In the IFN-γ1b-treated group, 75 of 162 patients (46.3%) experienced death or disease progression compared to 87 of 168 patients in the placebo group (51.8%; $p = .53$). Exploratory analyses suggested that there was less dyspnea after 48 weeks of treatment and less oxygen use in the IFN-γ1b-treated group versus placebo. There was no significant effect on lung function or gas exchange at 48 weeks of treatment. In the overall "intent-to-treat" patient population, there were 16 of 162 deaths in the IFN-γ1b-treated group (9.9%) compared to 28 of 168 deaths in the placebo group (16.7%), representing a 40% decrease in mortality in favor of IFN-γ1b ($p = .084$). An analysis of the estimated reduction in the risk of death by baseline FVC in the "intent-to-treat" population suggested that the survival benefit depends on baseline FVC ($p = .048$, Cox proportional hazard regression analysis). In those patients with FVC >60% (the median baseline FVC in the study population was 60%), there were 3 of 90 deaths in the IFN-γ1b-treated group (3.3%) versus 12 of 92 deaths in the placebo group (13%), representing a 75% decrease in mortality in favor of IFN-γ1b ($p = .02$). In contrast, in patients with FVC <60% there were 13 of 72 deaths in the IFN-γ1b-treated group (18%) versus 16 of 76 in the placebo group (21%); ($p = .75$). These secondary analyses suggest that patients with mild to moderate impairment in lung function at study entry may be more likely to benefit from IFN-γ1b. Most deaths were secondary to respiratory failure and occurred more acutely in the placebo group. IFN-γ1b was generally well-tolerated with few discontinuations due to adverse events, though there was an unexplained excess of non-fatal pneumonias in the IFN-γ1b-treated group versus placebo.

Mechanism of Action.   Interferon-γ1b is a naturally occurring human protein secreted primarily by T cells (CD4⁺ T cells, CD8⁺ T cells, and natural killer cells). Interferon-γ is a type 1 T-helper cell (Th₁) cytokine with multiple actions. Interferon-γ plays a critical role in host defense by inducing the differentiation of CD4⁺ T cells to the Th₁ phenotype.[426] Interferon-γ has been shown to inhibit the proliferation of fibroblasts and reduce the synthesis of connective tissue matrix proteins by fibroblasts. Interferon-γ appears to exert this effect by downregulating the expression of TGF-β₁, a Th₂ cytokine that provokes fibroblast proliferation and synthesis of connective tissue matrix proteins (see Chapter 8, "Inflammation in the Pathogenesis of Intersititial Lung Diseases").[427,428] TGF-β₁ activates a series of processes that uniformly contribute to the accumulation of collagen, and it may be the master switch for fibrotic events in the lung. TGF-β₁ down-regulates the expression of interferon-γ in a reciprocal manner (ie, a negative feedback loop).[423] Interferon-γ is a potent antagonist of TGF-β activity in vitro.[272] Also, it has been shown that interferon-γ decreases the expression of α-smooth muscle actin and alters the spindle morphologic characteristics of fibroblasts pretreated with TGF-β; these findings suggest that interferon-γ is able to reduce the number of myofibroblasts.[126,429]

The rationale for the use of interferon-γ in IPF comes, in part, from the hypothesis that an acquired deficiency of interferon-γ exists and may be necessary for the exaggerated wound healing process characteristic of this disease to take place.[430] Interferon-γ is found at high levels in granulomatous diseases that rarely progress to end-stage fibrosis (eg, sarcoidosis).[431] Studies of lung tissue from patients with IPF have shown deficits in interferon-γ and increased levels of TGF-β₁.[432–434] Impaired interferon-γ release may be a potentiating factor in the pathogenesis of IPF.[423] In the bleomycin model of lung fibrosis, TGF-β increases before the development of fibrosis, and if this is prevented by treatment with interferon-γ, the fibrosis is less (see Chapter 8, "Inflammation in the Pathogenesis of Interstitial Lung Diseases" Figure 8–3).[435] It has been shown that TGF-β activity in the lungs of patients with IPF is altered by interferon-γ treatment.[436]

Dosage and Administration.   Interferon-γ1b is administered via subcutaneous injection three times per week (200 μg). The ideal duration of therapy remains unknown. Ziesche and Block recommend that the treatment not be stopped because of the risk of the slow reappearance of fibrosis. In several patients, they found that the amount of interferon-γ that is required to maintain the degree of improvement gradually decreased.[430]

Adverse Effects.   The most frequent side effects associated with interferon-γ1b therapy include flulike symptoms, such as fever, headache, muscle soreness, malaise, fatigue, and chills. Acetaminophen (≥ 500 mg) or ibuprofen (≥ 400 mg with food) is to be taken at the time of injection to lessen these side effects. Other side effects reported include diarrhea, vomiting, nausea, abdominal pain, injection site erythema or tenderness, and depression.

Pirfenidone

Raghu and colleagues reported the results of a phase II open-label study evaluating pirfenidone.[437] The study found that pirfenidone was well tolerated, with minimal side effects. Additionally, treatment with pirfenidone appeared to allow discontinuation or tapering of prednisone and immunosuppressive therapy without loss of lung function. A multicenter randomized double-blind, placebo-controlled study of pirfenidone (1,800 mg/day) versus placebo was carried out in 107 Japanese patients with IPF.[438] The diagnosis was made using clinical and HRCT criteria (only 14 underwent lung biopsy). Ninety-one had findings consistent with definite IPF, and 16 had findings consistent with probable IPF. The subjects were enrolled at a ratio of 2:1 (pirfenidone, $n = 72$; placebo, $n = 35$), and the treatment period was 48 weeks. The primary endpoint was a comparison of SaO_2 at maximal exercise during a 6-minute treadmill test. Pirfenidone was effective in stabilizing the lung function and reducing the number of patients who experienced acute exacerbation of their disease (one in the pirfenidone group and five in the placebo group) (Figure 25–38). It has been suggested that pirfenidone may slow the progression of lung impairment in patients with pulmonary fibrosis and Hermansky-Pudlak syndrome.[439]

Mechanism of Action.   Pirfenidone is a pyridone molecule, 5-methyl-1-phenyl-2-(1H)-pyridone. In hamsters, pirfenidone has been shown to ameliorate

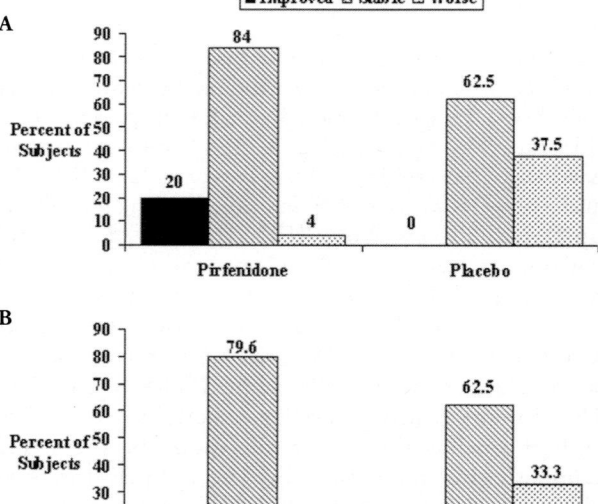

Figure 25–38   Pirfenidone ($n = 55$) vs placebo ($n = 25$): Change in lung function in patients that completed baseline and follow-up treadmill walk testing. *A*, Minimal oxygen saturation (SaO_2) during the exercise. Pirfenidone-treated patients had significantly better outcomes, $p = .006$ by Wilcoxon test for the 3 variables. *B*, FVC. Pirfenidone-treated patients had significantly better outcomes; $p = .019$ by Wilcoxon test for the 3 variables. Data are from Azuma A et al.[438]

bleomycin-induced pulmonary fibrosis. In vitro, this compound inhibits TGF-β-stimulated collagen synthesis, decreases the extracellular matrix, and blocks the mitogenic effect of profibrotic cytokines in adult human lung fibroblasts derived from patients with IPF.[439]

Dosage and Administration. The recommended course is oral administration of up to 40 mg/kg/day (to a maximum of 3,600 mg/day) in divided doses.

Adverse Effects. The most common side effects include rash (photosensitivity), abdominal discomfort, dyspepsia, anorexia, nausea, fatigue, and lethargy.[437,438] Other potential side effects include diarrhea, constipation, itching, dry skin, hyperpigmentation, headache, and weakness.

Penicillamine

Two retrospective studies of patients with ILD associated with scleroderma reported that penicillamine therapy was associated with an improvement in DL_{CO} but not in other lung function parameters.[440,441] Penicillamine has been used in the treatment of IPF mainly in isolated case reports or in very small series. Penicillamine plus prednisolone has been reported to be more effective than prednisolone alone or prednisolone plus azathioprine.[442] In one study, penicillamine was given to 18 patients with ILD in whom treatment with high-dose corticosteroids and/or immunosuppressive drugs had been unsuccessful. Median survival was improved when compared with historic controls.[443] In another report, penicillamine was given to 12 patients with "end-stage" fibrosis.[444] All patients improved clinically and functionally during the first year of treatment, and overall survival rates were felt to compare favorably with historic controls. The results of Selman and colleagues showed no improvement in survival with this therapy.[262] Thus, the usefulness of this therapy in the management of IPF is unknown, and treatment with this agent is probably not warranted until additional studies on its effectiveness are available.[233,258,443,445]

Cyclosporine

There are few published reports on the use of cyclosporine in ILD. All have been anecdotal and are less than encouraging.[446–448] A specific role for cyclosporine in patients with IPF who are awaiting lung transplantation has been proposed.[448] In these patients, the addition of cyclosporine may allow reduction in the dose of corticosteroids without precipitating clinical deterioration and may result in improvement in the native lung.

Other Treatments

A number of other agents have been reported in individual cases or in small case series of patients with IPF.[126] Also, in vitro studies and animal models have suggested several possible agents (see Chapter 13, "The Future of Medical Ther-

apy for Lung Fibrosis"). Further studies are required to evaluate the potential benefit of any of these approaches.

In vitro, interferon-β1a has been shown to reduce fibroblast migration and proliferation and inhibit collagen production by fibroblasts.[126] A prospective multicenter randomized double-blind, placebo-controlled trial examining the efficacy of interferon-β1a in IPF in the United States and Canada showed that it was not effective in reducing the decline in lung function or improving survival.[449,450]

Inhaled nitric oxide, an endothelium-dependent relaxing factor that is a potent pulmonary vasodilator, has been shown to reduce the pulmonary vascular resistance and improve cardiac output and arterial oxygenation in patients with end-stage pulmonary fibrosis and pulmonary hypertension.[451,452]

Chlorambucil and vincristine sulfate given alone or with corticosteroids has shown no substantial benefit.[249]

Relaxin is a pregnancy-related hormone that has tissue remodeling and antifibrotic effects. Relaxin inhibits the TGF-β-mediated overexpression of collagens and fibronectin and stimulates the expression of collagenase-1 by human lung fibroblasts in vitro.[453] It has been shown to block bleomycin-induced fibrosis in mice.[453] Relaxin also alters angiogenesis via the induction of vascular endothelial growth factor and basic fibroblast growth factor in wound macrophages.[444] A multicenter parallel-group randomized double-blind, placebo-controlled trial of relaxin (administered by continuous subcutaneous infusion over 24 weeks) in patients with scleroderma showed that it improved function (including FVC, functional status, and global assessment).[455] No clinical trials are available or ongoing in IPF.

Oxygen damage leads to fibrosis. *N*-Acetylcysteine prevents epithelial cell injury mediated by oxygen radicals and has been shown to attenuate fibrosis in animal models of lung fibrosis.[126,456–458] IPF is characterized by a huge alveolar oxidant burden and a deficiency of glutathione, a major antioxidant, in the pulmonary epithelial lining fluid. Therefore, a rational therapeutic strategy is to increase lung glutathione to augment the pulmonary antioxidant protective screen.[459–463] However, clinical studies with oral *N*-acetylcysteine have not shown it to be more effective than glucocorticoids.[456] A prospective double-blind, placebo-controlled study is underway in several European countries. The objective is to evaluate 150 patients given 1,800 mg of oral *N*-acetylcysteine daily, in addition to prednisone and azathioprine.[464]

Captopril inhibits the angiotensin-converting enzyme and completely abrogates Fas-induced apoptosis in human alveolar epithelial cells. It also inhibits fibroblast proliferation in vitro and reduces the fibrotic lung response in vivo.[126] A trial is ongoing at the National Institute of Respiratory Diseases in Mexico.[126,465]

Tumor necrosis factor (TNF)-α is associated with pulmonary inflammation and/or fibrosis and is present in the lungs of patients with UIP, possibly leading to up-regulation and overexpression of other fibrogenic cytokines, such as TGF-β. Two new anti-TNF agents, etanercept and infliximab, have been suggested as possible treatment agents for IPF. Tumor necrosis factor receptor: Fc (etanercept) was given (25 μg subcutaneously twice a week) along with oral prednisone (10 mg daily) in a pilot study of nine patients with severe IPF.[466,467] Patients were followed for 7 to 30 months (average = 19 months). The vital capacity improved in two, decreased in one, and remained unchanged in six patients, with an average decline of 1%. The DL_{CO} improved in two patients, declined in four, and was unchanged in two (measurement was unobtainable in one), with an average improvement of 9%. The $P(A-a)O_2$ gradient improved in three and was unchanged in six, with an average improvement of 17%. Two patients died, one from an acute pulmonary embolism and the other from postoperative hemorrhage at the site of a colon cancer resection. These data are encouraging in that they indicate that etanercept may reduce or prevent the loss of lung function in patients with IPF/UIP. Clinical trials in the ILDs are planned for these agents.

Several experimental agents have been suggested for future trials, including lovastatin (which blocks formation of granulation tissue by induction of fibroblast apoptosis in vitro and in vivo); antisense therapy (an antisense gene-specific oligonucleotide against the c-Ki-ras protein substantially inhibits the proliferation of diploid human fibroblasts); beractant (a natural bovine lung extract containing phospholipids, neutral lipids, fatty acids, and surfactant-associated SPs B and C that promotes apoptosis of normal human lung fibroblasts); keratinocyte growth factor (which induces proliferation of type II pneumocytes); soluble receptor to TGF-β (has reduced bleomycin-induced lung fibrosis); and TGF-α (a transgenic model in which overexpression led to fibrosis, and a knockout mouse deficient in this cytokine was protected from bleomycin injury).

ATS/ERS Treatment Recommendations for IPF

The ATS/ERS consensus statement recommends that treatment offered to a patient with IPF should be combined therapy, including corticosteroids and either azathioprine or cyclophosphamide.[230] This treatment should be limited to those patients who have been given adequate information regarding the merits and pitfalls of treatment and who possess features consistent with a more favorable outcome. Initial corticosteroid therapy (prednisone or equivalent) for IPF is as follows. (Lean body weight is the ideal weight expected for a patient of this age, sex, and height.)

- 0.5 mg/kg (lean body weight [LBW]) per day orally for 4 weeks, then
- 0.25 mg/kg (LBW) per day for 8 weeks, and
- taper to 0.125 mg/kg (LBW) daily or 0.25 mg/kg (LBW) every other day

PLUS one of the following:

Azathioprine
- 2 to 3 mg/kg LBW per day
- maximum dose of 150 mg/day orally
- beginning dose of 25 to 50 mg/day, increased by 25 mg increments every 7 to 14 days until maximum dose is reached

Cyclophosphamide
- 2 mg/kg LBW per day
- maximum dose of 150 mg/day orally
- beginning dose of 25 to 50 mg/day, increased by 25 mg increments every 7 to 14 days until maximum dose is reached

In the absence of complications or adverse effects of the medications, combined therapy should be continued for at least 6 months.[230] At that time, a repeat evaluation should be performed, using symptoms, radiologic findings, and physiological findings to determine the response to therapy (Table 25–16). Close monitoring for potential adverse effects is important. If the patient is found to be worse, the therapy should be stopped or changed (eg, continue prednisone at the present dose and switch to a different cytotoxic agent or consider an alternative therapy or lung transplantion). If the patient is found to be improved or stable, the combined therapy should be continued, using the same doses of the medications. The committee recommended that the therapy be continued indefinitely only in individuals with objective evidence of continued improvement or stabilization.[230]

Other Problems in Management

Clinical deterioration in patients with IPF is expected. Most patients experience episodes of worsening shortness of breath, decreased exercise tolerance, or other decline in functional status during the course of their illness. In evaluating the clinical deterioration in patients with IPF, disease progression may be difficult to distinguish from disease-associated complications and adverse effects of therapy[468] The clinical manifestations of disease progression are multiple and often nonspecific (see Table 25–8). End-stage IPF frequently leads to incapacitating respiratory insufficiency, with patients unable to carry out activities of daily life without extreme distress. Death usually results from intractable hypoxemia and respiratory failure (Figure 25–39).

Acute Exacerbation of IPF

Some patients have acute or rapidly progressive disease ("acute exacerbation" or "accelerated stage" of IPF), generally characterized by severe worsening dyspnea or cough. Occasionally, systemic symptoms such as fever, fatigue, and weight loss are present. Usually, the illness

TABLE 25–16   Assessment of Response to Treatment

Clinical Improvement *

Symptoms   Decreased level of dyspnea, specifically an increase in level of exertion required before patient must stop because of breathlessness, or severity of cough

Radiology   Reduced parenchymal abnormalities on chest radiograph or HRCT scan

Physiology   Improvement defined by changes in 2 or more of the following:
> 10% increase in TLC or FVC (minimum > 200 mL)
> 15% increase in DL_{CO} (minimum > 3 mL/min/mm Hg)
Significant improvement (≥ 4 percentage points, ≥ 4 mm Hg) or normalization of O_2 saturation or PaO_2 during formal exercise testing

Clinically Stable

Symptoms   No significant changes

Radiology   No significant changes

Physiology   Stable defined by 2 or more of the following:
< 10% change in TLC or FVC
< 15% change in DL_{CO}
No significant change in O_2 saturation or PaO_2 during formal exercise testing

Clinical Deterioration (after 6 months of therapy)

Symptoms   Increase in dyspnea or severity of cough not caused by another concomitant process

Radiology   Increased parenchymal abnormalities or development of honeycombing or pulmonary hypertension on chest radiograph or HRCT scan

Physiology   Deterioration defined by 2 or more of the following:
> 10% decrease in TLC or FVC
> 15% increase in DL_{CO}
Significant worsening (a fall of ≥ 4 percentage points, ≥ 4 mm Hg) of O_2 saturation or PaO_2 during formal exercise testing

*Two or more of the following, documented on 2 consecutive visits over a 3- to 6-months period)
DL_{CO} = diffusing capacity of the lung for carbon monoxide; FVC = forced vital capacity; HRCT = high-resolution computed tomography; PaO_2 = partial pressure of oxygen in arterial blood; TLC = total lung capacity.

duration prior to presentation is 4 to 8 weeks, normally accompanied by progressive worsening of symptoms.[469–471] It is important to rule out other causes of the acute decline, such as infection, pneumothorax, pulmonary embolism, and heart failure (see below).

New or progressive diffuse pulmonary opacities are found on chest radiography. Akira and colleagues examined the CT findings in 17 patients.[471] Peripheral parenchymal opacification ($n = 6$), multifocal parenchymal opacification ($n = 6$), and diffuse parenchymal opacification ($n = 5$) were the major patterns found.[471] The peripheral parenchymal opacifications corresponded pathologically to active fibroblastic foci. The multifocal parenchymal opacifications and diffuse parenchymal opacifications corresponded pathologically to acute diffuse alveolar damage. Three of the six patients with a multifocal pattern responded to corticosteroid therapy. All patients with a peripheral pattern showed various degrees of improvement following corticosteroid therapy.[471]

Lung function worsens as the disease progresses, especially gas exchange (usually a decrease in arterial oxygen tension of > 10 mm Hg compared to baseline).[471]

Most patients who have had surgical lung biopsies following the acute exacerbation of their IPF have been found to have histologic findings typical of the late or organizing stage of diffuse alveolar damage, in addition to the features of their chronic UIP pattern (ie, acute on chronic changes).[469] In addition, it appears that in some cases there is a prominence of active fibroblastic foci, suggesting an acceleration of the underlying UIP pattern of injury.[471] Other lesions that may be seen in association with acute exacerbations of IPF include OP, vasculitis and diffuse alveolar hemorrhage. By definition, no other identifiable cause for this acute injury is found.

Many of these patients will require admission to the hospital and treatment in an Intensive Care Unit (ICU) because repiratory failure often associated with hemodynamic instability (hypovolemia or sepsis), significant concomitant medical disease (usually cardiovascular disease or renal failure), or severe hypoxemia requiring frequent monitoring of arterial blood gases or mechanical ventila-

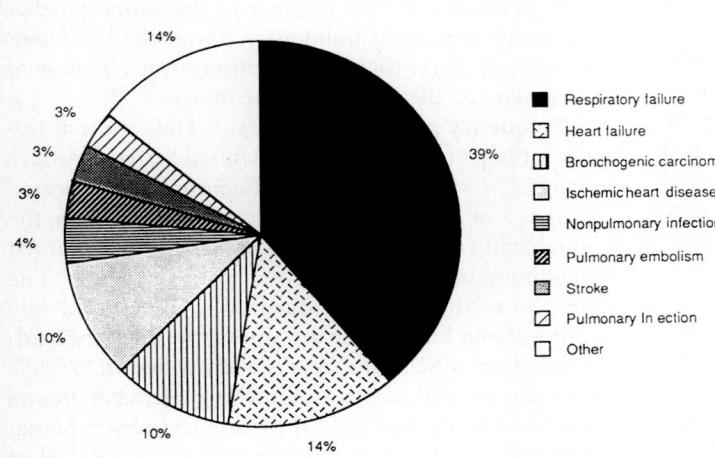

14%
3%
3%
3%
4%
10%
10%
14%
39%

■ Respiratory failure
▨ Heart failure
▥ Bronchogenic carcinoma
▢ Ischemic heart disease
▤ Nonpulmonary infection
▨ Pulmonary embolism
▨ Stroke
▨ Pulmonary In ection
▢ Other

Figure 25–39   Causes of death in IPF. Patients with IPF inevitably experience declines in functional status, most frequently due to progressive pulmonary fibrosis. This figure summarizes six studies that reported the clinical course of nearly 550 patients with IPF. Approximately 60% of the patients died during the study periods, which ranged from 1 to 6.8 years. Mean survival varied from 3.2 to 5 years, and between 65 and 100% of the patients received corticosteroids. The major cause of death was respiratory failure due to IPF progression. Cardiovascular conditions, including heart failure, ischemic heart disease, and stroke, accounted for nearly 27% of deaths, and over 10% of patients died of bronchogenic carcinoma. Less than 10% of deaths were due to pulmonary embolism and infections. Other, usually nonfatal disease-associated complications, include pneumothorax, corticosteroid-induced metabolic side effects and myopathy and therapy-related immunosuppression. Data are from Panos RJ et al.[468]

tion. Introduction of mechanical ventilation should come only after carefully weighing the patient's long term prognosis. Patients with endstage lung fibrosis from any cause are difficult to ventilate and are rarely successfully weaned from mechanical ventilation. Mortality during the hospitalization is high (up to 65%) and those who survive have a very poor prognosis (i.e., with a > 90% mortality rate in the 6 months following discharge from the hospital).

Pulmonary Physical Rehabilitation

Patients with IPF are usually so dyspneic with exertion that they discontinue any program of routine exercise. This discontinuation of exercise should not be encouraged because exercise increases the sense of well-being and improves muscle strength and ambulation. Daily walks or the use of a stationary bicycle are excellent routines. Supplemental oxygen may be required during exercise. Severe hypoxemia (PaO_2 < 55 mm Hg) at rest or during exercise should be managed by supplemental oxygen. Higher flow rates than those frequently used in chronic obstructive pulmonary disease may be required.

Cardiovascular Disease

Heart failure and ischemic heart disease are common problems in patients with IPF, accounting for nearly one-third of deaths. Right ventricular failure may develop as a result of pulmonary hypertension (present in ~70% of patients). Compression or destruction of pulmonary vessels by inflammation or fibrotic processes, vasoconstriction due to hypoxemia or acidemia, and pulmonary emboli are causes of the pulmonary hypertension and right heart failure. With the appearance of cor pulmonale, diuretic therapy and, rarely, phlebotomy is indicated. The use of pulmonary vasodilators in the treatment of IPF is only theoretic, and to date, no clinical trials are available. Left ventricular dysfunction occurs as a result of ischemic heart disease or uncontrolled systemic arterial hypertension.

Pneumothorax

Pneumothorax, which is characteristic of eosinophilic granuloma of the lung, may also occur in IPF. This complication may be extremely difficult to treat, because the lung is stiff and difficult to reexpand; and prolonged chest tube drainage, with high levels of negative pressure (20 to 40 mm Hg), may be necessary. Some patients may require thoracotomy, bleb resection, and pleurectomy.

Pulmonary Embolism

Acute pulmonary embolism, in my experience, is an occasional cause of clinical deterioration in this group of patients. Sudden worsening of dyspnea, with unexplained deterioration in arterial blood gases and without evidence of superimposed infection, should prompt the clinician to consider lung scan and/or pulmonary angiography. Pulmonary embolism causes 3 to 7% of deaths in IPF. Risk factors for pulmonary embolism in these patients include inactivity, heart disease (including right, left, or biventricular failure), cancer, and possibly corticosteroid-induced Cushing's disease.

Pulmonary Infection

The incidence of pulmonary infections is somewhat increased in IPF. Pulmonary infection is a major factor in the death of 2 to 4% of patients. Therapeutic interventions, especially corticosteroids and cytotoxic agents, may further increase the risk of infection and reactivation of latent infections by suppression of cell-mediated immunologic processes.

Lung Cancer

Bronchogenic carcinoma (adenocarcinoma, squamous cell carcinoma, small-cell carcinoma, and alveolar cell carcinoma) has been identified with increased frequency in IPF.[16,61,62,232,472–490] Most reports regarding the association of diffuse pulmonary fibrosis and lung cancers come from Japan; only a few clinical studies of this issue are available from other countries of the world, including the United States.[16,479–486,489–492] Despite these reports suggesting a relationship between lung fibrosis and cancer, Well and colleagues recently presented compelling data that seriously question the prevalent attitude about the correlation of IPF and lung cancer.[492–494] Date from a large analysis of death certificates in the United States (26,866,600 deaths in a 13-year period, with 107,312 deaths in patients with pulmonary fibrosis) showed that lung cancer occurred less frequently in patients with pulmonary fibrosis (4.8%) than in patients with obstructive pulmonary disease (10%) and asbestosis (27%) compared to the general population (6%).[493] There are concerns about this data because it is well known that death certificates are a poor source of information about the role of lung fibrosis as a cause of death. Furthermore, it is difficult to determine whether long-term survivors of pulmonary fibrosis had different rates of lung cancer than short-term survivors, because of missing data on the duration of the disease.[492,494]

Frequency and Risk Factors.   The reported frequency ranges from 4.8% in the United States to 48.2% in Japan.[485,486,491,492] The large differences in the reported frequency of lung cancer associated with IPF in the United States compared with that in Japan or the United Kingdom may result from several possible factors. The criteria or methods used for diagnosing IPF, clinical only or clinical plus histologic, vary among the different studies; therefore, misclassification is likely common.[487,491,492] There can be difficulty distinguishing adenocarcinoma from severely atypical type II pneumocyte hyperplasia, goblet cell metaplasia, and squamous metaplasia, all of which can be seen in association with IPF.[491] This can lead to false diagnoses of adenocarcinoma.[491]

Most of the patients are men with a history of cigarette smoking.[19,476,482,485,486] Ill-defined occupational and environmental exposures may increase the risk for both IPF and lung cancer.[19,494] The diffuse lung injury itself may increase the risk of lung cancer. It is postulated that carcinoma arises from the metaplastic bronchiolar epithelium that develops in these patients.[486] Interestingly, a number of the reported cases occurred in patients with familial IPF.

Location and Histologic Type.   Most lung cancers in IPF (79%) arise in peripheral areas involving fibrosis and are located in the lower lobes.[482,485,486] This finding is similar to the distribution of the fibrotic lesions in patients with IPF, implicating the inflammatory process and bronchiolar squamous metaplasia in the pathogenesis of lung cancer.[492] It is not certain if any histologic type of cancer is predominant in these patients. Squamous cell carcinoma was the most common histologic type (47%) in male patients, and adenocarcinoma was most common in female patients (64%).[489,492] Small cell-carcinoma was common in patients with synchronous multiple lung cancer and lung fibrosis.[482]

Possible Mechanisms.   The mechanisms underlying the apparent association of IPF and cancer are unclear.[492,494] Kuwano and coworkers performed immunohistochemistry and in situ detection of DNA strand breaks or apoptosis in the tissues of IPF patients for the tumor suppressor p53 protein (a transcription factor that plays a central role in the cellular response to DNA damage; it can cause either G1 arrest or apoptosis) and tumor suppressor p21$^{Waf1/Cip1/Sdi1}$ (p21; shown to inhibit cyclin-CDK complex kinase activity).[495] The p53 and p21 were especially expressed in hyperplastic bronchial and alveolar epithelial cells of lung tissues from all patients with IPF. In normal lung parenchyma and specimens of pulmonary emphysema, p53 and p21 were not detected except in scattered alveolar macrophages and in the epithelial cells within localized fibrotic regions. These results suggest that p53 and p21 are up-regulated in association with chronic DNA damage, resulting in either G1 arrest or apoptosis, so that the DNA damage can be repaired in IPF. These researchers (and others) speculated that chronic DNA damage and repair may lead to mutation of the p53 gene and tumorigenesis in IPF.[489,496] Recent findings suggest that allelic loss of the fragile histidine triad (*FHIT*) gene may be involved in carcinogenesis in the peripheral lung of patients with IPF.[497]

Management and Outcome.   It is possible that with the increasing use of screening CT scans in asymptomatic smokers, there will be an increased identification of localized cancers in patients with mild or early ILD[498] Localized tumors should be resected if the patient can tolerate the surgical procedure but this is frequently not possible because of the severity of the pulmonary dysfunction likely to exist after the surgery.

The prognosis for patients with IPF and lung cancer was very poor.[484]

Gastroesophageal Reflux Disease

Tobin and coworkers showed that patients with IPF have a high prevalence of gastroesophageal reflux (GER).[499] The episodes of GER tended to occur at night and often extended into the proximal esophagus. Most patients with IPF and GER did not have typical symptoms of heartburn or regurgitation. Further studies are needed to see if aggressive, chronic treatment of GER in these patients might be able to improve or halt further progression of their pulmonary disease. Tobin and coworkers advocated the use of ambulatory esophageal pH monitoring in patients with IPF to document the presence or absence of abnormal GER and to guide aggressive treatment of such reflux if it is found.[499]

Risk Factors for Progressive Disease and Survival in IPF

Several studies suggest that patients with IPF can be placed into lower- and higher-risk categories for progressive lung disease based on several factors. Higher-risk cases are males and those with mucus hypersecretion, moderate to severe dyspnea with exertion, a smoking history (the higher the number of pack-years, the worse the prognosis), moderate to severe loss in lung function at presentation (as assessed by DL_{CO} and gas exchange with exercise), neutrophilia or eosinophilia on cellular analysis of BAL fluid at presentation, decreased SP-A content and SP-A:PL ratio, and mixed ground-glass and reticular opacities or a predominance of reticular or honeycomb changes on HRCT scan. Survival is much worse with increasing age (Figure 25–33).[27,329,330,401,402,500,501]

Favorable indicators of survival that would encourage aggressive therapy in patients with IPF include younger age (< 50 years), a shorter symptomatic period (< 1 year) before initiating therapy, being in an earlier stage of disease (less dyspnea, more normal lung function, less parenchymal disease on chest radiograph or HRCT scan), showing a beneficial initial response to corticosteroid therapy, and being female.[196,408,500,502–504] Unfortunately, it does not appear that the extent of honeycombing on HRCT scan is very useful in predicting a favorable outcome in IPF (Figure 25–40).[274]

King and coworkers used hierarchical multivariable analysis of clinical, radiologic, and extensive physiological variables to develop a model that would allow clinicians to make more precise prognostic estimations about patients with IPF. This analysis yielded a CRP model that can be used to estimate the survival time in a patient with IPF. The model included the following parameters: age, smoking history; clubbing; extent of profusion of interstitial opacities, and presence or absence of pulmonary

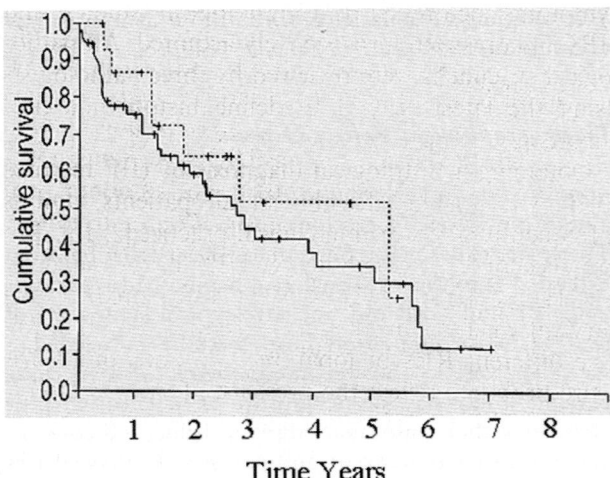

Figure 25–40   Kaplan-Meier survival curves in patients with UIP, grouped by HRCT scan fibrotic score of > 2 in at least one lobe (solid line) compared with CT scan fibrotic score in which no lobe has a score > 2 (broken line). Reproduced with permission from Flaherty et al.[274]

hypertension on the chest radiograph; %predicted TLC; and PaO_2 at the end of maximal exercise (Table 25–17). This model was superior to the originally reported CRP score in predicting survival in IPF (Figure 25–41).

The clinical course is invariably one of gradual deterioration. Occasionally, these patients may experience periods of rapid decline. (see "Acute exacerbation of IPF" above). The median length of survival from time of diagnosis varies between 2.5 and 3.5 year. In more recent studies that used the revised diagnostic cri-

teria for UIP, only 20 to 30% of subjects were alive 5 years after diagnosis.[274,398,410–412,505.]

NONSPECIFIC INTERSTITIAL PNEUMONIA

The term "nonspecific interstitial pneumonia" originated to allow pathologists a way to label a difficult-to-classify surgical lung biopsy specimen that did not demonstrate a clearly identifiable pattern (eg UIP, DIP).[399,506] However, the increasing use of surgical lung biopsy to confirm the diagnosis of IPF and the subsequent careful review of these cases allowed the identification of a reproducible classification scheme for the common patterns found (see "Katzenstein and Meyers classification" above) (see Table 25–2)[11] In addition, it was shown that this subclassification of idiopathic interstitial pneumonia had considerable clinical relevance (see Table 25–4).[11,398] Importantly, the NSIP pattern identified a group of ILDs with a more favorable prognosis than UIP.[274,398,399,410–413,507–511]

Idiopathic NSIP does appear to be a discrete entity (see Table 25–4). However, the current definition of NSIP remains somewhat troublesome because there are no distinctive clinical, radiographic or histopathological descriptions and to date, this condition has been largely "…defined more in terms of what it is not rather than what it is."[512] In the past, many cases now called NSIP were called "cellular interstitial pneumonia, not otherwise specified" or cellular UIP.[137,235,310,398] In addition, many of the published cases are likely misclassified because of failure to rigorously rule out secondary causes (especially hypersensitivity pneumonitis and connective tissue disease) and because of the difficulty distinguish-

TABLE 25–17   CRP Scoring System for Predicting Survival Time in IPF

		Clinical				Radiographic				Physiological			
Age		Smoking Status		Clubbing		Profusion		Pulmonary Hypertension		TLC (% predicted)		PaO_2 at Maximal Exercise	
Category	Score	Category	Score	Category	Score	Category	Score	Category	Score	Category	Score	Category	Score
< 40	0	current	0	no	0	< 15	0	no	0	≥ 80	0	≥ 65	0
40–44.9	3.2	former	10.2	yes	10.7	15–17.49	9.15	yes	10.3	70–79.9	2.75	60–64.9	1.5
45–49.9	6.4	never	13.6			≥ 17.5	18.30			60–69.9	5.50	55–59.9	3.0
50–54.9	9.6									50–59.9	8.25	50–54.9	4.5
55–59.9	12.8									< 50	11.00	45–49.9	6.0
60–64.9	16.0											40–44.9	7.5
65–69.9	19.2											35–39.9	9.0
70–74.9	22.4											< 35	10.5
≥ 75	25.6												
Maximum score possible	25.6	+	13.6	+	10.7	+	18.3	+	10.3	+	11.0	+	10.5
Total	100												

Reproduced with permission from King TE Jr et al.[28]

ing some cases of fibrotic NSIP from UIP.[2] Until further definition is available, the consensus of experts is that the diagnosis of NSIP should remain provisional.[2]

Etiology and Epidemiology

The etiology of NSIP remains to be defined. In immunocompetent individuals, both idiopathic and secondary forms of NSIP are found. The secondary forms are seen in patients with drug reactions, collagen-vascular diseases, hypersensitivity pneumonitis, and in survivors of ARDS.[513–519] In immunocompromised persons (eg, individuals with acquired immunodeficiency syndrome, bone marrow transplant recipients, and persons receiving various chemotherapeutic agents), a similar histologic reaction may occur.[520,521] However, Katzenstein and Myers suggest that many of these cases represent manifestations of difficult-to-diagnose viral or other infections or result from lung injury of various causes and suggest that this term not be used to classify such cases.[11]

The incidence and prevalence of NSIP are unknown. Several groups have reevaluated the surgical lung biopsy specimens from their centers over the past 10 to 25 years that were previouly diagnosed as IPF or idiopathic interstitial pneumonia. They show that the UIP pattern is most commonly found (47 to 63%) and the NSIP is second most common (14 to 36%), depending on the study design (see Table 25–10).[274,398,410,411,413,505] Most patients are middle-aged adults (mean age at onset varies between 39 and 60 years in most series). Among cases reported to date, there are more women then men but this varies considerably from center to center.[274,398,399,410–413,507–511] The majority of the patients are current or former cigarette smokers.

Clinical Findings

Table 25–18 summarizes the clinical characteristics at presentation in reported clinical series.[274,398,399,410–413,507–511] The illness onset is subacute, with an average duration of symptoms before diagnosis of approximately 11 months (range 2 to 44 months) (see Table 25–4). Dyspnea (80 to 100% of cases) and cough (33 to 85% of cases) are the most common presenting complaints. Fever and systemic flulike symptoms, fatigue, and weight loss are also common clinical findings.

Bibasilar crackles are frequently heard on chest examination. Inspiratory squeaks have also been found

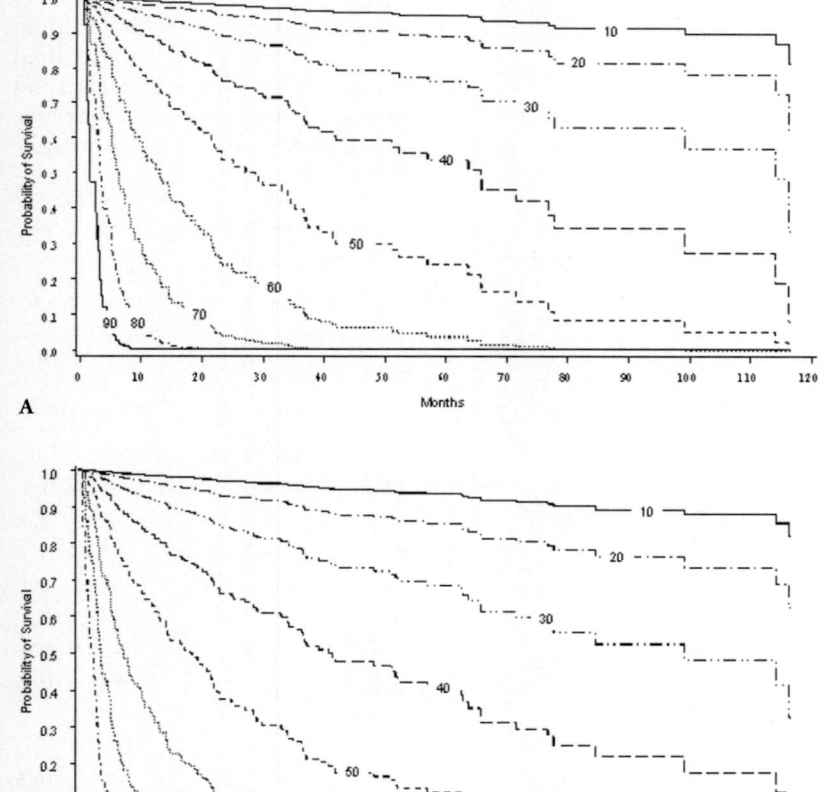

Figure 25–41 Clinical-radiologic-physiological (CRP) scoring system. King and coworkers used a hierarchical multivariable analysis of clinical, radiologic, and extensive physiological variables to develop a model that would allow clinicians to make more precise prognostic estimations about patients with IPF. The model includes the following parameters: age, smoking history, clubbing, extent of profusion of interstitial opacities, and presence or absence of pulmonary hypertension on the chest radiograph; %predicted TLC; and PaO$_2$ at the end of maximal exercise. *A,* Predicted survival curves for patients with a given CRP score, using the complete model. Researchers used data generated to predict survival curves for patients with IPF and a CRP score at 10-point intervals, as shown. For example, the calculated 5-year survival at CRP scores of 20, 40, 60, and 80 were 89, 53, 4, and < 1%, respectively (see Table 25–17). *B,* Predicted survival curves for patients with a given CRP score, using the abbreviated model that excluded the PaO$_2$ during maximal exercise. The investigators used the data generated to predict survival curves for patients with IPF and a CRP score at 10-point intervals as shown. For example, the calculated 5-year survival at CRP scores of 20, 40, 60, and 80 were 85, 41, 1, and < 1%, respectively. Reproduced with permission from King TE Jr et al.[28]

TABLE 25–18   Clinical Characteristics in Published Cases of NSIP

Study, Date, Number of Subjects

Characteristic	Katzenstein and Fiorelli 1994[399] n = 64*	Park and colleagues 1995[507,649] n = 7	Bjoraker and colleagues 1998[398] n = 14	Nagai and colleagues 1998[410] n = 31	Cottin and colleagues 1998[508] n = 12‖	Kim and colleagues 1998[509] n = 23#	Fujita and colleagues 1999[510] n = 24**	Daniil and colleagues 1999[412] n = 15	Travis and colleagues 2000[411] Fibrotic NSIP n = 22	Travis and colleagues 2000[411] Cellular NSIP n = 7	Nicholson and colleagues 2000[413] n = 28	Flaherty and colleagues 2002[274,511]§ Fibrotic NSIP n = 28	Flaherty and colleagues 2002[274,511]§ Cellular NSIP n = 5
Age (years; range)	46 9–78	55 43–61	57 ± 8.3 40–73	58 ± 8.2	53 31–68	55 43–69	60 44–74	43 31–66	50 30–71	39 26–50	53.5 ± 9.5	56 ± 11	50 ± 9
Sex M/F	26/38	1/6	8/6	15/16	6/6	1/22	7/17	7/8	15/7	5/2	28/8	16/12	3/2
Smoking Status (%)													
Current		NR	6	42	17	4	7	0	–	–	64	–	–
Former		NR	50	16	33	–	2	60	68†	60†	4	71%†	40%†
Never		NR	43	42	50	96	15	40	32	40	32	39%	60%
Symptoms													
Duration of (months; range)	8 0.25–60	9 1–36	15 ± 23	2 0–32	44 1–164	8 1–60	3 1–8	18 7–84			11 0–180	2.8 ± 2.9	1.8 ± 2
Dyspnea, %	80	100	100	100‡	100	83	100	100	100‡	100‡	NR	100	100
Cough, %	33	43	85	NR	67	83	67	60			NR	NR	NR
Signs													
Fever, %	22	NR	NR	32	8	NR	33%	NR			NR	NR	NR
Crackles, %	NR	NR	79	81	100	NR	62%	80			NR	NR	NR
Clubbing, %	NR	NR	21	10		NR	83%	40			NR	NR	NR
Outcome	5 of 48 (11%) with follow-up died (mean length of survival 16 months)	6 of 7 improved after 1–15 months of follow-up	Median survival 13.5 years	23 of 31 improved; 2 died (6%)	10 of 12 improved, 100% alive; mean duration of follow 50 months (range 10–159)	NR	20 of 24 improved; 4 died	3 of 12 improved; 4 died (27%)	90% 5-year and 35% 10-year survival; 9 died	No deaths	6 of 21 improved; 17 died (61%)	3 died	No deaths

*Ten cases had associated connective tissue disease; †current vs former smoking status not reported (NR); ‡cough and dyspnea were combined; §it appears that the same cases are reported in both papers; ‖3 had collagen vascular diseases, 3 had organic exposure or acute lung injury; #2 had collagen vascular diseases; **8 had collagen vascular diseases.

in a few subjects. Digital clubbing is less common than in IPF but was reported in 10 to 40% of cases.[398,410,412]

Findings in BAL Fluid

An increase in the percentage of lymphocytes (often > 50% of the cells) is common and strengthens the suspicion of NSIP, in conjunction with other findings including HRCT and pulmonary function test results (see Table 25–6).[2]

Physiological Findings

Many patients show moderate to severe physiological abnormalities. Lung function tests show a restrictive ventilatory defect in most of the patients with NSIP. Gas exchange abnormalities are common. The DL_{CO} is reduced in almost all subjects. Resting hypoxemia is not uniformly present, but more than two-thirds of these patients will develop hypoxemia during exercise (Figure 25–42).[2]

Lung Imaging Studies

Chest Radiograph

The chest radiograph usually shows bilateral hazy opacities in the lower lung zone (Figure 25–43). The CT scan may reveal far more extensive abnormalities than are suggested by the chest radiograph.

HRCT

HRCT scan findings in NSIP include bilateral patchy ground-glass attenuation, bilateral areas of consolidation, irregular lines, and bronchial dilatation. Ground-glass attenuation is the predominant finding in the majority of cases and is the sole abnormality in about one-third of cases (Figure 25–44). It is most commonly bilateral and symmetrical with subpleural predominance, although it appears to often spare the lung immediately adjacent to the pleura. This is often associated with lower lobe volume loss. The ground-glass attenuation in NSIP corresponds to interstitial thickening due to varying amounts of interstitial inflammation and fibrosis as seen on lung biopsy. Irregular linear or reticular opacities are seen in approximately half of all cases and may be associated with traction bronchiectasis. In general, honeycombing and marked consolidation are relatively infrequent.[274] The irregular linear opacities and bronchial dilatation present in areas of ground-glass attenuation suggest histologic interstitial fibrosis and microscopic honeycombing. Areas of consolidation on HRCT scan likely correspond to histologic areas of OP, with or without microscopic honeycombing.[2] Therefore, these findings should suggest another diagnosis, specifically hypersensitivity pneumonitis, and OP.

Fibrosing NSIP may be associated with HRCT scan evidence of honeycombing and cannot be distinguished from UIP without a surgical lung biopsy. Of the limited number of patients with NSIP who have had follow-up CT examinations after treatment, the abnormalities of NSIP have generally improved in the majority. Depending on the stage of the disease, the CT differential diagnosis of NSIP most often includes DIP, UIP, hypersensitivity pneumonitis, and OP.[2]

Histopathologic Findings

A surgical lung biopsy is required to confirm the diagnosis. NSIP is characterized by varying degrees of inflammation and fibrosis, with some forms being primarily inflammatory (cellular NSIP) and the most prevalent cases being primarily fibrotic (fibrotic NSIP) (see Chapter 2, Figures 2–14, 2–15, 2–16).[2,11] The changes are temporally uniform (ie, they lack fibroblastic foci and honeycombing), but the process may be patchy, with intervening areas of unaffected lung (Figure 25–45). The process is frequently accentuated in the peribronchiolar interstitium, and the density of the inflammatory infiltrate is considerably greater than that occurring in other idiopathic interstitial pneumonias, in particular, UIP.

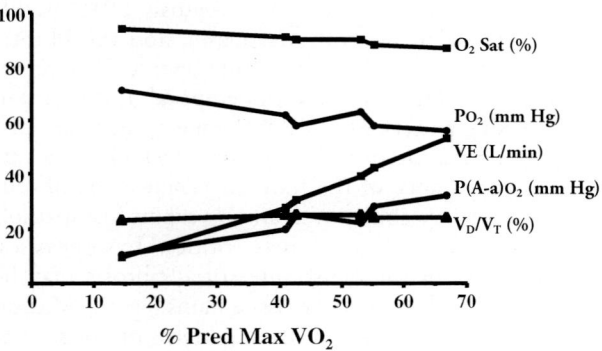

Figure 25–42 Exercise testing in nonspecific interstitial pneumonia (NSIP). A 28-year-old woman presented for evaluation of dyspnea on walking > 1 mile or up 2–4 flights of stairs. Chest radiograph revealed a reduction in lung volume without convincing evidence of other abnormality. Her physiological studies at presentation revealed FVC, 2.18 L (59% of predicted); FEV_1, 1.98 L (60% of predicted); FEV_1:FVC, 91%; TLC, 3.3 L (68% of predicted); DL_{CO}:V_A, (93% of predicted). Her resting room air arterial blood gases (elevation 5,000 feet) revealed PO_2, 78; PCO_2, 34; pH 7.43; oxygen saturation, 94%; $P(A-a)O_2$, 3.8. The patient performed an exercise test on a cycle ergometer. The work rate was increased 10 W/minute to her symptom-limited maximum. Blood was sampled serially from an indwelling arterial catheter. Her resting and exercise echocardiograms were normal. The patient achieved 94 W (65% of predicted). This study confirmed restrictive lung disease as the major pathophysiological disorder. The PO_2 and SaO_2 (measured by pulse oximetry) decreased, $P(A-a)O_2$ increased, and minute ventilation (V_E) increased systematically with work rate (shown as %predicted maximal VO_2). The dead space to tidal volume (V_T) ratio remained unchanged. The study was stopped because of shortness of breath and leg fatigue.

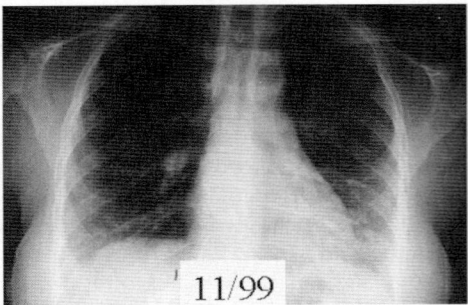
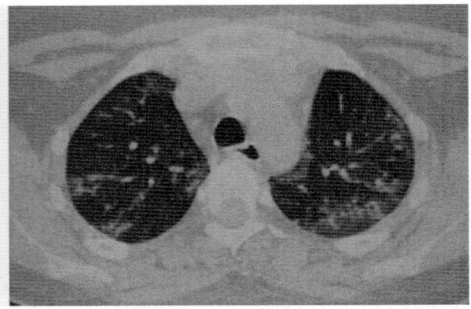

Figure 25–43   NSIP in a 25-year-old previously healthy woman. Left: chest radiograph with hazy opacities over both lower lung zones, greater on left than on the right, with reduced lung volumes. There appear to be air bronchograms in the left lower lobe. Right: CT scan showed diffuse air space opacities in all lung zones, more prominent in the mid to lower lung zones. There is no evidence of honeycombing. CT scan was more abnormal than suggested by the chest radiograph and fit with the patient's severe physiological impairment.

The fibrotic cases of NSIP have dense interstitial fibrosis with a diffuse or patchy pattern and can be difficult to distinguish reliably from UIP. Type II cell hyperplasia often accompanies the interstitial inflammation and may be quite prominent. Rarely, fibroblastic foci may be seen, but they are far less frequent than in UIP. Few foci of microscopic honeycomb fibrosis may be present.

The fibrosing-pattern NSIP presents more difficulty for pathologists. The differential diagnosis includes the UIP pattern and fibrotic forms of other types of interstitial pneumonitis, including chronic hypersensitivity pneumonitis, Langerhans cell histiocytosis, DIP, OP, diffuse alveolar damage (fibrotic phase), and the fibrotic stage of sarcoidosis.[2] It remains unknown if NSIP represents an early form of UIP. The temporal uniformity in the fibrosing pattern of NSIP is the most important distinguishing feature from UIP patterns, which has a variegated appearance of the fibrosis.[2] There is significant interobserver variability even among expert histopathologists in the recognition of these entities.[2] In some cases, the character of the dense interstitial fibrosis may be highlighted with connective tissue stains (eg, the Masson trichrome or Movat stain).[2] Both patterns can be seen in multiple biopsies from the same patient, even in multiple biopsies from the same lobe.[511] Importantly, when the UIP pattern and the NSIP pattern are found in one or more of the other lobes in the same patient, the clinical behavior is similar to that of IPF (Figure 25–46).[511] For

this reason cases with UIP in any lobe should be called UIP pattern and managed as one would manage IPF.[2]

The histologic differential diagnosis for cases of NSIP with a cellular pattern includes the patterns of infections, hypersensitivity pneumonitis, OP, LIP, resolving diffuse alveolar damage, eosinophilic pneumonia, and fibrosing NSIP.[2] Special stains for fungi, *P. carinii*, and acid-fast bacilli are useful to help exclude infections. The presence of even a rare, difficult-to-find, ill-formed granuloma (especially if near an airway) should suggest the diagnosis of hypersensitivity pneumonitis (also, infection, collagen vascular disease, or drug-induced pneumonitis need to be considered).

Management and Outcome

Unlike patients with IPF, the majority of patients with NSIP have a good prognosis, with most showing improvement and some patients experiencing almost complete recovery after treatment with corticosteroids. The corticosteroid treatment regimen is similar to that described in this chapter for IPF/UIP. However, because of the increased chance that these patients will respond to aggressive therapy, the treatment course is much longer. The prognosis appears to depend on the extent of fibrosis at the time of diagnosis. Relapse may occur. A minority of patients progress and die, usually 5 to 10 years after diagnosis.

Figure 25–44 NSIP. Left: HRCT through the lower lung shows bilateral ground-glass abnormality, with associated reticular abnormality. Histology showed a combination of inflammation and mild fibrosis (fibrotic NSIP). Right: HRCT through the lower lung shows marked clearing of the bilateral ground-glass abnormality.

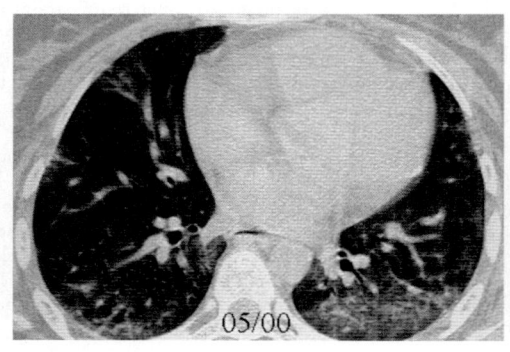
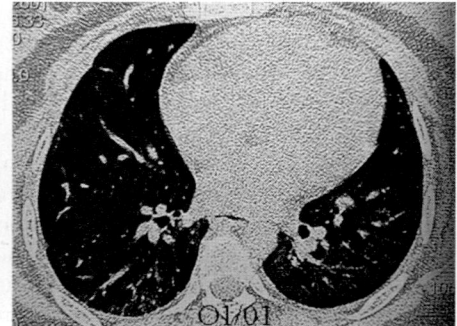

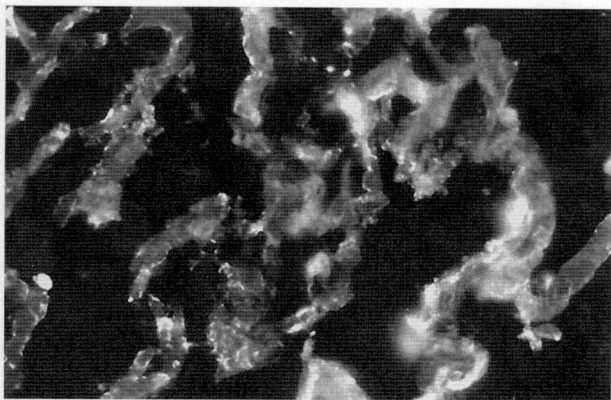

Figure 22–45 Immunofluorescence studies of lung tissue. A patient with a cellular form of NSIP, demonstrating granular deposition of IgG along alveolar walls and capillaries. Several interstitial and intra-alveolar mononuclear cells show positive.

DESQUAMATIVE INTERSTITIAL PNEUMONIA

The term desquamative interstitial pneumonia describes both an idiopathic clinicopathologic entity and a histologic pattern.[181] Previously, under the clinical concept of IPF, the cellular DIP was considered the early stage of the fibrotic UIP. Today, idiopathic DIP and UIP are viewed as separate clinicopathologic entities.[2] The radiographic and histologic patterns of UIP are required for the diagnosis of IPF.[2,230]

The histologic criteria for diagnosis of DIP have been narrowed following the description of the histologic pattern of RB-ILD and refinement of the criteria for UIP (see Table 25–2).[11,522] In addition, the ATS/ERS consensus panel, despite concern that doing so presented several problems, retained the term desquamative interstitial pneumonia in the new classification (see Table 25–1).[2] The ATS/ERS consensus panel seriously considered changing this term to "alveolar macrophage pneumonia," which is a more accurately descriptive term.[2] They also considered using the term RB-ILD for all of these cases because these two processes appear to represent the ends of a spectrum,

and it is more anatomically accurate and conveys important pathogenetic implications compared to the older term, desquamative interstitial pneumonia.[39,46,47,523] The clinicopathologic entity of DIP is very rare; RB-ILD and UIP are more common (see Table 25–4).[17,24]

This chapter will discuss these entities separately, but I believe they are most likely one disease process and that the term desquamative interstitial pneumonia will eventually be dropped. It should be emphasized from the outset that the histologic differential diagnosis of DIP and RB-ILD is very broad because intra-alveolar macrophage accumulation or a focal nonspecific "DIP-like" reaction is an expected finding in all cigarette smokers.[2] Consequently, because many patients with ILDs are smokers, these patterns often overlie the histologic patterns of these processes. For example, UIP, NSIP, pulmonary Langerhans cell histiocytosis, chronic hemorrhage or hemosiderosis, and veno-occlusive disease. A DIP-like reaction can occur in nonsmokers as a nonspecific reaction adjacent to a variety of pathologic lesions: interstitial lung disease associated with drug reactions (eg, amiodarone), chronic alveolar hemorrhage, pneumoconioses (eg, talcosis, hard metal disease, asbestosis), obstructive pneumonias, exogenous lipoid pneumonia, histiocyte-rich infections (eg, *Mycobacterium avium intracellulare*, human immunodeficiency virus).[34,36,524–530] Chronic eosinophilic pneumonia without eosinophils may resemble DIP (usually occurs when the patient has been treated with corticosteroids prior to the biopsy).

Etiology and Epidemiology

The etiology of idiopathic DIP and RB-ILD remains unknown. However, both are seen almost exclusively in cigarette smokers or persons exposed to passive cigarette smoke. Desquamative interstitial pneumonia was found in only 8% of cases in a recent review from the Mayo Clinic and was seen in less than 3% of the cases entered into the National Jewish Medical and Research Center/University of Colorado specialized center for research

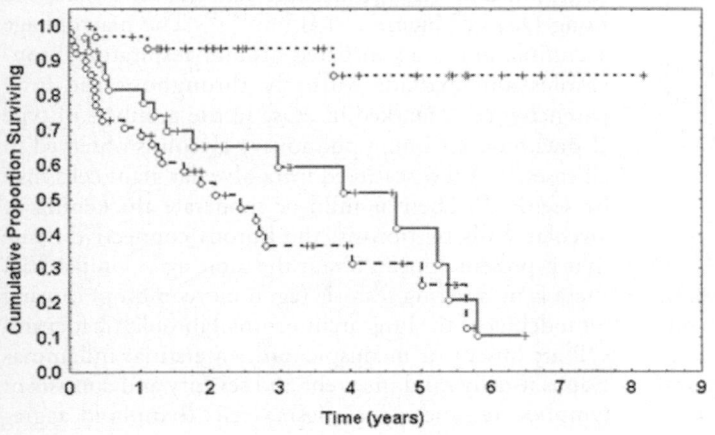

Figure 25–46 Kaplan-Meier survival curves for patients grouped by histologic classification. Marked differences in survival were noted among the different histologic groups, ie, patients with: UIP pattern in all lobes (broken line: concordant UIP; n = 51); UIP pattern in at least one lobe but a non-UIP pattern in at least one lobe, ie, intrapatient lobar variability (solid line: discordant UIP; n = 28); and NSIP in all lobes (dotted line: concordant NSIP; n = 30; p < .0003). + = last last follow-up visit; o = death). Patients with NSIP had better survival rates than did either UIP group. Reproduced with permission from Flaherty et al.[511]

(SCOR) in ILD program in Denver, CO.[398,531] Most patients are in the fourth to fifth decade of life. It is more common in men, at a ratio of 2:1. There does not appear to be any racial predilection, although the majority of reported cases have been in Whites.[532] It is rare that cases of DIP are reported in children.[529,533–537] These cases probably represent a disorder other than DIP in adults, and some may have been confused with other entities such as surfactant deficiency or alveolar proteinosis, which can show prominent alveolar macrophage accumulation.[538]

Rare cases of DIP have been reported in persons not exposed to cigarette smoke, especially in children and in cases of familial pulmonary fibrosis (see Chapter 6, "Pediatric Interstitial Lung Disease" Figure 6–4).[32,113,539] Mutations in the surfactant protein C gene are associated with familial DIP.[32]

Clinical Findings

Although the disease is occasionally recognized in an asymptomatic individual, most patients present with a subacute (weeks to months) illness that is characterized by dyspnea and cough.[540] Chest pain and weight loss can be present.[541] Pleural complications and spontaneous pneumothorax are unusual manifestations.[33,541] Occasionally, patients may present in respiratory failure. The chest examination may be normal but most often it reveals crackles, mostly at the bases. Digital clubbing is common (up to 42% of reported cases) and may resolve with treatment.[540] Cyanosis is uncommon.[541] Laboratory results are usually unremarkable.

Findings in BAL Fluid

BAL fluid from these patients shows a marked increase in the numbers of all cell types: neutrophils, eosinophils, lymphocytes, and, in particular, alveolar macrophages. The alveolar macrophages have granules of "smoker's pigment," consisting of intracellular yellow, golden, brown, or black smoke particulates.

Physiological Findings

Lung function testing in DIP shows a restrictive pattern with reduced DL_{CO} and hypoxemia on blood gas analysis.

Chest Imaging Findings

Chest Radiograph

The chest radiograph may be normal in up to 20% of cases.[33,137,181,542,543] The chest radiograph often shows diffuse ground-glass opacity in the middle and lower lung zones (see Chapter 1, "Approach to the Evaluation and Diagnosis of Interstitial Lung Disease" Figures 1–9,

1–10). A granular or nodular texture to ground-glass opacification has been reported.[544] The opacities are often triangular, radiating from the hilus to the lung base.[33,545]

HRCT

Ground-glass opacification is present on CT scan in all cases of DIP (see Chapter 4, "Imaging of Diffuse Parenchymal Lung Diseases" Figure 4–24).[385,546] In the majority of cases, there is a peripheral (59% of cases) and lower zone distribution (73%). The process can be patchy (23% of cases) or diffuse and uniform (18%). The ground-glass attenuation, which is the hallmark of this disease, is presumed to be due to a combination of diffuse intra-alveolar cells and diffuse mild septal fibrosis. Irregular linear opacities and reticular pattern are frequent (59%) but limited in extent and usually confined to the lung bases. Mild peripheral lower lung zone honeycombing is found in less than one-third of cases. The irregular linear opacities and honeycombing are presumed to correlate with evidence of lung fibrosis.

Patients who quit smoking or receive treatment often show a partial or nearly complete resolution of areas of ground-glass opacification.[385,547] Progression of ground-glass opacification to a reticular pattern occurs infrequently (< 20% of cases).[385,547]

Conditions that may be indistinguishable from DIP and RB-ILD include acute or subacute hypersensitivity pneumonitis, sarcoidosis, and infections such as *P. carinii* pneumonia.[2]

Histologic Findings

Grossly, the lung may appear normal, or the involved lung is multinodular, airless, and shows confluent consolidation.[33,181] Involved areas vary from red-gray to pasty yellow. The histologic hallmark of DIP is diffuse marked intra-alveolar macrophage accumulation of smoker's macrophages of a golden brown pigment with frequent tiny black particles; these cells may show fine granular positivity with iron stains (see Chapter 2, "Anatomic Distribution and Histopathologic Patterns of Interstitial Lung Disease" Figure 2–13).[2,137,181,523] The macrophage accumulation is accentuated around respiratory bronchioles and extends diffusely throughout the lung parenchyma. A marked increase in the numbers of type II pneumocytes lining pulmonary alveoli is observed in all cases.[539] A few scattered intra-alveolar giant cells may be seen.[38,181] There is mild or moderate thickening of alveolar walls by fibrosis; the fibrous connective tissue that is present appears about the same age.[2] Unlike UIP, there is no scarring fibrosis (eg, honeycombing) causing remodeling of the lung architecture. Fibroblastic foci and OP are absent or inconspicuous. Interstitial inflammation is usually mild in extent and severity and consists of lymphocytes and a few plasma cells (lymphoid aggregates).[2] Deposits of IgG and the third component of complement have been found in distal air spaces and on the surfaces of the accumulated macrophages.[539]

Management and Outcome

Smoking cessation is the primary treatment for DIP, often leading to spontaneous regression of the disease (Figure 25–47).[548] In those with moderate to severe symptoms and gas exchange abnormalities, corticosteroid therapy may be indicated.[547] A greater percentage of patients with DIP respond to steroid therapy than do patients with UIP. Recurrences may occur, especially if the patient starts smoking cigarettes or is exposed to passive smoke (Figure 25–48)

The prognosis of DIP is much better than that for other idiopathic interstitial pneumonias, especially UIP. In the classic study by Carrington and coworkers, the 5- and 10-year survivals were 95.2 and 69.6% for DIP in contrast to 65.4 and 28.5% for UIP.[137] However, in this study, honeycombing was present in 12.5% of the cases of DIP. In the more recent study by Travis and colleagues in which cases with honeycombing were excluded, the 5- and 10-year survival was 100%.[412] Nevertheless, DIP is known to progress, and a small number of patients may do poorly. Fulminant DIP, leading to death, is rare.[549] Lung transplantation has been performed successfully in patients with end-stage lung from DIP. Disease recurrence in the transplanted lung has been reported.[297,298,550]

RESPIRATORY BRONCHIOLITIS–INTERSTITIAL LUNG DISEASE

Respiratory bronchiolitis has been demonstrated in patients and in asymptomatic, otherwise healthy persons exposed to cigarette smoke.[17,24,551,552] The inflammation and fibrosis lead to distortion and narrowing of small airways. Because respiratory bronchiolitis was initially found at autopsy in young cigarette smokers without known disease, the lesions were considered to be clinically insignificant. Later, it was hypothesized that the lesions in the respiratory bronchioles could explain the mild abnormalities in lung function seen in cigarette smokers, so-called "small airway disease" (ie, elevated airflow resistance, airway hyperresponsiveness, and subsequent airflow limitation). More recently, RB-ILD has been recognized as a distinct clinical syndrome found in current or previous cigarette smokers.[2,522,540,543–556] RB-ILD and DIP appear to be linked, representing the ends of a spectrum of smoking-related processes (see "Desquamative Interstitial Pneumonia" above). Desquamative interstitial pneumonia is considered to be a more extensive form of RB-ILD in which the pigmented macrophages fill alveolar spaces diffusely throughout larger areas of the lung.[2] RB-ILD may be confused with eosinophilic granuloma of the lung (pulmonary histiocytosis X).

Etiology and Epidemiology

The incidence and prevalence of RB-ILD is unknown. In a recent study of 156 consecutive surgical lung biopsy and resection specimens, Fraig and colleagues found respiratory bronchiolitis in 70%; all but 2 had a history of smoking (although both of these cases had environmental exposure to passive smoke).[17] Among these 109 cases, peribronchiolar fibrosis was identified in 9 cases and alveolar septal fibrosis in 47 cases. However, based on clinical findings, only one case each of RB-ILD and DIP was identified.[17] Respiratory bronchiolitis can be found in the lungs of ex-smokers many

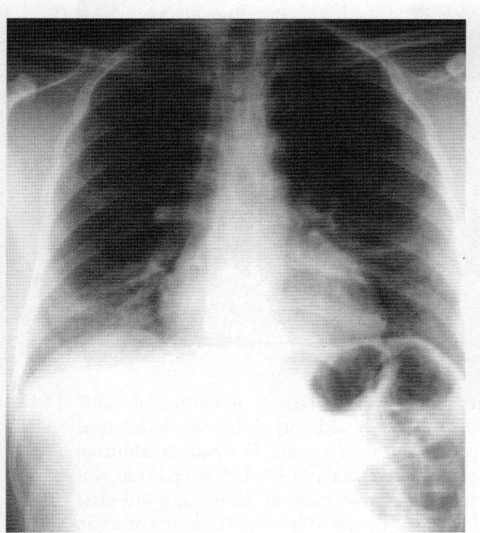
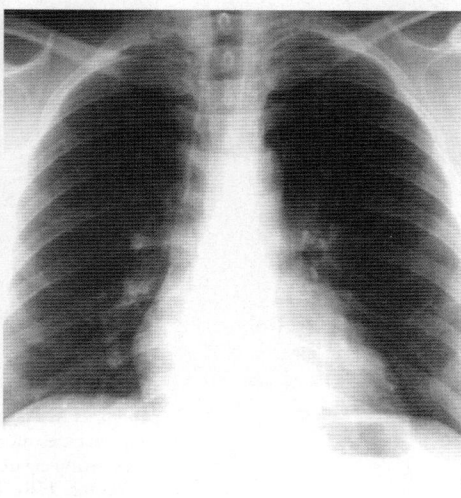

Figure 25–47 Desquamative interstitial pneumonia confirmed by surgical lung biopsy. Chest radiograph shows bilateral hazy opacities more prominent on the right (*A*). Chest radiograph 5 months later shows marked clearing following smoking cessation (*B*). The patient was asymptomatic and had normal lung function.

A   B

years after they stopped smoking, although the extent and severity is relatively worse in current smokers compared with ex-smokers.[17,553] Moon and colleagues found that 13 of 168 retrospectively reviewed patients from whom biopsy specimens were taken for suspected diffuse lung disease were identified with a histopathologic pattern of RB-ILD.[24] Histopathologically, four cases of RB-ILD overlapped with the pattern of DIP, and nine also had microscopic evidence of centrilobular emphysema.[24] In other studies examining surgical lung biopsies from patients with idiopathic interstitial pneumonias, RB-ILD and DIP were found in up to 17% of the cases (see Table 25–10).

Clinical Findings

RB-ILD is more common in men; the male to female ratio is 1.6:1.[23,540] However, recent data show an equal number of men and women affected.[557] Most are current or former smokers in the fourth or fifth decade of life, but it can occur at any age. The average exposure is over 30 pack-years of cigarette smoking. Patients commonly present with dyspnea (70%) and cough (58%). Coarse rales are often heard (33%) and occur throughout inspiration; sometimes they continue into expiration. Finger clubbing has been reported rarely.[23,24,540,556] Routine laboratory studies usually yield normal results.

Findings in BAL Fluid

BAL fluid findings are similar to those discussed for DIP. Interestingly, smoker's macrophages may persist in BAL fluid for three or more years after smoking cessation.[558–560] Similarly, the histologic lesion of respiratory bronchiolitis may also take three or more years to resolve.[17] Importantly, an absence of smoker's macrophages in BAL fluid should alert the clinician to another possible diagnosis.

Physiological Findings

Pulmonary function tests may be normal, and obstructive or restrictive patterns may be found.[557] An isolated increase in residual volume may also be noted.[522,556] A normal or slightly reduced DL_{CO} is frequently present, and hypoxemia may be present at rest or with exercise.

Chest Imaging Findings

Chest Radiograph

The chest radiograph is normal in up to 28% of patients (Figure 25–49).[540,557] Bronchial wall thickening in central bronchi (76% of cases) or peripheral bronchi (67%) is the most common abnormality.[557] Park and colleagues showed that ground-glass opacity is seen in 57% of subjects, without zonal predominance.[557] Areas of emphysema are present in 48% of the patients, with upper lung predominance in 38%.[557] Decreased lung volumes were noted in 3 of 21 patients.[557] Prominence of the peribronchovascular interstitium, small regular and irregular opacities, and small peripheral ring shadows are other uncommon features of respiratory bronchiolitis.[561] Diffuse, fine reticular or nodular interstitial opacities have been described on the chest radiograph, usually with normal lung volumes, in some studies.[522,540,556]

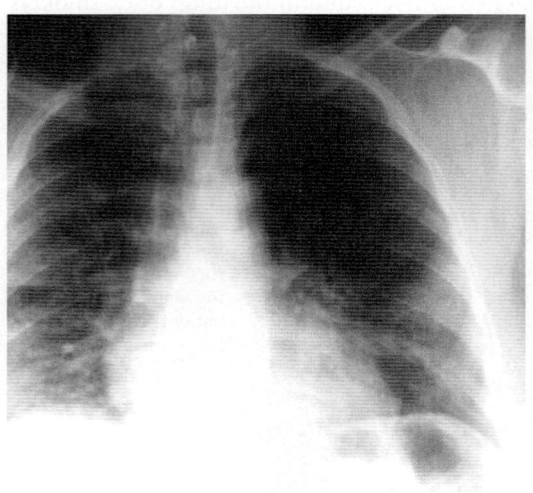

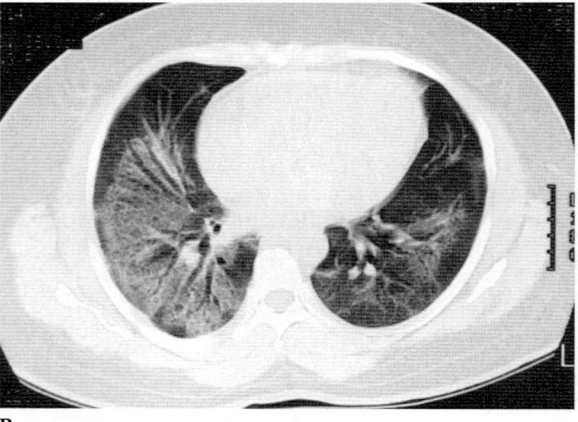

B

A

Figure 25–48 Desquamative interstitial pneumonia, same patient as in Figure 25–47. Chest radiograph (*A*) shows bilateral hazy opacities more prominent on the right. The patient admitted to restarting cigarette smoking several months before recurrence of symptoms. HRCT scan (*B*) shows marked diffuse ground-glass abnormalities. A follow-up CT scan following smoking cessation showed marked clearing of the ground-glass abnormalities

HRCT

Park and coworkers reported the most common finding on HRCT scan was bronchial wall thickening (19 of 21 patients), seen in the central bronchi in 19 patients (90%) and in the peripheral bronchi in 18 patients (86%). Other important features on HRCT included centrilobular nodules, ground-glass opacity and emphysema with air trapping (Figure 25–49).

Centrilobular nodules were seen without a zonal predominance in 71% of patients, in the upper lung zone in 67%, in the middle lung zone in 63%, and in the lower lung zone in 48% of patients. The nodules were more profuse in the upper lung zones in 53% of the patients. There was an even distribution of nodules in 27% of patients, more nodules in the middle lung in 13%, and more in the lower lung in 5%.[557]

Areas of ground-glass opacity were present in 67% of the patients without a zonal predominance. The areas of ground-glass opacity involved the lung zone diffusely in 50% of patients and were patchy in 50%.[557]

Centrilobular emphysema, detected in 12 of 21 patients (57%), was observed in the upper lung zones in all patients, with additional involvement of the middle and lower lung zones in 4 patients (33%).

Patchy areas of hypoattenuation were found in the lower lung zone (without central or subpleural predominance) in 38% of the patients.[557] These geographic areas of decreased attenuation were usually associated with decreased size of pulmonary blood vessels, suggesting that the decreased attenuation was due to air trapping.[557]

Reticular and septal lines were each noted in seven patients (33%) without zonal predominance. A mild degree of lower lung zone honeycombing was seen in one patient.[557]

Histopathologic Findings

Respiratory bronchiolitis is a highly sensitive and relatively specific morphologic marker of cigarette smoking; it is present in virtually all current smokers.[17,24,562] An inflammatory process involving the membranous and respiratory bronchioles is the characteristic histopathologic feature of RB-ILD. Tan-brown pigmented macrophages within respiratory bronchioles, neighboring alveolar ducts, and alveoli dominate the pathologic finding (a DIP-like reaction) (Figure 25–50). These macrophages stain strongly with diastase-predigested periodic acid-Schiff.[540] The bronchiole may be ectatic with mucus stasis; the walls are mildly thickened. There is frequently evidence of extension of the bronchiolar metaplastic epithelium into the immediately surrounding alveoli. Usually, most of the interstitium is normal; alternatively, it may demonstrate mild hyperinflation. The findings are sometimes so subtle as to be missed during routine evaluation. On occasion, examination of multiple-step sections may be required. Many cases of respiratory bronchiolitis reported in the last few years were actually misclassified as DIP in earlier studies. The histologic differential diagnosis is the same as that noted above for DIP.

CT—Pathologic Correlations. The key findings on CT scan have been correlated with the pathologic findings in a small number of cases of respiratory bronchiolitis.[23,558,564–566] Areas of ground-glass attenuation

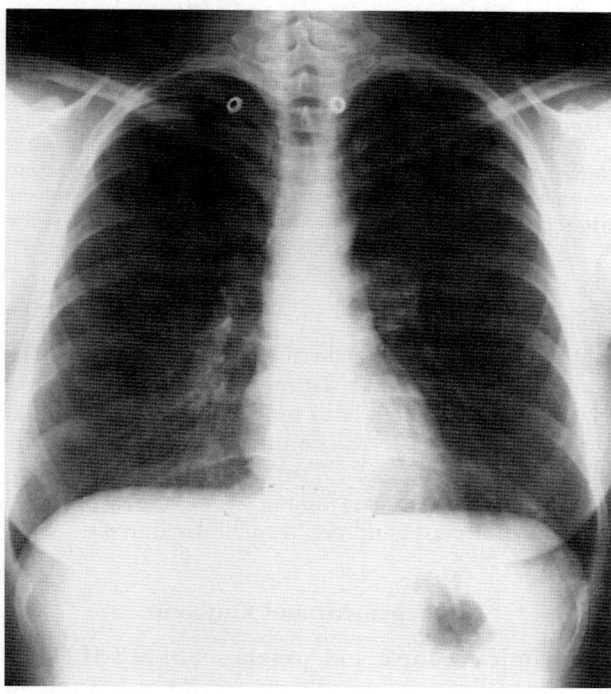

A

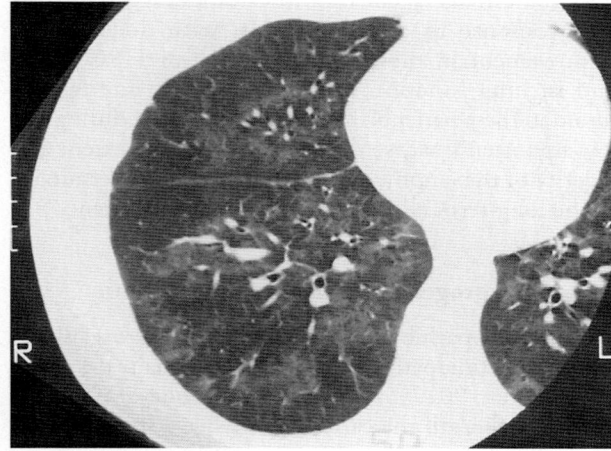

B

Figure 25–49 Respiratory bronchiolitis-associated ILD (RB-ILD). *A,* Posteroanterior chest radiograph from a woman with a heavy smoking history and complaints of progressive shortness of breath with exertion. This film was considered normal. *B,* HRCT scan from the same patient shows extensive ground-glass opacities. The diagnosis was confirmed by thoracoscopic lung biopsy. Symptoms improved following smoking cessation.

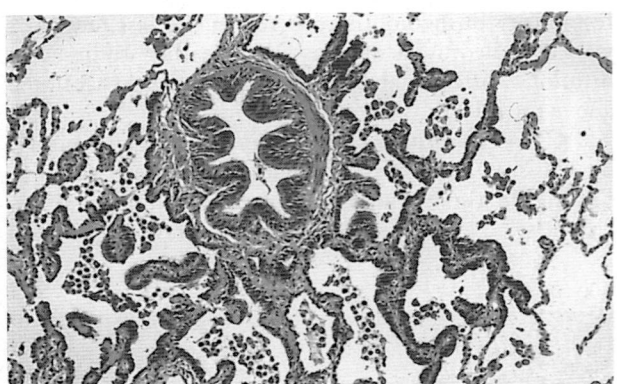

Figure 25–50   RB-ILD. Photomicrograph shows inflammatory process involving the respiratory bronchioles. Bronchiole wall is thickened, and bronchiolar metaplastic epithelium extends into immediately surrounding alveoli. Macrophages are present within the peribronchiolar alveolar spaces (diffuse interstitial pneumonia-like reaction). Hematoxylin-eosin stain was used.

appear related to three main histologic features: (1) accumulation of pigmented macrophages and mucus in alveolar spaces, associated with mild interstitial inflammation or fibrosis; (2) thickening of alveolar walls by inflammatory cells; and (3) presence of organizing alveolitis. Parenchymal micronodules appear to correspond to bronchiolectases and peribronchiolar fibrosis.

Management and Outcome

The clinical course and prognosis of RB-ILD are unknown. Because smoking appears to play a role in pathogenesis, smoking cessation is considered to be important in management. Most studies suggest a favorable response to corticosteroids, with documented improvement in the chest radiograph or HRCT scan and in lung function.[557] Emphysema is one feature found in these patients that does not decrease during follow-up; often it worsens. Consequently, the extent and severity of the emphysema may be a major determinant in the long-term clinical outcome of these patients.[557]

Cryptogenic Organizing Pneumonia

COP, or idiopathic bronchiolitis obliterans organizing pneumonia (idiopathic BOOP), was originally described by Lange in 1901.[566] However, recognition of COP did not increase until the early 1980s when several investigators highlighted the characteristic clinical course and suggested that COP is a distinct entity with features of a community-acquired pneumonia, rather than a primary airway disorder.[567–569] COP is included in the classification of the idiopathic interstitial pneumonias because of its idiopathic nature and its tendency, on occasion, to be confused with other forms of idiopathic interstitial pneumonia.[2]

Etiology and Epidemiology

The cause of COP is not known. The lesion of OP can be found in many settings (Table 25–19).[570–573] The true incidence and prevalence of COP are unknown. A prevalence of 6 to 7 cases per 100,000 admissions has been suggested.[574]

Clinical Findings

Disease onset is usually in the fifth or sixth decade, with a mean age of 58 years; men and women are affected equally (Table 25–20).[572] The duration of symptoms prior to diagnosis is typically less than 2 months; few have symptoms for more than 6 months prior to diagnosis (Figure 25–51). Cigarette smoking is not a precipitating factor, because approximately 50% of subjects are never smokers, 25% are ex-smokers, and only 25% are current smokers.[572,575] Lazor and coworkers suggest an actual putative protective effect of smoking on the development of COP.[576]

The clinical presentation often mimics that of community-acquired pneumonia. A persistent and usually nonproductive cough is the most common presenting symptom (72% of subjects). Frequently, patients experience dyspnea with exertion (66%). Disease onset is usually described as a flulike illness with fever (51%), malaise (48%), fatigue, and cough. Weight loss of more than 10 pounds is a common complaint (57%). Hemoptysis is a very rare presenting manifestation of COP.[577]

Physical examination reveals inspiratory crackles (74%). Wheezing is rare and is usually present in conjunction with crackles. Clubbing is rare (< 5%). Twenty-eight percent of patients in one series had normal lung examinations.[569]

Laboratory Findings

Routine laboratory studies are nonspecific. A leukocytosis is seen in approximately half of patients. The initial erythrocyte sedimentation rate is elevated, frequently reaching or exceeding 100 mm per hour; a positive C-reactive protein is observed in 70 to 80% of patients.[578,579] Autoantibodies are usually negative or only slightly positive.

Findings in BAL Fluid

Studies of BAL fluid have been reported in only a few subjects with COP (see Table 25–6). The percentage of instilled fluid recovered from patients with COP is lower than that from healthy volunteers. However, the total number of cells recovered is greater in patients with COP. The proportion of macrophages is lower in COP, whereas the proportion of lymphocytes, neutrophils, and eosinophils is higher.[572,580,581] Patients with COP tend to have higher lymphocyte counts than those similar to those in hypersensitivity pneumonitis. However, in hypersensitivity pneumonitis, CD25 expression is normal, and CD57⁺ cells are increased. This mixed

TABLE 25–19   Conditions Associated with BOOP Histopathology

Idiopathic BOOP (cryptogenic organizing pneumonitis)

Organizing diffuse alveolar damage/ adult respiratory distress syndrome (ARDS)[4]

Hypersensitivity pneumonitis[3]

Chronic eosinophilic pneumonia[3]

Collagen vascular diseases[3,298-301]
 Ankylosing spondylitis
 Behçet disease
 Essential mixed cryoglobulinemia
 Polyarteritis nodosa
 Polymyositis/dermatomyositis
 Rheumatoid arthritis
 Scleroderma
 Sjögren's syndrome
 Systemic lupus erythematosus

Infection[3]

Viral
 HIV infection[302,303]
 Adenovirus
 Influenza[304]

Bacterial
 Nocardia asteroides
 Mycoplasma pneumoniae[293,305,306]
 Legionella pneumophila[294]
 Chlamydial infection[307]

Protozoa
 Plasmodium vivax[308]
 Pneumocystis carinii pneumonia[309]

Fungal
 Aspergillus[310]

Drug-induced reactions (see Table 25–12)

Inhalation injury
 Sulfur dioxide

Lung irradiation[311]
 Breast cancer

Chronic thyroiditis[312]

Ulcerative colitis[313]

Aspiration of gastric contents[312]

Neoplasms/myeloproliferative disorders

Bone marrow transplantation

Lung transplantation/rejection

Wegener's granulomatosis[220]

Distal to bronchial obstruction, "obstructive pneumonitis"[3]

Chronic heart or renal failure

Common variable immunodeficiency syndrome[314]

Essential mixed cryoglobulinemia[315]

TABLE 25–20   Clinical Manifestations of Cryptogenic Organizing Pneumonitis*

Age of onset (n = 157)	58 (range 21 to 80) yrs	
Sex	54% men, 46% women	
Smoking history	27 smokers	
	28 exsmokers	
	48 nonsmokers	
	54 smoking history unknown	
Duration of symptoms	72% less than 2 mos	
	28% greater than 3 mos	
Symptoms	Cough	72%
	Dyspnea	66%
	Fever	51%
	Malaise	48%
	Flu-like illness	40%
	Weight loss	57%
Physical findings	Rales	74%
	Wheezes	"rare"
	Clubbing	Absent

*Data identification and data extraction. Eight major published reports that included five or more subjects with the diagnosis confirmed by lung biopsy from centers in North America, Europe, and Japan were reviewed.[554,569,574,588,589,604,611,656] In addition, patients with cryptogenic organizing pneumonitis (COP) studied at our institution were included in the patient population.[586] These works were critically reviewed for information on the clinical, physiologic, radiographic, and pathologic findings of COP. Each variable was analyzed to provide an accurate composite description of COP.

with IPF.[582] Other BAL fluid abnormalities in COP include the presence of foamy macrophages and, occasionally, mast cells and plasma cells; a decreased ratio of CD4 to CD8 cells; normal percentage of CD57⁺ cells; and increased activated T cells, as reflected in human HLA-DR expression CD3⁺HLA-DR⁺ cells (ie, activated T cells); CD8⁺HLA-DR⁺ cells (ie, activated suppressor/cytotoxic T cells); CD8⁺CD57⁺ cells and CD8⁺CD11b⁻ cells (ie, cytotoxic T cell); and occasionally, interleukin-2 receptor (CD25) expression.[583,584,] The findings are

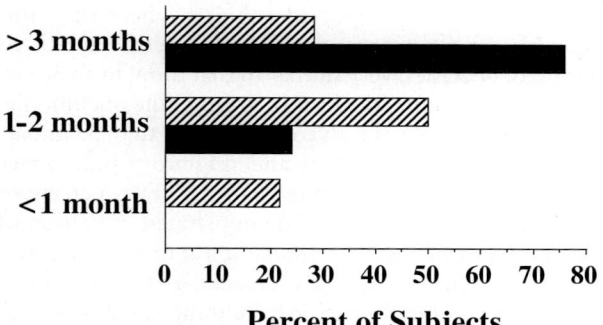

Figure 25–51   Adapted from King TE Jr and Mortenson RL.[555] Cryptogenic organizing pneumonitis (COP): duration of illness prior to diagnosis. A duration of illness < 3 months was found in 72% of patients with COP (*n* = 92). In contrast, 76% of patients with IPF (*n* = 25) had a duration of symptoms prior to diagnosis of > 3 months. Solid bars represent patients with COP; hatched bars are patients with IPF.

pattern of increased cellularity is thought to be characteristic of COP, especially when associated with multiple alveolar opacities on the chest radiograph.[578]

Matrix metalloproteinases (MMPs) and a tissue inhibitor of metalloproteinases (TIMP) are known to regulate remodeling of the extracellular matrix and thus to be important in the process of lung fibrosis. BAL fluid results from patients with COP were found to be consistent with an overproduction of MMP-9 and TIMP-1 and an imbalance between MMP-9 and TIMP-1 when compared with normal volunteers and patients with UIP. These may play a role in the pathogenesis of the disease.[585]

Physiological Findings

Pulmonary function is usually impaired; a restrictive defect is the most common finding (Figure 25–52).[586] An obstructive defect (FEV_1:FVC% < 70%) is found uncommonly (< 21%) and is seen mostly in patients who are current or former smokers. Lung function is occasionally normal. The pressure–volume curve is shifted downward and to the right, consistent with noncompliant lungs. The maximal transpulmonary pressure and the coefficient of elastic recoil (maximal transpulmonary pressure divided by total lung capacity) are increased. Gas exchange abnormalities are extremely common. The DL_{CO} is reduced in the majority of patients (72%). Widening of the resting $P(A-a)O_2$ gradient (> 20 mm Hg) and exercise-related hypoxemia are common abnormalities (83%).

Chest Imaging Studies

Chest Radiograph

The radiographic manifestations of classic COP are quite distinctive and have been well described: bilateral, diffuse alveolar opacities in the presence of normal lung volume (Figure 25–53).[554,568,569,573,576,578,587–594] This pattern was present in 79% of reported subjects where the radiographic appearance was detailed.[575] A peripheral distribution of opacities, very similar to that thought to be virtually pathognomic for chronic eosinophilic pneumonia, is also seen. Rarely, the alveolar opacities may be unilateral. In addition, recurrent and migratory pulmonary opacities are common (Figure 25–54).[595] Fifty percent of Japanese patients with COP demonstrated migration of radiographic shadows.[596] Irregular linear or nodular interstitial opacities were rarely present as the sole radiographic manifestation. Honeycombing is rarely seen at presentation and is discussed only as a late manifestation in the few patients who have progressive disease. Other radiographic abnormalities, such as pleural effusion, pleural thickening, hyperinflation, and lung cavities, occur uncommonly. Severity of the radiographic abnormalities correlates with the extent of histologic involvement of the respiratory bronchioles and alveolar ducts

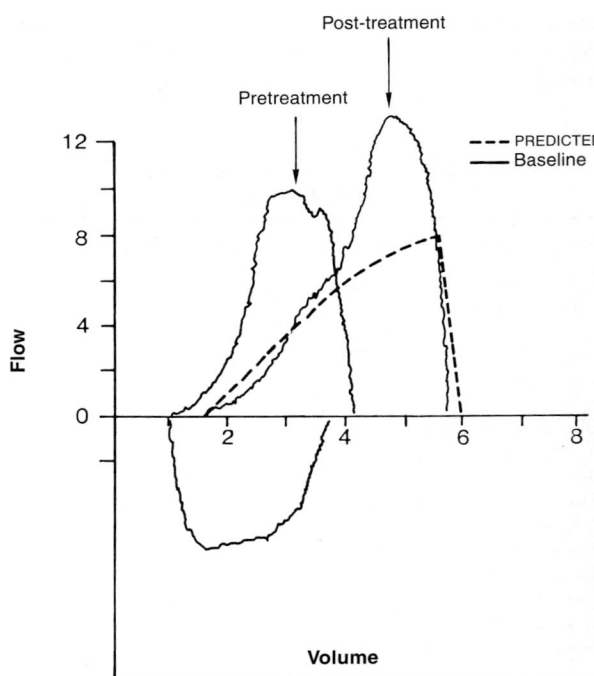

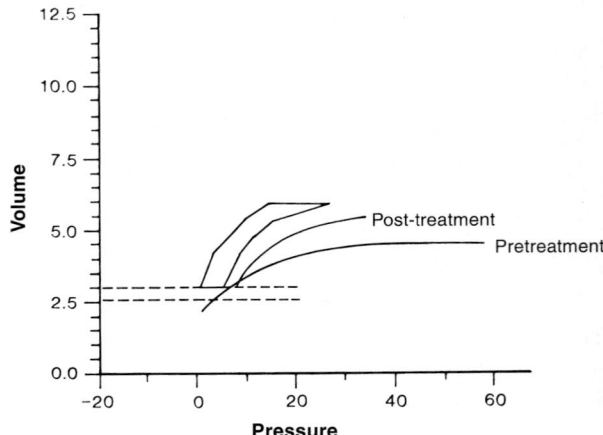

Figure 25–52 Lung function testing in COP. Pre- and post-treatment MEFV curve shows a restrictive defect that improves after treatment (*A*). Pre- and post-treatment static pressure-volume curve in the same patient shows a marked lung stiffness that improved after treatment (*B*). Reproduced with permission from Badesch D et al.[655]

but not of the larger terminal bronchioles. Focal OP can closely resemble lung cancer on a chest radiograph, and the exclusion of malignancy cannot be made on the basis of the radiographic appearances alone.[597]

HRCT

A CT scan of the lung reveals patchy air space consolidation in most cases (approximately 90% of cases) (see Chapter 4, Figure 4–25).[598] The consolidation is predominantly subpleural and/or peribronchovascular in dis-

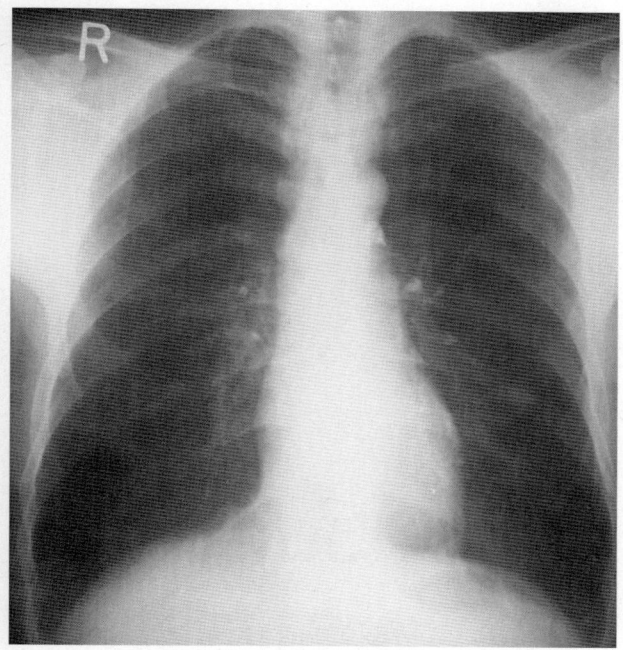

A

Figure 25–53 Cryptogenic organizing pneumonia in a 53-year-old Hispanic man with a 4-month history of progressive severe dyspnea with exertion and nonproductive cough that followed an acute upper respiratory tract infection. Posteroanterior radiograph taken at the time of patient's acute upper respiratory tract infection. The lung parenchyma is normal (*A*). Posteroanterior radiograph taken 4 months after previous film reveals alveolar opacities that are throughout all lung zones but most prominent in both lower lung zones (*B*). Follow-up posteroanterior radiograph after 3 months of corticosteroid therapy reveals marked improvement (*C*).

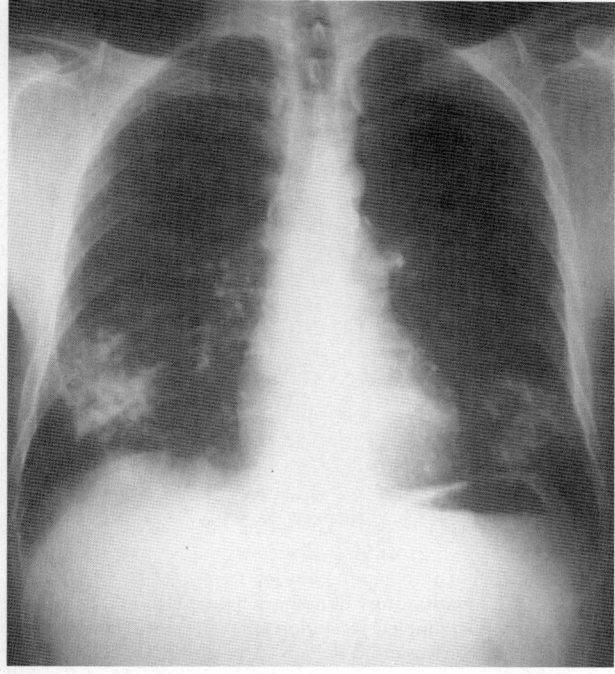

B

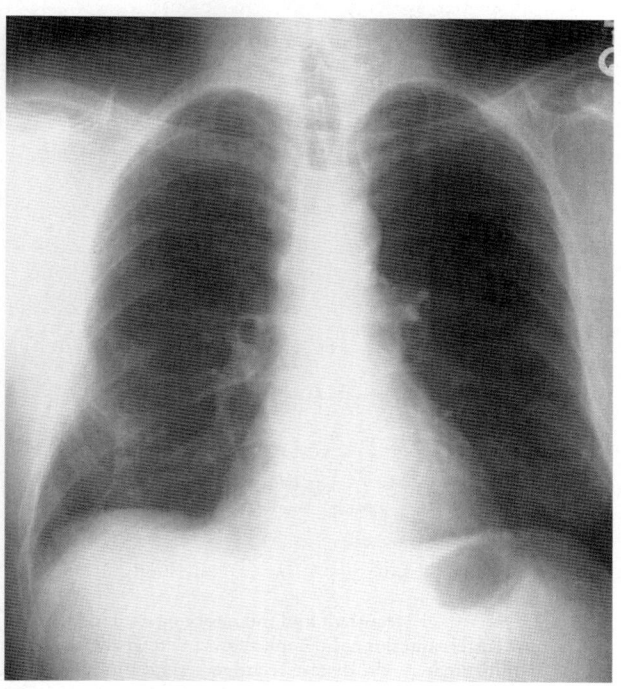

C

tribution (Figures 25–55, 25–56). Unilateral involvement is rare.[599] Ground-glass opacities (usually associated with lung consolidation) are seen in up to 60% of cases. Bronchial wall thickening and dilation are commonly evident in areas of consolidation.[594] Spontaneous regression of some focal areas of consolidation is a striking feature.[597]

Many variants of the typical CT patterns have now been described (see Chapter 4, Figure 4–25) (Table 25–21).[573,576,578,590–594,597] Small nodules (< 10 mm) are usually seen along bronchovascular bundles and are evident in up to 50% of cases (Figure 25–57, 25–58).[2] These patchy opacities occur more frequently in the periphery of the lung and are often in the lower lung zones.[600] Multiple large nodules may be found in approximately 15% of patients with COP at presentation.[2,601] These nodules usually have an irregular mar-

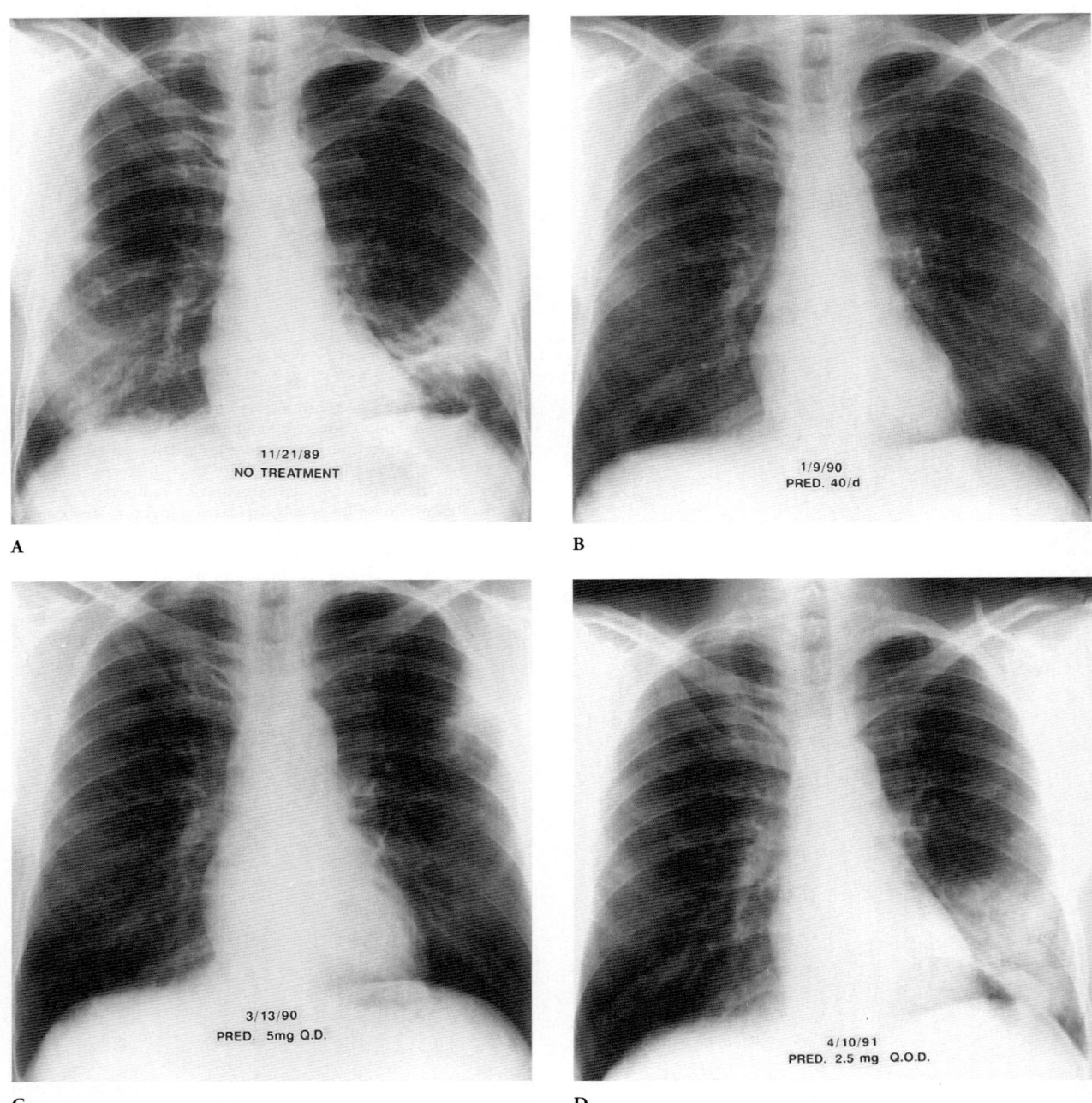

A

B

C

D

Figure 25–54   COP: recurrent and migratory opacities. A 55-year-old man with a 1-month history of dyspnea with exertion, fatigue, and weight loss. Posteroanterior radiograph shows bilateral alveolar opacities (*A*), but there was complete resolution following corticosteroid therapy (*B*). Unfortunately, the disease recurred several times following withdrawal of the corticosteroid therapy. A patchy alveolar subpleural opacity is present in the left upper lung (*C*). A final posteroanterior radiograph shows alveolar opacities in the left lower lung zone following tapering dose of prednisone (*D*).

gin (88%) with air bronchograms (45%). A perilobular pattern of OP has been described. This is characterized by opacification around the periphery of individual secondary lobules resembling poorly defined thickened interlobular septa (Figure 25–59). OP can, on occasion, progress to interstitial fibrosis and end-stage honeycomb lung (Figures 25–60, 25–61).[602] On the CT scan, a bibasal reticular pattern may be super-imposed on a background of areas of hazy opacities, frank consolidation, or acinar nodules. Ancillary findings include pleural tags (38%), spicules (35%), pleural thickening (33%), and parenchymal bands (25%). Crescentic and ring-shaped opacities have been reported in two cases of COP.[603] CT may reveal much more extensive disease than is expected from review of the plain chest radiograph. Pleural effusions are rare.

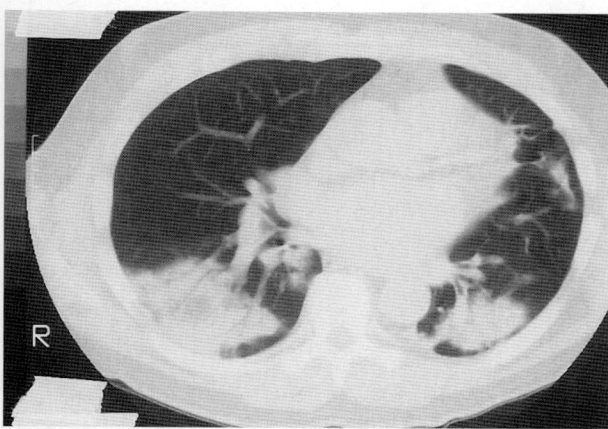

Figure 25–55   COP. HRCT scan shows patchy air space consolidation in the lower lobes (multiple similar opacities were seen in both lungs). Air bronchograms are present.

Histopathologic Findings

The histopathologic lesion characteristic of COP is an excessive proliferation of granulation tissue within small airways (ie, proliferative bronchiolitis) and alveolar ducts, along with chronic inflammation in surrounding alveoli (see Chapter 2, "Anatomic Distribution and Histopathologic Patterns of Interstitial Lung Disease" Figure 2–11). This OP is the most important basis underlying the clinical and radiographic manifestations of COP. Several additional key features are notable (see Table 25–2).[578,604,605] (1) The distribution of lesions is usually patchy and peribronchiolar; (2) the lesions are usually located predominantly within the air space (Figure 25–62); (3) there is a uniform recent temporal appearance to the changes in that all the lesions look similar, with an inflamed, edematous-appearing stroma with little collagen deposition; (4) the intraluminal buds of granulation tissue consist of loose, collagen-embedding fibroblasts and myofibroblasts that extend through the pores of Kohn from one alveolus to another, giving rise to the characteristic butterfly pattern (Figure 25–61);

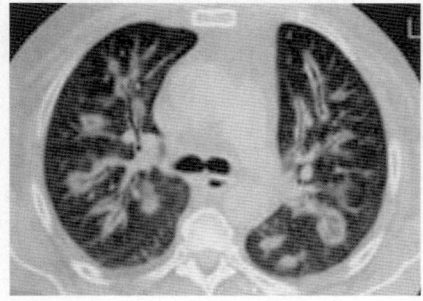

Figure 25–56   Bronchocentric pattern of organizing pneumonia: a strikingly peribronchovascular distribution in a diabetic patient with biopsy-proven organizing pneumonia. Reproduced with permission from Oikonomou A et al.[598]

(5) the bronchiolar lesions are usually secondary to intraluminal plugs of granulation tissue that occur in association with plugs in the alveolar ducts and alveolar spaces; (6) severe fibrotic changes (honeycombing) are unusual at the time of diagnosis; (7) foamy macrophages are very common in alveolar spaces, presumably secondary to the bronchiolar occlusion; the mitogen, platelet-derived growth factor (PDGF), and one of its receptors, PDGFR-β; PDGF+ cells and CD68+ macrophages were found in greater numbers in lungs with the BOOP pattern. In addition, an increased expression of PDGFR-β epitopes was observed in some patients. This has led to speculation that these molecules may play an important role in the pathogenesis of the destructive fibroproliferative process that characterizes this disease.[606] Further features are the fact that (8) giant cells are rare or absent, and no granuloma or vasculitis is present; and (9) the lung architecture is not severely disrupted. In patients with severe or progressive disease, we have shown that, in the initial stages of the acute respiratory illness, the lung lesions are characterized pathologically by florid BOOP. With progression, the biopsy may show features that are more consistent with a fibrotic NSIP-like pattern with interstitial inflammation and fibrosis (Figure 25–61).

Diagnosis

An open or thoracoscopic lung biopsy is recommended to confirm the diagnosis. Transbronchial lung biopsies are generally inadequate in confirming COP and in ruling out other disorders.[607] It has been suggested that the combination of bronchoalveolar (a lymphocytosis of > 25% with a CD4 to CD8 ratio greater than 0.9, combined with foamy macrophages of > 20%, or neutrophils of > 5%, or eosinophils of >2% and < 25%) and transbronchial lung biopsy specimens appears to be an effective method for the initial investigation in COP patients presenting with patchy radiographic shadows.[608] However, the histopathologic features of OP can be seen in a number of settings; therefore, small biopsies increase the chance of missing the central diagnosis. Multiple-step sectioning of transbronchial biopsy specimens may be useful in identifying the lesions of COP.

The biopsied tissue must be reviewed by an experienced lung pathologist who has been given adequate clinical information to guide the search for specific lesions to support the diagnosis. Once the characteristic findings of proliferative bronchiolitis are confirmed, the clinician must ensure that a thorough search has been performed to rule out the many other diagnostic considerations. Indeed, the presence of OP histopathology is not a diagnosis, but suggests that a search for an underlying etiology be pursued, because the pathologic appearance may be a response to injury from many disorders (see Table 25–19). Most frequently, a secondary cause is not found, although a variety of specific causes and disease associa-

TABLE 25–21   CT Patterns in Organizing Pneumonia

CT Pattern	CT Features	Reference
Classic COP pattern	Bilateral patchy air-space consolidation Volume loss may be present	554,568,569,573, 576,578,587–594
Focal pattern	Focal solitary organizing pneumonia Commonly found in upper lobes	597,650
Nodular pattern	Acinar pattern with nodules ~8 mm in diameter Subtle poorly defined (micro)nodular pattern Multiple large nodules or masses	590–592,594,597, 601,610,648
Bronchocentric pattern	Areas of consolidation surrounding bronchovascular bundles Appears commonly in patients with polymyositis and dermatomyositis	590,594,597, 610,651

Linear and band-like pattern	Lines or bands > 2 cm, smooth or irregular sometimes forming arcades
	    and/or containing air bronchograms. Usually at least 8 mm in width. They
	    are rarely the only finding.
	Some extend in a radial manner along the line of the bronchi towards the pleura,
	    usually intimately related to bronchi
	Some occur in a peripheral location bearing no relationship to the bronchi
		597,652

Perilobular pattern	Localization of parenchymal disease at the level of the secondary pulmonary lobule Usually associated with areas of consolidation or near nodules and masses	590,597,600, 601,652
Progressive fibrotic pattern	Bibasal reticular pattern may be superimposed on a background of areas of frank consolidation or acinar nodules Most frequently seen with connective tissue diseases; carries a poorer prognosis	597,601,602, 650,653

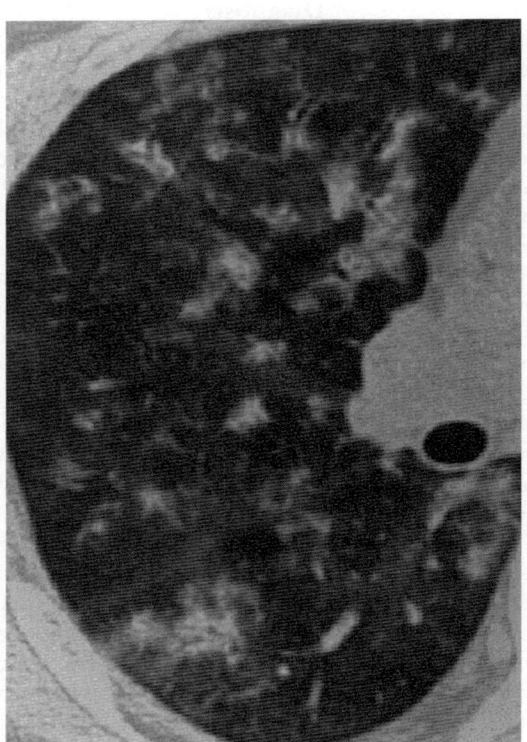

Figure 25–57 Peribronchial distribution of ground-glass opacity in 44-year-old man with bronchiolitis obliterans with organizing pneumonia (BOOP). HRCT scan shows multiple patchy areas of ground-glass opacity in right lung. Opacities are noted along bronchi and are seen in both peripheral and central zones. Reproduced with permission from Arakawa H et al.[610]

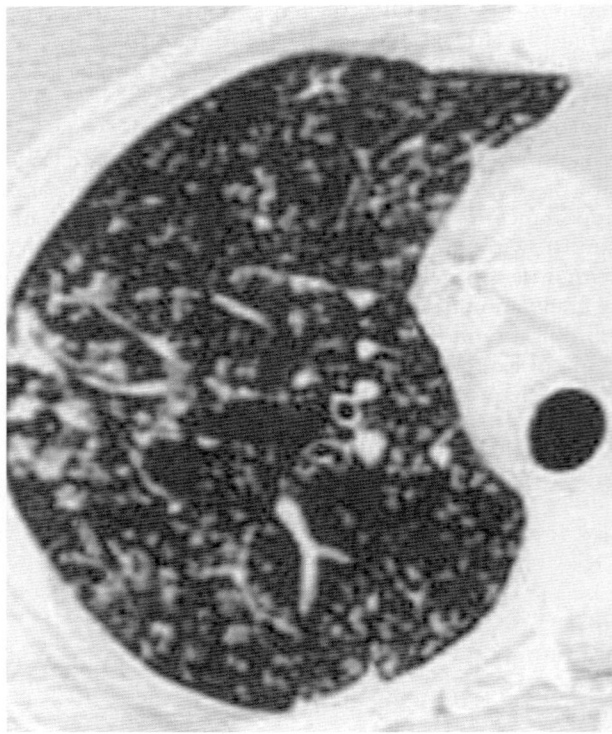

Figure 25–58 Biopsy-proven organizing pneumonia. CT scan of the right upper lobe of a patient with a 10-day history of dyspnea and suspected community-acquired pneumonia. There is a combined pattern of peripheral acinar nodules and smaller nodules, some of which resemble a tree-in-bud pattern. Reproduced with permission from Oikonomou A et al.[597]

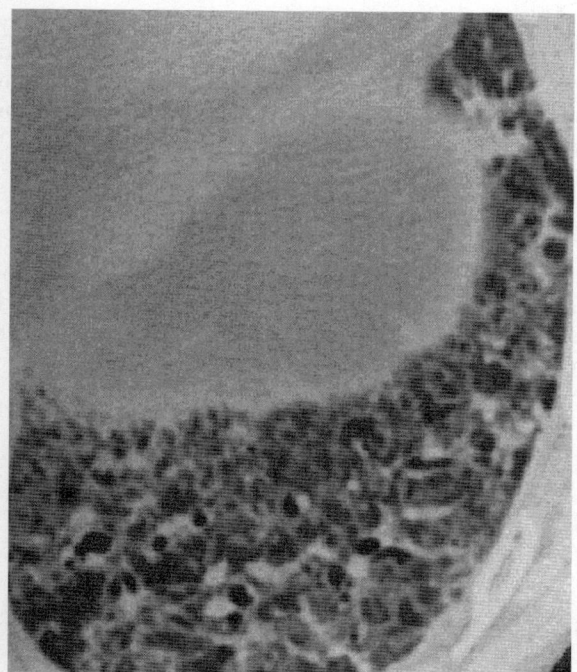

Figure 25–59 Intralobular reticular opacity in 68-year-old man with BOOP. HRCT scan shows fine reticular opacity at left lung base, associated with ground-glass opacity and dilatation of bronchi. Reproduced with permission from Arakawa H et al.[610]

tions are known. Thus, COP is a diagnosis of exclusion; infections, collagen vascular diseases, inhalation injuries, and lung irradiation are most frequently associated.[570,597,609] It is particularly important to rule out chronic eosinophilic pneumonia and hypersensitivity pneumonitis (extrinsic allergic alveolitis).[610]

Management and Outcome

Corticosteroid therapy is the most common treatment. Complete clinical recovery, physiological improvement, and normalization of the chest film are seen in two-thirds of patients (Figure 25–63).[2,571] Approximately one-third demonstrate persistent disease. In general, clinical improvement is rapid, within several days or a few weeks. Occasionally, recovery is quite dramatic. Delay in treatment increases the risk of more severe disease and relapses.[576] The rate of relapse varies from 9 to 58%.[576] Relapses occur commonly when corticosteroids are withdrawn too soon (after 1 to 2 months). At first relapse, 68% of patients are still under treatment for the initial episode.[576] Mild cholestasis identifies a subgroup of patients with multiple relapses.[576] Most patients who relapse improve when they are re-treated with corticosteroids. Spontaneous improvement in a few patients appears to occur over the course of 3 to 6 months.[569,611] Patients with air space opacities on the chest radiograph have a much better outcome than those with interstitial opacities. The overall prognosis for COP is much better than for other ILDs (eg, IPF). Five-year survival is higher in patients with COP (73%) than in those with secondary OP (44%), and respiratory-related deaths were more frequent in patients with secondary OP. Rapidly fatal COP is uncommon.

The dose of oral corticosteroids needed to treat patients with COP is not known. The author's experience is with high-dose oral corticosteroid therapy as described for other idiopathic interstitial pneumonias. High-dose parenteral corticosteroid therapy (eg, methylprednisolone, 125 to 250 mg intravenously every 6 hours for 3 to 5 days) has been recommended as initial treatment in patients with rapidly progressive COP.

For the stable or improved patient, the prednisone is gradually tapered to zero after 3 to 6 months of therapy. A chest radiograph or HRCT scan and pulmonary function tests should probably be performed every 6 to 8 weeks during the first year, and therapy should be reinstituted aggressively with any sign of recurrence. Although therapy with corticosteroids is usually well tolerated, side effects are common; some patients develop side effects more readily than others.

If the patient deteriorates despite corticosteroid therapy, a cytotoxic agent should be considered while low-dose (0.25 mg/kg/day) therapy with prednisone is continued.[612] Cyclophosphamide and azathioprine have both been used successfully, although the optimal dose in COP is unknown.[573]

Ichikawa and coworkers administered erythromycin at a low dose (600 mg daily) for 3 to 4 months to six patients with COP and obtained good CRP improvement.[613] They suggest that erythromycin can be successfully used instead of corticosteroids in the treatment of COP. I have no personal experience with this therapy for COP.

ACUTE INTERSTITIAL PNEUMONIA

AIP is a rare and fulminant form of lung injury that presents acutely (days to weeks from the onset of symptoms) and most commonly occurs in a previously healthy individual.[2,614–617] The cases of pulmonary fibrosis originally reported by Hamman and Rich had clinical and histopathologic features of AIP rather than UIP.[2,4,618] AIP needs to be distinguished from ARDS of known cause; the accelerated decline of UIP (see "Acute Exacerbation of IPF" above); diffuse alveolar damage, acute OP or acute alveolar hemorrhage in patients with collagen vascular diseases; infection (especially that due to *P. carinii* pneumonia and cytomegalovirus); and drug-induced hypersensitivity or acute eosinophilic pneumonia.[2]

Etiology and Epidemiology

The etiology and pathogenesis of AIP is unknown and appears to involve a complex array of cellular events associated with diffuse alveolar damage. Unfortunately, most case series fail to distinguish between those patients with a putative cause and those with idiopathic causes.[2] A major pathway of cellular damage involves neutrophil-mediated lung injury via toxic oxygen species and proteases.[617,619] Other cells likely play a role in the lung injury, such as epithelial, endothelial, and smooth muscle cells and histiocytes, fibroblasts, and the extracellular matrix.[11,614,620,621] (See "Histopathologic findings" below.)

Clinical Findings

AIP occurs over a wide age range; most patients are over the age of 40 years, with a mean age of 50 to 55 years.[2,614,616,622,623] There is no gender predominance, and there is no known association with cigarette smoking. The onset of AIP is usually abrupt, with the patient experiencing a prodromal illness that lasts 7 to 14 days before presentation. The most common clinical signs and symptoms are fever, cough, and shortness of breath.[622] Crackles are often heard on physical examination. Finger clubbing is rare.

Laboratory Findings

Routine laboratory studies in AIP are nonspecific and generally not helpful. A peripheral leukocytosis is common, and most patients have moderate to severe hypoxemia.

Findings in BAL Fluid

BAL fluid usually contains increased total cells, especially neutrophils and, occasionally, lymphocytes.[2,624]

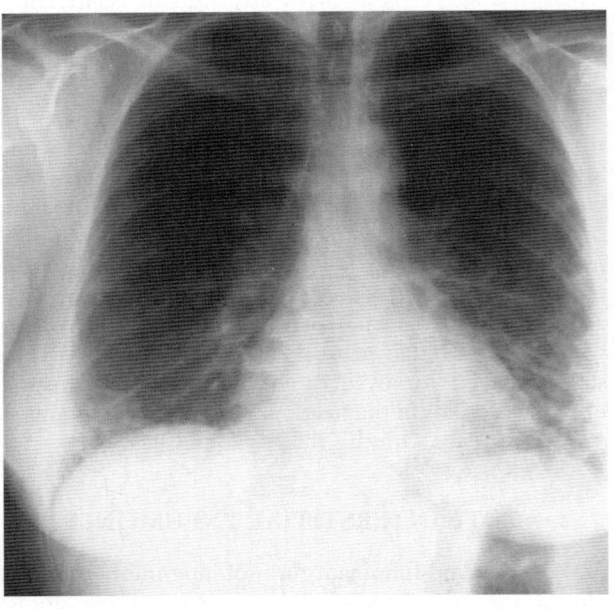

A

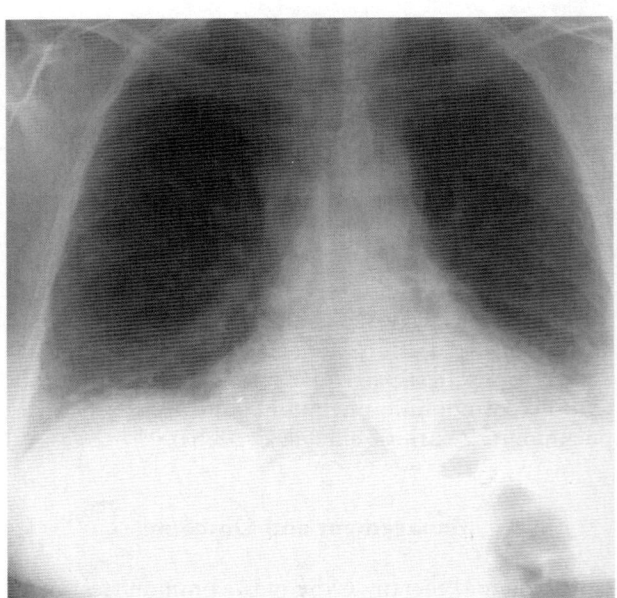

B

Figure 25–60 Progressive COP. A 48-year old woman with an 8-week history of cough, dyspnea with exertion, fatigue, and slight weight loss. *A,* This posteroanterior radiograph shows bilateral reticular and ground-glass opacities in the lower lung zones. There was improvement following corticosteroid therapy, but the patient did not return to normal lung function or exercise capacity. *B,* This follow-up posteroanterior radiograph shows bilateral, predominantly reticular, opacities in the lower lung zones, with associated volume loss. *C,* HRCT scan shows right lower lobe reticular and hazy opacities that are subpleural. This CT pattern is most common in patients with chronic progressive disease and looks similar to that usually seen in IPF.

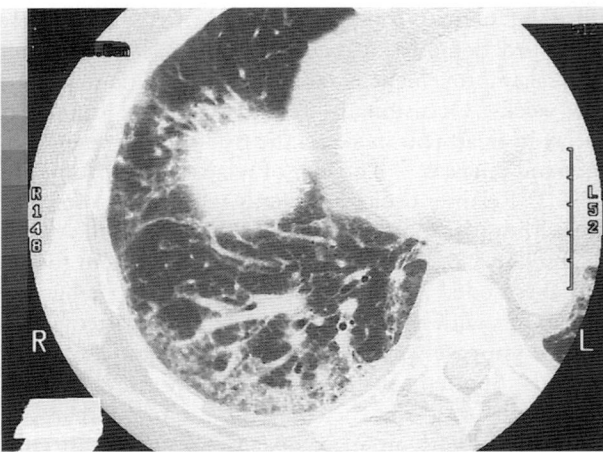

C

Signs of hemorrhage (red blood cells and/or hemosiderin) are common.[2,624] Atypical reactive pneumocytes and fragments of hyaline membranes may be seen.[2]

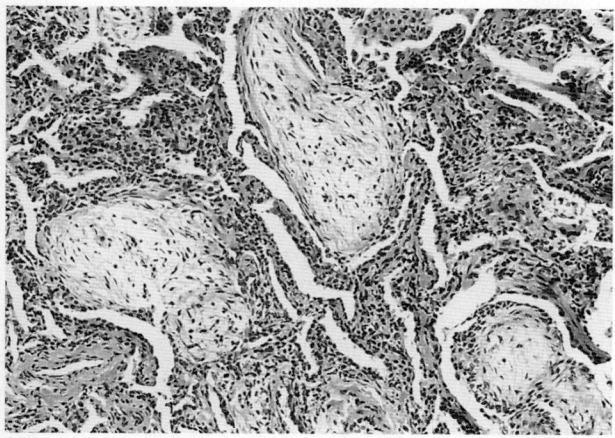

A

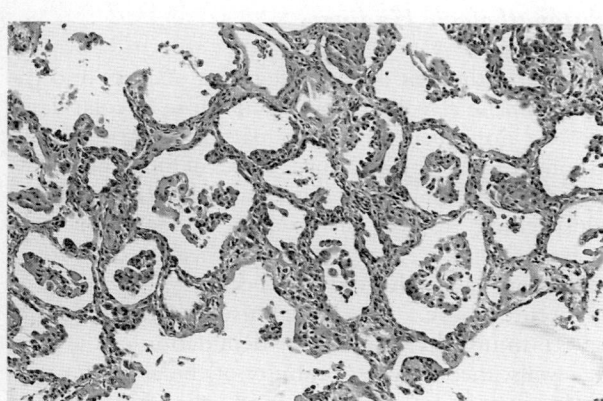

B

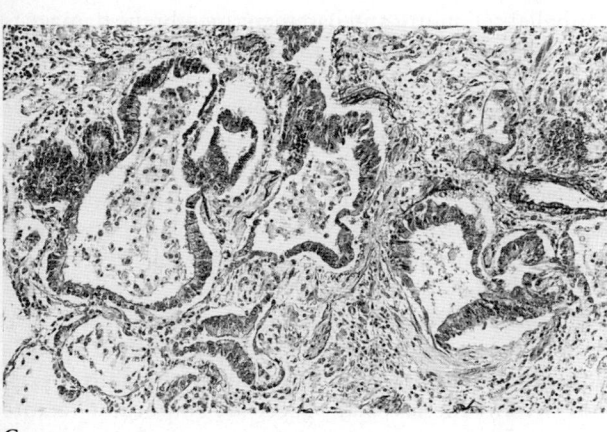

C

Figure 25–61 Rapidly progressive COP. Photomicrograph of lung biopsy in patient with acute respiratory failure. *A,* Photomicrograph shows a florid BOOP pattern. *B,* Another photomicrograph from the same patient, from a second open-lung biopsy obtained 7 months later, shows a NSIP-like pattern. *C,* A third photomicrograph, from the postmortem examination of the lungs, was obtained 9 months after the initial biopsy and shows honeycombing of the lung. All samples were stained with hematoxylin and eosin.

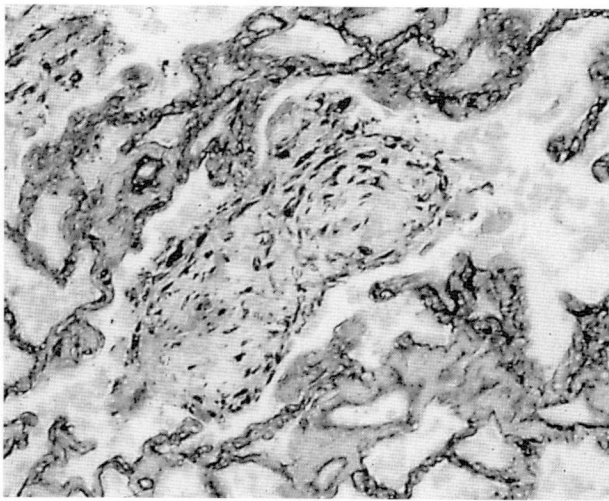

Figure 25–62 Masson bodies of organizing pneumonia. Fibroblasts with procollagen are within air spaces. The interstitium, delineated by basal limina, is minimally thickened (immunoperoxidase for procollagen type I and immunoalkaline phosphatase for type IV collagen; 3230). Reproduced with permission from Kuhn C III.[621]

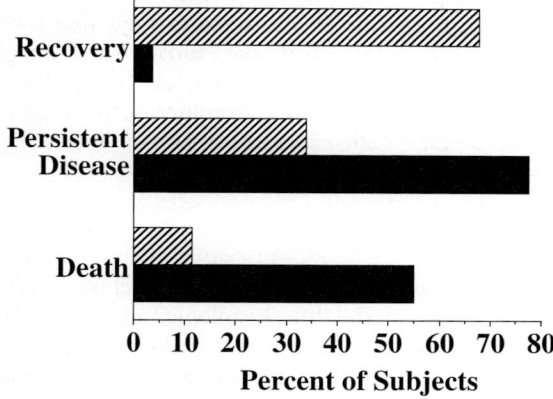

Figure 25–63 Treatment outcome and prognosis in COP. Nine major published reports that included 5 or more subjects with diagnosis confirmed by lung biopsy (total of 157 subjects) were reviewed.[554,569,586,588,589,604,656] These works were critically reviewed for information on the CRP and pathological findings of COP. Each variable was analyzed to provide an accurate composite description of COP. In addition, these data were compared to similar findings from 3 published reports of patients with IPF (*n* = 74).[315,554,604] The diagnosis of IPF was established on the basis of a compatible history, physical examination, chest radiograph, pulmonary physiological evaluation, and a confirmatory open lung biopsy. The mean age was 57 years, range 29 to 77 years. There were 20 women and 39 men. The smoking history was available in 39 subjects, of whom 16 were never smokers and 23 were current smokers or ex-smokers. Clinical improvement represents resolution of cough and/or dyspnea, normalization of lung function, or clearing of the chest film. Patients with IPF rarely improved completely following treatment; in fact, most had persistent disease with progression to death in 55% of subjects reported in these studies (*n* = 58). The solid bar represents patients with COP, and the hatched bar represents patients with IPF. Adapted from King TE Jr and Mortenson RL.[555]

Physiological Findings

A restrictive pattern is commonly found. Gas exchange abnormalities are very prominent. The diffusing capacity may be markedly reduced. Hypoxemia develops early and progresses rapidly to respiratory failure, which may be refractory to supplemental oxygen.[2] The majority of patients fulfill the clinical diagnostic criteria for ARDS: acute onset, a PaO$_2$ to fraction of inspired oxygen ratio equal to or less than 200 mm Hg, diffuse bilateral opacities on chest radiograph, and a pulmonary capillary wedge pressure of less than 18 mm Hg when measured or no clinical evidence of left atrial hypertension.[2]

Chest Imaging Studies

Chest Radiograph

The chest radiograph reveals diffuse bilateral air space opacification.[614,622,623] The lung volumes are usually normal, and the distribution of the air space opacities may be patchy, with sparing of the costophrenic angles.[2] The cardiac silhouette and vascular pedicle are normal, and interstitial abnormalities such as septal lines and peribronchial cuffing are usually absent.[2] During the acute stage, the lungs tend to become diffusely consolidated as the disease progresses.[2,623] As recovery begins (and the pathologic features move from the exudative to the organizing stage), the radiograph shows less consolidation and more of a ground-glass appearance, with irregular linear opacities.[2,623] Pleural effusions are uncommon.

HRCT

Ichikado and coworkers have described a close correlation in AIP between the three histologic stages of the disease (exudative, proliferative, and fibrotic phases) and patterns seen on HRCT scan (increased ground-glass attenuation, increased ground-glass attenuation with traction bronchiectasis, and honeycomb change, respectively).[625,626] The CT scan typically shows bilateral patchy symmetric areas of ground-glass attenuation, often accompanied by air space consolidation and traction bronchiectasis (Figure 25–64).[623,627,628] Other findings that may be seen include bilateral areas of air space consolidation, a predominantly subpleural distribution of disease, and mild honeycombing (usually involving < 10 percent of the lung). The distribution is most often basilar (either in the subpleural or central regions) (Figure 25–65). Occasionally, a diffuse pattern or upper lobe predominance is found. In patients with classic AIP, the areas of consolidation are most often in the dependent area of the lung, suggesting alveolar closure from the weight and hydrostatic pressure of the more superior lung tissue.[2] Hansell hypothesizes that the consolidation not associated with traction of the airways (a find-

ing more extensive in survivors of AIP) might correspond to areas of OP.[625,626] Intralobular linear opacities and subpleural honeycombing are seen in a minority of cases.[2] As the disease progresses, there may be distortion of the bronchovascular bundles, and traction bronchiectasis is seen (Figure 25–66).[2] The areas of consolidation tend to be replaced by ground-glass opacities. Cysts and other lucent areas of the lung become more common in the late stages of AIP.[2] The patients with AIP who die have CT scan findings suggestive of the fibroproliferative phase of diffuse alveolar damage, particularly findings of architectural distortion and ground-glass attenuation or consolidation associated with traction bronchiectasis.[627] The few patients who survive show progressive clearing of the ground-glass attenuation and consolidation. The most common residual HRCT scan findings are areas of hypoattenuation, lung cysts, reticular abnormality, and associated parenchymal distortion, occurring mainly in the nondependent lung.[2,629,630]

Histopathologic Findings

The histopathologic appearance is that of acute or organizing diffuse alveolar damage.[622] Diffuse alveolar damage is a nonspecific reaction pattern that occurs in response to a number of known causes of lung injury. The key pathologic features of diffuse alveolar damage are its nonspecificity and the characteristic temporal phases in its evolution: acute, organizing, and healed (or fibrotic) phases that vary in histologic appearance.[614,622]

Acute Phase.   The initial insult results in epithelial cell injury characterized by denudation of the alveolar walls, increased permeability of the alveolar capillaries, interstitial edema, and the presence of intra-alveolar hyaline membranes.[620,621] The extent of epithelial cell injury and basement membrane damage is important in modulating the nature and extent of the fibroblastic response in AIP (Figure 25–64).

Organizing Phase.   A stage of organizing follows the acute phase. The organizing phase is characterized by fibroblast proliferation and connective tissue synthesis.[11,614,620,621] The hyaline membranes are resorbed or incorporated into the alveolar septa and become overgrown with proliferating type II epithelial cells (Figures 25–66, 25–67).

Fibrotic Phase.   A severe, progressive fibrotic response may occur. Alveolar wall collapse and apposition, associated with reepithelization of the fibrotic exudate within the alveolar space, are important factors affecting the severity and extensiveness of the fibrotic process (Figure 25–66).[11,614,620,621] Lung biopsies are rarely performed during the acute exudative stage of the injury. An important feature of AIP is the presence of a temporally uniform lesion, which reflects an episode of acute lung injury occurring at a single time point. This differs from UIP in which pathologic lesions are of different ages. Therefore, the most characteristic features reported in most studies of lung biopsy specimens from patients with AIP are those found during the organizing proliferative stage of diffuse alveolar damage and include marked thickening of the alveolar septa due to interstitial edema, inflammatory cell infiltration, fibroblast proliferation (within the interstitium and air spaces), and type II cell hyperplasia. Collapse and apposition of adjacent alveolar septa is evident in most sections, and the hyaline membranes (most prominent during the acute phase) are less obvious, appearing only in focal areas along alveolar septa. Thrombi may be seen in small arteries.[617] During the healing phase of AIP, there may be no apparent residue or variable degrees of nonprogressive interstitial fibrosis and/or airway scarring may be seen.

Diagnosis and Differential Diagnosis

The diagnosis of AIP is based on two findings: (1) the presence of a clinical syndrome of idiopathic ARDS and (2) pathologic confirmation of organizing diffuse alveolar damage. Thus, an open or thoracoscopic lung biopsy is required to confirm the diagnosis. The differential diagnosis of AIP includes a number of pulmonary diseases. Among the disorders that may be confused with AIP are diffuse alveolar hemorrhage syndromes, acute eosinophilic pneumonia, rapidly progressive ILD associated with connective tissue disease (especially rheumatoid arthritis and polymyositis), or diffuse alveolar damage of known cause (sepsis, drug-induced toxicity, toxins, radiation pneumonitis, shock, or viral infection).[617] There is considerable overlap in HRCT scan appearance among patients with AIP and ARDS. However, Tomiyama and coworkers reported that patients with AIP tended to have more honeycombing and a more symmetrical and lower zone distribution of abnormalities than patients with ARDS.[631]

In most cases, AIP should be readily distinguished from other forms of idiopathic interstitial pneumonia. Distinguishing features among these clinicopathologic entities include the types of prodromal illness, radiographic and histopathologic findings, the clinical

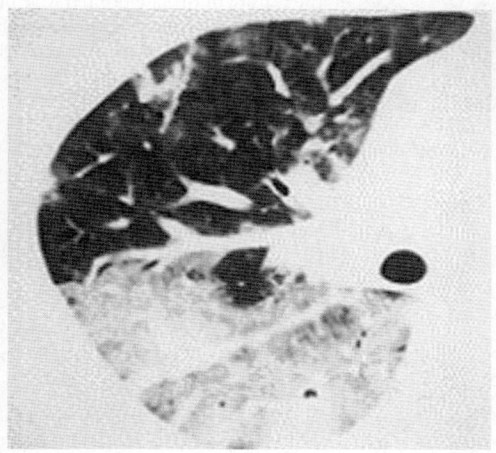

A

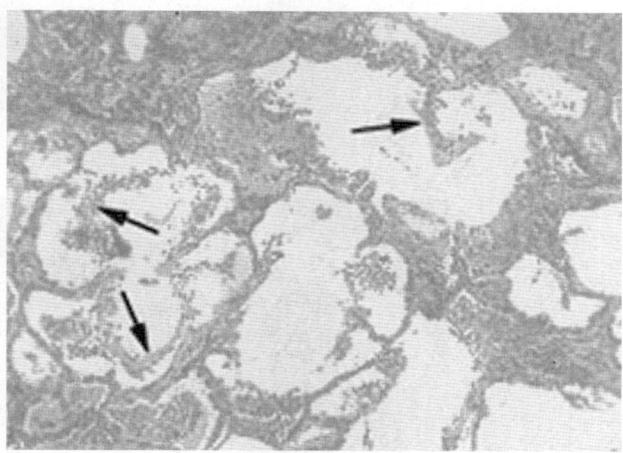

B

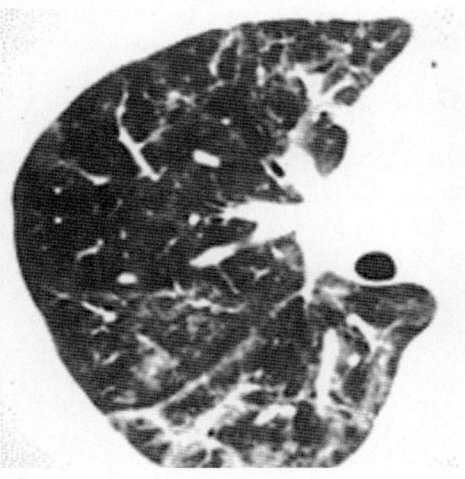

C

Figure 25–64 Findings in 29-year-old woman with acute interstitial pneumonia (AIP) who survived. *A,* HRCT scan of the right lung at the level of intermediate bronchus before high-dose corticosteroid therapy shows ground-glass attenuation and patchy consolidation, predominantly in the posterior lung regions. Relatively spared areas extend into the ventral zone of the lung. No associated traction bronchiolectasis or bronchiectasis is seen. *B,* Histologic section of right lung specimen obtained from open lung biopsy, which corresponds to the areas of ground-glass attenuation at HRCT scan, shows hyalinous membranes (arrows) within the air spaces and interstitial mononuclear infiltrates, which are the features of the exudative phase of diffuse alveolar damage (hematoxylin and eosin stain; ×25 original magnification). *C,* CT scan obtained 3 months after the initial one (A) shows a marked decrease of ground-glass attenuation and consolidation. Reproduced with permission from Ichikado K et al.[627]

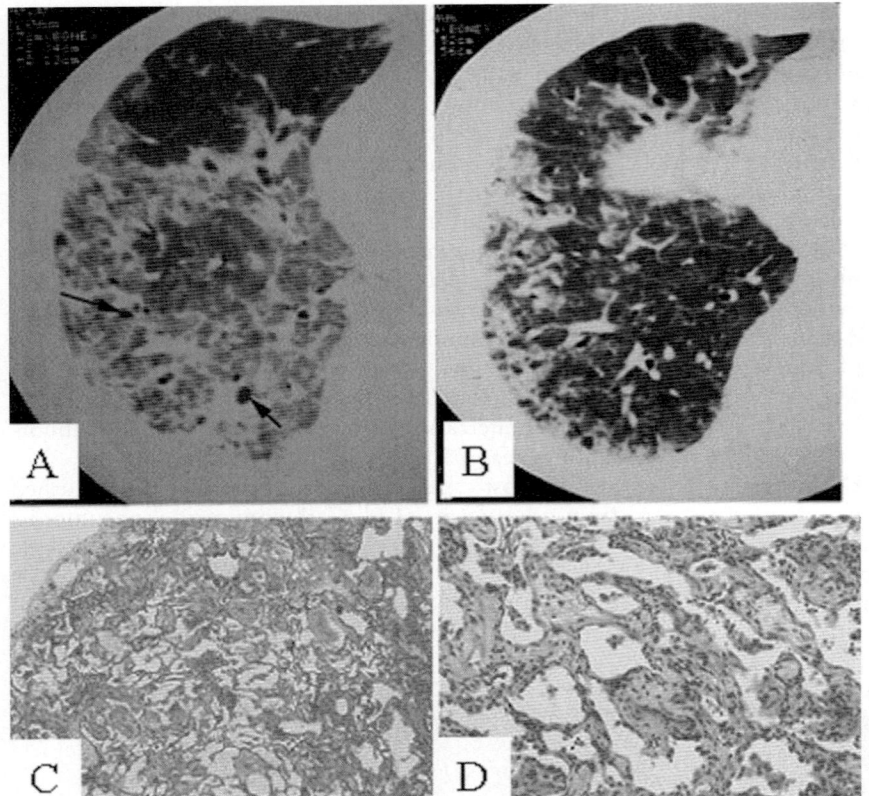

Figure 25–65 Findings in a 68-year-old-woman with AIP who survived. HRCT scan of the right lower lobe shows area of increased attenuation with traction bronchiectasis (*A, arrows*). CT scan obtained 18 days after the initial CT (*A*) shows decrease of the areas of increased attenuation (*B*). *C,* Photomicrograph of right lung obtained from open lung biopsy, which corresponds to area of increased attenuation (seen in *A*), shows diffuse thickening of alveolar walls (hematoxylin and eosin stain; ×5 original magnification). *D,* Histologic findings show diffuse interstitial fibroblastic proliferation, which is the feature of the late proliferative phase of diffuse alveolar damage (hematoxylin and eosin stain; ×200 original magnification). Reproduced with permission from Ichikado K et al.[627]

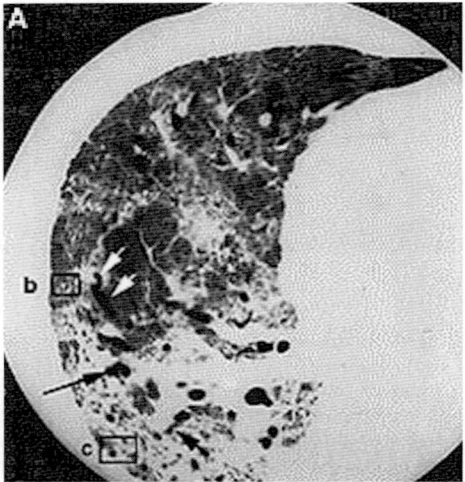

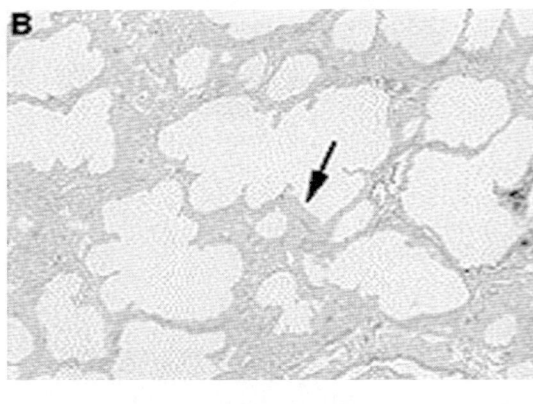

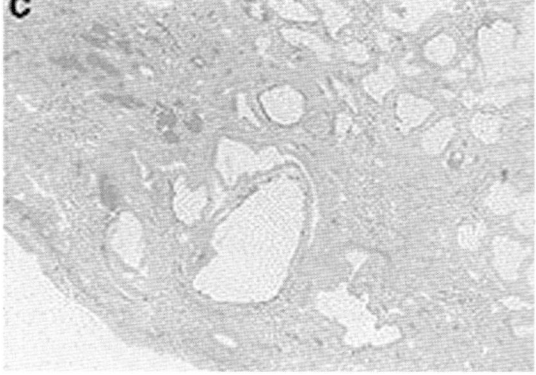

Figure 25–66 Findings in a 77-year-old man with AIP who did not survive. *A,* HRCT scan at the level of right intrapulmonary vein shows ground-glass attenuation and consolidation associated with traction bronchiolectasis and bronchiectasis (arrows) and architectural distortion, which is shown as displacement of bronchi (white arrows). *B,* Histologic section of autopsy specimen, corresponding to area of ground-glass attenuation with traction bronchiectasis (seen in *A*) shows organized hyalinous membrane (arrow) and interstitial collagenous deposition, which is the feature of the fibrotic phase of diffuse alveolar damage (hematoxylin and eosin stain; ×10 original magnification). *C,* Histologic section, corresponding to area of consolidation with traction bronchiolectasis and bronchiectasis (seen in *A*), shows interstitial and intra-alveolar collagenous deposition, which is the feature of the fibrotic phase (hematoxylin and eosin stain; ×5 original magnification). Reproduced with permission from Ichikado K et al.[627]

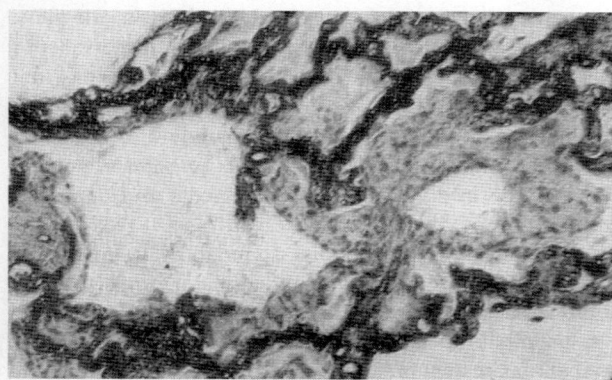

Figure 25–67   Reparative phase of diffuse alveolar damage. Distribution of matrix containing active fibroblasts (staining for procollagen) follows alveolar ducts in a distribution similar to that of hyaline membranes in acute diffuse alveolar damage (immunoperoxidase stain for procollagen type I and immunoglucose oxidase for type IV collagen (×230 original magnification). Reproduced with permission from Kuhn C III.[621]

course, and the response to therapy. A major clinical difference at presentation is disease duration; AIP is an acute disease of abrupt onset, DIP and COP have a subacute course over weeks to months, and UIP has a chronic course over more than 1 year.[616]

Management and Outcome

The main therapy for AIP is supportive care. Mechanical ventilation is often required because most patients develop respiratory failure. It is not clear if corticosteroid therapy is effective in AIP.[615,616,622] Meduri and colleagues, in studies conducted in patients with ARDS, showed that corticosteroids accelerated the repair process during the proliferative phase of diffuse alveolar damage and that they were most effective during the early proliferative phase before the development of acellular fibrosis with deranged alveolar architecture, which is seen in the late proliferative and the fibrotic phases.[632–635] When prescribed, they are given as described earlier in this chapter.

The mortality from AIP is high (> 60%), and the majority of patients die within 6 months of presentation.[614–616,622,624] Those who recover, however, usually do not have recurrence of the disease, and most have substantial or complete recovery of lung function. However, some series have documented both recurrence of the process and the development of chronic ILD among a substantial fraction of those who survive AIP.[615,616] No features have been shown to predict the course of disease among AIP survivors.[616] Ichikado and coworkers, in a retrospective study, showed that the extent of ground-glass attenuation or consolidation associated with traction bronchiolectasis or bronchiectasis and that the extent of architectural distortion was more extensive in those patients who died than in those who survived.[627]

REFERENCES

1. British Thoracic Society. The diagnosis, assessment and treatment of diffuse parenchymal lung disease in adults. Thorax 1999;54 Suppl 1:S1–S28.
2. Travis WD, King TE Jr, Bateman ED, et al. American Thoracic Society/European Respiratory Society international multidisciplinary consensus classification of the idiopathic interstitial pneumonias. Am J Respir Crit Care Med 2002;165:277–304.
3. Osler W. The principles and practice of medicine. New York: D Appleton; 1892. p. 1079.
4. Hamman L, Rich AR. Acute diffuse interstitial fibrosis of the lungs. Bull Johns Hopkins Hosp 1944;74:177–212.
5. Rubin EH, Lubliner R. Hamman-Rich syndrome. Review of literature and analysis of 15 cases. Medicine 1957;36:397–463.
6. Wagley PF. A new look at the Hamman-Rich syndrome. Johns Hopkins Med J 1972;131:412–24.
7. Turner-Warwick M. A perspective view on widespread pulmonary fibrosis. Br Med J 1974;2:371–6.
8. Liebow AA, Carrington DB. The interstitial pneumonias. In: Simon M, Potchen EJ, LeMay M, editors. Frontiers of pulmonary radiology. New York: Grune & Stratton; 1969. p. 102–41.
9. Liebow AA. Definition and classification of interstitial pneumonias in human pathology. Prog Respir Res 1975;8:1–33.
10. Katzenstein AL. Idiopathic interstitial pneumonia: classification and diagnosis. In: Katzenstein AL, Askin FB, editors. Surgical pathology of non-neoplastic lung disease. Philadelphia (PA): W.B. Saunders; 1997. p. 1–31.
11. Katzenstein ALA, Myers JL. Idiopathic pulmonary fibrosis. Clinical relevance of pathologic classification. Am J Respir Crit Care Med 1998;157:1301–15.
12. Crystal RG, Bitterman PB, Rennard SI, et al. Interstitial lung disease of unknown cause. Disorders characterized by chronic inflammation of the lower respiratory tract. N Engl J Med 1984;310:154–66, 235–44.
13. Scott J, Johnston I, Britton J. What causes cryptogenic fibrosing alveolitis? A case-control study of environmental exposure to dust. Br Med J 1990;301:1015–7.
14. Coultas DB, Zumwalt RE, Black WC, Sobonya RE. The epidemiology of interstitial lung disease. Am J Respir Crit Care Med 1994;150:967–72.
15. Mannino DM, Etzel RA, Parrish RG. Pulmonary fibrosis deaths in the United States, 1979–1991. An analysis of multiple-cause mortality data. Am J Respir Crit Care Med 1996;153:1548–52.
16. Iwai K, Mori T, Yamada N, et al. Idiopathic pulmonary fibrosis. Epidemiologic approaches to occupational exposure. Am J Respir Crit Care Med 1994;150:670–75.
17. Fraig M, Shreesha U, Savici D, Katzenstein AL. Respiratory bronchiolitis: a clinicopathologic study in current smokers, ex-smokers, and never-smokers. Am J Surg Pathol 2002;26:647–53.
18. Hubbard R, Lewis S, Richards K, et al. Occupational exposure to metal or wood dust and aetiology of cryptogenic fibrosing alveolitis. Lancet 1996;347:284–9.
19. Baumgartner KB, Samet J, Stidley CA, et al. Cigarette smoking: a risk factor for idiopathic pulmonary fibrosis. Am J Respir Crit Care Med 1997;155:242–8.
20. Begin R, Masse S, Cantin A, et al. Airway disease in a subset of nonsmoking rheumatoid patients. Characterization of the disease and evidence for an autoimmune pathogenesis. Am J Med 1982;72:743–50.
21. de Cremoux H, Bernaudin JF, Laurent P, et al. Interactions between cigarette smoking and the natural history of idiopathic pulmonary fibrosis. Chest 1990;98:71–6.
22. Hanley ME, King TE Jr, Schwarz MI, et al. The impact of smoking on mechanical properties of the lungs in idio-

pathic pulmonary fibrosis and sarcoidosis. Am Rev Respir Dis 1991;144:1102–6.

23. Heyneman LE, Ward S, Lynch DA, et al. Respiratory bronchiolitis, respiratory bronchiolitis-associated interstitial lung disease, and desquamative interstitial pneumonia: different entities or part of the spectrum of the same disease process? AJR Am J Roentgenol 1999;173:1617–22.

24. Moon J, du Bois RM, Colby TV, et al. Clinical significance of respiratory bronchiolitis on open lung biopsy and its relationship to smoking-related interstitial lung disease. Thorax 1999;54:1009–14.

25. Nagai S, Hoshino Y, Hayashi M, Ito I. Smoking–related interstitial lung disease. Curr Opin Pulm Med 2000;6:415–9.

26. Ryu JH, Colby TV, Hartman TE, Vassallo R. Smoking-related interstitial lung disease: a concise review. Eur Respir J 2001;17:122–32.

27. Schwartz DA, Merchant RK, Helmers RA, et al. The influence of cigarette smoking on lung function in patients with idiopathic pulmonary fibrosis. Am Rev Respir Dis 1991;144:504–6.

28. King TE Jr, Tooze JA, Schwarz MI, et al. Predicting survival in idiopathic pulmonary fibrosis. Scoring system and survival model. Am J Respir Crit Care Med 2001;164:1171–81.

29. King TE Jr, Schwarz MI, Brown K, et al. Idiopathic pulmonary fibrosis. Relationship between histopathologic features and mortality. Am J Respir Crit Care Med 2001;164:1025–32.

30. Mapel DW, Coultas DB. The environmental epidemiology of idiopathic interstitial lung disease, including sarcoidosis. Semin Respir Crit Care Med 1999;20:521–9.

31. Crystal RG, Fulmer JD, Roberts WC, et al. Idiopathic pulmonary fibrosis: clinical, histologic, radiographic, physiologic, scintigraphic, cytologic and biochemical aspects. Ann Intern Med 1976;85:769–88.

32. Thomas AQ, Lane K, Phillips J III, et al. Heterozygosity for a surfactant protein C gene mutation associated with usual interstitial pneumonitis and cellular nonspecific interstitial pneumonitis in one kindred. Am J Respir Crit Care Med 2002;165:1322–8.

33. Gaensler EA, Goff AM, Prowse CM. Desquamative interstitial pneumonia. N Engl J Med 1966;274:113–28.

34. Kuisk H, Sanchez JS. Desquamative interstitial pneumonia and idiopathic diffuse pulmonary fibrosis with their advanced final stages as "muscular cirrhosis of the lungs" (diffuse bronchiolectasis with muscular hyperplasia). AJR Am J Roentgenol 1969;107:258–79.

35. Tubbs RR, Benjamin SP, Osborne DG, Barenberg S. Surface and transmission ultrastructural characteristics of desquamative interstitial pneumonitis. Hum Pathol 1978;9:693–703.

36. Patchefsky AS, Banner M, Freundlich IM. Desquamative interstitial pneumonia significance of intranuclear viral-like inclusion bodies. Ann Intern Med 1971;74:322–7.

37. Kawanami O, Ferrans VJ, Fulmer JD, Crystal RG. Nuclear inclusions in alveolar epithelium of patients with fibrotic lung disorders. Am J Pathol 1979;94:301–12.

38. Shortland JR, Darke CS, Crane WAJ. Electron microscopy of desquamative interstitial pneumonia. Thorax 1969;24:192–208.

39. McNary WFJ, Gaensler EA. Intranuclear inclusion bodies in desquamative interstitial pneumonia. Electron microscopic observations. Ann Intern Med 1971;74:404–7.

40. Egan JJ, Woodcock AA, Stewart JP. Viruses and idiopathic pulmonary fibrosis. Eur Respir J 1997;10:1433–7.

41. Pinsker KL, Schneyer B, Becker N, Kamholz SL. Usual interstitial pneumonia following Texas A2 influenza infection. Chest 1981;80:123–6.

42. Jiwa M, Steenbergen RD, Zwaan FE, et al. Three sensitive methods for the detection of cytomegalovirus in lung tissue of patients with interstitial pneumonitis. Am J Clin Pathol 1990;93:491–4.

43. Irving WL, Day S, Johnston IDA. Idiopathic pulmonary fibrosis and hepatitis C virus infection. Am Rev Respir Dis 1993;148:1683–4.

44. Vergnon JM, Vincent M, De The G, et al. Cryptogenic fibrosing alveolitis and Epstein-Barr virus: an association? Lancet 1984;ii:768–71.

45. Egan JJ, Stewart JP, Hasleton PS, et al. Epstein-Barr virus replication within pulmonary epithelial cells in cryptogenic fibrosing alveolitis. Thorax 1995;50:1234–9.

46. Brewer DB, Heath D, Asquith P. Electron microscopy of desquamative interstitial pneumonia. J Pathol 1969;97:317–23.

47. Farr GH, Harley RA, Henninagr GR. Desquamative interstitial pneumonia. An electron microscopic study. Am J Pathol 1970;60:347–70.

48. O'Shea PA, Yardley JH. The Hamman-Rich syndrome in infancy: report of a case with virus-like particles by electron microscopy. Johns Hopkins Med J 1970;126:320–36.

49. Sutinen S, Rainio P, Sutinen S, et al. Ultrastructure of terminal respiratory epithelium and prognosis in chronic interstitial pneumonia. Eur J Respir Dis 1980;61:325–36.

50. Coalson JJ. The ultrastructure of human fibrosing alveolitis. Virchows Arch (Pathol Anat) 1982;395:181–99.

51. Corrin B, Dewar A, Rodriquez-Roisin R, Turner-Warwick M. Fine structural changes in cryptogenic fibrosing alveolitis and asbestosis. J Pathol 1985;147:107–19.

52. Ueda T, Ohta K, Suzuki N, et al. Idiopathic pulmonary fibrosis and high prevalence of serum antibodies to hepatitis C virus. Am Rev Respir Dis 1992;146:266–8.

53. Meliconi R, Andreone P, Fasano L, et al. Incidence of hepatitis C virus infection in Italian patients with idiopathic pulmonary fibrosis. Thorax 1996;51:315–7.

54. Kuwano K, Nomoto Y, Kunitake R, et al. Detection of adenovirus E1A DNA in pulmonary fibrosis using nested polymerase chain reaction. Eur Respir J 1997;10:1445–9.

55. Watters LC. Genetic aspects of idiopathic pulmonary fibrosis and hypersensitivity pneumonitis. Semin Respir Med 1986;7:317–25.

56. Rosenberg DM. Inherited forms of interstitial lung disease. Clin Chest Med 1982;3:635–41.

57. Marshall RP, McAnulty RJ, Laurent GJ. The pathogenesis of pulmonary fibrosis: is there a fibrosis gene? Int J Biochem Cell Biol 1997;29:107–20.

58. Lympany PA, du Bois RM. Diffuse lung disease: product of genetic susceptibility and environmental encounters. Thorax 1997;52:92–4.

59. Verleden GM, du Bois RM, Bouros D, et al. Genetic predisposition and pathogenetic mechanisms of interstitial lung disease of unknown origin. Eur Respir J 2001;32 Suppl:17S–29S.

60. Marshall RP, Puddicombe A, Cookson WO, Laurent GJ. Adult familial cryptogenic fibrosing alveolitis in the United Kingdom. Thorax 2000;55:143–6.

61. Beaumont F, Jansen HM, Elema JD, et al. Simultaneous occurrence of pulmonary interstitial fibrosis and alveolar cell carcinoma in one family. Thorax 1981;36:252–8.

62. McDonnel L, Sweeney EC, Jagoe WS, et al. Familial pulmonary fibrosis and lung cancer. Ir J Med Sci 1982;151:315–7.

63. Sandoz E. Uber zwei falle von fotaler bronchektasie. Beitr Pathol Anat 1907;41:495–516.

64. MacMillan JM. Familial pulmonary fibrosis. Dis Chest 1951;20:426–36.

65. Donohue WL, Laski B, Uchida I, Munn JD. Familial fibrocystic pulmonary dysplasia and its relation to the Hamman-Rich syndrome. Pediatrics 1959;24:786–813.

66. Appelman AC, Buytendijk HJ. Chronische interstitiele pneumonie/syndroom van Hamman-Rich/in een familie. Ned Tijdsch Geneeskd 1961;105:1928–30.

67. Resek PHP, Tolbert WM. Kongenitale/familiare/zystischc fibroses der lunge. Wien Klin Wochenschr 1962;74:869–73.

68. Davies GM, Potts MW. Chronic diffuse interstitial pulmonary fibrosis in brothers. Guys Hosp Rep 1964;113:36–44.

69. Hughes EW. Familial incidence of diffuse interstitial fibrosis. Postgrad Med J 1965;41:150–2.

70. Ellis RH. Familial incidence of diffuse interstitial fibrosis. Postgrad Med J 1965;41:150–2.

71. Young WA. Familial fibrocystic dysplasia. Can Med Assoc J 1966;94:1059–61.

72. Adelman AG, Chertkow G, Hayton RC. Familial fibrocystic pulmonary dysplasia. A detailed family study. Can Med Assoc J 1966;95:603–10.

73. Koch B. Familial fibrocystic pulmonary dysplasia: observations in one family. Can Med Assoc J 1967;92:801–8.

74. Swaye P, Van Ordstrand HS, McCormack LJ, Wolpaw SE. Familial Hamman-Rich syndrome. Report of eight cases. Dis Chest 1969;55:7–12.

75. Perry KMA, Benson MK, Hughes DT. Fibrosis pulmonar intersticial familiar. Pneu Med Argent 1971;58:495–500.

76. Nezelof C, Brien A, Beal G, et al. Fibropulmonaire familiale. Ann Pediatr (Paris) 1974;21:135–44.

77. Evans CC. HLA antigens in diffuse fibrosing alveolitis [abstract]. Thorax 1976;31:483.

78. Strimlan CV, Taswell HF, DeRemee RA, Keuppers F. HLA antigens and fibrosing alveolitis. Am Rev Respir Dis 1977;116:1120–1.

79. Fulmer JD, Sposovska MS, von Gal ER, et al. Distribution of HLA antigens in idiopathic pulmonary fibrosis. Am Rev Respir Dis 1978;118:141–7.

80. Varpela E, Tiilikainen A, Varpela M, Tukiainen P. High prevalences of HLA-BI5 and HLA-Dw6 in patients with cryptogenic fibrosing alveolitis. Tissue Antigens 1979;14:68–71.

81. O'Brodovich HM, Moser MM, Lu L. Familial lymphoid interstitial pneumonia: a long-term follow-up. Pediatrics 1980; 65:523–8.

82. Bitterman PB, Crystal RG. Is there a fibrotic gene? Chest 1980;78:549–50.

83. Murphy A, O'Sullivan BJ. Familial fibrosing alveolitis. Ir J Med Sci 1981;150:204–9.

84. Manigand G, Oury M, Faux N, et al. Familial diffuse interstitial pulmonary fibrosis [letter]. Nouv Presse Med 1982;11:50–1.

85. Libby DM, Gibofsky A, Fotino M, et al. Immunogenetic and clinical findings in IPF association with the B-cell alloantigen HLA-DR2. Am Rev Respir Dis 1983;127:618–22.

86. Prichard MG, Musk AW. Adverse effect of pregnancy on familial fibrosing alveolitis. Thorax 1984;39:319–20.

87. Tal A, Maor E, Bar-Ziv J, Gorodischer R. Fatal desquamative interstitial pneumonia in three infant siblings. J Pediatr 1984;104:873–6.

88. Barzo P. Familial idiopathic fibrosing alveolitis. Eur J Respir Dis 1985;66:350–2.

89. Musk AW, Zilko PJ, Manners P, et al. Genetic studies in familial fibrosing alveolitis possible linkage with immunoglobulin allotypes (Gm). Chest 1986;89:206–10.

90. Bitterman PB, Rennard SI, Keogh BA, et al. Familial idiopathic pulmonary fibrosis. Evidence of lung inflammation in unaffected family members. N Engl J Med 1986;314:1343–7.

91. Schechter MM. Diffuse interstitial fibrosis of the lungs. Am Rev Tuberc 1953;69:603–14.

92. Peabody JW, Peabody JW Jr, Hayes EW, Hayes EW Jr. Idiopathic pulmonary fibrosis; its occurrence in identical twin sisters. Dis Chest 1950;18:330–44.

93. Bonanni PP, Frymoyer JW, Jacox RF. A family study of idiopathic pulmonary fibrosis. A possible dysproteinemic and genetical determined disease. Am J Med 1965;39:411–21.

94. Solliday NH, Williams JA, Gaensler EA, et al. Familial chronic interstitial pneumonia. Am Rev Respir Dis 1973;108:193–204.

95. Javaheri S, Lederer DH, Pella JA, et al. Idiopathic pulmonary fibrosis in monozygotic twins. The importance of genetic predisposition. Chest 1980;78:591–4.

96. Renzi GD, Lopez-Majano V. Early diagnosis of interstitial fibrosis. Respiration 1976;33:294–302.

97. Riccardi VM. Von Recklinghausen neurofibromatosis. N Engl J Med 1981;305:1617–27.

98. DePinho RA, Kaplan KL. The Hermansky-Pudlak syndrome. Report of three cases and review of pathophysiology and management considerations. Medicine 1985;64:192–202.

99. Hermansky F, Pudlak P. Albinism associated with hemorrhagic diatheses and unusual pigmented reticular cells in the bone marrow. Report of two cases of histochemical studies. Blood 1959;14:162–9.

100. Hoste P, Willems J, Devriendt J, et al. Familial diffuse interstital pulmonary fibrosis associated with oculocutaneous albinism. Report of two cases with a family study. Scand J Respir Dis 1970;60:128–34.

101. Garay SM, Gardella JE, Fazzini EP, Goldring RM. Hermansky-Pudlak syndrome: pulmonary manifestations of a family study. Am J Med 1979;66:219–32.

102. Davies BH, Tuddenham EGD. Familial pulmonary fibrosis associated with oculocutaneous albinism and platelet function defect. QJM 1976;65:219–32.

103. Dwyer JM, Hickie JB, Garvan J. Pulmonary tuberous sclerosis. Report of three patients and a review of the literature. QJM 1971;40:115–25.

104. Berg G, Vejlens G. Maladie kystique du poumon et sclerose tubereuse du cerveau. Acta Paediatr 1939;26:16–30.

105. Makle SK, Pardee N, Martin CJ. Involvement of the lung in tuberous sclerosis. Chest 1970;58:538–40.

106. Harris JO, Waltuck BL, Swenson EW. The pathophysiology of the lungs in tuberous sclerosis. A case report and literature review. Am Rev Respir Dis 1969;100:379–87.

107. Master K, Ting EY, Katz M. Pathophysiology in pulmonary tuberous sclerosis. N Y State J Med 1974;74:2000–3.

108. Schneider EL, Epstein CJ, Kaback MJ, Brandes D. Severe pulmonary involvement in adult Gaucher's disease. Report of three cases and review of the literature. Am J Med 1977; 63:475–80.

109. Wolson AH. Pulmonary findings in Gaucher's disease. AJR Am J Roentgenol 1975;123:712–5.

110. Carrington CB, Cergell DW, Gaensler EA, et al. Lymphangioleiomyomatosis. Physiologic-patholog-radiolog correlations. Am Rev Respir Dis 1977;116:977–95.

111. Demedts M, Auwerx J, Goddeeris P, et al. The inherited association of interstitial lung disease, hypocalciuric hypercalcemia, and defective granulocytic function. Am Rev Respir Dis 1985;131:470–5.

112. Hodgson U, Laitinen T, Tukiainen P. Nationwide prevalence of sporadic and familial idiopathic pulmonary fibrosis: evidence of founder effect among multiplex families in Finland. Thorax 2002;57:338–42.

113. Buchino JJ, Keenan WJ, Algren JT, Bove KE. Familial desquamative interstitial pneumonitis occurring in infants. Am J Med Genet Suppl 1987;3:285–91.

114. Wright JA, Pennington JE. Familial lymphoid interstitial pneumonitis [abstract]. J Pediatr 1987;111:638.

115. Nogee LM, Dunbar AE III, Wert SE, et al. A mutation in the surfactant protein C gene associated with familial interstitial lung disease. N Engl J Med 2001;344:573–9.

116. Nogee LM, Dunbar AE III, Wert S, et al. Mutations in the surfactant protein C gene associated with interstitial lung disease. Chest 2002;121:20S–1S.

117. Amin RS, Wert SE, Baughman RP, et al. Surfactant protein deficiency in familial interstitial lung disease. J Pediatr 2001;139:85–92.

118. Whitsett JA. Genetic basis of familial interstitial lung disease: misfolding or function of surfactant protein C? Am J Respir Crit Care Med 2002;165:1201–2.

119. Marney A, Lane KB, Phillips JA III, et al. Idiopathic pulmonary fibrosis can be an autosomal dominant trait in some families [abstract]. Chest 2001;120:56S.

120. Turton CWG, Morris LM, Lawler SD, Turner-Warwick M. HLA in cryptogenic fibrosing alveolitis. Lancet 1978;i: 507–8.

121. Geddes DM, Brewerton DA, Webley M, et al. α1-antitrypsin phenotypes in fibrosing alveolitis and rheumatoid arthritis. Lancet 1977;ii:1049–51.

122. Briggs DC, Vaughan RW, Welsh KI, et al. Immunogenetic prediction of pulmonary fibrosis in systemic sclerosis. Lancet 1991;338:661–2.

123. Keogh BA, Crystal RG. Alveolitis: the key to the interstitial lung disorders [editorial]. Thorax 1982;37:1–10.

124. Rosan RC. Alveolitis. A functional tip for the morphologic crutch. Chest 1977;72:134–5.

125. Sheppard D. Pulmonary fibrosis: a cellular overreaction or a failure of communication? J Clin Invest 2001;107:1501–2.

126. Selman M, King TE Jr, Pardo A. Idiopathic pulmonary fibrosis: prevailing and evolving hypotheses about its pathogenesis and implications for therapy. Ann Intern Med 2001;134:136–51.

127. Gauldie J, Kolb M, Sime PJ. A new direction in the pathogenesis of idiopathic pulmonary fibrosis? Respir Res 2002;3:1–3.

128. Strieter RM, Belperio JA, Keane MP. Cytokines in innate host defense in the lung. J Clin Invest 2002;109:699–705.

129. Keane MP, Strieter RM. The importance of balanced pro-inflammatory and anti-inflammatory mechanisms in diffuse lung disease. Respir Res 2002;3:5.

130. Crystal RG, Gadek JE, Ferrans VJ, et al. Interstitial lung disease: current concepts of pathogenesis, staging, and therapy. Am J Med 1981;70:542–68.

131. Haslam PL, Thompson B, Mohammed I, et al. Circulating immune complexes in patients with cryptogenic fibrosing alveolitis. Clin Exp Immunol 1979;37:381–90.

132. Gelb AF, Dreisin RB, Epstein JD, et al. Immune complexes, gallium lung scans, and bronchoalveolar lavage in idiopathic interstitial pneumonitis-fibrosis. Chest 1983;84:148–153.

133. Davis GS, Brody AR, Craighead JE. Analysis of airspace and interstitial mononuclear cell populations in human diffuse interstitial lung disease. Am Rev Respir Dis 1978;118:7–15.

134. Haslam PL, Turton CWG, Heard B, et al. Bronchoalveolar lavage in pulmonary fibrosis: comparison of cells obtained with lung biopsy and clinical features. Thorax 1980;35:9–18.

135. Haslam PL, Turton CWG, Lukoszek A, et al. Bronchoalveolar lavage fluid cell counts in cryptogenic fibrosing alveolitis and their relation to therapy. Thorax 1980;35:328–39.

136. Haslam P. Bronchoalveolar lavage. Semin Respir Med 1984; 6:55–70.

137. Carrington CB, Gaensler EA, Coutu RE, et al. Natural history and treated course of usual and desquamative interstitial pneumonia. N Engl J Med 1978;298:801–9.

138. Dreisin RB, Schwarz MI, Theofilopoulos AN, Stanford RE. Circulating immune complexes in the idiopathic interstitial pneumonias. N Engl J Med 1978;298:353–7.

139. Hunninghake GW, Gadek JE, Lawley TJ, Crystal RG. Mechanisms of neutrophil accumulation in the lungs of patients with idiopathic pulmonary fibrosis. J Clin Invest 1981; 68:259–69.

140. Keogh BA, Bernardo J, Hunninghake GW, et al. Effect of intermittent high dose parenteral corticosteroids on the alveolitis of idiopathic pulmonary fibrosis. Am Rev Respir Dis 1983;127:18–22.

141. Winterbauer RH, Hammar SP, Hallman KO, et al. Diffuse interstitial pneumonitis. Clinicopathologic correlations in 20 patients treated with prednisone/azathioprine. Am J Med 1978;65:661–72.

142. Borzone G, Moreno R, Urrea R, et al. Bleomycin-induced chronic lung damage does not resemble human idiopathic pulmonary fibrosis. Am J Respir Crit Care Med 2001; 163:1648–53.

143. Usuki J, Fukuda Y. Evolution of three patterns of intra-alveolar fibrosis produced by bleomycin in rats. Pathol Int 1995;45:552–64.

144. Fukuda Y, Mochimaru H, Terasaki Y, et al. Mechanism of structural remodeling in pulmonary fibrosis. Chest 2001; 120:41S–43S.

145. Schwarz MI, King TE. Pleuropulmonary manifestation of the collagen vascular disorders. In: Mitchell RS, Petty TP, editors. Synopsis of clinical pulmonary diseases. St. Louis (MO): CV Mosby; 1982. p. 296.

146. Davis WB, Crystal RG. Chronic interstitial lung disease. In: Simmons ED, editor. Current pulmonary. Vol. 5. New York: John Wiley & Sons; 1984. p. 347.

147. Mackay IR, Ritchie B. Diffuse fibrosing alveolitis (diffuse interstitial fibrosis of the lungs): two cases with autoimmune features. Thorax 1965;20:200–5.

148. Williams AJ, Marsh J, Stableforth DE. Crytogenic fibrosing alveolitis; chronic active hepatitis and autoimmune haemolytic anaemia in the same patient. Br J Dis Chest 1985;79:200–3.

149. Weissman E, Becker NH. Interstitial lung disease in primary biliary cirrhosis. Am J Med Sci 1983;285:21–7.

150. Turner-Warwick M. Fibrosing alveolitis and chronic liver disease. QJM 1968;37:133–49.

151. May JJ, Schwarz ME, Driesin RB. Idiopathic thrombocytopenic purpura occurring with interstitial pneumonitis. Ann Intern Med 1979;90:199–200.

152. Bombardieri S, Paoletti P, DiMunno O, et al. Lung involvement in essential mixed cryoglobulinemia. Am J Med 1979;66:748–56.

153. Heatley RV, Thomas P, Prokipchuk EJ, et al. Pulmonary function abnormalities in patients with inflammatory bowel disease. QJM 1982;51:241–50.

154. McFadden RG, Craig ID, Paterson NAM. Interstitial pneumonitis is myasthenia gravis. Br J Dis Chest 1984;78: 187–91.

155. Mason AMS, McIllMurray MD, Golding PL, Hughes DTD. Fibrosing alveolitis associated with renal tubercular acidosis. Br J Dis Chest 1970;4:596–9.

156. Hodson ME, Haslam PL, Spiro SG, et al. Digital vasculitis in patients with cryptogenic fibrosing alveolitis. Br J Dis Chest 1984;78:140–8.

157. Campbell EJ, Harris B. Idiopathic pulmonary fibrosis (clinical conference). Arch Intern Med 1981;141:771–4.

158. Schwarz MI, Dreisin RB, Pratt DS, Stanford RE. Immunofluorescent patterns in the idiopathic interstitial pneumonias. J Lab Clin Med 1978;91:929–38.

159. Gadek J, Hunninghake G, Zimmerman R, Killman J. Pathogenetic studies in idiopathic pulmonary fibrosis. Control of neutrophil migration by immune complexes. Chest 1979;2:264–5.

160. Jansen JM, Schutte AJH, Elema ID, Giessen MVD. Local immune complexes and inflammatory response in patients with chronic interstitial pulmonary disorders associated with collagen vascular diseases. Clin Exp Immunol 1984;56:311–20.

161. King TE, Schwarz MI, Dreisin RB, et al. Circulating immune complexes in pulmonary eosinophilic granuloma. Ann Intern Med l979;91:397–9.

162. King TE, Christopher KL, Zeballos J, et al. Bronchoalveolar lavage, gallium-67 citrate lung scanning and circulating immune complexes in the staging of idiopathic pulmonary fibrosis: correlation with physiologic and morphologic features [abstract]. Clin Res 1984;32:63A.

163. Cocchiara R, Giallongo A, Amoroso S, et al. Circulating immune complexes in patients with usual interstitial pulmonary fibrosis: partial characterization and relationship with *Thermoactinomyces vulgaris*. Immunology 1981;44:817–25.

164. Daniele RP, Henson PM, Fantone JCI, et al. Symposium. Immune complexes injury of the lung. Am Rev Respir Dis 1981;124:738–55.

165. Scadding JG, Hinson KFW. Diffuse fibrosing alveolitis (diffuse interstitial fibrosis of the lungs): correlation of histology at biopsy with prognosis. Thorax 1967;22:291–304.

166. Nagaya H, Buckley CE, Sieher HO. Positive antinuclear factor in patients with unexplained pulmonary fibrosis. Ann Intern Med 1969;76:1135–45.

167. Nagaya H, Sieker HO. Pathogenetic mechanisms of interstitial pulmonary fibrosis in patients with serum antinuclear factor. A histologic and clinical correlation. Am J Med 1972;52:51–62.

168. Turner-Warwick M, Haslam P, Weeks J. Antibodies in some chronic fibrosing lung diseases II. Immunofluorescent studies. Clin Allergy 1971;1:209–19.

169. Chapman JR, Charles PJ, Venables PJW, et al. Definition and clinical relevance of antibodies to nuclear ribonucleoprotein and other nuclear antigens in patients with cryptogenic fibrosing alveolitis. Am Rev Respir Dis 1984;130:439–43.

170. Gottlieb AJ, Spiera H, Teirstein AS, Siltzbach LE. Serologic factors in idiopathic diffuse interstitial pulmonary fibrosis. Am J Med 1965;39:405–10.

171. Haslam P, Turner-Warwick M, Lukoszek A. Antinuclear antibody and lymphocyte responses to nuclear antigens in patients with lung disease. Clin Exp Immunol 1975;20:379–95.

172. Hunninghake GW, Kawanami O, Ferrans VJ, et al. Characterization of the inflammatory and immune effector cells in the lung parenchyma of patients with interstitial lung disease. Am Rev Respir Dis 1981;123:407–12.

173. Paradis IL, Dauber JH, Rabin BS. Lymphocyte phenotypes in bronchoalveolar lavage and lung tissue in sarcoidosis and idiopathic pulmonary fibrosis. Am Rev Respir Dis 1986;133:855–60.

174. Daniele RP, Elias JA, Epstein PE, Rossman MD. Bronchoalveolar lavage: role in the pathogenesis, diagnosis, and management of interstitial lung disease. Ann Intern Med 1985;102:93–108.

175. Mathieson JR, Mayo JR, Staples CA, Muller NL. Chronic diffuse infiltrative lung disease: comparison of diagnostic accuracy of CT and chest radiography. Radiology 1989;171:111–6.

176. Swensen SJ, Aughenbaugh GL, Brown LR. High-resolution computed tomography of the lung. Mayo Clin Proc 1989;64:1284–94.

177. Livingstone JL, Lewis JG, Reid L, Jefferson KE. Diffuse interstitial pulmonary fibrosis. A clinical, radiological, and pathological study based on 45 patients. QJM 1964;33:71–103.

178. Felson B. A new look at pattern recognition of diffuse pulmonary disease. AJR Am J Roentgenol 1979;133:183–9.

179. Watters LC, King TE, Schwarz MI, Waldron JA, et al. A clinical, radiographic, and physiologic scoring system for the longitudinal assessment of patients with idiopathic pulmonary fibrosis. Am Rev Respir Dis 1986;133:97–103.

180. McLoud TC, Carrington CB, Gaensler EA. Diffuse infiltrative lung disease: a new scheme for description. Radiology 1983;149:353–63.

181. Liebow AA, Steer A, Billingsley JG. Desquamative interstitial pneumonia. Am J Med 1965;39:369–404.

182. Epler GR, McLoud TC, Gaensler EA, et al. Normal chest roentgenograms in chronic diffuse infiltrative lung disease. N Engl J Med 1978;298:934–9.

183. Galko B, Grossman RF, Day A, et al. Hypertrophic pulmonary osteoarthropathy in four patients with interstitial pulmonary disease. Chest 1985;88:94–7.

184. Massaro D, Katz S. Fibrosing alveolitis: its occurrence, roentgenographic and pathologic features in von Recklinghausen's neurofibromatosis. Am Rev Respir Dis 1966;93:934–42.

185. Hargreave F, Hinson KF, Reid L, et al. The radiological appearances of allergic alveolitis due to bird sensitivity (bird fancier's lung). Clin Radiol 1972;23:1–10.

186. Unger GF, Scanlon GT, Fink JN, Unger JD. A radiologic approach to hypersensitivity pneumonias. Radiol Clin North Am 1973;11:339–56.

187. Soutar CA, Simon G, Turner-Warwick M. The radiology of asbestos-induced disease of the lungs. Br J Dis Chest 1974;68:235–52.

188. Webb RW. High-resolution CT of the lung parenchyma. Radiol Clin North Am 1989;27:1085–97.

189. Staples C, Muller N, Vedal S, et al. Usual interstitial pneumonia: correlation of CT with clinical, functional, and radiographic findings. Radiology 1987;162:377–81.

190. Muller N, Staples C, Miller R, et al. Disease activity in idiopathic pulmonary fibrosis: CT and pathologic correlation. Radiology 1987;165:731–4.

191. Muller NL, Miller RR, Webb WR, et al. Fibrosing alveolitis CT–pathologic correlation. Radiology 1986;160:585–8.

192. Bergin CJ, Muller NL. CT of interstitial lung disease: a diagnostic approach. AJR Am J Roentgenol 1987;148:9–15.

193. Bergin CJ, Muller NL. CT in the diagnosis of interstitial lung disease. AJR Am J Roentgenol 1985;145:505–10.

194. Bergin CJ, Coblentz CL, Chiles C, et al. Chronic lung disease: specific diagnosis by using CT. AJR Am J Roentgenol 1989;152:1183–8.

195. Wells AU, Rubens MB, du Bois RM, Hansell DM. Serial CT in fibrosing alveolitis: prognostic significance of the initial pattern. AJR Am J Roentgenol 1993;161:1159–65.

196. Wells AU, du Bois RM. Prediction of disease progression in idiopathic pulmonary fibrosis. Eur Respir J 1994;7:637–9.

197. Remy-Jardin M, Giraud F, Remy J, et al. Importance of ground-glass attenuation in chronic diffuse infiltrative lung disease: pathologic–CT correlation. Radiology 1993;189:693–8.

198. Lynch DA, Newell JD, Logan PM, et al. Can CT distinguish idiopathic pulmonary fibrosis from hypersensitivity pneumonitis? AJR Am J Roentgenol 1995;165:807–11.

299. Kreel L. Computed tomography of interstitial pulmonary disease. J Comput Assist Tomogr 1982;6:181–99.

200. Solomon A, Kreel L, McNicol M, Johnson N. Computed tomography in pulmonary sarcoidosis. J Comput Assist Tomogr 1979;3:754–8.

201. Steinberg DL, Webb WR. CT appearances of rheumatoid lung disease. J Comput Assist Tomogr 1984;8:881–4.

202. Wright PH, Buxton-Thomas M, Kreel L, Steel SJ. Cryptogenic fibrosing alveolitis: pattern of disease in the lung. Thorax 1984;39:857–61.

203. Zerhouni E, Naidich D, Stitik F, et al. Computed tomography of the pulmonary parenchyma. Part 2: interstitial disease. J Thorac Imag 1985;1:54–64.

204. Nakata H, Kimoto T, Nakayama T, et al. Diffuse peripheral lung disease: evaluation by high-resolution computed tomography. Radiology 1985;157:181–5.

205. Raghu G, Mageto YN, Lockhart D, et al. The accuracy of the clinical diagnosis of new-onset idiopathic pulmonary fibrosis and other interstitial lung disease: a prospective study. Chest 1999;116:1168–74.

206. Hunninghake G, Zimmerman MB, Schwartz DA, et al. Utility of lung biopsy for the diagnosis of idiopathic pulmonary fibrosis. Am J Respir Crit Care Med 2001;164:193–6.

207. Grenier P, Chevret S, Beigelman C, et al. Chronic diffuse infiltrative lung disease: determination of the diagnostic value of clinical data, chest radiography, and CT with Bayesian analysis. Radiology 1994;191:383–90.

208. Tung KT, Wells AU, Rubens MB, et al. Accuracy of the typical computed tomographic appearances of fibrosing alveolitis. Thorax 1993;48:334–8.

209. Wells AU, Hansell DM, Corrin B, et al. High resolution computed tomography as a predictor of lung histology in systemic sclerosis. Thorax 1992;47:508–12.

210. Leung AN, Miller RR, Muller NL. Parenchymal opacification in chronic infiltrative lung disease: CT–pathologic correlation. Radiology 1993;188:209–14.

211. Braude AC, Chamberlain DW, Rebuck AS. Pulmonary disposition of gallium-67 in humans: concise communication. J Nucl Med 1982;23:574–6.

212. Higasi T, Nakayam Y, Mureta A. Clinical evaluation of ^{67}Ga-citrate scanning. J Nucl Med 1972;13:196–201.

213. Lavender PJ, Lowe J, Barker JR, et al. Gallium-67 citrate scanning in neoplastic and inflammatory lesions. Br J Radiol 1971;44:361–6.

214. Van der Schoot JB, Groen AS, deJong J. Gallium-67 scintigraphy in lung diseases. Thorax 1972;27:543–6.

215. Dige-Peterson H, Heckscher T, Hertz M. ^{67}Ga-scintigraphy in nonmalignant lung diseases. Scand J Respir Dis 1972; 53:314–9.

216. Line BR, Fulmer JD, Reynolds HY, et al. Gallium-67 citrate scanning in the staging of idiopathic pulmonary fibrosis correlation with physiologic and morphologic features and bronchoalveolar lavage. Am Rev Respir Dis 1978;118:355–65.

217. Line BR, Hunninghake GW, Keogh BA, et al. Gallium-67 scanning to stage the alveolitis of sarcoidosis: correlation with clinical studies, pulmonary function studies and bronchoalveolar lavage. Am Rev Respir Dis 1981;123:440–6.

218. Wesselius LJ, Witztum KF, Taylor AT, et al. Computer-assisted versus visual lung Gallium-67 index in normal subjects and in patients with interstitial lung disorders. Am Rev Respir Dis 1983;128:1084–9.

219. Johnson DG, Johnson SM, Harris CC, et al. Ga-67 uptake in the lung in sarcoidosis. Radiology 1984;150:551–5.

220. Niden AH, Mishkin FS, Khurana MML. [67]Gallium citrate lung scans in interstitial lung disease. Chest 1976; 69 Suppl:266–8.

221. Beaumont D, Herry JY, Sapene M, et al. Gallium-67 in the evaluation of sarcoidosis: correlations with serum angiotension-converting enzyme and bronchoalveolar lavage. Thorax 1982;37:11–8.

222. Wallaert B, Ramon P, Fournier E, et al. Bronchoalveolar lavage, serum angiotension-converting enzyme, and gallium-67 scanning in extrathoracic sarcoidosis. Chest 1982;82:553–5.

223. Schoenberger CI, Line BR, Keogh BA, et al. Lung inflammation in sarcoidosis: comparison of serum angiotension-converting enzyme levels with bronchoalveolar lavage and gallium-67 scanning assessment of the T lymphocyte alveolitis. Thorax 1982;37:19–25.

224. Collard HR, King TE Jr. Lung biopsy in patients with usual interstitial pneumonia. Eur Respir J 2001;18:895–8.

225. Bensard DD, McIntyre RC Jr, Waring BJ, Simon JS. Comparison of video thoracoscopic lung biopsy to open lung biopsy in the diagnosis of interstitial lung disease. Chest 1993;103:765–70.

226. Gaensler EA, Carrington CB. Open biopsy for chronic diffuse infiltrative lung disease clinical, roentgenographic, and physiological correlations in 502 patients. Ann Thorac Surg 1980;30:411–26.

227. Ray JF III, Lawton BR, Myers WO, et al. Open pulmonary biopsy. Nineteen-year experience with 416 consecutive operations. Chest 1976;69:43–7.

228. Newman SL, Michel RP, Wang NS. Lingular lung biopsy: is it representative? Am Rev Respir Dis 1985;132:1084–6.

229. Wall CP, Gaensler EA, Carrington CB, Hayes JA. Comparison of transbronchial and open biopsies in chronic infiltrative lung diseases. Am Rev Respir Dis 1981;123:280–5.

230. King TE Jr, Costabel U, Cordier J-F, et al. American Thoracic Society. Idiopathic pulmonary fibrosis: diagnosis and treatment. International consensus statement. American Thoracic Society (ATS), and the European Respiratory Society (ERS). Am J Respir Crit Care Med 2000;161:646–64.

231. Johnston IDA, Prescott RJ, Chalmers JC, Rudd RM, for the Fibrosing Alveolitis Subcommittee of the Research Committee of the British Thoracic Society. British Thoracic Society study of cryptogenic fibrosing alveolitis: current presentation and initial management. Thorax 1997;52:38–44.

232. Stack BHR, Choo-Kang YEJ, Heard BE. The prognosis of cryptogenic fibrosing alveolitis. Thorax 1972;27:535–42.

233. Cegla UH, Kroidl RF, Meier-Sydow J, et al. Therapy of the idiopathic fibrosis of the lung. Experiences with three therapeutic principles corticosteroids in combination with azathioprine, D-penicillamine, and para-amino-benzoate. Pneumonologie 1975;152:75–92.

234. Turner-Warwick M, Burrows B, Johnson A. Cryptogenic fibrosing alveolitis: clinical features and their influence on survival. Thorax 1980;35:171–80.

235. Turner-Warwick M, Burrows B, Johnson A. Cryptogenic fibrosing alveolitis: response to corticosteroid treatment and its effect on survival. Thorax 1980;35:593–9.

236. Costabel U, Matthys H. Different therapies and factors influencing response to therapy in idiopathic diffuse fibrosing alveolitis. Respiration 1981;42:141–9.

237. Tukiainen P, Taskinen E, Holsti P, et al. Prognosis of cryptogenic fibrosing alveolitis. Thorax 1983;38:349–55.

238. Davis GS. Idiopathic pulmonary fibrosis. In: Cherniack RM, editor. Current therapy of respiratory disease–2. Toronto: BC Decker; 1986. p. 161.

239. Mapel DW, Samet JM, Coultas DB. Corticosteroids and the treatment of idiopathic pulmonary fibrosis. Past, present, and future. Chest 1996;110:1058–67.

240. Lynch JP III, White E, Flaherty K. Corticosteroids in idiopathic pulmonary fibrosis. Curr Opin Pulm Med 2001;7:298–308.

241. Kovacs WJ. Molecular mechanisms of glucocorticoid action. In: Rose BD, editor. UpToDate. Wellesley, MA: UpToDate; 2002.

242. Ozaki T, Nakayama T, Ishimi H, et al. Glucocorticoid receptors in bronchoalveolar cells from the patients with idiopathic pulmonary fibrosis. Am Rev Respir Dis 1982;127: 968–71.

243. Lacronique JG, Rennard SI, Bitterman PB, et al. Alveolar macrophages in idiopathic pulmonary fibrosis have glucocorticoid receptors, but glucocorticoid therapy does not suppress alveolar macrophage release of fibronectin and alveolar macrophage derived growth factor. Am Rev Respir Dis 1984;130:450–6.

244. Walsh LJ, Wong CA, Oborne J, et al. Adverse effects of oral corticosteroids in relation to dose in patients with lung disease. Thorax 2001;56:279–84.

245. Flaherty KR, Toews GB, Lynch JP III, et al. Steroids in idiopathic pulmonary fibrosis: a prospective assessment of adverse reactions, response to therapy, and survival. Am J Med 2001;110:278–82.

246. Turner-Warwick M, Haslam PL. The value of serial bronchoalveolar lavages in assessing the clinical progress of patients with cryptogenic fibrosing alveolitis. Am Rev Respir Dis 1987;135: 26–34.

247. Weese WC, Levine BW, Kazemi H. Interstitial lung disease resistant to corticosteroid therapy. Report of three cases treated with azathioprine or cyclophosphamide. Chest 1975;67:57–60.

248. Meuret G, Fueter R, Gloor F. Early stage of fulminant idiopathic pulmonary fibrosis cured by intense combination therapy using cyclophosphamide, vincristine, and prednisone. Respiration 1978;36:228–33.

249. Johnson MA, Kwan S, Snell NJC, et al. Randomized controlled trial comparing prednisolone alone with cyclophosphamide and low dose prednisolone in combination in cryptogenic fibrosing alveolitis. Thorax 1989;44:280–8.

250. Brown CH, Turner-Warwick M. The treatment of cryptogenic fibrosing alveolitis with immunosuppressant drugs. QJM 1971;40:289–302.

251. Topilow AA, Ruthenberg SP, Cottrell TS. Interstitial pneumonia after prolonged treatment with cyclophosphamide. Am Rev Respir Dis 1973;108:114–7.

252. Baughman RP, Lower EE. Use of intermittent, intravenous cyclophosphamide for idiopathic pulmonary fibrosis. Chest 1992;102:1090–4.

253. Zisman DA, Lynch JP III, Toews GB, et al. Cyclophosphamide in the treatment of idiopathic pulmonary fibrosis: a prospective study in patients who failed to respond to corticosteroids. Chest 2000;117:1619–26.

254. Burke DA, Stoddart JC, Ward MK, Simpson CGB. Fatal pulmonary fibrosis occurring during treatment with cyclophosphamide. Br Med J 1982;285:696.

255. Mark GJ, Lehingor-Zadeh A, Ragsdale BD. Cyclophosphamide pneumonitis. Thorax 1978;33:89–93.

256. Malik SW, Myers JL, DeRemee RA, Specks U. Lung toxicity associated with cyclophosphamide use. Two distinct patterns. Am J Respir Crit Care Med 1996;154:1851–6.

257. Segura A, Yuste A, Cercos A, et al. Pulmonary fibrosis induced by cyclophosphamide. Ann Pharmacother 2001;35:894–7.

258. Meier-Sydow J, Rust M, Kronenberger H, et al. Long-term follow-up of lung function parameters in patients with idiopathic pulmonary fibrosis treated with prednisone and azathioprine or D-penicillamine. Prax Pneumol 1979;33:680–8.

259. Dubrawsky C, Dubravsky NB, Withers HR. The effect of colchicine on the accumulation of hydroxyproline and on lung compliance after irradiation. Radiat Res 1978;73:111–20.

260. Zhang L, Zhu Y, Luo W. The protective effect of colchicine on bleomycin-induced pulmonary fibrosis in rats. Chin Med Sci J 1992;7:58–60.

261. Rennard SI, Bitterman PB, Ozaki T, et al. Colchicine suppresses the release of fibroblast growth factors from alveolar macrophages in vitro. The basis of a possible therapeutic approach to the fibrotic disorders. Am Rev Respir Dis 1988;137:181–5.

262. Selman M, Carrillo G, Salas J, et al. Colchicine, D-penicillamine, and prednisone in the treatment of idiopathic pulmonary fibrosis: a controlled clinical trial. Chest 1998;114:507–12.

263. Pesci A, Bertorelli G, Manganelli P, Ambanelli U. Bronchoalveolar lavage analysis of interstitial lung disease in CREST syndrome. Clin Exp Rheumatol 1986;4:121–4.

264. Lacher MJ. Spontaneous remission response to methotrexate in sarcoidosis. Ann Intern Med 1968;69:1247–8.

265. Lower EE, Baughman RP. The use of low dose methotrexate in refractory sarcoidosis. Am J Med Sci 1990;299:153–7.

266. Lower EE, Baughman RP, Winget D. The long-term use of methotrexate in patients with chronic symptomatic sarcoidosis. Sarcoidosis 1992;9:465S–466S.

267. Scott DGI, Bacon PA. Response to methotrexate in fibrosing alveolitis associated with connective tissue disease. Thorax 1980;35:725–31.

268. Ward WF, Shih-Heollwarth A, Tuttle RD. Collagen accumulation in irradiated rat lung: modification by D-penicillamine. Radiology 1983;146:533–7.

269. Ekimoto H, Aikawa M, Ohnuki T. Immunological involvement in pulmonary fibrosis induced by peplomycin. J Antibiot 1985;38:94–8.

270. Molteni A, Ward WF, Ts'ao C. Monocrotaline-induced pulmonary fibrosis in rats: amelioration by captotril and penicillamine. Proc Soc Exp Biol Med 1985;180:112–20.

271. Geismar LS, Hennessey SH, Reiser KM, Last JA. D-Penicillamine prevents collagen accumulation in lungs of rats given bleomycin. Chest 1986;89:153S–154S.

272. Eickelberg O, Pansky A, Koehler E, et al. Molecular mechanisms of TGF-β antagonism by interferon-γ and cyclosporine A in lung fibroblasts. FASEB J 2001;15:797–806.

273. Gay SE, Kazerooni EA, Toews GB, et al. Idiopathic pulmonary fibrosis: predicting response to therapy and survival. Am J Respir Crit Care Med 1998;157:1063–72.

274. Flaherty KR, Toews GB, Travis WD, et al. Clinical significance of histological classification of idiopathic interstitial pneumonia. Eur Respir J 2002;19:275–83.

275. Doud JR, McCabe MM, Montoya A, et al. The Loyola University lung transplant experience. Arch Intern Med 1993;153:2769–73.

276. Grossman RF, Frost A, Zamel N, et al. Results of single-lung transplantation for bilateral pulmonary fibrosis. N Engl J Med 1990;322:727–33.

277. American Thoracic Society. Lung transplantation. Am Rev Respir Dis 1993;147:772–6.

278. Toronto Lung Transplant Group. Experience with single-lung transplantation for pulmonary fibrosis. JAMA 1988;259:2258–62.

279. Sulica R, Teirstein A, Padilla ML. Lung transplantation in interstitial lung disease. Curr Opin Pulm Med 2001;7:314–22.

280. Doig JC, Corris PA, Hilton CJ, et al. Effect of single-lung transplantation on pulmonary hypertension in patients with end stage fibrosing lung disease. Br Heart J 1991;66:431–4.

281. Davis RD, Pasque MK. Pulmonary transplantation. Ann Surg 1995;221:14–28.

282. Johnson B, Duncan S, Ohori N, et al. Recurrence of sarcoidosis in pulmonary allograft recipients. Am Rev Respir Dis 1993;148:1373–7.

283. Kazerooni EA, Jackson C, Cascade PN. Sarcoidosis: recurrence of primary disease in transplanted lungs. Radiology 1994;192:461–4.

284. Padilla ML, Schilero GJ, Teirstein AS. Sarcoidosis and transplantation. Sarcoidosis Vasc Diffuse Lung Dis 1997;14:16–22.

285. Klemen H, Husain AN, Cagle PT, et al. Mycobacterial DNA in recurrent sarcoidosis in the transplanted lung–a PCR-based study on four cases. Virchows Arch 2000;436:365–9.

286. Nunley DR, Hattler B, Keenan RJ, et al. Lung transplantation for end-stage pulmonary sarcoidosis [see comments]. Sarcoidosis Vasc Diffuse Lung Dis 1999;16:93–100.

287. Kiatboonsri C, Resnick SC, Chan KM, et al. The detection of recurrent sarcoidosis by FDG-PET in a lung transplant recipient. West J Med 1998;168:130–2.

288. Nine JS, Yousem SA, Paradis IL, et al. Lymphangioleiomyomatosis: recurrence after lung transplantation. J Heart Lung Transplant 1994;13:714–9.

289. O'Brien JD, Lium JH, Parosa JF, et al. Lymphangiomyomatosis recurrence in the allograft after single-lung transplantation. Am J Respir Crit Care Med 1995;151:2033–6.

290. Boehler A, Speich R, Russi EW, Weder W. Lung transplantation for lymphangioleiomyomatosis. N Engl J Med 1996;335:1275–80.

291. Bittmann I, Dose TB, Muller C, et al. Lymphangioleiomyomatosis: recurrence after single lung transplantation. Hum Pathol 1997;28:1420–3.

292. Etienne B, Bertocchi M, Gamondes JP, et al. Relapsing pulmonary Langerhans cell histiocytosis after lung transplantation. Am J Respir Crit Care Med 1998;157:288–91.

293. Habib SB, Congleton J, Carr D, et al. Recurrence of recipient Langerhans' cell histiocytosis following bilateral lung transplantation [see comments]. Thorax 1998;53:323–5.

294. Gabbay E, Dark JH, Ashcroft T, et al. Recurrence of Langerhans' cell granulomatosis following lung transplantation. Thorax 1998;53:326–7.

295. Frost AE, Keller CA, Brown RW, et al. Giant cell interstitial pneumonitis. Disease recurrence in the transplanted lung. Am Rev Respir Dis 1993;148:1401–4.

296. Barberis M, Harari S, Tironi A, Lampertico P. Recurrence of primary disease in a single-lung transplant recipient. Transplant Proc 1992;24:2660–2.

297. King MB, Jessurun J, Hertz MI. Recurrence of desquamative interstitial pneumonia after lung transplantation. Am J Respir Crit Care Med 1997;156:2003–5.

298. Verleden GM. Recurrence of desquamative interstitial pneumonia after lung transplantation. Am J Respir Crit Care Med 1998;157:1349–50.

299. Lok SS, Smith E, Doran HM, et al. Idiopathic pulmonary fibrosis and cyclosporine: a lesson from single-lung transplantation. Chest 1998;114:1478–81.

300. Robinson DS, Geddes DM, Hansell DM, et al. Partial resolu-

tion of acute interstitial pneumonia in native lung after single lung transplantation. Thorax 1996;51:1158–9,1164–9.

301. Chan-Yeung M, Müller N. Cryptogenic fibrosing alveolitis. Lancet 1997;350:651–6.

302. Coultas DB. Epidemiology of idiopathic pulmonary fibrosis. Semin Respir Med 1993;14:181–96.

303. Smith C, Feldman C, Levy H, et al. Cryptogenic fibrosing alveolitis: a study of an indigenous African population. Respiration 1990;57:364–71.

304. Crystal RG, Bitterman PB, Mossman B, et al. Future research directions in idiopathic pulmonary fibrosis. Summary of a National Heart, Lung and Blood Institute working group. Am J Respir Crit Care Med 2002;166:236–46.

305. Barbas-Filho JV, Ferreira MA, Sesso A, et al. Evidence of type II pneumocyte apoptosis in the pathogenesis of idiopathic pulmonary fibrosis (IFP)/usual interstitial pneumonia (UIP). J Clin Pathol 2001;54:132–8.

306. Fukuda Y, Ishizaki M, Kudoh S, et al. Localization of matrix metalloproteinases-1, -2, and -9 and tissue inhibitor of metalloproteinase-2 in interstitial lung disease. Lab Invest 1998;78:687–98.

307. Zuo F, Kaminski N, Eugui E, et al. Gene expression analysis reveals matrilysin as a key regulator of pulmonary fibrosis in mice and humans. Proc Natl Acad Sci U S A 2002;99: 292–7.

308. Tablan OC, Reyes MP. Chronic interstitial pulmonary fibrosis following *Mycoplasma pneumoniae* pneumonia. Am J Med 1985;79:268–70.

309. Mufson MS, Sanders V, Wood SC, Chanock RM. Primary atypical pneumonia due to *Mycoplasma pneumoniae*. N Engl J Med 1963;268:1109–11.

310. Wright PH, Heard BE, Steel SJ, Turner-Warwick M. Cryptogenic fibrosing alveolitis: assessment by graded trephine lung biopsy histology compared with clinical, radiographic, and physiological features. Br J Dis Chest 1981;75:61–70.

311. Laros CD, Bergstein PGM. Relief of breathlessness in a case of progressive pulmonary fibrosis. Respiration 1982;43:452–7.

312. Picado C, Gomez de Almeida R, Xaubet A, et al. Spontaneous pneumothorax in cryptogenic fibrosing alveolitis. Respiration 1985;48:77–80.

313. Matusiewicz SP, Williamson IJ, Sime PJ, et al. Plasma lactate dehydrogenase: a marker of disease activity in cryptogenic fibrosing alveolitis and extrinsic allergic alveolitis? Eur Respir J 1993;6:1282–6.

314. Fulmer JD. Bronchoalveolar lavage. Am Rev Respir Dis 1982;126:961–3.

315. Watters LC, Schwarz MI, Cherniack RM, et al. Idiopathic pulmonary fibrosis: pretreatment bronchoalveolar lavage cellular constituents and their relationships with lung histopathology and clinical response to therapy. Am Rev Respir Dis 1987;135:696–704.

316. Peterson MW, Monick M, Hunninghake GW. Prognostic role of eosinophils in pulmonary fibrosis. Chest 1987;92:51–6.

317. Hawgood S, Benson BJ, Schilling J, et al. Nucleotide and amino acid sequences of pulmonary surfactant protein SP-18 and evidence for cooperation between SP-18 and SP 28-36 in surfactant lipid adsorption. Proc Natl Acad Sci U S A 1987;84:66–70.

318. Wright JR, Wager RE, Hawgood S, et al. Surfactant apoprotein Mr = 26,000–36,000 enhances uptake of liposomes by type II cells. J Biol Chem 1987;262:2888–94.

319. Dobbs LG, Wright JR, Hawgood S, et al. Pulmonary surfactant and its components inhibit secretion of phosphatidylcholine from cultured rat alveolar type II cells. Proc Natl Acad Sci U S A 1987;84:1010–4.

320. Rice WR, Ross GF, Singleton FM, et al. Surfactant-associated protein inhibits phospholipid secretion from type II cells. J Appl Physiol 1987;63:692–8.

321. Kuroki Y, Mason RJ, Voelker DR. Pulmonary surfactant apoprotein A structure and modulation of surfactant secretion by rat alveolar type II cells. J Biol Chem 1988;263:3388–94.

322. Cockshutt A, Weitz J, Possmayer F. The effects of surfactant-associated protein A on surface tension reduction and blood protein inhibition in two surfactant preparations [abstract]. FASEB J 1990;4:A2147.

323. Hughes DA, Haslam PL. Phosphatidylglycerol levels in bronchoalveolar lavage fluid from patients with cryptogenic fibrosing alveolitis in relation to response to prednisolone. Am Rev Respir Dis 1987;135:30.

324. Haslam PL, Hughes DA, Dewar A, Pantin CFA. Lipoprotein macroaggregates in bronchoalveolar lavage fluid from patients with diffuse interstitial lung disease comparison with idiopathic alveolar lipoproteinosis. Thorax 1988;43: 140–6.

325. Robinson PC, Watters LC, King TE, Mason RJ. Idiopathic pulmonary fibroisis: abnormalities in bronchoalveolar lavage fluid phospholipids. Am Rev Respir Dis 1988;137:585–91.

326. Honda Y, Tsunematsu K, Suzuki A, Akino T. Changes in phospholipids in bronchoalveolar lavage fluid of patients with interstitial lung disease. Lung 1988;166:293–301.

327. Low RB. Bronchoalveolar lavage lipids in idiopathic pulmonary fibrosis. Chest 1989;95:3–5.

328. Hughes DA, Haslam PL. Changes in phosphatidylglycerol in bronchoalveolar lavage fluids from patients with cryptogenic fibrosing alveolitis. Chest 1989;95:82–9.

329. McCormack FX, King TE Jr, Voelker DR, et al. Idiopathic pulmonary fibrosis: abnormalities in the bronchoalveolar lavage content of surfactant protein A. Am Rev Respir Dis 1991;144:160–6.

330. McCormack FX, King TE Jr, Bucher BL, et al. Surfactant protein A predicts survival in idiopathic pulmonary fibrosis. Am J Respir Crit Care Med 1995;152:751–9.

331. Kawada H, Horiuchi T, Shannon JM, et al. Alveolar type II cells, surfactant protein A (SP-A), and the phospholipid components of surfactant in acute silicosis in the rat. Am Rev Respir Dis 1989;140:460–70.

332. Horiuchi T, Mason RJ, Kuroki Y, Cherniack RM. Surface and tissue forces, surfactant protein A, and the phospholipid components of pulmonary surfactant in bleomycin-induced pulmonary fibrosis in the rat. Am Rev Respir Dis 1990;141:1006–13.

333. Miller YE, Walker SR, Spencer JS, et al. Monoclonal antibodies specific for antigens expressed by rat type II alveolar epithelial and nonciliated bronchiolar cells. Exp Lung Res 1989;15:635–49.

334. Thrall RS, Swendsen CL, Shannon TH, et al. Correlation of changes in pulmonary surfactant phospholipids with compliance in bleomycin-induced pulmonary fibrosis in the rat. Am Rev Respir Dis 1987;136:113–8.

335. Voelker DR, Mason RJ. Alveolar type II epithelial cells. In: Massaro D, editor. Lung cell biology. New York: Marcel Dekker; 1989. p. 487–538.

336. Kuroki Y, Tsutahara S, Shijubo N, et al. Elevated levels of lung surfactant protein A in sera from patients with idiopathic pulmonary fibrosis and pulmonary alveolar proteinosis. Am Rev Respir Dis 1993;147:723–9.

337. Greene KE, King TE Jr, Kuroki Y, et al. Serum surfactant proteins-A and -D as biomarkers in idiopathic pulmonary fibrosis. Eur Respir J 2002;19:439–46.

338. Honda Y, Kuroki Y, Matsuura E, et al. Pulmonary surfactant protein D in sera and bronchoalveolar lavage fluids. Am J Respir Crit Care Med 1995;152:1860–6.

339. Honda Y, Kuroki Y, Shijubo N, et al. Aberrant appearance of lung surfactant protein A in sera of patients with idiopathic pulmonary fibrosis and its clinical significance. Respiration 1995;62:64–9.

340. Takahashi H, Fujishima T, Koba H, et al. Serum surfactant proteins A and D as prognostic factors in idiopathic pulmonary fibrosis and their relationship to disease extent. Am J Respir Crit Care Med 2000;162:1109–14.

341. Kornbluth RS, Turino GM. Respiratory control in diffuse

interstitial lung disease and diseases of the pulmonary vasculature. Clin Chest Med 1980;1:91–102.

342. Renzi G, Milic-Emili J, Grassino AE. The pattern of breathing in diffuse lung fibrosis. Bull Eur Physiopathol Respir 1982;18:461–72.

343. Lourenco RV, Turino GM, Davidson LAG, Fishman AP. The regulation of ventilation in diffuse pulmonary fibrosis. Am J Med 1965;38:199–216.

344. Patton JMS, Freedman S. The ventilatory response to CO_2 of patients with diffuse pulmonary infiltration or fibrosis. Clin Sci 1972;43:55–69.

345. Bradley GW, Crawford R. Regulation of breathing during exercise in normal subjects and in chronic lung disease. Clin Sci Mol Med 1976;51:575–82.

346. VanMeerhaeghe A, Scano G, Sergyseils R, et al. Respiratory drive and ventilator pattern during exercise in interstitial lung disease. Bull Eur Physiopathol Respir 1981;17:15–26.

347. Savoy J, Dhingra S, Anthonisen NR. Role of vagal airway reflexes in control of ventilation in pulmonary fibrosis. Clin Sci 1981;61:781–4.

348. Dimarco AF, Kelsen SG, Cherniack NS, Gothe B. Occlusion pressure and breathing pattern in patients with interstitial lung disease. Am Rev Respir Dis 1983;127:425–30.

349. Burton JGW, Killian KJ, Jones NL. Pattern of breathing during exercise in patients with interstitial lung disease. Thorax 1983;38:778–84.

350. Renzi G, Milic-Emili J, Grassino AE. Breathing pattern in sarcoidosis and idiopathic pulmonary fibrosis. Ann N Y Acad Sci 1986;465:482–90.

351. Ostrow D, Cherniack RM. Resistance to airflow in patients with diffuse interstitial lung disease. Am Rev Respir Dis 1973;108:205–10.

352. Yernault JC, deJonghe M, deCoster A, Englert M. Pulmonary mechanics in diffuse fibrosing alveolitis. Bull Physiopathol Respir 1975;11:231–44.

353. Fulmer JD, Roberts WC, von Gal ER, Crystal RG. Small airways in idiopathic pulmonary fibrosis. Comparison of morphologic and physiologic observations. J Clin Invest 1977;60:595–610.

354. Schofield NM, Davies RJ, Cameron IR, Green M. Small airways in fibrosing alveolitis. Am Rev Respir Dis 1978; 113:729–35.

355. McCarthy DS, Ostrow DN, Hershfield ES. Chronic obstructive pulmonary disease following idiopathic pulmonary fibrosis. Chest 1980;77:473–7.

356. Englert M, Yernault JC, deCoster A, Clumeek N. Diffusing properties and elastic properties in interstitial diseases of the lung. Prog Respir Res 1975;8:177–85.

357. Gibson GJ, Pride NB. Lung distensibility. The static pressure-volume curve of the lungs and its use in clinical assessment. Br J Dis Chest 1976;70:143–83.

358. Gibson GJ, Pride NB. Pulmonary mechanics in fibrosing alveolitis. The effects of lung shrinkage. Am Rev Respir Dis 1977;116:637–47.

359. Gibson GJ, Pride NB, Davis J, Schroter RC. Exponential description of the static pressure–volume curve of normal and diseased lungs. Am Rev Respir Dis 1979;120:799–811.

360. Fulmer JD, Roberts WC, von Gal ER, Crystal RG. Morphologic-physiologic correlates of the severity of fibrosis and degree of cellularity in idiopathic pulmonary fibrosis. J Clin Invest 1979;63:665–76.

361. Holland RAB, Blacket RB. Pulmonary function in the Hamman-Rich syndrome. The abnormalities of ventilation, blood gases and diffusion at rest and on exercise. Am J Med 1960;28:955–66.

362. Austrian R, McClement JH, Renzetti AD Jr, et al. Clinical and physiologic features of some types of pulmonary diseases with impairment of alveolar capillary diffusion. The syndrome of "alveolar–capillary blocks." Am J Med 1951; 11:667–85.

363. Miller WC, Heard JG, Unger KM, Suich DM. Anatomical lung shunting in pulmonary fibrosis. Thorax 1986; 41:208–9.

364. Wagner PD, Dantzker DR, Dueck R, et al. Distribution of ventilation-perfusion ratios in patients with interstitial lung disease. Chest 1976;69:256–7.

365. West JB. Ventilation-perfusion relationships. Am Rev Respir Dis 1977;116:919–43.

366. Jernudd-Wilhelmsson Y, Hoernblad Y, Hedenstierna G. Ventilation-perfusion relationships in interstitial lung disease. Eur J Respir Dis 1986;68:39–49.

367. Keogh BA, Lakatos E, Price D, Crystal RG. Importance of the lower respiratory tract in oxygen transfer. Exercise testing in patients with interstitial and destructive lung disease. Am Rev Respir Dis 1984;129:S76–S80.

368. Kelley MA, Daniele RP. Exercise testing in interstitial lung disease. Clin Chest Med 1984;5:145–56.

369. Keogh BA, Crystal RG. Pulmonary function testing in interstitial pulmonary disease. What does it tell us? Chest 1980;78:856–65.

370. Jones NL, Rebuck AS. Tidal volume during exercise in patients with diffuse fibrosing alveolitis. Bull Eur Physiopathol Respir 1979;15:321–7.

371. Widimsky J, Riedel M, Stanek V. Central haemodynamics during exercise in patients with restrictive pulmonary disease. Bull Eur Physiopathol Respir 1977;13:369–79.

372. Hawrylkiewicz I, Izdebska-Makosa Z, et al. Pulmonary haemodynamics at rest and on exercise in patients with idiopathic pulmonary fibrosis. Bull Eur Physiopathol Respir 1982;18:403–10.

373. Jezek V, Fucik J, Michaejanic A, Jezkova L. The prognostic significance of functional tests in cryptogenic fibrosing alveolitis. Bull Eur Physiopathol Respir 1980;16:711–20.

374. Lupi-Herrera E, Seoane M, Verdejo S, et al. Hemodynamic effect of hydralazine in interstitial lung disease patients with cor pulmonale immediate and short term evaluation at rest and during exercise. Chest 1985;87:564–73.

375. Enson Y, Thomas HM, Bosken CH, et al. Pulmonary hypertension in interstitial lung disease: relation of vascular resistance to abnormal lung structure. Trans Assoc Am Phys 1975;88:248–55.

376. Sturani C, Papiris S, Galavotti V, Gunella G. Pulmonary vascular responsiveness at rest and during exercise in idiopathic pulmonary fibrosis: effects of oxygen and nifedipine. Respiration 1986;50:117–29.

377. Kennedy JI, Fulmer JD. Pulmonary hypertension in the interstitial lung disease. Chest 1985;87:558–60.

378. Todisco T, Cegla VH, Mattys H. Oxygen breathing during exercise in patients with diffuse interstitial lung fibrosis. Bull Eur Physiopathol Respir 1977;13:387–97.

379. Bye PTP, Anderson SD, Woolcock AJ, et al. Bicycle endurance performance of patients with interstitial lung disease breathing air and oxygen. Am Rev Respir Dis 1982;126:1005–12.

380. Bye PTP, Issa F, Berthon-Jones M, Sullivan CE. Studies of oxygenation during sleep in patients with interstitial lung disease. Am Rev Respir Dis 1984;129:27–32.

381. Perez-Padilla R, West P, Lertzman M, Kryger MH. Breathing during sleep in patients with interstitial lung disease. Am Rev Respir Dis 1985;132:224–9.

382. Terriff BA, Kwan SY, Chan-Yeung MM, Mueller NL. Fibrosing alveolitis: chest radiology and CT as predictors of clinical and functional impairment at follow-up in 26 patients. Radiology 1992;184:445–9.

383. Johkoh T, Muller NL, Ichikado K, et al. Respiratory change in size of honeycombing: inspiratory and expiratory spiral volumetric CT analysis of 97 cases. J Comput Assist Tomogr 1999;23:174–80.

384. Akira M, Sakatani M, Ueda E. Idiopathic pulmonary fibrosis: progression of honeycombing at thin-section CT. Radiology 1993;189:687–91.

385. Hartman TE, Primack SL, Kang EY, et al. Disease progression in usual interstitial pneumonia compared with desquamative interstitial pneumonia. Assessment with serial CT. Chest 1996;110:378–82.

386. Mino M, Noma S, Kobashi Y, Iwata T. Serial changes of cystic air spaces in fibrosing alveolitis: a CT-pathological study. Clin Radiol 1995;50:357–63.

387. Chopra SK, Taplin GV, Tashkin DP, Elam D. Lung clearance of soluble radioaerosols of different molecular weights in systemic sclerosis. Thorax 1979;34:63–7.

388. Rinderknecht J, Shapiro L, Krauthammer M, et al. Accelerated clearance of small solutes from the lungs in interstitial lung disease. Am Rev Respir Dis 1980;121:105–17.

389. Wells AU, Hansell DM, Harrison NK, et al. Clearance of inhaled ^{99m}Tc-DTPA predicts the clinical course of fibrosing alveolitis. Eur Respir J 1993;6:797–802.

390. Mogulkoc N, Brutsche MH, Bishop PW, et al. Pulmonary (99m)Tc-DTPA aerosol clearance and survival in usual interstitial pneumonia (UIP). Thorax 2001;56:916–23.

391. Winterbauer RH, Hammar SP. Sarcoidosis and idiopathic pulmonary fibrosis: a review of recent events. In: Simmons DH, editor. Current pulmonology. Vol. 7. Chicago: Year Book Medical; 1987. p. 117.

392. Baglio CM, Michel RD, Hunter WC. Primary interstitial pulmonary fibrosis: diffuse and circumscribed forms. Review of the literature and report of eleven cases. J Thorac Cardiovasc Surg 1960;40:695–715.

393. Fraire AE, Greenberg SD, O'Neal RM, et al. Diffuse interstitial fibrosis of the lung. Am J Clin Pathol 1973;59:636–47.

394. Cherniack RM, Colby TV, Flint A, et al. Quantitative assessment of lung pathology in idiopathic pulmonary fibrosis. Am Rev Respir Dis 1991;144:892–900.

395. Cherniack RM, Colby TV, Flint A, et al. Correlation of structure and function in idiopathic pulmonary fibrosis. Am J Respir Crit Care Med 1995;151:1180–8.

396. Gauldie J. Pro: Inflammatory mechanisms are a minor component of the pathogenesis of idiopathic pulmonary fibrosis. Am J Respir Crit Care Med 2002;165:1205–6.

397. Hyde DM, King TE Jr, McDermott T, et al. Idiopathic pulmonary fibrosis: the quantitative assessment of lung pathology. Comparison of a semi-quantitative versus a morphometric histopathologic scoring system. Am Rev Respir Dis 1992;146:1042–7.

398. Bjoraker JA, Ryu JH, Edwin MK, et al. Prognostic significance of histopathologic subsets in idiopathic pulmonary fibrosis. Am J Respir Crit Care Med 1998;157:199–203.

399. Katzenstein AL, Fiorelli RF. Nonspecific interstitial pneumonia/fibrosis. Histologic features and clinical significance. Am J Surg Pathol 1994;18:136–47.

400. Nicholson AG, Fulford LG, Colby TV, et al. The relationship between individual histologic features and disease progression in idiopathic pulmonary fibrosis. Am J Respir Crit Care Med 2002;166:173–7.

401. Schwartz DA, Helmers RA, Galvin JR, et al. Determinants of survival in idiopathic pulmonary fibrosis. Am J Respir Crit Care Med 1994;149:450–4.

402. Schwartz DA, Van Fossen DS, Davis CS, et al. Determinants of progression in idiopathic pulmonary fibrosis. Am J Respir Crit Care Med 1994;149:444–9.

403. Dayton CS, Schwartz DA, Helmers RA, et al. Outcome of subjects with idiopathic pulmonary fibrosis who fail corticosteroid therapy. Implications for further studies. Chest 1993;103:69–73.

404. Hay JH, Turner-Warwick M. Interstitial pulmonary fibrosis. In: Murray JF, Nadel JA, editors. Textbook of respiratory medicine. Philadelphia (PA): Harcourt Brace Jovanovich; 1988. p. 1445–61.

405. Hunninghake GW, Kalica AR. Approaches to the treatment of pulmonary fibrosis. Am J Respir Crit Care Med 1995;151:915–8.

406. Mason RJ, Schwarz MI, Hunninghake GW, Musson RA. NHLBI workshop summary. Pharmacological therapy for idiopathic pulmonary fibrosis. Past, present, and future. Am J Respir Crit Care Med 1999;160:1771–7.

407. Rudd RM, Haslam PL, Turner-Warwick M. Cryptogenic fibrosing alveolitis relationships of pulmonary physiology and bronchoalveolar lavage to treatment and prognosis. Am Rev Respir Dis 1981;124:1–8.

408. Sullivan E. Idiopathic pulmonary fibrosis: treatment with corticosteroids. In: Rose BD, editor. UpToDate in Medicine. Wellesley (MA): BDR; 2002.

409. Collard HR, King TE Jr. Clinical significance of histopathologic subgroups in the idiopathic interstitial pneumonias: is surgical lung biopsy essential? Semin Respir Crit Care Med 2001;22:347–56.

410. Nagai S, Kitaichi M, Itoh H, et al. Idiopathic nonspecific interstitial pneumonia/fibrosis: comparison with idiopathic pulmonary fibrosis and BOOP. Eur Respir J 1998;12:1010–9.

411. Travis WD, Matsui K, Moss J, Ferrans VJ. Idiopathic nonspecific interstitial pneumonia: prognostic significance of cellular and fibrosing patterns: survival comparison with usual interstitial pneumonia and desquamative interstitial pneumonia. Am J Surg Pathol 2000;24:19–33.

412. Daniil ZD, Gilchrist FC, Nicholson AG, et al. A histologic pattern of nonspecific interstitial pneumonia is associated with a better prognosis than usual interstitial pneumonia in patients with cryptogenic fibrosing alveolitis. Am J Respir Crit Care Med 1999;160:899–905.

413. Nicholson AG, Colby TV, Dubois RM, et al. The prognostic significance of the histologic pattern of interstitial pneumonia in patients presenting with the clinical entity of cryptogenic fibrosing alveolitis. Am J Respir Crit Care Med 2000;162:2213–7.

414. Fort JG, Scovern H, Abruzzo JL. Intravenous cyclophosphamide and methylprednisolone for the treatment of bronchiolitis obliterans and interstitial fibrosis associated with crysotherapy. J Rheumatol 1988;15:850–4.

415. Silver RM, Warrick JH, Kinsella MB, et al. Cyclophosphamide and low-dose prednisone therapy in patients with systemic sclerosis (scleroderma) with interstitial lung disease. J Rheumatol 1993;20:838–44.

416. Kolb M, Kirschner J, Riedel W, et al. Cyclophosphamide pulse therapy in idiopathic pulmonary fibrosis. Eur Respir J 1998;12:1409–14.

417. Raghu G, Depaso WJ, Cain K, et al. Azathioprine combined with prednisone in the treatment of idiopathic pulmonary fibrosis: a prospective, double-blind randomized, placebo-controlled clinical trial. Am Rev Respir Dis 1991;144:291–6.

418. Peters SG, McDougall JC, Douglas WW, et al. Colchicine in the treatment of pulmonary fibrosis. Chest 1993;103:101–4.

419. Douglas WW, Ryu JH, Bjoraker JA, et al. Colchicine versus prednisone as treatment of usual interstitial pneumonia. Mayo Clin Proc 1997;72:201–9.

420. Douglas WW, Ryu JH, Swensen SJ, et al. Colchicine versus prednisone in the treatment of idiopathic pulmonary fibrosis. A randomized prospective study. Members of the Lung Study Group. Am J Respir Crit Care Med 1998;158:220–5.

421. Douglas WW, Ryu JH, Schroeder DR. Idiopathic pulmonary fibrosis. Impact of oxygen and colchicine, prednisone, or no therapy on survival. Am J Respir Crit Care Med 2000; 161:1172–8.

422. Ziesche R, Hofbauer E, Wittmann K, et al. A preliminary study of long-term treatment with interferon-γ1b and low-dose prednisolone in patients with idiopathic pulmonary fibrosis. N Engl J Med 1999;341:1264–9.

423. Raghu G, Noble PW, Brown KK, Colby TV. Interferon-γ1b in idiopathic pulmonary fibrosis: reanalysis of a published study. In: King TE Jr, editor. ATS continuing education monograph series: new approaches to managing idiopathic pulmonary fibrosis. New York: American Thoracic Society; 2000. p. 36–43.

424. Kalra S, Utz JP, Ryu JH. Interferon-gamma 1b in the treatment of advanced IPF. Chest 2001;120:184S–185S.

425. Raghu G, Spada C, Otaki Y, Hayes J. IFN-γ in the treatment of advanced IPF and fibrotic nonspecific interstitial pneumonia: prospective, preliminary clinical observations in one center. Chest 2001;120:185S.

426. Gaviria JM, Root RK. Clinical use of recombinant human interferon-gamma. In: Rose BD, editor. UpToDate. Wellesley (MA): UpToDate; 2002.

427. Okada T, Sugie I, Aisaka K. Effects of γ-interferon on collagen and histamine content in bleomycin-induced lung fibrosis in rats. Lymphokine Cytokine Res 1993;12:87–91.

428. Cornelissen AM, Von den Hoff JW, Maltha JC, et al. Effects of interferons on proliferation and collagen synthesis of rat palatal wound fibroblasts. Arch Oral Biol 1999;44:541–7.

429. Yokozeki M, Baba Y, Shimokawa H, et al. Interferon-gamma inhibits the myofibroblastic phenotype of rat palatal fibroblasts induced by transforming growth factor-beta1 in vitro. FEBS Lett 1999;442:61–4.

430. Ziesche R, Block LH. Interferon gamma-1b: mechanism of action, preclinical studies, and clinical experience. In: King TE Jr, editor. ATS continuing education monograph series: new approaches to managing idiopathic pulmonary fibrosis. New York: American Thoracic Society; 2000. p. 36–43.

431. Prior C, Haslam PL. Increased levels of serum interferon-gamma in pulmonary sarcoidosis and relationship with response to corticosterod therapy. Am Rev Respir Dis 1991;143:53–60.

432. Majumdar S, Li D, Ansari T, et al. Different cytokine profiles in cryptogenic fibrosing alveolitis and fibrosing alveolitis associated with systemic sclerosis: a quantitative study of open lung biopsies. Eur Respir J 1999;14:251–7.

433. Prior C, Haslam PL. In vivo levels and in vitro production of interferon-gamma in fibrosing interstitial lung disease. Clin Exp Immunol 1992;88:280–7.

434. Broekelmann TJ, Limper AH, Colby TV, McDonald JA. Transforming growth factor-β1 is present at sites of extracellular matrix gene expression in human pulmonary fibrosis. Proc Natl Acad Sci U S A 1991;88:6642–6.

435. Baughman RP, Alabi FO. Nonsteroidal therapy for idiopathic pulmonary fibrosis. Curr Opin Pulm Med 2001;7:309–13.

436. Ziesche R, Block LH. Mechanisms of antifibrotic action of interferon gamma-1b in pulmonary fibrosis. Wien Klin Wochenschr 2000;112:785–90.

437. Raghu G, Johnson WC, Lockhart D, Mageto Y. Treatment of idiopathic pulmonary fibrosis with a new antifibrotic agent, pirfenidone: results of a prospective, open-label phase II study. Am J Respir Crit Care Med 1999;159:1061–9.

438. Azuma A, Tsuboi E, Abe S, et al. A placebo control and double blind phase II clinical study of pirfenidone in patients with idiopathic pulmonary fibrosis in Japan [abstract]. Am J Respir Crit Care Med 2002;165:A729.

439. Brantly ML, Troendle J, Avila N, et al. A randomized, placebo-controlled trial of oral pirfenidone for the pulmonary fibrosis of Hermansk-Pudlak syndrome [abstract]. Am J Respir Crit Care Med 2002;165:A728.

440. Steen VD, Owens GR, Redmond C, et al. The effect of D-penicillamine on pulmonary findings in systemic sclerosis. Arthritis Rheum 1985;28:882–8.

441. DeClerk LS, Dequeker J, Francx L, Demedts M. D-Penicillamine therapy and interstitial lung disease in scleroderma: a long-term followup study. Arthritis Rheum 1987;30:643–50.

442. Cegla UH. Treatment of idiopathic fibrosing alveolitis. Therapeutic experiences with azathioprine-prednisolone and D-penicillamine-prednisolone combination therapy. Schweiz Med Wochenschr 1977;107:184–7.

443. Goodman M, Turner-Warwick M. Pilot study of penicillamine therapy in corticosteroid failure patients with widespread pulmonary fibrosis. Chest 1978;74:338.

444. Chapela R, Zuniga G, Selman M. D-Penicillamine in the ther-

apy of fibrotic lung diseases. Int J Clin Pharmacol Ther Toxicol 1986;24:16–7.

445. Liebetrau G, Pielesch W, Ganguin HG, et al. Therapy of pulmonary fibrosis with D-penicillamine. Z Gesamte Inn Med 1982;37:263–6.

446. Alton EW, Johnson M, Turner-Warwick M. Advanced cryptogenic fibrosing alveolitis: preliminary report on treatment with cyclosporin A. Respir Med 1989;83:277–9.

447. Venuta F, Rendina EA, Ciriaco P, et al. Efficacy of cyclosporine to reduce steroids in patients with idiopathic pulmonary fibrosis before lung transplantation. J Heart Lung Transplant 1993;12:909–14.

448. Moolman JA, Bardin PG, Rossouw DJ, Joubert JR. Cyclosporin as a treatment for interstitial lung disease of unknown aetiology. Thorax 1991;46:592–5.

449. Raghu R, Bozic CR, Brown K, et al. Trial of interferon-β1a (IFN-β1a) in idiopathic pulmonary fibrosis (IPF): characteristics of patients with and without surgical lung biopsy [abstract]. Am J Respir Crit Care Med 2000;161:A527.

450. Raghu R, Bozic CR, Brown K, et al. Feasibility of a trial of interferon-β1a (IFN-β1a) in the treatment of idiopathic pulmonary fibrosis (IPF) [abstract]. Am J Respir Crit Care Med 2001;163:A707.

451. Channick RN, Hoch RC, Newhart JW, et al. Improvement in pulmonary hypertension and hypoxemia during nitric oxide inhalation in a patient with end-stage pulmonary fibrosis. Am J Respir Crit Care Med 1994;149:811–4.

452. Yung GL, Kriett JM, Jamieson SW, et al. Outpatient inhaled nitric oxide in a patient with idiopathic pulmonary fibrosis: a bridge to lung transplantation. J Heart Lung Transplant 2001;20:1224–7.

453. Unemori EN, Pickford LB, Salles AL, et al. Relaxin induces an extracellular matrix-degrading phenotype in human lung fibroblasts in vitro and inhibits lung fibrosis in a murine model in vivo. J Clin Invest 1996;98:2739–45.

454. Unemori EN, Lewis M, Constant J, et al. Relaxin induces vascular endothelial growth factor expression and angiogenesis selectively at wound sites. Wound Repair Regen 2000;8:361–70.

455. Seibold JR, Korn JH, Simms R, et al. Recombinant human relaxin in the treatment of scleroderma. A randomized, double-blind, placebo-controlled trial. Ann Intern Med 2000;132:871–9.

456. Behr J, Maier K, Degenkolb B, et al. Antioxidative and clinical effects of high-dose N-acetylcysteine in fibrosing alveolitis. Adjunctive therapy to maintenance immunosuppression. Am J Respir Crit Care Med 1997;156:1897–901.

457. Cortijo J, Cerda-Nicolas M, Serrano A, et al. Attenuation by oral N-acetylcysteine of bleomycin-induced lung injury in rats. Eur Respir J 2001;17:1228–35.

458. Hagiwara SI, Ishii Y, Kitamura S. Aerosolized administration of N-acetylcysteine attenuates lung fibrosis induced by bleomycin in mice. Am J Respir Crit Care Med 2000;162:225–31.

459. Drost E, Lannan S, Bridgeman MM, et al. Lack of effect of N-acetylcysteine on the release of oxygen radicals from neutrophils and alveolar macrophages. Eur Respir J 1991;4:723–9.

460. Bridgeman MM, Marsden M, MacNee W, et al. Cysteine and glutathione concentrations in plasma and bronchoalveolar lavage fluid after treatment with N-acetylcysteine. Thorax 1991;46:39–42.

461. Bridgeman MM, Marsden M, Selby C, et al. Effect of N-acetyl cysteine on the concentrations of thiols in plasma, bronchoalveolar lavage fluid, and lung tissue. Thorax 1994;49:670–5.

462. Meyer A, Buhl R, Magnussen H. The effect of oral N-acetylcysteine on lung glutathione levels in idiopathic pulmonary fibrosis. Eur Respir J 1994;7:431–6.

463. Meyer A, Buhl R, Kampf S, Magnussen H. Intravenous N-

acetylcysteine and lung glutathione of patients with pulmonary fibrosis and normals. Am J Respir Crit Care Med 1995;152:1055–60.

464. Demedts M, Behr J, Costabel U, et al. IFEGENIA: An international study of *N*-acetylcysteine (NAC) in IPF [abstract]. Am J Respir Crit Care Med 2001;163:A708.

465. Carrillo G, Estrada A, Mejya M, et al. Inhaled beclomethasone and colchicine (IBC) versus inhaled beclomethasone, colchicine and captopril (IBCCAP) in patients with idiopathic pulmonary fibrosis [abstract]. Am J Respir Crit Care Med 2000;161:A528.

466. Niden AH, Koss M, Boylen CT, et al. An open label pilot study to determine the potential efficacy of TNFR: FC (Enbrel®, Etanercept) in the treatment of usual interstitial pneumonitis (UIP) [abstract]. Am J Respir Crit Care Med 2001;163:A43.

467. Niden AH, Koss M, Boylen CT, Wilcox A. An open label pilot study to determine the potential efficacy of TNFR: FC (Enbrel®, Etanercept) in the treatment of usual interstitial pneumonitis (UIP) [abstract]. Am J Respir Crit Care Med 2002;165:A728.

468. Panos RJ, Mortenson R, Niccoli SA, King TE Jr. Clinical deterioration in patients with idiopathic pulmonary fibrosis. Causes and assessment. Am J Med 1990;88:396–404.

469. Kondoh Y, Taniguchi H, Kawabata Y, et al. Acute exacerbation in idiopathic pulmonary fibrosis. Analysis of clinical and pathologic findings in three cases. Chest 1993;103:1808–12.

470. Hiwatari N, Shimura S, Takishima T, Shirato K. Bronchoalveolar lavage as a possible cause of acute exacerbation in idiopathic pulmonary fibrosis patients. Tohoku J Exp Med 1994;174:379–86.

471. Akira M, Hamada H, Sakatani M, et al. CT findings during phase of accelerated deterioration in patients with idiopathic pulmonary fibrosis. AJR Am J Roentgenol 1997;168:79–83.

472. Spain D. The association of terminal bronchiolar carcinoma with chronic interstitial inflammation and fibrosis of the lungs. Am Rev Tuberc 1957;76:559–67.

473. Haddad R, Massaro D. Idiopathic diffuse interstitial pulmonary fibrosis (fibrosing alveolitis), atypical epithelial proliferation and lung cancer. Am J Med 1968;45:211–9.

474. Jones AW. Alveolar cell carcinoma occurring in idiopathic interstitial pulmonary fibrosis. Brit J Dis Chest 1970;64:78–84.

475. Driessen APPM, Scherpenisse LA. Familiair voorkomende diffuse interstitiele langfibrose gecompliceerd door alveolaire-cellencarcinoom. Ned Tijdschr Geneeskd 1970;114:2041–5.

476. Turner-Warwick M, Lebowitz M, Burrows B, Johnson A. Cryptogenic fibrosing alveolitis and lung cancer. Thorax 1980;35:496–9.

477. Blaha H, Korg O, Cujnik F. Coincidence of pulmonary fibrosis and bronchial carcinoma. MMWR 1981;123:289–94.

478. Lipton JR, Winstanley J, Carroll K, et al. Treatment of small cell lung carcinoma in association with cryptogenic fibrosing alveolitis. Postgrad Med J 1982;58:160–4.

479. Kitamura H, Kitamura H, Tsugu S. Combined epidermoid and adenocarcinoma in diffuse interstitial pulmonary fibrosis. Hum Pathol 1982;13:580–3.

480. Kawai T, Yakumaru K, Suzuki M, Kageyama K. Diffuse interstitial pulmonary fibrosis and lung cancer. Acta Pathol Jpn 1987;37:11–9.

481. Nagai A, Chiyotani A, Nakadate T, Konno K. Lung cancer in patients with idiopathic pulmonary fibrosis. Tohoku J Exp Med 1992;167:231–7.

482. Mizushima Y, Kobayashi M. Clinical characteristics of synchronous multiple lung cancer associated with idiopathic pulmonary fibrosis. A review of Japanese cases. Chest 1995;108:1272–7.

483. Matsushita H, Tanaka S, Saiki Y, et al. Lung cancer associated with usual interstitial pneumonia. Pathol Int 1995;45:925–32.

484. Takeuchi E, Yamaguchi T, Mori M, et al. Characteristics and management of patients with lung cancer and idiopathic interstitial pneumonia. Jpn J Thorac Dis 1996;34:653–8.

485. Ogura T, Kondo A, Sato A, Ando M, Tamura M. [Incidence and clinical features of lung cancer in patients with idiopathic interstitial pneumonia]. Nihon Kyobu Shikkan Gakkai Zasshi 1997;35:294–9.

486. Hironaka M, Fukayama M. Pulmonary fibrosis and lung carcinoma: a comparative study of metaplastic epithelia in honeycombed areas of usual interstitial pneumonia with or without lung carcinoma. Pathol Int 1999;49:1060–6.

487. Hubbard R, Venn A, Lewis S, Britton J. Lung cancer and cryptogenic fibrosing alveolitis. A population-based cohort study. Am J Respir Crit Care Med 2000;161:5–8.

488. Park J, Kim DS, Shim TS, et al. Lung cancer in patients with idiopathic pulmonary fibrosis. Eur Respir J 2001;17:1216–9.

489. Kawasaki H, Ogura T, Yokose T, et al. p53 Gene alteration in atypical epithelial lesions and carcinoma in patients with idiopathic pulmonary fibrosis. Hum Pathol 2001;32:1043–9.

490. Kawasaki H, Nagai K, Yokose T, et al. Clinicopathological characteristics of surgically resected lung cancer associated with idiopathic pulmonary fibrosis. J Surg Oncol 2001;76:53–7.

491. Ma Y, Seneviratne CK, Koss M. Idiopathic pulmonary fibrosis and malignancy. Curr Opin Pulm Med 2001;7:278–82.

492. Bouros D, Hatzakis K, Labrakis H, Zeibecoglou K. Association of malignancy with diseases causing interstitial pulmonary changes. Chest 2002;121:1278–89.

493. Wells C, Mannino DM. Pulmonary fibrosis and lung cancer in the United States: analysis of the multiple cause of death mortality data, 1979 through 1991. South Med J 1996;89:505–10.

494. Samet JM. Does idiopathic pulmonary fibrosis increase lung cancer risk? Am J Respir Crit Care Med 2000;161:1–2.

495. Kuwano K, Kunitake R, Kawasaki M, et al. p21Waf1/Cip1/Sdi1 and p53 expression in association with DNA strand breaks in idiopathic pulmonary fibrosis. Am J Respir Crit Care Med 1996;154:477–83.

496. Oshikawa K, Sugiyama Y. Serum anti-p53 autoantibodies from patients with idiopathic pulmonary fibrosis associated with lung cancer. Respir Med 2000;94:1085–91.

497. Uematsu K, Yoshimura A, Gemma A, et al. Aberrations in the fragile histidine triad (FHIT) gene in idiopathic pulmonary fibrosis. Cancer Res 2001;61:8527–33.

498. Ellis JR, Gleeson FV. New concepts in lung cancer screening. Curr Opin Pulm Med 2002;8:270–4.

499. Tobin RW, Pope CE II, Pellegrini CA, et al. Increased prevalence of gastroesophageal reflux in patients with idiopathic pulmonary fibrosis. Am J Respir Crit Care Med 1998;158:1804–8.

500. Brown K, King TE Jr. Recent advances in interstitial lung disease. In: Bone RC, Petty TL, editors. 1995 Year Book of pulmonary disease. St. Louis (MO): Mosby Year Book; 1995. p. 396–406.

501. Hiwatari N, Shimura S, Sasaki T, et al. Prognosis of idiopathic pulmonary fibrosis in patients with mucous hypersecretion. Am Rev Respir Dis 1991;143:182–5.

502. van Oortegem K, Wallaert B, Marquette CH, et al. Determinants of response to immunosuppressive therapy in idiopathic pulmonary fibrosis. Eur Respir J 1994;7:1950–7.

503. Lee JS, Im JG, Ahn JM, et al. Fibrosing alveolitis: prognostic implication of ground-glass attenuation at high-resolution CT. Radiology 1992;184:451–4.

504. Wells AU, Hansell DM, Rubens MB, et al. The predictive value of appearances on thin-section computed tomography in fibrosing alveolitis. Am Rev Respir Dis 1993;148:1076–82.

505. Park CS, Chung SW, Ki SY, et al. Increased levels of interleukin-6 are associated with lymphocytosis in bronchoalveolar lavage fluids of idiopathic nonspecific interstitial pneumonia. Am J Respir Crit Care Med 2000;162:1162–8.

506. Kitaichi M. Pathologic features and the classification of interstitial pneumonia of unknown etiology. Bull Chest Dis Res Inst Kyoto Univ 1990;23:1–18.

507. Park CS, Jeon JW, Park SW, et al. Nonspecific interstitial pneumonia/fibrosis: clinical manifestations, histologic and radiologic features. Korean J Intern Med 1996;11:122–32.

508. Cottin V, Donsbeck AV, Revel D, et al. Nonspecific interstitial pneumonia. Individualization of a clinicopathologic entity in a series of 12 patients. Am J Respir Crit Care Med 1998;158:1286–93.

509. Kim TS, Lee KS, Chung MP, et al. Nonspecific interstitial pneumonia with fibrosis: high-resolution CT and pathologic findings. AJR Am J Roentgenol 1998;171:1645–50.

510. Fujita J, Yamadori I, Suemitsu I, et al. Clinical features of nonspecific interstitial pneumonia. Respir Med 1999;93:113–8.

511. Flaherty KR, Travis WD, Colby TV, et al. Histopathologic variability in usual and nonspecific interstitial pneumonias. Am J Respir Crit Care Med 2001;164:1722–7.

512. Myers JL. Nonspecific interstitial pneumonia, UIP, and the ABCs of idiopathic interstitial pneumonias. Eur Respir J 1998;12:1003–4.

513. Kern DG, Durand KTH, Crausman RS, et al. Nonspecific interstitial pneumonia in the synthetic textile industry [abstract]. Am J Respir Crit Care Med 1997;155:A810.

514. Fujita J, Yoshinouchi T, Ohtsuki Y, et al. Non-specific interstitial pneumonia as pulmonary involvement of systemic sclerosis. Ann Rheum Dis 2001;60:281–3.

515. Douglas WW, Tazelaar HD, Hartman TE, et al. Polymyositis-dermatomyositis-associated interstitial lung disease. Am J Respir Crit Care Med 2001;164:1182–5.

516. King TE Jr. Nonspecific interstitial pneumonia and systemic sclerosis. Am J Respir Crit Care Med 2002;165:1578–9.

517. Vourlekis JS, Schwarz MI, Cool CD, et al. Nonspecific interstitial pneumonitis as the sole histologic expression of hypersensitivity pneumonitis. Am J Med 2002;112:490–3.

518. Lantuejoul S, Brambilla E, Brambilla C, Devouassoux G. Statin-induced fibrotic nonspecific interstitial pneumonia. Eur Respir J 2002;19:577–80.

519. Kim DS, Yoo B, Lee JS, et al. The major histopathologic pattern of pulmonary fibrosis in scleroderma is nonspecific interstitial pneumonia. Sarcoidosis Vasc Diffuse Lung Dis 2002;19:121–7.

520. Sattler F, Nichols L, Hirano L, et al. Nonspecific interstitial pneumonitis mimicking *Pneumocystis carinii* pneumonia. Am J Respir Crit Care Med 1997;156:912–7.

521. Siddiqui MT, Garrity ER, Husain AN. Bronchiolitis obliterans organizing pneumonia-like reactions: a nonspecific response or an atypical form of rejection or infection in lung allograft recipients? Hum Pathol 1996;27:714–9.

522. Myers JL, Veal CF, Shin MS, Katzenstein ALA. Respiratory bronchiolitis causing interstitial lung disease: a clinicopathologic study of six cases. Am Rev Respir Dis 1987; 35:880–4.

523. Singh G, Katyal SL, Whiteside TL, Stachura I. Desquamative interstitial pneumonitis. The intra-alveolar cells are macrophages. Chest 1981;79:128.

524. Patchefsky AS, Israel HL, Hoch WS, Gordon G. Desquamative interstitial pneumonia: relationship to interstitial fibrosis. Thorax 1973;28:680–93.

525. Bedrossian CW, Kuhn MC, III, Luna MA, et al. Desquamative interstitial pneumonia-like reaction accompanying pulmonary lesions. Chest 1977;72:166–9.

526. Herbert A, Sterling G, Abraham J, Corrin B. Desquamative interstitial pneumonia in an aluminum welder. Hum Pathol 1982;13:694–9.

527. Freed JA, Miller A, Gordon RE, et al. Desquamative interstitial pneumonia associated with chrysotile asbestos fibres. Br J Ind Med 1991;48:332–7.

528. Lougheed MD, Roos JO, Waddell WR, Munt PW. Desquamative interstitial pneumonitis and diffuse alveolar damage in textile workers. Potential role of mycotoxins. Chest 1995;108:1196–200.

529. Schroten H, Manz S, Köhler H, et al. Fatal desquamative interstitial pneumonia associated with proven CMV infection in an 8-month-old boy. Pediatr Pulmonol 1998;25:345–7.

530. Travis WD, Colby TV, Koss MN, et al. Non-neoplastic disorders of the lower respiratory tract. Washington, DC: Armed Forces Institute of Pathology and American Registry of Pathology; 2002.

531. King TE Jr, Schwarz MI. Chronic diffuse parenchymal lung diseases. In: Davis G, editor. Medical management of pulmonary diseases. New York: Marcel Dekker; 1999. p. 487–529.

532. Persaud V, Bateson EM, Ling JA, Hayes JA. Desquamative interstitial pneumonia. Br J Dis Chest 1967;61:159–62.

533. Tsukahara M, Yoshii H, Imamura T, et al. Desquamative interstitial pneumonia in sibs. Am J Med Genet 1995;59:431–4.

534. Balasubramanyan N, Murphy A, O'Sullivan J, O'Connell EJ. Familial interstitial lung disease in children: response to chloroquine treatment in one sibling with desquamative interstitial pneumonitis [see comments]. Pediatr Pulmonol 1997;23:55–61.

535. Paul K, Klettke U, Moldenhauer J, et al. Increasing dose of methylprednisolone pulse therapy treats desquamative interstitial pneumonia in a child. Eur Respir J 1999; 14:1429–32.

536. Lynch DA, Hay T, Newell JD Jr, et al. Pediatric diffuse lung disease: diagnosis and classification using high-resolution CT. AJR Am J Roentgenol 1999;173:713–8.

537. Nicholson AG, Kim H, Corrin B, et al. The value of classifying interstitial pneumonias in childhood according to defined histological patterns. Histopathology 1998;33:203–11.

538. Cutz E, Wert SE, Nogee LM, Moore AM. Deficiency of lamellar bodies in alveolar type II cells associated with fatal respiratory disease in a full-term infant. Am J Respir Crit Care Med 2000;161:608–14.

539. Stachura I, Singh G, Whiteside TL. Mechanisms of tissue injury in desquamative interstitial pneumonitis. Am J Med 1980;68:733–40.

540. Yousem SA, Colby TV, Gaensler EA. Respiratory bronchiolitis-associated interstitial lung disease and its relationship to desquamative interstitial pneumonia. Mayo Clin Proc 1989;64:1373–80.

541. Ansari A, Buechner HA, Brown M. Desquamative interstitial pneumonia: report of a case and review of the literature. Dis Chest 1968;53:511–6.

542. Goldberg NM, Mostyn EM. Desquamative interstitial pneumonia: a brief review of the literature and a discussion of treatment with oxygen and corticosteroids. Dis Chest 1967;52:245–50.

543. Sahn SA, Schwarz MI. Desquamative interstitial pneumonia with a normal chest radiograph. Br J Dis Chest 1974;68: 228–34.

544. Feigin DS, Friedman PJ. Chest radiography in desquamative interstitial pneumonitis: a review of 37 patients. AJR Am J Roentgenol 1980;134:91–9.

545. Klocke RA, Augerson WS, Berman HH, et al. Desquamative interstitial pneumonia. A disease with a wide clinical spectrum. Ann Intern Med 1967;66:498–506.

546. Hartman TE, Primack SL, Swensen SJ, et al. Desquamative interstitial pneumonia: thin-section CT findings in 22 patients. Radiology 1993;187:787–90.

547. Vedal S, Welsh EV, Miller RR, Mueller NL. Desquamative interstitial pneumonia computed tomographic findings before and after treatment with corticosteroids. Chest 1988;93:215–7.

548. Matsuo K, Tada S, Kataoka M, et al. Spontaneous remission of desquamative interstitial pneumonia [see comments]. Intern Med 1997;36:728–31.

549. Gould TH, Buist MD, Meredith D, Thomas PD. Fulminant

desquamative interstitial pneumonitis. Anaesth Intensive Care 1998;26:677–9.

550. Verleden GM, Sels F, Van Raemdonck D, et al. Possible recurrence of desquamative interstitial pneumonitis in a single lung transplant recipient. Eur Respir J 1998;11:971–4.

551. Niewoehner D, Kleinerman J, Rice D. Pathologic changes in the peripheral airways of young cigarette smokers. N Engl J Med 1974;291:755–8.

552. Cosio MG, Hale KA, Niewoehner DE. Morphologic and morphometric effects of prolonged cigarette smoking on the small airways. Am Rev Respir Dis 1980;122:265–71.

553. Wright JL, Lawson LM, Pare PD, et al. Morphology of peripheral airways in current smokers and ex-smokers. Am Rev Respir Dis 1983;127:474–7.

554. Guerry-Force ML, Mueller NL, Wright JL, et al. A comparison of bronchiolitis obliterans with organizing pneumonia, usual interstitial pneumonia, and small airways disease. Am Rev Respir Dis 1987;135:705–12.

555. King TE Jr, Mortenson RL. Syndromes that mimic idiopathic pulmonary fibrosis. Immunol Allergy Clin North Am 1992;12:461–89.

556. King TE Jr. Respiratory bronchiolitis-associated interstitial lung disease. Clin Chest Med 1993;14:693–8.

557. Park JS, Brown KK, Tuder RM, et al. Respiratory bronchiolitis-associated interstitial lung disease: radiologic features with clinical and pathologic correlation. J Comput Assist Tomogr 2002;26:13–20.

558. Agius RM, Rutman A, Knight RK, Cole PJ. Human pulmonary alveolar macrophages with smokers' inclusions: their relation to the cessation of cigarette smoking. Br J Exp Pathol 1986;67:407–13.

559. BAL Cooperative Group. Bronchoalveolar lavage constituents in healthy individuals, idiopathic pulmonary fibrosis, and selected comparison groups. Am Rev Respir Dis 1990;141:S169–S202.

560. Marques LJ, Teschler H, Guzman J, Costabel U. Smoker's lung transplanted to a nonsmoker. Long-term detection of smoker's macrophages. Am J Respir Crit Care Med 1997;156:1700–2.

561. Lynch DA, Schwarz MI, Heinig MT, et al. Respiratory bronchiolitis: radiographic assessment. Presented at Society of Thoracic Radiology; 1990 Jan 7.

562. Cottin V, Streichenberger N, Gamondès JP, et al. Respiratory bronchiolitis in smokers with spontaneous pneumothorax. Eur Respir J 1998;12:702–4.

563. Holt RM, Schmidt RA, Godwin D, et al. High resolution CT in respiratory bronchiolitis-associated interstitial lung disease. J Comput Assist Tomogr 1993;17:46–50.

564. Gruden JF, Webb WR. CT findings in a proved case of respiratory bronchiolitis. AJR Am J Roentgenol 1993;161:44–6.

565. Remy-Jardin M, Remy J, Gosselin B, et al. Lung parenchymal changes secondary to cigarette smoking: pathologic–CT correlations. Radiology 1993;186:643–51.

566. Lange W. Ueber eine eigenthumliche erkrankung der kleinen bronchien und bronchiolen (bronchitis et bronchiolitis obliterans). Dtsch Arch Klin Med 1901;70:342–64.

567. Grinblat J, Mechlis S, Lewitus Z. Organizing pneumonia-like process. An unusual observation in steroid responsive cases with features of chronic interstitial pneumonia. Chest 1981;80:259–63.

568. Davison AG, Heard BE, McAllister WAC, Turner-Warwick MEH. Cryptogenic organizing pneumonitis. QJM 1983;52:382–94.

569. Epler GR, Colby TV, McLoud TC, et al. Bronchiolitis obliterans organizing pneumonia. N Engl J Med 1985;312:152–8.

570. Lohr RH, Boland BJ, Douglas WW, et al. Organizing pneumonia. Features and prognosis of cryptogenic, secondary, and focal variants. Arch Intern Med 1997;157:1323–9.

571. Chang J, Han J, Kim DW, et al. Bronchiolitis obliterans organizing pneumonia:clinicopathologic review of a series of 45 Korean patients, including rapidly progressive form. J Korean Med Sci 2002;17:179–86.

572. Cazzato S, Zompatori M, Baruzzi G, et al. Bronchiolitis obliterans-organizing pneumonia: an Italian experience. Respir Med 2000;94:702–8.

573. Cordier JF. Organising pneumonia. Thorax 2000;55:318–28.

574. Alasaly K, Muller N, Ostrow D, et al. Cryptogenic organizing pneumonia. A report of 25 cases and a review of the literature. Medicine 1995;74:201–11.

575. King TE Jr. Bronchiolitis obliterans. In: Schwarz MI, King TE Jr, editors. Interstitial lung disease. Philadelphia (PA): Mosby-Year Book; 1993. p. 463–95.

576. Lazor R, Vandevenne A, Pelletier A, et al. Cryptogenic organizing pneumonia. Characteristics of relapses in a series of 48 patients. The Groupe d'Etudes et de Recherche sur les Maladies "Orphelines" Pulmonaires (GERM"O"P). Am J Respir Crit Care Med 2000;162:571–7.

577. Mroz BJ, Sexauer WP, Meade A, Balsara G. Hemoptysis as the presenting symptom in bronchiolitis obliterans organizing pneumonia. Chest 1997;111:1775–8.

578. Cordier JF. Cryptogenic organizing pneumonitis. Clin Chest Med 1993;14:677–92.

579. Izumi T. The global view of idiopathic bronchiolitis obliterans organizing pneumonia. In: Epler GR, editor. Diseases of the bronchioles. New York: Raven Press; 1994. p. 307–12.

580. Poletti V, Castrilli G, Romagna M, et al. Bronchoalveolar lavage, histological and immunohistochemical features in cryptogenic organizing pneumonia. Monaldi Arch Chest Dis 1996;51:289–95.

581. Forlani S, Ratta L, Bulgheroni A, et al. Cytokine profile of bronchoalveolar lavage in BOOP and UIP. Sarcoidosis Vasc Diffuse Lung Dis 2002;19:47–53.

582. Mukae H, Kadota J, Kohno S, et al. Increase of activated T-cells in BAL fluid of Japanese patients with bronchiolitis obliterans organizing pneumonia and chronic eosinophilic pneumonia. Chest 1995;108:123–8.

583. Pesci A, Majori M, Piccoli ML, et al. Mast cells in bronchiolitis obliterans organizing pneumonia. Mast cell hyperplasia and evidence for extracellular release of tryptase. Chest 1996;110:383–91.

584. Costabel U, Teschler H, Guzman J. Bronchiolitis obliterans organizing pneumonia (BOOP): the cytological and immunocytological profile of bronchoalveolar lavage. Eur Respir J 1992;5:791–7.

585. Choi KH, Lee HB, Jeong MY, et al. The role of matrix metalloproteinase-9 and tissue inhibitor of metalloproteinase-1 in cryptogenic organizing pneumonia. Chest 2002;121:1478–85.

586. King TE Jr, Mortenson RL. Cryptogenic organizing pneumonia. The North American experience. Chest 1992;102:8S–13S.

587. Davison AG, Heard BE, McAllister WAC, Turner-Warwick MEH. Steriod-responsive relapsing cryptogenic organising pneumonitis. Thorax 1982;37:785–6.

588. Muller NL, Guerry-Force ML, Staples CA, et al. Differential diagnosis of bronchiolitis obliterans with organizing pneumonia and usual interstitial pneumonia clinical, functional, and radiologic findings. Radiology 1987;162:151–6.

589. Chandler PW, Shin MS, Friedman SE, et al. Radiographic manifestations of bronchiolitis obliterans with organizing pneumonia versus usual interstitial pneumonia. AJR Am J Roentgenol 1986;147:899–906.

590. Muller NL, Staples CA, Miller RR. Bronchiolitis obliterans organizing pneumonia: CT features in 14 patients. AJR Am J Roentgenol1990;154:983–7.

591. Haddock JA, Hansell DM. The radiology and terminology of cryptogenic organizing pneumonia. Br J Radiol 1992;65:674–80.

592. Nishimura K, Itoh H. High-resolution computed tomographic features of bronchiolitis obliterans organizing pneumonia. Chest 1992;102:26S–31S.

593. Flowers JR, Clunie G, Burke M, Constant O. Bronchiolitis obliterans organizing pneumonia: the clinical and radiological features of seven cases and a review of the literature. Clin Radiol 1992;45:371–7.

594. Lee KS, Kullnig P, Hartman TE, Muller NL. Cryptogenic organizing pneumonia: CT findings in 43 patients. AJR Am J Roetngenol 1994;162:543–6.

595. Reich J, Scott D. Levitating lung lesions due to bronchiolitis obliterans organizing pneumonia. Chest 1993;103:623–4.

596. Izumi T, Kitaichi M, Nishimura K, Nagai S. Bronchiolitis obliterans organizing pneumonia. Clinical features and differential diagnosis. Chest 1992;102:715–9.

597. Oikonomou A, Hansell DM. Organizing pneumonia: the many morphological faces. Eur Radiol 2002;12:1486–96.

598. Bouchardy LM, Kuhlman JE, Ball WC Jr, et al. CT findings in bronchiolitis obliterans organizing pneumonia (BOOP) with radiographic, clinical, and histologic correlation. J Comput Assist Tomogr 1993;17:352–7.

599. Kanwar BA, Shehan CJ, Campbell JC, et al. A case of unilateral bronchiolitis obliterans organizing pneumonia (BOOP). Nebr Med J 1996;81:149–51.

600. Preidler KW, Szolar DM, Moelleken S, et al. Distribution pattern of computed tomography findings in patients with bronchiolitis obliterans organizing pneumonia. Invest Radiol 1996;31:251–5.

601. Akira M, Yamamoto S, Sakatani M. Bronchiolitis obliterans organizing pneumonia manifesting as multiple large nodules or masses. AJR Am J Roentgenol 1998;170:291–5.

602. Cohen AJ, King TE Jr, Downey GP. Rapidly progressive bronchiolitis obliterans with organizing pneumonia. Am J Respir Crit Care Med 1994;149:1670–5.

603. Voloudaki AE, Bouros DE, Froudarakis ME, et al. Crescentic and ring-shaped opacities. CT features in two cases of bronchiolitis obliterans organizing pneumonia (BOOP). Acta Radiologica 1996;37:889–92.

604. Katzenstein ALA, Myers JL, Prophet DW, et al. Bronchiolitis obliterans and usual interstitial pneumonia. Am J Surg Pathol 1986;10:373–81.

605. Colby TV, Myers JL. The clinical and histologic spectrum of bronchiolitis obliterans including bronchiolitis obliterans organizing pneumonia (BOOP). Semin Respir Med 1992;13:119–33.

606. Aubert JD, Paré PD, Hogg JC, Hayashi S. Platelet-derived growth factor in bronchiolitis obliterans-organizing pneumonia. Am J Respir Crit Care Med 1997;155:676–81.

607. Azzam ZS, Bentur L, Rubin AH, et al. Bronchiolitis obliterans organizing pneumonia. Diagnosis by transbronchial biopsy. Chest 1993;104:1899–901.

608. Poletti V, Cazzato S, Minicuci N, et al. The diagnostic value of bronchoalveolar lavage and transbronchial lung biopsy in cryptogenic organizing pneumonia. Eur Respir J 1996;9:2513–6.

609. Mihara N, Johkoh T, Ichikado K, et al. Can acute interstitial pneumonia be differentiated from bronchiolitis obliterans organizing pneumonia by high-resolution CT? Radiat Med 2000;18:299–304.

610. Arakawa H, Kurihara Y, Niimi H, et al. Bronchiolitis obliterans with organizing pneumonia versus chronic eosinophilic pneumonia: high-resolution CT findings in 81 patients. AJR Am J Roentgenol 2001;176:1053–8.

611. Yamamoto M, Ina Y, Kitaichi M. Bronchiolitis obliterans organizing pneumonia (BOOP): profile in Japan. In: Harasawa M, Fukuchi Y, Morinari H, editors. Interstitial pneumonia of unknown etiology. Tokyo: University of Tokyo Press; 1989. p. 61–70.

612. Purcell IF, Bourke SJ, Marshall SM. Cyclophosphamide in severe steroid-resistant bronchiolitis obliterans organizing pneumonia. Respir Med 1997;91:175–7.

613. Ichikawa Y, Ninomiya H, Katsuki M, et al. Low-dose/long-term erythromycin for treatment of bronchiolitis obliterans organizing pneumonia (BOOP). Kurume Med J 1993;40:65–7.

614. Katzenstein ALA, Myers JL, Mazur MT. Acute interstitial pneumonia. A clinicopathologic, ultrastructural, and cell kinetic study. Am J Surg Pathol 1986;10:256–67.

615. Bouros D, Nicholson AC, Polychronopoulos V, du Bois RM. Acute interstitial pneumonia. Eur Respir J 2000;15:412–8.

616. Vourlekis JS, Brown KK, Cool CD, et al. Acute interstitial pneumonitis: case series and review of the literature. Medicine 2000;79:369–78.

617. King TE Jr. Acute interstitial pneumonia (Hamman-Rich syndrome). In: Rose BD, editor. UpToDate. Wellesley (MA): UpToDate; 2002.

618. Hamman L, Rich AR. Fulminating diffuse interstitial fibrosis of the lungs. Trans Am Clin Climatol Assoc 1935;51:154–63.

619. Fulmer JD, Katzenstein ALA. The interstitial lung diseases. In: Bone RC, editor. Pulmonary and critical care medicine. Vol. 2. St. Louis (MO): Mosby Year Book; 1993.p. M1–1–15.

620. Kuhn C III, Boldt J, King TE Jr, et al. An immunohistochemical study of architectural remodeling and connective tissue synthesis in pulmonary fibrosis. Am Rev Respir Dis 1989;140:1693–1703.

621. Kuhn C III. Patterns of lung repair. A morphologist's view. Chest 1991;99:11S–14S.

622. Olson J, Colby TV, Elliott CG. Hamman-Rich syndrome revisited. Mayo Clin Proc 1990;65:1538–48.

623. Primack SL, Hartman TE, Ikezoe J, et al. Acute interstitial pneumonia: radiographic and CT findings in nine patients. Radiology 1993;188:817–20.

624. Nagai S, Kitaichi M, Izumi T. Classification and recent advances in idiopathic interstitial pneumonia. Curr Opin Pulm Med 1998;4:256–60.

625. Ichikado K, Johkoh T, Ikezoe J, et al. Acute interstitial pneumonia: high-resolution CT findings correlated with pathology. AJR Am J Roentgenol 1997;168:333–8.

626. Hansell DM. Acute interstitial pneumonia: clues from the white stuff. Am J Respir Crit Care Med 2002;165:1465–6.

627. Ichikado K, Suga M, Muller NL, et al. Acute interstitial pneumonia: comparison of high-resolution computed tomography findings between survivors and nonsurvivors. Am J Respir Crit Care Med 2002;165:1551–6.

628. Johkoh T, Muller NL, Taniguchi H, et al. Acute interstitial pneumonia: thin-section CT findings in 36 patients. Radiology 1999;211:859–63.

629. Desai SR, Wells AU, Rubens MB, et al. Acute respiratory distress syndrome: CT abnormalities at long-term follow-up. Radiology 1999;210:29–35.

630. Desai SR. Acute respiratory distress syndrome: imaging of the injured lung. Clin Radiol 2002;57:8–17.

631. Tomiyama N, Muller NL, Johkoh T, et al. Acute respiratory distress syndrome and acute interstitial pneumonia: comparison of thin-section CT findings. J Comput Assist Tomogr 2001;25:28–33.

632. Meduri GU, Belenchia JM, Estes RJ, et al. Fibroproliferative phase of ARDS. Clinical findings and effects of corticosteroids. Chest 1991;100:943–52.

633. Meduri GU, Tolley EA, Chrousos GP, Stentz F. Prolonged methylprednisolone treatment suppresses systemic inflammation in patients with unresolving acute respiratory distress syndrome: evidence for inadequate endogenous glucocorticoid secretion and inflammation-induced immune cell resistance to glucocorticoids. Am J Respir Crit Care Med 2002;165:983–91.

634. Meduri GU, Headley AS, Golden E, et al. Effect of prolonged methylprednisolone therapy in unresolving acute respiratory distress syndrome: a randomized controlled trial. JAMA 1998;280:159–65.

635. Meduri GU, Chinn AJ, Leeper KV, et al. Corticosteroid rescue treatment of progressive fibroproliferation in late ARDS. Patterns of response and predictors of outcome. Chest 1994;105:1516–27.

636. Katzenstein AL, Askin FB. Surgical pathology of non-neoplastic lung disease. Philadelphia (PA): W.B. Saunders, 1997.

637. Suga M, Iyonaga K, Okamoto T, et al. Characteristic elevation of matrix metalloproteinase activity in idiopathic interstitial pneumonias. Am J Respir Crit Care Med 2000;162:1949–56.

638. Wells AU, Cullinan P, Hansell DM, et al. Fibrosing alveolitis associated with systemic sclerosis has a better prognosis than lone cryptogenic fibrosing alveolitis. Am J Respir Crit Care Med 1994;149:1583–90.

639. Kuhn C III, McDonald JA. The roles of the myofibroblast in idiopathic pulmonary fibrosis: ultrastructural and immunohistochemical features of sites of active extracellular matrix synthesis. Am J Pathol 1991;138:1257–65.

640. Peyrol S, Cordier JF, Grimaud JA. Intra-alveolar fibrosis of idiopathic bronchiolitis obliterans-organizing pnemonia. Cell-matrix patterns. Am J Pathol 1990;137:155–70.

641. Lappi-Blanco E, Soini Y, Pääkkö P. Apoptotic activity is increased in the newly formed fibromyxoid connective tissue in bronchiolitis obliterans organizing pneumonia. Lung 1999;177:367–76.

642. Selman M, Ruiz V, Cabrera S, et al. TIMP-1, -2, -3, and -4 in idiopathic pulmonary fibrosis. A prevailing nondegradative lung microenvironment? Am J Physiol Lung Cell Mol Physiol 2000;279:L562–74.

643. Hayashi T, Stetler-Stevenson WG, Fleming MV, et al. Immunohistochemical study of metalloproteinases and their tissue inhibitors in the lungs of patients with diffuse alveolar damage and idiopathic pulmonary fibrosis. Am J Pathol 1996;149:1241–56.

644. Raghu G, Striker LJ, Hudson LD, Striker GE. Extracellular matrix in normal and fibrotic human lungs. Am Rev Respir Dis 1985;131:281–9.

645. Uhal BD, Joshi I, True AL, et al. Fibroblasts isolated after fibrotic lung injury induce apoptosis of alveolar epithelial cells in vitro. Am J Physiol Lung Cell Mol Physiol 1995;269:L819–28.

646. Uhal BD, Joshi I, Hughes WF, et al. Alveolar epithelial cell death adjacent to underlying myofibroblasts in advanced fibrotic human lung. Am J Physiol Lung Cell Mol Physiol 1998;275:L1192–9.

647. Lappi-Blanco E, Kaarteenaho-Wiik R, Soini Y, et al. Intraluminal fibromyxoid lesions in bronchiolitis obliterans organizing pneumonia are highly capillarized. Hum Pathol 1999;30:1192–6.

648. Johkoh T, Müller NL, Cartier Y, et al. Idiopathic interstitial pneumonias: diagnostic accuracy of thin-section CT in 129 patients. Radiology 1999;211:555–60.

649. Park JS, Lee KS, Kim JS, et al. Nonspecific interstitial pneumonia with fibrosis: radiographic and CT findings in seven patients. Radiology 1995;195:645–8.

650. Cordier JF, Loire R, Brune J. Idiopathic bronchiolitis obliterans organizing pneumonia. Definition of characteristic clinical profiles in a series of 16 patients. Chest 1989;96:999–1004.

651. Ikezoe J, Johkoh T, Kohno N, et al. High-resolution CT findings of lung disease in patients with polymyositis and dermatomyositis. J Thorac Imaging 1996;11:250–9.

652. Murphy JM, Schnyder P, Verschakelen J, et al. Linear opacities on HRCT in bronchiolitis obliterans organising pneumonia. Eur Radiol 1999;9:1813–7.

653. Gosink BB, Friedman PJ, Liebow AA. Bronchiolitis obliterans: roentgenologic-pathologic correlation. Am J Roentgenol Radium Ther Nucl Med 1973;117:816–32.

654. DeRemee RA. Facets of the algorithmic synthesis. In: DeRemee RA, ed. Clinical profiles of diffuse interstitial pulmonary disease. Mount Kisco (NY): Futura Publishing Company; 1990. p. 9–44.

655. Badesch D, Collins T, King TE Jr. Rapidly progressive interstitial lung disease in a 58-year old man. Semin Respir Med 1989;10:101–4.

656. Bartter T, Irwin RS, Nash G, et al. Idiopathic bronchiolitis obliterans organizing pneumonia with peripheral infiltrates on chest roentgenogram. Arch Intern Med 1989;149:273–9.

26

BRONCHIOLITIS

TALMADGE E. KING JR

Bronchiolitis is a fibrotic lung disease that primarily affects the small conducting airways, often sparing a considerable portion of the interstitium (Figures 26–1 and 26–2). The small airways of the lung are those airways 3 mm or less in diameter, the vast majority of which are bronchioles. Bronchioles are divided into terminal (membranous) and respiratory bronchioles. Terminal bronchioles are constructed of ciliated cuboidal epithelium, thin discontinuous bands of smooth muscle, and submucosal connective tissue. Terminal bronchioles function purely as an air-conducting system. Respiratory bronchioles contain alveoli within their walls, allowing them to play a role in respiration. The small airways represent a relatively silent portion of the lung. Because of their large number and resulting overall cross-sectional area, small airways contribute very little to resistance. Therefore, there may be considerable damage to the small airways before the patient is symptomatic or before there are any detectable abnormalities on lung function testing.

Bronchiolitis results from damage to the bronchiolar epithelium. The repair process leads to excessive proliferation of granulation tissue in the airway walls, the lumen, or both. The alveoli adjacent to the small airways are almost always involved. Because of the variable course, etiology, and histologic appearance, it has been difficult to derive a clear understanding of this disease. Consequently, there remain many uncertainties regarding the epidemiology, pathophysiology, pathogenesis, long-term sequelae, and treatment of bronchiolitis.

Bronchiolitis was probably first recognized in the 1800s, but it was not described well until 1901.[1] Interest in "bronchiolar syndromes" has increased in the last two decades because of the recognition that bronchiolar injury (bronchiolitis with or without obliterans) frequently accompanies infections, organ transplantation, drug reactions, connective tissue diseases, and toxic gas or fume exposure. In addition, several syndromes that involve the small airways have been identified and better clarified. Finally, bronchiolocentric lesions affecting mainly the small airways may present with manifestations that are more suggestive of an interstitial lung disease (see Chapter 2, "Anatomic Distribution and Histopathologic Patterns of Interstitial Lung Disease"). This chapter reviews the clinical, radiographic, and histopathologic findings of the bronchiolar syndromes.[2] Bronchiolar injury and repair are important features of asthma and bronchitis/emphysema, but because of the limited scope of this chapter they will not be discussed.

This chapter is divided into two sections: (1) an overview of the definitions, approach to diagnosis, and common features of bronchiolitis and (2) a discussion of the specific disease entities.

GENERAL CONSIDERATIONS

Definitions

The nomenclature applied to the bronchiolar syndromes has been confusing. The following terms have been used: bronchiolitis obliterans, bronchiolitis fibrosa obliterans, bronchiolitis obliterans and interstitial pneumonia, bronchiolitis obliterans organizing pneumonia (BOOP), cryptogenic organizing pneumonia (COP), and follicular bronchiolitis. Unfortunately, the terms are frequently used interchangeably to describe what are now believed to be separate and distinct clinical entities. In the past, the common clinical use of the term "bronchiolitis obliterans" was to describe a morphologically heterogeneous group of lesions that resulted in airflow limitation on lung function testing. However, pathologists generally used the term to describe a distinct form of intraluminal fibrosis that was most likely to be associated clinically

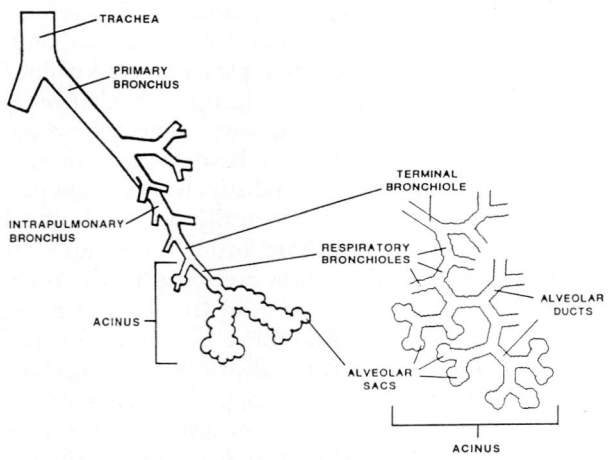

Figure 26–1 The tracheobronchial airway tree: the trachea, primary bronchi, intrapulmonary bronchi, terminal bronchioles, and air passages of the pulmonary acinus. Reproduced with permission from Plopper et al.[296]

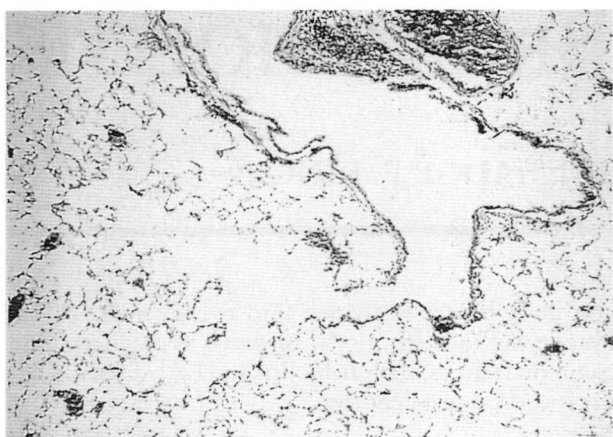

Figure 26–2   Junctional area between the purely conductive airways and the respiratory portion of the lung. The terminal (nonrespiratory) bronchiole has a continuous cuboidal epithelium, whereas alveoli open off the respiratory bronchiole (hematoxylin and eosin stain). Reproduced with permission from Corrin B.[297]

with a restrictive lung function abnormality on lung function testing. Prior to the description of BOOP in 1985, most cases described as idiopathic bronchiolitis obliterans were probably examples of BOOP.

In an effort to clarify our discussion of bronchiolitis, we have chosen the following definitions.

- Bronchiolitis: the broad spectrum of histopathologic processes that show some degree of inflammation, narrowing, or obliteration of the small airways.
- Bronchiolitis obliterans: the histologic lesion characterized by polypoid obliteration of the lumen of bronchioles, without involvement of the distal lung parenchyma, by inflammation or organizing pneumonia, ie, constrictive bronchiolitis. Constrictive bronchiolitis is, in general, a rare finding in isolation.
- Bronchiolitis obliterans syndrome: a clinical term that refers to the progressive airflow limitation secondary to small airway obstruction, which commonly complicates lung transplantation. It is defined not by histology but by lung function changes.[3,4] However, not all lung transplant recipients in whom airflow obstruction develops have this syndrome.[4]
- Organizing pneumonia: a distinctive reaction pattern characterized histologically by intraluminal polyps in the respiratory bronchioles, alveolar ducts, and alveolar spaces accompanied by organizing pneumonia in the more distal parenchyma (see Chapter 2, "Anatomic Distribution and Histopathologic Patterns of Interstitial Lung Disease" and Chapter 24, "Eosinophilic Pneumonias"). In organizing pneumonia, the alveolar walls show a mild to moderate chronic inflammatory infiltrate, type II cell hyperplasia, and foamy macrophages in the alveolar spaces; a proliferative bronchiolitis is present. Because only a minority of cases showing the organizing pneumonia pattern represent the

idiopathic syndrome described in 1985, and because patients with idiopathic BOOP manifest a distinctive clinical syndrome, this group is referred to as cryptogenic organizing pneumonia in order to distinguish this syndrome from other causes of the organizing pneumonia pattern.

- Cryptogenic organizing pneumonia: according to the American Thoracic Society/European Respiratory Society consensus statement, the term COP is preferred over the term BOOP. COP conveys the essential features of the syndrome and avoids confusion with airway diseases such as constrictive bronchiolitis obliterans that can be problematic with the term BOOP.[5] Although in organizing pneumonia the majority of the histopathologic changes are centered on small airways, the major feature is a patchy process characterized by organizing pneumonia involving alveolar ducts and alveoli, with or without bronchiolar intraluminal polyps (see Chapter 25, "Idiopathic Interstitial Pneumonias").

Classification of Bronchiolitis

Three classification schemes appear useful in defining cases of bronchiolitis: (1) a clinical classification based on the etiology; (2) a histopathologic classification, which includes two major morphologic types (proliferative bronchiolitis and constrictive bronchiolitis), and (3) a radiologic classification based on the findings of thin-section high-resolution computed tomography (HRCT).[6,7] The histopathologic–radiologic classification appears most useful, because the histopathologic–radiologic changes correlate best with clinical manifestations.

Clinical Classification

The clinical classification of bronchiolitis is based on etiology (Table 26–1): inhalation injury, infections, drug reactions, and idiopathic causes. The first three categories are frequently recognized by their association with an acute illness or known exposure prior to the onset of disease. Idiopathic cases often have a more insidious onset, characterized by cough or dyspnea; initially, they may be confused with more common problems, such as chronic obstructive pulmonary disease (COPD) or interstitial lung disease, depending on the predominant histopathologic pattern.

Radiologic Classification

HRCT is an excellent way to examine the morphology of small airways diseases (Figure 26–3). Consequently, it has become the method of choice for assessing these airways, often replacing the need for surgical lung biopsy. Several studies have examined the patterns found on computed tomography (CT) scans and correlated these patterns with histopathologic findings.[8–10] Based on radiologic features, Müller and Miller classified bronchiolar diseases into three predominant CT patterns: (1) nodules and branching lines; (2) ground-glass opacification (hazy increased attenuation, ie, increased density of the lung with preservation of bronchial and vascular margins) and consolidation (hazy increased parenchymal attenuation in which the bronchial and vascular margins are obscured); and (3) low attenuation (ie, decreased density of lung or "black lung") and mosaic perfusion (a patchwork of regions of varied attenuation, interpreted as secondary to regional differences in perfusion) (Table 26–2).[8,11] They showed that these patterns correlated with certain histopathologic features and clinical syndromes.

Histopathologic Classification

The histopathologic classification of bronchiolitis includes the proliferative and constrictive varieties (Table 26–3). Each type, including the presumed pathogenesis, is described below.

Proliferative Bronchiolitis. Proliferative bronchiolitis is characterized by an organizing intraluminal exudate and is found, to some degree, in a variety of pulmonary disorders.[7] It is particularly extensive and prominent in COP (also called idiopathic BOOP). The intraluminal fibrotic buds (Masson bodies) are seen in respiratory bronchioles, alveolar ducts, and alveoli (Figure 26–4). Proliferative bronchiolitis is most frequently associated with diffuse alveolar opacities on chest radiograph and CT scan. A restrictive defect is found on pulmonary function testing, especially when COP is present.

Constrictive Bronchiolitis. Constrictive bronchiolitis is characterized by alterations in the walls of membranous and respiratory bronchioles that cause concentric narrowing or complete obliteration of the airway lumen (Figure 26–5). The changes of constrictive bronchiolitis may be extremely subtle, and frequently they are identified only after step-sectioning and special staining (eg, the use of stains to identify remnants of airway walls) of the lung biopsy specimen. Often these lesions occur without extensive changes in alveolar ducts or alveolar walls. The range of histopathologic changes includes (1) subtle cellular infiltrates around the small airways; (2) extensive cellular infiltrates and smooth muscle hyperplasia; (3) bronchiolectasia with mucus stasis, distortion, and fibrosis; and (4) total obliterative bronchiolar scarring.[7] These lesions are seen most often in patients with progressive obstructive lung disease. The chest radiograph may be normal. Cases of constrictive bronchiolitis are very rare. It is useful to further divide constrictive bronchiolitis into five main groups: (1) cellular bronchioli-

TABLE 26–1   Clinical Syndromes Associated with Histologic Bronchiolitis, with or without Obliterans

Inhalation injury
   Toxic fume inhalation
   Irritant gases
   Mineral dusts
   Organic dusts
   Volatile flavoring agents[76,77]

Postinfectious
   Diffuse lesions
   Localized lesions

Drug-induced reactions

Idiopathic
   No associated diseases
      Cryptogenic bronchiolitis
      Respiratory bronchiolitis-associated interstitial lung disease
      Cryptogenic organizing pneumonia
   Associated with other diseases
      Associated with organ transplantation
      Associated with connective tissue disease
         De novo process
         Drug reaction
      Idiopathic pulmonary fibrosis
      Hypersensitivity pneumonitis
      Malignant histiocytosis
      Chronic eosinophilic pneumonia
      Adult respiratory distress syndrome
      Vasculitis, especially Wegener's granulomatosis
      Chronic thyroiditis
      Primary biliary cirrhosis[303]
      Ulcerative colitis[304]
      Irradiation pneumonitis
      Aspiration pneumonitis[305,306]
      Diffuse panbronchiolitis
      Lysinuric protein intolerance[307]
      Ataxia-telangiectasia[308]
      Kartagener's syndrome[309]
      Pulmonary capillaritis[310]
      Paraneoplastic pemphigus[294]

tis, (2) follicular bronchiolitis, (3) diffuse panbronchiolitis, (4) respiratory (smoker's) bronchiolitis, and (5) cryptogenic constrictive bronchiolitis (see Table 26–3).

Cellular Bronchiolitis. Cellular bronchiolitis is a descriptive histologic term that refers to inflammatory infiltrates that involve the lumen, the walls of bronchioles, or both.[12] The inflammation may be acute, chronic, or both.

Follicular Bronchiolitis. Follicular bronchiolitis is a distinctive subset of cellular bronchiolitis characterized by the dramatic proliferation of lymphoid follicles with germinal centers along the airways and an infiltration of the epithelium by lymphocytes.[12] Follicular bronchitis and bronchiolitis may occur in patients with rheumatoid arthritis, Sjögren's syndrome, juvenile rheumatoid arthritis, immunodeficiency syndromes, familial lung disorders, chronic infection, and a heterogeneous group of patients with a hypersensitivity-type reaction.[13,14]

Diffuse Panbronchiolitis. Diffuse panbronchiolitis is an inflammatory process characterized by mononuclear cell inflammation of the respiratory bronchioles

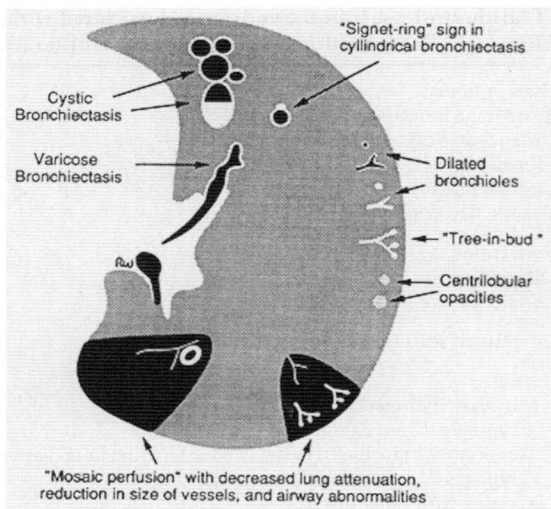

Figure 26–3 High-resolution computed tomography (HRCT) findings in airway diseases. Reproduced with permission from Webb WR.[298]

and the presence of foamy macrophages in the bronchiolar lumina and adjacent alveoli. These findings often produce nodular lesions.[12]

Respiratory Bronchiolitis.   Respiratory bronchiolitis is characterized by a cellular reaction in and around respiratory bronchioles. There is mild inflammation of the walls of the respiratory bronchioles, which extends to involve the adjacent alveoli.[12] Slight fibrosis may be present. There is often a prominent increase in pigmented macrophages in the airway lumina and alveolar spaces (see Chapter 25, "Idiopathic Interstitial Pneumonias").

Cryptogenic Constrictive Bronchiolitis.   Cryptogenic constrictive bronchiolitis (bronchiolitis obliterans) is characterized by submucosal and peribronchial fibrosis that causes concentric extrinsic narrowing of the bronchiolar lumen with little, if any, active inflammation.[9,12] A variety of other histologic changes can be seen: smooth muscle hyperplasia, bronchiolectasis with mucus stasis, distortion and fibrosis of the walls of small airways with bronchial metaplasia extending to peribronchiolar alveolar septa, and complete irreversible luminal obliteration with ultimate replacement of the bronchiole by an acellular scar.[12]

Epidemiology of Bronchiolitis

The epidemiology of bronchiolitis is not completely understood. Bronchiolitis in infants and children is recognized worldwide. Because of its association with infection, bronchiolitis predictably occurs with outbreaks of infection, depending on the specific etiologic agent.[15] For example, respiratory syncytial virus (RSV) is the most common agent in infant bronchiolitis; therefore, outbreaks in this age group tend to mirror epidemics of RSV infection. The overall average rate of bronchiolitis for all pathogens and all ages is 16 per 100 children less than 18 years of age.[15]

Adult bronchiolitis (with or without obliterans) is rare and has not been well studied. Many cases are associated with accidents that result in inhalation injuries. The estimated annual incidence of silo filler's disease is 5 cases per 100,000 silo-associated farm workers.[16] Most cases occur during the harvest period (September to October).

TABLE 26–2   Radiologic Classification of Bronchiolitis

Predominant CT Pattern*	Predominant Histopathologic Pattern	Common Diseases
Nodules and branching lines	Cellular bronchiolitis	Infectious bronchiolitis, acute *Aspergillus* infection, diffuse panbronchiolitis, bronchial disease (asthma chronic bronchitis, bronchietasis)
Low attenuation and mosaic perfusion	Constrictive bronchiolitis	Viral infections, *Mycoplasma pneumoniae*, toxic fume inhalation, connective tissue disease (especially rheumatoid arthritis), bone marrow, lung, or heart-lung transplantation, inflammatory bowel disease
Ground-glass opacification and consolidation	Bronchiolitis obliterans organizing pneumonia	Cryptogenic organizing pneumonia, secondary bronchiolitis obliterans organizing pneumonia
	Respiratory bronchiolitis	Smoker's bronchiolitis, respiratory bronchiolitis-associated interstitial lung disease, desquamative interstitial pneumonia
Mixed patterns	Chronic infiltrative lung diseases with bronchiolocentric infiltrates	Hypersensitivity pneumonitis, sarcoidosis, pneumoconiosis (asbestosis and silicosis), hard metal pneumoconiosis (giant cell interstitial pneumonia)
	Follicular bronchiolitis	Connective tissue disease, immunodeficiency disease, hypersensitivity reaction with eosinophilia

Adapted from Müller and Miller.[8]
*Most diseases have additional features on computed tomography (CT) scan, but these are the predominant patterns.

TABLE 26–3   Pathologic and Radiologic Features of Various Forms of Constrictive Bronchiolitis

Pathologic Diagnosis	Pathologic Features	HRCT Features	Prototype Clinical Entity	Other Causes
Cryptogenic constrictive bronchiolitis	Circumferential thickening of bronchiolar wall with obliteration of lumen	Diffuse or geographic mosaic pattern, bronchial dilatation, air trapping	Prior toxic fume exposure, Chronic rejection (bone marrow, heart-lung, or lung transplantation)	Rheumatoid lung disease, Prior viral/*Mycoplasma* infection, Swyer-James syndrome, Inflammatory bowel disease, Neuroendocrine cell hyperplasia
Respiratory bronchiolitis	Mild chronic bronchiolar inflammation, macrophage accumulation in bronchiolar lumen and adjacent alveoli	Poorly defined centrilobular nodules, patchy ground-glass attenuation	Smoker's lung	None
Cellular bronchiolitis	Inflammatory infiltration of bronchiolar wall	Centrilobular nodules, centrilobular branching lines, tree-in-bud pattern	Acute infection (viral, *Mycoplasma*)	Chronic infection (mycobacterial), Invasive aspergillosis, Hypersensitivity pneumonitis
Follicular bronchiolitis	Lymphoid follicles adjacent to bronchioles	Centrilobular nodules, peribronchial nodules, ground-glass opacity	Rheumatoid lung disease	Other collagen vascular diseases Immunodeficiency
Diffuse panbronchiolitis	Severe transmural inflammation of bronchiolar wall, foamy macrophages in bronchiolar lumen	Centrilobular nodules, centrilobular branching lines, tree-in-bud pattern, bronchiolectasis, bronchiectasis	Difuse panbronchiolitis	Cystic fibrosis, Immune deficiency, Atypical mycobacterial infection

Adapted from Müller and Miller,[8] Worthy and Müller,[9] and Colby and Leslie.[12]
HRCT = high-resolution computed tomography.

In a search of the pathology and interstitial lung disease databases for the years 1993 to 2000 at the University of Colorado, only 19 patients with bronchiolitis were identified (excluding those post-transplantion or with respiratory bronchiolitis or diffuse panbronchiolitis). In the case of bone marrow, heart-lung, and lung transplant recipients, bronchiolitis is a relatively common complication (see below). Bronchiolitis obliterans occurs in 50 to 60% of lung or heart-lung recipients by 5 years post-transplantation.

Pathogenesis

In some diseases associated with bronchiolitis, varying degrees of both proliferative and constrictive bronchiolitis can be found on histologic examination. Thus, it appears that a similar sequence of events may lead to both histopathologic patterns of bronchiolitis. The particular type and severity of bronchiolitis that develops appear to relate to the type of insult, the extent and severity of the initial insult, and predominant site of the injury (bronchioles, alveolar ducts, or both).

The initial lesion in constrictive bronchiolitis likely involves airway epithelial injury and destruction. An inflammatory response follows, with accumulation of neutrophils at the site of injury. Neutrophils cause further injury to the airway epithelium and matrix by release of inflammatory mediators. The persistence of the injury may determine whether there is resolution and recovery or progression to a less reversible state, manifested by intramural and intraluminal fibrosis. The repair process results in the characteristic obliterative bronchiolar lesions.

Studies of bronchiolitis following transplantation have provided additional insight into the potential pathogenetic mechanism that leads to some forms of small airway injury. Bronchiolitis following transplantation is thought to be primarily a result of chronic lung rejection.[17] Alloimmunologic injury to endothelial and epithelial structures is a key feature.[4] Donor-specific alloreactivity of bronchoalveolar lavage (BAL) fluid lymphocytes, manifested by a proliferative response to donor spleen cells, appears to be a useful marker for this process.[18] DiGiovine and colleagues have suggested that the pathogenesis of bronchiolitis obliterans is mediated, in part, by neutrophils.[19] Bronchiolitis obliterans is associated with an increased oxidative burden and activation of inflammatory and growth-stimulating mediators. These subjects have significantly elevated neutrophil counts and levels of interleukin (IL)-8 compared to lung transplant recipients without bronchiolitis obliterans. Furthermore, they demonstrate immunolocalization of IL-8 associated with α-smooth muscle actin-positive cells in the peribronchial region of bronchiolitis obliterans. Belperio and coworkers found that elevated levels of the

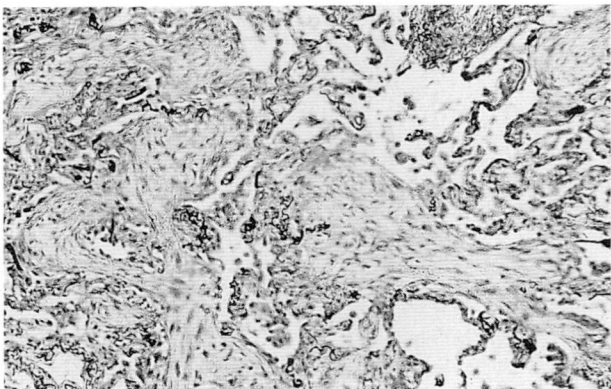

Figure 26–4   Bronchiolitis obliterans organizing pneumonia. Photomicrograph of thoracoscopic lung biopsy specimen from a patient with cryptogenic organizing pneumonia. Polypoid masses of granulation tissue fill the lumens of a respiratory bronchiole and alveolar ducts. Adjacent alveolar interstices are broadened by a lymphoplasmacytic inflammatory infiltrate (pentachrome stain; ×10 original magnification).

CXC chemokines (monokine induced by interferon [IFN]-γ [MIG]/CXC chemokine ligand [CXCL]9, IP-10/CXCL10, and IFN-inducible T-cell α-chemoattractant [ITAC]/CXCL11) in human BAL fluid were associated with the continuum from acute to chronic rejection.[20] Because the CXC chemokines are potent leukocyte chemoattractants and are involved in other inflammation and/or fibroproliferative diseases, it has been suggested that the expression of these chemokines during an allogeneic response promotes the persistent recruitment of mononuclear cells, leading to chronic lung rejection and bronchiolitis obliterans.

The levels of Clara cell secretory protein (a differentiation marker for the bronchiolar epithelium with both antioxidative and antiinflammatory/

immmunomodulatory effects) in serum and BAL fluid is lowered in bronchiolitis obliterans syndrome.[21] The correlation between decreased Clara cell secretory protein levels and increased neutrophils in BAL fluid suggests a loss of local airway defense capacity in bronchiolitis obliterans syndrome.[21]

Duncan and coworkers showed that T-cell responses in lung transplant recipients were marked by highly selective clonal expansions, presumably driven by indirect recognition of a limited number of immunodominant alloantigens.[22] These processes are exaggerated among allograft recipients with bronchiolitis obliterans, implying that cognate immune mechanisms are important in the pathogenesis of this process.[22]

Finally, data suggest a potential role for genotypic susceptibility in the development of bronchiolitis in this setting. Cytokine gene polymorphisms of tumor necrosis factor-α, IFN-γ, IL-10, IL-6, or transforming growth factor [TGF]-β genes may play a role.[4]

Chest Imaging Studies in Bronchiolitis

Chest Radiograph

The chest radiograph is of limited usefulness in the diagnosis and follow-up of patients with bronchiolitis. In patients with constrictive bronchiolitis, the chest radiograph may be normal or may show varying combinations and degrees of any of the following: hyperinflation, peripheral attenuation of the vascular markings, and nodular or reticular opacities.[8] In cases of proliferative bronchiolitis, the chest radiograph shows unilateral or bilateral areas of consolidation. The consolidation is often patchy and peripheral (see Chapter 25, "Idiopathic Interstitial Pneumonias").

HRCT

An understanding of the anatomy of the small airway is useful in recognizing the changes that might be present on HRCT scans in patients with bronchiolitis. The smallest functioning subunit of the lung is the secondary pulmonary lobule. The secondary pulmonary lobule is supplied by a central bronchiole and accompanying pulmonary arteriole and is drained by pulmonary veins and lymphatics in the interlobular septa. In a normal subject, the centrilobular pulmonary arterioles are visible on HRCT scan as short branching structures located 2 to 3 mm from the pleural surface. The accompanying terminal bronchiole is not usually visible because it is filled with air. Only scattered interlobular septa are identified on HRCT. Therefore, any additional centrilobular opacities seen with HRCT are abnormal findings.[9] There are important technical considerations that must be handled for the proper imaging of the small airways by HRCT.[8,9,23,24]

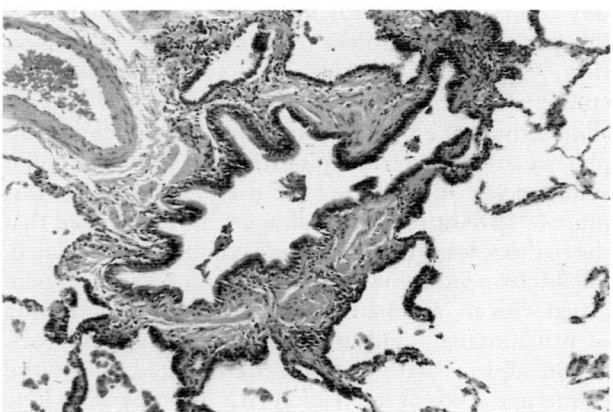

Figure 26–5   Constrictive bronchiolitis. Photomicrograph of lung biopsy specimen shows bronchial smooth muscle hyperplasia, thickening and mild scarring of the bronchiolar wall, and scarring of the adjacent alveoli, which are lined by metaplastic bronchiolar epithelium (hematoxylin and eosin stain; ×10 original magnification).

Inspiratory CT.   Bronchiolitis is suggested on inspiratory CT scans by the presence of centrilobular thickening, bronchial wall thickening, bronchiolar dilatation, the tree-in-bud pattern, and the mosaic perfusion pattern.[8,25–30] Cylindrical bronchiectasis is frequently associated with bronchiolitis.[27] Air trapping (retention of excess gas or "air" in all or part of the lung as a result of complete or partial airway obstruction) is an indirect sign of bronchiolitis.[11] Small peripheral centrilobular nodular parenchymal densities are nonspecific indirect signs of small airways disease.[30] These hazy nodular opacities appear as focal rounded areas of increased ground-glass attenuation, measuring less than 1 cm in size.[30]

Expiratory CT.   Expiratory CT scans are important in the assessment of air trapping, which is a characteristic finding of partial airway obstruction.[89] The presence of air trapping is an accurate indicator of the presence of small airways disease and may be a better means for detecting bronchiolitis than findings with inspiratory CT scanning.[29,31–34] In patients with normal airways, the pulmonary lobules increase in density during the expiratory phase (homogeneous increase in attenuation). However, if there is partial obstruction of the small airways by bronchiolitis, they cannot empty normally during maximal expiration; therefore, the lobule(s) remains radiolucent (decreased attenuation).[29,31–34] Adjacent inflammatory infiltration may result in peribronchiolar ground-glass abnormality. The pattern of centrilobular thickening and the presence of associated features such as ground-glass attenuation assist in the differential diagnosis of bronchiolitis (see Table 26–3). Most of these findings lack sensitivity in isolation, and surgical lung biopsy is required to confirm the diagnosis.

The CT findings associated with proliferative bronchiolitis and organizing pneumonia are described in Chapter 4, "Imaging Diffuse Parenchymal Lung Diseases" and Chapter 25, "Idiopathic Interstitial Pneumonias." The predominant CT findings are bilateral areas of consolidation. These are usually found in a predominantly peribronchial or subpleural distribution of the consolidation.[29] The findings are asymmetric and vary over time. Nodules related to focal organizing pneumonia surrounding bronchioles may be seen.[29]

BAL

BAL has frequently been used to sample the alveolar regions of the lung. However, BAL studies are limited in most forms of bronchiolitis. The comparison of the first portion, called "bronchial wash," with subsequent BAL fluid retrieved has demonstrated a gradient in cellular composition, with more neutrophils and fewer macrophages in the peripheral airways (ie, bronchial wash) compared with alveoli (ie, distal lavage).[35] Table 26–4 shows the BAL fluid cellular profile in several bronchiolar diseases. BAL cellular analysis may be useful in the early recognition of bronchiolitis obliterans syndrome in lung transplant recipients.

CLINICAL SYNDROMES ASSOCIATED WITH BRONCHIOLITIS

Bronchiolitis Secondary to Inhalational Lung Injury

The inhalation of fumes, gases, mists, mineral dusts, or organic material constitutes a significant industrial and environmental hazard (Table 26–5). Exposure can result in either a subtle or severe clinical illness. Massive exposure can lead to death from bronchiolar spasm, laryngeal spasm, reflex respiratory arrest, or simple asphyxia.[36–42] Lesser levels of exposure can be associated with the immediate development of pulmonary edema and the late development of constrictive bronchiolitis with airflow limitation (Table 26–6). Desgranges is credited with the first report of "nitrous fume" poisoning in 1804.[43] It is now recognized that nitrous fume exposure is a significant industrial and environmental hazard that occurs in many settings: agriculture, fire fighting, the chemical industry, the munitions and missile industries, gold and coal mining, and arc welding in confined spaces. Exposure to oxides of nitrogen is common and can lead to acute and chronic lung injury. Silo filler's disease is a well-studied example.[16,44]

Silo Filler's Disease

Silo filler's disease is a form of lung injury that results from the inhalation of nitrogen dioxide and dinitrogen

TABLE 26–4   **BAL Fluid Cellular Profile in Bronchiolar Diseases**

	Macrophages	Lymphocytes	Neutrophils	Eosinophilis	CD4/CD8 Ratio
Cigarette-related bronchiolitis	↑↑↑		↑	(↑)	↓
Diffuse panbronchiolitis			↑↑↑		ND*
Idiopathic bronchiolitis obliterans			↑↑↑	↑	ND*
Transplant bronchiolitis obliterans			↑↑	↑	↓
Idiopathic BOOP	↑↑↑		↑↑	↑	↓

Reproduced with permission from Costabel.[311]
BAL = bronchoalveolar lavage; BOOP = bronchiolitis obliterans organizing pneumonia; ND = not determined.

TABLE 26–5 Inhalational Exposures Associated with Development of Bronchiolitis

Toxic gases
Grain dusts
Irritant gases (eg, chlorine)
Mineral dusts
Organic dusts (hypersensitivity pneumonitis)
Cigarette smoke
Free-base cocaine
Fire smoke

TABLE 26–6 Toxic Exposures Associated with Bronchiolitis, with or without Obliterans

Nitrogen dioxide* ("nitrous fume")[43,46,47,312]
  Spillage of nitric acid (component of jet and missile fuels)[48,313]
  Metal pickling[40,314]
  Silo gas[37,45,46,49,315–318]
  Chemical manufacturing (explosives, dyes, lacquers, celluloid)[319]
  Detonation of explosives[36,319–321]
  Electric arc or acetylene gas welding
  Contamination of anesthetic gases (nitrous oxide gas cylinder)[40]
  Nitrocellulose combustion[322]
  Tobacco smoke[323]
  Fire smoke*† (firemen, astronauts, others exposed to burning materials)[46,53,55,324–330]
Sulfur dioxide†[328–331]
  Burning of sulfur-containing fossil fuels
  Bleaching of wool, straw, wood pulp[329,332]
  Sugar refining, fruit preserving
  Fungicides
  Refrigerants
  Ore smelting
  Acid production
Ammonia†[41]
  Fertilizer and explosives, production, refrigeration
Chlorine‡[332,333]
  Bleaching, disinfectant and plastic making
Chloramine gas[334]
Phosgene*
  Chemical industry, dye and insecticide manufacturing
Chloropicrin
Trichlorethylene
Ozone[63]
  Arc welding and air, sewage and water treatment
Cadmium oxide
  Ore: smelting, alloying, welding
Methyl sulfate
Hydrogen sulfide
  Natural gas making, paper pulp, sewage treatment, tannery work
Hydrogen fluoride
  Etching, petroleum industry, silk-working
Talcum powder (hydrous magnesium silicate)[335]
Stearate of zinc powder[336]
Oxygen toxicity[337]
Asbestos (chrysotile and amphibole)[63]
Iron oxide§[63]
Aluminum oxide§[63]
Silica§[63]
Sheet silicates (talc, mica, etc.)§[63]
Coal§
Activated charcoal[338]
Talc[339]
Free-base cocaine*
Incinerator fly ash[340]
Thionyl-chloride (production of lithium batteries)[341]

*These agents have been associated with the development of proliferative bronchiolitis (intraluminal polyps).
†These agents have been associated with the development of constrictive bronchiolitis.
‡These agents have been associated with the development of histologic focal bronchiolitis without significant clinical disease.
§These agents have been associated with the development of respiratory bronchiolitis.

tetroxide from air on the surface of the silage in agricultural silos. Most exposed workers have mild and self-limited symptoms. Severe pulmonary reactions can occur, usually after accidental exposures in unventilated farm silos. Nitrogen dioxide is relatively insoluble. Unlike highly water-soluble gases such as chlorine, ammonia, and sulfur dioxide, nitrogen dioxide is less irritating to the mucus membranes of the nasal and upper airways. The gas produces a yellowish to brownish haze and an acrid, ammonia-like odor that is irritating and suffocating to heavily exposed individuals.[45] Following inhalation, the gas reaches the periphery of the lung where it combines with water to form nitric and nitrous acids and nitric oxide, which are powerful oxidants capable of causing severe tissue injury.

Clinical Findings. Clinical manifestations of exposure to nitrogen dioxide depend on the concentration of the inhaled gas and the duration of exposure.[46–49] Three clinical patterns or phases may follow exposure (Table 26–7); these phases are not directly related to time from exposure. All phases may not appear in an individual patient.[50] Progression to death may be an outcome at any stage.

Acute (Upper Airway Injury and Pulmonary Edema). The clinical presentation following low-level exposure includes acute upper airway and visual disturbances, cough, dyspnea, fatigue, cyanosis, vomiting, hemoptysis, hypoxemia, vertigo, somnolence, headache, emotional difficulties, and/or loss of consciousness. These findings usually resolve within hours, but some may persist for several days or weeks.

In the acute phase, patients who develop pulmonary edema (so-called chemical pneumonitis) and adult respiratory distress syndrome (ARDS) have significant pulmonary dysfunction. Hypoxemia occurs and is secondary to ventilation-perfusion mismatching as a result of altered airway dynamics and interstitial and alveolar edema, impaired diffusing capacity, and methemoglobinemia that occurs when nitrate ions react with hemoglobin.[43,46] Severe metabolic acidosis occurs because of the dissolution of nitrogen dioxide in body fluids, resulting in formation of nitrous and nitric acid, as well as the lactic acidosis resulting from tissue hypoxia. Systemic hypertension may be present.

The radiographic manifestations during the acute stage include pulmonary edema (ie, alveolar filling). In survivors, these changes clear rapidly.

TABLE 26–7   Course of Illness Following Accidental Nitrogen Dioxide Exposure

Time Course of Disease Following Exposure	Clinical Presentation	Chest Roentgenogram	Routine Laboratory Tests and Physiology	Outcome
Immediate	Acute bronchitis, bronchiolar spasm, laryngospasm, respiratory arrest. May occasionally be asymptomatic	Pulmonary edema	May develop severe ARDS with hypoxemia, impaired DL_{CO}, methemoglobinemia, metabolic acidosis, obstructive and/or restrictive pulmonary defect	Recovery usual. Death may occur
Hours, days, or a few weeks (2–6 weeks)	Asymptomatic period	Normal	Normal	May progress to next phase
Hours, days, or weeks (usually)	Progressive dyspnea, cough, hypoxemia, cyanosis, and rales on chest examination	May be normal. Most commonly exhibit miliary or discretely nodular pattern. Hyperinflation may be the only abnormality in some cases	Irreversible obstructive changes most characteristic, but restrictive or mixed disease is often present	Chronic pulmonary insufficiency. Death may result from progressive disease

ARDS = adult respiratory distress syndrome; DL_{CO} = Diffusing capacity of the lung for carbon monoxide.
Reproduced with permission from King TE Jr.[50]

Physiological studies reveal the simultaneous occurrence of restrictive and obstructive ventilatory defects; the former is manifest as a shift in the static pressure-volume curve downward and to the right. These abnormalities gradually resolve in survivors.

Histopathologic findings, as determined from autopsy studies, include marked intra-alveolar edema and exudation as well as thickening of the alveolar walls with lymphocytic cellular infiltrates.

Complete recovery without obvious sequelae is usually observed.[36,46,48] At higher concentrations of nitrogen dioxide exposure, sudden death may occur.

Subacute (Adult Respiratory Distress Syndrome). Uncommonly, some patients may remain asymptomatic or experience only minimal clinical manifestations at the time of exposure; later (in 3 to 30 hours) they develop the clinical picture of severe ARDS. Recovery without long-term sequelae is usual, but death may occur at this stage.

Chronic (Bronchiolitis Obliterans). After recovery from the acute illness, or in patients with no symptoms following exposure, recurrence or new onset of clinical illness may be seen 2 to 6 weeks later. This phase is characterized by the progressive onset of cough and dyspnea associated with mild hypoxemia.[40,48] Tachypnea is present, and rales are usually heard. The radiographic pattern in this late stage may vary. A normal chest film may be seen; however, a miliary or discretely nodular pattern is thought to be characteristic of bronchiolitis obliterans (Figure 26–6).

In those patients who progress to the chronic phase, physiological disturbances include hypoxemia at rest or with exercise and associated restrictive or obstructive pulmonary function abnormalities.[38,40,51,52] With lung function testing, a progressive and irreversible obstructive ventilatory defect is noted; occasionally, only changes consistent with pulmonary hyperinflation are seen.

Widespread proliferative bronchiolitis with marked intraluminal fibrous tissue proliferation arising in the bronchiolar wall (without organizing pneumonia) is found, especially in those with preceding pulmonary edema; however, these findings may occur as the initial manifestation of previous exposure (Figure 26–7).

Management. The treatment of patients exposed to nitrogen dioxide or other toxic gases or fumes should include observation in the hospital for 48 hours, followed by weekly or biweekly evaluations for 6 to 8 weeks. When respiratory dysfunction is present, treatment with corticosteroids should be started immediately.[44] The usefulness of corticosteroid therapy has been demonstrated in the management of both the acute phase (pulmonary edema) and the late phase (bronchiolitis obliterans).[87,46–49,53,54] Corticosteroids should be continued for a minimum of 8 weeks because relapses have been reported with earlier cessation of therapy.[39,46,55] Bronchodilators are occasionally helpful, but antibiotics should be used only when clinically indicated; they should be directed at a specific pathogen. If methemoglobinemia is present, methylene blue should be administered at a dose of 2 mg/kg intravenously, followed by doses titrated according to the concentration of methemoglobin in the blood. For patients in whom this diagnosis is suspected and for whom open lung biopsy or general anesthesia is planned, it has been suggested that nitrous oxide not be used as an anesthetic because of concern that it might lead to disease progression.[56]

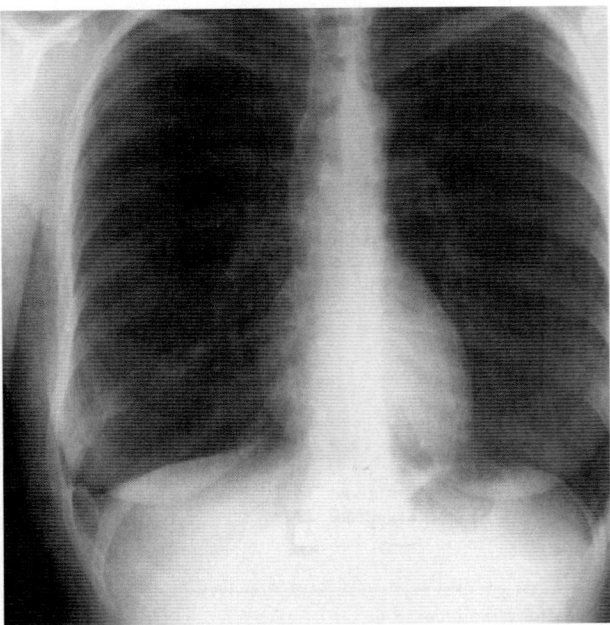

Figure 26–6 Bronchiolitis obliterans as seen on a posteroanterior chest radiograph. Only pulmonary hyperinflation is seen. Serial lung function testing in this patient showed progressive severe airflow obstruction with marked air trapping. A biopsy was performed in the right lung.

Prognosis.   In general, the prognosis for survivors (one-third die acutely) of toxic fume inhalation is good. Some authors have suggested that lasting pulmonary disability is uncommon in silo filler's disease; whereas others have identified a wide variety of functional derangements.[38,46,57] The disease entity described previously results from acute and moderate to severe exposure. It is not entirely clear what functional abnormalities result from chronic low-level exposure to nitrogen dioxide. Education is the key in prevention of this disease; simple measures to reduce nitrogen dioxide levels are recognized, and approved respiratory protection equipment is available.

Other Irritant Gases

A number of irritant gases have occasionally been associated with bronchiolitis, with or without obliterans (see Table 26–6). Because lung biopsies were not performed in all of the cases studied, it is not always clear that the pulmonary injury associated with these inhalation exposures is bronchiolitis obliterans alone. However, sulfur dioxide, chlorine gas, "smoke inhalation" or inhalation burns, hydrogen chloride, ammonia, phosgene, and chloropicrin produce a disease with clinical, physiological, and radiographic manifestations similar to those described for nitrogen dioxide. Respiratory bronchiolitis following exposure to photochemical air pollutants, ozone, and nitrogen dioxide have recently been reviewed.[58–62]

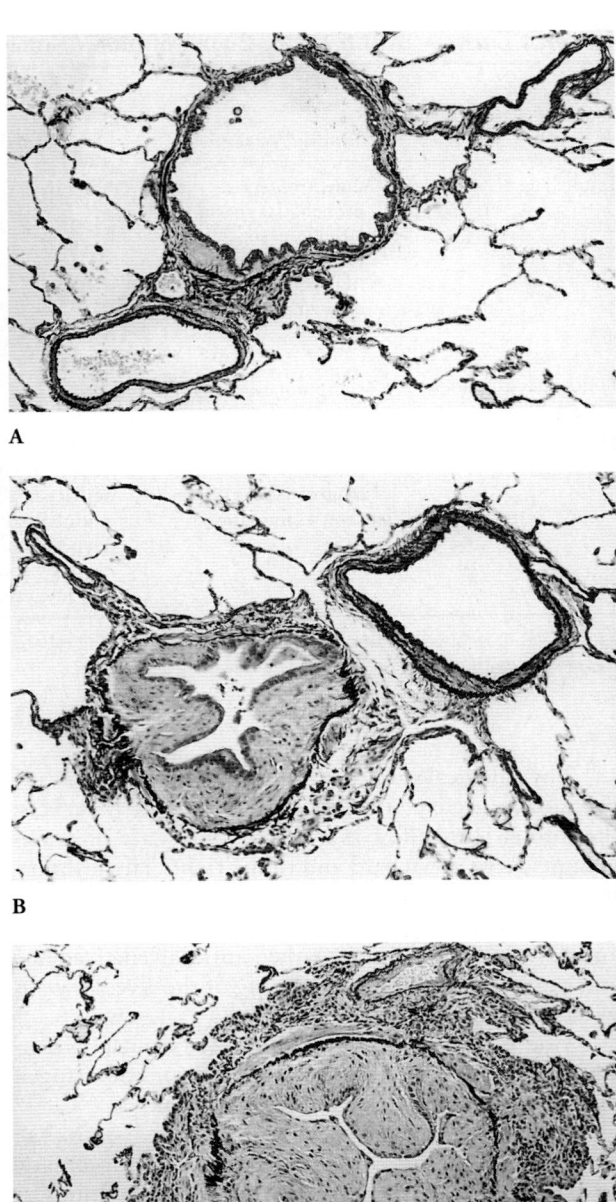

Figure 26–7 Photomicrograph of open lung biopsy specimen from the same patient depicted in Figure 26–6, a bronchiolitis obliterans patient with constrictive bronchiolitis following toxic gas exposure. Initial review of the biopsy failed to identify any significant abnormality. Step-sectioning of the tissue specimen was necessary to better show the lesions. *A*, Slightly dilated but otherwise normal bronchiole with normal intervening lung (pentachrome stain; ×156 original magnification). *B*, Step-section of specimen. Marked concentric narrowing of the bronchiolar lumen due to fibrosis is apparent (pentachrome stain; ×156 original magnification). *C*, Step-section of specimen. There is complete obliteration of the bronchiolar lumen due to fibrosis. In some areas of this biopsy, the airway could only be identified because of the staining of the basement membrane (pentachrome stain; ×156 original magnification).

Mineral Dusts

Churg and Wright have written extensively about the development of pathologic changes in the small airways (respiratory bronchiolitis) secondary to exposure to inorganic mineral dusts, including asbestos, silica, iron oxide, aluminum oxide, several different sheet silicates, and coal.[63–68] The clinical relevance of the lesions found in these subjects awaits better definition. Nevertheless, the development of airflow obstruction, rather than the classic restriction, is increasingly recognized in subjects with inorganic mineral dust exposure.

Pathologically, these lesions are characterized by marked abnormalities in the small airways, particularly the membranous and respiratory bronchioles (see Chapter 2, Figure 2–22).[69] The basic lesion consists of fibrosis in the walls of these small airways and, occasionally, the alveolar ducts.[63] It appears that the lesions extend down into the airway. Often, the lesions are accompanied by pigment deposition. These lesions occur most commonly in heavily exposed workers. The role of cigarette smoke is unclear, but a synergistic role appears likely. The lesions are also seen in workers who are nonsmokers.[70–73] The pathogenesis of these lesions is not well defined. They appear to result from the inflammatory response that follows deposition of mineral particles or fibers in the walls of the small airways.[63]

Organic Dusts

Numerous agents are associated with the development of hypersensitivity pneumonitis (see Chapter 19, "Hypersensitivity Pneumonitis"). Although interstitial pneumonitis is seen in virtually 100% of patients with hypersensitivity pneumonitis and granulomas are seen in approximately 70%, bronchiolar lesions are seen in essentially all cases.[74,75] The bronchioles contain granulomata within the walls or lumina or show tufts of granulation tissue as seen in bronchiolitis obliterans (Figure 26–8). A reversible restrictive process is the most common physiological abnormality in hypersensitivity pneumonitis. However, small airway dysfunction may be present in patients with early hypersensitivity pneumonitis. As the disease progresses, either obstructive or restrictive physiology may arise, depending on the predominant histopathologic process present.

Volatile Flavoring Agents

Eight former employees of a microwave popcorn factory were found to have severe fixed obstructive lung disease.[76,77] Four of the patients were on lung transplant lists. All eight had a respiratory illness resembling bronchiolitis obliterans, with symptoms of cough and dyspnea on exertion.[76,77] Employment duration ranged from 8 months to 9 years. Other investigators have reported cases with a similar illness.[78] On the basis of the reported eight cases, the calculated rate of illness was 28 to 70 cases per 10,000 person-years.[76,77,79] If correct, this would represent a 5- to 11-fold excess over the expected number of reported occupational respiratory conditions attributed to toxins.

The ages of the patients ranged from 29 to 53 years (median age 43 years).[80] Cough, shortness of breath, and wheezing were the presenting symptoms.[78,80] The forced expiratory volume in 1 second (FEV_1) % predicted ranged from 14 to 68%; FEV_1/forced vital capacity (FVC) from 22.6 to 75%, and all had high residual volumes.[80] Six of eight workers had normal single-breath carbon monoxide diffusing capacity. Bronchiolitis obliterans was also found in another cluster of cases in workers employed by a flavoring manufacturing plant.[78] Most patients identified had normal preplacement spirometry results.[78] These values subsequently demonstrated a precipitous drop with the development of moderate to severe nonreversible airway obstruction.[78]

Chest radiographs showed hyperinflation in three cases. Few patients had chest CT scans. HRCT findings included diffuse cylindrical bronchiectasis and a mosaic pattern suggestive of air trapping.[81] This pattern suggests a predominant constrictive bronchiolitis pattern. Two patients had pathology consistent with obliterative bronchiolitis; one of these had granulomas.[80]

The presumed exposure was to a mixture of soybean oil, salt, flavorings, and coloring agents that was mixed in a large heated tank. This process produced visible dust, aerosols, and vapors with a strong buttery odor. More than 100 volatile organic compounds were identified in the air samples from the mixing room area of this popcorn plant.[82] Diacetyl (2,3)-butanedione, a ketone with butter-flavor characteristics, was the pre-

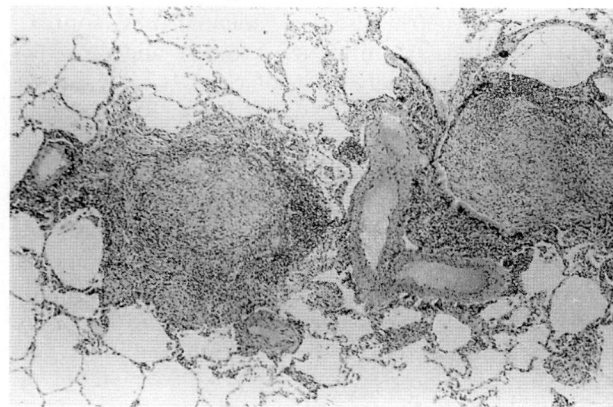

Figure 26–8 Bronchiolitis obliterans in bird fancier's lung. An intraluminal polypoid mass, covered by respiratory epithelium and completely encroaching on the lumen of the bronchiole, is shown at upper right. The left bronchiole is completely obliterated. Note the peribronchial and mural infiltration by mononuclear cells and lymphocytes. Other regions of the lung biopsy specimen showed the classic features of hypersensitivity pneumonitis.

dominant compound isolated.[82] The highest incidence of the illness occurred in workers who worked nearest the mixing tank and were more likely to have inhaled mixing tank substances. Preliminary animal studies at the Division of Respiratory Disease Studies, National Institute for Occupational Safety and Health, suggest severe damage to airway epithelium after inhalation exposure to high air concentrations of butter-flavoring vapors (diacetyl) used at one of the worksites.[76,77]

After removal from exposure, the patients did not recover, but they did appear to have no further loss of lung function.[78] However, the National Institute for Occupational Safety and Health is investigating whether other cases of fixed obstructive lung disease have occurred in workers at other microwave popcorn factories or in work with food flavoring agents that might be heated and aerosolized.[76,77] It does not appear that there is any risk to the general population using microwave popcorn products.[83]

Infectious Causes of Bronchiolitis

Infection is the most common cause of acute bronchiolitis. Infectious causes of bronchiolitis are more commonly found in children than in adults. The agents most commonly associated with bronchiolitis include viruses and *Mycoplasma pneumoniae*.[84,85] These agents have a propensity to infect and injure epithelial cells of the respiratory tract. Constrictive bronchiolitis is the most common histopathologic pattern found following infection.

Infectious Bronchiolitis in Children

Acute bronchiolitis is a common illness in infants and young children, occurring primarily as a result of a viral infection.[84,85] Pathogens include RSV (approximately 34% of cases), parainfluenza virus types 1, 2, and 3 (approximately 30% of cases), adenoviruses (approximately 7% of cases), influenza A and B, and *M. pneumoniae* (approximately 11% of cases) (Table 26–8). Males are more commonly affected with RSV than are females (1.5–1.8 males:1 female). Recently, reviews of bronchiolitis in children have been published.[15,86,87]

Infectious bronchiolitis obliterans is rarely seen in individuals older than 2 years of age. Adenovirus types 3, 7, and 21 are the most common etiologic agents. Other causes include measles, whooping cough due to *Bordetella pertussis*, *M. pneumoniae*, and influenza A. Severe infectious bronchiolitis obliterans leading to hospitalization and death is rare.

Clinical Findings. The usual presentation is an acute viral-like illness with mild coryza and sneezing, occurring during the winter months. Several days later, cough, dyspnea, tachypnea, tachycardia, fever, chest wall retractions, sibilant and sonorous rales, expiratory wheezing, and, in severe cases, cyanosis, develop. Prostration and respiratory failure are unusual.

Radiographic Findings. The radiographic pattern of childhood bronchiolitis is variable. It may be normal or show hyperinflation with increased bronchial markings. Subsegmental consolidation and collapse may be seen.[88] A pattern similar to that of diffuse interstitial pneumonia, often in association with hyperinflation, is seen. Some patients demonstrate a diffuse nodular or reticulonodular pattern, whereas others may have patchy alveolar or ground-glass opacities.[89,90] Those with a nodular pattern frequently have "pure" bronchiolitis obliterans on lung biopsy, whereas those with the reticulonodular pattern are likely to have more interstitial inflammation and scarring.[84,89,90] The role of HRCT has not been adequately defined, but it is thought to be important in ruling out other diagnoses, especially bronchiectasis. Ventilation-perfusion lung scans may be very helpful, because a markedly abnormal pattern of patchy, matched ventilation and perfusion defects is often seen, even when the plain chest film is unremarkable.[91] Bronchography may reveal saccular bronchiectasis and ballooning of the airways at the blind end when the airways are distended by positive pressure; passage of contrast medium into the alveoli does not occur. Bronchography has largely been abandoned with the advent of HRCT.[91]

TABLE 26–8   Postinfectious Causes of Bronchiolitis*

Acute bronchiolitis
  Common
    Respiratory syncytial virus[84,342]
    Parainfluenza (types 1, 2, and 3)[343]
    Adenovirus (types 1, 2, 3, 5, 6, 7, and 21)[88]
    Mycoplasma pneumoniae[344]
  Uncommon
    Coronavirus
    Rubeola[345]
    Mumps
    Varicella zoster[346]
    Influenza[347,348]
    Rhinovirus
    Parvovirus B19
    Enteroviruses

Bronchiolitis obliterans[91]
  Herpes simplex virus
  Human immunodeficiency virus[349]
  Cytomegalovirus[350]
  Rubeola
  Parainfluenza (type 3)
  Adenovirus
  Mycoplasma pneumoniae[351]
  Klebsiella
  Hemophilus influenzae
  Legionella pneumophila[352]
  Serratia marcescens[353]
  Bordetella pertussis
  Streptococcus group B, beta hemolytic
  Cryptococcus neoformans
  Nocardia asteroides
  Pneumocystis carinii
  Aspergillus[354]

*This applies mostly to children.

Physiological Findings. Tests of lung function may be normal. However, obstructive changes with air trapping can often be documented. Pulmonary function testing has not been well studied in infants with this disease. Resting hypoxemia is frequently present.[84,92,93] Whether or not bronchiolitis in infancy predisposes the patient to asthma or COPD in later life remains unproven, but data suggesting such an association have appeared in the literature.[92,94–96]

Histopathologic Findings. In this setting, open or thoracoscopic lung biopsy is the gold standard for the diagnosis of bronchiolitis obliterans. The earliest change is necrosis of the respiratory epithelium, followed by epithelial proliferation.[84,89,100,101] Dense plugs of alveolar debris and strands of fibrin are seen in small bronchi and bronchioles, causing partial or complete obstruction. These findings may develop as soon as 8 days after the onset of the illness. A lymphocytic infiltrate, including collections with germinal centers, may be seen in the airway wall. Severe and widespread destruction of the respiratory epithelium may cause denudation and a pronounced inflammatory response that involves the adjacent peribronchial space and alveolar walls. Depending on the stage at which the biopsy is obtained, findings consistent with proliferative bronchiolitis (early), constrictive bronchiolitis (late), or both may be seen. Mauad and Dolhnikoff examined the histopathologic features of lung biopsies from 34 pediatric patients with a diagnosis of childhood bronchiolitis obliterans.[102] Ninety-seven percent had the constrictive type, with variable degrees of airway obstruction.[102] The pathogenetic mechanisms involved in the development of obliterative bronchiolitis secondary to infection and the reason for the predilection in infants are unknown.[84,103]

Management. Treatment is symptomatic, including the administration of supplemental oxygen and adequate hydration. Bronchodilators, antibiotics, antiviral agents, and corticosteroids are frequently used in management, but few controlled clinical trials of their efficacy have been performed.[104–107] Mechanical ventilation is rarely required; it may be necessary if progressive respiratory failure ensues.[84,103,108] Lung transplantation has been performed in severe cases.

Prognosis. Recovery is usual and occurs in days or weeks.[84,85,92] Whether or not bronchiolitis in infancy predisposes to asthma or COPD in later life remains unproved.

Swyer-James Syndrome. This syndrome, also known as unilateral hyperlucent lung, is a long-term complication of bronchiolitis in children, especially following adenoviral infection occurring in infancy. The affected child may be asymptomatic, but more often, he or she has recurrent pulmonary infections and eventually develops bronchiectasis. Dyspnea on exertion, hemoptysis, and chronic productive cough are seen. Patients may have localized, unilateral, or bilateral involvement. The chest radiograph demonstrates lobar or unilateral hyperlucent lung; normal or reduced volume of the involved lung is noted on full inspiration.

Severe airway obstruction occurs during expiration. The involved lung has a diminished pulmonary vascular bed, decreased pulmonary blood flow, and reduced peripheral vascular markings. Bronchography demonstrates diffuse bronchiectasis with absence of filling of the terminal bronchioles (a "pruned tree" appearance). HRCT is the procedure of choice for identifying the characteristic changes in Swyer-James syndrome.[109]

The final size of the involved lung in Swyer-James syndrome relates to the age of the patient at the time bronchiolitis occurs. If the onset is early in life, the lung fails to grow normally and appears smaller than the opposite lung. If the bronchiolitis occurs later in childhood, the lung may be of normal size. Pulmonary function tests reveal airflow obstruction and a reduced total lung capacity in cases in which concomitant pulmonary fibrosis exists. The syndrome has been reported with a number of etiologic agents and must be distinguished from the congenital absence of the pulmonary artery, pulmonary arterial occlusion, partial obstruction of a lobar or main bronchus, and congenital lobar emphysema. CT and pulmonary angiography are helpful in distinguishing among these conditions.

Infectious Bronchiolitis in Adults

Acute bronchiolitis in older children and young adults has been associated primarily with *M. pneumoniae*; however, a number of other viruses (eg, RSV, especially in the elderly) and bacterial agents have been identified. Only sporadic cases of bronchiolitis obliterans secondary to infection have been reported in the adult population.[15,110]

The clinical presentation of infectious bronchiolitis in adults is not well defined, and no systematic study has been reported. Most have a history of an upper respiratory tract illness that precedes the onset of dyspnea with exertion, cough, tachypnea, fever, and wheezing. Measles, varicella zoster, and pertussis have been reported to cause bronchiolitis obliterans in adults. A number of adults have developed an acute or subacute diffuse ventilatory obstruction that has occasionally been fatal.[111–114]

Idiopathic Forms of Bronchiolitis

Several idiopathic clinicopathologic syndromes associated with prominent involvement of the bronchioles have recently been reported. Although no specific etiology has been identified for these syndromes, the constellation of findings in reported cases suggest that these are unique syndromes that must be distinguished from more common problems, such as COPD, pneumonia, or pulmonary fibrosis.

Cryptogenic "Adult" Bronchiolitis

Cryptogenic adult bronchiolitis is a rare clinicopathologic syndrome that must be distinguished from asthma, chronic bronchitis, emphysema, cystic fibrosis, bronchiectasis, and α_1-antitrypsin deficiency.[115–118] Few cases have been reported, and it is not entirely clear that all of those reported are the same entity. For example, many patients have had a significant cigarette smoking history and may represent examples of smoker's bronchiolitis. Despite these concerns, the constellation of findings in reported cases appears unique and suggests that adult bronchiolitis represents a distinct definable clinicopathologic entity that is a diagnostic challenge to clinicians and pathologists.[116,117,119,120]

The pathogenesis of cryptogenic adult bronchiolitis is unknown. The true incidence of the disease is also unknown, but it has been estimated to be the cause of approximately 4% of all obstructive lung diseases. The disorder is largely diagnosed by exclusion and requires a high index of suspicion, along with an awareness of its unique clinical features.

Clinical Findings.   Most patients are middle-aged women who have a nonproductive cough, shortness of breath, or other nonspecific chest complaints, usually of relatively short duration (6 to 24 months). Most are identified because of an accelerated severe obstructive respiratory disorder, which is clinically distinct from the more commonly encountered obstructive disorders. There is no history of cigarette smoking, chronic sputum production, frequent chest infections, wheezing, known connective tissue disorder, or immunoglobulin deficiency. No association with inhalation injury or viral infection has been identified. Physical findings are unremarkable, although wheezing or crackles may be heard.

Diagnostic Studies.   The chest radiographic findings are normal or nonspecific. Increased bronchial wall thickening may be seen. Hyperinflation (without marked flattening or hyperlucent areas) may be the only abnormality noted.[90] HRCT scans are normal or show airway dilatation.

Pulmonary function testing yields a variety of results. Most patients have increased lung volumes and airflow limitation. A few patients who have had pressure-volume curves performed show an upward shift and a normal slope consistent with airflow limitation. The diffusing capacity is reduced, and resting hypoxemia may be present. Exercise testing shows gas exchange abnormalities associated with an abnormal deadspace volume to tidal volume ratio (V_D/V_T).

BAL studies demonstrate marked neutrophilia associated with an increase in the specific neutrophil products collagenase and myeloperoxidase. The majority of patients have a neutrophil level higher than 25% (normal for nonsmokers is < 4%); some have levels exceeding 90%.

Pathologic Findings.   Lung biopsies reveal a cellular constrictive bronchiolitis, often quite subtle, with both acute and chronic inflammatory changes, primarily in the membranous bronchioles (Figure 26–9). Few cases examined have shown airway obliteration and mucus stasis. The pulmonary parenchyma is normal or shows only mild hyperinflation. Mild focal interstitial fibrosis has been identified in a few subjects. Vascular lesions have been well described (Figures 26–10 and 26–11).

Treatment.   Steroids may be of benefit in many patients with adult bronchiolitis. Early treatment may be important, because irreversible structural changes and persistent progressive breathlessness may develop, often with recurrent bouts of respiratory infection. BAL fluid neutrophilia returns toward normal in patients who respond to treatment. Thus, recognition of these cases and distinction from other small airway disorders (eg, respiratory bronchiolitis-associated interstitial lung disease, asthma, chronic bronchitis, emphysema, bronchiolitis associated with connective tissue disease, and diffuse panbronchiolitis) are possible and important.

Connective Tissue Diseases

Pulmonary involvement is common in many of the connective tissue disorders. In most cases, the pulmonary dysfunction involves alveolar rather than airway pathology. Bronchiolitis appears to occur infrequently and varies in its manifestations among the connective tissue diseases. Furthermore, most of the current understanding of bronchiolar disease in this setting is from anecdotal case reports or small case series. Bronchiolitis is most common in patients with rheumatoid arthritis, both constrictive bronchiolitis and follicular bronchiolitis.

Rheumatoid Arthritis

Bronchiolitis obliterans with airway obstruction is an increasingly recognized complication in rheumatoid arthritis.[115,121–142] The basic lesion is fibrous narrowing and obliteration of the bronchioles and smallest bronchi. Several reports have appeared demonstrating this association and have further suggested a role for penicillamine in the pathogenesis of this disorder.[89,121,125,131,133,134,139,143–146] The role of previous penicillamine therapy as an etiologic factor in the development of bronchiolitis obliterans in rheumatoid arthritis remains to be confirmed.[121,125,129,134,139,144] Cooney also suggests that there might be a relationship among chronic eosinophilic pneumonia and rheumatoid arthritis in the development of bronchiolitis obliterans.[123]

Clinical Findings.   The clinical manifestations of bronchiolitis obliterans associated with rheumatoid arthritis help to distinguish it from other pulmonary processes associated with rheumatoid arthritis. There is an abrupt onset of dyspnea and dry cough, often associated with inspiratory rales and a midinspiratory squeak. Interestingly, the majority of patients are middle-aged women with seropositive rheumatoid arthritis. This is consistent with the increased incidence of rheumatoid arthritis in women but not consistent with the reported increased frequency of pulmonary disease associated

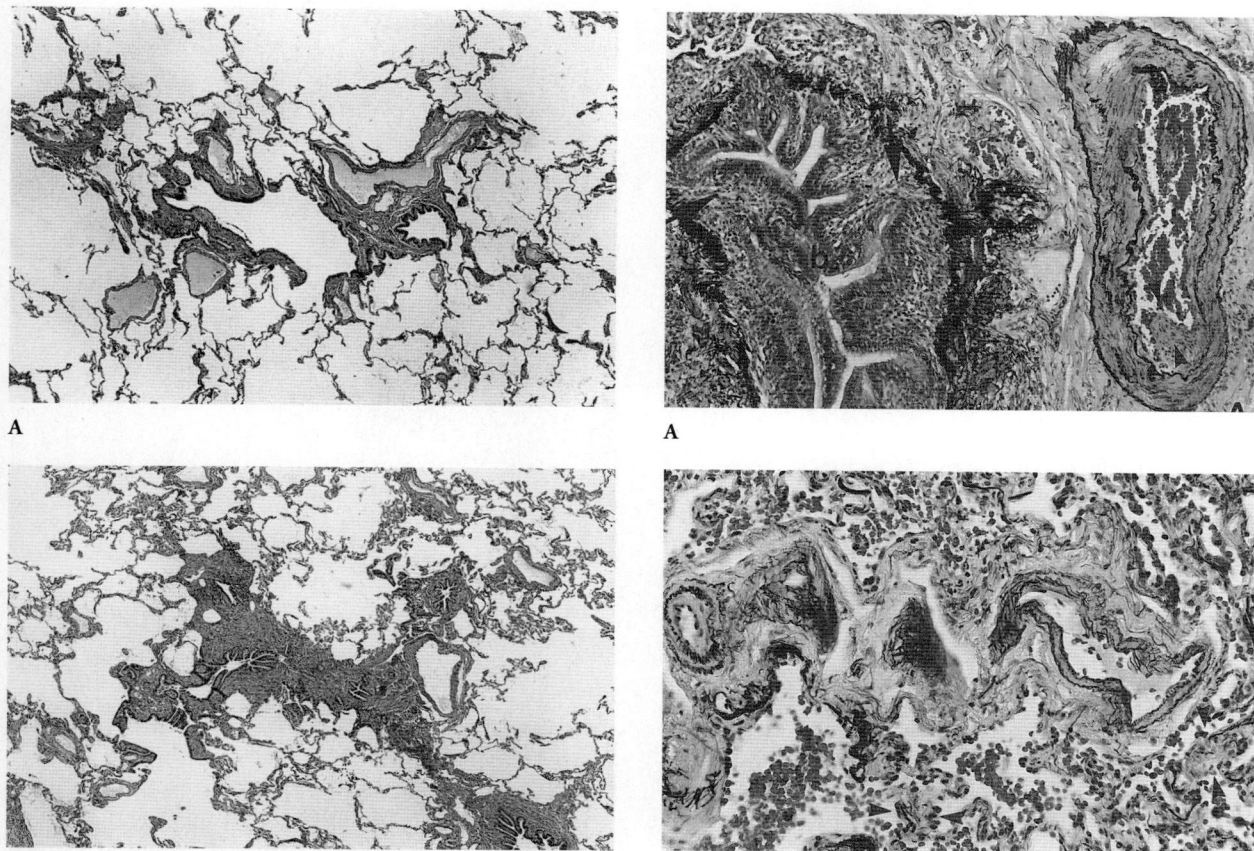

A

B

A

B

Figure 26–9 Cryptogenic constrictive bronchiolitis. *A*, Constrictive bronchiolitis manifesting as bronchiolar scarring, dilatation and distortion, and mild extension of the metaplastic bronchiolar epithelium into a few surrounding air spaces is evident. The adjacent lung parenchyma is otherwise normal (hematoxylin and eosin stain). *B*, Constrictive bronchiolitis with bronchiolar scarring, smooth muscle hypertrophy, and marked irregularity in the shape of the bronchioles. There is mild extension of the bronchiolar epithelium into the surrounding alveoli (hematoxylin and eosin stain). Reproduced with permission from Kraft et al.[120]

with rheumatoid arthritis in men.[147–149] A recent study demonstrated that five of six patients with this process had definite evidence of an advanced autoimmune exocrinopathy (Sjögren's syndrome).

Diagnostic Studies.   The chest radiograph is usually normal but can show signs suggestive of air trapping (Figure 26–12). One case report demonstrated bronchiolitis as the cause of bilateral consolidation in the upper zone on chest radiograph.[137] Expiratory CT often shows multiple scattered areas of air trapping consistent with small airway obstruction.[150] Pulmonary function studies usually reveal airflow obstruction, mild to moderate arterial hypoxemia and respiratory alkalosis, and a normal pulmonary compliance (Figure 26–13). The rapid rate of progression of the airflow obstruction would be atypical for COPD.[131,133,140]

Histopathologic Findings.   Pathologically, a constrictive bronchiolitis is most common (Figure 26–14A).

Figure 26–10 Pulmonary vascular remodeling in a case of obliterative bronchiolitis, inflammatory stage. These micrographs are from a 40-year-old woman, a heavy smoker who presented with florid right heart failure. Her chest radiograph demonstrated cardiomegaly, prominent central pulmonary arteries, and diffuse parenchymal opacities. The chest CT scan also showed bilateral pleural effusions and confirmed the cardiomegaly and enlarged pulmonary arteries. Right heart catheterization documented the pulmonary hypertension and demonstrated a reactive vascular bed, because the infusion of the vasodilator iloprost significantly reduced the pulmonary arterial pressure and vascular resistance. *A*, A terminal bronchiole (b) shows severe infiltration of chronic inflammatory cells between the lining epithelium and the elastic layer. This inflammatory process imparts a polypoid obstructive morphology to the lining bronchiolar mucosa. The accompanying blood vessel, pulmonary artery (a), exhibits eccentric intimal growth (*arrowhead*), irregular intimal fibrosis, focal disruption of the internal elastica, and hypertrophy of the media. Note the marked thickening of the adventitia by collagen, which is continuous with the bronchiolar inflammation (pentachrome stain; ×40 original magnification). *B*, Pulmonary artery profile with thickening of the intima, media, and adventitia (v). Note the fibrotic thickening of alveolar septa as part of the interstitial component of the lung disease (*arrowheads*) and alveolar hemosiderin-laden macrophages (m) (pentachrome stain; ×40 original magnification). Reproduced with permission from Tuder et al.[299]

There is often a lymphoplasmocytic infiltration of small airway walls. The lumens are gradually obliterated, and the bronchiolar wall is destroyed by granulation tissue (Figure 26–14B). The lesions are usually confined to the small bronchi and bronchioles. Parenchymal involve-

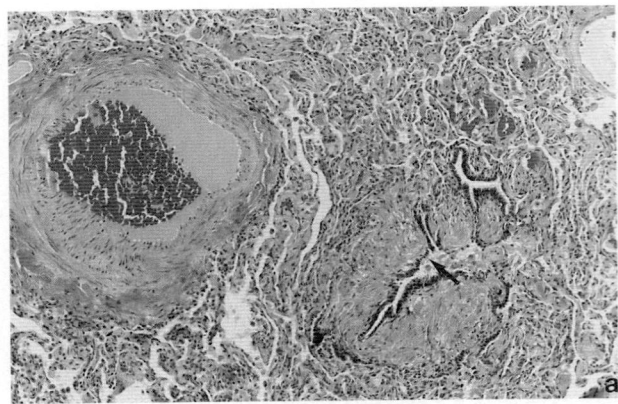

A

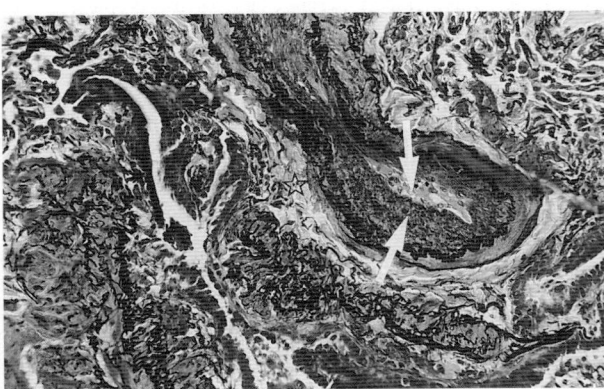

B

Figure 26–11   Pulmonary vascular remodeling in a case of obliterative bronchiolitis, scarring stage. These micrographs are from a 58-year-old man who presented with bronchiolitis obliterans. The chest CT scan showed an enlarged main pulmonary artery. *A*, The respiratory bronchioles show ingrowths of connective tissue in the subepithelial layer, with displacement of the lining cells. The inner lining appears fenestrated due to formation of polypoid projections toward the lumen (*arrow*) (hematoxylin and eosin stain; ×100 original magnification). *B*, The accompanying pulmonary artery exhibits intimal fibrosis (*arrow*), which is best appreciated with the pentachrome-stained slide. *, The peribronchial connective tissue shows continuity between the bronchiole and the pulmonary vessel (×200 original magnification).

ment is generally localized to the area surrounding the bronchiolitis. The lesions may be at different stages of development or appear uniform.[14,131] Immunofluorescence studies showed granular IgM depositions along the alveolar septa in one case and a striking linear IgG alveolar wall staining in another, both suggesting a possible direct immune-mediated lung injury.[135,143]

Treatment and Prognosis.   Treatment with antibiotics and bronchodilators is ineffective.[133] Corticosteroid therapy appears effective in some patients. The use of intravenous cyclophosphamide and oral prednisone has recently been suggested.[144,151] Erythromycin may be useful for the management of this process, but it has not been adequately studied.[152] The prognosis is poor, with early deaths reported.[129] Most patients have a chronic course.

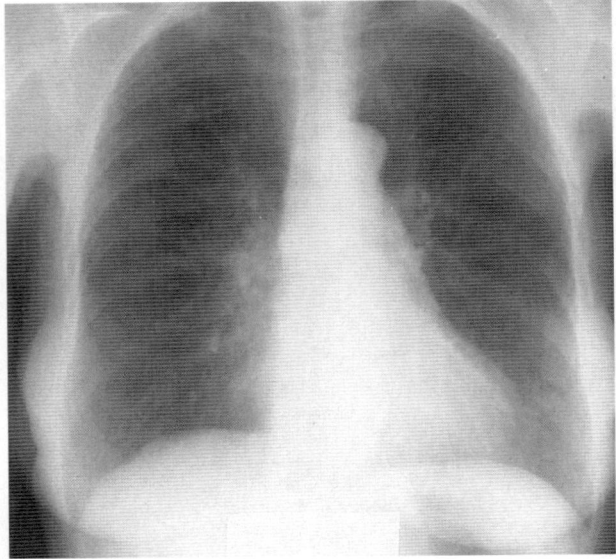

A

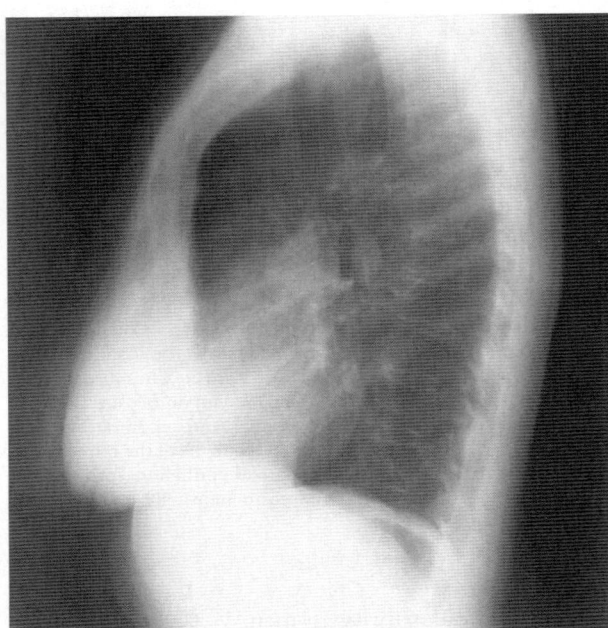

B

Figure 26–12   Bronchiolitis obliterans in a 61-year-old woman with a 9-year history of deforming rheumatoid arthritis, who presented with a 1-year history of progressive dyspnea. Her room-air arterial blood gases (elevation 5,280 feet) were PaO_2 53, $PaCO_2$ 37, and pH 7.47. Shown are the posteroanterior (*A*) and lateral (*B*) chest radiographs that reveal overdistension and peribronchial thickening. The patient died of respiratory failure despite aggressive treatment with corticosteroids and immunosuppressive drugs.

Follicular Bronchiolitis

Patients with rheumatoid arthritis usually present with dyspnea (100%); fever and cough occur occasionally. A positive rheumatoid factor is present, often at high lev-

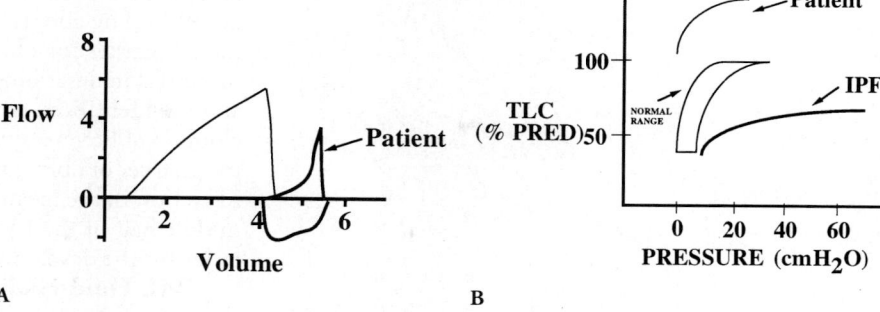

TLC 5.43 L (123% of predicted)
TGV 4.82 L (191% of predicted)
FVC 1.12 L (33% of predicted)
FEV$_1$ 0.59 (24% of predicted)
RAW 314% of predicted
SGAW 18% of predicted
DL$_{CO}$ 59% of predicted

Figure 26–13   Bronchiolitis obliterans in same patient (with rheumatoid arthritis) depicted in Figure 26–12. *A*, Flow–volume relationship and lung volume determination revealed severe airflow limitation and overdistension. The diffusing capacity for carbon monoxide (DL$_{CO}$) was reduced. *B*, The relationship of the static deflation volume and transthoracic pressure in the same patient is compared to the normal range. This patient's curve is shifted up and to the left due to hyperinflation. The coefficient of elastic retraction (P$_{ST}$ max/total lung capacity[TLC]) was 3.22 cmH$_2$O/L; which is within the normal range. Shown for comparison is the pressure-volume curve of a patient with idiopathic pulmonary fibrosis (IPF) and severe restriction. TVG = thoracic gas volume; FVC = forced vital capacity; FEV$_1$ = forced expiratory volume in 1 second; RAW = airway resistance; SGAW = specific airway conductance.

els (1:640 to 1:2,560). The chest film is abnormal, showing bilateral reticular or nodular opacities. Arterial blood gases demonstrate hypoxemia, hypocapnia, and a widened alveolar–arterial oxygen gradient. Both obstructive and restrictive patterns have been identified by spirometry, but the restrictive pattern appears to be more common. Immunofluorescence studies are negative.

The lesions of follicular bronchiolitis produce obstruction by external compression of the bronchioles rather than by direct luminal occlusion as is characteristic for proliferative bronchiolitis obliterans. In almost all cases, a concentric inflammatory infiltrate of lymphocytes and plasma cells surrounds the bronchioles (Figure 26–15). Abundant germinal centers in the peribronchiolar regions are present and are characterized by hyperplastic follicles located between bronchioles and pulmonary arteries. The bronchiolar lumen is often compressed into a slitlike or fish-mouth shape. Some have suggested that follicular bronchiolitis may be the precursor of interstitial lymphoid pneumonia or pseudolymphoma. Treatment with corticosteroids has yielded variable results. Erythromycin may be useful for the management of this process.[152]

Organ Transplantation

Pulmonary disease is a common complication of organ transplantation and consequently is a significant source of morbidity and mortality in transplant recipients. Bronchiolitis, manifested by progressive airflow obstruction, is increasingly becoming the most frequent noninfectious post-transplantation respiratory complication. The BOOP pattern has also been reported in transplant recipients.[153]

Lung Transplantation

Initially, lung transplant recipients were thought not to develop bronchiolitis obliterans. However, this complication is now recognized as the major factor limiting long-term success with this procedure.[154] The incidence of bronchiolitis obliterans among single-lung recipients is approximately 20%; in double or bilateral sequential single-lung recipients, the incidence is 12%.[155] The prevalence has been estimated to be as high as 65% at 5 years.[156–159]

Bronchiolitis Obliterans Syndrome

Progressive airflow limitation, secondary to small airway obstruction, is the hallmark of the bronchiolitis obliterans syndrome. This syndrome has a variable clinical course. Some patients experience rapid loss of lung function and respiratory failure.[4] Others experience either slow progression or intermittent loss of function with plateaus during which pulmonary function is stable for prolonged periods of time. Bronchiolitis obliterans syndrome likely reflects more than one process.[160] The diagnostic criteria for the bronchiolitis obliterans syndrome have recently been updated (Table 26–9).[4]

Risk Factors.   Many factors have been reported as risk factors for bronchiolitis obliterans syndrome.[155,161–164] Based on a review of the literature, a committee sponsored by the International Society for Heart and Lung Transplantation proposed that these risk factors be divided into three groups (probable, potential, and hypothetic) because a causal relationship has not been proven in most cases.[4]

- Probable risk factors include acute rejection, lymphocytic bronchitis/bronchiolitis, medication noncompliance, and cytomegalovirus infection-associated pneumonitis.
- Potential risk factors include cytomegalovirus infection without pneumonitis; organizing pneumonia; bacterial, fungal, and non-cytomegalovirus viral infection; older donor age; longer graft ischemic time; and persistent donor antigen-specific reactivity.

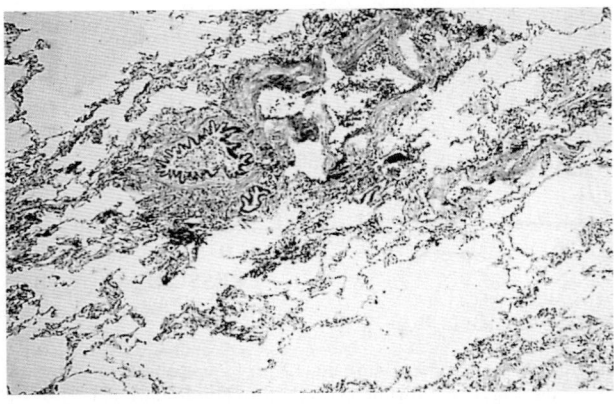

A

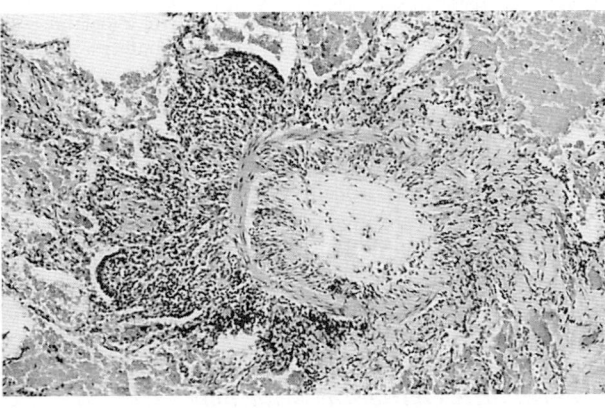

B

Figure 26–14   Rheumatoid arthritis: bronchiolitis obliterans. *A*, Mild bronchiolar inflammation and a luminal cellular infiltrate of chronic inflammatory cells. The normal bronchiolar epithelium has been partially replaced by metaplastic epithelium. *B*, Complete obliteration of a small airway. An area of lymphoid hyperplasia is noted on the right. These histologic findings were quite subtle, affecting only the small airways, and multiple step-sections were required to demonstrate the occlusive lesions.

- Hypothetic risk factors include underlying disease, the genotype of the recipient for certain cytokine gene polymorphisms, human leukocyte antigen (HLA) mismatching, and gastroesophageal reflux with aspiration.

Clinical Findings.   The clinical presentation is similar to that described in heart-lung transplantation: nonproductive cough, mild malaise, and fatigue are common symptoms. Eventually, all subjects develop dyspnea. Physical examination is usually normal, but inspiratory squeaks may be heard. Crackles are uncommon.

Physiological Findings.   Pulmonary function tests show largely irreversible airflow obstruction; however, total lung capacity is reduced (Figure 26–16). A reduction in the diffusing capacity of the lung for carbon monoxide (DL_{CO}) is common. Hypoxemia and hypocapnia are almost always present. Spirometric criteria have been developed for the diagnosis and staging

of bronchiolitis obliterans in this setting (see Table 26–9).[158] The adoption of FEV_1 as a physiological surrogate marker for obliterative bronchiolitis has proved successful in describing the pattern of functional decline and the identification of the main risk factors for bronchiolitis obliterans syndrome. In addition, it is a sensitive marker of obliterative bronchiolitis.[160] A permanent reduction in the mean forced expiratory flow during the middle half of the FVC appears to be an early sensitive index for the development of bronchiolitis obliterans.[165]

BAL Fluid Findings.   BAL fluid cellular analysis shows an association between the bronchiolitis obliterans syndrome and lavage fluid neutrophilia in lung transplant recipients.[4,19,21] This finding may precede the development of lung function impairment.[4,21,166,167] In addition, after lung transplantation, persistent lavage fluid neutrophilia is associated with a poor outcome.[168] Preliminary studies suggest that BAL may be a useful tool for assessing the pathogenesis of bronchiolitis in this setting of chronic allograft rejection. Elevated levels of cytokines have been identified in lavage fluid from these patients (eg, IL-8, markers of oxidative stress, neutrophil elastase, TGF-β, platelet-derived growth factor, collagen I/III, insulin-like growth factor-1).[4] However, none is specific or sensitive enough to be used reliably for diagnosing bronchiolitis obliterans syndrome.[4]

Radiographic Findings.   Decreased peripheral vascular markings, slight volume loss, and subsegmental atelectasis may be early changes. A common radiographic finding in longstanding disease is the gradual progression of pleural-based densities in the middle and upper lung zones. Biopsy reveals subpleural parenchymal fibrosis without active inflammation. The scarring may result from relative ischemia in areas of affected lung.

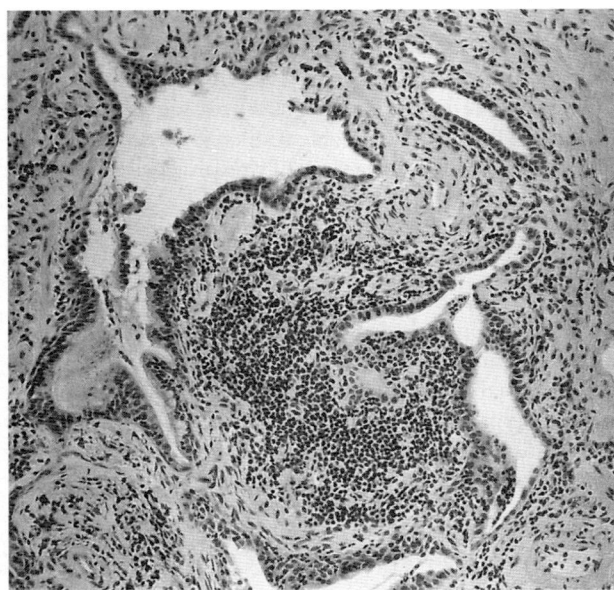

Figure 26–15   Follicular bronchiolitis in rheumatoid arthritis. Prominent lymphoid follicle adjacent to and impinging on the distal airway.

TABLE 26–9   Staging System for Bronchiolitis Obliterans Syndrome Following Lung Transplantation*

Stage[†]	Original Classification System		Proposed Classification System	
	$DFEV_1$, %[‡]	FEV_1, % of Baseline[§]	FEV_1, % of Baseline	FEF_{25-75}, % of Baseline
0	<–20%	>80%	>90%	>75%
0-p			81 to 90%	<75%
1	–20 to –35%	66 to 80%	66 to 80%	
2	–35 to –50%	51 to 65%	51 to 65%	
3	>50%	<50%	<50%	

*Adapted from Cooper et al, Estenne et al, and Trulock EP.[3,4,158]
[†]Subcategories a and b, without and with bronchiolitis obliterans as defined by histology, respectively.
[‡]$DFEV_1$ = ([current FEV_1 – baseline FEV_1] [baseline FEV_1]) × 100%. A 10 to 15% decrease in FEV_1 may be more appropriate for early detection of bronchiolitis obliterans syndrome.[4]
[§]Baseline FEV_1 is the average of the two best FEV_1 measurements, 3 to 6 weeks apart; for the purpose of staging. A significant decrease in FEV_1 or FEF_{25-75} is determined by the average of 2 measurements made at least 3 weeks apart, without patient use of an inhaled bronchodilator.[4] FEV_1 = forced expiratory volume in 1 second; FEF_{25-75} = midexpiratory flow rate; 0-p = potential-bronchiolitis obliterans syndrome stage.

HRCT scanning in cases of bronchiolitis obliterans usually shows lobular or segmental areas of lung attenuation and narrowing of pulmonary vessels, representing regions of air trapping and oligemia.[169] Worthy and colleagues showed that the two most sensitive and specific findings on HRCT scans of patients with bronchiolitis obliterans following lung transplantation were air trapping and bronchial dilatation.[29] CT performed in patients during suspended full expiration has been shown to reveal air trapping. Lung regions that retain air during exhalation (air trapping) remain more lucent than normal lung regions do. Detection of air trapping can provide clues to an otherwise unsuspected or underappreciated small airway disease.[170]

Histopathologic Findings.   Three major kinds of airway injury may be seen in lung allografts: acute rejection, bronchiolitis obliterans, and lymphocytic bronchitis or bronchiolitis.[161] The lesions of bronchiolitis obliterans involve the membranous and respiratory bronchioles. Histologically, bronchiolitis obliterans can take the form of dense subepithelial fibrous plaques, looser fibromyxoid tissue, or a combination of both.[160] If a submucosal mononuclear cell infiltrate is present, the lesions are considered active. Their absence may indicate inactive disease. Vascular changes are often found and usually consist of fibrointimal thickening of arteries and veins, with or without an active inflammatory component.

A BOOP pattern, with patchy organizing pneumonia and granulation tissue plugs extending into the alveolar ducts, has been reported in some lung transplant recipients.[171] It was present in 13% of double-lung and 5% of single-lung transplant patients.[172] BOOP was most often associated with acute rejection.[172] The clinical and radiographic features are progressive respiratory failure, acute or subacute alveolar opacities noted on chest radiograph, and a restrictive pattern of pulmonary function tests. Usually, known causes of this lesion are identifiable, especially infection. Patients respond well to corticosteroid therapy.

Management.   Approximately 50% of all deaths after the first year post-transplantation are due to bronchiolitis obliterans. Except for retransplantation, no effective treatment has been successfully employed.[173] Prevention of repeated episodes of rejection appears important. Prompt diagnosis and treatment of acute rejection and infectious complications is key. Jackson and colleagues have reported that the acute onset of bronchiolitis obliterans syndrome, defined by a sharp, steep, and irreversible decline in FEV_1, is associated with episodes of acute rejection in the first 6 months. These episodes are often triggered by an acute event, and the prognosis is poor, with bronchiolitis obliterans being the main cause of death.[160] These investigators also noted that those lung transplant recipients who develop bronchiolitis obliterans syndrome following a smooth linear decline in lung function are less likely to be subject to acute events and have a better prognosis.[160]

A regimen of immunosuppression, which includes azathioprine, cyclosporine, and prednisone, is most commonly employed. This regimen appears to slow the rate of decline in lung function; however, the overall prognosis remains poor. Cytolytic therapy with an antilymphocyte preparation has been used as treatment, but there is little data documenting its efficacy.[174] The addition of mycophenolate mofetil (3 g/day) was shown to allow the reduction in the dose of prednisone in a patient with bronchiolitis obliterans following lung transplantation.[175] It is unknown if this will be effective therapy. Methotrexate has been used to treat persistent or progressive bronchiolitis obliterans with limited success.[176] Inhaled steroids added to systemic immunosuppression after lung transplantation was ineffective in the prevention of bronchiolitis obliterans syndrome after lung transplantation.[177]

Heart-Lung Transplantation

Heart-lung transplantation has been used for the management of chronic lung and/or heart disease (eg, end-

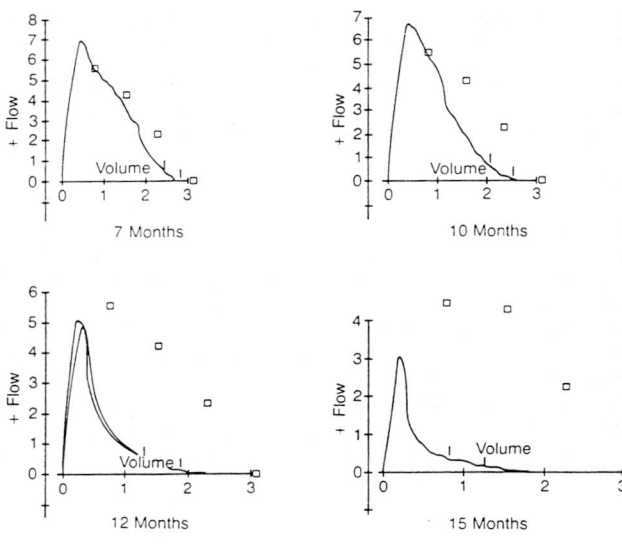

Figure 26–16   Bronchiolitis obliterans associated with heart-lung transplantation. Data curves from a 33 year-old woman 7, 10, 12, and 15 months following transplantation show the sequential changes that typically occur in the forced expiratory flow–volume curve with the development of bronchiolitis obliterans. *A,* Upper left figure shows an essentially normal curve. *B,* Upper right curve shows early "coving" of the expiratory flow limb over the middle 50% of the forced vital capacity (FEV). *C,* Progressive obstruction was present 12 months post-transplantation (lower left). *D,* Airflow obstruction was worse at 15 months (lower right). Small boxes in each panel represent normal flow. Flow is expressed in liters per second; volume is expressed in liters. Reproduced with permission from Theodore et al.[300]

stage pulmonary vascular disease, idiopathic cardiomyopathy, coronary artery disease, congenital heart disease, terminal pulmonary lymphangiomyomatosis, cystic fibrosis, and end-stage Eisenmenger's syndrome).[178–184] The main pulmonary complication in long-term survivors of heart-lung transplantation is a life-threatening obstructive ventilatory defect, bronchiolitis obliterans.[178–181] The incidence of obliterative bronchiolitis in this setting appears to have declined in recent years from 50% to between 10 and 23%.[185] However, in a recent study, 65% of lung transplant recipients (n = 74; 48 heart-lung, 18 single-lung, and 8 bilateral-lung recipients) who survived longer than 90 days, and who underwent transplantation more than 15 months before the data analysis, developed bronchiolitis obliterans syndrome.[186]

Clinical Findings

Bronchiolitis obliterans is noted clinically several months to several years following heart-lung transplantation. A cough producing mucopurulent sputum is most often seen. Progressive dyspnea follows. Most patients experience repeated upper respiratory tract infections, both viral and bacterial in origin. Occasionally, disease onset is identified only by abnormalities in routine pulmonary function testing (Figure 26–17). With advanced disease, wheezing on exertion is common.

The development of bronchiolitis obliterans is frequently preceded by early, severe, poorly controlled organ rejection.[187] Often, patients have a history of previous lung infection with cytomegalovirus, *Pneumocystis carinii,* or Epstein-Barr virus. Chest examination reveals diffuse coarse crackles and expiratory rhonchi.

On physical examination, scattered late-inspiratory, high-pitched rhonchi (inspiratory squeaks) are frequently heard. Bibasilar crackles are uncommon, but they may be heard late in the course of the disease. The

classic signs of severe airflow obstruction and hyperinflation are seen in advanced end-stage disease.

Radiographic Findings

The chest radiograph may be normal in early stages of the disease, but it frequently reveals diffuse nonspecific peribronchial and interstitial infiltrates and variable pleural thickening. Bronchography and CT scanning reveal central bronchiectasis.

Physiological Findings

Pulmonary function tests show largely irreversible airflow obstruction; however, the total lung capacity is reduced. The DL_{CO} is moderately depressed. Hypoxemia and hypocapnia are universally present.

Histopathologic Findings

Histopathologic changes involve all areas of the lung, but they are frequently patchy. Inspissated mucus and distal obstructive airway changes are noted frequently. Diffuse increases in peribronchial and interstitial fibrosis are present in most biopsies. Pleural, venous, and arteriosclerotic vascular changes are common. These changes are different from those in acute pulmonary rejection, which is characterized by perivascular lymphocytic cuffing and diffuse alveolar damage.[183] Clinical acute rejection predisposes recipients to the subsequent development of bronchiolitis obliterans.

Occasionally, classic BOOP with patchy organizing pneumonia and granulation tissue plugs extending into the alveolar ducts is observed as the predominant lesion. The clinical and radiographic features are those seen with BOOP (discussed earlier in this chapter). Usually, known causes of this lesion are identified (eg, infection, aspiration, and drug reaction).

Pathogenesis

Increasing evidence suggests that the key pathogenetic factor is a form of alloreactive injury to the bronchial epithelium.[18] A number of other possible causes or associations of bronchiolitis obliterans in heart-lung transplantation have been described: (1) recurrent persistent bacterial or viral infections; (2) immunoreaction to the transplanted lung (eg, host-versus-graft disease or transplant rejection); (3) altered mucociliary clearance and impaired ciliary function from injury to the pulmonary nerve supply or from abnormal mucus chemistry and viscosity; (4) bronchial artery ligation and resulting alteration in repair of injured bronchi and bronchioles; (5) reaction to immunosuppressive drugs, especially cyclosporine, which has been shown to have fibroproliferative properties that could cause progressive narrowing and obliteration of affected bronchioles; and (6) loss of cough reflex and aspiration, creating a milieu favorable to continued growth of infectious agents. Increasing frequency and severity of acute rejection episodes are strongly associated with the development of bronchiolitis obliterans syndrome.[183,186–189] Organizing pneumonia, bacterial or fungal pneumonia, and increasing severity and frequency of cytomegalovirus infections potentiate the effect of acute rejection.[186] Late episodes of acute rejection and younger recipient age increase the risk for development of advanced disease.

Diagnosis

Open or thoracoscopic lung biopsy is required to confirm the diagnosis of bronchiolitis obliterans and to rule out other causes of pulmonary dysfunction in patients who have undergone heart-lung transplantation.[190] With increased recognition of this potential complication, early detection of the disorder, through use of serial pulmonary function tests, bronchoalveolar lavage, and repeated transbronchial lung biopsies, can be achieved; this may decrease the need for surgical lung biopsy to confirm the diagnosis. The value and role of serial surveillance transbronchial lung biopsies in the absence of clinical symptoms and signs remain unknown.[191] Guilinger and coworkers found unsuspected rejection or infection that required therapy in 25% of all surveillance bronchoscopy procedures after lung transplantation.[192] Most episodes (68%) of unsuspected rejection and/or infection occurred in the first 6 months after lung transplantation.[192]

Management

No clearly useful treatment protocol has been established. Efforts to prevent repeated episodes of rejection seem most important. Prompt diagnosis and treatment of acute rejection and any infectious complications is paramount. Routine serial lung function testing and fiberoptic bronchoscopy with transbronchial biopsy and bronchoalveolar lavage are helpful. The best medical regimen for prevention of bronchiolitis obliterans remains to be defined. Nevertheless, current experience suggests that optimal maintenance of immunosuppression requires a regimen that includes azathioprine and cyclosporine. Prednisone is also commonly included. Use of corticosteroids, bronchodilators, antibiotics, antithymocyte globulin, or OKT3 monoclonal antibodies has resulted in documented stabilization or reversal of disease in some patients. Retransplantation has been successful. Spontaneous improvement does not occur.

Bone Marrow Transplantation

Acute (20 to 100 days after transplantation) or chronic (> 100 days following transplantation) graft-versus-host

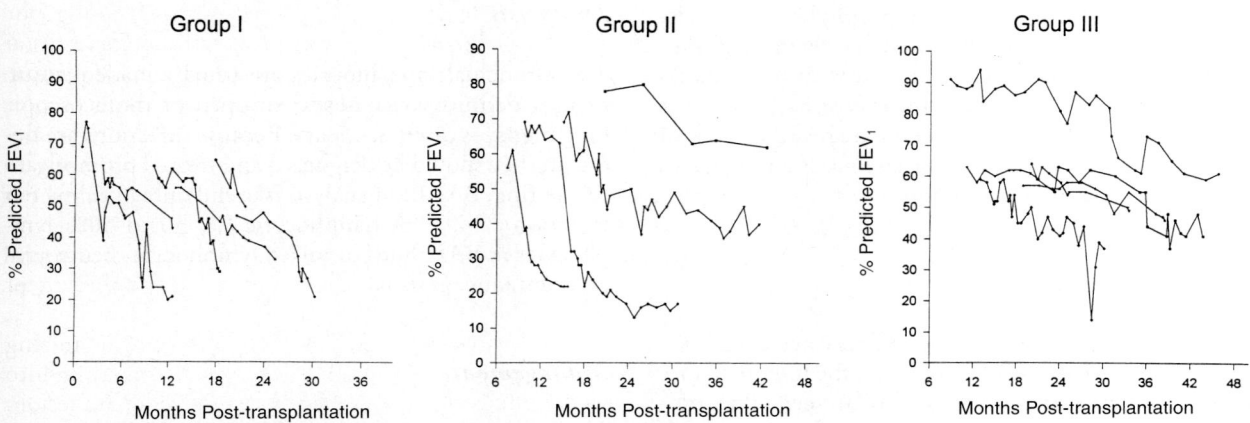

Figure 26–17   Patterns of decrement in the forced expiratory volume in 1 second (FEV$_1$) during the clinical course of bronchiolitis obliterans in single -lung transplant recipients. In group I, patients (*n* = 6) had a rapid onset and a relentless progressive course In group II, this pattern (*n* = 5) was also characterized by a rapid onset and initial rapid decline but was followed by stabilization in lung function. The third pattern, group III (*n* = 4), was characterized by an insidious onset and course. Reproduced with permission from Nathan et al.[165]

disease frequently complicates the course of patients undergoing allogeneic bone marrow transplantation. Acute graft-versus-host disease affects 30 to 60% of patients.[193–195] The disease involves the skin, liver, and gut, and 90% of patients with this complication survive.[196–198] The syndrome of chronic graft-versus-host disease occurs in 33% of long-term allogeneic transplant survivors. The protean manifestations of this disorder include scleroderma-like skin lesions, Sjögren's syndrome, oral and esophageal mucositis, malabsorption, chronic liver disease, generalized wasting, infections, and disorders of immunoregulation.[197,199–203]

Pulmonary disease is a common complication of bone marrow transplantation, occurring in 40 to 60% of patients. Furthermore, pulmonary complications are a significant source of morbidity and mortality in transplant recipients. Disease usually results from an infectious pneumonia (bacterial, fungal, or viral, especially cytomegalovirus) or idiopathic interstitial pneumonitis. Lymphocytic bronchitis and lymphoplasmacytic infiltrates of the trachea and large bronchi are among the earliest pulmonary problems encountered after bone marrow transplantation.[196,197,201,203–205] Progressive airflow obstruction secondary to bronchiolitis obliterans is the most frequent noninfectious post-transplantation respiratory complication.[196,201,203,206–212] Cases appear after the first 100 days post-transplantation, usually in the setting of chronic graft-versus-host disease. Graft-versus-host disease has been postulated to play a role in the development of this lung disease.[196,203,206,208,209,213,214] Bronchiolitis obliterans is most prevalent in patients following allogeneic transplantation, but recently it has been reported with autologous bone marrow transplantation as well.

Clinical Findings

Approximately 10 to 17% of long-term survivors with chronic graft-versus-host disease develop severe obstructive pulmonary disease.[215] Risk factors include older age, recurrent sinusitis, methotrexate prophylaxis for graft-versus-host disease, and acquired hypogammaglobulinemia.[216,217] Patients usually present with nonproductive cough (60%), dyspnea with exertion (51%), and nasal congestion. Scattered wheezes are heard in 40% of patients; expiratory squeaks are also frequently noted. Bibasilar crackles are uncommon.

Radiographic Findings

The chest radiograph may show diffuse interstitial infiltrates; in approximately 80% of cases, the lung fields are normal. Hyperventilation may also be seen. Pneumothoraces may complicate the course of patients with advanced disease. HRCT can be helpful in supporting the diagnosis. In established bronchiolitis obliterans, the most striking CT feature is lobular or segmental areas of lung attenuation associated with narrowing of pulmonary vessels.[218] The attenuation is presumed to represent areas of air trapping and oligemia.[169]

Physiological Findings

The development of a new obstructive pattern on pulmonary function testing is a significant signal that bronchiolitis obliterans is developing, especially when noted in the presence of graft-versus-host disease.[212,214] Reduced flow, often with hyperinflation and air trapping, is the most common manifestation. Bronchial hyperreactivity also has been identified in some patients following transplantation, but the majority have fixed obstruction that is unresponsive to bronchodilators. The presence of bronchial hyperreactivity before transplantation has not been associated with the subsequent development of clinically or pathologically proven post-transplantation broncholitis obliterans. The diffusing capacity is reduced, and hypoxemia is common.[201,211,213,219–221]

Histopathologic Findings

Lung biopsy findings are quite variable. The major changes are in and around the bronchioles. In most patients with rapidly progressive obstruction, marked lymphocytic, plasmacytic, or neutrophilic infiltration of the walls of the terminal respiratory bronchioles and obliteration of the bronchiolar lumina with fibrous tissue and surrounding interstitial fibrosis (ie, "pure" bronchiolitis obliterans) are found. A moderate lymphocytic infiltrate may involve the adjacent pulmonary parenchyma. Other changes characteristic of constrictive bronchiolitis are frequently noted. The BOOP pattern has been found after bone marrow transplantation.[222]

Diagnosis

Transbronchial lung biopsies are usually inadequate to make a definitive diagnosis. An open or thoracoscopic lung biopsy is often necessary. Because infections are frequent, they should be diagnosed and treated promptly. In this setting, BAL fluid analysis is useful only in ruling out infection.[207,223,224] A lymphocytic (ie, 30 to 50% lymphocytes in BAL fluid) or mixed lymphocyte–neutrophil predominance is usual.

Management

The appropriate treatment of bronchiolitis obliterans associated with bone marrow transplantation is questionable. In the majority of cases, bronchodilators and corticosteroids have not improved airflow limitation.

Furthermore, use of immunosuppressive agents for the treatment of chronic graft-versus-host disease has had no consistent beneficial effect on pulmonary function. Consequently, it appears that early recognition and management of rejection are required if treatment is to be successful.

The prognosis is variable. A significant number of reported patients have had progressive or persistent disease; many have died secondary to respiratory failure (40 to 65% of subjects) (Figure 26–18). Increasing recognition, early treatment, and the introduction of cyclosporine A have resulted in a reduction of the incidence of post-transplantation obstructive airway disease.

Drug-Induced Bronchiolitis

Bronchiolitis, usually with organizing pneumonia, has been reported in association with a number of drugs (Table 26–10). Most reports are of single cases or small case series.

Bronchiolitis Associated with Gold Compounds

Gold compounds have been used for the treatment of rheumatoid arthritis for over 50 years. More recently, gold has been used to treat other disorders such as pemphigus, bronchial asthma, psoriatic arthritis, ankylosing spondylitis affecting peripheral joints, and juvenile rheumatoid arthritis. Unfortunately, the benefit of gold treatment has been limited by the high incidence of adverse effects. Most complications are minor, consisting of local dermatitis, stomatitis, transient hematuria, and mild proteinuria. More serious reactions are rare and involve the hematopoietic system (eosinophilia, thrombocytopenia, granulocytopenia, aplastic anemia), kidneys (nephrotic syndrome, renal insufficiency), and liver (cholestatic jaundice).[225] Several forms of pulmonary disease occur among patients treated with gold, including chronic interstitial pneumonitis, organizing pneumonia, and bronchiolitis obliterans.[226,227] Chronic interstitial pneumonitis is the most common presentation of gold-induced lung disease. Bronchiolitis accompanies the chronic interstitial pneumonitis in a few cases. Some of these cases are recognized as gold-related BOOP.[228]

Pure bronchiolitis obliterans, with airflow obstruction, has been associated with gold therapy.[136] Because patients with rheumatoid arthritis are prone to develop pure bronchiolitis obliterans, it is difficult to state that these cases resulted from gold-induced airway injury. All four cases of gold-induced bronchiolitis obliterans were identified in middle-aged females with seropositive rheumatoid arthritis. Although in one case a smoking history was not available, the remaining three were nonsmokers. One case was treated with penicillamine 3 years before gold therapy was started.[138] In addition to dysp-

nea and cough, two of them had wheezing. Skin rash was observed in one case. Peripheral eosinophilia was not mentioned in these four cases. On pulmonary function testing, three cases showed decreases in both vital capacity and the FEV_1 to FVC ratio; the remaining one revealed marked hyperinflation, although the results from spirometer tests were completely normal.[138] They were treated with corticosteroids. Two cases recovered completely, and one survived with residue of cough and dyspnea on mild exertion. One patient died of bronchiolitis.[136] Interestingly, three of these four cases had active rheumatoid arthritis when bronchiolitis developed (ie, active arthritis, subcutaneous nodules [1 case], and high titers of rheumatoid factor). Gold salts may act as a cofac-

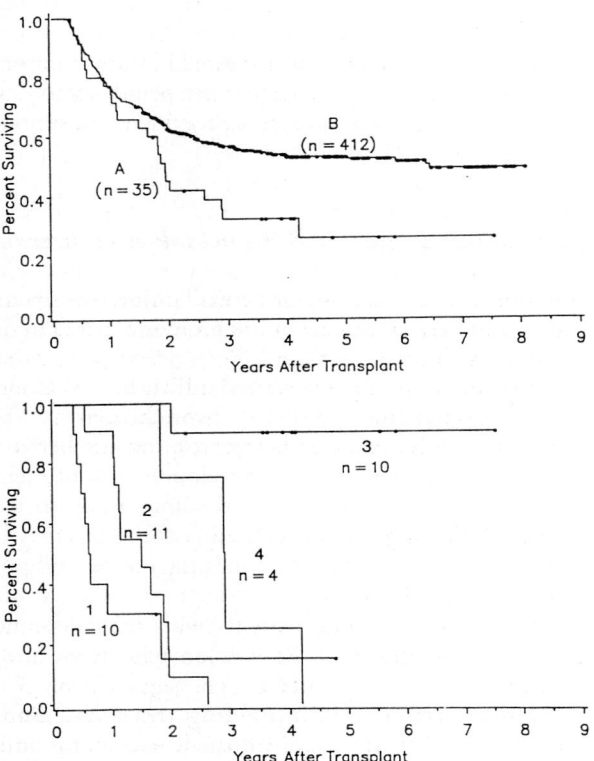

Figure 26–18 Bronchiolitis obliterans associated with bone marrow transplantation. *Top,* Curve A shows survival after bone marrow transplantation in 35 patients with obstructive lung disease. Curve B shows survival of 412 concurrent allogeneic marrow recipients, aged 16 years or more, with chronic graft-versus-host disease who survived at least 80 days after transplantation, with no evidence of obstructive lung disease. Filled circles indicate surviving patients as of 30 June 1988. *Bottom,* Survival after marrow transplantation is shown for 35 patients with obstructive lung disease categorized by time of onset and rate of progression. Category 1 patients (*n* = 10) had early onset (<150 days after transplantation) of rapidly progressive (>30% decrease in FEV_1) obstruction. Patients in category 2 (*n* = 11) had later onset (>150 days after transplantation) of rapidly progressive disease; category 3 patients (*n* = 10) had later onset of slowly progressive (< 30% decrease in FEV_1) disease; and those in category 4 (*n* = 4) showed early onset of slowly progressive disease. Reproduced with permission from Clark et al.[301]

TABLE 26–10   Drug-Induced Reactions Associated with Development of Bronchiolitis

Penicillamine[231]
Gold[226,335,356]
Amiodarone[238,241,354–359]
Hexamethonium
L-tryptophan[360]
Busulfan
Free-base cocaine use[361]
Cephalosporin[362]
Sulfasalazine[363]
Acebutolol[238]
Sulindac[364]
Bleomycin
Interferon[365]
Minocycline[366]
Sauropus androgynus[243,245,246]
Paraquat poisoning

tor in the disease process (as discussed in the sections on bronchiolitis obliterans associated with penicillamine and rheumatoid arthritis) but there is no evidence to support this hypothesis.[136]

Penicillamine-Associated Bronchiolitis Obliterans

Pulmonary complications of penicillamine therapy are uncommon. Use of this agent has been implicated in the pathogenesis of four diffuse lung processes: (1) bronchiolitis obliterans, (2) interstitial infiltrates, (3) Goodpasture's syndrome, and (4) bronchospasm.[229,230] Whether there is a cause and effect relationship between penicillamine therapy and the development of bronchiolitis obliterans in patients with rheumatoid arthritis is unclear.[231] This form of bronchiolitis obliterans may be characterized by a rapidly deteriorating course and pulmonary insufficiency.

The majority of the patients with penicillamine-associated bronchiolitis are women who have never smoked. Breathlessness and cough begin within 3 to 14 months after initiation of drug treatment. Radiographic abnormalities are unusual, except for mild hyperinflation. Pulmonary function abnormalities are characteristically obstructive. The histopathology is thought to be distinct from other causes of bronchiolitis obliterans, because penicillamine-associated cases usually show a concentric, constrictive form of bronchiolar obstruction. Death from progressive respiratory failure occurs in one-third of patients.

The implication of penicillamine as the etiologic agent is less tenable because bronchiolitis obliterans has not been reported in other diseases treated with penicillamine for prolonged periods (eg, Wilson's disease).[134,232] Although conclusive proof of an association between bronchiolitis obliterans and penicillamine therapy is lacking, when confronted with a dyspneic patient with rheumatoid arthritis on penicillamine therapy, one

should stop the drug, consider open lung biopsy, and then administer corticosteroids to prevent disease progression. Cyclophosphamide and prednisone may constitute a useful treatment approach.

Amiodarone-Induced Bronchiolitis

Amiodarone is an iodinated benzofuran derivative that is highly effective in suppressing ventricular and supraventricular tachyarrhythmias. Adverse side effects are common and include photosensitivity, blue-gray discoloration of the skin, thyroid dysfunction, corneal deposits, abnormal liver function tests, and bone marrow suppression.[233] The most serious adverse reaction is pulmonary toxicity, which occurs in 5 to 15% of patients.[234] Although there are exceptional cases, the total cumulative dose is more likely to correlate with pulmonary toxicity than are serum drug levels.[234] Preexisting pulmonary abnormalities may increase the likelihood of developing toxicity, and the clinical manifestations of pulmonary toxicity may be worse, based on the decreased pulmonary reserve.[234]

One characteristic finding in all patients exposed to amiodarone is the presence of numerous foamy macrophages in the air spaces. These cells are filled with amiodarone–phospholipid complexes. Like other amphilic compounds, amiodarone has a tendency to cause an accumulation of phospholipids within lysosomes in the lungs and other tissues due to the inhibition of phospholipase A.[233] Ultrastructural studies show myelinoid inclusion bodies in the affected tissue.

Several patterns of presentation of pulmonary disease occur in patients treated with amiodarone. Chronic interstitial pneumonitis is the most common presentation and is characterized by an insidious onset of nonproductive cough, dyspnea, weight loss, and a chest radiograph revealing focal or diffuse interstitial opacities. This chronic variety usually begins after 2 months of therapy and when the daily treatment dose exceeds 400 mg/day.[234] ARDS is a rare but potentially fatal form of pulmonary toxicity. A fulminant course of ARDS has been noted in patients who had undergone surgery or pulmonary angiography while on amiodarone. A solitary pulmonary mass, simulating a pulmonary malignancy, can be seen.[235–237]

An organizing pneumonia with or without bronchiolitis obliterans (BOOP pattern) is seen in approximately 25% of cases.[238–240] This presentation is acute and is characterized by cough, fever, dyspnea, and patchy alveolar opacities on the chest radiograph. The findings mimic those of an infectious pneumonitis.[241] Pleuritic chest pain and nonproductive cough are common. Crackles and pleural rub are typically evident on auscultation. Treatment consists primarily of stopping the drug, provided that alternative treatment options are made for potentially life-threatening arrhythmia. Corticosteroid therapy (prednisone 40 to 60 mg/day, tapered over 2 to 6 months) can be life-saving for severe cases and for patients in whom withdrawal of amiodarone is not advisable. Because of its accumulation in fatty tissues and long elimination half-life (approximately 45 days), pulmonary toxicity may progress despite drug discontinuation and may recur upon steroid withdrawal.

Sauropus Androgynus-Induced Bronchiolitis

An outbreak of rapidly progressive respiratory distress associated with the consumption of uncooked *Sauropus androgynus*, a vegetable, was recently reported in Taiwan.[242–246] *S. androgynus* is claimed to be effective in weight control. Most of the patients were young and middle-aged women. They took uncooked *S. androgynus* juice, generally mixed with guava or pineapple juice, for a mean duration of 10 weeks. Progressive dyspnea and persistent cough were the main symptoms on presentation.

Pulmonary function testing uniformly revealed moderate to severe airflow obstruction with a mean FEV_1 of 0.66 L (26% of predicted). No bronchodilator response was observed. Room-air arterial blood gas analysis showed hypoxemia.

Chest radiographs were essentially normal. HRCT showed bilateral bronchiectasis and patchy low attenuation of the lung parenchyma with mosaic perfusion. Air trapping was more important than findings of bronchiectasis when correlating pulmonary function.[246] Ventilation-perfusion scintigraphic findings were compatible with those of obstructive lung disease.

Histopathology of open lung biopsy specimens confirmed the presence of bronchiolitis obliterans.[243] The spectrum of histologic changes ranged from slight bronchiolar inflammation and fibrosis to marked submucosal fibrosis, causing complete cicatricial obliteration of the lumen.[247] An obliterative arteriopathy with segmental necrosis of small bronchi may also be seen.[247,248] A dense eosinophil infiltrate was noted in the bronchiolar submucosa or fibrotic tissue of the completely obliterated bronchioles in two patients.[245] In one case, an open lung biopsy disclosed BOOP.[242] Immunohistochemical stains of the open lung biopsy specimens showed a predominance of T cells over B cells. Immunofluorescent stains for IgG, IgM, IgA, C1q, C3, and C4 were negative.[243]

BAL was performed prior to administration of medication in two women who had regularly ingested this vegetable.[244] Both patients showed a significant increase in neutrophils and, to a lesser extent, of eosinophils in the lavage fluid compared with two unrelated controls. Augmented expression of the IL-10 gene was detected in the two patients who had regularly ingested *S. androgynus*.[244] Papaverine has been previously identified in this vegetable, but it is unlikely to be responsible for the full range of toxicity seen.[242]

No effective treatment has been reported because the clinical response to prednisolone was limited.[243]

Malignant Histiocytosis

Colby and colleagues described the clinicopathologic spectrum of pulmonary involvement in malignant histiocytosis.[249] The tumor was systemic and composed of malignant cells with the morphologic and functional characteristics of histiocytes. The clinical presentation was variable. Fever, cough, lymphadenopathy, hepatosplenomegaly, and pancytopenia were common. The chest radiograph was frequently abnormal and revealed diffuse bilateral infiltrates (reticular and reticulonodular) or discrete nodules, with or without pleural effusions. Three of five patients in this study died within 10 months of presentation. The predominant histologic feature was a nondestructive nodular infiltrate within pulmonary lymphatics that showed a tendency to invade adjacent structures. Invasion and occlusion of small airways, as well as bronchiolitis obliterans, were identified in three of the five cases reported.

Chronic Eosinophilic Pneumonia

Eosinophilic pneumonia is a nonspecific term that refers to several entities that have in common pulmonary infiltration with lung and/or blood eosinophilia (see Chapter 24, "Eosinophilic Pneumonias"). The syndrome of chronic eosinophilic pneumonia is characterized by fever, cough, dyspnea, weight loss, and malaise. The disease often waxes and wanes. Physical examination reveals wheezes in some patients. The chest radiograph typically shows dense progressive consolidation that frequently appears in the periphery of the lungs but has no clear relationship to segmental and lobar anatomy. The histopathologic features are characterized primarily by the infiltration of many mature eosinophils and a small number of lymphocytes and plasma cells into the pulmonary parenchyma. Multinucleated giant cells, Charcot-Leyden crystals, sarcoidlike granulomata, mild angiitis, edema, and proteinaceous exudates also occur. Bronchiolitis obliterans is a rare abnormality in this process.[250,251]

Wegener's Granulomatosis

Necrotizing granulomatous inflammation and necrotizing vasculitis are the classic histologic features of Wegener's granulomatosis (WG) (see Chapter 22, "Pulmonary Vasculitis").[252] Recently, several histologic variants have been recognized, including cases characterized by bronchocentric inflammation, a marked eosinophilic infiltrate, alveolar hemorrhage, and capillaritis or interstitial fibrosis.[253] It has also been recognized that the BOOP pattern may be seen on biopsy in WG.[254] Uner and coworkers reported 16 cases of WG with BOOP-like fibrosis as the main histologic finding. The extensive geographic necrosis characteristic of WG was absent in all cases, although small suppurative granulomas, minute

812 Part 3: Clinical Entities

foci of bland necrosis, and microabscesses were common. All cases showed the typical necrotizing vasculitis of WG. Other frequent findings included darkly stained multinucleated giant cells, prominent acute inflammation, aggregates of epithelioid histiocytes, hemosiderin-filled macrophages, and areas of nonspecific parenchymal fibrosis. The clinical and radiographic features of this variant of WG appear to be indistinguishable from the classic type.[255]

Diffuse Panbronchiolitis

Diffuse panbronchiolitis is a distinctive form of small airways disease that is relatively common in Japan, China, and Korea; it is rare in other parts of the world.[256–259] A few case reports of the disease in non-Asians have appeared in the literature.[260–264] A familial occurrence has been described, with a significant increase in HLA-Bw54 (63% frequency).[265] Because HLA-Bw54 or its related haplotype are confined primarily to some mongoloid races (eg, Japanese, Chinese, and Koreans), the genetic and ethnic background observed with this unique syndrome may be explained. HLA-Bw54 may also be a useful marker in the differential diagnosis of diffuse panbronchiolitis, because the frequency of this antigen in the general population is very low (11.8%).[265] A similar pulmonary lesion has been demonstrated in ulcerative colitis, rheumatoid arthritis, and adult T-cell leukemia.[266,267] Environmental factors also appear important, because the disorder is very uncommon in persons of Asian ancestry living abroad.

Clinical Findings

Diffuse panbronchiolitis is more prevalent in men, with a 2:1 male to female ratio. The peak incidence occurs between the fourth and seventh decades of life; the mean age at presentation is 50 years. Chronic sinusitis is present in 75 to 100% of cases. Sinus symptoms often precede chest symptoms by years or decades. Chronic cough with expectoration of copious purulent sputum, exertional dyspnea, and wheezing are the most common clinical manifestations. Cigarette smoking or occupational exposures have not been shown to be predisposing factors. Physical examination reveals coarse crackles; clubbing is not a feature.

The most characteristic laboratory abnormality is persistent marked elevation of serum cold agglutinins; *Mycoplasma* antibody titers are negative. Rheumatoid factor may be elevated. Immunoglobulin levels are usually normal.

BAL

BAL fluid studies reveal marked neutrophilia in patients with diffuse panbronchiolitis.[268] However, Kawakami and coworkers identified T-cell subsets in patients with diffuse panbronchiolitis, before and after long-term treatment with macrolide antibiotics. They found that the percentages of lymphocytes and CD3$^+$ gamma delta$^+$ cells in the BAL fluid of patients with diffuse panbronchiolitis were similar to those in control subjects, but the absolute number of these cells was higher in patients with diffuse panbronchiolitis. Treatment resulted in a significant reduction in the absolute number of these cells. A further two-color analysis of T-cell subsets in BAL fluid showed a significantly higher ratio and number of CD8$^+$ HLA-DR$^+$ cells in patients with diffuse panbronchiolitis. Treatment resulted in a significant reduction of activated T cells. Most BAL fluid CD8$^+$ cells were CD8$^+$ CD11b- cytotoxic T cells. The number of CD4$^+$ cells was also higher in patients with diffuse panbronchiolitis than in control patients, and most were CD4$^+$ CD29$^+$ memory T cells. However, treatment did not influence the number of these cells. The number of lymphocytes, CD3$^+$ gamma delta$^+$, CD8$^+$ CD11b−, CD8$^+$ HLA-DR$^+$, and CD4$^+$ CD29$^+$ cells was higher in patients with bacterial infection than in those without bacterial infection, and interestingly, macrolide therapy reduced the number of lymphocytes, CD3$^+$ gamma delta$^+$, CD8$^+$ CD11b− and CD8$^+$ HLA-DR$^+$ cells, irrespective of bacterial infection. In peripheral blood, the percentage of CD8$^+$ HLA-DR$^+$ cells was also higher in patients with diffuse panbronchiolitis than in healthy subjects and significantly decreased after treatment. The expression of the adhesion molecules CD11a/CD18 (α/β-chains of lymphocyte function-associated antigen 1 [LFA-1]) on lung CD3$^+$ cells and CD49d (α-chain of very late antigen [VLA]) on lung CD4$^+$ cells was enhanced compared with that on peripheral blood in patients with diffuse panbronchiolitis.[269]

Radiographic Findings

The chest radiograph often reveals small nodular opacities up to 2 mm in diameter; the opacities are seen diffusely throughout the lung fields (Figures 26–19 and 26–20). A reticular "airway" pattern may be evident with more advanced disease. Hyperinflation may also be present (see Figure 26–20).

HRCT yields more information about the location and distribution of the pulmonary disease than do conventional radiographic techniques.[270] HRCT also better reflects the clinical stages and pathology (Figure 26–21). On HRCT scans, the nodular shadows are distributed in a centrilobular fashion, often extending to small branching linear areas of attenuation (Figure 26–22). The nodular and linear densities correspond to thickened and dilated bronchiolar walls with intraluminal mucus plugs (Figure 26–23). Inhomogeneity in lung density may be apparent as a result of peripheral air trapping. Bronchiectasis may be prominent in advanced disease.

Physiological Findings

Pulmonary function tests reveal marked obstruction. Arterial blood gases show hypoxemia, with or without hypercapnia. Rarely, a restrictive ventilatory defect may be present. The diffusing capacity is variably reduced. In general, patients with diffuse panbronchiolitis exhibit less bronchodilator responsiveness than do patients with COPD. Reduced nasal nitric oxide has been found in diffuse panbronchiolitis.[271]

Histopathologic Findings

Diffuse panbronchiolitis is characterized histologically by chronic inflammation, principally affecting the respiratory bronchioles. Few pathologists outside Japan are familiar with this entity.[272] The most distinctive pathologic feature of diffuse panbronchiolitis is chronic inflammation and an accumulation of foamy cells in the walls of the respiratory bronchioles, adjacent alveolar ducts, and alveoli (panbronchiolitic unit lesion).[272] Thickening of the walls of the respiratory bronchioles; infiltration with lymphocytes, plasma cells, and histiocytes; and extension of the inflammatory changes to peribronchiolar tissue are noted in biopsy specimens. Advanced disease is manifested by secondary ectasia of proximal bronchioles. The differential diagnosis is important both clinically and histologically because of the similarity of diffuse panbronchiolitis to other chronic airway diseases.

Management and Outcome

The optimal therapy for diffuse panbronchiolitis is unclear. Low-dose erythromycin (200 to 600 mg/day) is adequate for most patients. Erythromycin impairs neutrophil chemotaxis, neutrophil superoxide production, and neutrophil-derived elastolytic activity, and it decreases the number of neutrophils in BAL fluid following challenge with gram-negative bacteria. Leukotriene B4, a potent proinflammatory mediator, is significantly higher in patients with diffuse panbronchiolitis than in control subjects, and the level is significantly reduced after erythromycin treatment.[273] Interestingly, the percent reduction of the level of leukotriene B4 was significantly correlated with neutrophil chemotactic activity and with neutrophil percentage before and after erythromycin treatment. In addition, erythromycin may cause a reduction in mucus production by decreasing glycoconjugate secretion. Finally, erythromycin has been shown to reduce the circulating pool of T lymphocytes bearing HLA-DR, a marker of cellular activation. In untreated patients, the centrilobular areas of high attenuation initially observed on HRCT scanning often show progression to dilatation of the proximal airway.[274] After erythromycin therapy, there often is a significant reduction

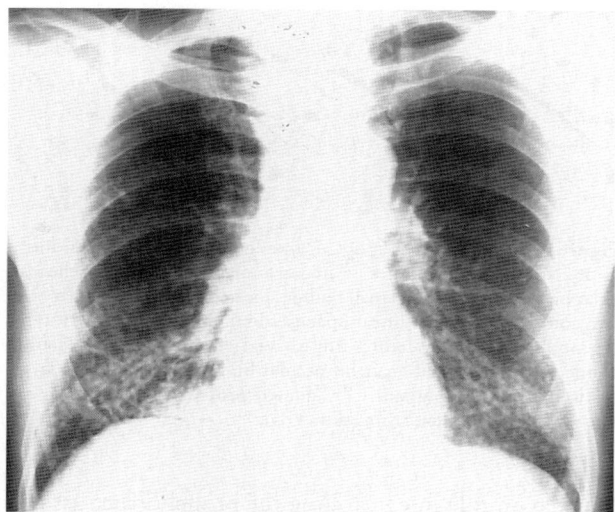

Figure 26–19   Posteroanterior chest radiograph of a patient with diffuse panbronchiolitis shows multiple small nodular shadows disseminated throughout both lungs. The lung volumes appear normal. Reproduced with permission from Dr. Yukihiko Sugiyama, Jichi Medical School, Tochigi, Japan.

in the extent of small nodular opacities, the severity of "periairway" thickening, and the extent of mucus plugging on CT scanning, with a corresponding significant improvement in lung function.[274]

Corticosteroids are commonly used in treatment regimens, but there is no evidence supporting their efficacy. Nonsteroidal antiinflammatory drugs (NSAIDs)

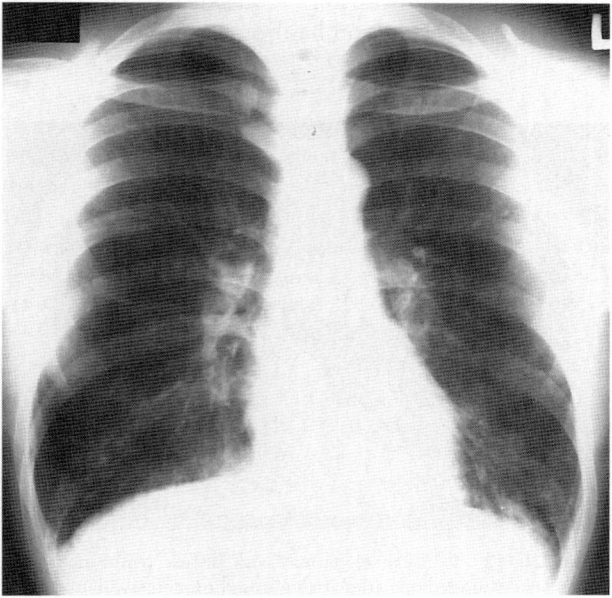

Figure 26–20   Posteroanterior chest radiograph of a patient with diffuse panbronchiolitis shows evidence of hyperinflation. Multiple small nodular shadows are most prominent in the left lower lungs.

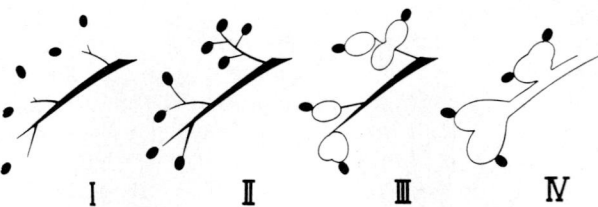

Figure 26–21 Schematics of CT types of diffuse panbronchiolitis. Type I shows small nodules located around the end of bronchovascular branchings; type II, small nodules located in a centrilobular area and connected to small linear opacities branching 1 mm apart, type III, nodules accompanied by ring-shaped or small ductal opacities connected to proximal bronchovascular bundles; and type IV, large cystic opacities accompanied by dilated proximal bronchi. Reproduced with permission from Akira et al.[302]

may have a role in controlling the bronchorrhea associated with this disease by altering airway epithelial ion and water transport. No controlled trials with NSAIDs have been performed. Routine use of β₂-agonists or ipratropium bromide should be encouraged to promote mucociliary clearance and bronchodilation in patients with a component of reversible airway disease and as a part of a routine pulmonary toilet. In addition, treatment of coexisting sinus disease may help in the control of airway disease.

Prompt treatment of bronchial infections is also important. The choice of antibiotics should be guided by results of sputum Gram's stain and culture. The disease progresses insidiously, and the prognosis is often poor, with fatalities resulting from repeated respiratory infections (particularly with *Pseudomonas aeruginosa*) that result in respiratory failure. Lung transplantation has been successfully performed in patients with diffuse panbronchiolitis. Unfortunately, recurrence of the disease after lung transplantation has been reported.[275]

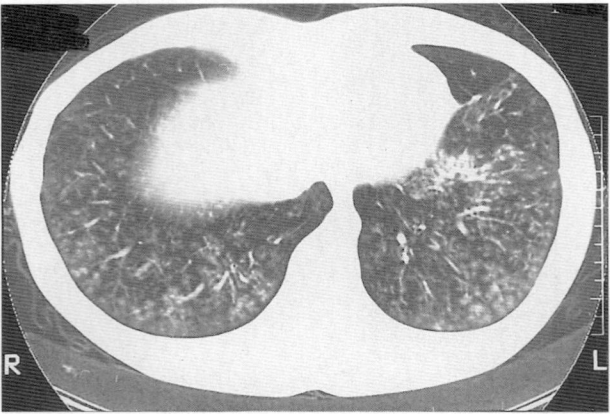

Figure 26–22 CT scan of patient with diffuse panbronchiolitis shows small rounded opacities arising from bronchovascular branchings. In addition, the scan demonstrates dilatation of airways and bronchial wall thickening, especially in the left lung. Reproduced with permission from Dr. Yukihiko Sugiyama, Jichi Medical School, Tochigi, Japan.

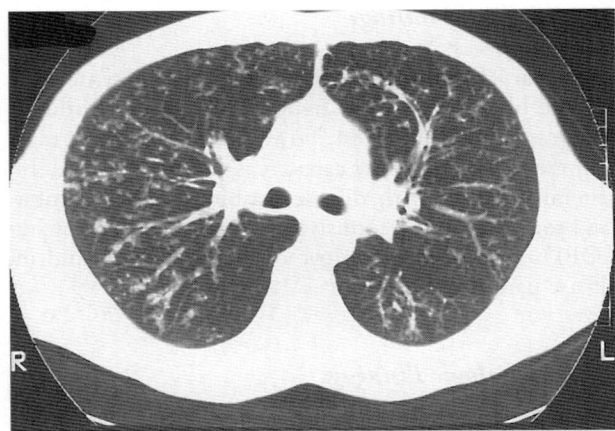

Figure 26–23 CT scan of patient with diffuse panbronchiolitis shows small rounded opacities arising from bronchovascular branchings. Reproduced with permission from Dr. Yukihiko Sugiyama, Jichi Medical School, Tochigi, Japan.

Primary Diffuse Hyperplasia of Pulmonary Neuroendocrine Cells

Foci of neuroendocrine cell hyperplasia is a common incidental finding in a number of lung disorders, particularly in patients with carcinoid tumors, bronchiectasis, lung fibrosis, and pulmonary arterial hypertension. In addition, Miller and Müller showed that multicentric neuroendocrine cell proliferation is common in patients with peripheral carcinoid tumors of the lung. Associated bronchiolar fibrosis was found in a high proportion of such patients, but it was usually asymptomatic.[276] Aguayo and colleagues reported the clinical and pathologic findings of six patients with diffuse neuroendocrine cell hyperplasia associated with symptomatic airflow obstruction due to bronchiolitis obliterans. Primary diffuse hyperplasia of pulmonary neuroendocrine cells is a clinicopathologic entity, characterized by diffuse hyperplasia and dysplasia of neuroendocrine cells, primarily involving the distal bronchi and bronchioles.[277] The disorder was seen primarily in women in their fifth or sixth decade. Clinical findings included nonproductive cough and longstanding dyspnea (usually of > 10 years duration). All reported cases were never-smokers. The chest examination was unremarkable.

The chest radiograph showed diffuse reticular or nodular opacities in most cases; multiple nodules were seen in a few cases. HRCT demonstrated diffuse small airway thickening with patchy areas of hyperlucency, suggesting air trapping. Brown and coworkers described air trapping, mosaic perfusion throughout both lungs, and occasional small nodules measuring 3 to 5 mm in diameter on HRCT scans of a patient with this syndrome.[278] The most common physiological abnormality was irreversible airflow obstruction.

Open or thoracoscopic lung biopsy is required for diagnosis. The spectrum of histopathologic changes includes diffuse hyperplasia and dysplasia of neuroendocrine cells, numerous neuroepithelial bodies, prominent carcinoid tumorlets, and even typical carcinoid tumors involving the distal bronchi and bronchioles (Figure 26–24).

The pathogenesis, treatment, and prognosis of this syndrome are unknown. Most patients have a relatively benign course characterized by many years of symptoms. Lung transplantation has been performed in one subject with a similar syndrome (ie, multiple peripheral tumorlets and microcarcinoids in close association with bronchioles causing an obliterative bronchiolitis).

Paraneoplastic Pemphigus

Pemphigus is a group of rare, chronic, potentially fatal, autoimmune vesiculobullous diseases of the mucous membranes and skin.[280] Three major types of pemphigus have been described, each of which has distinct clinical and pathologic features: pemphigus vulgaris, pemphigus foliaceus, and paraneoplastic pemphigus.[280] Paraneoplastic pemphigus occurs in patients with a known or occult neoplasm, including lymphoreticular malignancies such as non-Hodgkin's lymphoma, chronic lymphocytic leukemia, Castleman's disease, thymoma, and Waldenström's macroglobulinemia.[280–282] Paraneoplastic pemphigus can be the initial presentation of malignancy or may occur in individuals with a known neoplastic process.

Severe painful mucosal erosions and polymorphous skin lesions, acantholysis with interface dermatitis or keratinocyte necrosis, and autoantibodies to various epidermal proteins characterize paraneoplastic pemphigus.[280–281] Distinctive clinical findings include severe painful oral erosions and ulcerations, with hemorrhagic crusting of the lips and polymorphous skin lesions that resemble erythema multiforme, bullous pemphigoid, or lichen planus pemphigoid.[283] Paraneoplastic pemphigoid is associated with autoantibodies directed against both the basement membrane and epithelial cell surface membranes.[280] Patients form anti-Dsg 1 and anti-Dsg 3 antibodies and also have pathogenic autoantibodies against plakin proteins.[280] The plakins are a group of sequence-related proteins that form the intracellular plaques of desmosomes and hemidesmosomes and mediate attachment of the cytoskeletal intermediate filaments to transmembrane adhesion molecules such as desmogleins.[284] The plakin proteins are found in numerous tissues, including respiratory epithelium.[284]

Recently, cases of paraneoplastic pemphigus with pulmonary involvement have been reported. These have been most often associated with Castleman's tumor.[283,285–294] Castleman's tumor has been found in approximately 10% of patients with paraneoplastic pemphigus. In general, Castleman's tumors are benign, except for physical displacement of other internal organs and the sporadic induction of severe paraneoplastic syndromes.[289] Pulmonary involvement occurs in approximately 30% of patients with paraneoplastic pemphigus.[284] The disease process can directly affect the tracheobronchial tree because the pathogenic autoantibodies against plakin proteins are known to be associated with or induce injury to the epithelium of large and small airways.[284] This causes constrictive bronchiolitis, resulting in severe lung impairment, which, in turn, leads to respiratory failure and death.

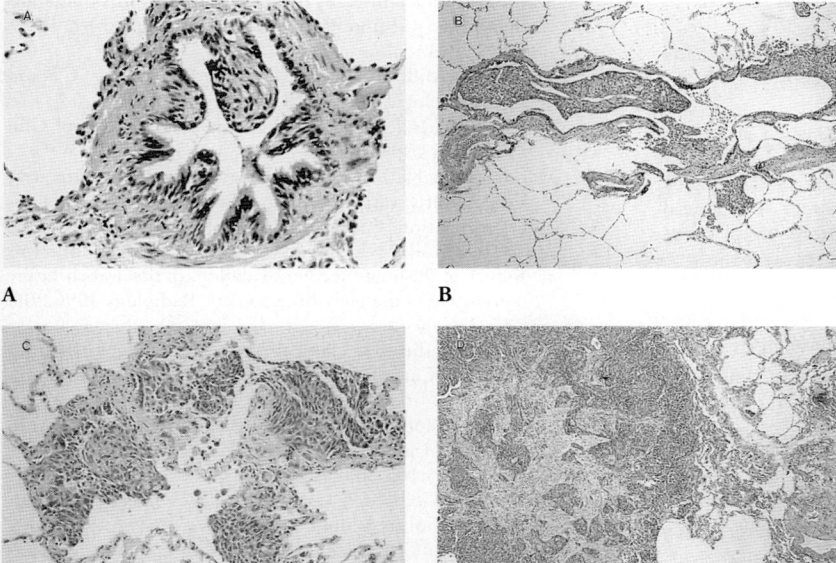

A

B

C

D

Figure 26–24   Primary diffuse hyperplasia of pulmonary neuroendocrine cells. All samples stained with hematoxylin and eosin. *A,* Neuroepithelial bodies are prominent within the bronchiolar mucosa. Often, numerous neuroendocrine cell tumorlets of varying size and morphology are adjacent to these lesions. *B,* Neuroendocrine cell cluster embedded in fibroelastic tissue within a small airway. The walls of this airway are abnormal as well *C,* Neuroendocrine cell cluster obliterating the walls of a terminal bronchiole and protruding into the lumen of associated air spaces. *D,* A well-circumscribed fibroelastic nodule with several irregularly sized neuroendocrine cell nests. No residual lumens could be described in these larger lesions. Reproduced with permission from Dr. Samuel M. Aguayo, Emory University, Atlanta, GA.

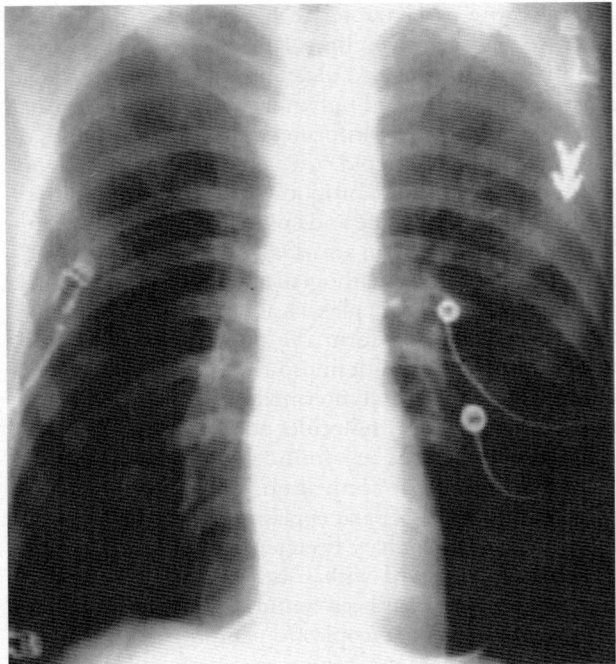

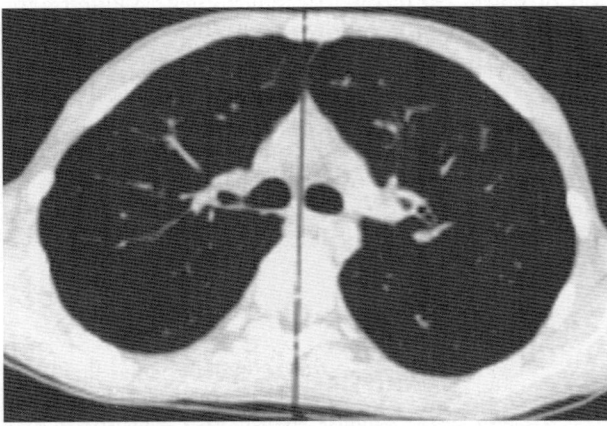

Figure 26–25   Bronchiolitis obliterans associated with Castleman's tumor. *A*, Chest radiograph shows severe hyperinflation. *B*, HRCT scan inspiratory and expiratory images show severe air trapping. A CT scan of the abdomen showed a Castleman's tumor. Reproduced with permission from Dr. Lawrence R. Goodman, Medical College of Wisconsin, Milwaukee, WI.

The condition often begins insidiously with dyspnea. Chest imaging studies are not specific for the diagnosis but eventually show features consistent with bronchiolitis obliterans (Figure 26–25). Bronchoscopic findings may include inflammation, vesiculation, or denudation of tracheobronchial epithelium, and pulmonary function testing may reveal an obstructive ventilatory defect.[295] Bronchial histopathology may show acantholysis, mixed inflammatory infiltrates, and apoptotic epithelial cell changes; direct immunofluorescence may

reveal immunoglobulin deposition along the epithelial cell surface as well as the basement membrane zone.[284,295]

When associated with a malignant neoplasm, paraneoplastic pemphigus tends to be progressive and fatal within 2 years.[280] Treatment of the underlying malignancy does not influence the skin disease, although treatment of associated benign neoplasms (eg, thymoma or Castleman's tumor) does lead to resolution of paraneoplastic pemphigus.[280] Systemic corticosteroids, often combined with cyclosporine or cyclophosphamide, are the mainstay of therapy but have not been effective in halting the progressive respiratory failure associated with bronchiolitis obliterans.[280]

REFERENCES

1. Epler GR. Historic perspectives of the bronchiolar disorders. In: Epler GR, editor. Diseases of the bronchioles. New York: Raven Press; 1994. p. 3–14.
2. Hartman TE, Primack SL, Lee KS, et al. CT of bronchial and bronchiolar diseases. Radiographics 1994;14:991–1003.
3. Cooper JD, Billingham M, Egan T, et al. A working formulation for the standardization of nomenclature and for clinical staging of chronic dysfunction in lung allografts. International Society for Heart and Lung Transplantation. J Heart Lung Transplant 1993;12:713–6.
4. Estenne M, Maurer JR, Boehler A, et al. Bronchiolitis obliterans syndrome 2001: an update of the diagnostic criteria. J Heart Lung Transplant 2002;21:297–310.
5. Travis WD, King TE Jr, Bateman ED, et al. American Thoracic Society/European Respiratory Society international multidisciplinary consensus classification of the idiopathic interstitial pneumonias. Am J Respir Crit Care Med 2002; 165:277–304.
6. Colby TV, Churg AC. Patterns of pulmonary fibrosis. In: Sommers SC, Rosen PP, Fechner RE, editors. 1986 Pathology annual. Vol. 21. Norwalk, CT: Appleton-Century-Crofts; 1986. p. 277–309.
7. Colby TV, Myers JL. The clinical and histologic spectrum of bronchiolitis obliterans including bronchiolitis obliterans organizing pneumonia (BOOP). Sem Respir Med 1992; 13:119–33.
8. Müller NL, Miller RR. Diseases of the bronchioles: CT and histopathologic findings. Radiology 1995;196:3–12.
9. Worthy SA, Müller NL. Small airway diseases. Radiol Clin North Am 1998;36:163–73.
10. Markopoulou KD, Cool CD, Elliot TL, et al. Obliterative bronchiolitis: varying presentations and clinicopathological correlation. Eur Respir J 2002;19:20–30.
11. Austin JH, Müller NL, Friedman PJ, et al. Glossary of terms for CT of the lungs: recommendations of the nomenclature committee of the Fleischner Society. Radiology 1996;200: 327–31.
12. Colby TV, Leslie KO. Clinical diagnosis of interstitial infiltrates. In: Cagle PT, editor. Diagnostic pulmonary pathology. New York: Marcel Dekker; 2000. p. 231–49.
13. Fortoul TI, Cano-Valle F, Oliva E, Barrios R. Follicular bronchiolitis in association with connective tissue diseases. Lung 1985;163:305–14.
14. Yousem SA, Colby TV, Carrington CB. Follicular bronchitis/bronchiolitis. Hum Pathol 1985;16:700–6.
15. Penn CC, Liu C. Bronchiolitis following infection in adults and children. Clin Chest Med 1993;14:645–54.
16. Zwemer FL, Pratt DS, May JJ. Silo filler's disease in New York state. Am Rev Respir Dis 1992;146:650–3.

17. Hausen B, Dwenger A, Gohrbandt B, et al. Early biochemical indicators of the obliterative bronchiolitis syndrome in lung transplantation. J Heart Lung Transplant 1994;13:980–9.

18. Rabinowich H, Zeevi A, Paradis IL, et al. Proliferative responses of bronchoalveolar lavage lymphocytes from heart-lung transplant patients. Transplantation 1990;49:115–21.

19. DiGiovine B, Lynch JP III, Martinez FJ, et al. Bronchoalveolar lavage neutrophilia is associated with obliterative bronchiolitis after lung transplantation: role of IL-8. J Immunol 1996;157:4194–202.

20. Belperio JA, Keane MP, Burdick MD, et al. Critical role for CXCR3 chemokine biology in the pathogenesis of bronchiolitis obliterans syndrome. J Immunol 2002;169:1037–49.

21. Nord M, Schubert K, Cassel TN, et al. Decreased serum and bronchoalveolar lavage levels of Clara cell secretory protein (CC16) is associated with bronchiolitis obliterans syndrome and airway neutrophilia in lung transplant recipients. Transplantation 2002;73:1264–9.

22. Duncan SR, Valentine V, Roglic M, et al. T cell receptor biases and clonal proliferations among lung transplant recipients with obliterative bronchiolitis. J Clin Invest 1996;97:2642–50.

23. Kazerooni EA. High-resolution CT of the lungs. AJR Am J Roentgenol 2001;177:501–19.

24. Hansell DM. High-resolution CT of diffuse lung disease: value and limitations. Radiol Clin North Am 2001;39:1091–113.

25. Morrish WF, Herman SJ, Weisbrod GL, Chamberlain DW. Bronchiolitis obliterans after lung transplantation—findings at chest radiography and high-resolution CT. Radiology 1991;179:487–90.

26. Lentz D, Bergin CJ, Berry GJ, et al. Diagnosis of bronchiolitis obliterans in heart-lung transplantation patients: importance of bronchial dilatation on CT. AJR Am J Roentgenol 1992;159:463–7.

27. Loubeyre P, Revel D, Delignette A, et al. Bronchiectasis detected with thin-section CT as a predictor of chronic lung allograft rejection. Radiology 1995;194:213–6.

28. Ikonen T, Kivisaari L, Harjula AL, et al. Value of high-resolution computed tomography in routine evaluation of lung transplantation recipients during development of bronchiolitis obliterans syndrome. J Heart Lung Transplant 1996;15:587–95.

29. Worthy SA, Park CS, Kim JS, Müller NL. Bronchiolitis obliterans after lung transplantation: high-resolution CT findings in 15 patients. AJR Am J Roentgenol 1997;169:673–7.

30. Waitches GM, Stern EJ. High-resolution CT of peripheral airways diseases. Radiol Clin North Am 2002;40:21–9.

31. Leung AN, Fisher K, Valentine V, et al. Bronchiolitis obliterans after lung transplantation: detection using expiratory HRCT. Chest 1998;113:365–70.

32. Lee ES, Gotway MB, Reddy GP, et al. Early bronchiolitis obliterans following lung transplantation: accuracy of expiratory thin-section CT for diagnosis. Radiology 2000;216:472–7.

33. Siegel MJ, Bhalla S, Gutierrez FR, et al. Post-lung transplantation bronchiolitis obliterans syndrome: usefulness of expiratory thin-section CT for diagnosis. Radiology 2001;220:455–62.

34. Bankier AA, Van Muylem A, Knoop C, et al. Bronchiolitis obliterans syndrome in heart-lung transplant recipients: diagnosis with expiratory CT. Radiology 2001;218:533–9.

35. Shaw RJ, Djukanovic R, Tashkin DP, et al. The role of small airways in lung disease. Respir Med 2002;96:67–80.

36. Becklake MR, Goldman HI, Bosman AR, Freed CC. The long-term effects of exposure to nitrous fumes. Am Rev Tuberc 1957;76:398–409.

37. Ramirez RJ, Dowell AR. Silo-filler's disease: nitrogen dioxide-induced lung injury: long-term follow-up and review of the literature. Ann Intern Med 1971;74:569–76.

38. Jones GR, Proudfoot AT, Hall JI. Pulmonary effects of acute exposure to nitrous fumes. Thorax 1973;28:61–5.

39. Clutton-Brock J. Two cases of poisoning by contamination of nitrous oxide with higher oxides of nitrogen during anesthesia. Br J Anaesth 1967;39:388–92.

40. Fleming GM, Chester EH, Montenegro HD. Dysfunction of small airways following pulmonary injury due to nitrogen dioxide. Chest 1979;75:720–1.

41. Sobonya R. Fatal anhydrous ammonia inhalation. Hum Pathol 1977;8:293–9.

42. Burns TR, Mace ML, Greenberg SD, Jachimczyk JA. Ultrastructure of acute ammonia toxicity in the human lung. Am J Forensic Med Pathol 1985;6:204–10.

43. Prowse K. Nitrous fume poisoning. Bull Eur Physiopathol Respir 1977;13:191–202.

44. Douglas WW, Norman G, Hepper G, Colby TV. Silo-filler's disease. Mayo Clin Proc 1989;64:291–304.

45. Troisi FM. Delayed death caused by gassing in a silo containing green forage. Br J Indust Med 1957;14:56–8.

46. Horvath EP, Colico DGA, Barbee RA, Dickie HA. Nitrogen dioxide-induced pulmonary disease. J Occup Med 1978;20:103–10.

47. Milne JEH. Nitrogen dioxide inhalation and bronchiolitis obliterans. J Occup Med 1969;11:538–47.

48. Yockey CC, Eden BM, Byrd RB. The McConnel missile accident: clinical spectrum of nitrogen dioxide exposure. JAMA 1980;244:1221–3.

49. Moskowitz RL, Lyons HA, Cottle HR. Silo-filler's disease: clinical, physiologic and pathologic study of patient. Am J Med 1964;36:457–62.

50. King TE Jr. Bronchiolitis obliterans. In: Schwarz MI, King TE Jr, editors. Interstitial lung disease. Philadelphia: Mosby-Year Book; 1993. p. 463–95.

51. Scott EU, Hunt WB. Silo-filler's disease. Chest 1973;63:701–6.

52. Rafii S, Godwin MD. Relapse following latent period. Arch Pathol 1961;72:424–33.

53. Woodford DM, Coutu RE, Gaensler EA. Obstructive lung disease from acute sulfur dioxide exposure. Respiration 1979;38:238–45.

54. Eichenberger A, Weber J, Hausser E. Pneumopathic des ensileus (silo-filler's disease). Schweiz Med Wschr 1966;96:1652–5.

55. Tse RL, Bockman AA. Nitrogen dioxide toxicity. Report of four cases in firemen. JAMA 1970;212:1341–4.

56. LaFleche LR, Boivin C, Leonard C. Nitrogen dioxide—a respiratory irritant. Can Med Assoc J 1961;84:1438–43.

57. Rigner KG, Swensson A. Late prognosis of nitrous fume poisoning and follow-up study. Acta Med Scand 1961;170:291–9.

58. Koren HS, Devlin RB, Graham DE, et al. Ozone-induced inflammation in the lower airways of human subjects. Am Rev Respir Dis 1989;139:407–15.

59. Graham DE, Koren HS. Biomarkers of inflammation of ozone-exposed humans. Comparison of the nasal and bronchoalveolar lavage. Am Rev Respir Dis 1990;142:152–6.

60. Paulo M, Gong HJ. Respiratory effects of ozone: whom to protect, when, and how? J Respir Dis 1991;12:482–99.

61. Tyler WS, Julian MD, Hyde DM. Respiratory bronchiolitis following exposures to photochemical air pollutants. Sem Respir Med 1992;13:94–113.

62. Wright JL. Inhalational lung injury causing bronchiolitis. Clin Chest Med 1993;14:635–44.

63. Churg A. Small airways disease associated with mineral dust exposure. Sem Respir Med 1992;13:140–5.

64. Churg A, Wright JL. Small airways disease and mineral dust exposure. Pathol Annu 1983;18:233–51.

65. Churg A, Wright JL. Small-airway lesions in patients exposed to nonasbestos mineral dusts. Hum Pathol 1983;14:688–93.

66. Wright JL, Churg A. Morphology of small-airway lesions in patients with asbestos exposure. Hum Pathol 1984;15:68–74.

67. Churg A, Wright JL, Wiggs B, et al. Small airways disease and

mineral dust exposure. Am Rev Respir Dis 1985;131: 139–43.

68. Wright JL, Churg A. Severe diffuse small airways abnormalities in long term chrysotile asbestos miners. Br J Indust Med 1985;42:556–9.

69. Kennedy SM, Wright JL, Mullen JB, et al. Pulmonary function and peripheral airway disease in patients with mineral dust or fume exposure. Am Rev Respir Dis 1985;132:1294–9.

70. Wright JL, Tron V, Wiggs B, Churg A. Cigarette smoke potentiates asbestos-induced airflow abnormalities. Exp Lung Res 1988;14:537–48.

71. Begin R, Boileau R, Peloquin S. Asbestos exposure, cigarette smoking, and airflow limitation in long-term Canadian chrysotile miners and millers. Am J Indust Med 1987; 11:55–66.

72. Becklake MR. Chronic airflow limitation: its relationship to work in dusty occupations. Chest 1985;88:608–17.

73. Becklake MR. Occupational exposures: evidence for a causal association with chronic obstructive pulmonary disease. Am Rev Respir Dis 1989;140:S85–S91.

74. Selman-Lama M, Perez-Padilla R. Airflow obstruction and airway lesions in hypersensitivity pneumonitis. Clin Chest Med 1993;14:699–714.

75. Pérez-Padilla R, Gaxiola M, Salas J, et al. Bronchiolitis in chronic pigeon breeder's disease. Morphologic evidence of a spectrum of small airway lesions in hypersensitivity pneumonitis induced by avian antigens. Chest 1996;110:371–7.

76. From the Centers for Disease Control and Prevention. Fixed obstructive lung disease in workers at a microwave popcorn factory—Missouri, 2000–2002. JAMA 2002;287:2939–40.

77. Fixed obstructive lung disease in workers at a microwave popcorn factory—Missouri, 2000–2002. MMWR Morb Mortal Wkly Rep 2002;51:345–7.

78. Lockey J, McKay R, Barth E, et al. Bronchiolitis obliterans in the food flavoring manufacturing industry [abstract]. Am J Respir Crit Care Med 2002;165:A461.

79. Kreiss K, Gomaa A, Kullman G, et al. Endemic bronchiolitis obliterans syndrome in microwave popcorn workers: a new occupational lung hazard [abstract]. Am J Respir Crit Care Med 2002;165:A461.

80. Akpinar-Elci M, Kanwal R, Kreiss K. Bronchiolitis obliterans syndrome in popcorn plant workers [abstract]. Am J Respir Crit Care Med 2002;165:A526.

81. Lynch DA. Imaging of small airway disease, Bronchiolitis obliterans in new occupational settings: developing a clinical and public health approach, Morgantown, WV, August 25, 2001, National Institute for Occupational Safety and Health (NIOSH).

82. Kreiss K, Gomaa A, Kullman G, et al. Clinical bronchiolitis obliterans in workers at a microwave popcorn plant. N Engl J Med 2002;347:330–8.

83. Schachter EN. Popcorn worker's lung. N Engl J Med 2002;347:360–1.

84. Wohl MEB, Chernick V. Bronchiolitis: state of the art. Am Rev Respir Dis 1978;118:759–81.

85. Smith CB, Overall CJJ. Clinical and epidemiologic clues to the diagnosis of respiratory infections. Radiol Clin North Am 1973;11:261–78.

86. Wohl MEB. Bronchiolitis in children. In: Epler GR, editor. Diseases of the bronchioles. New York: Raven Press; 1994. p. 397–407.

87. Hardy KA. Childhood bronchiolitis obliterans. In: Epler GR, editor. Diseases of the bronchioles. New York: Raven Press; 1994. p. 415–26.

88. Wenman WM, Pagtakhan RD, Reed MH, et al. Adenovirus bronchiolitis in Manitoba: epidemiologic, clinical and radiologic features. Chest 1982;81:605–9.

89. Gosink BB, Friedman PJ, Liebow AA. Bronchiolitis obliterans: roentgenologic-pathologic correlation. Am J Roentgenol Radium Ther Nucl Med 1973;117:816–32.

90. Breatnach E, Kerr I. The radiology of cryptogenic obliterative bronchiolitis. Clin Radiol 1982;33:657–61.

91. Hardy KA, Schidlow DV, Zaeri N. Obliterative bronchiolitis in children. Chest 1988;93:460–6.

92. Green M. Bronchiolitis. In: Sadaul P, Milic-Emili J, Simonsson BG, Clark TJH, editors. Small airways in health and disease. Amsterdam: Excerpta Medica (ICS 485); 1979. p. 90–4.

93. Wohl ME. Present capacity to evaluate pulmonary function relevant to bronchiolitis. Pediatr Res 1977;11(3 Pt 2):252–3.

94. Hall WJ, Hall CB. Clinical significance of pulmonary function tests. Alterations in pulmonary function following respiratory vital infection. Chest 1979;76:458–65.

95. McConnochie KM, Roghmann KJ. Predicting clinically significant lower respiratory tract illness in childhood following mild bronchiolitis. Am J Dis Child 1985;139(6): 625–31.

96. McIntosh K. Bronchiolitis and asthma: Possible common pathogenetic pathways. J Allergy Clin Immunol 1976;57: 595–604.

97. Twiggs JT, Larson LA, O'Connell EJ, Ilstrup DM. Respiratory syncytial virus infection: ten-year follow-up. Clin Pediatr (Phila) 1981;20:187–90.

98. Weiss ST, Tager IB, Munoz A, Speizer FE. The relationship of respiratory infections in early childhood to the occurrence of increased levels of bronchial responsiveness and atopy. Am Rev Respir Dis 1985;131:573–8.

99. McConnochie KM, Mark JD, McBride JT, et al. Normal pulmonary function measurements and airway reactivity in childhood after mild bronchiolitis. J Pediatr 1985;107: 54–8.

100. McLean KH. The pathology of acute bronchiolitis: a study of its evolution. II. The repair phase. Aust Ann Med 1957; 6:29–43.

101. McLean KH. The pathology of acute bronchiolitis: a study of its evolution. I. The exudative phase. Aust Ann Med 1956;5:254–67.

102. Mauad T, Dolhnikoff M. Histology of childhood bronchiolitis obliterans. Pediatr Pulmonol 2002;33:466–74.

103. Mellins RB. Bronchiolitis—comments on pathogenesis and treatment. Pediatr Res 1977;11:268–9.

104. Friis B, Andersen P, Brene E, et al. Antibiotic treatment of pneumonia and bronchiolitis. A prospective randomised study. Arch Dis Child 1984;59:1038–45.

105. Klassen TP, Rowe PC, Sutcliffe T, et al. Randomized trial of salbutamol in acute bronchiolitis. J Pediatr 1991;118: 807–11.

106. Caramia G, Palazzini E. Efficacy of ribavirin aerosol treatment for respiratory syncytial virus bronchiolitis in infants. J Int Med Res 1987;15:227–33.

107. Hefelfinger DC. Bronchiolitis: a clearer picture is emerging. J Respir Dis 1986;7:17–27.

108. Ellis EF. Therapy of acute bronchiolitis. Pediatr Res 1977; 11:263–4.

109. Marti-Bonmati L, Perales FR, Catala F, et al. CT findings in Swyer-James syndrome. Radiology 1989;172:477–80.

110. Coultas DB, Funk LM. Postinfectious bronchiolitis obliterans. In: Epler GR, editor. Diseases of the bronchioles. New York: Raven Press; 1994. p. 215–29.

111. Ham JC. Acute infectious obstructing bronchiolitis: a potentially fatal disease in the adult. Ann Intern Med 1964;60:47–60.

112. Harris C. Acute obstructive bronchiolitis. Presentation of a fatal case. JAMA 1965;194:203–5.

113. Dines DE. Acute bronchiolitis as a cause of chronic obstructive lung disease in adults. Report of two cases. Lancet 1967;87:281–2.

114. Marinopoulos GC, Huddle KR, Wainwright H. Obliterative bronchiolitis: virus induced? Chest 1991;99:243–5.

115. Turton CW, William G, Green M. Cryptogenic obliterative bronchiolitis in adults. Thorax 1981;36:805–10.

116. Dorinsky PM, Davis WB, Lucas JG, et al. Adult bronchioli-

tis. Evaluation by bronchoalveolar lavage and response to prednisone therapy. Chest 1985;88:58–63.

117. Kindt GC, Weiland JE, Davis WB, et al. Bronchiolitis in adults. A reversible cause of airway obstruction associated with airway neutrophils and neutrophil products. Am Rev Respir Dis 1989;140:483–92.

118. Meier-Sydow J, Schneider M, Rust M. Chronic bronchiolitis in adults. Eur J Respir Dis 1986;69 Suppl 146:337–44.

119. Edwards C, Cayton R, Bryan R. Chronic transmural bronchiolitis: non-specific lesion of small airways. J Clin Pathol 1992;45:993–8.

120. Kraft M, Mortenson RL, Colby TV, et al. Cryptogenic constrictive bronchiolitis. Am Rev Respir Dis 1993;148:1093–101.

121. Murphy KC, Atkins CJ, Offer RC, et al. Obliterative bronchiolitis in two rheumatoid arthritis patients treated with penicillamine. Arthritis Rheum 1981;24:557–60.

122. Green M, Turton CW. Bronchiolitis and its manifestations. Eur J Respir Dis 1982;53 Suppl 121:36–42.

123. Cooney TP. Interrelationship of chronic eosinophilic pneumonia, bronchiolitis obliterans, and rheumatoid disease: a hypothesis. J Clin Pathol 1981;34:129–37.

124. Jacobs P, Bonnyns M, Depierreux M, et al. Rapidly fatal bronchiolitis obliterans with circulating antinuclear and rheumatoid factors. Case report. Eur J Respir Dis 1984;65:384–8.

125. Stein HB, Patterson AC, Offer RC, et al. Adverse effects of D-penicillamine in rheumatoid arthritis. Ann Intern Med 1980;92:24–9.

126. Penny WJ, Knight RK, Rees AM, et al. Obliterative bronchiolitis in rheumatoid arthritis. Ann Rheum Dis 1982;41:469–72.

127. Chebat J, Seigneur F, Lechien J, et al. Obliterating bronchiolitis during D-penicillamine treatments [letter]. Nouv Presse Med 1980;9:2655.

128. Chebat J, Seigneur F, Lechien J, et al. Bronchiolite severe au cour de trois cas de polyarterite rhumatoide traitee por D-penicillamine. Rev Fr Mal Respir 1981;9:147–9.

129. Wolfe F, Shurle DR, Lin JJ, et al. Upper and lower airway disease in penicillamine-treated patients with rheumatoid arthritis. J Rheumatol 1983;10:406–10.

130. Yousem SA, Colby TV, Carrington CB. Lung biopsy in rheumatoid arthritis. Am Rev Respir Dis 1985;131:770–7.

131. Begin R, Masse S, Cantin A, et al. Airway disease in a subset of nonsmoking rheumatoid patients. Characterization of the disease and evidence for an autoimmune pathogenesis. Am J Med 1982;72:743–50.

132. Collins RL, Turner RA, Johnson AM, et al. Obstructive pulmonary disease in rheumatoid arthritis. Arthritis Rheum 1976;19:623–8.

133. Geddes DM, Corrin B, Brewerton DA, et al. Progressive airway obliteration in adults and its association with rheumatoid disease. Q J Med 1977;46:427–44.

134. Epler GR, Snider GL, Gaensler EA, et al. Bronchiolitis and bronchitis in connective tissue disease. A possible relationship to the use of penicillamine. JAMA 1979;242:528–32.

135. Herzog CA, Miller RR, Hoidal JR. Bronchiolitis and rheumatoid arthritis. Am Rev Respir Dis 1981;124:636–9.

136. Holness I, Tenebaum J, Cooter NB, Grossman RF. Fatal bronchiolitis obliterans associated with chrysotherapy. Ann Rheum Dis 1983;42:593–6.

137. McCann BG. Obliterative bronchiolitis and upper zone pulmonary consolidation in rheumatoid arthritis. Thorax 1983;38:73–4.

138. Lahdensuo A. Bronchiolitis in rheumatoid arthritis. Chest 1984;85:705–8.

139. Lyle WH. D-penicillamine and fatal obliterative bronchiolitis. Br Med J 1977;1:105.

140. Geddes DM, Webley M, Emerson PA. Airways obstruction in rheumatoid arthritis. Ann Rheum Dis 1979;38:222–5.

141. Vest JV, Smith TW, Gorman JC, et al. Airways abnormalities in non-smokers with rheumatoid arthritis [abstract]. Am Rev Respir Dis 1980;121:202A.

142. Schwarz MI, Lynch DA, Tuder R. Bronchiolitis obliterans: the lone manifestation of rheumatoid arthritis? Eur Respir J 1994;7:817–20.

143. Jansen HM, Elema JD, Hylkema BS, et al. Progressive obliterative bronchiolitis in a patient with rheumatoid arthritis. Eur J Respir Dis 1982;121:43–52.

144. van de Laar MA, Westerman CJ, Wagenaar SS, Dinant HJ. Beneficial effect of intravenous cyclophosphamide and oral prednisone on D-penicillamine-associated bronchiolitis obliterans. Arthritis Rheum 1985;28:93–7.

145. Brewerton DA. D-penicillamine [letter]. Br Med J 1976;2:1507.

146. Cordier JF, Falconnet M, Moulin J, et al. Bronchiolile severe et polyarthrite rhumatoide: role tres prohohle de la D-penicillamine dan deux observations. Lyon Med 1980;244:113–4.

147. Brannen HM, Good CA, Divertie MB, Baggenstoss AH. Pulmonary disease associated with rheumatoid arthritis. JAMA 1964;189:914–8.

148. Scadding JG. The lungs in rheumatoid arthritis. Proc R Soc Med 1969;62:227–38.

149. MacFarlane JD, Dieppe PA, Rigden BG, Clark TJH. Pulmonary and pleural lesions in rheumatoid disease. Br J Dis Chest 1978;72:288–300.

150. Aquino SL, Webb WR, Golden J. Bronchiolitis obliterans associated with rheumatoid arthritis: findings on HRCT and dynamic expiratory CT. J Comput Assist Tomogr 1994;18:555–8.

151. Fort JG, Scovern H, Abruzzo JL. Intravenous cyclophosphamide and methylprednisolone for the treatment of bronchiolitis obliterans and interstitial fibrosis associated with crysotherapy. J Rheumatol 1988;15:850–4.

152. Hayakawa H, Sato A, Imokawa S, et al. Bronchiolar disease in rheumatoid arthritis. Am J Respir Crit Care Med 1996;154:1531–6.

153. Verberckmoes R, Verbeken E, Verschakelen J, Vanrenterghem Y. BOOP (bronchiolitis obliterans organizing pneumonia) after renal transplantation. Nephrol Dial Transplant 1996;11:1862–3.

154. Ohori NP, Iacono AT, Grgurich WF, Yousem SA. Significance of acute bronchitis/bronchiolitis in the lung transplant recipient. Am J Surg Pathol 1994;18:1192–204.

155. Maurer JR. Lung transplantation bronchiolitis obliterans. In: Epler GR, editor. Diseases of the bronchioles. New York: Raven Press; 1994. p. 275–89.

156. Bando K, Paradis IL, Similo S, et al. Obliterative bronchiolitis after lung and heart-lung transplantation. An analysis of risk factors and management. J Thorac Cardiovasc Surg 1995;110:4–13.

157. Girgis RE, Tu I, Berry GJ, et al. Risk factors for the development of obliterative bronchiolitis after lung transplantation. J Heart Lung Transplant 1996;15:1200–8.

158. Trulock EP. Lung transplantation. Am J Respir Crit Care Med 1997;155:789–818.

159. Heng D, Sharples LD, McNeil K, et al. Bronchiolitis obliterans syndrome: incidence, natural history, prognosis, and risk factors. J Heart Lung Transplant 1998;17:1255–63.

160. Jackson CH, Sharples LD, McNeil K, et al. Acute and chronic onset of bronchiolitis obliterans syndrome (BOS): are they different entities? J Heart Lung Transplant 2002;21:658–66.

161. Paradis I, Yousem S, Griffith B. Airway obstruction and bronchiolitis after lung transplantation. Clin Chest Med 1993;14:751–63.

162. Kshettry VR, Kroshus TJ, Savik K, et al. Primary pulmonary hypertension as a risk factor for the development of obliterative bronchiolitis in lung allograft recipients. Chest 1996;110:704–9.

163. Kroshus TJ, Kshettry VR, Savik K, et al. Risk factors for the development of bronchiolitis obliterans syndrome after

lung transplantation. J Thorac Cardiovasc Surg 1997;114: 195–202.

164. Fiser SM, Tribble CG, Long SM, et al. Ischemia-reperfusion injury after lung transplantation increases risk of late bronchiolitis obliterans syndrome. Ann Thorac Surg 2002;73: 1041–8.

165. Nathan SD, Ross DJ, Belman MJ, et al. Bronchiolitis obliterans in single-lung transplant recipients. Chest 1995;107:967–72.

166. Riise GC, Williams A, Kjellstrom C, et al. Bronchiolitis obliterans syndrome in lung transplant recipients is associated with increased neutrophil activity and decreased antioxidant status in the lung. Eur Respir J 1998;12:82–8.

167. Riise GC, Andersson BA, Kjellstrom C, et al. Persistent high BAL fluid granulocyte activation marker levels as early indicators of bronchiolitis obliterans after lung transplant. Eur Respir J 1999;14:1123–30.

168. Henke JA, Golden JA, Yelin EH, et al. Persistent increases of BAL neutrophils as a predictor of mortality following lung transplant. Chest 1999;115:403–9.

169. Eber CD, Stark P, Bertozzi P. Bronchiolitis obliterans on high-resolution CT: a pattern of mosaic oligemia. J Comput Assist Tomogr 1993;17:853–6.

170. Stern EJ, Frank MS. Small-airway diseases of the lungs: findings at expiratory CT. AJR Am J Roentgenol 1994;163:37–41.

171. Milne DS, Gascoigne AD, Ashcroft T, et al. Organizing pneumonia following pulmonary transplantation and the development of obliterative bronchiolitis. Transplantation 1994;57:1757–62.

172. Chaparro C, Chamberlain D, Maurer J, Winton T, et al. Bronchiolitis obliterans organizing pneumonia (BOOP) in lung transplant recipients. Chest 1996;110:1150–4.

173. Novick RJ, Andréassian B, Schäfers HJ, et al. Pulmonary retransplantation for obliterative bronchiolitis. Intermediate-term results of a North American-European series. J Thorac Cardiovasc Surg 1994;107:755–63.

174. Snell GI, Esmore DS, Williams TJ. Cytolytic therapy for the bronchiolitis obliterans syndrome complicating lung transplantation. Chest 1996;109:874–8.

175. Speich R, Boehler A, Thurnheer R, Weder W. Salvage therapy with mycophenolate mofetil for lung transplant bronchiolitis obliterans: importance of dosage. Transplantation 1997;64:533–5.

176. Dusmet M, Maurer J, Winton T, Kesten S. Methotrexate can halt the progression of bronchiolitis obliterans syndrome in lung transplant recipients. J Heart Lung Transplant 1996;15:948–54.

177. Whitford H, Walters EH, Levvey B, et al. Addition of inhaled corticosteroids to systemic immunosuppression after lung transplantation: a double-blind, placebo-controlled trial. Transplantation 2002;73:1793–9.

178. McGregor CG, Hamieson SW, Baldwin JC, et al. Combined heart-lung transplantation for end-stage Eisenmenger's syndrome. J Thorac Cardiovasc Surg 1986;91:443–50.

179. Burke CM, Theodore J, Baldwin JC, et al. Twenty-eight cases of human heart-lung transplantation. Lancet 1986;i: 17–9.

180. Wellens F, Estenne M, deFrancquen P, et al. Combined heart-lung transplantation for terminal pulmonary lymphangioleiomyomatosis. J Thorac Cardiovasc Surg 1985;89:872–6.

181. Dawkins KD, Jamieson SW, Hunt SA, et al. Long-term results, hemodynamics, and complications after combined heart and lung transplantation. Circulation 1985;71:919–26.

182. Burke CM, Theodore J, Dawkins KD, et al. Post-transplant obliterative bronchiolitis and other late lung sequelae in human heart-lung transplantation. Chest 1984;86:824–9.

183. Yousem SA, Burke CM, Billingham ME. Pathologic pulmonary alterations in long-term human heart-lung transplantation. Hum Pathol 1985;16:911–23.

184. Modry DL, Oyer PE, Jamieson SW, et al. Cyclosporine in heart and heart-lung transplantation. Can J Surg 1985;28: 274–80,282.

185. Burke CM, Yousem SA, Corris PA. Heart-lung transplantation. In: Epler GR, editor. Diseases of the bronchioles. New York: Raven Press; 1994. p. 259–74.

186. Girgis RE, Tu I, Berry GJ, et al. Risk factors for the development of obliterative bronchiolitis after lung transplantation. J Heart Lung Transplant 1996;15:1200–8.

187. Scott JP, Wallwork J, Stewart S, et al. Risk factors for obliterative bronchiolitis in heart-lung transplant recipients. Transplantation 1991;51:813–7.

188. Sharples LD, Tamm M, McNeil K, et al. Development of bronchiolitis obliterans syndrome in recipients of heart-lung transplantation--early risk factors. Transplantation 1996;61:560–6.

189. Tamm M, Sharples L, Higenbottam T, et al. Bronchiolitis obliterans syndrome (BOS) following heart-lung transplantation. Transplant International 1996;9 Suppl 1: S299–302.

190. Kramer MR, Stoehr C, Whang JL, et al. The diagnosis of obliterative bronchiolitis after heart-lung and lung transplantation: low yield of transbronchial lung biopsy. J Heart Lung Transplant 1993;12:675–81.

191. Tamm M, Sharples LD, Higenbottam TW, et al. Bronchiolitis obliterans syndrome in heart-lung transplantation: surveillance biopsies. Am J Respir Crit Care Med 1997;155: 1705–10.

192. Guilinger RA, Paradis IL, Dauber JH, et al. The importance of bronchoscopy with transbronchial biopsy and bronchoalveolar lavage in the management of lung transplant recipients. Am J Respir Crit Care Med 1995;152:2037–43.

193. Ettinger NA, Trulock EP. Pulmonary considerations of organ transplantation, Part 1. Am Rev Respir Dis 1991;143: 1386–405.

194. Ettinger NA, Trulock EP. Pulmonary considerations of organ transplantation, Part 2. Am Rev Respir Dis 1991;144: 213–23.

195. Ettinger NA, Trulock EP. Pulmonary considerations of organ transplantation, Part 3. Am Rev Respir Dis 1991;144: 433–51.

196. Ostrow D, Buskard N, Hill RS, et al. Bronchiolitis obliterans complicating bone marrow transplantation. Chest 1985;87:828–30.

197. Atkinson K, Storb R, Prentice RL, et al. Analysis of late infections in 89 long-term survivors of bone marrow transplantation. Blood 1979;53:720–31.

198. Thomas ED, Storb R, Clift RA, et al. Bone marrow transplantation. N Engl J Med 1975;292:832–43,895–902.

199. Graze PR, Gale RP. Chronic graft versus host disease: a syndrome of disordered immunity. Am J Med 1979;66:611–20.

200. LeBourgeois JP, Vernant JP, Thiellet A, et al. Unusual incidence of localized pneumonitis after total body irradiation for bone marrow transplantation. Exp Hematol 1984;15 Suppl 12:23.

201. Shulman HM, Sullivan KM, Weiden PL, et al. Chronic graft-versus-host syndrome in man. A long-term clinicopathological study of 20 Seattle patients. Am J Med 1980;69: 204–17.

202. Sullivan KM, Shulman HM, Storb R, et al. Chronic graft-versus-host disease in 62 patients: adverse natural course and successful treatment with combination immunosuppression. Blood 1981;57:267–76.

203. Ralph DD, Springmeyer SC, Sullivan KM, et al. Rapidly progressive air-flow obstruction in marrow transplant recipients: possible association between obliterative bronchiolitis and chronic graft-versus-host disease. Am Rev Respir Dis 1984;129:641–4.

204. Beschorner WE, Saral R, Hutchins LM, et al. Lymphocytic bronchitis associated with graft-versus-host disease in recipients of bone-marrow transplants. N Engl J Med 1978;299:1030–6.

205. Hackman RC, Sale GE. Large airway inflammation as a possible manifestation of a pulmonary graft-versus-host reaction on bone marrow allograft recipents [abstract]. Lab Invest 1981;44:26A.

206. Rodriguez-Roisin R, Roca J, Marin P, et al. Pulmonary follow-up in patients with bone marrow transplantation (BMT) and graft-versus-host disease (GVHD). Exp Hematol 1985;17 Suppl 13:145.

207. Rodriguez–Roisin R, Roca S, Granena A, et al. Obliterative bronchiolitis: a distinct pathophysiological form of pulmonary involvement in bone marrow transplantation. Exp Hematol 1984;15 Suppl 12:12–4.

208. Roca J, Granena A, Rodriguez-Roisin R, et al. Fatal airway disease in an adult with chronic graft-versus-host disease. Thorax 1982;37:77–8.

209. Link H, Reinhard D, Neithammer D, et al. Obstructive ventilation disorders as a severe complication of chronic graft-versus-host disease after bone marrow transplantation. Exp Hematol 1982;10:92–3.

210. Wyatt SE, Nunn P, Hows JM, et al. Airways obstruction in association with graft-versus-host disease following bone marrow transplantation. Exp Hematol 1984;15 Suppl 12:17–8.

211. Johson FL, Stokes DC, Ruggiero M, et al. Chronic obstructive airways disease after bone marrow transplantation. J Pediatr 1984;105:370–6.

212. Rosenberg ME, Vercellotti GM, Snover DC, et al. Bronchiolitis obliterans after bone marrow transplantation. Am J Hematol 1985;18:325–8.

213. Link H, Ostendorf P, Wilms K, et al. Pulmonary complications after bone marrow transplantation. Exp Hematol 1983;13 Suppl 11:125–7.

214. Link H, Ostendorf P, Wernet P, et al. Pulmonary complication after allogeneic bone marrow transplantation. The Tubingen experience. Exp Hematol 1984;15 Suppl 12:21–2.

215. Keane TJ, Van Dyk J, Rider WD. Idiopathic interstitial pneumonia following bone marrow transplantation: the relationship with total body irradiation. Int J Radiat Oncol Biol Phys 1981;7:1365–70.

216. Crawford SW, Clark JG. Bronchiolitis associated with bone marrow transplantation. Clin Chest Med 1993;14:741–9.

217. Chan CK. Bone marrow transplantation bronchiolitis obliterans. In: Epler GR, editor. Diseases of the bronchioles. New York: Raven Press; 1994. p. 247–57.

218. Hansell DM, Rubens MB, Padley SP, Wells AU. Obliterative bronchiolitis: individual CT signs of small airways disease and functional correlation. Radiology 1997;203:721–6.

219. Schmeiser T, Heymer B, Arnold R, et al. A clinicopathological study of bone-marrow transplant associated pulmonary disease. Exp Hematol 1985;17 Suppl 13:149.

220. Buckner CD, Meyers JD, Springmeyer SC, et al. Pulmonary complications of marrow transplantation. Review of the Seattle experience. Exp Hematol 1984;15 Suppl 12:1–5.

221. Sorensen PG, Ernst P, Panduro J, Moller J. Reduced lung function in leukemia patients undergoing bone marrow transplantation. Scand J Haematol 1984;32:253–7.

222. Kanda Y, Takahashi T, Imai Y, et al. Bronchiolitis obliterans organizing pneumonia after syngeneic bone marrow transplantation for acute lymphoblastic leukemia. Bone Marrow Transplantation 1997;19:1251–3.

223. Cordonnier C, Bernaudin JF, Feuilhade M, et al. Diagnostic value of bronchoalveolar lavage (BAL) in pneumonitis occurring after allogeneic bone marrow transplantation (BMT). Exp Hematol 1984;15 Suppl 12:26.

224. Leskinen R, Tukiainen P, Taskinen E, et al. Bronchoalveolar lavage in the diagnosis of pulmonary complications in bone marrow transplant recipients. Preliminary experience. Exp Hematol 1984;15 Suppl 12:24–5.

225. Gordon DA. Gold compounds in the rheumatic diseases. In: Kelley WN, Harris ED, Ruddy S, Sledge CB, editors. Text book of rheumatology. Philadelphia: Saunders; 1993. p. 743–59.

226. Winterbauer RH, Wilske KR, Wheelis RF. Diffuse pulmonary injury associated with gold treatment. N Engl J Med 1976;294:919–21.

227. Tomioka H, King TE Jr. Gold-induced pulmonary disease: clinical features, outcome, and differentiation from rheumatoid lung disease. Am J Respir Crit Care Med 1997; 155:1011–20.

228. Hollingsworth HM. Drug-related bronchiolitis obliterans organizing pneumonia. In: Epler GR, editor. Diseases of the bronchioles. New York: Raven Press; 1994. p. 367–76.

229. Turner-Warwick M. Adverse reactions affecting the lung: possible association with D-penicillamine. J Rheumatol 1981; 7:166–8.

230. Camus P. The respiratory complications of D-penicillamine therapy (author's translation). Rev Fr Mal Respir 1982;10:7–20.

231. Yam LY, Wong R. Bronchiolitis obliterans and rheumatoid arthritis. Report of a case in a Chinese patient on D-penicillamine and review of the literature. Ann Acad Med, Singapore 1993;22:365–8.

232. Sternlieb I, Bennet B, Scheinberg IH. D-penicillamine-induced Goodpasture's syndrome in Wilson's disease. Ann Intern Med 1975;82:673–6.

233. Mason JW. Amiodarone. N Engl J Med 1987;316:455–66.

234. Martin WJ, Rosenow EC. Amiodarone pulmonary toxicity. Recognition and pathogenesis (Pt 1). Chest 1988;93: 1067–75.

235. Greenspon AJ, Kidwell GA, Hurley W, Mannion J. Amiodarone-related postoperative adult respiratory distress syndrome. Circulation 1991;3 Suppl 84:407–15.

236. Wood DL, Osborn MJ, Rooke J, Holmes DR Jr. Amiodarone pulmonary toxicity: report of two cases associated with rapidly progressive fatal respiratory distress syndrome after pulmonary angiography. Mayo Clin Proc 1985;60:601–3.

237. Piccione W Jr, Faber LP, Rosenberg MS. Amiodarone-induced pulmonary mass. Ann Thorac Surg 1989;47:18–9.

238. Camus P, Lombard JN, Perrichon M, et al. Bronchiolitis obliterans organising pneumonia in patients taking acebutolol or amiodarone. Thorax 1989;44:711–5.

239. Dean PJ, Groshart KD, Porterfield JG, et al. Amiodarone-associated pulmonary toxicity. A clinical and pathologic study of eleven cases. Am J Clin Pathol 1987;87:7–13.

240. Valle JM, Alvarez D, Antunez J, Valdes L. Bronchiolitis obliterans organizing pneumonia secondary to amiodarone: a rare etiology. Eur Resp J 1995;8:470–1.

241. Zitnik RJ. Drug-induced lung disease: antiarrhythmic agents. J Respir Dis 1996;17:254–70.

242. Lin TJ, Lu Lu CC, Chen KW, Deng JF. Outbreak of obstructive ventilatory impairment associated with consumption of Sauropus androgynus vegetable [comments]. J Toxicol Clin Toxicol 1996;34:1–8.

243. Lai RS, Chiang AA, Wu Wu MT, et al. Outbreak of bronchiolitis obliterans associated with consumption of Sauropus androgynus in Taiwan. Lancet 1996;348:83–5.

244. Chen CW, Hsiue TR, Chen KW, et al. Increased IL-5 and IL-10 transcription in bronchial cells after Sauropus androgynus ingestion. J Formos Med Assoc 1996;95:699–702.

245. Chang H, Wang JS, Tseng HH, et al. Histopathological study of Sauropus androgynus-associated constrictive bronchiolitis obliterans: a new cause of constrictive bronchiolitis obliterans. Am J Surg Pathol 1997;21:35–42.

246. Yang CF, Wu MT, Chiang AA, et al. Correlation of high-resolution CT and pulmonary function in bronchiolitis obliterans: a study based on 24 patients associated with consumption of Sauropus androgynus. AJR Am J Roentgenol 1997;168:1045–50.

247. Wang JS, Tseng HH, Lai RS, et al. Sauropus androgynus-constrictive obliterative bronchitis/bronchiolitis--histopathological study of pneumonectomy and biopsy

specimens with emphasis on the inflammatory process and disease progression. Histopathology 2000;37:402–10.

248. Chang YL, Yao YT, Wang NS, Lee YC. Segmental necrosis of small bronchi after prolonged intakes of *Sauropus androgynus* in Taiwan. Am J Respir Crit Care Med 1998;157:594–8.

249. Colby TV, Carrington CB, Mark GJ. Pulmonary involvement of malignant histiocytosis: a clinicopathologic spectrum. Am J Surg Pathol 1981;5:61–73.

250. Fox B, Seed WA. Chronic eosinophilic pneumonia. Thorax 1980;35:570–80.

251. Morrissey WL, Gaensler EA, Carrington CB, Turner HG. Chronic eosinophilic pneumonia. Respiration 1975;32:453–68.

252. Travis WD, Hoffman GS, Leavitt RY, et al. Surgical pathology of the lung in Wegener's granulomatosis. Review of 87 open lung biopsies from 67 patients. Am J Surg Pathol 1991;15:315–33.

253. Myers JL, Katzenstein ALA. Wegener's granulomatosis presenting with massive pulmonary hemorrhage and capillaritis. Am J Surg Pathol 1987;11:895–8.

254. Mark EJ, Flieder DB, Matsubara O. Treated Wegener's granulomatosis: distinctive pathological findings in the lungs of 20 patients and what they tell us about the natural history of the disease. Hum Pathol 1997;28:450–8.

255. Uner AH, Rozum-Slota B, Katzenstein AL. Bronchiolitis obliterans-organizing pneumonia (BOOP)-like variant of Wegener's granulomatosis. A clinicopathologic study of 16 cases. Am J Surg Pathol 1996;20:794–801.

256. Homma H, Yamanaka A, Tanimoto S, et al. Diffuse panbronchiolitis: a disease of the transitional zone of the lung. Chest 1983;83:63–9.

257. Izumi T. A nation-wide survey of diffuse panbronchiolitis in Japan. In: Grassi C, Rizzato G, Pozzi E, editors. Sarcoidosis and other granulomatous disorders. New York: Elsevier Science Publishers; 1988. p. 753–7.

258. Sugiyama Y. Diffuse panbronchiolitis. Clin Chest Med 1993;14:765–72.

259. Fisher MS Jr, Rush WL, Rosado-de-Christenson ML, et al. Diffuse panbronchiolitis: histologic diagnosis in unsuspected cases involving North American residents of Asian descent. Arch Pathol Lab Med 1998;122:156–60.

260. Randhawa P, Hoagland MH, Yousem SA. Diffuse panbronchiolitis in North America. Report of three cases and review of the literature. Am J Surg Pathol 1991;15:43–7.

261. Poletti V, Patelli M, Poletti G, et al. Diffuse panbronchiolitis observed in an Italian [letter]. Chest 1990;98:515–6.

262. Homer R, Khoo L, Walker Smith G. Diffuse panbronchiolitis in a Hispanic man with travel to Japan. Chest 1995;107:1176–8.

263. Fitzgerald JE, King TE Jr, Lynch DA, et al. Diffuse panbronchiolitis in the United States. Am J Respir Crit Care Med 1996;154:497–503.

264. Martinez JA, Guimaraes SM, Ferreira RG, Pereira CA. Diffuse panbronchiolitis in Latin America. Am J Med Sci 2000;319:183–5.

265. Sugiyama Y, Kudoh S, Maeda H, et al. Analysis of HLA antigens in patients with diffuse panbronchiolitis. Am Rev Respir Dis 1990;141:1459–62.

266. Yamanishi Y, Maeda H, Hiyama K, et al. Rheumatoid arthritis associated with diffuse panbronchiolitis. Intern Med 1998;37:338–41.

267. Ono K, Shimamoto Y, Matsuzaki M, et al. Diffuse panbronchiolitis as a pulmonary complication in patients with adult T-cell leukemia. Am J Hematol 1989;30:86–90.

268. Koga T. Neutrophilia and high level of interleukin 8 in the bronchoalveolar lavage fluid of diffuse panbronchiolitis. Kurume Med J 1993;40:139–46.

269. Kawakami K, Kadota J, Iida K, et al. Phenotypic characterization of T cells in bronchoalveolar lavage fluid (BALF) and peripheral blood of patients with diffuse panbronchi-

olitis; the importance of cytotoxic T cells. Clin Exp Immunol 1997;107:410–6.

270. Sueyasu Y. Diffuse panbronchiolitis—a thin-section CT scoring system. Kurume Med J 1996;43:63–71.

271. Nakano H, Ide H, Imada M, et al. Reduced nasal nitric oxide in diffuse panbronchiolitis. Am J Respir Crit Care Med 2000;162:2218–20.

272. Iwata M, Colby TV, Kitaichi M. Diffuse panbronchiolitis: diagnosis and distinction from various pulmonary diseases with centrilobular interstitial foam cell accumulations. Hum Pathol 1994;25:357–63.

273. Oda H, Kadota J, Kohno S, Hara K. Leukotriene B4 in bronchoalveolar lavage fluid of patients with diffuse panbronchiolitis. Chest 1995;108:116–22.

274. Akira M, Higashihara T, Sakatani M, Hara H. Diffuse panbronchiolitis: follow-up CT examination. Radiology 1993;189:559–62.

275. Baz MA, Kussin PS, Trigt PV, et al. Recurrence of diffuse panbronchiolitis after lung transplantation. Am J Respir Crit Care Med 1995;151:895–8.

276. Miller RR, Müller NL. Neuroendocrine cell hyperplasia and obliterative bronchiolitis in patients with peripheral carcinoid tumors. Am J Surg Pathol 1995;19:653–8.

277. Aguayo SA, Miller YE, Waldron JA Jr, et al. Idiopathic diffuse hyperplasia of pulmonary neuroendocrine cells and airway disease. N Engl J Med 1992;327:1285–8.

278. Brown MJ, English J, Müller NL. Bronchiolitis obliterans due to neuroendocrine hyperplasia: high-resolution CT–pathologic correlation. AJR Am J Roentgenol 1997;168:1561–2.

279. Sheerin N, Harrison NK, Sheppard MN, et al. Obliterative bronchiolitis caused by multiple tumourlets and microcarcinoids successfully treated by single lung transplantation. Thorax 1995;50:207–9.

280. Goldstein BG, Goldstein AO. Pemphigus and bullous pemphigoid. In: Rose BD, editor. UpToDate. Wellesley, MA: UpToDate; 2002.

281. Anhalt GJ, Kim SC, Stanley JR, et al. Paraneoplastic pemphigus: an autoimmune mucocutaneous disease associated with neoplasia. N Engl J Med 1990;323:1729–35.

282. Kimyai-Asadi A, Jih MH. Paraneoplastic pemphigus. Int J Dermatol 2001;40:367–72.

283. Kim SC, Chang SN, Lee IJ, et al. Localized mucosal involvement and severe pulmonary involvement in a young patient with paraneoplastic pemphigus associated with Castleman's tumour. Br J Dermatol 1998;138:667–71.

284. Nousari HC, Deterding R, Wojtczack H, et al. The mechanism of respiratory involvement in paraneoplastic pemphigus. N Engl J Med 1999;340:1406–10.

285. Fullerton SH, Woodley DT, Smoller BR, Anhalt GJ. Paraneoplastic pemphigus with autoantibody deposition in bronchial epithelium after autologous bone marrow transplantation. JAMA 1992;267:1500–2.

286. Saito K, Morita M, Enomoto K. Bronchiolitis obliterans with pemphigus vulgaris and Castleman's disease of hyaline-vascular type: an autopsy case analyzed by computer-aided 3-D reconstruction of the airway lesions. Hum Pathol 1997;28:1310–2.

287. Chorzelski T, Hashimoto T, Maciejewska B, et al. Paraneoplastic pemphigus associated with Castleman tumor, myasthenia gravis and bronchiolitis obliterans. J Am Acad Dermatol 1999;41:393–400.

288. Hasegawa Y, Shimokata K, Ichiyama S, Saito H. Constrictive bronchiolitis obliterans and paraneoplastic pemphigus. Eur Respir J 1999;13:934–7.

289. Wolff H, Kunte C, Messer G, et al. Paraneoplastic pemphigus with fatal pulmonary involvement in a woman with a mesenteric Castleman tumour. Br J Dermatol 1999;140:313–6.

290. Takahashi M, Shimatsu Y, Kazama T, et al. Paraneoplastic

pemphigus associated with bronchiolitis obliterans. Chest 2000;117: 603–7.

291. van der Waal RI, Pas HH, Nousari HC, et al. Paraneoplastic pemphigus caused by an epithelioid leiomyosarcoma and associated with fatal respiratory failure. Oral Oncol 2000;36:390–3.

292. Chin AC, Stich D, White FV, et al. Paraneoplastic pemphigus and bronchiolitis obliterans associated with a mediastinal mass: a rare case of Castleman's disease with respiratory failure requiring lung transplantation [abstract]. J Pediatr Surg 2001;36:E22.

293. Cordel N, Ringeisen F, Antoine M, et al. Paraneoplastic pemphigus with constrictive bronchiolitis obliterans[abstract]. Dermatology 2001;202:145.

294. Fujimoto W, Kanehiro A, Kuwamoto-Hara K, et al. Paraneoplastic pemphigus associated with Castleman's disease and asymptomatic bronchiolitis obliterans. Eur J Dermatol 2002;12:355–9.

295. Osmanski JP II, Fraire AE, Schaefer OP. Necrotizing tracheobronchitis with progressive airflow obstruction associated with paraneoplastic pemphigus. Chest 1997;112:1704–7.

296. Plopper CG, Ten Have-Opbrock AAW. Anatomical and histological classification of the bronchioles. In: Epler GR, editor. Diseases of the bronchioles. New York: Raven Press; 1994. p. 15–25.

297. Corrin B. Development and structure of the normal lung. In: Turner-Warwick M, Hodson ME, Corrin B, Kerr IH, editors. Clinical atlas of respiratory diseases. London: JB Lippincott; 1989. p. 1.1–1.14.

298. Webb WR. High-resolution computed tomography of obstructive lung disease. Radiol Clin North Am 1994; 32:745–57.

299. Tuder RM, Cool C, Jennings C, Voelkel NF. Diffuse alveolar hemorrhage. In: Schwarz MI, King TE Jr, editors. Interstitial lung diseases. Hamilton, ON: BC Decker; 1998. p. 251–63.

300. Theodore J, Starnes VA, Lewiston NJ. Obliterative bronchiolitis. Clin Chest Med 1990;11:309–21.

301. Clark JG, Crawford SW, Madtes DK, Sullivan KM. Obstructive lung disease after allogeneic marrow transplantation. Clinical presentation and course. Ann Intern Med 1989; 111:368–76.

302. Akira M, Kitatani J, Yong-Sik L, et al. Diffuse panbronchiolitis: evaluation with high-resolution CT. Radiology 1988;168:433–8.

303. Chatté G, Streichenberger N, Boillot O, et al. Lymphocytic bronchitis/bronchiolitis in a patient with primary biliary cirrhosis. Eur Respir J 1995;8:176–9.

304. Camus P, Piard F, Ashcroft T, et al. The lung in inflammatory bowel disease. Medicine 1993;72:151–83.

305. Matsuse T, Oka T, Kida K, Fukuchi Y. Importance of diffuse aspiration bronchiolitis caused by chronic occult aspiration in the elderly. Chest 1996;110:1289–93.

306. Janoski MM, Raymond GS, Puttagunta L, et al. Psyllium aspiration causing bronchiolitis: radiographic, high-resolution CT, and pathologic findings. AJR Am J Roentgenol 2000;174:799–801.

307. Parto K, Svedström E, Majurin ML, et al. Pulmonary manifestations in lysinuric protein intolerance. Chest 1993;104: 1176–82.

308. Ito M, Nakagawa A, Hirabayashi N, Asai J. Bronchiolitis obliterans in ataxia-telangiectasia. Virchows Arch 1997;430: 131–7.

309. Homma S, Kawabata M, Kishi K, et al. Bronchiolitis in Kartagener's syndrome. Eur Respir J 1999;14:1332–9.

310. Schwarz MI, Mortenson RL, Colby TV, et al. Pulmonary capillaritis. The association with progressive irreversible airflow limitation and hyperinflation. Am Rev Respir Dis 1993;148:507–11.

311. Costabel U. Bronchoalveolar lavage characteristics of the bron-

chiolar diseases. In: Epler GR, editor. Diseases of the bronchioles. New York: Raven Press; 1994. p. 59–76.

312. Von Oettingen WF. The toxicity and potential dangers of nitrous fumes. Public Health Bull 1941;272:1–34.

313. Clancy PJ, Watson SL, Reardon JR. Nitrogen tetroxide exposure in the missile industry. J Occup Med 1962;4:691–7.

314. Darke CS, Warrack AJN. Bronchiolitis from nitrous fumes. Thorax 1958;13:327–33.

315. Schell NW. Chronic silo-filler's disease. Conn State Med J 1958;22:546–52.

316. Hayhurst ER, Scott E. Four cases of sudden death in a silo. JAMA 1914;63:1570–2.

317. Grayson RR. Silage gas poisoning: nitrogen dioxide pneumonia, a new disease in agricultural workers. Ann Intern Med 1956;45:393–408.

318. Cornelius EA, Betlach EH. Silo-filler's disease. Radiology 1960;74:232–8.

319. Kennedy MCS. Nitrous fumes and coal miners with emphysema. Ann Occup Hyg 1972;15:285–300.

320. Muller B. Nitrogen dioxide intoxication after a mining accident. Respiration 1969;26:249–61.

321. Kroenenberger FL. Bronchiolitis after shot-firing in a colliery. Br J Dis Chest 1959;53:308–13.

322. Nichols BH. Clinical effects of inhalation of nitrogen dioxide. Am J Roentgenol Radiat Ther 1930;23:516–20.

323. Haagen-Smit AJ, Brunelle MF, Hava J. Nitrogen oxide content of smoke from different types of tobacco. Arch Ind Health 1959;20:399–400.

324. Space medicine. Noxious descent. Med World News 1975;16:6.

325. Galea M. Fatal sulfur dioxide inhalation. Can Med Assoc J 1964;91:345–7.

326. Lepine C, Soucy R. La bronchopneumopathic d'origini toxique. Un ed Can 1962;91:7–11.

327. Prugger F. Ein fall von subletaler, akuter schwefeldioxydvergiftung und deren folgeerscheinungen auf die lungenfunktion. Pneumonologie 1974;156:97–8.

328. Charan NB, Myers CG, Lakshminarayan S, Spencer TM. Pulmonary injuries associated with acute sulfur dioxide inhalation. Am Rev Respir Dis 1979;119:555–60.

329. Arora NS, Aldrich TK. Bronchiolitis obliterans from a burning automobile. South Med J 1980;73:507–10.

330. Editorial. The hazard of toxic gases from combustion roentgenry films. JAMA 1929;92:1764.

331. Newhall HH, Brahim SA. Chronic obstructive airway disease in patients with Sjögren's syndrome. Am Rev Respir Dis 1977;115:295–304.

332. Murphy DMF, Fiarman RP, Lapp NL, Morgan KC. Severe airway disease due to inhalation of fumes from cleansing agents. Chest 1976;69:372–6.

333. Chester EH, Gillespie DG, Krause FD. The prevalence of chronic obstructive pulmonary disease in chlorine gas workers. Am Rev Respir Dis 1969;99:365–73.

334. Tanen DA, Graeme KA, Raschke R. Severe lung injury after exposure to chloramine gas from household cleaners. N Engl J Med 1999;341:848–9.

335. Molnars JJ, Nathenson G, Edberg S. Fatal aspiration of talcum powder by child: report of case. New Engl J Med 1962; 266:36–7.

336. Heiman H, Aschner PW. Aspiration of stearate of zinc in infancy, a clinical and experimental study. Am J Dis Child 1922;23:503–10.

337. Anderson WR, Strickland MB. Pulmonary complications of oxygen therapy in the neonate. Postmortem study of bronchopulmonary dysplasia with emphasis on fibroproliferative obliterative bronchitis and bronchiolitis. Arch Pathol 1971;91:506–14.

338. Elliott CG, Colby TV, Kelly TM, Hicks HG. Charcoal lung. Bronchiolitis obliterans after aspiration of activated charcoal. Chest 1989;96:672–4.

339. Reijula K, Paakko P, Kerttula R, et al. Bronchiolitis in a patient with talcosis. Br J Ind Med 1991;48:140–2.

340. Mukae H, Kadota J, Kohno S, et al. Increase of activated T-cells in BAL fluid of Japanese patients with bronchiolitis obliterans organizing pneumonia and chronic eosinophilic pneumonia. Chest 1995;108:123–8.

341. Konichezky S, Schattner A, Ezri T, et al. Thionyl-chloride-induced lung injury and bronchiolitis obliterans. Chest 1993;104:971–3.

342. Stuart-Harris CH. Acute respiratory diseases. J Clin Pathol 1968;Suppl 2:1–5.

343. O'Reilly JF. Adult bronchilitis and parainfluenza type 2. Postgrad Med J 1980;56:787–8.

344. Chan ED, Welsh CH. Fulminant *Mycoplasma pneumoniae* pneumonia [clinical conference]. West J Med 1995;162:133–42.

345. Pianzola LE, Drut R. Giant cell bronchialveolitis (measles?). Report of 8 cases in adults. Rev Clin Esp 1972;124:151–62.

346. Nikki P, Meretoja O, Valtonen V, et al. Severe bronchiolitis probably caused by varicella zoster virus. Crit Care Med 1982;10:344–6.

347. Laraya-Cuasay LR, DeForest A, et al. Chronic pulmonary complications of early influenza virus infection in children. Am Rev Respir Dis 1977;116:617–25.

348. Stuart-Harris CH. Influenza and its complications. Br Med J 1966;5480:149–50.

349. Díaz F, Collazos J, Martinez E, Mayo J. Bronchiolitis obliterans in a patient with HIV infection. Respir Med 1997;91:171–3.

350. Case records of the Massachusetts General Hospital. Weekly clinicopathological exercises. Case 37–1981. N Engl J Med 1981;305:627–35.

351. Coultas DB, Samet JM, Butler C. Bronchiolitis obliterans due to *Mycoplasma pneumonia*. West J Med 1986;144:471–4.

352. Sato P, Madtes DK, Thorning D, Albert RK. Bronchiolitis obliterans caused by *Legionella pneumophila*. Chest 1985;87:840–2.

353. Goldstein JD, Godleski JJ, Balikian JP, Herman PG. Pathologic patterns of *Serratia marcescens* pneumonia. Hum Pathol 1982;13:479–84.

354. Sieber SC, Cole SR, McNab JM, Shore E. Bronchiolitis associated with the finding of the fungus *Aspergillus*. Report of two cases. Conn Med 1994;58:13–7.

355. Paakko P, Sutinen S, Anttila S, et al. Bronchial alveolitis with pulmonary basal lamina injury in a rheumatoid patient during gold treatment. Pathol Res Pract 1988;183:46–53.

356. Schwartzman KJ, Bowie DM, Yeadon C, et al. Constrictive bronchiolitis obliterans following gold therapy for psoriatic arthritis. Eur Respir J 1995;8:2191–3.

357. Conte SC, Pagan V, Murer B. Bronchiolitis obliterans organizing pneumonia secondary to amiodarone: clinical, radiological and histological pattern. Monaldi Arch Chest Dis 1997;52:24–6.

358. Jessurun GA, Hoogenberg K, Crijns HJ. Bronchiolitis obliterans organizing pneumonia during low-dose amiodarone therapy. Clin Cardiol 1997;20:300–2.

359. Oren S, Turkot S, Golzman B, et al. Amiodarone-induced bronchiolitis obliterans organizing pneumonia (BOOP). Respir Med 1996;90:167–9.

360. Tazelaar HD, Viggiano RW, Pickersgill J, Colby TV. Interstitial lung disease in polymyositis and dermatomyositis. Clinical features and prognosis as correlated with histologic findings. Am Rev Respir Dis 1990;141:727–33.

361. Patel RC, Dutta D, Schonfeld SA. Free-base cocaine use associated with bronchiolitis organizing pneumonia. Ann Intern Med 1987;107:186–7.

362. Dreis DF, Winterbauer RH, Van Norman GA, et al. Cephalosporin-induced interstitial pneumonitis. Chest 1984;86:138–40.

363. Williams T, Eidus L, Thomas P. Fibrosing alveolitis, bronchiolitis obliterans and sulfasalazine therapy. Chest 1982;81:766–8.

364. Takimoto CH, Lynch D, Stulbarg MS. Pulmonary infiltrates associated with sulindac therapy. Chest 1990;97:230–2.

365. Ogata K, Koga T, Yagawa K. Interferon-related bronchiolitis obliterans organizing pneumonia. Chest 1994;106:612–3.

366. Piperno D, Donne C, Loire R, Cordier JF. Bronchiolitis obliterans organizing pneumonia associated with minocycline therapy: a possible cause. Eur Respir J 1995;8:1018–20.

27 LYMPHOPLASMOCYTIC INFILTRATIONS OF THE LUNG

GREGORY P. COSGROVE
MICHAEL B. FESSLER
MARVIN I. SCHWARZ

Lymphocytic interstitial pneumonitis (LIP) was first described by Carrington and Liebow in 1966.[1] It is distinguishable from the desquamative and usual interstitial pneumonias (UIPs) by the presence of monotonous sheets of lymphocytes that expand the interstitium and compress the alveolar spaces (Figure 27–1).[2] Although it was originally described as an exclusively interstitial infiltrate, this is not the case because it is also characterized by alveolar space collections. The infiltration can either be diffuse or more localized in nature. Lymphoid aggregates with or without germinal centers are distributed along lymphatic routes but can be angiocentric as well (Figures 27–2 and 27–3).[3,4] The lymphocytes in LIP are polyclonal; reports of monoclonal lymphocyte populations in cases diagnosed as LIP highlight that LIP and low-grade pulmonary lymphoma are very likely pathogenetically related and that it can be difficult to discriminate histopathologically between them.[5–7] Immunocytochemical techniques reveal that the polyclonal lymphocytes in LIP are either B cells, particularly those in the lymphoid nodules, or T cells, which are primarily located in the lung interstitium.[2,8,9] In human immuno-

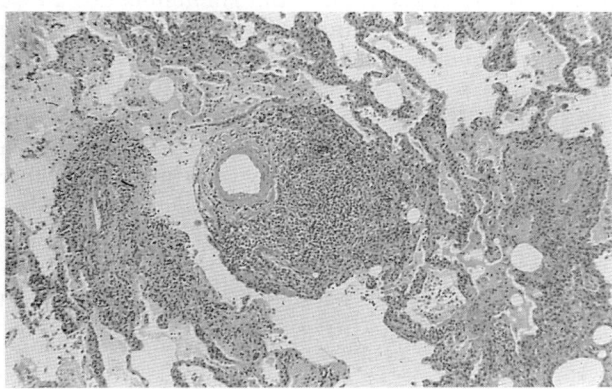

Figure 27–2 Lymphocytic interstitial pneumonitis (idiopathic variety). Lymphocyte infiltration of alveolar walls (interstitium). An angioconcentric collection of lymphocytes adjacent to a small muscular pulmonary artery. The wall of the vessel is intact.

deficiency virus (HIV)-associated LIP, T cells with an increased CD4 to CD8 ratio are found in the bronchoalveolar lavage (BAL) fluid.[10] Smaller numbers of

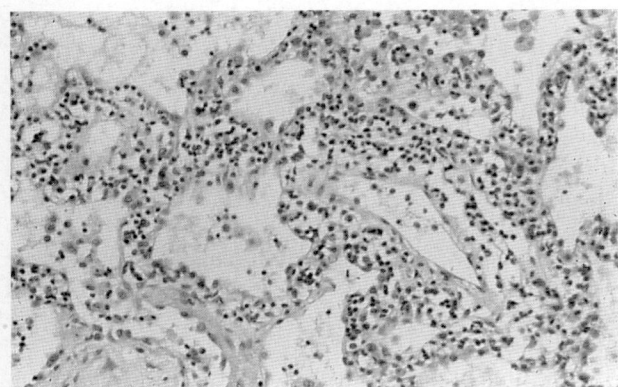

Figure 27–1 Lymphocytic interstitial pneumonitis (Sjögren's syndrome). Broadening of the alveolar interstitium by an infiltrate that consists primarily of mature lymphocytes.

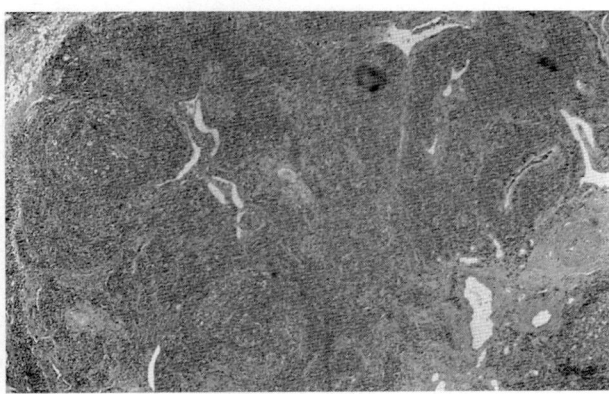

Figure 27–3 Lymphocytic interstitial pneumonitis (idiopathic variety). A dense infiltrate of lymphocytes involving the interstitium in a bronchiolocentric location, forming germinal centers.

plasma cells, immunoblasts, and macrophages are also found in the interstitial lymphocytic infiltrates. Other essential histopathologic features that characterize LIP include (1) type II cell hyperplasia; (2) the accumulation of large interstitial reticuloendothelial cells, mononuclear cells, and giant cells forming noncaseating granulomas (Figure 27–4); (3) perivascular and paraseptal amyloid deposition; and (4) well-formed lymphoid germinal centers.[1,9–14]

LIP has been described as a hyperplastic disorder of the bronchus-associated lymphoid tissue, lying on a spectrum that extends from follicular bronchiolitis to pseudolymphoma to LIP.[5] LIP must be differentiated from other lymphocytic infiltrations of the lung, such as primary lymphomas and lymphomatoid granulomatosis (LG), because it is potentially malignant, and benign lymphocytic angiitis and granulomatosis are an uncommon form of pulmonary vasculitis.[10,15–25] The so-called pseudolymphoma is another lymphocytic lung infiltration with histologic characteristics similar to those of LIP, but it is localized and often presents as a single mass or several masses on the chest radiograph rather than as a diffuse interstitial infiltrate. Most authors agree that pulmonary pseudolymphoma represents a localized form of LIP.[10] Pseudolymphoma is not only associated with the same predisposing conditions as diffuse LIP, but it also has the potential to convert to a lymphoma.[17,23,24]

ETIOLOGY

It is difficult to determine the incidence of LIP, but it appears to be an uncommon cause of interstitial lung disease (ILD). In one series from the Mayo Clinic, only 13 cases were found in a 10-year period.[26] Although it occurs infrequently, LIP is associated with other disease states, many of which are associated with some form of dysproteinemia or with putative autoimmunity, as shown in Table 27–1. The literature confirms that 50 to 77% of patients with LIP, including those with the idiopathic variety, have some associated serum protein abnormality.[2,24] The dysproteinemia is most often polyclonal, but monoclonal gammopathies (IgG or IgM) also occur.[11,26–29] Paradoxically, LIP also occurs with hypogammaglobulinemia in both adults and children.[2,30]

Sjögren's syndrome, either the primary or secondary forms (ie, those associated with a collagen vascular disease, most often rheumatoid arthritis) accounts for at least 25% of the cases of reported LIP.[8,10,11,13,15,27] It is likely that the idiopathic variety, with or without an associated dysproteinemia, and the acquired immunodeficiency syndrome (AIDS) in both children and adults account for the majority of LIP.[10,31–35] Other pulmonary manifestations of Sjögren's syndrome include tracheobronchiolitis, bronchiectasis, lymphocytic bronchitis, and other forms of ILD, such as usual interstitial pneumonitis.[36,37] Furthermore, several cases of common variable hypogammaglobulinemia have been complicated by Sjögren's syndrome and LIP.[11] Hypogammaglobulinemia-associated LIP has a high incidence of conversion to a lymphoreticular malignancy.[38] Both pernicious anemia and agammaglobulinemia were reported in an unusual case of LIP.[39] Other diseases associated with a dysproteinemia and LIP and believed to be autoimmune in origin include chronic active hepatitis, myasthenia gravis, autoimmune thyroid disease, anemia, hemolytic anemia, multiple sclerosis, juvenile rheumatoid arthritis, and systemic lupus erythematosus without Sjögren's syndrome.[11,24,40–47] Retroviruses (HIV-I, human T-cell leukemia virus type I [HTLV-I]) and infections with the Epstein-Barr virus (EBV) have been identified in some patients with LIP.[10,35,48–51]

CLINICAL PRESENTATION

When dysproteinemia is present, it may precede, occur simultaneously with, or follow the onset of the pulmonary disease (LIP). Although patients with Sjögren's syndrome often have the classic triad of keratoconjunctivitis sicca, xerostomia, and a collagen vascular disease such as rheumatoid arthritis, the lung disease can precede the more typical manifestations.[19] Approximately 10% of patients with either the primary or secondary collagen vascular disease types of Sjögren's syndrome have pulmonary complications that result from bronchitis, bronchiectasis, and pneumonia due to drying and inspissation of secretions. Less frequently, bronchiolitis obliterans, diffuse interstitial fibrosis, pulmonary vasculitis, lymphoma, pseudolymphoma, and lymphocytic interstitial pneumonia occur.[10,21,22,38,52–54] In one series of 343 patients with Sjögren's syndrome, 16 had diffuse lung disease, and in only 3 was LIP the cause.[13,16] Because many of these patients did not undergo pulmonary function testing and because pathologic material was available in only a few instances, this study probably underestimated the incidence of this complication.

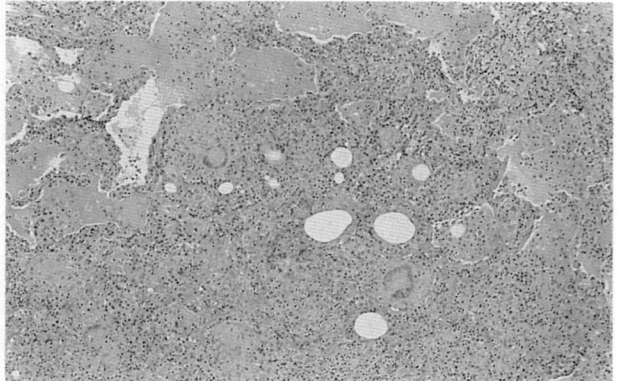

Figure 27–4   Lymphocytic interstitial pneumonitis (AIDS). Diffuse lymphocytic infiltrates with granuloma formation. Note the giant cells.

TABLE 27–1   Lymphocytic Interstitial Pneumonitis Disease Associations

Idiopathic without dysproteinemia[2,8]

With dysproteinemia
   Hypogammaglobulinemia[11]
      Adults[26]
      Children[30]
   Monoclonal gammopathy[11,16,48,162]
   Polyclonal gammopathy[11,28,29,40]
   Sjögren's syndrome[9,162]
      Connective tissue disease associated[26]
      Primary[21,26]
   Chronic active hepatitis[9,40,41]
   Primary biliary cirrhosis[9,163]
   Myasthenia gravis[40]
   Autoimmune thyroiditis[11,24,42]
   Pernicious anemia[39]
   Autoimmune hemolytic anemia[43]
   Pulmonary immune complexes[73,84]
   Systemic lupus erythematosus[46,47]
   Multiple sclerosis[44]
   Multicentric Castleman's disease[164]
   Benign hypergammaglobulinemic purpura of Waldenström[44]
   Juvenile rheumatoid arthritis[45]

Allogeneic bone marrow transplantation (graft-vs-host disease)[87,165]

Viral infections
   Acquired immunodeficiency syndrome
      Children[31,55]
      Adults[10,33-35]
   Epstein-Barr virus[51]
   Human T-cell lymphotrophic virus type 1 (HTLV-1)[48]

Miscellaneous
   Tuberculosis[166]
   Celiac sprue[74]
   Dilantin[167]
   Post-Legionnaires' pneumonia[168]
   Surfactant protein C deficiency[169]

Familial forms[58,59,169]

LIP occurs more commonly in women and appears between the fourth and seventh decades in the majority of adult cases; the mean age at onset is 56 years.[9,11,16,26] LIP also occurs in children, particularly those with hypogammaglobulinemia or AIDS.[12,55-57] A familial form of LIP has also been reported in children.[58,59] The most common presenting symptoms are dyspnea and cough, which are progressive if untreated.[11,15,24] In many cases, these symptoms are present for months or years before diagnosis. Other associated symptoms include weight loss, pleuritic pain, arthralgias, and fever. A woman with AIDS-associated LIP presented with recurrent pneumothoraces.[60] Clubbing and bibasilar rales are the most frequent physical findings and are usually the only findings in the idiopathic variety. Finger clubbing, initially reported to occur in 50% of cases, is a far less frequent finding.[11,26] Other physical findings may include associated conditions such as hepatosplenomegaly, lymphadenopathy, and parotid gland enlargement, symmetrical arthritis in rheumatoid arthritis, generalized lymphadenopathy due to lymphoma, as well as keratoconjuctivitis sicca in Sjögren's syndrome.

Historically, these patients experience repeated episodes of pneumonia secondary to either hypo- or agammaglobulinemia or complications associated with inspissation of respiratory secretions in Sjögren's syndrome.[11,26]

Bibasilar reticulonodular infiltrates are characteristically seen in LIP (Figure 27–5). The chest radiograph and computed tomographic lung scan in LIP are nonspecific; in pseudolymphoma there may be single or multiple well-circumscribed masses, which often coalesce and characteristically have air bronchograms that must be differentiated from a pulmonary lymphoma or an alveolar cell carcinoma.[61] A mixed alveolar-interstitial pattern appears when infiltrates coalesce as a result of underlying dense lymphocytic infiltration of the lung parenchyma and cause compression of alveoli (Figures 27–6 and 27–7). A case of lymphocytic bronchiolitis associated with AIDS demonstrated a micronodular pattern on the chest radiograph.[62] Radiographic honeycomb lung appears, along with signs of pulmonary hypertension, in chronic, progressive disease.[14,26,62] Although pleural effusions can occur, they are infrequent except in AIDS-related LIP.[61] In fact, the presence of pleural effusion, large nodules, and consolidation, with or without hilar and mediastinal adenopathy, are suggestive of a primary pulmonary lymphoma (Figure 27–8), wheareas cysts are suggestive of LIP.[2,11,15,63,64] A computed tomography (CT) series that followed 14 LIP patients over a median of 13 months reported predominant findings of ground-glass attenuation, thickening of interlobular septae, centrilobular nodules, cystic air spaces, and consolidation; all parenchymal abnormalities were reported to be reversible, with the exception of the cysts, and interval development of new cysts was noted mainly in areas of previous centrilobular nodularity.[65] Other features reported on CT scans include lymph node enlargment in 68% of patients, subpleural small nodules in 86%, and thickening of bronchovascular bundles in 86%.[66]

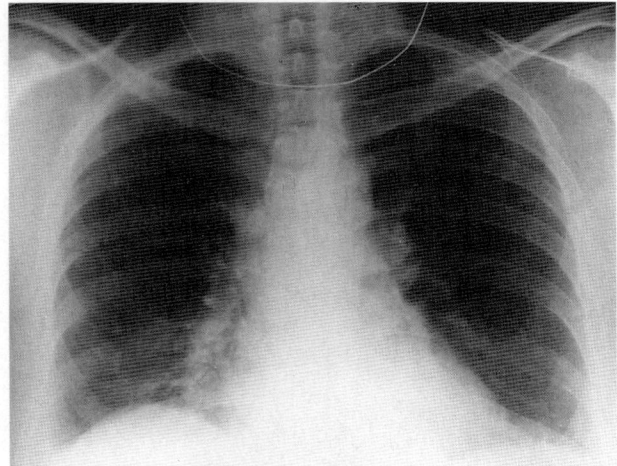

Figure 27–5   Lymphocytic interstitial pneumonitis. Chest radiograph demonstrating lower-zone diffuse reticular infiltrates.

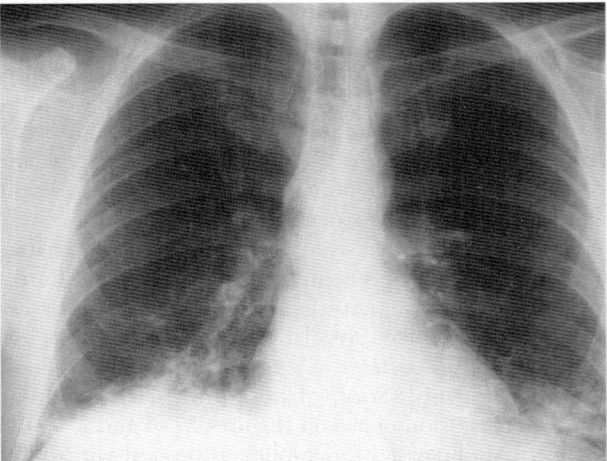

Figure 27–6   Lymphocytic interstitial pneumonitis. Chest radiograph demonstrating patchy lower-zone alveolar infiltrates.

The physiological disturbances are very similar to those seen in the other ILDs and include reduction of lung volumes, preservation of air flow parameters, a reduction of the diffusing capacity of the lung for carbon monoxide (DL_{CO}), and hypoxemia.[11,13,16,26,29] Compared with idiopathic pulmonary fibrosis, in LIP, the forced expiratory volume in 1 second (FEV_1) is lower, and respiratory volume and the DL_{CO}/VA ratio is higher.[67]

The few BAL fluid studies conducted in LIP patients show striking increases in both numbers and

percentages of lymphocytes.[28,68,69] Church and colleagues, in characterizing the lymphocyte subsets in the lung parenchyma of children with hypogammaglobulinemia, found a predominance of CD4[+] cells.[30] The CD8[+] cells predominate in adults with AIDS-associated LIP.[10] In a case in which CD8[+] cells were measured, the gallium scan was positive, and the serum angiotensin-converting enzyme was elevated.[70] Importantly, the use of Southern blotting or polymerase chain reaction (PCR) to detect the monoclonality of immunoglobulin gene rearrangement of BAL fluid lymphocytes may sometimes indicate a diagnosis of pulmonary lymphoma.[71,72] Other abnormal laboratory findings reflect the underlying disease state (ie, antinuclear antibody and rheumatoid factors in Sjögren's syndrome associated with a collagen vascular disease, low immunoglobulin levels in acquired hypogammaglobulinemia, and a poly- or monoclonal gammopathy that can occur with or without Sjögren's syndrome). Note, however, that LIP is often idiopathic and not always associated with a serum protein abnormality. When this occurs, it presents as an ILD of unknown etiology. Open lung biopsy is required for diagnosis in almost all cases.

PROGNOSIS AND TREATMENT

Although it is difficult to predict the outcome in LIP, there are four distinct possibilities: (1) resolution following corticosteroid therapy, alone or in combination with other immunosuppressive drugs; (2) progression to pulmonary fibrosis, cor pulmonale, and death; (3) a superimposed pulmonary or systemic infection leading to death; or (4) the development of a complicating lymphoma.[2,8,11,14,26,30,73] The median survival rate for patients with LIP has been reported as 11.51 years.[67] The data regarding response to corticosteroid therapy are uncontrolled and often unaccompanied by objective physiological testing, and the dosage schedules differ among reports. Although some patients experience excellent therapeutic outcomes, there are no clinical, laboratory, or histologic parameters to help predict the outcome in individual cases. Five of the patients studied by Liebow and Carrington demonstrated complete resolution following corticosteroid therapy, and several others stabilized during treatment.[11] In the series by Strimlan and colleagues, 6 of 13 subjects were considered improved following treatment with oral corticosteroids.[26] Of these six patients, four were treated with corticosteroids alone and two also received chlorambucil. The follow-up period ranged from 1 to 14 years. Two patients were considered stable at 32 and 42 months, respectively, and the five who died did so within 2 years of their diagnosis. Other authors have documented corticosteroid responsiveness in individual cases.[16,17,39,46,74] Cyclophosphamide has not been rigorously evaluated as a therapy for LIP. A series of primary Sjögren's syndrome patients with assorted pulmonary

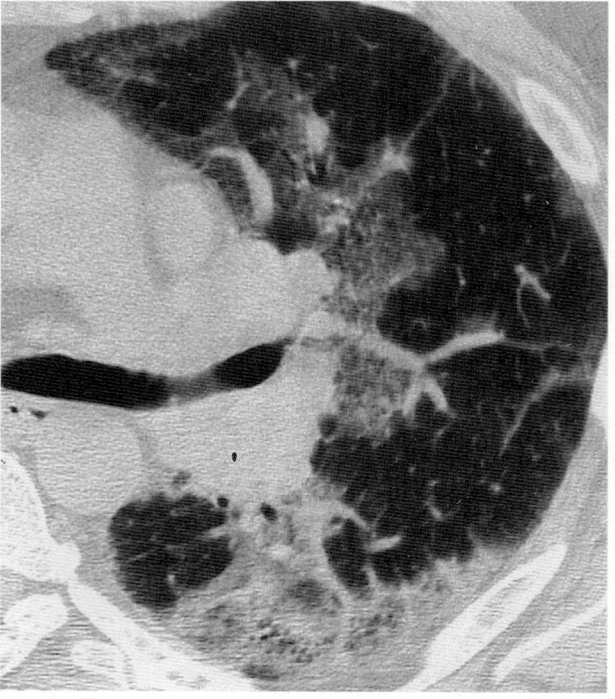

Figure 27–7   Lymphocytic interstitial pneumonitis. High resolution CT scan indicating patchy air space filling.

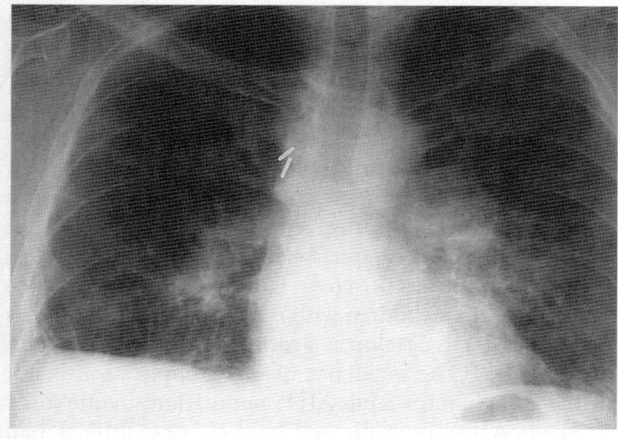

A

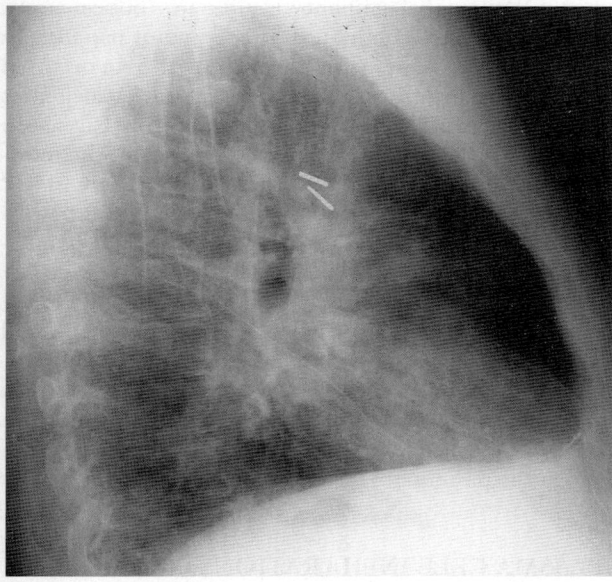

B

Figure 27–8 *A* and *B,* Lymphocytic interstitial pneumonitis conversion to B-cell lymphoma. Note the bilateral hilar adenopathy and right-sided pleural disease as well as the pulmonary infiltration. Diagnosis was established by right paramediastinal lymph node biopsy.

pathology, including 5 patients with LIP, reported symptomatic and physiological improvement in 7 of 11 patients treated with azathioprine; however, histopathologic diagnosis was not reported for these improved patients.[36] Cyclosporin A was reported to be effective in a case of common variable immunodeficiency-associated LIP.[75] In HIV-associated LIP, reports of the effect of zidovudine therapy have been variable, with one report describing improvement in two patients and another reporting no change in a single patient.[76,77] Bacterial superinfection is a common cause of death in patients with dysproteinemias, especially those with hypogammaglobulinemia.[11,26,30] In other reported cases, LIP progressed to fibrosis and end-stage honeycomb lung despite therapeutic intervention.[11,26]

Although three large series[2,11,26] do not support the evolution of LIP into a pulmonary and/or systemic lymphoma, many individual reports document this progression.[2,10,11,15,18,20,23,26,78–80] A single case report describes progression of LIP to lymphomatoid granulomatosis (LG) in a patient with suspected Sjögren's syndrome.[81] Lymphomas complicating either LIP or the related pulmonary pseudolymphoma are often difficult to diagnose by routine methods because they are well differentiated, may appear years after the LIP has been diagnosed, and are associated with slow growth and prolonged survival.[16,74] In fact, 20 to 69% of primary pulmonary lymphomas have germinal centers, and up to 50% have noncaseating granulomas, both of which are characteristic histopathologic features of LIP.[5] LIP is readily differentiated from LG, which is now considered to be an angiocentric lymphoma, by the absence of angiocentricity and vascular necrosis in the former. Sjögren's syndrome is associated with primary lymphomas of the parotid gland that arise from a specific clone of cells, the IgM-κ type.[82] A monoclonal B-cell lymphoma of the lung has also been found in a patient with pre-existing LIP associated with Sjögren's syndrome and in a patient with LIP without an associated dysproteinemia.[10,25] The standard criteria for determining the malignant transformation of LIP are listed in Table 27–2; Turner and colleagues, however, have put forth more specific cytologic criteria.[20] They propose that lymphocytic pulmonary infiltrations that follow a lymphangitic rather than an interstitial distribution are more likely to be malignant. The monocellular lymphocytic infiltrates are distributed along bronchovascular bundles and pulmonary veins, in contrast to the alveolar walls as is seen in LIP. The second criterion proposed by these authors is that the small lymphocytic infiltrate is monoclonal as opposed to polyclonal. Evidence suggests that there is little difference in survival between patients with LIP and well-differentiated pulmonary lymphoma, even when all the criteria are used in distinguishing a benign from a malignant infiltration. Of interest, Kurosu and colleagues used a two-step PCR and sequencing analysis of the immunoglobulin heavy-chain gene to demonstrate

TABLE 27–2   Criteria for Differentiation of Malignant Infiltrates from LIP or Pseudolymphoma

1. Involvement of hilar and mediastinal lymph nodes
2. Invasion of bronchial mucosa and erosion of bronchial cartilage
3. Seeding of the parietal pleura
4. Absence of lymphoid germinal centers
5. Extrapulmonary involvement
6. Mitotic figures
7. Monotypic lymphocytes
8. Absence of corticosteroid response?

See references.[8,18,19]

that a subset of patients diagnosed with LIP have minor monoclonal lymphocyte nests hidden on a polyclonal background. In one patient diagnosed with primary pulmonary lymphoma, the same clone was detected in a lung biopsy specimen diagnosed as LIP years previously.[7,8] In another study, the same methodology demonstrated two or three oligoclonal populations in each of five HIV-associated LIP biopsy specimens, suggesting the coexistence of several occult clonal B-cell populations in HIV-related LIP.[6] Such studies indicate a pathogenetic connection between LIP and low-grade pulmonary lymphoma and suggest that a subset of diagnosed LIP may actually represent early stage low-grade lymphoma.

PATHOGENESIS

An autoimmune pathogenesis of LIP is supported by its association with primary or secondary Sjögren's syndrome, pernicious anemia, autoimmune hemolytic anemia, myasthenia gravis, primary biliary cirrhosis, and chronic active hepatitis.[9–13,31,39,40] Similar lymphocytic infiltrates in the parotid gland in Sjögren's syndrome, the gastric mucosa in pernicious anemia, and the thyroid in Hashimoto's thyroiditis further support this notion.[11,24,39] Abnormal lymphocyte trafficking in LIP may be due to high expression levels of vascular cell adhesion molecule-1 in venular endothelium.[83] In addition, pulmonary immune complexes have been found in two cases.[73,74,78–80,82,84] In one, the presence of pulmonary immune complexes was also associated with the autoerythrocyte sensitization syndrome.[40] In the other, a patient with LIP without an associated dysproteinemia or autoimmune disease had increased levels of circulating immune complexes in addition to pulmonary immune complexes.[84] This latter patient responded dramatically to corticosteroid therapy. Although the autoimmune theory is an attractive one, particularly in lieu of the B-cell monoclonal lymphomas that may develop, immune complexes have not been found routinely in other cases.[16]

Virus-like particles within the bronchial epithelium have been documented in a single patient with Sjögren's syndrome and LIP.[85] This patient had increased levels of serum IgM, and electron microscope studies revealed electron-dense material, thought to be immunoglobulin, within plasma cells adjacent to the bronchial epithelium. Recently, a retrovirus-type particle that is similar to the AIDS virus was found in salivary tissue homogenates from patients with Sjögren's syndrome.[86] LIP also develops as a result of the chronic graft-versus-host reaction, a late complication of allogeneic bone marrow transplantation occurring between 200 and 400 days after transplantation.[87,88] In both reported cases, there was also evidence of Sjögren's syndrome, a clinical feature commonly seen in chronic graft-versus-host disease. Although mono- or polyclonal gammopathies are found in the majority of patients with LIP, further supporting the autoimmune theory of pathogenesis, this does not explain the occurrence of LIP in subjects with hypo- or agammaglobulinemia.[3,26,30]

AIDS offers the most recent association between LIP and a disease state that features hypergammaglobulinemia, autoimmune manifestations, and, most prominently, a depressed cellular immune system. This complication occurs in both children and adults.[10,31–35,38,55–57,68] LIP is a common disease-defining pulmonary complication of AIDS in children. Dyspnea without fever and a reticulonodular infiltrate on chest radiograph are pathognomonic for LIP in children with AIDS.[57] Bronchiectasis has been reported to develop as a consequence of LIP in pediatric AIDS.[89] The incidence of this complication is not nearly as high in the adult AIDS population. In one study of adult AIDS complicated by LIP, one subject had parotid enlargement and another had the sicca syndrome;[33] extranodal lymphocytic infiltrates (bone marrow, kidney) were also common in this group of patients. In nine adult AIDS cases with associated LIP, eight occurred in subjects with African ancestry.[33,34,38] Other associations between idiopathic LIP and viral infections have been inferred. In the southwestern region of Japan, the retrovirus HTLV-I has been linked to the development of LIP by an 84% seropositivity for HTLV-I in patients with LIP. BAL fluid cells indicate that the lymphocyte population consists primarily of $CD8^+/CD11^+$-cytotoxic cells.[48] One study indicated that 6 of 11 patients with HTLV-I uveitis, but without evidence of lung involvement, had BAL fluid lymphocytosis with a decreased $CD4^+$ to $CD8^+$ ratio.[90] EBV, a herpes virus, was found by in situ hybridization in the lymphocytes of 9 of 14 subjects with LIP of various etiologies and in only 2 of 10 subjects with idiopathic pulmonary fibrosis.[51]

PLASMA CELL INFILTRATIONS OF THE LUNG

Plasma cell interstitial pneumonia (PIP), a variant of LIP, was first described by Moran and Toten.[28] The histologic appearance of PIP resembles that of LIP, but plasma cells predominate as the cell type infiltrating the alveolar interstitium; lymphocytes and giant cells are interspersed among the plasma cell infiltrates. Unlike LIP, however, progression to fibrosis and/or lymphoma has not been documented.[91] Only a few cases have been reported in the literature, and the clinical-physiological-radiologic presentation is similar to that of LIP.[23,29,92] Two of these patients had a polyclonal gammopathy.[28] One had a remarkable response to corticosteroids, and the other died of a superimposed infection. In another unique case, there was an IgM monoclonal spike and a hyperviscosity syndrome in addition to PIP. In this case, the bone marrow examination did not support a diagnosis of multiple myeloma or Waldenström's macroglobulinemia, and the patient's radiographic and physiological abnormalities improved markedly after a course of corticosteroids on one occasion and after a combination of corticosteroids and cyclophosphamide on another.

PIP must be distinguished from plasma cell granuloma, which appears as an isolated mass or masses in the lung. The prognosis for patients with plasma cell granuloma, a benign lesion, is excellent following resection. Plasma cell granuloma is not associated with dysproteinemia or a systemic disease, and it usually occurs in children and young adults.[92] Plasma cell granulomas are most often discovered after routine chest radiography and are resected because the nature of the lesion is undefined. Histologically, plasma cell granuloma resembles PIP but, like pseudolymphoma, it is not a diffuse disease. Plasma cell granulomas must be differentiated from plasmacytomas, which are malignant monoclonal plasma cell proliferations that occur in patients with systemic multiple myeloma.[93,94] The majority of the extramedullary plasmacytomas that complicate multiple myeloma occur in the respiratory tract, the skin, the gastrointestinal tract, and the lymphatic system.[95] Thoracic involvement for the most part refers to extramedullary rib destruction or an infectious pneumonia.[96,97] A malignant plasmacytoma, which presents as an isolated lung parenchymal mass, is unusual. When present, however, it is often accompanied by pleural effusions and mediastinal lymphadenopathy.[98–101] The other form of pulmonary involvement in myeloma is a diffuse pulmonary infiltration that is usually found during the terminal phases of multiple myeloma and plasma cell leukemia.[102] In one case, alveolar–septal amyloidosis was also present, in addition to the myelomatous diffuse lung infiltration.[103] A form of primary amyloidosis also occurs with multiple myeloma and appears to be caused by interstitial paraprotein deposition.[103] In diffuse plasma cell infiltration of the lung parenchyma in multiple myeloma, plasma cells predominate in the BAL fluid.[94] These patients also have a myeloma-type protein in the serum or pleural fluid.[99,100]

Primary pulmonary plasmacytomas, plasmacytomas occurring in the absence of radiographic or hematologic evidence of multiple myeloma, are extremely rare, with only 22 cases reported in the literature.[104–106] Pulmonary nodular lesions have been reported in most cases.[104] A recent report, however, also documented diffuse pulmonary infiltrates as the initial presentation of primary pulmonary plasmacytoma.[105] There is some doubt as to whether or not these lesions are truly primary. Identical aneuploidy has been demonstrated in plasma cells from primary pulmonary plasmacytomas and histologically normal bone marrow, suggesting that systemic involvement is present but below the level of detection when standard criteria for multiple myeloma are used.[106]

Waldenström's macroglobulinemia, a disease characterized by a monoclonal IgM spike in the serum, anemia, and bone marrow infiltration with lymphoplasmacytic cells, is frequently complicated by a diffuse pulmonary disease resulting from plasmacytoid lymphocytic infiltration of the alveolar walls and pleura.[107–109] The infiltrating cell can be differentiated histologically from the mature plasma cell found in PIP; note that there is no bone marrow involvement in PIP. Pulmonary parenchymal involvement occurs in 69% of patients with Waldenström's macroglobulinemia; in 66%, thoracic involvement is the initial manifestation of the disease.[108] However, the pulmonary component may also appear many years after the diagnosis has been made.[110] Mediastinal adenopathy has been reported in 25% of cases; pleural effusion occurs in approximately half of all patients.[107,109] BAL fluid examination in one patient revealed 10% plasma cells, lymphocytes, and a monoclonal protein spike.[111] The pleural effusions not only contain the specific cell type, but also demonstrate a monoclonal IgM spike as seen in the serum.[112] The chest radiograph may show diffuse reticulonodular infiltrates, masslike homogenous lesions, pleural effusions, and hilar lymphadenopathy.[113] As in PIP, the usual onset is in the fifth or sixth decade. Chlorambucil in combination with corticosteroids is the preferred therapy.[114] Recently, nucleoside analogs such as 2-chlorodeoxyadenosine and fludaribine, which may accelerate apoptosis, have proven to be effective alternative treatments in therapeutically naïve patients.[115,116] Rituximab, a chimeric monoclonal antibody directed against CD20, is an additional therapy currently being investigated.[117]

ANGIOIMMUNOBLASTIC LYMPHADENOPATHY

Angioimmunoblastic lymphadenopathy (AILD) was first described in 1974 by Frizzera and colleagues and later by Lukes and Trindle.[118,119] These authors described a disease with features of both a lymphoma and a systemic autoimmune disorder. More recently, the disease has been reclassified and is now considered a non-Hodgkin's T-cell lymphoma.[120] The systemic manifestations of the disease are characterized by hyperreactivity of the B cell immune system resulting in a polyclonal gammopathy, and clinical and laboratory features that suggest a collagen vascular disease. The morphologic changes in the lymph nodes typify this disease (Figure 27–9). Examination of lymphatic tissue reveals disruption of lymph node architecture by infiltrating plasma cells, lymphocytes, and immunoblasts. Multinucleated giant cells must be distinguished from the Reed-Sternberg cells.[119,121] Other characteristic findings necessary for the diagnosis are the proliferation of finely arborizing blood vessels among the immunoblasts and amorphous collections of eosinophilic material within the intracellular spaces. The pulmonary parenchymal histopathologic findings, on the other hand, are not specific and consist of interstitial infiltration with immunoblasts, lymphocytes, and plasma cells. Other findings include alveolar type II cell hyperplasia with minimal alveolar wall fibrosis. Arborization and proliferation of blood vessels are not found within the lung parenchyma, but the entire spectrum of histologic features can be found in the hilar and mediastinal lymph nodes, reflecting the neoplastic nature of the disease.[119,121–123]

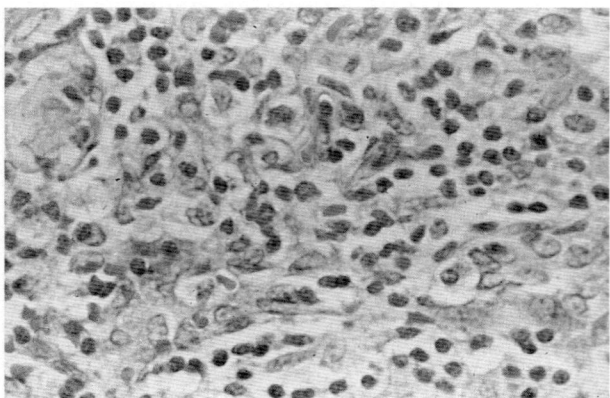

Figure 27–9 Angioblastic lymphadenopathy. Lymph node with defacement of the normal architecture by immunoblasts and proliferating blood vessels.

AILD appears in the 50- to 70-year-old age group and affects both sexes equally. Most often, these patients present with fever, chills, weight loss, generalized lymphadenopathy, hepatosplenomegaly, and occasionally a skin rash.[111,112,118,119,121,124,125] Hypergammaglobulinemia is the hallmark of this disease; a Coombs-positive hemolytic anemia, eosinophilia, cryoglobulinemia, and leukocytosis may also be present[118,119,121–126]

Pulmonary parenchymal involvement has been present in approximately 20 of the 200 reported cases of AILD, and hilar and/or mediastinal lymphadenopathy without parenchymal involvement occurs in as many as 40% of AILD cases.[118,122,123,125,127–130] The pulmonary parenchymal involvement is often accompanied by hilar and mediastinal lymphadenopathy; pleural effusions are present in 10% of these patients.[123,131,132] The radiographic appearance of the lung disease is primarily a reticulonodular infiltrate with basilar predominance. Coalescence of the nodular component can occur, producing a mixed alveolar interstitial pattern.[118,122,123] Pulmonary function testing usually reveals a mixed restrictive-obstructive pattern with evidence of involvement of the small airways. As with other diffuse lung diseases, hypoxemia with an increased alveolar–arterial oxygen gradient, a reduction in DL_{CO}, and a reduced pulmonary compliance are frequently seen.[122,123,129] Other than the subacute onset of cough and dyspnea, the clinical picture is similar to that seen in patients without pulmonary involvement. The laboratory findings are also similar, but Weisenburger and colleagues reported four patients with pulmonary involvement and AILD who had a dermatologic vasculitis and hypocomplementemia.[130]

B lymphocyte proliferation in AILD initially suggested that the disease was of B-cell origin. Although lymphocyte subtyping of lavaged lung cells or tissue is not available, one study supports enhanced B cell activity in the lung.[111] Iseman and colleagues demonstrated polyclonal immunoglobulin immunofluorescence on the surface of mononuclear cells infiltrating alveolar walls.[122]

There have also been reports of an apparent association between the development of AILD and certain pharmacologic and infectious agents. These include griseofulvin, sulfonamides, diphenylhydantoin, methyldopa, pyrimethamine, and penicillin.[119,132–136] However, more sophisticated molecular techniques have demonstrated that the underlying derangement in AILD is due to T-cell clonal disorders.[137,138] The hyperactive B-cell response seen in the disease is likely secondary and a result of the marked increase in cytokine production from T cells within lymph nodes with the elaboration of interleukins (ILs)-2, -4, -5, -6, and13 and interferon-γ.[139]

Although the occasional patient with AILD has a prolonged survival time, the majority die within 1 year after diagnosis. The most common cause of death is intercurrent infection, which includes bacterial sepsis with both gram-positive and gram-negative organisms, fungal sepsis, *Pneumocystis carinii* pneumonia, and systemic herpes simplex infection.[118,119,121,123,124,140] This is likely a function of the altered immune response seen in these patients with ineffective humoral and cell-mediated immunity. Despite aggressive treatment with combined chemotherapy used in cyclophosphamide, hydroxydaunomycin, oncovin, and prednisone (CHOP)-like regimens, a complete or sustained remission is seen in only 25% of patients.[137] Treatment with cyclosporin A induced a dramatic remission in one patient.[141] This observed response to cyclosporin A may reflect the immunologic nature of the disease and the prominent T-cell activity of cyclosporin A.

LYMPHOMATOID GRANULOMATOSIS (ANGIOCENTRIC LYMPHOMA)

LG was first described by Liebow and colleagues in 1972 as a distinct clinicopathologic entity characterized by an angiocentric lymphoproliferative process, the most prominent clinical feature being lung involvement.[142] The characteristic histologic triad was a polymorphic lymphoid infiltrate composed of small lymphocytes, plasma cells, and immunoblasts. The other distinguishing features included angiitis and granulomatosis (Figure 27–10). Although originally classified by some to be one of the granulomatous vasculitides, its clinical nature, response to therapy, and poor outcome in some patients established that this disease was a form of angiocentric lymphoma with vascular destruction and systemic manifestations. It is also termed angiocentric lymphoma and angiocentric immunoproliferative lesion as a result of its angiodestructive course.[143,144] In LG, T lymphocytes are of the T helper-CD4 variety; there is also evidence for a monoclonal B-cell proliferation in which EBV RNA and EBV-encoded nuclear proteins have been detected.[145–148] The progression of LIP and Sjögren's syndrome to LG has been documented.[149]

Men are more frequently affected than women; the usual age of onset is between 40 and 60 years. Rarely, it may also affect children.[150–152] Cough, dyspnea, and

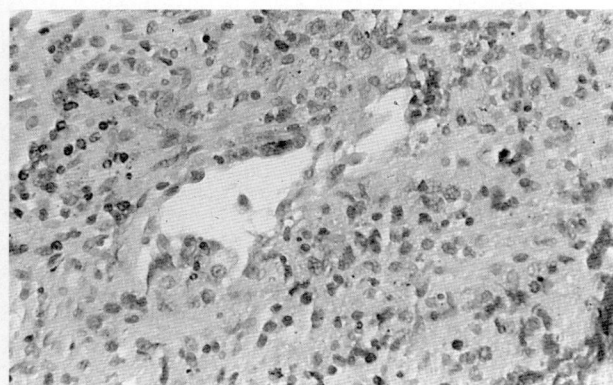

Figure 27–10 Lymphomatoid granulomatosis (angiocentric lymphoma). Destruction of a small pulmonary artery by proliferating immunoblasts.

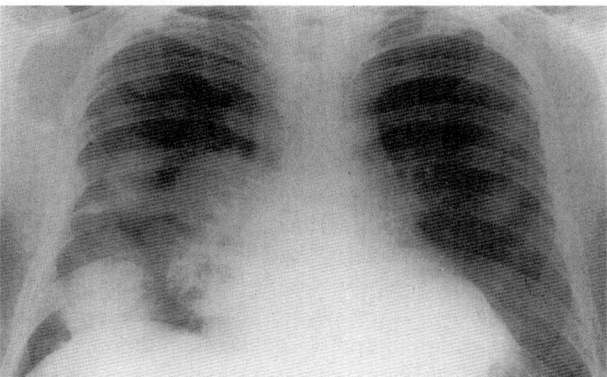

Figure 27–11 Lymphomatoid granulomatosis. Chest radiograph with multiple masslike lesions in both lungs.

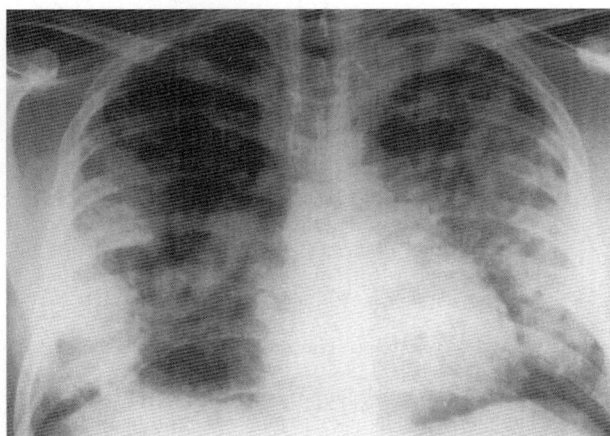

Figure 27–12 Lymphomatoid granulomatosis. Chest radiograph demonstrating dense alveolar infiltrates superimposed on diffuse reticulonodular infiltrates.

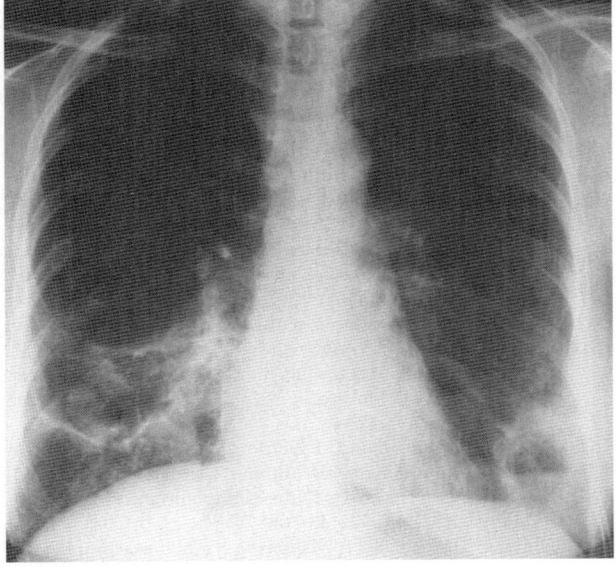

Figure 27–13 Lymphomatoid granulomatosis. Chest radiograph demonstrating bilateral lower-zone cavitary lesions.

chest pain are present in most patients as a result of prominent involvement of the lung. Systemic symptoms include weight loss, fever, and night sweats. Occasionally, skin lesions are the only presenting manifestation, but they are found in conjunction with the pulmonary disease in 20 to 40% of cases. These lesions are both dermal and subcutaneous and can be tender and accompanied by erythema. They may resemble erythema nodosum. Neurologic involvement occurs in up to 33% of cases and can result in either peripheral neuropathy, cranial nerve palsies, or direct involvement of the brain. Destructive diseases of the nasopharynx and paranasal sinuses, reminiscent of lethal midline granuloma or Wegener's granulomatosis, may also occur. Less commonly, involvement of other organ systems such as the kidneys, liver, and spleen may be found at autopsy. It is, however, unusual for patients to exhibit clinical dysfunction of these organs. The presence of clinical manifestations in organ systems other than the lungs implies advanced lymphomatous disease with a poor prognosis. Lymphadenopathy occurs rarely in LG.[153–155]

There are no characteristic laboratory abnormalities. The chest radiograph shows primarily middle- and lower-zone involvement by multiple nodules, which have a tendency to coalesce and cavitate and occasionally produce alveolar infiltrates (Figures 27–11, 27–12, and 27–13).[153] Diffuse interstitial infiltration also occurs, and unilateral disease is possible.[154] In contrast to other primary pulmonary lymphomas, hilar and mediastinal adenopathy almost never occurs. In Hodgkin's disease with lung involvement, on the other hand, radiographically apparent adenopathy is expected. Cavitation is probably due to the angiodestructive nature of this lesion, which results in pulmonary infarct.

The 5-year survival rate is 50%, and therapy consists of combinations of corticosteroid drugs and cyclophosphamide or multiagent cytotoxic therapy. Poor prognostic features include central nervous system involvement and hepatosplenomegaly. A subset of patients, particularly those without extensive systemic involvement and primarily pulmonary involvement, may enjoy prolonged survival.

Other primary lymphomas of the lung can present with diffuse pulmonary infiltration that suggests diffuse ILD. These lymphomas include angiotropic large-cell lymphoma, formerly known as malignant angioendothiomatosis, which appears as proliferating mononuclear cells in the lumens of arterioles, venules, capillaries, and small pulmonary arteries.[156] Rapidly spreading T-cell lymphomas have been reported to produce the picture of the acute respiratory distress syndrome as well as a more gradual onset of cough, dyspnea, and diffuse pulmonary infiltration.[157,158] Lymphoma subtypes can be differentiated by immunohistologic staining and by the newly developed PCR techniques to detect the gene arrangements and clonality of lung tissue cells or lavaged cells.[159–161]

REFERENCES

1. Carrington B, Liebow A. Lymphocytic interstitial pneumonia [abstract]. Am J Pathol 1966;48:36a.
2. Koss M, Hochholzer L, Langloss J, et al. Lymphoid interstitial pneumonia: clinicopathological and immunopathologic findings in 18 cases. Pathology 1987;19:178–85.
3. Colby T, Yousem S. Pulmonary lymphoid lesions. Semin Diagn Pathol 1985;2:183–96.
4. Colby T. Lymphoproliferative diseases. In: Dail D, Hammar S, editors. Pulmonary pathology. New York: Springer-Verlag; 1988. p. 711–26.
5. Koss MN. Pulmonary lymphoid disorders. Semin Diagn Pathol 1995;12:158–71.
6. Kurosu K, Yumoto N, Rom WN, et al. Aberrant expression of immunoglobulin heavy chain genes in Epstein-Barr virus-negative, human immunodeficiency virus-related lymphoid interstitial pneumonia. Lab Invest 2000;80:1891–903.
7. Kurosu K, Yumoto N, Furukawa M, et al. Third complementarity-determining-region sequence analysis of lymphocytic interstitial pneumonia: most cases demonstrate a minor monoclonal population hidden among normal lymphocyte clones. Am J Respir Crit Care Med 1997;155:1453–60.
8. Kaufman S, Long J. Parotid mass and pulmonary nodules in a 36-year-old woman. N Engl J Med 1977;297:652–60.
9. Kohler P, Cook R, Brown W, et al. Common variable hypogammaglobulinemia with T cell nodular interstitial pneumonitis and B cell nodular hyperplasia: different lymphocyte populations with a similar response to prednisone therapy. J Allergy Clin Immunol 1982;20:299–305.
10. Travis W, Fox C, Devany K, et al. Lymphoid pneumonitis in 30 adult patients infected with the human immunodeficiency virus: lymphocytic interstitial pneumonitis versus nonspecific interstitial pneumonitis. Hum Pathol 1992;23:529–41.
11. Liebow A, Carrington C. Diffuse pulmonary lymphoreticular infiltrations associated with dysproteinemia. Med Clin North Am 1973;57:809–43.
12. Bonner HJ, Ennis R, Greelhoed G, et al. Lymphoid infiltration and amyloidosis of lung in Sjögren's syndrome. Arch Pathol 1973;95:42–4.
13. Strimlan C, Rosenow EI, Divertie M, et al. Pulmonary manifestations of Sjögren's syndrome. Chest 1976;70:354–61.
14. MacFarland A, Davies D. Diffuse lymphoid interstitial pneumonia. Thorax 1973;28:768–76.
15. Banerjee D, Ahmad D. Malignant lymphoma complicating lymphocytic interstitial pneumonia: a monoclonal B-cell neoplasm arising in a polyclonal lymphoproliferative disorder. Hum Pathol 1982;13:780–2.

16. Halprin G, Ramirez R, Pratt P. Lymphoid interstitial pneumonia. Chest 1972;62:418–23.
17. Reich N, McCormack L, Van Orstand H. Pseudolymphoma of the lung. Chest 1974;65:424–7.
18. Greenberg S, Heisler J, Gyorkey F, et al. Pulmonary lymphoma versus pseudolymphoma: a perplexing problem. South Med J 1972;65:775–84.
19. Case records of the Massachusetts General Hospital (case 41–1984). N Engl J Med 1984;311:969–78.
20. Turner R, Colby T, Doggett R. Well differentiated lymphocytic lymphoma. A study of 47 patients with primary manifestation in the lung. Cancer 1984;54:2088–96.
21. Talal N, Bunim J. The development of malignant lymphoma in the course of Sjögren's syndrome. Am J Med 1964;36:529–40.
22. Anderson I, Talal N. The spectrum of benign to malignant lymphoproliferation in Sjögren's syndrome. Clin Exp Immunol 1972;10:199–204.
23. Salzstein S. Extranodal malignant lymphoma and pseudolymphomas. Pathol Annu 1969;4:159–84.
24. Salzstein S. Pulmonary malignant lymphomas and pseudolymphomas: classification, therapy and prognosis. Cancer 1963;16:928–55.
25. Seldana M, Israel H. Necrotizing sarcoidal granulomatosis, benign lymphocytic angiitis, and granulomatosis: do they exist? Semin Respir Med 1989;10:182–8.
26. Strimlan C, Rosenow EI, Weiland L, et al. Lymphocytic interstitial pneumonia: a review of 13 cases. Ann Intern Med 1978;68:616–21.
27. Alkhayer M, McCann B, Harrison B. Lymphocytic interstitial pneumonitis in association with Sjögren's syndrome. Br J Dis Chest 1988;82:305–9.
28. Moran T, Totten R. Lymphoid interstitial pneumonia with dysproteinemia: report of two cases with plasma cell predominance. Am J Clin Pathol 1970;54:747–56.
29. Young R, Tillman R, Burton A, et al. Lymphoid interstitial pneumonia with polyclonal gammopathy. J Natl Med Assoc 1969;61:310–4.
30. Church J, Hart I, Saxon A, et al. Lymphoid interstitial pneumonitis and hypogammaglobulinemia in children. Am Rev Respir Dis 1981;124:491–6.
31. Case records of the Massachusetts General Hospital (case 9–1986). N Engl J Med 1986;314:629–40.
32. Zuckier LS, Ongseng F, Goldfarb C. Lymphocytic interstitial pneumonitis: a cause of pulmonary gallium-67 uptake in a child with acquired immunodeficiency syndrome. J Nucl Med 1988;29:707–11.
33. Solal-Celigny P, Couderc L, Herman D, et al. Lymphoid interstitial pneumonitis in acquired immunodeficiency syndrome-related complex. Am Rev Respir Dis 1985;131:956–60.
34. Oldham S, Costillo M, Jacobsen F, et al. HIV associated lymphocytic interstitial pneumonia: radiologic manifestations and pathologic correlation. Radiology 1989;170:883–7.
35. Morris J, Rosen M, Marchevsky A, et al. Lymphocytic interstitial pneumonitis in patients at risk for the acquired immunodeficiency syndrome. Chest 1987;91:63–7.
36. Deheinzelin D, Capelozzi VL, Kairalla RA, et al. ILD in primary Sjögren's syndrome. Clinical-pathological evaluation and response to treatment. Am J Respir Crit Care Med 1996;154:794–9.
37. Gardiner P. Pleuropulmonary abnormalities in primary Sjögren's syndrome. J Rheumatol 1993;20:831–7.
38. Grieco M, Chinoy-Acharya P. Lymphocytic interstitial pneumonia associated with the acquired immunodeficiency syndrome. Am Rev Respir Dis 1985;31:952–5.
39. Levinson A, Hopewell P, Stites D, et al. Co-existent lymphoid interstitial pneumonia, pernicious anemia and agammaglobulinemia: comment on autoimmune pathogenesis. Arch Intern Med 1976;136:213–6.
40. Helman C, Keeton G, Benatar S. Lymphoid interstitial pneu-

monia with associated chronic active hepatitis and renal tubular acidosis. Am Rev Respir Dis 1977;115:161–4.

41. Ramos-Casals M, Garcia-Carrasco M, Cervera R, et al. Hepatitis C virus infection mimicking primary Sjögren syndrome. A clinical and immunologic description of 35 cases. Medicine (Baltimore) 2001;80:1–8.

42. Khardori R, Eagleton L, Soler N, et al. Lymphocytic interstitial pneumonitis in autoimmune thyroid disease. Am J Med 1991;90:649–52.

43. Steinberg D, Andrews J. Lymphocytic interstitial pneumonitis and other immunologic disorders. Ann Intern Med 1978;89:1011.

44. Miller RM, Weedon D, Robertson IM. Benign hypergammaglobulinaemic purpura of Waldenstrom associated with lymphoid interstitial pneumonitis. Australas J Dermatol 1998;39:238–40.

45. Uziel Y, Hen B, Cordoba M, et al. Lymphocytic interstitial pneumonitis preceding polyarticular juvenile rheumatoid arthritis. Clin Exp Rheumatol 1998;16:617–9.

46. Benisch B, Peison B. The association of lymphocytic interstitial pneumonia and systemic lupus erythematosus. Mt Sinai J Med 1979;46:398–401.

47. Yum M, Ziegler V, Walker P, et al. Pseudolymphoma of the lung in a patient with systemic lupus erythematosus. Am J Med 1979;66:172–6.

48. Setoguchi Y, Takahashi S, Nukiwa T, et al. Detection of human T-cell lymphotropic virus type I-related antibodies in patients with lymphocytic interstitial pneumonia. Am Rev Respir Dis 1991;144:1361–5.

49. Malamou-Mitsi V, Tsai M, Greer J, et al. Lymphoid interstitial pneumonitis not associated with HIV infection: role of Epstein-Barr virus. Mod Pathol 1992;5:487–91.

50. Kramer M, Saldana M, Ramos M, et al. High titers of Epstein-Barr virus antibodies in adult patients with lymphocytic interstitial pneumonitis associated with AIDS. Respir Med 1992;86:49–52.

51. Barbera J, Hiayashi S, Hegele R, et al. Detection of Epstein-Barr virus in lymphocytic interstitial pneumonia by in situ hybridization. Am Rev Respir Dis 1992;145:940–6.

52. Newhall H, Brahim S. Chronic obstructive airway disease in patients with Sjögren's syndrome. Am Rev Respir Dis 1977;115:295–304.

53. Bloch K, Buchanan W, Wohl M, et al. Sjögren's syndrome. A clinical, pathological and serological study of 62 cases. Medicine 1965;44:187–99.

54. Gumpel J. Sjögren's syndrome with pulmonary fibrosis. Waldenström's hypergammaglobulinemic purpura and immune paresis. Proc R Soc Med 1971;64:397–401.

55. Joshi V, Oleske J, Minnelor A, et al. Pathologic pulmonary findings in children with the acquired immunodeficiency syndrome: a study of ten cases. Hum Pathol 1985;16:241–6.

56. Scott G, Buck B, Leterman J, et al. Acquired immunodeficiency syndrome in infants. N Engl J Med 1984;310:76–81.

57. Goldman H, Ziprkowski M, Charytan M, et al. Lymphocytic interstitial pneumonitis in children with AIDS: a perfect radiographic-pathologic correlation [abstract]. AJR Am J Roentgenol 1985;145:868A.

58. O'Brodovich H, Moser M, Lu I, et al. Familial lymphoid pneumonia: a long term follow-up. Pediatrics 1980;63:523–8.

59. Wrighth J, Pennington P. Familial lymphoid interstitial pneumonitis [letter]. J Pediatr 1987;111:638.

60. Parker J, Shellito V, Pei L, et al. Lymphocytic interstitial pneumonitis presenting as recurrent pneumothoraces. Chest 1991;100:1733–5.

61. Buchwald I. Pulmonary pseudolymphoma presenting as a solitary nodular density with an air bronchogram. Chest 1974;65:691–3.

62. Ettensohn D, Mayer K, Kaassismian N, et al. Lymphocytic bronchiolitis associated with HIV infection. Chest 1988;93:201–2.

63. Ichikawa Y, Kinoshita M, Koga T, et al. Lung cyst formation in lymphocytic interstitial pneumonia: CT features. J Comput Assist Tomogr 1994;18:745–8.

64. Honda O, Johkoh T, Ichikado K, et al. Differential diagnosis of lymphocytic interstitial pneumonia and malignant lymphoma on high-resolution CT. AJR Am J Roentgenol 1999;173:71–4.

65. Johkoh T, Ichikado K, Akira M, et al. Lymphocytic interstitial pneumonia: follow-up CT findings in 14 patients. J Thorac Imaging 2000;15:162–7.

66. Johkoh T, Muller NL, Pickford HA, et al. Lymphocytic interstitial pneumonia: thin-section CT findings in 22 patients. Radiology 1999;212:567–72.

67. Fessler MB, Schwarz MI, King TJ Jr, et al. Lymphocytic interstitial pneumonitis vs. IPF: comparison of outcome, clinical, and physiological variables. Ann J Resp Crit Care Med 2001;163:A706.

68. Anderson V, Lee H. Lymphocytic interstitial pneumonitis in pediatric AIDS. Pediatr Pathol 1988;8:417–21.

69. Montes M, Tomasi T, Noehren T, et al. Lymphoid interstitial pneumonia with monoclonal gammopathy. Am Rev Respir Dis 1968;98:277–80.

70. Harrison W, Mathers J, Glauser F. Gallium scans and serum angiotension converting enzyme levels in talc granulomatosis and lymphocytic interstitial pneumonia. South Med J 1980;73:1663–7.

71. Pisani RJ, Witzig TE, Li CY, et al. Confirmation of lymphomatous pulmonary involvement by immunophenotypic and gene rearrangement analysis of bronchoalveolar lavage fluid. Mayo Clin Proc 1990;65:651–6.

72. Philippe B, Delfau-Larue MH, Epardeau B, et al. B-cell pulmonary lymphoma: gene rearrangement analysis of bronchoalveolar lymphocytes by polymerase chain reaction. Chest 1999;115:1242–7.

73. DeCoteau W, Tourville D, Ambrus J, et al. Lymphoid interstitial pneumonia and autoerythrocyte sensitization syndrome. Arch Intern Med 1974;134:519–22.

74. Neil G, Lukie B, Cockcroft D, et al. Lymphocytic interstitial pneumonia and abdominal lymphoma complicating coeliac sprue. J Clin Gastroenterol 1986;8:282–5.

75. Davies CW, Juniper MC, Gray W, et al. Lymphoid interstitial pneumonitis associated with common variable hypogammaglobulinaemia treated with cyclosporin A. Thorax 2000;55:88–90.

76. Bach MC. Zidovudine for lymphocytic interstitial pneumonia associated with AIDS. Lancet 1987;ii:796.

77. Helbert M, Stoneham C, Mitchell D, et al. Zidovudine for lymphocytic interstitial pneumonitis in AIDS. Lancet 1987;ii:1333.

78. Case records of the Massachusetts General Hospital (13–1980). N Engl J Med 1980;302:795–895.

79. Gibbs A, Seal R. Primary lymphoproliferative conditions of the lung. Thorax 1978;33:140–52.

80. Herbert A, Walters M, Cawley M, et al. Lymphocytic interstitial pneumonia identified as lymphoma of mucosa associated lymphoid tissue. J Pathol 1985;146:129–38.

81. Weisbrot IM. Lymphomatoid granulomatosis of the lung, associated with a long history of benign lymphoepithelial lesions of the salivary glands and lymphoid interstitial pneumonitis. Report of a case. Am J Clin Pathol 1976;66:792–801.

82. Zulman J, Jaffe R, Talal N. Evidence that the malignant lymphoma of Sjögren's syndrome is a monoclonal B-cell neoplasm. N Engl J Med 1978;299:1215–20.

83. Brodie SJ, de la Rosa C, Howe JG, et al. Pediatric AIDS-associated lymphocytic interstitial pneumonia and pulmonary arterio-occlusive disease: role of VCAM-1/VLA-4 adhesion pathway and human herpesviruses. Am J Pathol 1999;154:1453–64.

84. Dreisin R, Schwarz MI, Theofilopoulos A, Stanford RE. Circulating immune complexes in the idiopathic interstitial pneumonias. N Engl J Med 1978;298:353–7.

85. Sutinen S, Huhti E. Ultrastructure of lymphoid interstitial pneumonia. Am J Clin Pathol 1977;67:328–33.
86. Garry R, Fermin C, Hart D, et al. Detection of a human intracisternal A-type retroviral particle antigenically related to HIV. Science 1990;250:1127–9.
87. Perreault C, Coosineau S, D'Angelo G, et al. Lymphoid interstitial pneumonia after allogeneic bone marrow transplantation. Cancer 1985;55:1–9.
88. Stein R, Hummel D, Bohn D, et al. Lymphocytic pneumonitis following bone marrow transplantation in severe combined immunodeficiency. Am Rev Respir Dis 1991;143:1406–8.
89. Amorosa J, Miller R, Laraya-Cuasay, et al. Bronchiectasis in children with lymphocytic interstitial pneumonia and acquired immune deficiency syndrome. Pediatr Radiol 1992;22:603–7.
90. Sugimoto M, Mita S, Tokunaga M, et al. Pulmonary involvement in human T-cell lymphotropic virus type-1 uveitis: T-lymphocytosis and high proviral DNA load in bronchoalveolar lavage fluid. Eur Respir J 1993;6:938–43.
91. Essig LJ, Timms E, Hancock E, Sharp GC. Plasma cell interstitial pneumonia and macroglobulinemia. A response to corticosteroid and cyclophosphamide therapy. Am J Med 1974;56:398–405.
92. Bahadori M, Liebow A. Plasma cell granulomas of the lung. Cancer 1973;31:191–208.
93. Helwig C. Extramedullary plasma cell tumors as observed in various locations. Arch Pathol 1943;36:95–111.
94. Menashe P, Stenson W, Reynoso G, et al. Bronchoalveolar lavage plasmacytosis in a patient with plasma cell dyscrasia. Chest 1989;95:221–7.
95. Wang J, Pandha HS, Treleaven J, et al. Metastatic extramedullary plasmacytoma of the lung. Leuk Lymphoma 1999;35:423–5.
96. Shin M, Carcelen M, Kang-Jey H. Diverse roentgenographic manifestations of the rare pulmonary involvement in myeloma. Chest 1992;102:946–8.
97. Kintzner J, Rosenow E, Kyle R. Thoracic and pulmonary abnormalities in multiple myeloma: a review of 958 cases. Arch Intern Med 1978;138:727–50.
98. Hill LI, White MJ. Plasmacytoma of the lung. J Thorac Surg 1953;25:187–93.
99. Herskovies T, Anderson H, Bayrd E. Intrathoracic plasmacytoma: presentation of 21 cases and review of the literature. Dis Chest 1965;47:1–20.
100. Gabriel S. Multiple myeloma presenting as a pulmonary infiltration. Dis Chest 1965;47:123.
101. Gupta R, Roy D, Gupta I, et al. Extramedullary plasmacytoma IgG type I presenting as a mediastinal syndrome. Br J Dis Chest 1974;68:65–70.
102. Suchman A, Coleman M, Mouradian J, et al. Aggressive plasma cell myeloma: a terminal phase. Arch Intern Med 1981;141:1315–20.
103. Morgan J, McCau lD, Rodriquez F, et al. Pulmonary immunologic features of alveolar septal amyloidosis associated with multiple myeloma. Chest 1987;92:704–8.
104. Joseph G, Pandit M, Korfhage L. Primary pulmonary plasmacytoma. Cancer 1993;71:721–4.
105. Horiuchi T, Hirokawa M, Oyama Y, et al. Diffuse pulmonary infiltrates as a roentgenographic manifestation of primary pulmonary plasmacytoma. Am J Med 1998;105:72–4.
106. Laso FJ, Tabernero MD, Iglesias-Osma MC. Extramedullary plasmacytoma: a localized or systemic disease? Ann Intern Med 1998;128:156.
107. Furgeson W, Bachman B, O'Toole W. Waldenström's macroglobulinemia with diffuse pulmonary infiltration: lung biopsy and response to chlorambucil therapy. Am Rev Respir Dis 1963;88:689–97.
108. Beumer H, Olislagers W, Djajadiningrat R, et al. Pleuropulmonary involvement in Waldenström's macroglobulinemia: case report. Respiration 1984;45:154–7.
109. Winterbauer R, Riggens R, Griesman F, et al. Pleuropulmonary manifestations of Waldenström's macroglobulinemia. Chest 1974;66:368–75.
110. Rausch P, Herion J. Pulmonary manifestations of Waldenström's macroglobulinemia. Am J Hematol 1980;9:201–9.
111. Filok R, Warren P. Bronchoalveolar lavage in Waldenström's macroglobulinemia with pulmonary infiltrates. Thorax 1986;41:409–12.
112. King T, Schwarz M, Mathew M. Waldenström's macroglobulinemia: report of a case with pulmonary involvement and recurrent pneumococcal sepsis after pneumococcal vaccination. JAMA 1984;76:184–9.
113. Bragg D. Lymphoproliferative disorders of the lung histopathology, clinical manifestations and imaging features. AJR Am J Roentgenol 1994;163:273–81.
114. Gertz MA, Fonseca R, Rajkumar SV. Waldenström's macroglobulinemia. Oncologist 2000;5:63–7.
115. Dimopoulos M, Kantarjian H, Estey E, et al. Treatment of Waldenström's macroglobulinemia with 2 chlorodeoxyadenosine. Ann Intern Med 1993;118:195–8.
116. Thalhammer-Scherrer R, Geissler K, Schwarzinger I, et al. Fludarabine therapy in Waldenström's macroglobulinemia. Ann Hematol 2000;79:556–9.
117. Treon SP, Agus DB, Link B, et al. CD20–directed antibody-mediated immunotherapy induces responses and facilitates hematologic recovery in patients with Waldenström's macroglobulinemia. J Immunother 2001;24:272–9.
118. Frizzera G, Moran E, Rappaport H. Angio-immunoblastic lymphadenopathy with dysproteinemia. Lancet 1974;i:1070–3.
119. Lukes R, Tindle B. Immunoblastic lymphadenopathy. A hyperimmune entity resembling Hodgkin's disease. N Engl J Med 1975;292:1–8.
120. Harris N, Jaffe ES, Stein H, et al. A revised European-American classification of lymphoid neoplasms: a proposal from the International Lymphoma Study Group. Blood 1994; 84:1361–92.
121. Frizzera G, Moran E, Rappaport H. Angio-immunoblastic lymphadenopathy: prognosis and clinical course. Am J Med 1975;59:803–18.
122. Iseman M, Schwarz MI, Stanford RE. Interstitial pneumonia in angio-immunoblastic lymphadenopathy with dysproteinemia: a case report with special histological studies. Ann Intern Med 1976;85:752–5.
123. Bradley S, Dines D, Burk P, et al. The lung in immunoblastic lymphadenopathy. Chest 1981;80:212–8.
124. Moore S, Harrison EJ, Wieland L. Angioimmunoblastic lymphadenopathy. Mayo Clin Proc 1976;51:273–80.
125. Kuijpers T, Shaw M, Croonen A. Pulmonary involvement in angio-immunoblastic lymphadenopathy (AILD): case report and review of the literature. Eur J Radiol 1983;3:155–7.
126. Neiman R, Dervan P, Haidenschild C, et al. Angioimmunoblastic lymphadenopathy: an ultrastructural and immunological study with review of the literature. Cancer 1978;41:266–71.
127. Pruzanski W. Lymphadenopathy associated with dysgammaglobulinemia. Semin Hematol 1980;17:44–7.
128. Price D, Dent R. Pulmonary involvement in angio-immunoblastic lymphadenopathy. Postgrad Med J 1983;59:728–9.
129. Zylak C, Banerjee R, Galbraith P, et al. Lung involvement in angioimmunoblastic lymphadenopathy (AILD). Radiology 1976;121:513–9.
130. Weisenburger D, Armitage J, Dick F. Immunoblastic lymphadenopathy with pulmonary infiltrates, hypocomplimentemia and vasculitis. Am J Med 1977;63:849–54.
131. Siegler D, Winner S. Pulmonary and pleural involvement in angio-immunoblastic lymphadenopathy. Br J Dis Chest 1980;74:296–9.
132. Cullen M, Stansfield A, Oliver R, et al. Angio-immunoblastic lymphadenopathy: report of ten cases and review of the literatuare. Q J Med 1979;189:151–77.

133. Boros L, Bhaskar A, D'Souza J. Monoclonal evolution of angioimmunoblastic lymphadenopathy. Am J Clin Pathol 1981;75:856–60.

134. Pay S, Dinc A, Simsek I, et al. Sulfasalazine-induced angioimmunoblastic lymphadenopathy developing in a patient with juvenile chronic arthritis. Rheumatol Int 2000;20:25–7.

135. Tsung S, Lin J. Angioimmunoblastic lymphadenopathy in a patient taking diphenylhydantoin. Ann Clin Lab Sci 1981; 2:542–5.

136. Weisenburger D. Immunoblastic lymphadenopathy associated with methyldopa therapy. Cancer 1978;42:2322–7.

137. Sallah S, Gagnon GA. Angioimmunoblastic lymphadenopathy with dysproteinemia: emphasis on pathogenesis and treatment. Acta Haematol 1998;99:57–64.

138. Serke S, van Lessen A, Hummel M, et al. Circulating CD4+ T lymphocytes with intracellular but no surface CD3 antigen in five of seven patients consecutively diagnosed with angioimmunoblastic T-cell lymphoma. Cytometry 2000; 42:180–7.

139. Ohshima KS, Suzumiya J, Kawasaki C, et al. Cytoplasmic cytokines in lymphoproliferative disorders: multiple cytokine production in angioimmunoblastic lymphadenopathy with dysproteinemia. Leuk Lymphoma 2000;38:541–5.

140. Abu-Zahra H, McDonald D, Horne W. Angio-immunoblastic adenopathy with dysproteinemia [letter]. Lancet 1975;i:114–5.

141. Takemori N, Kodaira J, Toyoshima N, et al. Successful treatment of immunoblastic lymphadenopathy-like T-cell lymphoma with cyclosporin A. Leuk Lymphoma 1999;35: 389–95.

142. Liebow A, Carrington C, Friedman P. Lymphomatoid granulomatosis. Hum Pathol 1972;3:457–533.

143. Lipford EJ, Margolick J, Longo D, et al. Angiocentric immunoproliferative lesions: a clinicopathologic spectrum of postthymic T-cell proliferations. Blood 1988;72:1674–87.

144. Jaffee E, Lipford E, Margolick J, et al. Lymphomatoid granulomatosis and angiocentric lymphoma. Semin Respir Med 1989;10:167–72.

145. Myers J, Kurtin P, Katzenstein A, et al. Lymphomatoid granulomatosis: evidence of immunophentotypic diversity and relationship to Epstein-Barr virus. Am J Surg Pathol 1995;19:1300–12.

146. Taniere P, Thivolet-Bejui F, Vitrey D, et al. Lymphomatoid granulomatosis—a report on four cases: evidence for B phenotype of the tumoral cells. Eur Respir J 1998;12: 102–6.

147. Fassas A, Jagannath S, Desikan KR, et al. Lymphomatoid granulomatosis following autologous stem cell transplantation. Bone Marrow Transplant 1999;23:79–81.

148. Haque AK, Myers JL, Hudnall SD, et al. Pulmonary lymphomatoid granulomatosis in acquired immunodeficiency syndrome: lesions with Epstein-Barr virus infection. Mod Pathol 1998;11:347–56.

149. Weisbrot I. Lymphomatoid granulomatosis of the lung: associated with a long history of benign lymphoepithelial lesions of the salivary glands and lymphoid interstitial pneumonia. Am J Clin Pathol 1976;66:792–801.

150. Karnak I, Ciftci AO, Talim B, et al. Pulmonary lymphomatoid granulomatosis in a 4 year old. J Pediatr Surg 1999;34: 1033–5.

151. LeSueur BW, Ellsworth L, Bangert JL, et al. Lymphomatoid granulomatosis in a 4–year-old boy. Pediatr Dermatol 2000;17:369–72.

152. Paspala AB, Sundaram C, Purohit AK, et al. Exclusive CNS involvement by lymphomatoid granulomatosis in a 12–year-old boy: a case report. Surg Neurol 1999;51:258–60.

153. Epstein D, Glickstein M. Pulmonary lymphoproliferative disorders. Radiol Clin North Am 1989;27:1077–84.

154. Pisani R, DeRemee R. Clinical complication of the histopathologic diagnosis of pulmonary lymphomatoid granulomatosis. Mayo Clin Proc 1990;65:151–63.

155. Fauci A, Haynes B, Costa J, et al. Lymphomatoid granulomatosis: prospective clinical and therapeutic experience over 10 years. N Engl J Med 1982;306:68–74.

156. Tan TB, Spaander PJ, Blaisse M, et al. Angiotropic large cell lymphoma presenting as ILD. Thorax 1988;43:578–9.

157. Eliasson AH, Rajagopal KR, Dow NS. Respiratory failure in rapidly progressing pulmonary lymphoma. Role of immunophenotyping in diagnosis. Am Rev Respir Dis 1990;141:231–4.

158. Harrison N, Twelves C, Addis B, et al. Peripheral T-cell lymphoma presenting with angioedema and diffuse pulmonary infiltrates. Am Rev Respir Dis 1988;138:976–80.

159. Subramaian D, Albrecht S, Gonzales J, et al. Primary pulmonary lymphoma: diagnosis by immunoglobulin gene rearrangement study using a novel polymerase chain reaction technique. Am Rev Respir Dis 1993;148:222–6.

160. Keicho N, Oka T, Takouchi K, et al. Detection of lymphomatous involvement of the lung by bronchoalveolar lavage: application of immunophenotypic and gene rearrangement analysis. Chest 1994;105:458–62.

161. Betsuyaku T, Munakata M, Yamaguchi E, et al. Establishing diagnosis of pulmonary malignant lymphoma by gene rearrangement analysis of lymphocytes in bronchoalveolar lavage fluid. Am J Respir Crit Care Med 1994;149:526–9.

28 PULMONARY LANGERHANS CELL HISTIOCYTOSIS

ROBERT VASSALLO
ANDREW H. LIMPER

The term histiocytosis describes a variety of proliferative disorders of histiocytes (cells that are morphologically similar to macrophages).[1] On one end of the spectrum is a group of aggressive malignant neoplasms, the histiocytic lymphomas, whereas on the other end of the spectrum there are simple reactive histiocytic proliferations that may be seen in lymph nodes in the course of a variety of conditions and are of no clinical consequence.[1–3] Between these two extremes are conditions characterized by proliferation and infiltration of organs by a particular histiocyte called the Langerhans' cell. The Langerhans cell histiocytoses are proliferative disorders of histiocytic infiltration of organs resulting in organ dysfunction.[4–6]

Commonly referred to as histiocytosis X, these histiocytic disorders were initially subdivided into three categories: *Letterer-Siwe* disease, *Hand-Schüller-Christian* disease, and eosinophilic granuloma. These conditions are now believed to represent different expressions of the same basic disorder (Table 28–1). In 1987, the Histiocyte Society proposed the use of the term Langerhans cell histiocytosis (LCH) to include the various clinicopathologic conditions previously known as *Hand-Schüller-Christian* disease, *Letterer-Siwe* disease, *Hashimoto-Pritzker* disease, and eosinophilic granuloma.[7] The term LCH was intentionally chosen to replace the term "histiocytosis X," which had been proposed in 1953, in order to acknowledge the central role of the Langerhans' cell in these diseases and to reflect the increased understanding of these disorders as part of a spectrum of diseases. The organs most commonly affected by LCH include the skeleton (especially skull and axial skeleton), the lungs, the central nervous system (especially the hypothalamic region), and skin.[6,8–11] The lungs may be involved alone or in the setting of multiple organ involvement by LCH (see Table 28–1).[12–14]

EPIDEMIOLOGY

The true incidence and prevalence of pulmonary Langerhans cell histiocytosis (PLCH) are not known.

Gaensler and Carrington reported that of 502 patients who underwent open lung biopsy for the evaluation of diffuse lung disease, 17 (3.4%) had eosinophilic granuloma.[15] This may underestimate the true prevalence of the condition because there are an unknown number of patients who do not undergo lung biopsy but are diagnosed by radiographic and clinical criteria. Biopsy of individuals with advanced disease may reveal burnt-out or nonspecific fibrotic changes rather than the characteristic histopathologic appearance, resulting in nondiagnostic biopsies. In addition, without the use of immunostaining, it is possible that a proportion of cases of PLCH are missed or misclassified in prior studies.

PLCH occurs predominantly in smokers between the ages of 30 and 50 years.[12,13,16–19] Although infrequent in elderly individuals, there are now several reports in the literature that document the diagnosis of PLCH in individuals older than 65 years of age (Table 28–2). The relative frequency in men and women is controversial. Although generally believed to affect men more often than women,[20,21] a number of recent studies indicate that PLCH may be equal or even more prevalent in women. This may reflect the changes in prevalence of cigarette smoking by women (see Table 28–2).[12,13,18]

Table 28–1 Simplified Classification of Langerhans Cell Histiocytosis in Adults.

Single-organ involvement
- Lung (occurs in isolation in > 85% of cases with lung involvement)
- Bone
- Skin
- Pituitary
- Lymph nodes
- Other sites: thyroid, liver, spleen, brain

Multisystem disease
- Multiorgan disease with lung involvement (in 5 to 15% of cases with lung involvement)
- Multiorgan disease without lung involvement
- Multiorgan histiocytic disorder

Reproduced with permission from Vassallo R et al.[32]

Considerable evidence suggests that PLCH is a smoking-related interstitial lung disorder.[16,19] The overwhelming majority of individuals with PLCH are active or former cigarette smokers (see Table 28–2). In a recent review of 102 adults with PLCH seen in a tertiary referral center, 98 patients were either smokers at the time of diagnosis or had recently quit smoking [Vassallo and colleagues, manuscript in preparation]. Similarly, over 90% of individuals with PLCH reported a history of cigarette smoking in other case series published in the literature (see Table 28–2). Interestingly, isolated pulmonary LCH is uncommon in children, although systemic LCH is more prevalent in children than adults.[14] A recent report described two patients with childhood LCH who developed pulmonary involvement only after initiation of smoking. This suggests that the relatively more common occurrence of LCH in the lung in adults (when compared with children) is related to smoking.[22] Further evidence linking smoking to PLCH comes from reports that PLCH may radiographically improve following smoking cessation,[23] and that PLCH may recur in transplanted lungs if the recipient resumes cigarette smoking.[24]

Most patients with PLCH tend to be heavy smokers, although the disease may certainly occur in individuals following a relatively brief history of cigarette smoking [unpublished observations]. Despite the close association between cigarette smoking and the incidence of PLCH, there are no data that correlate the amount of daily cigarette consumption with the severity of the disease. In addition, although smoking seems to be the predominant causative factor linked with the development of PLCH, the effect of smoking cessation on the natural course of the disease is not clear.

There are no other known inhalational or other exposures linked to the development of PLCH. Whether genetic factors play a role in the development of PLCH is unclear. A number of studies have reported families with more than one affected relative with LCH.[25–27] A case of familial PLCH presenting in childhood has been reported,[26] but to date it appears that virtually all cases of adult PLCH are sporadic. For unknown reasons, PLCH occurs mainly in Caucasians and is distinctly uncommon in African Americans and other ethnic groups.

PATHOGENESIS

The Langerhans' cell plays a central role in the pathogenesis of PLCH. Langerhans' cells are derived from $CD34^+$ mononuclear cells that also are precurors of dendritic cells.[28] Dendritic and Langerhans' cells are specialized immune cells found in a variety of tissues and are extremely potent antigen presenting cells that are far more capable of inducing lymphocyte proliferation compared to equivalent numbers of macrophages.[29,30] Following exposure to antigens in the lung, dendritic cells and Langerhans' cells migrate to regional lymphoid tis-

Table 28–2   Summary of Clinical Features and Pulmonary Function Test Abnormalities in Adults with Pulmonary Langerhans Cell Histiocytosis

	Freidman et al[13]	Basset et al[21]	Travis et al[18]	Schonfeld et al[17]	Delobbe et al[7]
Number	100	78	48	42	45
Gender M:F	40/60	61/17	19/29	24/18	32/13
Age (range in years)	1 to 60	1 to 69	15 to 54	16 to 74	12 to 62
Nonsmokers	2 out of 69	22 out of 53	None	1 out of 42	2 out of 45
Symptoms (%)					
Cough	50	N/A	58	N/A	N/A
Dyspnea	35	N/A	48	N/A	44
Weight loss	9	N/A	15	N/A	N/A
Chest pain	18	N/A	10	N/A	N/A
Fever	15	N/A	17	N/A	N/A
Pneumothorax	11	N/A	4	5	16
Hemoptysis	6	N/A	N/A	N/A	N/A
Asymptomatic	23	N/A	6	36	22
Extrapulmonary disease (N)					
Bone	4	19	4	4	1
Diabetes insipidus	5	N/A	4	1	1
Skin	N/A	N/A	2	1	N/A
Lymph nodes	2	N/A	N/A	N/A	2
PFT findings (N)	N/A	42	39	26	45
Normal study (%)	33	15	N/A	"None"	35
Restriction (%)	30	N/A	23	N/A	27
Obstruction (%)	59	21	28	N/A	33
Mixed pattern (%)	N/A	N/A	23	N/A	5

PFT = pulmonary function tests; N/A = data not available.

sues and mature into cells that lose the capacity to process new antigens but have the required molecular signals (such as upregulation of members of the B7 costimulatory family of molecules on the surface) that enable appropriate lymphocyte responses to occur in response to antigens.[29] In the normal lung, Langerhans' cells are found almost exclusively within the tracheobronchial epithelium, suggesting that Langerhans' cells act as a primary line of defense surveying antigens deposited in the airway following inspiration and processing these antigens.[31] In view of the constant exposure of the airway to inhaled antigens from a large variety of sources, it becomes evident that Langerhans' cells play a critical role in orchestrating the immune response to a vast array of different antigenic challenges. The details of how Langerhans' cells coordinate immune responses following exposure to an immense variety of antigenic peptides is not known, but it is a mechanism that may hold the key to understanding why this disease develops in a small proportion of individuals who smoke.

Cigarette smoke is the most important exposure associated with the development of PLCH.[16,19,32] Although only a small proportion of smokers develop PLCH, a number of studies have demonstrated that smoking induces the accumulation of Langerhans' cells in the lung suggesting that some component/s in cigarette smoke may facilitate recruitment of precursors of Langerhans' cells into the lung or alternately, may induce the maturation of local cells into Langerhans' cells. In this context, cytokines such as tumor necrosis factor-alpha (TNF-α), granulocyte-macrophage colony–stimulating factor (GM-CSF), and transforming growth factor-beta (TGF-β) may have an important role.[33–35] Immunohistochemical techniques demonstrate that GM-CSF is abundant in the epithelium of bronchioles affected by the inflammatory lesions of PLCH and is associated with the presence of numerous CD1a+ Langerhans' cells, whereas in bronchioles not affected by disease, the expression of GM-CSF is less.[36] The pulmonary lesions of patients with PLCH also demonstrate abundant expression of TGF-β,[37] a cytokine that serves in both autocrine and paracrine modes to control the differentiation, proliferation, and state of activation of immune cells and has profound effects on the process that leads to lung fibrosis and scarring.[38,39] TGF-β, TNF-α, and GM-CSF enhance the in vitro generation of Langerhans' cells from CD34+ hematopoietic stem cells and are likely to be local factors produced at the site of inflammatory lesions that perpetuate and regulate the immune response that ultimately leads to the characteristic changes seen in the course of this disease. Alveolar macrophages, airway epithelial cells, and fibroblasts may be the source of these and other cytokines that are involved in sustaining the local inflammatory response.

The nature by which cigarette smoke leads to PLCH is unknown. It has been suggested that cigarette smoke–induced secretion of bombesin-like peptides (BLP) by neuroendocrine cells in the airway may play

a prominent role.[40,41] BLPs are known to induce a variety of pharmacologic effects on the lung, including bronchoconstriction, induction of cytokine secretion by macrophages, promotion of growth of lung fibroblasts, and modulation of T cell responses.[42,43] Patients with PLCH have cells with bombesin-like immunoreactivity, therefore, it is possible that BLPs may be important in the pathogenesis of PLCH.[40,44] However, other studies have demonstrated that in experimental models of murine lung fibrosis induced by bleomycin, administration of exogenous bombesin by infusion resulted in attenuation of the development of pulmonary fibrosis.[45] Other components of cigarette smoke, such as tobacco glycoprotein (TGP), have been implicated in the pathogenesis.[46] TGP is an immunostimulant that causes T and B lymphocyte differentiation and stimulates lymphokine production.[47,48] Lymphocytes obtained from patients with PLCH respond abnormally to TGP when compared with normal lymphocytes with decreased proliferation and cytokine release (especially interleukin-2).[46] Because of the role of interleukin-2 (IL-2) in regulating histiocyte proliferation, it has been suggested that the relative lack of IL-2 favors local proliferation of Langerhans' cells in the lung, a contention supported by an anecdotal report of clinical remission of LCH in a child treated with intravenous IL-2.[49]

Although the link between smoking and PLCH appears strong, the disease occurs in a very small percentage of smokers, indicating that in addition to exogenous factors, there clearly must be some inherent genetic factor (or additional environmental factors) that leads to PLCH. A genetic factor that may be associated with susceptibility to LCH is the TNF-2 genotype (a genotype with a TNF-α promoter sequence having a G-A transition in position 308), which has been identified in some patients with systemic forms of LCH.[50]

Recent studies have indicated that systemic forms of LCH are clonal proliferative disorders, a finding that has sparked controversy regarding the natural biology of LCH.[51–53] Although the monoclonal proliferation of Langerhans' cells was demonstrated convincingly in both childhood and adult forms of LCH, a recent study reported that 71% of nodules from patients with PLCH were nonclonal, and only in a minority of cases was clonal expansion of CD1a positive Langerhans' cells demonstrated.[54] This suggests that in contrast to LCH involving other sites, PLCH is more likely to be a reactive process secondary to some inciting stimulus, most likely cigarette smoking. This important observation implies that PLCH is inherently different from other forms of LCH and accordingly, the management and natural course of this disease does not necessarily follow that observed for other forms of LCH. However, one cannot exclude the possibility that following sustained and persistent exposure to cigarette smoking, a reactive nonclonal process may progress into a clonal proliferative process. This is similar to what is seen in patients with gluten sensitive enteropathy that is accompanied by clonal lymphoid proliferations, which may disappear with the avoidance of gluten or may progress to a lymphomatous transformation if the inciting stimulus is not removed.

PATHOLOGY

The gross appearance of PLCH is distinctive but nonspecific. Gross inspection of the lung may demonstrate cysts on the lung surface, and upon sectioning the lung, one appreciates the presence of nodules that may be up to 2 cm in diameter (although usually are 1 cm or less in size), are firm, and may be associated with cavitation.[12,21] In advanced cases, the predominant finding is a hyperinflated and fibrotic lung with honeycomb change.[21]

The histopathologic appearance of the lung depends on the stage of the disease. In early disease there are loose cellular nodules composed of a mixed population of cells with variable numbers of Langerhans' cells, eosinophils, lymphocytes, plasma cells, fibroblasts, and pigmented alveolar macrophages. Importantly, these loose collections of cells are bronchiolocentric in location.[12,18,55] Eosinophils are dispersed throughout the nodules in variable numbers.[12,18] Some cases have minimal eosinophil infiltration whereas others show pools of eosinophils surrounded by the histiocytic reaction.[12] The term eosinophilic granuloma is thus not an accurate descriptive term because the lesions that occur are not typical granulomas and some cases may be devoid of eosinophil infiltration.

The lesions of PLCH are bronchiolocentric and discrete, described classically as roughly symmetric stellate lesions with central scarring scattered throughout the pulmonary parenchyma with the accumulation of pigmented alveolar macrophages in the adjacent air spaces forming "pseudodesquamative interstitial pneumonia" (pseudo-DIP) changes.[12,13,18] The stage of evolution of the process has an important influence on the pathologic findings. In the early stages, numerous cells accumulate adjacent to terminal or respiratory bronchioles, resulting in destruction of the bronchiolar wall and the adjacent alveolar structures. Clusters of Langerhans' cells and lymphocytes occupy the center of these lesions. Cellular infiltrates extending into the parenchyma for variable distances may produce thickening of the alveolar walls adjacent to the granulomas. Typically, these nodular lesions center around small airways (peribronchiolar distribution), although in large lesions, the point of origin may be difficult to ascertain (Figure 28–1).[12,18] Occasionally, the visceral pleura is involved. In one series of twelve adults with PLCH, all of the open biopsy specimens demonstrated the presence of nodular and/or reticular lesions that ranged from 0.4 to 13 mm in maximal diameter, with an average median diameter of 2.5 mm.[55]

The ultrastructural features of Langerhans' cells in these lesions are similar to those described for normal pulmonary Langerhans' cells. In areas where lymphocytic infiltrates are present, close contact between Langerhans' cells and lymphocytes occur, which may be representative of the presentation of antigens by the Langerhans' cells to T cells in these regions.[56] Definitive identification of Langerhans' cells is possible by the recognition of Birbeck granules (pentalaminar rod-shaped intracellular structures), which may be visualized by electron microscopy[4,57] and by immunohistochemical staining for the CD1a antigen on the cell surface, a feature not seen with other cells of histiocytic origin.[56] Identification of Langerhans' cells in biopsy specimens using monoclonal antibody staining to the CD1a surface antigen is recommended for definitive diagnosis, although expert pathologists may be able to make a confident diagnosis on the basis of the morphologic appearance alone. S-100 protein detection by immunostaining is also employed to detect the presence of Langerhans' cells in tissue specimens.[55] Although the identification of Langerhans' cells is required to enable a definitive diagnosis, the mere presence of these cells in pulmonary lesions is not equivalent to PLCH, because Langerhans' cells may be identified in a variety of other lesions.

The cystic lesions are not a direct consequence of necrosis of the nodular lesions. Cystic lesions probably form as peribronchiolar lesions destroy the cellular and connective tissue components of the bronchiolar walls causing progressive dilatation of the lumen. Eventually the bronchiole is encased by fibrous tissue, resulting in the bizarre-shaped irregular cystic lesions that are so characteristic of PLCH. In addition, as seen in other fibrotic disorders, traction emphysema of alveoli adjacent to stellate scars and peribronchiolar fibrotic rings are commonly observed, which contributes to the cystic appearance of the tissue.

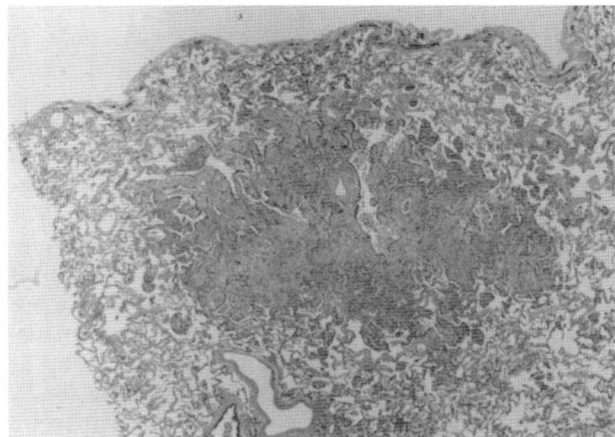

Figure 28–1 Lung biopsy specimen from a patient with pulmonary Langerhans cell histiocytosis under low magnification microscopy demonstrating a typical bronchiolocentric stellate/nodular lesion (hematoxylin and eosin ×100 original magnification). (Specimen provided by Dr. T Colby, Mayo Clinic, Scottsdale.)

Involvement of accompanying vascular structures is common. In one study, vascular medial thickening was found in 82% of biopsy specimens.[18] Interestingly, in the same study, 70% of biopsy specimens demonstrated vascular mural inflammation consisting predominantly of lymphocytes and occasionally eosinophils and plasma cells.[18]

PLCH is sometimes confused with DIP because of accumulation of microphages in adjacent airspaces.[12,55] These changes are common in PLCH and are reflective of the spectrum of varying degrees of lung injury that may be encountered in the same individual exposed to cigarette smoke.[16] The pseudo-DIP reaction may be so extensive as to overshadow the bronchiolar lesions of PLCH. Indeed, we have observed patients with high-resolution computed tomography (HRCT) evidence of an alveolar filling process who were eventually found to have PLCH on open lung biopsy, which was accompanied by extensive involvement with DIP-like changes. Thus the possibility of PLCH should be considered in any biopsy specimen that suggests DIP. Other histologic entities that may sometimes be confused with PLCH include usual interstitial pneumonia, bronchiolitis obliterans, eosinophilic pneumonia, eosinophilic pleuritis, pulmonary lymphoma, and nonspecific scars and subpleural blebs.[12]

Sampling error is another problem in the histologic diagnosis of PLCH. This is a significant problem with the transbronchial biopsy approach for histologic diagnosis due to the focal nature of the lesions. In addition, due to the focal nature of the process, lesions may not be present in every biopsy, and cases may be missed or misdiagnosed depending on how careful and meticulous the pathologic examination is. For this reason, experienced pathologists recommend that the possibility of PLCH be considered in all cases of interstitial lung disease in which biopsy findings are either normal or nondiagnostic.

CLINICAL FEATURES

Patients with PLCH have several clinical presentations. Review of the published literature suggests that up to a third of patients are asymptomatic at the time of diagnosis and present to the pulmonologist because of incidental abnormalities found on chest radiography [although our experience is that only about 15% of patients are truly asymptomatic at the time of diagnosis; unpublished observation].[13,17,21] When symptomatic, most individuals with PLCH complain of a nonproductive cough and dyspnea on exertion (see Table 28–2). A substantial proportion of patients (approximately a third) complain of constitutional symptoms such as weight loss (up to 20 to 30 pounds), fever, night sweats, and anorexia. Presentation with a spontaneous pneumothorax is considered a classic presentation, although it occurs only in 10 to 15% of patients at the time of initial diagnosis. Pleuritic pain and recurrent pneumothorax may be encountered in 20 to 25% of patients during the course of the disease. Some patients also complain of severe chest wall pain, which may be unrelated to rib involvement with disease or prior pneumothorax. Hemoptysis is infrequent and is reported in less than 5% of patients in most series (see Table 28–2). The occurrence of hemoptysis in an adult with PLCH may indicate the development of a fungus ball in a cavity or the development of bronchogenic carcinoma.

In addition to the symptoms as secondary to respiratory tract involvement, approximately 15% of adults with PLCH also report symptoms related to the involvement of other organ systems. These include pain due to bony involvement; polyuria and polydipsia as a consequence of hypothalamic involvement (with diabetes insipidus); skin rashes due to cutaneous LCH; adenopathy from superficial lymph node involvement, a mass in the neck due to involvement of the thyroid gland; and abdominal discomfort due to infiltration of the liver and spleen.

The physical examination is generally unremarkable.[13,21] Finger clubbing is unusual, and auscultation of the chest is often normal, although may at times reveal evidence of airflow limitation.[13] There are no diagnostically useful serum biochemical or hematologic tests, and most individuals with PLCH have normal hematologic indices (including circulating eosinophil counts) and serum angiotensin converting enzyme levels. A proportion of patients will have a modest elevation of the sedimentation rate, and, very occasionally, a sedimentation rate greater than 100 mm/h occurs in this disease [unpublished observation]. The presence of low titers of various autoantibodies and circulating immune complexes have been reported but are of no diagnostic significance.[58]

DIAGNOSTIC STUDIES

Chest Radiography

The chest radiograph (CXR) is abnormal in most patients with PLCH. In the early stages, bilateral, poorly demarcated micronodular or reticulonodular interstitial infiltrates with sparing of the lung bases are characteristic (Figure 28–2).[13,17,21,59] Cystic changes may be found, either as the predominant finding or more commonly superimposed on a background of reticular/nodular changes.[60] In the later stages, nodular lesions tend to be less frequent and cystic changes become more prominent. Contiguous cystic cavities (up to 2 cm in size) may occur in advanced stages of PLCH resulting in a radiographic appearance that is indistinguishable from that seen with advanced emphysema or lymphangioleiomyomatosis (LAM). The finding of cystic change on the CXR should always prompt the clinician to think of PLCH as one cause. Honeycombing (multiple ring shadows 5 to 10 mm in diameter) is often seen on the CXR.[13,60]

Lung volumes as judged by the CXR tend to be normal or increased, even in the presence of extensive parenchymal abnormalities, a finding that is helpful in distinguishing PLCH from other interstitial lung diseases, which are commonly associated with reduced lung volumes.[13,59,60] The costophrenic angles are typically spared in PLCH, and their involvement has been suggested to portend an adverse prognosis.[60]

Rarely, PLCH can present as a solitary pulmonary nodule on the CXR.[61–63] In three reported cases of PLCH presenting as a solitary nodule, the affected individuals were smokers, did not complain of any pulmonary symptoms at the time of diagnosis, and remained free of radiographic interstitial lung involvement on follow-up that ranged from 2[61] to 24 years.[62] Although in the series by Friedman and colleagues, 8 out of 100 patients had evidence of pleural involvement on CXR,[13] in our experience, pleural involvement and effusions are very uncommon in PLCH. In a retrospective review of 102 adults with PLCH, we identified only one case of pleural effusion that was identified on the chest radiograph [unpublished observation]. Other unusual chest radiographic findings reported include alveolar infiltrates, prominent pulmonary arteries,[13] and hilar adenopathy.[64] Very infrequently, the CXR may also be normal.[65]

High-Resolution Computed Tomography

High-resolution CT scan of the chest is very useful for this diagnosis. HRCT is helpful in providing the radiographic correlate of the changes seen on surgical lung biopsy.[66] HRCT is also useful to assist the surgeon in choosing an optimal site for the lung biopsy. Several descriptive studies illustrate the utility of HRCT diagnostically for delineating the nodules and cysts that often have a characteristic appearance and distribution.[66–72] Similar to histopathology, the HRCT findings are dictated by the course of the disease.

Early on, the most common finding is that of small nodules, some showing cavitation.[72] They vary from a few millimeters to 2 cm in size.[71] As the disease progresses, cystic changes predominate, and in advanced disease, cystic change, fibrosis, and honeycombing tend to supervene.[72] In a number of patients the HRCT demonstrates both nodular and cystic changes occurring predominantly in a middle and upper lobe distribution (Figure 28–3) with sparing of the lung bases.[59,69–71,73,74] Although the combination of cystic and nodular changes is most frequently described as the classic changes associated with PLCH, the most frequent CT abnormality reported in the published literature is the presence of lung cysts, which are generally (but not always) less than 20 mm in size and typically have a thin (1 mm or less) wall.[18,69–72,75,76] The cysts seen in PLCH are often bizarre shaped unlike the more uniform cystic abnormalities seen in LAM.

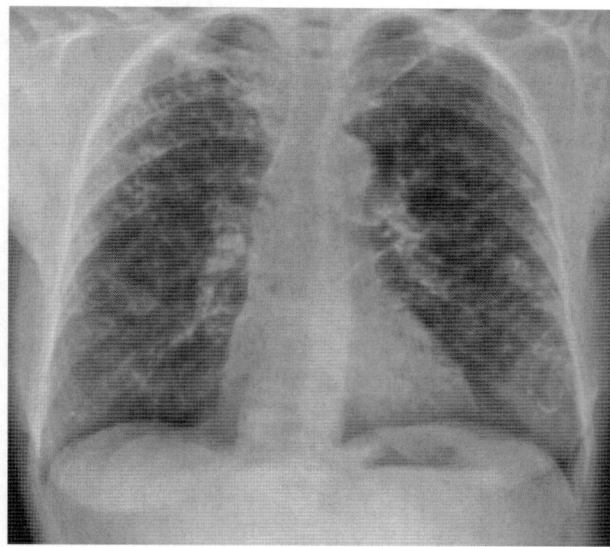

Figure 28–2   Chest radiograph in pulmonary Langerhans cell histiocytosis. 46-year-old smoker who complained of a cough. Chest radiograph demonstrated bilateral nodular and reticular infiltrates with upper and middle lobe predominance and sparing of the costophrenic angles.

The pattern of abnormalities on HRCT are useful for diagnosis, and, in a substantial proportion of cases, the combination of cystic lesions and nodules with sparing of the lung bases results in a radiographic pattern that is so characteristic of PLCH that a presumptive diagnosis of PLCH may be established.[70] When the HRCT shows these changes and the radiologist is confident of the diagnosis, our practice is to avoid further invasive testing with lung biopsy unless a definitive diagnosis is required.

In addition to lung cysts and nodules, other radiographic findings are seen and may cause diagnostic confusion with other conditions. Ground-glass attenuation may be observed in a proportion of patients with PLCH.[71] Although in most cases the presence of ground-glass infiltrates are discreet and do not obscure the more classic changes, rarely the extent of ground-glass attenuation may be sufficiently extensive to render the radiographic picture similar to hypersensitivity pneumonitis, bronchiolitis obliterans with obstructing pneumonia (BOOP), or chronic eosinophilic pneumonia [unpublished observations] Similarly, mild mediastinal or paratracheal adenopathy may be detected on the HRCT in one-third of cases [unpublished observations] and may present diagnostic confusion with sarcoidosis.

Pulmonary Function Testing and Exercise Physiology

Pulmonary function testing (PFT) should be performed in all individuals suspected or known to have PLCH because helpful prognostic indicators can be found on spirometry and lung volume measurement at the time of diagnosis.[77] A variety of abnormalities in pulmonary function testing have been described (see Table 28–2). PFTs are either normal or demonstrate obstructive, restrictive, or mixed abnormalities depending on when the test is performed during the course of the disease.[13,18,77,78] The most consistent abnormality reported in the literature is a reduction in the diffusing capacity of carbon monoxide (DL_{CO}), which occurs in about two-thirds of patients at the time of diagnosis.[17,18,78] The degree of impairment in DL_{CO} appears to correlate with the limitation in exercise performance.[78] Crausman and colleagues reported on 23 adult patients with PLCH who presented with either normal or predominantly restrictive pulmonary physiology.[78] In contrast, a combination of both restrictive and obstructive physiology has been reported in other studies, with the predominant abnormality being obstruction.[13,18,77] We recently reviewed 81 PFT studies performed in our institution on adults with PCLH within 6 months of diagnosis and found restriction in 45.7%, obstruction in 27.2%, mixed abnormalities in 4.9%, isolated reduction in diffusing capacity in 8.6%, and normal findings in 13.6% [Vassallo and colleagues, manuscript in preparation].

Just as variable PFT patterns may be seen in the initial stages of disease, advanced disease may also be accompanied by a variable expression of physiologic impairment. Some patients develop predominantly cystic and bullous disease at the late stages, which results in air trapping, increased lung volumes, increased residual volume/total lung capacity (RV/TLC) ratios, and variable degrees of obstruction.[13,21] Others may develop severe honeycombing and fibrotic changes, which result in severe restriction with decreased lung volumes.

Although the physiologic changes are nonspecific, the finding of obstructive physiology together with a reduced DL_{CO} in a patient with interstitial infiltrates on the chest radiograph should suggest the possibility of PLCH. PFTs are also useful for follow-up and monitoring of disease progression in PLCH. Monitoring the change in forced expiratory volume and DL_{CO} may prove to be useful as prognostic markers.[77]

Patients with PCLH also have reduced exercise capacity. Exercise testing indicates strong correlation between overall exercise performance and indices of vascular involvement such as DL_{CO} and baseline and exercise dead-space volume/tidal volume (VD/VT), suggesting that the exercise impairment commonly found in these patients reflects pulmonary vascular dysfunction rather than abnormalities in ventilatory function or gas exchange.[78]

Role of Brochoscopy, Bronchoalveolar Lavage, Transbronchoscopic Biospy, and Surgical Lung Biopsy

Surgical lung biopsy is considered the gold standard for the diagnosis of PLCH. However, it is possible to establish a diagnosis of PLCH using less invasive measures

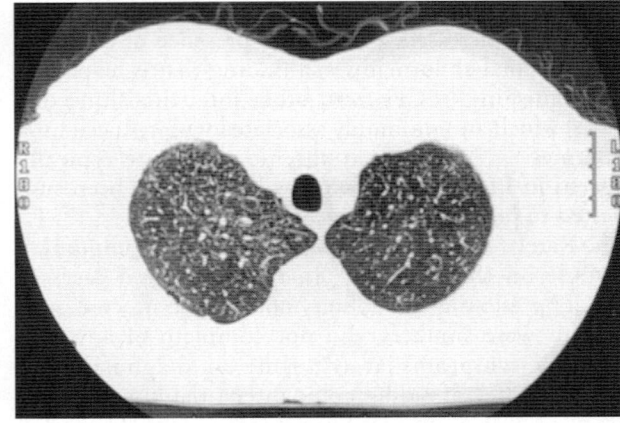

A

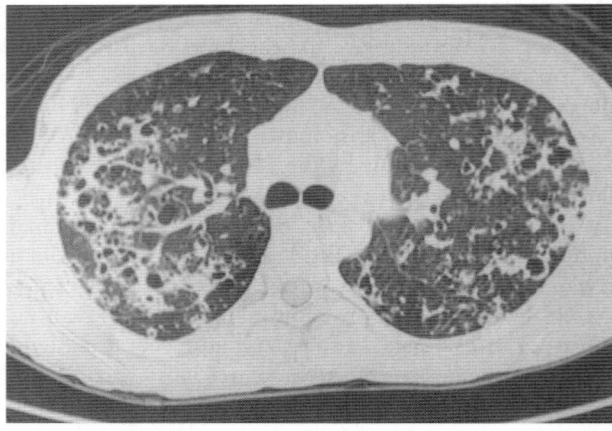

B

C

Figure 28–3 High-resolution computed tomography (HRCT) findings in pulmonary Langerhans cell histiocytosis. A, A 61-year-old white male with a 50- to 60-pack-year history of cigarette smoking. He complained of a dry cough, fatigue, and weight loss. HRCT revealed numerous tiny miliary nodules throughout both lungs. Cystic change was not identified. B, A 46-year-old white male smoker who complained of a very mild cough at presentation. HRCT shows multiple thick-walled cystic lesions associated with nodularity. C, A 35-year-old woman with a 20-pack-year history of smoking presented with intractable cough. HRCT showed multiple cystic spaces and nodular infiltrates that follow a bronchovascular distribution.

(Figure 28–4). Bronchoscopy with transbronchoscopic lung biopsy (TBLB) has a low yield (10 to 40%).[18,55,79] This is in part due to the patchy nature of the disease and an insufficient amount of tissue obtained. It is not clear whether staining of TBLB specimens with antibodies to CD1a improves the yield, although one study suggests that little is added by immunostaining of tissue.[55] TBLB may prove useful by providing an alternative diagnosis in individuals with suspected PLCH, such as sarcoidosis, hypersensitivity pneumonitis, infections, or LAM. It is possible that the risk of pneumothorax complicating TBLB is higher in these patients due to cystic lung disease, although there are no data in the literature to support this.

Bronchoalveolar lavage (BAL) should be considered in all patients suspected of having PCLH. The total number of cells recovered in BAL fluid is typically increased, as expected in smokers. A reduction in the CD4/CD8 ratio of T cells and an increase in eosinophil counts have also been reported, but these findings are inconsistent and nonspecific.[80] The diagnosis of PLCH may be established by detecting increased numbers of CD1a positive cells (Langerhans' cells) in both children and adults with PCLH (see Figure 28–4).[81–84] Although the percentage of BAL Langerhans' cells needed to establish a diagnosis is unknown, it is generally accepted that levels of CD1a positive BAL cells of 5% or greater render PLCH very likely in the appropriate clinical setting.[19,81–84] We and others believe that a cutoff of 5% is required for a presumptive diagnosis of PLCH rather than 3%, because increased numbers of CD1a positive cells may be detected in the BAL fluid of heavy smokers without disease and have also been reported in patients with other interstitial lung diseases.[19,85,86] In our experience, few patients are found with greater than 5% CD1a positive cells in the BAL fluid (ie, the sensitivity of this test using this cutoff is low), and, in the majority of cases, an indeterminate elevation (2 to 5%) in CD1a positive cells is found.

Diagnostic Evaluation

Pulmonary Langerhans cell histiocytosis should be considered in the differential diagnosis of any smoker presenting for evaluation of lung infiltrates, especially if the

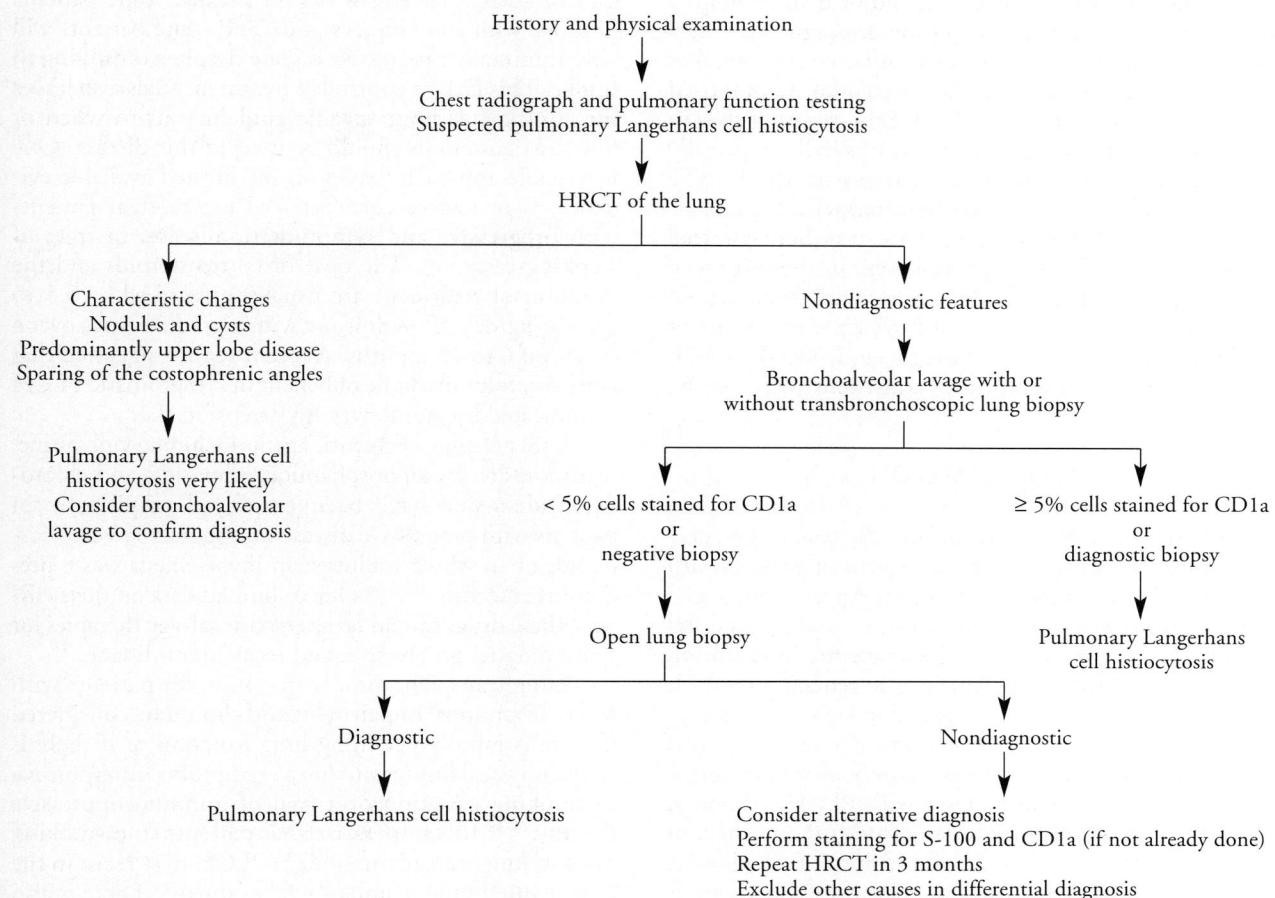

Figure 28–4 Suggested diagnostic algorithm for the evaluation of patients with suspected pulmonary Langerhans cell histiocytosis. HRCT = high-resolution computed tomography; S-100 = protein expressed by histiocytes. Reproduced with permission from Vassallo R et al.[32]

infiltrates occur predominantly in an upper lobe distribution and spare the lung bases. Although there are no specific clues in the history or physical examination, the absence of a history of cigarette smoking, age greater than 65 years, and the presence of basilar crackles on physical examination render the diagnosis of PLCH unlikely. A number of clinical scenarios should alert the clinician to the possibility of PLCH as a diagnosis. These include the history of a spontaneous pneumothorax in any smoker with lung infiltrates, the presence of diffuse bilateral lung infiltrates in a smoker with minimal symptoms (chest radiograph looking much worse than anticipated from the history), the presence of cysts on the chest radiograph, the presence of upper lobe predominant infiltrates on chest radiography, bilateral lung infiltrates with evidence of obstruction on pulmonary function testing, and any individual with a history of diabetes insipidus or skin rash who also presents with bilateral lung infiltrates. Although the disease may mimic other lung diseases, the main differential diagnostic considerations include sarcoidosis, silicosis, hypersensitivity pneumonia, vasculitides, and LAM.

HRCT is the most useful noninvasive test in the evaluation of patients with suspected PCLH (see Figure 28–4). The presence of typical changes on the HRCT scan render the diagnosis almost certain and, in many situations, obviate the need for surgical lung biopsy. Bronchoscopy and BAL rarely provide diagnostic information but are useful to rule out other conditions that are frequently considered in the differential. As discussed previously, the finding of ≥ 5% CD1a–staining cells in the BAL fluid is virtually diagnostic of PLCH, especially if associated with compatible changes on the HRCT scan. Surgical lung biopsy may be necessary if the HRCT scan or BAL/TBLB is nondiagnostic or if there is a need to establish a definitive diagnosis (eg, in the setting of transplant evaluation). In the patient with documented Langerhans cell histiocytosis and systemic involvement (such as skin or bone), the diagnosis is usually established if HRCT shows features consistent with PLCH.

TREATMENT

Due to the rarity of the disease and the lack of prospective controlled studies, the management of patients with PLCH has traditionally been based on expert opinion, evidence from retrospective studies, and anecdotal reports.[17,87] To date, there is no therapeutic intervention shown prospectively to be effective in reducing morbidity or mortality. Because of this, and in view of the strong association with cigarette smoking, it is recommended that smoking cessation be the first component of the management strategy for all patients with PLCH. Although there are no controlled trials demonstrating the effect of smoking cessation on the natural history of the disease, several lines of evidence indicate that this intervention is critical. Abstinence from tobacco leads to stabilization of symptoms in many patients, and, in a substantial proportion of patients, smoking cessation alone represents the only intervention required for improvement or stabilization of symptoms.[23,88] Indeed, some reports document objective radiographic and physiologic improvement in lung function following smoking cessation.[23,89] This is not the case for all individuals with PLCH, and there are clearly some patients who develop progressive disease in spite of smoking cessation, and, conversely, some patients tend to be minimally symptomatic and suffer little progression of disease in spite of continued smoking. In addition to beneficial effects on the course of PLCH, smoking cessation is essential to limit the progression of any accompanying obstructive airway disease and the eventual risk of development of lung carcinoma, which may be more prevalent in these individuals.[90]

Corticosteroids have been the primary pharmacologic agent used in the management of PLCH, in spite of limited data supporting their efficacy.[13,17] The evidence in favor of corticosteroid use in PLCH comes from retrospective studies and case reports that indicated symptomatic or radiographic improvement following a therapeutic trial of corticosteroids.[13,17] Unfortunately, there are no prospective or randomized trials that compare the efficacy of corticosteroid treatment to smoking cessation alone. For this reason, it is difficult to establish the efficacy of corticosteroids in PLCH because some patients improve with smoking cessation and some patients will have minimally progressive disease despite continuing to smoke. This lack of controlled treatment trials also leaves the clinician without specific guidelines as to when or how corticosteroids should be used in this disease. One reasonable approach, based on the limited available evidence, is to reserve corticosteroid use to treat patients with progressive and symptomatic disease, in spite of smoking cessation. The dose of corticosteroids and the duration of treatment are usually prescribed at 0.5 to 1.0 mg/kg/day of prednisone with a gradual taper over a period of 6 to 12 months. A recent report suggested that corticosteroids might be of benefit in symptomatic PLCH complicated by pulmonary hypertension.[91]

Other chemotherapeutic agents including vinblastine, methotrexate, cyclophosphamide, etoposide, and chlorodeoxyadenosine have been employed empirically in patients with progressive disease unresponsive to corticosteroids or in which multisystem involvement was a predominant feature.[10,92–94] Due to limited data on their efficacy, these drugs should be reserved as salvage therapies for symptomatic, progressive, and recalcitrant disease.

Lung transplantation is an option for patients with severe respiratory impairment and should be considered if there is rapidly declining lung function or if there is severe physical limitation due to symptoms unresponsive to smoking cessation or a trial of immunosuppressive therapy.[95–98] It is imperative that patients stop smoking prior to lung transplantation, as PLCH may recur in the transplanted lung if smoking is resumed.[24] There is also a report of recurrence of PCLH in the transplanted lung, in spite of presumed abstinence from tobacco use.[94,99]

Pneumothoraces are managed in a standard fashion, although pleurectomy is generally avoided in patients for whom lung transplantation is an option. Similarly, the development of cor pulmonale is managed in a standard fashion with diuretics. There is no specific treatment for the pulmonary hypertension that frequently accompanies advanced forms of the disease.[100] The responsiveness of this form of pulmonary hypertension to prostacyclin or other vasodilators is not known, although it is reasonable to consider anticoagulation in all patients with moderate to severe pulmonary hypertension.

Outcomes and Prognosis

Definitive longitudinal information on patient outcomes in PLCH is limited. Patients who are asymptomatic at presentation seem to have the best prognosis, with some reports indicating spontaneous resolution of radiographic abnormalities without any specific treatment.[13,21] These patients constitute a minority of affected individuals. Generally speaking, retrospective studies imply that the majority of patients afflicted with PLCH demonstrate some improvement or only minimal progression over time.[12,13,21] More recent studies suggest that the outcomes of adults with PLCH may be worse than previously suggested and a substantial proportion of patients die prematurely from this disease.[77] As mentioned previously, the role of smoking cessation or immunosuppressive therapy on the course of disease or outcomes is not known. Although a substantial proportion seem to improve or stabilize, there are patients who develop progressive disease resulting in substantial respiratory impairment and premature mortality from respiratory failure. We and others have also observed occasional cases of PLCH that progress relatively slowly over several decades.

A variety of factors have been associated with adverse clinical outcome including: extremes of age, multisystem involvement, prolonged constitutional disturbance, extensive cysts and honeycombing on CXR, markedly reduced diffusing capacity, low forced expiratory volume in 1 second/forced vital capacity (FEV_1/FVC) ratio, corticosteroid therapy at time of follow-up, and a high RV/TLC ratio.[21,77] Although collectively these factors may be helpful to identify patients at risk of poor outcomes, their use is limited due to the lack of effective therapeutic options.

Due to the lack of longitudinal studies, the incidence of respiratory failure, pulmonary hypertension, and cor pulmonale related to PLCH is unknown. The incidence of these complications is likely more common than previously thought. A pulmonary vasculopathy occurs in virtually all patients with advanced PLCH and is associated with severe pulmonary hypertension.[100,101] The management of pulmonary hypertension is unknown, but anecdotal reports suggest that there may be a significant response to corticosteroid therapy.[91] A

proportion of patients develop progressive disease with respiratory failure. It is difficult to determine how many patients with PLCH progress to respiratory failure because a proportion of these patients have associated emphysema due to long-standing tobacco abuse.

The effect of pregnancy on lung function of women with PLCH has never been reported. Anecdotally, complete remission of cutaneous and lymph node involvement by LCH during pregnancy has been reported.[102] Opinion seems to indicate that in the absence of significant respiratory impairment, PLCH is not a contraindication to pregnancy.[103]

Several case reports and series describe a variety of neoplasms in association with adult and childhood LCH, including lymphoma, multiple myeloma, myelodysplastic syndrome, adenocarcinoma of the lung, and a variety of solid organ cancers.[90,104-113] The increased prevalence of malignant neoplasms in patients with LCH may reflect heavy cigarette smoking, the use of chemotherapeutic agents to treat LCH, or inherent chromosomal or genetic abnormalities. We have observed that adults with PLCH have a substantially increased prevalence of malignant hematologic cancers, especially myeloproliferative disorders, although we were unable to demonstrate a significant increase in lung cancer prevalence. These cancers may either predate or occur after the diagnosis of LCH. It is important for clinicians to recognize this association due to implications in follow-up and counseling of these patients.

REFERENCES

1. Cline MJ. Histiocytes and histiocytosis. Blood 1994;84: 2840–53.
2. Nezelof C, Barbey S. Histiocytosis: nosology and pathobiology. Pediatr Pathol 1985;3:1–41.
3. Lampert F. Langerhans cell histiocytosis. Historical perspectives. Hematol Oncol Clin North Am 1998;12:213–9.
4. Nezelof C, Basset F, Rousseau MF. Histiocytosis X histogenetic arguments for a Langerhans cell origin. Biomedicine 1973;18:365–71.
5. Berry DH, Becton DL. Natural history of histiocytosis-X. Hematol Oncol Clin North Am 1987;1:23–34.
6. Baumgartner I, von Hochstetter A, Baumert B, et al. Langerhans'-cell histiocytosis in adults. Med Pediatr Oncol 1997;28:9–14.
7. Favara BE, Feller AC, Pauli M, et al. Contemporary classification of histiocytic disorders. The WHO Committee On Histiocytic/Reticulum Cell Proliferations. Reclassification Working Group of the Histiocyte Society. Med Pediatr Oncol 1997;29:157–66.
8. Malpas JS, Norton AJ. Langerhans cell histiocytosis in the adult. Med Pediatr Oncol 1996;27:540–6.
9. Malpas JS. Langerhans cell histiocytosis in adults. Hematol Oncol Clin North Am 1998;12:259–68.
10. Giona F, Caruso R, Testi AM, et al. Langerhans' cell histiocytosis in adults: a clinical and therapeutic analysis of 11 patients from a single institution. Cancer 1997;80:1786–91.
11. Howarth DM, Gilchrist GS, Mullan BP, et al. Langerhans cell histiocytosis: diagnosis, natural history, management, and outcome. Cancer 1999;85:2278–90.
12. Colby TV, Lombard C. Histiocytosis X in the lung. Hum Pathol 1983;14:847–56.

13. Friedman PJ, Liebow AA, Sokoloff J. Eosinophilic granuloma of lung. Clinical aspects of primary histiocytosis in the adult. Medicine (Baltimore) 1981;60:385–96.

14. Carlson RA, Hattery RR, O'Connell EJ, Fontana RS. Pulmonary involvement by histiocytosis X in the pediatric age group. Mayo Clin Proc 1976;51:542–7.

15. Gaensler EA, Carrington CB. Open biopsy for chronic diffuse infiltrative lung disease: clinical, roentgenographic, and physiological correlations in 502 patients. Ann Thorac Surg 1980;30:411–26.

16. Ryu JH, Colby TV, Hartman TE, Vassallo R. Smoking-related interstitial lung diseases: a concise review. Eur Respir J 2001;17:122–32.

17. Schonfeld N, Frank W, Wenig S, et al. Clinical and radiologic features, lung function and therapeutic results in pulmonary histiocytosis X. Respiration 1993;60:38–44.

18. Travis WD, Borok Z, Roum JH, et al. Pulmonary Langerhans cell granulomatosis (histiocytosis X). A clinicopathologic study of 48 cases. Am J Surg Pathol 1993;17:971–86.

19. Tazi A, Soler P, Hance AJ. Adult pulmonary Langerhans' cell histiocytosis. Thorax 2000;55:405–16.

20. Lewis J. Eosinophilic granuloma and its variants with special reference to lung involvement. QJM 1964;33:337–59.

21. Basset F, Corrin B, Spencer H, et al. Pulmonary histiocytosis X. Am Rev Respir Dis 1978;118:811–20.

22. Bernstrand C, Cederlund K, Ashtrom L, Henter JI. Smoking preceded pulmonary involvement in adults with Langerhans cell histiocytosis diagnosed in childhood. Acta Paediatr 2000;89:1389–92.

23. Mogulkoc N, Veral A, Bishop PW, et al. Pulmonary Langerhans' cell histiocytosis: radiologic resolution following smoking cessation. Chest 1999;115:1452–5.

24. Etienne B, Bertocchi M, Gamondes JP, et al. Relapsing pulmonary Langerhans cell histiocytosis after lung transplantation. Am J Respir Crit Care Med 1998;157:288–91.

25. Arico M, Nichols K, Whitlock JA, et al. Familial clustering of Langerhans cell histiocytosis. Br J Haematol 1999;107: 883–8.

26. Hirsch MS, Hong CK. Familial pulmonary histiocytosis-X. Am Rev Respir Dis 1973;107:831–5.

27. Shapiro DN, Hutchinson RJ. Familial histiocytosis in offspring of two pregnancies after artificial insemination. N Engl J Med 1981;304:757–9.

28. Galy A, Travis M, Cen D, Chen B. Human T, B, natural killer, and dendritic cells arise from a common bone marrow progenitor cell subset. Immunity 1995;3:459–73.

29. Banchereau J, Steinman RM. Dendritic cells and the control of immunity. Nature 1998;392:245–52.

30. Banchereau J, Briere F, Caux C, et al. Immunobiology of dendritic cells. Annu Rev Immunol 2000;18:767–811.

31. Holt PG, Haining S, Nelson DJ, Sedgwick JD. Origin and steady-state turnover of class II MHC-bearing dendritic cells in the epithelium of the conducting airways. J Immunol 1994;153:256–61.

32. Vassallo R, Ryu JH, Colby TV, et al. Pulmonary Langerhans'-cell histiocytosis. N Engl J Med 2000;342:1969–78.

33. de Graaf JH, Tamminga RY, Dam-Meiring A, et al. The presence of cytokines in Langerhans' cell histiocytosis. J Pathol 1996;180:400–6.

34. Kannourakis G, Abbas A. The role of cytokines in the pathogenesis of Langerhans cell histiocytosis. Br J Cancer Suppl 1994;23:S37–40.

35. Tazi A, Moreau J, Bergeron A, et al. Evidence that Langerhans cells in adult pulmonary Langerhans cell histiocytosis are mature dendritic cells: importance of the cytokine microenvironment. J Immunol 1999;163:3511–5.

36. Tazi A, Bonay M, Bergeron A, et al. Role of granulocyte-macrophage colony stimulating factor (GM-CSF) in the pathogenesis of adult pulmonary histiocytosis X. Thorax 1996;51:611–4.

37. Asakura S, Colby TV, Limper AH. Tissue localization of transforming growth factor-beta1 in pulmonary eosinophilic granuloma. Am J Respir Crit Care Med 1996;154: 1525–30.

38. Letterio JJ, Roberts AB. Regulation of immune responses by TGF-beta. Annu Rev Immunol 1998;16:137–61.

39. Jaksits S, Kriehuber E, Charbonnier AS, et al. CD34+ cell-derived CD14+ precursor cells develop into Langerhans cells in a TGF-beta 1-dependent manner. J Immunol 1999;163:4869–77.

40. Aguayo SM, Kane MA, King TE Jr, et al. Increased levels of bombesin-like peptides in the lower respiratory tract of asymptomatic cigarette smokers. J Clin Invest 1989;84: 1105–13.

41. Aguayo SM, King TE Jr, Kane MA, et al. Urinary levels of bombesin-like peptides in asymptomatic cigarette smokers: a potential risk marker for smoking-related diseases. Cancer Res 1992;52:2727S–31S.

42. Del Rio M, Hernanz A, de la Fuente M. Bombesin, gastrin-releasing peptide, and neuromedin C modulate murine lymphocyte proliferation through adherent accessory cells and activate protein kinase C. Peptides 1994;15:15–22.

43. Lemaire I. Bombesin-related peptides modulate interleukin–1 production by alveolar macrophages. Neuropeptides 1991;20:217–23.

44. Aguayo SM, King TE Jr, Waldron JA Jr, et al. Increased pulmonary neuroendocrine cells with bombesin-like immunoreactivity in adult patients with eosinophilic granuloma. J Clin Invest 1990;86:838–44.

45. Piguet PF, Vesin C, Thomas F. Bombesin down modulates pulmonary fibrosis elicited in mice by bleomycin. Exp Lung Res 1995;21:227–37.

46. Youkeles LH, Grizzanti JN, Liao Z, et al. Decreased tobacco-glycoprotein-induced lymphocyte proliferation in vitro in pulmonary eosinophilic granuloma. Am J Respir Crit Care Med 1995;151:145–50.

47. Francus T, Klein RF, Staiano-Coico L, et al. Effects of tobacco glycoprotein (TGP) on the immune system. II. TGP stimulates the proliferation of human T cells and the differentiation of human B cells into Ig secreting cells [published erratum appears in J Immunol 1988;140:4413]. J Immunol 1988;140:1823–9.

48. Francus T, Manzo G, Canki M, et al. Two peaks of interleukin 1 expression in human leukocytes cultured with tobacco glycoprotein. J Exp Med 1989;170:327–32.

49. Hirose M, Saito S, Yoshimoto T, Kuroda Y. Interleukin-2 therapy of Langerhans cell histiocytosis. Acta Paediatr 1995;84:1204–6.

50. Wu WS, McClain KL. DNA polymorphisms and mutations of the tumor necrosis factor-alpha (TNF- alpha) promoter in Langerhans cell histiocytosis (LCH). J Interferon Cytokine Res 1997;17:631–5.

51. Willman CL. Detection of clonal histiocytes in Langerhans cell histiocytosis: biology and clinical significance. Br J Cancer Suppl 1994;23:S29–33.

52. Willman CL, Busque L, Griffith BB, et al. Langerhans'-cell histiocytosis (histiocytosis X)—a clonal proliferative disease [see comments]. N Engl J Med 1994;331:154–60.

53. Yu RC, Chu C, Buluwela L, Chu AC. Clonal proliferation of Langerhans cells in Langerhans cell histiocytosis. Lancet 1994;343:767–8.

54. Yousem SA, Colby TV, Chen YY, et al. Pulmonary Langerhans' cell histiocytosis: molecular analysis of clonality. Am J Surg Pathol 2001;25:630–6.

55. Housini I, Tomashefski JF Jr, Cohen A, et al. Transbronchial biopsy in patients with pulmonary eosinophilic granuloma. Comparison with findings on open lung biopsy. Arch Pathol Lab Med 1994;118:523–30.

56. Tazi A, Bonay M, Grandsaigne M, et al. Surface phenotype of Langerhans cells and lymphocytes in granulomatous

lesions from patients with pulmonary histiocytosis X. Am Rev Respir Dis 1993;147:1531–6.

57. Chu T, Jaffe R. The normal Langerhans cell and the LCH cell. Br J Cancer Suppl 1994;23:S4–10.

58. King TE Jr, Schwarz MI, Dreisin RE, et al. Circulating immune complexes in pulmonary eosinophilic granuloma. Ann Intern Med 1979;91:397–9.

59. Moore AD, Godwin JD, Muller NL, et al. Pulmonary histiocytosis X: comparison of radiographic and CT findings. Radiology 1989;172:249–54.

60. Lacronique J, Roth C, Battesti JP, et al. Chest radiological features of pulmonary histiocytosis X: a report based on 50 adult cases. Thorax 1982;37:104–9.

61. Fichtenbaum CJ, Kleinman GM, Haddad RG. Eosinophilic granuloma of the lung presenting as a solitary pulmonary nodule. Thorax 1990;45:905–6.

62. Khoor A, Myers JL, Tazelaar HD, Swensen SJ. Pulmonary Langerhans cell histiocytosis presenting as a solitary nodule. Mayo Clin Proc 2001;76:209–11.

63. ten Velde GP, Thunnissen FB, van Engelshoven JM, Wouters EF. A solitary pulmonary nodule due to eosinophilic granuloma. Eur Respir J 1994;7:1539–40.

64. Pomeranz SJ, Proto AV. Histiocytosis X. Unusual-confusing features of eosinophilic granuloma. Chest 1986;89:88–92.

65. Epler GR, McLoud TC, Gaensler EA, et al. Normal chest roentgenograms in chronic diffuse infiltrative lung disease. N Engl J Med 1978;298:934–9.

66. Soler P, Bergeron A, Kambouchner M, et al. Is high-resolution computed tomography a reliable tool to predict the histopathological activity of pulmonary Langerhans cell histiocytosis? Am J Respir Crit Care Med 2000;162:264–70.

67. Kulwiec EL, Lynch DA, Aguayo SM, et al. Imaging of pulmonary histiocytosis X. Radiographics 1992;12:515–26.

68. Seely JM, Effmann EL, Muller NL. High-resolution CT of pediatric lung disease: imaging findings. AJR Am J Roentgenol 1997;168:1269–75.

69. Webb WR. High-resolution computed tomography of obstructive lung disease. Radiol Clin North Am 1994;32:745–57.

70. Bonelli FS, Hartman TE, Swensen SJ, Sherrick A. Accuracy of high-resolution CT in diagnosing lung diseases. AJR Am J Roentgenol 1998;170:1507–12.

71. Brauner MW, Grenier P, Mouelhi MM, et al. Pulmonary histiocytosis X: evaluation with high-resolution CT. Radiology 1989;172:255–8.

72. Brauner MW, Grenier P, Tijani K, et al. Pulmonary Langerhans cell histiocytosis: evolution of lesions on CT scans [see comments]. Radiology 1997;204:497–502.

73. Bergin CJ, Coblentz CL, Chiles C, et al. Chronic lung diseases: specific diagnosis by using CT. AJR Am J Roentgenol 1989;152:1183–8.

74. Hartman TE, Tazelaar HD, Swensen SJ, Muller NL. Cigarette smoking: CT and pathologic findings of associated pulmonary diseases. Radiographics 1997;17:377–90.

75. Bernstrand C, Cederlund K, Sandstedt B, et al. Pulmonary abnormalities at long-term follow-up of patients with Langerhans cell histiocytosis. Med Pediatr Oncol 2001;36:459–68.

76. Stern EJ, Webb WR, Golden JA, Gamsu G. Cystic lung disease associated with eosinophilic granuloma and tuberous sclerosis: air trapping at dynamic ultrafast high-resolution CT. Radiology 1992;182:325–9.

77. Delobbe A, Durieu J, Duhamel A, Wallaert B. Determinants of survival in pulmonary Langerhans' cell granulomatosis (histiocytosis X). Groupe d'Etude en Pathologie Interstitielle de la Societe de Pathologie Thoracique du Nord. Eur Respir J 1996;9:2002–6.

78. Crausman RS, Jennings CA, Tuder RM, et al. Pulmonary histiocytosis X: pulmonary function and exercise pathophysiology. Am J Respir Crit Care Med 1996;153:426–35.

79. Vassallo R, Ryu JH, Limper AH. Pulmonary Langerhans cell histiocytosis: a 22 year experience at the Mayo Clinic. Am J Resp Crit Care Med 1999;159:A63.

80. Hance AJ, Basset F, Saumon G, et al. Smoking and interstitial lung disease. The effect of cigarette smoking on the incidence of pulmonary histiocytosis X and sarcoidosis. Ann N Y Acad Sci 1986;465:643–56.

81. Auerswald U, Barth J, Magnussen H. Value of CD-1-positive cells in bronchoalveolar lavage fluid for the diagnosis of pulmonary histiocytosis X. Lung 1991;169:305–9.

82. Chollet S, Soler P, Dournovo P, et al. Diagnosis of pulmonary histiocytosis X by immunodetection of Langerhans cells in bronchoalveolar lavage fluid. Am J Pathol 1984;115:225–32.

83. Danel C, Israel-Biet D, Costabel U, et al. The clinical role of BAL in pulmonary histiocytosis X. Eur Respir J 1990; 3:949–50, 961–9.

84. Xaubet A, Agusti C, Picado C, et al. Bronchoalveolar lavage analysis with anti-T6 monoclonal antibody in the evaluation of diffuse lung diseases. Respiration 1989;56:161–6.

85. Kawanami O, Basset F, Ferrans VJ, et al. Pulmonary Langerhans' cells in patients with fibrotic lung disorders. Lab Invest 1981;44:227–33.

86. Casolaro MA, Bernaudin JF, Saltini C, et al. Accumulation of Langerhans' cells on the epithelial surface of the lower respiratory tract in normal subjects in association with cigarette smoking. Am Rev Respir Dis 1988;137:406–11.

87. Nondahl SR, Finlay JL, Farrell PM, et al. A case report and literature review of "primary" pulmonary histiocytosis X of childhood. Med Pediatr Oncol 1986;14:57–62.

88. Von Essen S, West W, Sitorius M, Rennard SI. Complete resolution of roentgenographic changes in a patient with pulmonary histiocytosis X. Chest 1990;98:765–7.

89. Morimoto T, Matsumura T, Kitaichi M. [Rapid remission of pulmonary eosinophilic granuloma in a young male patient after cessation of smoking]. Nihon Kokyuki Gakkai Zasshi 1999;37:140–5.

90. Lombard CM, Medeiros LJ, Colby TV. Pulmonary histiocytosis X and carcinoma. Arch Pathol Lab Med 1987;111:339–41.

91. Benyounes B, Crestani B, Couvelard A, et al. Steroid-responsive pulmonary hypertension in a patient with Langerhans' cell granulomatosis (histiocytosis X). Chest 1996;110:284–6.

92. Saven A, Burian C. Cladribine activity in adult Langerhans-cell histiocytosis. Blood 1999;93:4125–30.

93. Dimopoulos MA, Theodorakis M, Kostis E, et al. Treatment of Langerhans cell histiocytosis with 2 chlorodeoxyadenosine. Leuk Lymphoma 1997;25:187–9.

94. Gabbay E, Dark JH, Ashcroft T, et al. Recurrence of Langerhans' cell granulomatosis following lung transplantation. Thorax 1998;53:326–7.

95. Egan TM, Detterbeck FC, Keagy BA, et al. Single lung transplantation for eosinophilic granulomatosis. South Med J 1992;85:551–3.

96. Yeatman M, McNeil K, Smith JA, et al. Lung transplantation in patients with systemic diseases: an eleven-year experience at Papworth Hospital. J Heart Lung Transplant 1996;15:144–9.

97. Loire R, Brune J. [Severe late stage lesions of pulmonary histiocytosis X. Report of 3 transplantations]. Rev Mal Respir 1993;10:223–8.

98. Montoya A, Mawulawde K, Houck J, et al. Survival and functional outcome after single and bilateral lung transplantation. Loyola Lung Transplant Team. Surgery 1994;116:712–8.

99. Habib SB, Congleton J, Carr D, et al. Recurrence of recipient Langerhans' cell histiocytosis following bilateral lung transplantation [see comments]. Thorax 1998;53:323–5.

100. Fartoukh M, Humbert M, Capron F, et al. Severe pulmonary hypertension in histiocytosis X. Am J Respir Crit Care Med 2000;161:216–23.

101. Harari S, Brenot F, Barberis M, Simmoneau G. Advanced pulmonary histiocytosis X is associated with severe pulmonary hypertension. Chest 1997;111:1142–4.

102. Scherbaum WA, Seif FJ. Spontaneous transient remission of disseminated histiocytosis X during pregnancy. J Cancer Res Clin Oncol 1995;121:57–60.

103. King TE Jr. Restrictive lung disease in pregnancy. Clin Chest Med 1992;13:607–22.

104. Burns BF, Colby TV, Dorfman RF. Langerhans cell granulomatosis (histiocytosis X) associated with malignant lymphomas. Am J Surg Pathol 1983;7:529–31.

105. Coli A, Bigotti G, Ferrone S. Histiocytosis X arising in Hodgkin's disease: immunophenotypic characterization with a panel of monoclonal antibodies. Virchows Arch A Pathol Anat Histopathol 1991;418:369–73.

106. Egeler RM, Neglia JP, Arico M, et al. The relation of Langerhans cell histiocytosis to acute leukemia, lymphomas, and other solid tumors. Hematol Oncol Clin North Am 1998;12:369–78.

107. Neumann MP, Frizzera G. The coexistence of Langerhans' cell granulomatosis and malignant lymphoma may take different forms: report of seven cases with a review of the literature. Hum Pathol 1986;17:1060–5.

108. Yamashita H, Nagayama M, Kawashima M, et al. Langerhans-cell histiocytosis in an adult patient with multiple myeloma. Clin Exp Dermatol 1992;17:275–8.

109. Surico G, Muggeo P, Rigillo N, Gadner H. Concurrent Langerhans cell histiocytosis and myelodysplasia in children. Med Pediatr Oncol 2000;35:421–5.

110. Churn M, Davies C, Slater A. Synchronous bilateral carcinoma of the breasts occurring in a young woman with a history of Langerhans' cell histiocytosis in infancy. Clin Oncol 1999;11:410–3.

111. Baikian B, Descamps V, Grossin M, et al. [Langerhans cell histiocytosis and myelomonocytic leukemia: a non-fortuitous association]. Ann Dermatol Venereol 1999;126:409–11.

112. Roufosse C, Lespagnard L, Sales F, et al. Langerhans' cell histiocytosis associated with simultaneous lymphocyte predominance Hodgkin's disease and malignant melanoma. Hum Pathol 1998;29:200–1.

113. Sartoris DJ, Resnick D. Myelofibrosis arising in treated histiocytosis X. Eur J Pediatr 1985;144:200–2.

29 LYMPHANGIOLEIOMYOMATOSIS

ARNOLD S. KRISTOF
JOEL MOSS

Lymphangioleiomyomatosis (LAM) is a rare, multi-system disease in which proliferation of abnormal smooth muscle cells leads to cystic lung disease and progressive respiratory failure.[1-4] LAM is also associated with angiomyolipomas primarily found in the kidney, and masses in the axial lymphatics termed lymphangioleiomyomas. In retrospect, the first cases of LAM were described in 1937, when patients with chylous effusion, proliferation of abnormal smooth muscle in the lymph nodes, and honeycomb lung were reported.[5,6] The first comprehensive descriptions of LAM patients were published in 1966 and 1975.[7-9] Several natural history studies and patient registries have since shed more light on the clinical characteristics, etiology, prognosis, and management of patients with LAM.[10-12]

Patients with pulmonary LAM can be grouped into those with sporadic disease or with LAM arising in the presence of tuberous sclerosis complex (TSC), an autosomal-dominant neurocutaneous syndrome resulting from mutations in the *TSC1* or *TSC2* genes. TSC is estimated to occur in 1 in 6,000 to 10,000 live births.[13] It is equally distributed among the genders and characterized by seizure disorder, widespread hamartomatous lesions, and mental retardation.[14] In recent screening studies, one-third of female patients with TSC had evidence of cystic lung disease consistent with the diagnosis of pulmonary LAM.[15-17]

EPIDEMIOLOGY

There are currently approximately 400 known patients with LAM in North America; however, based on a 30% prevalence, at least 7,000 women with TSC would be predicted to have LAM. The majority of cases of sporadic LAM have been reported in North America, Europe, and Japan. Although this may reflect a true geographic distribution, it is more likely due to a higher likelihood of diagnosis in countries with greater health care resources. The mean age at diagnosis was in the midthirties with peak prevalence in the third and fourth decade; mean time from onset of symptoms to diagnosis was approximately 3 years.[18-21] There was no apparent relationship between race, ethnicity, or smoking and disease prevalence. Phenomena such as point epidemics, occupation-related outbreaks, and horizontal/vertical disease transmission have not been reported, suggesting that infectious and inflammatory agents are not likely to cause the disease.

Both sporadic LAM and LAM in patients with TSC affect primarily women of childbearing age. Lung disease has been reported to worsen or present during pregnancy or with the use of exogenous estrogens.[22-25] However, patients have carried normal children to term without overt deterioration in lung function [unpublished observations]. These observations, along with early case reports of favorable responses to androgen therapy, led to the hypothesis that estrogens play a role in disease onset and/or progression. However, well-established cases of LAM in males or postmenopausal women have been described,[20,21,26,27] suggesting that cystic lung destruction can progress in the absence of high levels of estrogens. Moreover, the use of oral contraceptive medication was not associated with an increased risk of LAM,[28] and a large proportion of patients with LAM have never taken exogenous estrogens.

ETIOLOGY

In patients with sporadic LAM, mutations in the *TSC2*, but not *TSC1*, gene have been identified in lesions that exhibit abnormal proliferation of smooth muscle cells.[29] *TSC1* on chromosome 9q34 encodes hamartin, a protein containing structural domains that predict a role in cytoskeletal architecture.[30] Hamartin regulated the Rho-dependent formation of focal adhesions and actin stress fiber assembly by interacting with specific actin-binding proteins (ezrin-radixin-moesin proteins).[31] Recent studies in *Drosophila* demonstrated cooperation between *TSC1* and *TSC2* homologues in the control of cell growth, proliferation, and organ size.[32-35] *TSC2*, located on chromosome 16p13, encodes tuberin, which, by functioning as a guanosine triphosphate (GTP)ase-activating protein, inhibits Rap1A and Rab5, proteins involved in endocytosis, cell proliferation, and control of the cell cycle.[36,37] Tuberin mutations led to the loss of its apparent tumor suppressor activity, an event that could contribute to the abnormal smooth muscle proliferation seen in LAM.[38] Since hamartin was shown to interact physically with tuberin,[39] and no phenotypic differences have been observed between patients with *TSC1* and

TSC2 mutations, a unique tumor-suppressing signaling pathway seems likely to play a major role in the pathogenesis of both sporadic LAM and LAM in patients with TSC.

Germline mutations are heterozygous in patients with TSC. There is no family history of TSC in approximately two-thirds of patients, suggesting a high rate of spontaneous mutations in the *TSC1* and *TSC2* genes. Loss of heterozygosity for TSC mutations is found in somatic tumors, providing evidence for a second mutation (second-hit hypothesis) necessary for the loss of *TSC1/2*-related tumor suppressor activity (Figure 29–1).[40] The second-hit hypothesis may partially explain the variability in disease severity and distribution of lesions. Although germline mutations were absent, mutations in the *TSC2* gene were identified in angiomyolipoma and parenchymal lung lesions in tissues from patients with sporadic LAM.[29] In several individuals, identical *TSC2* mutations were found in both lung and abdominal angiomyolipomas, suggesting that the abnormal cells may be capable of metastasis.[29] Apart from genetic factors, there is little evidence that infectious, carcinogenic, or inflammatory agents play a role in the pathogenesis of LAM.

PATHOLOGY

Lung

Typical gross anatomic findings are enlargement of the lungs with bilateral cysts each of 0.5 to 2.0 cm in diameter.[41] Microscopic examination of lung tissue shows distinctive foci of abnormal smooth muscle cells (LAM nodules) abutting areas of cystic change (Figure 29–2A). Cystic spaces are lined with hyperplastic type II pneumocytes, which are readily demonstrated on scanning electron microscopy and have numerous microvilli. The abundance of type II epithelial cells distinguishes LAM-related cysts from emphysematous spaces, which are primarily lined with type I epithelial cells.[41] LAM foci can appear to invade adjacent pleura, small airways, and blood vessels. Involvement of distal vascular structures may be accompanied by evidence of hemosiderosis, perhaps reflecting chronic, recurrent hemorrhage.

LAM foci consist of two distinct populations of irregularly arranged abnormal smooth muscle cells (Figure 29–2B). Small spindle-shaped cells are typically located at the center of LAM foci, whereas large epithelioid cells with abundant cytoplasm are located at the periphery. Both cell types react with antibodies to smooth muscle–specific antigens (ie, α-actin, vimentin, desmin, smooth muscle myosin heavy chains I and II).[41] The peripheral epithelioid cells are more likely to react with HMB45,[42] a monoclonal antibody that was originally reported to recognize gp100, a premelanosomal protein present in certain melanoma cells (Figure 29–2C). Inflammatory cells are notably absent in and around LAM foci.

In sporadic LAM and TSC, type II pneumocyte hyperplasia may be observed in areas apparently lacking LAM cells. In TSC, multifocal micronodular pneumocyte hyperplasia (MMPH) describes clusters of type II pneu-

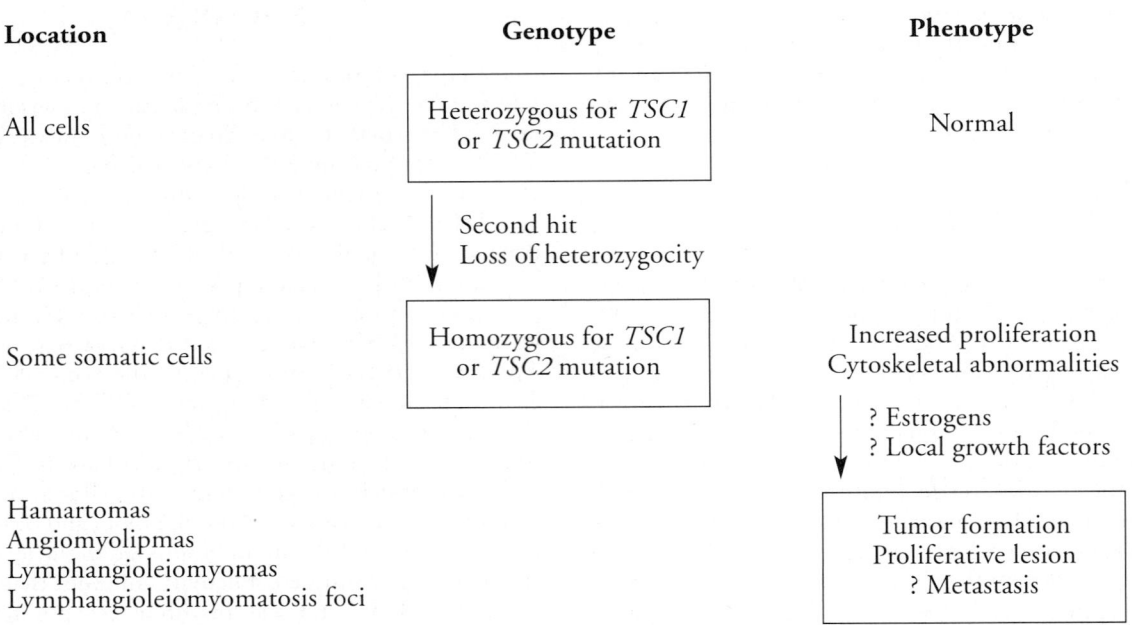

Location	Genotype	Phenotype
All cells	Heterozygous for *TSC1* or *TSC2* mutation	Normal
	↓ Second hit Loss of heterozygocity	
Some somatic cells	Homozygous for *TSC1* or *TSC2* mutation	Increased proliferation Cytoskeletal abnormalities
		↓ ? Estrogens ? Local growth factors
Hamartomas Angiomyolipmas Lymphangioleiomyomas Lymphangioleiomyomatosis foci		Tumor formation Proliferative lesion ? Metastasis

Figure 29–1   The cell biology of tuberous sclerosis complex and lymphangioleiomyomatosis. In subjects with heterozygous *TSC1* or *TSC2* germline mutations, second somatic mutations (second hits), possibly from loss of heterozygosity, can occur in selected anatomic locations leading to tumors.

mocytes that form small nodular lesions within alveolar spaces. These lesions occur only in patients with TSC and can arise regardless of the presence of pulmonary LAM. Loss of heterozygosity of the *TSC2* gene was found in LAM-cell foci but not in MMPH nodules in microdissected lung tissue from a patient with TSC, suggesting distinct mechanisms in the genesis of each lesion.[43]

Extrapulmonary LAM and Angiomyolipomas

Extrapulmonary LAM is characterized by the presence of encapsulated abnormal smooth muscle masses up to 20 cm in size that arise from axial lymphatic structures.[44] The masses contain irregularly arranged bundles of abnormal smooth muscle cells of the small spindle-shaped and large epithelioid variety. In tissue sections from select patients, LAM cells appeared to invade the lymph node capsule and were found in the surrounding adipose tissue. Cystic dilatation of lymphatic vessels can result from obstruction by LAM lesions.

Angiomyolipomas are tumors that contain LAM cells, fragments of poorly developed blood vessels, and varying amounts of adipose tissue (Figure 29–3).[45] These masses are usually located in the kidney but can be present in other intra-abdominal organs. Extra-abdominal lesions have also been reported.[46]

Immunohistochemistry

Immunohistochemical characterization of abnormal smooth muscle cells has furnished insights into the pathogenesis of sporadic LAM as well as LAM in patients with TSC. As noted earlier, abnormal antibodies to smooth muscle cells found in lymphangioleiomyomas, lymph nodes, angiomyolipomas, and pulmonary LAM foci react with the HMB45 antibody, as well as with smooth muscle markers. Other proteins detected in abnormal levels in LAM cells can be grouped into those that are involved in cell proliferation and apoptosis, extracellular matrix proteolysis, and sex hormone binding. LAM cells contained higher levels of *Bcl-2, MCL1, cMYC,* and proliferating cell nuclear antigen (PCNA) than did normal lung tissue, or normal smooth muscle cells.[42,47] These proteins are involved in inhibition of

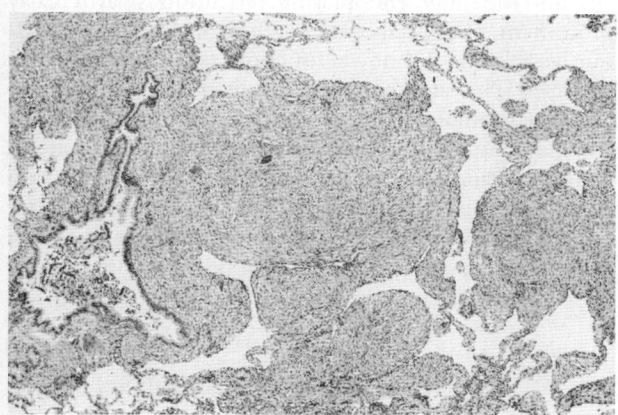

A

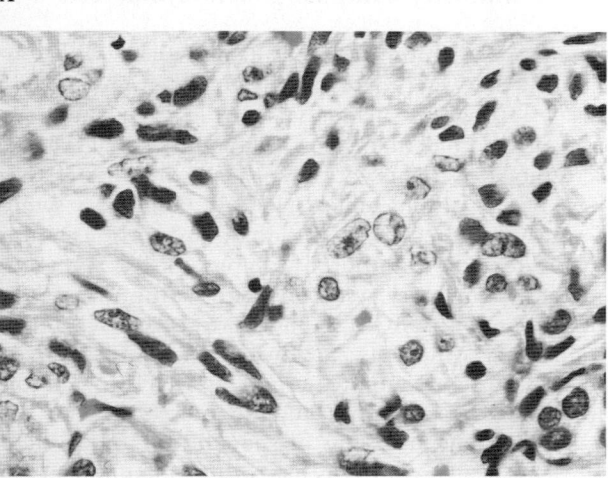

B

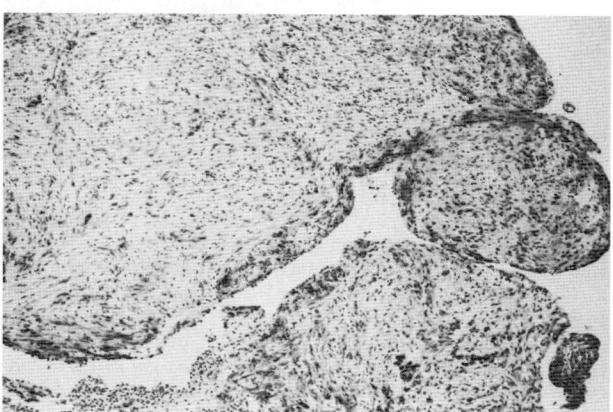

C

Figure 29–2   Histologic characteristics of lymphangioleiomyomatosis (LAM). *A,* Low-power section demonstrating foci of abnormal smooth muscle cells abutting a cystic space (hematoxylin and eosin stain; ×50 original magnification). *B,* High-power section showing spindle-shaped and epithelioid cells arranged in a haphazard fashion within a LAM focus (hematoxylin and eosin stain; ×1,000 original magnification). *C,* Brown coloration depicts LAM cells immunoreactive with anti-HMB45 antibody, located mainly in the periphery of a LAM nodule (peroxidased-iaminobenzidine [DAB] method with hematoxylin and eosin counterstaining; ×250 original magnification).

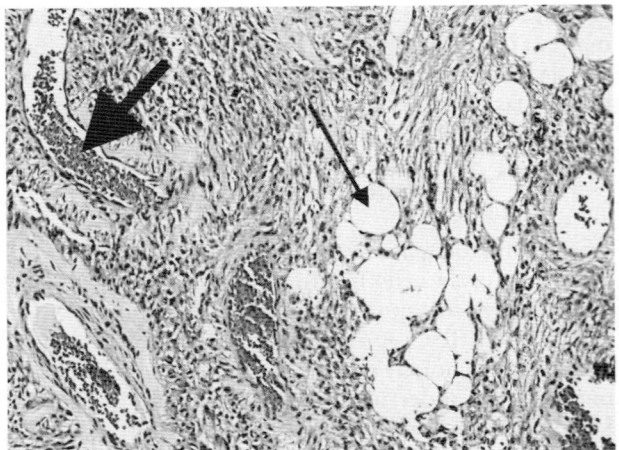

A

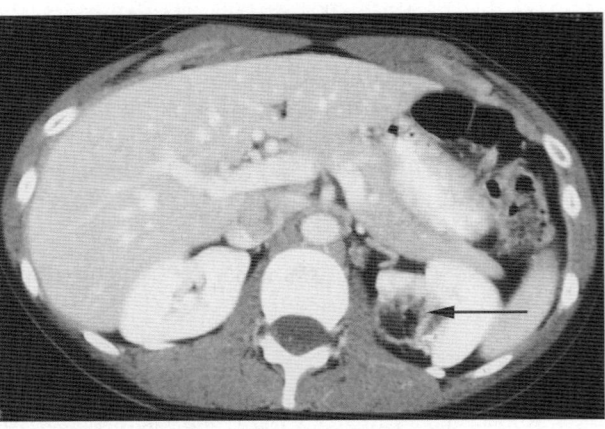

B

Figure 29–3 Angiomyolipoma. *A*, Tissue sections show clusters of blood vessels (*large arrow*), abnormal smooth muscle cells arranged in a haphazard fashion, and adipose tissue (*small arrow*) within an angiomyolipoma (hematoxylin and eosin; ×200 original magnification). *B*, Abdominal computed tomography scan demonstrates an angiomyolipoma of the left kidney (*arrow*) containing areas of contrast enhancement, as well as hypodense regions consistent with the presence of fat.

tivity colocalized with that of collagen type IV, and was frequently associated with disruption of the basement membrane. Amounts of tissue inhibitors of metalloproteases (TIMPs) were not greater in LAM cells than in the surrounding normal tissue.

Estrogen and progesterone receptors were found in the nuclei of the peripherally located large epithelioid LAM cells.[49] Because these cells failed to express markers of high proliferative potential (ie, PCNA, *Bcl-2*, *cMYC*), it is unclear whether sex hormone receptor overexpression is necessary for LAM cell proliferation or invasiveness. However, these receptors appear to be downregulated by high concentrations of exogenous progesterone, suggesting that they play a role in the pathogenesis of LAM.[50]

Electron Microscopy

Transmission electron microscopy of LAM cells demonstrates many of the ultrastructural features of smooth muscle cells, such as F-actin filaments with dense bodies, desmin filaments, and vimentin. Nuclei are typically elongated with normally dispersed chromatin. Organelle structure is generally intact, however mitochondria are few, and the rough endoplasmic reticulum is particularly prominent. LAM cells contain electron-lucent cytoplasmic vesicles of unknown function as well as glycogen particles. The large epithelioid cells in the periphery of LAM foci contain cytoplasmic vesicles that are filled with lamellar material and resemble premelanosomes found in certain melanoma cells. Extracellular matrix destruction is seen surrounding LAM cells, as evidenced by fragmented elastin fibers and spiraling collagen fibrils. A model of the pathogenesis of LAM based on histopathologic evidence is presented in Figure 29–4.

CLINICAL MANIFESTATIONS

Pulmonary Lymphangioleiomyomatosis

The most common presentation in patients with sporadic LAM was progressive dyspnea or pneumothorax.[18–21] Cough and hemoptysis were less frequent. However, due to modern imaging techniques, as well as active screening of patients with TSC, a large number of cases have been found in subjects without pulmonary symptoms. A retrospective evaluation of lung sections visible on abdominal computed tomography (CT) scans revealed pulmonary cysts consistent with LAM in 26% of patients with TSC.[15] In 38 women with TSC and no pulmonary symptoms, 34% had evidence of LAM on high-resolution computed tomography (HRCT) of the lung, and all had normal lung function.[16]

Symptoms and signs of sporadic LAM as well as LAM associated with TSC may be due to pulmonary or extrapulmonary disease. Dyspnea, cough, and recurrent

apoptosis, enhancement of cell proliferation, and cell cycle control. On nick end-labeling studies of histologic sections, cellular apoptosis was less common in LAM foci than in surrounding tissue.[47] Within LAM foci, PCNA immunoreactivity was observed in the central spindle-shaped cells, as opposed to the peripheral epithelioid type, suggesting functional heterogeneity among LAM cell morphologic subtypes and greater proliferation at the center of the nodule.

Several observations support a role for protease/antiprotease imbalance in the pathogenesis of LAM. Consistent with their invasive nature, pulmonary LAM cells reacted with antibodies to matrix metalloproteases (MMP-2 and MMP-9), proteins involved in the breakdown of collagen and elastin.[48] MMP-2 immunoreac-

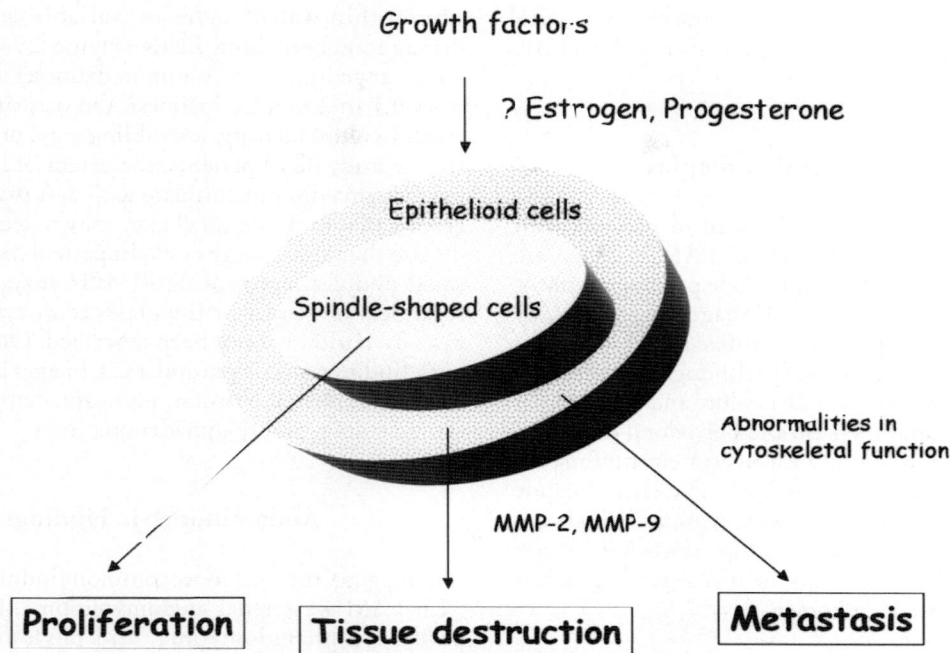

Figure 29–4   The pathogenesis of lymphangioleiomyomatosis (LAM). A diagram depicting the cut surface of a pulmonary LAM lesion (LAM nodule) is shown. Central spindle-shaped cells express markers of cell proliferation, whereas peripheral epithelioid cells, perhaps via expression of matrix metalloproteases (eg, [matrix metalloproteinase] MMP-2, MMP-9), may be responsible for tissue destruction and metastasis.

pneumothoraces are the most common manifestations. Dyspnea may also result from chylothorax, which can be present without significant parenchymal disease. Although nonspecific crackles are frequently heard on physical examination, clubbing and wheezes are rare.[18–21] In patients with chronic respiratory failure, signs of right-sided heart failure may be present.

Patients with LAM are at increased risk of developing osteoporosis. In a survey of 104 patients, 61% had osteoporosis (22%) or osteopenia (39%) on bone densitometry.[51] Bone density improved when patients were treated with bisphosphonates. To what extent osteoporosis in patients with LAM occurs as a complication of therapy or as a feature of the underlying disease is unknown. Aggressive treatment of patients with LAM with bisphosphonates is recommended for patients when bone densitometry shows reduced bone density.

Extrapulmonary Lymphangioleiomyomatosis

Manifestations of extrapulmonary LAM arise from expansion of lymphatic masses and the accumulation of fluid due to lymphatic obstruction. Accumulation of lymph results in chylous ascites or pleural effusions in 5 to 30 % of patients.[18,20,21] Accumulation of chyle tends to be persistent; symptoms, including abdominal discomfort and dyspnea, may be relieved by periodic fluid aspiration or pleurodesis. Patients can also develop

peripheral lymphedema,[52,53] which tends to worsen during the day and can be relieved by leg elevation [unpublished observations]. Swelling of perineal tissues, urinary frequency and urgency, fecal incontinence, tenesmus, and dyspareunia have also been ascribed to lymphatic obstruction.[54] Rarely, patients can experience chyloptysis, chyluria, or pericardial effusion.

Angiomyolipomas

Angiomyolipomas range from 0.5 to 20 cm in size, most commonly arise in the kidney, and can lead to hematuria and flank pain. Hematuria or intra-abdominal hemorrhage may be life threatening. Angiomyolipomas can also be found in other locations, including the liver and retroperitoneum. Angiomyolipomas, more commonly unilateral, are present in 30 to 50% of patients with sporadic LAM and have not been reported to display malignant features. Angiomyolipomas occur in approximately 70% of patients with TSC. In contrast to findings in patients with sporadic LAM, in patients with TSC, angiomyolipomas tend to be multiple and bilateral, can occur in males, and are more likely to be associated with renal cysts.[45] The latter is of interest because the *TSC2* gene is located immediately adjacent to *PKD1*, abnormalities in which cause polycystic kidney disease. In patients with TSC, a malignant variant of angiomyolipoma (monotypic epithelioid tumor) can occur. These are frequently immunoreactive with HMB45 and should be considered during diagnostic evaluation.[55,56]

Tuberous Sclerosis Complex

A variety of skin lesions may be seen in patients with TSC, regardless of the presence of LAM.[57] These are commonly asymptomatic and include periungual fibromas, facial angiofibromas, and Shagreen patches. In addition, patients may develop cardiac rhabdomyomas, which can resolve spontaneously, although patients may require medical therapy for heart failure and arrhythmias or surgical resection.[14] Seizure and behavioral disorders, as well as low grade central nervous system tumors, are also common in patients with TSC. The latter include cortical tubers and low grade astrocytomas, which can also involve the eye. The relationship between the severity of the TSC phenotype and the incidence or progression of lung disease is unknown.

LABORATORY TESTS

In patients with LAM, arterial blood gas analysis most often reveals respiratory alkalosis. Hypercapnic respiratory failure is rare, even in patients with end-stage disease. On electrolyte analysis, a compensatory metabolic acidosis may be observed. In patients with chronic hypoxia, polycythemia may be present.

Endobronchial lesions related to LAM have not been described on bronchoscopy. Total and differential bronchoalveolar lavage cell counts in patients with sporadic LAM were similar to those in healthy volunteers.[18] Hemosiderin-laden macrophages were observed in 81% of patients with LAM, perhaps consistent with vascular invasion by LAM cells or bleeding into the cystic spaces.[18]

IMAGING STUDIES

Lung

The chest radiograph in patients with sporadic LAM demonstrates increased bilateral reticular interstitial markings with normal or increased lung volume (Figure 29–5A). In some cases, small nodules may predominate. Other findings include pneumothorax and pleural effusion. The latter may be unilateral or bilateral. In patients with severe disease, cysts and bullae may be visualized. Because parenchymal lung disease is mild in many patients at presentation, the chest radiograph is often normal.[58]

Because the plain chest radiograph is nonspecific, HRCT scanning of the chest is the modality of choice for the evaluation of patients with LAM and demon-

strates thin-walled cysts of variable size scattered throughout both lung fields (Figure 29–5B, and C). Cysts range from 2 to 40 mm in diameter and cyst walls from 0.1 to 2 mm in thickness. On occasion, cyst walls are difficult to identify, resembling areas of emphysema. In one study of 39 patients, the extent of involved lung parenchyma did not correlate with cyst diameter,[59] suggesting that multiple small cysts may reflect more severe disease than fewer large cysts. In patients with TSC, the small nodules representing MMPH may be visualized regardless of gender or the presence of cystic lung disease; cavitation has not been described. Other less common findings on conventional CT images include pneumothorax, pleural effusion, pericardial effusion, dilated thoracic duct, and lymphadenopathy.

Abdominopelvic Findings

On imaging, the four most common findings in patients with LAM were renal angiomyolipoma, lymphadenopathy, lymphangiomyoma, and chylous ascites.[60,61] Abdominal manifestations were identified in 76% of patients with LAM. Angiomyolipomas contain areas of low attenuation representing fat (see Figure 29–3B) that are best visualized by thin-section non-enhanced helical CT.[60] Retroperitoneal adenopathy was present in 39% of patients, and the extent correlated with the severity of lung disease.[60] Lymphangioleiomyomas, or cystic spaces filled with low attenuation fluid, were observed in 13 patients and were thought to arise from lymphatic obstruction.[60] Consistent with their clinical manifestations, these lesions were shown by consecutive abdominal CT scans to increase in size during the day [unpublished observations]. Enlarged lymph nodes and lymphangioleiomyomas may involve large areas of the abdomen and/or pelvis. Although these tumors can displace intra-abdominal and pelvic structures, in general, they were not characterized as invasive. Finally, 9% of patients exhibited chylous ascites, which in most cases was associated with pleural effusion.

Other Imaging Modalities

Patients with presumed sporadic LAM should be screened for TSC via magnetic resonance imaging (MRI) of the head. Findings might include hamartomatous lesions (tubers) and low-grade astrocytomas. In addition, the prevalence of meningioma was higher in patients with sporadic LAM than in the general population.[62]

Almost all patients with LAM exhibit ventilation and perfusion abnormalities on scanning. A speckling pattern, perhaps due to trapping of radionuclide in cysts, was seen in 74% of patients, the severity of which correlated with severity of the CT scan and pulmonary function abnormalities.[18,59] The location of ventilation/perfusion abnormalities was rarely mismatched.

Bone densitometry should be performed in all patients with LAM. The mean lateral lumbar density was a sensitive indicator of changes in bone density when following patients with LAM.[51]

PULMONARY FUNCTION TESTS

The classic pattern of pulmonary function abnormalities in patients with LAM is an obstructive ventilatory defect with or without superimposed restriction.[18,20,21] However, in a survey of 80 patients with LAM, 42% had normal lung function.[21] Although LAM is primarily a disease of the lung parenchyma, a significant bronchodilator response was observed in 20 to 25% of patients.[18,63] Low forced expiratory volume in 1 second (FEV$_1$) and FEV$_1$/forced vital capacity (FVC) ratio are usually accompanied by an increased residual volume (RV)/total lung capacity (TLC) ratio, indicating thoracic gas trapping. Airway obstruction was found to be due to increased pulmonary flow resistance rather than a loss of lung elastic recoil.[64] Despite the fact that LAM involves the pulmonary interstitium, there was no evidence for the loss of lung compliance when lung mechanics were assessed.[64] However, since none of the patients in this study had a decreased TLC, it is unclear whether the restrictive ventilatory abnormality seen in some patients with LAM is due to changes in lung elasticity or chest wall abnormalities.

The DL$_{CO}$ was reduced in 66 to 97% of patients with LAM, which is the most common pulmonary function test abnormality.[19,21,63] DL$_{CO}$ can be disproportionately reduced in patients with relatively preserved flow rates and lung volumes, suggesting a role for ventilation-perfusion abnormalities in the pathogenesis of LAM [unpublished observations]. An endogenous vasodilator, nitric oxide, was increased in the exhaled air in patients with LAM.[65] Moreover, many patients exhibited significant hypoxemia at rest or during exercise in the absence of evidence of significant parenchymal or airway disease.

A comprehensive study of 15 patients was undertaken to assess exercise physiology in patients with LAM.[66] Most patients exhibited mild to moderate resting hypoxemia (PaO$_2$ > 65 mm Hg), reduced DL$_{CO}$, and diminished FEV$_1$, reflecting relatively severe disease. Fourteen of 15 patients had an abnormally low exercise capacity, most commonly associated with diminished or absent ventilatory reserve. However, significant exercise

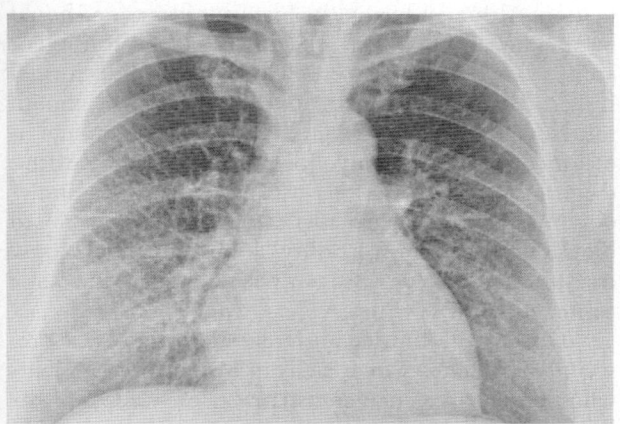

A

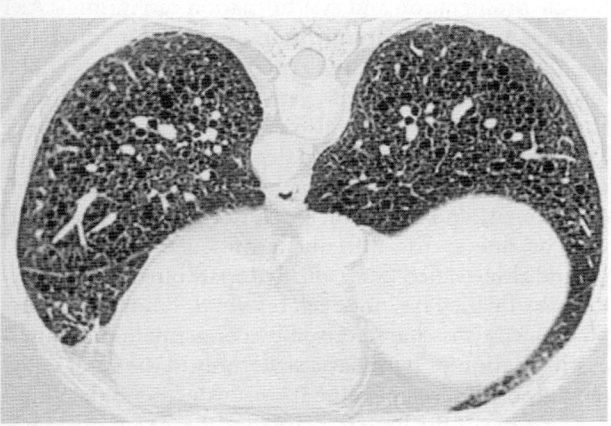

B

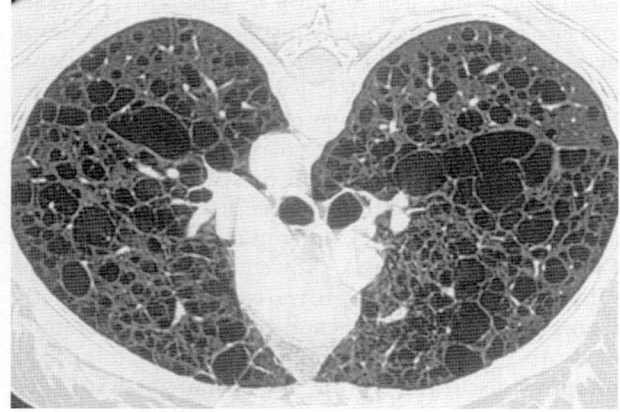

C

Figure 29–5 Imaging of the chest in patients with lymphangioleiomyomatosis. *A*, Plain chest radiograph shows bilateral increased interstitial marking without volume loss. High-resolution computed tomography of the chest may demonstrate *B*, multiple small parenchymal cysts or *C*, fewer large cysts; in both cases, cyst walls are well-demarcated.

limitation occurred in some patients who had only a mild to moderate reduction in FEV_1. Heart rate reserve and oxygen pulse at end exercise were also diminished in the majority of patients, suggesting a cardiac component to exercise limitation, perhaps due to pulmonary hypertension, or less likely, to intrinsic cardiac disease.

In a separate study of 134 patients, both DL_{CO} and FEV_1, independently, correlated with diminished exercise capacity [manuscript in preparation]. The 57 patients with a normal FEV_1 and DL_{CO} exhibited a normal exercise capacity. In the 44 patients with both diminished DL_{CO} and FEV_1, average breathing reserve was in the normal range (23 ± 3 L/min $\pm$ SEM), significant desaturation occurred during exercise, and oxygen pulse at end exercise was diminished. In addition, patients who were given supplemental oxygen during exercise demonstrated persistent cardiac dysfunction and exercise limitation. These findings suggest a pulmonary vascular abnormality despite the absence of resting hypoxemia or significant mechanical dysfunction.

PATHOLOGIC, RADIOLOGIC, AND PHYSIOLOGIC CORRELATION

Several tools have been introduced to provide outcome variables for the identification of prognostic markers and etiologic factors. A lung histology score (LHS) was developed to grade the severity of disease in patients with sporadic LAM or LAM with TSC.[63,67] The score encompasses the presence of airway inflammation, number of cysts, and degree of smooth muscle proliferation. The LHS represents the percentage of lung parenchyma involved by abnormal smooth muscle cells, cystic spaces, and airway inflammation. Thirty-four of 74 histologic specimens showed a predominance of solid smooth muscle proliferative lesions over cystic spaces. A significant bronchodilator response was more likely to be present in patients with a predominant smooth muscle pattern on biopsy and in those with decreased FEV_1/FVC and increased RV/TLC ratios. There was not significantly more airway inflammation in the responders than in nonresponders.[63] Furthermore, consistent with an important role for a gas exchange defect in the pathophysiology of LAM, the DL_{CO} was the best predictor of severity of disease, as assessed by a lung histology score.[63] These observations suggest that the type of anatomic lesion in patients with LAM may determine the degree of bronchial hyperresponsiveness and gas exchange abnormality.

Two radiologic approaches have been useful in gauging disease severity in patients with LAM. Severity of lung destruction as determined by HRCT scan was assessed by a scoring system that reflects the proportion of lung parenchyma involved by cysts.[58,59,68] There was little interobserver variability, and the lung severity score correlated well with indices of lung function. In patients with sporadic LAM and LAM with TSC, there was a sig-

nificant relationship between the overall extent of disease or average cyst size with the FEV_1/FVC ratio as well as the DL_{CO}.[16,59] Furthermore, parenchymal destruction as assessed by HRCT of the lung correlated inversely with exercise capacity in 10 patients.[69]

To eliminate interobserver variability, a quantitative CT technique was used to assess the degree of lung occupied by cystic spaces.[69] After acquisition, scans were reconstructed with a computer algorithm, and the proportion of lung parenchyma with Hounsfeld Units (HU) less than -900 (air) to that with HU less than -300 (the value representing total lung) was calculated and used to derive a quantitative CT index of cystic involvement. The quantitative CT index correlated inversely with FEV_1, FEV_1/FVC ratio, DL_{CO}, and exercise capacity.[69]

DIAGNOSIS

The gold standard for the diagnosis of LAM remains the open lung biopsy showing the characteristic histologic pattern and immunoreactivity of LAM cells with the HMB45 antibody. Transbronchial biopsy has been used successfully,[70–73] although larger sections may be required for accurate diagnosis and to derive prognostic information. Although histopathologic confirmation should be obtained, cytologic examination of pleural effusion or ascites has sometimes revealed clusters of abnormal smooth muscle cells that are immunoreactive for smooth muscle actin.[74] Fine-needle aspiration of lymphangioleiomyomas or angiomyolipomas may yield a positive diagnosis[75-78]; however, the vascular nature of angiomyolipomas mandates particular care in performing closed biopsies. The diagnostic utility of transbronchial biopsy or aspiration cytology has not been evaluated in a large cohort of patients with LAM.

Due to the limited differential diagnosis, a presumptive diagnosis of LAM can be made in patients who demonstrate characteristic cysts on HRCT of the lung and who have evidence of extrapulmonary LAM and/or angiomyolipoma. Several diseases of smooth muscle proliferation and cyst formation can mimic LAM (Table 29–1). Eosinophilic granuloma occurs in young women who smoke, causes predominantly upper lobe disease with thick-walled cysts and cavitating nodules, and has a characteristic histologic pattern. Birt-Hogg-Dubé syndrome is a recently described autosomal dominant disease characterized by benign skin tumors, renal carcinomas, and recurrent pneumothoraces. The latter may be due to the infrequent presence of small subpleural thin-walled cysts, the histopathologic characterization of which has not been reported. Pulmonary lymphangiectasis is characterized by congenital or acquired cystic dilation of lymphatic structures in the lung without smooth muscle proliferation.[79] Mesenchymal cystic hamartoma of the lung is a rare syndrome that can cause hemoptysis, hemothorax, and/or pneumothorax.[80] It

**Table 29–1   The Differential Diagnosis of Patients With
Chronic Lung Disease Involving Cyst Formation or Smooth Muscle Proliferation.**

Disease	Distinguishing Features		
	Clinical	*Radiology*	*Pathology*
Cyst formation			
Eosinophilic granuloma	Smokers	Upper lobe predominance with thick-walled cysts and cavitating nodules.	Characteristic pattern on hematoxylin and eosin stain
Emphysema	Smokers	Upper lobe predominance Well-defined cyst walls are rarely visualized	Type I epithelial cells predominate No abnormal smooth muscle cell proliferation
Birt-Hogg-Dubé syndrome	Hereditary disease associated with mesenchymal tumors and renal cell carcinoma	Patients tend to have few peripherally located parenchymal cysts	Not well-characterized
Pulmonary lymphangiectasis	Congenital or acquired due to lymphatic congestion	Localized or diffuse cystic lesions with pulmonary infiltrates	Absence of smooth muscle proliferation
Lymphangiomas	Congenital localized tumors confined to the neck and mediastinum	Cystic lesions of the neck and mediastinum that arise from lymphatic structures	Endothelium-lined cysts surrounded by lymphoid tissue, fibroblasts, and smooth muscle cells
Diffuse pulmonary lymphangiomatosis	Usually diagnosed in late childhood	Interstitial infiltrates with pleural and pericardial effusions No cysts	Endothelium-lined anastomosing lymphatic spaces along bronchovascular structures surrounded by collagen and spindle-shaped cells Less marked smooth muscle cell proliferation than LAM. Preserved lung parenchyma HMB45 negative.
Smooth muscle proliferation			
Mesenchymal cystic hamartoma of the lung	Rare syndrome of benign multifocal mesenchymal lung tumors that may cause hemoptysis, pneumothorax, or hemothorax	Nodules that evolve into cysts with time May be difficult to distinguish from LAM in patients with TSC who exhibit MMPH	Cysts have outer layer of mesenchymal cells and are lined by normal or metaplastic respiratory epithelium.
Benign metastasizing leiomyomata	May develop after removal of uterine leiomyoma May respond to hormonal manipulation	Multiple 0.5 to 1.0 cm nodules Cavitation and interstitial pattern have been described No cysts	Regularly arranged fascicles of smooth muscle cells that tend to stain positive for estrogen and progesterone receptors and are HMB45 negative.

LAM = lymphangioleiomyomatosis; HMB45 = a monoclonal antibody; TSC = tuberous sclerosis complex; MMPH = multifocal micronodular pneumocyte hyperplasia

may be difficult to distinguish the radiologic pattern from that of LAM; on histopathology, however, cysts are characterized by an outer cambium layer lined with normal or metaplastic respiratory epithelium. One case of cystic pulmonary metastasis of endometrial stromal sarcoma was found to stain positive for HMB45.[81]

Certain rare disorders of proliferation of abnormal smooth muscle can affect the lung. Benign metastasizing uterine leiomyomata are nodular lung lesions that are identified after the resection of uterine leiomyomata.[82-84] Pulmonary cysts, however, are not a feature, and histopathologic examination shows well-organized fascicles of smooth muscle cells that are not immunoreactive with HMB45.

Uterine leiomyosarcoma and multiple pulmonary fibroleiomyomatosis hamartomas are lung diseases with smooth muscle proliferation that can be excluded based on the radiologic and histologic appearance.

TREATMENT

Pulmonary Lymphangioleiomyomatosis

Most information regarding therapy for sporadic LAM or LAM in TSC comes from case reports or series. Due to the small number of patients and variable progression of the disease, low statistical power has limited the feasibility of randomized placebo-controlled trials. Given the putative role of estrogens in LAM, treatment regimens have included the use of androgenic hormones such as medroxyprogesterone and luteinizing hormone–releasing hormone (LH-RH) agonist. Although some reports indicated significant treatment responses,[85,86] other retrospective studies suggested that disease progression was unaffected by hormonal manipulation.[21] Further studies may identify subgroups of patients who are more likely to respond to progesterone, enhancing the feasibility of a randomized controlled trial. Other hormonal therapies, including danazol, surgical oophorectomy, and tamoxifen, have fallen out of favor as first-line therapies because their efficacy has not been corroborated in larger studies. In addition, tamoxifen is a mixed estrogen agonist/antagonist and may worsen the disease in patients with LAM.

Presently, the treatment of patients with LAM is directed toward the alleviation of symptoms and the prevention of complications. Patients with chronic respiratory failure should be treated with supplemental oxygen. Because patients with LAM can experience profound dyspnea and hypoxemia during exercise, oxygen requirements should be determined both at rest and during physical exertion. It is not known whether patients with LAM are more prone than others to sleep-disordered breathing.

Recurrent pneumothoraces can be treated conservatively with tube thoracostomy but often require chemical pleurodesis using doxycycline or bleomycin. Although talc pleurodesis may be more effective at preventing recurrence in patients with secondary pneumothorax, the resulting pleural scarring can complicate later lung transplantation and perhaps should be avoided as a first approach.

Chylous effusions can be aspirated for the relief of symptoms, although pleurodesis is often necessary due to their persistent nature. In addition, frequent thoracentesis and paracentesis can lead to large fluid and protein losses. Other approaches to the management of effusions in patients with LAM, including dietary management, somatostatin analogues, or thoracic duct ligation or irradiation have not been proven effective. Diuretic therapy is sometimes useful, presumably by reducing central venous pressure.

Due to progressive respiratory failure, patients with LAM eventually may require lung transplantation. Selection criteria for candidates and outcomes are similar to those for other chronic lung diseases.[87,88] Colonization of the lungs with pathogenic microorganisms, however, does not usually complicate the pre- and post-transplant clinical course of LAM patients,[21] as it does for patients with cystic fibrosis and bronchiectasis. Overall actuarial survival at 1 and 2 years post-transplantation was approximately 70 and 60%, respectively.[87,88] Consistent with a role for a metastatic mechanism in the pathogenesis of LAM, recurrence of disease in the transplanted lung has been demonstrated.[89–91]

Certain special circumstances dictate an individualized approach to the transplant evaluation of LAM patients. Although not a contraindication to transplantation, pleural adhesions as a result of previous pleurodesis or pleural involvement by LAM lesions may increase the likelihood of hemorrhage, prolonged duration of surgery, and phrenic nerve injury. The location of a previous pleurodesis as well as the presence of chylous effusion may influence the side chosen for transplantation.

Patients who underwent double lung transplantation may have had slightly higher survival rates at 2 years than those who received a single lung, but the benefit was not apparent at 5 years.[88] Given the lack of clear indications and the paucity of donor lungs, the decision of single versus double lung transplantation should be based on individual evaluation. In terms of clinical outcomes, the effect of hyperinflation of the remaining native lung on the transplanted lung is unknown. Heart-lung transplantation has been performed in patients with right heart failure.[87,88] Because of the requirement for cardiopulmonary bypass, surgical outcomes can be affected by factors that prolong the procedure. Combined kidney-lung transplants have been performed in selected patients with respiratory failure who had unrelenting symptoms secondary to renal angiomyolipomas as well as in patients with TSC who had reduced renal function.

The variability and poor predictive value of pulmonary function measures has limited their use in identifying candidates for lung transplantation. Many patients have severe airflow obstruction; however, other patients with marked hypoxemia and right heart failure seem to predominantly exhibit gas exchange abnormalities, and transplantation is performed when oxygen requirements exceed the capability of exogenous delivery systems. The DL_{CO} correlated best with the LHS and may be a better predictor of the need for transplantation. Moreover, the degree of cystic lung destruction on HRCT of the lung may not reflect the severity of the gas exchange abnormality and should not be used to gauge the need for transplantation in an individual patient.

Extrapulmonary Lymphangioleiomyomatosis

In patients with sporadic LAM, angiomyolipomas are typically benign and should be treated conservatively. In patients with TSC, hemorrhage was more likely from angiomyolipomas of greater than 3.5 cm in size.[92] Because for any given tumor, the risk of bleeding is not known, prophylactic nephrectomy is not recommended. Occasionally, excessive bleeding, obstruction of adjacent abdominal structures, or persistent pain may prompt intervention, but conservation of renal function is critical, and total nephrectomy should be avoided unless absolutely necessary. The current standard of care includes subtotal nephrectomy or vascular embolization for the treatment of significant renal hemorrhage.[45,93–95]

Counseling

Appropriate counseling of patients is necessary for the prevention of specific disease-related complications. The presence of resting hypoxemia may require the use of supplemental oxygen during air travel. It is unclear whether patients with pulmonary LAM are at greater risk than other passengers of developing pneumothorax during air travel. However, pneumothoraces that do occur can be more severe, or the lung can fail to re-expand due to the low cabin pressure. In general, air travel has not been contraindicated in patients with LAM unless a pneumothorax is present.

The potential risks of pregnancy should be addressed on an individual basis. Some case reports had suggested a risk of exacerbation of the disease in pregnant women with LAM. In one study, the onset of pulmonary symptoms during pregnancy occurred in 9 of 46 patients, but symptoms worsened during pregnancy in only 2 of the 9.[21] It is unclear to what extent the presence of symptoms was due to underlying disease progression rather than changes that normally occur during pregnancy (ie, anemia, increased minute ventilation, decreased functional residual capacity). Patients with LAM, however, have carried full-term infants with no changes in lung function [unpublished observations]. In the absence of a cohort study assessing the effects of pregnancy on clinical outcomes, patients should be told that pregnancy is not contraindicated, but the possibility of an increased risk of pneumothorax, deterioration in lung function, and disease progression should be considered in their decision-making and prenatal care.

Genetic counseling should be provided for patients with LAM who are found to have TSC. There is a 50% chance of TSC in the offspring of affected parents, even in the absence of a prior family history. In addition, unaffected parents of an affected child, have a slightly increased risk (~2%) of having a second child with TSC.[13] Finally, when patients who present with LAM are found to have TSC, careful screening of other family members may reveal affected individuals who are potentially at risk for medical complications.

NATURAL HISTORY AND PROGNOSIS

Although original reports suggested that most patients with LAM die within 10 years of diagnosis,[8,9] recent studies revealed significant variability in disease progression and actuarial survival. Perhaps due to the availability of transplantation, earlier diagnosis, improved supportive therapy, and identification of patients with milder disease, the 10-year actuarial survival probability after diagnosis was approximately 75%.[20,21] In a study from Japan, survival probability was lower at 40%.[19] In nine patients with TSC and LAM, survival was not significantly different from that of patients with TSC who did not have pulmonary LAM (78% with an average follow-up of 17 years).[96] The presence of chylothorax was once thought to indicate a better prognosis; however, the longer survival was more likely due to the earlier detection of patients with mild parenchymal lung disease.

A concerted effort has been made to develop prognostic indicators derived from pathologic, radiologic, or physiologic parameters. By histopathology, the predominance of cysts was a better predictor of mortality than was LAM-cell proliferation.[19,67] However, the lung histology score, which encompasses the degree of cystic destruction and smooth muscle proliferation, was the best predictor of mortality and time to transplantation (Figure 29–6).[67] One study suggested that the degree of obstruction, as assessed by the FEV_1/FVC ratio, predicted the mortality at 2 and 5 years after diagnosis.[19] Because the DL_{CO} was the best predictor of radiologic and pathologic disease severity, it may represent a more appropriate indicator of mortality or time to transplantation, particularly in patients in whom a gas exchange abnormality is the predominant physiologic manifestation.[59,63,68,69] Parameters derived from cardiopulmonary exercise testing such as the degree of oxygen desaturation and ventilatory limita-

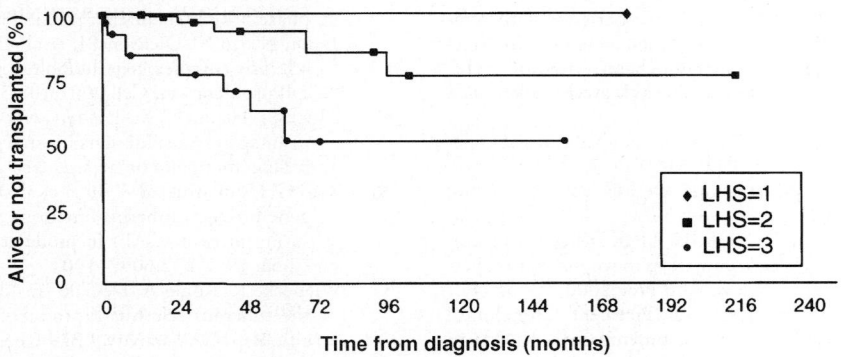

Figure 29–6 Prognosis in patients with lymphangioleiomyomatosis. A Kaplan-Meier plot shows that the risk of death or transplantation decreases with increasing lung histology score (LHS). Adapted from Matsui K et al.[67]

tion, exercise capacity, and cardiac performance might represent more sensitive indicators of disease-related functional impairment and better prognostic indicators.

Because LAM is a rare disease, little information has been obtained regarding changes in lung function or radiologic severity over time. In a group of 43 patients, rates of decline in the FEV_1 and DL_{CO} were highly variable but greater than in the general population.[85] Patients with a predominant pattern of smooth muscle proliferation ('solid') were more likely to have a more rapid rate of decline in FEV_1.[63] In the same study, the rate of decline in DL_{CO} was highly variable and did not correlate with histologic severity.

REFERENCES

1. Moss J. LAM and other diseases characterized by smooth muscle proliferation. In: Lenfant C, editor. Lung biology in health and disease. New York: Marcel Dekker.

2. Kalassian KG, Doyle R, Kao P, et al. Lymphangioleiomyomatosis: new insights. Am J Respir Crit Care Med 1997; 155:1183–6.

3. Sullivan EJ. Lymphangioleiomyomatosis: a review. Chest 1998;114:1689–703.

4. Kelly J, Moss J. Lymphangioleiomyomatosis. Am J Med Sci 2001;321:17–25.

5. Burrell LST, Ross JM. A case of chylous effusion due to leiomyosarcoma. Br J Tuberc 1937;31:38–9.

6. von Stossel E. Uber musculare cirrose der lunge. Beitr Klin Tuberk 1937;90:432–42.

7. Cornog JL Jr, Enterline HT. Lymphangiomyoma, a benign lesion of chyliferous lymphatics synonymous with lymphangiopericytoma. Cancer 1966;19:1909–30.

8. Corrin B, Liebow AA, Friedman PJ. Pulmonary lymphangiomyomatosis. A review. Am J Pathol 1975;79:348–82.

9. Silverstein EF, Ellis K, Wolff M, et al. Pulmonary lymphangiomyomatosis. Am J Roentgenol Radium Ther Nucl Med 1974;120:832–50.

10. Izumi T, Kitaichi M, Nagai S. Perspectives on lymphangioleiomyomatosis in Japan. In: Moss J, editor. LAM and other diseases characterized by proliferation of smooth muscle. New York: Marcel Dekker, Inc.; 1999. p. 1–8.

11. Cordier JF, Lazor R, the Groupe d'Etudes et de Recherche sur les Maladies "Orphelines" Pulmonaires. Perspectives on lymphangioleiomyomatosis in France. In: Moss J, editor. LAM and other diseases characterized by proliferation of smooth muscle. New York: Marcel Dekker, Inc.; 1999. p. 9–31.

12. Lipman MCI, duBois RM. Clinical experience with lymphangioleiomyomatosis in the United Kingdom. In: Moss J, editor. LAM and other diseases characterized by proliferation of smooth muscle. New York: Marcel Dekker, Inc.; 1999. p. 33–43.

13. Osborne JP, Fryer A, Webb D. Epidemiology of tuberous sclerosis. Ann N Y Acad Sci 1991;615:125–7.

14. Webb DW, Osborne JP. Tuberous sclerosis. Arch Dis Child 1995;72:471–4.

15. Costello LC, Hartman TE, Ryu JH. High frequency of pulmonary lymphangioleiomyomatosis in women with tuberous sclerosis complex. Mayo Clin Proc 2000;75:591–4.

16. Moss J, Avila NA, Barnes PM, et al. Prevalence and clinical characteristics of lymphangioleiomyomatosis (LAM) in patients with tuberous sclerosis complex. Am J Respir Crit Care Med 2001;164:669–71.

17. Franz DN, Brody A, Meyer C, et al. Mutational and radiographic analysis of pulmonary disease consistent with lymphangioleiomyomatosis and micronodular pneumocyte hyperplasia in women with tuberous sclerosis. Am J Respir Crit Care Med 2001;164:661–8.

18. Chu SC, Horiba K, Usuki J, et al. Comprehensive evaluation of 35 patients with lymphangioleiomyomatosis. Chest 1999;115:1041–52.

19. Kitaichi M, Nishimura K, Itoh H, et al. Pulmonary lymphangioleiomyomatosis: a report of 46 patients including a clinicopathologic study of prognostic factors. Am J Respir Crit Care Med 1995; 151(2 Pt 1):527–33.

20. Taylor JR, Ryu J, Colby TV, et al. Lymphangioleiomyomatosis. Clinical course in 32 patients. N Engl J Med 1990; 323:1254–60.

21. Urban T, Lazor R, Lacronique J, et al. Pulmonary lymphangioleiomyomatosis. A study of 69 patients. Groupe d'Etudes et de Recherche sur les Maladies "Orphelines" Pulmonaires (GERM"O"P). Medicine (Baltimore) 1999;78:321–37.

22. Yockey CC, Riepe RE, Ryan K. Pulmonary lymphangioleiomyomatosis complicated by pregnancy. Kans Med 1986;87:277–8, 293.

23. Urban T, Kuttenn F, Gompel A, et al. Pulmonary lymphangiomyomatosis. Follow-up and long-term outcome with antiestrogen therapy; a report of eight cases. Chest 1992; 102:472–6.

24. Brunelli A, Catalini G, Fianchini A. Pregnancy exacerbating unsuspected mediastinal lymphangioleiomyomatosis and chylothorax. Int J Gynaecol Obstet 1996;52:289–90.

25. Shen A, Iseman MD, Waldron JA, et al. Exacerbation of pulmonary lymphangioleiomyomatosis by exogenous estrogens. Chest 1987;91:782–5.

26. Aubry MC, Myers JL, Ryu JH, et al. Pulmonary lymphangioleiomyomatosis in a man. Am J Respir Crit Care Med 2000;162(2 Pt 1):749–52.

27. Kang HW, Kim CJ, Kang SK, et al. Pulmonary lymphangioleiomyomatosis in a male. J Korean Med Sci 1991;6:83–5.

28. Johnson SR, Tattersfield AE. Clinical experience of lymphangioleiomyomatosis in the UK. Thorax 2000;55:1052–7.

29. Carsillo T, Astrinidis A, Henske EP. Mutations in the tuberous sclerosis complex gene TSC2 are a cause of sporadic pulmonary lymphangioleiomyomatosis. Proc Natl Acad Sci U S A 2000;97:6085–90.

30. Fukuhara S, Gutkind JS. A new twist for the tumour suppressor hamartin. Nat Cell Biol 2000;2:E76–8.

31. Lamb RF, Roy C, Diefenbach TJ, et al. The TSC1 tumour suppressor hamartin regulates cell adhesion through ERM proteins and the GTPase Rho. Nat Cell Biol 2000;2:281–7.

32. The European Chromosome 16 Tuberous Sclerosis Consortium. Identification and characterization of the tuberous sclerosis gene on chromosome 16. Cell 1993;75:1305–15.

33. Soucek T, Pusch O, Wienecke R, et al. Role of the tuberous sclerosis gene-2 product in cell cycle control. Loss of the tuberous sclerosis gene-2 induces quiescent cells to enter S phase. J Biol Chem 1997;272:29301–8.

34. Tapon N, Ito N, Dickson BJ, et al. The Drosophila tuberous sclerosis complex gene homologs restrict cell growth and cell proliferation. Cell 2001;105:345–55.

35. Potter CJ, Huang H, Xu T. Drosophila tsc1 functions with tsc2 to antagonize insulin signaling in regulating cell growth, cell proliferation, and organ size. Cell 2001;105:357–68.

36. Xiao GH, Shoarinejad F, Jin F, et al. The tuberous sclerosis 2 gene product, tuberin, functions as a Rab5 GTPase activating protein (GAP) in modulating endocytosis. J Biol Chem 1997;272:6097–100.

37. Wienecke R, Konig A, DeClue JE. Identification of tuberin, the tuberous sclerosis-2 product. Tuberin possesses specific Rap1GAP activity. J Biol Chem 1995;270:16409–14.

38. Aicher LD, Campbell JS, Yeung RS. Tuberin phosphorylation regulates its interaction with hamartin: two proteins involved in tuberous sclerosis. J Biol Chem 2001;276:21017–21.

39. Nellist M, van Slegtenhorst MA, Goedbloed M, et al. Char-

acterization of the cytosolic tuberin-hamartin complex. Tuberin is a cytosolic chaperone for hamartin. J Biol Chem 1999;274:35647–52.

40. Sampson JR, Harris PC. The molecular genetics of tuberous sclerosis. Hum Mol Genet 1994;3 Spec No:1477–80.

41. Ferrans VJ, Yu ZX, Nelson WK, et al. Lymphangioleiomyomatosis (LAM): a review of clinical and morphological features. J Nippon Med Sch 2000;67:311–29.

42. Matsumoto Y, Horiba K, Usuki J, et al. Markers of cell proliferation and expression of melanosomal antigen in lymphangioleiomyomatosis. Am J Respir Cell Mol Biol 1999; 21:327–36.

43. Maruyama H, Seyama K, Sobajima J, et al. Multifocal micronodular pneumocyte hyperplasia and lymphangioleiomyomatosis in tuberous sclerosis with a TSC2 gene. Mod Pathol 2001;14:609–14.

44. Matsui K, Tatsuguchi A, Valencia J, et al. Extrapulmonary lymphangioleiomyomatosis (LAM): clinicopathologic features in 22 cases. Hum Pathol 2000;31:1242–8.

45. Neumann HP, Schwarzkopf G, Henske EP. Renal angiomyolipomas, cysts, and cancer in tuberous sclerosis complex. Semin Pediatr Neurol 1998;5:269–75.

46. Wu K, Tazelaar HD. Pulmonary angiomyolipoma and multifocal micronodular pneumocyte hyperplasia associated with tuberous sclerosis. Hum Pathol 1999;30:1266–8.

47. Usuki J, Horiba K, Chu SC, et al. Immunohistochemical analysis of proteins of the Bcl-2 family in pulmonary lymphangioleiomyomatosis: association of Bcl-2 expression with hormone receptor status. Arch Pathol Lab Med 1998; 122:895–902.

48. Hayashi T, Fleming MV, Stetler-Stevenson WG, et al. Immunohistochemical study of matrix metalloproteinases (MMPs) and their tissue inhibitors (TIMPs) in pulmonary lymphangioleiomyomatosis (LAM). Hum Pathol 1997;28:1071–8.

49. Brentani MM, Carvalho CR, Saldiva PH, et al. Steroid receptors in pulmonary lymphangioleiomyomatosis. Chest 1984;85:96–9.

50. Matsui K, Takeda K, Yu ZX, et al. Downregulation of estrogen and progesterone receptors in the abnormal smooth muscle cells in pulmonary lymphangioleiomyomatosis following therapy. An immunohistochemical study. Am J Respir Crit Care Med 2000;161(3 Pt 1):1002–9.

51. Taveira-DaSilva AM, Hedin CM, Chen CC, et al. Bone mineral density (BMD) studies in 104 patients with lymphangioleiomyomatosis (LAM). Am J Respir Crit Care Med 2001;163:A560.

52. van Lith JM, Hoekstra HJ, Boeve WJ, et al. Lymphoedema of the legs as a result of lymphangiomyomatosis. A case report and review of the literature. Neth J Med 1989;34:310–6.

53. Abe R, Kimura M, Airosaki A, et al. Retroperitoneal lymphangiomyomatosis with lymphedema of the legs. Lymphology 1980;13:62–7.

54. Johnson SF, Davey DD, Cibull ML, et al. Lymphangioleiomyomatosis. Am Surg 1993;59:395–9.

55. Pea M, Bonetti F, Martignoni G, et al. Apparent renal cell carcinomas in tuberous sclerosis are heterogeneous: the identification of malignant epithelioid angiomyolipoma. Am J Surg Pathol 1998;22:180–7.

56. Cibas ES, Goss GA, Kulke MH, et al. Malignant epithelioid angiomyolipoma ("sarcoma ex angiomyolipoma") of the kidney: a case report and review of the literature. Am J Surg Pathol 2001;25:121–6.

57. Roach ES, Delgado MR. Tuberous sclerosis. Dermatol Clin 1995;13:151–61.

58. Muller NL, Chiles C, Kullnig P. Pulmonary lymphangiomyomatosis: correlation of CT with radiographic and functional findings. Radiology 1990;175:335–9.

59. Avila NA, Chen CC, Chu SC, et al. Pulmonary lymphangioleiomyomatosis: correlation of ventilation-perfusion scintigraphy, chest radiography, and CT with pulmonary function tests. Radiology 2000;214:441–6.

60. Avila NA, Kelly JA, Chu SC, et al. Lymphangioleiomyomatosis: abdominopelvic CT and US findings. Radiology 2000; 216:147–53.

61. Bernstein SM, Newell JD Jr, Adamczyk D, et al. How common are renal angiomyolipomas in patients with pulmonary lymphangiomyomatosis? Am J Respir Crit Care Med 1995;152(6 Pt 1):2138–43.

62. Moss J, DeCastro R, Patronas NJ, et al. Meningiomas in lymphangioleiomyomatosis (LAM). JAMA 2001;286:1879–81.

63. Taveira-DaSilva AM, Hedin CM, Stylianou MP, et al. Reversible airflow obstruction, proliferation of abnormal smooth muscle cells and impairment of gas exchange as predictors of outcome in lymphangioleiomyomatosis. Am J Respir Crit Care Med 2001;164:1072–6.

64. Burger CD, Hyatt RE, Staats BA. Pulmonary mechanics in lymphangioleiomyomatosis. Am Rev Respir Dis 1991; 143(5 Pt 1):1030–3.

65. Dweik RA, Laskowski D, Ozkan M, et al. High levels of exhaled nitric oxide (NO) and NO synthase III expression in lesional smooth muscle in lymphangioleiomyomatosis. Am J Respir Cell Mol Biol 2001;24:414–8.

66. Crausman RS, Jennings CA, Mortenson RL, et al. Lymphangioleiomyomatosis: the pathophysiology of diminished exercise capacity. Am J Respir Crit Care Med 1996; 153(4 Pt 1):1368–76.

67. Matsui K, Beasley MB, Nelson WK, et al. Prognostic significance of pulmonary lymphangioleiomyomatosis histologic score. Am J Surg Pathol 2001;25:479–84.

68. Aberle DR, Hansell DM, Brown K, et al. Lymphangiomyomatosis: CT, chest radiographic, and functional correlations. Radiology 1990;176:381–7.

69. Crausman RS, Lynch DA, Mortenson RL, et al. Quantitative CT predicts the severity of physiologic dysfunction in patients with lymphangioleiomyomatosis. Chest 1996; 109:131–7.

70. Naalsund A, Johansen B, Foerster A, et al. When to suspect and how to diagnose pulmonary lymphangioleiomyomatosis. Respirology 1996;1:207–12.

71. Delgrange E, Delgrange B, Wallon J, et al. Diagnostic approach to pulmonary lymphangioleiomyomatosis. J Intern Med 1994;236:461–4.

72. Guinee DG Jr, Feuerstein I, Koss MN, et al. Pulmonary lymphangioleiomyomatosis. Diagnosis based on results of transbronchial biopsy and immunohistochemical studies and correlation with high-resolution computed tomography findings. Arch Pathol Lab Med 1994;118:846–9.

73. Bonetti F, Chiodera PL, Pea M, et al. Transbronchial biopsy in lymphangiomyomatosis of the lung. HMB45 for diagnosis. Am J Surg Pathol 1993;17:1092–102.

74. Yamauchi M, Nakahara H, Uyama K, et al. Cytologic finding of chyloascites in lymphangioleiomyomatosis. A case report. Acta Cytol 2000;44:1081–4.

75. Matthews LM. Fine needle aspiration diagnosis of lymphangiomyomatosis. A case report. Acta Cytol 1999;43:1155–8.

76. Ackley CD, Heineman L, Dodd LG. Utility of fine-needle aspiration in the diagnosis of recurrent pulmonary lymphangioleiomyomatosis: a case report. Diagn Cytopathol 1998;19:458–61.

77. Berner A, Franzen S, Heilo A. Fine needle aspiration cytology as a diagnostic approach to lymphangioleiomyomatosis. A case report. Acta Cytol 1997;41:877–9.

78. Buhl L, Larsen KE, Bjorn-Hansen L. Lymphangioleiomyomatosis. Is fine needle aspiration cytodiagnosis possible? Acta Cytol 1988;32:559–62.

79. Faul JL, Berry GJ, Colby TV, et al. Thoracic lymphangiomas, lymphangiectasis, lymphangiomatosis, and lymphatic dysplasia syndrome. Am J Respir Crit Care Med 2000; 161(3 Pt 1):1037–46.

80. Mark EJ. Mesenchymal cystic hamartoma of the lung. N Engl J Med 1986;315:1255–9.

81. Itoh T, Mochizuki M, Kumazaki S, et al. Cystic pulmonary metastases of endometrial stromal sarcoma of the uterus, mimicking lymphangiomyomatosis: a case report with immunohistochemistry of HMB45. Pathol Int 1997;47: 725–9.

82. Abramson S, Gilkeson RC, Goldstein JD, et al. Benign metastasizing leiomyoma: clinical, imaging, and pathologic correlation. AJR Am J Roentgenol 2001;176:1409–13.

83. Kayser K, Zink S, Schneider T, et al. Benign metastasizing leiomyoma of the uterus: documentation of clinical, immunohistochemical and lectin-histochemical data of ten cases. Virchows Arch 2000;437:284–92.

84. Esteban JM, Allen WM, Schaerf RH. Benign metastasizing leiomyoma of the uterus: histologic and immunohistochemical characterization of primary and metastatic lesions. Arch Pathol Lab Med 1999;123:960–2.

85. Johnson SR, Tattersfield AE. Decline in lung function in lymphangioleiomyomatosis: relation to menopause and progesterone treatment. Am J Respir Crit Care Med 1999;160: 628–33.

86. Eliasson AH, Phillips YY, Tenholder MF. Treatment of lymphangioleiomyomatosis. A meta-analysis. Chest 1989;96: 1352–55.

87. Boehler A, Speich R, Russi EW, et al. Lung transplantation for lymphangioleiomyomatosis. N Engl J Med 1996;335: 1275–80.

88. Trulock EP. Lung transplantation: special considerations and outcome in LAM. In: Moss J, editor. LAM and other diseases characterized by smooth muscle proliferation. New York: Marcel Dekker, Inc.; 1999. p. 65–78.

89. Bittmann I, Dose TB, Muller C, et al. Lymphangioleiomyomatosis: recurrence after single lung transplantation. Hum Pathol 1997;28:1420–3.

90. O'Brien JD, Lium JH, Parosa JF, et al. Lymphangiomyomatosis recurrence in the allograft after single-lung transplantation. Am J Respir Crit Care Med 1995;151:2033–6.

91. Nine JS, Yousem SA, Paradis IL, et al. Lymphangioleiomyomatosis: recurrence after lung transplantation. J Heart Lung Transplant 1994;13:714–9.

92. van Baal JG, Smits NJ, Keeman JN, et al. The evolution of renal angiomyolipomas in patients with tuberous sclerosis. J Urol 1994;152:35–8.

93. Mourikis D, Chatziioannou A, Antoniou A, et al. Selective arterial embolization in the management of symptomatic renal angiomyolipomas. Eur J Radiol 1999;32:153–9.

94. Kessler OJ, Gillon G, Neuman M, et al. Management of renal angiomyolipoma: analysis of 15 cases. Eur Urol 1998;33: 572–5.

95. Soulen MC, Faykus MH Jr, Shlansky-Goldberg RD, et al. Elective embolization for prevention of hemorrhage from renal angiomyolipomas. J Vasc Interv Radiol 1994;5: 587–91.

96. Castro M, Shepherd CW, Gomez MR, et al. Pulmonary tuberous sclerosis. Chest 1995;107:189–95.

30 PULMONARY ALVEOLAR PROTEINOSIS

JASON S. VOURLEKIS
KELLY E. GREENE

Pulmonary alveolar proteinosis (PAP) represents a heterogeneous group of diseases that share the common histopathology of a granular, lipoproteinaceous exudate within alveolar spaces. Recent advances in the understanding of surfactant biology have shed new light on this poorly understood syndrome. In particular, the identification of surfactant protein B deficiency as the primary cause of congenital PAP coupled with the discovery of the major role that the hematopoietic growth factor, granulocyte-macrophage colony–stimulating factor (GM-CSF), plays in surfactant clearance have provided greater insight into the pathogenetic mechanisms of PAP. This chapter provides an overview of PAP with particular reference to surfactant biology and the known perturbations that result in the disease state.

PULMONARY SURFACTANT

Overview

Pulmonary surfactant is produced by type II alveolar epithelial cells (type II cells). It functions to lower surface tension within alveoli, thereby facilitating lung expansion and preventing atelectasis.[1] Chemically, 90 to 95% of surfactant is composed of lipid and 5 to 10% is protein. Phospholipids, in particular saturated phosphatidylcholines such as dipalmitoyl phosphatidylcholine (DPPC), constitute over 80% of the lipid fraction. The protein portion is largely composed of surfactant proteins A, B, C, and D (SP-A, SP-B, SP-C, SP-D) with serum proteins contributing a small fraction.

Surfactant Protein A

Surfactant protein A constitutes 50% of the total surfactant protein.[2] It is a large, hydrophilic protein. In the mature form, SP-A is composed of six trimers that form an octadecameric bouquetlike structure.[3] Within the alveolus, SP-A functions to enhance the adsorption of surfactant to the air-liquid interface and is essential to the formation of tubular myelin. Tubular myelin repre-

sents a conglomerate structure enriched in SP-A, SP-B, and surfactant lipid, which serves as an intermediate form of surfactant between its secretion by the type II cell and its full incorporation into the lipid monolayer. Targeted deletion of the SP-A gene in mice results in a decrease in the number of tubular myelin structures visible on electron microscopy and minimal increases in the relative amount of saturated phosphatidylcholines in both alveolar and lung tissue.[4,5] Histologically and physiologically, however, there are no differences between the SP-A knockout mouse and the wild-type mouse.[6]

Surfactant Protein B

Surfactant protein B is a small hydrophobic protein necessary for surfactant function.[7] SP-B facilitates the surface spreading of phospholipids within the surfactant monolayer, which is critical to the reduction of surface tension between the air-liquid interface and to the prevention of atelectasis. Targeted deletion of SP-B in mice results in acute respiratory failure and death shortly following birth.[8] In humans, SP-B deficiency is similarly lethal.[9,10] Microscopic examination of the lung in SP-B deficient mice reveals an absence of both lamellar bodies and tubular myelin.[8] In addition, they show abnormal processing of SP-C, manifest by the accumulation of proSP-C fragments and decreased mature SP-C peptide within the alveolar spaces. Functionally, SP-B–deficient mice have a diminished lung compliance and an absence of hysteresis on performance of pressure-volume curves.[11] However, compared to wild-type littermates, there are no differences in SP-A, SP-D, or lipid concentration.

Surfactant Protein C

Surfactant protein C is a hydrophobic protein that is synthesized exclusively by type II cells.[7] SP-C is believed to stabilize the surface activity of surfactant, particularly during the expansion and compression associated with tidal breathing.[1] SP-C–deficient mice do not show any abnormalities in development or lung histology.[12] However, the physiologic study of SP-C–deficient mice reveals abnormalities in surfactant surface tension at low lung volumes.

Surfactant Protein D

Surfactant protein D is a large, hydrophilic protein with a molecular mass of approximately 43 kD.[1] The mature protein represents an aggregate of four trimers (dodecamer), forming a cruciform-shaped molecule.[3] The development of an SP-D–deficient mouse has greatly elucidated the function of SP-D.[13] SP-D appears to regulate the surfactant lipid pool. Metabolic studies indicate that SP-D–deficient mice accumulate saturated phosphatidylcholine within the alveolar spaces and lung tissue due to diminished catabolism relative to wild-type mice.[14] However, alveolar macrophage degradation of DPPC is normal, suggesting that SP-D deficiency may interfere with type II cell uptake of surfactant lipid.[15]

Surfactant Production and Catabolism

Type II cells are responsible for surfactant production.[16] Precursor molecules including glucose and fatty acids are derived from three general sources: the systemic circulation, recycling of alveolar surfactant, and de novo synthesis within the type II cells. Regulation of surfactant production has been studied mainly in neonatal lung tissue and appears to be under the control of several hormones, most notably corticosteroids.[17] Surfactant lipid is synthesized within the endoplasmic reticulum and subsequently transported through the Golgi apparatus into lamellar bodies. Surfactant proteins also are transported through the Golgi apparatus where they are exported in transport vesicles.[18] The transport vesicles merge with multivesicular bodies within the cell cytoplasm. Final processing of the surfactant proteins occurs at this stage. The fusion of multivesicular bodies results in the formation of lamellar bodies, the final form of secreted surfactant. This latter step appears critically dependent on proper SP-B processing as SP-B–deficient mice accumulate multivesicular bodies and fail to make lamellar bodies.[8]

Traditionally it was believed that type II cells accounted for 80% of surfactant turnover and alveolar macrophages processed the remainder.[19,20] However, recent work with the genetically engineered GM-CSF–deficient mouse has provided new information, suggesting that the contribution of the alveolar macrophage may be greater. Mice lacking either the gene encoding for GM-CSF or the GM-CSF-beta receptor develop pulmonary alveolar proteinosis.[21–24] Metabolic studies indicate that the rate of surfactant synthesis is unchanged from wild-type mice and that the surfactant

accumulation occurs due to a defect in clearance.[22] The effects of GM-CSF on surfactant catabolism are believed to be mediated through its effects on the alveolar macrophage.[25] Bone marrow transplantation, which reconstitutes only the alveolar macrophage population, corrects PAP in GM-CSF-receptor–deficient mice.[26] Further GM-CSF deficiency does not appear to affect the binding of surfactant protein and lipid to the alveolar macrophage but rather results in decreased degradation relative to wild-type mice.[27] It is possible that the type II cell, which expresses the GM-CSF receptor on its surface, also is a target of GM-CSF.[28] A PAP-like lesion due to increased surfactant production also has been reported in mice overexpressing interleukin-4 (IL-4).[29] In this case, IL-4 appears to regulate type II cell surfactant synthesis via an unknown mechanism.

CLINICAL SYNDROMES OF PULMONARY ALVEOLAR PROTEINOSIS

The clinical, radiographic, and pathologic features of PAP are quite similar regardless of etiology. In the absence of a clear predisposing etiology such as chronic myelogenous leukemia, the diagnosis of idiopathic PAP is made. This section focuses on idiopathic PAP as the paradigm and then reviews the secondary forms of PAP (Table 30–1) for which an etiology is reasonably well established.

Table 30–1   Exposures and Conditions Associated with Alveolar Proteinosis

Environmental exposures
  Aluminum[41]
  Cement[42]
  Insulation[44]
  Silica[149–153,155]
  Titanium[43]
Hematologic and neoplastic disorders
  Acute lymphocytic leukemia[133,134,161]
  Acute myelogenous leukemia[133–135,161,162]
  Amyloidosis[163]
  Chronic myelogenous leukemia[133,134,161,164–168]
  Essential thrombocythemia[169–171]
  Fanconi's anemia[172]
  Hairy cell leukemia[134]
  Hodgkin's disease[134,161]
  Non-Hodgkin's lymphoma[134]
  Melanoma[173]
  Multiple myeloma[174]
  Myelodysplastic syndrome[164]
  Polycythemia vera[175,176]
Immunologic disorders
  Monoclonal gammopathy[177]
  Selective IgA deficiency[138–140]
  Severe combined immunodeficiency[138,144,145]
Miscellaneous
  Dermatomyositis[178]
  Lung transplantation[179,180]

Idiopathic PAP

Epidemiology

Alveolar proteinosis has been recognized worldwide, although the majority of reported cases are in Caucasian and Oriental populations.[30] The male to female ratio is 2.4:1. Most patients present in early to midadulthood. The mean age at diagnosis in 7 series totaling 151 patients was 36 years and the range 1 to 87 years.[31–37] In North America, the incidence of PAP is estimated to be 2 per 10,000,000 per year.[38] A comparable incidence was reported in Israel.[39]

Etiology

In most cases of PAP, an etiology is never identified. The association of PAP with other systemic diseases, both genetic and acquired, suggests that there is likely more than one etiology.[40] Dust exposures, particularly to crystalline silica, may be an important precipitant of PAP.[41–44] Analysis of lung tissue in idiopathic PAP reveals tenfold greater alveolar particulate counts compared with control subjects.[45] Whether the dust accumulation results from alveolar macrophage dysfunction associated with PAP or whether it results in surfactant accumulation is unknown. It is also possible that there are subtle, genetic defects that are unmasked by the appropriate environmental exposure, as has been described with SP-B deficiency.[46]

Pathogenesis

The GM-CSF and GM-CSF-beta-receptor knockout mice clearly have established a role for GM-CSF in the regulation of alveolar macrophage surfactant clearance. The applicability of these models to the human disease is uncertain. Kinetic studies in human PAP using radiolabeled surfactant are consistent with defective clearance as the mechanism for surfactant accumulation.[47,48] However, whether the defect in clearance is due to an alteration in GM-CSF biology is unknown. Defects in both GM-CSF production and receptor signaling have been demonstrated in human PAP.[49–54] A point mutation in the GM-CSF-receptor beta-chain gene was associated with diminished cellular receptor expression in a 20-month-old infant with PAP.[49] In another patient, a mutation in the GM-CSF gene was associated with diminished cellular protein production following in vitro stimulation.[54] Another possible, pathogenetic mechanism is the presence of a circulating GM-CSF inhibitor. Circulating anti-GM-CSF antibodies have been found in both serum and bronchoalveolar lavage fluid in 100% of patients tested.[37,53,55,56] The role of this antibody is uncertain, however, as it is not clear that the antibody alone is sufficient to cause PAP. Taken as a whole, these studies suggest that PAP may represent a syndrome with multiple biologic defects that culminate in a common histopathologic lesion.

Alveolar macrophage dysfunction has been cited as one reason for the apparent susceptibility to opportunistic infections, particularly from intracellular pathogens, seen in PAP.[40,57] Microscopically, the macrophages appear swollen and their cytoplasm is filled with surfactant lipid. Compared with alveolar macrophages harvested from normal controls, PAP alveolar macrophages show impairments in chemotaxis, phagocytosis, adherence, and proliferation.[58] The addition of PAP alveolar exudate to healthy alveolar macrophages in vitro, results in the cells assuming a vacuolated phenotype similar to PAP alveolar macrophages.[58,59] Further, the cells become less viable in cell culture and show diminished phagocytosis.[59,60] These data coupled with the finding that alveolar macrophage chemotaxis normalizes following whole lung lavage in PAP, suggest that the surfactant accumulation leads to defects in macrophage biology.[61] In this regard, it has been shown in vitro that administration of either synthetic or natural surfactant to alveolar macrophages has a general suppressive effect.[62–66]

Histology

Pathologically, as shown in Figure 30–1, PAP is very distinct.[67] The lung architecture is well preserved but there is a diffuse alveolar exudate composed of a granular, eosinophilic material that readily stains with periodic acid–Schiff (PAS) and is diastase resistant. Foamy alveolar macrophages are often present within the alveolar spaces and ghost cells may be seen. Ghost cells are remnant cells in which the cell membrane is still visible but the nucleus has dissolved. Type II cell hyperplasia is a common finding. The presence of inflammation or necrosis suggests a secondary process such as associated

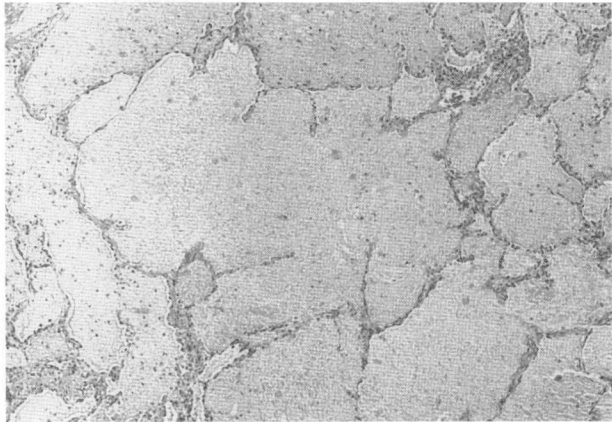

Figure 30–1 Photomicrograph of pulmonary alveolar proteinosis lung tissue showing a diffuse, acellular, granular material within the alveolar spaces. The alveolar septa appear normal (hematoxylin and eosin stain, ×100).

infection. Ultrastructurally, electron microscopy demonstrates numerous lamellar bodies within type II cells and tubular myelin within alveolar spaces.[68] Analysis of alveolar lavage fluid reveals an abundance of all surfactant proteins, which helps distinguish idiopathic PAP from surfactant protein-B deficiency.[69–73]

Clinical Manifestations

Most patients will present with a subacute or insidious onset of symptoms, particularly cough and exertional dyspnea.[74] A preceding upper respiratory tract illness has been reported in up to 50% of patients.[31] The cough may be productive of a "chunky" material.[31] Rarely is there purulent sputum and hemoptysis has been reported in up to 25% of patients.[34] An ill-defined chest discomfort, sometimes pleuritic in nature, is present in 30% of cases.[34] Systemic symptoms, particularly a fever greater than 38.5°C and weight loss, are uncommon and should arouse suspicion of an associated infection or possible underlying systemic illness.[34] On physical examination most patients appear well.[40] Mild tachypnea and low-grade fever may be present and cyanosis can be seen in advanced cases.[34,36] Chest examination often is normal.[30] When abnormal, a combination of coarse breath sounds and crackles may be auscultated. Clubbing has been reported in up to 25% of patients.[36] Pulmonary function assessment reveals exertional and, sometimes, resting hypoxemia.[40] The hypox-

emia results from both ventilation-perfusion mismatch and physiologic shunting.[75] Most patients manifest reductions in total lung capacity, vital capacity, and diffusing capacity consistent with a restrictive physiology.[32,36]

PAP patients appear to have increased susceptibility to opportunistic infections, particularly *Nocardia asteroides* and mycobacterial infections.[35,76,77] Fungal infections with *Cryptococcus neoformans*, *Aspergillus*, *Mucor*, and *Pneumocystis carinii* also have been reported.[78] This susceptibility may be a direct consequence of the alveolar macropage dysfunction or it may represent another defect in cell-mediated immunity. GM-CSF is critical to controlling infection with *Pneumocystis carinii* in an experimental animal model, and GM-CSF deficient mice are more susceptible to bacterial pneumonia.[79,80] Therefore, GM-CSF deficiency may lead to defects in microbial immunity.

Diagnosis

The diagnosis of PAP should be considered in any previously healthy individual who presents with exertional dyspnea and an alveolar filling pattern on a chest radiograph. On standard chest radiography (Figure 30–2), a combination of ground-glass opacities and consolidation are the main findings, often in a midlung zone and perihilar (batwing) distribution.[81] Sparing of the diaphragms is frequently noted. On high-resolution computed tomography (HRCT) similar findings are present along with irregular reticular opacities, which represent septal thickening (Figure 30–3).[82] The reticular lines outline the secondary pulmonary lobule, forming polygonal structures that have the appearance of patio flagstone, referred to as "crazy paving." Crazy paving is

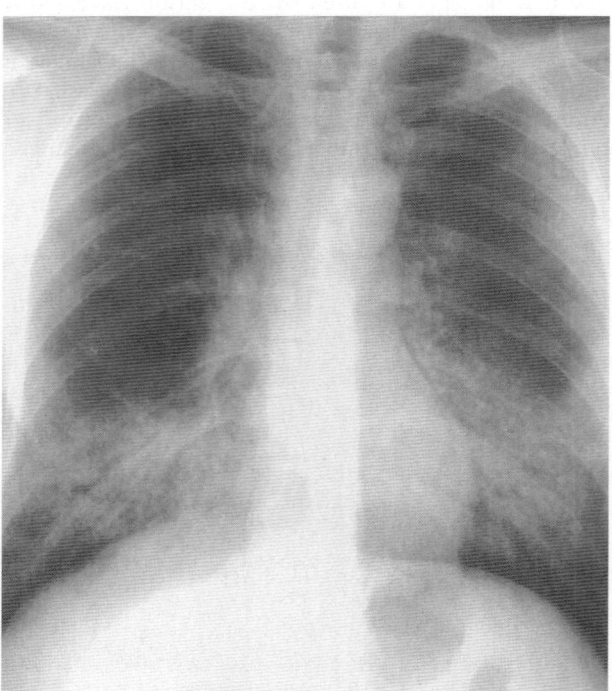

Figure 30–2   Standard posterior-anterior chest radiograph of a patient with pulmonary alveolar proteinosis showing bilateral, ground-glass abnormalities in a perihilar distribution.

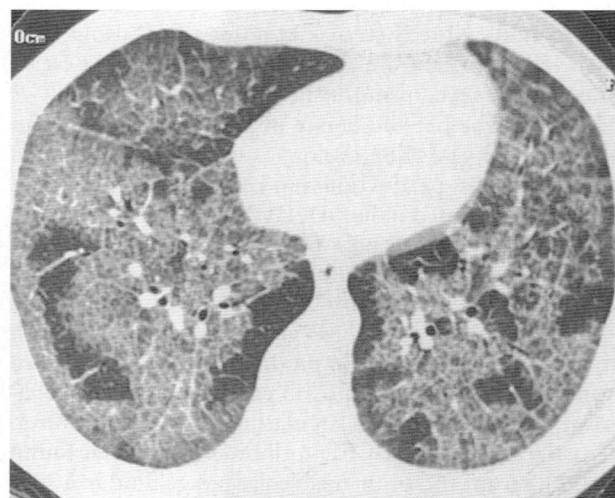

Figure 30–3   High-resolution computed tomography of the chest in pulmonary alveolar proteinosis showing bilateral, diffuse ground-glass abnormalities and reticular opacities. The reticular lines form polygons giving the radiographic appearance of "crazy paving."

highly suggestive but not diagnostic of PAP. A similar pattern may be seen with several other interstitial lung diseases, including lymphangitic carcinomatosis and acute respiratory distress syndrome.[83,84]

Bronchoscopy is an important diagnostic tool in PAP. It has been suggested that bronchoalveolar lavage alone in conjunction with a characteristic clinical presentation provide sufficient evidence for diagnosis.[40] Cytologic examination of PAS-stained lavage exudate reveals a typical amorphous, granular, lipoproteinaceous exudate and simultaneously, with the use of appropriate staining, allows the exclusion of infection.[85] Electron microscopy, if available, adds an additional degree of diagnostic certainty but may be impractical.[86] When studied, the use of combined cytologic and ultrastructural examination showed high sensitivity but poor specificity.[87] Recently, the use of Papanicolaou's staining of bronchoalveolar exudate has been shown to be highly sensitive and specific for PAP.[88] The presence of large numbers of green-orange staining globular densities helped distinguish PAP from other lung diseases. Given the relative safety of transbronchial biopsy, we advocate its performance along with bronchoalveolar lavage as an initial first step. The sensitivity of transbronchial biopsy ranges from 37 to 83%.[36,89] The use of HRCT to guide the location of biopsy sampling may increase the diagnostic yield. In cases where diagnostic uncertainty persists, a surgical lung biopsy may be safely obtained for definitive diagnosis.[36]

A neutralizing antibody against GM-CSF has been isolated from the serum of 100% of PAP patients studied.[53,55,56,90] Similar findings have been reported by 3 different groups of investigators working on different continents. Detection of the antibody also appears to have high specificity as it was found in only 5% of healthy control subjects and in none of 46 diseased control subjects, including 6 subjects with secondary PAP.[90] When applied only to patients with diffuse lung disease, the positive and negative predictive values of the antibody were 100%. Should further testing confirm these initial results, the detection of an anti-GM-CSF antibody in conjunction with a high clinical suspicion and characteristic HRCT may supplant bronchoscopy as the diagnostic test of choice.

Bronchoalveolar lavage and serum levels of SP-A and SP-D are both elevated in PAP.[48,70–72,91,92] This finding is not specific as similar results have been reported for the acute respiratory distress syndrome and idiopathic pulmonary fibrosis.[91–93] In established cases of PAP, serum surfactant protein levels may function as surrogate markers of disease activity.[72,91] Monitoring of serum lactate dehydrogenase (LDH) levels also has been advocated as a means to assess disease activity.[94]

Treatment

The decision to treat should be based on careful assessment of a patient's symptoms and functional limitations.[95] Whole lung lavage is the mainstay of therapy for PAP and remains the treatment of choice for patients with severe disease.[40] Whole lung lavage has been shown to result in immediate improvements in gas exchange and lung function.[96] In the experience of one center, 60% of patients experience a sustained remission following the performance of two lung lavages.[40] Goldstein and colleagues found that roughly 50% of patients required lavage beyond the first year following diagnosis but only 1 of 11 patients required lavage beyond 10 years.[36] Generally, whole lung lavage is a safe procedure. Intraoperative hypoxemia and postlavage unilateral pulmonary edema are the most common complications.[97]

Published data regarding open label use of GM-CSF for the treatment of idiopathic PAP are available for 21 patients.[37,98–101] Twelve (57%) have shown clinical improvement. In Seymour and colleagues' series of 14 patients, the development of peripheral eosinophilia in response to GM-CSF therapy was predictive of clinical improvement.[37] They found that 5 of the 6 responders improved on the initial dosage of 5 μg/kg/day subcutaneously within 12 weeks of therapy and only 1 of 4 not responsive to this dose, responded to a higher dose. Five patients subsequently relapsed off therapy but all three retreated with GM-CSF again responded. Overall, GM-CSF was well tolerated and treatment was stopped due to side effects in only one patient. Based on these data, it is reasonable to consider GM-CSF as an alternative therapy to whole lung lavage in patients with chronic, persistent PAP. It is possible that the "apparent" response to GM-CSF in some cases, actually reflects the variable natural history of PAP. Ultimately, the performance of a randomized, blinded study of GM-CSF therapy in PAP should allow a more definitive evaluation of the potential therapeutic role of GM-CSF.

Outcome

Prior to the widespread use of whole lung lavage, PAP often was a progressive and fatal disease with crude mortality approaching 30%.[30,102] In contrast, recent case series are notable for the absence of reported deaths.[97] It frequently is stated that 30% of PAP patients will experience a spontaneous remission. However, Seymour and colleagues reviewed the available literature through 1997 and found that clinical remission was documented in only 8% of 303 published cases.[37] Part of the variability likely lies in how remission is defined. Most investigators have used the absence of symptoms as a proxy for clinical remission.[33] It is likely that more detailed analyses including radiographic and physiologic assessment would reveal persistence of disease. Given the low mortality associated with PAP and the lack of proven interventions other than whole lung lavage, routine monitoring of disease activity is not advocated. Rather, patients should be seen on an as-needed basis with annual follow-up for asymptomatic patients. In our experience, the patients' sense of shortness of breath is as reliable as an indicator of disease activity and hence the need for treatment as any physiologic or radiographic study.

Hereditary Surfactant Protein B Deficiency (Congenital PAP)

Hereditary surfactant protein B deficiency is caused by mutations in the SP-B gene.[103] The observation of congenital PAP clustering within families suggested a genetic basis to this disease.[104,105] In 1993, Nogee and colleagues reported two siblings who died from congenital PAP in whom SP-B protein was undetectable in lung tissue.[9] Further investigation revealed the index patient to have a frameshift mutation at position 375 of the SP-B gene, referred to as the 121ins2 mutation, resulting in premature termination of gene transcription and the absence of detectable messenger ribonucleic acid (mRNA).[106] His sister was found to be heterozygous for this mutation. Three siblings who died of congenital PAP from an unrelated family were also found to be homozygous for the same mutation.[105] Further, two healthy siblings from the second family were heterozygous for the 121ins2 mutation as were both parents. The unrelated parents of another neonate who died from congenital PAP were also found to be heterozygous for 121ins2. These landmark reports established a linkage between SP-B deficiency and congenital PAP. Further investigation of these original cases and of new cases has greatly improved our understanding of this rare disease.

Genetics

The SP-B gene is located on chromosome 2.[18] There are 11 exons. The preproprotein is encoded on exons 1 through 10, whereas the active protein is encoded by exons 6 and 7. The 121ins2 mutation is located within exon 4 but leads to a premature stop codon in exon 6.[103] Congenital PAP is associated with both homozygosity and heterozygosity for the 121ins2 SP-B gene mutation.[106,107] In some heterozygotes, no other mutations were identified whereas others showed unique mutations.[107,108] In the largest study to date, 32 infants with congenital PAP were screened for the 121ins2 mutation.[108] Fifty percent were homozygous for this mutation, 31% carried the 121ins2 mutation on one allele and a second mutation on the other allele, and the remaining 19% were homozygous for novel SP-B mutations. In all, 15 different SP-B gene mutations were identified. One important implication of this study is that most, if not all, cases of congenital PAP are related to SP-B protein deletions or mutations. A second important finding is that, when systemically studied, all affected infants had mutations in both SP-B alleles. This latter finding coupled with the normal physical development and lung function present in 121ins2 heterozygotes, suggests that heterozygosity alone may not be sufficient to cause congenital PAP.[109]

Homozygosity for the 121ins2 mutation is associated with the absence of both SP-B mRNA and protein. In contrast, proSP-B protein, mature SP-B protein, and near normal levels of SP-B mRNA have been reported in association with 121ins2 heterozygosity and other mutations.[108,110] Transient SP-B deficiency was reported in an infant heterozygous for a guanine to adenine substitution at position 417 within exon 5 of the SP-B gene.[46] As the infant showed clinical recovery, immunoblotting of transtracheal aspirates revealed mature SP-B protein.

Pathogenesis

Within the lung, SP-B protein is synthesized within type II cells and Clara cells that line the bronchiolar epithelium. Following translation of the 381 amino acid preproprotein, the nascent peptide is directed into the secretory pathway and packaged, along with other surfactant apoproteins, into transport vesicles within the trans-Golgi network. The transport vesicles merge with multivesicular bodies where final processing of the SP-B precursor to the active form occurs. Within type II cells, the multivesicular bodies fuse and form lamellar bodies that are secreted into the alveolus. Analysis of human lung tissue in SP-B deficiency reveals an abundance of multivesicular bodies within type II cells but very few lamellar bodies and no tubular myelin.[107,111] Further, there is an abnormal accumulation of multivesicular bodies along with SP-A and SP-C between the basolateral border of type II cells and the epithelial basement membrane, indicating that SP-B may be important to the directional movement of surfactant.[111] SP-B also appears essential to proper SP-C processing.[112,113] In human SP-B deficiency, there is a relative paucity of mature SP-C and accumulation of an abnormal intermediate form of SP-C, which is approximately three times larger than the mature protein.[112]

The consequence of SP-B deficiency is the accumulation of abnormal surfactant within the alveolar space, leading to reduced lung compliance. In vitro study of surfactant isolated from SP-B–deficient infants shows increased surface tension relative to normal surfactant, suggesting that it is less protective from atelectasis.[113] Why surfactant accumulates in the alveolus in SP-B deficiency is unknown. The absence of SP-B protein may retard alveolar clearance of phosphatidylglycerol.[113] A third, potential consequence of SP-B deficiency is a lack of protection from hyperoxic lung injury associated with mechanical ventilation. Heterozygote SP-B–deficient mice are more susceptible to hyperoxic lung injury than their SP-B replete littermates.[114] This susceptibility may also explain the association of certain SP-B genetic polymorphisms with neonatal respiratory distress syndrome.[115]

Histology

Histologically, congenital PAP resembles the adult form.[116] There is diffuse, granular eosinophilic material within the alveolar spaces, often associated with type II cell hyperplasia and lipid-laden macrophages. The granular eosinophilic material avidly stains with PAS. In some cases, the alveolar exudate may be quite minimal and even focal.[117] A chronic mononuclear cellular infiltration of alveolar septa is variably present as is interstitial fibrosis.[111] Immunostaining of surfactant proteins typically reveals abundant SP-A.[118] Depending on the specific SP-B genetic mutation, pro-SP-B staining and even light staining for mature SP-B protein may be present.[107,110] SP-C staining usually indicates the presence of both mature protein and the previously described abnormal variant.[10]

Clinical Manifestations, Treatment, and Outcome

Congenital PAP generally is recognized in full-term infants of uncomplicated pregnancies.[116] Symptoms and signs of respiratory distress typically develop within a few hours following birth. Most are diagnosed initially with neonatal pneumonia. However, with a failure of response to antibiotics and persistent infiltrates, the diagnosis of congenital PAP is entertained. In premature infants, neonatal respiratory distress syndrome must also be considered. This latter disease is dramatically responsive to surfactant therapy, whereas congenital PAP is not.[119]

The specific SP-B genotype may influence the clinical presentation.[103] SP-B gene mutations within exon 5 have been associated with milder disease and survival beyond infancy.[46,120] In contrast, most patients homozygous for the 121ins2 mutation will succumb within 3 months of birth.[116] Congenital PAP has been reported in infants heterozygous for the 121ins2 mutation, but most seem to develop normally and have normal lung function.[109]

The diagnosis of SP-B deficiency is established by analysis of transtracheal aspirate for SP-B and SP-C protein. In 121ins2 homozygotes, no detectable SP-B is found and an "abnormally" sized SP-C variant is present. The absence of detectable SP-B protein or mRNA on lung tissue obtained by surgical biopsy is confirmatory. Unfortunately, these techniques are not commercially available and, to date, can be performed only in specialized research laboratories. In cases of suspected congenital PAP, referral to medical centers with expertise in neonatalogy is indicated.

There is no effective medical treatment for SP-B deficiency. Administration of exogenous surfactant does not appear to ameliorate the disease course and, in fact, may even be harmful.[121] In one infant, exogenous surfactant therapy was associated with the development of granulomatous inflammation.[121] Exogenous SP-B protein was centered within the granulomas, suggesting

that it may have been the target of a cell-mediated immune response.

Lung transplantation provides a therapeutic option in some cases.[122] SP-B deficiency represents an attractive disease for gene therapy. Based on animal model data, the SP-B gene will need to be reconstituted in type II cells as reconstitution in bronchiolar Clara cells does not correct murine SP-B deficiency.[123]

Infection-Associated Pulmonary Alveolar Proteinosis

Secondary alveolar proteinosis is associated with *Pneumocystis carinii*, particularly in acquired immunodeficiency syndrome (AIDS) patients.[124,125] An association with cytomegalovirus pulmonary infection has also been described.[126] In these cases, the infection is diagnosed simultaneously or even prior to PAP, suggesting a potential causality. Clinically, these cases must be distinguished from opportunistic infection developing in a patient with established PAP.

Lysinuric Protein Intolerance

Lysinuric protein intolerance (LPI) is an autosomal recessive disease predominantly affecting Fins, which is caused by defective cationic amino acid transport in epithelial cells.[127,128] Most patients present in infancy following weaning from breast feeding. Clinically, the disease is manifest by failure to thrive. Physical characteristics include osteoporosis, hepatosplenomegaly, and hyperammonemia. PAP has been reported in approximately 10% of LPI patients.[129,130] Concomitant alveolar hemorrhage was present in two cases.[131] The mechanism of PAP in LPI is unknown. Recent investigation showed impairment in humoral immunity in most patients, with deficiencies in IgG subclasses being the most common abnormality.[132] IgA deficiency was not present and studies of cell-mediated immunity showed normal results. With proper dietary therapy, most patients will grow to adulthood. Whole lung lavage has been advocated for treatment of associated PAP.[130]

Malignancy-Associated Pulmonary Alveolar Proteinosis

Pulmonary alveolar proteinosis is associated with several different malignancies, most consistently acute and chronic myelogenous leukemia (AML, CML). It is estimated that PAP develops in 10% of AML patients and 5% of patients with hematologic malignancies.[133] In some cases, associated infection with *Pneumocystis carinii* or cytomegalovirus has been reported.[134] The alveolar proteinosis appears to be a direct consequence of the leukemia as the pulmonary lesions often regress following successful treatment of the malignancy. Dirksen and colleagues reported three cases of AML associated with PAP where the leukemic clones lacked either one or both subunits of the GM-CSF receptor.[135] These same clones were harvested from the lung of all three patients by bronchoalveolar lavage. Following chemotherapy-induced remission, the PAP resolved and the cells of the myeloid lineage showed normal expression of both GM-CSF-receptor subunits. AML also is associated with circulating GM-CSF-alpha receptor, which, theoretically, may function as a circulating inhibitor.[136]

Selective Immunoglobulin A Deficiency

Low serum IgA levels, consistent with selective IgA deficiency, also have been reported in association with PAP.[137–140] Whether this association represents cause-and-effect is unknown. PAP has not been associated with the more severe humoral immunodeficiency syndrome, common variable immunodeficiency, which may share genetic determinants with selective IgA deficiency.[141]

Severe Combined Immunodeficiency

Severe combined immunodeficiency (SCID) represents an inherited group of immunologic disorders characterized by profound defects in both cell-mediated and humoral immunity, resulting in frequent infections with both common and opportunistic pathogens.[142] The most common type of SCID is X-linked, which is caused by a mutation in the common cytokine receptor gamma chain (γ_c). γ_c is essential to signaling of interleukins 2, 4, 7, 9, and 15 (IL-2, IL-4, IL-7, IL-9, IL-15).[143] Phenotypically, affected individuals have thymic and lymph node hypoplasia.[142] There are several, well-documented reports of PAP associated with SCID.[138,144,145] In less than 10% of cases, *Pneumocystis carinii* pneumonia was concomitantly diagnosed. Most patients died from complications of SCID.

The mechanism of PAP in SCID is uncertain. Recent reports of PAP in SCID mice have confirmed these earlier investigations.[146,147] Microscopically, there were no evident defects in surfactant composition as immunostaining readily identifies both SP-A and SP-B and electron microscopy reveals normal-appearing lamellar bodies and tubular myelin.

Silicosis

Silicoproteinosis is an acute, severe form of silicosis that pathologically resembles PAP and has a high mortality.[148] It is caused by exposure to high concentrations of fine silica dust, such as occurs with sandblasting.[149–151] Silicoproteinosis also has been reported with quartz milling, coal mining, uranium mining, and sandblasting

of dental prostheses.[152–155] Patients may present with concomitant infections including nontuberculous mycobacterial disease.[149,151] The chest radiograph shows a combination of features including air space consolidation with air bronchograms, fine nodular densities, upper lobe volume loss, and mediastinal adenopathy.[156] HRCT findings include fine centrilobular nodules, ground-glass opacification, and air space consolidation. Pathologically, silicotic nodules in addition to alveolar proteinosis are often present.[150] Birefringent silica particles can be identified in most cases.[150,151,157] Most patients die within 2 years of disease onset. Whole lung lavage may be helpful.[152] Unilateral lung transplantation has been performed successfully.[155]

Surfactant Protein C Mutations

Interstitial lung disease associated with an inherited mutation in the SP-C gene has been described.[158] In the index case of a 6-week-old infant, there was an absence of detectable SP-C protein in the alveolar lavage fluid but immunostaining clearly showed SP-C precursor protein within type II cells.[158] Pathologically, a lesion resembling nonspecific interstitial pneumonitis was present.[159] The infant's mother had been diagnosed with desquamative interstitial pneumonitis in childhood and died of acute respiratory failure following delivery. Diffuse alveolar damage in association with honeycomb fibrosis were the major findings on autopsy of her lung. Separately, two siblings with lymphocytic interstitial pneumonitis were reported to have undetectable SP-C protein by immunohistochemistry of lung tissue and by immunoblot analysis of bronchoalveolar lavage fluid.[160] However, a mutation in the SP-C gene was not detected in either sibling.

REFERENCES

1. Griese M. Pulmonary surfactant in health and human lung diseases: state of the art. Eur Respir J 1999;13:1455–76.
2. Johansson J, Curstedt T, Robertson B. The proteins of the surfactant system. Eur Respir J 1994;7:372–91.
3. Mason RJ, Greene KE, Voelker DR. Surfactant protein A and surfactant protein D in health and disease. Am J Physiol 1998;275:L1–13.
4. Korfhagen TR, Bruno MD, Ross GF, et al. Altered surfactant function and structure in SP-A gene targeted mice. Proc Natl Acad Sci U S A 1996;93:9594–9.
5. Ikegami M, Korfhagen TR, Bruno MD, et al. Surfactant metabolism in surfactant protein A deficient mice. Am J Physiol 1997;272:L479–85.
6. Ikegami M, Jobe AH, Whitsett JA, Korfhagen TR. Tolerance of SP-A-deficient mice to hyperoxia or exercise. J Appl Physiol 2000;89:644–8.
7. Weaver TE, Conkright JJ. Functions of surfactant proteins B and C. Annu Rev Physiol 2001;63:555–78.
8. Clark JC, Wert SE, Bachurski CJ, et al. Targeted disruption of the surfactant protein B gene disrupts surfactant homeostasis, causing respiratory failure in newborn mice. Proc Natl Acad Sci U S A 1995;92:7794–8.

9. Nogee LM, deMello DE, Dehner LP, Colten HR. Brief report: deficiency of pulmonary surfactant B in congenital alveolar proteinosis. N Engl J Med 1993;328:406–10.

10. Williams GD, Christodoulou J, Stack J, et al. Surfactant protein B deficiency: clinical, histological, and molecular evaluation. J Paediatr Child Health 1999;35:214–20.

11. Tokieda K, Whitsett JA, Clark JC, et al. Pulmonary dysfunction in neonatal SP-B-deficient mice. Am J Physiol 1997;273:L875–82.

12. Glasser SW, Burhans MS, Korfhagen TR, et al. Altered stability of surfactant in SP-C deficient mice. Proc Natl Acad Sci U S A 2001;98:6366–71.

13. Korfhagen TR, Sheftelyevich V, Burhans MS, et al. Surfactant protein D regulates surfactant phospholipid homeostasis in vivo. J Biol Chem 1998;273:28438–43.

14. Ikegami M, Whitsett JA, Jobe AH, et al. Surfactant metabolism in SP-D gene-targeted mice. Am J Physiol 2000;279: L468–76.

15. Ikegami M, Hull WM, Yoshida M, et al. SP-D and GM-CSF regulate surfactant homeostasis via distinct mechanisms. Am J Physiol 2001;281:L697–703.

16. Hawgood S. Surfactant: composition, structure, and metabolism. In: Crystal RG, West JB, editors. The lung: scientific foundations. Vol. 1. Philadelphia: Lippincott-Raven Publishers; 1997. p. 557–71.

17. Rooney SA, Young SL, Mendelson CR. Molecular and cellular processing of lung surfactant. FASEB J 1994;8:957–67.

18. Hawgood S. Surfactant protein genes and human disease: the plot thickens. J Pediatr 1998;132:198–200.

19. Wright JR. Clearance and recycling of pulmonary surfactant. Am J Physiol 1990;259:L1–L12.

20. Rider ED, Ikegami M, Jobe AH. Localization of alveolar surfactant clearance in rabbit lung cells. Am J Physiol 1992;263:L201–9.

21. Stanley E, Lieschke GJ, Grail D, et al. Granulocyte/macrophage colony-stimulating factor-deficient mice show no major perturbation of hematopoiesis but develop a characteristic pulmonary pathology. Proc Natl Acad Sci U S A 1994;91:5592–6.

22. Dranoff G, Crawford AD, Sadelain M, et al. Involvement of granulocyte-macrophage colony-stimulating factor in pulmonary homeostasis. Science 1994;264:713–6.

23. Nishinakamura R, Nakayama N, Hirabayashi Y, et al. Mice deficient for the IL-3/GM-CSF/IL-5 β_c receptor exhibit lung pathology and impaired immune response, while β_{IL3} receptor-deficient mice are normal. Immunity 1995;2:211–22.

24. Robb L, Drinkwater CC, Metcalf D, et al. Hematopoietic and lung abnormalities in mice with a null mutation of the common β subunit of the receptors for granulocyte-macrophage colony-stimulating factor and interleukins 3 and 5. Proc Natl Acad Sci U S A 1995;92:9565–9.

25. Carraway MS, Piantadosi CA, Wright JR. Alveolar proteinosis: a disease of mice and men. Am J Physiol 2001;280:L377–8.

26. Nishinakamura R, Wiler R, Dirksen U, et al. The pulmonary alveolar proteinosis in granulocyte macrophage colony-stimulating factor/interleukins 3/5 β_c receptor-deficient mice is reversed by bone marrow transplantation. J Exp Med 1996;183:2657–62.

27. Yoshida M, Ikegami M, Reed JA, et al. GM-CSF regulates protein and lipid catabolism by alveolar macrophages. Am J Physiol 2001;280:L379–86.

28. Huffman-Reed JA, Rice WR, Zsengeller ZK, et al. GM-CSF enhances lung growth and causes alveolar type II epithelial cell hyperplasia in transgenic mice. Am J Physiol 1997;273: L715–25.

29. Ikegami M, Whitsett JA, Chroneos ZC, et al. IL-4 increases surfactant and regulates metabolism in vivo. Am J Physiol 2000;278:L75–80.

30. Davidson JM, Macleod WM. Pulmonary alveolar proteinosis. Br J Dis Chest 1969;63:13–28.

31. Rosen SH, Castleman B, Liebow AA. Pulmonary alveolar proteinosis. N Engl J Med 1958;258:1123–42.

32. DuBois RM, McAllister WAC, Branthwaite MA. Alveolar proteinosis: diagnosis and treatment over a 10-year period. Thorax 1983;38:360–3.

33. Kariman K, Kylstra JA, Spock A. Pulmonary alveolar proteinosis: prospective clinical experience in 23 patients for 15 years. Lung 1984;162:223–31.

34. Prakash UBS, Barham SS, Carpenter HA, et al. Pulmonary alveolar phospholipoproteinosis: experience with 34 cases and a review. Mayo Clin Proc 1987;62:499–518.

35. Witty LA, Tapson VF, Piantadosi CA. Isolation of mycobacteria in patients with pulmonary alveolar proteinosis. Medicine 1994;73:103–9.

36. Goldstein LS, Kavuru MS, Curtis-McCarthy P, et al. Pulmonary alveolar proteinosis: clinical features and outcomes. Chest 1998;114:1357–62.

37. Seymour JF, Presneill JJ, Schoch OD, et al. Therapeutic efficacy of granulocyte-macrophage colony-stimulating factor in patients with idiopathic acquired alveolar proteinosis. Am J Respir Crit Care Med 2001;163:524–31.

38. Hoffman RM, Rogers RM. Pulmonary alveolar proteinosis. In: Bone RC, Dantzker DR, editors. Pulmonary and critical care medicine. Vol. 2. St. Louis: Mosby Year Book; 1993. p. 1–7.

39. Ben-Dov I, Kishinevski Y, Roznman J, et al. Pulmonary alveolar proteinosis in Israel: ethnic clustering. Isr Med Assoc J 1999;1:75–8.

40. Shah PL, Hansell D, Lawson PR, et al. Pulmonary alveolar proteinosis: clinical aspects and current concepts on pathogenesis. Thorax 2000;55:67–77.

41. Miller RR, Churg AM, Hutcheon M, Lam S. Pulmonary alveolar proteinosis and aluminum dust exposure. Am Rev Respir Dis 1984;130:312–5.

42. McCunney RJ, Godefroi R. Pulmonary alveolar proteinosis and cement dust: a case report. J Occup Environ Med 1989;31:233–7.

43. Keller CA, Frost A, Cagle PT, Abraham JL. Pulmonary alveolar proteinosis in a painter with elevated pulmonary concentrations of titanium. Chest 1995;108:277–80.

44. McDonald JW, Alvarez F, Keller CA. Pulmonary alveolar proteinosis in association with household exposure to fibrous insulation material. Chest 2000;117:1813–7.

45. McEuen DD, Abraham JL. Particulate concentrations in pulmonary alveolar proteinosis. Environ Res 1978;17:334–9.

46. Klein JM, Thompson MW, Snyder JM, et al. Transient surfactant protein B deficiency in a term infant with severe respiratory failure. J Pediatr 1998;132:244–8.

47. Ramirez-R J, Harlan WR Jr. Pulmonary alveolar proteinosis: nature and origin of alveolar lipid. Am J Med 1968;45: 502–12.

48. Alberti A, Luisetti M, Braschi A, et al. Bronchoalveolar lavage fluid composition in alveolar proteinosis: early changes after therapeutic lavage. Am J Respir Crit Care Med 1996; 154:817–20.

49. Dirksen U, Nishinakamura R, Groneck P, et al. Human pulmonary alveolar proteinosis associated with a defect in GM-CSF/IL-3/IL-5 receptor common β chain expression. J Clin Invest 1997;100:2211–7.

50. Seymour JF, Begley CG, Dirksen U, et al. Attenuated hematopoietic response to granulocyte-macrophage colony-stimulating factor in patients with acquired pulmonary alveolar proteinosis. Blood 1998;92:2657–67.

51. Tchou-Wong KM, Harkin TJ, Chi C, et al. GM-CSF gene expression in normal but protein release is absent in a patient with pulmonary alveolar proteinosis. Am J Respir Crit Care Med 1997;156:1999–2002.

52. Carraway MS, Ghio AJ, Carter JD, Piantadosi CA. Detection of granulocyte-macrophage colony-stimulating factor in patients with pulmonary alveolar proteinosis. Am J Respir Crit Care Med 2000;161:1294–9.

53. Thomassen MJ, Yi T, Raychaudhuri B, et al. Pulmonary alveolar proteinosis is a disease of decreased availability of GM-CSF rather than an intrinsic cellular defect. Clin Immunol 2000;95:85–92.

54. Bewig B, Wang X-D, Kirsten D, et al. GM-CSF and GM-CSF βc receptor in adult patients with pulmonary alveolar proteinosis. Eur Respir J 2000;15:350–7.

55. Tanaka N, Watanabe J, Kitamura T, et al. Lungs of patients with idiopathic pulmonary alveolar proteinosis express a factor which neutralizes granulocyte-macrophage colony stimulating factor. FEBS Lett 1999;442:246–50.

56. Kitamura T, Tanaka N, Watanabe J, et al. Idiopathic pulmonary alveolar proteinosis as an autoimmune disease with neutralizing antibody against granulocyte/macrophage colony-stimulating factor. J Exp Med 1999;190:875–80.

57. Golde DW. Alveolar proteinosis and the overfed macrophage. Chest 1979;76:119–20.

58. Golde DW, Territo M, Finley TN, Cline MJ. Defective lung macrophages in pulmonary alveolar proteinosis. Ann Intern Med 1976;85:304–9.

59. Gonzalez-Rothi RJ, Harris JO. Pulmonary alveolar proteinosis: further evaluation of abnormal alveolar macrophages. Chest 1986;90:656–61.

60. Nugent KM, Pesanti EL. Macrophage function in pulmonary alveolar proteinosis. Am Rev Respir Dis 1983;127:780–1.

61. Hoffman RM, Dauber JH, Rogers RM. Improvement in alveolar macrophage migration after therapeutic whole lung lavage in pulmonary alveolar proteinosis. Am Rev Respir Dis 1989;139:1030–2.

62. Thomassen MJ, Meeker DP, Antal JM, et al. Synthetic surfactant (Exosurf) inhibits endotoxin-stimulated cytokine secretion by human alveolar macrophages. Am J Respir Cell Mol Biol 1992;7:257–60.

63. Thomassen MJ, Antal JM, Connors MJ, et al. Characterization of Exosurf (surfactant)-mediated suppression of stimulated human alveolar macrophages cytokine responses. Am J Respir Cell Mol Biol 1994;10:399–404.

64. Thomassen MJ, Antal JM, Divis LT, Wiedemann HP. Regulation of human alveolar macrophage inflammatory cytokines by tyloxapol: a component of the synthetic surfactant Exosurf. Clin Immunol Immunopathol 1995;77:201–5.

65. Antal JM, Divis LT, Erzurum SC, et al. Surfactant suppresses NF-κB activation in human monocytic cells. Am J Respir Cell Mol Biol 1996;14:374–9.

66. Berger A, Havet N, Vial D, et al. Dioleylphosphatidylglycerol inhibits the expression of type II phospholipase A2 in macrophages. Am J Respir Crit Care Med 1999;159:613–8.

67. Katzenstein AA. Miscellaneous: specific diseases of uncertain etiology. In: Katzenstein AA, editor. Katzenstein and Askin's surgical pathology of non-neoplastic lung disease. Philadelphia: W.B. Saunders Co.; 1997. p. 393–416.

68. Schober R, Bensch KG, Kosek JC, Northway WH. On the origin of the membranous intraalveolar material in pulmonary alveolar proteinosis. Exp Mol Pathol 1974;21:246–58.

69. Voss T, Schafer KP, Nielsen PF, et al. Primary structure differences of human surfactant-associated proteins isolated from normal and proteinosis lung. Biochim Biophys Acta 1992;1138:261–7.

70. Crouch E, Persson A, Chang D. Accumulation of surfactant protein D in human pulmonary alveolar proteinosis. Am J Pathol 1993;142:241–8.

71. Honda Y, Takahashi H, Shijubo N, et al. Surfactant protein A concentration in bronchoalveolar lavage fluids of patients with pulmonary alveolar proteinosis. Chest 1993;103:496–9.

72. Honda Y, Kuroki Y, Matsuura E, et al. Pulmonary surfactant protein D in sera and bronchoalveolar lavage fluids. Am J Respir Crit Care Med 1995;152:1860–6.

73. Doyle IR, Davidson KG, Barr HA, et al. Quantity and structure of surfactant proteins vary among patients with alveolar proteinosis. Am J Respir Crit Care Med 1998;157:658–64.

74. Wang BM, Stern EJ, Schmidt RA, Pierson DJ. Diagnosing pulmonary alveolar proteinosis: a review and an update. Chest 1997;111:460–6.

75. Martin RJ, Rogers RM, Myers NM. Pulmonary alveolar proteinosis: shunt fraction and lactic acid dehydrogenase concentration as aids to diagnosis. Am Rev Respir Dis 1978;117:1059–62.

76. Burbank B, Marrione TG, Cutler SS. Pulmonary alveolar proteinosis and nocardiosis. Am J Med 1960;28:1002–7.

77. Reyes JM, Putong PB. Association of pulmonary alveolar lipoproteinosis with mycobacterial infection. Am J Clin Pathol 1980;74:478–85.

78. Jones CC. Pulmonary alveolar proteinosis with unusual complicating infections. Am J Med 1960;29:713–22.

79. Paine R III, Preston AM, Wilcoxen S, et al. Granulocyte-macrophage colony-stimulating factor in the innate immune response to *Pneumocystis carinii* pneumonia in mice. J Immunol 2000;164:2602–9.

80. LeVine AM, Reed JA, Kurak KE, et al. GM-CSF-deficient mice are susceptible to pulmonary group B streptococcal infection. J Clin Invest 1999;103:563–9.

81. Lynch DA, Brown KK, Lee JS, Hale VAE. Imaging of diffuse infiltrative lung disease. In: Lynch DA, Newell JD Jr, Lee JS, editors. Imaging of diffuse lung disease. Hamilton-London: B.C. Decker Inc.; 2000. p. 57–140.

82. Lee KN, Levin DL, Webb WR, et al. Pulmonary alveolar proteinosis: high-resolution CT, chest radiographic, and functional correlations. Chest 1997;111:989–95.

83. Tan RT, Kuzo RS. High-resolution CT findings of mucinous bronchoalveolar carcicoma: a case of pseudopulmonary alveolar proteinosis. AJR Am J Roentgenol 1997;168:99–100.

84. Johkoh T, Itoh H, Muller NL, et al. Crazy-paving appearance at thin-section CT: spectrum of disease and pathologic findings. Radiology 1999;211:155–60.

85. Burkhalter A, Silverman JF, Hopkins MB III, Geisinger KR. Bronchoalveolar lavage cytology in pulmonary alveolar proteinosis. Am J Clin Pathol 1996;106:504–10.

86. Costello JF, Moriarty DC, Branthwaite MA, et al. Diagnosis and management of alveolar proteinosis: the role of electron microscopy. Thorax 1975;30:121–32.

87. Martin RJ, Coalson JJ, Rogers RM, et al. Pulmonary alveolar proteinosis: the diagnosis by segmental lavage. Am Rev Respir Dis 1980;121:819–25.

88. Chou C, Lin F, Tung S, et al. Diagnosis of pulmonary alveolar proteinosis: usefulness of Papanicolaou-stained smears of bronchoalveolar lavage fluid. Arch Intern Med 2001;161:562–6.

89. Rubenstein I, Mullen BM, Hoffstein V. Morphologic diagnosis of idiopathic pulmonary alveolar lipoproteinosis—revisited. Arch Intern Med 1988;148:813–6.

90. Kitamura T, Uchida K, Tanaka N, et al. Serological diagnosis of idiopathic pulmonary alveolar proteinosis. Am J Respir Crit Care Med 2000;162:658–62.

91. Kuroki Y, Tsutahara S, Shijubo N, et al. Elevated levels of lung surfactant protein A in sera from patients with idiopathic pulmonary fibrosis and pulmonary alveolar proteinosis. Am Rev Respir Dis 1993;147:723–9.

92. Honda Y, Kuroki Y, Shijubo N, et al. Aberrant appearance of lung surfactant protein A in sera of patients with idiopathic pulmonary fibrosis and its clinical significance. Respiration 1995;62:64–9.

93. Greene KE, Wright JR, Steinberg KP, et al. Serial changes in surfactant-associated proteins in lung and serum before and after onset of ARDS. Am J Respir Crit Care Med 1999;160:1843–50.

94. Hoffman RM, Rogers RM. Serum and lavage lactate dehydrogenase isoenzymes in pulmonary alveolar proteinosis. Am Rev Respir Dis 1991;143:42–6.

95. Claypool WD, Rogers RM, Matuschak GM. Update on the

clinical diagnosis, management, and pathogenesis of pulmonary alveolar proteinosis. Chest 1984;85:550–8.

96. Rogers RM, Levin DC, Gray BA, Moseley LW Jr. Physiologic effects of bronchopulmonary lavage in alveolar proteinosis. Am Rev Respir Dis 1978;118:255–64.

97. Walsh FW, Rumbak MJ. The technique of whole lung lavage. J Crit Illness 1996;11:191–7.

98. Kavuru MS, Sullivan EJ, Piccin R, et al. Exogenous granulocyte-macrophage colony-stimulating factor administration for pulmonary alveolar proteinosis. Am J Respir Crit Care Med 2000;161:1143–8.

99. Wylam ME, Ten RM, Katzmann JA, et al. Aerosolized GM-CSF improves pulmonary function in idiopathic pulmonary alveolar proteinosis. Am J Respir Crit Care Med 2000;161:A889.

100. Barraclough RM, Gillies AJ. Pulmonary alveolar proteinosis: a complete response to GM-CSF therapy. Thorax 2001; 56:664–5.

101. Alkins SA, Niven A, Hurwitz KM. Unique associations and novel treatment of pulmonary alveolar proteinosis. Chest 1999;116:428S–9S.

102. Larson RK, Gordinier R. Pulmonary alveolar proteinosis: reports of six cases, review of the literature, and formulation of a new theory. Ann Intern Med 1965;62:292–312.

103. Thompson MW. Surfactant protein B deficiency: insights into surfactant function through clinical surfactant protein deficiency. Am J Med Sci 2001;321:26–32.

104. Teja K, Cooper PH, Squires JE, Schnatterly PT. Pulmonary alveolar proteinosis in four siblings. N Engl J Med 1981;305:1390–2.

105. Moulton SL, Krous HF, Merritt TA, et al. Congenital pulmonary alveolar proteinosis: failure of treatment with extracorporeal life support. J Pediatr 1992;120:297–302.

106. Nogee LM, Garnier G, Dietz HC, et al. A mutation in the surfactant protein B gene responsible for fatal neonatal respiratory disease in multiple kindreds. J Clin Invest 1994; 93:1860–3.

107. deMello DE, Nogee LM, Heyman S, et al. Molecular and phenotypic variability in the congenital alveolar proteinosis syndrome associated with inherited surfactant protein B deficiency. J Pediatr 1994;125:43–50.

108. Nogee LM, Wert SE, Proffit SA, et al. Allelic heterogeneity in hereditary surfactant protein B (SP-B) deficiency. Am J Respir Crit Care Med 2000;161:973–81.

109. Yusen RD, Cohen AH, Hamvas A. Normal lung function in subjects heterozygous for surfactant protein-B deficiency. Am J Respir Crit Care Med 1999;159:411–4.

110. Ballard PL, Nogee LM, Beers MF, et al. Partial deficiency of surfactant protein B in an infant with chronic lung disease. Pediatrics 1995;96:1046–52.

111. deMello DE, Heyman S, Phelps DS, et al. Ultrastructure of lung in surfactant protein B deficiency. Am J Respir Cell Mol Biol 1994;11:230–9.

112. Vorbroker DK, Profitt SA, Nogee LM, Whitsett JA. Aberrant processing of surfactant protein C in hereditary SP-B deficiency. Am J Phsyiol 1995;268:L647–56.

113. Beers MF, Hamvas A, Moxley MA, et al. Pulmonary surfactant metabolism in infants lacking surfactant protein B. Am J Respir Cell Mol Biol 2000;22:380–91.

114. Tokieda K, Iwamoto HS, Bachurski CJ, et al. Surfactant protein-B-deficient mice are susceptible to hyperoxic lung injury. Am J Respir Cell Mol Biol 1999;21:463–72.

115. Floros J, Veletza SV, Kotikalapudi P, et al. Dinucleotide repeats in the human surfactant protein B gene and respiratory distress syndrome. Biochem J 1995;305:583–90.

116. Nogee LM. Surfactant protein-B deficiency. Chest 1997; 111:129S–35S.

117. Mildenberger E, deMello DE, Lin Z, et al. Focal congenital alveolar proteinosis associated with abnormal surfactant protein B messenger RNA. Chest 2001;119:645–7.

118. Lin Z, deMello DE, Batanian JR, et al. Aberrant SP-B mRNA in lung tissue of patients with congenital alveolar proteinosis. Clin Genet 2000;57:359–69.

119. Jobe AH. Pulmonary surfactant therapy. N Engl J Med 1993; 328:861–8.

120. Dunbar AE III, Wert SE, Ikegami M, et al. Prolonged survival in hereditary surfactant protein B (SP-B) deficiency associated with a novel splicing mutation. Pediatr Res 2000; 48:275–82.

121. Hamvas A, Cole FS, deMello DE, et al. Surfactant protein B deficiency: antenatal diagnosis and prospective treatment with surfactant replacement. J Pediatr 1994;125:356–61.

122. Hamvas A, Nogee LM, Mallory GB Jr, et al. Lung transplantation for treatment of infants with surfactant protein B deficiency. J Pediatr 1997;130:231–9.

123. Lin S, Na C, Akinbi HT, et al. Surfactant protein B -/- mice are rescued by restoration of SP-B expression in alveolar type II cells but not Clara cells. J Biol Chem 1999;274:19168–74.

124. Ruben FL, Talamo TS. Secondary pulmonary proteinosis occurring in two patients with acquired immune deficiency syndrome. Am J Med 1986;80:1187–90.

125. Katzenstein AA. Infection. I. Unusual pneumonias. In: Katzenstein AA, editor. Katzenstein and Askin's surgical pathology of non-neoplastic lung disease. Philadelphia: W.B. Saunders; 1997. p. 247–85.

126. Ranchod M, Bissell M. Pulmonary alveolar proteinosis and cytomegalovirus infection. Arch Pathol Lab Med 1979; 103:139–42.

127. Simell O, Perheentupa J, Rapola J, et al. Lysinuric protein intolerance. Am J Med 1975;59:229–40.

128. Borsani G, Bassi MT, Sperandeo MP, et al. SLC7A7, encoding a putative permease-related protein, is mutated in patients with lysinuric protein intolerance. Nat Genet 1999;21:297–301.

129. Parto K, Svedstrom E, Majurin M, et al. Pulmonary manifestations of lysinuric protein intolerance. Chest 1993; 104:1176–82.

130. Santamaria F, Parenti G, Guidi G, et al. Early detection of lung involvement in lysinuric protein intolerance: role of high-resolution computed tomography and radioisotopic methods. Am J Respir Crit Care Med 1996;153:731–5.

131. Parto K, Kallajoki M, Aho H, Simell O. Pulmonary alveolar proteinosis and glomerulonephritis in lysinuric protein intolerance: case reports and autopsy findings of four pediatric patients. Hum Pathol 1994;25:400–7.

132. Lukkarinen M, Parto K, Ruuskanen O, et al. B and T cell immunity in patients with lysinuric protein intolerance. Clin Exp Immunol 1999;116:430–4.

133. Cordonnier C, Fleury-Feith J, Escudier E, et al. Secondary alveolar proteinosis is a reversible cause of respiratory failure in leukemic patients. Am J Respir Crit Care Med 1994; 149:788–94.

134. Bedrossian CWM, Luna MA, Conklin RH, Miller WC. Alveolar proteinosis as a consequence of immunosuppression. Human Pathol 1980;11:527–35.

135. Dirksen U, Hattenhorst U, Schneider P, et al. Defective expression of granulocyte-macrophage colony-stimulating factor/interleukin-5 receptor common β chain in children with acute myeloid leukemia associated with respiratory failure. Blood 1998;92:1097–103.

136. Sayani F, Montero-Julian FA, Ranchin V, et al. Identification of the soluble granulocyte-macrophage colony stimulating factor receptor protein in vivo. Blood 2000;95:461–9.

137. Hammarstrom L, Vorechovsky I, Webster D. Selective IgA deficiency and common variable immunodeficiency. Clin Exp Immunol 2000;120:225–31.

138. Colon AR, Lawrence RD, Mills SD, O'Connell EJ. Childhood pulmonary alveolar proteinosis. Am J Dis Child 1970; 121:481–5.

139. Bell DY, Hook GER. Pulmonary alveolar proteinosis: analy-

sis of airway and alveolar proteins. Am Rev Respir Dis 1979;119:979–90.

140. Webster JR Jr, Battifora H, Furey C, et al. Pulmonary alveolar proteinosis in two siblings with decreased immunoglobulin A. Am J Med 1980;69:786–9.

141. Eisenstein EM, Sneller MC. Common variable immunodeficiency: diagnosis and management. Ann Allergy 1994; 73:285–92.

142. Fischer A. Primary T-lymphocyte immunodeficiencies. Clin Rev Allergy Immunol 2001;20:3–26.

143. Leonard WJ. X-linked severe combined immunodeficiency: from molecular cause to gene therapy within seven years. Mol Med Today 2000;6:403–7.

144. Haworth JC, Hoogstraten J, Taylor H. Thymic alymphoplasia. Arch Dis Child 1967;42:40–54.

145. Symchych PS, Flynn DM. Pulmonary alveolar proteinosis in an infant. Arch Dis Child 1969;44:769–72.

146. Jennings VM, Dillehay DL, Webb SK, Brown LS. Pulmonary alveolar proteinosis in SCID mice. Am J Respir Cell Mol Biol 1995;13:297–306.

147. Warner T, Balish E. Pulmonary alveolar proteinosis: a spontaneous and inducible disease in immunodeficient germ-free mice. Am J Physiol 1995;146:1017–24.

148. Beckett W, Abraham JL, Becklake M, et al. Adverse effects of crystalline silica exposure. Am J Respir Crit Care Med 1997;155:761–5.

149. Buechner HA, Ansari A. Acute silicoproteinosis: a new pathologic variant of acute silicosis in sandblasters, characterized by histologic features resembling alveolar proteinosis. Chest 1969;55:274–84.

150. Suratt PM, Winn WC Jr, Brody AR, et al. Acute silicosis in tombstone sandblasters. Am Rev Respir Dis 1977;115: 521–9.

151. Owens MW, Kinasewitz GT, Gonzalez E. Case report: sandblaster's lung with mycobacterial infection. Am J Med Sci 1988;295:554–7.

152. Xipell JM, Ham KN, Price CG, Thomas DP. Acute silicoproteinosis. Thorax 1977;32:104–11.

153. Banks DE, Bauer MA, Castellan RM, Lapp NL. Silicosis in surface coalmine drillers. Thorax 1983;38:275–8.

154. Rubin E, Weisbrod GL, Sanders DE. Pulmonary alveolar proteinosis. Radiology 1980;135:35–41.

155. Orriols R, Ferrer J, Tura JM, et al. Sicca syndrome and silicoproteinosis in a dental technician. Eur Respir J 1997;10: 731–4.

156. Dee P, Suratt PM, Winn WC Jr. The radiographic findings in acute silicosis. Radiology 1978;126:359–63.

157. Abraham JL, McEuen DD. Inorganic particulates associated with pulmonary alveolar proteinosis: SEM and x-ray microanalysis results. Appl Pathol 1986;4:138–46.

158. Nogee LM, Dunbar AE III, Wert SE, et al. A mutation in the surfactant protein C gene associated with familial interstitial lung disease. N Engl J Med 2001;344:573–9.

159. Katzenstein AA, Myers JL. Idiopathic pulmonary fibrosis: clinical relevance of pathologic classification. Am J Respir Crit Care Med 1998;157:1301–15.

160. Amin RS, Wert SE, Baughman RP, et al. Surfactant protein deficiency in familial interstitial lung disease. J Pediatr 2001;139:85–92.

161. Carnovale R, Zornoza J, Goldman AM, Luna M. Pulmonary alveolar proteinosis: its association with hematologic malignancy and lymphoma. Radiology 1977;122:303–6.

162. Lakshminarayan S, Schwarz MI, Stanford RE. Unsuspected pulmonary alveolar proteinosis complicating acute myelogenous leukemia. Chest 1976;69:433–5.

163. Merino-Angulo A, Periz-Marti M, de Otazu RD. Pulmonary alveolar lipoproteinosis associated with amyloidosis. Chest 1990;98:1048.

164. Doyle AP, Baclcerzak SP, Wells CL, Crittenden JO. Pulmonary alveolar proteinosis with hematologic disorders. Arch Intern Med 1963;112:940–6.

165. Green D, Dighe P, Ali NO, Katele GV. Pulmonary alveolar proteinosis complicating chronic myelogenous leukemia. Cancer 1980;46:1763–6.

166. Aymard J, Gyger M, Lavallee R, et al. A case of pulmonary alveolar proteinosis complicating chronic myelogenous leukemia. A peculiar aspect of busulfan lung? Cancer 1984;53:954–6.

167. Rguez-Luaces M, Lafuente A, Martin MP, et al. Haematopoietic transplantation in pulmonary alveolar proteinosis associated with chronic myelogenous leukaemia. Bone Marrow Transplant 1997;20:507–10.

168. Tsushima K, Shigeru K, Hirosi S, et al. Pulmonary alveolar proteinosis in a patient with chronic myelogenous leukemia. Respiration 1999;66:173–5.

169. Levinson B, Jones RS, Wintrobe MM, Cartwright GE. Thrombocythemia and pulmonary intra-alveolar coagulum in a young woman. Blood 1958;13:959–71.

170. Payseur CR, Knowaler BE, Hyde R. Pulmonary alveolar proteinosis. Am Rev Tuberc 1958;78:906–15.

171. Plenk HP, Swift SA, Chambers WL, Peltzer WE. Pulmonary alveolar proteinosis—a new disease? Radiology 1960;74: 928–38.

172. Steens RD, Summers QA, Tarala RA. Pulmonary alveolar proteinosis in association with Fanconi's anemia and psoriasis: a possible common pathogenetic mechanism. Chest 1992; 102:637–8.

173. Schiller V, Aberle DR, Aberle AM. Pulmonary alveolar proteinosis: occurrence with metastatic melanoma to lung. Chest 1989;95:466–7.

174. Meijer WG, Van Marwijk Kooy M, Ladde BE. A patient with multiple myeloma and respiratory insufficiency due to accumulation of paraprotein in the alveolar space. Br J Haematol 1994;87:663–5.

175. Edmonson WR, Gere JB. Pulmonary alveolar proteinosis. Ann Intern Med 1960;52:1310–8.

176. Fraimow W, Cathcart RT, Kirshner JJ, Taylor RC. Pulmonary alveolar proteinosis: a correlation of pathological and physiological findings in a patient followed up with serial biopsies of the lung. Am J Med 1960;28:458–67.

177. Mork JN, Johnson JR, Zinneman HH, Bjorgen J. Pulmonary alveolar proteinosis associated with IgG monoclonal gammopathy. Arch Intern Med 1968;121:278–83.

178. Samuels MP, Warner JO. Pulmonary alveolar lipoproteinosis complicating juvenile dermatomyositis. Thorax 1988;43: 939–40.

179. Parker LA, Novotny DB. Recurrent alveolar proteinosis following double lung transplantation. Chest 1997;111:1457–8.

180. Yousem SA. Alveolar lipoproteinosis in lung allograft recipients. Hum Pathol 1997;28:1383–6.

31

MISCELLANEOUS INTERSTITIAL LUNG DISEASES

MARVIN I. SCHWARZ

RESPIRATORY TRACT AMYLOIDOSIS

Amyloidosis is the result of extracellular accumulation of amyloid fibrils. In tissue it appears as a cellular amorphous eosinophilic material that stains positively with congo red dye. Examination of this stain with polarized light reveals a typical green birefringence. Amyloid material is composed of fibrillary proteins arranged in twisted beta-pleated sheets.[1] Two amyloid proteins, AA and AL, have been identified. AA, the major component of secondary amyloidosis, is probably derived from an acute serum protein of hepatic origin. The AL protein originates from the variable portion of the immunoglobulin light chain, usually the lambda rather than the kappa light chain. This monoclonal immunoglobulin light chain is present in both urine and serum of patients with systemic primary amyloidosis and the amyloidosis associated with multiple myeloma.[2–4] Up to 15% of cases of multiple myeloma have AL or primary amyloidosis.[5] Moreover, several cases of AL amyloidosis with lung involvement have been reported in Waldenströms macroglobulinemia, another monoclonal disease.[6]

Primary amyloidosis is a plasma cell dyscrasia resulting from an abnormal proliferation of plasma cells that produce both a monoclonal gammopathy and excessive light chain deposition in the extracellular matrix of various tissues. In addition to respiratory tract involvement, nephrotic syndrome is seen in 33% of patients with primary amyloidosis, myocardiopathy in 25%, neuropathy in 17%, and gastrointestinal involvement in 8% of cases.[1,7]

Primary amyloidosis can be systemic in nature or sometimes can affect only one organ system, such as the respiratory tract. Thus, respiratory tract involvement can be the sole manifestation of primary amyloidosis, or it may be one component of a systemic disease. Various reports have estimated that some form of respiratory tract involvement, although sometimes asymptomatic and discovered for the first time at autopsy, occurs in 30 to 90% of cases of primary amyloidosis.[8,9] A recent series reported an 18% incidence of clinically apparent respiratory tract involvement in primary amyloidosis.[10] Secondary amy-

loidosis (AA), with incidental lung involvement, appears with other diffuse lung diseases such as tuberculosis, lupus erythematosus, alveolar proteinosis, bronchiectasis, Sjögren's syndrome, rheumatoid arthritis, lymphocytic interstitial pneumonia, pulmonary lymphoma, hypersensitivity pneumonitis, cystic fibrosis, and Crohn's disease.[11–19] Cases of diffuse interstitial secondary amyloidosis have been found in scleroderma and ankylosing spondylitis as well.[20,21] Secondary amyloidosis involving the lungs, but without an accompanying primary interstitial lung disease or underlying chronic inflammatory state such as bronchiectasis, is unusual. Even in this case it is most often an incidental finding at autopsy. There are two recorded cases of AA amyloid causing a diffuse interstitial lung disease. In one there was no evidence of a predisposing condition,[22] and in the other, a patient with rheumatoid arthritis, AA amyloid was the sole cause of the interstitial lung disease.[23] In one series of 14 patients with secondary amyloidosis, but without a predisposing lung condition, no patient had pulmonary complaints or premortem evidence of lung involvement.[24] A form of amyloidosis identical to primary amyloidosis (AL) can complicate multiple myeloma. There is also a senile form of amyloidosis that is not immunoglobulin derived and is most often discovered at postmortem examination. As with most cases of secondary amyloidosis involving the lung, senile amyloidosis is clinically silent, occurring in 10 to 20% of the population over the age of 80 years. The most frequent sites of deposition of senile amyloid are the myocardium and the pulmonary vessels.[25]

Lesser[26] recorded the first case of pulmonary involvement by amyloid in 1887. More than 300 cases of respiratory tract amyloidosis have been reported since Lesser's observations.[27–29] Table 31–1 lists the various presentations of respiratory tract amyloidosis.

Tracheobronchial Amyloidosis

Tracheobronchial amyloidosis is a form of primary amyloidosis (AL) that is localized to the respiratory tract and

TABLE 31–1   Presentation of Respiratory Tract Amyloidosis

Oropharyngeal
    Macroglossia (obstructive sleep apnea)

Tracheobronchial
    Localized polyp
    Diffuse involvement

Nodular parenchymal
    Single nodule
    Multiple nodular lesion
    Miliary

Diffuse alveolar-septal (interstitial)

Hilar and/or mediastinal lymph nodes

Pleural

Pulmonary vascular

not associated with other systemic involvement.[30–33] One case with a serum monoclonal immunoglobulin (Ig)G spike of the lambda type has been reported.[34] This condition usually does not produce symptoms until the fifth or sixth decade. It presents as either an isolated endobronchial or tracheal tumor or as diffuse constricting plaques that involve major portions of or the entire tracheobronchial tree. The symptoms relate to the severity, extent, and location of the lesions. A single endobronchial polyp may cause lobar atelectasis and obstructive pneumonia. Wheezing and hemoptysis often occur, and tracheobronchial amyloid is often misdiagnosed as asthma.[35] It is difficult to differentiate between localized endobronchial amyloidosis and endobronchial malignancy on bronchoscopic inspection. Endobronchial resection, if possible, or lobectomy yields an excellent therapeutic result; laser ablation also appears to be an effective therapeutic modality.[34]

The diffuse form of tracheobronchial amyloidosis produces cough, wheezing, dyspnea, and hemoptysis; these symptoms are often present for several years before a diagnosis is established. At bronchoscopy, submucosal shiny pale plaques are visible as are regions of localized bronchostenosis.[36–38] Computed tomography demonstrates marked tracheal thickening and narrowing of the main lobar and segmental bronchi. Patients with tracheobronchial amyloidosis have frequent episodes of pneumonia that often lead to bronchiectasis. Mortality from respiratory failure and/or infection is not infrequent in patients with the diffuse forms of tracheobronchial amyloidosis.[27] Treatment, except for endobronchial resection when possible, is generally unsatisfactory. Repeated endobronchial laser ablation offers a new therapeutic alternative.[27–34,37,38] Hemorrhage may occasionally complicate an endobronchial resection.[35] Tracheopathia osteoplastica, calcification, and ossification of subcutaneous nodules throughout the tracheobronchial tree may be the end result of diffuse endobronchial amyloidosis.[39]

Nodular Parenchymal Amyloidosis

As in the tracheobronchial form, nodular parenchymal amyloidosis, although associated with local light-chain deposition, is not a component of a systemic disease.[25] Approximately 33% of the recorded cases of nodular amyloidosis present as a single rounded "coin" lesion that is usually asymptomatic and discovered following screening chest radiography (Figures 31–1 and 31–2). Malignancy and infectious granuloma must be excluded. The low intensity of the lesion on T_2 weighted images by computed tomography (CT) and magnetic resonance imaging (MRI) may help in the differentiation from bronchogenic carcinoma.[40] Recurrence of an amyloidoma rarely, if ever, occurs following resection.[41] Diagnosis is often established by ultrasound-guided transthoracic needle aspiration.[42,43]

The multinodular form of this disease must be differentiated from metastatic malignancy or miliary tuberculosis (Figure 31–3). These nodules are slow growing, can cavitate and calcify, but are rarely the cause of sig-

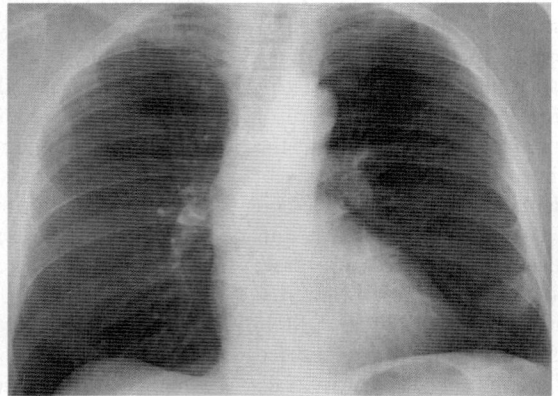
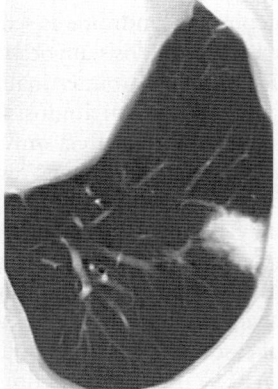

Figure 31–1 Amyloidoma. *A*, Chest radiograph of a slow-growing nodule in a 60-year-old man. *B*, Computed tomography of same lesion.

A

B

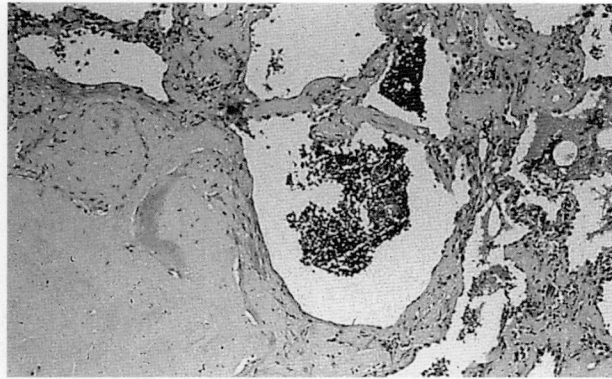

A

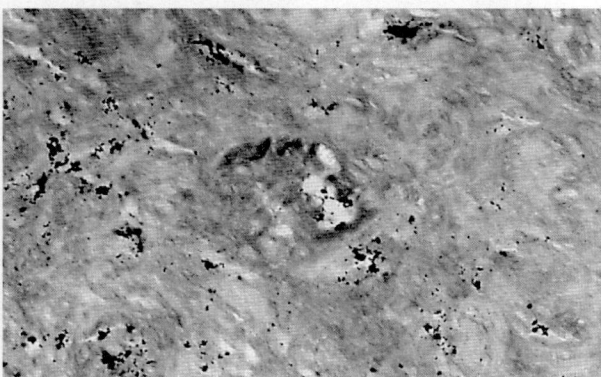

B

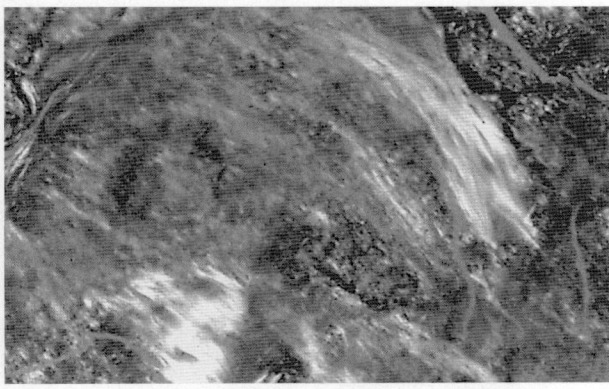

C

Figure 31–2   Resected amyloidoma. Same patient as in Figure 31–1. *A*, There is a cellular amorphous extracellular material replacing the lung parenchyma (hematoxylin and eosin stain; ×40 original magnification). *B*, Positive congo red stain. *C*, Apple-green birefringence with polarized light.

nificant symptoms or physiologic impairment (Figure 31–4). An exception to this is a case in which nodular compression of small bronchi resulted in bronchiectasis and massive pulmonary hemorrhage.[44] The multinodular form has also been reported to occur with Sjögren's syndrome, hypergammaglobulinemic purpura, human immunodeficiency virus (HIV) infection, Crohn's disease, intravenous drug abuse, and asbestos exposure and

can be accompanied by hilar adenopathy.[45–51] Histology indicates focal calcification and ossification in addition to the amorphous eosinophilic material (see Figure 31–4). A cellular infiltrate of lymphocytes, histiocytes, and multinucleated giant cells frequently surrounds these lesions.[41] Multifocal nodular pulmonary amyloidosis, although not a surgically treatable disease, has an excellent prognosis and rarely is associated with significant functional impairment.[48]

Diffuse Alveolar Septal Amyloidosis

Diffuse alveolar septal or interstitial amyloidosis occurs in conjunction with either primary amyloidosis or multiple myeloma. In primary amyloidosis it also can appear without evidence of systemic involvement.[52] Although the incidence of diffuse pulmonary involvement is high in primary amyloidosis with systemic involvement, in only 5 to 10% of cases does it significantly contribute to mortality.[33,53] Once respiratory symptoms occur, however, survival has been reported to be less than 2 years. Data from a large series indicates a better prognosis for some cases.[54] Diffuse alveolar septal amyloidosis is often associated with cardiac muscle and pulmonary vascular involvement. Pleural disease and, less commonly, hilar and mediastinal adenopathy have been described. Electron microscopic studies demonstrate that the amyloid is deposited within the interstitium, within the walls of small blood vessels, and the alveolar capillary basement membranes.[55]

Progressive dyspnea and cough are the most prominent symptoms, which, due to their frequent association with an amyloid cardiomyopathy, must be differentiated from left ventricular failure. Recurrent hemoptysis can result from the dissection of involved pulmonary vessels,[56] and severe pulmonary hypertension can appear secondary to diffuse vascular involvement.[57–59] The chest radiograph shows diffuse reticulonodular infiltrates and occasionally hilar and mediastinal lymph nodes (Figure 31–5).[60] High-resolution computed tomography (HRCT) scans occasionally demonstrate calcification within the interstitial infiltrates (Figure 31–6).[61] Diffuse parenchymal cyst formation has also been seen on HRCT.[62] Pleural effusions result from direct involvement of the pleura or from congestive heart failure.[63,64] Pulmonary function tests indicate a reduction in lung volumes and the diffusing capacity for carbon monoxide. Diagnosis is established on lung biopsy, revealing an eosinophilic, amorphous substance within alveolar walls as well as vessels that exhibit an apple-green birefringence with congo red stain (Figure 31–7). Corticosteroids, melphalan, and colchicine have been used with variable results for the treatment of primary systemic amyloidosis.[65] One case of diffuse alveolar septal amyloidosis showed a response to intradermal dimethyl sulfoxide (DMSO) treatments.[66] Intensive intravenous melphalan coupled with blood stem cell transplantation

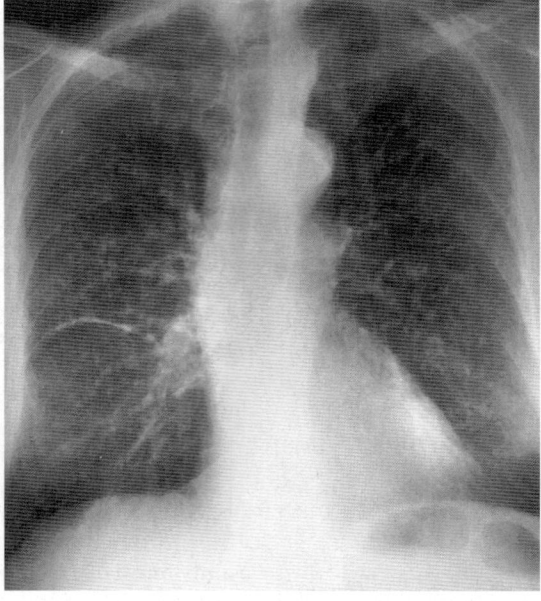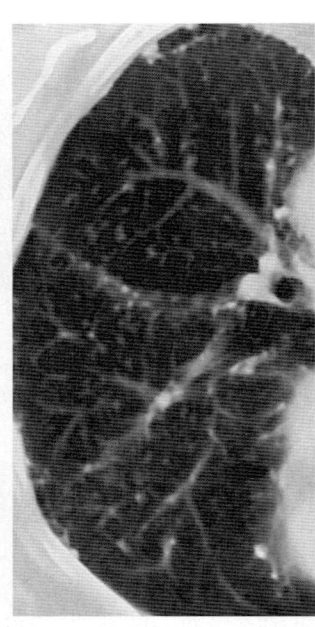

Figure 31–3   Multinodular amyloidosis. *A,* Note the diffuse interstitial nodules of varying size on the chest radiograph. This patient was asymptomatic with a normal physiology. *B,* High-resolution computed tomography scan showing an area of miliary nodulation.

A   **B**

eradicates the underlying plasma cell dyscrasia and improves the nephrotic syndrome.[67] The effect of this therapy on the diffuse lung involvement is unknown.

Pulmonary Vascular Amyloidosis

Although vascular wall involvement is common in diffuse alveolar septal amyloidosis, the resultant physiologic disturbances are usually attributed to the amyloid interstitial lung disease or concomitant myocardial amyloid with left ventricular dysfunction.[26,54] With extensive involvement of the interstitial capillaries as well as the small and muscular pulmonary arteries, however, a syndrome suggestive of primary pulmonary hypertension evolves (Figure 31–8).[57–59] This is accompanied by an inordinate reduction of the diffusing capacity for carbon monoxide and an increase in the mean pulmonary artery pressure out of proportion to the severity of the reduction in lung volumes.[59]

INTERSTITIAL LUNG DISEASE FOLLOWING ASPIRATION

Several pulmonary syndromes may develop following the accidental aspiration of gastric contents: *acute respiratory distress syndrome* occurs secondary to a chemical pneumonitis; asthma; infectious pneumonia; lung abscess; and, with repeated episodes, bronchiectasis and possibly interstitial fibrosis. If the acute aspiration is recognized, the above consequences do not usually present a diagnostic challenge. The appearance of lower zone pulmonary alveolar infiltrates following aspira-

tion of gastric contents or the development of the acute respiratory distress syndrome with more massive aspirations is a well recognized clinical sequence.[69] The acute alveolar filling process resolves after a large aspiration, but it may be replaced by interstitial infiltrates

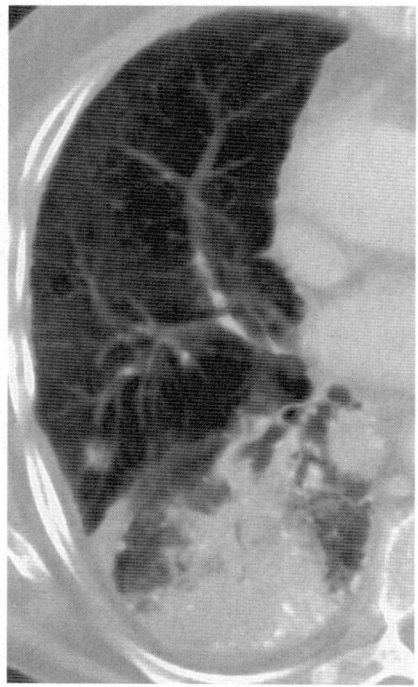

Figure 31–4   Amyloidosis. High-resolution computed tomography showing focal stippled calcification in a large amyloidoma.

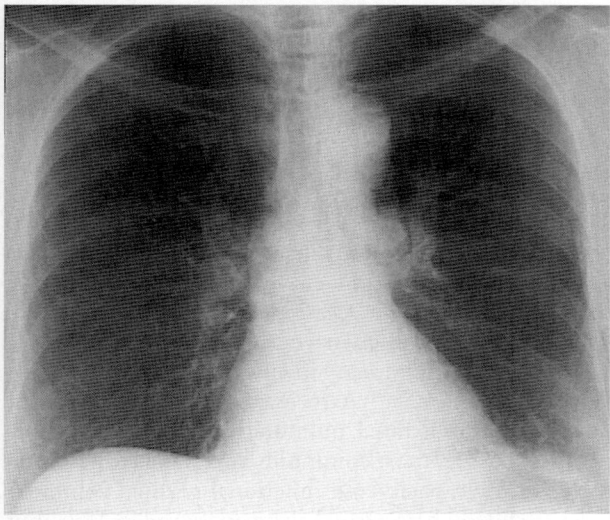
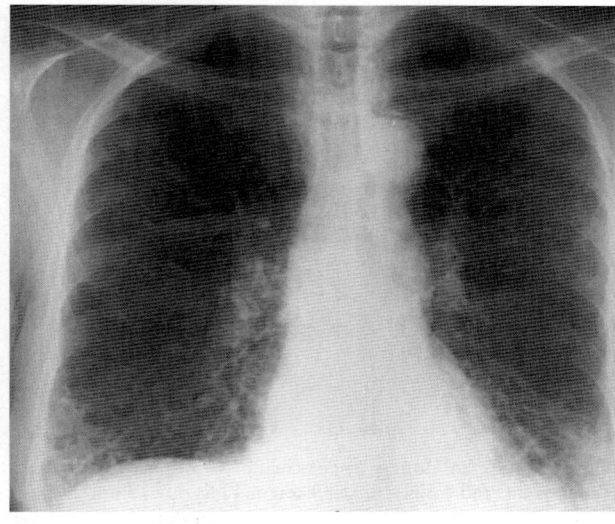

A   B

Figure 31–5   Alveolar-septal amyloidosis. *A*, Chest radiograph of patient with multiple myeloma demonstrating ill-defined interstitial infiltrates most prominent at the left base. *B*, Chest radiograph of the same patient 4 years later with severe respiratory symptoms and a marked increase in the reticulonodular infiltrates. Kerley's B lines are also visible.

on the chest radiograph and dyspnea reappears within the first week.

Histologically, a fibrinoid inflammatory exudate involves the alveolar walls and spaces. Hyaline membranes form within the alveolar spaces and indicate diffuse alveolar damage. The inflammatory exudate consists of both lymphocytes and polymorphonuclear leukocytes. The exudative reaction is thought to be the result of exposure of the alveolar epithelium and endothelium to the acid environment. In addition, interstitial foreign body granulomas appear as a reaction to the aspirated meat or vegetable fiber. One report suggests a favorable response of this reaction to corticosteroids.[68]

A more insidious form of pulmonary fibrosis has been reported to occur with recurrent subclinical aspirations of gastric contents that usually occur during sleep and are associated with hiatal hernia, gastroesophageal reflux, and other esophageal and neurologic problems.[68,69] One study of 143 patients with hiatal hernia and reflux detected lower zone pulmonary interstitial infiltrates in 4%.[68] Another study in patients with interstitial lung disease of unknown cause reported that 54% had gastroesophageal reflux as compared with 8.5% in a normal control population.[70] Both studies postulated that repeated small aspirations produce inflammatory damage to small bronchiolar and alveolar

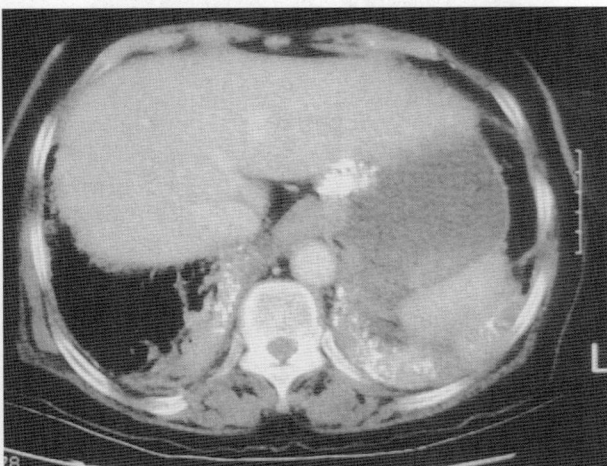

Figure 31–6   High-resolution computed tomography of a patient with alveolar septal amyloidosis demonstrated interstitial calcium deposition.

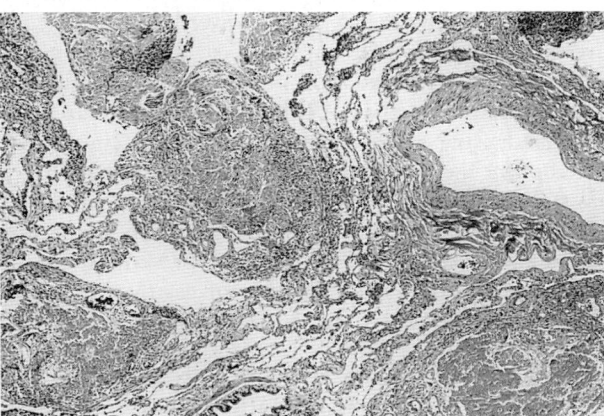

Figure 31–7   Alveolar-septal amyloidosis. Nodular masses of amorphous eosinophilic amyloid material expanding the interstitium. There is also a mononuclear cell infiltrate. This patient had primary systemic amyloidosis (AL) (hematoxylin and eosin stain; ×40 original magnification).

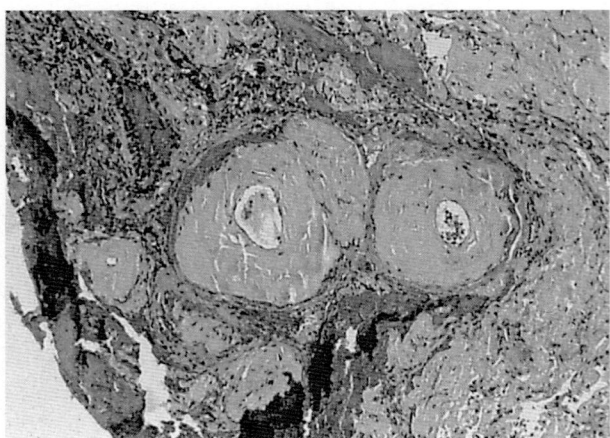

Figure 31–8   Pulmonary hypertension in primary amyloidosis (hematoxylin and eosin stain; ×40 original magnification).

structures, which in turn initiates the fibrotic response. Using dual-channel ambulatory esophageal pH monitoring, 16 of 17 patients with idiopathic pulmonary fibrosis (IPF) had evidence of esophageal acid exposure, and only 4 of these had reflux symptoms. Because of the high incidence of esophageal reflux, the authors concluded that this may be a contributing factor in the pathogenesis of IPF.[71] Animal models support the concept of gastric acid–induced pulmonary parenchymal cell damage as do autopsy series in patients who have died following massive gastric aspiration.[72] Clinically, patients with insidious aspiration of gastric contents are usually over 50 years of age; are often overweight; report symptoms of reflux; and have recurrent episodes of nocturnal asthma, bronchitis, and pneumonia. They complain of being awakened from sleep by bronchospasm or paroxysms of coughing. Severe, progressive dyspnea and clubbing are not seen. Slowly progressive reticulonodular densities appear on the chest radiograph and are located primarily in the lower lung zones (Figures 31–9 and 31–10).

A diagnosis of aspiration-induced interstitial fibrosis is often difficult to establish. A technique has been described using a semiquantitative lipid-laden alveolar macrophage index.[73] Bronchoalveolar lavage macrophages are stained with oil red O and graded according to the intensity of cellular staining. A high mean index was found in the aspirators. Techniques to prevent aspiration and pharmacologic neutralization of gastric acid is the recommended therapy.

GAUCHER'S DISEASE

Adult Gaucher's disease is characterized by hepatosplenomegaly, bone marrow infiltration resulting in anemia and thrombocytopenia, long bone erosions, and an elevated serum acid phosphatase.

There are three types of Gaucher's disease: the adult form that is relatively benign (type 1); an infantile form that is uniformly fatal due to involvement of the central nervous system (type 2); and a juvenile form for those cases that do not conform to the first two (type 3).[74] Gaucher's disease is an autosomally recessively inherited deficiency of the lysosomal enzyme glucocerebrosidase. The disease prevalence is between 1:30,000 and 1:50,000 with a high incidence in Ashkenazi Jews.[75,76] There is also a decreased activity of the enzyme glucocerebrosidase in the involved organs.[75] Occasionally the lung is involved.

Until recently, there have been fewer than 25 documented cases of pulmonary involvement in type 1 (adult) Gaucher's disease.[77–81] A review of 95 Israeli patients, however, demonstrated pulmonary physiologic abnormalities in 68%, most commonly this was a reduction in the diffusing capacity and functional residual volume.[82] Chest radiograph abnormalities were found in 17%, but in only 4% were there extensive interstitial changes. Patients with this disorder also have an increased risk of pulmonary infections.[83] The primary pulmonary disease first becomes apparent during childhood, and in only two of the previously recorded cases did it first appear in young adults. The survival following onset of the pulmonary disease is variable, ranging from months to years. Chest radiographs demonstrate either a diffuse miliary or reticulonodular pattern; in one case, radiographic evidence of mediastinal adenopathy was found.[84] Histologic examination of the lung reveals masses of Gaucher's cells (alveolar macrophages filled with aggregated glucocerebroside) infiltrating alveolar walls and filling air spaces producing a histologic appearance reminiscent of desqua-

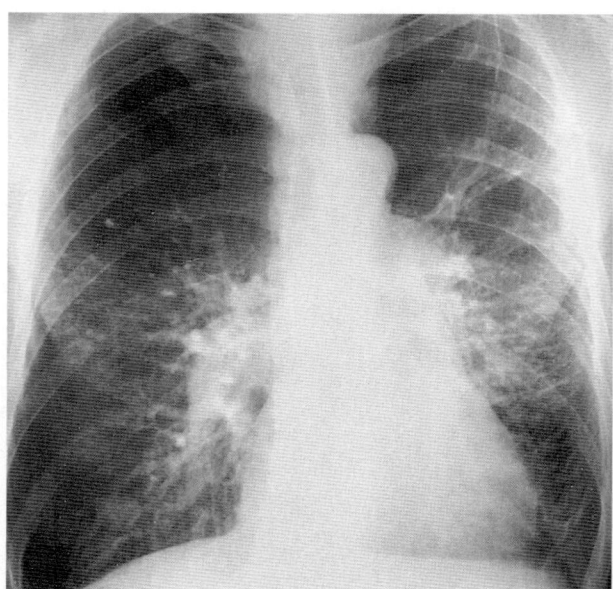

Figure 31–9   Chest radiograph of interstitial lung disease in a patient with Zenker's diverticulum. Note the interstitial infiltrates and the air-fluid level in the left superior mediastinum.

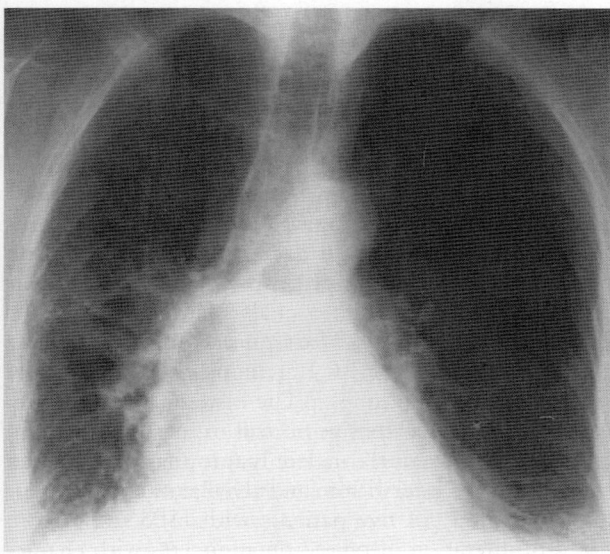

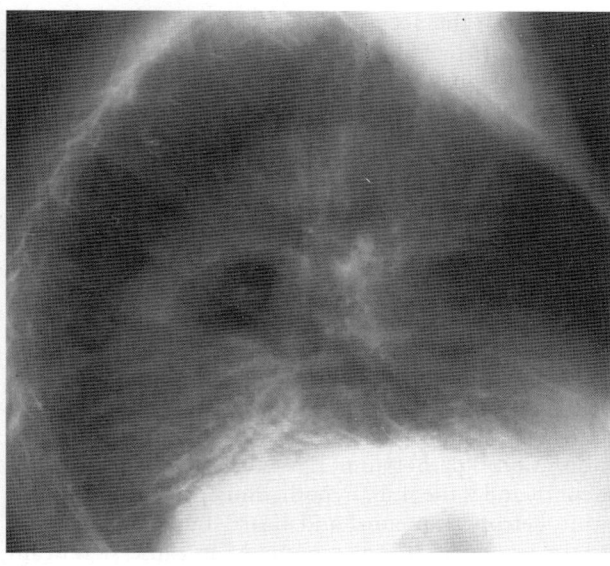

A   **B**

Figure 31–10   Chest radiograph of mixed interstitial alveolar infiltrates thought to be due to a large hiatal hernia. *A, B,* Note the lower zone prominence of the infiltrates and the hiatal hernia on both views of the chest.

mative interstitial pneumonia. These cells are autofluorescent and stain positively with periodic acid–Schiff (PAS). Gaucher's cells can also be identified by their abundant cytoplasm and "rumpled tissue paper appearance" in the bronchoalveolar lavage (BAL) fluid.[79] In addition to the desquamative pattern, patchy interstitial infiltrates following a lymphatic distribution and interstitial thickening also occur. The most common finding is involvement of the interstitial capillaries indicating the systemic nature of this disease.[85] HRCT findings consist of reticular change and ground-glass density. Pseudo-Gaucher's cells have been reported in a fatal case of pulmonary tuberculosis.[86]

Enzyme replacement with alglucerase, a placental enzyme preparation, or imiglucerase, a recombinant preparation, are effective therapies for the systemic disease.[77] Enzyme replacement has resulted in significant improvement in gas exchange in two pulmonary cases and radiograph improvement in one.[79,82] There is one case of Gaucher's cells obstructing small pulmonary vessels resulting in pulmonary hypertension and cor pulmonale.[87] In another patient with pulmonary hypertension from Gaucher's disease, continuous intravenous prostacyclin reduced pulmonary pressures.[88] There is also a case describing vertebral extramedullary hematopoiesis producing a postmediastinal mass on the chest radiograph in a 75-year-old woman with Gaucher's disease.[89]

NIEMANN-PICK DISEASE

This lipid storage disorder is characterized by the accumulation of sphingomyelin in the cells of the reticuloendothelial and central nervous systems. It results from a deficiency of sphingomyelinase. The infantile form is rapidly fatal due to neurologic involvement whereas the adult form is relatively benign and uncommon. Several cases of pulmonary interstitial involvement with the typical foamy-appearing macrophage containing sphingomyelin have been reported. This produces either a miliary or reticulonodular appearance on the chest radiograph, and honeycombing may result.[90,91] Niemann-Pick cells (sea-blue histiocytes) are seen in BAL fluid.[92]

FABRY'S DISEASE

Fabry's disease is an X-linked inborn error of glycosphingolipid catabolism, which results from a deficiency of lysosomal galactosidase A activity. This results in the accumulation of glycosphingolipids in the kidney, heart, skin, and brain.[93] It begins in childhood, but the mean age of survival is 41 years. Adult patients with less pronounced disease can survive to older ages and are discovered primarily because of cardiac involvement causing a cardiomyopathy. Primary clinical manifestations include acroparesthesias, angiokeratoma, corneal and lenticular opacities, and hypohidrosis. Because of endothelial accumulation of the glycosphingolipids, renal failure, cardiac failure, and cerebrovascular accidents lead to an early death.[93] Pulmonary involvement has occasionally been reported. There is one case of diffuse alveolar hemorrhage associated with renal failure.[94] This pulmonary renal syndrome was due to microvascular endothelial dysfunction in both organs. In another case of Fabry's disease, typical lamellar inclusion bodies representing the accumulated glycosphingolipids were seen on bronchial biopsy specimens and in induced sputum.[95] Previously a universally fatal disease, the recent development of human recombinant α-galactosidase A, has been shown to reverse the clinical manifestations of this disease.[96,97]

ERDHEIM-CHESTER DISEASE

Erdheim-Chester disease is a rare lipidosis of unknown etiology resulting from xanthogranulomatous tissue deposition. Monocytic cells, which infiltrate the affected tissues, appear as foamy histiocytes. Symmetric sclerosis of the meta and diaphysis of long bones due to histiocytic infiltration is pathognomonic.[98,99] Extraskeletal involvement includes the skin, hypothalmus/posterior pituitary, orbit, retroperitoneum, and heart. Lung involvement occurs in up to 20% of cases and can cause significant morbidity and mortality. There are diffuse interstitial infiltrates sometimes with an upper lobe predominance on the chest radiograph. The CT scan shows thickening of the visceral pleura and interlobular septa with patchy reticular and centrilobular opacities, as well as ground-glass attenuation.[100,101] Histologic features in the lung include involvement of the visceral pleura, interlobular septa, and bronchovascular bundles. The infiltrate consists of foamy histiocytes, lymphocytes, and scattered giant cells in a lymphatic distribution.[101,102] Surface markers are negative for CDla and electronmicroscopy does not reveal Birbeck granules, which differentiate this disease from the Langerhans' cell of eosinophilic granuloma.[103] There is no effective treatment.

HERMANSKY-PUDLAK SYNDROME

Hermansky-Pudlak syndrome (HPS) is a recessively inherited disease with dysfunction of several subcellular organelles, including platelet dense granules, melanosomes, and lysosomes.[104,105] Therefore, it is characterized by partial oculocutaneous albinism, a hemorrhagic defect due to platelet dysfunction; and the accumulation of ceroid, a chromolipid related to lipofuscin in the reticuloendothelial system of various tissues.[104,105] The ceroid-like material is also found in the buccal mucosa and the urine. The underlying biochemical defect is unknown. However, two HPS-causing genes have been identified. *HPS1*, whose function is unknown, and *ADTB3A*, which codes for the beta 3A subunit of adaptor complex 3 and is responsible for vesicle formation in the transgolgi network.[106]

The oculocutaneous albinism is tyrosine positive as opposed to true albinism and may be difficult to detect in dark-skinned races. The disease appears to be autosomal recessive, and the majority of cases originate from southern Holland and northwestern Puerto Rico.[107] In addition to the albinism and platelet defect, both an inflammatory granulomatous colitis and progressive pulmonary fibrosis can occur.[108] The pulmonary fibrosis is more common in women and affects 30% of all cases with HPS. It usually appears between the second and fourth decades.[108,109] Familial cases have been reported infrequently.[110,111] The lung disease is slowly progressive and unresponsive to therapy resulting in debilitating dyspnea and restrictive pulmonary function tests. The fibrosis is thought to be due to the accumulation of ceroid, an insoluble fluorescent lipoprotein, which is extracellular and present in the lysosomes of alveolar macrophages.[106] The mean age of onset of dyspnea is 35 years.[111] The chest radiograph and HRCT are nonspecific and usually reveal a honeycomb lung.[112] The histologic appearance, in addition to the extensive fibrosis of the alveolar walls, reveals ceroid-material-filled macrophages scattered throughout the interstitium and alveolar spaces. A recent histologic study of five patients with HPS indicated a florid proliferation of type 2 pneumocytes with characteristic foamy swelling and patchy fibrosis with lymphocytic and histiocytic infiltration around bronchioles occasionally causing obliterative bronchiolitis. There was lower lobe honeycombing, but this was not subpleural as is the case in usual interstitial pneumonia.[113] This study also indicated that there was a defect in the formation and secretion of surfactant protein from the type 2 pneumocyte. Ultrastructural studies indicated cytoplasmic lamellar bodies compressing the cell nucleus. These macrophages can be identified by the Fontana-Masson silver reduction technique in the lung lavage of a patient with HPS.[107] The cellular differential count in the BAL fluid was within normal range. There is no effective treatment for this disorder and lung disease is the most frequent reason for decreased survival.

HYPOCALCIURIC HYPERCALCEMIA AND INTERSTITIAL LUNG DISEASE

This is a rare syndrome recognized by the presence of familial hypercalcemia with hypocalciuria, granulocyte dysfunction, and an interstitial lung disease.[114] The inheritance pattern is autosomal dominant. The disease begins in infancy, the hypercalcemia is asymptomatic and does not response to parathyroidectomy. In contrast to other granulomatous interstitial lung diseases such as sarcoidosis or berylliosis, the urine calcium is normal or low, and the level of 1,25-dihydroxyvitamin D_3 is within normal limits. The lung disease is granulomatous, revealing foreign body giant cells and mononuclear cells infiltrating the alveolar interstitium. There are, however, no well-formed circumscribed granulomas as occur in sarcoidosis or berylliosis. In chronic cases, the lung becomes fibrotic and honeycomb changes appear. Survival is approximately 10 years, once the lung disease is discovered. The third feature of this syndrome is granulocyte dysfunction due to a myeloperoxidase deficiency and reduced antistaphylococcal killing.[115] Affected families may have one or all three of the primary manifestations of this syndrome.

LYMPHANGITIC CARCINOMATOSIS

Lymphangitic carcinomatosis is a form of metastatic lung disease producing an interstitial pattern on the chest radiograph. It originates from adenocarcinomas of the breast, lung, stomach, pancreas, prostate, ovary, and kidney. Metastases from squamous cell carcinomas of the cervix and oropharynx can, in rare instances, cause lymphangitic carcinomatosis.[116,117] Sarcomas occasionally spread to the lung producing a lymphangitic pattern, referred to as lymphangitis sarcomatosis.[118] In one large series, lymphangitic carcinomatosis accounted for 8% of all metastatic malignancies to the lung; the most frequent primary sites were breast and stomach.[119,120]

The syndrome is characterized by the insidious onset of dyspnea although in unusual circumstance patients present with acute respiratory failure.[121] An irritating cough due to submucosal endobronchial lymphatic involvement is seen in most cases. Bronchorrhea resulting from diffuse lymphangitic metastasis of colon carcinoma and diffuse infiltration of mucus-secreting adenocarcinoma cells into the lung has been described, but this event rarely occurs in lymphangitic carcinomatosis.[122] Lymphangitic carcinomatosis progresses rapidly and typically results in cor pulmonale and death within 3 to 6 months after diagnosis.[123] Because lymphangitic carcinomatosis is often accompanied by tumor emboli, death may be accelerated or may occur suddenly from acute cor pulmonale. The pulmonary symptoms may also precede symptoms referable to the primary tumor site and thus present as dyspnea and an interstitial lung disease of unknown etiology. The presence of lymphangitic carcinomatosis in a young adult without an apparent primary site, should lead one to search for gastric adenocarcinoma.[124] Occasionally, patients with lymphangitic carcinomatosis, in addition to the progressive dyspnea and cough, have asthmatic symptoms.[125]

The chest radiograph typically demonstrates lower zone Kerley's B lines and reticulonodular infiltrates; extensive involvement of all lung fields occurs over time (Figure 31–11). The appearance of chest radiographic Kerley's B lines in a patient with interstitial lung disease with normal left ventricular function, should raise the suspicion for lymphangitic carcinomatosis. In addition, pleural effusions and hilar and mediastinal adenopathy may be present (Figures 31–12 and 31–13). Infrequently, the chest radiograph appears normal in a symptomatic patient with histologic evidence of lymphangitic carcinomatosis. This has been reported to occur with carcinoma of the breast.[126] It is not unusual to see pulmonary lymphangitic spread at postmortem examination in breast cancer patients who were not symptomatic prior to death.[120] In some patients with primary bronchogenic carcinoma, unilateral lymphangitic spread

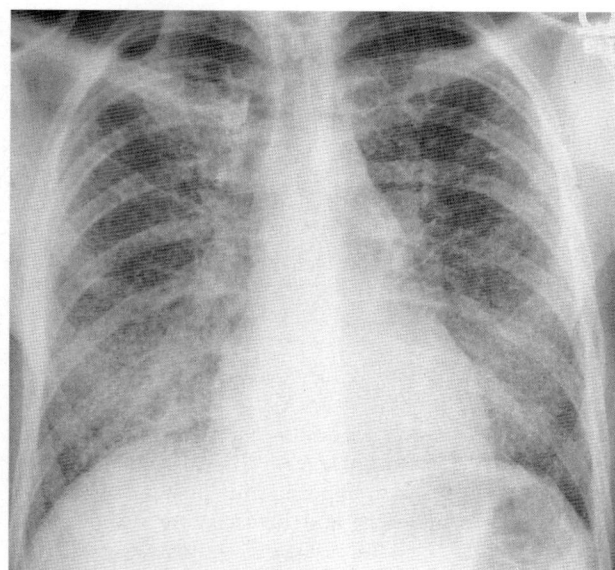

Figure 31–11   Chest radiograph of lymphangitic carcinomatosis. A 23-year-old man with reticulonodular infiltrates and Kerley's B lines best seen in the left lower lobe. The primary site was a gastric carcinoma.

that is often associated with mediastinal and/or hilar adenopathy may occur (Figure 31–14).

Lymphangitic carcinomatosis produces a restrictive ventilatory impairment with stiff noncompliant lungs, a reduction in the diffusing capacity for carbon monoxide, and marked gas exchange abnormalities resulting in severe hypoxemia and eventually subacute cor pulmonale. HRCT scans show uneven thickening of the bronchovascular bundles, isolated thickening of interstitial lines, and polygonal or septal lines (Figure 31–15).[127] In one study of chest CT findings comparing lymphangitic carcinomatosis with sarcoidosis and diffuse lymphoma, there was greater involvement of the interlobular septa and subpleural interstitium in lymphangitic carcinomatosis.[128]

Microscopically, the lungs reveal tumor cells filling peribronchial, perivascular, and subpleural lymphatics (Figure 31–16). In addition, an associated fibrotic reaction in the adjacent alveolar septae accounts for the majority of the parenchymal radiographic findings.[129] The most intriguing histologic feature is an extensive obliterative endarteritis that involves the small muscular pulmonary arteries (Figure 31–17). Malignant cells are visible within the vessel lumens. This vascular obstruction probably accounts for the development of subacute corpulmonale. Lymphangitic carcinomatosis may actually result from small-vessel tumor emboli that lodge distally and then spread to the lymphatics directly through the vascular walls.[130] This obstructs the subpleural lymphatics accounting for the Kerley's B lines and pleural effusions that are visible on radiographic studies. The hilar and mediastinal lymph nodes become involved with tumor by retrograde

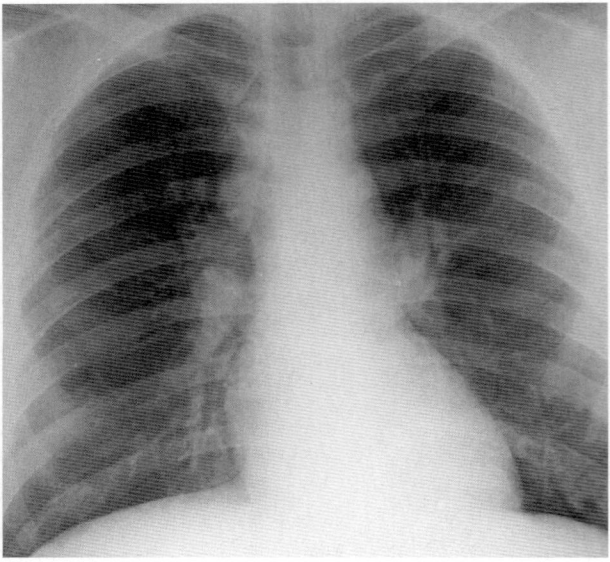

A

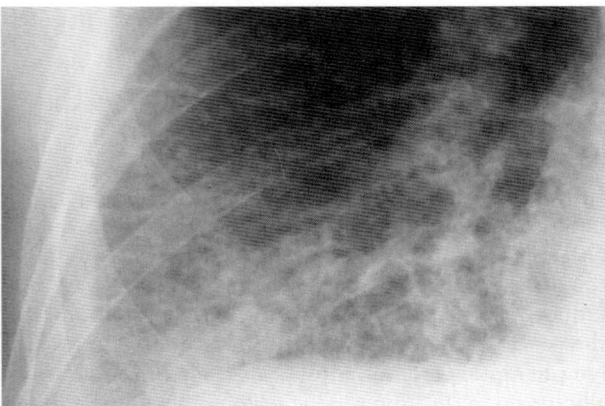

Figure 31–13   Chest radiograph of lymphangitic carcinomatosis. Note the Kerley's B lines and pleural effusion.

tumor to other organs as well as the bone marrow. Although survival is dismal in lymphangitic carcinomatosis, endocrine manipulation and chemotherapy are effective for some cases, particularly those that originate from the prostate and breast.[132–134]

NEUROFIBROMATOSIS (VON RECKLINGHAUSEN'S DISEASE)

Neurofibromatosis (NF) results from an abnormal proliferation of neural crest cells and therefore can affect any organ system. Neurofibromatosis occurs in 1 out of

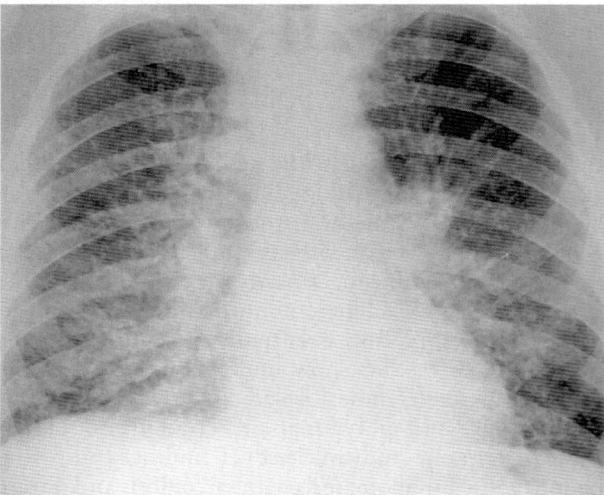

B

Figure 31–12   Lymphangitic carcinomatosis. *A*, Chest radiograph of a central adenocarcinoma of the lung with bilateral hilar and mediastinal adenopathy and diffuse linear interstitial infiltrates. *B*, Chest radiograph taken two months later demonstrating progression of the lymphangitic spread and loss of lung volume.

lymphatic spread.[130] Transbronchial biopsy and bronchial washings are usually positive and obviate the need for an open or video-assisted thoracoscopic lung biopsy. In addition, endobronchial lymphatic involvement is common, and the diffuse plaque-like infiltrate visible at bronchoscopy is highly accessible to endobronchial biopsy. Although rarely necessary, microvascular cytology of mixed venous blood may also yield this diagnosis.[131]

A microangiopathic hemolytic anemia, thrombocytopenia, and a leukoerythroblastic peripheral blood picture may appear due to diffuse endovascular spread of

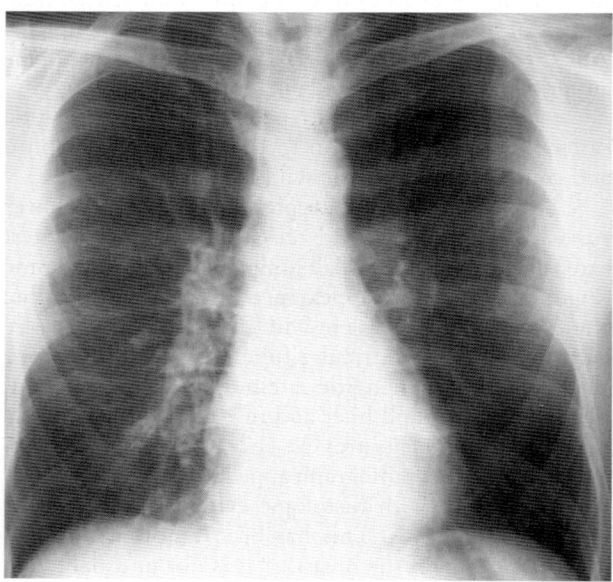

Figure 31–14   Chest radiograph of unilateral lymphangitic carcinomatosis. Note the reticular (linear) infiltrates involving the right lung. Bronchoscopy revealed a right lower lobe endobronchial adenocarcinoma.

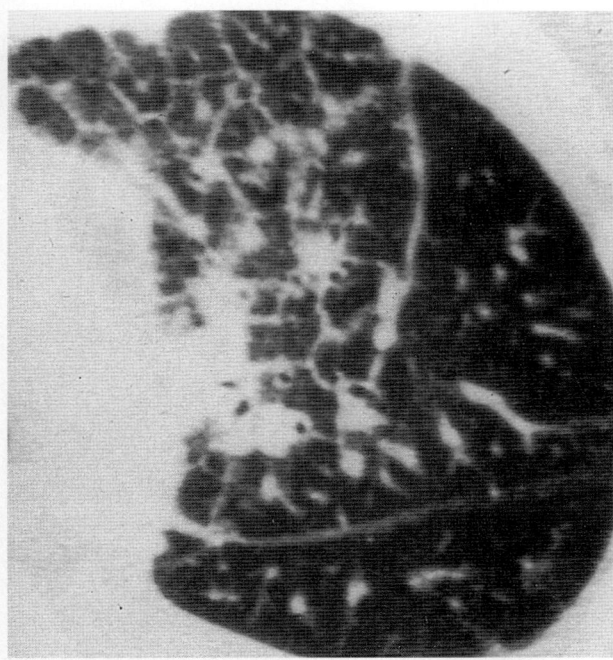

Figure 31–15 High-resolution computed tomography demonstrating polygonal septal lines extending to the pleural surface (Kerley's B) representing peripheral lymphatic obstruction.

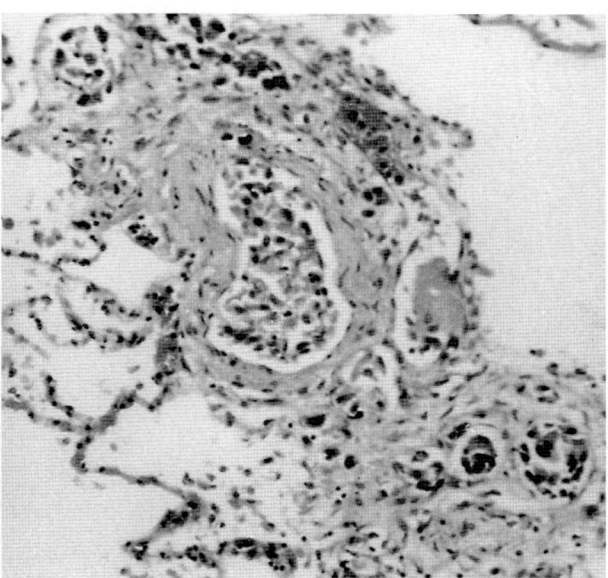

Figure 31–17 Lymphangitic carcinomatosis. There is an obliterative endarteritis due to malignant cells occluding the lumens of small muscular pulmonary arteries (hematoxylin and eosin; ×40 original magnification).

3,500 births, and its inheritance pattern is autosomal dominant,[135,136] but as many as 50% of cases are spontaneous, making it one of the most common gene mutations in man.[137–139] The gene for neurofibromatosis 1 is found on chromosome 17 and represents a tumor-suppressor gene.[140] Neurofibromatosis type 1 (NF1) or von Recklinghausen's disease is recognized by the appearance of multiple café-au-lait spots and cutaneous neu-

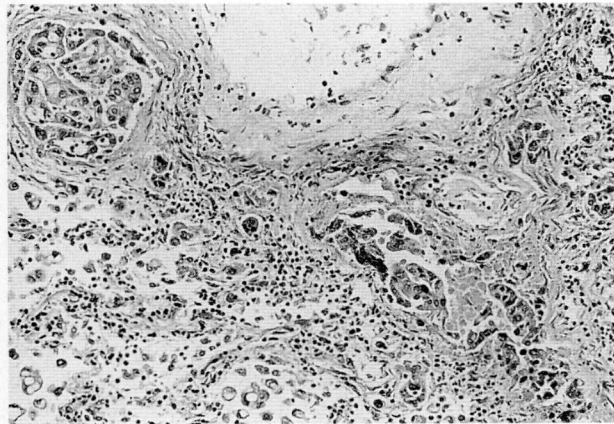

Figure 31–16 Lymphangitic carcinomatosis. Patient with gastric carcinoma demonstrating malignant cells within lymphatic channels of the interlobular septum. Also note the malignant cells lying free within the alveolar spaces (hematoxylin and eosin; ×10 original magnification).

rofibromas. The Lisch nodule, a hamartoma of the iris, is present in over 90% of patients. Internal neurofibromatous tumors are most commonly found in the central nervous system. A second type of NF, neurofibromatosis 2 (NF2), occurs in 1 out of 50,000 births and the genetic locus is on chromosome 22. The manifestations of NF2 appear later in life (puberty, young adulthood). They have neurofibromatous tumors, but without the dermatologic manifestations. Typically, lung disease does not occur in NF2 patients.[139]

Interstitial lung disease has been reported to occur in 20% of patients with type 1 neurofibromatosis.[143] The interstitial lung disease appears between the ages of 35 and 60 years, and dyspnea is the most common presenting symptom. The chest radiograph demonstrates lower zone reticulonodular infiltrates with the eventual appearance of bullous changes in the upper zones (Figure 31–18).[138–141] The physiologic abnormality is characterized by the gradual appearance and slow progression of a mixed obstructive and restrictive ventilatory impairment. Alveolar septal fibrosis is the major histopathologic change, but an alveolitis consisting of a mononuclear cell infiltration is found in earlier disease.[135,136] Scar carcinoma can complicate the fibrotic lung disease.[142] Severe bullous lung disease with airflow limitation also occurs (Figure 31–19).[143] Primary lung cancer can develop in the walls of emphysematous cysts.[144] In one case, immunofluorescent studies of lung tissue failed to reveal immune complex deposition.[145] It has been postulated that the interstitial lung disease in neurofibromatosis results from excessive collagen deposition rather than from a postinflammatory scarring process.[141]

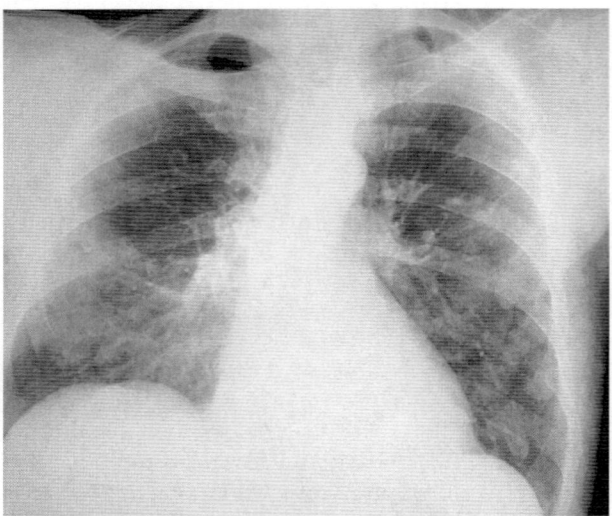

Figure 31–18   Neurofibromatosis. Chest radiograph demonstrating diffuse reticulonodular infiltrates. The rounded lesions seen in the left hemithorax are actually subcutaneous neurofibromas. Also note the subcutaneous neurofibromas along the left chest wall.

Other pulmonary complications of NF1 are listed in Table 31–2. Involvement of the phrenic nerve roots by neurofibroma resulted in bilateral diaphragmatic paralysis resulting in exertional dyspnea and severe orthopnea in a 36-year-old man.[146] Vascular involvement consisting of extensive intimal fibrosis and neurofibromas can result in severe pulmonary hypertension.[147] In this case, the pulmonary angiogram was compatible with chronic thrombotic pulmonary hypertension. Spontaneous hemothorax secondary to neurofibromatous involvement of the subclavian or intercostal arteries with dissection into the pleural space can also occur.[148,149]

LYSINURIC PROTEIN INTOLERANCE

Lysinuric protein intolerance (LPI) is an autosomal recessive disease caused by the defective transport of lysine, arginine, and ornithine with excessive loss of the proteins in the urine.[150] These individuals demonstrate failure to thrive, growth retardation, hepatosplenomegaly, hypertonicity, and osteoporosis. Fewer than 100 patients, primarily from Finland, have been reported.[151] Pulmonary complications have been reported in children and adults with LPI.[151–154] Acute respiratory insufficiency is the only life-threatening complication of LPI. Alveolar proteinosis is the interstitial lung disease most commonly seen and can appear acutely; pulmonary hemorrhage has also been described. Prior to the episodes of acute respiratory insufficiency, affected patients have interstitial infiltrates on the chest radiograph and HRCT scan. In fact, most adult patients with LPI demonstrate clinically silent and physiologically unimportant interstitial lung disease.[154]

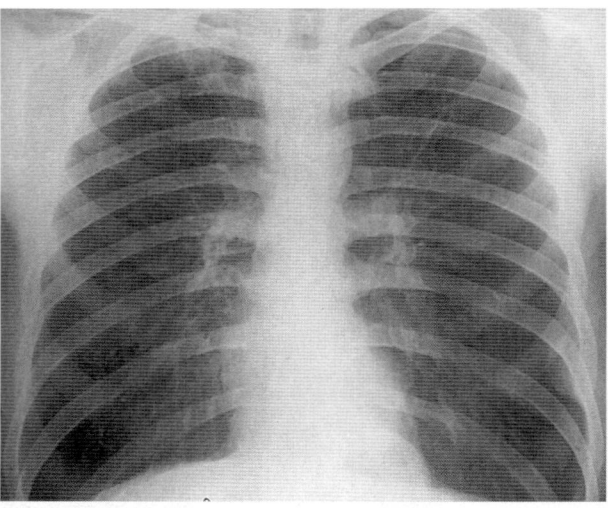

A

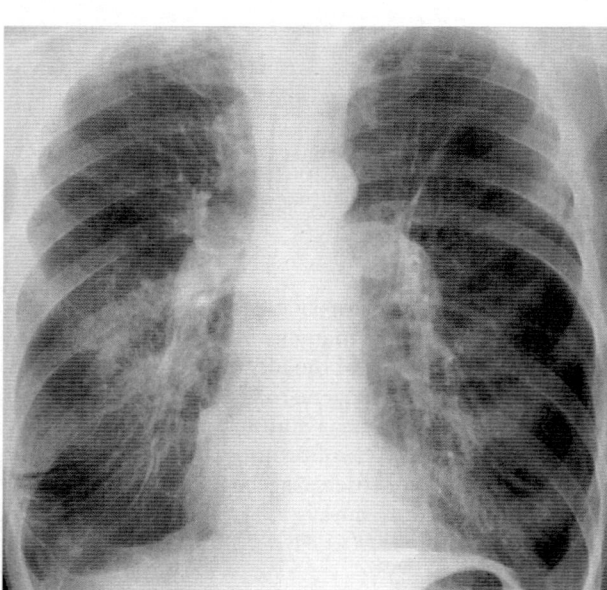

B

Figure 31–19   Neurofibromatosis. *A*, Chest radiograph demonstrating hyperinflation and an extrapleural mass in the left lower lung field, which represents a cutaneous neurofibroma. *B*, Chest radiograph of same patient 10 years later with further hyperinflation, lower zone interstitial infiltrates, and pulmonary hypertension.

DIABETES MELLITUS

It is no surprise that due to the extensive microcirculation of the lung and the microangiopathic process that typifies diabetes mellitus, that lung dysfunction has the potential for occurring in this metabolic disorder.[155] Postmortem studies of diabetic patients show broadening of epithelial cell and capillary basement membranes of the lungs.[156] Another postmortem study comparing 61 diabetic with 50 nondiabetic subjects did not find statistically significant differences in the incidence of

**TABLE 31–2   Thoracic Manifestations
of Neurofibromatosis**

Thoracic cage
   Subcutaneous chest wall neurofibromas or rarely
      neurofibrosarcoma (single or multiple)
   Inferior rib notching from intercostal neurofibroma
   Kyphoscoliosis
   Apical intercostal neurofibromas simulating a thickened pleura
      or a Pancoast's tumor
Mediastinal masses
   Posterior
      Lateral meningocele
      Neurofibromas or schwannomas of the vagus nerve
      Pheochromocytoma (rare)
   Middle
      Neurofibromatous mass probably originating from vagus
        nerve
Lung parenchyma
   Bullous emphysema
   Interstitial lung disease
   Malignant masses
      Metastatic neurofibrosarcoma
      Scar carcinoma
      Primary neurogenic tumor
Others
   Bilateral diaphragmatic paralysis
   Hemothorax
   Pneumothorax
   Pulmonary hypertension

alveolar wall fibrosis and medial thickening of small blood vessels. They did find a nodular form of fibrosis, which they felt was specific for this disorder, that was present within the alveolar walls of the diabetic subjects. Areas of pulmonary hemorrhages were also more frequent in the lungs of diabetic subjects.[157]

Although the data is conflicting, abnormal lung physiologic testing has been documented in 60% of a diabetic population; however, the abnormalities were subclinical in most cases.[158] The most consistent finding is an impaired diffusing capacity primarily due to a reduction in the pulmonary capillary blood volume.[159] In juvenile diabetics, low lung volumes and reduced elastic recoil have been described.[160,161] There is evidence suggesting that long-term normoglycemia with intensive insulin therapy in type 1 diabetics is beneficial in preventing deterioration of pulmonary function.[162]

AGNOGENIC MYELOID METAPLASIA

Agnogenic myeloid metaplasia (myelofibrosis with myeloid metaplasia) is a myeloproliferative syndrome in which the bone marrow becomes fibrotic and hematopoiesis takes place in extramedullary sites, most notably in the spleen and the liver. Other extramedullary sites are, however, occasionally affected.[163] Five cases of pulmonary extramedullary hematopoiesis associated with interstitial, peribronchiolar, and pleural fibrosis

have been reported.[164] This presents as diffuse infiltration on the chest radiograph.

GRANULOMATOUS PNEUMONITIS INDUCED BY BACILLE CALMETTE-GUÉRIN

Bacille Calmette-Guérin (BCG) is an attenuated but variable strain of the tubercle bacillus that is used in the immunotherapy of cancer, particularly bladder carcinoma.[165] On rare occasions, occurring in less than 1% of cases receiving intravesical BCG, a disseminated granulomatous process that affects the liver, bone marrow, and the lung can occur. Patients develop fever, cough, and dyspnea, and the chest radiographs show reticulonodular or miliary infiltrates. Bronchoalveolar lavage reveals a T-cell lymphocytosis with a preponderance of T helper (CD4) cells.[166] Cultures and direct staining of the granulomatous pneumonitis that develops are negative for BCG. It is believed that the granulomatous pneumonitis represents a hypersensitivity reaction. Corticosteroid treatment is effective.[167]

PULMONARY FIBROSIS AS A CONSEQUENCE OF THE ACUTE RESPIRATORY DISTRESS SYNDROME

The acute respiratory distress syndrome (ARDS) refers to a constellation of clinical, radiologic, and physiologic abnormalities that result from a number of acute injuries to the alveolar lining epithelium and capillary basement membrane. This results in the leakage of serum contents into the alveolar spaces. It most often occurs after shock, sepsis, trauma, aspiration, and some infectious diseases. A similar picture and pathologic consequences can occur in systemic lupus erythematosus (SLE), polymyositis, acute interstitial pneumonitis (Hamman-Rich syndrome), toxic gas exposure, and drug-induced (IP), particularly from the cytotoxic drugs employed in cancer chemotherapy. Although it remains controversial, this common pathway and the subsequent lung injury results from a combination of the following: neutrophil accumulation with the release of toxic oxygen products and proteolytic enzymes; the loss of pulmonary surfactant; intravascular platelet aggregation; intravascular complement activation; and the release from various inflammatory cells of proinflammatory and profibrotic cytokines such as tumor necrosis factor.[168–174] The critical injury is to the alveolar epithelial surface resulting in a loss of integrity of the alveolar-capillary basement membrane, and subsequent leakage of serum contents into the alveolar spaces, which, in turn, can initiate the fibroproliferative response. Between 40 to 60% of patients survive the episode of ARDS. Survival depends not only on the severity and eventual control of the initial injury but on the prevention of further injury during the course of the illness. Such further morbidity often results from a secondary infection and/or the development of multiorgan system failure.

Exudation of serum products that contain fibronectin and fibrinogen into the air spaces follows alveolar epithelial damage. This appears as alveolar edema and intra-alveolar hyaline membrane formation that accounts for the early inflammatory histology of diffuse alveolar damage. With control of the primary process there will be a slow resolution of this stage. With continuing injury, fibroblasts and myofibroblasts migrate into the intra-alveolar exudate, possibly partially due to the chemotactic properties of serum fibronectin. If nothing interferes with this process, intra-alveolar and interstitial fibrosis will result. This is referred to as the proliferative or organizing phase of ARDS (organizing phase of diffuse alveolar damage).

Multiple studies have shown that corticosteroids are ineffective during the early phase of ARDS.[175–178] However, during the fibroproliferative phase, corticosteroid preparations appear to have an effect on the reversal of this process.[179–181] There is clinical evidence to suggest that the failure of the prone position to improve oxygenation in ARDS coincides with the fibroproliferative phase of disease.[182] During the early fibroproliferative phase type III collagen is deposited. This new collagen is more susceptible to digestion by collagenase and to the anti-inflammatory effects of corticosteroid drugs. Type 1 collagen, the primary collagen found in most forms of pulmonary fibrosis, appears during the latter fibroproliferative phase. An increase in type I collagen is first reflected by an increase in type I procollagen production, as measured in BAL fluid.[183] Moreover, if there is a shift in the balance between type I collagen and collagenase, as measured by collagen breakdown products, this favors fibroproliferation and pulmonary fibrosis. Another marker of fibroproliferation and decreased survival are elevated bronchoalveolar lavage levels of transforming growth factor alpha, a potent mitogen in ARDS patients.[184] The transforming growth factors also inhibit the interstitial collagenases and the apoptosis of fibroblasts. Clinically, this is seen as a failure to improve gas exchange 1 week following the diagnosis of ARDS and is associated with a mortality rate in excess of 90%.[178] One study showed a 75% survival in eight patients who received corticosteroid therapy an average of 15 days after the diagnosis of ARDS. Seven of these patients underwent open lung biopsy to document the fibroproliferative phase.[181] In another study of ten patients with ARDS, there was worsening gas exchange and stiff lungs 10 to 20 days postinitial injury. Open lung biopsy revealed interstitial fibroproliferation, inflammation, organizing pneumonia, and air space obliteration. Eight subjects survived following intravenous administration of methylprednisolone.[185]

During the fibrotic stage, there is collapse and apposition of the alveolar walls[174] likely due to the loss or failure of the production of surfactant.[173] This, in turn, prevents both re-epithelialization, a critical step in the repair process, as well as the subsequent reconstitution of the alveolar epithelium by differentiating type II cells, thereby promoting extracellular matrix accumulation. This causes severe gas exchange disturbances and a noncompliant, difficult-to-ventilate respiratory system. It is clear from postmortem studies that the predominant histologic changes include alveolar hyaline membrane formation, edema, and alveolar septal inflammation (exudative phase), which can evolve to severe alveolar wall and air space fibrosis (fibroproliferative phase) (Figure 31–20).[170] Fibrosis is most frequently noted in the lungs of patients who expired 3 to 4 weeks postinitial injury. In these individuals, there is biochemical evidence of increased lung collagen production. These findings are in contrast to those for patients who survived less than 10 days, in whom the collagen content is not increased and in whom anatomic studies of lung tissue do not reveal significant amounts of fibrosis.[171] Other studies have raised the question as to whether high inspired oxygen fractions are pathogenetic in the interstitial and air space fibrosis of ARDS. These studies demonstrated increased collagen content in the lungs of those nonsurvivors who had inspired oxygen fractions of at least 40% for twice the time, compared with a group with normal collagen contents.[172] A pulmonary lesion, radiographically and morphologically similar to bronchopulmonary dysplasia of newborns, has been reported in adults with ARDS who require high oxygen concentrations for prolonged periods of time and survive.[178] In these patients, the lungs become hyperinflated and cystic-type honeycomb changes occur (Figure 31–21). Histologic examination of lung tissue reveals marked disruption of the alveolar architecture with cystic dilation of air spaces and broad bands of alveolar septal fibrous tissue.[186]

The appearance of collagenase activity directed against types I and III collagen, as well as increased neutrophil elastase activity, and increased neutrophil num-

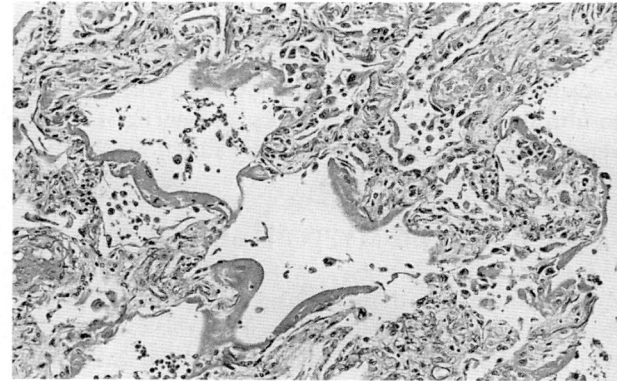

Figure 31–20   Acute respiratory distress syndrome—organizing stage. Hyaline membranes are becoming incorporated into the interstitium. The interstitium is broadened due to fibroblastic proliferation and the elaboration of collagen fibers (hematoxylin and eosin; ×40 original magnification).

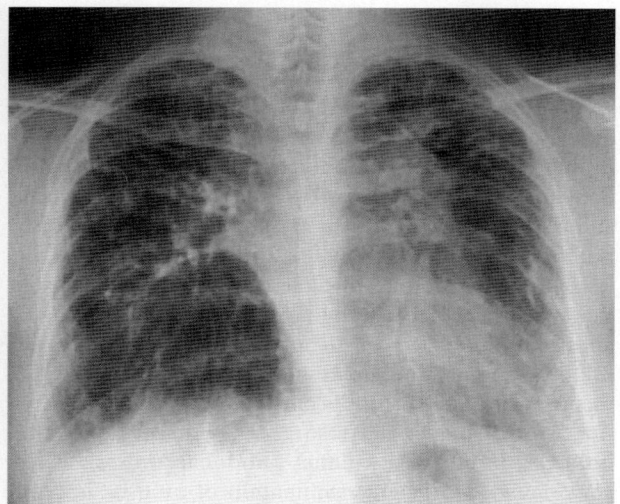

Figure 31–21   Acute respiratory distress syndrome (ARDS). Chest radiograph taken 2 years following an episode of sepsis and ARDS requiring prolonged ventilation with high oxygen concentrations.

bers in the BAL fluid of ARDS patients support the role of neutrophils in the pathogenesis of ARDS-associated fibrosis.[187-188] Others have drawn attention to seemingly common features in the pathogenesis of idiopathic pulmonary fibrosis and the fibrotic phase of ARDS.[189]

What becomes of those who survive an episode of ARDS? It is clear that the majority of these patients do quite well but often have residual physiologic disturbances that have a tendency to improve with time.[190] This conclusion was, however, based on only 129 surviving patients recorded in the literature. Forty to 60% of ARDS survivors are asymptomatic (after the episode).[191] Several symptomatic patients demonstrated residual interstitial infiltrates on the chest radiograph, and biopsy material revealed variable degrees of a lymphoplasmocytic infiltration of the alveolar walls, alveolar wall fibrosis, and type II cell hyperplasia, a nonspecific interstitial pneumonitis.[192] A study of 52 surviving ARDS patients indicated that maximum improvement in pulmonary function occurs within 6 months following an ARDS episode.[193] This evidence supports the contention that the fibrosis that follows an acute episode of ARDS is at least partially reversible.[194]

Expected physiologic disturbances include a reduction in both total lung and diffusing capacities that improves throughout the first year in 25 to 33% of ARDS survivors. Residual physiologic disturbances after 6 months to 1 year are rarely severe but tend to persist if present.[193,195] Symptomatic bronchial hyperactivity following both methacholine challenge and exercise have been described in several ARDS survivors.[196] Which factors predict persistent pulmonary functional impairment in survivors of ARDS?[197-199] One report described pulmonary function testing in 39 survivors at 6 months,[194] noting persistent abnormalities of the diffusing capacity

for carbon monoxide, forced vital capacity, and total lung capacity in 61%, 43%, and 21% of the patients, respectively. A low diffusing capacity for carbon monoxide correlated with higher pulmonary artery pressures, more severe gas-exchange disturbances, and the occurrence of sepsis during the acute episode. A reduction of the vital capacity and lung volumes appeared to correlate with peak airway pressures exceeding 50 cm H_2O during the period of mechanical ventilation of the acute episode. Another study described 16 survivors studied at 1 year after ARDS[198] and found correlation between abnormalities of diffusing capacity, forced vital capacity, and total lung capacity with the initial severity of the thoracic compliance, shunt fraction, pulmonary artery pressure, level of positive end-expiratory pressure, and total ventilator time. In addition, ventilatory support requiring a fraction of inspired oxygen (FiO_2) greater than 0.6 for more than 24 hours predicted a reduced diffusing capacity at 1 year.[196] Another study devised an ARDS severity score in which the duration of ventilation and the lowest static thoracic compliance predicted persistent physiologic impairment 1 year after the episode.[199]

INTERSTITIAL LUNG DISEASE FOLLOWING PULMONARY INFECTIONS

It is clear that bacterial pneumonias, tuberculosis, and fungal infections, particularly if there is delay in treatment, can lead to pulmonary fibrosis, however, in these instances the fibrosis is not diffuse. There is also data to support the concept that an acute diffuse infectious pneumonia causing diffuse alveolar inflammation can result in diffuse fibrosis.

An infectious agent (virus) has been proposed as a possible inciting event for IPF. There is, however, little support for this concept. It is not unusual for patients with IPF, bronchiolitis obliterans organizing pneumonia (BOOP), or nonspecific interstitial pneumonia (NSIP) to date the onset of their symptoms to an upper respiratory tract infection or viral-like syndrome. These patients, particularly those with BOOP, report low-grade fever, myalgias, and arthralgias prior to the onset of cough and dyspnea.[200,201] However, attempts at isolating a virus from the lungs of patients with these disorders are generally unsuccessful, and, when evidence for prior viral infection is present, the data are difficult to interpret. There is no question that viral pneumonias, which are complicated by diffuse alveolar damage and acute respiratory distress syndrome, can result in fibroproliferation. When attempting to assign a viral pathogenesis to the more chronic indolent interstitial lung diseases, there is little scientific support.[202] In one case of IPF, using immunofluorescent and ultrastructural methods, adenoviral particles were demonstrated.[203] This finding was probably coincidental. Ultrastructural studies of lungs of several patients with desquamative interstitial pneumonia revealed intranuclear inclusions that were originally thought to represent viral particles but most likely were nuclear debris.[204,205] One study reported that 10 of 13 patients with IPF had serum antibodies to the Epstein-Barr (EB) virus but not herpes simplex or cytomegalovirus. A serum viral-capsid antigen was also present in all 13, indicating recent infection. These results were compared to 12 patients with a variety of other interstitial lung diseases, and EB virus was not detected.[206] These studies have not been duplicated. Two additional patients developed a chronic syndrome characterized by fever, an ill-defined interstitial pneumonitis (IP), pancytopenia, and other systemic manifestations.[207] Both of their illnesses followed an acute EB virus infection that resolved with acyclovir therapy. Lung histology indicated interstitial lymphocytes as well as intra-alveolar macrophage accumulation. The appearance of diffuse pulmonary infiltrates in well-established cases of infectious mononucleosis, another EB virus–related disease, are well described.[208] In some cases of infectious mononucleosis, hilar lymph nodes, diffuse or localized pneumonitis, pleural effusions, and respiratory insufficiency occurred during the acute phase.[209] Lung tissue revealed lymphoplasmacytic interstitial infiltrates but alveolar wall fibrosis was not seen. Patients who recover from the acute phase resolve without residual interstitial lung disease.[208,210]

The EB virus has been implicated in several other interstitial lung diseases.[211–214] Viral replication was present in the epithelial cells of the lower respiratory tract in patients with IPF.[211–213] This occurred in 14 of 20 patients studied. More specifically, this study provided immunocytochemical evidence that type II epithelial cells contained proteins encoded by the EB virus that usually appear during a time of active infection. As pointed out by Hogg,[211] however, this does not necessarily show that replication of the virus was taking place at the time of biopsy. In another study, the EB virus genome was found by in situ hybridization in lung epithelial cells in 9 of 14 patients with lymphocytic interstitial pneumonia (LIP).[212] These investigators compared the LIP patients with 10 IPF patients and only two IPF patients demonstrated the EB virus genome. The EB virus has also been found in the acute interstitial lung disease that occurs with polymyositis (organizing diffuse alveolar damage) by both in situ hybridization and the polymerase chain reaction.[214] This type of acute IP is identical to the Hamman-Rich syndrome, however, similar findings have not been reported.

The hepatitis C virus (HCV) was also implicated as a cause of IPF. A study from Japan of 66 IPF cases found HCV serum antibodies in 19 subjects using enzyme-linked immunosorbent assay (ELISA). Twelve of these were also positive when the recombinant immunoblotting assay (RIBA) was employed.[215] On the other hand, a study from the United Kingdom indicated that only 1 of 62 patients with IPF demonstrated antibodies to HCV.[216] There is no question, however, that HCV is implicated in hepatic inflammation, which can progress to fibrosis and end-stage cirrhosis,[217] and has been implicated in mixed cryoglobulinemia, which can be associ-

ated with diffuse alveolar hemorrhage and a small vessel vasculitis of the lungs.[218]

Animal models used to study the more chronic consequences of inhaled influenza virus document the development of a persistent interstitial inflammatory cellular infiltrate composed of mononuclear cells. In addition to the septal inflammation, collagen deposition was detected and viral antigen was present in these lungs.[219–221] Increased numbers of lymphocytes and neutrophils were persistently lavaged from the lungs of these mice. These data suggest that viral infection can lead to generalized fibrosis either by an autoimmune mechanism (antigen-antibody complexes) or due to an inflammatory response to the virus. Moreover, this response can be amplified by a superimposed bacterial infection or oxidant exposure.[220,221] The evidence that influenza virus causes human pulmonary fibrosis is less convincing. Pathologic examination of lung tissue from fatal cases of human influenza pneumonia reveal diffuse alveolar damage with alveolar hemorrhage and edema, intra-alveolar inflammatory cells, and bronchial and bronchiolar ulceration. Alveolar wall fibrosis is an infrequent finding.[222,223] Two cases of usual interstitial pneumonia (UIP) following a confirmed influenza A_2 infection have been described.[224,225] The first patient had an open lung biopsy procedure 16 days after the onset of his illness. In addition he received high concentrations of inspired oxygen. A favorable response to corticosteroids was obtained. The other recovered from the acute infection and then complained of increasing dyspnea. The chest radiograph revealed a progressive interstitial lung disease. An open lung biopsy procedure, performed 4 months after the acute episode, revealed both usual and desquamative interstitial pneumonitis. There was no response to corticosteroid therapy.[224] Other studies have reported the presence of variable degrees of alveolar wall fibrosis and septal inflammation resulting from viral pneumonias.[225,226]

There is an association between HIV, the causative agent of acquired immunodeficiency syndrome (AIDS), and NSIP.[227–234] NSIP also occurs as an idiopathic disorder in the immunocompetent host, in hypersensitivity pneumonitis, in collagen vascular diseases, and after hypersensitivity to certain medicatons.[231] In NSIP with AIDS, the patients may be dyspneic with physiologic abnormalities in the face of a normal radiograph or have diffuse interstitial infiltrates on the chest radiograph without evidence of pulmonary infection.[232–234] The question remains whether this represents a primary response to the HIV infection, or is it residual of *Pneumocystis carinii* or some other infectious agent. Cases of NSIP are found to occur in HIV-positive individuals even when the CD4 and total lymphocyte counts are still preserved.[230] One group reported NSIP in 27 of 110 AIDS cases in which infection or drug toxicity were excluded.[233] Open lung biopsies of AIDS-related NSIP reveal a lymphoplasmocytic alveolar wall infiltration and evidence of diffuse alveolar damage. Extensive fibrosis may also occur.[233,234] Presenting symptoms include dyspnea and cough of varying duration and crackles on auscultation. The chest radiograph may be normal or may demonstrate diffuse infiltrates being indistinguishable from *P. carinii* pneumonia.[229] Reduction of the diffusing capacity for carbon monoxide occurs in patients with both normal and abnormal chest radiographs and as many as 50% of dyspneic AIDS patients have normal chest radiographs.[227,235] Corticosteroids are of benefit in patients with progressive symptoms and physiologic disturbances, but a number of cases resolve spontaneously.[230]

Lymphocytic interstitial pneumonitis (See Chapter 27, "Lymphoplasmacytic Infiltrations of the Lung") is another noninfectious interstitial pneumonia occurring in AIDS, and it is more likely to affect children compared with adults.[236] Lymphocytic interstitial pneumonitis has also been associated with human T-cell lymphotrophic virus type I (HTLV-I).[237] In five adult cases of LIP in AIDS, high serum titers of EB virus were found.[238] Another interstitial pneumonia, BOOP, has also appeared in several cases of AIDS.[239,240] Corticosteroid drugs reversed this process. Acute eosinophilic pneumonia has also been described in this patient population.[241]

Mycoplasma pneumoniae infections, the great majority of which have a benign self-limiting course, may infrequently evolve into a severe interstitial pneumonitis that can result in death.[242,243] There are several well-documented cases of progressive end-stage pneumonitis caused by mycoplasma resulting in diffuse interstitial fibrosis.[244,245] The first demonstrated rapid evolution into an interstitial process requiring mechanical ventilation and high inspired oxygen concentrations.[244] The patient was 31 days postpartum and expired 17 days following the onset of acute pneumonitis. Complement fixation antibody titers for *Mycoplasma pneumoniae* rose during the second week of the illness. At autopsy, extensive alveolar wall fibrosis, in addition to a mononuclear cell interstitial infiltrate and alveolar desquamation, were present. The second revealed the presence of a mycoplasma antigen within alveolar macrophages.[245] A case of IP, which developed one year following a documented erythromycin-sensitive mycoplasma pneumonia, responded to corticosteroid treatment.[246]

Pulmonary fibrosis following *Legionella pneumophila* pneumonia has also been described.[247–251] Most data comes from autopsied cases. The prominent features include interstitial fibrosis and intra-alveolar organization and fibrosis. Ultrastructural studies revealed disruption of the alveolar epithelial lining and basement membranes. There are also survivors of acute legionnaires' disease in whom chest radiographic and physiologic evidence of interstitial lung disease persists.[248] There are two cases of well-documented *L. pneumophila* without erythromycin response, but with rapid clinical improvement after corticosteroids were initiated.[251]

There is evidence, in non-AIDS patients, that *P. carinii* pneumonia results in diffuse interstitial fibrosis.[252,253] It is not unusual for patients who recover from

this infection to have residual restrictive ventilatory impairment and a reduction in the diffusing capacity that slowly resolves.[254] The sequelae of varicella pneumonia in adults including pulmonary fibrosis and persistent diffusion abnormalities has been described.[255,256] Years following the acute event, diffuse interstitial micronodular calcifications appear on the chest radiograph but without physiologic consequence (Figure 31–22).[256]

INTERSTITIAL PNEUMONITIS AFTER TRANSPLANTATION

Allogeneic Bone Marrow Transplantation

Allogeneic or unrelated bone marrow transplantation (BMT) is employed for the treatment of acute

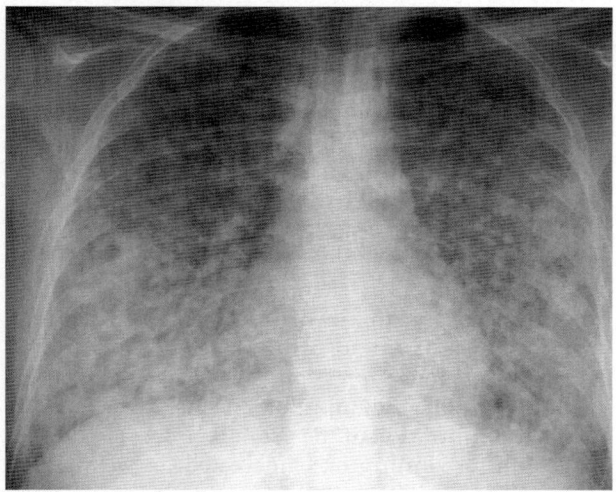

A

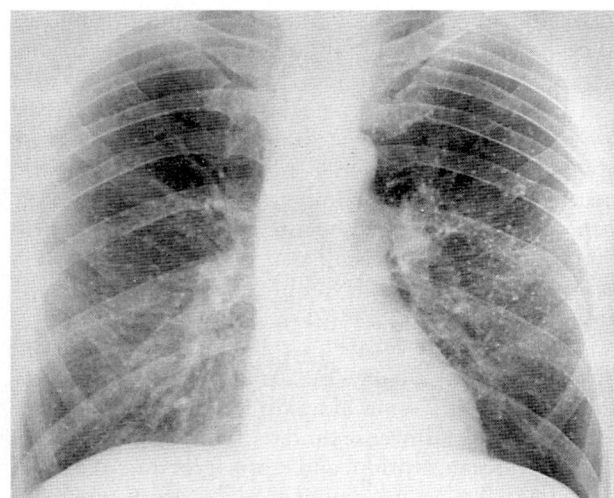

B

Figure 31–22   Chest radiographs of chickenpox (varicella) pneumonia. *A*, Diffuse alveolar infiltrates. *B*, Ten years later, miliary diffuse calcification.

leukemia, chronic myelogenous leukemia, aplastic anemia, and Hodgkin's and non-Hodgkin's lymphomas and offers an improved survival in some individuals.[257–259] Pulmonary complications occur in 20 to 60% of BMT recipients and, depending on the causes, are associated with a fatality rate of up to 50%.[260,261] Within the first 100 days post-BMT, the interstitial pneumonias are more heterogeneous and result from either human cytomegalovirus (CMV), herpes zoster, *P. carinii* (infrequent due to prophylaxis), or herpes simplex.[262,263] Viral pneumonia is the leading infectious cause of death post-BMT.[264] The incidence of CMV pneumonia, for example, is 25%, if the recipient is seropositive prior to transplant.[261] If both the recipient and donor are seronegative, the incidence of CMV is still 10% due to the use of blood products.[264] It is less common to see diffuse IP from an infectious cause beyond 1 year post-BMT.[263] Human herpesvirus 6 (HHV-6) can coexist with CMV or be the sole pathogen of post-BMT infectious IP.[265]

In approximately 50% of the cases of interstitial pneumonitis occurring within the first 100 days post-BMT, an infectious etiology cannot be established; this has been termed the idiopathic pneumonia syndrome (IPS).[259,266–269] The incidence of this complication ranges between 12 to 20% of all patients receiving a BMT. Several factors play a role in the appearance of noninfectious IP including induction total body irradiation; preinduction chemotherapy with combinations of lung cytotoxic drugs such as cyclophosphamide, busulfan, and carmustine; post-transplant chemotherapy for suppression of the chronic graft-versus-host reaction; and multiple transfusions. Recurrent malignant infiltration of the primary process is another cause of diffuse infiltrates. Undetected CMV infection is also an issue.[270] Idiopathic pneumonia syndrome appears 2 to 7 weeks post-transplant. The onset is usually acute with cough, dyspnea, fever, and the appearance of diffuse patchy air space filling to a varying degree on the chest radiograph. The histopathologic features of cytotoxic drug- and radiation-induced IP are similar. The histologic appearance is that of diffuse alveolar damage showing edematous interstitium, intra-alveolar hyaline membranes and a cellular interstitial reaction, followed by interstitial fibroblastic proliferation and mature collagen deposition. Although some patients respond favorably to corticosteroid therapy, the mortality rate is 70%.[271]

Chronic graft-versus-host disease (GVHD) develops from 100 to 500 days post-transplantation and presents with scleroderma-like skin lesions, Sjögren's syndrome, liver failure secondary to primary biliary cirrhosis, malabsorption, and esophageal mucositis that leads to aspiration pneumonia.[272,273] Diffuse parenchymal lung diseases, which complicate chronic GVHD, include obliterative bronchiolitis, a progressive obstructive airways disease,[274,275] lymphocytic IP,[276] a cellular NSIP,[277] and BOOP.[278,279]

The appearance of cough, dyspnea, bronchospasm, and physiologic evidence of airflow limitation and air trapping occurring in BMT patients from 3 to 24 months after transplant has several etiologies.[280] A follicular lymphocytic bronchitis with infiltration of the bronchial mucosa, submucosa, and muscularis layer by small lymphocytes results in necrosis and loss of the mucociliary clearance mechanism and increases the risk of infectious complications.[280,281] In addition, obliterative bronchiolitis occurring as a complication of GVHD has a variable response to bronchodilators and corticosteroid treatment.[282] It is estimated that at least 10% of patients surviving BMT will develop irreversible airflow limitation. The risk is increased if GVHD is present. In a prospective study of 281 adult patients alive 1 year after allogeneic BMT, factors associated with the presence of airflow limitation included increased gender, the male gender, smoking, the presence of GVHD, and methotrexate prophylaxis.[282] In this study, 20% of patients with GVHD had airflow limitation.

Two patients who developed LIP 242 and 632 days post-transplant, as demonstrated on an open lung biopsy, are described. The BAL fluid revealed an increased lymphocyte content consisting primarily of CD8 suppressor T lymphocytes.[276] The chest radiographs revealed bilateral reticulonodular infiltrates, and both patients responded to a combination of azathioprine and corticosteroids.

A NSIP with both overt and subclinical GVHD occurs. This parenchymal process could be the result of prior infection or therapeutic intervention, however, it may also represent a GVHD reaction involving the lung parenchyma and be independent of obliterative bronchiolitis.[263] There is progressive reduction of the diffusing capacity for carbon monoxide but with preservation of flow rates and lung volumes. NSIP is particularly prone to occur in subjects receiving BMT for chronic myelogenous leukemia (CML).[283] In this study, lung tissue was not available for examination. A case of NSIP also demonstrated organizing pneumonitis and was reversed with corticosteroids and cyclosporine.[271] The incidence of NSIP as a late complication of BMT is reduced with intravenous immunoglobulin therapy.[284] Another unusual complication of allogeneic BMT is the development of pulmonary hypertension secondary to pulmonary veno-occlusive disease several months post-transplantation.[285]

Cyclosporin A, which is used for prophylaxis of the chronic GVHD syndrome, has been implicated in the production of a fatal noncardiogenic capillary leak pulmonary edema syndrome.[286]

Autologous Bone Marrow Transplantation

Autologous bone marrow transplantation eliminates the need for a human leukocyte antigen (HLA)-identical donor, in which case GVHD is not seen. The incidence of interstitial pneumonia (infectious or noninfectious) is less than that seen in allogeneic BMT and ranges from 7.6 to 40%.[287–289] In a study of 143 subjects, 20 developed interstitial pneumonitis. In the cases in which tissue was available, IPS was present in half, and the mortality rate was as high as 50%. The median time of onset was 41 days post-BMT (5 to 624 days). It should be kept in mind that autologous BMT recipients may receive different preinduction chemotherapies and irradiation doses, depending on the underlying malignancy being treated. This difference in treatment probably explains the difference in the development of IPS. The high incidence of CMV pneumonitis seen in allogeneic BMT is not the case for the autologous BMT group.

A diffuse alveolar hemorrhage syndrome is another early complication of autologous BMT.[290] Twenty-nine of 141 patients developed dyspnea, hypoxia, cough, and diffuse alveolar infiltrates on the chest radiograph between 7 and 40 days after bone marrow rescue. Hemoptysis is not necessarily one of the presenting symptoms, but BAL fluid reveals a bloody return and contains hemosiderin-laden macrophages. Twenty-three of these patients died, and postmortem examination confirmed the diagnosis of diffuse alveolar hemorrhage as well as morphologic changes compatible with acute respiratory distress syndrome with underlying diffuse alveolar damage. Again, preinduction chemotherapy is thought to be the most likely cause. High-dose intravenous methylprednisolone may in some cases provide effective treatment for this complication.[291] Diffuse alveolar hemorrhage developed in one long-term survivor of an autologous BMT. The patient developed a systemic vasculitis with elevated antineutrophil cytoplasmic antibody titers and underlying pulmonary capillaritis to account for the pulmonary hemorrhage. An excellent response was achieved with anti-inflammatory and immunosuppressive therapy.[292]

DISEASES OF AUTOIMMUNITY ASSOCIATED WITH INTERSTITIAL LUNG DISEASE

Several of the idiopathic interstitial pneumonias (IIP), such as NSIP, are considered to be inflammatory lung diseases that can lead to fibrosis and are possibly initiated by altered immunity in response to some unknown antigen that injures the lung epithelium. In others, such as UIP, inflammation is minimal and fibroproliferation predominates. There is evidence to support a localized immune response of the lung parenchyma to account for the development of some IIP. Autoantibodies (rheumatoid and antinuclear factors) and immune complexes are found in the serum of some of these patients.[293–295] In addition, immune complexes are present in lung tissue in some cases, particularly in those with NSIP as opposed to UIP.[296,297] The clinicopathologic similarity between NSIP and UIP and the interstitial lung diseases that complicate the collagen vascular diseases lend further support to this hypothesis.

Table 31–3 lists other systemic disease states thought to be autoimmune in nature and sometimes associated with an interstitial pneumonia.

Hematologic Diseases

The association of interstitial lung disease and autoimmune hemolytic anemia was first described by Scadding.[298] Open lung biopsy specimens demonstrated a combination of desquamative interstitial pneumonia (DIP) and UIP. The authors postulated that antibody and complement-coated erythrocytes were trapped within the small vessels of the lung resulting in immune-complex-initiated inflammation. The hematologic disorder and the pulmonary disease resolved after treatment with corticosteroids. Another report described the simultaneous occurrence of LIP, chronic hepatitis, and autoimmune hemolytic anemia, which also responded to corticosteroid treatment.[299]

The occurrence of purpura and interstitial lung disease was first described by Turner-Warwick[300] in 2 of 154 subjects with IIP. There is an interesting case describing the simultaneous occurrence of idiopathic thrombocytopenic purpura (ITP) and a cellular NSIP.[301] This individual had marked elevation of circulating immune complexes and platelet-bound IgG. Immune complexes were also seen in the lung parenchyma, and an excellent

---

TABLE 31–3   Interstitial Lung Disease Associations in Autoimmune Diseases other than Collagen Vascular Diseases

Hematologic diseases
    Autoimmune hemolytic anemia
    Idiopathic thrombocytopenic purpura
    Essential cryoglobulinemia
Gastrointestinal diseases
    Ulcerative colitis
    Crohn's disease
    Celiac disease
    Whipple's disease
Hepatic diseases
    Primary biliary cirrhosis
    Chronic active hepatitis
    Cryptogenic cirrhosis
Endocrine diseases
    Hashimoto's thyroiditis
    Riedel's thyroiditis
Renal diseases
    Renal tubular acidosis
Neurologic diseases
    Peripheral neuropathy
Muscular diseases
    Myasthenia gravis
Vascular diseases
    Takayasu's arteritis
    Giant cell arteritis

response to corticosteroids was obtained. A case of interstitial pneumonitis and ITP was described in which tissue immune complexes were located in the walls of vessels, as opposed to the interstitium; this patient also responded to corticosteroid therapy.[302] A patient underwent splenectomy for ITP and in the ensuing 6 years developed an interstitial lung disease, as well as chronic active hepatitis and Coombs-positive hemolytic anemia.[303]

Mixed cryoglobulinemia (MC) is a systemic disease recognized by a dermatologic leukocytoclastic vasculitis, arthritis, hepatitis, systemic vasculitis, and glomerulonephritis. Cryoglobulins consist of either a monoclonal (type I) or mixed polyclonal and monoclonal IgM rheumatoid factors (type II) IgG or polyclonal IgG and rheumatoid factor (type III). In addition IgG, IgA, and complement are components of the cryoglobulin complex.[304] It was believed that essential mixed cryoglobulinemia represented an immune-complex-induced disease in which the hepatitis B virus played a causative role.[305] This hypothesis has always been problematic, because hepatitis B surface antigen (HBsAg) or antibodies are infrequently found in the serum of MC patients.[306] It has, however, become clear that hepatitis C accounts for a number of patients with MC.[307] Although this is a systemic process, in most series pulmonary involvement is only occasionally mentioned. In one study of 34 patients with MC, however, chest radiographic interstitial infiltrates were present in all cases.[308] In only nine subjects were there complaints of dyspnea or abnormalities of pulmonary function testing. Histologic material was not available in this series. Lung tissue has been studied in a limited number of cases and demonstrates an active cellular infiltration of the alveolar walls and arterioles with both acute and chronic inflammatory cells. In one case, immunofluorescent studies revealed IgG and IgM deposition in the alveolar structures.[309] Mixed cryoglobulinemia can also be responsible for diffuse alveolar hemorrhage secondary to pulmonary capillaritis, a small vessel vasculitis of the lungs.[310,311]

Gastrointestinal Diseases

Inflammatory Bowel Disease

Extracolonic manifestations such as uveitis, arthritis, skin lesions, and liver disease often complicate the inflammatory bowel diseases (IBD). The lung, however, is generally not considered a frequent secondary site of extragastrointestinal involvement. Multiple expressions of lung disease accompany ulcerative colitis and Crohn's disease. These include pulmonary vasculitis[312,313]; pleuropericarditis[314]; NSIP, which may progress to fibrosis and honeycomb lung[315,316]; BOOP[317,318]; pulmonary suppuration[318]; sulfasalazine (Azulfidine)-induced lung disease[319–321]; DIP[322]; and the full range of bronchial diseases, including bronchitis, bronchiectasis, follicular bronchiolitis, panbronchiolitis, colobronchial fistula, and bronchial stenosis.[323–329] Respiratory symptoms can predate the onset of IBD.[330] In a study of 33 patients with IBD, most cases representing ulcerative colitis indicated that bronchiectasis, often asymptomatic, and BOOP were the most frequent pulmonary complications.[330] Conditions more likely to accompany Crohn's disease included a sarcoid-like granulomatous disease of the upper and lower airways and subclinical lymphocytic alveolitis.[331,332] Women with IBD are more apt to have pulmonary complications.

Pulmonary vasculitis in ulcerative colitis appears acutely, often coinciding with exacerbations of the bowel disease and produces diffuse alveolar filling with a lower lobe predilection. Hemoptysis, fever, and dyspnea are the usual symptoms. It can recur, and in the few reported cases it has been responsive to both corticosteroid treatment and colectomy. Cavitating masses reminiscent of Wegener's granulomatosis have also been seen.

The IP and fibrosis that occur in ulcerative colitis are clinically insidious, and their incidence is difficult to determine.[315] When Eade and colleagues[316] compared 36 patients with either ulcerative colitis or Crohn's disease with age-matched controls, they found that the diffusing capacity for carbon monoxide was significantly lower in the patient group, although there was preservation of lung volumes. Heatley and colleagues[333] studied 102 patients with IBD and found pulmonary function abnormalities in 50% including a reduction of the diffusing capacity in 25%. Six of these had radiographic evidence of interstitial lung disease. A correlation between pulmonary abnormalities and the site or activity of bowel disease, length of illness, or the presence or absence of circulating immune complexes was not present. Another study of 29 patients with Crohn's disease failed to demonstrate radiographic abnormalities, but lower diffusing capacities for carbon monoxide and forced expiratory volumes were detected.[334] One series reported 22 patients with Crohn's disease who were devoid of pulmonary symptoms and had normal chest radiographs, but BAL lymphocytosis was present in more than 50% of patients, demonstrating the potential for latent pulmonary disease.[332,335]

It is important to consider sulfasalazine-induced lung disease in patients being treated for IBD. In most reported cases of this drug-induced lung disease, the pulmonary infiltrates cleared after withdrawal of the drug or with the addition of corticosteroids.[319] Occasionally there is a history of sulfa sensitivity and peripheral eosinophilia often accompanies the pneumonitis, which histologically is either eosinophilic and/or organizing pneumonia.[320,321]

Celiac Disease

An association between celiac disease and an IP was found in 3 of 21 patients determined by clinical, radiologic, and physiologic criteria.[336] An increase in serum avian antigens has been found in celiac disease patients, suggesting hypersensitivity pneumonitis as the cause of the lung disease.[336,337] Serum precipitens to avian antigens, however, were found in only 12% of patients with celiac disease.[338,339] This is similar to the general population. Other reports have suggested that lung involvement in celiac disease can represent sarcoid-like granulomatous lesions, LIP, idiopathic pulmonary hemosiderosis, or bronchiectasis.[340–342]

Whipple's Disease

Whipple's disease is a multisystemic disorder most often occurring in middle-aged white males and characterized by arthritis, diarrhea, weight loss, and fever.[343] Pleuropulmonary manifestations include pleuritis,[344,345] mediastinal lymphadenopathy,[346,347] parenchymal sarcoid-like granulomas,[348,349] and diffuse interstitial infiltrates[350,351] that appear either prior to, concurrently with, or follow the onset of the gastrointestinal manifestations. The Whipple's bacillus (*Tropheryma whippelii*) is not found in the granulomatous reaction. In one case, diffuse perivascular and peribronchial lung inflammation consisting of mononuclear cells contained bacilliform cytoplasmic inclusions.[350] The pleuropulmonary and other extragastrointestinal manifestations may be a consequence of immune complexes formed in response to the bacterial antigen.[350] Convincing anecdotal clinical and physiologic evidence suggests that cough, dyspnea, and pleurisy may resolve following antibiotic treatment.[351]

Liver Disease

Primary biliary cirrhosis (PBC), an inflammatory and cholestatic liver disease characterized by antibodies to mitochondrial antigen and circulating immune complexes, frequently has extrahepatic manifestations including Sjögren's syndrome, autoimmune thyroiditis, renal tubular acidosis, scleroderma, and rheumatoid arthritis.[352–355] Lung involvement in the form of an IP (lymphocytic or UIP) and fibrosis,[356] organizing pneumonitis,[357] and sarcoid-like granuloma formation are well documented.[358,359] In PBC patients without clinical or radiographic evidence for pulmonary involvement, BAL fluid reveals a lymphocytosis implying subclinical alveolitis.[360] The clinical, radiologic, and physiologic manifestations of IP may precede the more hepatic manifestations of PBC.[361] Weekly methotrexate (10 to 20 mg) used in the treatment of PBC and primary sclerosing cholangitis caused a drug-induced pneumonitis in 14% of patients.[362]

Both chronic hepatitis from hepatitis C virus and cryptogenic cirrhosis can occur concurrently with IP and fibrosis. Disease activity and response to therapy is similar for both organs.[363–365] In one study of chronic hepatitis, a reduction in the diffusing capacity was found in 25% of the patients,[366] although not all prospective studies have reported such a high incidence.[367]

Thyroid Disease

The lung disease that occurs with Hashimoto's thyroiditis, which is usually accompanied by another immunologic condition such as Sjögren's syndrome, usually represents LIP. Riedel's thyroiditis, a disease characterized by dense fibrosis of the thyroid gland and associated mediastinal fibrosis, sclerosing cholangitis, and retroperitoneal fibrosis, may have contiguous inflammation and fibrosis of both upper lung zones.[368] Four cases of BOOP have been reported with various thyroid diseases, including hyperthyroidism, thyroiditis, and hypothyroidism.[369]

Neurologic Disease

A peripheral neuropathy (mixed motor and sensory) has been reported to occur in IPF.[370] In one series of IPF and peripheral neuropathy (8 patients), one patient developed rheumatoid arthritis 7 years after the diagnosis; the others, however, had no other evidence of a systemic connective tissue disease.[370] Two patients presented with neuropathy, and in the remaining six neuropathy appeared between 6 months and 8 years following the pulmonary diagnosis.

Muscular Disease

Myasthenia gravis can cause respiratory failure due to respiratory muscle dysfunction and often coexists with systemic lupus erythematosus, rheumatoid arthritis, scleroderma, Sjögren's syndrome, Hashimoto's thyroiditis, and pernicious anemia, all of which can be associated with an interstitial lung disease (UIP, NSIP, and LIP). An interstitial lung disease can also complicate primary myasthenia gravis.[371,372] LIP and UIP have been described. The incidence of this complication is unknown, but it is interesting in light of the occurrence of antibodies to both skeletal muscle and acetylcholine receptors as well as autoantibodies present in myasthenic serum. There is also one report of a patient with ocular myasthenia gravis who developed a systemic vasculitis with glomerulonephritis and renal failure, dermatologic leukocytoclastic vasculitis, as well as diffuse alveolar hemorrhage with underlying pulmonary capillaritis.[373]

Vascular Disease

Dyspnea is a common symptom in patients with Takayasu's arteritis, most likely due to obstruction of the pulmonary arterial system.[374] A single case documented the presence of dense pulmonary fibrosis associated with a neutrophilic BAL and an immune complex glomerulonephritis.[375] Giant cell (temporal) arteritis classically presenting with symptoms of headache and jaw claudication may also manifest systemic manifestations, including fever, anemia, and polymyalgia rheumatica. There is a 9% incidence of cough and throat pain in these patients.[376] Vascular pathology reveals giant cell noncaseating granuloma with destruction of the internal elastic lamina. There are several case reports and postmortem studies that indicate the presence of an interstitial granulomatous process that are both peribronchial and occasionally noted within small vessels of the lung. In one well-documented case, an interstitial pattern was present on the chest radiograph, which represented granuloma invading both vessel walls and the alveolar interstitium.[377] The response of the pulmonary disease to corticosteroid therapy was not mentioned. Another report describes the presence of interstitial fibrosis in addition to the granulomatous vascular lesions.[378] The question of the simultaneous occurrence of sarcoidosis and giant cell arteritis has been raised.[379,380] There is some evidence to suggest that the pulmonary lesions are corticosteroid responsive.[381]

Pulmonary Calcification

Metastatic calcification of the lung is a well-known complication of chronic renal failure, particularly in those patients who require chronic hemodialysis.[382,383] However, hyperparathyroidism[384] and other hypercalcemic states, such as the milk-alkali syndrome, hypervitaminosis D,

and malignancies involving bone including multiple myeloma and leukemia, may also predispose patients to this complication.[385,386] It is more frequently a postmortem finding but can sometimes be detected by chest radiographs and HRCT during life and confirmed by technetium-99m lung scanning.[383–387] Although most patients are asymptomatic, some develop progressive dyspnea and even respiratory failure.[382–388] The chest radiograph is often confused with pneumonia or pulmonary edema,[389] and the radiographic infiltrates often have an upper lobe predelection (Figure 31–23).[390] Computed tomographic scanning shows the presence of high-attenuation parenchymal consolidation. The majority of cases occur in patients on chronic hemodialysis, and in up to 75% of hemodialyzed patients there is pre- or postmortem evidence of metastatic calcification to the lungs.[390]

Histologically, deposition occurs in all tissues of the lung including the interstitium, vascular walls, and bronchioles. The calcium deposition is thought to elicit a fibrotic response by the lung interstitium (Figure 31–24).[390] An unusual case of progressive pulmonary calcification following successful renal transplantation has been described.[391,392]

PULMONARY ALVEOLAR MICROLITHIASIS

Pulmonary alveolar microlithiasis (PAM) is a rare disease of unknown etiology in which lamellar concretions composed of calcium and phosphorus form within the alveolar spaces. The clinicophysiologic consequences depend on the proportion of alveoli that are filled with these calcium microspheres. It was originally described in 1918,

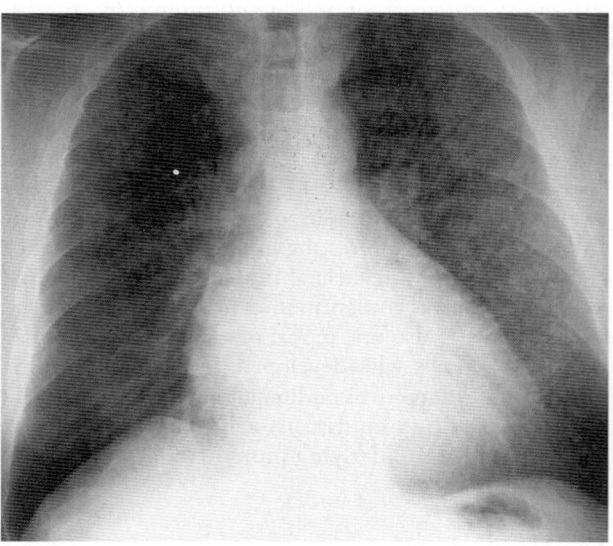

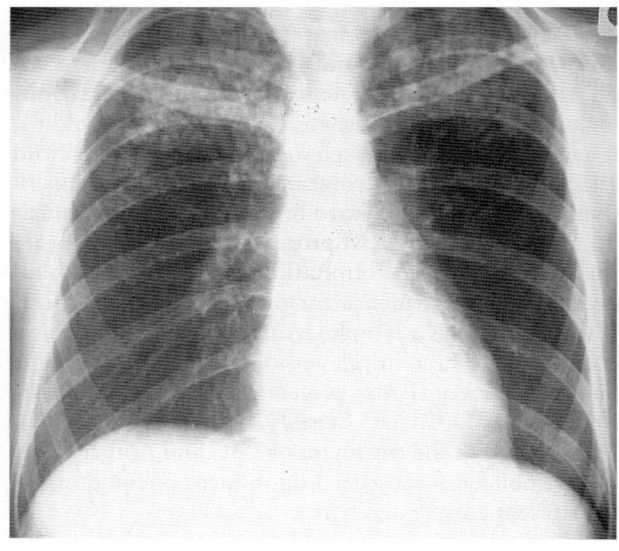

A   **B**

Figure 31–23   Chest radiographs of metastatic pulmonary calcification. *A, B,* There is diffuse nodulation with upper and midzone predominance. There is a striking upper lung zone localization with coalescence of the nodules resulting in an alveolar filling pattern. Both patients were receiving chronic hemodialysis.

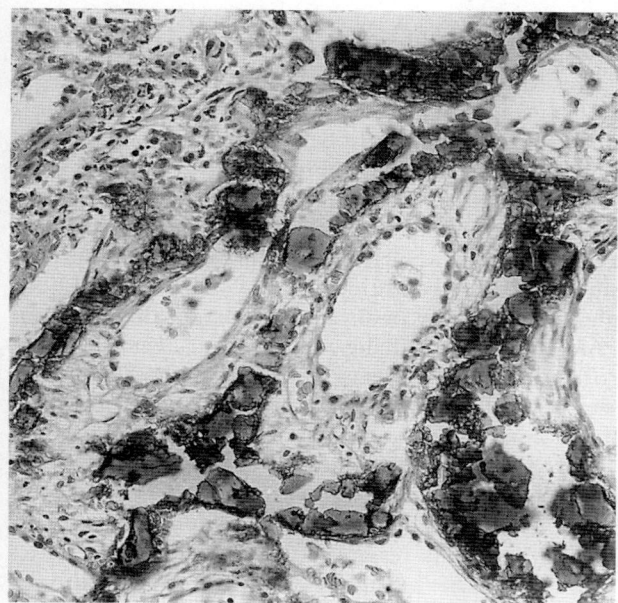

Figure 31–24 Metastatic pulmonary calcification. In addition to the calcium deposits in the interstitium and around pulmonary blood vessels, there is also interstitial fibrosis (hematoxylin and eosin stain; ×40).

and since then less than 200 cases have been described in the literature.[392–394]

The concretions or calcium-phosphorus microspheres are between 0.01 and 3.0 mm in diameter and can fill up to 80% of the air spaces.[395–399] These remain unattached to the alveolar walls, lying free in the alveolar space (Figure 31–25). Over time, a fibroproliferative response with elaboration of collagen fibers supervenes, and interstitial fibrosis results.[396–399] The calcium-phosphorus microspheres are occasionally found within the alveolar wall and bronchial submucosa.[408] There are reports of extrapulmonary deposition of concretions in the sympathetic nervous system, the gonads, and the kidney.[401,402]

The pathogenesis of PAM remains unknown. Most believe that it represents an inborn error of calcium metabolism confined to the lung. There are also local changes in pH that produce an alkaline environment and allow for precipitation of calcium salts in the alveoli.[402–406] The familial occurrence of this disease in over 50% of reported cases lends some credence to this hypothesis.[394,397,403,404–409]

Clinical Presentation

Most cases are diagnosed between the ages of 30 to 50 years, but initially diagnosed newborn, pediatric, and adult cases over 50 years have been described.[404,405,410] There is an equal gender predeliction.[394,400,407] There is no racial predisposition, and cases have been reported from all parts of the world.[394,397,398,411–414] There does,

however, appear to be an excessive number of cases reported from Turkey,[415] representing approximately 33% of the world literature.[413] As previously stated, at least 50% of cases are familial and usually occur in siblings, suggesting an autosomal recessive trait.[400,416] Patients may be asymptomatic when first discovered (usually by chest radiograph) and remain so for 20 to 30 years.[417] There is a gradual onset of cough and dyspnea sometimes with expectoration of the microliths.[396,397,410] The delay in or the eventual appearance of symptoms in the face of an abnormal chest radiograph is determined by the extent of the alveolar involvement, the size of the microliths, and the superimposition of interstitial fibrosis.[396–406] Crackles, clubbing, and cor pulmonale appear with interstitial fibrosis.[395–397,410–418]

The chest radiograph shows diffuse bilateral, varying-sized, calcified nodular densities. The greatest concentration is in the lower two-thirds of the lung (Figure 31–26). The cardiac and diaphragmatic borders are usually not visible. The nodules for the most part are calcified and air bronchograms and air alveolograms are visible.[418–420] In long-standing cases, hyperinflation due to bullous emphysema appears in the upper lobes; reticulonodular infiltrates and Kerley's B lines due to interstitial fibrosis also are seen.[395–398] Computed tomographic scans demonstrated calcific densities, pleural calcification, and subpleural cysts that appear as a black line between the pleural surface and the involved lung.[421,422] Pulmonary uptake of technetium 99m occurs in PAM, but this cannot be differentiated from metastatic calcification to the lung.[423–425] A case of sarcoidosis showing profuse micronodular calcification in radiographic studies indentical to microlithiasis has been described.[426]

Lung physiologic testing often shows no or only mild abnormalities when the disease is first discovered. With time, there are gradual reductions of lung volumes and diffusing capacity and gas exchange abnormalities appear. These changes occur gradually and progress to

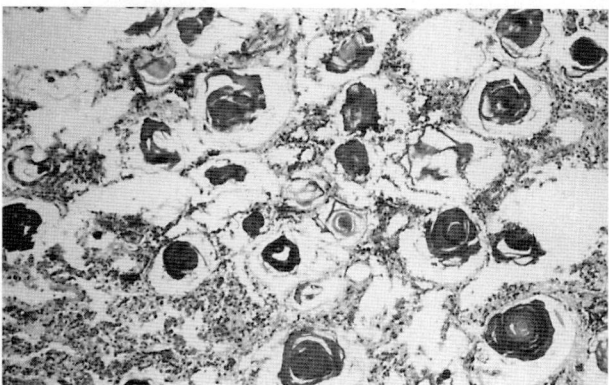

Figure 31–25 Pulmonary alveolar microlithiasis. Note the laminar nature of the calcium-phosphorus microliths lying free within the alveolar spaces. There is also some broadening of the alveolar walls due to inflammation and collagen deposition.

hypoxemia at rest, pulmonary hypertension, and cor pulmonale.[397,398,402,407,427–429]

There are no detectable abnormalities of systemic calcium metabolism or other laboratory tests. Microliths occasionally are seen in the sputum or in the cell pellet of the BAL, but this is not necessarily specific for PAM.[417,430]

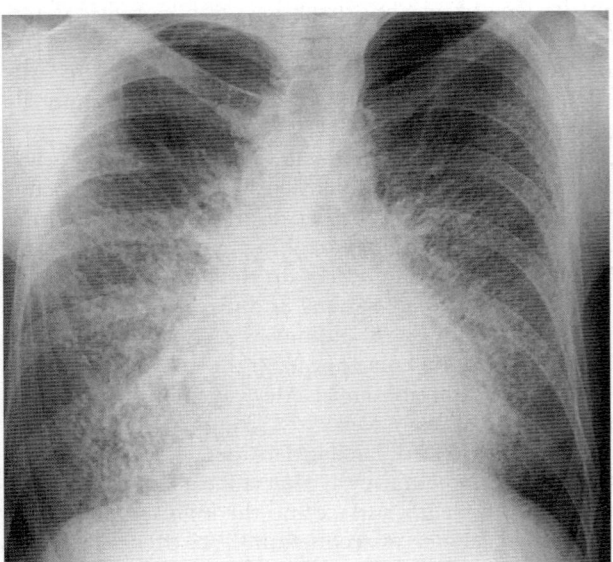

A

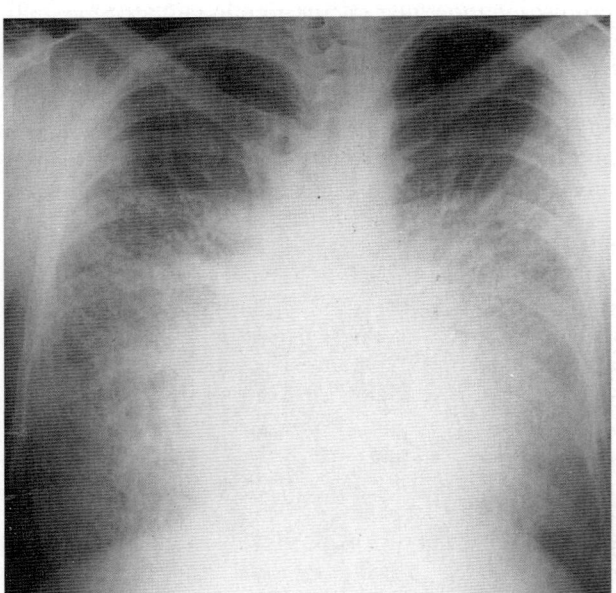

B

Figure 31–26 Pulmonary alveolar microlithiasis. Chest radiograph demonstrating nodular densities with the greatest concentration in the middle and lower lung fields. *A*, The cardiac shadow is partially obliterated as well as the medial portions of the diaphragm. *B*, Chest radiograph taken 10 years later with progression of the disease. Clinically, the patient had cor pulmonale.

The diagnosis is usually established from both the chest radiograph and CT scan appearances.[394,418,431] Transbronchial biopsy will confirm the diagnosis.[398,432] The differentiation between PAM and diffuse pulmonary ossification must be made. Pulmonary ossification occurs secondary to mitral stenosis or pulmonary fibrosis as well as following ARDS, amyloidosis, and any cause of chronic left ventricular dysfunction. There is also an idiopathic variety. The chest radiograph can be similar in these conditions.[400,433–435] The calcified nodules of pulmonary ossification are larger than those in PAM, and the underlying condition usually points to the correct diagnosis. Metastatic pulmonary calcification seen primarily in patients on chronic hemodialysis rarely if ever confounds the differential diagnosis.[436,437]

There is no medical therapy. Corticosteroids, chelating agents, and whole lung lavage are ineffective.[398,429,438] One case of PAM complicated by lymphocytic interstitial pneumonitis responded to corticosteroid treatment.[439] Another advanced case was treated with nasal continuous positive airway pressure, which improved oxygenation by reducing intrapulmonary shunting. Follow-up was only three months.[440] In general, lack of effective therapy notwithstanding, an asymptomatic state or lack of significant deterioration in symptoms or physiology has been reported to persist for up to 30 years after diagnosis. When symptoms do occur, they progress slowly. Significant physiologic deterioration implies superimposition of pulmonary fibrosis.[396] Acute deterioration has been attributed to pulmonary embolism or to spontaneous pneumothorax.[405,421,441] Successful bilateral sequential lung transplantation has been performed and offers the only potential treatment.[442–444]

BRONCHIOLOALVEOLAR CELL CARCINOMA

Bronchioloalveolar cell carcinoma (BACC) or alveolar cell carcinoma accounts for less than 10% of primary lung tumors.[445–449] It presents either as an isolated coin lesion, multiple coin lesions, a localized nonresolving pneumonic infiltrate, or the more diffuse variety, which can be pneumonic in appearance or appear as diffuse alveolar nodules.[445,450,451] This discussion will be confined to the diffuse form of BACC. In diffuse BACC, it is proposed that a multifocal origin rather than endobronchial or lymphangitic spread explains its appearance.[450]

Type A or the well-differentiated form of diffuse BACC is recognized by tall columnar cells with vacuolated cytoplasms that line the alveoli. These cells produce mucin which fill air spaces (Figure 31–27).[445,452–459] Type A diffuse BACC must be differentiated from bronchioloalveolar metastasis due to well-differentiated adenocarcinomas arising from the breast, ovary, pancreas, and stomach.[447,460] In type B BACC the cells are more cuboidal, producing a hobnailed appearance; they also secrete less mucin than type A BACC (see Figures 31–27 and 31–28).[447,456,461,462] Type A BACC elicits a B-lymphocyte response in the lung, and type B BACC elicits a T-lymphocyte and Langerhans' cell response. Bronchioloalveolar cell carcinomas are often a mixture of types A and B. It is likely that BACC arises from one of the following cell lines: the type II pneumocyte, the Clara cell, or the bronchiolar goblet cell.[458,463–470]

Up to 50% of BACC develops in lung scars, either a localized scar producing a "scar carcinoma" or arising from diffuse fibrotic lung disease. Diffuse fibrotic processes such as idiopathic pulmonary fibrosis,[470,471] rheumatoid lung,[472,473] scleroderma,[474] mitral stenosis,[475] busulfan-induced fibrosis,[476] Hodgkin's disease,[477] radiation fibrosis,[478] eosinophilic granuloma of the lung,[479] asbestosis,[480,481] lipoid pneumonia,[482] and angioimmunoblastic lymphadenopathy[483] can develop either localized or diffuse BACC. A viral hypothesis for diffuse BACC is attractive because of the morphologic similarity to a disease seen in sheep known as jaagsiekte or pulmonary adenomatosis caused by a retrovirus.[484–486] No viral agent has been identified in BACC.[461]

Patients with the diffuse form of BACC present with progressive dyspnea, cough, fatigue, and weight loss.[445–447,461] Most patients are between the ages of 50 and 70 years.[446,461] There is no race or gender predilection and in older studies, no relationship to tobacco use was reported.[462,463,487–492] Recent data indicates that tobacco may be a factor in the development of BACC in up to 75% of patients.[493,494] BACC has been reported in identical twins and in several members of a family who also had familial idiopathic pulmonary fibrosis.[495,496] Occasionally, sputum production is copious (bronchorrhea) due to excessive secretion of mucus by the malignant cells. Daily production of 30 mL to several liters of sputum has been reported, resulting in volume depletion and prerenal azotemia.[446,447,456,457,487,488,497,498] A case of pulmonary

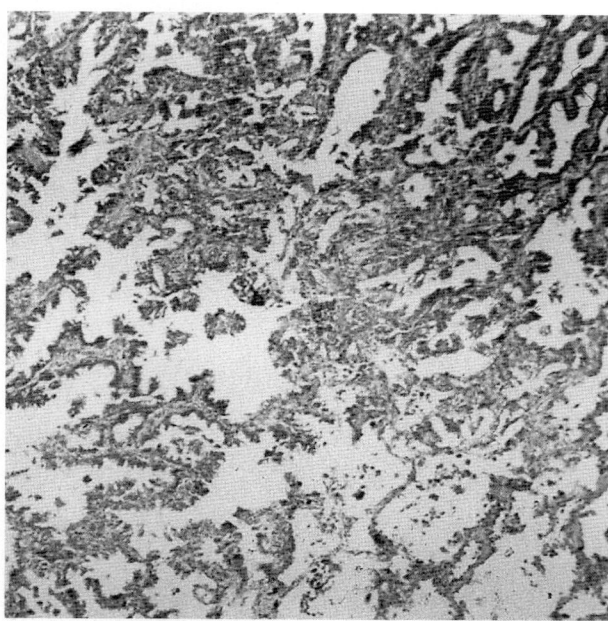

Figure 31–28 Bronchioloalveolar cell carcinoma (diffuse type B). There is a hobnailed appearance to the cuboidal cells lining the alveolar spaces (hematoxylin and eosin stain; ×40 original magnification).

hypertension due to direct involvement of the lymphatic channels of the pulmonary arterial walls that resulted in impingment of the vascular lumens has been described.[499]

The chest radiographic findings in diffuse BACC are in the form of either a pneumonic consolidation (Figure 31–29) or diffuse alveolar nodules (Figure 31–30). The radiographic appearance may resemble a nonresolving pneumonia or other diffuse alveolar filling disease.

A restrictive ventilatory defect with a low diffusing capacity and hypoxemia characterizes diffuse BACC. As in pulmonary alveolar proteinosis, the shunt fraction is increased.[461,499–502]

Prerenal azotemia, hyponatremia, and hypochloremia may result from bronchorrhea.[497,498] Carcinoembryonic antigen and serum CA19-9, a marker of pancreatic cancer, may be elevated in BACC.[503] Diagnosis is established by either sputum cytology, BAL, and/or transbronchial lung biopsy.[461,504–506] Open or thoracoscopic biopsy are rarely necessary in the diffuse forms of BACC.[507]

Outcomes for diffuse BACC are dismal. The tumor is generally resistant to any form of chemotherapy or radiation therapy.[446,447,461,508–510] The mean survival in diffuse BACC is 3 to 4 months.[447] Bronchorrhea responded with a marked reduction in sputum volume following erythromycin therapy in one case of BACC.[511,512]

LIPOID PNEUMONIA

Lipoid pneumonia is a mixed alveolar interstitial process induced by either the inhalation or aspiration of an oil-based product derived from vegetable, animal, or min-

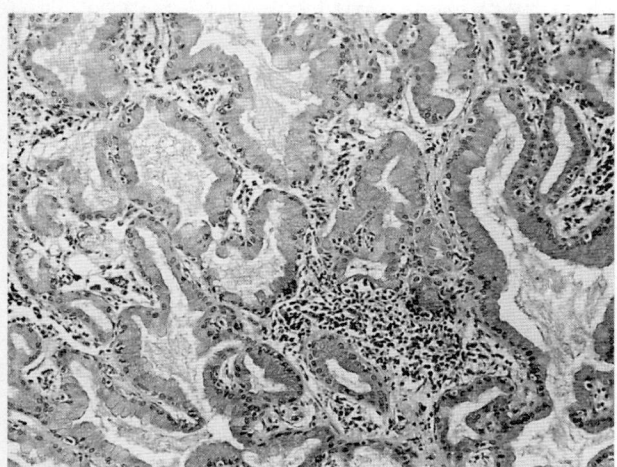

Figure 31–27 Bronchioloalveolar cell carcinoma (diffuse type A). The alveoli are lined by well-differentiated columnar cells with vacuolated cytoplasms. Also note the mucus accumulation in the air spaces (hematoxylin and eosin stain; ×40 original magnification).

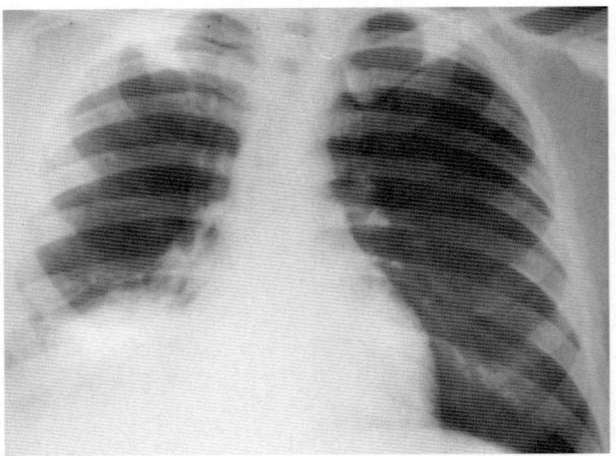

A

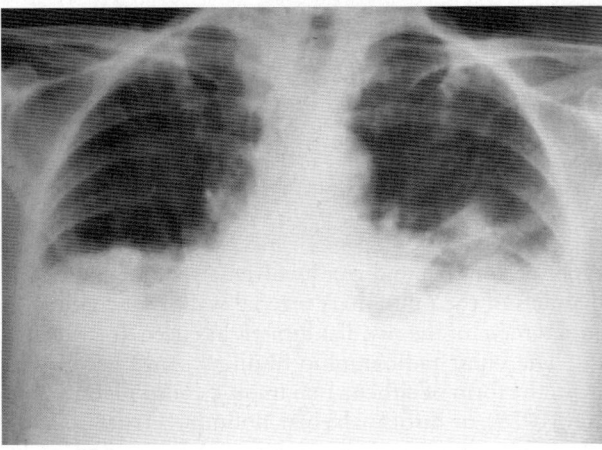

B

Figure 31–29   Bronchioloalveolar cell carcinoma. *A*, Chest radiograph demonstrating right lower lobe consolidation unresponsive to antibiotics. *B*, Chest radiograph taken 6 months later demonstrating more diffuse consolidation. Transbronchial biopsy established the diagnosis.

eral sources. It is also referred to as exogenous lipoid pneumonia differentiating it from endogenous lipoid pneumonia also referred to as cholesterol pneumonia. The latter refers to a histologic change distal to a bronchiolar or endobronchial air obstruction or suppurative process. In these cases, macrophages have a foamy appearance due to the accumulation of lipids in their cytoplasms. The origin of lipids in endogenous lipoid pneumonia is the fat and cholesterol derived from necrotic alveolar tissue.[513,514] This discussion will be confined to exogenous lipoid pneumonia.

The majority of cases of exogenous lipoid pneumonia are secondary to mineral oil aspiration and occur in patients with esophageal disorders, gastroesophageal reflux, and neurologic problems. Another common way to acquire lipoid pneumonia is by aspiration of petroleum jells, which are inserted in the nasal passages for lubrication, oily nose drops, or oil-based sprays. There are, however, a number of other unusual sources reported including motor oil sprays,[515,516] industrial oil sprays,[516–520] the feeding of animal fats (ghee) to babies,[521,522] accidental intravenous injection of olive oil in an attempt to enlarge the genitals,[523] suicide by mineral oil emersion,[524] petroleum jell used for the lubrication of an endotracheal tube,[525] liquid paraffin aspiration in fire eaters,[526] the use of lip gloss,[527] and baby oil aspiration.[528]

Histology

In general, vegetable oils do not cause much reaction in the lung. On the other hand, animal oils are hydrolyzed after aspiration, causing the release of free fatty acids resulting in inflammation and necrosis.[529] Mineral oils are phagocytosed by alveolar macrophages and this with repeated aspiration can eventually lead to fibrosis. Because they are bland, mineral oils do not stimulate a gag reflex or cough, but they do inhibit ciliary function.[530,531] Mineral oil floats to the top of a column of undigested food in the esophagus, therefore, it is the first to be aspirated in patients with esophageal disorders.[532] Once in the lung, mineral oil is engulfed by alveolar macrophages, but the damage done by the oil to the phagocytic cells results in release of the oil into the alveolar environment.[533] This results in inflammation, primarily by monocytic cells, the development of foreign body granulomas with the giant cells, and eventually in fibroblastic proliferation and collagen deposition. Early on there is broadening of the alveolar walls by edema, fibroblastic proliferation, and monocytic cells (Figure 31–31).[529] Intra-alveolar lipid-laden macrophages and giant cells are also present. In more advanced (chronic) lipoid pneumonia, there is a chronic granulomatous pneumonitis with fibroblastic proliferation, fibrosis, masses of foamy macrophages, and foreign-body giant cells. Various histologic stages of exogenous lipoid pneumonia are present in the same biopsy speciman because this process is usually ongoing and spans months to years before discovery.[532]

Clinical Picture

The populations that develop lipoid pneumonia are often elderly patients taking mineral oil at bedtime to prevent constipation, particularly those with gastroesophageal or neurologic problems that lead to reflux and aspiration. Another common predisposing cause is the use of petroleum-based products (eg, Vaseline) at bedtime for nasal lubrication.[533–536] Other environmental or occupational exposures such as mineral oil or petroleum sprays in the lubrication of industrial machinery,[517–520] fire eating,[526] and laxative abuse in women with anorexia nervosa[537] should be considered as appropriate causes.

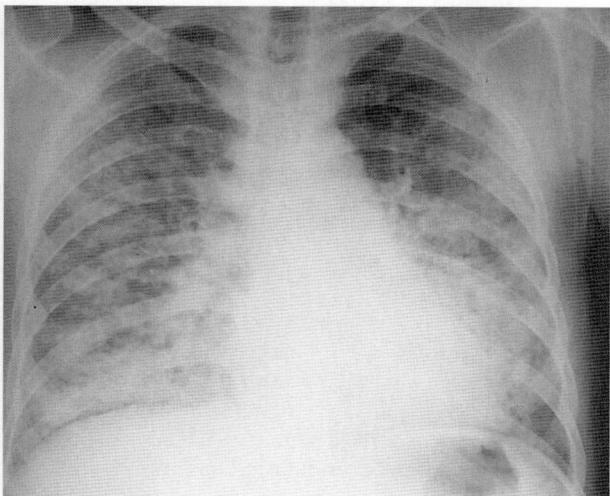

A

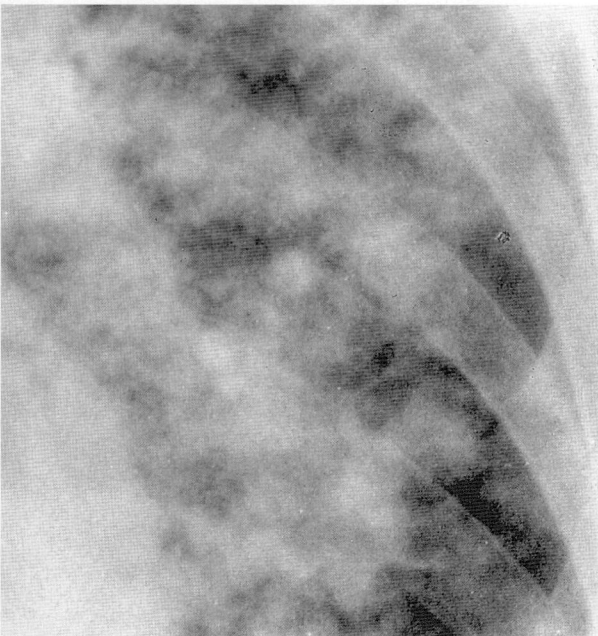

B

Figure 31–30   Bronchioloalveolar cell carcinoma. *A,* Chest radiograph demonstrating a diffuse alveolar filling process. *B,* Close-up view illustrating the coalescing alveolar nodules.

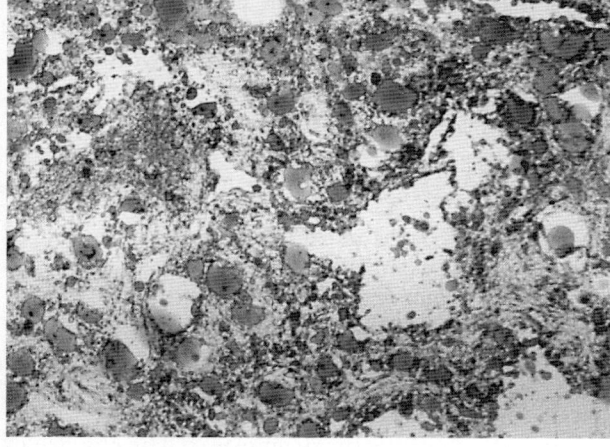

Figure 31–31   Lipoid pneumonia. Fat globules are present within alveolar spaces and alveolar macrophages. There is also interstitial edema (hematoxylin and eosin strain; ×40 original magnification).

Lipoid pneumonia can present as one of three clinical scenarios: (1) an incidental finding on the chest radiograph in an asymptomatic patient; (2) an acute or subacute presentation with cough, sputum, fever, and basilar alveolar infiltrates on the chest radiograph; and (3) cough and dyspnea of some duration with reticulonodular bibasilar infiltrates.[533,534,536,538] There may be superimposition of a community-acquired pneumonia that responds to antibiotics but is followed by a failure to clear the chest radiograph.[534,536,538] Physical findings include bibasilar crackles, rhonchi, wheezing, and bronchial breath sounds. Pulmonary function testing reveals restrictive ventilatory impairment, hypoxemia, and a reduced diffusing capacity. Bronchial inflammation and hyper-reactivity may result in reversible airflow limitation.[533–535,539] One unusual laboratory abnormality reported with lipoid pneumonia is hypercalcemia, which may be due to the production of vitamin D by the granulomatous cells similar to that which occurs in sarcoidosis. This results in increased gut absorption of dietary calcium.[540,541]

The chest radiograph is variable. Lipoid pneumonia is seen at postmortem examination in asymptomatic patients with normal premortem chest radiographs.[521] In the more acute forms, alveolar infiltrates and occasionally consolidation are evident. This usually occurs in the lower lobes and represent a combination of oil filling the alveolar spaces, an influx of phagocytic macrophages, and sometimes a superimposed infectious pneumonia producing bibasilar or patchy alveolar infiltrates with air bronchograms (Figure 31–32).[539,542,543] Over time and with repeated bouts of aspiration, a granulomatous and fibrotic reaction occurs, producing reticulonodular infiltrates and contraction of the involved lobes (Figure 31–33).[539,542] The lower lobes, right greater than left, and the middle lobes are most commonly affected. Radiographic infiltrates in the upper lobes are less likely to represent lipoid pneumonia.[536–538] Because this is an ongoing process in most cases, it would not be unusual to have alveolar superimposed on interstitial infiltrates. Hilar adenopathy, pleural effusions, and cavitation in a known case of lipoid pneumonia should raise suspicion of a complicating bronchogenic carcinoma or superinfection with cryptococcus or an atypical mycobacterium.[544–549] Computed tomography demonstrating alveolar infiltrates with fat density (low attenuation) is highly suggestive of this diagnosis.[550–552] A "crazy paving pattern" similar to that described in alveolar proteinosis was reported in five of seven patients with tissue-confirmed lipoid pneumonia.[553,554] This consists of well-defined areas of ground-glass attenuation with superimposed septal thickening (Figure 31–34).

Diagnosis

The diagnosis is based on clinical suspicion in the proper clinical setting, accompanied by supporting historic information. Confirmation is obtained from the chest radiograph, CT scans, and evaluation of the sputum or BAL for the presence of fat-containing macrophages.[533,539,555–559] The identification of alveolar macrophages with foamy cytoplasms or abundant free-lipid material in the sputum or BAL confirms the diagnosis.[555] The absence of these findings does not, however, exclude the diagnosis.[533] In one series, sputum evaluation for fat confirmed the diagnosis in 85%.[555] Diagnostic BAL shows alveolar macrophages with vacuolated cytoplasms that stain positively with Sudan or oil red O stains demonstrating the fat vacuoles.[556–559] Alveolar macrophages with vacuolated cytoplasms are also seen in two phospholipoidoses: pulmonary alveolar proteinosis and drug-induced lung disease due to amiodarone. These do not, however, stain positively with the Sudan or oil red O stains.[560] Although not necessary, biochemical analysis of lavage can identify the inhaled material.[557] Lung biopsy is sometimes necessary. If a case of unknown interstitial lung disease proves to be lipoid pneumonia on the biopsy specimen, careful questioning of the patient will reveal the source.

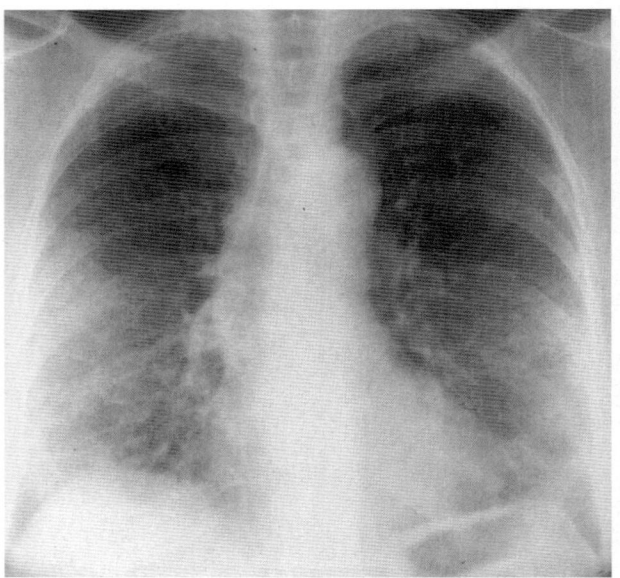

A

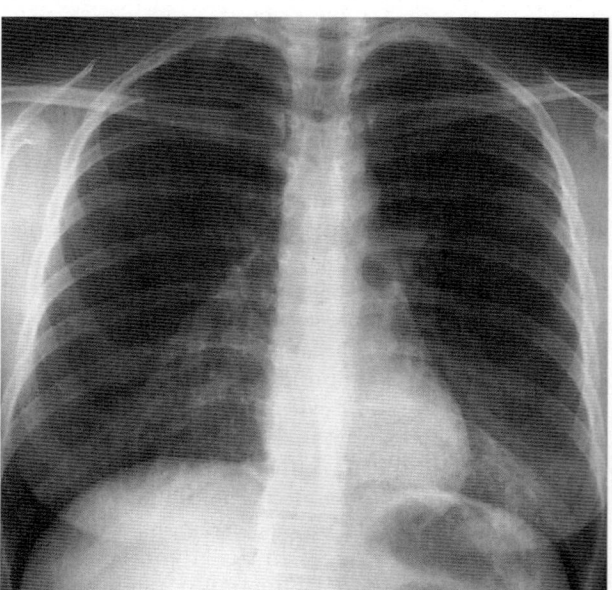

Figure 31–32   Lipoid pneumonia. Chest radiograph showing the acute phase with bibasilar alveolar infiltrates.

B

Figure 31–33   Lipoid pneumonia. *A,* Chest radiograph of a patient with chronic aspiration of oily nose drops demonstrating diffuse reticulonodular infiltrates with mid and lower zone distribution. *B,* Computed tomography showing basilar honeycomb change.

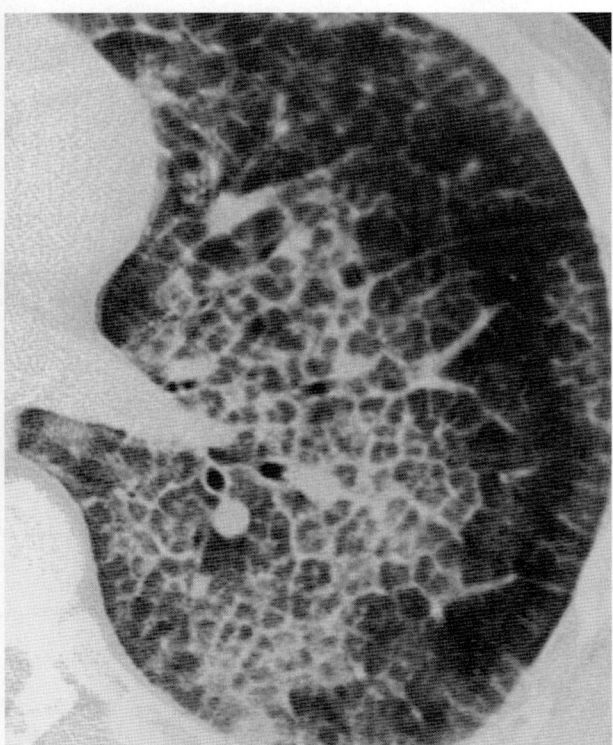

Figure 31–34 High-resolution computed tomography of chronic lipoid pneumonia demonstrating a "crazy paving" pattern.

Treatment and Prognosis

If discovered in time and if the offending oil is discontinued, the prognosis for these patients is good. Death, when it occurs, is either due to an overwhelming aspiration, a superimposed infection, or a comorbid illness. Corticosteroid medication is effective for the acute pneumonitis and also in some chronic cases.[561–563] Cases also resolve spontaneously. The decision to use corticosteroids depends on the degree of physiologic disturbance and the failure to improve following a period of observation. There have been several cases in which whole lung lavage was used successfully, presumably by removing the oil from the alveolar environment.[564,565]

REFERENCES

1. Glenner GC. Amyloid deposits and amyloidosis: the B-fibrillosis. N Engl J Med 1980;302:1283–92,1333–43.
2. Kisilevsky R, Axelrad M, Corbett W, et al. The role of inflammatory cells in the pathogenesis of amyloidosis. Lab Invest 1977;37:544–53.
3. Isersky C, Ein D, Page DL, et al. Immunochemical cross reactions of human amyloid proteins with immunoglobulin light polypeptide chains. J Immunol 1972;108:752–4.
4. Kyle RA. Primary systemic amyloidoses. J Intern Med 1992;232:523–4.
5. Tan SY, Pepys MB. Amyloidosis. Histopathology 1994;25:403–14.
6. Zathoukal P, Bezdicek P, Schimonova M, et al. Waldenströms macroglobulinemia with pulmonary amyloidosis. Respiration 1998;65:414–6.
7. Menke DM, Kyle RA, Fleming CR, et al. Symptomatic gastric amyloidosis in a patient with primary systemic amyloidosis. Mayo Clin Proc 1993;68:763–7.
8. Smith RL, Hutchins GM, Moore GW, Humphrey RL. Type and distribution of pulmonary parenchymal and vascular amyloid: correlation with cardiac amyloid. Am J Med 1979;66:96–104.
9. Toriumi J. The lung in generalized amyloidosis. Acta Pathol Jpn 1972;22:141–52.
10. Skinner M, Anderson JJ, Simmon SR, et al. Treatment of 100 patients with primary amyloidosis: a randomized trial of melphalan, prednisone, and colchicine versus colchicine alone. Am J Med 1996;100:290–8.
11. Biberstein M, Wolf P, Pettross B, et al. Amyloidosis complicating cystic fibrosis. Am Soc Clin Pathol 1983;80:752–4.
12. Gallney K, Gibbons D, Keogh B, Fitzgerald MX. Amyloidosis complicating cystic fibrosis. Thorax 1993;48:949–50.
13. Suzuki A, Ohosone Y, Obana M, et al. Cause of death in 81 autopsied patients with rheumatoid arthritis. J Rheumatol 1994;21:33–6.
14. Wing BC, Wong KL, Ip MS, et al. Sjögren's syndrome with amyloid A presenting as multiple pulmonary nodules. J Rheumatol 1994;21:165–7.
15. Marenco JL, Sanchez-Burson J, Ruiz Campos J, et al. Pulmonary amyloidosis and unusual lung involvement in SLE. Clin Rheumatol 1994;13:525–7.
16. Davis CJ, Butchart EG, Gibbs AR. Nodular pulmonary amyloidosis occurring in association with pulmonary lymphoma. Thorax 1991;46:217–8.
17. Merino-Angulo A, Perez-Marti M, Diaz de Otaru R. Pulmonary alveolar phospholipoproteinosis associated with amyloidoses. Chest 1990;98:1048–52.
18. Sumi AM, Ohya N, Shinoura H, et al. Diffuse interstitial pulmonary amyloidosis in rheumatoid arthritis. J Rheumatol 1996;23:933–6.
19. Orriols R, Aliaga JL, Rodrigo MJ, et al. Localized alveolar septal amyloidosis with hypersensitivity pneumonitis. Lancet 1992;i:1261–2.
20. Btavia R, Toda MR, Vidal F. Pulmonary diffuse amyloidosis and ankylosing spondylitis—a rare association. Chest 1992;102:1608–10.
21. Benharroch D, Sukenik S, Sachs M. Bronchioloalveolar carcinoma and generalized amyloidosis complicating progressive systemic sclerosis. Hum Pathol 1992;23:839–41.
22. Planes C, Kleinkneiht D, Brauner M, et al. Diffuse interstitial lung disease due to AA amyloidosis. Thorax 1992;47:323–4.
23. Sumiya M, Ohya N, Shinovra H, et al. Diffuse interstitial pulmonary amyloidosis in rheumatoid arthritis. J Rheumatol 1996;23:933–6.
24. Gertz MA, Kyle RA. Secondary systemic amyloidosis: response and survival in 64 patients. Medicine 1991;70:246–56.
25. Kunze WP. Senile pulmonary amyloidosis. Pathol Res Pract 1979;164:413–22.
26. Lesser A. Ein fall von Enchondroma osteiodes mixtum der lunge mit patieller amyloid entortung. Virchows Arch (Pathol Anat) 1887;69:404–8.
27. Thompson PJ, Citron KM. Amyloid and the lower respiratory tract. Thorax 1983;38:84–7.
28. Gertz MA, Greipp PR. Clinical aspects of pulmonary amyloidosis. Chest 1986;90:790–1.
29. Utz JP, Swensen SJ, Gertz MA. Pulmonary amyloidosis: the Mayo Clinic experience from 1980–1993. Ann Intern Med 1996;124:407–13.
30. Costa P, Corrin B. Amyloidosis localized to the lower respiratory tract: probable immunoamyloid nature of the tracheobronchial and nodular pulmonary forms. Histopathology 1985;9:703–10.

31. Toyoda M, Ebihaia Y, Kato H, Kita S. Tracheobronchial A2 amyloidosis: histologic, immunohistochemical, ultrastructural and immunoelectron microscopic observations. Hum Pathol 1993;24:970–6.

32. Hiu AN, Koss MN, Hochholzer L, Wehunt WD. Amyloidosis presenting in the lower respiratory tract. Arch Pathol Lab Med 1986;110:212–8.

33. Cordier JF, Loire R, Brane J. Amyloidosis of the lower respiratory tract: clinical and pathologic features in a series of 21 patients. Chest 1986;90:827–31.

34. Nugent AM, Elliott H, McGuigan JA, Varghese G. Pulmonary amyloidosis: treatment with laser therapy and systemic steroids. Respir Med 1996;90:433–5.

35. Rajan KG, Reynolds SP, McConnochie K, White JP. Localized amyloid—presenting as bronchial asthma. Eur J Respir Dis 1987;71:213–5.

36. Attwood HD, Price CG, Riddell RJ. Primary diffuse tracheobronchial amyloidosis. Thorax 1972;27:620–4.

37. Russchen GH, Wouters B, Meinesz AF, et al. Amyloid tumor resected by laser therapy. Eur Respir J 1990;3:932–3.

38. Yap JL, Wang H, Poh JC. A case of primary diffuse tracheobronchial amyloidosis treated by laser therapy. Singapore Med J 1992;33:198–200.

39. Alroy GG, Lichtig C, Kaftori JK. Tracheobronchopathia osteoplastica: endstage of primary lung amyloidosis? Chest 1972;61:465–8.

40. Matsumoto K, Ueno M, Matsuo V, et al. Primary solitary amyloidoma of the lung: findings on CT and MRI. Eur Radiol 1997; 7:586–8.

41. Schoen FJ, Alexander RW, Hood CI, Dunn LJ. Nodular pulmonary amyloidosis. Arch Pathol Lab Med 1980;104:66–9.

42. Liaw YS, Kuo SH, Yang PC, et al. Nodular amyloidosis of the lung and heat mimicking breast carcinoma with pulmonary metastasis. Eur Respir J 1995;5:871–3.

43. Mollers MJ, van Schaik JP, vander Putte SC. Pulmonary amyloidoma: histologic proof yielded by transthoracic coaxial fine needle biopsy. Chest 1992;102:1597–8.

44. Lee AB, Bogaars HA, Passero MA. Nodular pulmonary amyloidosis: a cause of bronchiectasis and fatal pulmonary hemorrage. Arch Intern Med 1983;143:603–4.

45. Batra P, Collin JD, Magidson JG. Pulmonary nodular amyloidosis presenting as Sjögren's syndrome. J Natl Med Assoc 1983;75:903–5.

46. Bignold L, Martyn M, Basten A. Nodular pulmonary amyloidosis associated with benign hypergammaglobulinemic purpura. Chest 1980;78:334–7.

47. Shah SP, Khine M, Anigbogu J, Miller A. Nodular amyloidosis of the lung from intravenous drug abuse: an uncommon cause of multiple pulmonary nodules. South Med J 1998; 91:402–4.

48. Beer TW, Edward CS. Pulmonary nodules secondary to reactive systemic anyloidosis (AA) in Crohn's disease. Thorax 1993;48:1287–8.

49. Stokes MB, Jagirdar J, Burchstein O, et al. Nodular pulmonary immunoglobulin light chain deposits with coexistant amyloid and non-amyloid features in an HIV infected patient. Mod Pathol 1997;10:1059–65.

50. Hiroshima K, Ohwada H, Fshibashi M, et al. Nodular pulmonary amyloidosis associated with asbestos exposure. Pathol Int 1996;46:66–70.

51. Daltin AR, Featherstone T, Athanasou N. Organ limited amyloidosis with lymphadenopathy. Postgrad Med J 1992;68: 47–50.

52. Kanada DJ, Sharma OP. Long term survival with diffuse interstitial pulmonary amyloidosis. Am J Med 1979;67:879–82.

53. Celli BR, Rubinow A, Cohen AS, Brody JS. Patterns of pulmonary involvement in systemic amyloidosis. Chest 1978; 74:543–7.

54. Celli BR, Falk RH, Cohen AS. Lung involvement in patients with primary amyloidosis. Its prevalence and clinical consequences [abstract]. Am Rev Respir Dis 1985;131:A74.

55. Eshun-Wilson K, Frandsen NE, Christensen HE. Pulmonary alveolar septal amyloidosis: a scanning and transmission electron microscopy study. Virchows Arch (Pathol Anat) 1976;371:89–99.

56. Road JD, Jacques J, Sparling JR. Diffuse alveolar septal amyloidosis presenting with recurrent hemoptysis and medial dissection of the pulmonary arteries. Am Rev Respir Dis 1985;132:1368–70.

57. Shiue ST, McNally DP. Pulmonary hypertension from prominent vascular involvement in diffuse amyloidosis. Arch Intern Med 1988;148:687–9.

58. Sullivan EJ, Schwarz MI. Pulmonary hypertension resulting from primary pulmonary amyloidosis. Semin Respir Crit Care Med 1994;15:238–42.

59. Veinot JP, Edwards WD, Kyle RA. Pulmonary vascular amyloid causing pulmonary hypertension: report of a case and review of the literature. Cardiovasc Pathol 1993;2:231–5.

60. Hiller N, Fisher D, Shmesh O, et al. Primary amyloidosis presenting as an isolated mediastinal mass: diagnosis by fine needle biopsy. Thorax 1995;50:908–9.

61. Graham C, Stearn EJ, Finkbeiner WE, Webb WR. High resolution CT appearance of diffuse alveolar septal amyloidosis. AJR Am J Roentgenol 1992;158:265–7.

62. Ohdama S, Akagawa S, Matsubara O, Yoshizawa Y. Primary diffuse alveolar septal amyloidosis with multiple cysts and calcification. Eur Respir J 1996;9:1569–71.

63. Kavuru MS, Adamo JP, Ahmad M, et al. Amyloidosis and pleural disease. Chest 1990;98:20–3.

64. Bontemp SF, Tillie-Leblond I, Coprin MC, et al. Pleural amyloidosis: thoracoscopic aspects. Eur Respir J 1995;8: 1025–7.

65. Merlini G. Treatment of primary amyloidosis. Semin Hematol 1995;32:60–79.

66. Iwasaki T, Hamano T, Aizawa K, et al. A case of pulmonary amyloidosis associated with multiple myelemia treated with dimethyl sulfoxide [review]. Acta Hematol 1994;91:91–4.

67. Dember LM, Sanchorawala V, Seldin DC, et al. Effect of dose-intensive intravenous melphalan and autologies blood stem-cell transplantation in AL amyloidosis-associated renal disease. Ann Intern Med 2001;134:746–53.

68. Coriat P, Labrousse J, Vilde F, et al. Diffuse interstitial pneumonitis due to aspiration of gastric contents. Anaesthesia 1984;39:703–5.

69. Pearson JEG, Wilson RSE. Diffuse pulmonary fibrosis and hiatus hernia. Thorax 1971;26:300–5.

70. Mays EE, Dubois JJ, Hamilton GB. Pulmonary fibrosis associated with tracheobronchial aspiration. Chest 1976;69:512–5.

71. Tobin RW, Pope CE, Pelligrini, et al. Increased prevalence of gastroesophogeal reflux in patients with idiopathic pulmonary fibrosis. Am J Respir Crit Care Med 1998;158: 1804–8.

72. Sladen A, Zanca P, Hadnott WH. Aspiration pneumonitis: the sequelae. Chest 1971;59:448–50.

73. Corwin WR, Irwin RS. The lipid-laden alveolar macrophage as a marker of aspiration in parenchymal lung disease. Am Rev Respir Dis 1985;132:576–81.

74. Schneider EL, Epstein CJ, Kaback MJ, et al. Severe pulmonary involvement in Gaucher's disease: report of three cases and review of the literature. Am J Med 1977;63:475–80.

75. Brady RO, Kanfer JN, Bradley RM, et al. Demonstration of a deficiency of glucocerebroside cleaving enzyme in Gaucher's disease. J Clin Invest 1966;45:1112–6.

76. Niederau C, Haussinger D. Gauchers disease: a review for the internist and hepatologist. Hepatogastroenterology 2000; 47:984–97.

77. Wolsen AH. Pulmonary findings in Gaucher's disease. AJR Am J Roentgenol 1975;123:712–5.

78. Pelini M, Boice D, O'Neil K, LaRocque J. Glucocerebrosidase treatment of type 1 Gaucher's disease with severe pulmonary involvement. Ann Intern Med 1994;121:196–7.

79. Carson KF, Williams CA, Rosenthal DL, et al. Bronchoalveolar lavage in a girl with Gaucher's disease: a case report. Acta Cytol 1994;38:597–600.

80. Tunaci A, Berkman YM, Gokmen E. Pulmonary Gaucher's disease: high resolution computed tomographic features. Pediatr Radiol 1995;25:237–8.

81. Beutler E, Kay A, Saven A, et al. Enzyme replacement therapy for Gaucher's disease. Blood 1991;78:1183–9.

82. Kerem K, Elstein D, Abrahamou A, et al. Pulmonary function abnormalities in type 1 Gaucher's disease. Eur Respir J 1996;9:340–5.

83. Terry RD, Sperry WM, Brodoff B. Adult lipoidosis resembling Niemann-Pick disease. Am J Pathol 1954;30:263–86.

84. Myers B. Gaucher's disease of the lungs. BMJ 1937;2:8–12.

85. Yassa NA, Wilcox AG. High resolution CT pulmonary findings in adults with Gauchers disease. Clin Imaging 1998; 22:339–42.

86. Links TP, Karrenbeld A, Steensma JT, et al. Fatal respiratory failure caused by pulmonary infiltration by pseudo-Gaucher cells. Chest 1992;101:265–6.

87. Roberts WC, Frederickson DS. Gaucher's disease of the lung causing severe pulmonary hypertension with associated acute recurrent pericarditis. Circulation 1967;35:783–9.

88. Baksta E, Gaine SP, Rubin LJ. Continuous intravenous epoprostenol therapy for pulmonary hypertension in Gauchers disease. Chest 2000;117:1821–9.

89. Chen IY, Lynch DA, Shroyer KR, Schwarz MI. Gaucher disease: an unusual cause of intrathoracic extramedullary hematopoiesis. Chest 1993;104:1923–4.

90. Lynn R, Terry RD. Lipid histiochemistry and electron microscopy in adult Niemann-Pick disease. Am J Med 1964;37:987–94.

91. Lachman R, Crocker A, Schulman J, et al. Radiologic findings in Niemann-Pick disease. Radiology 1973;108:659–64.

92. Gogus S, Gocmen A, Kocak N, et al. Lipoidosis with sea-blue histiocytes: report of two siblings with lung involvement. Turk J Pediatr 1994;36:139–44.

93. Desnick RJ, Iuannou YA, Eng C. Fabry disease. In: Scriver CR, Beaudet AL, Sly WS, Valle D, editors. The metabolic and molecular basis of inherited disease. Vol 3. 8th ed. New York: McGraw Hill; 2001. p. 3733–74.

94. Shirai T, Ohtake T, Kimura M, et al. Atypical Fabry's disease presenting with cholesterol crystal embolization. Intern Med 2000;39:601–2.

95. Kelly MM, Leigh R, McKenzie R, et al. Induced sputum examination: diagnosis of pulmonary involvement in Fabry's disease. Thorax 2000;55:720–1.

96. Eng CM, Guffon N, Wilcox WR, et al. Safety and efficiency of recombinant human alpha galactosidase. A replacement therapy in Fabry's disease. N Engl J Med 2001;345: 9–16.

97. Frustaci A, Chimenti L, Ricci R, et al. Improvement of cardiac function in the cardiac variant of Fabry's disease with galactose infusion therapy. N Engl J Med 2001;345:25–32.

98. Rush WL, Andriko JA, Talatea-Salle F, et al. Pulmonary pathology or Erdheim-Chester disease. Mod Pathol 2000; 13:747–54.

99. Kenn W, Stabler A, Zachoval R, et al. Erdheim-Chester disease: a case report and literature overview. Eur Radiol 1999; 9:153–8.

100. Egan AJ, Boardman LA, Tazelar HD, et al. Erdheim-Chester disease: clinical, radiologic and histopathologic findings in five patients with interstitial lung disease. Am J Surg Pathol 1999;23:17–26.

101. Wittenberg KIT, Svensen SJ, Myers JL. Pulmonary involvement with Erdheim-Chester disease: radiographic and CT findings. AMJ Am J Roentgenol 2000;174:1327–31.

102. Devouassoux G, Lantuejoul S, Chatelain P, et al. Erdheim-Chester disease: a primary macrophage disorder. Am J Respir Crit Care Med 1998;157:650–3.

103. Kenn W, Eck M, Allolio B, et al. Erdheim-Chester disease: evidence for a disease entity different from Langerhans cell histiocytoses? Three cases with detailed radiologic and immunohistochemical analysis. Hum Pathol 2000;31:734–9.

104. Hermansky F, Pudlak P. Albinism associated with hemorrhagic diathesis and unusual pigmented cells in the bone marrow. Report of two cases with histochemical studies. Blood 1959;14:162–8.

105. Hurzing M, Anikster Y, Gahl WA. Hermansky-Pudlak syndrome and related disorders or organelle formation. Traffic 2000;1:823–35.

106. Armstrong LW, Rom WN, Martiniuk FT. The gene for lysosomal protein CD63 is normal in patient with Hermansky-Pudlak syndrome. Lung 1998;176:249–56.

107. Garcy SM, Gardella JE, Fazzini EP, et al. Hermansky-Pudlak syndrome. Pulmonary manifestations of a ceroid storage disorder. Am J Med 1979;66:737–47.

108. White DA, Walker Smith GJ, Cooper JAD, et al. Hermansky-Pudlak syndrome and interstitial lung disease: report of a case with lavage findings. Am Rev Respir Dis 1984;130: 138–41.

109. Shinella RA, Greco MA, Garcy SM, et al. Hermansky-Pudlak syndrome: a clinicopathologic study. Hum Pathol 1985;16:366–76.

110. Wockel W, Hubner G, Arnholt H, et al. Hermansky-Pudlak Syndrome mit lungen fibrose be zwei Brudern. Pathologie 1992;13:82–9.

111. Hoste P, Willems J, Devriendt J, et al. Familial diffuse interstitial fibrosis associated with oculocutaneous albinism: report of two cases with a family study. Scand J Respir Dis 1979;60:128–34.

112. Brantly M, Avila NA, Scholelersuk V, et al. Pulmonary function and high resolution CT findings in patients with an inherited form of pulmonary fibrosis, Hermansky-Pudlak syndrome, due to mutations in HPS-1. Chest 2000;117: 129–36.

113. Nakatani Y, Nakamura N, Jano J, et al. Interstitial pneumonia in Hermansky-Pudlak syndrome: significance of florid foamy swelling/degeneration (giant lamellar body degeneration) of type 2 pneumocytes. Virchows Arch 2000;437:304–13.

114. Auwerx J, Demedts M, Bouillin R, et al. Coexistence of hypocalciuric hypercalcemia and interstitial lung disease in a family: a cross sectional study. Eur J Clin Invest 1985;15:6–14.

115. Demedts M, Auwerx J, Godderis P, et al. The inherited association of interstitial lung disease, hypocalciuric hypercalcemia and defective granulocyte function. Am Rev Respir Dis 1985;131:470–5.

116. Maulitz RM, Sahn SA. Pulmonary lymphangitic carcinomatosis from the cervix. Arch Intern Med 1979;134:708–9.

117. Yamamoto T, Nakane T, Kimura T, et al. Pulmonary lymphangitic carcinomatosis from an oropharyngeal squamous cell carcinoma. Oral Oncol 2000;36:125–8.

118. Liau CT, Jung SM, Lim KE, et al. Pulmonary lymphangitic sarcomatosis from cutaneous angiosarcoma: an unusual presentation of diffuse interstitial lung disease. Jpn J Clin Oncol 2000;30:37–9.

119. Harold JT. Lymphangitis carcinomatosa of the lungs. QJM 1952;21:353–60.

120. Goldsmith HS, Baily HD, Callahan EL, et al. Pulmonary lymphangitic carcinomatosis from breast cancer. Arch Surg 1967;94:483–8.

121. Sood N, Bandarenko N, Paradowski LV. Acute respiratory failure secondary to lymphangitic carcinomatosis. J Clin Oncol 2000;18:229–32.

122. Shimura S, Takishima T. Bronchorrhea from diffuse lymphangitic metastasis of colon carcinoma to the lung. Chest 1994;105:308–10.

123. Yang SP, Lin CC. Lymphangitic carcinomatosis of the lung: the clinical significance of its roentgenographic classification. Chest 1972;62:179–87.

124. Case records of the Massachusetts General Hospital. N Engl J Med 1983;309:477–86.

125. Sweigert CF, McLaughlin EF, Heath EM. Carcinoma of the pancreas with pulmonary lymphangitic carcinomatosis simulating bronchial asthma: case report. Ann Intern Med 1947;27:301.

126. Alkalay I, Fairfax CW, Bullard JC. Lymphangitic carcinomatosis of the lungs with normal appearing chest x-ray films. Chest 1972;62:229–30.

127. Munk PL, Muller NL, Miller RR, et al. Pulmonary lymphangitic carcinomatosis: CT and pathologic findings. Radiology 1988;166:705–9.

128. Hinda O, Johkoh T, Ichikado K, et al. Comparison of high resolution CT findings of sarcoidosis, lymphoma and lymphangitic carcinomatosis: is there any difference of involved interstitium? J Comput Assist Tomogr 1999;23:374–9.

129. Trapnell DH. Radiologic appearances of lymphangitis carcinomatosa of the lung. Thorax 1964;19:251–61.

130. Spencer H. Secondary tumors of the lung. In: Pathology of the lung excluding pulmonary tuberculosis. Vol 2. 3rd ed. New York: McGraw Hill; 1977. p. 1000–1.

131. Masson RG, Krikorian J, Lukl P, et al. Pulmonary microvascular cytology in the diagnosis of lymphangitic carcinomatosis. N Engl J Med 1989;321:71–6.

132. Schwarz MI, Waddell LC, Dombeck DH, et al. Prolonged survival in lymphangitic carcinomatosis. Ann Intern Med 1969;71:779–83.

133. Heffner JE, Duffey DJ, Schwarz MI. Massive pleural effusions from prostatic lymphangitic carcinomatosis. Resolution with endocrine therapy. Arch Intern Med 1982;42:375–6.

134. Schimmel DH, Julien PJ, Gamsu GG. Resolution of pulmonary lymphangitic carcinoma of the breast. Chest 1976;69:106–8.

135. Rosenberg DM. Inherited forms of interstitial lung disease. Clin Chest Med 1982;3:635–41.

136. Riccardi VM. von Recklinghausen's neurofibromatosis. N Engl J Med 1981;305:1616–27.

137. Messner RL, Messner MR, Lewis SJ. Neurofibromatosis: a familial and family disorder. J Neurosci Nurs 1985;17:221–9.

138. Klatte EC, Franken EA, Smith JA. The radiographic spectrum of neurofibromatosis. Semin Roentgenol 1976;11:17–33.

139. Riccardi VM. Neurofibromatosis update. Neurofibromatosis 1989;2:284–91.

140. Lazaro C, Ravella A, Gaona A, et al. Neurofibromatosis type 1 due to germ-line mosaicism in a clinically normal father. N Engl J Med 1994;331:1403–7.

141. Webb WR, Goodman PC. Fibrosing alveolitis in patients with neurofibromatosis. Radiology 1977;122:289–93.

142. Scheerder ID, Elinck W, Renterghem DV, et al. Desquamative interstitial pneumonia and scar cancer of the lung complicating generalized neurofibromatosis. Eur J Respir Dis 1984;65:623–6.

143. Volpini E, Conuertino G, Fulgoni P, et al. Pulmonary changes in a man affected by von-Recklinghausen's disease. Monaldi Arch Chest Dis 1996;51:123–4.

144. Shimizu Y, Tsuchiya A, Watanabe S, Saitoh R. von-Recklinghausen's disease with lung cancer derived from the wall of emphysematous bullae. Intern Med 1994;33:167–71.

145. Patchefsky AS, Atkinson WG, Hoch WS, et al. Interstitial pulmonary fibrosis and von-Recklinghausen's disease: an ultrastructural and immunofluorescent study. Chest 1973;64:459–64.

146. Hassoun PM, Celli BR. Bilateral diaphragmatic paralysis secondary to central von Recklinhausen's disease. Chest 2000;117:1196–200.

147. Samuels N, Berkman N, Milgalter E, et al. Pulmonary hypertension secondary to neurofibromatosis: intimal fibrosis vs. thromboembolism. Thorax 1999;54:858–9.

148. Griffiths AP, White J, Dawson A. Spontaneous hemothorax: a cause of sudden death in von Recklinghausen's disease. Thorax 1998;53:679–81.

149. Miura H, Taira O, Uchida O, et al. Spontaneous hemothorax associated with von Recklinghausen's disease: review of occurrence in Japan. Thorax 1997;52:577–8.

150. Smell O, Perheentupa J, Rapola J, et al. Lysinuric protein intolerance. Am J Med 1975;559:229–40.

151. Parto K, Kallajoki A, Heikki A, Smell O. Pulmonary alveolar proteinosis and glomerulonephritis in lysinuric protein intolerance: case reports and autopsy findings of four pediatric patients. Hum Pathol 1994;25:400–7.

152. DiRocco M, Garibotto G, Rossi GA, et al. Role of hematological, pulmonary, and renal complications in the long term prognosis of patients with lysinuric protein intolerance. Eur J Pediatr 1993;152:437–40.

153. Santamaria F, Parenti G, Guidi G, et al. Early detection of lung involvement in lysinuric protein intolerance: role of high resolution computed tomography and radioisotopic methods. Am J Respir Crit Care Med 1996;153:731–5.

154. Parto K, Svedstrom E, Majurin ML, et al. Pulmonary manifestations in lysinuric protein intolerance. Chest 1993;104:1176–82.

155. Sandler M. Is the lung a "target organ" in diabetes mellitus? Arch Intern Med 1990;150:1385–8.

156. Vracko R. A comparison of the microvascular lesions in diabetes mellitus with those of normal aging. J Am Geriatr Soc 1982;30:201–5.

157. Farina J, Fumo V, Fernandez-Acenero MJ, Muzas MA. Nodular fibrosis of the lung in diabetes mellitus. Virchows Arch 1995;427:61–3.

158. Sandler M, Bunn AS, Stewart RI. Cross-section study of pulmonary function in patients with insulin-dependent diabetes mellitus. Am Rev Respir Dis 1987;135:223–9.

159. Asunuma Y, Fujiya S, Ide H, Agishi Y. Characteristics of pulmonary function in patients with diabetes mellitus. Diabetes Res Clin Pract 1985;1:95–101.

160. Primhak RA, Whincup G, Tsanakas JN, Miher RDG. Reduced vital capacity in insulin-dependent diabetes. Diabetes 1987;36:324–6.

161. Schuyler MR, Niewoehner DE, Inkley SR, Kohm R. Abnormal lung elasticity in juvenile diabetes mellitus. Am Rev Respir Dis 1976;113:37–41.

162. Ramirez LC, Dal Nogare A, Hsia C, et al. Relationship between diabetes control and pulmonary function in insulin dependent diabetes mellitus. Am J Med 1991;91:371–6.

163. Beckman EN, Oehrle JS. Fibrous hematopoietic tumors arising in agnogenic myeloid metaplasia. Hum Pathol 1982;13:804–10.

164. Asakura S, Colby TV. Agnogenic myeloid metaplasia with extramedullary hematopoiesis and fibrosis in the lung. Chest 1994;105:1866–8.

165. Reinhert KU, Sybrecht GW. T-helper cell alveolitis after bacillus Calmette-Guérin immunotherapy for superficial bladder tumor. J Urol 1994;151:1634–7.

166. Israel-Biet D, Venet A, Sandron D, et al. Pulmonary complications of intravesical Bacille Calmette-Guérin immunotherapy. Am Rev Respir Dis 1987;135:763–5.

167. LeMense GP, Strange C. Granulomatous pneumonitis following intravesical BCG: what therapy is needed? Chest 1994;106:1624–6.

168. Petty TL. Acute respiratory distress syndrome ARDS. Dis Mon 1990;Jan:1–58.

169. Hudson LD. Adult respiratory distress syndrome. Semin Respir Med 1981;2:99–174.

170. Pratt PC, Vollmer RT, Shelburns JD, et al. Pulmonary morphology in a multihospital collaborative extracorporeal membrane oxygenation project. 1. Light microscopy. Am J Pathol 1979;276:357–68.

171. Zapol WM, Trelstad RL, Coffey JW, et al. Pulmonary fibrosis in severe acute respiratory failure. Am Rev Respir Dis 1979;119:547–54.

172. Collins JF, Smith JD, Coalsen JD, et al. Variability in lung collagen amounts after prolonged support of acute respiratory failure. Chest 1984;85:641–6.

173. Hallman W, Spragg R, Harrell JH, et al. Evidence of lung surfactant abnormalities in respiratory failure. J Clin Invest 1982;70:673–83.

174. Burkhardt A. Alveolitis and collapse in the pathogenesis of pulmonary fibrosis. Am Rev Respir Dis 1989;140:513–24.

175. Weigelt JA, Norcross JR. Borman KR, et al. Early steroid therapy for respiratory failure. Arch Surg 1985;120:536–40.

176. Luce JM, Montgomery B, Marks JD, et al. Ineffectiveness of high dose methylprednisolone in preventing parenchymal lung injury and improving mortality in patients with septic shock. Am Rev Respir Dis 1988;138:62–8.

177. Bone RC, Fisher CJ, Clemmer TP, et al. Early methylprednisolone treatment for septic syndrome and the adult respiratory distress syndrome. Chest 1987;92:1032–6.

178. Bernard GR, Luce JM, Sprung CL, et al. High dose corticosteroids in patient with the adult respiratory distress syndrome. N Engl J Med 1987;317:1565–70.

179. Meduri GW. Pulmonary fibroproliferation and death in patients with late ARDS. Chest 1995;107:5–6.

180. Hooper RG, Kearl RA. Established ARDS treated with a sustained course of adrenocortical steroids. Chest 1990;97:138–43.

181. Meduri GU, Chinn AJ, Leeper KV, et al. Corticosteroid rescue treatment of progressive fibroproliferation in late ARDS: patterns of response and predictors of outcome. Chest 1994;105:1516–27.

182. Nakos G, Tsangaris I, Kostanti E, et al. Effect of the prone position on patients with hydrostatic pulmonary edema compared with acute respiratory distress syndrome and pulmonary fibrosis. Am J Respir Crit Care Med 2000;161:360–8.

183. Armstrong L, Thickett DR, Mansell JP, et al. Changes in collagen turnover in early acute respiratory distress syndrome. Am J Respir Crit Care Med 1999;160:1910–5.

184. Madtes D, Rubenfeld G, Klima LD, et al. Elevated transforming growth factor-alpha levels in bronchoalveolar lavage fluid of patients with acute respiratory stress syndrome. Am J Respir Crit Care Med 1998;158:424–30.

185. Ashbough DG, Maier RV. Idiopathic pulmonary fibrosis in adult respiratory distress syndrome. Arch Surg 1985;120:530–3.

186. Churg A, Golden J, Fligiel S, et al. Bronchopulmonary dysplasia in the adult. Am Rev Respir Dis 1983;127:117–20.

187. Christner P, Fein A, Goldberg S, et al. Collagenase in the lower respiratory tract of patients with adult respiratory distress syndrome. Am Rev Respir Dis 1985;131:690–5.

188. Lee CT, Fein AM, Lippman ML, et al. Elastolytic activity in pulmonary lavage fluid from patients with adult respiratory distress syndrome. N Engl J Med 1981;304:192–6.

189. Rinaldo JE, Rogers RM. Adult respiratory distress syndrome: changing concepts of lung injury and repair. N Engl J Med 1982;306:900–9.

190. Albert WM, Priest GR, Moser KM. The outlook for survivors of ARDS. Chest 1983;84:272–4.

191. Hert R, Albert RK. Sequelae of the adult respiratory distress syndrome. Thorax 1994;49:8–13.

192. Lakshminarayan S, Stanford RE, Petty TL. Prognosis after recovery from adult respiratory distress syndrome. Am Rev Respir Dis 1976;113:7–15.

193. McHugh LG, Milberg JA, Whitcomb ME, et al. Recovery of function in survivors of the acute respiratory distress syndrome. Am J Crit Care Med 1994;150:90–4.

194. Mittermayer CH, Hassenstein J, Riede VN. Is shock-induced lung fibrosis reversible? A report on recovery from shock lung. Pathol Res Pract 1978;10:73–87.

195. Vahov V, Lieberman P, Molho M. Pulmonary function following the adult respiratory distress syndrome. Chest 1978;74:247–50.

196. Simpson DL, Goodman M, Spector SL, et al. Long-term follow-up and bronchial reactivity testing in survivors of the adult respiratory distress syndrome. Am Rev Respir Dis 1978;117:449–54.

197. Peters JI, Bell RC, Prihoda TJ, et al. Clinical determinants of abnormalities in pulmonary functions in survivors of the adult respiratory distress syndrome. Am Rev Respir Dis 1989;139:1163–8.

198. Elliot CG, Rasmusson BY, Crapo RO, et al. Prediction of pulmonary function abnormalities after adult respiratory distress syndrome (ARDS). Am Rev Respir Dis 1987;135:634–8.

199. Suchyta MR, Elliot CG, Jensen RL, Crapo R. Predicting the presence of pulmonary function impairment in adult respiratory distress syndrome survivors. Respiration 1993;60:103–8.

200. Schwarz MI. The idiopathic interstitial pneumonias. Semin Respir Med 1979;1:47–54.

201. Cross KR. Diffuse interstitial pneumonitis; acute, fibrosing, and focal healing patterns; etiology and malignant potentiality. AMA Arch Pathol 1957;63:132–7.

202. Read J. The pathogenesis of the Hamman-Rich syndrome. A review from the stand point of possible allergic etiology. Am Rev Tuberc Pulmonol Dis 1958;78:353–67.

203. Kawal T, Fujiwara T, Aoyama Y, et al. Diffuse interstitial fibrosing pneumonitis and adenovirus infection. Chest 1976;69:692–4.

204. Patchefsky AS, Banner M, Freundlich IM. Desquamative interstitial pneumonia: significance of intranuclear viral-like inclusion bodies. Ann Intern Med 1971;74:322–7.

205. McNary WE, Gaensler EA. Internuclear inclusion bodies in desquamative interstitial pneumonia: electron microscopic observations. Ann Intern Med 1971;74:404–7.

206. Vergnon JM, Dethe G, Weynants P, et al. Cryptogenic fibrosing alveolitis and Epstein-Barr virus: an association? Lancet 1984;ii:768–71.

207. Schooley RT, Carey RW, Miller G, et al. Chronic Epstein-Barr virus infection associated with fever and interstitial pneumonitis. Ann Intern Med 1986;104:636–43.

208. Veal CF, Carr MB, Briggs DD. Diffuse pneumonia and acute respiratory failure due to infectious mononucleosis in a middle-aged adult. Am Rev Respir Dis 1990;141:502–4.

209. Lander P, Palayew MJ. Infectious mononucleosis: a review of chest roentgenographic manifestations. J Can Assoc Radiol 1974;25:303–6.

210. Dorman JM, Glich TH, Shannon D, et al. Complications of infectious mononucleosis: a fatal case in a two year old child. Am J Dis Child 1974;128:239–43.

211. Hogg JC. Epstein-Barr virus and cryptogenic fibrosing alveolitis. Thorax 1995;50:1232–8.

212. Barbera JA, Hayashi S, Hegele RG, Hogg JC. Detection of Epstein-Barr virus in lymphocytic interstitial pneumonia by in situ hybridization. Am Rev Respir Dis 1992;145:940–6.

213. Egan JJ, Stewart JP, Haselton PS, et al. Ebstein-Barr virus replication within pulmonary epithelial cells in cryptogenic fibrosing alveolitis. Thorax 1995;50:1234–9.

214. Hashimoto Y, Nawata Y, Kurasawa K, et al. Investigation of EB virus and cytomegalovirus in rapidly progressive interstitial pneumonitis in polymyositis/dermatomyositis by in situ hybridization and polymerase chain reaction. Clin Immunol Immunopathol 1995;77:298–306.

215. Veda T, Ohta K, Suzuki N, et al. Idiopathic pulmonary fibrosis and high prevalence of serum antibodies to hepatitis C virus. Am Rev Respir Dis 1992;146:266–8.

216. Irving WL, Day S, Johnston IDA. Idiopathic pulmonary fibrosis and hepatitis C virus infection. Am Rev Respir Dis 1993;148:1683–4.

217. Lauer GM, Walker BD. Hepatitis C virus infection. N Engl J Med 2001;345:41–52.

218. Phillips PE, Dougherty RM. Hepatitis C virus and mixed cryoglobulinemia. Clin Exp Immunol 1991;9:551–5.

219. Jakab GJ, Astry CL, Warr GA. Alveolitis induced by influenza virus. Am Rev Respir Dis 1983;128:730–9.

220. Jakab GJ, Bassett DJP. Influenza virus infection ozone exposure, and fibrogenesis. Am Rev Respir Dis 1990;141:1307–15.

221. Jakab GJ. Sequential virus infections, bacterial superinfections and fibrogenesis. Am Rev Respir Dis 1990;142:374–9.

222. Oseasohn R, Anderson L, Kaji M. Clinicopathologic study of thirty three fatal cases of Asian influenza. N Engl J Med 1959;260:509–18.

223. Lindsay MI, Herman EC, Morrow GW, et al. Hong Kong influenza: clinical, microbiologic, and pathologic features in 127 cases. JAMA 1970;214:1825–32.

224. Pinsker KL, Schneyer B, Becker N, et al. Usual interstitial pneumonitis following Texas A2 influenza infection. Chest 1981;80:123–6.

225. Laraya-Cuassay LR, DeFrost A, Huff D, et al. Chronic pulmonary complications of early influenza virus infection in children. Am Rev Respir Dis 1977;116:617–25.

226. Conte P, Heitzman ER, Markarian B. Viral pneumonia, roentgen pathologic correlations. Radiology 1970;95:267–72.

227. Ognibene FP, Masur H, Rogers P, et al. Nonspecific interstitial pneumonitis without evidence of *Pneumocystis carinii* in asymptomatic patients infected with human immunodeficiency virus. Ann Intern Med 1988;109:874–9.

228. White DA, Matthay RA. Noninfectious complications of infection with the human immunodeficiency virus. Am Rev Respir Dis 1989;140:1763–87.

229. Simmons JT, Suffredini AF, Lack EE, et al. Non-specific interstitial pneumonitis in patients with AIDS: radiographic features. AJR Am J Roentgenol 1987;149:265–8.

230. Griffiths MH, Miller RF, Semple SJG. Interstitial pneumonitis in patients infected with the human immunodeficiency virus. Thorax 1995;50:1141–6.

231. Katzenstein ALA, Fiorelli RF. Non-specific interstitial pneumonitis/fibrosis: histologic features and clinical significance. Am J Surg Pathol 1994;18:136–47.

232. Stover DE, White DA, Romano PA, et al. Spectrum of pulmonary diseases associated with the acquired immune deficiency syndrome. Am J Med 1985;78:429–37.

233. Suffredini AF, Ognibene FP, Lack EE, et al. Non-specific interstitial pneumonitis: a common cause of pulmonary disease in the acquired immunodeficiency syndrome. Ann Intern Med 1987;107:7–13.

234. Ramaswamy G, Jagadhu V, Tchertkoff V. Diffuse alveolar damage and interstitial fibrosis in acquired immunodeficiency syndrome patients without concurrent infection. Arch Pathol Lab Med 1985;109:408–12.

235. Shaw RJ, Roussak C, Forster SM, et al. Lung function abnormalities in patients infected with the human immunodeficiency virus with and without overt pneumonitis. Thorax 1988;43:436–40.

236. Pahwa S, Kaplan M, Fikrig S, et al. Spectrum of human T-cell lymphocytic virus type III infection in children. JAMA 1986;255:2299–305.

237. Setoguchi V, Takahashi S, Nukiwa T, Kira S. Dectection of human T-cell lymphotropic virus type I-related antibodies in patients with lymphocytic interstitial pneumonia. Am Rev Respir Dis 1991;144:1361–5.

238. Kramer MR, Saldana MJ, Ramos M, Pitchenik AE. High titers of Epstein-Barr virus antibodies in adult patients with lymphocytic interstitial pneumonitis associated with AIDS. Respir Med 1992;86:49–52.

239. Allen JN, Wewers MD. HIV-associated bronchiolitis obliterans organizing pneumonia. Chest 1989;96:192–7.

240. Sanito NJ, Morley TF, Condoluci DV. Bronchiolitis obliterans organizing pneumonia in an AIDS patient. Eur Respir J 1995;8:1021–4.

241. Glazer C, Cohen L, Schwarz MI. Acute eosinophilic pneumonia in acquired immunodeficiency syndrome. Chest 2001;120:1732–5.

242. Vastro JA, Littner MR, Tashkin DP, et al. Diffuse pulmonary interstitial infiltrate and mycoplasmal pneumonia. Am Rev Respir Dis 1974;110:659–62.

243. Meyers BR, Hirschman SZ. Fatal infections associated with mycoplasmal pneumonia: discussion of three cases with autopsy findings. Mt Sinai J Med 1972;36:258–64.

244. Kaufman JM, Cuvelier CA, Van Der Statten M. Mycoplasma pneumonia with fulminent evolution into diffuse interstitial fibrosis. Thorax 1980;35:140–4.

245. Reigner PH, Domenighetti G, Feihl F, et al. Syndrome de detresse respiratore aigu sur infection a mycoplasme. Schweiz Med Wochenschr 1980;110:220–3.

246. Tablan OC, Reyes MP. Chronic interstitial pulmonary fibrosis following mycoplasma pneumonia. Am J Med 1985;79:268–70.

247. Kuriman K, Shelboorne JD, Googh W, et al. Pathologic findings and long term sequelae in Legionnaires disease. Chest 1979;75:736–9.

248. Hernandez FJ, Kirby BD, Stanley TM, et al. Legionnaires disease: postmortem pathologic findings in 20 cases. Am J Pathol 1977;73:488–95.

249. Blackman JA, Harley RA, Hicklin MD, et al. Pulmonary sequelae of Legionnaire's disease with pneumonia. Ann Intern Med 1979;90:552–4.

250. Chastre J, Raghu G, Soler P, et al. Pulmonary fibrosis following pneumonia due to acute legionnaire's disease. Chest 1987;91:57–62.

251. Hurter T, Rumpelt HJ, Ferlinz R. Fibrosing alveolitis responsive to corticosteroids following Legionnaire's disease. Chest 1992;101:281–3.

252. Nowak J. Late pulmonary changes in the course of infection with *Pneumocystis carinii*. Acta Med Pol 1966;7:23–41.

253. Whitcomb ME, Schwarz MI, Charles MA, et al. Interstitial fibrosis after *Pneumocystis carinii* pneumonia. Ann Intern Med 1970;73:761–5.

254. Sanyal SK, Mariencheck WC, Hughes WT, et al. Course of pulmonary dysfunction in children surviving *Pneumocystis carinii* pneumonia: a prospective study. Am Rev Respir Dis 1964;60:183.

255. Bocles JS, Ehrenkranz NJ, Marks A. Abnormalities of respiratory function in varicella pneumonia. Ann Intern Med 1964;60:183–6.

256. Abrahams EW, Evans C, Knyvett AF, et al. Varicella pneumonia: a possible cause of subsequent pulmonary calcification. Med J Aust 1964;2:781–5.

257. Storb R, Santos GW. Application of bone marrow transplantation in leukemia and aplastic anemia. Clin Haematol 1983;12:721–37.

258. Prentice HG. A review of the current status and techniques of allogeneic bone marrow transplantation for treatment of leukemia. J Clin Pathol 1983;36:1207–14.

259. Noble PW. The pulmonary complications of bone marrow transplantation in adults. West J Med 1989;150:443–9.

260. Meyers JD, Flournoy N, Thomas ED. Non-bacterial pneumonia after allogeneic bone marrow transplantation: a review of ten year's experience. Rev Infect Dis 1982;4:1119–32.

261. Krowka MJ, Rosenow EC, Hoagland HC. Pulmonary complications of bone marrow transplant. Chest 1985;87:237–46.

262. Crawford SW, Hackman RC, Clark JG. Open lung biopsy diagnosis of diffuse pulmonary infiltrates after marrow transplantation. Chest 1988;94:949–53.

263. Wingard JR, Santos GW, Soral R. Late onset interstitial pneumonia following allogeneic bone marrow transplantation. Transplantation 1985;39:21–3.

264. Crawford SW. Detecting occult viral infection after marrow transplantation. Eur Respir J 1996;9:1115–7.

265. Buchbinder S, Elmaagatci AH, Schaefer OW, et al. Human herpes virus 6 is an important pathogen in infectious lung

disease after allogeneic bone marrow transplantation. Bone Marrow Transplant 2000;26:639–44.

266. Cardozo BL, Hagenbee RA. Interstitial pneumonitis following bone marrow transplantation: pathogenesis and therapeutic considerations. Eur J Cancer Clin Oncol 1985;21:43–51.

267. Wingard JR, Mellits DE, Sostrin MB, et al. Interstitial pneumonitis after allogeneic bone marrow transplantation. Medicine 1988;67:175–86.

268. Weiner RS, Bortin MM, Gale RP, et al. Interstitial pneumonitis after bone marrow transplantation: assesment of risk factors. Ann Intern Med 1986;104:168–75.

269. Khouri NF, Saral R, Armstrong EM, et al. Pulmonary interstitial changes following bone marrow transplantation: a complex multifactor disorder. Radiology 1979;133:587–92.

270. Barbera JA, Martin-Campos JM, Ribalata T, et al. Undetected viral infection in diffuse alveolar damage associated with bone marrow transplantation. Eur Respir J 1996;9:1195–200.

271. Raschko JW, Cottler-Fox M, Abbondanzo SL, et al. Pulmonary fibrosis after bone marrow transplantation responsive to treatment with prednisone and cyclosporin. Bone Marrow Transplant 1989;4:201–5.

272. Wick MR, Moore SB, Gastineau DA, et al. Immunologic, clinical and pathologic aspects of human graft versus host disease. Mayo Clin Proc 1983;58:603–12.

273. Sullivan KM, Parkiman R. The pathophysiology and treatment of graft versus host disease. Clin Haematol 1983;12:775–89.

274. Kurzrock R, Zander A, Kanojia M, et al. Obstructive lung disease after allogeneic bone marrow transplantation. Transplantation 1984;37:156–60.

275. Ralph DD, Springmeyer SC, Sullivan KM, et al. Rapidly progressive airflow obstruction in marrow transplant recipients. Am Rev Respir Dis 1984;129:641–4.

276. Perreault C, Cousineau S, d'Angelo G, et al. Lymphoid interstitial pneumonia after allogeneic bone marrow transplantation: a possible manifestation of chronic graft versus host disease. Cancer 1985;55:1–9.

277. Yousem SA. The histological spectrum of pulmonary graft vs. host disease in bone marrow transplant recipients. Hum Pathol 1995;26:668–75.

278. Palmas A, Teffin A, Meyers JL, et al. Late onset non-infectious pulmonary complications after allogeneic bone marrow transplant. Br J Haematol 1998;100:680–7.

279. Baron FA, Hermanne JP, Dowlati A, et al. Bronchiolitis obliterans organizing pneumonia and ulcerative colitis after allogeneic bone marrow transplantation. Bone Marrow Transplant 1998;21:951–4.

280. Barret AJ, Kendra JR, Lucas CF, et al. Cyclosporin A as prophylaxis against graft versus host disease. BMJ 1982;285:162–6.

281. Beschorner WE, Saral R, Hutchins GM, et al. Lymphocytic bronchitis associated with graft versus host disease in recipients of bone marrow transplants. N Engl J Med 1978;299:1030–6.

282. Clark JG, Schwartz DA, Flourneg N, et al. Risk factors for airflow obstruction in recipients of bone marrow transplants. Ann Intern Med 1987;107:648–56.

283. Prince DS, Wingard JR, Saral K, et al. Longitudinal changes in pulmonary function following bone marrow transplantation. Chest 1989;96:301–6.

284. Kawada K, Terasaki PI. Evidence of immunosuppression by high dose gamma-globulin. Exp Hematol 1987;15:133–6.

285. Hackman RC, Madtes DK, Peterson FB, et al. Pulmonary venoocclusive disease following bone marrow transplantation. Transplantation 1989;47:989–92.

286. Sloane JP, Depledga MH, Powles RL, et al. Histopathology of the lung after bone marrow transplantation. J Clin Pathol 1983;36:346–54.

287. Wingard JR, Sostrin MB, Vtiesendorp HM, et al. Interstitial pneumonitis following autologous bone marrow tranplantation. Transplantation 1988;46:61–5.

288. Pecego R, Hill R, Applebaum FR, et al. Interstitial pneu-

monitis following autologous bone marrow transplantation. Transplantation 1986;42:515–8.

289. Jochelson M, Tarbell NJ, Freedman AS, et al. Acute and chronic pulmonary complications following autologous bone marrow transplantation in non-Hodgkins lymphoma 8. Bone Marrow Transplant 1990;6:329–31.

290. Robbins RA, Linder J, Stahl MG, et al. Diffuse alveolar hemorrhage in autologous bone marrow transplant recipients. Am J Med 1989;87:511–8.

291. Chao NJ, Duncan SR, Long GD, et al. Corticosteroid therapy for diffuse alveolar hemorrhage in autologus bone marrow transplant recipients. Ann Intern Med 1991;114:145–6.

292. Seiden MV, O'Donnell WJ, Weinblatt M, Licht J. Vasculitis with recurrent pulmonary hemorrhage in a long-term survivor after autologous bone marrow transplantation. Bone Marrow Transplant 1990;6:345–7.

293. Gottlieb AJ, Spiera A, Tierstein AS, et al. Serologic factors in idiopathic diffuse pulmonary fibrosis. Am J Med 1965;39:405–10.

294. Turner-Warwick M, Haslam P. Antibodies in some chronic fibrosing lung disease 1: non-organ specific autoantibodies. Clin Allergy 1971;1:83–95.

295. Dreisen RB, Schwarz MI, Theophilopoulos AN, et al. Circulating immune complexes in the idiopathic interstitial pneumonias. N Engl J Med 1978;299:353–7.

296. Turner-Warwick M, Haslam P. Antibodies in some chronic fibrosing lung diseases II: immunofluorescent studies. Clin Allergy 1971;1:209–19.

297. Schwarz MI, Dreisen RB, Pratt DS, Stanford RE. Immunofluorescent patterns in the idiopathic interstitial pneumonias. J Lab Clin Med 1978;91:929–38.

298. Scadding JW. Fibrosing alveolitis with autoimmune hemolytic anemia: two case reports. Thorax 1977;32:134–9.

299. Williams AJ, Marsh J, Stableforth DE. Cryptogenic fibrosing alveolitis, chronic active hepatitis, and autoimmune hemolytic anemia in the same patient. Br J Dis Chest 1905;79:200–3.

300. Turner-Warwick M. Cryptogenic fibrosing alveolitis. Br J Hosp Med 1972;7:697–704.

301. May JJ, Schwarz MI, Dreisen RB. Idiopathic thrombocytopenia purpura and interstitial pneumonitis. Ann Intern Med 1979;90:199–200.

302. Meduri GV, Reynoso G. Idiopathic interstitial pneumonitis occurring with idiopathic thrombocytopenic purpura. Chest 1989;96:A253S.

303. Kleiner-Baumgarten A, Schlaeffer F, Kaynan A. Multiple autoimmune manifestations in a spleenectomized subject with HLA-BB. Arch Intern Med 1983;143:1987–9.

304. Barnett EV, Bluestone R, Gracchiolo A, et al. Cryoglobulinemia and disease. Ann Intern Med 1970;73:95–100.

305. Levo Y, Gorevic P, Kassab H, et al. Association between hepatitis B virus and essential mixed cryoglobulinemia. N Engl J Med 1977;296:1501–4.

306. Popp JW, Dionstag JL, Wavels JR, Block KJ. Essential mixed cryoglobulinemia without evidence for hepatitis B virus infection. Ann Intern Med 1980;92:379–83.

307. Levey JM, Bjordsson B, Banner B, et al. Mixed cryoglobulinemia in chronic hepatitis C infection: a clinicopathologic analysis of 10 cases and review of the literature. Medicine 1994;73:53–67.

308. Bombardieri S, Paoletti P, Ferri C, et al. Lung involvement in essential mixed cryoglobulinemia. Am J Med 1979;66:748–56.

309. Clinicopathological conference: mixed cryoglobulinemia. Am J Med 1976;61:95–9.

310. Leatherman JW. Immune alveolar hemorrhage. Chest 1987;91:891–7.

311. Gomez-Tello V, Onoro-Canaveral JJ, de la Casa Monje RM, et al. Diffuse recidivant alveolar hemorrhage in a patient

with hepatitis C virus-related mixed cryoglubulinemia. Intensive Care Med 1999;319–22.

312. Isenberg JI, Goldstein H, Korn AR, et al. Pulmonary vasculitis—an uncommon complication of ulcerative colitis. N Engl J Med 1968;279:1376–7.

313. Forrest JAH, Shearman DJC. Pulmonary vasculitis and ulcerative colitis. Dig Dis 1975;20:482–6.

314. Patwardhan RV, Heilpern RJ, Brewster AC, et al. Pleuropericarditis: an extraintestinal complication of inflammatory bowel diseases. Report of three cases and review of the literature. Arch Intern Med 1983;143:94–6.

315. McKee AL, Rajapksa A, Kalish PE, et al. Severe interstitial pulmonary fibrosis in a patient with chronic ulcerative colitis. Am J Gastroenterol 1983;78:86–9.

316. Eade OE, Smith CL, Alexander JR, et al. Pulmonary function in patients with inflammatory bowel disease. Am J Gastroenterol 1980;73:154–6.

317. Swinburn CR, Jackson GJ, Cobden I, et al. Bronchiolitis obliterans organizing pneumonia in a patient with ulcerative colitis. Thorax 1988;43:435–6.

318. Butland RJA, Cole P, Citron KM. Chronic bronchial suppuration and inflammatory bowel disease. QJM 1981;197: 3–5.

319. Jones GR, Malone DNA. Sulphasalazine induced lung diseases. Thorax 1972;27:713–7.

320. Davies D, MacFarland A. Fibrosing alveolitis and treatment with sulfasalazine. Gut 1974;15:185–8.

321. Williams T, Eidus L, Thomas P. Fibrosing alveolitis, bronchiolitis obliterans and sulfasalazine therapy. Chest 1982;81: 766–8.

322. Case records of the Massachusetts General Hospital #12-1993. N Engl J Med 1993;328:869–76.

323. Higgenbottam T, Cochrane GM, Clark TJH, et al. Bronchial disease in ulcerative colitis. Thorax 1980;35:581–5.

324. Shneerson JM. Lung bullae, bronchiectasis, and Hashimotos thyroiditis associated with ulcerative colitis treated by colectomy. Thorax 1981;36:313–4.

325. Gibb WRG, Dhillon DP, Zilkha KJ, et al. Bronchiectasis with ulcerative colitis and myelopathy. Thorax 1987;42:155–6.

326. Desau SJ, Gephardt GN, Stoller JK. Diffuse panbronchiolitis preceding ulcerative colitis. Chest 1989;45:1342–4.

327. Wolfgang D, Kullnig P, Wolfgang P, et al. Colobronchial fistula: a rare complication of Crohn's colitis. Am Rev Respir Dis 1990;142:1225–7.

328. Rickli H, Fretz C, Hoffman M, et al. Severe inflammatory upper airway stenosis in ulcerative colitis. Eur Respir J 1994;7:1899–902.

329. Lamblin C, Copin MC, Billaut L, et al. Acute respiratory failure due to tracheobronchial involvement in Crohn's disease. Eur Respir J 1996;9:2176–8.

330. Camus P, Piard F, Ashugt T, et al. The lung in inflammatory bowel disease. Medicine 1993;72:157–83.

331. Shah SM, Texter EC, White HS. Inflammatory bowel disease associated with granulomatous lung disease: report of a case with endoscopic findings. Gastrointest Endosc 1976;23:98–9.

332. Wallart B, Colomed JF, Tonnel AB, et al. Evidence of lymphocytic alveolitis in Crohn's disease. Chest 1985;87: 363–7.

333. Heatley RV, Thomas P, Prokipchuk EJ, et al. Pulmonary function abnormalities in patients with inflammatory bowel disease. QJM 1982;203:241–50.

334. Neilly JB, Main ANH, Murray J, et al. Pulmonary abnormalities in Crohn's disease. Respir Med 1989;83:487–91.

335. Bonniere P, Walaert B, Cortot A, et al. Latent pulmonary involvement in Crohn's disease; biological, functional, bronchoalveolar lavage and sarcoidosis studies. Gut 1986; 27:919–25.

336. Lancaster Smith MJ, Benson MK, Strickland ID. Coeliac disease and diffuse interstitial lung disease. Lancet 1971;i:473–6.

337. Berrill WT, Fitzpatrick PF, MacLeod WM, et al. Bird fancier's lung and jejunal villous atrophy. Lancet 1975;ii:1000–8.

338. Hendrick DJ, Fauz JA, Anand B, et al. Is bird fancier's lung associated with coeliac disease? Thorax 1978;33:425–8.

339. Tarlo SM, Broder I, Prokipchuk EJ, et al. Association between celiac disease and lung disease. Chest 1981;80:715–8.

340. Neil GA, Lukie BE, Cockcroft DW, et al. Lymphocytic pneumonia and abdominal lymphoma complicating celiac sprue. J Clin Gastroenterol 1986;8:282–5.

341. Wright PH, Menzies IS, Pounder RE, et al. Adult idiopathic pulmonary hemosiderosis and coeliac disease. QJM 1981;197:95–102.

342. Mahadeva R, Flower C, Shneerson J. Bronchiectasis in association with coeliac disease. Thorax 2000;53:527–9.

343. Maizel H, Ruffin JM, Dobbins WO. Whipple's disease: a review of 19 patients from one hospital and a review of the literature since 1950. Medicine 1970;49:175–205.

344. Enzinger FM, Hehwig EB. Whipple's disease: a review of the literature and report of 15 cases. Virchows Arch (Pathol Anat) 1963;336:238–69.

345. Pollack JJ. Pleuropulmonary Whipple's disease. South J Med 1985;78:216–7.

346. Eyler WR, Doub HP. Extraintestinal roentgen manifestations of intestinal lipodystrophy. JAMA 1956;150:534–6.

347. Samuels T, Hamilton P, Shaw P. Whipple disease of the mediastinum. AJR Am J Roentgenol 1990;154:1187–8.

348. Rodarte JR, Garrison CO, Holly KE, et al. Whipple's disease simulating sarcoidosis: a case with unique clinical and histologic features. Arch Intern Med 1972;129:479–82.

349. Cho C, Linscheer WG, Hirschkorn MA, et al. Sarcoidlike granulomas as an early manifestation of Whipple's disease. Gastroenterology 1984;87:941–7.

350. Winberg C, Rose M, Rapport H. Whipple's disease of the lung. Am J Med 1978;65:873A.

351. Symmons DPM, Shepherd AN, Boardman PL, et al. Pulmonary manifestations of Whipple's disease. QJM 1985; 220:497–504.

352. Goldring PL, Smith M, Williams R. Multisystem disease in chronic liver disease. Am J Med 1973;1:959–62.

353. Mason AMS, McIllmurray MB, Goldring PL. Fibrosing alveolitis associated with renal tubular acidosis. BMJ 1970;4:596–9.

354. Rodriguez-Roisin R, Pares A, Bruguere M, et al. Pulmonary involvement in primary biliary cirrhosis. Thorax 1981;36: 208–12.

355. Clark AK, Galbraith RM, Hamilton EBD, et al. Rheumatic disorders in primary biliary cirrhosis. Ann Rheum Dis 1978;37:42–7.

356. Wallace JG, Tong MJ, Weki BH, et al. Pulmonary involvement in primary biliary cirrhosis. J Clin Gastroenterol 1987;9: 431–5.

357. Davison AG, Epstein O. Relapsing organizing pneumonitis in a man with primary biliary cirrhosis with CREST syndrome and chronic pancolitis. Thorax 1983;38:316–7.

358. Keefe EB. Sarcoidosis and primary biliary cirrhosis: literature review and illustrative case. Am J Med 1987;85:977–80.

359. Leff JA, Ready JB, Repetto C, et al. Coexistence of primary biliary cirrhosis and sarcoidosis. West J Med 1990;153: 439–41.

360. Wallert B, Bonnjere P, Prin L, et al. Primary biliary cirrhosis: subclinical inflammatory alveolitis in patients with normal chest roentgenograms. Chest 1986;90:842–8.

361. Izdebska-Makosa Z, Zielinski U. Primary biliary cirrhosis in a patient with interstitial lung fibrosis. Chest 1987;92:766–7.

362. Sharma A, Provenzale D, Mukusick A, Kaplan MM. Interstitial pneumonitis after low dose methotrexate therapy in primary biliary cirrhosis. Gastroenterology 1994;107:266–70.

363. Turnick-Warwick M. Fibrosing alveolitis and chronic liver disease. QJM 1968;37:133–7.

364. Helman CA, Keoton GR, Benatar SR. Lymphoid interstitial pneumonia with associated chronic active hepatitis and

renal tubular acidosis. Am Rev Respir Dis 1977;115: 161–4.

365. Capron JP, Martic R, Rey JL, et al. Fibrosing alveolitis and hepatitis B surface antigen in a patient with immunoglobulin A deficiency. Am J Med 1979;66:874–8.

366. Golding PL, Smith M, Williams R. Multisystem involvement in chronic liver disease. Am J Med 1973;55:772–82.

367. Krowka MJ, Cortese DA. Pulmonary aspects of chronic liver disease and liver transplantation. Mayo Clin Proc 1985;60: 407–18.

368. Ward MJ, Davies D. Riedel's thyroiditis with invasion of the lungs. Thorax 1981;36:956–7.

369. Watanabe K, Senju S, Maeda F, et al. Four cases of bronchiolitis obliterans organizing pneumonia associated with thyroid disease. Respiration 2000;67:572–6.

370. Turton C, Jacobs JM. Cryptogenic fibrosing alveolitis associated with peripheral neuropathy. QJM 1983;207:417–23.

371. Montes M, Tomasi TB, Noehren TH, et al. Lymphoid interstitial pneumonia with monoclonal gammopathy. Am Rev Respir Dis 1968;98:277–80.

372. Adner MM, Sherman JD, Ise C, et al. An immunologic survey of forty-eight patients with myasthenia gravis. New Engl J Med 1964;271:1327–33.

373. Kradin RL, Kiprov D, Dickersin GR, et al. Immune complex disease with fatal pulmonary hemorrhage: its occurence in a patient with myasthenia gravis. Arch Pathol Lab Med 1981;105:582–5.

374. Kawai C, Ishikawa K, Kato M, et al. "Pulmonary pulseless disease:" pulmonary involvement in so-called Takayasu's disease. Chest 1978;73:651–7.

375. Greene NB, Baugham RP, Kim CK. Takayasu's arteritis associated with interstitial lung disease and glomerulonephritis. Chest 1986;89:605–6.

376. Larsen TS, Hall S, Heppern GG, et al. Respiratory tract symptoms as a clue to giant cell arteritis. Ann Intern Med 1984;101:594–7.

377. Karam GTT, Fulmer JD. Giant cell arteritis presenting as interstitial lung disease. Chest 1982;82:781–4.

378. Doyle L, McWilliam L, Hasleton PS. Giant cell arteritis with pulmonary involvement. Br J Dis Chest 1988;82:88–92.

379. Bradley JD, Pinals RS, Blumfeld AB, et al. Giant cell arteritis with pulmonary nodules. Am J Med 1984;77:135–9.

380. Marcussen N, Lund C. Combined sarcoidosis and disseminated visceral giant cell vasculitis. Pathol Res Pract 1989;184:325–30.

381. Kramer MR, Melzer E, Nesher G, et al. Pulmonary manifestations of temporal arteritis. Eur J Respir Dis 1987;71:430–3.

382. Conger JD, Hammond WS, Alfrey AC, et al. Pulmonary calcification in chronic dialysis patients. Ann Intern Med 1975;83:330–6.

383. Faubert PF, Shapiro WB, Porush JG. Pulmonary calcification in haemodialyzed patients detected by technetium-99m diphosphonate scanning. Kidney Int 1980;18:95–102.

384. Khafif RA, Delima C, Silverberg A, et al. Acute hyperparathyroidism with systemic calcinosis. Arch Intern Med 1989;149:681–4.

385. Mulligan RM. Metastatic calcification. Arch Pathol Lab Med 1947;43:177–230.

386. Kaltrieder HB, Baum GL, Bogaty G, et al. The so-called metastatic calcification of the lung. Am J Med 1969;46:188–96.

387. Nogee LM, Garnier G, Dietz HC, et al. A mutation in the surfactant protein B gene responsible for fatal neonatal respiratory disease in multiple hundreds. J Clin Invest 1994;93:1860–3.

388. Firoozia H, Pudlowski R, Golimba, et al. Diffuse interstitial calcification of the lungs in chronic renal failure mimicking pulmonary edema. AJR Am J Roentgenol 1977;129: 1103–5.

389. Bonin M, Miyai K. Metastatic pulmonary calcification: morphology, chemical and x-ray microanalysis. Lab Invest 1977;36:331–7.

390. Kuzela DC, Huffer WE, Conger JD, et al. Soft tissue calcification in chronic dialysis patients. Am J Pathol 1977;86: 403–21.

391. Breitz HB, Sirotta PS, Nelp WB, et al. Progressive pulmonary calcification complicating successful renal transplantation. Am Rev Respir Dis 1987;136:1480–2.

392. Harbitz F. Extensive calcification of the lungs as a distinct disease. Arch Intern Med 1918;21:139–46.

393. Puhr L. Mikrolithiasis alveolaris pulmonum. Virchows Arch 1933;290:156–60.

394. Sosman MC, Dodd GD, Jones WD, Pillmore GU. The familial occurrence of pulmonary alveolar microlithiasis AJR Am J Roentgenol 1957;77:947–1012.

395. Meyer HH, Gilbert ES, Kent G. A clinical review of pulmonary microlithiasis. JAMA 1956;161:1153–7.

396. Balikian JP, Fuleihan FJD, Nucho CN. Pulmonary alveolar microlithiasis. Report of five cases with special reference to roentgen manifestations. AJR Am J Roentgenol 1968;103: 509–18.

397. Prakash UBS, Barham SS, Rosenow EC III, et al. Pulmonary alveolar microlithiasis. A review including ultrastructural and pulmonary function studies. Mayo Clin Proc 1983;58: 290–300.

398. Mitro JM, Moreno A, Coca A, et al. Pulmonary alveolar microlithiasis with an unusual radiological pattern. Br J Dis Chest 1982;76:91–6.

399. Chang AR. Test and teach. Pulmonary alveolar microlithiasis. Pathology 1980;12:164–7, 282–3.

400. Katzenstein AA, Askin FB. Surgical pathology of non-neoplastic lung disease. Philadelphia: WB Saunders; 1982. p. 368.

401. Coetzee T. Pulmonary alveolar microlithiasis with involvement of the sympathetic nervous system and gonads. Thorax 1970;25:637–42.

402. Badger TL, Gottlieb L, Gaensler EA. Pulmonary and alveolar microlithiasis, or calcinosis of the lungs. N Engl J Med 1955;253:709–15.

403. Caffrey PR, Altman RS. Pulmonary alveolar microlithiasis occurring in premature twins. J Pediatr 1965;66:758–63.

404. Palombini BC, Porto ND, Wallau CU, Camargo JJ. Bronchopulmonary lavage in alveolar microlithiasis. Chest 1981;80:423–4.

405. Sears MR, Chang AR, Taylor AJ. Pulmonary alveolar microlithiasis. Thorax 1971;26:704–11.

406. Yang SP, Lin CC. Pulmonary alveolar microlithiasis. A report of two youngest cases in a family. Dis Chest 1963;44:163–7.

407. O'Neil RP, Cohn JE, Pellegrino ED. Pulmonary alveolar microlithiasis—a family study. Ann Intern Med 1967;67: 957–67.

408. al-Damluji SJ, al-Omari MM, al-Fakhri S. Pulmonary alveolar microlithiasis in two siblings from Iraq. Br J Dis Chest 1973;67:246–52.

409. Kino T, Kohara Y, Tsuji S. Pulmonary alveolar microlithiasis: a report of two young sisters. Am Rev Respir Dis 1972; 105:105–10.

410. Fuleihan FJD, Abboud RT, Balikian JP, Nucho CKN. Pulmonary alveolar microlithiasis: lung function in five cases. Thorax 1969;24:84–90.

411. Chinachoti N, Tangchai P. Pulmonary alveolar microlithiasis associated with the inhalation of snuff in Thailand. Dis Chest 1957;32:687–9.

412. Onadeko BO, Beetlestone CA, Cooke AR, et al. Pulmonary alveolar microlithiasis. Postgrad Med J 1977;53:165–7.

413. Shama SK, Sharma S, Mukhopadhyaya S, et al. Pulmonary alveolar microlithiasis: report of three cases with pulmonary function and exercise studies. Indian J Chest Dis Allied Sci 1992;34:205–15.

414. Nouh MS. Pulmonary alveolar microlithiasis: a report of four cases. East Afr Med J 1991;68:39–42.

415. Ucan ES, Keyf AI, Aydilek R, et al. Pulmonary alveolar microlithiasis: review of Turkish reports. Thorax 1993;48: 171–3.

416. Biary MS, Abdullah MA, Assaf HM, Wazzan A. Pulmonary alveolar microlithiasis in a Saudi child and two cousins. Ann Trop Pediatr 1993;13:409–13.

417. Macie-Taylor BH, Waroman AG, Madden CA, Page RL. A case of alveolar microlithiasis: observation over 22 years and recovery of material by lavage. Thorax 1985;40:952–3.

418. Schraufnagel DE, Pate JAP, Wang NS. Micronodular pulmonary pattern: association with inhaled aerosol. AJR Am J Roentgenol 1981;137:57–63.

419. Saputo V, Zocchi M, Mancosu M, et al. Pulmonary alveolar microlithiasis: a case with a discussion of differential diagnosis. Helv Paediatr Acta 1979;34:245–55.

420. Fraser RG, Pate JAP. Diagnosis of disease of the chest. Vol 2. Philadelphia: W.B. Saunders; 1979. p. 1741.

421. Winselberg GG, Boller M, Sachs M, Weinberg J. CT evaluation of pulmonary alveolar microlithiasis. J Comput Assist Tomogr 1984;8:1029–31.

422. Pant K, Shah A, Mathur RK, et al. Pulmonary alveolar microlithiasis with pleural calcification and nephrolithiasis. Chest 1990;98:245–6.

423. Coolens J, Devos P, DeRoo M. Diffuse pulmonary uptake of Tc-99m bone imaging agents: case report and survey. Eur J Nucl Med 1985;11:36–42.

424. Shigeno C, Fukunaga M, Morita R, et al. Bone scintigraphy in pulmonary alveolar microlithiasis. Clin Nucl Med 1982;7:103–7.

425. Brown ML, Swee RG, Olson RJ, Bender E. Pulmonary uptake of Tc-99m diphosphonate in alveolar microlithiasis. AJR Am J Roentgenol 1978;131:703–4.

426. Seinstein DS. Pulmonary sarcoidosis: calcified micronodular pattern simulating pulmonary alveolar microlithiasis. J Thorac Imag 1999;14:218–20.

427. Oka S, Shiraishi K, Ogata K, et al. Pulmonary alveolar microlithiasis. Report of 3 cases. Am Rev Respir Dis 1966;93:612–6.

428. Brown J, Leon W, Felton C. Hemodynamic and pulmonary studies in pulmonary alveolar microlithiasis. Am J Med 1984;77:176–8.

429. Thomason WB. Pulmonary alveolar microlithiasis. Thorax 1959;14:76–81.

430. Tao LC. Microlithiasis in sputum specimens and their relationship to pulmonary alveolar microlithiasis. Am J Clin Pathol 1978;69:482–5.

431. Korn MA, Schurawitzki H, Klepetko W, Burghuber OC. Pulmonary alveolar microlithiasis: findings on high resolution CT. AJR Am J Roentgenol 1992;158:981–2.

432. Cale WF, Petsonk EL, Boyd CB. Transbronchial biopsy of pulmonary alveolar microlithiasis. Arch Intern Med 1983;143:358–9.

433. Daugavietis HE, Mautner LS. Disseminated nodular pulmonary ossification with mitral stenosis. Arch Pathol 1957;63:7–12.

434. Popelka CG, Kleinerman J. Diffuse pulmonary ossification. Arch Intern Med 1977;137:523–5.

435. Fried ED, Godwin TA. Extensive diffuse pulmonary ossification. Chest 1992;102:1614–5.

436. Firooznia H, Pudlowski R, Golimbu C, et al. Diffuse interstitial calcification of the lungs in chronic renal failure mimicking pulmonary edema. AJR Am J Roentgenol 1977;129:1103–5.

437. Conger JD, Hammond WS, Alfrey AC, et al. Pulmonary calcification in chronic dialysis patients. Clinical and pathologic studies. Ann Intern Med 1975;83:330–5.

438. Thind GS, Bhatia JL. Pulmonary alveolar microlithiasis. Br J Dis Chest 1978;72:151–4.

439. Ratjen FA, Schoenfeld B, Wiesemann HG. Pulmonary alveolar microlithiasis and lymphocytic interstitial pneumonitis in a ten year old girl. Eur Respir J 1992;5:1283–5.

440. Freiberg DB, Young IH, Laks H, et al. Improvement in gas exchange with nasal continuous positive airway pressure in pulmonary alveolar microlithiasis. Am Rev Respir Dis 1992;145:1215–6.

441. Waters MH. Microlithiasis alveolaris pulmonum. Tubercle 1960;41:276–80.

442. Stamatis G, Zerkowski HR, Doetsch N, et al. Sequential bilateral lung transplantation for pulmonary alveolar microlithiasis. Ann Thorac Surg 1993;56:972–5.

443. Bonnette P, Bisson A, el Kadi NB, et al. Bilateral single lung transplantation: complications and results in 14 patients. Eur J Cardiothorac Surg 1992;6:550–4.

444. Cluzel P, Grenier P, Bernadac P, et al. Pulmonary alveolar microlithiasis: CT findings. J Comput Assist Tomogr 1991;15:938–42.

445. Liebow AA. Bronchiolo-alveolar carcinoma. Adv Intern Med 1960;10:329–58.

446. Ludington LG, Verska JJ, Howard T, et al. Bronchilar carcinoma (alveolar cell), another great imitator. A review of 41 cases. Chest 1972;61:622–8.

447. Edgerton F, Rao U, Takita H, Vincent RG. Bronchioalveolar carcinoma. A clinical overview and bibliography. Oncology 1981;38:269–73.

448. Berkman YM. The many faces of bronchiolo-alveolar carcinoma. Semin Roentgenol 1977;12:207–14.

449. Hewlett TH, Gomex AC, Aronstam EM, Steer A. Bronchiolar carcinoma of the lung. Review of 39 patients. J Thorac Cardiovasc Surg 1964;48:614–24.

450. Bennett DE, Sasser WF. Bronchiolar carcinoma: a valid clinicopathologic entity? Cancer 1969;24:876–87.

451. Miller WT, Husted J, Freiman D, et al. Bronchioloalveolar carcinoma: two clinical entities with one pathologic diagnosis. AJR Am J Roentgenol 1978;130:905–12.

452. Donaldson JC, Kaminsky DB, Elliott RC. Bronchiolar carcinoma. Report of 11 cases and review of the literature. Cancer 1978;41:250–8.

453. McNamara JJ, Kingsley WB, Paulson DL, et al. Alveolar cell (bronchiolar) carcinoma of the lung. J Thorac Cardiovasc Surg 1969;57:648–56.

454. Wormer DC. Cavitary bronchiolar carcinoma. A case report. Am Rev Respir Dis 1969;99:773–6.

455. Manning JT Jr, Spjut HJ, Tschen JA. Bronchioloalveolar carcinoma: the significance of two histopathologic types. Cancer 1984;54:525–34.

456. Dunn D, Hertel B, Norwood W, Nicoloff DM. Bronchioloalveolar cell carcinoma of the lung: a clinicopathological study. Ann Thorac Surg 1978;26:241–7.

457. Marco M, Galy P. Bronchioloalveolar carcinoma. Clinicopathologic relationships, natural history, and prognosis in 29 cases. Am Rev Respir Dis 1973;107:621–9.

458. Kimula Y. A histochemical and ultrastructural study of adenocarcinoma of the lung. Am J Surg Pathol 1978;2:253–63.

459. Nash G, Langlinais PC, Greenwald KA. Alveolar cell carcinoma: does it exist? Cancer 1972;29:322–6.

460. Rosenblatt MB, Lisa JR, Collier F. Primary and metastatic bronchioloalveolar cell carcinoma. Dis Chest 1967;52:147–52.

461. Edwards CW. Alveolar carcinoma: a review. Thorax 1984;39:166–74.

462. Greenberg SD, Smith MN, Spjut HJ. Bronchioloalveolar carcinoma—cell of origin. Am J Clin Pathol 1975;63:153–67.

463. Sidhu GS, Forrester EM. Glycogen-rich Clara cell-type bronchioloalveolar carcinoma: light and electron microscopic study. Cancer 1977;40:2209–15.

464. Axiotis CA, Jennings TA. Observations on bronchioloalveolar carcinomas, with special emphasis on localized lesions. Am J Surg Pathol 1988;12:918–31.

465. Singh G, Katyal SL, Torikata C. Carcinoma of type II pneumocytes. Immunodiagnosis of a subtype of bronchioloalveolar carcinomas. Am J Pathol 1981;102:195–208.

466. Morningstar WA, Hassan MO. Bronchioloalveolar carcinoma with nodal metastases. An ultrastructural study. Am J Surg Pathol 1979;3:273–8.

467. Espinoza CG, Balis JU, Saba SR, et al. Ultrastructural and immunohistochemical studies of bronchioloalveolar carcinoma. Cancer 1984;54:2182–9.

468. Bonikos DS, Hendrickson M, Bensch KG. Pulmonary alveolar cell carcinoma. Am J Surg Pathol 1977;1:93–108.

469. Eimoto T, Teshima K, Shirakusa T, Kikuchi M. Ultrastructure of well-differentiated adenocarcinomas of the lung with special reference to bronchioloalveolar carcinoma. Ultrastruct Pathol 1985;8:177–90.

470. Genereux GP, Merriman JE. Desquamative interstitial pneumonia: progression to the end-stage lung and the unusual complication of alveolar cell carcinoma. J Can Assoc Radiol 1973;24:144–9.

471. Schorn D, DeKock JJ. Carcinoma in a Hamman-Rich lung. A case report. S Afr Med J 1973;47:644–6.

472. Moolten SE. Scar cancer of lung complicating rheumatoid lung disease. Mt Sinai J Med 1973;40:636–43.

473. Blodgett RC Jr, Cera PJ Jr, Jones FL Jr. Alveolar cell carcinoma associated with rheumatoid nodule. Chest 1972;62:625–7.

474. Talbott JH, Barocas M. Carcinoma of the lung in progressive systemic sclerosis: a tabular review of the literature and a detailed report of the roentgenographic changes in two cases. Semin Arthritis Rheum 1980;9:191–217.

475. Fox H. Alveolar adenocarcinoma complicating pulmonary fibrosis due to mitral stenosis. Br J Dis Chest 1973;67:253–6.

476. Min KW, Gyorkey F. Interstitial pulmonary fibrosis: atypical epithelial changes, and bronchiolar cell carcinoma following busulfan therapy. Cancer 1968;22:1027–32.

477. Lutwyche VU. Another presentation of fibrosing alveolitis and alveolar cell carcinoma. Chest 1976;70:292–3.

478. Lesser M, Chang JC, Yoo OH, Roswit B. Bronchioloalveolar (sic) carcinoma arising in areas previously irradiated for Hodgkin's disease. South Med J 1983;76:689–91.

479. Hammer SP, Bochus D, Remington F, et al. Langerhans' cells and serum precipitating antibodies against fungal antigens in bronchioloalveolar cell carcinoma: possible association with pulmonary eosinophilic granuloma. Ultrastruct Pathol 1980;1:19–37.

480. Demy NG, Adler H. Asbestosis and malignancy. AJR Am J Roentgenol 1967;100:597–602.

481. DuVuyst P, Dumortier P, Jacobouitz D, et al. Environment asbestosis complicated by lung cancer. Chest 1994;105:1593–5.

482. Felson B, Ralaisomay G. Carcinoma of the lung complicating lipoid pneumonia. AJR Am J Roentgenol 1983;141:901–7.

483. Cremers S, Dutrieux-Fauchet MC, Dutrieux C. Bronchioalveolar carcinoma in angio-immunoblastic lymphadenopathy. Eur J Respir Dis 1983;64:222–8.

484. Bonne C. Morphological resemblance of pulmonary adenomatosis (jaagsiekte) in sheep and certain cases of cancer of the lung in man. Am J Cancer 1939;35:491–501.

485. Perk K, Hod I. Sheep lung carcinoma: an endemic analogue of a sporadic human neoplasm. J Natl Cancer Inst 1982;69:747–9.

486. Nodel TA, Perk K. Bronchioloalveolar cell carcinoma. Am J Pathol 1978;90:783–6.

487. Schraufnagel D, Peloquin A, Pare JAP, Wang NS. Differentiating bronchioloalveolar carcinoma from adenocarcinoma. Am Rev Respir Dis 1982;125:74–9.

488. Storey CF, Kudtson KP, Lawrence BJ. Bronchiolar "alveolar cell" carcinoma of the lung. J Thorac Cardiovasc Surg 1953;26:331–406.

489. Weiss W, Altan S, Rosenzweig M, Weiss WA. Lung cancer type in relation to cigarette dosage. Cancer 1977;39:2568–72.

490. Thomas JS, Tullett WM, Stack BHR. Bronchioloalveolar cell carcinoma: a 21 year retrospective study of cases at the Western Infirmary, Glasgow. Br J Dis Chest 1985;79:132–40.

491. Vincent RG, Pickren JW, Lane WW, et al. The changing histopathology of lung cancer. A review of 1682 cases. Cancer 1977;39:1647–55.

492. Watson WL, Farpour A. Terminal bronchiolar or alveolar cell cancer of the lung. Cancer 1966;19:776–80.

493. Falk RT, Pickle LW, Fantham ET, et al. Epidemiology of bronchioloalveolar carcinoma. Cancer Epidemiol Biomarkers Prev 1992;1:339–44.

494. Morabia A, Wynder FL. Relation of bronchioloalveolar carcinoma to tobacco. BMJ 1992;242:541–3.

495. Joishy SK, Cooper RA, Rowley PT. Alveolar cell carcinoma in identical twins. Ann Intern Med 1977;87:477–80.

496. Beaumont F, Jansen HM, Elema JD, et al. Simultaneous occurrence of pulmonary interstitial fibrosis and alveolar cell carcinoma in one family. Thorax 1981;36:252–8.

497. Homma H, Kira S, Takahashi Y, Imai H. A case of alveolar cell carcinoma accompanied by fluid and electrolyte depletion through production of voluminous amounts of lung liquid. Am Rev Respir Dis 1975;111:857–62.

498. Dwek JH, Charytan C, Stachura I, Kaganowicz A. Salt-wasting bronchorrhea and its mechanisms. Arch Intern Med 1977;137:791–4.

499. Singh PS, Nath H, Pinkard NB, Alexander CB. Bronchioloalveolar carcinoma causing pulmonary hypertension: a unique manifestation. AJR Am J Roentgenol 1994;162:30–2.

500. Sarlin RF, Schillaci RF, Georges TN, Wilcox JR. Focal increased lung perfusion and intrapulmonary veno-arterial shunting in bronchioloalveolar cell carcinoma. Am J Med 1980;68:618–23.

501. Fishman HC, Danon J, Koopot N, et al. Massive intrapulmonary venoarterial shunting in alveolar cell carcinoma. Am Rev Respir Dis 1974;109:124–8.

502. Dyer NH, Hughes DTD, Thompson JMA. Bronchiolar carcinoma: a case report with pulmonary function studies. Thorax 1967;22:260–4.

503. Heikkila L, Suomalainen RJ, Lindgren J, et al. Carcinoembryonic antigen and gastrointestinal cancer associated antigen CA-19-9 in bronchioloalveolar carcinomas and pulmonary adenocarcinomas. Ann Chir Gynaecol 1986;75:260–5.

504. Shin MS, Bailey WC. Alveolar cell carcinoma: diagnostic pitfalls in evaluating the chest roentgenogram. South Med J 1985;78:193–5.

505. Epstein DM, Gefter WB, Miller WT. Lobar bronchioloalveolar cell carcinoma. AJR Am J Roentgenol 1982;139:463–8.

506. Springmeyer SC, Hackman R, Carlson JJ, McClellan JE. Bronchioloalveolar cell carcinoma diagnosed by bronchoalveolar lavage. Chest 1983;83:278–9.

507. Case 22-1994. Case records of the Massachussetts General Hospital. N Engl J Med 1994;330:1599–606.

508. Delarue NC, Anderson W, Sanders D, Starr J. Bronchioloalveolar caracinoma. A reappraisal after 24 years. Cancer 1972;29:90–7.

509. Dhingra HM, Valdivieso M, Carr DT, et al. Randomized trial of three combinations of cisplatin with vindesine and/or VP-16-213 in the treatment of advanced non-small-cell lung cancer. J Clin Oncol 1985;3:176–82.

510. Miller TP, Livingston RB. Phase II trial of 5-FU, vincristine, and mitomycin in metastatic bronchioloalveolar cell lung cancer: a Southwest Oncology Group study. Cancer Treat Rep 1985;69:1313–4.

511. Suga T, Sugiyama Y, Fujii T, Kitannura S. Bronchioloalveolar carcinoma with bronchorrhea treated with erythromycin. Eur Respir Dis 1994;7:2249–51.

512. Barsky SH, Grossman DA, Ho J, Holmes EC. The multifocality of bronchioloalveolar lung carcinoma: evidence and implications of a multiclonal origin. Mod Pathol 1994;7:633–40.

513. Woodheap M, Parkes WR. Disorders caused by other organic agents: oil granuloma (lipoid pneumonia). In: Parks WD, editor. Occupational lung disorders. Oxford: Butterworth-Heineman; 1994. p. 778–82.

514. Verbeken EK, Demedts M, Vanwing J, et al. Pulmonary phospholipid accumulation distal to an obstructed bronchus. Arch Pathol Lab Med 1989;113:886–90.

515. Van den Plas O, Trigaux JP, Van Beers B, et al. Gravity-dependent infiltrates in a patient with lipoid pneumonia. Chest 1990;98:1253–4.

516. Glynn KP, Gale NA. Exogenous lipoid pneumonia due to inhalation of spray lubricant (WD-40 lung). Chest 1990;97:1265–6.

517. Skorodin MS, Chandrasekar AJ. An occupational cause of exogenous lipoid pneumonia. Arch Pathol Lab Med 1983;107:610–1.

518. Kizer KW, Golden JA. Lipoid pneumonitis in a commercial balance diver. Undersea Biomed Res 1987;14:545–52.

519. Penes MC, Vallon JJ, Sabot JF, Vallon C. GC/MS detection of paraffins in a case of lipoid pneumonia following occupational exposure to oil spray. Anal Toxicol 1990;14:372–4.

520. Cullen MR, Balmes JR, Robins JM, Smith GJ. Lipoid pneumonia caused by oil mist exposure from a steel rolling tandem mill. Am J Ind Med 1981;2:51–8.

521. Annobil SH, Mirad NA, Khurama P, et al. Reaction of human lungs to aspirated universal fat (ghee): a clinicopathologic study. Virchows Arch 1995;426:301–5.

522. Annobil SH, Ogunbiy AO, Benjamin R. Chest radiographic findings in childhood lipoid pneumonia following aspiration of animal fat. Eur J Radiol 1993;16:217–20.

523. Bhagat R, Holmes IH, Kulaga A, et al. Self injection with olive oil. A cause of lipoid pneumonia. Chest 1995;107:875–6.

524. Hussain IR, Edenborough FP, Wilson RS, Stableforth DE. Severe lipoid pneumonia following attempted suicide by mineral oil ingestion. Thorax 1996;51:652–3.

525. Gold MI. Use of petroleum jelly [letter]. Anesthesiology 1985;63:339–40.

526. Beerman B, Christensson T, Moller P, Stillstrom A. Lipoid pneumonia: an occupational hazard of fire eaters. BMJ 1984;289:1728–9.

527. Becton DL, Lowe JE, Falletta JM. Lipoid pneumonia in an adolescent girl secondary to use of lip gloss. J Pediatr 1984;105:421–3.

528. de la Rocha SR, Cunningham JC, Fox E. Lipoid pneumonia secondary to baby oil aspiration: a case report and review of the literature. Pediatr Emerg Care 1985;1:74–80.

529. Pinkerton H. Reaction to oils and fats in the lung. Arch Pathol 1928;5:380–401.

530. Proetz AW. The effects of certain drugs upon living nasal ciliated epithelium. Ann Otol Rhinol Laryngol 1934;43:450–63.

531. Ikeda K. Lipoid pneumonia of the adult type. Arch Pathol 1937;23:470–92.

532. Hughes RL, Freilich RA, Bytell DE, et al. Aspiration and occult esophageal disorders. Chest 1981;80:489–95.

533. Freidman DG, Engelberg H, Merritt WH. Oil aspiration (lipoid) pneumonia in adults: a clinical pathological study of 47 cases. Arch Intern Med 1940;66:11–38.

534. Miller A, Bader RA, Bader ME, et al. Mineral oil pneumonia. Ann Intern Med 1962;57:627–34.

535. Buechner HA, Strug LH. Lipoid granuloma of the lung of exogenous origin. Dis Chest 1956;29:402–4.

536. Volk BW, Nathanson L, Losner S, et al. Incidence of lipoid pneumonia in a survey of 389 chronically ill patients. Am J Med 1951;10:316–24.

537. Ferguson GT, Miller YE. Occult mineral oil pneumonitis in anorexia nervosa. West J Med 1988;148:211–3.

538. Sodeman WA, Stuart BM. Lipoid pneumonia in adults. Ann Intern Med 1946;24:241–53.

539. Weill H, Ferrans VJ, Gay RM, Ziskind MM. Early lipoid pneumonia. Roentgenologic, anatomic, and physiologic characteristics. Am J Med 1964;36:370–6.

540. Grenaway TM, Caterson ID. Hypercalcemia and lipoid pneumonia. Aust N Z J Med 1989;19:713–15.

541. Rolla AR, Granfone A, Balogh K, et al. Granuloma related hypercalcemia in lipoid pneumonia. Am J Med Sci 1986;292:313–6.

542. Genereux GP. Lipoids in the lungs: radiologic-pathologic correlation. J Can Assoc Radiol 1970;21:2–15.

543. Lipinski JK, Weisbrod GL, Sanders DE. Exogenous lipoid pneumonitis: pulmonary patterns. AJR Am J Roentgenol 1981;136:931–4.

544. Guest JL, Arean VM, Brenner HA. Group IV atypical mycobacterium infection occurring in association with mineral oil granuloma of lungs. Am Rev Respir Dis 1967;95:656–62.

545. Hutchins GM, Boitnott JK. Atypical mycobacterial infection complicating mineral oil pneumonia. JAMA 1978;240:539–41.

546. Dixon C, Bolivar R, Katz R, McMurtrey M. Lipoid pneumonia and *Mycobacterium fortuitum* pulmonary infection: successful treatment with sulfisoxazole. Tex Med 1985;81:57–60.

547. Subramanian S, Kherdekar SS, Babu PG, Christian CS. Lipoid pneumonia with *Cryptococcus neoformans* colonization. Thorax 1982;37:319–20.

548. Felson B, Ralaisomay G. Carcinoma of the lung complicating lipoid pneumonia. AJR Am J Roentgenol 1983;141:901–7.

549. Bryan CS, Boitnott JK. Adenocarcinoma of the lung with chronic mineral oil pneumonia. Am Rev Respir Dis 1969;99:272–4.

550. Wheeler PS, Stitik FP, Hutchins GM, et al. Diagnosis of lipoid pneumonia by computed tomography. JAMA 1981;245:65–6.

551. Joshi RR, Cholankeril JV. Computed tomography in lipoid pneumonia. J Comput Assist Tomogr 1985;9:211–3.

552. Leek S, Muller NL, Hale V, et al. Lipoid pneumonia: CT findings. J Comput Assist Tomogr 1995;19:48–51.

553. Laurent F, Philippe JC. Vergier B, et al. Exogenous lipoid pneumonia: HRCT, MR, and pathologic findings. Eur Radiol 1999;9:1190–6.

554. Franquet T, Gimenez A, Bordes R, et al. The crazy paving pattern in exogenous lipoid pneumonia: CT-pathologic correlation. AJR Am J Roentgenol 1998;170:315–7.

555. Losner S, Volk BW, Slade WR, et al. Diagnosis of lipoid pneumonia by sputum examination. Am J Clin Pathol 1950;20:539–45.

556. Levade T, Salvayre R, Dongay G, et al. Chemical analysis of the bronchoalveolar washing fluid in the diagnosis of liquid paraffin pneumonia. J Clin Chem Clin Biochem 1987;25:45–8.

557. Spatafora M, Bellia V, Ferrara G, Genova G. Diagnosis of a case of lipoid pneumonia by bronchoalveolar lavage. Respiration 1987;52:154–6.

558. Silverman JF, Turner RC, West RL, Dillard TA. Bronchoalveolar lavage in the diagnosis of lipoid pneumonia. Diagn Cytopathol 1989;5:3–8.

559. Lauque D, Dongay G, Levade T, et al. Bronchoalveolar lavage in liquid paraffin pneumonitis. Chest 1990;98:1149–55.

560. Stein B, Zaartari GS, Pine JF. Amiodarone pulmonary toxicity: clinical, cytologic, and ultrastructural findings. Acta Cytol 1987;31:357–61.

561. Ayvazian LF, Steward DS, Merkel CG, Frederick WW. Diffuse lipoid pneumonitis successfully treated with prednisone. Am J Med 1967;43:930–4.

562. Mayo WP, Foster GL, Jernigan CL. Lipoid pneumonia. J Ky Med Assoc 1983;81:881–4.

563. Chin NK. Hui KP, Sinniah R, Chan TB. Idiopathic lipoid pneumonia in an adult treated with prednisolone. Chest 1994;105:956–7.

564. Wong CA, Wilsher ML. Treatment of exogenous lipoid pneumonia by whole lung lavage. Aust N Z J Med 1994;24:734–735.

565. Chang HY, Chen CW, Chen CY, et al. Successful treatment of diffuse lipoid pneumonitis with whole lung lavage. Thorax 1993;48:947–8.

INDEX

AAT, 191
Abciximab-induced alveolar hemorrhage, 508
ABMA, 8
ABPA, 677–679
  vs. Churg-Strauss syndrome, 617
  CT, *679*
Accelerated silicosis, 391
Acebutolol-induced eosinophilic pneumonia
  infiltrate, *500*
Acebutolol-induced interstitial pneumonitis, *498*
ACEI
  pulmonary fibrosis, 327
ACEI-induced eosinophilic pneumonia, 494
Acetylcysteine
  idiopathic pulmonary fibrosis, 743
  pulmonary fibrosis, 328
Acetylsalicylic acid (ASA)-induced pulmonary edema, 506, 507
ACR
  1990 criteria
    Wegener's granulomatosis, *601,* 601–602
  vasculitides classification, 599–600
ACTH
  hypersensitivity pneumonitis, 476
Acute eosinophilic pneumonia
  HRCT
    septal thickening, *101*
Acute hypersensitivity pneumonitis
  differential diagnosis, 470
  methotrexate-induced, 494
Acute idiopathic pulmonary hemorrhage of infancy (AIPHI), 138–139
  Stachybotrys chartarum, 139
Acute interstitial pneumonia (AIP), 765–771
  BAL, 766–767
  chest imaging, 768
    HRCT, 768, *769–770*
    radiograph, 768
  clinical findings, 766
  CT, 90–91
  diagnosis, 769–780
  epidemiology, 765–766
  etiology, 765–766
  histopathologic findings, 768–769
  laboratory findings, 766
  management and outcome, 771
  mortality, 771
  physiological findings, 768

Acute lung allograft rejection
  diffuse alveolar hemorrhage, 641
Acute lupus pneumonitis, 548–550
Acute progressive (subacute) hypersensitivity pneumonitis
  differential diagnosis, 470–471
  micrography, *473*
Acute pulmonary syndrome
  diffuse alveolar hemorrhage, 640
Acute reactive arthritis
  sarcoidosis, 351
Acute respiratory distress syndromes (ARDS), 278, 880
  alcoholics, 284
  chest radiography, *891*
  drug-induced, *514*
  organizing stage, *890*
  pulmonary fibrosis, 889–891
  Silo filler's disease, 795
Acute reversible hypoxemia syndrome
  in systemic lupus erythematosus, 551–552
Acute silicosis, 391, *393*
Adenocarcinoma
  BAL, 120, *121*
  pancreatic sarcoid masses mimicking, 355
Adenovirus
  children, 135
  IIP, 707
  pediatric interstitial lung disease, 135
Adhesion molecules
  expression, 233
  sarcoidosis, 344
Adolescent
  hypersensitivity pneumonitis
    CT, *136*
    radiography, *136*
Adrenaline-induced transient pulmonary infiltrates, *506*
Adrenocorticotropic hormone (ACTH)
  hypersensitivity pneumonitis, 476
Advanced multiple-beam equalization radiography (AMBER), 76
Aedes, 672
African Americans
  sarcoidosis, 335
Age, 6
  sarcoidosis, 334–335
Agnogenic myeloid metaplasis, 889
AIDS
  NSIP, 892
AILD, 831–832
AIP. *See* Acute interstitial pneumonia

AIPHI, 138–139
  Stachybotrys chartarum, 139
Airway function, 55–56
Alcoholics
  acute respiratory distress syndromes, 284
Alglucerase
  Gaucher's disease, 883
Allergic bronchopulmonary aspergillosis (ABPA), 677–679
  vs. Churg-Strauss syndrome, 617
  CT, *679*
Allergic bronchopulmonary candidiasis
  Churg-Strauss syndrome, 669
Allogeneic bone marrow transplantation
  interstitial pneumonitis after, 893–894
Allogeneic single lung transplantation
  chronic beryllium disease, 446
All-trans-retinoic acid, 505, 516
Alpha1-antitrypsin (AAT), 191
Alpha-galactosidase A
  Fabry's disease, 884
Alveolar epithelium
  normal, 221–222
  progenitors
    circulating stem cells, 223–225
  pulmonary fibrosis, 221–237
  repair, 222–225
    hypothetical model, *223*
Alveolar fibrosis
  animal models, 201–209
  inflammatory cells, 188–189
Alveolar filling
  radiographs, *10–14*
Alveolar hemorrhage
  drug-induced, 508–509
  drug-induced pneumonitis, 508
  drug-induced thrombocytopenia, 508
  Golde score, *121*
  induction, 509
  phenytoin-induced, 508
  propylthiouracil-induced, 508
  rodenticide-induced, 509
  tretinoin-induced, 508
  Wegener's granulomatosis, 604, *607*
Alveolar macrophage derived growth factor (AMDGF), 556
  coal workers' pneumoconiosis, 411
Alveolar macrophages
  host factors, 305–307
Alveolar proteinosis
  conditions associated with, *866*
  congenital, 139–140
  radiography, *11*

Alveolar sarcoidosis
CT, 100
Alveolar septal amyloidosis
chest radiography, *881*
HRCT, *881*
Alveolitis
sarcoidosis, *309*
AMBER, 76
AMDGF, 556
coal workers' pneumoconiosis, 411
American College Rheumatology (ACR)
1990 criteria
Wegener's granulomatosis, *601,*
601–602
vasculitides classification, 599–600
American Thoracic Society/European
Respiratory Society (ATS/ERS)
classification
classification, 702–703
Amiodarone, 208
pharmacology, 511–512
Amiodarone-induced acute respiratory
distress syndromes (ARDS)
clinical and radiographic pattern, 514
Amiodarone-induced alveolar hemorrhage
clinical and radiographic pattern, 514
Amiodarone-induced bronchiolitis,
810–811
Amiodarone-induced diffuse alveolar
hemorrhage (DAH), 644
Amiodarone-induced interstitial lung
disease (ILD), 485
CT, 101
dose-related toxicity, 494
HRCT, *102*
incidence, 494
Amiodarone-induced organizing
pneumonia, 501
Amiodarone-induced organizing
pneumonitis, 513–514
HRCT, *513*
Amiodarone-induced pulmonary fibrosis
chest radiography, *505*
clinical and radiographic pattern, 513
Amiodarone lung. *See* Amiodarone
pneumonitis
Amiodarone pneumonitis, 511–516
clinical and radiographic pattern,
512–514
clinical features, 512
diagnostic and therapeutic
management, 514–515
foam cells, *515*
mortality, 515
vacuolated macrophages, *515*
Amphiboles, 419
Amyloidoma
chest radiography, *878*
Amyloidosis
alveolar septal
chest radiography, *881*

ankylosing spondylitis, 579
diffuse alveolar septal, 879–880
HRCT, *880*
multinodular, *880*
nodular parenchymal, 878–879
primary
pulmonary hypertension in, *882*
pulmonary vascular, 880
respiratory tract, 877–880
presentation, *878*
with rheumatoid arthritis, 543
Sjögren's syndrome, 572
tracheobronchial, 877–878
ANA
coal workers' pneumoconiosis, 411
Anaphylatoxin, 189
ANCA. *See* Antineutrophil cytoplasmic
antibodies
Ancylostoma braziliense
eosinophilic pneumonia, 674–675
Ancylostoma duodenale
eosinophilic pneumonia, 676
Anemia, 8
Angioblastic lymphadenopathy, *832*
Angiocentric lymphoma, 832–834
chest radiograph, *833*
Angioimmunoblastic lymphadenopathy
(AILD), 831–832
Angiomyolipoma, *854*
kidney, *157*
Angiomyolipomas, 855–856
Angiotensin-converting enzyme inhibitor
(ACEI)-induced eosinophilic
pneumonia, 494
Angiotensin-converting enzyme inhibitors
(ACEI)
pulmonary fibrosis, 327
Animal models
extracellular matrix
lung injury, 279–280, *280*
Ankylosing spondylitis, 574–579
definition, 574–575
fibrocavitary disease, *578*
infectious complications, 578
interstitial lung disease, 575–577
malignancy, 579
obstructive lung disease, 579
pleuropulmonary manifestations,
575–579
respiratory muscle mobility, 577–578
Anopheles, 672
Anterior uveitis, *353*
Anthracosis, 402
Antibasement membrane antibodies
(ABMA), 8
Antibasement membrane antibody
disease. *See* Goodpasture's
syndrome
Anticoagulant-induced alveolar
hemorrhage, 508
Antigenic stimulus, 211

Antigens
hypersensitivity pneumonitis, 457–458
Antineutrophil cytoplasmic antibodies
(ANCA), 618–620
Churg-Strauss syndrome, 617, 668
clinical utility, 618–619
diffuse alveolar hemorrhage, 8, 632–633
methodology, 618
perinuclear, 614
target antigens, *615,* 618
terminology, *615,* 618
vasculitis pathogenesis, 619–620
Antinuclear factor (ANA)
coal workers' pneumoconiosis, 411
Antiphospholipid syndrome
pulmonary vasculitis associated with,
621
Antisense therapy
idiopathic pulmonary fibrosis, 744
Antitrypsin, 191
Anti-tumor growth factor- beta 1
(TGF-beta-1)
pulmonary fibrosis, 326
Arava
sarcoidosis, 317
ARDS. *See* Acute respiratory distress
syndromes
Arterial CO_2 tension ($PaCO_2$), 56
Arterial oxygen tension gradient ($P_{(A-a)}O_2$),
56
Arthralgia
sarcoidosis, 351
ASA-induced pulmonary edema, 506, 507
Asbestos, *423*
cell signal transduction pathways,
424–425
cellular and molecular effects,
422–425
characteristics, 418–419
lung epithelium, 422–423
RNS, 424
ROS, 423
Asbestos-induced lung disease
clinical aspects, 419–422
mechanisms, 425–429
Asbestos-induced pleural fibrosis, *421,*
421–422
Asbestosis, 15, *50,* 207
clinical aspects, 419–422
CT, *84,* 95–98
curvilinear subpleural line, 83
focal pulmonary masses, 97–98
HRCT, *86, 419*
mechanisms, 425–428
prognosis, 429
radiography, 96, *419*
smoking, 6
treatment, 429
Asbestosis model, 207
Asbestos-related disease, 387
BAL, 121

Ascaris
Churg-Strauss syndrome, 669
Ascaris lumbricoides, 674
Ascaris pneumonia, 674
Ascaris suum, 674
Ashkenazi Jews
Gaucher's disease, 882
Asians
sarcoidosis, 335
Takayasu's arteritis, 620
Aspergillus, 523
Churg-Strauss syndrome, 669
PAP, 868
pulmonary alveolar proteinosis, 168
sarcoidosis, 301
Aspergillus fumigatus, 677
ankylosing spondylitis, 578
Aspergillus umbrosus
hypersensitivity pneumonitis, 459
Aspergillus versicolor
hypersensitivity pneumonitis, 459
Aspiration
pediatric BAL, 143
Aspiration pneumonia
scleroderma, 559
Aspiration pneumonitis
polymyositis and dermatomyositis,
566–567
Asthma, 475
Churg-Strauss syndrome, 667–668
CT, *79*
eosinophils, 683
mimicking Wegener's granulomatosis,
603
Ataxia telangiectasia
eosinophils, 684
Atelectasis
rounded, 422
radiography, *422*
sarcoidosis
radiography, 357
in systemic lupus erythematosus, 553
Atomic Energy Commission
beryllium exposure limits, 436
ATRA, 505, 516
ATS/ERS classification
classification, 702–703
Auranofin-induced interstitial lung disease
(ILD), 518–519
Autoimmune disease
gastrointestinal, 896–898
hematologic, 895–896
interstitial lung disease, *3*
interstitial lung disease associations in,
895
Autoimmune hemolytic anemia, 895
Autoimmunity diseases, 895–898
Autologous bone marrow transplantation
interstitial pneumonitis after, 894–895
Avian albumin
hypersensitivity pneumonitis, 458

Avian antigens
hypersensitivity pneumonitis, 458
Avian gamma globulin
hypersensitivity pneumonitis, 458
Avian-related hypersensitivity
pneumonitis, 458
Azathioprine
acute lupus pneumonitis, 549
bronchiolitis obliterans syndrome, 805
idiopathic pulmonary fibrosis, 739–740
IIP, 717
interstitial lung disease
in rheumatoid arthritis, 541
sarcoidosis, 370
Wegener's granulomatosis, 612

BACC, 900–901, *901*
BAL, 120
chest radiograph, *902–903*
Bacille Calmette-Guerin (BCG)
complications of, 516
granulomatous pneumonitis, 889
Bacillus subtilis
hypersensitivity pneumonitis, 458
BAL. *See* Bronchoalveolar lavage
Basal lamina
exposure, 211
Basic fibroblast growth factor (bFGF),
254–255, 440
fibrosis, *255*
B cells, 200
BCG
complications of, 516
granulomatous pneumonitis, 889
BCNU
induced ILD, 6
CT, 101, *104*
toxicity, 516
Behcet's disease, 579–580, 621
diffuse alveolar hemorrhage, 634, 640
Belgium
beryllium, 436
BeLPT, 438
Beractant
idiopathic pulmonary fibrosis, 744
Berylliosis, 338
Beryllium
cutaneous contact, 436
diagnostic criteria, *436*
exposure, 436–437
standard, 436
immunopathogenesis, 438–440
lung cancer, 446
sensitization, 441
toxicology, 438–440
Beryllium disease, 339, 435–447
clinical features, 440–442
historic perspective, 435
pathology, 437–438
Beryllium lymphocyte proliferation test
(BeLPT), 438

Beta-agonist
shrinking lung syndrome, 553
Beta2-agonist-induced pulmonary edema,
506–507
Beta-glucosidase
Gaucher's disease, 164
BFGF, 254–255, 440
fibrosis, *255*
Bipolaris
allergic bronchopulmonary syndromes,
678
Bipolaris australiensis
eosinophilic pneumonia, 676
Bipolaris spicifera
eosinophilic pneumonia, 676
Bird fancier's lung
bronchiolitis obliterans, *797*
Birds. *See* Avian
Bleomycin
recurrent pneumothoraces, 860
Bleomycin-induced interstitial lung
disease (ILD), 485
CT, 100–101
dose-related toxicity, 494
HRCT, *101*
Bleomycin-induced lung fibrosis, 709
Bleomycin-induced lung injury, 279
Bleomycin-induced pulmonary fibrosis
IL-1ra, 248
Bleomycin lung, 516–518
BAL, 517
chest radiography, *517*
HRCT, *518*
incidence, 517
pulmonary metastases, *518*
Bleomycin model, 203–207
ameliorating fibrosis, 205–207
mechanisms of fibrosis, 204–205
mechanisms of injury, 203–204
Blood eosinophilia
Churg-Strauss syndrome, 668
tropical eosinophilia, 673
Blood tests
sarcoidosis, 363–365
BMPI, 161
BMPRII gene, 152
Bone marrow transplantation, 807–809
allogeneic
interstitial pneumonitis after,
893–894
autologous
interstitial pneumonitis after,
894–895
bronchiolitis obliterans, *809*
Bone marrow transplantation-induced
alveolar hemorrhage, 508–509
Bone marrow transplantation-induced
pulmonary edema, 505
Bone morphogenetic protein I (BMPI), 161
Bone morphogenetic protein receptor II
(BMPRII) gene, 152

BOOP. *See* Bronchiolitis obliterans organizing pneumonia
Bordetella pertussis, 798
Borellia burgdorferi
sarcoidosis, 301
Borg scale values, 69
Breast cancer
radiation-induced interstitial lung disease, 522
radiation-induced organizing pneumonia, 523
Bronchial biopsy
sarcoidosis, 362
Bronchial hyperreactivity, 475
Bronchiectasis
CT, *679*
HRCT, 106
with rheumatoid arthritis, 542
in systemic lupus erythematosus, 550
Bronchiolar disease
BAL, *793*
CT, 102–103
Bronchiolitis, 787–816
BAL, 793
chest imaging studies, 792–793
HRCT, 792–793
radiography, 792
classification, 788–790
clinical syndromes associated with, *789,* 793–799
CT, *84*
definition, 787–788
drug-induced, 809–811
drug-induced reactions associated with, *810*
eosinophilic, 683
epidemiology, 790–791
idiopathic forms, 799–800
infant
respiratory syncytial virus, 790
infants, 138
infectious causes, 798–799
inhalational exposures associated with, *794*
organ transplantation, 803–805
pathogenesis, 791–792
pediatric infectious, 798–799
postinfectious causes, *798*
proliferative, 789
radiologic classification, *790*
smoking, 6
smoking-related respiratory
CT, 102
in systemic lupus erythematosus, 550
Bronchiolitis obliterans
bird fancier's lung, *797*
chest radiography, *796*
children, 135
CT, 102
mixed obstructive-restrictive ventilatory deficit, 68

pediatric, 135 . *See also* Children.
photomicrograph, *796*
rheumatoid arthritis
CT, *105*
radiography, *105*
with rheumatoid arthritis, 542
Silo filler's disease, 795
Bronchiolitis obliterans organizing pneumonia (BOOP), *39,* 195, 682–683
BAL, 128
collagen, 278
extracellular matrix, *280*
HRCT, *764, 765*
photomicrograph, *792*
radiography, *12*
Bronchiolitis obliterans syndrome, 803–805
Bronchioloalveolar cell carcinoma (BACC), 900–901, *901*
BAL, 120
chest radiograph, *902–903*
Bronchoalveolar lavage (BAL), 19–20, 114–129
cell differentials, *126*
cellular patterns, *124, 125*
chronic eosinophilic pneumonia, 664
cigarette smoking, 118
coal workers' pneumoconiosis, 411
diagnosis
adjunct, 125–128
differential diagnosis, 118–125, *119*
diffuse parenchymal lung disease, 128–129
foamy macrophages, *121*
in healthy adults, 117–118
cell differentials, *118*
HRCT, 117
hypersensitivity pneumonitis, 454, *468,* 468–470
laboratory processing, 116–117
cell studies, 116–117
cytology interpretation, 117
soluble components, 117
new drug development, 129
NSIP *vs.* UIP, *128*
PAP, 869
pediatric
immunocompromised host, 143
technical principles, 115
prognosis, 129
rheumatoid arthritis, *540*
sarcoidosis, 360–362
silicosis, 395
technical principles, 114–117
bronchoscopic procedure, 114–115
children, 115
side effects, 115–116, *116*
tropical eosinophilia, 673
Bronchocentric granulomatosis, 679
ankylosing spondylitis, 578

Bronchodilator therapy
coal workers' pneumoconiosis, 413
Bronchogenic carcinoma
idiopathic pulmonary fibrosis, 746–747
scleroderma, 562
Bronchopneumonia
recurrent
Sjögren's syndrome, 572
Bronchopulmonary dysplasia
premature neonates, 135
Bronchoscopy
PAP, 869
Bronchospasm
BAL, *116*
Brugia malayi, 672
Budgerigars
hypersensitivity pneumonitis, 458
Butylated hydroxytoluene-oxygen, 209

Cadmium chloride, 208
Calcification
radiography, *17*
Canada
beryllium, 436
Candida albicans
allergic bronchopulmonary syndromes, 678
Candidate genes
sarcoidosis, 339–340
Capillaria aerophila
eosinophilic pneumonia, 676
Capillaritis, 38
Capillary hemangiomatosis, *647*
Caplan's syndrome
coal workers' pneumoconiosis, 410, 413
Captopril
idiopathic pulmonary fibrosis, 743
Carbamate-induced interstitial lung disease (ILD), 494
Carbamazepine-induced interstitial lung disease (ILD), 681
Carmustine (BCNU)
induced ILD, 6
CT, 101, *104*
toxicity, 516
Castleman's tumor, 815, *816*
Cathepsin G, 191, 192
Cavitary lung disease
Sjögren's syndrome, 572
Wegener's granulomatosis, 603–604
Cavitation
sarcoidosis
radiography, 357
CBD. *See* Chronic beryllium disease
CC chemokine, 263
pulmonary fibrosis, 264–266
sarcoidosis, 308
CC chemokine receptors, 263–264, *264*
Celiac disease, 896–897
differentiation from sarcoidosis, 355

Cellular bronchiolitis, 789
    CT, 102
    HRCT
        centrilobular thickening, 103, *106*
    micrography, *473*
    mycoplasma infection
        CT, *106*
Cellular interstitial pneumonia, 43
Cellular interstitial pneumonitis
    infants, 138
Cellulose, 208
Central nervous system
    sarcoidosis, 350
Centrilobular emphysema
    coal workers' pneumoconiosis, 409–410
    HRCT, *86*
Centrilobular nodules, *81*
Ceramics
    silicosis, 388
Chapel Hill nomenclature
    Churg-Strauss syndrome, 667
    microscopic polyangiitis, 614
    systemic vasculitis, 600, *600*
    Wegener's granulomatosis, 601–602
Chemokines, 257–263
    sarcoidosis, 308, 344
Chemoreceptors
    dyspnea, 65–66
Chemotactic cytokines, 257–266, *258*
    chemokines, 257–263
Chemotherapy lung, 501–504
    chest radiography, *503*
    histopathologic features, *504*
    HRCT, *504*
    incidence, 503–504
    risk factors, 501–502
    time to onset, 502
Chest pain, 7
Chest radiographs, 9–19
    alveolar opacities, 10–12
    interstitial opacities, 12–19
Chickenpox
    chest radiograph, *893*
Chickens
    hypersensitivity pneumonitis, 458
Children. *See also* Adolescent; Infants;
    Pediatric
    HRCT, 78, 106
    Swyer-James syndrome, *143*
    UIP, 136–137
China
    eosinophilic pneumonia, 676
Chlamydia
    pediatric interstitial lung disease, 135
Chlorambucil
    idiopathic pulmonary fibrosis, 743
    LIP, 829
    sarcoidosis, 370–371
Chlorine gas, 796
Chlorodeoxyadenosine
    PLCH, 846

Chloroquine
    lupus pernio, 349
    sarcoidosis, 354
Chronic air space diseases
    CT, 100
Chronic aspiration
    BAL, 124
Chronic aspiration pneumonitis
    mixed connective tissue disease, 574
Chronic beryllium disease (CBD), 435,
    439, 441–442
    diagnosis, 442–445
        BAL, 122, 442–443
        biologic samples, 444
        evaluation, 444–445
        imaging, 442
        laboratory abnormalities, 443–444
        lung biopsy, 444
    follow-up, 445–446
    immunopathogenesis, *437*
    natural history, 445
    prevention, 447
    pulmonary physiology, 442
    radiography, *443*
    signs and symptoms, 441–442
    surveillance, 446–447
    treatment, 445–446
Chronic bronchitis
    silicosis, 396
Chronic cough
    HRCT, 106
Chronic eosinophilic pneumonia, 660,
    661–665
    bronchiolitis, 811
    vs. Churg-Strauss syndrome, 617
    cutaneous mycosis fungoides, *684*
    eosinophilic alveolitis, *124*
Chronic hypersensitivity pneumonitis
    micrography, *474*
Chronic interstitial pneumonia, 549–550
Chronic lung disease
    with cyst formation or smooth muscle
        proliferation
        differential diagnosis, *859*
Chronic pneumonitis
    infants, 139
Chronic silicosis, 391
Churg-Strauss syndrome, 123, 615–618,
    667, 667–670, *668*
    ANCA, 617
    BAL, 668
    cause, 669
    clinical manifestations, 616–617
    diagnosis, 669
        criteria, 615–616
        differential, 616–617
    epidemiology, 616
    histopathologic features, *615*
    leukotriene receptor antagonists, 617
    organ involvement frequency, *614*
    pathogenesis, 617

    prognosis, 617–618
    pulmonary infiltrates, 668
    treatment, 617–618
    vs. Wegener granulomatosis, 669
Cigarette smoking
    BAL, 118
    idiopathic pulmonary fibrosis, *722*
    IIP, 706, *707*
    obstructive lung disease, 106
    PLCH, 840
    restrictive lung disease, 106
CIMDLs
    vs. Wegener's granulomatosis, 610–611
Circulating stem cells
    alveolar epithelial progenitors, 223–225
Clonorchis sinensis
    eosinophilic pneumonia, 676
Clopidogrel-induced alveolar hemorrhage,
    508
Closing volume, 56
Clubbing
    fingers, *711*
Coagulation disorders
    diffuse alveolar hemorrhage, 645
Coal
    characteristics, 403
    formation, 403
Coal mining, 403–404
Coal workers' pneumoconiosis (CWP),
    95, 402–414
    clinical features, 412–413
    epidemiology, 405–408
    histology, *409*
    history, 402–403
    HRCT, 95
    incidence, 407–408
    management, 413–414
    mortality, 408–409
    pathogenesis, 410–412
    pathology, 409–410
    prevalence, 407–408
    radiography, 411, 412
Cobalt pneumoconiosis
    anatomic distribution, 49
Cobblestoning
    Wegener's granulomatosis, 608–609
Cocaine
    Churg-Strauss syndrome, 669
Cocaine-induced midline destructive
    lesions (CIMDLs)
    vs. Wegener's granulomatosis, 610–611
Coccidioides immitis
    eosinophilic pneumonia, 676
Coesite, 387
Colchicine
    Behcet's disease, 580
    diffuse alveolar septal amyloidosis, 879
    idiopathic pulmonary fibrosis, 739
    IIP, 717–718
Collagen
    degradation, 192–193

scleroderma, 554, 556
synthesis
    interference, 328
Collagenase, 190, 192
    sarcoidosis, 365
Collagens, 277
Collagen vascular disease
    BAL, 128
    CT, *84*
Collagen vascular disease-associated
    interstitial lung disease (ILD)
    age, 6
Colony stimulating factors
    adverse effects, 518
    alveolar macrophages, 306–307
Community-acquired pneumonia
    vs. acute noninfectious interstitial
        pneumonia, 5
Complicated pneumoconiosis. *See*
    Progressive massive fibrosis
Computed radiography
    thorax, 75
Computed tomography (CT)
    normal patients, 79–80
Congenital alveolar proteinosis, 139–140
Congenital pulmonary alveolar proteinosis
    (PAP), 870–871
Conglomerate pneumoconiosis. *See*
    Progressive massive fibrosis
Conjunctiva
    sarcoidosis, 353
Conjunctivitis
    granulomatous, *353*
Connective tissue disease-related
    interstitial lung disease
    polymorphism, 175
Connective tissue diseases, 535–581
    BAL, *539*
    bronchiolitis, 800–802
    pleural lesions and effusions in,
        545–546
    pulmonary vasculitis associated with,
        621
Connective tissue growth factor, 255
    fibrosis, *255*
Constrictive bronchiolitis, 789–790
    CT, 102
    pathogenesis, 791
    pathologic and radiologic features, *791*
    photomicrograph, *792*
Contact dermatitis, 436
Continuous mining, 404
Coombs-positive hemolytic anemia, 896
COP. *See* Cryptogenic organizing
    pneumonia
Corticosteroids, 22
    acute eosinophilic pneumonia, 499
    acute lupus pneumonitis, 549
    amiodarone pneumonitis, 515
    Ascaris pneumonia, 674
    Behcet's disease, 580

bleomycin lung, 517–518
chronic beryllium disease, 446
chronic eosinophilic pneumonia,
    664–665
Churg-Strauss syndrome, 618, 670
COP, 765
diffuse alveolar septal amyloidosis, 879
eosinophilic pneumonia in larva
    migrans syndrome, 674
hypersensitivity pneumonitis, 476
idiopathic pulmonary fibrosis, 246,
    736–737
interstitial lung disease
    polymyositis and dermatomyositis,
        565
LIP, 829
lipoid pneumonia, 905
lupus pernio, 349
lymphomatoid granulomatosis,
    833–834
methotrexate lung, 520
pediatric interstitial lung disease, 145
PLCH, 846
relapsing polychondritis, 581
rheumatoid bronchiolitis, 802
rheumatoid pleural effusions, 546
sarcoidosis, 316, 355, 366–369
silicosis, 397
Silo filler's disease, 795
Sjögren's syndrome, 571
tuberculin skin test, 716
Corynebacterium pseudotuberculosis
    eosinophilic pneumonia, 677
Costovertebral ankylosis, 577
Cough, 7
Coumadin-induced alveolar hemorrhage,
    509
Crackles
    BAL, *116*
    hypersensitivity pneumonitis, 461
Crazy paving pattern
    HRCT
        diffuse parenchymal lung disease,
            87
    lipoid pneumonia, 903–904
    PAP, 868–869
CREST syndrome, 553, 557
Cricoarytenoid arthritis, 541–542
    ankylosing spondylitis, 578
Cricopharyngeal achalasia, 566–567
Cristobalite, 387
Crohn's disease
    differentiation from sarcoidosis, 355
Cryoglobulinemia
    diffuse alveolar hemorrhage, 641
Cryptococcus
    pulmonary alveolar proteinosis, 168
Cryptococcus albidus
    hypersensitivity pneumonitis, 459
Cryptococcus neoformans
    PAP, 868

Cryptogenic
    definition, 1
Cryptogenic adult bronchiolitis, 799–800
Cryptogenic bronchiolitis obliterans
    CT, 102, *105*
    radiologic classification, *104*
Cryptogenic constrictive bronchiolitis,
    801
Cryptogenic organizing pneumonia
    (COP), 90, 703, 758–765
    anatomic distribution, 48
    BAL, 759–760
    BOOP histology, *759*
    chest imaging studies, 760–762
        HRCT, 760–761, *763*
        radiography, 760, *761–762, 766*
    clinical findings, 759
    diagnosis, 763–765
    epidemiology, 759
    etiology, 759
    histopathologic findings, 763
    laboratory findings, 759
    management and outcome, 765
    migratory opacity
        HRCT, *92*
    physiological findings, 760
Cryptogenic pulmonary eosinophilia, 659
Cryptostroma corticale, 474
Culex, 672
Curvilinear subpleural line
    asbestosis, 83
Curvularia lunata
    allergic bronchopulmonary syndromes,
        678
Cutaneous mycosis fungoides
    chronic eosinophilic pneumonia, *684*
Cutaneous sarcoidosis, 348
CWP. *See* Coal workers' pneumoconiosis
CXC chemokine receptors, 259–260, *260*
CXC chemokines, 258–259
    angiogenic activity, *259*
    pulmonary fibrosis, 260–261
    sarcoidosis, 308
CyA
    AILD, 832
    LIP, 830
    sarcoidosis, 317, 371
Cyclophosphamide
    acute lupus pneumonitis, 549
    Behcet's disease, 580
    Churg-Strauss syndrome, 618
    idiopathic pulmonary fibrosis, 129,
        739
    IIP, 716–717
    interstitial lung disease
        in rheumatoid arthritis, 541
    LIP, 829
    lymphomatoid granulomatosis,
        833–834
    microscopic polyangiitis, 615
    pediatric interstitial lung disease, 145

PLCH, 846
pulmonary vascular disorders in
    scleroderma, 560
rheumatoid bronchiolitis, 802
toxicity, 611–612
Wegener's granulomatosis, 611, 612
Cyclophosphamide-induced interstitial
    lung disease (ILD), 518
CT, 101
Cyclosporin
Behcet's disease, 580
pediatric interstitial lung disease, 145
Cyclosporin A (CyA)
AILD, 832
LIP, 830
sarcoidosis, 317, 371
Cyclosporine
bronchiolitis obliterans syndrome, 805
idiopathic pulmonary fibrosis,
    743–744
interstitial lung disease
    in rheumatoid arthritis, 541
Cystic lung disease
CT, 98–99
Cysts
HRCT
    diffuse parenchymal lung disease,
        84–85
Cytokines, 245–267
extracellular matrix, 283–284
fibroblast, 315–316
growth factors, 253–255
matrix components, 316
sarcoidosis, 343–344
scleroderma, 556
Cytomegalovirus
IIP, 707
pediatric interstitial lung disease, 135
Cytomegalovirus pneumonia, 125

DAD, 635, 635
diffuse alveolar hemorrhage, 645–646
DAH. See Diffuse alveolar hemorrhage
Decorin
pulmonary fibrosis, 326
Deflazacort
for sarcoidosis, 352
Delayed pulmonary toxicity syndrome,
    502
Delayed-type hypersensitivity skin tests
sarcoidosis, 363
15-deoxyspergualin
sarcoidosis, 317
Dermatomyositis. See also Polymyositis
    and dermatomyositis
chest roentgenogram, 567
survival, 567
Desquamative interstitial pneumonia
    (DIP), 37–38, 41–42, 42, 753–771
BAL, 754
chest imaging, 754

HRCT, 754
    radiography, 754, 755–756
children, 137
    prognosis, 145
clinical findings, 754
CT, 84, 90
epidemiology, 753–754
etiology, 753–754
histologic findings, 754–755
management and outcome, 755
patchy ground-glass opacity
    HRCT, 91
pediatric, 137
    prognosis, 145
physiological findings, 754
radiography, 12
Desquamative interstitial pneumonitis
familial
    infants, 140
DHSS, 497
Diabetes mellitus, 888–889
Diaphragmatic dysfunction
in systemic lupus erythematosus,
    552–553
Dietary food supplement-induced
    interstitial lung disease (ILD), 494
Diethylcarbamazine
tropical eosinophilia, 674
Diffuse alveolar damage (DAD), 635, 635
diffuse alveolar hemorrhage, 645–646
Diffuse alveolar filling
acute silicosis, 394
Diffuse alveolar hemorrhage (DAH),
    632–647
acute lung allograft rejection, 641
acute pulmonary syndrome, 640
ANCA, 632–633
Behcet's disease, 640
bland alveolar hemorrhage, 633
cause, 633
clinical presentation, 635–637
coagulation disorders, 645
cryoglobulinemia, 641
diagnosis, 637–638
diffuse alveolar damage, 645–646
fibrillary glomerulonephritis, 647
Goodpasture's syndrome, 641–643
Henoch-Schonlein purpura, 640
histology, 632–633
idiopathic pulmonary hemosiderosis,
    643–644
immunoglobulin A nephropathy, 640
isolated pulmonary capillaritis, 639
lymphangioleiomyomatosis, 646
malignancy, 647
microscopic polyangiitis, 638–639
mitral stenosis, 644–645
obstructive sleep apnea, 647
penicillamine, 644
polymyositis and dermatomyositis,
    567

primary antiphospholipid syndrome,
    640
pulmonary capillaritis, 641
pulmonary capillary hemangiomatosis,
    647
pulmonary veno-occlusive disease,
    646–647
pyromellitic dianhydride, 644
revolving phase, 633
syndromes
    anemia, 8
    BAL, 119–120, 120
systemic lupus erythematosus, 639–640
trimellitic anhydride, 644
tuberous sclerosis, 646
Wegener's granulomatosis, 638
Diffuse alveolar septal amyloidosis,
    879–880
Diffuse panbronchiolitis, 789–790,
    812–814
chest radiograph, 813
CT, 814
radiologic classification, 104
with rheumatoid arthritis, 542
Diffuse parenchymal lung disease. See also
    Interstitial lung disease
BAL, 128, 128–129
chest radiographs, 75–76
    pattern recognition, 80–88
CT, 77–79
HRCT, 77–79
    pattern recognition, 81–82
magnetic resonance, 79
nuclear, 76–77
surgical lung biopsy, 21
Diffuse pulmonary disease
anatomic distribution, 31–35, 32
    angiocentric, 32
    bronchocentric/bronchiolocentric,
        32, 33
    diffuse interstitial infiltrates,
        34–35, 36
    lymphatic, 32–33, 33
    nodular, 34
    parenchymal consolidation, 34, 35
    peripheral acinar, 33–34, 34
    pleural, 32
    septal, 34
Diffusion capacity (DL$_{co}$), 56, 65
asbestosis, 97
measurement, 69
sarcoidosis, 359
silicosis, 397
Digital clubbing, 8
Dimethyl sulfoxide (DMSO)
diffuse alveolar septal amyloidosis,
    879–880
DIP. See Desquamative interstitial
    pneumonia
Dirofilaria immitis
eosinophilic pneumonia, 676

DKC1 gene, 174
DL$_{co}$, 56, 65
    asbestosis, 97
    measurement, 69
    sarcoidosis, 359
    silicosis, 397
DMSO
    diffuse alveolar septal amyloidosis,
        879–880
Double negative (CD4-CD8-) alpha beta+
    T cells, 199–200
Doxycycline
    recurrent pneumothoraces, 860
D-penicillamine
    pulmonary vascular disorders in
        scleroderma, 560–561
DRESS, 497
Drug-induced acute respiratory distress
    syndromes (ARDS), *514*
Drug-induced alveolar hemorrhage, 508
Drug-induced alveolitis
    patterns, 496
Drug-induced angiitis, *510*
Drug-induced antisynthetase syndrome,
    511
Drug-induced bronchiolitis, 809–811
Drug-induced cellular pneumonitis
    patterns, 496
Drug-induced Churg-Strauss syndrome,
    509–510
Drug-induced eosinophilic pneumonia,
    496–500, 679–682, *681*
Drug-induced hypersensitivity
    pneumonitis
    patterns, 496
Drug-induced hypersensitivity syndrome
    (DHSS), 497
Drug-induced interstitial lung disease
    (ILD), *2, 6,* 485–524
    BAL, *127*
    CT, 100–101
    diagnostic criteria, 495–496
    patterns of, *486–493,* 496–511
    risk factors, 494
Drug-induced lung disease
    ankylosing spondylitis, 579
    polymyositis and dermatomyositis,
        567
    rheumatoid arthritis, 544
Drug-induced organizing pneumonia
    connective tissue, *502*
    opacity, *501*
    patterns, 500–501
Drug-induced pneumonitis
    alveolar hemorrhage, 508
    BAL, 127
Drug-induced polyarteritis, 509
Drug-induced polymyalgia, 511
Drug-induced polymyositis, 511
Drug-induced pulmonary edema,
    505–508

Drug-induced pulmonary fibrosis,
    504–505
Drug-induced pulmonary infiltrate (PIE),
    496–500
Drug-induced pulmonary vasculitis, 509
Drug-induced pulmonary veno-occlusive
    disease, 510
Drug-induced systemic lupus
    erythematosus (SLE), 510–511
    infiltrates, *511*
Drug-induced thrombocytopenia
    alveolar hemorrhage, 508
Drug-induced transient pulmonary
    infiltrate (PIE), 505
Drug-induced Wegener's granulomatosis,
    509
Drug-rash and eosinophilia systemic
    syndrome (DRESS), 497
Ducks
    hypersensitivity pneumonitis, 458
Dust exposure
    coal workers' pneumoconiosis, 405–406
    IIP, 706–707
Dust masks
    hypersensitivity pneumonitis, 476
Dyspnea, 7
    chemoreceptors, 65–66
    exertional, 64–66
    mechanisms, 64–66
    slopes, 69
Dysproteinemia, 826

Early response proinflammatory cytokines,
    247–251
    IL-1, 247–249
    tumor necrosis factor-alpha, 249–251
EBV
    idiopathic pulmonary fibrosis, 892
    IIP, 707
    LIP, 826
    pediatric interstitial lung disease, 135
ECG
    sarcoidosis, 351, 366
Echocardiography
    sarcoidosis, 366
EELV, 61
EGF, *226,* 229–230
Eicosanoid, 232
EILV, 60
Elastase, 190, 191
Elastin, 277
    digestion, 190
Elderly
    amiodarone pneumonitis, 512
Electrocardiogram (ECG)
    sarcoidosis, 351, 366
Embolization
    Behcet's disease, 621
Emphysema, 16
    coal workers' pneumoconiosis,
        409–410

HRCT, 106, *106*
    silica, 95
End-expiratory lung volume (EELV), 61
End-inspiratory lung volume (EILV), 60
Endobronchial brachytherapy
    adverse effects, 523–524
Endobronchial laser ablation
    tracheobronchial amyloidosis, 878
Endomyocardial biopsy
    sarcoidosis, *363*
Endothelin
    pulmonary fibrosis, 327
End-stage renal disease
    renal transplantation, 613
    silicosis, 397
Environmental exposure
    interstitial lung disease, *3*
Eosinophilia-myalgia syndrome
    L-tryptophan, 681
Eosinophilia pneumonia
    malignancies, 683–684
Eosinophilic bronchiolitis, 683
Eosinophilic bronchitis, 683
Eosinophilic granuloma
    age, 6
    smoking, 6
Eosinophilic lung disease, 657–658
    BAL, 122–123
Eosinophilic-myalgia syndrome
    L-tryptophan-induced, 511, 681
Eosinophilic pneumonia, 657–685
    acebutolol-induced
        infiltrate, *500*
    acute
        HRCT, *101*
    anatomic distribution, 48
    Ancylostoma braziliense, 674–675
    Ancylostoma duodenale, 676
    angiotensin-converting enzyme
        inhibitor (ACEI)-induced, 494
    chest radiography, *83*
    chronic, 660, 661–665
        bronchiolitis, 811
        vs. Churg-Strauss syndrome, 617
        cutaneous mycosis fungoides, *684*
        eosinophilic alveolitis, *124*
    classification, 658–659, *659*
    CT, *84*
    definition, 658
    of determined origin, 672–676
    diagnostic criteria, 658
    drug-induced, 496–500, 679–682, *681*
    heroin-induced
        chest radiography, *682*
    HRCT, *500*
    idiopathic, 661–667
    idiopathic acute, 660–661, 665–667
        chest radiograph, *666*
    idiopathic chronic, *657, 660*
        chest radiograph, *662–663*
    in larva migrans syndrome, 674–675

L-tryptophan-induced, 496
l-tryptophan-induced, 496
minocycline-induced, 680
    chest radiography, *499*
Necator americanus, 676
NSAID-induced, 494
of parasitic origin, 672–676
pathology, 659–661
radiography, *12*
of undetermined origin, 661–672
Eosinophils, 192
Epithelial cells
    factors, *224*
    fibroblast growth, 231–233
    injury
        basal lamina exposure, 211
        wound healing and remodeling,
            233–236
Epithelial growth factors (EGF), *226,*
    229–230
Epithelioid cell granulomas
    sarcoidosis, 347
Epstein-Barr virus (EBV)
    idiopathic pulmonary fibrosis, 892
    IIP, 707
    LIP, 826
    pediatric interstitial lung disease, 135
Erdheim-Chester disease, 884
Ergoline-induced pleural fibrosis, 494
ERV, 60
Erythema nodosum
    disease associations with, *348*
    sarcoidosis, 348
Erythrocyte sedimentation
    chronic eosinophilic pneumonia, 663
    hypersensitivity pneumonitis, 467
Erythromycin
    COP, 765
    rheumatoid bronchiolitis, 802
Etanercept
    idiopathic pulmonary fibrosis, 744
    Wegener's granulomatosis, 612
Ethnicity
    pulmonary vasculitis, 601
Etoposide
    PLCH, 846
Eurotium amstelodami
    hypersensitivity pneumonitis, 459
Exercise
    cardiovascular responses to, 61–62
    intolerance, 62
    neurogenic mechanisms, 59
    pathophysiology, *57–58,* 57–64
    ventilatory responses to, 57–61
Exercise electrocardiogram (ECG)
    sarcoidosis, 366
Exercise-induced hypoxemia, 59
Exercise testing
    clinical utility, 68, *68*
Exertional dyspnea, 64–66, *65*
Expiratory reserve volume (ERV), 60

Expiratory timing (TE), 60
Extracellular matrix, 276–293
    animal models
        lung injury, 279–280, *280*
    biologic effects, 284–286
    cell functions, 284–286, *285*
    cellular origin, 282–283
    clinical implications, 290–292
    cytokines, 283–284
    destruction, 288–290
    distribution, *281*
    healthy adult lungs, 277
    human lung disease, *279*
    interstitial lung disease, 277–279
        mechanisms, 282–284
    receptors, 286–287
    schematic representation, *278*
Extrapulmonary
        lymphangioleiomyomatosis
    and angiomyolipomas
        pathology, 853
    treatment, 860–861
Extrinsic allergic alveolitis. *See*
    Hypersensitivity pneumonitis

Fabry's disease, 173–174, 883–884
Familial desquamative interstitial
        pneumonitis
    infants, 139, *140*
Familial hypocalciuric hypercalemia
        (FHH), 172–173
    cellular basis, 172
    genetic basis, 172
    murine models, 172–173
Familial idiopathic pulmonary fibrosis
        (IPF), 174
Familial pulmonary fibrosis
    chest radiography, *708*
Familial sarcoidosis, 174
Family history, 7
Farmer's lung
    Japan, 460
    prevalence, 459
    thermophilic actinomycetes, 474
    treatment, 476
Fauci classification
    pulmonary vasculitis, 599
FBN1, 170
FEF, 55
Felty's syndrome
    veno-occlusive disease in, 544
FEV, 63
FEV1
    CWP, 404
    pediatric interstitial lung disease, 142
    silicosis, 393
Fever
    BAL, *116*
FEV1/FVC ratio, 55, 67
    pediatric interstitial lung disease, 142
    silicosis, 393

FGF, 226–229, *227*
    collagen synthesis, 197–198
    epithelium, 231–233
FHH, 172–173
    cellular basis, 172
    genetic basis, 172
    murine models, 172–173
Fibers
    mineralogic classification, *419*
Fibrillary glomerulonephritis
    diffuse alveolar hemorrhage, 647
Fibrillin gene (FBN1), 170
Fibroblast growth factors (FGF),
        226–229, *227*
    collagen synthesis, 197–198
    epithelium, 231–233
Fibroblasts, 315
    collagen breakdown, 193
    cytokines, 315–316
    scleroderma, 556
    TGF-beta, 256
    TNF-alpha, 250
Fibrobullous disease
    with rheumatoid arthritis, 543
Fibronectin, 277
    digestion, 190
Fibrosing alveolitis, 562
    children
        prognosis, 145
Fibrosis
    bFGF, *255*
    connective tissue growth factor, *255*
    HRCT, 75
    IL-1, *248*
    ILGF-I, *254*
    PDGF, *253*
    TGF-beta, *256*
    TNF-alpha, *250*
Fibrotic cytokines, 255–257
15-deoxyspergualin
    sarcoidosis, 317
Finches
    hypersensitivity pneumonitis, 458
Fingers
    clubbing, *711*
Firefighters
    sarcoidosis, 338
FITC, 201
FK506
    Behcet's disease, 580
Fleischner Society, 82
Flow-volume curves, *63*
Fluid instillation
    BAL, 115
Fluid recovery
    BAL, 115
Fluorescein isothiocyanate (FITC), 201
Fluorescent light factories
    sarcoidosis, 338
Focal pulmonary masses
    asbestosis, 97–98

Follicular bronchiolitis, 789
    rheumatoid arthritis, 802–803, *804*
    with rheumatoid arthritis, 542
Follicular bronchitis
    infants, 138
Forced expiratory flow (FEF), 55
Forced expiratory volume (FEV), 63
Forced expiratory volume in 1 second
        (FEV1)
    CWP, 404
    pediatric interstitial lung disease, 142
    silicosis, 393
Forced expiratory volume in 1
        second/forced vital capacity
        (FEV1/FVC) ratio, 55, 67
    pediatric interstitial lung disease, 142
    silicosis, 393
Forced vital capacity (FVC)
    asbestosis, 97
    CWP, 404
    pediatric interstitial lung disease, 142
Foundry work
    silicosis, 387–388, 390
France
    beryllium, 436
Franconi's disease
    Sjögren's syndrome, 569
FRC, 55
    pediatric interstitial lung disease, 142
FRC/TLC
    pediatric interstitial lung disease, 142
Functional residual capacity (FRC), 55
    pediatric interstitial lung disease, 142
Functional residual capacity /total lung
        capacity (FRC/TLC)
    pediatric interstitial lung disease, 142
Fusarium vasinfectum
    allergic bronchopulmonary syndromes,
        678
FVC
    asbestosis, 97
    CWP, 404
    pediatric interstitial lung disease, 142

Galactosidase A
    Fabry's disease, 884
Gallium 67 lung scan
    chronic eosinophilic pneumonia, 663
    idiopathic pulmonary fibrosis, *713*
Gallium scans
    hypersensitivity pneumonitis, 466
    sarcoidosis, 358, *360*
Gamma delta resident pulmonary
        lymphocytes, 199–200
Gamma delta T cells
    colonization, 200
Gamma globulin
    pediatric interstitial lung disease,
        144–145
Gas exchange
    abnormalities, 56–57

histiocytosis X, 67–68
    idiopathic pulmonary fibrosis,
        67–68
    impaired diffusion, 56–57
    right-to-left shunting, 57
    sarcoidosis, 67–68
    ventilation-perfusion inequalities,
        57
Gastroesophageal reflex (GERD), 6
    idiopathic pulmonary fibrosis, 747
Gastrointestinal autoimmune disease,
        896–898
Gaucher's cells
    electron micrograph, *163*
    light micrograph, *162*
Gaucher's disease, 152, 162–164, 882–883
    age, 6
    animal model, 163
    clinical presentation, 163
    genetic basis, 162–163
    lung, *164*
    physiological abnormalities, 163–164
    radiographic abnormalities, 163–164
    treatment, 164
Gauley Bridge Tunnel, 387
Gelatinase, 192
Gender, 6
    sarcoidosis, 334–335
    Takayasu's arteritis, 620
Genetics, 152–178
    extrapulmonary
        lymphangioleiomyomatosis, 861
    Fabry's disease, 173–174
    familial hypocalciuric hypercalcemia,
        172–173
    future directions, 176–178
    IIP, 707–709
    lipoid proteinosis, 173
    metabolic pulmonary disease, 162–170
    PAM, 173
    pulmonary fibrosis, 175–176
    pulmonary matrix disorders, 170
    sarcoidosis, 302–303, 339–340
    scleroderma, 553–554
    surfactant protein-C mutations,
        160–162
    tumor suppressor syndromes, 153–160
GERD, 6
    idiopathic pulmonary fibrosis, 747
Germany
    beryllium, 436
Giant cell arteritis, 620
    incidence, 600–601
Giant cell interstitial pneumonia, *50*
    anatomic distribution, 49
Glomerulonephritis
    idiopathic
        diffuse alveolar hemorrhage, 641
GM-CSF, 152, 191
    PAP, 869
    pediatric interstitial lung disease, 145

GM1 gangliosidosis, 167
GnRH agonists, 158
Gold
    bronchiolitis associated with, 809–810
Golde score, 119, *121*
Gold-induced interstitial lung disease
        (ILD), 518–519
Gold lung, 518–519
Gonadotropin releasing hormone (GnRH)
        agonists, 158
Goodpasture's syndrome, 637, *637*
    diffuse alveolar hemorrhage, 634,
        641–643
    mimicking Wegener's granulomatosis,
        604–605
    smoking, 6
Graft-*versus*-host disease (GVHD), 894
Granulocyte-macrophage colony-
        stimulating factor (GM-CSF), 152,
        191
    PAP, 869
    pediatric interstitial lung disease, 145
Granuloma formation, *347, 347*–348
    sarcoidosis, 309–312
        immune regulation, 310–314
Granulomatous conjunctivitis, *353*
Granulomatous inflammation
    in rheumatoid arthritis, 541
Granulomatous interstitial lung disease
        (ILD)
    polymorphism, 175
Granulomatous interstitial pneumonia
    etiology, 44
Granulomatous interstitial pneumonitis,
        473
Granulomatous lung disease
    causes, *367*
Granulomatous nephritis, 354
Granulomatous pneumonitis
    Bacille Calmette-Guerin, 889
Growth factors, 253–255
    sarcoidosis, 344
Guillain-Barre syndrome
    sarcoidosis resembling, 350
GVHD, 894

Halfuginone
    pulmonary fibrosis, 328
Hamartin gene (TSC1), 153, 155
Hamman-Rich syndrome, 5, 701
Hand-Schuller-Christian disease, 838
Hard metal (cobalt) pneumoconiosis
    anatomic distribution, 49
Hard metal lung disease
    BAL, 122
Hashimoto-Pritzker disease, 838
Hashimoto's thyroiditis, 897
Health professionals
    sarcoidosis, 338
Heart
    coal workers' pneumoconiosis, 413

Heart failure
   idiopathic pulmonary fibrosis, 746
Heart-lung transplantation, 805–807
   bronchiolitis obliterans, *806*
Heerfordt's syndrome, 353
Helminthosporium
   allergic bronchopulmonary syndromes,
      678
Hematologic autoimmune disease,
      895–896
Hemodynamic instability, 745
Hemoptysis, 7
   HRCT, 106
Henoch-Schonlein purpura
   diffuse alveolar hemorrhage, 633, 640
Heparin growth factor (HGF), 230–231,
      231
Hepatitis C
   idiopathic pulmonary fibrosis, 892
   IIP, 707
Hepatocellular carcinoma
   radiation pneumonitis, *524*
Herb-induced interstitial lung disease
      (ILD), 494
Hereditary surfactant protein B deficiency,
      870–871
Hermansky-Pudlak syndrome, 152,
      164–167, 884
   clinical presentation, 166
   electron micrography, *165*
   family history, 7
   genetic basis, 164–165
   genotype-phenotype, 166
   HRCT, *166*
   macrophages, *165*
Heroin-induced eosinophilic pneumonia
   chest radiography, *682*
Heroin-induced pulmonary edema,
      505
HGF, 230–231, 231
High-resolution computed tomography
      (HRCT), 9–10, 19, 51
   asbestosis, 419, *419*
   BAL, 117
   children, 78, 106
   clinical applications, 103–107
   clinical indications for, *106*
   differential diagnosis
      anatomical distribution, *82*
   diffuse parenchymal lung disease,
      77–79
      anatomic distribution, 81–88
   fibrosis, 75
   idiopathic pulmonary fibrosis
      honeycomb, *83*
   silicosis, 394
Hilar lymph nodes
   enlargement, 394
      radiography, *394*
Histamine
   rheumatoid arthritis, 539

Histiocytosis X
   anatomic distribution, 48
   gas exchange abnormalities, 67–68
Histoplasma capsulatum
   pulmonary alveolar proteinosis, 168
HIV
   NSIP, 892
HIV-I
   LIP, 826
HLA-DR
   epithelial expression, 222
HLA-DR14
   sarcoidosis, 339–340
HLA-DR15
   sarcoidosis, 339–340
HMG-CoA reductase inhibitors
   pulmonary fibrosis, 327
Hodgkin's disease
   radiation
      paramediastinal fibrosis following,
         523
   radiation-induced interstitial lung
      disease, 522
   radiography, *11, 18*
Hodgkin's lymphoma, 518
Honeycomb
   UIP, *324*
Honeycomb lung
   defined, 85
   idiopathic pulmonary fibrosis, *729*
      HRCT, *83*
   radiography, *15*
   usual interstitial pneumonia, *41*
Host factors
   inflammatory response, 303–309
Host promoting factor, 455
Hot tub lung, 44
24-hour electrocardiogram (ECG)
   sarcoidosis, 366
HRCT. *See* High-resolution computed
      tomography
HTLV-I
   LIP, 826
Human T-cell leukemia virus type I
      (HTLV-I)
   LIP, 826
Hyalinosis cutis et mucosae, 173
Hydrochlorothiazide-induced pulmonary
      edema, 507
   time to onset, 495
Hydroxychloroquine
   interstitial lung disease
      in rheumatoid arthritis, 541
   pediatric interstitial lung disease, 145
   sarcoidosis, 354, 369, 372
3-hydroxy-3-methylglutaryl (HMG)-CoA
      reductase inhibitors
   pulmonary fibrosis, 327
Hypercalciuria, 354
Hypereosinophilic syndrome
   vs. Churg-Strauss syndrome, 617

Hyperinflation
   radiography, *17*
Hypersensitivity chronic bronchitis
   vs. hypersensitivity pneumonitis,
      461–462
Hypersensitivity pneumonitis, 5, *46, 439,*
      452–477, 475
   acute, 461
      vs. chronic, 462
      differential diagnosis, 470
      HRCT, *84*
   acute progressive (subacute)
      differential diagnosis, 470–471
      micrography, *473*
   adolescent
      CT, *136*
      radiography, *136*
   anatomic distribution, 48
   antigens, 457–458
   avian-related, 458
   BAL, 126, 454, *468,* 468–470
   bird antigens, 458
   chronic, 461
      micrography, *474*
      radiography, *85, 99*
   clinical features, 460–462
   CT, *84,* 98, 463–465, *464*
   differential diagnosis, *471*
   drug-induced
      patterns, 496
   etiologic agents, *453–454*
   fungi, 458–459
   ground-glass attenuation, 464
   histology, 473–475
   historical background, 452–454
   HRCT, *463*
   vs. hypersensitivity chronic bronchitis,
      461–462
   vs. idiopathic pulmonary fibrosis, 6
   inhalation challenge, 471–472
   laboratory tests, 467–468
   lung biopsy, 472
   lymphocytic alveolitis, *124*
   moldy hay, 457–458
   MRI, *465,* 465–466
   neutrophils, *469*
   pathogenesis, 454–457, *455*
   pigeon fanciers, 459–460
   prevalence, 459–460
   prognosis, 476–477
   pulmonary circulation, 467
   pulmonary function tests, 466–467
   radiography, *18,* 98, 462–463, *462–463*
   scintigraphic studies, 466
   smoking, 460
   subacute, 461
   summer-type
      Japan, 460
   survival, 476–477
   thermophilic actinomycetes, 457–458
   treatment, 475–476

Hypersensitivity pneumonitis2 locus, 165
Hypocalciuric hypercalcemia
  interstitial lung disease, 884–885
Hypovolemia, 745
Hypoxemia
  coal workers' pneumoconiosis, 413
  diffuse alveolar hemorrhage, 637
  exercise-induced, 59
  idiopathic acute eosinophilic
    pneumonia, 666

IAEP, 660–661, 665–667
  chest radiograph, *666*
IBD, 896
IC, 55
ICAM-1, 456
Idiopathic
  definition, 1
Idiopathic acute eosinophilic pneumonia
    (IAEP), 660–661, 665–667
  chest radiograph, *666*
Idiopathic bronchiolitis obliterans
    organizing pneumonia (BOOP). *See*
    Cryptogenic organizing pneumonia
Idiopathic chronic eosinophilic
    pneumonia, *657, 660*
  chest radiograph, *662–663*
Idiopathic eosinophilic pneumonia,
    661–667
Idiopathic glomerulonephritis
  diffuse alveolar hemorrhage, 641
Idiopathic hypereosinophilic syndrome,
    670–672
Idiopathic interstitial pneumonia (IIP),
    160, 701–771
  age, 6
  BAL, 710
  chest imaging studies, 710–714
    gallium 67 lung scan, 712–713,
      713
    HRCT, 712
    radiography, 710–711
  classification, *702*
  clinical manifestations, 710, *710*
  contrasting pathologic features, *703*
  CT, 88–91
  diagnosis, 704–705
  diffuse lung diseases mimicking
    distinguishing features of, 704–705
  distinguishing clinical features, *706*
  environmental and occupational
    exposure, 706–707
  eosinophils, 683
  epidemiology, 703–704
  genetic factors, 707–709
  histopathologic diagnosis, *721*
  historical perspective, 701
  inflammatory, fibrotic and immune
    processes, 709–710
  interstitial lung disease, *3, 5*
  pathogenesis, 705–710

physiological testing, 710
radiography, *89*
redefining pathologic classification,
    701–703
smoking, 6
surgical lung biopsy, 713–714
treatment, 714–720
  azathioprine, 717
  colchicine, 717–718
  corticosteroids, 714–716
  cyclophosphamide, 716–717
  cyclosporine, 718
  lung transplantation, 719–720
  methotrexate, 718
  patient selection, 714
  penicillamine, 718
  response assessment, 719
viral factors, 707
Idiopathic pneumonia syndrome, 502
Idiopathic pulmonary alveolar proteinosis
    (PAP), 867–870
  clinical manifestations, 868
  diagnosis, 868–869
  epidemiology, 867
  etiology, 867
  histology, 867–868
  pathogenesis, 867
Idiopathic pulmonary fibrosis (IPF)
  acute exacerbation, 744–745
  anatomic distribution, 47
  BAL, 127, 723–724
  cardiovascular disease, 746
  clinical findings, 722–723
  collagen
    degradation dysregulation,
      193–194
    synthesis, 194–195
  corticosteroids, 246
  CT
    accuracy, *731*
  diagnosis, *736*
    confirmation, 734
  diffuse coarse reticular, *729*
  disease progression, *719*
  electron micrography, *187*
  epidemiology, 720–722
  Epstein-Barr virus, 892
  etiology, 721–722
  familial, 174
  fibrosis, *210*
  gallium 67 lung scan, *713*
  gas exchange, 725
    abnormalities, 67–68
  HCV, 892
  histopathology, 730–731
    and physiology, 731–732
      quantitative assessment, 731
    and survival, 733–734
  honeycombing, *729*
  HRCT, *83, 106,* 729–730
  hyperexpanded, *729*

vs. hypersensitivity pneumonitis, 6
infants, 139
inflammation, 246
laboratory findings, 723
lung imaging studies, 727–730
  HRCT, 727–730
  radioaerosol studies, 730
  radiography, 727
  ventilation and perfusion
    scintiphotography, 730
lung volumes, 725
management and outcome, 734–736,
    738–739
  assessment, *744*
  ATS/ERS recommendations,
    744–745
mimicking hypersensitivity
    pneumonitis, 461
mortality
  cause, *745*
natural history, 734
neutrophilic alveolitis, *124*
pathogenesis, 721–722
physiological findings, 724–725
progressive
  risk factors, 747–748
pulmonary hemodynamics, 726
pulmonary infection, 746
pulmonary physical rehabilitation, 746
radiography, *16*
sleep disturbance, 726–727
smoking, 68, *722*
survival, 747–748
  CRP scoring, *748*
usual interstitial pneumonia, 40
Idiopathic pulmonary hemosiderosis
  diffuse alveolar hemorrhage, 643–644
Idiopathic thrombocytopenic purpura
    (ITP), 895
IFN alpha
  Churg-Strauss syndrome, 670
  pediatric interstitial lung disease, 145
IFN-beta1
  idiopathic pulmonary fibrosis, 743
IFN-gamma. *See* Interferon-gamma
IgA
  coal workers' pneumoconiosis, 411
  deficiency, 872
  hypersensitivity pneumonitis, 458
  nephropathy, 633
    diffuse alveolar hemorrhage, 640
  silicosis, 396
IgE
  tropical eosinophilia, 673
IgG
  coal workers' pneumoconiosis, 411
  hypersensitivity pneumonitis, 467
  silicosis, 396
IIP. *See* Idiopathic interstitial pneumonia
IL-1, 247–249
  alveolar macrophages, 306

fibrosis, *248*
lymphocytes, 189
IL-2
    host factors, 304
IL-4
    host factors, 304
IL-6
    alveolar macrophages, 306
    hypersensitivity pneumonitis, 455
IL-8
    bronchiolitis, 791
    neutrophils, 189
    scleroderma, 556
IL-9
    host factors, 304
IL-10, 253
    host factors, 304
IL-12
    alveolar macrophages, 306
IL-13
    host factors, 304–305
IL-15
    alveolar macrophages, 306
IL-17
    host factors, 305
IL-18
    alveolar macrophages, 306
IL-8/CSCL8, 261–262
ILD. *See* Interstitial lung disease
ILO
    classification
        silicosis, 393
    criteria, 95
IL-2R
    sarcoidosis, 365
IL-2 receptor (IL-2R)
    sarcoidosis, 365
Immune complexes
    scleroderma, 556
Immune granulomas
    sarcoidosis, 347
Immune-mediated model, 208
Immunocompromised host
    pediatric BAL, 143
Immunoglobulins. *See* Ig
Immunoglobulins (IVIG)-induced
    pulmonary edema, 507
Immunosuppressive drugs
    bronchiolitis obliterans syndrome, 805
    relapsing polychondritis, 581
    Sjögren's syndrome, 571
Inducing factor, 455
Industrial bronchitis
    coal workers' pneumoconiosis, 405
Industries
    using beryllium, *435*
Infants
    acute idiopathic pulmonary
        hemorrhage, 138–139
    bronchiolitis
        respiratory syncytial virus, 790

cellular interstitial pneumonitis, 138
chronic pneumonitis, 139
familial desquamative interstitial
    pneumonitis, 139, *140*
follicular bronchitis, 138
idiopathic pulmonary fibrosis, 139
interstitial lung disease
    unique forms, *135*, 135–141
lipoid pneumonia, *135*
NEHI
    prognosis, 145
pulmonary vascular disorders,
    140–141
surfactant protein abnormalities,
    139–140
Infection-associated pulmonary alveolar
    proteinosis (PAP), 871
Infectious bronchiolitis
    in adults, 799
    children, 798–799
Infiltrative lung disease
    differential diagnosis
        chest radiography, *80*
        lobule evaluation, *81*
Inflammation, 187–211
    eosinophils, 192
    idiopathic pulmonary fibrosis, 246
    lymphocytes, 198–202
    macrophages, 192
    neutrophils, 190–192
Inflammatory bowel disease (IBD), 896
Inflammatory pseudotumor
    trachea, *605*
Inflammatory response
    host factors, 303–309
Infliximab
    idiopathic pulmonary fibrosis, 744
    Wegener's granulomatosis, 612
Influenza
    pediatric interstitial lung disease, 135
Inhalational lung injury
    bronchiolitis secondary to, 793–799
Inhalation challenge
    hypersensitivity pneumonitis,
        471–472
Inhalation provocation test
    diagnosis, 472
    hypersensitivity pneumonitis, *471*
Inhaled steroids
    hypersensitivity pneumonitis, 476
Inspiratory capacity (IC), 55
Inspiratory timing (TI), 60
Insulin-like growth factor-I, 254
    collagen synthesis, 196–197
    fibrosis, *254*
Integrins, 286
    receptor, *287*
    signaling pathway, 287
    signal transduction, *288*
Intercellular adhesion molecule (ICAM)-
    1, 456

Interferon alpha (IFN alpha)
    Churg-Strauss syndrome, 670
    pediatric interstitial lung disease, 145
Interferon-beta1 (IFN-beta1)
    idiopathic pulmonary fibrosis, 743
Interferon-gamma (IFN-gamma)
    BAL, 129
    host factors, 305
    idiopathic pulmonary fibrosis,
        739–742
    pulmonary fibrosis, 326
    sarcoidosis, 365
Interferon-induced interstitial lung disease
    (ILD), 519
Interleukin. *See* IL
International Labor Office (ILO)
    classification
        silicosis, 393
    criteria, 95
Interstitial fibrosis
    alveolar cells, 188–189
    animal models, 201–209
    HRCT, 106
    inflammatory cells, 188–189
    usual interstitial pneumonia, *41*
Interstitial infiltrates
    radiography, *15*
Interstitial lung disease (ILD)
    associated genetic polymorphisms,
        174–175
    characterization of, 104–105
    children, 4
    classification, 2–4
        collagen vascular disease associated,
            1
        drug and treatment-induced, *2*
        histologic, *3–4*
        idiopathic interstitial pneumonia
            and autoimmune disease, *3*
        occupational and environmental
            exposure related, *3*
        primary or unclassified disease
            related, *2*
    clinical evaluation, 5–21
        history, 5–7
        laboratory investigation, 8
        physical examination, 8
        physiologic testing, 8–9
        radiographic features, 9–19, *16*
        respiratory symptoms and signs,
            7–8
    clinicopathologic correlation, 46–47
    drugs causing
        patterns of, *486–493*
    epidemiology, 4–5
    following aspiration, 880–882
    following pulmonary infection,
        891–893
    follow-up, 22–23
    HRCT
        early detection, 103–104

idiopathic interstitial pneumonia, 5
laboratory results, *9*
morphologic clues, *47*
naturally occurring murine models, 175–176
normal biopsy, 46, *47*
pathogenesis, 5, 245–267
pathology correlated with radiology, 47
peripheral predominance, 82
physiology, 54–70
   clinical utility, 66–70
   differential diagnosis, 67–68
   exercise pathophysiology, *57–58,*
     57–64
   gas exchange abnormalities, 56–57
   prognosis, 69–70
   pulmonary mechanics, 54–56
   therapy, 68–69
quantification, 105–106
radiation-induced, 522
   dose-related toxicity, 494
   incidence, 494
reaction patterns, *36,* 36–45
   alveolar hemorrhage, 37–38, *38*
   bronchiolitis obliterans organizing
     pneumonia, *39,* 39–40
   cellular interstitial infiltrates, 41–45
   desquamative interstitial
     pneumonia, 41–42, *42*
   diffuse alveolar damage, 36–37, *37*
   granulomatous inflammation,
     44–45
   interstitial fibrosis, 40–41
rheumatoid arthritis, 4
rodenticide-induced, 494
sarcoidosis, 4
scleroderma, 4
systemic signs, *8*
thioglucose-induced, 518–519
thiomalate-induced, 518–519
treatment, 22–23
Interstitial nodules
   radiography, *13–14, 14*
Interstitial pneumonia
   animal models, 162
   definition, 1
   genetic basis, 161–162
Interstitial pneumonitis
   acebutolol-induced, *498*
   after transplantation, 893–895
   cellular
     infants, 138
   familial desquamative
     infants, 139
   granulomatous, 473
   lymphocytic, *825*
     child
       radiography, *138*
     children, 137
   lymphoid
     CT, *84,* 91

methotrexate-induced
   granuloma, *498*
   HRCT, *498*
   pediatric lymphocytic, 137
   radiography, *138*
Interstitial pulmonary edema
   mitral valve disease, *82*
Interstitial pulmonary fibrosis (IPF)
   Epstein-Barr virus, 892
   HCV, 892
Intravenous gammaglobulin
   pediatric interstitial lung disease, 145
Intravenous immunoglobulin
   Wegener's granulomatosis, 612
IPF. *See* Idiopathic pulmonary fibrosis
Ischemic heart disease
   idiopathic pulmonary fibrosis, 746
Isolated pulmonary capillaritis
   diffuse alveolar hemorrhage, 639
Isovolume pressure-flow, 56
Israel
   beryllium, 436
   sarcoidosis, 335
ITP, 895
IVIG-induced pulmonary edema, 507

Japan
   beryllium, 436
   Farmer's lung, 460
   sarcoidosis, 335
   summer-type hypersensitivity
     pneumonitis, 460
Juvenile chronic arthritis
   sarcoidosis mimicking, 352
Juxtacapillary receptors, 66

Kaolinite, 387
Katzenstein and Meyers classification
   idiopathic interstitial pneumonia,
     702
Kazhakstan
   beryllium, 436
Keratinocyte growth factor (KGF), 199,
   231
   VgVd 1 murine T cells, 199
Keratoconjunctivitis
   Sjögren's syndrome, 569
Kerley's B lines, 13
Ketoconazole
   sarcoidosis, 354, 371
KGF, 199, 231
   VgVd 1 murine T cells, 199
Kidney
   angiomyolipoma, *157*
Klebsiella, 538
Knockout mice, 209
Kveim-Siltzbach test
   development, 332
   sarcoidosis, 302
Kveim test
   sarcoidosis, 363

Lacrimal glands
   sarcoidosis, 353
Lactate dehydrogenase (LDH)
   amiodarone pneumonitis, 514
   hypersensitivity pneumonitis, 467
LAM. *See* Lymphangioleiomyomatosis
Laminin, 277
Langerhans cell histiocytosis, *49*
   BAL, 123
   classification, *838*
   CT, *84*
   eosinophils, 683
   HRCT, 98–99
Larva migrans syndrome
   eosinophilic pneumonia in, 674–675
Laryngeal sarcoidosis, 347
Lavage lymphocytosis, 361
LDH
   amiodarone pneumonitis, 514
   hypersensitivity pneumonitis, 467
Leflunomide (Arava)
   sarcoidosis, 317
Legionella, 5
Legionella pneumophilia pneumonia, 893
Leptomeninges
   sarcoidosis, 350
Lethal neonatal hyperparathyroidism
   (LNH), 172
Letterer-Siwe disease, 838
Leukocytes, 188
   adhesion, 189
   deformability, 188–189
   injurious potential, 188–189
Leukocytoclastic vasculitis, *607*
Leukocytosis, 8
Leukotriene B4 (LTB4)
   neutrophils, 189
Leukotriene inhibitors-induced
   pulmonary infiltrate (PIE), 496
LH-RH agonist
   pulmonary
     lymphangioleiomyomatosis, 860
Lidocaine-induced transient pulmonary
   infiltrates (PIE), *506*
Liebow and Carrington classification
   idiopathic interstitial pneumonia, 701
Lines
   HRCT
     diffuse parenchymal lung disease, 83
LIP. *See* Lymphocytic interstitial
   pneumonia
Lipoid pneumonia, 901–905, *903*
   BAL, 20
   chest radiograph, *904*
   clinical picture, 902–904
   CT, *103*
   diagnosis, 904
   histology, 902
   infant, *135*
   radiography, *103*
   treatment and prognosis, 905

Lipoid proteinosis, 173
Lipopolysaccharide (LPS), 190
Lisch nodule, 887
Liver biopsy
    sarcoidosis, 362
Liver function tests
    sarcoidosis, 364
LNH, 172
Loa loa
    eosinophilic pneumonia, 676
Löffler's syndrome, 659, 676
Löfgren's syndrome, 372
Long-wall mines, 404–405
Lovastatin
    idiopathic pulmonary fibrosis, 744
LPI, 169, 871, 888
LPS, 190
L-selectin
    neutrophils, 189
LTB4
    neutrophils, 189
L-tryptophan-induced eosinophilic-
    myalgia syndrome, 511, 681
L-tryptophan-induced eosinophilic
    pneumonia, 496
Lumber industry
    sarcoidosis, 338
Lung
    development, 225–231
    epithelial-mesenchymal interactions
        mediation, 225–226
    fibroblast growth factors, 227–229
    inflammation
        genetic manipulation, 176
    injury
        events triggered, *291*
        and repair, *277, 278*
    repair, *224*
        epithelial-mesenchymal
            interactions, 225–233
    static expiratory pressure-volume
        curve, 54
Lung allografts
    lymphangioleiomyomatosis, 158
    rejection
        acute, 641
Lung attenuation
    HRCT
        diffuse parenchymal lung disease, 87
Lung biopsy, 21
    hypersensitivity pneumonitis, 472
Lung cancer
    beryllium, 446
    idiopathic pulmonary fibrosis,
        746–747
    radiation-induced, 523
    radiation-induced interstitial lung
        disease, 522
    silicosis, 396
Lung disease
    CT, *84*

Lung epithelium
    asbestos, 422–423
Lung fibrosis. *See also* Pulmonary fibrosis
    unclassifiable, *714*
Lung function tests
    chronic eosinophilic pneumonia, 664
    tropical eosinophilia, 673
Lung injury
    immune activation, 314–315
Lung transplantation
    allogeneic single
        chronic beryllium disease, 446
    bronchiolitis, 803
    bronchiolitis obliterans syndrome
        staging system, *805*
    congenital PAP, 871
    IIP, 719–720
    lymphangioleiomyomatosis, 158
    pediatric interstitial lung disease, 145
    PLCH, 846–847
    recipient selection guidelines, *720*
Lupus pernio, *349*
    sarcoidosis, 348
Lupus pneumonitis
    acute, 548–550
Luteinizing hormone-releasing hormone
    (LH-RH) agonist
    pulmonary
        lymphangioleiomyomatosis, 860
Lymphangioleiomyomatosis (LAM), 152,
    851–862
    age, 6
    anatomic distribution, 50–51
    and angiomyolipomas
        pathology, 853
    cell accumulation, 156
    cell biology, *852*
    clinical manifestations, 854–857
        angiomyolipomas, 855–856
        extrapulmonary, 855
        pulmonary, 854–856
        tuberous sclerosis complex, 856
    clinical presentation, 156–157
    CT, *84, 99*
    diagnosis, 858–859
    differential diagnosis, 156–157
    diffuse alveolar hemorrhage, 646
    electron microscopy, 854
    epidemiology, 851
    etiology, 851–852
    extrapulmonary
        and angiomyolipomas
            pathology, 853
        treatment, 860–861
    genetic basis, 154–155
    histologic characteristics, *853*
    imaging studies, 856–857
        abdominopelvic, 856
        chest radiography, *857*
        lung, 856
    immunohistochemistry, 853–854

laboratory tests, 856
lung allografts, 158
lung transplantation, 158
natural history and prognosis, *861,*
    861–862
pathogenesis, *855*
pathologic, radiologic, and physiologic
    correlation, 858
pathology, 852–854
    extrapulmonary
        lymphangioleiomyomatosis and
        angiomyolipomas, 853
    lung, 852–853
pulmonary cyst, 156
pulmonary function tests, 857–858
radiography, 15
treatment, 157–158, 859–861,
    860–861
Lymphangiomyomatosis
    HRCT, *86*
Lymphangitic carcinoma, 885–886
    anatomic distribution, 50
    chest radiograph, *885–886*
Lymphangitic carcinomatosis
    BAL, 120
    compute tomography, 94
    HRCT, *85*
    radiography, *15*
Lymph node calcification, 884–885
    sarcoidosis
        radiography, 357
Lymphocytes, 198–202
    gamma delta resident pulmonary,
        199–200
    IL-1, 189
    pulmonary fibrosis
        animal models, 200–201
    sarcoidosis, 341–342
Lymphocytic interstitial pneumonia (LIP),
    825, *825,* 826
    chest radiograph, *827–828*
    children, 137
        radiography, *138*
    clinical presentation, 826–828
    conversion to beta-cell lymphoma,
        829
    CT, *828*
    disease associations, *827*
    etiology, 826
    malignant infiltrates differentiation
        from, *829*
    pathogenesis, 830
    prognosis, 829–830
    in rheumatoid arthritis, 540
    treatment, 829–830
Lymphocytic T-helper predominant
    alveolitis, 438
Lymphoid interstitial pneumonitis
    CT, *84,* 91
Lymphoid tissue
    sarcoidosis, 347

Lymphokines
  sarcoidosis, 344
Lymphomatoid granulomatosis, 832–834
  chest radiograph, *833*
Lysinuric protein intolerance (LPI), 169,
    871, 888

Macrophage inflammatory protein 1alpha
    (MIP-1alpha)
  scleroderma, 556
Macrophages, 192
  coal workers' pneumoconiosis, 411
  collagen degradation, 192–193
Macrophages-T-cell
  granuloma formation, 310–312
Malignancy-associated pulmonary alveolar
    proteinosis (PAP), 871–872
Malignant disease
  BAL, 120–121
Malignant histiocytosis
  bronchiolitis, 811
Malignant lymphoma
  anatomic distribution, 50
Man-made mineral fibers (MMMF), 419
Mansonia, 672
Mantle irradiation
  thoracic changes, *522*
Marfan syndrome, 170
  biochemical basis, 170
  gene identification, 170
Matrix metalloproteinase (MMP), 288,
    289
  idiopathic pulmonary fibrosis, *194*
Matrix metalloproteinase-1 (MMP)-1, 193
Matrix metalloproteinase-3 (MMP-3), 193
Matrix metalloproteinase-9 (MMP-9), 193
Maximal voluntary ventilation (MVV), 63
MEA, 172
Mechanical ventilation
  AIP, 771
  introduction, 746
Mediastinal lymphadenopathy
  HRCT
    diffuse parenchymal lung disease, 88
Mediastinal lymphoma
  radiation
    paramediastinal fibrosis following,
      523
Mediastinoscopy
  sarcoidosis, 362
Medroxyprogesterone
  pulmonary
    lymphangioleiomyomatosis, 860
Melkersson-Rosenthal syndrome, 349
Melphalan
  diffuse alveolar septal amyloidosis, 879
Mercury
  self-injection, 485
Metabolic acidosis, 59
Metabolic disorders
  genetic basis, *171*

Metabolic pulmonary disease, 162–170
  Gaucher's disease, 152, 162–164
    age, 6
  GM1 gangliosidosis, 167
  Hermansky-Pudlak syndrome, 152,
    164–167
    family history, 7
  lysinuric protein intolerance, 169
  Niemann-Pick disease, 152, 167
  pulmonary alveolar proteinosis, *51*,
    167–169
    BAL, 119, *120*
    CT, *84*, 100
    ground-glass opacity
      HRCT, *101*
  SP-B mutations, 169–170
Metal miners
  silicosis, 390
Metastatic cancer
  CT, *84*
Metastatic pulmonary calcification
  chest radiograph, *898*
Methotrexate
  acute lupus pneumonitis, 549
  IIP, 718
  interstitial lung disease
    in rheumatoid arthritis, 541
  lupus pernio, 349
  pediatric interstitial lung disease, 145
  PLCH, 846
  sarcoidosis, 316–317, 369–370, 372
  Wegener's granulomatosis, 612
Methotrexate-induced acute
    hypersensitivity pneumonitis, 494
Methotrexate-induced interstitial lung
    disease (ILD), 485
  CT, 101
Methotrexate-induced interstitial
    pneumonitis
  granuloma, *498*
  HRCT, *498*
Methotrexate-induced pneumonitis,
    519–520
  chest radiography, *497*
  with rheumatoid arthritis, 544
Methotrexate lung, 519–520
Metschnikowia pulcherrima
  ankylosing spondylitis, 578
Micronodular pneumocyte hyperplasia
    (MMPH), 160
Microscopic polyangiitis (MPA), 613–615
  diffuse alveolar hemorrhage, 638–639
  incidence, 600
  organ involvement frequency, *614*
Mikulicz's syndrome, 353
Miliary granulomatous infections, *35*
Miliary nodules
  radiography, *13*
Mineral dusts, 797
Miners
  silicosis, 391

Miners' asthma, 402
Miners' black lung, 402
Mining
  silicosis, 387
Minocycline-induced eosinophilic
    pneumonia, 680
  chest radiography, *499*
Minocycline-induced pulmonary infiltrate
    (PIE), 494
MIP-1alpha
  scleroderma, 556
Mitomycin-induced alveolar hemorrhage,
    508
Mitomycin-induced hemolytic uremic
    syndrome, 520–521
Mitomycin-induced interstitial lung
    disease (ILD), 485
Mitomycin-induced pulmonary fibrosis
  basilar changes, *506*
Mitomycin lung, 520–521
Mitomycin pneumonitis, 520
Mitral stenosis
  diffuse alveolar hemorrhage, 644–645
Mitral valve disease
  interstitial pulmonary edema, *82*
Mixed connective tissue disease, 572–574
  chest roentgenogram, *575*
  definition, 572–573
  HRCT, *576*
  interstitial lung disease, 573
  obstructive lung disease, 573–574
  pleuropulmonary manifestations,
    573–574, *574*
  respiratory response to exercise, *577*
Mixed cryoglobulinemia, 896
Mixed dust pneumoconiosis
  BAL, 121–122
Mixed interstitial alveolar infiltrates
  chest radiograph, *883*
MMMF, 419
MMP, 288, *289*
  idiopathic pulmonary fibrosis, *194*
MMP-1, 193
MMP-3, 193
MMP-9, 193
MMPH, 160
Moldy hay
  hypersensitivity pneumonitis, 457–458
Monoclonal antibodies
  BAL, 129
Monocrotaline, 209
Monocyte chemoattractant protein, 231
Monocyte chemotactic peptide-1, 189
  scleroderma, 556
Monocyte-macrophage
    compartmentalization
  granuloma formation, 310
Monokines
  sarcoidosis, 343–344
Mononuclear phagocytes
  sarcoidosis, 342–343

Morquio's syndrome, 167
Mosaic pattern
    HRCT
        diffuse parenchymal lung disease,
            87
Mouth
    sarcoid plaques, *349*
MPA, 613–615
    diffuse alveolar hemorrhage, 638–639
    incidence, 600
    organ involvement frequency, *614*
(99mTc-)diethylenetriamine pentaacetate
        (DTPA), 423
    epithelial permeability scanning
        sarcoidosis, 359
    hypersensitivity pneumonitis, 466
Mucin
    hypersensitivity pneumonitis, 458
Mucor
    PAP, 868
Multinodular amyloidosis, *880*
Multiple endocrine adenomatosis (MEA),
        172
MVV, 63
Myasthenia gravis, 897
Mycobacterium avium-intracellulare, 35, 44
    hypersensitivity pneumonitis, 459
Mycobacterium bovis, 516
Mycobacterium chelonae
    CT, *677*
Mycobacterium hominis
    sarcoidosis, 333
Mycobacterium simiae
    eosinophilic pneumonia, 677
Mycobacterium tuberculosis
    pulmonary alveolar proteinosis, 168
    sarcoidosis, 301, 333
Mycophenolate mofetil
    sarcoidosis, 317
Mycoplasma, 5
    pediatric interstitial lung disease, 135
Mycoplasma infection
    cellular bronchiolitis
        CT, *106*
Mycoplasma pneumoniae, 470, 893
Mycosis fungoides
    cutaneous
        chronic eosinophilic pneumonia,
            684
Myofibroblast, 282

N-acetylcysteine
    idiopathic pulmonary fibrosis, 743
    pulmonary fibrosis, 328
Necator americanus
    eosinophilic pneumonia, 676
Necrotizing angiitis
    Zeek classification, 599
Necrotizing sarcoid granulomatosis,
        621–622
NEHI, 135–136

prognosis, 145
Nephritis
    granulomatous, 354
Neuroendocrine cell hyperplasia of
        infancy (NEHI), 135–136
    prognosis, 145
Neurofibromatosis, 158–160, 886–888
    chest radiograph, *888*
    family history, 7
    pulmonary presentation, 160
    thoracic manifestations, *889*
Neurofibromatosis 1 (NF1), 158–160
    animal models, 159
    molecular basis, 159
Neurofibromatosis 2 (NF2), 158–160
    animal models, 159–160
    molecular basis, 159
Neuromechanical coupling, *66*
Neurosarcoidosis, 349–350
    MRI, *350*
    treatment, 373
Neutrophils, 188, 190–192
    attraction, *189*
    hypersensitivity pneumonitis, *469*
    IL-8, 189
    leukotriene B4, 189
    L-selectin, 189
    rheumatoid arthritis, 539
New drug development
    BAL, 129
NF1, 158–160
    animal models, 159
    molecular basis, 159
NF2, 158–160
    animal models, 159–160
    molecular basis, 159
NF-kb, 287
Niemann-Pick disease, 152, 167, 883
    clinical presentation, 167
    genetic basis, 167
    molecular basis, 167
    murine models, 167
    pathologic presentation, 167
    radiographic presentation, 167
Nitric oxide
    idiopathic pulmonary fibrosis, 743
Nitrofurantoin-induced interstitial lung
        disease (ILD), 485
    incidence, 494
Nitrofurantoin lung, 521
Nitrogen dioxide, 793–796
    accidental exposure, *795*
Nitrosourea-induced interstitial lung
        disease (ILD)
    dose-related toxicity, 494
    incidence, 494
Nitrous fume poisoning, 793
Nocardia
    pulmonary alveolar proteinosis, 168
    sarcoidosis, 301, 333
    Wegener's granulomatosis, 604

Nocardia asteroides
    PAP, 868
Nodular parenchymal amyloidosis,
        878–879
Non-Hodgkin's lymphoma
    radiation-induced interstitial lung
        disease, 522
Noninfectious interstitial pneumonia
    vs. community-acquired pneumonia, 5
    radiography, *6*
Nonpulmonary sarcoidosis
    treatment, *368*
Nonspecific interstitial pneumonia
        (NSIP), 42–45, *43,* 748–753
    AIDS, 892
    anatomic distribution, 47
    BAL, *128, 712,* 751
    clinical findings, 749–751, *750*
    CT, *84,* 88–90
    epidemiology, 749
    etiology, 749
    exercise testing, *751*
    histopathologic findings, 751–752
    HIV, 892
    lung imaging studies, 751
        HRCT, 751
        radiography, 751
    management and outcome, 752–753
    mortality, 43, *44*
    physiological findings, 751
    progressive systemic sclerosis
        HRCT, *90*
    scleroderma, 559
Nonsteroidal antiinflammatory drugs
        (NSAID)
    Löfgren's syndrome, 372
Nonsteroidal antiinflammatory drugs
        (NSAID)-induced asthma, 494
Nonsteroidal antiinflammatory drugs
        (NSAID)-induced eosinophilic
        pneumonia, 494
Nose
    sarcoid plaques, *349*
NSAID
    Löfgren's syndrome, 372
NSAID-induced asthma, 494
NSAID-induced eosinophilic pneumonia,
        494
NSIP. *See* Nonspecific interstitial
        pneumonia
Nuclear factor-kb (NF-kb), 287
Nuclear imaging
    diffuse parenchymal lung disease, 76–77

Obliterative bronchiolitis
    pulmonary vascular remodeling,
        801–802
Obstructive lung disease
    cigarette smoking, 106
Obstructive sleep apnea
    diffuse alveolar hemorrhage, 647

Occupational exposure
   beryllium, *435*
   silica, 387–388
Occupational interstitial lung disease
   (ILD), *3, 6*
Ocular sarcoidosis, 353
ODC
   asbestos, 424
   signal transduction
      oncogene expression, 425
ODTS, 470
Open lung biopsy
   lymphangioleiomyomatosis, 858
Ophthalmologic review
   sarcoidosis, 366
Opportunistic infections
   BAL, 124–25
Organic dusts, 797
Organic dust toxic syndrome (ODTS),
   470
Organizing pneumonia. *See also*
   Bronchiolitis obliterans organizing
      pneumonia
   ankylosing spondylitis, 578–579
   CT, 90, *764*
   drug-induced, 501–502
   vs. fibroblast foci
      morphological differences, *723*
   HRCT, *502*
   polymyositis and dermatomyositis,
      566
   radiation-induced
      breast cancer, 523
   in rheumatoid arthritis, 540–541
Ornithine decarboxylase (ODC)
   asbestos, 424
   signal transduction
      oncogene expression, 425
OSHA
   beryllium exposure limits, 436
Osteopenia, 352
Osteoporosis, 352–353
   Wegener's granulomatosis, 611
Ovarian hyperstimulation syndrome
   with pulmonary edema, 507
Oxygen
   paraquat model, 207
Oxygen therapy
   inducing pulmonary infiltrates, 494

PAM, 173, 898–900, *899*
   chest radiograph, *900*
Panbronchiolitis
   CT, 102–103
   diffuse, 789–790, 812–814
      with rheumatoid arthritis, 542
Pancreatic sarcoid masses
   mimicking adenocarcinoma, 355
Panlobular emphysema
   CT, *84*
Panlobular ground-glass attenuation, 81, *82*

PAP. *See* Pulmonary alveolar proteinosis
Papillary adenomas
   type II pneumocytes, 160
Paragonimus westermani
   eosinophilic pneumonia, 676
Parakeets
   hypersensitivity pneumonitis, 458
Paramediastinal fibrosis
   radiation-induced, 523
Paraneoplastic pemphigus, 815–816
Paraquat-induced interstitial lung disease
   (ILD), 494
Paraquat model, 207
Parenchymal opacification
   HRCT
      diffuse parenchymal lung disease,
         87
Partial pressure arterial oxygen (PaO2)
   silicosis, 397
Parvovirus, 135
PDGF, 232, 253–255
   alveolar macrophages, 307
   fibrosis, *253*
Pediatric bronchiolitis obliterans, 135. *See
   also* Children
Pediatric bronchoalveolar lavage (BAL)
   immunocompromised host, 143
   technical principles, 115
Pediatric desquamative interstitial
      pneumonia (DIP), 137
   prognosis, 145
Pediatric fibrosing alveolitis
   prognosis, 145
Pediatric infectious bronchiolitis, 798–799
Pediatric interstitial lung disease (ILD), 4,
      134–146
   BAL, 143–144
   classification, 134–141
   clinical presentation, 141
   deaths, *145*
   diagnosis, 141–144, *142*
   HRCT, 142–143
   infection, 135
   of known etiology, *134,* 134–136
      aspiration, 134–135
   lung biopsy, 144
   physical findings, *141*
   prognosis, 145–146
   pulmonary function tests, 142
   severity of illness
      classification, *142*
      prognosis, *145*
   symptoms, *141*
   treatment, 144–145
   of unknown etiology, *134,* 136–137
Pediatric lymphocytic interstitial
      pneumonitis, 137
   radiography, *138*
Penicillamine
   idiopathic pulmonary fibrosis, 743
   IIP, 718

interstitial lung disease
   in rheumatoid arthritis, 541
Penicillamine-associated bronchiolitis
   obliterans, 810
Penicillamine-induced alveolar
   hemorrhage, 509
Penicillamine-induced Goodpasture's
   syndrome, 644
Penicillium citreonigrum
   hypersensitivity pneumonitis, 459
Penicillum brevicoompactum, 476
Percutaneous liver biopsy
   sarcoidosis, 363
Perinuclear antineutrophil cytoplasmic
   antibodies (ANCA), 614
Peripheral blood counts
   sarcoidosis, 363
Peripheral eosinophilia, 8
Peripheral neuropathy
   idiopathic pulmonary fibrosis, 897
Persistent tachypnea of infancy (PTI),
   135–136, 138
Phenytoin-induced alveolar hemorrhage,
   508
Phenytoin-induced pulmonary vasculitis,
   681
Photophobia
   Sjögren's syndrome, 569
Phthisis, 402
Physiologic deadspace, 57–59
PIE
   diagnosis, 498
   drug-induced, 496–500
Pigeon breeder's lung, 460
Pigeon fanciers
   hypersensitivity pneumonitis,
      459–460
Pirfenidone
   idiopathic pulmonary fibrosis, *742,*
      742–743
   pulmonary fibrosis, 326–327
Pituitary gland
   sarcoid mass
      CT, *351*
Plant dust-induced (Scadding's) fibrosing
   alveolitis, 208
Plant-induced interstitial lung disease, 494
Plasma cell interseptal pneumonia (PIP),
   830–831
Plasmodium vivax, 260
Platelet-derived growth factors (PDGF),
   232, 253–255
   alveolar macrophages, 307
   fibrosis, *253*
PLCH. *See* Pulmonary Langerhans cell
   histiocytosis
Plethysmography, 55–56
Pleural abnormalities
   HRCT
      diffuse parenchymal lung disease,
         86

Pleural disease
    ankylosing spondylitis, 578
    polymyositis and dermatomyositis, 568
    sarcoidosis
        radiography, 356–357
    scleroderma, 562
    Sjögren's syndrome, 572
Pleural fibrosis
    mechanisms, 429–429
Pleural mesothelioma
    radiation-induced, 523
Pleurisy
    mixed connective tissue disease, 574
PMF, 391. See also Coal workers'
        pneumoconiosis
    coal workers' pneumoconiosis, 410
    conglomerate silicosis, 392
Pneumoconiosis, 388. See Coal workers'
        pneumoconiosis
    BAL, 121–122, 122
    CT, 95
    hard metal (cobalt)
        anatomic distribution, 49
Pneumocystis carinii
    eosinophilic pneumonia, 676
    PAP, 868
    pneumonia
        AILD, 832
        Wegener's granulomatosis, 612
    pulmonary alveolar proteinosis, 168
Pneumonia
    definition, 1
    pulmonary alveolar proteinosis
        mimicking, 168
Pneumonitis
    definition, 1
Pneumothorax, 15
    coal workers' pneumoconiosis, 414
    idiopathic pulmonary fibrosis, 746
    sarcoidosis
        radiography, 357
Pneumotox
    web site, 495
Polyarteritis
    drug-induced, 509
Polychondritis
    relapsing, 580–581, 611
Polymyalgia
    drug-induced, 511
Polymyositis
    chest roentgenogram, 566
    drug-induced, 511
    pulmonary vasculitis associated with,
        621
Polymyositis and dermatomyositis,
        562–568
    chest roentgenogram, 568
    classification, 563
    definition, 562–563
    interstitial lung disease, 563–566
        BAL, 565

clinical features, 564
    epidemiology, 563–564
    frequency, 565
    histopathologic findings, 565
    laboratory findings, 564
    pathogenesis, 564
    physiologic testing, 565
    prognosis and management,
        565–566
    roentgenographic findings, 564
    malignancy with, 568
    pleuropulmonary manifestations,
        563–568, 564
Polyvinyl pyridine N-oxide (PVNO)
    silicosis, 397
Prednisone
    bronchiolitis obliterans syndrome, 805
    COP, 765
    microscopic polyangiitis, 615
    pulmonary vascular disorders in
        scleroderma, 560
    rheumatoid bronchiolitis, 802
    Wegener's granulomatosis, 611
Pregnancy
    sarcoidosis, 355
Premature neonates
    bronchopulmonary dysplasia, 135
Primary amyloidosis
    pulmonary hypertension in, 882
Primary antiphospholipid syndrome
    diffuse alveolar hemorrhage, 640
Primary biliary cirrhosis, 897
Primary diffuse hyperplasia
    pulmonary neuroendocrine cells,
        814–815
Primary pulmonary plasmacytomas, 831
Progesterone
    lymphangioleiomyomatosis, 157–158
Programmed cell death
    sarcoid granuloma, 313–314
Progressive massive fibrosis (PMF), 391.
        See also Coal workers'
        pneumoconiosis
    coal workers' pneumoconiosis, 410
    conglomerate silicosis, 392
Progressive systemic sclerosis (PSS),
        553–562. See Scleroderma
    nonspecific interstitial pneumonia
        HRCT, 90
Proliferative bronchiolitis, 789
Promoting factor, 455
Propionibacterium acnes
    sarcoidosis, 301
Propranolol
    sarcoidosis, 355
Propylthiouracil-induced alveolar
        hemorrhage, 508
Propylthiouracil-induced Wegener's
        granulomatosis, 509
Proteases, 191
Proteoglycans, 277

P-selectin
    endothelial cells, 189
Pseudallescheria boydii
    allergic bronchopulmonary syndromes,
        678
Pseudoalveolar sarcoidosis, 91
Pseudolymphoma
    malignant infiltrates differentiation
        from, 829
Pseudomonas fluorescens
    hypersensitivity pneumonitis, 458
Psoriatic arthritis, 579
PSS, 553–562. See Scleroderma
    nonspecific interstitial pneumonia
        HRCT, 90
PTI, 135–136, 138
Puerto Ricans
    sarcoidosis, 335
Pulmonary alveolar microlithiasis (PAM),
        173, 898–900, 899
    chest radiograph, 900
Pulmonary alveolar proteinosis (PAP), 51,
        167–169, 865–871
    animal models, 168
    BAL, 119, 120
    chest radiograph, 868
    circulating anti-GM-CSF
        autoantibodies, 169
    clinical presentation, 168
    clinical syndromes of, 866–867
    congenital, 870–871
    CT, 84, 100
    GM-CSF/IL-3/IL-5 receptor common
        beta-chain defects, 169
    ground-glass opacity
        HRCT, 101
    HRCT, 868
    idiopathic . See Idiopathic pulmonary
        alveolar proteinosis.
    infection-associated, 871
    malignancy-associated, 871–872
    mimicking pneumonia, 168
    outcome, 869–870
    photomicrograph, 867
    treatment, 869
Pulmonary artery pressures, 62
Pulmonary calcification, 898
Pulmonary capillaritis
    associated with diffuse alveolar
        hemorrhage, 632
    diffuse alveolar hemorrhage, 634, 634,
        641
Pulmonary capillary hemangiomatosis
    diffuse alveolar hemorrhage, 647
Pulmonary cyst
    lymphangioleiomyomatosis, 156
Pulmonary edema
    BAL, 116
    drug-induced, 505–508
    interstitial
        mitral valve disease, 82

pulmonary vasodilator-induced, 508
Silo filler's disease, 794–795
Pulmonary embolism
CT, *84*
idiopathic pulmonary fibrosis, 746
Pulmonary fibrosis, 314–316. *See also*
Idiopathic pulmonary fibrosis
acute respiratory distress syndromes,
889–891
alveolar epithelium, 221–237
CC chemokines, 264–266
CXC chemokines, 260–261
cytokine networks, *266*
development, 209–211
drug-induced, 504–505
familial
chest radiography, *708*
genetic manipulation, 175–176,
175–176
lymphocytes
animal models, 200–201
mortality
age stratification, *704*
murine models, 175–176
radiography, *19*
risk factors, *708*
scleroderma, *76*
silica-induced
IL-1ra, 248
T cells, 201–202
therapy, 323–328
current problems, 323
etiology, 323–328
future, *326*
organ-specific, 328
type1/type 2 paradigm, 251–255
vital statistics, 704
Pulmonary gamma delta T cells
polymorphic self-ligands, 199
Pulmonary hemorrhage
mixed connective tissue disease, 574
pediatric BAL, 143
in systemic lupus erythematosus, 552
Pulmonary hemosiderosis
idiopathic
diffuse alveolar hemorrhage,
643–644
Pulmonary histiocytosis Z
HRCT, *100*
radiography, *100*
Pulmonary hypertension
mixed connective tissue disease, 574
polymyositis and dermatomyositis, 567
in systemic lupus erythematosus, 551
Pulmonary infection
in systemic lupus erythematosus, 553
Pulmonary infiltrate (PIE)
diagnosis, 498
drug-induced, 496–500
Pulmonary Langerhans cell histiocytosis
(PLCH), 838–847

anatomic distribution, 48
clinical features, *839,* 842
diagnostic studies, 842–846
algorithm, *845*
BAL, 844–845
bronchoscopy, 844–845
chest radiography, 842–843, *843*
evaluation, 845–846
HRCT, 843, *844*
pulmonary function testing,
843–844
surgical lung biopsy, 844–845
transbronchoscopic biopsy,
844–845
epidemiology, 835–836
lung biopsy, *841*
outcomes and prognosis, 847
pathogenesis, 839–841
pathology, 841–842
pulmonary function test abnormalities,
839
treatment, 846–847
Pulmonary lymphangioleiomyomatosis,
854–855
treatment, 859–860
Pulmonary lymphocytes, 199–200
host factors, 303–305
Pulmonary lymphoplasmocytic
infiltrations, 825–834
Pulmonary matrix disorders, 170
Marfan syndrome, 170
Pulmonary neuroendocrine cells
primary diffuse hyperplasia, 814–815,
815
Pulmonary nodules
sarcoidosis
radiography, 356
Pulmonary plasma cell infiltrations,
830–831
Pulmonary sarcoidosis
treatment, *368*
Pulmonary surfactant, 865–866
Pulmonary tuberculosis
silicosis, 395
Pulmonary vascular amyloidosis, 880
Pulmonary vascular disorders
infants, 140–141
in rheumatoid arthritis, 544
scleroderma, 560–562
Sjögren's syndrome, 572
Pulmonary vascular resistance (PVR),
61–62
Pulmonary vasculitis, 599–622
associated with connective tissue
disorders, 621
classification, 599–600
definition, 599–600
drug-induced, 509
epidemiology, 600–601
nomenclature, 599–600
phenytoin-induced, 681

Pulmonary vasodilator-induced
pulmonary edema, 508
Pulmonary veno-occlusive disease, *646*
diffuse alveolar hemorrhage, 646–647
drug-induced, 510
Purpura, 895
Wegener's granulomatosis, *607*
PVNO
silicosis, 397
PVR, 61–62
Pyoderma grangrenosum
Wegener's granulomatosis, *607*
Pyromellitic dianhydride
diffuse alveolar hemorrhage, 644

Quartz, 387

Race
sarcoidosis, 335
Radiation-induced interstitial lung disease
(ILD), 522
dose-related toxicity, 494
incidence, 494
Radiation-induced lung cancer, 523
Radiation-induced organizing pneumonia
breast cancer, 523
Radiation-induced paramediastinal
fibrosis, 523
Radiation-induced pleural mesothelioma,
523
Radiation pneumonitis, 485, 523
hepatocellular carcinoma, *524*
Radiation therapy
heart damage, *523*
thoracic complications of, 521–524,
522
Radiography, *96*
Radiotherapy
sarcoidosis, 372
Rapid eye movement (REM) sleep, 64
Raynaud's phenomenon, 557
Sjögren's syndrome, 569
RB-ILD. *See* Respiratory bronchiolitis-
interstitial lung disease
Reactive arthritis
acute
sarcoidosis, 351
Reactive nitrogen species (RNS)
asbestos, 424
Reactive oxygen species (ROS)
asbestos, 423
paraquat model, 207
Recirculating lymphocytes, 200
Recombinant soluble TNF receptor
(rsTNFR), 251
Recurrent bronchopneumonia
Sjögren's syndrome, 572
Red spider allergens
eosinophils, 684
Regression factor, 455
Relapsing polychondritis, 580–581, 611

Relaxin, 292
  idiopathic pulmonary fibrosis, 743
  pulmonary fibrosis, 328
REM sleep, 64
Renal biopsy
  sarcoidosis, 366
Renal sarcoidosis, 354
Renal transplantation
  end-stage renal disease, 613
Renal ultrasound
  sarcoidosis, 366
Resected amyloidoma, *879*
Resident pulmonary lymphocytes,
  199–200
Residual volume (RV), 55, 67
  coal workers' pneumoconiosis, 410
  pediatric interstitial lung disease, 142
Residual volume /total lung capacity
  (RV/TLC)
  pediatric interstitial lung disease, 142
Respiratory bronchiolitis
  smoking-related
    CT, 102
Respiratory bronchiolitis-interstitial lung
  disease (RB-ILD), *51,* 755–758
  anatomic distribution, 47–48
  chest radiography, *757*
  CT, *85,* 90
Respiratory motion artifact, 78
Respiratory muscle dysfunction
  polymyositis and dermatomyositis,
    568
Respiratory syncytial virus (RSV)
  infant bronchiolitis, 790
Respiratory tract amyloidosis, 877–880
  presentation, *878*
Restrictive lung disease
  cigarette smokers, 106
Reticular (linear) interstitial infiltrates
  radiography, *14*
Reticulonodular interstitial infiltrates
  radiography, *14*
Retinoic acid syndrome, 516
Reverse transcriptase polymerase chain
  reaction (RT-PCR), 161, 194
Rheumatoid arthritis, 535–546
  airway disease in, 541–543
  BAL, *540*
  bronchiolitis, 800–802, *802*
  bronchiolitis obliterans, *804*
    CT, *105*
    radiography, *105*
  chest radiograph, *538*
  clinical and pathologic pulmonary
    manifestations, *536*
  follicular bronchiolitis, 802–803, *804*
  HRCT, *539*
  interstitial lung disease, 4, 536–546
    BAL, 539–540
    clinical manifestations, 538
    epidemiology, 536–537

histopathology features, 540–541
  pathogenesis, 537–538
  physiologic features, 539
  prognosis and management, 541
  roentgenographic features, 538
methotrexate reaction in
  anatomic distribution, 48
pleural disease in, 544–546
pleuropulmonary manifestations,
  536–546, *537*
pulmonary infection with, 543
radiography, *16, 19*
rheumatoid nodules with, 543, *543*
silicosis, 396
thoracic cage immobility, 546
Rheumatoid arthritis-associated diffuse
  alveolar hemorrhage (DAH), 633
Rheumatoid disease
  radiologic classification, *104*
Rheumatoid factor
  coal workers' pneumoconiosis, 411
  hypersensitivity pneumonitis, 467
Rhinitis
  Churg-Strauss syndrome, 668
Rhizopus
  allergic bronchopulmonary syndromes,
    678
Riedel's thyroiditis, 897
Right ventricular hypertrophy (RVH)
  coal workers' pneumoconiosis, 413
RNS
  asbestos, 424
Rodenticide-induced alveolar hemorrhage,
  509
Rodenticide-induced interstitial lung
  disease (ILD), 494
Room and pillar mines, 404
ROS
  asbestos, 423
  paraquat model, 207
Rounded atelectasis, 422
  radiography, *422*
RsTNFR, 251
RSV
  infant bronchiolitis, 790
RT-PCR, 161, 194
Russia
  beryllium, 436
RV, 55, 67
  coal workers' pneumoconiosis, 410
  pediatric interstitial lung disease, 142
RVH
  coal workers' pneumoconiosis, 413
RV/TLC
  pediatric interstitial lung disease, 142

SACE, 339
  chronic beryllium disease, 444
  sarcoidosis, 364–365
Saddle nose deformity
  therapy, 613

of Wegener's granulomatosis, *604*
Salem sarcoid, 338
Salivary glands
  sarcoidosis, 353
Sandblasting
  silicosis, 388
Sarcoid-affected lymph nodes
  in nonsarcoid disease, 355
Sarcoid arthritis, 351–352
Sarcoid bone cysts, 332
Sarcoid bone disease, 352, *352*
Sarcoid granuloma
  programmed cell death, 313–314
Sarcoid myositis, 352
Sarcoidosis, 300–318, 332–373, 372, *439*
  age, 6
  alveolar
    CT, 100
  anatomic distribution, 48
  antigenic factors, 301–303
  atypical pulmonary involvement
    radiography, 356–357
  BAL, 125–126, 360–362
  biopsy, 362
  clinical presentation, 347–355
    calcium metabolism, 354
    cardiovascular involvement,
      350–351
    eye disease, 353
    gastrointestinal and hepatic
      involvement, 354–355
    lymphoreticular involvement, 354
    musculoskeletal involvement,
      351–352
    nonspecific constitutional
      symptoms, 347
    pulmonary involvement, 347
    renal disease, 353–354, *354*
    skin involvement, 348–349
    upper respiratory tract, 347–348,
      348
  CT, *84,* 91–94
  cutaneous, 348
  differential diagnosis, *471*
  disease activity and prognosis, 365
  eosinophils, 684
  familial, 174
  gas exchange abnormalities, 67–68
  genetic factors, 302–303
  granulomas, *45*
  imaging, 355–359
    CT, 356–358, *358*
    radiography, 355–357, *356–357*
    radionuclide, 358–358
  immunologic abnormalities, *301*
  immunosuppressive drugs
    molecular targets, 316–318
  infection, 301–302
  inflammatory cells
    granuloma formation, 309–310
  interstitial lung disease, 4

investigation algorithm, 366
laryngeal, 347
lymphocytic alveolitis, *124*
milestones, 332
nonpulmonary
    treatment, *368*
ocular, 353
pathogenesis, 333–345
    age and gender, 334–335
    asymptomatic, *334*
    clustering, 337–338
    disease frequency, 334–335
    epidemiology, 333–339
    etiology, 333, *333*
    genetic factors, 339–340
    geography, 335–336
    immune processes, 340–345
    occupation, 338–339
    race, 335
    smoking, 338
    symptoms, *334*
pathology, 346–347
pediatric BAL, 144
polymorphonuclear cells, 307–309
pseudoalveolar, 91
pulmonary
    treatment, *368*
pulmonary function tests, 359–360
radiography, *11, 93*
    eggshell nodal calcification, *94*
renal, 354
smoking, 68, *338*
treatment, 366–372
    algorithm, 372
Sarcoidosis of the upper respiratory tract
    (SURT), 347–348
Sauropus androgynus-induced
    bronchiolitis, 811
Scadding's fibrosing alveolitis, 208
Scatter factor (SF). *See* HGF
Schistosomiasis, 676
SCID, 872
Scleroderma, 413, 553–562
    airways disease in, 559–560
    BAL, 558–559, *560*
    chest roentgenogram, *558*
    clinical classification, *554*
    clinical manifestations, 557
    collagen, 554
    CREST syndrome, *561*
    definition, 553
    genetics, 553–554
    histopathologic features, 559
    interstitial lung disease, 4, 555–559
        epidemiology, 555
        immune complexes, 556
        pulmonary fibrosis pathogenesis,
            555–556
    outcome predictors, *555*
    pathogenesis, 553–554
    physiologic features, 557–558

pleuropulmonary manifestations,
    554–555, *556*
prognosis, 561–562
pulmonary fibrosis, *76*
pulmonary vasculitis associated with,
    621
roentgenographic features, 557
Scorpion sting
    eosinophils, 684
Self-induced alveolar hemorrhage, 509
Sepsis, 745
Serpentine asbestos, 419
Serum angiotensin converting enzyme
    (SACE), 339
    chronic beryllium disease, 444
    sarcoidosis, 364–365
Serum markers
    scleroderma, 556–557
Severe combined immunodeficiency
    (SCID), 872
Shrinking lungs syndrome
    Sjögren's syndrome, 572
    in systemic lupus erythematosus,
        552–553
Silica
    emphysema, 95
    forms of, 387
    inhalation
        biologic consequences, 388–389
        occupational health exposure to,
            387–388
Silica-induced pulmonary fibrosis
    IL-1ra, 248
Silica model, 207
Silicates, 387
Silicon dioxide, 387
Silicosis, 95, 387–398, 872
    accelerated, 391
    acute, 391, *393*
    airway obstruction, 396
    anatomic distribution, 48–49
    BAL, 121–122, 395
    chronic, 391
    chronic bronchitis, 396
    complications, 395–397
        immune-mediated, 395–396
        mycobacterial infection, 395
        renal, 397
    CT, *84*
    diagnosis, 394–395
    epidemiology, 390–391
    histologic pattern
        acute *vs.* chronic, 390
    ILO classification, 393–394
    lung cancer, 396
    pathology, 389–390
    physical findings, 392
    prevention, 397–398
    progressive massive fibrosis, 95
    pulmonary function, 393
    radiographic patterns, 391

diseases mimicking, 395
radiography, *18,* 393–394
recommended exposure limit, 398
simple
    CT, *84*
symptoms, 392
transbronchial lung biopsy, 395
treatment, 397
types, 391–392
Silo filler's disease, 793–796
Simple silicosis, 391
    radiograph, *391*
Single nucleotide polymorphisms (SNPs)
    silicosis, 389
Site
    BAL, 115
Sjögren's syndrome, 347, 568–572, *825,*
    826
    definition, 568–569
    interstitial lung disease, 570–572
    LIP, 826
    pleuropulmonary manifestations,
        570–572, *571*
    tracheobronchial tree desiccation,
        571–573
Skin biopsy
    sarcoidosis, 366
S-LAM, 153–154
    cystic changes, *157*
    epidemiology, 154
SLE. *See* Systemic lupus erythematosus
Sleep, 64
Sleep apnea
    obstructive
        diffuse alveolar hemorrhage, 647
Sleep disturbance
    idiopathic pulmonary fibrosis,
        726–727
Small airways diseases
    radiologic classification, *104*
Smoke inhalation, 796
Smokers
    pulmonary fibrosis, 323
Smoker's lung
    radiologic classification, *104*
Smoking, 6–7. *See also* Cigarette smoking
    coal workers' pneumoconiosis, 406–207
    hypersensitivity pneumonitis, 460
    idiopathic pulmonary fibrosis, 68
    sarcoidosis, 68, 338, *338*
Smoking cessation
    coal workers' pneumoconiosis, 413
    desquamative interstitial pneumonia,
        755
    PLCH, 846
Smoking-related respiratory bronchiolitis
    CT, 102
SNPs
    silicosis, 389
Somatostatin receptor scintigraphy (SRS)
    sarcoidosis, 359

SP-A, 865
  silicosis, 389
SP-B, 865
  mutations, 169–170
SP-C. *See* Surfactant protein C
SP-D, 866
Spontaneous pneumomediastinum
  complicating rheumatoid arthritis, 546
Spontaneous pneumothorax
  complicating rheumatoid arthritis, 546
Sporadic lymphangioleiomyomatosis (S-
    LAM), 153–154
  cystic changes, *157*
  epidemiology, 154
Sprue
  differentiation from sarcoidosis, 355
Sputum eosinophilia
  chronic eosinophilic pneumonia, 663
SRS
  sarcoidosis, 359
Stachybotrys chartarum, 139
Static lung compliance, *54,* 54–56
Static lung volumes, 55
  measurement, 69
Statins
  pulmonary fibrosis, 327
Stemphylium
  allergic bronchopulmonary syndromes,
    678
Steroids
  cryptogenic adult bronchiolitis, 800
  hypersensitivity pneumonitis, 476
  sarcoidosis, 348
Stishovite, 387
Stop ventilation, 78
Strongyloides stercoralis, 674
  BAL, *676*
Subacute amiodarone pneumonitis
  clinical and radiographic pattern, 512
Subclinical amiodarone pneumonitis
  clinical and radiographic pattern, 514
Subglottic stenosis
  Wegener's granulomatosis, *606*
Sulfasalazine-induced lung disease
  IBD, 896
Sulfites
  eosinophils, 684
Sulfur dioxide, 796
Summer-type hypersensitivity
    pneumonitis
  Japan, 460
Supplemental oxygen, 66
  chronic beryllium disease, 446
Surfactant
  production and catabolism, 866
Surfactant protein abnormalities
  infants, 139–140
Surfactant protein A (SP-A), 865
  silicosis, 389
Surfactant protein B (SP-B), 865
  mutations, 169–170

Surfactant protein C (SP-C), 152,
    865–866
  interstitial lung disease
    genetic basis, *161*
  misprocessing, 160
  mutations, 160–162, 872
    idiopathic interstitial pneumonia,
      160
  structure and function, 160
Surfactant protein D (SP-D), 866
Surfactants
  disease epithelial markers, 236–237
Surgical lung biopsy
  parenchymal lung disease, *21*
SURT, 347–348
Sweden
  beryllium, 436
Swyer-James syndrome, 799
  children, 135, *143*
  radiograph, *88*
Systemic lupus erythematosus (SLE),
    546–553
  acute lupus pneumonitis, 548–550
  airway disease in, 550
  BAL, *551*
  chronic interstitial pneumonia,
    549–550
  clinical manifestations by organ
    system, *547*
  diffuse alveolar hemorrhage, 633,
    639–640
    chest radiograph, *636*
  drug-induced, 510–511
  HRCT, *550*
  infiltrate, *552*
  interstitial lung disease in, 547–550
    epidemiology, 547
    pathogenesis, 547–548
  lung immunofluorescence, *637*
  pleural disease in, 550–551
  pleuropulmonary manifestations, *547,*
    547–553
  pulmonary vascular disease, 551–552

Tachypnea
  hypersensitivity pneumonitis, 461
Tacrolimus
  sarcoidosis, 317
Takayasu's arteritis, 620–621, 897–898
Talc, 387
Talc pleurodesis
  recurrent pneumothoraces, 860
Taurine-niacin
  pulmonary fibrosis, 328
T-cells
  antigen receptors
    sarcoidosis, 340–341
  clones
    sarcoid granuloma, 312–313
  compartmentalization
    granuloma formation, 309

  pulmonary fibrosis, 201–202
TDM, 279
Technetium-labeled pentetic acid
    (DTPA), 77
Technetium 99m glucoheptonate
  chronic eosinophilic pneumonia, 663
Teenager
  hypersensitivity pneumonitis
    CT, *136*
    radiography, *136*
Teleradiology, 75
Tenosynovitis, 352
TGF-beta. *See* Tumor growth factor-beta
TGF-beta-1
  profibrotic properties, *326*
  pulmonary fibrosis, 325
Thalidomide
  pulmonary fibrosis, 327
Theophylline
  shrinking lung syndrome, 553
Thermophilic actinomycetes
  farmer's lung, 474
  hypersensitivity pneumonitis,
    457–458
Thiabendazole
  Strongyloides stercoralis, 674
Thiamazole-induced Wegener's
    granulomatosis, 509
Thioglucose-induced interstitial lung
    disease (ILD), 518–519
Thiomalate-induced interstitial lung
    disease (ILD), 518–519
Thoracentesis
  rheumatoid pleural effusions, 546
Thorax
  computed radiography, 75
Thrombocytopenia
  drug-induced
    alveolar hemorrhage, 508
Thromboembolism
  in systemic lupus erythematosus, 551
Th1/Th2
  granuloma formation, *312*
  host factors, 305
  sarcoidosis, 308
Tidal flow-volume curve, 55
TIMPs, 194, 288
  idiopathic pulmonary fibrosis, *194*
TIMPs-4, 194
Tissue inhibitors of metalloproteinases
    (TIMPs), 194, 288
  idiopathic pulmonary fibrosis, *194*
Tissue inhibitors of metalloproteinases-4
    (TIMPs-4), 194
TLC, 54, 56
  pediatric interstitial lung disease, 142
T lymphocyte CD4:CD8 ratios
  sarcoidosis, 361–362
TNF-alpha. *See* Tumor necrosis factor-
    alpha
Tobacco glycoprotein, 840

Torulopsis
  allergic bronchopulmonary syndromes, 678
Total lung capacity (TLC), 54, 56
  pediatric interstitial lung disease, 142
Toxic oil syndrome, 682
Toxocara, 674
  pediatric interstitial lung disease, 135
Trachea
  inflammatory pseudotumor, *605*
Tracheobronchial amyloidosis, 877–878
Tracheobronchial tree, *787*
  desiccation of, 571–572
Traction bronchiectasis
  HRCT
    diffuse parenchymal lung disease, 85–86
    IFP, *87*
Traction bronchiolectasis
  HRCT
    diffuse parenchymal lung disease, 85–86
TRALI, 507
Transbronchial biopsy, *21*
  sarcoidosis, 362, *363*
  silicosis, 395
Transforming growth factor-beta, 255–256
  alveolar macrophages, 307
  collagen synthesis, 195–196, 198
Transfusion-related acute lung injury (TRALI), 507
Transgenic mice, 209
Transplantation
  sarcoidosis, 371–372
Trehalose-6,6'-dimycolate (TDM), 279
Tretinoin-induced alveolar hemorrhage, 508
Trichomonas tenax
  eosinophilic pneumonia, 676
Trichosporon cutaneum
  hypersensitivity pneumonitis, 458–459
Trichosporon terrestre
  allergic bronchopulmonary syndromes, 678
Tridymite, 387
Trimellitic anhydride
  diffuse alveolar hemorrhage, 644
Trimethoprim-sulfamethoxazole
  Wegener's granulomatosis, 613
Tropheryma whippelii, 897
Tropical eosinophilia, 672–674
TSC. *See* Tuberous sclerosis complex
TSC2, 153, 155
Tuberculin skin test
  corticosteroids, 716
Tuberculosis
  differential diagnosis, *471*
Tuberin gene (TSC2), 153, 155
Tuberous sclerosis
  diffuse alveolar hemorrhage, 646

family history, 7
HRCT1, *156*
radiography, 15
Tuberous sclerosis complex (TSC), 153–158, 856
  animal models, 155
  cell biology, *852*
  lungs, 153–154
  MMPH, 153
Tuberous sclerosis complex (TSC)-lymphangioleiomyomatosis (LAM), 153–154
  epidemiology, 154
Tumor growth factor-beta (TGF-beta), 231–232
  fibroblasts, 256
  fibrosis, *256, 283*
  lung injury, *283*
  silica model, 207
  silicosis, 389
Tumor growth factor- beta 1 (TGF-beta-1)
  profibrotic properties, *326*
  pulmonary fibrosis, 325
Tumor necrosis factor-alpha (TNF-alpha), 191, 231, 249–251
  alveolar macrophages, 307
  blockade
    sarcoidosis, 371
  fibroblasts, 250, 315
  fibrosis, *250*
  idiopathic pulmonary fibrosis, 743–744
  pulmonary fibrosis, 327
  rheumatoid arthritis, 540
  sarcoidosis, 365
  scleroderma, 556
  silica model, 207
  silicosis, 389
Tumor suppressor syndromes, 153–160
  genetic basis, *153*
  neurofibromatosis, 158–160
  tuberous sclerosis complex, 153–158
Tunneling
  silicosis, 387
Turkeys
  hypersensitivity pneumonitis, 458
24-hour electrocardiogram
  sarcoidosis, 366
Type I cells, 222
Type II cells, 222
  idiopathic pulmonary fibrosis, *224*
  migration, 233
  secretions, 231
Type II pneumocytes
  papillary adenomas, 160

UIP. *See* Usual interstitial pneumonia
Unilateral postinfectious constrictive b
  bronchiolitis. *See* Swyer-James
  syndrome

United Kingdom
  beryllium, 436
Urback-Wiethe disease, 173
Ureaplasma urealyticum
  pediatric interstitial lung disease, 135
Urine tests
  sarcoidosis, 365
US National Coal Workers' Autopsy, 390
Usual interstitial pneumonia (UIP), 40
  BAL, *128, 712*
  children, 136–137
  CT, *84,* 88
    accuracy, *731*
  fibroblastic focus, 324, *324–325*
  heterogeneity, *44*
  honeycomb, *324*
  interstitial fibrosis, *41*
  Kaplan-Meier survival curves, *748*
  mediastinal lymphadenopathy
    CT, 88
  in rheumatoid arthritis, 540
  scleroderma, 559
Uveitis, 353

Vasculitis
  in systemic lupus erythematosus, 551
VC, 54, 55
  sarcoidosis, 359
Veno-occlusive disease
  with Felty's syndrome, 544
Ventilatory capacity
  reduced, 62–64
Ventilatory muscles
  function, 61
Ventricular arrhythmias
  sarcoidosis, 350–351
Vermont granite industry
  silicosis, 391
VgVd 1 murine T cells
  keratinocyte growth factor, 199
Vinblastine
  PLCH, 846
Vincristine sulfate
  idiopathic pulmonary fibrosis, 743
Vital capacity (VC), 54, 55
  sarcoidosis, 359
Volatile flavoring agents, 797–798
Von Recklinghausen's disease, 886–888
V_T/IC, 60
V_T/VC, 60

Waldenstrom's macroglobulinemia, 831
Wallernia sebi
  hypersensitivity pneumonitis, 459
Wegener granulomatosis, 601–605
  anatomic distribution, 49–50
  bronchiolitis, 811–812
  vs. Churg-Strauss syndrome, 669
  classification, 601–602
  clinical manifestations, 602–608
    nervous system, 605–606

ophthalmic, 603, *603*
otolaryngologic, 603
pulmonary, 603–604
renal, 606–607
diagnosis, 608–611
    bronchoscopic manifestations,
        608–609
    chest radiography, *608*
    differential, 610–611
    imaging studies, 608
    laboratory testing, 610
diffuse alveolar hemorrhage, 638
drug-induced, 509
histopathologic features, *609,*
    609–610
historic background, 601–602
incidence, 600
inflammatory pseudotumor, *609*
necrotizing glomerulonephritis, *608*
necrotizing granulomatous
    lung lesions, *606*

skin lesions, *607*
organ involvement frequency, *614*
organ manifestations, *602*
pleural effusion, 605
post-obstructive pneumonia, *604*
propylthiouracil-induced, 509
saddle nose deformity, *604*
skin manifestations, *607*
therapy, 611–613
    disease sequelae, 613
    historic background, 611
    remission, 611–612
    salvage, 611–612
thiamazole-induced, 509
Wheezing, 7
    BAL, *116*
    hypersensitivity pneumonitis, 461
Whipple's disease, 897
    differentiation from sarcoidosis, 355
Whole lung lavage (WLL)
    PAP, 869

silicosis, 397
WLL
    PAP, 869
    silicosis, 397
Wound
    healing and remodeling
        epithelial functions, 233–236
Wuchereria bancrofti, 672

X-linked dyskeratosis congenita, 174

Yersinia enterocolitica
    sarcoidosis, 301

Zeek classification
    necrotizing angiitis, 599
Zenker's diverticulum
    chest radiograph, *882*